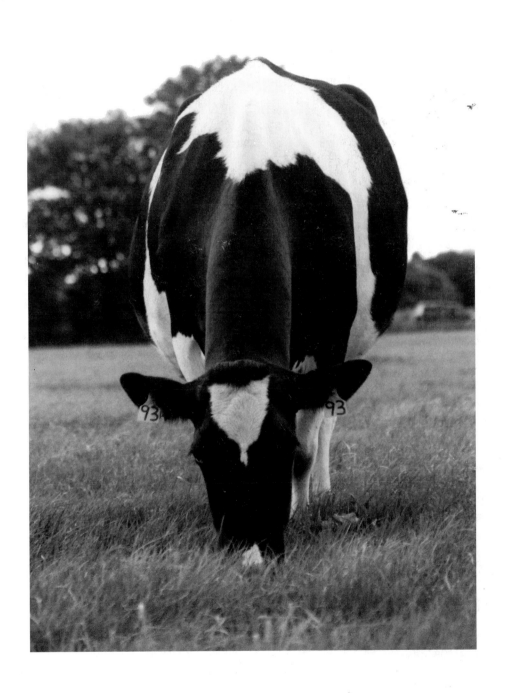

Bovine Medicine
Diseases and Husbandry of Cattle

Second edition

Edited by

A.H. Andrews
with
R.W. Blowey
H. Boyd
R.G. Eddy

Blackwell
Science

© 2004 by Blackwell Science Ltd
a Blackwell Publishing Company

Editorial Offices:
Blackwell Science Ltd, 9600 Garsington Road, Oxford OX4
2DQ, UK
   Tel: +44 (0)1865 776868
Iowa State Press, a Blackwell Publishing Company, 2121
State Avenue, Ames Iowa 50014-8300 USA
   Tel: +1 515 292 0140
Blackwell Science Asia Pty Ltd, 550 Swanston Street,
Carlton, Victoria 3053, Australia
   Tel: +61 (0)3 8359 1011

First published 1992 by Blackwell Science
Second edition published 2004 by Blackwell Publishing

Library of Congress Cataloging-in-Publication Data
Bovine medicine : diseases and husbandry of cattle / edited
by A.H. Andrews ... [et al.].
   2nd ed.
      p. cm.
   Includes bibliographical references (p.).
   ISBN 0-632-05596-0 (alk. paper)
   1. Cattle–Diseases. 2. Cattle. I. Andrews, A.H.

SF961.B78 2003
636.2'0896–dc22
                                              2003063030

ISBN 0-632-05596-0

A catalogue record for this title is available
from the British Library

Set in 9.5 on 12 pt Times
by SNP Best-set Typesetter Ltd., Hong Kong
Printed and bound in the UK using acid-free paper
by CPI Bath

For further information on
Blackwell Publishing, visit our website:
www.blackwellpublishing.com

Contents

List of Colour Plates   vi

List of Contributors   vii

Preface   xi

Preface to the First Edition   xii

PART 1: MANAGEMENT   **1**

1   Calf Rearing   3
    D.M. Allen

2   Suckler Herds   7
    D.M. Allen

3   Beef Finishing Systems   14
    D.M. Allen

4   Dairy Farming   22
    A.H. Andrews and A. Poole

5   Heifer Rearing – 12 Weeks to Calving   54
    B. Drew

6   Tropical Cattle Management   68
    R.D. Fielding and R.W. Matthewman

7   Ethnoveterinary Medicine in the Tropics   83
    R.D. Fielding

8   Heat Stress in Dairy Cattle   88
    J.K. Shearer

9   Nutrition   95
    J.M. Wilkinson

10   Alternative Forages   123
    M. Tame and the late P.S. Jarvis

PART 2: DISEASE   **133**

11   Diagnosis and Differential Diagnosis in
    the Cow   135
    R.G. Eddy and P.J.N. Pinsent

The Calf   **159**

12   Outline of Clinical Genetics   161
    G.B. Young

13   Congenital Conditions   172
    A.H. Andrews

14   Calf Diarrhoea   185
    P.R. Scott, G.A. Hall, P.W. Jones and
    J.H. Morgan

15   Salmonellosis   215
    P.W. Jones, P.R. Watson and T.S. Wallis

16   Digestive Disorders of Calves   231
    R.W. Blowey

17   Calf Respiratory Disease   239
    A.H. Andrews

18   Other Calf Problems   249
    A.H. Andrews

Growing Cattle   **265**

19   Endoparasites   267
    S.M. Taylor and A.H. Andrews

20   Respiratory Diseases   286
    A.H. Andrews

21   Trace Element Disorders   294
    N.F. Suttle

Adult Cattle
Mastitis and Teat Conditions   **309**

22   Anatomy, Physiology and Immunology
    of the Udder   311
    K.G. Hibbitt, N. Craven and E.H. Batten

23   Mastitis   326
    P.W. Edmondson and A.J. Bramley

24   Summer Mastitis   337
    J.E. Hillerton

25   Bulk Milk Testing and Mastitis Monitoring   341
    D.J. O'Rourke and R.W. Blowey

26   The Milking Machine   353
    D.J. O'Rourke

27   Skin Infections of the Bovine Teat and
    Udder and Their Differential Diagnosis   363
    J.K. Shearer, J.R. Townsend and
    E.P.J. Gibbs

28 Factors Affecting Milk Quality   373
    R.W. Blowey and R.A. Laven

29 The Enhancement of Bovine Mammary
    Gland Immunity Through Vaccination   379
    *K.P. Kenny, T. Tollersrud and
    F.D. Bastida-Corcuera*

30 Antimicrobial Therapy of Mastitis   391
    D.J. O'Rourke and J.D. Baggot

Lameness   **407**

31 Lameness in the Foot   409
    R.W. Blowey

32 Lameness Above the Foot   435
    A.D. Weaver

Fertility   **469**

33 Reproductive Physiology in Cattle   471
    P.J. Hartigan

34 The Postpartum Period   508
    I.M. Sheldon, D.C. Barrett and H. Boyd

35 Problems Associated with Oestrous
    Cyclicity   530
    H. Boyd, D.C. Barrett, and M. Mihm

36 Failure to Conceive and Embryonic Loss 552
    D.C. Barrett, H. Boyd and M. Mihm

37 Fetal Loss   577
    G. Caldow and D. Gray

38 Bull Infertility   594
    D.N. Logue and W.M. Crawshaw

39 Artificial Insemination and Diseases
    Transmitted by Semen   627
    G.H. Wentink

40 Embryo Transfer   634
    A.K. Smith

41 Herd Fertility Management   652
    (a) Beef herds   652
    S. Borsberry

    (b) Dairy herds   662
    D.C. Barrett and H. Boyd

42 Pharmacological Manipulation of
    Reproduction   678
    J.G. Allcock and A.R. Peters

Major Infectious Diseases   **689**

43 Viral Diseases   691

    (a) Bluetongue   691
    R.P. Kitching

    (b) Enzootic bovine leukosis   693
    C. Venables and M.H. Lucas

    (c) Foot-and-mouth disease   700
    R.P. Kitching

    (d) Rinderpest   707
    E.C. Anderson

    (e) Vesicular stomatitis   710
    R.P. Kitching

    (f) Bovine immunodeficiency virus   713
    A.H. Andrews

44 Bacterial Conditions   717
    A.H. Andrews and the late B.M. Williams

45 Ectoparasites, Tick and Arthropod-borne
    Diseases   740
    *S.M. Taylor, A.G. Hunter and
    A.H. Andrews*

Metabolic Problems   **779**

46 Major Metabolic Disorders   781
    R.G. Eddy

47 Metabolic Profiles   804
    D.A. Whitaker

System and Miscellaneous Conditions   **819**

48 Alimentary Conditions   821
    R.G. Eddy

49 Respiratory Conditions   860
    A.H. Andrews and R.S. Windsor

50 Skin Conditions   875
    L.R. Thomsett

51 Neurological Disorders   890
    P.R. Scott

52 Ocular Diseases   917
    P.G.C. Bedford

53 Other Conditions   927
    A.H. Andrews

54 Major Poisonings   937
    C.J. Giles and A.H. Andrews

Welfare   **953**

55 Welfare   955
    D.M. Broom

Therapy and Disease Prevention   **969**

56 Health, Housing and Hygiene   971
    D.W.B. Sainsbury

57 Biosecurity   987
    D.C. Barrett and A.J. Taylor

58 Immunological Fundamentals   996
    W.P.H. Duffus

59 Vaccines and Vaccination of Cattle   1004
    I.D. Baker

60 Antiparasitics   1019
    M.A. Taylor

61 Antimicrobial Agents   1035
    A.H. Andrews

62 Inflammation and Pain   1045
    J.L. Fitzpatrick, A.M. Nolan, P. Lees and
    S.A. May

63 Growth Promoters in Cattle   1067
    K. Lawrence

64 Injection Damage   1078
    J.H. Pratt

65 Alternative Medicine   1081
    C.E.I. Day

66 Aspects of Bovine Surgery   1105
    G. Wyn-Jones

*The Interaction of the Animal, Environment
and Management*   **1131**

67 Stress and the Pathogenesis of Disease   1133
    P.J. Hartigan

Global Variation in Cattle Practice   **1149**

68 Diseases Related to Management
    in Europe   1151
    G.H. Wentink and A. de Kruif

69 Cattle Disease in Africa   1156
    R.S. Windsor

70 Rabies   1164
    R.S. Windsor

71 Dairy Farming in Saudi Arabia   1172
    J.C. Fishwick

72 Bovine Medicine in New Zealand and
    Australia   1177
    N.D. Sargison and J.J. Vermunt

73 North American Dairy Production and
    Veterinary Involvement   1183
    T.W. Graham

74 The North American Beef Industry   1188
    D. Sjeklocha and S. Sweiger

Index   1193

Colour plates appear between pages 468 and 469

List of Colour Plates

All colour plates appear between 468 and 469.

16.1 Hair loss over legs and perineum associated with steatorrhea and diarrhoea.
16.2 Alopecia due to poorly dispersed fats from milk subsitute.
16.3 Rumen bloat and chronic scour.
16.4 Calf *in extremis*.
16.5 Abomasum at necropsy.
16.6 Chronic peri-weaning calf diarrhoea.
23.1 Lumen and keratinized lining in teat duct.
23.2 Signs of clinical mastitis.
27.1 Early stages of bovine herpes mammillitis.
27.2 Bovine herpes mammillitis (two days).
27.3 Bovine herpes mammillitis (four days).
27.4 Bovine herpes mammillitis and scab formation.
27.5 Bovine herpes mammillitis (about seven days).
27.6 Bovine herpes mammillitis (about two weeks).
27.7 Bovine herpes mammillitis (two to three weeks).
27.8 Bovine herpes mammillitis – teat after shedding necrotic tissue.
27.9 Pseudocowpox.
27.10 Pseudocowpox lesion (seven days).
27.11 Pseudocowpox (10–12 days).
27.12 Pseudocowpox scab.
27.13–16 Atypical Pseudocowpox lesions.
27.17 Cowpox showing vesicle development.
27.18 Cowpox following vesicle rupture.
27.19 Cowpox with scab formation.
27.20 Severe cowpox.
27.21 *Staphylococcus aureus* infection of teat.
27.22 Teat chaps.
27.23 Photosensitization of the teat.
27.24 Foot-and-mouth disease – vesiculation of the teat.
27.25 Pseudocowpox infection with cowpox infection.
27.26 Pseudocowpox infection with bovine herpes mammillitis.
27.27 Blackspot of a teat orifice.
27.28 Mud abrasion of the teat.
27.29 Ringworm lesions.
27.30 Thelitis and serous exudate in peractute mastitis.
27.31 Filamentous papillomatosis of the teat.
27.32 Nodular papillomatosis of the teat.
31.1 Hoof with corium removed.
31.2 Cross-section of white line.
31.3 Gross claw overgrowth.
31.4 Overgrowth from the sole.
31.5 White line across a square-ended toe.
31.6 Haemorrhage at the sole ulcer site and in white line.
31.7 Typical sole ulcer.
31.8 Heel ulcer and early sole ulcer haemorrhage.
31.9 Typical white line separation with impacted stone.
31.10 Rings on a cow's horns demonstrate disruption of horn formation in the periparturient animal.
31.11 Cows prefer to walk on the soft surface of a rubber mat.
31.12 Cows walking along the grass verge to avoid the stony track.
31.13 Digital dermatitis and slurry heel.
31.14 A vertical fissure.
31.15 Axial wall fissure.
31.16 Interdigital necrobacillosis.
31.17 The chronic 'hairy wart' form of digital dermatitis.
31.18–19 Necrosis of the apex of the pedal bone.
31.20 Insertion of a tube to flush and drain deep pedal infections.
40.1 Classification and grading of embryos.
44.1 *Anthrax bacillium*.
44.2 Blackleg due to *Clostridium chauveoi*.
44.3 Endocarditis.
50.1 Generalized *Trichophyton verrucosum* infection.
50.2 *Trichophyton verrucosum* infection on calf's head.
50.3 *Linognathus vituli* lice and ova on calf.
50.4 *Sarcoptes scabiei* infection.
50.5–6 Generalized sarcoptic scabies.
50.7 Nodular lesions of demodicosis.
50.8–9 Viral papillomatosis.
50.10 Pruritis/pyrexia/haemorrhagic syndrome.
50.11–12 Severe photodermatitis.
50.13–14 Dermatophilosis.
52.1 Cyclopia.
52.2 Esotropia: (a) early; (b) marked.
52.3 Epibulbar dermoid.
52.4 Infectious bovine keratoconjunctivitis.
52.5 Squamous cell carcinoma.
52.6 Anterior uveitis secondary to septicaemia of undetermined aetiology.
52.7 Congenital cataract.
52.8 Lens discision.
52.9 Papillary coloboma.
52.10 Normal bovine fundus.
52.11 Severe papilloedema with disc haemorrhages.
65.1 Acupuncture to treat anoestrus.
65.2 Stomach 36 acupuncture point.

List of Contributors

James G. Allcock BVM&S CertCHP MRCVS, Intervet UK Ltd, Milton Keynes, UK

David M. Allen BSc PhD MBIAC, Beef Industry Consultant, formerly Head of Beef Improvement Services, Meat and Livestock Commission, Milton Keynes, UK

Euan C. Anderson BVM&S PhD MRCVS, formerly Veterinary Research Laboratory, Harare, Zimbabwe

Anthony H. Andrews BVetMed PhD MBIAC MRCVS, Independent Veterinary Consultant, formerly Senior Lecturer, Royal Veterinary College, UK

J. Desmond Baggot BSc MVM PhD DSc FACVPT DipECVPT FRCVS, School of Veterinary Medicine, St George's University, Grenada, West Indies

Ian D. Baker BVSc MRCVS, Hampden Veterinary Hospital, Aylesbury, UK

David C. Barrett BSc(Hons) BVSc(Hons) DBR DCHP MRCVS, Senior Lecturer, Division of Farm Animal Medicine and Production, Department of Veterinary Clinical Studies, University of Glasgow, UK

Felix D. Bastida-Corcuera DVM, PhD, University of California, Los Angeles, USA

E. Hamish Batten BSc PhD, formerly School of Veterinary Sciences, University of Bristol, UK

Peter G. C. Bedford BVetMed PhD DipECVO DVOphthal MRCVS, Small Animal Medicine and Surgery Group, Department of Clinical Sciences, Royal Veterinary College, UK

Roger W. Blowey BSc BVSc FRCVS, Wood Veterinary Group, Gloucester, UK

Steve Borsberry BVSc CertCHP DBR MRCVS, 608 Veterinary Clinic, Solihull, UK

Hugh Boyd VMD MRCVS, formerly Senior Lecturer, Veterinary School, University of Glasgow, UK

A. John Bramley BSc PhD, Department of Animal Sciences, College of Agriculture and Life Sciences, Vermont, USA

Donald M. Broom MA PhD Hon DSc, Department of Clinical Veterinary Medicine, University of Cambridge, UK

George L. Caldow BVM&S MSc CertCHP MRCVS, Scottish Agricultural College, Veterinary Science Division, Melrose, UK

Neil Craven BVSc BSc PhD MRCVS, Pfizer Ltd, Sandwich, UK

W. Mark Crawshaw BVetMed DCHP MRCVS, Scottish Agricultural College, Veterinary Science Division, Ayr, UK

Christopher E. I. Day MA VetMB MRCVS Chinham House, Stanford in the Vale, UK

Bridget Drew BSc PhD, Royal Agricultural College, Cirencester, UK

W. Philip H. Duffus BVSc MA PhD MRCVS, School of Veterinary Science, University of Bristol, UK

Roger G. Eddy BVetMed FRCVS, formerly at Shepton Veterinary Group, Shepton Mallet, UK

Peter W. Edmondson MVB CertCHP FRCVS, Shepton Veterinary Group, Shepton Mallet, UK

R. Denis Fielding BSc MSc PhD, Faculty of Veterinary Medicine, Royal (Dick) School of Veterinary Studies, University of Edinburgh, Easter Bush, UK

John Fishwick MA VetMB DCHP MRCVS, Department of Veterinary Clinical Science, Royal Veterinary College, Hatfield, UK

Julie L. Fitzpatrick BVMS PhD MRCVS, Division of Farm Animal Medicine, University of Glasgow, UK

E. Paul J. Gibbs BVSc PhD MRCVS, Department of Pathobiology, University of Florida, Gainsville, USA

Colin J. Giles BVetMed PhD MRCVS, Vice President Medicine Pharmaceuticals R&D, Pfizer Inc., Kalamazoo, Michigan, USA

Thomas W. Graham BSc DVM MPVM PhD, Veterinary Consulting Services, Davis, USA

Douglas Gray BVM&S MSc MRCVS, Scottish Agricultural College, Veterinary Services, Bucksburn, Aberdeen, UK

Graham A. Hall BVSc PhD FRCPath DipECVP MRCVS, CAMR, Porton Down, UK

Pat J. Hartigan BSc MA MVM PhD MRCVS, Honorary Fellow, Department of Physiology, Trinity College, Dublin, Ireland

Ken G. Hibbitt BVSc PhD MRCVS, formerly Head of Division, Institute for Animal Health, Compton, UK

J. Eric Hillerton BSc PhD FRES, Division of Environmental Microbiology, Institute for Animal Health, Compton, UK

Archibald G. Hunter BVM&S DTVM MRCVS, Centre for Tropical Veterinary Medicine, Royal (Dick) School of Veterinary Studies, University of Edinburgh, Easter Bush, UK

The late **Peter S. Jarvis** BSc, formerly of the Milk Marketing Board and Senior Adviser, Genus

Philip W. Jones BSc PhD CBiol MIBiol, Department of Environmental Microbiology, Institute for Animal Health, Compton, UK

Kevin P. Kenny MVB PhD MRCVS, Department of Agriculture, Dublin, Ireland

R. Paul Kitching BVetMed PhD MRCVS, National Centre for Foreign Animal Disease, Winnipeg, Canada

Aart de Kruif DVM PhD DipECAR, Clinic of Obstetrics, Ghent University, Belgium

Richard A. Laven BVetMed PhD MRCVS, Scottish Agricultural College, Veterinary Science Division, Dumfries, UK

Keith Lawrence BVSc PhD FRCVS, Elanco Animal Health, Basingstoke, UK

Peter Lees CBE BPharm PhD CBiol FIBiol Dr(hc)Ghent Hon Assoc. RCVS Hon Dip ECVPT, Department of Veterinary Basic Studies, Royal Veterinary College, Hatfield, UK

David N. Logue BVM&S PhD FRCVS, Scottish Agricultural College, Veterinary Science Division, Ayr

Margaret H. Lucas BVSc BSc DipBact MRCVS, formerly of the Central Veterinary Laboratory, Weybridge, UK

Richard W. Matthewman BSc MAgSc PhD, formerly of the Centre for Tropical Veterinary Medicine, Royal (Dick) School of Veterinary Studies, University of Edinburgh, Easter Bush, UK

Stephen A. May MA VetMB PhD DEO DipECVS DVR MRCVS, Department of Veterinary Clinical Studies, Royal Veterinary College, Hatfield, UK

Monika Mihm PhD MRCVS, Division of Veterinary Physiology and Pharmacology, Department of Veterinary Preclinical Studies, University of Glasgow, UK

Jeremy H. Morgan MA VetMB PhD MRCVS, formerly of the Institute for Animal Health, Compton, UK

Andrea M. Nolan MVB PhD DVA DipECVA DipECVPT MRCVS, Dean of Veterinary Faculty, Department of Veterinary Preclinical Studies, University of Glasgow, UK

Declan J. O'Rourke MVB FRCVS, Pfizer Ltd, Sandwich, UK

Andrew R. Peters BA PhD BVetMed DVetMed FRCVS, formerly Professor of Animal Health and Production, Royal Veterinary College, University of London, UK

P. Jim N. Pinsent BVSc FRCVS, formerly Senior Lecturer, School of Veterinary Science, University of Bristol, UK

Anthony Poole NDA CDA, formerly of Farm Management Services Information Unit, Milk Marketing Board, UK

John H. Pratt BVM&S DVSM MRCVS, formerly Head of Veterinary Services, Meat and Livestock Commission, Milton Keynes, UK

David W. B. Sainsbury BSc MA PhD MRCVS FRSH CBiol FIBiol, formerly Lecturer, Animal Science Division, Department of Clinical Veterinary Medicine, University of Cambridge, UK

Neil D. Sargison BA VetMB DSHP MRCVS, Faculty of Veterinary Medicine, Royal (Dick) School of Veterinary Studies, University of Edinburgh, Easter Bush, UK

Philip R. Scott DVM&S DSHP CertCHP FRCVS, Faculty of Veterinary Medicine, Royal (Dick) School of Veterinary Studies, University of Edinburgh, Easter Bush, UK

Jan K. Shearer DVM MS, College of Veterinary Medicine, University of Florida, Gainesville, USA

I. Martin Sheldon BVSc DCHP DBR DipECAR PhD ILTM MRCVS, Unit of Veterinary Reproduction, Royal Veterinary College, Hatfield, UK

David Sjeklocha DVM, Curtis, Nebraska, USA

Alistair K. Smith BVM&S DBR MRCVS, Ovaflo Bovine Embryo Transfer, Skene, Aberdeen, UK

Neville F. Suttle BSc PhD, formerly of the Moredun Research Institute, Penicuik, UK

Shaun Sweiger DVM MS, Edmond, Oklahoma, USA

Mike Tame BSc PhD Principle Associate, Abacus Organic Associates, East Stour, Dorset, UK

Andrew J. Taylor MA VetMB MRCVS, formerly Senior Veterinary Surgeon, Genus Breeding Limited, Chippenham, UK

Mike A. Taylor BVMS PhD MRCVS, VLA Veterinary Surveillance Unit, Central Science Laboratory, York, UK

Stuart M. Taylor BVM&S MRCVS, formerly Senior Veterinary Research Officer, Stormont, Northern Ireland

Lovell R. Thomsett DVD FRCVS, formerly Senior Lecturer, Royal Veterinary College, Hatfield, UK

Tore Tollersrud DVM PhD, National Veterinary Institute, Oslo, Norway

J. R. Townsend DVM, College of Veterinary Medicine, University of Florida, Gainsville, USA

Chris Venables BSc MIBiol CBiol, Veterinary Laboratories Agency, Addlestone, UK

Jos J. Vermunt Institute of Veterinary, Animal & Biomedical Sciences, Massey University, New Zealand

Timothy S. Wallis BSc PhD, Division of Environmental Microbiology, Institute for Animal Health, Compton, UK

Patricia R. Watson BSc PhD, Division of Environmental Microbiology, Institute for Animal Health, Compton, UK

A. David Weaver BSc DrVetMed PhD Dr(hc) FRCVS, Emeritus Professor, University of Missouri, Columbia, USA

G. Henk Wentink DVM PhD, Research Institute of Animal Husbandry, Lelystad, The Netherlands

David A. Whitaker MA VetMB MVSc MRCVS, Department of Veterinary Clinical Studies, Royal (Dick) School of Veterinary Studies, University of Edinburgh, Easter Bush, UK

J. Mike Wilkinson BSc PhD CBiol MIBiol, Chalcombe Publications, Welton, Lincoln, UK

The late **Bernard M. Williams** DVSM PhD MRCVS, formerly Head of the Veterinary Investigation Service, Ministry of Agriculture, Fisheries and Food (now DEFRA), Tolworth, UK

Roger S. Windsor MBE BVM&S BSc MA MRCVS, formerly Veterinary Centre Manager, Scottish Agricultural College, Veterinary Science Division, Dumfries

Geraint Wyn-Jones BVSc Hons DVR MRCVS, Meadowbank Veterinary Centre, Northop, UK

Gilbert B. Young PhD MRCVS, formerly Director, Animal Breeding Research Organisation, Edinburgh, UK

Preface

It is now about ten years since the first edition of *Bovine Medicine* was published. While it was originally anticipated that it would be used mainly in Britain and Europe, it is pleasing to note that a good proportion of the sales have been in other parts of the world. In recognition of this, more emphasis has been placed on conditions and their treatment in areas other than temperate regions. Additionally, a new section gives an insight to the differences in bovine medicine as practised in various parts of the world.

Almost all parts of the book have been updated or completely rewritten. There are some new chapters, including one which integrates the various problems which occur in cattle, another on basic surgical techniques and others on artificial insemination and embryo transfer. An effort has been made to encompass all the main subjects which occur in the husbandry and diseases of cattle.

I wish to thank all the authors and co-editors for their hard work. Roger Blowey, Hugh Boyd and Roger Eddy have provided advice and assistance despite their many commitments. I would also like to thank John Sproat for supplying the photographs of cattle used on the end papers.

Every effort has been made to identify copyright holders of material reproduced in this book. Any inadvertent omissions will be rectified in any future reprint or edition of this work.

I hope that everyone reading the new edition will find it to be an interesting source of information.

Readers' note

Inevitably, when it comes to therapies, medicines and vaccines, each country has different needs and requirements. The laws concerning the use of particular therapeutic and preventative agents may vary and the reader is reminded that it is his or her duty to ensure that any preparation prescribed conforms with all relevant national legislation where the preparation is to be used. It is also essential to ensure that dosages and routes of administration are determined according to any national or local directions and other product information which has been provided with the medicine. While every effort has been made to ensure that the uses suggested and doses recommended are correct they should always be checked with currently available information. It must also be remembered that any meat withdrawal time or milk witholding time for drugs should follow the guidelines of the country in which a drug is used.

A.H. Andrews

Preface to the First Edition

Bovine Medicine aims to provide, within the covers of one book, much of the practical information available on cattle disease and production. Such an objective is admirable in sentiment but very difficult to achieve in practice. It involves the concentration of effort by a large number of different, and often very busy, experts into one volume. For the present part it is hoped that what we have produced will not only be a source of information but, in many areas, it will be an enjoyable, educational read. It is hoped that it will be used as a working guide rather than a reference book and that it will be of particular help to those at the 'sharp end' of the veterinary profession, i.e. in practice. Bearing this in mind, this work does not contain every detail concerning each disease, organism or clinical entity.

Inevitably there are some areas of subject overlap as might be expected with skin conditions and ectoparasites and 'downer cow', etc. Where possible each author has provided his or her own perspective on the subject.

In addition, references have been kept to a minimum to ensure a less disjointed read. In consequence, we would be pleased to receive comments from readers on any deficiencies or difficulties encountered in presentation or content.

It has taken approximately 2 years to complete a work of this magnitude. The continual expansion in veterinary knowledge and expertise may well mean that in certain areas some recent developments have been omitted. Again, we would be pleased for any such deficiencies to be pointed out to us.

There has been considerable recent interest in alternative medicine for animals. Mindful of this, a section is included on the subject to help readers make up their own minds on its relevance to cattle therapy.

I must thank Blackwell Science, and particularly Peter Saugman for his patience during the production of this book. Much work has also fallen on my coeditors Hugh Boyd, Roger Blowey and Roger Eddy. However, the book would not have been completed but for the dedicated secretarial and managerial help of Mrs Rosemary Forster.

A.H. Andrews

Part 1
MANAGEMENT

Chapter 1
Calf Rearing

D.M. Allen

Introduction   3
Calf reception   3
Rearing systems   3
    Early weaning: bucket feeding   4
    Early weaning: machine feeding   5
Follow-on rearing   5
Performance targets   5
Veal production   5
Calf identification   6

Introduction

Whether calves from the dairy herd are being reared as dairy herd replacements or for beef production, a good start in life is essential. Calves of subnormal weight at three months of age tend to lag behind throughout the growing period.

The starting point for good calf rearing is the consumption of at least 2 litres of colostrum by suckling or bucket feeding within the first six hours of life and a further 2 litres within 12 hours. The passive immunity conferred on the calves by the immune lactoglobulin in colostrum is vital to disease resistance, especially if calves are transferred to another farm for rearing, probably via a collection centre or auction. Mortality among calves deprived of colostrum is high. Therefore, it is advisable to keep some colostrum in a freezer in case of emergencies.

Colostrum is a rich feed and a good source of the fat soluble vitamins A, D and E. Therefore it is sensible to feed all available colostrum even to calves that are beyond the stage when they can gain passive immunity.

Calf reception

Dairy-bred calves for beef rearing are usually purchased at about two weeks of age, often from a calf group or dealer. When they arrive at the farm, calves should be inspected individually and any showing signs of ill health returned to the supplier or isolated. Navels should be dipped in a concentrated iodine or phenol solution to guard against navel ill and joint ill. Any calves with signs of lice should be treated with an approved ectoparasite product. A multivitamin injection containing vitamins A, D and E is good value for money.

The calves should be housed in pens bedded liberally with dry straw and clean, fresh water should be made available. Milk is best withheld for a few hours after arrival but any calves that appear stressed may be given a warm drink of 1 litre of a proprietary electrolyte solution.

If calves are housed individually, which is permissible up to eight weeks of age, pens should be at least 1.8 × 1.0 metres and should permit visual and physical contact with at least one other calf. Group-housed calves up to 150kg liveweight need a minimum space allowance of 1.5 m^2, rising to 2.0 m^2 at 150–200 kg. Pen floors should have a slope from back to front of at least 1 in 20 to permit good drainage.

Calves do not mind cold weather but need good ventilation without drafts. The modern trend in temperate climates is to erect simple monopitch buildings in which calves can be housed until they are 12 weeks or older. In the coldest weather straw bales or wooden sheets can be placed above the rear half of pens to provide more insulation. Where calves are single-penned, the pens are dismantled at weaning and the calves left where they are as a rearing group. If buildings and pens are used continuously for calf rearing, after each batch they should be power washed or steam cleaned, disinfected and left empty for at least two weeks before restocking.

Rearing systems

In high yielding dairy herds, calves are weaned off their dams as soon as possible after they have received colostrum and are reared by the early weaning system pioneered in the UK but also applicable worldwide. Calves can be weaned off milk replacer after five to seven weeks, which makes the system convenient and saves money compared to weaning at an older age. The secret of success is to ensure that individual calves are eating at least 1 kg per day of a palatable early weaning concentrate before they are weaned.

The commonest rearing system is a twice daily bucket feed of milk replacer, but some rearers use computer-controlled machines that mix milk replacer and provide it to the calves via teats from which they suckle.

In the EU, where milk production is subject to milk quotas, milk produced over the quota has no market value so it is sensible to feed it to calves rather than purchase a milk replacer. However, if milk production is at or under quota, a milk replacer should be used. Feeding whole milk needs just the same attention to temperature and feeding level as milk replacer.

The high cost of dried skimmed milk on which milk replacers used to be based has led to the development of so-called 'zero' milk replacers. These are based on dried whey supplemented with fats and lactose to equate as closely as possible to cow's milk. Whey-based replacers are up to 25 per cent cheaper than skimmed milk products but can give equally good results.

For bucket feeding, replacers are mixed at 125–150 g/l, according to the manufacturer's recommendation. The mix is made up with water at 45–50°C so that the temperature at feeding is 42°C. Automatic feeding machines mix replacer at 100–125 g/l but can be set to vary reconstitution rates according to the stage of rearing. It is essential to keep all feeding equipment scrupulously clean.

Scouring and pneumonia are the twin scourges of calf rearing. Typically, calf mortality is 5 per cent, mainly due to these two causes, but it can rise to 10 per cent. The target in a well-managed calf rearing unit should be to keep mortality below 3 per cent.

Scouring is most likely in the first two weeks following removal from the dam and may be simply because the calf has been overfed or the milk replacer is at the wrong temperature. However, it may also be caused by pathogenic organisms. *E. coli* is the classic cause but a survey of calf units by practising veterinarians identified a number of other pathogens responsible for scouring. The immediate reaction to scouring is to take the calf off milk and feed a warm electrolyte solution. If the scouring does not start to clear up within 24 hours veterinary advice should be sought. Antibiotics should only be used on veterinary prescription.

If salmonella infection is suspected, veterinary advice should be sought straight away and rectal swabs taken for laboratory analysis so that the appropriate antibiotic can be prescribed. Infected calves should be isolated. Many *Salmonella* species are transmissible to humans so during an outbreak special attention needs to be paid to personal hygiene. Salmonellosis usually occurs in the first two or three weeks of life but can occur later, even beyond the milk feeding period (Chapter 15).

Pneumonia can occur at any time but is most prevalent in still, damp winter weather and is exacerbated if calves are moved at this time. Frequent observation is needed to identify the early symptoms of pneumonia – listlessness, holding back at feeding time, a runny nose, rapid breathing or coughing. Veterinary advice should be sought straight away. Not only is pneumonia a major cause of calf mortality but also infected calves that recover often fail to thrive due to lung damage.

Dehorning and castration are stressful and so should not be done together, nor should they coincide with the stress of weaning. Healthy calves can be dehorned three weeks into the rearing period using a hot air or hot iron disbudder, with castration at four weeks.

Early weaning: bucket feeding

The commonest early weaning rearing method is twice daily bucket feeding with weaning at five to seven weeks. With milk replacer mixed at 125 g/l, the first full feed for a purchased calf is 1 litre. Home-bred calves are fed this level twice daily until they are about five days old, then the feeding level per feed is increased by 0.25 litres every other day up to a maximum of 2 litres per feed, that is 4 litres per day.

Some expert calf rearers have found a useful saving in labour, without detriment to calf performance, by feeding the calves milk replacer once daily after the first seven to ten days. In this case the feeding level is built up gradually to 3 litres per day. However, the saving in labour should not compromise calf inspection, which should continue frequently to detect health problems.

From the start calves are fed an early weaning concentrate containing 18 per cent crude protein and with a good amino acid profile, since the calf needs some of its protein intake to escape fermentation and degradation in the forestomachs. The energy value should be at least 12.5 MJ ME/kg DM.

Even the youngest calves crave some roughage in their diet and, rather than letting them pick up straw from the bedding, it is better to feed hay or straw from a rack. Hay is rarely of good enough quality for calves and, even if it is, they eat too much of it at the expense of concentrates and become pot-bellied. Instead, feed bright, dry barley or oat straw.

As previously mentioned, calves must be eating at least 1 kg concentrate per day before they can be weaned. Weaning may be abrupt after about 35 days, or a gradual weaning procedure may be used in which the level of milk replacer is reduced gradually over an additional 5–10 days to encourage concentrate consumption. Gradual weaning avoids the check to growth that accompanies abrupt weaning.

The early weaning concentrate should be fed *ad libitum* until it is replaced by a cheaper follow-on concentrate, or until it is rationed as forage feeds are introduced (p. 5).

The consumption of milk powder is 15–20 kg and the target daily gain to weaning is 0.5–0.6 kg/day, depending on breed type and sex.

Early weaning: machine feeding

Feeding milk *ad libitum* to group-housed calves can be the preferred choice where the buildings used for calf rearing do not lend themselves to the erection of individual pens or, as in dairy herds, where calves are born over a long period.

The saving in labour is not as great as might be supposed because, although mixing is automatic and cleaning is quicker, handling the calves is more time consuming, especially teaching them to suckle.

The most sophisticated machines are computer controlled and recognize individual calves fitted with an electronic tag. So mixing rates and feeding levels can be varied from calf to calf, including a gradual weaning procedure. Some machines can feed whole milk as well as milk replacer and even dispense a small quantity of concentrates to encourage calves to eat dry feed immediately after suckling. Of course these machines are expensive but the cost is spread over up to 80 calves that can be reared at a time, so the annual depreciation per calf may be reasonable.

A cheaper approach to *ad libitum* feeding held sway for a time but is little used now. This was to feed cold acidified milk which stays fresh for two to three days stored in a simple plastic bin and is led to a teat through a tube fitted with a non-return valve. The equipment is cheap but lacks the sophisticated control of individual calves achieved by computer-controlled feeders.

Calves are trained to suckle about 1 litre of milk replacer and then the milk supply is removed until the next feed. The procedure is repeated twice in the next 24 hours and then calves are allowed to suckle *ad libitum*, with not more than six calves per teat. Intake may be depressed in the coldest winter weather and then it is advisable to use an immersion heater to take the chill off the milk replacer. The feeding equipment should be cleaned thoroughly between mixes.

A trough containing early weaning concentrates should be placed near the teats, but far enough away to avoid spoilage by saliva or spilt milk.

Calves fed *ad libitum* consume more milk replacer than restricted bucket-fed calves. This manifests itself as rather loose faeces that must be differentiated from scouring. The high replacer intake inhibits early concentrate consumption and may delay weaning. Therefore, it is important to employ a gradual weaning programme to allow weaning at five to seven weeks. Even at these high intakes of milk replacer, it is essential that fresh water should always be available.

Consumption of milk replacer powder is 25–30 kg and the target daily gain to weaning is 0.6–0.7 kg/day, depending on breed type and sex.

Follow-on rearing

When calves are weaned at five to seven weeks the early weaning concentrate must continue to be fed *ad libitum*. In the case of calves going into intensive beef systems, concentrate feeding continues to appetite through to 12 weeks, although the finishing diet is introduced gradually from eight to ten weeks.

Where calves are designated for forage-based beef systems, forage is introduced by the tenth week and the early weaning concentrate is replaced by a cheaper mix. When calves reared through the winter are to be grazed in the next summer, it is important to hold gains at 0.6–0.8 kg/day until turnout in the spring or the ability of the calves to exhibit extra rapid compensatory growth on high quality grazed grass will be inhibited. To achieve this the follow-on concentrate needs to be rationed at about $2\frac{1}{2}$ kg/day with forage fed to appetite.

Performance targets

Performance targets for early weaned bull calves fed concentrates *ad libitum* to three months are shown in Table 1.1.

Veal production

Veal production is a specialized system of calf rearing designed to produce a white meat that is especially popular in Italy and Germany. Traditionally, calves were housed in narrow crates and fed milk only until slaughter at 14–16 weeks, producing a carcass of 100–110 kg. Subsequently the feeding period was extended to 22 weeks or more to produce a carcass of 160+ kg.

Consumer revulsion at the unnatural production method has brought about considerable changes in the way veal is produced, sanctioned by EU and national legislation. For example, veal crates have been banned in Britain since 1990, although EU legislation does not ban existing crated housing in continental Europe until 2006. Similarly, legislation stipulates a minimum iron content for calf milks and insists that calves over two weeks of age have access to digestible solid food. The effect has been to promote the production of veal that is pink in colour rather than white.

A welfare-friendly veal production system has been demonstrated experimentally in Britain with group-housed calves fed milk replacer from a machine and

Table 1.1 Calf rearing targets to three months of age for bull calves fed concentrates *ad libitum*. Source: Meat and Livestock Commission (MLC).

	Bucket feeding		Machine feeding	
	Holstein–Friesian Hereford × F	Charolais × F Simmental × F	Holstein–Friesian Hereford × F	Charolais × F Simmental × F
Feeds (kg)				
Milk powder	15–20	15–20	25–30	25–30
Concentrates	170	185	160	180
Liveweight (kg)				
Purchase	50	55	50	55
Weaning	68	76	71	80
3 months	110	120	115	130
Daily gain (kg)				
Preweaning	0.5	0.6	0.6	0.7
Post weaning	0.9	1.0	0.9	1.0

F = Holstein–Friesian.

supplemented with barley straw as a source of roughage. Carcasses were acceptable to the veal trade but variability of performance was an unsolved problem.

In the Netherlands, the main EU veal producer, there are now two approaches to veal production. First there is a white veal system in which group-housed calves are fed largely on milk replacer but with limited access to maize silage (which does not affect meat colour). The calves are slaughtered at about six months of age at around 285 kg liveweight. A pink veal system is also employed by some producers in which calves are fed about 40 kg milk replacer powder plus 500 kg concentrates and 500 kg maize silage. The calves are slaughtered at about 32 weeks at a weight of around 320 kg.

Calf identification

A beneficial consequence of the BSE crisis and subsequent foot-and-mouth disease epidemic is a realization that being able to trace the whereabouts of cattle throughout their lives is an essential requirement of food safety for people and disease control in cattle.

Traceability is subject to EU legislation. The British Cattle Tracing System (CTS) is administered by the British Cattle Movement Service (BCMS) that commenced operations in September 1998. This fully computerized system was preceded by a paper passport system that started in July 1996. A one-off survey was undertaken of all cattle in 2000, including older cows and bulls which did not have passports, so that all cattle could be included in the BCMS database.

Calves must be double tagged within 36 hours of birth unless they are being sent for immediate slaughter. An application for a passport must normally be made within seven days of tagging but calves can be moved twice during the first 28 days of life, using the reverse of the cattle passport application form as a temporary passport. An all-numeric numbering system has replaced the former alpha numeric identity.

Chapter 2
Suckler Herds

D.M. Allen

Introduction	7
Planning the suckler herd	7
Choice of bull	7
Choice of cow breed type	8
Rearing replacement heifers	9
Suckler herd management	10
Suckled calf management	11
Grassland management	12
Targets of performance	13

Introduction

The key indicator of profitability and technical efficiency in suckler herds is the calf output produced annually from each cow that is bulled. The most profitable herds owe their success to producing a large number of live calves per 100 cows bulled, with low calf mortality, rapid growth to weaning and a high sale value per kg for well-reared calves. This is as true under dry range conditions as it is on productive temperate grassland.

Suckler herd management is not the simple matter it may seem at first sight, with a cow suckling a single calf. The linked components are reproductive efficiency, milk production and growth. However, in practice the body condition of cows is a simple and sensitive barometer of their nutritional status and potential performance. Controlling body condition through the year is the key to high herd output at low cost.

Most beef suckler cows are kept on marginal land in upland or range areas where winter (or dry season) feeds are scarce. So it is common for calves to be sold at weaning, or after a period of further feeding, to finishers on better land. However, increasingly in UK upland herds where suitable buildings are available, male calves are finished as bull beef on purchased concentrates.

Planning the suckler herd

Fitting a suckler enterprise into farm resources is as important to profitable production as herd management. Can the herd be integrated with a sheep flock? Are there arable crop residues that can be used to cheapen cow feeding? Are buildings and feeds available to add value to calves by feeding them beyond weaning? The answers to these and other relevant questions provide the framework on which a profitable enterprise can be built.

Particularly important is the choice of season of calving. Most herds calve in the spring or at the start of the rainy season because this minimizes cow feeding costs. The cow is working hardest suckling her calf on low cost, high quality grazed forage. On productive grassland autumn calving is an option, the extra cost of winter feeding cows suckling calves being offset by greater calf weaning weight. Autumn calving usually achieves the highest financial gross margin per cow, but spring calving rivals its gross margin per hectare. The need to reduce production costs has forced many former autumn-calving herds to change to spring calving.

The decision on calving season may be forced by the availability of housing and labour, regardless of feed availability. Housing allows a choice of calving season and avoids poaching of land by outwintered stock. However, the provision of housing increases fixed costs on the farm.

Choice of bull

The bull contributes half the genes of all the calves sired by him and so choice of breed and individual bull are both critical to herd performance. Even at weaning, when maternal effects are expressed at their maximum, sire breed has a greater effect on weaning weight than dam type.

Heavy breeds such as Charolais and Simmental are generally used as terminal sires, that is to produce the slaughter generation. They sire calves with the highest weaning weights (Table 2.1) and the rapid gains are carried through into the post-weaning period. However, the cost of this extra growth performance is a higher proportion of assisted calvings and greater neonatal calf mortality (Table 2.2). Overall, nevertheless, calves sired by heavier breeds produce the greatest annual output of weaning weight per cow.

It is several years since these survey data were collected and there may have been subsequent changes in the relative performance of breeds. Also, breeds such as the double-muscled Belgian Blue are now available to commercial producers in the UK. This breed is just below the Charolais in growth performance but has greater dystokia. Belgian Blue crosses have exceptional carcass characteristics with high killing out and meat yield percentages. Limousin crosses are also outstanding for these characteristics.

Most commercial suckler herds in Britain have opted for continental terminal sire breeds, especially Charolais, Limousin and Simmental. However, some producers prefer local breeds or use Angus bulls to gain quality premiums that offset poorer growth performance. Easy care Angus and Herefords are often selected in pastoral and range countries where large numbers of cattle are managed by a single stockworker. Breed choice would

also be affected if herd replacements are home bred. Then easy calving breeds with good maternal abilities would be preferred (see p. 9).

The selection of an individual bull within a breed is just as important as breed choice. In recent years bull selection has been transformed by the development of a sophisticated statistical method of analysing breeding records from pedigree herds, known by its acronym BLUP (best linear unbiased predictor). The analysis of records from all related cattle, whatever herd they are in, effectively disentangles management and genetic effects on performance to calculate estimated breeding values (EBVs) that can be used with confidence to select bulls of above average genetic merit.

In Britain the recording agency Signet combines EBVs for selected performance characters into selection indices of overall genetic merit. There are two such indices. The calving value is used where ease of calving is paramount, for example for heifer matings and in the selection of bulls to breed female replacements. The beef index is used for bull selection when growth rate and carcass quality are the objectives, for example for terminal sires in suckler herds. Signet publishes EBVs and selection indices for participating breeds. A maternal index is under development.

Choice of cow breed type

In range countries the tradition was to keep purebred herds of Angus, Hereford, Shorthorn or local breed cattle. To some extent that tradition still exists. For example, French suckler cows are still largely purebred. However, crossbred cows have a considerable advantage over purebreds due to hybrid vigour (or heterosis), which is most pronounced for improved reproductive efficiency. The outcome is that the weaning weight of calves from crossbred cows is 15–25 per cent above the average of the parent breeds. Add to this an

Table 2.1 Effects of sire breed on calf 200-day weights. Source: Meat and Livestock Commission (MLC).

Sire breed	Type of farm		
	Lowland	Upland	Hill
Hereford 200-day weight (kg)	208	194	184
Difference from Hereford (+/– kg)			
Charolais	+32	+33	+21
Simmental	+24	+28	+14
South Devon	+23	+27	+16
(North) Devon	+17	+21	+7
Lincoln Red	+14	+20	+5
Sussex	+7	+13	+2
Limousin	+7	+10	+2
Aberdeen Angus	–14	–12	–8

Table 2.2 Effects of sire breed on calving ease and annual productivity. Source: Meat and Livestock Commission (MLC).

Sire breed	Assisted calvings (%)	Calf mortality (%)	Calving interval (days)	Calf weaning weight per cow per year (kg)
Charolais	9.0	4.8	374	208
Simmental	8.9	4.2	374	203
South Devon	8.7	4.0	375	203
(North) Devon	6.4	2.6	373	200
Limousin	7.4	3.8	375	199
Lincoln Red	6.7	2.0	373	198
Sussex	4.5	1.5	372	196
Hereford	4.0	1.6	372	189
Aberdeen Angus	2.4	1.3	370	179

improvement in longevity and the lifetime advantage to crossbreds is considerable.

Recognition of the benefits of crossbreeding in Britain is as old as the development of breeds themselves. Traditional crossbreds include the celebrated Blue Grey (White Shorthorn bull × Galloway cow), Shorthorn × Highland and Irish-bred Blue Grey (Angus × Dairy Shorthorn). As supplies of these traditional crosses started to become scarce some 30 years ago, beef breed × dairy cows started to be used as suckler cows, notably Hereford × Friesian and Angus × Friesian. It was later still that US ranchers discovered the heterosis advantage of Hereford × Angus and the reciprocal cross over either of the pure breeds.

The Hereford × Friesian was, and still is, widely used as a suckler cow. It produces more milk than the Blue Grey and weans a heavier calf; however, the Blue Grey has better reproductive efficiency and, overall, performance of the two crosses is similar. Both crosses share the advantage of medium body size. Heavy cows such as Charolais × Friesian need more feed but are unable to translate enough of their greater weight into heavier calf weaning weight to rival the efficiency of a lighter breed type. Nonetheless, many British suckled calf producers use these heavier cows and are prepared to trade a theoretical reduction in efficiency (that may not be apparent at farm level) for the improved conformation of calves which commands a premium at the calf sales and later in carcass value.

The penetration of the Friesian breed by extreme dairy Holstein genes from North America has caused such a deterioration in beef breed × Friesian cow conformation that it shows through in the calf. This has sparked off a search for alternative suckler herd replacements that are crossbred with good maternal qualities and have acceptable conformation. Moreover, in the wake of the BSE crisis many herd owners wish to breed their own replacements so that they can maintain a closed cow herd.

Merely saving heifer calves from terminal sire breeds such as Charolais increases cow size progressively and reduces maternal performance – the worst of all worlds. The simplest planned approach to breeding replacements is to breed about half the herd to a sire breed of medium size with good maternal qualities, for example Angus or Salers. In smaller herds this is best done by artificial insemination (AI). In the next generation, Angus cross females, for example, might be mated to Salers whose female progeny are in turn mated back to Angus. This two-breed rotation is known as crisscrossing. The other half of the herd would usually be mated to terminal sire breeds.

Bulls for breeding herd replacements should be selected to have a good calving value index (which incorporates EBVs for calf birth weight, ease of calving

score and gestation length) and a high EBV for 200-day milk (an estimate of the genetic merit for milk production that the sire passes to his female offspring).

In some parts of the world, notably the US, sophisticated breeding programmes have been used to create composite breeds combining the best features of three or four foundation breeds. A composite may be bred to feature maternal qualities, terminal sire qualities, heat tolerance and so on. A four-breed composite is effectively a purpose-bred pure breeding population that retains up to 75 per cent of the hybrid vigour of the initial first (F1) crosses between the original four breeds.

The creation of composite breeds needs very large numbers of cattle. However, commercial suckled calf producers with relatively small herds will have access to composites from international genetics companies with large-scale breeding operations involving thousands of cattle. The main demand will be for purpose-bred suckler herd replacements of good maternal ability.

Rearing replacement heifers

The replacement policy in a suckler herd should involve culling cows that are persistently barren, calve unacceptably late or are on the verge of the emaciation commonly associated with old age. A typical replacement rate is 16 per cent which indicates an average herd life of seven years.

In the UK, culling policies have been disrupted in the wake of the BSE crisis by the Over Thirty Month Scheme (OTMS) in which the carcasses of cattle over 30 months old are removed from human consumption. Compensation payments for culls are much lower than cull cow values before the BSE crisis and this will continue to inhibit planned culling until the scheme is eventually wound down.

Replacements may be purchased as calves from dairy herds, as bulling heifers or, less frequently nowadays, as heifers on the point of calving. With calves and bulling heifers it is prudent to purchase a surplus of 15–20 per cent to allow selection. Heifers that prove unsuitable as replacements are slaughtered for beef.

In most situations heifers should be calved for the first time at two years of age to optimise lifetime performance. However, autumn-born calves from the dairy herd would usually be calved at $2\frac{1}{2}$ years in a spring-calving suckler herd. In either case, good management is necessary to achieve target mating and post calving weights (Table 2.3).

Heifers are best calved at the start of the herd calving period to allow for an almost inevitable slippage in time to the second calving. Also, since dystokia is worst in

Table 2.3 Rearing targets for replacement heifers.

	Mating weight (kg)	Post calving weight (kg)
Two-year calving		
British breed crosses	325	510
Continental breed crosses	350	550
Calving at 2½ years		
British breed crosses	400	540
Continental breed crosses	435	575

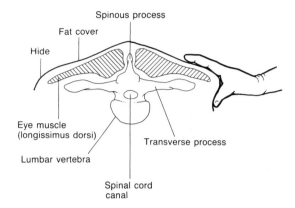

Fig. 2.1 Technique for condition scoring.

heifers, it is desirable to mate them to an easy calving breed such as Angus or Hereford. Difficult calving is a cause of delayed rebreeding.

Suckler herd management

Suckler herd management aims for a high proportion of cows producing live calves in a calving period of 12 weeks or less. The advantages of a compact calving period are, firstly, that herd rationing matches closely the nutritional needs of individual cows, saving feed costs. Secondly, calvings can be supervised closely to provide assistance when needed, reducing calf mortality. Finally, calf performance is uniform with few of the late-born calves that are so difficult to utilize profitably.

Generally, a long drawn out calving period is a sure sign of low herd conception rate. Late calvers have too little time to rebreed by the end of the mating season and get later and later, eventually failing to get in calf altogether. The only solutions to an over-long calving period are to cull late calvers or switch them between spring- and autumn-calving herds so that they calve on time. The danger of the latter strategy is that cows shuttle from one herd to the other without the underlying causes of low conception rate being tackled.

The main reason why cows fail to conceive is that they are too thin. Under UK conditions, body condition at mating, scored on a scale from 0 (emaciated) to 5 (grossly overfat), needs to be 2½ in winter but can be as low as 2 if cows are grazing high quality forage and current nutrient intake is high. The key targets that achieve the necessary body condition at mating are a score of 3 in the autumn and 2 at turnout to grazing in the spring. The time to carry out condition scoring is in mid pregnancy, while there is still time to adjust feeding management before calving.

The method of condition scoring (Fig. 2.1) is to grip the loin between the thumb and forefinger mid-way between the hip (hook) bone and the last rib on the left side of the cow. The thumb curls over the ledge formed by the transverse processes of the spine to feel the overlying fat cover. It is best to handle cows until experience of the technique has been gained but, thereafter, a skilled stockworker can use close visual inspection to obtain a working guide to condition.

Descriptions of condition score classes are presented in Table 2.4. One possible confusion is with continental crosses of good conformation. Their thick muscling may overhang the transverse processes of the spine and confuse handling or visual assessments. If this is the case, condition should also be assessed by handling the ribs with the flat of the hand. If the score is above 3 in the autumn, autumn-calving cows are put at the risk of a difficult calving. If spring calvers score less than 3 in the autumn, the permissible winter weight loss is reduced and feed costs increase.

Feeding spring-calving cows through the winter that are at target condition score 3 in the autumn allows the loss of one unit of condition score, which equates to about 100 kg liveweight or 0.5 kg daily. Autumn calvers, on the other hand, must be fed through the winter for the additional strain of lactation and must be at condition score 2½ when mated in mid-winter. Therefore, in cows at condition score 3 in the autumn a weight loss of only 0.25 kg/day is permissible until they are safely in calf. If there is a time to feed suckler cows generously, this is it. Thereafter, the rate of weight loss can increase to 0.5 kg/day. Autumn-calved heifers are still growing as well as milking and should not be allowed to lose weight through the winter.

These guidelines are translated into daily metabolizable energy (ME) allowances expressed as megajoules (MJ) for cows fed a typical moderate quality ration in Table 2.5.

It is all too easy during the grazing season to concentrate on calf performance and forget that cows at target condition score 2 in the spring need to gain

Table 2.4 Condition scoring of suckler cows.

Condition score	Description
0	Spine very prominent with no detectable fat cover over the sharp transverse processes of the spine
1	Spine still prominent but transverse processes no longer sharp
2	Transverse processes can still be felt, but now rounded with a thin covering of fat
3	Individual transverse processes can now only be felt with firm pressure by the thumb
4	Transverse processes can hardly be felt, even with firm pressure
5	Transverse processes completely obscured with a thick layer of soft fat and puffy fat deposits around the tail head

Table 2.5 Metabolizable energy (ME) allowances for winter feeding suckler cows. Reproduced from Allen (2001) with permission of Chalcombe Publications.

Liveweight (kg)	Daily weight loss (kg)	Milk yield (kg)	ME (MJ/day)
Spring calver			
(a) Precalving[a]			
500	−0.5	0	55
600			62
700			69
(b) Post calving[a]			
500	−0.5	10	89
600			97
700			105
Autumn calver			
(a) Premating[b]			
500	−0.25	10	99
600			107
700			115
(b) Post mating[b]			
500	−0.5	7	74
600			81
700			88

[a] If no weight loss is permissible add 20 MJ ME per day.
[b] If no weight loss is permissible add 10 MJ ME per day.

100 kg liveweight by the autumn. If by mid-season there is any doubt that the whole herd or individual cows may not attain the required total gain, action must be taken to rectify the situation. The provision of more selective grazing of fresh pasture may suffice. Alternatively, it may be necessary to take more drastic action with autumn calvers and wean calves early to remove the strain of lactation.

Suckled calf management

If cow performance is good, calf performance is usually also good. This is not to say that calf performance looks after itself. Nevertheless, a compact calving means fewer of the late-born calves have subnormal weaning weights. In addition, achieving target body condition scores in cows is conducive to high milk yield.

In most situations the cow is capable of producing as much milk as the calf can suckle. This can lead to problems early in the suckling period, especially with spring-calving beef × dairy cows of high milk potential, when calves consume too much milk and scour. If the cause of scouring is viral or bacterial it is worth considering an appropriate scour vaccine.

Milk consumption increases quickly during the first month of suckling and, although calves pick at solid food early in life, milk intake dominates calf performance in the first three months. With a cow type of moderate yield potential, milk still accounts for half the calf gain in the third month and in higher yielding beef breed × Friesians this balance is not reached until the fourth month. Nevertheless, by this time the intake of solid food by the calf is increasing rapidly.

Milk intake is especially important to the spring-born calf that has a relatively short suckling period of six to seven months. The nutritional requirements of the calf and seasonal grass growth are well matched, although supplementary feeding helps to sustain daily gain from late summer onwards as grass growth and quality decline.

Management of the autumn-born calf is more complicated because the suckling period is longer and peak milk yield must be supported on winter rations. The most cost-effective approach over the winter is to feed the cow well in the early months until she is safely in calf and then to rely increasingly on creep feeding calves concentrates and the highest quality conserved forage available. It is energetically much more efficient to feed the calf directly than to increase cow feeding to stimulate milk yield.

When autumn-calved cows are turned out to grass in the spring there is a boost to milk yield, but by late summer calves require creep feeding to sustain daily gains. It is wise to wean the calves sooner rather than

Table 2.6 Performance targets for lowland and upland suckler herds.

	Continental breed sire[a]			British breed sire[a]		
	Autumn	Spring (silage)	Spring (straw)	Autumn	Spring (silage)	Spring (straw)
Calves reared/cow	0.92	0.92	0.92	0.95	0.95	0.95
Calf gain (kg/day)	1.0	1.1	1.1	0.9	1.0	1.0
Weaning (months)	10	7	7	10	7	7
Calf autumn weight (kg)	350	280	280	320	260	260
Cow concentrate (tonnes)	0.25	0.12	0.3	0.25	0.12	0.3
Calf concentrate (tonnes)	0.25	0.08	0.08	0.1	0.05	0.05
Silage (tonnes @ 22% DM)	6.5	5.0	—	6.5	5.0	—
Feeding straw (tonnes)	0.5	1.0	2.5	0.5	1.0	2.5

[a] Mated to suckler cows of average weight 550–600 kg.

later so that they can be managed separately and the cows left to gain condition before housing. The least stressful way of breaking the bond between calf and dam at weaning is to house the calves. An alternative approach is to put the cows and calves in well-fenced adjacent fields within sight and sound of each other.

In most ranching and pastoral countries bull calves are castrated for the convenience of herd management and a preference for steer beef over bull beef. However, in France, Italy and Spain it has become the custom to rear male calves entire because they grow faster and leaner than steers and are more profitable. In the UK, suckler bull beef is increasing and finds a ready market. The most common approach is to wean spring-born bulls in late summer and transfer them gradually over a period of about three weeks to an all-concentrate diet (Chapter 3).

For the system to be successful it is a considerable advantage to have a compact calving period so that older bull calves do not pester late-calving cows when they are in oestrus. In any case, cows with bull calves need to be separated from those with heifers by six months of age or there is a risk of premature pregnancy in the heifer calves. For this reason the system works best in spring-calving herds because there is no need to split the herd.

Grassland management

Grazed grass is the cheapest and one of the most nutritious feeds available on the farm. With financial margins under pressure, the key to profitable production is to utilize grazing to the full. This involves good grazing management and extending the grazing season where practicable.

Grassland management for suckler herds does not necessarily mean using the levels of nitrogen fertilizer employed by dairy farmers, although this may be the right policy on some productive lowland farms. In practice, especially on the upland farms where most suckler cows are kept in the UK, farmers use only moderate levels of nitrogen fertilizer and rely more on clover to increase sward productivity. Moreover, extensive grassland management is encouraged in the EU by the payment of extensification premiums for stocking lightly.

Whatever the type of sward, grazing management should aim to control the average sward height of grazed and ungrazed areas. Cows gain most weight early in the grazing season when average sward height is maintained at 8–10 cm. However, they graze selectively leaving patches that go to seed and are of poor nutritional quality when they have to be grazed later on. So until mid season it is necessary to graze swards more tightly at an average sward height of 6–8 cm to inhibit seed heading. Thereafter, when the risk of seed heading is less and there is an inevitable build-up of dead herbage in the base of the sward, average sward height can be relaxed to 8–10 cm to allow selective grazing.

In the period of peak grass growth in early summer, high stocking rates of three autumn calving cows per hectare or four spring calvers are needed to exert the necessary control of sward height. At these relatively high stocking rates it is important to have a reserve grazing buffer in case of reduced grass growth in dry weather. This can be achieved by setting aside an additional 25 per cent of grassland that is conserved as silage if possible, but grazed if necessary.

As the season progresses beyond mid season the grazing area needs to increase and this is achieved by grazing aftermaths on fields cut previously for silage or hay.

Parasitic worms causing gastroenteritis and bronchitis are less of a problem in suckled calves than in young dairy-bred calves in their first grazing season. Nevertheless, it is advisable to treat autumn-born calves at weaning. In any case, both autumn- and spring-born calves should be treated at yarding to guard against winter scour (Chapter 19).

With silage making the priority is a feed with high intake characteristics rather than the highest possible ME per kg dry matter (DM). Cutting can be delayed for a week or so to await dry sunny weather that allows an effective 24-hour wilt for clamp silage, longer for big bales, and produces silage with the best fermentation quality.

Targets of performance

The objectives of suckler herd management outlined in this chapter have been compiled into suckler herd targets appropriate to lowland and upland herds in the UK and other European countries with similar climatic conditions (Table 2.6). For the predominant spring-calving herds targets are shown for herds both on grass farms, where silage is the basic winter feed, and on arable farms, where winter diets are based on straw and concentrates. Achieving the physical targets is a prerequisite of profitable production.

Reference

Allen, D. (2001) *Rationing Beef Cattle*, 2nd edn. Chalcombe Publications, Lincoln.

Chapter 3
Beef Finishing Systems

D.M. Allen

Introduction	14
Planning and budgeting	14
Finishing suckled calves and stores	15
Winter finishing	15
Grass finishing	17
Dairy beef systems	18
Cereal (barley) beef	19
Grass and maize silage beef	19
Eighteen-month beef	20
Grass beef	20

Introduction

A whole range of overlapping beef finishing systems is applicable to cattle bred in suckler and dairy herds. The higher the lifetime daily gain of the beef system, the younger is the slaughter age and the lighter the slaughter weight at a stated carcass fat cover. Also, within a given beef system, bulls grow faster and are leaner than steers which, in turn, grow faster and are leaner than heifers.

These characteristics of beef systems make it possible to chart average relationships between slaughter age and slaughter weight, illustrated in Fig. 3.1 for Charolais crosses. It is possible to construct similar graphs for other breed types and to predict the likely slaughter weight of cattle slaughtered at a particular age and vice versa. Note that as long as the Over Thirty Month Scheme (OTMS) is in place as a BSE control measure in the UK, beef from cattle over 30 months old at slaughter is destroyed, although this will change from 2004 onwards.

Cattle remain in an EU fat class for several weeks. The main EU fat class for bull carcasses is 3 on a five-point scale from 1 (ultra lean) to 5 (grossly overfat) and 4L for steers and heifers, which is the average fat class for all carcasses in Britain.

Calves from beef suckler herds on marginal land usually have to be sold in the autumn for finishing on farms with more productive land. However, spring-born calves may be overwintered for sale in spring, if buildings and feed are available, and bull calves may be finished on purchased concentrates as suckler bull beef.

The heaviest yearling steer calves purchased by fin- ishers in the autumn may be finished through the ensuing winter for sale at 16–18 months old. Heifers and lighter steer calves are fed a store ration over the winter in preparation for grazing the following summer. Any that fail to finish off grass are yarded for a further winter finishing period.

Still, all too many cattle are managed aimlessly with no particular finishing system in mind and are sold finished or in store condition when prices seem favourable. This approach leads to a good deal of trading in suckled calves and stores, some of which may change ownership three or four times in their lifetime. Farm assurance schemes now limit the number of times an animal can be traded within the scheme.

Under range conditions in the USA, the growth rate of suckled calves is poorer than on European grass farms. However, feed grains are cheap and a special approach to finishing has been adopted in beef feed lots. Weaned calves from range herds are sold to 'back grounding' farms where they are grown on forage at moderate store rates of gain as feeder cattle. They then enter feed lots at 12–18 months of age for rapid finishing over a five-month period on a 'hot' high-grain ration.

In the case of dairy-bred calves, several distinctive beef systems have been developed. At one extreme is cereal (barley) beef in which bulls fed an all-concentrate diet grow rapidly to slaughter at 11–13 months of age. At the other extreme are forage-based systems in which steers and heifers are either winter finished off silage supplemented with concentrates for slaughter at 16–20 months of age or grass finished in summer at 20–24 months old.

In reality, cattle passport statistics indicate that more than a third of steers do not follow any of the production systems described here and are slaughtered at 24–30 months of age. The reason is thought to be that farmers delay slaughter until after they have obtained the second beef subsidy (p. 15), paid from 22 months of age. It demonstrates how subsidy rules manipulate production and marketing decisions.

Planning and budgeting

The fall in market prices for beef cattle in the aftermath of the BSE crisis has focused attention on beef system

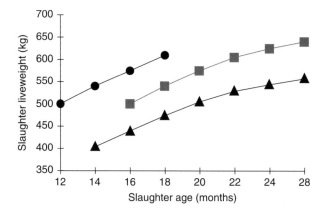

Fig. 3.1 Average relationships between slaughter age and slaughter weight for Charolais cross cattle. (Bulls were slaughtered at EU fat class 3, steers and heifers at EU fat class 4L.) ● = Bulls; ■ = steers; ▲ = heifers.

plans and budgets. Formerly, too many beef farmers were preoccupied by the margin between buying and selling prices, or even just the sale price achieved regardless of cost. Now controlling costs, whilst achieving performance targets, is very important. Also essential is maximizing eligibility for EU subsidies, without which profitable production is difficult.

The EU beef regime that came into effect in January 2000 is more complex than previous schemes. As before, bulls may qualify for a single Bull Premium and steers for one or both Beef Special Premiums (BSP), the first of which is paid at 9–20 months of age and the second at over 22 months. There is no upper limit on the number of claims provided the stocking rate does not exceed 1.8 Livestock Units (LU) per forage hectare, otherwise claims are scaled back. If a national ceiling of claims is exceeded, payments are also scaled back. Cattle must be retained for at least 2 months after the claim is made. All slaughter cattle, including cull cows, qualify for a slaughter premium provided they have been on the farm for at least two months. Suckler Cow Premiums are paid up to a farm quota and a minimum of 5 per cent and maximum of 40 per cent of claims can be made on heifers over 8 months of age. Complex rules apply to Extensification Premiums paid on farms practising extensive production methods. Detailed rules and rates of payment can be found in official publications. In 2003 discussions were in progress to alter fundamentally the basis of subsidy payments with headage subsidies replaced by area payments.

The starting point for planning is a decision on which beef system fits farm resources best, setting performance targets and drawing up a budget to evaluate margin potential. Figure 3.2 presents a budget format that can be used to evaluate finishing systems and shows as an example cereal bull beef from purebred Holstein–Friesian bulls.

If production is based on borrowed capital, it is important to calculate the interest on working capital that must be paid. The conventional method of calculation is the cost of the calf or store plus half the variable costs multiplied by the monthly bank interest rate for the number of months cattle are fed.

Sale returns are highly dependent on the quality of cattle produced, especially their conformation. Figure 3.3 illustrates differentials for steer carcasses classified by the EU method, in a conformation range from E (excellent), U+, –U, R (average), O+, –O and P (very poor). Note the severe discount for poor –O conformation, especially for carcasses that stray into what is regarded by most buyers as overfat class 4H. Holstein–Friesian carcasses fall into the poorest conformation classes –O and P and a high proportion of the beef is used for manufacturing. Good conformation classes –U and better contain mainly continental breed crosses.

Generally, young bulls sell for the same price per kg carcass or slightly less than steers in deadweight sales, but command a premium at selected live auction markets. Heifers usually sell at a small discount. There is a steady move towards deadweight selling under pressure from supermarket buying specifications.

Finishing suckled calves and stores

At the start of a winter feeding period there are two options for steers and heifers. Either the cattle are fed to gain at least 0.9 kg/day, often higher, for finishing that winter. Or they are fed a store ration to gain 0.6–0.8 kg/day in preparation for grazing the following summer.

It is generally held that the profitability of finishing depends mainly on buying and selling skills. It is perfectly true that the feeder's margin – the difference between the purchase and sale price – determines the average gross margin. However, finishers with the best margins owe much of their success to achieving high standards of cattle performance.

Winter finishing

Winter finishing has a feeding period of four to eight months, depending on breed, sex category and individual performance. At the start of the winter the cattle may be yearling suckled calves or older store cattle. Commonly, they are fed rationed concentrates with silage to appetite, but on arable farms arable byproducts may partly or wholly replace grass silage.

Steers of all breed types are well suited to winter finishing. Early maturing heifers are less suitable because they finish too quickly at light weights. Nevertheless, continental cross heifers can be winter finished at around 0.9 kg/day on a high forage diet.

	Budget (£/head)	Example: cereal beef[a] (£/head @ 2003 prices)
A Calf or store cost		40
B Calf rearing to 3 months: dairy-bred calf		58
C Forage costs . . . cattle/ha @ . . . £/ha[b]		0
D Concentrate costs *1.9* tonnes @ *£100*/t		190
E Other feeds: straw *0.3* tonnes @ *£30*/t		9
straights . . . tonnes @ . . . /t		
by-products . . . tonnes @ . . . /t		
F Other variable costs: veterinary		10
bedding		20
marketing		8
Miscellaneous		10
Total		**48**
G Total calf + variable costs		
(A + B + C + D + E + F)		**345**
H Sale weight (kg liveweight or carcass)		475 kg
I Forecast sale price (£/kg)		0.8 £/kg
J Returns: weight **H** × sale price **I**		**380**
K Gross margin (excluding premiums)		35
L Premiums: 1st beef special premium		0
2nd beef special premium		0
bull premium		130
slaughter premium		50
extensification premium		0
Total		**180**
Overall gross margin (including premiums) **K + L**		**215**

[a] Holstein–Friesian bull beef.
[b] Guidelines on forage costs at 2003 prices:
    intensive (350 kg N fertilizer/ha) £210/ha
    semi-intensive (250 kg N/ha) £150/ha
    extensive (75 kg N or less/ha) £70/ha.

Fig. 3.2 Budget format for beef finishing systems.

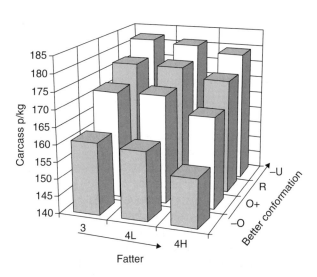

Fig. 3.3 Price differentials for steer carcasses of different EU conformation and fat classes. Source: Meat and Livestock Commission price report 1999.

Standards for winter finishing suckled calves and stores are shown in Table 3.1. Continental cross steers slaughtered at two years old or more may be too heavy for some buyers.

Suckler bull beef is still relatively new to the UK, but has been commonplace in France for many years. Production is expanding in the UK but demand is limited and it is important to secure a market before commencing production. The system is simplest for spring-born calves which are weaned in the autumn and transferred gradually over about three weeks to an all-concentrate diet containing 16 per cent crude protein. However, autumn-born calves weaned in the spring can also be used. The British safety code for bull beef production recommends no more than 20 bulls to a pen but much larger groups are housed in continental Europe.

Maize silage is short of protein but has good feed intake characteristics and is an excellent source of energy. In continental Europe maize silage is widely

Table 3.1 Standards for winter finishing.

	Yearling suckled calf			18-month store		
	British	Continental		British	Continental	
	Steer	Steer	Heifer	Steer	Steer	Heifer
Feeding period (months)	5	6	5	5	5	5
Start weight (kg)	320	350	310	420	475	400
Daily gain (kg)	0.9	1.0	0.8	0.8	0.9	0.8
Silage (tonnes, 22% DM)	3.6	3.6	4	5.7	5.9	5.5
Concentrates (kg)	300	450	220	135	265	200
Slaughter weight (kg)	455	525	430	540	610	525
Carcass (kg)	250	295	235	300	340	290

Table 3.2 Standards for suckler bull beef using continental crosses.

	Spring-born		Autumn-born	
	Concentrates	Maize silage	Concentrates	Maize silage
Start age (months)	6	6	6	6
Feeding period (months)	6	7	6	7
Start weight (kg)	245	245	230	230
Daily gain (kg)	1.4	1.3	1.4	1.3
Concentrates (tonnes)	1.4	1.0	1.4	1.0
Maize silage (tonnes)[a]	—	3.3	—	3.1
Slaughter weight (kg)	500	525	485	510
Carcass (kg)	280	295	270	285

[a] Maize silage at 30% DM.

used as the forage base for intensive bull beef production. The medium-sized feed lots of the Po valley in northern Italy with a few hundred to a few thousand cattle are a good example. In these maize silage comprises 30–50 per cent of ration DM.

Maize silage has not been used much for bull beef production in Britain but there is potential for systems in which maize silage forms up to 30 per cent of the dry matter of the diet, producing daily gains not far short of all-concentrate diets. Where suckled calf producers on marginal land have suitable buildings available, bull beef fed purchased concentrates can be a useful way of adding value to herd output.

Standards for suckler bull beef are shown in Table 3.2. Achieving the target daily gains is a prerequisite of profitable production. In practice many producers extend the feeding period and take bulls to slaughter weights in excess of 600 kg. At these high slaughter weights there is a danger of feed cost exceeding the value of daily gain and carcasses being too heavy for buyers.

Grass finishing

Grazed grass is the cheapest and potentially the highest quality home grown feed. There is a growing realization of the need to exploit grass better by managing swards to maximize daily gains and, where practicable, to extend the grazing season.

In grass finishing systems, achieving high daily gains is especially important so that marketing begins in midseason and reduces cattle numbers in step with declining grass production and quality.

Two aspects of management are crucial. Firstly, in the winter preceding grass finishing, gains are held down at a store level so that cattle exhibit rapid compensatory growth when they are turned out onto spring grass. Secondly, grazing should be managed to get the best

Table 3.3 Specimen winter store rations.

Weight (kg)	British cross steer/heifer @ 0.6 kg/day		Continental cross steer @ 0.8 kg/day	
	Silage (kg/day)	Straw + concentrate (kg/day)	Silage + concentrate (kg/day)	Straw + concentrate (kg/day)
200	18	3.5 + 2.0	16 + 1	3.5 + 3.0
250	21	4.0 + 2.5	19 + 1	4.5 + 3.0
300	23	4.5 + 3.0	22 + 1	4.5 + 3.5
350	26	5.0 + 3.5	20 + 2	5.0 + 4.0
400	28	5.0 + 4.0	23 + 2	5.0 + 4.5

combination of daily gains in cattle and regrowth of high quality grass.

Grass finishing may commence with stores purchased in the spring or with suckled calves or stores purchased in the autumn that are overwintered before grass finishing. Specimen low cost rations for overwintering cattle are shown in Table 3.3. The lower gain of 0.6 kg/day is optimum for British cross steers and heifers of all breed types. The higher gain of 0.8 kg/day is suitable for continental cross steers.

During the grazing season on set stocked pastures, the provision of a continuous supply of nutritious grass is achieved by controlling sward height (the average of grazed and ungrazed grass). In the first half of the season sward height is controlled at 6–8 cm to inhibit seed heading. Then in the second half of the season, when there is less risk of seed heading and dead herbage begins to accumulate in the base of the sward, grazing height is relaxed to 8–10 cm to allow more selective grazing.

The confidence to manage cattle at the high early summer stocking rates needed to achieve this degree of control is helped by adding 25 per cent to the main grazing area as a buffer that can be grazed if grass runs short but is conserved if not needed. From mid-season grazing needs to expand onto aftermath regrowths on areas previously cut for silage or hay.

Grazing performance is undermined if cattle, especially those in their first season of independent grazing, become infected with parasitic worms that cause gastro-enteritis and bronchitis. Effective control programmes include early season treatment to inhibit the build-up of infective larvae on the sward, mid-season treatment accompanied by a move to fresh aftermaths on fields previously conserved or mid-season treatment with a long-acting bolus to control infection even though pastures carry infective larvae. The choice depends on farm circumstances (Chapter 19).

Standards for an overwintering and grass finishing system are presented in Table 3.4. Because the second

Table 3.4 Standards for overwintering and grass finishing suckler-bred steers and heifers.

	British cross		Continental cross	
	Steer	Heifer	Steer	Heifer
Winter store period				
Feeding period (months)	6	6	6	6
Start weight (kg)	270	235	300	260
Daily gain (kg)	0.6	0.6	0.8	0.6
Concentrates (kg)	90	90	500	90
Silage (tonnes)	4.5	4.3	5.2	4.5
Grass finishing				
Turnout weight (kg)	375	345	445	370
Feeding period (months)	5	5	6	5
Daily gain (kg)	0.8	0.7	0.9	0.8
Concentrates (kg)	50	0	150	50
Slaughter weight (kg)	500	450	600	490
Carcass (kg)	275	245	335	270

BSP is paid from 22 months of age, steers that are close to this age at the end of the grazing season are often yarded for winter finishing just to claim the subsidy. It is a strategy that needs to be costed carefully.

Dairy beef systems

In the UK the main dairy herd calving season is in late summer and autumn, which contrasts with many other countries where cows calve in the spring. It reflects the high proportion of milk produced used for year-round liquid consumption.

Intensive indoor dairy beef systems can utilize calves born at any time of year. However, grass-based systems work best utilizing calves from the main calving season. At turn-out in the spring these calves are old enough to make effective use of grazed grass.

Cereal (barley) beef

Cereal beef is a housed bull beef system feeding an all-concentrate diet to slaughter at 11–13 months of age. Carcasses have a creamy white fat which is popular with some supermarkets and independent butchers. However, it is advisable to secure market outlets before commencing production, especially if poor conformation Holstein–Friesians are reared. The system is at its most profitable when it adds value to home-grown grain or home-bred calves.

Profitable production is heavily dependent on achieving high target daily gains. The protein content of the diet is reduced progressively from 18 per cent crude protein in the calf ration to 14 per cent in the final finishing ration. From six months of age part of the protein can be supplied by urea. Rumen enhancers such as monensin sodium improve feed conversion efficiency by about 10 per cent, but their continued use in the EU is controversial.

Standards for cereal beef are shown in Table 3.5.

Grass and maize silage beef

Grass silage bull beef was popular in the 1980s as a beef system that made very intensive use of grass, all of which was made into silage. Its flaw was that it was a system designed for its production capabilities rather than market demand. In the original system bulls were 16–18 months old at slaughter, by which time the carcasses were too heavy for many buyers and the fat was coloured by carotene. There are also question marks over the eating quality of beef from bulls over 14 months of age.

There is still a place for grass silage bull beef up to 14 months of age and the standards in Table 3.6 are for slaughter at this age. The system could also be used for steers and heifers but, for reasons that have been enumerated already, grass-based systems now place emphasis on the utilization of grazed grass.

The section on winter finishing (see p. 15) has already discussed the potential for maize silage in beef production. With up to 30 per cent of the ration DM as maize

Table 3.5 Standards for cereal bull beef.

	Breed type			
	Holstein–Friesian	Limousin × Friesian	Belgian Blue × Friesian	Charolais × Friesian/ Simmental × Friesian
Slaughter age (months)	11.5	12.5	12.5	12.5
Daily gain (kg)[a]	1.3	1.3	1.35	1.4
Concentrates (tonnes)[a]	1.8	1.9	1.9	2.0
Slaughter weight (kg)	460	500	510	530
Carcass (kg)	250	285	290	295

[a] From 3 months of age.

Table 3.6 Standards for grass silage bull beef.

	Breed type				
	Holstein– Friesian	Hereford × Friesian	Limousin × Friesian	Belgian Blue × Friesian	Charolais × Friesian/ Simmental × Friesian
Daily gain (kg)[a]	1.15	1.05	1.3	1.25	1.3
Slaughter age (months)	14	14	14	14	14
Concentrates (tonnes)[a]	1.1	0.63	0.63	0.94	1.3
Silage (tonnes @ 22% DM)[a]	5.7	6.8	6.7	6.1	5.4
Cattle/ha	7.9	6.6	6.7	7.4	8.3
Slaughter weight (kg)	495	465	513	535	555
Carcass (kg)	270	255	290	300	305

[a] From 3 months of age.

Table 3.7 Standards for maize silage bull beef production.

	Breed type				
	Holstein–Friesian	Hereford × Friesian	Limousin × Friesian	Belgian Blue × Friesian	Charolais × Friesian/ Simmental × Friesian
Daily gain (kg)[a]	1.25	1.2	1.25	1.3	1.3
Slaughter age (months)	13	12.5	13.5	13.5	13.5
Protein concentrate (tonnes)[a]	0.50	0.47	0.52	0.52	0.52
Cereal (tonnes)[a]	1.0	0.7	0.7	0.7	0.75
Silage (tonnes @ 30% DM)[a]	3.8	4.0	4.4	4.4	4.4
Cattle/hectare	8.7	8.3	7.5	7.5	7.5
Slaughter weight (kg)	490	455	510	530	535
Carcass (kg)	265	245	285	300	300

[a] From 3 months of age.

silage there is little decline in daily gain from cereal beef levels. Experience of the system is limited and so the bull beef system presented in Table 3.7 is somewhat speculative. It is based on 25 per cent of the ration DM as maize silage supplemented with a protein concentrate and cereal. Profitable production is heavily dependent on a high yield of good quality maize silage and achieving target daily gains. Continental × Friesian heifers may be suitable for maize silage beef fed to gain about 1.0 kg/day and slaughtered at 435–450 kg liveweight.

Eighteen-month beef

Eighteen-month beef is a grass-based system that utilizes dairy-bred steers born in the autumn. It is the original planned system of production in the UK. Calves are reared through their first winter, grazed from six to twelve months of age and then finished in their second winter on rationed concentrates with silage to appetite. Heifers may be used for eighteen-month beef, but are better suited to grass finishing.

Profitability depends heavily on achieving good grazing performance. In farm practice this has taken second priority to making a large tonnage of first-cut silage. This partly explains the poor financial margins achieved in recent years. In addition, the system has a relatively high concentrate requirement, a high silage requirement and, at best, steers only qualify for a single BSP payment.

The principles of good grazing management described for grass finishing (see p. 17) apply equally to eighteen-month beef. The cattle graze for the full season and so, from mid-season, there is a need to expand onto fresh aftermath grazing on areas previously cut for silage as the cattle grow heavier, but grass production and quality decline. In addition, there is a strong case for supplementing calves with about 1 kg concentrate daily for two or three weeks after turn-out in the spring until they become accustomed to grazing. Also, supplementation should be reintroduced in late summer to counter rapidly declining grass quality, starting at 1 kg daily and building up to 2 kg daily for a month before housing.

Standards for the system are shown in Table 3.8. The overall daily gain of 0.9 kg for Limousin × Friesian steers is made up of 0.8 kg/day through the rearing winter, 0.8 kg/day during grazing and 1.1 kg/day in the finishing winter. The finishing gain would be achieved at an average concentrate consumption of about 2.5 kg cereal or concentrate with good quality grass silage to appetite. Limousin × Friesian heifers would be managed at an overall daily gain of 0.8 kg/day to a slaughter weight of 450 kg.

Grass beef

Grass beef is the most extensive of the planned dairy beef systems. Farmers see it as a low cost system that maximizes subsidy income. At best, steers qualify for both BSP payments, an extensification premium and the slaughter premium. Carcasses from continental cross steers may be too heavy for some buyers. Heifers are well suited to the system and can be more profitable than unsubsidized steers.

Good grazing gains are essential for profitable production. If first season gains are below target, winter store feeding costs are increased to catch up lost ground. Ideally, winter gains should be 0.5–0.6 kg/day for heifers and early maturing Hereford × Friesian steers and 0.7–0.8 kg/day for continental cross steers.

Table 3.8 Standards for steers in eighteen-month beef.

	Breed type				
	Holstein–Friesian	Hereford × Friesian	Limousin × Friesian	Belgian Blue × Friesian	Charolais × Friesian/Simmental × Friesian
Daily gain (kg)	0.85	0.85	0.9	0.95	0.95
Slaughter age (months)	18	17	18	18	18
Concentrates (tonnes)[a]	1.3	0.9	1.0	1.1	1.2
Silage (tonnes @ 22% DM)[a]	5.8	5.1	6.0	5.7	5.5
Cattle/hectare	3.4	3.9	3.3	3.5	3.6
Slaughter weight (kg)	500	460	520	525	540
Carcass (kg)	270	250	290	295	300

[a] From 3 months.

Table 3.9 Standards for steers in grass beef production.

	Breed type				
	Holstein–Friesian	Hereford × Friesian	Limousin × Friesian	Belgian Blue × Friesian	Charolais × Friesian/Simmental × Friesian
Daily gain (kg)	0.73	0.68	0.75	0.80	0.83
Slaughter age (months)	22+	22+	22+	22+	22+
Concentrates (tonnes)[a]	0.4	0.3	0.5	0.5	0.6
Silage (tonnes @ 22% DM)[a]	7.0	5.7	6.7	6.7	6.7
Cattle/ha	1.6	1.7	1.6	1.6	1.6
Slaughter weight (kg)	555	515	585	595	610
Carcass (kg)	300	280	330	335	340

[a] From 3 months of age.

In the second grazing season steers need to be marketed as soon as possible after they qualify for the second BSP to reduce stocking rate as the season progresses. Marketing of heifers should start in mid-season. This need to reduce stock numbers from mid-season in step with declining grass production favours early maturing types of cattle. So early maturing Hereford × Friesian steers fit the system better than late maturing Holstein–Friesians or Charolais × Friesians that may fail to finish off grass and have to be housed for a period of winter finishing. Similarly, early maturing heifers have advantages over later maturing steers. Nonetheless, all the breed types, steers and heifers can be utilized in the system provided their performance characteristics are understood and managed accordingly.

Grazing management is complicated by the fact that there are two age groups of cattle on the farm. A complex leader–follower grazing system was developed in which the younger cattle graze selectively ahead of the older age group. Despite its merits, it is rarely adopted by farmers who prefer to keep the two age groups separate.

The principles of good grazing management described for grass finishing (see p. 17) are applicable to grass beef. As with eighteen-month beef there is a strong case for supplementing calves with about 1 kg concentrate daily for two or three weeks after turn-out in the spring and reintroducing supplementation in late summer to counter declining grass production and quality.

Standards for steers in the system are presented in Table 3.9. As an example of standards for heifers, Limousin × Friesians would have a lifetime gain of around 0.6 kg/day to slaughter at 20 months of age weighing 500 kg.

Chapter 4
Dairy Farming

A.H. Andrews and A. Poole

Structure in Europe and the world	22
Trends of structure in the United Kingdom	24
Milk utilization	26
Dairy breeds	27
Feeding dairy cows	30
Dry matter intake	30
Energy	31
Protein	31
Feeding strategies	32
Minerals and vitamins	33
Grassland farming	33
Grassland production	33
Grassland utilization	35
Winter feeding systems	37
Dairy farm buildings	38
Parlour and dairy	39
Cow housing and feeding barn	40
Feed storage area	41
Calving and isolation boxes	42
Slurry	42
Herd records	44
Physical records	44
Breeding records	45
Milk records	45
Financial records	47
Management	47
Labour	47
Breeding	47
Culling	47
Age at first calving	48
Breed of sire used	48
Genetic worth of the sire	48
Health	49
Economics of dairy farming	50
Measures of efficiency	50
Farm assurance and herd health schemes	52
Organic farming	52
The future	52

Structure in Europe and the world

Dairy farming in Europe and elsewhere is a very diverse industry and ranges from high-yielding cows in Israel, the USA and Canada as well as within European countries such as the Netherlands, Denmark and the UK to the small, low-yielding herds of Greece, Portugal, Spain and Italy. In many parts of the world milking herds consist of a single cow, often with a calf at foot, or very small numbers of low-yielding cows. This occurs in many parts of Africa and Asia, and in Europe smallish herds are seen in countries such as Greece, Portugal, Spain and Italy. While there have been very gradual changes in the last half-century in Europe and the United Kingdom, the introduction of milk quotas in 1984 accelerated these. In the last decade since the first edition of *Bovine Medicine* was published the changes have been faster and at the start of the new twenty-first century they have become very rapid indeed. There are increasing trends towards a so-called 'global market' with a lowering of tariff barriers. If this continues this will mean that many areas where milk price is directly or indirectly subsidized will have to deal with lowered price for the product. Many areas with low labour costs and good weather to grow crops are starting to gear themselves up to the challenge of producing low cost milk for export to other parts of the world. This is at present particularly occurring in North and South America.

Over the past few years much thought has been invested by the World Trade Organization, among others, about increasing the flow of milk and dairy products across the globe. However, the dairy markets are some of the most protected of agricultural products and the Organization for Economic Co-operation and Development estimated in the late 1990s that member states producer support arrangements were, in absolute terms, higher than for all other commodities. It is this background which is causing international trade organizations to find ways to reduce export subsidies paid by countries and to alter tariff quotas for imported products.

The introduction of milk production quotas had a very profound effect on the European milk industry. Its aim was to reduce overall European milk production and the changes undertaken by producers to accommodate this altered many milk parameters. The structure in 1983 prior to the change is given in Table 4.1a and the present situation within the enlarged EU is shown in Table 4.1b. The position presented in Table 4.1a was reached over the previous 23 years by each country expanding its milk production through an expanded herd size and increased yield per cow. Total

Table 4.1a EEC dairy structure (pre milk quotas).

	Cows ('000)	Herds ('000)	Average herd size	Yield (l/cow)	Total production ('000t)	Self-sufficiency BF (%)	SNF (%)
Germany	5451	363	15.3	4650	26007	116	136
France	6506	367	19.8	3950	33337	122	128
Italy	3120	424	7.3	3540	11030	66	63
Netherlands	2333	58	40.8	5330	12550	256	116
Belgium	946	45	21.7	3930	4145	104	116
Luxembourg	70	2	29.7	4274	320		
UK	3257	54	58.2	4906	17680	86	104
Irish Republic	1528	77	19.9	3910	6480	298	175
Denmark	913	35	28.2	5585	5205	212	142
Greece	219	77	3.1	3200	770	–	–
Portugal	369	115	3.2	3021	1115	–	–
Spain	1885	–	–	3382	6375	–	–

Source: Milk Marketing Board (1986).

Table 4.1b EU dairy structure in 2000 (post milk quotas).

Country	Cows (2000) ('000)	Herds (1997) ('000)	Average herd size (1997)	Yield (2000) (kg/cow)	Total production (2000) ('000t)	Butterfat content (2000) (% by weight)	Protein content (2000) (% by weight)
Germany	4539	186	27.9	6157	28332	4.22	3.41
France	4413	146	30.7	5844	24775	4.08	3.19
Italy	2172	102	20.5	5113	10774	3.66	3.26
Netherlands	1532	37	44.0	7302	11155	4.40	3.46
Belgium	629	20	32.3	5420	3383	4.09	3.34
Luxembourg	44	1	36.5	6030	265	4.19	3.34
United Kingdom	2339	36	68.8	6133	14489	4.01	3.30
Irish Republic	1238	39	32.4	4191	5280	3.70	3.23
Denmark	644	13	50.8	7272	4720	4.28	3.44
Greece	173	24	7.7	4756	805	3.67	3.22
Spain	1141	106	11.9	5007	5900	3.75	3.09
Portugal	355	70	5.2	5819	2057	3.84	3.19
Austria	621	86	8.4	4977	3340	4.13	3.33
Finland	358	29	13.3	6916	2524	4.22	3.29
Sweden	426	16	29.6	7748	3348	4.18	3.31
EU Fifteen	20624	911	24.0	5885	121146	4.07	3.31

Sources: various including mainly National Dairy Council (2001).

cow population did not increase to the same extent as the number of dairy producers gradually declined. The reasons for this were due to both individual national policies and the then EC requirements.

The Common Agricultural Policy (CAP) set out to increase food production, maintain farm incomes and prevent rural depopulation. This encouraged the very small farms of much of Europe to survive and expand,

Table 4.2 Production and milk quota ('000 tonnes) for EU Member States.

	Production		Milk quota	
	1983	1983–84	1991–92	2000–2001
Germany	26 429	23 792	22 927	27 865
France	33 230	26 768	24 613	24 236
Italy	11 310	9 914	9 221	10 314
Netherlands	12 782	12 197	11 213	11 075
Belgium	4 149	3 643	3 364	3 310
Luxembourg	319	294	272	269
UK	17 878	15 950	14 789	14 602
Irish Republic	6 380	5 599	5 301	5 342
Denmark	5 361	4 933	4 525	4 455
Greece	765	588	581	675
Spain				5 917
Portugal				1 872
Austria				2 749
Finland				2 407
Sweden				3 303
EU Fifteen				118 391

Sources: Milk Marketing Board (1990); National Dairy Council (2001).

while for the larger producers, financial help made dairy farming relatively profitable compared with other sectors of agriculture. Thus total milk production for the 10 members of the EC at that time rose from 87.5 million tonnes in 1965 to 120.7 million tonnes in 1983. The success of the EU milk quota in controlling production is demonstrated by the fact that even in the expanded Union total milk production was 120.9 million tonnes in 1998.

While the CAP was proving very satisfactory for dairy farmers, the financial support they were receiving was increasingly threatening the whole EU budget. Most of this aid was provided through intervention buying of surplus products. In fact, sale into intervention became the accepted market rather than the market of last resort. Thus by 1983, self-sufficiency levels rose within the EC to 125 per cent for butterfat (BF) and 166 per cent for solids-not-fats (SNF) (Table 4.1a) and the cost of dairy support made up one quarter of the whole EC agricultural budget. Thus at this stage, milk quotas were imposed to control milk production and each member country had to take a cut of varying proportions (Table 4.2).

If national production exceeded the allocated quota then a super-levy was imposed. This super-levy was to be calculated either on a dairy basis or on an on-farm basis. On a dairy basis, if national production and the supplying dairy were over quota, then levy was imposed on the dairy and hence back to the individual over-

quota producers at a rate of 100 per cent of the target price for milk. On an on-farm basis, provided national production exceeded quota, each farm paid super-levy on excess production above its individual quota at a rate of 75 per cent of the target price for milk. In 1987–88 further changes to the means of determining super-levy liability were made so that those producers most over quota paid the highest proportion of the levy, again provided the national quota was exceeded.

Quota has been transferable between individual farmers within a member state, either on a sale (attached to land or without, but both are complex) or lease basis (a much simpler procedure) or else on an administratively based system where unused quota reverts to an authority and is re-allocated. Further regulation in 1987 imposed a butterfat ceiling on quotas, thereby giving a reduction in national quota if the average butterfat of 1985–86 was exceeded. Also in 1987 further quota cuts were announced, resulting in a further fall by 1989 of 8 per cent. The calculation of any liability for excess production for a farmer is extremely complex. It depends on the amount of milk over quota and on the average butterfat content of the milk. Each producer has a butterfat reference figure. If a levy is to be charged then the farmer's production volume will be adjusted up or down by the amount that the butterfat average differs from his/her reference figure. Again levies only arise when national production is too high.

The objective of reducing milk production has been achieved. Initially it was envisaged that milk quotas would be phased out in the early 2000s. However, this has not been the case and the CAP reform has extended milk quota until 2006. Special increases in quota were allocated to Italy, Spain, Greece, Ireland and Northern Ireland in 2000 and 2001 in addition to the increase of 1.5 per cent given to all countries in three stages from 2005. The intervention price will be gradually cut from 2005 and it is expected that the system will have been re-examined in detail by then.

Trends of structure in the United Kingdom

Changes to the structure in dairy farming in the United Kingdom have mirrored the trends over the last 25 years in Europe. Thus there are fewer producers and slightly fewer cows, but in larger herds and with a higher yield per cow (Table 4.3). This has been brought about by the virtual elimination of the small herd. In 1972, 20 per cent of cows were in herds of less than 30 cows, but by 1997 it was about 5 per cent. This acceleration has increased at the beginning of the new century as milk prices dropped, causing most farms either just to break even or to lose money. The foot and mouth disease outbreak of 2001 has caused more producers to cease milk production, and present numbers of herds are likely to decrease sharply.

The December 2001 census showed UK dairy cows down to 2.203 million with in-calf heifers down to 0.442 million. While beef cows were down to 1.673 million, in-calf beef heifer numbers rose.

The changes to larger herds have been facilitated by new technology and mechanization and a consequent loss of labour. In 1972, 67 per cent of farms milked through a cowshed, with only 28 per cent in 1990.

Table 4.3 The structure of dairying in England and Wales, 1965 to 2001.

Year	Producers ('000)	Cows (millions)	Average herd size	Yield (l/cow)
1965	100.5	2.65	26	3545
1970	80.3	2.71	33	3755
1975	60.3	2.70	46	4070
1980	43.4	2.67	58	4715
1984	39.3	2.70	67	4950
1988	31.7	2.38	69	4870
1990	31.5	2.33	70	5020
1995	28.1	2.10	74	5380[a]
1998	24.7	1.92	77	5770[a]
1999	23.3	1.94	82	5955[a]
2000	21.8	1.84	85	5940[a]
2001	20.2	1.76		

[a] United Kingdom figures.
Source: Milk Marketing Board, 1990; National Dairy Council, 2001.

Herringbone parlours accounted for only 11 per cent of milking installations in 1972, but made up over 45 per cent in 1990 (Fig. 4.1), and are the main system today.

The increased yields have been realized by improved feeding (see Chapter 9), breeding and management techniques. The breed of cow in the UK has altered, 64 per cent Friesian in 1965 moving to over 91 per cent Holstein–Friesian by 1990, which has also made a major contribution.

Milk purchase has also undergone some very fundamental changes in the last century. Initially farmers sold direct to dairy companies. However, as the latter became larger the individual farmer had problems in obtaining a fair price. This resulted in Agricultural Marketing Acts in 1931 and 1933, which set up a framework whereby all the milk produced was taken by the Milk Marketing Boards who then had to sell it on the producer's behalf. The Agricultural Act of 1993 allowed the abolition of the Milk Marketing Boards in Great Britain and from 1 November 1994 the Milk Marketing Scheme was revoked (Northern Ireland from 1 March 1995). In the deregulated market, producers are free to sell their milk wherever they choose including direct to dairy companies, or via intermediary organizations managed jointly by the dairy company and producers, or independent producer groups, usually co-operatives, who either then sell to the dairy companies or process the milk themselves. Many sold milk via Milk Marque, which was considered in 1999 to be a monopoly, resulting in its division into three new regionally based co-operatives, namely Axis, Milklink and Zenith, which

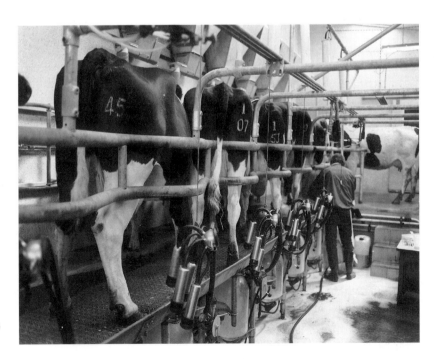

Fig. 4.1 Milking in the herringbone parlour.

Table 4.4 Utilization of milk in England and Wales (%) to 1989–90 and in the United Kingdom (%) to 2000.

	Liquid milk	Butter	Cheese	Condensed milk	Cream	Others
1964–65	73	3	11	5	5	3
1969–70	66	10	10	4	7	3
1974–75	62	8	16	4	8	2
1979–80	50	23	15	3	7	2
1982–83	45	31	14	2	6	2
1983–84	45	30	14	2	6	3
1984–85	48	27	15	2	5	3
1987–88	49	23	19	2	3	4
1989–90	51	20	18	2	4	4
1993–94[a]	86	2	4	2	3	3
2000[a]	50	2	22	4	2	20

Source: Milk Marketing Board (1986); National Dairy Council (2001).
[a] Figures on a different basis to previously.

began to operate as fully independent businesses from 1 April 2000. There has since been more rationalization and mergers, with one group involved in milk purchase in Scotland, England and Wales becoming known as British Milk. Some milk purchasers now have their headquarters outside the UK.

The last few years have seen many milk purchasers buying milk from individual farmers or small groups or farmer clubs. In the early part of the twenty-first century the number of purchasers has been reducing and farmers are starting to combine in co-operatives to provide more negotiating power with the purchasers. Milk is now purchased in varying ways, but is usually paid for according to its composition, cell count and bacterial count (undertaken in the UK by a Bactoscan, see Chapter 25). There are also seasonality payments.

Milk utilization

While milk production has increased over the last 25 years, milk consumption has slightly reduced. The amount used as liquid milk has declined from 73 to 45 per cent. However, because of quotas this percentage has increased again (Table 4.4). Self-sufficiency in 1999 compared with 1996 in the UK was 74 per cent (68 per cent) for butter, 64 per cent (69 per cent) for cheese, 128 per cent (129 per cent) for condensed milk, 147 per cent (147 per cent) for cream and 187 per cent (112 per cent) for skim milk powder.

Prior to the EU, the UK was mainly concerned with supplying the liquid market, with Commonwealth countries supplying butter and cheese requirements.

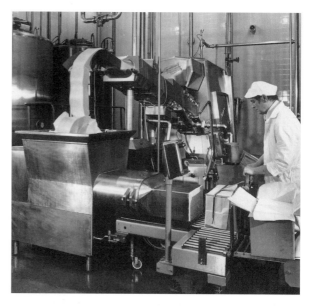

Fig. 4.2 A modern butter-making creamery produces and packs 5 tonnes of butter an hour.

This changed with increasing amounts of milk being used for manufacturing. At one stage (Table 4.4) butter manufacture increased (Fig. 4.2) with much intervention producing the so-called 'butter mountain'. With liquid milk sales realizing the highest return to the producer, the producers in England and Wales should be in a more favourable position than the rest of the EU, as shown in Table 4.5. The large quantities of other uses constitute mainly milk powder and milk fed to livestock, which is common practice in some countries.

Table 4.5 Utilization of whole milk, 1984–1989 (%).

	Liquid Milk		Butter		Cheese		Condensed milk		Cream		Others	
	'84	'89	'84	'89	'84	'89	'84	'89	'84	'89	'84	'89
Germany	13	14	46	34	13	17	4	3	9	13	15	19
France	9	17	38	36	22	28	1	1	4	5	26	13
Italy	29	28	14	14	44	43	–	–	4	5	9	10
Netherlands	6	6	42	36	27	32	8	6	3	4	14	16
Belgium	15	16	55	51	5	7	–	1	5	8	20	17
Luxembourg	11	13	56	53	3	4	–	–	9	13	21	17
UK	41	48	26	20	14	19	2	3	4	3	13	7
Irish Republic	10	11	62	58	9	13	2	2	3	4	14	12
Denmark	8	6	38	37	30	32	–	–	5	8	19	17
Greece	29	30	3	2	47	53	–	–	2	3	19	12

Source: Milk Marketing Board (1986, 1990).

Table 4.6 Dairy herd breed distribution.

	Approximate percentage of national herd	Yield (kg/cow)	Butterfat (%)	Protein (%)
Ayrshire	2.0	5887	4.04	3.34
Holstein/Friesian	90.0	6960	3.98	3.27
Guernsey	1.8	4899	4.76	3.58
Jersey	1.6	4708	5.40	3.29
Dairy Shorthorn	0.3	5589	3.88	3.30
Others and crosses	4.3	–	–	–

Sources: various, including National Dairy Council (2001).

While this table relates to the 1980s, proportions are relatively similar today. The surplus situation in Europe was at one time exacerbated by much of the liquid milk consumed being skimmed milk, or semi-skimmed milk, allowing the release of milk for butter production. The last 20 years have also seen a similar trend in the UK, with about 20 per cent of liquid milk consumed as skim or semi-skim in the 1980s, 55 per cent in 1994 and 62 per cent in 1998. The further quota restrictions have taken this into account.

Dairy breeds

The principal dairy breeds of the United Kingdom are given in Table 4.6. These breeds or their local variations are now becoming very similar in many other parts of the world. While every breed has its enthusiasts, the vast majority of herds are mainly Holstein–Friesian type (Fig. 4.3). These black and white cows are renowned for their high yields of average quality milk. As they become more extreme, the surplus males are of less use for beef. Recently the input costs have been examined by some farmers and there is a slight tendency for those who wish low input production to favour animals of a less extreme Holstein type. These animals are also often favoured by the organic milk producers. However, those aiming at the very high yielding herd are still pursuing a Holstein type of animal. The main drawback of such animals is that any surplus calves produced are of limited use in beef production. Such problems in the future may be overcome by the use of sexed semen and then possibly by the one of embryo transfer in those

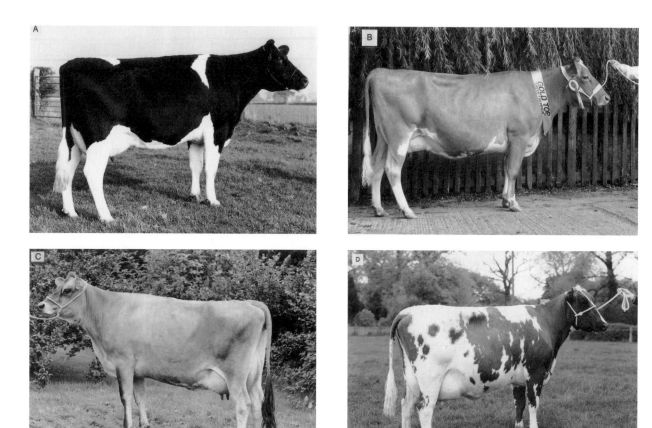

Fig. 4.3 (a) A Friesian cow, (b) a Guernsey cow, (c) a Jersey cow, (d) an Ayrshire cow.

cows not required to produce dairy herd replacements. The increased interest in organic farming and sustainable agriculture is likely to be reflected in an increase in usage of Friesian-type animals, which are more adjusted to such production systems than the Holstein.

The Channel Island breeds, Guernseys and Jerseys, are still popular with a minority of breeders. They are docile cows producing lower yields of very high quality 'gold top' milk. This sells at a premium to the liquid milk or cream markets. The milk is now often sold homogenized. The breed does produce very efficiently on the basis of weight of milk constituents produced. The beefing qualities are low and the fat tends to be yellow, but the meat can be acceptable when crossed with one of the continental beef breeds such as Charolais, Limousin, Simmental or Belgian Blue. Dystokia problems in the Channel Island breeds are few because of a broad and pliable pelvis that allows delivery of viable live calves when crossed with the large beef breeds.

The Ayrshire is still regionally very popular in a few parts of its native Scotland. While its numbers have decreased, the breed has currently been given a boost as its milk is being specifically retailed by some chain food stores. A smaller cow than the Friesian, it produces lower milk yields but of higher quality. It is a breed renowned for the dairy type and so is not very suitable for beef.

The Dairy Shorthorn has suffered from the demise of being the major breed pre World War II, now slipping to almost insignificance. With good beefing qualities, it tended to fall between two stools, with neither the milk quantity of the Friesian nor the quality of the Channel Island breeds. Types of the breed are used in some countries. Its use may also increase on farms practising sustainable or organic agriculture.

The beefing characteristics of the dairy breeds are of importance in England and Wales as the majority of the beef produced originates from the dairy herd. Until March 1996, the origin of British beef was as in Fig. 4.4. The Over Thirty Month Scheme (OTMS), which prevented the sale of older animals for human consumption, plus the Calf Processing Aid Scheme (CPAS), which paid a premium for calves slaughtered before 20

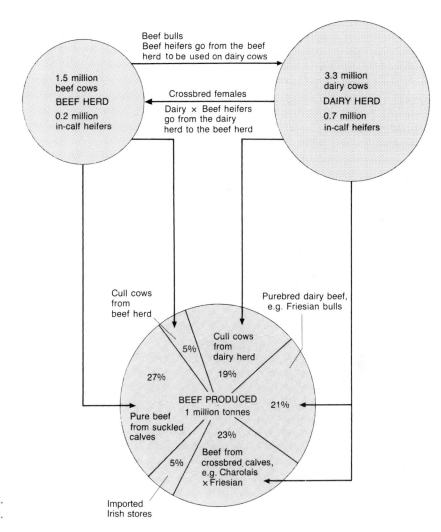

Fig. 4.4 Sources of beef in the UK.
Source: Meat and Livestock Commission.

Table 4.7 Sources of home-produced beef. Reproduced with permission from Meat and Livestock Commission (1999).

	1993 (%)	1995 (%)	1996 (%)	1998 (%)
UK-bred steers, heifers and young bulls	78	76	92	100
beef herd	34	35	43	52
dairy herd	44	41	49	48
Cull cows	19	22	8	0
beef herd	8	6	3	0
dairy herd	11	16	5	0
Adult bulls	1	1	0	0
Irish cattle	1	1	0	0

days of age, payable from May 1996 until 31 July 1999, altered these proportions so that in the early twenty-first century the origins are as in Table 4.7. These are likely to alter with an increase in the amount of beef derived from the dairy herd. Recent BSE problems in other parts of Europe are also altering the types of animal which are entering the meat industry for use both directly and in manufacturing. In Britain, should the OTMS be removed, it will cause another alteration in the constituents of beef which is consumed. At present, increased proportions of total beef production are being used for manufacturing and catering and so if human consumption of over thirty-month-old beef is again allowed, there should be a market for the product.

The Friesian breed has played an important part in beef production with most farmers producing sufficient of their cows pure to provide the heifer replacements for the dairy herd, with the remainder being bred to a beef bull to maximize calf returns. Figure 4.5 shows that, in most years, 60–70 per cent of inseminations have been to a dairy bull, with the remainder to beef breeds. These data cannot at present be updated, but the most numerous breeds of bull used for artificial insemination (AI) in 1986 are shown in Table 4.8. While the dairy inseminations follow the pattern of breed distribution,

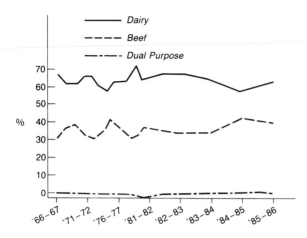

Fig. 4.5 Dairy, dual purpose and beef inseminations as percentages of total inseminations. Source: *Report of Breeding and Production Organization*, MMB (1986).

Table 4.8 AI breed demand in MMB areas, 1986 (%).

Ayrshire	0.7
Friesian/Holstein	57.8
Guernsey	0.8
Jersey	1.2
Shorthorn	0.2
Total dairy breeds	*60.7*
Aberdeen Angus	2.8
Belgian Blue	1.1
Charolais	7.4
Hereford	12.0
Limousin	12.7
Simmental	1.7
Others	1.6
Total beef breeds	*39.3*

Source: *Report of the Breeding and Production Organization*, MMB (1986).

with beef the continental breeds are replacing the traditional British beef breeds, especially the Hereford. The Belgian Blue is more widely used in the UK than shown in Table 4.8, but again recent figures are unobtainable. The Aberdeen Angus continues to enjoy some support because of the ease of calving, particularly when used on maiden heifers or small cows. It also has some marketing advantages in that Angus beef can demand a premium.

While there is an increasing amount of embryo transfer occurring and costs have reduced, it is still an uncommon procedure. However, the possible use of sexed semen does appear to offer considerable possibilities over the next few years. Its uptake will be very

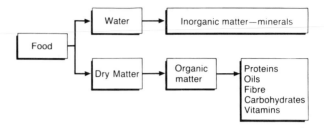

Fig. 4.6 Food components.

dependent on the price and the quality of the bulls offered.

Feeding dairy cows (see also Chapter 9)

A vital feature of dairy cow management is correct feeding. Food, either purchased or home produced, amounts to 60 per cent of the variable costs of production so the efficiency of feed use is extremely important. In the past, most high-energy feeds were purchased as concentrates from feed manufacturing companies. The onset of bigger herds, access to machinery to mix up feeds and the ability to buy feed constituents at competitive prices have meant that many dairy and beef farmers now produce their own rations, often feeding them as complete feeds or total mixed rations (TMR).

The main components of feed are shown in Fig. 4.6. All feeds contain water in varying amounts. Dry feeds such as cereals will only have about 14 per cent water, while other feeds such as mangels and other root crops will be up to 90 per cent water. While all cows require water it is the dry matter proportion of the total food that supplies the nutrients for maintenance and production. In general, the higher the dry matter of the overall diet, the higher will be the dry matter intake (DMI). Apart from the need for minerals and vitamins, the main aspects to consider in dairy cow feeding are DMI and energy and protein levels.

Dry matter intake

Dry matter intake (DMI) is affected by the liveweight of the cow, stage of lactation, milk yield, type of feed and frequency of feeding. As a guide for estimating DMI the following equation is used:

$$\text{DMI (kg/day)} = 0.025 \times \text{liveweight (kg)} + 0.1 \times \text{milk yield (kg/day)}$$

At calving DMI will be 2–3 kg/day lower than calculated, but it will then increase to peak at three to five

Table 4.9 Energy requirements of dairy cows.

Breed	Liveweight (kg)	Maintenance (MJ/day)	Production (MJ/kg milk)	Liveweight gain (MJ/kg gain)	Pregnancy (MJ/day)
Ayrshire	500	54	5.3	34	23
Friesian	600	63	5.2	34	23
Guernsey	450	49	5.8	34	23
Jersey	350	40	5.9	34	23
Shorthorn	550	59	5.1	34	23

Table 4.10 Digestible crude protein requirements of dairy cows.

Breed	Liveweight (kg)	Maintenance (g/day)	Production (g/kg milk)	Pregnancy (g/day)
Ayrshire	500	300	60	150
Friesian	600	350	55	150
Guernsey	450	275	70	150
Jersey	350	225	70	150
Shorthorn	550	325	55	150

months after calving. After peak milk production, intake decreases slowly through lactation and is lower during the dry period. DMI can be increased by feeding highly or more digestible feeds such as maize silage. Thus cows will eat greater quantities of a 70 per cent digestibility (D) silage then one of 64 D. Also succulent feeds such as brewers' grains, kale and roots considerably enhance intakes in an otherwise dry diet of hay or silage with concentrates. When feeding large quantities of concentrates, splitting the feed into three or four feeds rather than the conventional two in the parlour will also increase intake and reduce rumen acidity. This is also why TMR can work well and again it will increase feed intake.

Energy (see Chapter 9)

The energy requirements of a dairy cow depend on her needs for maintenance, lactation, pregnancy and whether she is increasing or decreasing weight (Table 4.9). Energy in diets in Britain is measured as metabolizable energy (ME) and the units are megajoules (MJ) per kilogramme dry matter (DM). If dairy cows are in energy deficit then body fat will be mobilized, causing liveweight loss to make up for some or all of the deficit. This will contribute about 28 MJ of ME per kg liveweight loss. Estimated energy requirements are shown in Table 4.9. Thus, for example, a 600 kg Friesian cow producing 20 kg/day of milk, in calf and gaining 0.5 kg/day liveweight would require:

Maintenance	63 MJ
Production (20 × 5.2)	104 MJ
Liveweight gain (0.5 × 34)	17 MJ
Pregnancy	23 MJ
Total energy required	*207 MJ/day*

Protein (see Chapter 9)

Protein is required for both maintenance and production. In contrast to the case for energy, body tissues cannot be used to make up a shortfall in protein and so milk yields will suffer if protein is in deficit, especially in early lactation. Protein is often measured as crude protein (CP) and is given as percentage of dry matter. In rations it used to be measured in grammes of digestible crude protein (DCP) per kilogram DM. Requirements for maintenance and production are shown in Table 4.10.

A refinement of the DCP system is the division of rumen degradable protein (RDP) and rumen undegradable protein (UDP). A dairy cow has a need for both types of protein. The system has been further refined into the metabolizable protein (MP) system. This looks at the rate at which protein becomes available within the rumen and is given as quickly degradable protein (QDP) and slowly degradable protein (SDP). These two (QDP + SDP) form what is known as the effective rumen degradable protein (ERDP). A cow has a need for both rumen degradable protein (both quick and slow) and rumen undegradable protein.

Different feeds contain different proportions or ratings of these. Thus silage is about 80 per cent degradable and soya is about 60 per cent degradable. Also, degradability does depend on the form of the feed, thus heating or formalin treatment reduces rumen degradability. The rate of passage out of the rumen also has an effect, with higher passage rates increasing the UDP.

In many instances, although the protein supplied may be sufficient in terms of its CP or DCP basis, it may still be deficient in either RDP or UDP. In early lactation on a predominantly grass silage diet, any shortfall is likely to be in UDP; this explains the observed good response when fishmeal or soya was added. Meat and bone meal are also a good source of UDP but were banned in Great Britain in 1988 for ruminants and in the rest of the EU finally in 2001. The EU also decided to ban the use of fishmeal in ruminant diets from 1 January 2001, resulting in the loss of a major practical source of UDP. However, it may return.

Feeding strategies

Many textbooks have been written on strategies for feeding dairy cows. The main principles are (i) to maximize DMI and (ii) to provide the cow's requirements as cheaply as possible. These two requirements are associated as the higher the DMI then the lower the energy concentration in the diet and hence the cheaper the production of the ration.

In early lactation of high-yielding cows, it will be difficult to satisfy their requirements within appetite. This will result in a loss of bodyweight, perhaps 0.5 kg/day,

for the first 120 days of lactation. As yield declines and appetite increases then balance should be reached and then any liveweight loss in early lactation can be replaced in mid to late lactation (see Fig. 4.7 and Chapter 9). As will be discussed later, a compromise has to be achieved between biological efficiency and economic efficiency.

Very approximately, the most common feeds for dairy cows (grazing grass, grass silage and concentrates) have a relative cost of 1:2:3. Therefore, greater profits will be shown as the proportion of grass and silage in the total diet increases provided performance does not suffer (see Fig. 4.8).

While flat rate feeding of concentrates is popular, particularly with total mixed rations (TMR), most farmers feed at least partly to yield. In most instances

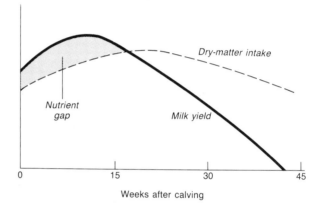

Fig. 4.7 Nutrient gap.

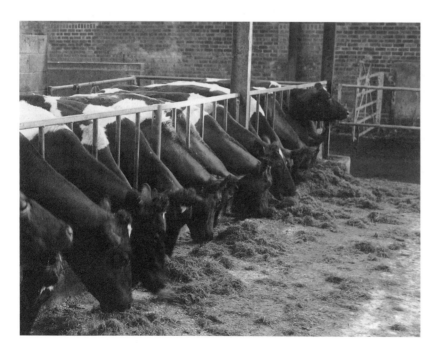

Fig. 4.8 Feeding silage at a barrier.

Table 4.11 Examples of possible cow diets.

	Stage of lactation		
	Early	Mid	Late
Concentrates (kg DM/day)	8	6	2
Silage (kg DM/day)	8	12	12
Total DMI (kg/day)	16	18	14
Energy supplied (MJ/day)	180	195	145
Energy required (MJ/day)	195	186	133

Table 4.12 Main mineral requirement of dairy cows.

	Ca	P	Mg	Na
Maintenance (g/day)				
Liveweight (kg)				
400	14	19	6	7
500	18	26	8	9
600	21	32	9	10
Production (g/10 kg milk)				
Fat content of milk (%)				
4.0	28	17	6	6
5.0	30	17	6	6

this is important as dairy cows are not similar enough in their genetic make-up to allow feeding as if a single animal. It also cannot work unless cows are all at the same stage of lactation rather than calving over widespread periods or all the year round. Thus most farmers do to a certain extent 'feed to yield' or requirements, whereby concentrates are allocated on an individual basis depending on the yield attained and/or condition loss. In consequence, more concentrates are fed early on in lactation and are reduced as lactation progresses. Appetite is dependent on DMI so as concentrate consumption increases, forage intake reduces. This has the effect of limiting forage intake in early lactation as concentrates are normally eaten in preference to forages. Table 4.11 shows the effect of this on the cow's diet. For correct digestion the dry matter ratio between concentrates and forage should be in the range 70:30 to 30:70 in early to mid lactation. Any lower and performance will suffer, any higher and digestion will suffer (see pages 829–32).

Minerals and vitamins

The daily requirements for these must be adequately met if the dairy cow is to remain healthy and produce effectively. The major essential elements are calcium, phosphorus, magnesium, sodium, potassium, chlorine and sulphur. Table 4.12 gives the daily requirements for four minerals. The main vitamins required are A, D and E. As milk yields increase the mineral and vitamin requirements become more critical. They should always form an integral part of the ration. When proprietary concentrates are fed these will usually produce sufficient of these nutrients for the productive cow. However, where rations are all or nearly all TMR then addition of adequate amounts of vitamins and minerals is essential.

Grassland farming

Grass and its derivatives, hay and silage, form an important part of dairy farming. The two major aspects to consider are grassland production and grassland utilization.

Grassland production

To get optimum production from grassland the basics must be correct. These include climate and soil type about which little can be done. Grass grows best on a medium loam soil with adequate summer rainfall. These conditions are most often found in the west of England and Wales. Where soil is heavy and waterlogged, then drainage can give good results. Conversely, in dry areas, irrigation has a part to play, although the economics of grassland irrigation in Britain are questionable on all except the driest farms. Soil acidity should be corrected to a pH of 5.5–6.5.

Having achieved as near optimum as possible with the basics the next area to consider is grass varieties. For grazing, most seed mixtures are based on varieties of perennial ryegrass (Fig. 4.9). There are many recommended varieties in the National Institute of Agricultural Botany (NIAB) lists. Timothy is often sown, which adds some palatability and midsummer growth. Older grass varieties such as meadow fescue and cocks-foot are not often sown now. Most mixtures will also include some white clover. This provides nutrients by fixing atmospheric nitrogen and also increases intake by improving the palatability of the sward. But clover is difficult to establish and maintain in grassland receiving high levels of fertilizer nitrogen.

Once established, and with good management, a grazing sward should remain highly productive for 10 years or more. The main enemy to this is grazing in too wet conditions, when treading and poaching will quickly destroy a sward and allow weed grasses to establish. Swards mainly for cutting are usually based on a shorter term perennial ryegrass or Italian ryegrass. These have a more erect growth habit and are easier to cut but are

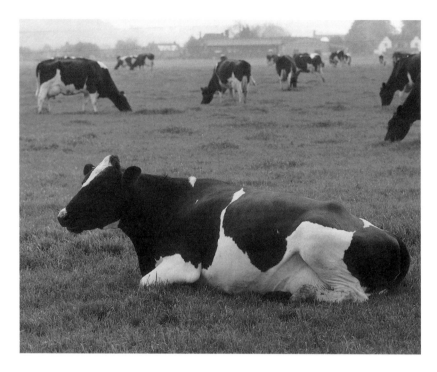

Fig. 4.9 Cow set stocking, grazing a rye-grass sward.

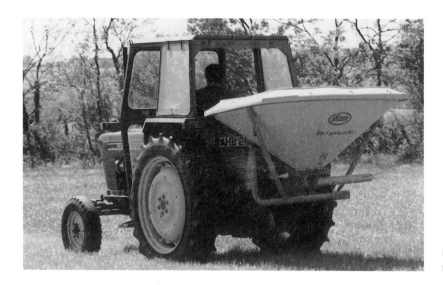

Fig. 4.10 A good response is shown from nitrogen fertilizer.

not so persistent. They are often grown as a grass break in an arable rotation for two to three years. Often the species are sown pure. If clover is required then red clover is more suited to a cutting regime than white clover. In between these extremes are many dual purpose mixtures that are both grazed and cut during a season.

The best time to sow grass is in August–September. This gives it a chance to establish before winter and to be in full production the following spring. A spring reseed in April–May will lose much of the first year's production and can be vulnerable to summer drought.

Having established the grass the fertilizer requirement must be satisfied. Normal recommendations for grazing would be an annual application of 300 kg/ha nitrogen, 40 kg/ha phosphate and 40 kg/ha potash. Under a cutting regime the nitrogen and potash would be increased to 350 and 150 kg respectively. Whilst phosphate and potash are essential for grass growth the main response is shown to nitrogen. Much trial work has been undertaken showing a good response up to 400 kg/ha, but the average nitrogen use is still under 200 kg/ha (Fig. 4.10). Researchers have defined a target nitrogen use as being the point in the response curve where 10 kg of grass dry

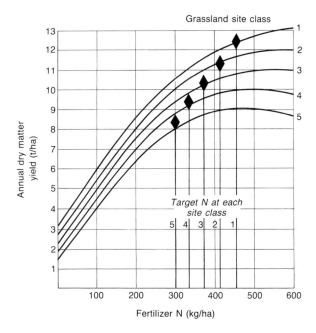

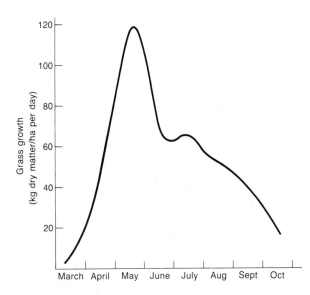

Fig. 4.12 Seasonal pattern of grass growth. Source: *Milk from Grass* (GRI and ICI).

Fig. 4.11 Target nitrogen on five site classes. Source: *Milk from Grass* (GRI and ICI).

matter are produced for each 1 kg of fertilizer nitrogen. Nitrogen use is now controlled in many areas.

Figure 4.11 shows the target point for five site classes, class 1 being the most suited to grass growth and class 5 the least suitable.

Grassland utilization

Grass growth is uneven through the year with a peak in the spring and then falling away through the growing season (Fig. 4.12). Grass growth will also vary greatly between seasons depending mainly on the summer rainfall. Nor are the animal requirements even over the season. For all these reasons any system of grassland utilization must be flexible and adaptable to cover any situation.

The overall aim is to provide the cow with her maintenance requirement and as much of her production as possible for each day of the year. This will be achieved with an integrated grazing and cutting system whereby in early season about one-third of the grass area is grazed and two-thirds is cut. This is reversed in mid season and then the whole farm is grazed in the autumn.

The most common systems of grazing management are either continuous grazing or rotational grazing with paddocks or strip grazing. There is little to choose between systems in terms of output so choice is down to personal preference and ease of management.

Under any system, cows should be stocked at a heavy density (6–8/ha) in the spring, which will allow a

maximum area to be cut without affecting milk production. Maintenance plus 20–25 l/day of milk can easily be obtained from spring grass. For an autumn-calving cow, as grass declines so milk yield declines and there should be no need to introduce supplementary feeding. Spring-calving cows may need supplementary feeding to sustain yields in the summer. This may be concentrates or forage crops such as rape or stubble turnips.

Efficient conservation is a vital part of grassland management. It both provides a feed for winter use by the cows and aids grassland management by utilizing grass surplus to the grazing requirement. The main options for conservation are either hay or silage. There is a continuing move away from hay towards silage on dairy farms because:

- it is more flexible and integrates better with grazing;
- silage is a better feed for dairy cows;
- silage can be made in poorer (not poor) weather conditions; and
- silage can respond to higher levels of fertilizer nitrogen use.

However, silage making does require a higher capital investment in both machinery and storage areas (Fig. 4.13). Much of this criticism has now been overcome by the use of contractors and with the advent of big bale silage. These have given even the smallest dairy farm the opportunity to improve grassland utilization and profitability by changing to silage making.

Whilst grass is the most important forage crop, reference must be made to other forage crops that may have

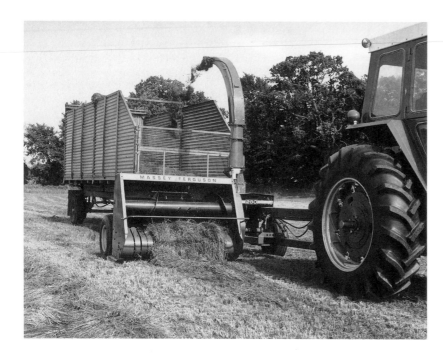

Fig. 4.13 Silage making with a precision chop forage harvester.

a place on dairy farms by producing heavier yields than grass or producing feed in a season when grass is not available. The most popular forage crops are maize, fodder beet, kale, lucerne, and stubble turnips and rape.

Maize

This is increasing in popularity in southern England and is normally made into silage but can be fed green. To be successful it requires high summer temperatures so even in southern England a sheltered field should be used. It produces a similar or heavier yield per hectare than grass and has the advantage of being harvested in one cut. The resultant silage is a very palatable, high energy, low protein feed that improves a winter ration. It is often mixed with grass silage in the proportion 1:1 to 1:4 maize: grass but can successfully be fed on its own.

Fodder beet

This has about the highest yield of dry matter per unit area of any fodder crop. It can be grown successfully anywhere but prefers a heavier soil. It is an arable crop and the farmer needs arable techniques to grow it successfully, especially for establishment, weed control and harvesting. It is harvested in October/November and stored for winter use. It provides a palatable high energy feed, which helps butterfat percentages.

Kale

This is a high protein green feed grown mainly for grazing in the autumn and early winter. It produces a high yield of succulent feed that stimulates milk production. It can be cut and fed to dairy cows in the yards but is more commonly grazed, which means that it should be grown in dry fields with good access. Mud, dirty cows and bad feet can be a problem. However, some have successfully made silage.

Lucerne

This is a drought-resistant legume that grows well on light chalky soils. Being a legume it fixes atmospheric nitrogen and hence is cheap to grow once established. Cut four or five times during the season it provides good yields of high protein silage, but it can be difficult to get a good fermentation in the silage. A useful crop for organic farms with suitable soils.

Stubble turnips and rape

Although these are not the same they are used for the same purpose – to provide a succulent green feed either in the summer or autumn. For summer use they need sowing in the spring but autumn grazing can be achieved by drilling after harvesting an early cereal crop. They both provide grazing when feed might otherwise be short.

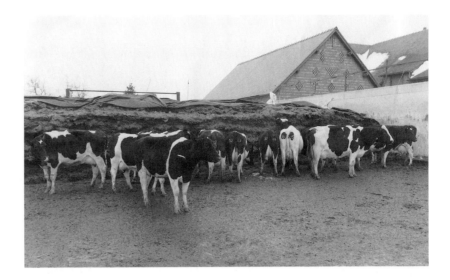

Fig. 4.14 Self-feeding silage.

Winter feeding systems

A winter feeding system will be partially dictated by the objectives, high or low milk yields, and by the facilities available.

In all cases the first requirement is to know the quantity of bulk feeds available. Over a 200-day winter a Friesian cow may well consume about 3.5 t of dry matter. If there are 2.2 t of silage dry matter per cow then this will leave 1.3 t to be made up with concentrates or other purchased feed. Provided there are about 1.8 t of forage dry matter for a 200-day winter then a reasonable feeding system can be devised. This equates to about 7 t/cow of fresh weight silage. Anything much less than this will create problems, not so much from the cow's point of view but from the economic side as it will tend to be an unprofitable winter. Anything more than this will be a bonus and an asset to the farm especially if of a high D value.

All feed changes should be done gradually to prevent digestive upsets. Thus silage should be gradually introduced on a limited access basis from calving or by mid-September, whichever is the earlier. The herd should be housed at night by some time in October depending on conditions and then housed continually from mid-October onwards, again depending on weather conditions. Over this period silage consumption will increase and other feeds can be gradually introduced. The same principle applies in the spring, when ideally the herd should be kept inside at night on silage for seven to ten days after turning out with grazing time gradually increased.

Silage will either be self-fed (Fig. 4.14) or fed mechanically behind a barrier or in a trough. Self-feeding works well for low yields, provided that the silage quality is even throughout the clamp, that the face is not more than 2 m high and that there is enough space at the face, 24 hour access of at least 40 cm/cow.

To avoid secondary fermentation the silage face needs to move back by at least 150 cm/day. Self-feeding is labour saving and requires no machinery. It is better but not essential to have a roof over the silo and intakes will improve if a light is left on at night. Keep cows back from the silage face with a barrier, either a solid rail or an electric wire. The latter, however, can often reduce intake. To prevent waste the face must be kept tidy and waste silage removed.

Mechanical feeding of silage will either involve putting the silage in a trough or behind a barrier with a tractor and fore-loader/blockcutter or else loading the silage into a forage wagon that will spread it behind the barrier. Many people claim that this will increase intake compared with self-feeding by 10 per cent or more. Two simple barrier designs are shown in Fig. 4.15.

For 24-hour access the herd will need a minimum feed space of 40 cm/cow, but space of up to 75 cm is now often recommended for best intakes. Again cleanliness is important and waste silage should be removed on a regular basis, preferably at least once daily. It is important to ensure that silage is always available *ad libitum*. Leaving the trough empty for two to three hours before feeding will suppress intake and can cause digestive problems. It is a tremendous advantage to a winter feeding system to have a trough or barrier available as almost any feed can be fed behind it, from silage to hay, roots, brewers grains, sugar beet pulp or concentrates. This gives a great flexibility. When feeds such as dried beet pulp or concentrates are fed it is essential to have at least 60 cm/cow of trough space to ensure a reasonably even intake among cows.

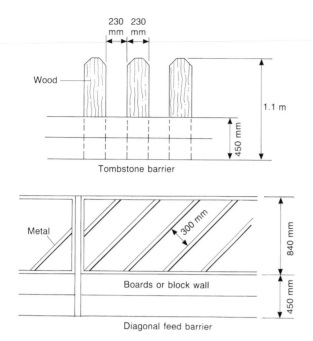

Wood

230 mm 230 mm

1.1 m

450 mm

Tombstone barrier

Metal

300 mm

840 mm

Boards or block wall

450 mm

Diagonal feed barrier

Fig. 4.15 Two types of feed barrier.

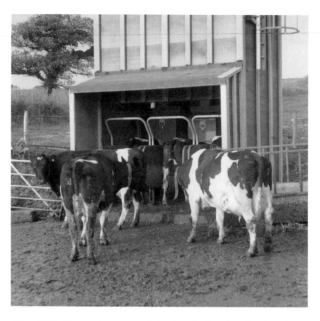

Fig. 4.16 Cows at a computerized out-of-parlour feed station.

A sophistication of this system is complete diet feeding or total mixed rations (TMR). Here all the feeds are placed in a mixer wagon, which mixes them together and delivers the diet behind a feeding barrier. Because of the degree of mixing the cow is unable to separate out, say, barley from silage and so eats the whole mixture uniformly. Ideally the wagon has weigh cells so giving a very accurate measurement of feeds. Use of a mixer wagon allows the feeding of a wide range of feeds that may represent a very economical buy, but which are normally either difficult to feed or unpalatable, e.g. molasses and rapeseed meal. It also allows much more satisfactory feed digestion within the rumen and further down the alimentary tract. Some farmers are now buying straights and producing their own complete diets, usually with the help of a nutritionist. Attention is being focused on straights and ensuring that they are stored in satisfactory containers which allow the feed to be kept dry, vermin and bird proof. The introduction of herd health and quality assurance schemes has drawn attention to how feeds are stored. On some farms forage boxes are used instead of mixer wagons, but these do not really mix up the feed.

Most milking parlours have facilities to feed concentrates and it is usual to feed these twice per day at milking time. A limit to be fed during each milking would be 4–5 kg. If anything above this is needed then an out-of-parlour feed at the barrier is beneficial. This not only splits the feeds, which helps digestion, but also allows a proportion of the concentrate to be replaced with alternative feeds such as cereals, maize gluten or sugar beet pulp.

A sophistication of this system is with computerized out-of-parlour feeders (Fig. 4.16). Each cow has a transponder identifying her to a feeder station. This is then programmed to allow a specified amount of feed per day in a number of feeds. The cow can then eat up to her allowance but no more. Although the capital cost of these installations is high they make for very accurate feeding, based on the sound principle of 'little and often'. They perhaps demonstrate the way dairying will go in the future. Printouts can be obtained for cows not consuming their allocated amounts.

In all feeding systems water must not be overlooked. With milk being 86 per cent water any shortage of water will quickly limit milk production. A dairy cow will need 60–100 kg of water per day and being creatures of habit tend to all want to drink at the same time, especially late afternoon. This makes a large reservoir and fast flow of water essential. The volume drunk will increase as milk yield increases and in dry hot weather, so that 120 litres or more is not uncommon.

Dairy farm buildings

Because of the diverse nature of dairy farming there are almost as many different designs of dairy building units as there are dairy farmers.

However, if starting from scratch the main needs are for a milking parlour and dairy, winter housing and

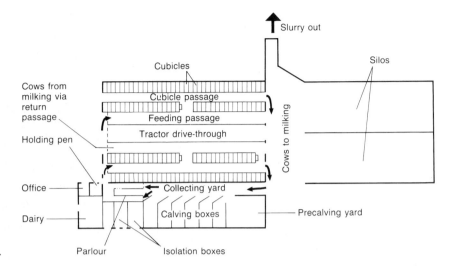

Fig. 4.17 Typical layout of a dairy unit.

feeding barn, food storage area, calving and isolation boxes, slurry handling area and various collecting yards and access concrete. A typical set of dairy buildings is shown in Fig. 4.17.

Important considerations when designing a dairy unit include the following.

- Cow-free access for the milk tanker so that collection can be made at any time.
- Good cow flow so that cows come from the bedded area through the parlour and back with a minimum of narrow passages and sharp corners.
- Good feeding access so that cows can be fed without having to work amongst them.
- Access to silage storage areas away from the cows so that silage making can take place while the cows are in the yards or in for milking.
- Good handling arrangements for veterinary treatment and AI.
- Adequate slurry storage as spreading may be restricted in nitrogen vulnerable zones.
- Thought should be given to the way the buildings blend in with the surroundings. Choice of materials and site are important.
- Adequate loose boxes for calving, sick animals, etc.

Parlour and dairy

This is the key to the whole dairy unit, being used twice (or three times) a day 365 days of the year. Cowsheds are very labour intensive and outdated while rotary parlours in the past have proved unreliable, with no benefits over a static parlour but are now becoming more common again. Automatic (robotic) parlours are also now being introduced. Figure 4.18 shows the most common parlours used, an abreast and a herringbone parlour.

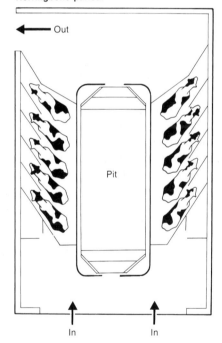

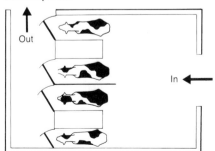

Fig. 4.18 An abreast and a herringbone parlour.

The most simple parlour is the abreast, which is particularly suitable for herds of up to 80 cows with one man milking either with three milking units and six standings or six units and six standings. The cows enter and leave one at a time so a degree of individual treatment for a slow milker or slow eater is possible. The parlour should have a loft above to hold the concentrates, which fall by gravity to the feeder situated between each pair of cows. Milking rate will be about 30–40 cows/hour.

In a herringbone parlour, by far the most common, the milker stands in a pit, which removes most of the bending required. The cows come in and out of the parlour in batches and stand at an angle to the pit on either side. A herringbone parlour is suitable for any sized herd and one man could comfortably milk 100 cows in two hours with a 10:10 herringbone, i.e. 10 milking units, 10 standings. For 300 cows or more larger herringbones with two or three milkers are common. A loft above the parlour will hold the concentrates and each standing will have a feeder. In some parlours feeding has been discontinued.

Automatic cluster removers (ACRs) are now available that make it possible for one man to handle more machines without the danger of overmilking.

In any parlour the work routine is to let the cow or group of cows in, feed them, dry wipe the udder or wash and dry if dirty, wash the udder, test the foremilk, attach the cluster, remove the cluster, teat dip or spray, transfer the milk and let the cows out. Pre-milking teat dipping is practised in some herds, especially those with high levels of environmental mastitis.

The dairy should be adjacent to the parlour and will contain some dairy equipment such as the vacuum regulator, milk pump, water heater and washing equipment. The bulk milk tank will also be situated here. The capacity of the bulk tank is important and must be sufficient to hold the likely peak milk production. Except in a herd with a very compact calving pattern about 30–35 litres/cow capacity is normally sufficient.

Both the parlour and dairy must be kept scrupulously clean and in Britain will be inspected regularly by the authorities. The motors and refrigeration unit should be housed separately in an engine house. It is also useful to have a small area near the parlour where the cowman can keep the records necessary for herd management.

Cow housing and feeding barn (Chapter 56)

The choice for cow housing will rest between housing in straw yards and cubicles.

Cows often appear more comfortable in a straw yard but if they are to keep clean they need about 6 m²/cow. They also use a lot of straw over a winter (about 2.5–

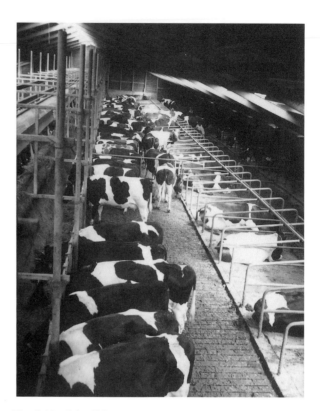

Fig. 4.19 A feed/sleep arrangement with metal cubicles.

3 tonnes per cow), which creates work to cart in and take out each day. But straw yards do help to alleviate a problem by reducing the volume of slurry produced.

Cubicles (see p. 422) have gained in popularity and, well designed, can be a very trouble-free system with a low demand on labour (Fig. 4.19). The main requirement for comfort is to make the cubicle large enough, about 1.2 m wide and 2.2 m long, with a good lying surface. They can be made of metal or timber and a typical design is shown in Fig. 4.20. This design is for Friesian cows and does not offer sufficient flexibility for many high-yielding cows and so ones such as in Figs 4.21 and 4.22 are used. Other new models are also available. The measurements of an ideal cubicle are given in Table 4.13.

The cubicle should slope from the head to tail end and the best surface is concrete with mattresses, mats or sand as a bed. A strategically placed headrail is essential to ensure the cow dungs in the scraper passageway. Passageways should be at least 2.4 m (8 ft) wide to allow for good cow flow and sufficient width for the scraper.

The whole cubicle and scraper passageway can either be situated within an open span building or be part of a purpose-built cubicle building. For all situations it is important to have a draught-free environment with plenty of ventilation. This is normally achieved by the use of Yorkshire boarding (vertical boarding with gaps to allow free movement of air) or with an open ridge to the building or kennel.

With either straw yards or cubicle beds, the feeding areas can be either inside or outside the building. An inside area is preferable but will add to the cost. An example of an arrangement with a centre feed passage is shown in Fig. 4.23.

The advantages of this type of arrangement are that the cows can be shut in the feed area while the cubicles are scraped and vice versa. Feed can be put out without driving through the cows and it is also possible to split the whole herd into groups, by milk yield or calving date, which can assist management.

There has been increasing emphasis on cow comfort, particularly from the point of view of preventing lameness and providing suitable conditions to ensure that cows lie down for similar lengths of time as they do when at grass. This is difficult or impossible to achieve with cubicles and so some farms have altered accommodation to straw yards (see Figs 4.24, 4.25 and 4.26). Such alterations do require sufficient space for each cow (see Table 4.14). They can result in rapid improvement of locomotion scores, and considerably reduce lameness due to white line disease and solar ulceration (Hughes, 2000). However, mastitis levels can rapidly increase, particularly due to *Strep. uberis* and *E. coli*, unless great care is taken in producing a satisfactory straw bed. The keys to success include making available a large quantity of straw for each cow (about 2.5–3 tonnes) and ensuring that it is kept dry when stored and the bed remains dry. Regular cleaning out every 4–6 weeks may help prevent mastitis problems, but this is possibly less important than the quality of the straw used. Good ventilation is also required to help keep the straw bed dry.

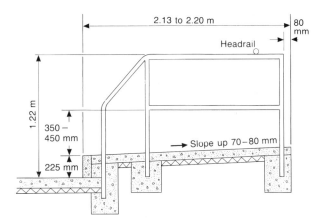

Fig. 4.20 A metal cubicle division.

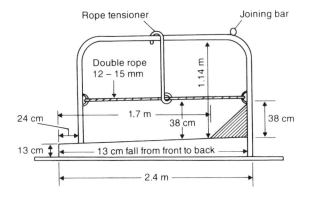

Fig. 4.21 A cubicle suitable for a Holstein cow (courtesy of J. Hughes).

Feed storage area

The major item here is the silage storage facility. This can range from a tower silo to a simple hardcore pad.

Construction of a simple silo is worthwhile to make handling easier and to prevent waste. Clamp silos are the most common and are usually constructed with a concrete base and walls of earth, sleepers or concrete. Safety is essential and in Britain walls must be up to DEFRA (Department for the Environment, Food and Rural Affairs) standards bearing in mind the walls have to contain not only the weight of the silage but also pressure from the tractor when consolidating the clamp. For open silos, guide rails must be provided 900 mm above the wall and for roofed silos sufficient height (5.5 m) must be allowed for tractor clearance. All effluent must be contained in a sealed tank that can be pumped out.

For self-feeding of silage the height of clamp must not be more than 2 m and capacity will need to be about 12–15 m³ per cow for a winter's storage. If other feeds

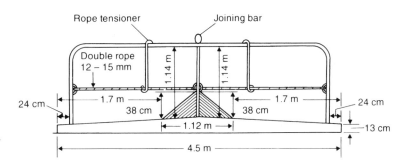

Fig. 4.22 A double fronted cubicle suitable for Holstein cows (courtesy of J. Hughes).

Table 4.13 Measurements of cubicles suitable for high yielding Holstein cattle as determined in Britain (adapted from Hughes, 2000).

Measurement	Metric (Imperial)
Length	2.4 m (8 ft)
If double fronted cubicles with concrete fillet so maximum forward lungeing space length can be reduced to 2.28 m (7 ft 6 inches)	
Width	1.2 m (4 ft)
If width 1.14 m (3 ft 9 in) there must be a flexible lower barrier	
Rear step	<150 mm (6 inches or less)
Fall (front to rear)	100–125 mm (4–5 inches)
Division height	1.14 m (3 ft 9 inches)
Lower division rail (flexible)	400 mm (1 ft 4 inches)
Barrier thickness ideally flexible – at least	19 mm ($^3/_4$ inch)
Brisket board	100 mm (4 inches)
Brisket board from front	0.75 m (2 ft 6 inches)
Brisket board from rear	1.7 m (5 ft 8 inches)
Sloped concrete fillet (instead of brisket board) height	38 cm (1 ft 3 inches)
Concrete fillet from heel stone	1.7 m (5 ft 8 inches)
Barrier (above fillet) if head to head cubicles	76 cm (2 ft 6 inches)
Head rail (below average wither height) $^1/_5$ cubicle length from front	150–250 mm (6–10 inches)

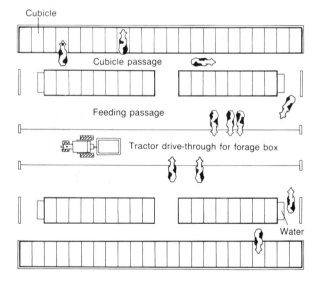

Fig. 4.23 Sleep and feed arrangements.

are to be stored they must be kept in buildings which can be made vermin-free so that the feed remains clean and dry.

Calving and isolation boxes

These need siting in a convenient position to allow for ease of entry and exit for cows. The area would also probably include a cow handling area where cows can be restrained for veterinary treatment or insemination. They require a separate air space.

Boxes should be reasonably spacious and must have a tying-up ring or some other method to aid cow restraint. Walls must be rendered so that disinfection can take place. It is also useful to have a water bowl and feed rack, tractor access for cleaning out and, maybe, a milking point so that cows can be milked in the box. Sick cows may die or have to be destroyed in the boxes so good access for the slaughterer's lorry is essential.

For a herd with spread calving pattern, one box for every 40–50 cows should suffice. Placing hinges and a swinging gate against a wall with the fixed end about 0.5 m (2 ft) from a corner is a useful method of restraint. It allows the gate to be swung round to restrain a cow between the gate and the wall.

Slurry

With more and more farmers using a loose housing and cubicle system, disposal of slurry is becoming an increasing problem. Also, water authorities are rightly demanding more control of pollution. A dairy cow will produce about 7000–8000 l (7–8 m³) of slurry over a winter. This has quite a high fertilizer value (10 000 l will contain 25 kg N, 10 kg P_2O_5, 45 kg K_2O) but much of this will be lost by leaching if it is spread during the winter when the soil is saturated. Also, the pollution risk is much increased. In the UK there are laws concerning application in nitrogen vulnerable zones (NVZs). Therefore, winter storage becomes almost essential.

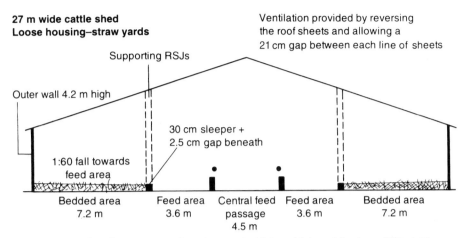

27 m wide cattle shed
Loose housing–straw yards

Ventilation provided by reversing
the roof sheets and allowing a
21 cm gap between each line of sheets

Supporting RSJs

Outer wall 4.2 m high

30 cm sleeper +
2.5 cm gap beneath

1:60 fall towards
feed area

| Bedded area 7.2 m | Feed area 3.6 m | Central feed passage 4.5 m | Feed area 3.6 m | Bedded area 7.2 m |

Fig. 4.24 A 27.5 m (90 ft) wide cattle shed with loose housing (reprinted from Hughes, 2000).

NB: The base of the feed manger should be made 62.5 cm high and the top rail fitted 65 cm above and inset 5 cm towards the forage

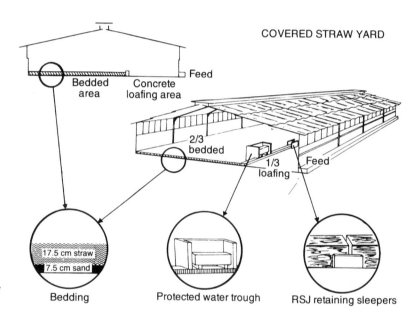

COVERED STRAW YARD

Bedded area · Concrete loafing area · Feed

2/3 bedded · 1/3 loafing · Feed

17.5 cm straw
7.5 cm sand

Bedding · Protected water trough · RSJ retaining sleepers

Fig. 4.25 Structures within a covered straw yard (reprinted from Hughes, 2000).

Slurry is usually scraped with a tractor-mounted squeegy to the store. The store must be able to cope with slurry, water, waste feed and bedding. It will reduce the volume considerably if clean water from roofs is diverted to a separate soak-away or drain.

Long-term storage can be provided in a sealed tower or a storage compound. With a slurry tower, the slurry is scraped into a reception pit and then pumped into the sealed tower. This is kept agitated to prevent settling or crusting of material. For emptying, the slurry runs back by gravity to the reception pit and is then pumped into the slurry spreader. It provides a good pollution-free system but is expensive to install and can create problems if management is not good leading to crusting and blockage of pumps.

By contrast the storage compound, although not cheap to construct, provides a simple-to-manage system with very few problems. The compound should be large

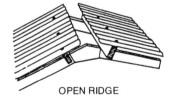

OPEN RIDGE

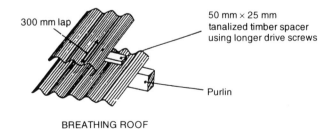

300 mm lap

50 mm × 25 mm tanalized timber spacer using longer drive screws

Purlin

BREATHING ROOF

Fig. 4.26 Ventilation for a covered straw yard (reprinted from Hughes, 2000).

44 • Chapter 4

enough to hold a winter's slurry, have a concrete or hard base to facilitate emptying and a shallow ramp to push the slurry up for filling. Slurry is pushed in all winter and then at a suitable time emptying takes place with a tractor and fore-loader direct into spreaders. A sophistication is a 'weepy wall' silo with walls constructed of timber or concrete sleepers with gaps between the

sleepers (Fig. 4.27). This allows water to drain from the slurry, which is collected and spread separately. This considerably reduces the volume of material needing to be stored for the winter and improves the handling of the remaining material.

Herd records

Herd records are essential for management of the herd but they must be simple to keep, understood by the farmer and his staff and of use in the herd management. Before records can be kept, cows must be individually identified. With herds becoming larger and to make identifying cows by relief staff possible, this identification must be permanent and clear.

Freeze branding with liquid nitrogen kills the pigment cells in hair and results in a clear white number on black cows but is not so successful with light coloured cows. Ear tags are also often used and can be very clear if large. However, there is always the possibility of losing tags. With the coming of new technology it is possible that most cow identification in the future will be by transponder, either implanted into the cow or worn on a collar or ear tag or placed in the rumen.

For short-term cow identification, e.g. for a cow needing treatment, etc., spray cans of different coloured paints or tail tape, sticky coloured tape, can be successfully used.

Computers are now used for keeping records for most large herds, but this is by no means essential and the capital cost will result in a place for manual recording in small herds for many years to come. Records kept will be either physical or financial. In many countries treatment records must also be kept.

Physical records

The notebook: The herdsman or farmer should always have a notebook in his pocket to record information

Table 4.14 Space allowances for straw yards suitable for high yielding Holstein cattle as determined in Britain (adapted from Hughes, 2000).

Space allocation	Metric
Strawed area	
Freshly calved cow	6.5 m² (70 ft²)
Mid lactation cow	5.6 m² (60 ft²)
Dry cow	4.6 m² (50 ft²)
Plus	
Loafing area	
All production stages minimum	2.3 m² (25 ft²)
Thus total minimum	
Freshly calved cow	8.8 m² (95 ft²)
Mid lactation cow	7.9 m² (85 ft²)
Dry cow	6.9 m² (75 ft²)
Optimum number per pen = 40 cows	
Area per pen of 40 cows	
Freshly calved cows	350 m² (450 yd²)
Mid lactation cows	320 m² (380 yd²)
Dry cow	275 m² (335 yd²)

- Maximum per pen with sufficient space = 60
- Drainage in feeding area = 1 in 60
- Straw usage = 2.5 t per cow

- Feeding passage never less than 3.7 m (12 ft) wide
- Easy access from bedded area
- Water – recess into bedded area but no access from bed
- Ventilation must allow moisture to escape – roof open ridged, possibly breathing or gap roof

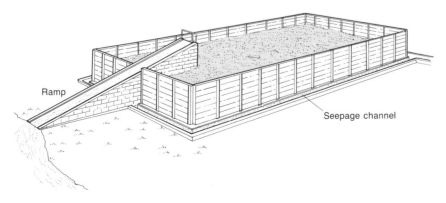

Fig. 4.27 A weeping-walled slurry compound.

Cow record card

Cow name ______________ Pedigree number ______________ Ear tag number ______________

Sire Date of birth ______________

Dam ______________

Lactation									
1	Calving date	Sex of calf	Sire	Milk yield	Days	Fat %	Protein %	Lactose %	Date dry
	Service dates				Veterinary treatment				
2	Calving date	Sex of calf	Sire	Milk yield	Days	Fat %	Protein %	Lactose %	Date dry
	Service dates				Veterinary treatment				
3	Calving date	Sex of calf	Sire	Milk yield	Days	Fat %	Protein %	Lactose %	Date dry
	Service dates				Veterinary treatment				

Fig. 4.28 Cow record card.

such as bulling cows when the event is observed, before transferring this to more permanent records.

Cow record cards: This will be the cow's 'log book' and will give a concise picture of each cow's history. It must contain basic details such as name, pedigree number, ear tag number, herd number, date of birth, service dates, calving dates, sex and sire of calf data, production details, health records and details of veterinary treatment. An example is shown in Fig. 4.28. Much of this information can now be computerized. Today in the UK each animal also has a Cattle Passport.

Breeding records

Apart from information kept on the cow record card a simple breeding record should be kept. This will be used to keep dates of calving, pre-service oestrus, services and identification of sire and expected calving dates. These records should allow the farmer or herdsman to quickly identify any problem cows, such as those not cycling or not holding to service, so that treatment can be carried out before the calving interval slips. These records can be successfully maintained with written entries on a card but often a more visual record is kept. This is usually a rotary board with pins or magnetic blocks of different colours used to identify cows. These are placed on the board to record events so any cow 'out of line' is quickly obvious and can be investigated. If this method is used it is important to have a more permanent back-up in case the pins are accidentally removed. Figure 4.29 shows examples of these records. Several computerized systems are now available and they are being increasingly used in larger herds. These will usually allow the creation of various action lists such as those cows to separate out for routine veterinary examination, those due to come on heat that week, those due to be served, those due to be dried off, those due to calve, etc.

Milk records

Whilst it is possible to record milk yields from cows personally, most farmers who wish to record milk use National Milk Records. The scheme supplies a milk recorder to measure the milk and take a sample, which is then sent to a laboratory for testing for the percent-

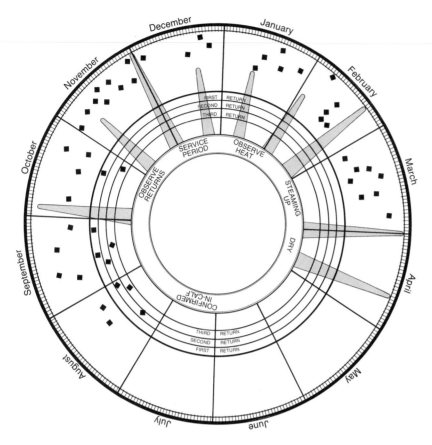

Fig. 4.29 Breeding board.

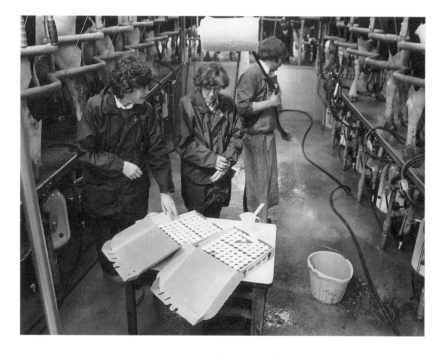

Fig. 4.30 The milk recorder sampling milk in the parlour.

age of butterfat, protein and lactose and cell count. The recorder also enters dates of calving, service, drying off and culling (Fig. 4.30). The results are sent back to the farmer within a week and contain records not only for that month but also on a cumulative basis from the commencement of lactation. At the end of the lactation a cow record card is produced. From the dates provided an action list is produced for the next month with lists of cows due to calve, to dry off, to serve or to pregnancy diagnose.

Milk records are used for pedigree purposes, to provide information to prepare Improved Contemporary Comparisons (ICC) for bulls and to assist with cow selection for breeding purposes.

Apart from this, milk records can be used for management purposes for individually rationing cows or for use in a milk prediction scheme.

Financial records

Farmers keep many financial records with varying degrees of sophistication to assist with the management of the herd. Many farmers use a bureau service provided by a firm supplying the feed or use a service provided by agricultural organizations or consultants. All of these measure the main output from the dairy herd, milk income, and relate this to the main variable cost of production, namely feed. This then gives a margin over feed analysis, expressed on the basis of per herd, per hectare, per cow or per litre. For example, the gross margin per litre in England and Wales in 1995–96 was 15.34 p/litre and 13.24 p/litre in 1997–98; and that per cow was £897/cow in 1995–96 and £809/cow in 1997–98. Margins in some of the next few years were considerably lower (e.g. £807 per cow and 14 pence per litre in November 2002, taking into account inflation).

These services are all computerized and rely on the farmer supplying information monthly on cow numbers, milk quantity and quality, feed used and price, fertilizer used and price, and land area used.

The farmer then has the results returned to him and often has a league table comparing his results with other farmers or comparing his results for this year with the previous year or budget.

Differences between the various schemes are small but some form of financial monitoring provides an essential part of the dairy herd management.

Management

Labour

No dairy system will work efficiently without good labour. In many cases this is supplied by the farmer and his family but for larger herds employing a herdsman is common. In the milk costs survey for 1986–87, 63 per cent of herds only used family labour. From the same survey there was an average labour use of 35 hours/cow per year. This ranged from 79 hours/cow for herds of below 30 cows to 27 hours/cow for those above 100 cows. About half of this time was spent milking the cows and the other half tending them. Labour costs will vary depending on factors such as herd size, facilities available and type of person employed but will range between £250 and £300/cow or about 4 pence per litre.

A herdsman will be one of the most skilled workers employed on the farm. He must enjoy working with cows and be prepared to work the long hours made necessary by milking twice a day, seven days a week. He must be observant to see signs of unhealthy cows, to see cows in oestrus or about to calve and to see signs of under- or overfeeding. He must be capable of keeping records accurately.

He must be clean, to produce high quality milk and to prevent a dirty environment. He must be strong as there is still considerable physical work involved in cow feeding and calving especially. Fortunately, the herdsman's job provides a high degree of job satisfaction and interest for a dedicated man.

Most herdsmen are paid a fixed wage for the job but may also have bonus schemes related to such things as milk yield per cow (less common since quotas), margin over feed costs, calving percentage or calves sold.

Apart from the main herdsman, relief will be needed for weekends, holidays and sickness. Often this relief will be provided by the farmer or another farm worker. Failing this, relief agencies exist which can provide a herdsman often at short notice. At present numbers of farm workers are decreasing rapidly, resulting in increased numbers of animals being cared for by each individual stock person.

Breeding

The aim of a breeding policy must be to get the cows in calf regularly and to provide sufficient replacements of high genetic potential to maintain the herd size at the optimum level. This will depend on the culling rate, the age at first calving, the breed of sire used and the genetic worth of that sire.

Culling

Studies have shown that the majority of culls are sold for reasons such as poor breeding, mastitis, bad feet, injury, etc. (Table 4.15). These might be termed

Table 4.15 Reasons for culling (%). Sources: Cull cow surveys 1984 – FMS Information Unit; Milk Development Council, 2000.

	1984	2000
Poor yield/quality	12	10
Poor breeder	21	28
Bad legs or feet	9	7
Mastitis/cell count	15	18
Udder	8	6
Old age	10	5
Injury	5	4
Others	20	22

unplanned reasons and will not lead to overall herd improvement.

With good management it should be possible to keep the annual culling rate to 20 per cent. But the national average is about 25 per cent. Also, because so much of that culling is for the unplanned reasons outlined above, the rate of genetic progress is considerably slowed. In some countries such as North America culling percentages tend to be higher, while in others such as New Zealand they are lower.

Age at first calving (see Chapter 5)

This is very much linked with culling rate. Table 4.16 shows the effect of three culling rates and three different ages of first calving. The number of heifer replacements needed more than doubles between options. Although heifers need a higher plane of nutrition to reach sufficient weight to calve at two years old their lifetime yield will exceed those calving at three years (Table 4.17).

Breed of sire used

Most dairy farmers breed sufficient cows pure to get the desired number of replacements, the remainder being put to a beef sire to maximize the value of the calf. Depending on the factors outlined above this can mean between 40 and 80 per cent of the herd will need to be bred pure.

Table 4.16 Number of replacement heifers needed per 100 cows.

Culling rate (%)	Age at first calving (years)		
	2	2½	3
15	30	38	45
20	40	50	60
25	50	63	75

With many first calf heifers still being bred to a beef bull this gives very limited scope to do other than breed pure with the dairy cows especially if management is below average. However, where choice is available then cows with the highest cow genetic index (CGI) should be used to breed replacements.

As pre-sexed semen becomes more available and affordable it will become increasingly possible to produce all high genetic merit heifers from those cows chosen to breed replacements. The remainder can then be bred to a beef bull and again it will be possible to choose the calf's sex. Otherwise embryo transfer can be used to solve both these management problems.

Genetic worth of the sire

The choice here will rest between using natural service and AI. The chances of being able to use a bull of high genetic merit which was referred to as 'ICC' for natural service are very remote, so AI is to be recommended. Also, AI gives choice for traits other than production such as ease of calving, conformation or size. Within the overall traits desired, bulls with the highest ICCs for weight of fat plus protein should be used. Also, it is important to choose bulls with a reliable proof, i.e. with a weighting of +40 or above, with daughters in over 20 herds and with less than 25 per cent of daughters in the two herds with most daughters. A wide selection of bulls are available meeting these requirements (Fig. 4.31) (see also Chapters 5, 12). Genetic merit has been converted into various numbers such as the production index number (PIN), which is a comparison of milk volume and weight of the milk constituents, and index of total economic merit (ITEM), which includes both production and conformation parameters.

It has always been difficult for farmers to assess a high genetic merit (HGM) bull in terms of their own herds. The advent of a large number of companies selling semen and the different methods used to express genetic merit in various countries have also not helped. It has resulted in the production of conversion formulae to predict performance. Production information is

Table 4.17 Production associated with age at first calving. Source: Rearing replacements for beef and dairy herds (MLC and MMB).

	Age at first calving (months)				
	23–25	26–28	29–31	32–34	35–37
Herd life (years)	4.0	4.0	3.8	3.8	3.8
Lifetime yield (kg)	18725	18708	17943	17970	17637
Yield/day in herd (kg)	13.1	13.2	13.1	13.1	13.2
Yield/day of life (kg)	8.8	8.4	7.9	7.5	7.3

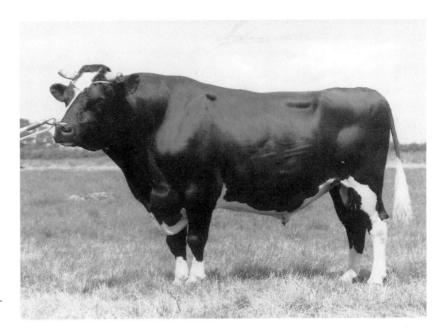

Fig. 4.31 Peckforton Citation River ET— a high ICC Friesian bull.

expressed as predicted transmitting abilities (PTAs). In the UK, production (profit) index number (PIN) has been used for several years, but was biased towards milk quantity and constituents. This was superseded by the index of total economic merit (ITEM) for a time, which included conformation traits as well as those of production. More recently the PLI (production plus lifespan index) has also been included to provide an indication of production and lifetime performance. Other indices have been introduced including mastitis and calving interval.

In 2001 a new genetic evaluation system was introduced for Holstein cattle in the UK. The system is based on the Swedish interbull evaluations for production and conformation. The procedure, developed in 1995, is known as the multiple trait across country evaluations (MACE) and involves the incorporation of data on a particular bull from its own country and also from anywhere else it has been used plus parent information from the home country and abroad. As a bull is used in different countries it reduces the evaluation contribution of the parents to the overall genetic levels such as PIN. This parental contribution can initially be up to a third when the bull has not produced daughters in another country, but reduces to about 1 per cent when it has been widely used in that country and two or more others. The information will still be expressed in PIN and PLI values.

The other objective of obtaining a calf per year will largely depend on herd management. Very few cows are infertile but many fail to breed regularly. Key management times are as follows:

(1) Post calving: ensure the cow is clean, has no discharges and is cycling regularly.

(2) At service: ensure the cow is on a rising plane of nutrition and not losing weight. Oestrous detection is a skill found in a good herdsman. Four observation periods during the day of at least 20 minutes each will aid oestrous detection. Oestrous detectors such as tail paint, dyes or vasectomized bulls can be used to help detection.

(3) Post service: cows should still be closely observed for repeat heats. Cows apparently in calf should be pregnancy tested at 24 days after service with a milk progesterone test or at six to eight weeks after service with a veterinary examination.

To achieve a regular 365-day calving interval, first service should be at 50–60 days from calving, which allows time for one repeat service before losing time.

An MMB report on Checkmate, the Board's fertility monitoring service, showed a wide difference between the top and bottom 10 per cent selected on the interval between calving and assumed conception (Table 4.18).

New techniques to improve the rate of genetic progress will doubtless be developed further over the next few years. These mainly revolve around embryo transplants and include possibilities with sexed embryos and super-ovulated cows producing many embryos for non-surgical transplants. As the cost comes down and the success rate improves these techniques will be used on more commercial farms.

Health

This subject will be dealt with very fully in the main text of the book. Suffice to say here that cow health is paramount to success in dairying.

Table 4.18 Example of overall herd fertility results. Source; Checkmate report, 1985 (FMS Information Unit, MMB).

	Whole sample	Top 10%	Bottom 10%
Average interval calving: assumed conception (days)	99	81	130
Average interval calving: first service (days)	71	64	80
Services/assumed conception	1.82	1.65	2.22

Table 4.19 Average, bottom 25% and top 25% of farms based on retained profit/litre. Source: ADAS and HSBC data to April 2000 (after Lott, 2000).

	Bottom 25%	Average	Top 25%
Farm size (hectares)	99	102	114
Herd size	146	157	180
Yield per cow (litres)	6860	6967	6863
Total milk produced (litres)	999977	1093000	1237000
Output (pence per litre)	20.31	20.55	21.26
Variable costs (ppl)	7.73	7.17	6.78
Gross margin (ppl)	12.58	13.37	14.40
Direct overhead costs (ppl)	8.01	7.23	6.87
Rent, finance and quota (ppl)	4.07	3.66	3.08
Total overheads	12.08	10.89	9.95
Profit before drawings/tax (ppl)	0.50	2.48	4.54
Drawings/tax (ppl)	2.90	2.58	2.45
Retained profit/loss (ppl)	−2.40	−0.09	+2.45
Total cost of production (ppl)	22.71	20.64	18.81

Veterinary and medicine charges are usually between £35–80/cow or 0.4–0.8 p/litre and are made up of drugs, particularly anthelmintics and antibiotics, and veterinary charges. The main diseases that cause losses to the farmer through loss of production, cost of treatment or even death of the cow are mastitis (see Chapter 23), hypocalcaemia (see p. 781), hypomagnesaemia (see p. 787), lameness (see Chapter 32) and calving problems.

Economics of dairy farming

Measures of efficiency

The overall measure of efficiency on any dairy farm is profit. Profit is calculated by deducting from the whole farm gross margin the overhead costs of the business. The gross margin (GM) is the output of milk, calves and cull cows less the herd replacement charge to give the gross output. From this are deducted the variable costs, of production, purchased feed, forage costs, veterinary costs, and medicine and sundry costs. The overhead costs are paid wages, power and machinery, sundries, property charges, interest and depreciation.

Each year various farm advisory services produce reports looking at the economics of specialist dairy farms. These analyse the average as well as the top and bottom 25% of farms selected by profit/hectare. The results in Table 4.19 are an example and highlight the differences. The system is now known as benchmarking, which compares or measures a level of achievement which is seen as the target for that individual or business.

For all the major factors those in the top group outperform the others showing the enormous range of results found on fairly similar farms. However, on very many farms full records are not available to carry out this type of analysis and simpler records must be used. There are many, such as margin over concentrates, margin over all purchased feed (MOPF) or gross margin, all per litre, per cow or per hectare. Statistical analysis shows none of these measures to be closely correlated to profit. The best measures are those where land area, and hence intensity of farming, are taken into

Table 4.20 Analysis by margin over purchased feeds (MOPF) (£/cow).

	MOPF (£/cow)				
	<575	575–625	625–675	675–725	>725
Milk yield (l/cow)	4741	5118	5414	5724	6245
Concentrate use (kg/l)	0.30	0.28	0.27	0.27	0.27
MOPF (p/l)	10.95	11.76	12.02	12.26	12.38
MOPF (£/cow)	519	602	651	702	773
Stocking rate[a] (LSU/ha)	2.24	2.15	2.18	2.18	2.27
MOPF (£/ha)	1079	1195	1314	1425	1634

[a] MOPF: margin over purchased feeds; LSU: livestock stocking units.

Table 4.21 Analysis by margin over purchased feeds (MOPF) (p/l).

	MOPF (p/l)				
	<10.5	10.5–11.1	11.1–11.7	11.7–12.3	>12.3
Milk yield (l/cow)	5730	5677	5621	5494	5270
Concentrate use (kg/l)	0.33	0.29	0.27	0.24	0.21
MOPF (p/l)	9.7	10.8	11.3	11.9	12.6
MOPF (£/cow)	616	663	686	697	700
Stocking rate[a] (LSU/ha)	2.30	2.24	2.20	2.14	2.11
MOPF (£/ha)	1275	1370	1401	1395	1398

[a] MOPF: margin over purchased feeds; LSU: livestock stocking units.

Table 4.22 Analysis by margin over purchased feeds (MOPF) (£/ha).

	MOPF (£/ha)				
	<1100	1100–1300	1300–1500	1500–1700	>1700
Milk yield (l/cow)	4975	5309	5538	5821	6172
Concentrate use (kg/l)	0.27	0.26	0.27	0.27	0.29
MOPF (p/l)	11.76	12.09	12.19	12.18	11.83
MOPF (£/cow)	585	642	675	709	730
Stocking rate[a] (LSU/ha)	1.73	2.02	2.23	2.42	2.80
MOPF (£/ha)	940	1195	1389	1598	1916

[a] MOPF: margin over purchased feeds; LSU: livestock stocking units.

account. Provided the overhead costs are not exceptionally high, then margin over feed/ha (Table 4.22) will have a large influence on profit.

However, with the quota system now limiting production on farms, many people are now saying that margin per quota volume and hence margin per litre has become the most important measure (see Table 4.19). Tables 4.20–4.22 show that, depending on the criteria chosen, very different methods of production give the best results. These tables are based on the 1986–87

Milkminder report, which analysed data from 2459 herds, and *Genus Management Costed Dairy Farming 1989–90*.

A high margin per cow results from a high yield per cow with modest concentrate use. Stocking rate does not change substantially over the range of results. Farms with a high margin per litre had a lower milk yield per cow but with a much lower concentrate usage. Stocking rate also fell so there was little improvement in margin per hectare. Those with a high margin per

Table 4.23 Details of spring- and autumn-calving systems.

	Spring	Autumn
Yield (l/cow)	5228	5634
Concentrate use (kg/cow)	946	1409
MOPF (p/l)	13.0	12.4
MOPF (£/cow)	678	698
Stocking rate (cows/ha)	2.29	2.30
MOPF (£/ha)	1553	1605

hectare had a higher yield produced with increased concentrate usage and with a much higher stocking rate. The intensity of farming was much greater.

All these different systems of producing milk can lead to good profits if carried out efficiently. Therefore, depending on the farm situation and the circumstances appertaining, different systems can suit different farms.

A vigorous debate also ensues about the merits of seasonality of calving and its effect on profits. Both spring calving and autumn calving are very defined systems that can be successful and profitable if operated efficiently. Table 4.23 shows the differences between the systems.

A British spring-calving herd (calving February–April) produces a lower yield with less purchased feed than an autumn-calving herd (September–December). This gives a higher margin per litre but lower margin per cow and per hectare.

Both systems can be equally profitable but as the margin per cow is lower for the spring calver then the overhead costs must also be lower to show the same profit.

Thus the level of overhead costs goes a long way to determining the farm system. Where overhead costs are very low (i.e. an owner-occupied farm with no rent, no borrowed money, no paid labour and little machinery), then a very extensive system with low yields and low outputs can be practised and still show a good profit. However, if the overhead costs are high then the farm must be intensively run with high yields and high stocking rates, putting surplus land into arable crops to generate a high gross output. Only then will a satisfactory profit be generated.

There are many ways of making a profit in dairy farming. The skilled operator and the one making the greatest profit will be the one managing the resources of land, labour, capital, stock and quota most efficiently.

Farm assurance and herd health schemes

These are another initiative to ensure high management and health standards on dairy farms. They help provide an audit and accountability trail from the animal to the end consumer. They will usually involve regular periodic inspections of the accommodation, management, health and record keeping of the farm. These visits may be undertaken by veterinary surgeons or other inspectors. The aim is to provide reports and, where necessary, to enforce improvements within given time periods. In Britain the schemes are mainly run or approved by the milk purchasers. While at present they are limited in their effectiveness they do provide the mechanisms to improve both animal health and welfare.

Organic farming

In the United Kingdom and other parts of Europe there has been rising interest in organic farming. At present in Great Britain only about 5 per cent of milk is produced in this way but the volume is growing. While there are strict criteria to follow, the farmer is at present rewarded with a higher milk price. However, as stocking rates are lower and also costs of organic feeds are high, margins tend not to be greater than in conventional farms.

This method of food production has been receiving increasing attention over the last 15 years. Its main aim is to ensure that production is undertaken in harmony with the environment and that as much is returned to the land as is removed from it. The system has been taken up in many countries especially those of Europe. Organic farming is defined in EU law under EU Regulation 1804/99. The system involves meeting various criteria before a farm can be defined as organic and this involves a conversion period which involves the land and, in Britain, usually takes about 2.5 years. The objectives of the system are to sustain the animals in good health by the use of effective management systems, good stockmanship and suitable diets and by preventing conditions where remedial treatments have previously been used. The use of alternative and complementary medicines is indirectly encouraged by the increase in stated withdrawal periods, usually by at least 100 per cent. The EU regulations only allow three 'synthetic drug treatments' a year (except for vaccines and antiparasitic preparations). At present a premium is paid for organic milk, which makes it an attractive proposition for some dairy farmers, but this is reducing.

The future

While milk quotas remain within the EU it is probable that they will be further reduced for most nations in the short term and then gradually or rapidly abandoned. The commodity price will eventually have to become closer to world milk prices under the direction of various World Trade Organization initiatives. In several parts of the world cow numbers and milk production are being geared up to meet this. In most European countries there will be a reduction in dairy cow numbers as yields increase. There will also be fewer farms with larger numbers of cattle and proportionately fewer people employed. This will inevitably lead to more cows or animals per stock person and an increased requirement for mechanisation. Feeding practices will continue to change to allow the expression of genetic merit with its increased yields per cow. Sexed semen will facilitate a reduction in the number of cows made pregnant to produce herd replacements and will also then allow poorer producing cows to be bred to beef bulls again, often with sexed semen.

Increasing movement of animal products may lead to more interest being paid to the methods of production in those countries which are primarily exporters. The global transportation of food will probably also result in increased levels of disease in those which are major importers of animals and animal products. Unless disease levels in importing countries are allowed to rise, increased emphasis must be placed on health control and monitoring in the exporting regions.

Dairy farm incomes are likely to be further squeezed, resulting in the formation of various producer groups to give improved bargaining power with milk buyers. Such milk producer groups will also be able to purchase creameries and milk processing plants to improve integration of the supply chain. Much of the price structure will still depend on the prices which the main supermarkets are prepared to pay. However, as prosperity increases more people will eat less at home and more outside the home. This will allow the development of the catering market at all levels and again will provide marketing initiatives. There will be more niche marketing, either direct to the public via farm shops, farmer markets and the internet, or indirectly via shops of all types.

Those doing the job well will survive although they will have to keep their eye very much on the various trends which develop concerning milk and its products. Whilst political decisions and the further reduction or demise of milk quotas will close many doors, it is probable that others will open and there will be good opportunities in dairy farming for many producers.

References

Farm Management Services Information (1990) Checkmate report. Milk Marketing Board, Thames Ditton, pp. 1–17.

Federation of United Kingdom Milk Marketing Board (1984) United Kingdom Dairy Facts and Figures, Thames Ditton, pp. 1–200.

Federation of United Kingdom Milk Marketing Board (1990) United Kingdom Dairy Facts and Figures, Thames Ditton, pp. 1–209.

Genus Management (1990) An Analysis of Genus Management Costed Dairy Farming 1989–90, Crewe, pp. 1–24.

Hughes, J. (2000) Internal cattle building design and cow tracks. In *The Health of Dairy Cattle* (ed. by A.H. Andrews), pp. 278–98. Blackwell Science, Oxford.

Lott, E. (2000) Benchmarking – a vital tool to British agriculture. *UK Vet*, **5**, No. 6, 28–31.

Meat and Livestock Commission (1999) Life after CPAS. *Beef Management Matters*, No. 6, 1–16.

Milk Development Council (2000) Longevity – Controlling Culling to Improve Herd Profitability. Publication 51 (03/00), Cirencester, pp. 1–12.

Milk Marketing Board (1986) EEC Dairy Facts and Figures, Thames Ditton, pp. 1–178.

Milk Marketing Board (1990) EEC Dairy Facts and Figures, Thames Ditton, pp. 1–210.

National Dairy Council (2001) Dairy Facts and Figures 2001 Edition, London, pp. 1–275.

Chapter 5
Heifer Rearing – 12 Weeks To Calving

B. Drew

Introduction	54
Age at calving	55
Month of calving	55
Rearing management, 3–6 months	55
Management and housing	55
Feeding	56
Rearing management, 6–12 months	56
Management at turnout	56
Supplementary feeding	56
Optimum growth rates	56
Grazing systems	57
Autumn management	58
Rearing management, 12–15 months	58
Housing and management	58
Feeding for fertility	58
Stress	59
Breeding policy	59
Sire selection: breeding replacements from heifers	60
Selecting a sire	60
Selecting for longevity	60
Selecting for a low incidence of dystokia	61
Service management	61
Controlled breeding	61
Rearing management, 15–18 months	62
Rearing management, 18–22 months	62
Rearing management, 22–24 months (2 months precalving)	62
Growth rates in pregnancy	62
Fly prevention	63
Cubicle training	63
Minerals and trace elements	63
Management factors affecting dystokia and calf mortality	64
Management prior to calving	64
Management at calving	65
Targets for growth for two-year calving	65
Management during the first lactation	65
Survival rates	66

Introduction

Dairy heifer rearing is generally considered to be a non-intensive, low-profit enterprise. Indeed, few farmers would rear heifers at all if it were not for their interest in herd improvement and disease control. However, planned heifer rearing is the starting point for profitable dairying. An increasing number of farmers now realize the importance of this and are adopting more intensive methods, particularly where the land involved could be used for alternative, more profitable, enterprises.

The low priority given to heifer rearing is supported by DAISY survey data (Kossaibati & Esslemont, 1996) which stated that in the average herd, 22 per cent of dairy heifers born were lost before they started their first lactation, with a further 14 per cent culled before they completed their first lactation, while in the worst herds, almost 60 per cent of heifers failed to calve for a second time.

Calving at two years is more profitable than calving at two and a half to three years as little over half the area of land is required, lifetime milk yield is greater and the amount of feed, housing, labour and working capital required for the rearing enterprise is reduced. A policy of calving at two years can only be achieved if the majority of cows calve within a relatively short period or a proportion of herd replacements are taken from heifers.

The management of a dairy heifer between 12 weeks old and calving has a considerable effect on her potential for milk yield, fertility, the incidence of dystokia and on longevity. Insufficient growth rates during the rearing period result in the production of small-framed heifers with disappointing milk yields due to their inability to compete with older cows during the first lactation. Poor growth rates at around the time of service result in low pregnancy rates and delayed entry into the herd.

The faster a heifer grows, the more efficient she is in converting feed into liveweight gain. This could suggest that heifers should be fed to grow as rapidly as possible, especially during the summer months when grass provides an abundant and relatively inexpensive source of feed. However, in some circumstances, high growth rates during the first year can result in lower milk yields due to the effect of rapid growth on the relative proportion of fat and milk secretory cells in the developing udder.

The potential of a heifer will only be maximized if she is reared to a plan with careful control over performance at all stages of the rearing period. Target growth rates and intermediate target weights should be set as soon as the predicted date of first calving has been decided. Optimal growth rates will depend on age at calving, estimated mature body size, management after calving and average herd yield.

Dairy heifer rearing is a specific farm enterprise involving capital, land and labour. It should be managed and recorded with the same attention to detail as that given to the other enterprises on the farm, with preplanned target rates of growth being achieved throughout the rearing period.

A detailed description of the management and targets required for autumn-born heifers reared to calve at two years is given in this chapter. The pattern of growth and targets for weight-for-age for spring-born heifers calving at two years are similar. There is less pressure to maintain steady weight gains when the aim is to calve at an older age and there are periods when lower growth rates are acceptable.

Age at calving

The younger a heifer is at calving the less land, housing and capital are required during her rearing period but heifers should not calve at less than 23 months because a higher incidence of calving problems can be expected and subsequent milk yields are disappointing. With a high stocking rate of 0.4 ha/livestock unit, the area of land required for each replacement unit is 0.4 ha for heifers calving at two years, 0.5 ha for heifers calving at two and a half years and 0.7 ha for heifers calving at three years. When the stocking rate is 0.5 ha/livestock unit the area required for heifers calving at three years is twice that required for heifers calving at two. The housing and capital required to sustain a two year system is also reduced. For instance, a 100 cow, autumn-calving herd calving at two years needs 40 replacements requiring accommodation for calves and yearling heifers. However, a similar herd calving at three years must maintain 60 heifers and house the third-year heifers during their third winter when space requirements are approaching those of adult cattle (Table 4.16).

The first lactation milk yields of heifers calving at two years are likely to be lower than if the age of first calving is delayed. Milk yields of two-year-old calving heifers at the ADAS Bridgets Research Centre averaged 4544 kg milk as compared with a yield of 4980 kg for heifers calving at three years (Furniss et al., 1986), However, when differences in the mean calving interval are taken into account the effect on yield was marginal (Table 5.1). This is supported by more recent research (Pirlo et al., 2000) which showed that as age of first calving increased there was generally an increase in milk yield and milk fat percentage, but at the same time rearing costs increased. The optimum age for first calving still appears to be approximately 23 to 24

Table 5.1 Effect of age at calving on first lactation milk yield. Source: Furniss et al. (1986).

	Age (years)	
	2	3
Milk yield (305 days) (kg)	4544	4980
Calving interval (days)	386	401

months. It is known that the average life expectancy of two-year calvers is greater and the lifetime milk production higher than heifers calving at three years (Table 4.17).

There are a few circumstances when it is preferable to adopt a policy of calving heifers at two and a half to three years. Calving at an older age reduces the management pressures imposed by the two-year system and permits the utilization of marginal land unsuitable for cropping. It also enables replacements to be taken from cows of high genetic merit even if they calve later in the season. Calving at three years can only be justified when there is a large area of outlying rough grazing.

Month of calving

Most dairy farmers plan to calve their heifers in a batch at one season of the year. Autumn-calving herds find difficulty in maintaining this seasonality in the pattern of calving unless either herd fertility is high or a proportion of the calves reared for replacements are taken from heifers. The optimum month of calving varies with the relative prices of milk and compound feed and with the management pressures from other enterprises. Once the optimum month of calving for a herd has been established the heifers should be mated to calve at the same time or shortly before the earliest calving cows.

Calving heifers before the cows reduces the stress imposed following introduction to the herd and allows for a longer interval between calving and service. However, some farmers prefer to calve heifers at the same time as the early calving cows as they find that they are then easier to manage in the parlour.

Rearing management, 3–6 months

Management and housing

Heifers should be housed in semi-covered yards such as that shown in Fig. 5.1. The calves should be given as much fresh air as possible with a draught-free lying

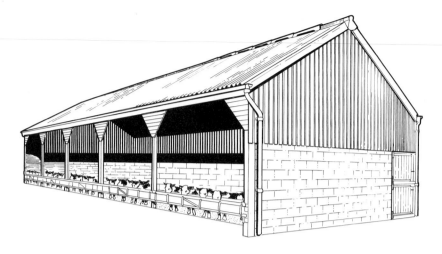

Fig. 5.1 Example of a well-ventilated calf house.

area. Autumn-born heifers should be housed throughout the period but spring-born heifers may be turned out towards the end of the period if aftermaths are available.

Feeding

Minimum target growth rates during the first year of life should be based on estimated mature body weight. A steady liveweight gain at a rate equivalent to the estimated mature body weight in g/day is required. Thus a Jersey heifer with a mature weight of 500 kg should be predicted to grow at 500 g/day (0.5 kg) while a Holstein should be expected to grow at a minimum of 700 g/day (0.7 kg).

It is important to maintain a constant rate of gain. Poor growth rates, whether caused by an inadequate diet or disease, are likely to lead to compensatory gain at grass, which can have an adverse effect on subsequent milk yield.

From 12 weeks of age the calves should be fed to achieve target growth rates, with either a silage, hay or straw based diet offered, supplemented with concentrate feed as either a rearing nut or home mix. The total diet at this stage would typically be approximately 16 per cent crude protein. The amount of concentrate feed offered should be varied according to forage quality and the growth rates required. Forage should be of high quality, fresh and palatable. Calves should not be given forage that would be unacceptable to cows. Calves fed silage should also be offered clean barley straw and can be expected to take about 5 per cent of their roughage in this form. Regular monthly weighings are essential to monitor progress and adjust nutrition. On infected farms consideration should be given to vaccination against lungworm prior to turnout (see p. 274).

Rearing management, 6–12 months

Management at turnout

Autumn-born heifers should be turned out to pasture when weather and soil conditions permit. After turnout the winter ration should be continued until the forage intake declines, generally within one to two weeks. The compound can then be withdrawn. Spring-born heifers are normally housed until aftermaths become available.

Supplementary feeding

Following withdrawal of compound feed soon after turnout, no supplementary feed should be required until late August or early September. Attention should be given to mineral and trace element supplementation, especially in areas of known deficiency (see Chapter 21).

Optimum growth rates

Stocking rates should be adjusted to maintain a steady rate of liveweight gain over the summer. During May and June when grass is of high quality it is not unusual for heifers to grow at 0.8–1.0 kg/day unless a tight stocking density is maintained. In the months leading up to puberty it is desirable to restrict daily liveweight gains to approximately 0.7 kg/day for Holsteins or equivalent for smaller breeds based on the animals' predicted mature weight.

It is known that high growth rates in prepubertal heifers are detrimental to milk production (Little & Kay, 1979; Drew & Altman, 1982). A typical relationship between early liveweight gain and the first lactation milk yield of heifers is shown in Fig. 5.2. Mammary growth and development is under hormonal control and serum concentrations of some of the hormones involved are affected by plane of nutrition (Sejrsen & Foldager, 1992; Sejrsen, 1994). It is likely that the negative influence of a high plane of nutrition on mammary growth is caused by changes in the secretion of these hormones. Rapid growth before puberty has been shown to coincide with impaired development of the mammary epithelium, decreased serum growth hormone and elevated serum prolactin concentrations (Foldager & Sejrsen, 1982). After puberty there is little or no effect (Fig. 5.3).

Summary evidence from recent studies at ADAS Bridgets suggests that there are production and economic benefits from restricting the rate of liveweight gain (to around 0.7 kg/day) in the prepubertal period, in terms of subsequent milk yield performance, with little or no loss in terms of onset of puberty or first calving age and weight. There is also a potential benefit to be gained from a period of cheaper feeding followed by compensatory growth.

Grazing systems

Ideally, calves should be turned out to pasture with a low level of parasite challenge. Up to late June this can be classified as land that falls into one of the following categories: new seeds after an arable rotation and grassland used only for conservation in the previous year. After mid July a pasture can be assumed clean if either it is an aftermath or not grazed by cattle earlier in the year (Chapters 19, 60).

If parasite-free calves are turned out to and remain on a clean pasture it should be safe to graze for the remainder of the season. Unfortunately, in intensive dairy systems it is seldom possible to provide clean grazing as such. On permanent pasture, helminth egg output can be suppressed by anthelmintic treatment.

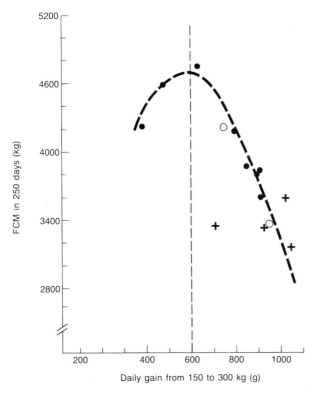

Fig. 5.2 First lactation milk production in relation to early life liveweight gain (after Foldager & Sejrsen, 1982).

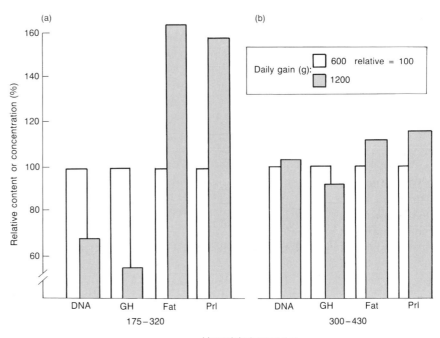

Fig. 5.3 Relative content of DNA and fat in mammary glands and serum growth hormone (GH) and prolactin (Prl) concentrations in (a) prepubertal and (b) post pubertal heifers raised on two planes of nutrition (after Foldager & Sejresen, 1982).

Overall it is important to reduce parasitic challenge in the heifers' first grazing season whilst allowing sufficient challenge for them to build up natural immunity. Individual parasitic control programmes should be drawn up for each herd (Chapter 19).

In continuous grazing systems the stocking rate should be adjusted to match the grass available and the required growth rate, aiming for a sward height of 5–6 cm in spring, 7–8 cm in mid summer and 9–10 cm in autumn. In what is known as the '1–2–3' grazing system the grazing area dedicated to the heifers is divided into three blocks. In spring the heifers graze one area while the other two blocks are cut for silage. Later the heifers graze the two silage aftermaths while the grazed block is cut for silage. At the end of the season all three blocks can be used for grazing.

An alternative grazing system is described as the 'leader–follower' system. This is a rotational grazing system of eight to twelve paddocks where the youngest heifers graze each paddock ahead of older heifers (Kossaibati & Esslemont, 1986).

Grass growth and supply should be monitored throughout the summer to achieve the required growth targets. Concentrate supplementation should be provided if required.

Autumn management

During the period May–August target liveweight gains should be achieved without difficulty. At the end of this period the heifers should be well grown for their age and breed without any obvious fatness (Table 5.9).

Heifers calving at two years require supplementary feeding from late August or early September depending on grass growth, soil and weather conditions. Growth rates decline rapidly from this time and if additional energy is not supplied liveweight gains will be low. A compound feed or home mixed cereal ration supplemented with minerals and vitamins should be fed.

Regular weighings are essential at this time for both autumn- and spring-born heifers programmed for calving at two years. Heifers being reared to calve at three years can be allowed a store period.

Autumn-born heifers should be assessed for size and suitability for service. Actual weights should be compared with targets. If any animal is found to be below target but, with additional feeding, could attain the minimum service weight, she should be housed at the beginning of September and fed an appropriate ration.

Rearing management, 12–15 months

Housing and management

Heifers reared for two-year calving should be housed at least six weeks prior to service and given any routine veterinary treatments required during the period. They should be housed in semi-covered yards with a total space allowance of approximately 6 m²/animal. A clean concrete loafing area should be included to encourage good hoof development. A special area of cubicles can be left to train the heifers.

Feeding for fertility

It is known that the level of nutrition over the service period is important in ensuring high pregnancy rates and entry into the herd at the optimum time. In a study undertaken on six commercial dairy farms, the fertility of heifers fed rations considered to be adequate by the farmers was compared with the fertility of heifers fed the same diets supplemented with cereal (Drew & Pointer, 1977). The supplemented diets were calculated to provide an additional 20 MJ/day metabolizable energy (ME) and were fed for a 12-week period commencing six weeks prior to service. Ovulation was controlled and the heifers were inseminated at a fixed time. Semen and inseminators were used equally over all groups.

The calving rates to fixed time insemination are shown in Table 5.2. There was a wide variation in fertility between farms, but on each farm a higher proportion of heifers fed the improved ration calved to the synchronized service. The calving rates to first service for the heifers on the farm ration ranged from 32 to 67 per cent and for the supplemented groups from 59 to 79 per cent. In this study, no significant relationship between body condition score and fertility was found. However, other workers have reported a relationship between body condition and fertility, with lower pregnancy rates occurring at each end of the score range.

It is likely that change in body condition score has a greater effect on fertility than the actual score at service. Holstein/Friesian heifers weighing 350 kg require to grow at a rate of approximately 0.8 kg/day in order to maintain body condition. As it has been shown

Table 5.2 The effect of level of nutrition on the fertility of dairy heifers.

Farm	Number of heifers	Percentage calved to the synchronized insemination	
		Control	Supplemented
1	62	40	67
2	58	59	75
3	56	32	59
4	37	67	79
5	78	54	69
6	73	53	67
Mean	61	50.0	68.9

that loss of body condition is associated with low pregnancy rates a ration calculated to provide for maintenance and at least 0.8 kg/day liveweight gain should be provided to Holstein/Friesian heifers over the service period. Rations for other breeds should be adjusted according to relative body size.

Attempts to reduce the period of supplementary feeding to three weeks before and after service have been only partially successful. Reducing the period of supplementary feeding to three weeks prior to service should only be considered if Friesian heifers are in condition score 2.5–3.0 (Holstein and Jersey 2.0–2.5), or heifers are to be mated by natural service or observed oestrus artificial insemination (AI) and the reduced period of feeding does not affect the time of housing. The period of supplementary feeding after service should not be shortened as it is likely to increase the incidence of early embryonic loss.

In addition to providing a ration to satisfy the above standards it is important to avoid major changes to the composition of the diet during the ten days before and after service. Changes in diet are almost always associated with disappointing pregnancy rates.

Stress

Stress, such as that caused by noise, physical trauma, overcrowding or some routine veterinary treatments, can alter the concentration and pattern of secretion of the reproductive hormones and is, therefore, potentially detrimental to fertility. In intensive management systems it is difficult to eliminate the possibility of stress, but with careful planning it can be reduced to a level at which pregnancy rates are not likely to be affected.

Housing should be undertaken six weeks prior to service as oestrous behaviour is suppressed during the first oestrous cycle after housing. It is important to ensure that sufficient trough space is provided to avoid competition. There should be an adequate loafing area, the building should be well ventilated and the floor such that animals in oestrus will not slip. If AI is to be used, the handling facilities should be designed to allow for quiet and efficient movement of animals. The heifer should be presented standing at the same level as the inseminator and restrained from sideways movement.

Breeding policy

Some farmers consider oestrous detection in heifers to be too difficult and time consuming for AI to be practical. This is likely to be a problem when groups of heifers graze outlying fields away from satisfactory handling facilities. Synchronization offers a possible solution to this problem but the management standards on farms

Table 5.3 The effect of the parity of the dam on lactation performance of heifers.

	Dam	
	Heifer	Cow
Weight at first service (kg)	370	360
Weight at calving (kg)	496	503
First lactation yield (305-day) (kg)	4977	4742
Proportion rebred	0.8	0.8

must be good to achieve acceptable results and avoid disappointment.

The cost of keeping a bull is often less than AI but the risk of disease and injury are greater. The increased cost of using AI can only be justified if a pure bred sire is used and the female calves reared for herd replacements. A few farmers are still reluctant to take replacements from heifers, preferring to use mature cows with a proven record of performance. The rate of genetic progress will be greater when replacements are taken from heifers, providing a sire of high genetic merit is used.

A study by Furniss et al. (1988) of the first lactation and breeding records of 569 heifers calving in a Friesian/Holstein-based herd showed that those heifers born to heifers yielded significantly more milk in 305-day lactation than those from cows (Table 5.3).

Rearing replacements from heifers and the earliest calving cows enables a two-year calving policy to be adopted, with herd replacements entering the herd at the optimum time. The management of the heifer rearing enterprise is simplified as it should only be necessary to rear calves born over a six to eight week period. It also assists in the maintenance of the optimum calving pattern as the later calving cows can be mated to a beef bull.

The incidence of dystokia need be no greater with a selected AI Holstein/Friesian bull, than a Hereford bull used in natural service. In a survey of 61 herds recording aspects of rearing and calving experience with heifer calvings, the incidence of dystokia associated with Hereford sires, averaged over all data, was almost identical to that associated with Friesians (Table 5.4). There was no difference between the breed in calf mortality rates. When using Holstein/Friesian AI bulls for heifer inseminations there is no need to restrict the selection to those noted to be easy calving although those recorded as having greater than average calving difficulties should generally be avoided. The most critical factor is overall heifer rearing management to ensure that they are large but not fat at the time of calving.

Sire selection: breeding replacements from heifers

A survey of farmers breeding replacements from heifers showed that the main selection criterion was 'ease of calving'. It would appear that it is not unusual for this issue completely to override all the principles taken into account when selecting replacements from cows. Any heifer mated to a pure-bred bull is potentially a dam of the next generation. The bull used must be at least as good as those used on the cows and should also be genetically superior to the sire of the heifer to which it is mated. Only by adopting these basic principles can genetic progress be made. When a bull is considered to be of sufficient merit to be a sire of the next generation, attention should be given to the effect that he may have on the incidence of dystokia.

Selecting a sire (see p. 48–9)

Genetic improvement has long-term effects on herd performance and profitability. The effect is cumulative, making the inclusion of heifers in the breeding of replacements important for maximizing genetic progress (Table 5.5). It is advisable to select a 'team' of several sires (typically three or four) for a herd, including two or more which are suitable for use on maiden heifers. Using several sires reduces risk, although too many can lead to unnecessary complication and lack of uniformity in the herd. There are two key economic indices used to describe the overall production potential of sires in the UK: these are profitable life index (£PLI) and production index (£PIN). £PLI and £PIN are used to describe the average net margin per cow per year which the bull is likely to pass to his daughters and bulls can be ranked on these values for comparison. A short list of sires based on their £PLI and their overall type merit can be produced as a starting point. The cut-off point for this list is likely to vary depending on the genetic merit of the existing herd, with high genetic merit herds having to apply higher standards of selection to ensure progress continues to be made. It must be ensured that the average £PLI of the bulls selected is higher than the average £PLI of the cows/heifers to be mated. The predicted (production) transmission ability (PTA) indicates the relative production potential in terms of milk volume and composition. The reliability of PTAs should be considered: the higher the reliability, the greater the confidence in the predicted values. Generally, sires with a PTA reliability of 70 per cent or greater should be selected. Once a short list of top production bulls has been produced, the selection should be refined using factors such as milk composition and functional conformation traits including udders, legs and feet, SCC and calving difficulty.

Selecting for longevity

Few studies have been undertaken in this country on the relationship between conformation (type), production and longevity. Many studies of these relationships have been undertaken in the USA and show that first lactation yield is the best early indicator of longevity and lifetime yield of dairy cattle. Type scores may add a little to the accuracy of prediction, but not nearly as much as is commonly assumed by breeders. To a great extent, longevity in cows depends on the management

Table 5.4 Effect of breed of sire on dystokia in heifers.

Breed of sire	Percentage of calvings		
(No. of heifers)	Unassisted	Assisted	Difficult
Friesian (1181)	63	25	12
Hereford (753)	63	24	13

Table 5.5 Example of accumulating genetic merit in younger animals.

Lactation No.	No. of animals	Average £PIN[a]	Average PTA[b]					Average reliability
			Milk (kg)	Fat (kg)	Prot (kg)	Fat (%)	Prot (%)	
Young stock	289	53	460	13.0	14.6	−0.08	−0.01	27
1	97	48	417	11.6	13.3	−0.07	−0.01	44
2	130	37	314	10.1	10.1	−0.04	0.00	51
3	90	34	312	9.3	9.5	−0.05	−0.01	54
4	73	23	224	5.6	6.5	−0.05	−0.01	59
5	31	10	148	4.1	3.1	−0.03	−0.03	61

[a] PIN, production (profit) index number.
[b] PTA, predicted (production) transmission ability.

decisions of the farmer. However, differences in longevity between cows within the same herd are now believed to be heritable and factors thought to influence longevity are being included in genetic selection parameters.

Selecting for a low incidence of dystokia

The service sire has a considerable effect on dystokia. The results of a detailed analysis of 1485 heifer calvings to six Friesian/Holstein bulls used equally on 58 farms showed that the differences between the bulls used in the percentage of assisted and difficult calvings were statistically highly significant (Table 5.6). However, the effect of the bull was far less marked than the management on the farm on which the heifer calved. Of the 58 farms in the study, 18 reported mean calf mortality rates of 1.3 per cent born dead or died within 24 hours and recorded a low incidence of dystokia with all bulls. Twelve farms reported mean calf mortality rates of 26.9 per cent, which on some farms was associated with a high incidence of dystokia. On the farms with low mortality, none of the bulls was associated with an incidence of dystokia of more than 4 per cent, while on the high mortality farms no bulls resulted in an incidence of less than 20 per cent. In this study the bulls used were known to be breed average or less for both dystokia on cows (<2.7 per cent) and gestation length (<281 days).

In Table 5.6 only bulls 1 and 3 were specifically recommended for ease of calving. This highlights the importance of ensuring that if a recommendation is based on heifer calvings, that the bull has been used on sufficient farms for the data to be reliable.

In general, bulls with short gestation lengths give easier calvings. The mean gestation lengths of bulls in this study ranged from 273 to 279 days. Providing a bull is not known to be above breed average for dystokia on cows, he can be considered for use on heifers, especially if the gestation length is also less than the mean for the breed. However, some farmers reported dystokia with

bulls that were the easiest calving overall, while other farmers reported that heifers calved without assistance to bulls that caused the most problems generally. In view of the considerable variation between farms and farm/bull interactions it is not possible to be certain whether dystokia will occur on an individual farm.

Heifer calves are generally smaller than bull calves and with the advent of sexed semen it is now possible to inseminate maiden heifers with 'female' Holstein semen to ensure maximum genetic progress in the herd and at the same time reduce calving difficulties.

Other factors involved in dystokia are discussed in the section on 'Management at calving' (see p. 65).

Service management

Controlled breeding (see also Chapter 42)

The introduction of synchronization techniques in the mid 1970s offered farmers a unique opportunity to exploit the use of AI without the time consuming and difficult task of oestrous detection or the need to separate individuals from a group for service. The results of numerous studies have shown that the pregnancy rates following prostaglandin or progestagen treatment are similar to those obtained with untreated controls inseminated at observed oestrus. Despite these findings, the uptake of commercial techniques to control the bovine oestrous cycle have fallen well short of expectations, as in the field results can be disappointing where herd management or supervision of the breeding programme are not of a sufficiently high standard.

There are many reasons why group synchronization of heifers has failed to become a technique in widespread use. Initially, farmer expectation was too high. Many had been accustomed to running heifers with a natural service bull for perhaps nine to twelve weeks. By this time around 90 per cent should have become pregnant, even with modest levels of performance. Farmers have, therefore, become used to finding the majority of heifers confirmed in calf when manually examined as a group and tend to expect similar results from a single AI mating.

Compared with natural service, the cost of a controlled breeding programme with AI is likely to be at least £25–£35 if a double insemination is given. If only 40 per cent of served heifers produce a calf and 50 per cent of those are male the service cost per heifer calf born could easily be in excess of £100.

Although pregnancy rates of 40 per cent are not unusual, the management factors affecting fertility in dairy heifers are generally well understood. Providing the recommendations given in the section 'Rearing management, 12–15 months' (see p. 58) are followed,

Table 5.6 The effect of bull on dystokia in heifers.

Bull (number of calvings)	Percentage calvings		
	Normal	Assisted	Difficult
1 (236)	52	37	11
2 (231)	70	25	5
3 (249)	79	19	2
4 (221)	71	24	5
5 (261)	79	19	2
6 (263)	63	31	6

pregnancy rates of 65–75 per cent should be achieved. At this level of fertility the use of synchronization becomes more attractive if used only for a proportion of the group.

Several synchronization techniques (p. 678) are now routinely used for controlled breeding of heifers, including the use of prostaglandins, progestagen and GnRH. The oestrous response following synchronization in heifers is generally precise and pregnancy rates to fixed time insemination satisfactory. However, a proportion of heifers do not show oestrus within the expected window after treatment and programmes may therefore recommend AI only at observed oestrus or AI at a fixed time followed by either AI at subsequent observed oestrus or natural service.

An example synchronization programme would be a system whereby the heifers are housed or moved to a field adjacent to the handling facilities six weeks before commencement of service. At the same time the heifers are weighed and the diet adjusted to ensure a minimum gain of 0.8 kg/day with adequate mineral supplementation. Any routine veterinary treatments necessary are undertaken and a check made to ensure that the heifers can be clearly and easily identified. After a minimum of four weeks all heifers are injected with prostaglandin and observed closely for standing oestrus. Heifers not inseminated after the first injection are given a second injection and inseminated at a fixed time, either once at around 84 hours after treatment or twice at 72 and 96 hours after injection. Following the synchronized mating either the heifers are observed for repeat AI, or a bull of another breed is turned in as soon as the period of intense oestrous behaviour has subsided, which is usually on the fifth or sixth day after the second injection.

Rearing management, 15–18 months

Housed heifers should be allowed approximately 7 m^2/head from this age. The preservice ration should be maintained for at least six weeks. As soon as it is known that pregnancy has been established in the majority of heifers, decisions can be taken on the level of nutrition for the remainder of the period. Their weights should be recorded and compared with target (Table 5.9). They should be grouped according to size. Required growth rates should be calculated using the target calving weight and feed adjusted accordingly, with higher levels of supplementary concentrate feed offered to the smaller heifers. Growth rates of up to 1 kg/day or more are not uncommon in Holstein heifers at this age. It is likely that, at this age, the variation in weights of heifers of similar age will be around 80–100 kg. Adjusting feed

levels according to size at this time enables the heifer group to become more evenly matched. High-quality silage and barley straw without further supplementation should be sufficient for well-grown heifers. A mineral mix should be fed to heifers given silage and straw alone.

Rearing management, 18–22 months

Autumn-born heifers should be turned out as soon as soil and weather conditions permit. Nitrogenous fertilizer with phosphate and potash according to soil requirements should be applied. The sward height should be maintained at about 6–8 cm. Target stocking rate at this stage should be six to seven livestock units/ha.

Rearing management, 22–24 months (2 months precalving)

In the two months before calving heifers should be housed or grazed with the dry cows of a similar stage of gestation as this reduces the stress of introducing them to the milking herd post calving. If heifers are to be managed and milked as a separate group during their first lactation, precalving heifers can be managed as a separate group. In the last two months of pregnancy the growth rate of heifers should be controlled to approximately 0.7 kg/day.

Growth rates in pregnancy

Target growth rates between the third to eighth month of pregnancy should be approximately 0.8 kg/day, but should be adjusted to ensure adequate calving weights. The target calving weight for a heifer depends on her estimated mature body size and the management routine during the first lactation. The target calving weight for a Holstein heifer is around 650 kg precalving. In management systems where heifers are fed as a heifer group in the first lactation there is obviously less competition than where heifers are competing with older cows.

Two-year calving heifers competing with cows in self-fed silage systems are at the greatest risk as not only are they relatively small in weight and stature but they are also changing their teeth at this time.

In an investigation involving Friesian/Holstein heifers calving at two years, Keown (1986) showed that growth rate during pregnancy has a significant effect on milk production, with the heavier heifers at calving producing the most milk (Fig. 5.4).

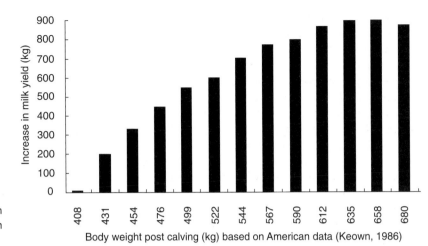

Fig. 5.4 The effect of weight at calving on first lactation yield (increase in first lactation milk yield). Data used with permission.

Weight, height and pelvic length at calving were found to affect milk yield. All these relationships were statistically significant and suggest that while rapid growth in the prepubertal heifer is detrimental to milk yield, the converse applies during pregnancy.

The initial results suggested that there is a positive relationship between body condition score and milk yield throughout the condition score range. However, a more detailed analysis showed that when heifers are fed adequately during the first lactation there is no beneficial effect on milk yield of feeding to calve them at body condition scores above 2.5 for Friesians or greater than 2.0 for Holsteins or the Channel Island breeds. This information is reassuring in view of the fact that an increased level of assistance at calving was required when heifers calved at condition scores of 3.0 or more (see pp. 10–11).

To a considerable extent, dystokia can be avoided by careful management in the ninth month of pregnancy. Growth rate should be restricted at this time.

Fly prevention

Summer mastitis can be a cause of loss in heifers (see Chapter 24). It is most likely to occur between the fifth and eighth month of pregnancy, usually in July, August and September. The incidence of summer mastitis can be reduced by grazing large open fields away from woods and streams and by the use of fly repellent measures. Impregnated ear tags, sprays and pour-ons have proved to be of benefit in preventing disturbance and irritation caused by flies and reducing the incidence of New Forest eye and summer mastitis. The incidence of the latter can also be reduced by regular (e.g. weekly) teat treatment with proprietary fly repellents.

Cubicle training

Some dairy heifers can show clinical signs of laminitis early in their first lactation. This is frequently a stress-related condition associated with changes in the environment, social grouping and feeding, which occur at the time of first calving. It has been shown that housing heifers for a few weeks during a period when cubicles are not occupied by cows has two advantages. Firstly, the heifers become accustomed to using cubicles and are less likely to reject them following introduction into the herd, and secondly, as one of the postparturient stresses is eliminated, the incidence of laminitis and other stress-related metabolic diseases is reduced. Providing a clean concrete loafing area whenever the animals are housed, throughout the heifer rearing phase, encourages better hoof formation and reduces problems when heifers move into cubicle yards post calving.

Minerals and trace elements

A detailed description of some of the minerals and trace elements of particular significance to the dairy heifer is given in Chapters 21, 46. In view of the fact that dairy heifers receive relatively little compound feed, deficiencies are more likely than with the milking herd. The advice given regarding minerals such as phosphorus, copper, cobalt, selenium and manganese fed to dairy cows applies equally to dairy heifers (Chapters 18, 21).

Although iodine deficiency may not be a widespread problem, it can be responsible for serious losses on individual farms (see pp. 253–60). If perinatal calf mortality in heifer calvings has exceeded 10 per cent in previous years an investigation into the iodine status of the herd is recommended early in the season and treatment undertaken during the fifth to eighth months of pregnancy.

Magnesium supplementation is normally given to dairy cows prior to calving in order to reduce the incidence of hypocalcaemia. As heifers are less prone to this condition, supplementary magnesium is not always provided (see Chapter 46). Data from ADAS trials suggest that magnesium supplementation in the month prior to calving reduces the incidence of dystokia. As the energy intake should be restricted at this time it is usually most convenient to provide this via the water.

Management factors affecting dystokia and calf mortality

Management at around the time of calving has a major effect on dystokia and calf mortality. Management prior to service and during the first eight months of pregnancy is generally considered to have little effect, although opinion is divided. The results of a large-scale investigation into the factors affecting dystokia showed a tendency for calf mortality and dystokia to be greater at each end of the growth rate range (Table 5.7).

On the basis of this study, high weight gains during pregnancy should not result in unacceptable levels of dystokia, especially if liveweight gain is restricted during the final month of pregnancy. An analysis of the precalving weight and height records showed there to be no significant relationships with dystokia.

In order to study the effect of management on the factors affecting calving difficulty and calf mortality, the performance of the 18 farms with calf mortality rates below 5 per cent was compared with the performance of the 12 farms with calf mortality rates over 20 per cent. There was no difference between the groups in the growth rates of the heifers (Table 5.8).

These figures suggest that growth rate of the heifer has little effect on dystokia. Equally, there appeared to be no differences between the groups in the size of the calves born, farmers with both low and high mortality rates recording a similar proportion of small, medium and large calves. The high mortality rate farms assisted a greater proportion of heifers in all of the size group categories and classified 58 per cent of large calves as difficult calvings compared with only 8 per cent of the large calves on the low mortality rate farms.

There is no evidence from these data to suggest that the management of the heifer during pregnancy accounted for the differences obtained. The differences would, therefore, appear to be due mainly to factors

Table 5.7 Effect of weight gain during pregnancy on dystokia.

Weight gain (kg/day)	Calf mortality (%)	Percentage calvings		
		Normal	Assisted	Difficult
<0.4 (49)	19	61	35	7
0.41–0.60 (348)	10	74	25	3
0.61–0.80 (854)	11	69	26	5
>8.0 (199)	14	64	28	8

Number of cattle recorded at each weight gain is given in brackets.

Table 5.8 Farms with calf mortality rates below 5 per cent compared with farms with calf mortality rates above 20 per cent.

Heifer measurements	Low mortality	High mortality
Number of farms	18	12
Number of heifers	447	212
Average number/farm	25	18
Mean age at calving (days)	731	734
Mean weight at service (kg)	330	323
Mean weight at calving (kg)	504	492
Mean height at service (cm)	117	118
Mean height at calving (cm)	128	127
Mean distance hook to pin at service (cm)	44	43
Mean distance hook to tail head at service (cm)	38	38

relating to the management of the heifer at around the time of calving.

Management prior to calving

Providing weather conditions permit, it is preferable to graze heifers in a field or paddock adjacent to the dairy complex, where the forage is naturally sparse or can be deliberately restricted to ensure that the optimum body condition at calving is achieved. The heifers should have the opportunity for exercise. The diet offered should be a correctly formulated transition diet which introduces the heifer to the main forages and feeds which she will be fed post calving. Mineral supplementation remains as for dry cows. Supplementary magnesium should be provided.

The group should be observed at least four to five times daily from three weeks prior to the estimated date of the first calving. Care should be taken to adjust the 'due to calve' dates for the gestation length of the bulls used.

Management at calving

Grazed heifers should calve in their allotted field or paddock if possible; housed heifers should calve in buildings with which they are familiar.

There is evidence to suggest that moving a heifer to a calving box increases the risk of dystokia and therefore it is preferable to avoid movement unless this is essential for adequate assistance (Chapter 67). The field should be well fenced to avoid the possibility of heifers rolling into positions from where it would be difficult to assist. The herdsman should be trained to recognize fear, abnormal pain or distress and instructed on the correct use of calving aids.

Targets for growth for two-year calving

The targets shown in Table 5.9 refer to heifers calving at two years. The target growth rates for heifers calving at 2.5 or 3.0 years are less as they can grow at a slower rate overall and during growth they can be allowed a store period. The maximum growth rates suggested for the first year and the minimum growth rates during the immediate preservice period apply.

Management during the first lactation

Heifers fed in competition with cows during their first lactation are likely to give less milk in the first lactation and have less chance of surviving to calve for a second time than when fed in a heifer group.

Table 5.9 Growth targets for two-year calving of Holstein heifers.

From	To	Daily liveweight gain (kg)	Target liveweight (kg) (at end of period)
Birth	Weaning	0.50	65
Weaning	4 months	0.90	150
4 months	10 months	0.65	280
10 months	13 months	0.80	350
13 months	17 months	0.90	460
17 months	22 months	0.90	595
22 months	Calving	0.65	630 (pre calving)

A study involving 179 small-framed Friesian heifers calving at two years, all the progeny of one sire, compared the milk yields and longevity of heifers fed with or without competition during their first lactation. The first lactation milk yields and survival rates to the end of the fifth lactation of heifers at a range of service weights are shown in Table 5.10.

On this farm no allowances were made for the size of heifer or the effect of competition on milk yield. A higher percentage of heifers in the group fed with cows were therefore culled on grounds of disappointing milk yields.

In a subsequent study, the lactation records of 1346 cows on 54 farms were examined to determine the extent to which heifers were affected by competition with cows. The farms were allocated to one of three groups according to the method of management during the first lactation:

Group 1: fed as a heifer group throughout the winter period.
Group 2: housed with cows. Fed a complete diet or manger fed.
Group 3: housed with cows. Fed on self-feed silage.

Heifers fed as a heifer group (group 1) gave more milk than those fed in competition with cows (Table 5.11).

Farmers electing to feed cows in groups are more likely to be aiming for high yields than those where the

Table 5.10 The effect of competition on first lactation milk yield and survival rates to the end of the fifth lactation.

Weight at service (kg)	Milk yield (kg)	
	Competition	No competition
225–259	2892 (33)[a]	3852 (37)
260–279	3334 (46)	4070 (73)
280–299	3639 (18)	3992 (52)
300–349	3131 (21)	3857 (32)

[a] Numbers in parentheses represent survival rate percentage.

Table 5.11 Mean first lactation milk yields.

Group (No.)	305-day yield			Total lactation yield	Lactation length
	Milk	Fat	Protein		
1 (207)	5200	209	170	5369	319
2 (580)	4504	180	146	4641	308
3 (559)	4274	174	140	4358	309

whole herd is managed as a single unit. When the milk yields are compared with the average herd yield it can be seen that the true effect in heifers between herds is some 5 per cent of mature potential (Table 5.12).

Although heifers fed in competition with cows during their first lactation are likely to yield less milk, it is not always possible, feasible or economic to manage, milk and feed them separately.

The effect of competition can be minimized by ensuring that heifers are well grown prior to calving. Size is important, but not the only factor determining the peck order within a group of cows.

Immediately after calving a heifer is maternally orientated and may be weakened by a prolonged and difficult calving. She is, therefore, least able to establish her place in the peck order. Bullying following introduction to the herd can be reduced by ensuring that the heifer has regained her strength after calving and by allowing her to join the herd in the late afternoon or early evening when there appears to be less aggressive behaviour. Competition for food can be reduced by providing access to 'easy'-feed silage in self-fed systems. It is as well to remember that heifers calving at two years of age are changing their teeth at this time and find difficulty in extracting silage from well-consolidated clamps. The problem is obviously most acute on farms where the width of the silage face is inadequate or where true 24-hour access is not provided. Silage or other forage should be fed in mangers or cut from clamps and fed behind an easy-feed barrier. The newly introduced heifers should be observed carefully to ensure that they are maximizing forage and concentrate intake. Sufficient loafing areas and loose housing or cubicles should be provided for all the cows in the herd. There is a tendency for farmers to provide 5 per cent fewer cubicles than cows in the group on the assumption that not all the animals will wish to lie down at the same time. Heifers will not always lie in empty cubicles between older cows and therefore it is recommended that one cubicle is provided for each cow and heifer in the group.

Survival rates

On average, cows in Britain fail to survive in the herd for sufficient time to fulfil their mature yield potential. The mean length of herd life is less than 3.5 lactations, while mature yields are not obtained until the fourth, fifth or even the sixth lactation. It is also estimated that some 40 per cent of all heifer calves born alive fail to calve for a second time. The main reasons for disposal are fertility and low milk production. It is evident that the rate of growth during the rearing period influences milk yield; the level of nutrition at around the time of service affects pregnancy rates and the management of the heifer at calving the incidence of dystokia and calf mortality. It must be emphasized that attention to detail and good management throughout the rearing period have a considerable effect on longevity and overall herd profitability.

References

Drew, S.B. (1988) The influence of management factors during rearing on the subsequent performance of Friesian heifers. *British Cattle Breeders Digest*, **43**, 41–8.

Drew, S.B. & Altman, J.F.B. (1982) The effect of weight at first insemination on the subsequent performance of Friesian dairy heifers. *Animal Production*, **34**, 371.

Drew, S.B. & Pointer, C.G. (1977) The effect of level of nutrition on fertility in Friesian heifers in autumn and early winter. EAAP 28th Annual Meeting, Brussels, 22–27 August 1977. Commission on Animal Health and Production Paper 77/8, pp. 1–3.

Foldager, J. & Sejrsen, K. (1982) Nutrition of replacement heifers affects mammary development and their ability to produce milk. World Congress on Diseases of Cattle, The Netherlands, vol. I, p. 45.

Furniss, S.J., Kirby, S.P.J. & Smith, G. (1988) The effect of dam's parity on the performance of daughters. *British Cattle Breeders Conference Digest*, **43**, 49–50.

Furniss, S.J., Stroud, A., Barrington, H., Kirby, S.P.J., Wray, J.P. & Dakin, P. (1986) The effect of dams' parity on first lactation performance of dairy heifers. *Animal Production*, **42**, 463.

Hafs, H.D., Manns, J.G. & Drew, S.B. (1975) The onset of oestrus and fertility of dairy heifers and suckled beef cows treated with prostaglandin. *Animal Production*, **21**, 13–28.

Keown, J.F. & Everett, R.W. (1986) Effect of days carried calf, days dry and weight of first calf heifers on yield. *Journal of Dairy Science*, **69**, 1891–6.

Kossaibati, M.A. & Esslemont, R.J. (1996) *Understanding the Rearing of Dairy Heifers – A Stockman's Guide*. BCVA, NMR, DAISY, Forte Dodge.

Little, W. & Kay, R.M. (1979) The effects of rapid rearing and early calving on the subsequent performance of dairy heifers. *Animal Production*, **29**, 131–42.

Table 5.12 Mean first lactation yields (kg) as percentage of mature yields in different management systems.

Group	Mean heifer yield	Mean cow yield	Yield difference	Heifer yield as percentage of cow yield
1	5200	6265	−1065	83
2	4504	5630	−1126	80
3	4274	5479	−1205	78

Pirlo, G., Miglior, F. & Speroni, M. (2000) Effect of age at first calving on production traits and on difference between milk yield returns and rearing costs in Italian Holsteins. *Journal of Dairy Science*, **83**, 603–8.

Sejrsen, K. (1994) Relationships between nutrition, puberty and mammary development in cattle. *Proceedings of the Nutrition Society*, **53**, 103–11.

Sejrsen, K. & Foldager, J. (1992) Mammary growth and milk production capacity of replacement heifers in relation to diet energy concentration and plasma hormone levels. *Acta Agricultura Scandinavica Section A. Animal Science*, **42**, 99–105.

Chapter 6
Tropical Cattle Management

R.D. Fielding and R.W. Matthewman

Introduction	68
Statistics	68
The productivity of tropical cattle	68
Production strategy	69
Calf management	69
Preweaning management	70
Weaning	71
Post weaning management	71
Onset of puberty	72
Monitoring growth	72
Adult production	72
Grass production	73
Systems of production	74
Management of dairy cows	77
Management of beef production	78

Introduction

In the following sections an overview is given of tropical cattle management and the tropical production systems in which cattle are found. Attention is paid to the main differences between tropical and temperate production systems in order to introduce them to the unfamiliar reader. The majority of tropical cattle are kept in extensive subsistence systems that differ fundamentally in their management objectives from commercial temperate enterprises. The latter tend to be specialized single product units whilst in the tropics livestock units are usually multi-purpose with important social as well as commercial objectives.

Statistics

Asia, Africa and South America contain approximately 74 per cent of the world's cattle (Table 6.1) and if other tropical areas are taken into account such as Central America then over 78 per cent are found in the tropics and subtropics. The same tropics produce only 59 per cent of the world's beef and veal and 55 per cent of the world's milk (Tables 6.2 and 6.3).

This discrepancy represents a challenge for those involved in tropical cattle management, since the tropics have many advantages for bovine production. These include: a potential year-round growing season in the absence of very low temperatures; grass species capable of greater energy capture and dry matter yields than temperate grasses; vast land areas un-utilized or underutilized; labour availability, much with strong animal keeping traditions; and many locally adapted breeds that have been selected for production in adverse environments.

Counteracting these advantages are several constraints, which include: high temperatures which depress production and food intake; long periods without rain when grass growth is impossible; animal diseases, such as trypanosomiasis and those transmitted by ticks; communal grazing systems that inhibit investment and the use of improved management techniques; and a lack of effective local demand and infrastructure to stimulate and support production. These advantages and constraints are discussed in greater detail in the subsequent sections.

The productivity of tropical cattle

The productivity of tropical cattle is sometimes said to be low. This is often untrue when total output is considered. Absolute production levels of milk or meat are usually low compared with temperate cattle, but capital inputs are also usually low. Productivity levels, in terms of use of capital as opposed to production levels, may therefore be relatively high.

The multiple outputs of tropical cattle systems include milk, meat, dung, hides and draught power (Fig. 6.1). Additional functions include acting as a saving mechanism, as a means of realizing emergency cash, as a means of fulfilling social obligations and as a symbol of wealth and status within the community. These outputs are not reflected in commonly used measurements of performance such as offtake, which refer only to products and animals that are sold. Social offtake, barter offtake, subsistence offtake, increases in herd size and the use of animals for draught power are not reflected in normal offtake measurements. The difference between the number of animals sold each year from subsistence systems and from commercial ranches of 8–10 per cent and 18–20 per cent respectively may be explained largely by these differences in objectives and products.

Production strategy

Some people have argued that the tropics are suited to multipurpose low input/low output systems. The environmental constraints on high producing animals and the lower quality forages and byproducts of the tropics

Table 6.1 World cattle numbers by continent (1000 head). Source: Food and Agriculture Organization (1998)

	1989–91	%	1998	%
World	1 294 020		1 318 386	(+1.9)
Africa	187 534	14.5	217 388	16.5
North and Central America	160 074	12.4	158 195	12.0
South America	272 829	21.1	299 947	22.8
Asia	400 563 (FMR)	31.0	450 389	34.2
Europe	123 383 (FMR)	9.5	156 212	11.8
Oceania	31 759	2.5	36 254	2.7
USSR	117 877	9.0	–	–

FMR: formerly; prior to break-up of USSR.
Number in brackets is the percentage change 1989–91 to 1998.

Table 6.2 World beef and veal production by continent (1000 t). Source: Food and Agriculture Organization (1998)

	1989–91	%	1998	%
World	52 718		53 695	(+1.9)
Africa	3 319	6.3	3 805	7.1
North and Central America	13 217	25.1	14 710	27.4
South America	9 044	17.2	9 886	18.4
Asia	5 269 (FMR)	10.0	10 023	18.7
Europe	11 056 (FMR)	21.0	12 726	23.7
Oceania	2 188	4.1	2 546	4.7
USSR	8 625	16.3	–	–

FMR: formerly; prior to break-up of USSR.
Number in brackets is the percentage change 1989–91 to 1998.

support this view. Intensification and specialization are certainly inhibited by the need for multi-purpose production. However, as development evolves it will probably promote the type of specialization that has taken place in temperate areas. The speed of this evolution will be determined by our ability to counteract the direct and indirect negative environmental effects on the production systems and to capitalize on the positive ones.

Calf management

In traditional cattle systems, such as pastoralism and settled extensive systems, reproductive cycles follow seasonal climatic variation. The peak of calving often occurs in the early wet season. In Sudan, in southern Darfur, most calvings occur in April, May and June. South of the Equator in Zambia the corresponding peak occurs in October and November. In humid areas where there is less seasonal nutritional stress, calvings occur throughout the year.

Table 6.3 World milk production from cows, by continent (1000 t, whole, fresh). Source: Food and Agriculture Organization (1998)

	1989–91	%	1998	%
World	475 154		466 347	(–1.9)
Africa	15 221	3.2	17 913	3.8
North and Central America	84 146	17.7	91 385	19.6
South America	32 013	6.7	45 325	9.7
Asia	56 674 (FMR)	11.9	82 871	17.8
Europe	167 194 (FMR)	35.2	207 768	44.6
Oceania	14 126	3.0	21 086	4.5
USSR	105 779	22.3	–	–

FMR: formerly; prior to break-up of USSR.
Number in brackets is the percentage change 1989–91 to 1998.

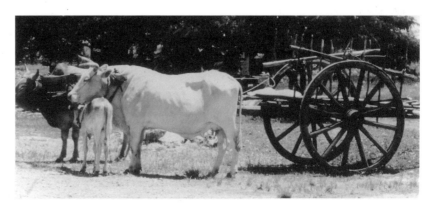

Fig. 6.1 Draught cows in Guadaloup.

Preweaning management

In pastoral systems, young calves are separated from the grazing herd during the day and kept in special calf areas. After evening suckling cows and calves may again be separated. In Nigeria, Fulani pastoralists allow calves to suckle briefly in the morning to induce milk let-down and then tether them until milking is completed. After milking the calves suckle until the herds move off for grazing. Calves seldom receive supplements and may not even receive adequate milk due to overmilking for human consumption. This is typical of pastoralism in Africa and the Middle East.

Calf management inputs in these systems are minimal and this is reflected in the levels of production. In arid areas gains may be as low as 200 g/day with liveweights of 60 kg and 150 kg at 6 and 18 months respectively. Calf mortality rates of 15–20 per cent in pastoral herds and of up to 40 per cent in sedentary herds are normally encountered.

Environmental stress, principally due to high ambient temperatures, is best minimized through correct time of grazing, use or planting of shade trees and provision of simple open houses that offer protection from the direct rays of the sun, but ensure maximum air flow.

As production systems improve indoor rearing systems may be adopted. Semi-intensive and intensive calf rearing systems found in the tropics include the following.

● Single suckling for beef calves where the objective is to achieve greatest calf growth rates and conversion of milk to meat.
● Dairy ranching where calves are separated at night and the cows are milked once in the morning and limited or restricted suckling is allowed throughout the day. If management will allow evening milking, suckling all night and separating the cow and calf during the day is a better option, as carried out by some pastoralists.

In the tropics calves may be reared inside, outside or a combination of both. Calves can be reared outside all year, though a number of disadvantages are associated with outside rearing on grass paddocks.

● It is difficult to keep grass sufficiently young and nutritious for calves.
● It is difficult to keep calves free from internal parasites if they are grazing in small enclosed areas.
● Environmental stress (temperature and radiation) can be high, even if good shading is available.

The combination of poor nutrition, parasites and climatic stress is a major constraint to calf rearing. Adequate nutrition is the key to success and to enabling a stable host–parasite relationship to be established.

For the first two months the calf should ideally be kept in an individual stall measuring about 2 × 1.5 m. In warmer areas, portable calf pens may be used. The most practical indoor system is a shed sited in a gravel or concrete yard where the calves may exercise. The house must provide shelter, be easily cleaned and should keep calves warm in cool weather and cool in warm weather. It may be no more than a simple roof over a concrete base. Slatted-floor houses have advantages, but are more expensive (Fig. 6.2). No walls are necessary in the humid tropics, but adequate overhangs are required in high rainfall areas.

Housed calves, if properly managed, tend to perform better than calves on pasture. A typical home mixed ration to accompany whole milk is a mixture of 50 per cent ground guinea corn and 50 per cent groundnut cake from two to three weeks of age.

The calf cannot utilize average quality tropical forage successfully until it is four or five months old. Consequently, it is desirable to suckle or bucket feed for as many months as possible and to feed concentrates and high-quality roughage. In intensive systems, the provision of some good quality forage is beneficial to stimulate rumen development.

Major calf diseases in intensive systems include scouring (gastroenteritis) (see Chapter 14), pneumonia (see Chapter 17) and worms (roundworms,

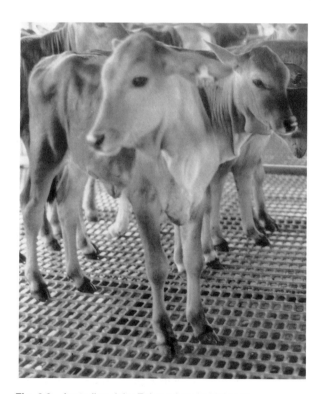

Fig. 6.2 Australian dairy Zebu calves in Malaysia.

thread-worms, hookworms, lungworms and tapeworms) (see Chapter 19). Suckling systems tend to have lower mortality rates than bucket feeding systems. The advantage is due to the avoidance of disease caused by incomplete sterilization of buckets and equipment, and suckled calves may receive more milk at more frequent intervals. In herds with many calves to be fed twice a day, maintenance of sanitation is difficult and the incidence of gastrointestinal disorders and indigestion in bucket-fed calves is often high (Chapter 16).

Restricted suckling can overcome many problems and is the system commonly practised in pastoral and semi-intensive systems. It is also widely used in the dairy ranching systems of South America. Calves are housed separately, either at night or during the day, and are then allowed to suckle for one minute to achieve let-down before the cows are milked in the morning or evening. The cows are fully milked-out and the calves then run with the cows for the rest of the day or night. When properly managed, restricted suckling systems have several advantages including better calf growth and health, higher milk yields including more saleable milk and are associated with reduced mastitis in the cows.

Weaning

In many systems calves are naturally weaned when the milk supply from the cows ceases due to the poorer nutrition of the dry season. This leaves calves at varying liveweights and different degrees of readiness for survival during the dry period. Where cows continue to produce milk, the chances of reconception are reduced, often to such an extent that a calving pattern of a calf every two years develops.

In some systems weaning is effected earlier by traditional methods. These may include thorns tied to the calf's head or sacks tied around the cows' udders. Dairy heifers in less extensive systems are best weaned at four to five months of age, depending on the availability of alternative feeds of adequate quality. Beef calves should have maximum benefit from the cows' milk and hence should be weaned as late as seven months. Heifer calves should be weaned early enough to prevent them conceiving to the bull running with the cows. Avoiding early conceptions is difficult in many extensive traditional systems, though in many zebu breeds maturity does not occur until a greater age (i.e. 18 months plus) when animals have reached approximately 66 per cent of their mature weight.

Post weaning management

Once weaned, calves usually encounter a period of suboptimal nutrition. Reasonable gains can be made in the rainy season, but weight loss frequently occurs in the dry season caused by combined energy and protein deficiencies. Of the two, protein is usually the more important. Levels of nitrogen in dry tropical grasses commonly fall to around 0.5 per cent, equivalent to 3–4 per cent digestible crude protein (DCP) in the dry matter. At this level of protein, grass digestibility is low and intake falls. The calf may enter a negative nitrogen balance as metabolic faecal nitrogen loss exceeds nitrogen intake. Young cattle allowed only poor quality roughages thus tend to develop a 'bloated' appearance.

Breeds differ in their ability to recover from weight loss. These differences include the ability to reduce metabolic rate during feed shortage and the efficiency of water conservation in periods of water shortage. The latter may lead to increases in feed digestibility due to slower rates of passage. The risk with major weight loss, in excess of 15–20 per cent, is permanent stunting and increased disease susceptibility.

During 'normal' dry seasons deaths are often rare, but once the rains begin, losses may occur due to the stresses of wetting, lower temperatures and highly succulent grasses causing digestive upsets.

Provided that the dry season weight loss is within the range of tolerance of the breed type, then rearing cattle usually show compensatory growth during the subsequent rainy season and make rapid gains (Hogg, 1991). Tropical cattle have been naturally selected to cope with recurring periods of undernutrition and then to compensate effectively. This is a characteristic of great importance which may be threatened by the increased introduction of exotic genes. The physiological mechanisms that allow compensation involve reduced metabolic rate, induced by a period of undernutrition, and increased voluntary food intake during realimentation. The period of realimentation and compensation is determined by the length of the rainy season. This is often short and animals again enter a period of undernutrition resulting in further weight loss. A 'zig-zag' pattern of animal growth thus characterizes many tropical rearing systems. Whilst dry season losses can be avoided by supplementation this is rarely justified economically.

An understanding of compensatory growth is important for reasons of rearing economy and in the management of feeding trials involving measurement of liveweight gain. Animals that are in a compensation phase may give a misleading result if compared with animals not in a compensation phase.

The consequences of the weight gain/weight loss pattern of growing tropical cattle are several and include delayed oestrus, reduced lifetime performance, reduced selection opportunities and also increased susceptibility to disease.

When rearing stock are housed or confined they may still suffer extended periods of poor nutrition when they are fed adult diets, such as sugar-cane tops or other low-quality byproduct feeds. In pastoral systems greater care is normally given to female stock because of their importance in producing calves and milk. Sub-optimal management of rearing stock is common in all ruminant systems, tropical or temperate. It is unfortunate that the consequences cannot be better communicated to the livestock owners and herders so as to motivate them to improve the management of their rearing stock.

Onset of puberty

Oestrus

In heifers, the period between weaning and calving can be divided into two phases: weaning to first service and first service to calving. The aim is to achieve optimum growth with the earliest maturity at the lowest cost. To achieve this small quantities of concentrate or supplement can be a great benefit. A check in growth occurs at weaning, but can be compensated for by the addition of concentrates.

The onset of oestrus occurs at a particular weight according to breed. Under good conditions regular cycling may be achieved at 13–14 months. In the tropics low nutritive quality of grasses, disease and environmental stresses usually result in delayed oestrus compared with temperate conditions. Whereas *Bos taurus* reach puberty at 30–40 per cent of mature weight, *B. indicus* reach puberty at around 60 per cent of mature weight (Macfarlane and Worrall, 1970).

The weight of the young heifer at first service and its rate of growth up to calving have an important effect on milk yield in later lactations. If early calving is combined with underfeeding in the rearing stage, heifers may be permanently stunted and milk production reduced.

Once heifers are cycling normally and have achieved an adequate body weight, mating or service should be timed to ensure calving at the optimum time of the year. This is often assumed to be the beginning of the rains, but it may be better to aim for calving just before the rainy season. This will allow the calves to start grazing during the rainy season before the quality of the herbage falls and as the dry season approaches.

Sperm production

The onset of sperm production is not as critical as the onset of oestrus. Only where conditions are very poor and liveweights low is the onset of sperm production delayed.

Castration is carried out in many traditional cattle systems, but is usually left until the animal's potential has been assessed. Inferior animals are castrated in order to stop them mating. However, sometimes the 'biggest and best' are castrated to produce draught oxen.

Monitoring growth

In traditional systems, monitoring of liveweight is by eye, but in more controlled systems regular weighing is desirable. If weighing facilities are not available on the farm, heart-girth measurements can be taken using a weigh-band. Attention should be paid to the breed for which the weigh-bands were initially designed, and if possible the accuracy should be checked against actual weighings and the bands calibrated appropriately. Direct weighing and heart-girths do not always fully define the state of the animal and condition scoring may be appropriate. Systems of condition scoring for *B. taurus* cattle (pp. 10, 11) may not be appropriate for *B. indicus* breeds, and scoring systems designed for tropical cattle should be used (Pullen, 1978; Nicholson and Butterworth, 1985). Pullen suggested a score range of 0–5 from emaciated to fattest while Nicholson and Butterworth suggested a nine-point scoring range.

Adult production

The different tropical cattle production systems are the result of differing levels of dry matter production per unit area available for grazing. This varies from very low levels in the arid areas (<1000 kg/ha per annum) to high levels (>10000 kg/ha per annum) in the humid areas, reducing again to low levels where intensive crop production limits grazing to roadside verges and intercrop areas.

Grazing utilization is often complicated by land ownership, which includes 'ownership' by nation, tribe, group or individual. Most grazing is communal and herders have the right to graze as many animals as they wish. Individual ownership and/or leasing of grazing land are increasing and this may stimulate intensification and improvement. Much depends on the availability of employment opportunities for those who are unsuccessful when land rights are allocated. If such opportunities are not available enforcement of land ownership is difficult and social pressure tends to result in the continuation of communal grazing.

Since grazing is crucial in cattle nutrition, the following sections highlight important aspects of grassland production.

Grass production

Grass represents the major link between the sun as the ultimate source of energy and the grazing animal. For the grass, however, the grazing animal can be regarded as a parasite. It is thus important that this relationship is not a destructive one for the grass. Animal productivity depends on a vigorous grass sward and management must safeguard the viability of the herbage above all else.

The factors that determine grassland dry matter productions are amount of light, leaf area, efficiency of species, amount of carbon dioxide, temperature, water and nutrients.

In the short term the manager can determine leaf area and nutrient level and in the longer term the species and possibly water level, through run-off control. Many tropical grasses are physiologically different from temperate grasses. They fix carbon as C_4 rather than C_3 compounds and are regarded as biologically more efficient than temperate grasses. This is partly the result of the structure of tropical grasses, which are taller and more effective in sunlight interception.

Tropical grasses have evolved to survive short rainy seasons. They grow quickly, reproduce and senesce. Whilst grass breeders have extended the growing period of many species, the short life cycle of grasses is still a problem when grazing animals require dry matter throughout the year.

Figure 6.3 illustrates the changes in the nutrient composition of grasses with time.

The fall-off in crude protein (CP) percentages reduces the rate of degradation of dry matter and rate of passage and thereby dry matter intake. While growing conditions are good in the wet season, CP levels can be as high as 12–14 per cent, but can be as low as 2–3 per cent in the dry season. The aim of the manager is to counteract low dry matter intake by appropriate management measures as discussed below.

Range monitoring

The interaction between animals and range is constantly changing and the result may be a long-term improvement or deterioration. A knowledge of the direction of this trend is very important and regular observation (monitoring) should be carried out using the following methods.

Remote sensing: This involves the use of satellites or aircraft to determine land use, land potential and changes in herbage production over time.

Soil and botanical trend monitoring: This involves establishing specific points or transects on the range

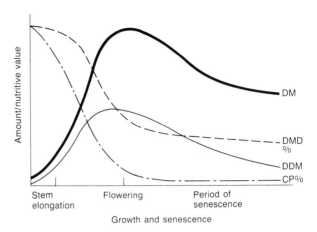

Fig. 6.3 Generalized changes in the amount and nutritive value of herbage during growth and senescence of the herbage. DM, dry matter available for grazing – determined by species and available nutrients; DMD, dry matter digestibility – falls from over 65% to around 40% largely as a result of changes in the crude protein level; DDM, available digestible dry matter – the resultant of DM and DMD; CP, crude protein – falls from over 12% to around 2%.

that can be visited annually to assess the degree of soil erosion and ground cover. The botanical species are identified and the increase or decrease in particular species is recorded. Botanical trend monitoring is appropriate for stable ecosystems where changes occur only slowly. In arid and semi-arid areas with variable rainfall changes can occur relatively quickly. When rains are adequate and grazing pressure reduced areas that appeared seriously overgrazed can recover dramatically through the germination of seeds of annual grasses (Behnke *et al.*, 1993).

Management to maximize voluntary food intake

Maximization of voluntary food intake is the underlying objective in ruminant feeding management. Tropical grasses are less digestible at the same stage of growth than temperate grasses, due to greater lignification. The lower digestibility reduces rate of passage and hence reduces food intake. Some breeds of tropical cattle may have evolved to cope with poor quality feeds through a greater dry matter intake capacity per unit body weight than temperate cattle.

Management strategies to maximize voluntary intake involve maximizing food production, avoiding food losses and stimulating intake as follows.

(1) Provision of adequate water and water harvesting through the use of pounds and micro terraces.
(2) Control of grazing time, intensity and frequency to maximize grass production, i.e. maintenance of

a sustainable carrying capacity according to the manager's objectives.

(3) Inclusion of legumes in the sward or as browse.
(4) Fire control to prevent destruction of accumulated standing hay in the dry season and in ranching systems to control bush encroachment.
(5) Exclusion of wildlife and non-authorized grazers.
(6) Provision of minerals and, in the long term, correction of soil mineral deficiencies.
(7) Simple rotation and grazing by appropriate herding, or use of fencing under intensive systems.
(8) Division of the herd into units of need, i.e. young stock, dry cows, lactating cows.
(9) Good herding practices, including choice of area to be grazed and duration of grazing.
(10) Routine health maintenance.

Systems of production

Management and production levels are determined by factors such as the herder's objectives, climate and land tenure. In communally owned dry areas that are marginal or exclude crops pastoral livestock systems are found with cattle (Fig. 6.4), sheep, goats and camels. In wetter areas small-scale mixed farming systems have developed where sheep and goats are important and where cattle and buffaloes may have a role for milk, meat, dung and draught power. In tropical highland areas where the climate is less severe milk production is often based on exotic cross cattle (Fig. 6.5). Where land is privately owned, particularly in South America, more intensive dairy farming methods occur in combination with large-scale dairy and beef ranching.

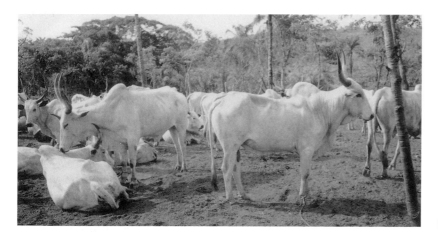

Fig. 6.4 Fulani cattle in Nigeria.

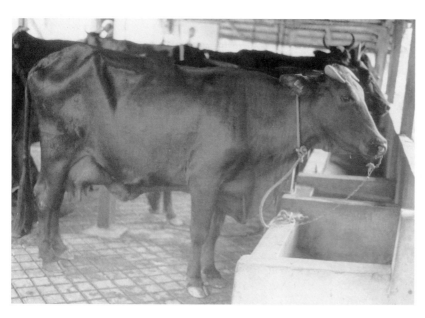

Fig. 6.5 Sahiwal × Friesian cattle in Malaysia.

*Pastoralism and settled extensive systems
of production*

Low and unpredictable rainfall coupled with communal land-use rights have led to migratory and seasonal patterns of grazing. Such systems are found throughout the Sahel from Mauritania to Sudan and through Ethiopia, Somalia, Kenya, Uganda and Tanzania. Cattle owners include the Fulani (Fulbe), Tuareg, Dinka, Borana, Karamajong and Masai. Pastoralists keep cattle to meet subsistence needs in areas unsuitable for crops. Milk is a major product that provides a daily source of food or tradeable produce and allows herders to exploit remote areas. Due to recurring droughts and increased population pressure resulting in loss of traditional grazing areas, these patterns are changing in many areas. Pastoralists are being forced to settle and engage in agriculture or some other activity.

Settled production occurs where cattle are combined with crop production. In Nigeria the term 'mixed farming' has been used to denote the use of cattle as draught animals for cultivation. Draught animals are common throughout the tropics and because of their vital role in the production of subsistence crops such as maize, sorghum, millet or rice their management is often better than that of cattle which are not used for draught.

Most settled farming is subsistence in nature and except where used for draught, livestock have a secondary role to crop farming. Management inputs are often relatively low. Land is seldom individually owned and communal grazing is a major method of food supply. The management and improvement of communally owned land are limited by the difficulties associated with getting people to cooperate.

Food inputs are natural pasture, browse, crop residues and supplements. Crop residue grazing is seasonal, but important for extensively managed cattle. Millet and sorghum residues provide early dry-season food and may be stored in stacks for use in the dry season, although they are often grazed off quickly in a 'free for all'.

One technology that has been proposed for improving the system as a whole is that of fodder banks. Fodder banks are fenced areas of high-quality forage that are made available for grazing for only a few hours per day and for only the most needy stock. The establishment of fodder banks has been described by Otsyina *et al.* (1987) using *Stylosanthes* species such as *S. guianensis* cv. Cook and *S. hamata* cv. Verano. Fodder banks have had limited success as has the oversowing of rangeland with legumes. The latter depends for success on the control of grazing, which with extensive grazing is virtually impossible.

Milk production

Milk is produced under a variety of systems, ranging from one-cow zero-grazed units in Mauritius where cows are fed on sugar-cane tops and roadside grasses, to large-scale extensive dairy ranching in Central and South America, intensive large-scale milk cooperatives in India, and very large, zero-grazed, environmentally controlled exotic cow units in Saudi Arabia.

Consumers in the tropics accord a high value to milk as a human food. The rate of increase in milk production has been considerably greater in tropical countries than in traditional milk producing and exporting nations (FAO, 1998). World milk production actually declined between 1989–91 and 1998, but increased by 18 per cent in Africa and 42 per cent in South America over the same period (FAO, 1998). Milk production can be an important enterprise in rural development for several reasons:

● it provides a year-round source of income for the farmer;
● it contributes to family nutrition;
● it can utilize crop byproducts;
● it serves to transfer money from urban to rural areas; and
● it creates rural employment opportunities.

These advantages have led to many development initiatives involving local/exotic crossbreds and sometimes pure exotics. There have been many disasters and failures, but also some notable successes as in India with Operation Flood, and in Kenya and Uganda with smallholder milk production schemes.

The major challenges for milk producers in the tropics include:

● achieving a high intake of good quality food throughout the year;
● coping with disease challenges;
● storage and transporting a bulky and perishable commodity.

Extensive systems: dairy ranching: Dairy ranching is an extensive system of milk and calf production particularly associated with South America, and countries such as Bolivia and Columbia. It is a flexible, dual purpose, low input low output system that depends for its success on the plentiful availability of low cost land and labour. Dairy ranching occurs particularly in those areas where conditions are hot and humid. There is enough moisture to produce sufficient food throughout the year but the temperature is too high to permit specialized high output milk production.

A wide range of genotypes are used in dairy ranching. Crossbreds between *Bos indicus* and *Bos taurus* are commonly encountered. In the more favourable environments high grade cattle are used whilst in the more difficult areas use is made of pure *Bos indicus* types. Similarly, there is a wide range of production systems. Some farmers milk their cattle twice a day whilst others milk their cattle only once a day. Some depend entirely on grazing whilst others use concentrates. In most cases the presence of the calf is used to stimulate milk let-down and one or more quarters are left for suckling by the calf after milking. The calves are allowed only limited access to the cows. However, much depends on the relative prices of meat and milk. If meat is in high demand then the calf may be allowed more milk in order to promote growth. If the price of fresh milk is high then the amount allowed for the calf may be severely restricted, which sometimes leads to increased calf mortality.

The total milk production from dairy ranching in South America is considerable and may represent half of the total milk consumed in a country such as Colombia. One of the great advantages of dairy ranching is its flexibility and the regular income from milk sales that it offers. It has been adopted as a system by many farmers throughout South America and clearly therefore must be meeting their needs.

Smallholder dairying: the Indian model: India is famous for its Anand pattern of dairy development. It is the fourth highest milk producer in the world after Europe, the Russian Federation and the USA and since 1950 it has more than doubled its output. This has involved the setting up of dairy cooperative societies which all milk producers are eligible to join. Farmers are usually paid for their milk within 12 hours of delivery to a collection point. Payment is based on quality and quantity.

The societies are formed into milk unions, which provide collection, processing and marketing services, and may market livestock feed and provide artificial insemination (AI), veterinary and other services.

Urban dairying in Africa: Recent years have seen a huge increase in urban dairying in and around cities and major towns throughout the tropics. Whilst such developments provide a regular income for producers and readily available fresh milk for the consumers they are also associated with a number of problems. These include urban pollution due to waste accumulation and undesirable smells and noises. Disposal of the carcasses of dead animals is a further problem as are the various threats to human health. The latter arise directly from the consumption of milk and meat containing organisms that cause diseases, such as tuberculosis and brucellosis, or indirectly from the increased activities of

flies and rats which multiply on the wastes associated with livestock farming in confined conditions (Waters-Bayer, 1995). Urban livestock farming, and dairying in particular, has largely developed without outside involvement in response to people's needs for income. They are undertakings that have usually been ignored by traditional ministries and organizations. However, if cities and towns in the tropics are to be developed in keeping with governments' aspirations and hopes then policies to limit and perhaps relocate urban dairying and livestock production are urgently needed.

Semi-intensive and intensive dairy production: In South America, exotic breeds are used intensively in highland areas. Highland areas are found throughout South America and also in Africa on the Jos Plateau in Nigeria, the Kenyan and Ethiopian Highlands and in parts of Tanzania such as Arusha.

Kenya Highlands: The smallholder dairy industry in Kenya has grown impressively over the last 25 years. There are now over 400 000 smallholder dairy farmers producing 70 per cent of milk sold. It is estimated that there are over 3 million dairy cattle in Kenya, concentrated for the most part in peri-urban areas. The majority include some amount of Friesian in their genetic make-up, but other breeds including Sahiwal, Brown Swiss, Ayrshire and Channel Islands have a significant role (Fig. 6.6). The pure exotics are found in the high potential areas in the highlands where lower temperatures and more dependable rains and food supplies make them a sustainable option. Dairy crosses with local Zebus are found in the harsher lower potential environments.

In the most fertile highland areas the production system is based on zero-grazing of Napier grass (*Pennisetum pupureum*) together with the use of roadside grasses and available byproducts such as maize stover, banana stems and sweet potato vines. The use of forage and tree legumes is being encouraged. So intensive is the system that 29 per cent of smallholders buy forage to feed their cows at some time during the year. Commercial concentrates are widely used. Grazing systems of varying intensity are encountered in less fertile areas. In these systems use is made of grasses such as Kikuyu grass (*Pennisetum clandestinum*) and Rhodes grass (*Chloris gayana*).

Yields of around 2500 kg per 10-month lactation period are commonly obtained. The median calving interval amongst the better smallholder herds has been estimated at 426 days. Fifty per cent of herds use artificial insemination with an approximate success rate of 50 per cent. Zero-grazed systems do not lend themselves to easy heat detection and this is an area for continuing extension inputs and training.

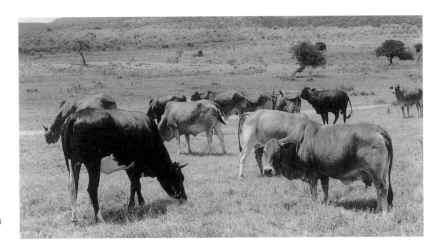

Fig. 6.6 Sahiwal and Sahiwal × Friesian cattle in Kenya.

East coast fever (pp. 750–53), transmitted by ticks, is the biggest threat to exotic breeds, although zero-grazing represents a significant tick avoidance strategy. Smallholders are increasingly adopting strategic hand-spraying methods of tick control rather than using government dips.

Many smallholder households in Kenya have benefited both nutritionally and financially from their dairying enterprises. Perhaps regrettably, intensification and commercialization of milk production tend to be associated with the control of income from milk moving from the women to the men. Nevertheless, it is hoped that the accumulated expertise and improved technologies will allow the continuing expansion of smallholder dairying into the low potential areas of the country (Reynolds *et al.*, 1996).

Beef production

In Africa and Asia beef has traditionally been a byproduct of milk and draught power production. Governments have often been disappointed with the level of beef production from their traditional herds. This has led to the mounting of many projects aimed at increasing beef output. These have included group ranching schemes as in Kenya and parastatal ranching initiatives as in Uganda and several other countries. Most of these projects have ultimately proved uneconomic, although private commercial ranches have usually been more successful.

Increased beef production from medium- to large-scale intensive feedlots has also been attempted with the aim of drawing immature stock from the rural areas for finishing to produce improved quality beef. These initiatives have not usually been successful and small-scale finishing schemes are proving a more successful form of intensification.

Beef may remain a byproduct of milk and draught power in Africa and Asia for the foreseeable future. It is appropriate therefore to focus research on ways of feeding and managing culled cows and oxen so as to maximize their value as meat animals.

In South America the situation is different and specialized high quality ranch beef from extensive systems has found a ready market in America, Europe and the Far East for many years.

There are indications that the demand for meat is growing rapidly in urban areas of the tropics. This represents a tremendous opportunity for beef producers, large and small, in tropical areas (Delgado *et al.*, 1999).

Management of dairy cows

The general objectives of management can be assumed to be broadly the same for all types of dairy cattle.

Ideally, dairy cows should produce a calf every year, since milk production is usually maximized with a 305-day lactation and yearly calving. Since gestation lengths vary between 275 and 287 days, it is necessary for the cow to conceive again within 80–90 days of calving. First service should be at about 50 days after calving. This is seldom achieved in tropical systems, and calving intervals of up to 500 days occur. The main reason is a delayed return to oestrus due to poor nutrition, suckling and other stresses including those of climate and disease.

Artificial insemination is not widespread in the tropics, but in some countries, such as Kenya and Pakistan, insemination services have been operational for many years. The benefits of genetic improvement from AI are constrained by the problems of detecting oestrus, which are especially acute in smallholder one cow units. The achievement of optimum breeding patterns and milk production also depends on the provision of suitable environmental conditions and proper feeding.

A major objective of the management of dairy cows in the tropics should be the reduction or the avoidance of environmental heat load. This can be achieved in a number of ways:

- Where possible animals should be grazed at night.
- Concentrates should be fed early in the morning and late in the afternoon.
- Adequate water should be provided.
- Natural and constructed shade should be provided.
- Buildings and shelters should be made of appropriate materials.
- Houses and yards should be sited so as to take full advantage of prevailing winds.
- Calving should occur in the coolest season, if nutrition allows.
- Animals should be managed indoors wherever possible, so as to reduce muscular work.
- Animals should be sprayed with water during the hottest periods to facilitate cooling.

The effect of adverse tropical environmental conditions can be overcome to a large extent if cost is not a constraint. In the Middle East, exotic breeds of dairy cattle are maintained in intensive systems and can achieve yields in excess of 8000 l/cow per year (Chapters 8, 71).

Feeding (see also Chapter 9)

Dairy cows require higher levels of feeding than growing or working animals. Energy inputs for lactation may equal or even exceed maintenance requirements, though in the tropics requirements for lactation will not usually exceed maintenance. For a 300 kg cow producing 1000 l in a 300-day lactation, average daily metabolisable energy (ME) requirements will be approximately 30 MJ for maintenance and 15–20 MJ for lactation depending on the butterfat (BF) content of the milk. Such levels of milk production can be achieved by a number of rations and feeds can be combined according to their degradability, ME content and their CP content. Some typical dairy rations used in southern Africa are shown in Table 6.4.

Other rations can be devised for different tropical regions based on a knowledge of locally available foods such as groundnut cake, wheat bran, maize, oats/barley, green grain, tapioca, rice bran, urea, molasses and cottonseed.

Health and hygiene

The two prime considerations of dairy cow health are the need to maintain optimum milk production

Table 6.4 Typical rations for dairy cows using combinations of feedstuffs. BF = butterfat.

Feedstuff	Diet (kg fresh weight)	
	360 kg cow	540 kg cow
	Diet 1	Diet 2
Legume hay (average)	1	1.6
Maize silage (average)	11	16
Grass hay (mature)	2	3.9
	Diet 3	Diet 4
Legume hay (average)	4	4
Maize silage (average)	18	27
Maintenance + 4 litres	(4.5% BF)	(3.5% BF)
	Diet 5	Diet 6
Green lucerne (early flower)	11	3
Grass hay (average)	3.5	18
Maize silage (average)	9	4.5
Maintenance + 4 litres	(4.5% BF)	(3.5% BF)

throughout lactation and optimum levels of fertility so that cows produce calves at regular intervals. In addition it is necessary to rear a healthy calf to weaning and to first calving. Attention must be given to a number of disease and general health problems.

Tick-borne infections, trypanosomiasis (Chapter 45), helminths and liver fluke (Chapter 19) are major problems in many areas, as is streptothricosis (see p. 886) in parts of Africa. Exotic animals are particularly susceptible to many of the endemic diseases.

Adequate attention to disease prevention is of primary importance in the tropics, where veterinary services are often unavailable (Chapter 69).

In hot climates it is better to milk at the cooler times of day. Milk cooling can present problems where constant electricity supplies are not present. Water supplies to local dairies are often poor and hygiene may be neglected.

Management of beef production

Ranching

In commercial ranching systems both land and animals are under the control of the same active management. This contrasts with pastoral systems where land is communally owned but rarely communally managed.

Table 6.5 Example of routine management programme for an East African cattle ranch.

Month	Approximate monthly rainfall (mm)	Operation
December/January/February	110	Calving; ear tagging, weighing and recording
February	100	Check breeding bulls and cows; cull and replace
March	160	Improved nutrition for breeding bulls and cows (bulls throughout mating season)
March/April/May	140	Brand, castrate, dehorn last year's calves
April/May/June	110	Join breeding bulls to herd of breeding cows
		Sell marketable stock; steers, surplus heifers, culls
May/June	60	Supplementation of lactating cows
		Conserve forage
July	10	Remove bulls from breeding herd
July/August/September	10	Wean
August	10	Pregnancy diagnosis; remove non-pregnant stock

Under some circumstances a system with two 70-day breeding seasons at four month intervals can be applied and may improve annual calving percentage and economic returns.

Animals are owned by individuals or groups of individuals who try to maximize rather than optimize their use of the communal land.

Ranching can operate throughout a range of intensity levels. Extensive systems may involve a one-herd system with little or no monetary investment other than in the cattle. Intensification may involve one or more of the following stages.

● Water development, e.g. boreholes or small dams.
● Routine health care.
● Mineral supplementation.
● Construction of handling and dipping facilities.
● Correct use of fire, e.g. creation of firebreaks.
● Multiple herd systems, e.g. young stock, steer herds, etc.
● Protein supplementation.
● Fencing, e.g. perimeter and paddock.
● Forage conservation.

An important aspect of ranch management is organizing routines. A routine approach means that the important husbandry tasks are designated to be carried out at particular times during the year. All concerned then know what should be done and when it should be carried out. Table 6.5 shows an example of a routine programme for a cattle ranch in East Africa. The programme of activities is determined by seasonal feed availability, which is determined by rainfall.

Government and parastatal companies have often involved themselves in ranching to intensify cattle production away from subsistence systems. The attempts have rarely been successful. The reasons have usually been economic, arising from indifferent managements, low meat prices and the high costs of intensification, which have rarely been justified. Most successful ranching is in the purely commercial sector.

Supplementation

Tropical cattle commonly suffer a period of weight loss during the dry season. Compensatory growth can overcome the worst effects, but feed supplementation may be feasible where it can be controlled. The practical approach should include the use of sustainable stocking rates, fire control, deferred grazing, seasonal control of breeding and tactical marketing. Once supplementation is accepted as a workable option two considerations arise: the nature of the supplement and the stock to be supplemented.

Nature of the supplementation: The supplement should improve the quality of the overall diet rather than act as a substitute for a part of that diet. The effective utilization of nitrogen supplementation in the form of urea mixed in a carrier such as molasses depends upon there being a deficiency of degradable protein in the rumen. This is not always the case and the response to urea supplementation has not always been as predictable as anticipated.

Other forms of background supplement such as minerals are important over the long term, but have no effect on reducing dry-season weight losses. The possible exception is salt, which may serve to stimulate the intake of poor-quality roughage. In Nigeria, a naturally occurring and renewable mineral supplement known as Kanwa is fed to both settled and transhumant cattle owned by Fulani and agropastoralists. Kanwa contains 1.5 per cent Na, 4.7 per cent K, 23.7 per cent Ca, 0.6 per cent P and trace amounts of Mg, Fe, Mn, Cu, Co and Zn.

Increased attention is being paid to the potential of small amounts of highly digestible cellulose as a supplement in the form of legume or browse material. Such material can stimulate cellulolytic bacteria and enable an improved utilization of a low quality diet. Browse usually contains over 10 per cent CP/unit DM and can often have as high as 25 per cent CP/unit DM. It thus forms a good supplement to poor-quality roughage.

Other forms of supplement in Nigeria include cottonseed cake, groundnut tops, cow pea stalks, groundnut cake and also salt, chaff, bran, cut branches and cut grass. In Sudan some livestock owners in the Gezira area provide daily supplement mixtures containing cottonseed cake, groundnut cake, bran and molasses. Where breweries are nearby, brewers' grains may also be available.

Animals to supplement: Not all animals have the same need for supplementation and optimum use of resources can be achieved by identifying an order of priority, e.g. weaned calves, late pregnancy/early lactation cows, breeding heifers. Lowest priority will normally be given to growing steers.

Drought: Drought conditions represent a special case for supplementation where survival is the objective. An early difficulty is establishing that drought, as opposed to a long dry season, exists. When the fact is established a number of options are available: (i) do nothing; (ii) sell some stock and buy feed; (iii) sell all stock and restock later; or (iv) move animals to an area with grazing.

Where supplementation is adopted it is important not to start supplementing too soon, but to allow animals to lose some weight to reduce their maintenance requirements. Bovines have adaptive mechanisms for dealing with drought, one of which involves a reduction in metabolic rate. Such mechanisms should be activated prior to survival supplementation.

Animals at greatest risk and females required to continue the herd after the drought should be given priority for drought feeding. Once a decision has been taken to provide survival feeding the feedstuff is usually determined by cost and availability. Infrequent feeding of large amounts is probably preferred so as to ensure every targeted animal gets some feed.

Feedlots

Feedlots have been set up in different forms and for a wide variety of reasons; as large- or small-scale units, as commercial or government sponsored ventures to produce export quality carcasses and as a means of trying to reduce overgrazing of communal areas. Initial developments tended to follow the large-scale pattern of North American feedlots, but it is now recognized that small-scale projects that demand more labour than capital are more sustainable.

Certain circumstances are required before intensification becomes an economic strategy, as follows.

- Beef is one of the most expensive meats within the country.
- Animals are economically available for feeding on a continuing basis.
- Above average quality feeds are economically available on a continuing basis.
- Adequate initial funding is available.
- Infrastructural factors such as transport, communications, husbandry and health services are available and adequate.
- There is an absence of restrictive factors, e.g. butcher cartels or legal restrictions on export.

A failure to satisfy these requirements has led to the limited success of many feedlots.

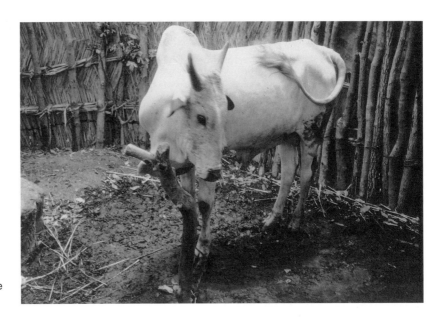

Fig. 6.7 Stall-fed fattening of Fulani cattle in Nigeria.

Smallholder fattening

In Malawi a smallholder fattening project was started as long ago as 1957 and has now expanded to other parts of the country. It has proved to have many benefits, as follows.

- Home-grown beef for the local market saving foreign exchange.
- A means of saving for farmers, which can be used to invest in crop production.
- The provision of manure for the maintenance of soil fertility.
- Stabilization of the farming system by providing an employment opportunity.

The participating farmer must build a suitable stall for one or two animals. Several farmers commonly build their stalls together. Farmers receive a credit steer of 260–280 kg with the assistance of the extension services. This is fed on maize stover, groundnut haulms and maize bran during the dry season and cut-and-carry Napier grass (*Pennisetum purpureum*) and/or Rhodes grass (*Chloris gayana*) during the rainy season. Average daily gain is about 0.5 kg and with approximately 200 days feeding total gains of 100 kg are achieved producing a final weight of 360–380 kg.

In Nigeria, stall feeding and fattening is also carried out and is a common method of cattle production in the subhumid zone and northern savannah areas (Fig. 6.7). Farmers often keep up to six animals, usually young bulls, for 18–24 months before selling them to urban traders. This method of production has been the subject of a major extension exercise by the National Livestock Projects Department in Nigeria, and has been of some success in Kano State where work bulls after 2–3 years are stall-fattened for 6–8 months and sold to butchers.

References

Behnke, R.E., Scoone, I. & Kerven, C. (eds) (1993) Range ecology at disequilibrium: new models of natural variability and pastoral adaptation in African savannas. Overseas Development Institute (ODI), London.

Delgado, C., Rosegrant, M., Steinfeld, H., Ehui, S. & Courbois, C. (1999) Livestock to 2020: the next food revolution. Brief 61. International Food Policy Research Institute (IFPRI), 2033 K Street, Washington.

Food and Agricultural Organization (1998) *Production Yearbook 52*, pp. 186–8, 195–7, 212–14.

Hogg, B.W. (1991) Compensatory growth in ruminants. In *Growth Regulation in Farm Animals* (ed. by A.M. Pearson & T.R. Dutson), pp. 103–34. Elsevier Applied Science, London.

Macfarlane, J.S. & Worrall, K. (1970) Observations on the occurrence of puberty in *Bos indicus* heifers. *East African Agricultural and Forestry Journal*, **35**, 409–10.

Nicholson, M.J. & Butterworth, M.H. (1985) *A Guide to Condition Scoring of Zebu Cattle*, International Livestock Centre for Africa, Addis Ababa, Ethiopia, pp. 3–30.

Otsyina, R.M., von Kaufman, R.R., Mohamed Saleem, M.A. & Suleiman, H. (1987) *Manual on Fodder Bank Establishment and Management*, International Livestock Centre for Africa, Addis Ababa, Ethiopia, pp. 8–12.

Pullen, N.B. (1978) Condition scoring of White Fulani Cattle. *Tropical Animal Health and Production*, **10**, 118–20.

Reynolds, L., Metz, T. & Kiptarus, J. (1996) Smallholder dairy production in Kenya. *World Animal Review* **87**, 66–73.

Waters-Bayer, A. (1995) Living with livestock in town: urban animal husbandry and human welfare. In *Livestock Production and Diseases in the Tropics: Livestock Production and Human Welfare: Proceedings of the VIII International Conference of Institutions of Tropical Veterinary Medicine* (ed. by K.H. Zessin), pp. 121–32. Deutsche Stiftung für Internationale Entwicklung, Zentralstelle für Ernährung und Landwirtschaft.

Wilson, R.T. (1995) *Livestock Production Systems*, pp. 1–141. MacMillan Education, London.

Chapter 7
Ethnoveterinary Medicine in the Tropics

R.D. Fielding

Introduction 83
Definition and examples of nature of EVM 83
Why ethnoveterinary medicine? 83
Advantages and disadvantages of EVM 84
The way forward – validation? 84
Discussion 85
Conclusions 86

Introduction

Over the last 30 to 40 years most 'top-down' rural development projects in the tropics have continued to have disappointing results. In response to this, and prompted largely by social scientists, there has been a growing awareness that an appreciation of rural people's local knowledge should be the starting point for discussing development interventions of any kind. This participatory 'bottom-up' approach is now being applied across all areas of natural resource use in the tropics. As regards the maintenance of health amongst the livestock resource it is Constance McCorkle, an anthropologist, and Evelyn Mathius-Mundy, a veterinarian, who have done most in the last 15 years or so to bring attention to that local knowledge in the tropics which deals with animal disease treatment. This body of knowledge is now commonly referred to as ethnoveterinary medicine (EVM). The objective of this chapter is to highlight the key issues and developments in EVM in the tropics.

Definition and examples of nature of EVM

For the purposes of this chapter ethnoveterinary medicine is defined simply as the traditional treatments and practices that livestock keepers are using now, other than modern synthetic drugs. The majority of the treatments are of plant origin. Some EVM involves magico-religious practices. Although these latter practices can be very important to those who use them, they are not discussed here.

There is an increasing amount of literature listing and describing EVM practices (Mathius-Mundy & McCorkle, 1989; Bizimana, 1994; IIRR, 1994), including various internet sites. Some examples of EVM from these and other sources are presented below.

The majority of ethnoveterinary practices are aimed at relatively chronic conditions such as internal and external parasites, digestive disorders such as inappetance, constipation, diarrhoea and bloat, wounds, lameness, non-specific 'fevers' and 'coughs and colds'.

In Ethiopia goatkeepers boil the leaves of the castor-oil plant (*Ricinus communis*) to provide a viscous liquid which they use to control mange in their goats. The active agent, ricin, is very poisonous for humans and provides an example of an EVM agent that must be handled with care (Peacock, 1996).

In many Mediterranean countries honey is used on wounds to promote healing (personal observation). The mode of action is believed to be partly achieved through an osmotic effect which draws fluid into the wound. This fluid serves to 'flush out' dirt and other contaminants and thus promotes healing.

There are many plants which appear to have some anthelmintic effect: *Artemisia maritima*, *Caesalpinia crista*, *Melia azedarach*, *Mallotus philippinensis*, *Chrysanthemum* spp., *Matteuccia orientalis*, *Carica papaya*, *Heracleum* spp., *Hedysarum coronarium*, *Aloe barteri*, *Terminalia avicennioides* and *Diospyros mollis* (Hammond *et al.*, 1997). Firing and bloodletting are widely used practices to treat problems such as lameness and inflammation. These practices are most commonly used by owners of horses and donkeys.

Why ethnoveterinary medicine?

In addition to the increasing appreciation of local knowledge as explained above there are several other reasons which have contributed to the recent growth in interest in EVM at farm, local, national and international levels.

Antibiotics, acaricides and anthelmintics can be dramatically effective when affordable and correctly used. However, the rising cost of these medicines and its consequences is now a major issue. If the cost of a treatment is a significant proportion of the value of the animal that is being treated then one or more things may happen:

- The animal is left untreated or a low cost EVM method is used.
- The seller of the chemical dilutes it to make it cheaper and so that it will 'go further'. Monteiro *et al.* (1998) in Kenya found that of seven anthelmintics marketed as containing levamisole, an effective anthelmintic agent, two contained none, whilst two others had levels of levamisole of 11.8 per cent and 78.7 per cent of the amount stated on the label.
- Livestock owners who buy costly drugs may also try to make them 'go further' by diluting them, by underdosing or by not completing the full recommended course of treatment. All abuses of drugs are associated with incomplete cures and with the promotion of organism resistance.

Even when properly administered the long-term regular use of drugs and chemicals such as anthelmintics and acaricides leads to the loss of an animal's natural resistance. If for whatever reason the anthelmintics/acaricides are suddenly unavailable the animal is totally exposed to the worst effects of the parasites and organisms which these drugs are keeping under control. For this reason the routine use of acaricides, for example, has been questioned for some time (Norval, 1983).

Farmers in the tropics rarely have any awareness of the environmental damage and pollution that may be caused by the incorrect disposal of chemicals and/or the associated packaging.

Globally there is a growing interest in 'alternative' and 'sustainable' approaches to disease treatment. In human medicine what were once regarded as 'odd', such as herbalism, acupuncture and homeopathy, are now taken seriously. Veterinary medicine is currently evolving, in a similar way (see Chapter 65).

Advantages and disadvantages of EVM

The advantages of EVM are as follows:

- Livestock keepers are already familiar with it, it is what they use now.
- A significant part of it appears to 'work'. For example, Bennet-Jenkins and Bryant (1996) tested the anthelmintic effect of *Eucalyptus grandis* leaves with feral goats. On autopsy these authors found 91

per cent fewer *Haemonchus contortus* in the treated group as compared to the control ($p < 0.05$).

- It is freely available or at a cost in proportion to the value of the animal.
- It is easily administered, usually topically or orally.
- EVM relieves the worry and concern of owners of sick animals in that it makes it possible to do something, effective or not, for their animals.

However, EVM is not without disadvantages and limitations:

- Particular methods are often geographically localized and the scope for their further dissemination is limited.
- Cures are variable in their effectiveness according to season, method of preparation, etc., and few if any have been validated in the same way in which synthetic drugs must be validated.
- From a technical standpoint some are totally ineffective.
- EVM has little to offer against the acute viral diseases of animals, other than treatments for the signs.
- EVM is not always practical on a large scale. A particular EVM method may require considerable amounts of leaves, seeds or even roots. Identifying a plant as certainly medicinal may lead to its total destruction. In Nepal people have been excluded from some forests because of the excessive collection of medicinal plants, albeit they were for use in human medicine.

In the new millenium the major arguments for giving greater attention to EVM include the following:

- It is what livestock keepers use now and, by definition therefore, should be the starting point for any animal health intervention.
- It would be unwise to rely on only one strategy for disease control, i.e. modern drugs, when the strategy has limitations, some of which have been highlighted above.
- In the long term the 'official' recognition of EVM empowers those who practise it, with potential benefits for increased participation in other areas of social and economic development.

The way forward – validation?

Over the last 15 years or so there have been many publications listing EVM medicines and practices, as indicated above. However, there have been very few trials and validations of EVM that stand up to rigorous scientific scrutiny. There may be a bias in favour of identifying treatment success with EVM, as has been observed in human ethnomedicine (Roscoe, 1991). Thus it is now timely to bring to EVM the rigour of objective assessment.

Hammond et al. (1997) have outlined one approach for the identification and validation of anthelmintic plants used in EVM. In brief this methodology involves the following stages:

- A wide-ranging survey to identify all relevant EVMs and the people involved.
- Selection of the 'best bet' anthelmintic plants being used against the most economically important diseases.
- Study of selected plants in terms of their use in human medicine, given that many plants are used in both human and animal medicine.
- Preparation of the test medicines in the ways used by the livestock owners/healers.
- Testing for activity against indicator helminths.
- Testing for toxic effects, probably on-station.
- Validation on-farm with livestock owners.

If the results of the above are positive it is logical to proceed to more detailed identification of the active principles and of how their effects might be extended, for example through improved storage.

It is relatively easy to list EVM practices and to review the literature in human and animal medicine. However, as soon as any attempt is made to test EVM in a quantitative way major problems arise. The ultimate one is cost, but this arises from the fact that so many EVM practices are locally specific and highly variable in their application and use.

One response to the above problem is a qualitative method of validation based on 'confidently used' EVM. IIRR (1994) produced a collection of EVM practices in Asia using a workshop brainstorming technique. The authors attempted to 'validate' practices on a scale of 1–6 as follows:

(1) Workshop participants agreed that the treatment would be useful.
(2) Treatment is widely used in a region or a country. (Some remedies were also validated against practices from outside Asia.)
(3) Workshop participants had first-hand knowledge of the remedy's use on-farm.
(4) Traditional healers are known to use the remedy.
(5) The remedy is cited in the literature in one of two ways: either it is used to treat the same problem in humans or another animal species or this plant has proven pharmacological activity to treat the problem in question (laboratory validation).

(6) The remedy has been scientifically validated as effective to treat the problem in the livestock species in question.

Of some 330 treatments listed by IIRR (1994) only five are designated as '6', i.e. as being scientifically validated. Of these five, one is for a pig sedative using the leaves of Mimosa pudica, the other four are for upper respiratory problems in poultry (leaves of Heliotropium indicum, Spondias pinnata and garlic, Allium sativum) and for internal parasites (garlic and the latex of papaya, Carica papaya).

Is validation of EVM important for the livestock owners who use it? Possibly 'no' if they are using practices that have been used 'successfully' for generations. But possibly 'yes' if they have seen the effectiveness of modern drugs as indicated above. Are users of EVM experimenting with/validating EVM medicines and methods now in any way at all? Until relatively recently the answer given by outsiders would have been 'no'. But following on from the work of van Veldhuizen et al. (1997) and others, it is now clear that much experimentation is done by ordinary farmers in the tropics although its extent remains to be fully documented. One example of an on-farm ethnoveterinary validation with farmers has been provided in Peru within the Project for the Validation of Technologies in Communities (McCorkle & Bazalar, 1996). In this instance the validation exercise proved to be very positive and beneficial for the community concerned.

If EVM is locally specific then validation probably has to be locally specific. In the past validation work has been something usually done on-station and in laboratories with the use of specialized equipment. The need for these has not gone away, but there are a number of tools such as weigh-bands and body condition scoring systems which serve to make validation on-farm more feasible. Van Wyk et al. (1997) have reported an eyelid colour system for measuring anaemia in sheep and relating this to worm burdens. This system could be used to help organize balanced groups of animals with similar worm burdens for the purposes of testing the efficacy of, for example, anthelmintic plants. The McMaster method for counting parasite eggs in animal faeces is one that can be learnt relatively easily and used at farmer group level. Although facilitated farmer validation may seem ambitious it seems unlikely that extensive validation of EVM in the tropics will be achieved in any other way.

Discussion

If it is assumed that validation trials can be organized and carried out, there are two possible outcomes. One is that the plant has no statistically significant effect on the targeted organism. For example, on the basis of a literature review, Hammond *et al.* (1997) suggested that *Mallotus philippensis*, widely used in EVM in Asia, could be effective as a broad spectrum anthelmintic. Following an actual validation of the dried powdered fruit of this plant, termed kamala, Jost *et al.* (1996) concluded that a particular sample of the dried fruit was ineffective against particular gastrointestinal nematodes in certain goats indigenous to Balochistan, Pakistan. If a medicinal plant is found to be ineffective in a validation it will be difficult to communicate the result to many livestock owners. There is unlikely to be any campaign, or funding, to stop livestock owners using it. Furthermore, livestock owners may not believe the negative result, and in any case there may be some medicinal effect albeit in different circumstances and at a biological but statistically insignificant level.

If a validation proves positive, what are the options? One obvious option is to encourage greater use of the medicine in question through extension services and publications. Even so it will be difficult to make universal recommendations as is possible with a synthetic drug, because of the underlying variability in EVM as arising, for example, from species, seasonal and method of preparation effects.

Thus, whether or not validation is carried out and whether or not it is positive seems unlikely to have much effect on the short-term use of ethnoveterinary medicines by livestock owners outwith the specific locality in question, although this is not necessarily the case for the long term.

Conclusions

The key issues highlighted above are as follows:

- If poverty and/or drug costs continue to increase then so will the use of EVM.
- Some EVM 'works' and is worth investigating/ validating objectively.
- The evolution of evidence-based EVM will be slow and may require a new participative approach to validation.

From the above points it can be further concluded that there is likely to be a continuing place for EVM in the tropics alongside modern methods of disease treatment and according to circumstances.

References

Bennet-Jenkins, E. & Bryant, C. (1996) Novel anthelmintics. *International Journal of Parasitology*, **26**, 937–47.

Bizimana, N. (1994) *Traditional Veterinary Practice in Africa*. Deutsche Gesellschaft für Technische Zusammenarbeit (GTZ) Gmbh, Eschborn.

Hammond, J.A., Fielding, D. & Bishop, S.C. (1997) Prospects for plant anthelmintics in tropical veterinary medicine. *Veterinary Research Communications*, **21**, 213–28.

IIRR (1994) *Ethnoveterinary Medicine in Asia: An Information Kit on Traditional Animal Health Care Practices*. International Institute of Rural Reconstruction, Silang, Cavite, Philippines.

Jost, C.C., Sherman, D.M., Thomson, E.F. & Hesselton, R.M. (1996) Kamala (*Mallotus philippinensis*) fruit is ineffective as an anthelmintic against gastro-intestinal nematodes in goats indigenous to Balochistan, Pakistan. *Small Ruminant Research*, **20**, 147–53.

McCorkle, C.M. & Bazalar, H. (1996) Field trials in ethnoveterinary research and development: lessons from the Andes. In *Ethnoveterinary Research and Development* (ed. by C.M. McCorkle, E. Mathias & T.W. Schillhorn van Veen), pp. 264–82. Intermediate Technology Publications, London.

Mathius-Mundy, E. & McCorkle, C.M. (1989) *Ethnoveterinary Medicine: An Annotated Bibliography*. Bibliographies in Technology and Social Change, No 6. Technology and Social Change Program, Iowa State University, Ames, Iowa.

Monteiro, A.M., Wanyangu, S.W., Kariuki, D.P., Bain, R., Jackson, F. & McKellar, Q.A. (1998) Pharmaceutical quality of anthelmintics sold in Kenya. *Veterinary Record*, **142**, 396–8.

Nichter, M. (1992) (ed.) *Anthropological Approaches to the Study of Ethnomedicine*. Gordon and Breach Sciences, San Antonio.

Norval, R.A.I. (1983) Arguments against intensive dipping. *Zimbabwe Veterinary Journal*, **14**, 19–25.

Peacock, C.P. (1996) *Improving Goat Production in the Tropics – A Manual for Development Workers*. Oxfam, Oxford.

Roscoe, P. (1991) *The Perils of 'Positivism': A Critique of the Image of 'Positivism' in Cultural Anthropology*. Unpublished manuscript, as cited by Nichter (1992).

van Veldhuizen, L., Waters-Bayer, A., Ramirez, R., Johnson, A. & Thompson, J. (eds) (1997) *Farmers' Research in Practice: Lessons from the Field*. Intermediate Technology Publications, London.

van Wyk, J.A., Malan, F.S. & Bath, G.F. (1997) Rampant anthelmintic resistance in sheep in South Africa – what are the options? In *Managing Anthelmintic Resistance in Endoparasites* (ed. by J. van Wyk & P.C. van Schalkwyk), pp. 51–63. Workshop held at the 116th International Conference of the World Association for the Advancement of Veterinary Parasitology, August 1997, Sun City, South Africa.

Further reading

Ibrahim, M.A., Nwude, N., Ogunsusi, R.A. & Aliu, Y.O. (1984) Screening of West African plants for anthelmintic activity. *International Livestock Centre for Africa Bulletin*, **17**, 19–23.

ITDG & IIRR (1996) *Ethnoveterinary Medicine in Kenya: A Field Manual of Traditional Animal Health Care Practices.* Intermediate Technology Development Group and International Institute of Rural Reconstruction, Nairobi.
Relevant internet site: http://pc4.sisc.ucl.ac.be/prelude/prelude_Homepage.html (17.11.99).

Relevant internet: http://www.rbgkew.org.uk/peopleplants/ (17.11.99).
Wanyama, J. (1997) *Confidently used Ethnoveterinary Knowledge among Pastoralists of Samburu, Kenya.* Intermediate Technology, Nairobi.

Chapter 8
Heat Stress in Dairy Cattle

J.K. Shearer

Introduction   88
Thermoregulation and the thermal comfort zone   88
Body heat production   89
Heat gain from the environment   89
Body heat loss   89
Effects of heat stress on performance   89
   Prepartum heat stress   89
   Peripartum heat stress   90
   Postpartum heat stress   90
Methods to reduce heat stress   90
   Natural shade   90
   Artificial shade   90
Cooling by reducing ambient air temperature   91
   Evaporative cooling pads and fans   92
   High pressure foggers   92
   Misters   92
Enhancing the cow's natural mechanisms of heat loss   92
   Sprinklers and fans   92
   Sprayers in parlour exit lanes   93
   Cooling ponds   93

Introduction

Cattle, like all mammals and birds, are homeotherms. Despite wide fluctuations in environmental temperature they are capable of maintaining a relatively constant body temperature. This ability to regulate or stabilize body temperature is essential to preserve the multitude of biochemical reactions and physiological processes that occur with normal metabolism. As environmental temperatures rise a series of thermoregulatory responses designed to stabilize body temperature are initiated. These include physiological, anatomical and behavioural changes which exhibit themselves as reduced feed intake, decreased activity, shade or wind seeking, increased peripheral blood flow, sweating and panting.

During periods when ambient air temperature and humidity are particularly high, thermoregulatory activities may not be sufficient to maintain normal body temperature. The result is a rise in body temperature and the induction of a series of thermoregulatory events whose objective is survival from a potentially life-threatening crisis. Performance is naturally a sec-ondary concern and almost always suffers. The specific thermoregulatory responses that impact performance are a reduction in feed intake and nutrient absorption, and a redirection of blood flow from internal organs to peripheral tissues. During the prepartum period, this results in lower calf birthweight and reduced milk yield in the subsequent lactation. Postpartum, hyperthermia depresses dry matter intake, reduces milk yield and decreases reproductive performance.

Methods to relieve heat stress include the provision of shade, forced air movement as with fans, and water in the form of a fog, mist or sprinkle droplet. In some areas of the world cooling of cows may be accomplished by permitting access to ponds which are managed for such purposes. Depending upon specific climatic conditions (i.e. hot dry or arid verses hot and humid) these can be used in combination to assist cows in the achievement of acceptable heat balance.

Thermoregulation and the thermal comfort zone

For lactating dairy cattle, the most comfortable environmental temperature range is between 5 and 25°C (41 and 77°F), otherwise known as the thermal comfort zone. Within this range of temperatures optimal animal performance can be expected. Temperatures that range outside this zone may require an alteration in the basal metabolic rate for the animal to maintain normal body temperature. The lower critical temperature is the point at which an animal will begin to feel cold and must increase body heat production. It varies with age, physiological status (lactating or non-lactating), degree of insulation, level of milk production and acclimatization. For example, the lower critical temperature for neonatal calves is reported to be 12.8°C (55°F). On the other hand, a mature cow in peak lactation may be comfortable at a temperature of −25°C (−13°F). The upper critical temperature is the point above which an animal begins to feel warm and must begin to compensate. Unlike the variability described for lower critical temperature, the upper critical temperature limit remains constant at about 25°C (77°F) regardless of age or physiological status.

Body heat production

Total body heat load is a combination of heat derived from metabolism and that obtained from environmental sources. Internal body heat associated with basal body functions (digestion and cellular biochemical reactions) accounts for 35–70 per cent of total daily heat production. In ruminants there is greater heat gain associated with the digestion of roughages as compared with concentrate feedstuffs. Other sources of body heat include that associated with daily physical activity and increased metabolic activity associated with lactational performance. Finally, it is significant to note that the increased respiratory rates and panting associated with evaporative cooling, while necessary to cool the cow, also account for an increase in daily maintenance requirements by 7–25 per cent.

Heat gain from the environment

The primary sources of heat gain from the environment are solar radiation and high ambient air temperature. The amount of heat absorbed by an animal exposed to direct sunlight is related to coat colour. Black cows absorb over twice as much heat from the sun as white cows. This is complicated by virtue of the fact that the flow of heat away from the cow's body is restricted by high ambient air temperature which narrows the thermal gradient between the cow's body and the surrounding air. Thus, solar radiation together with high ambient air temperature are important sources of heat gain from the environment. Since little can be done to reduce air temperature, efforts to provide shade should be a high priority.

Body heat loss

The release of heat from any object to the environment is proportional to its exposed surface area. Further, the ratio of surface area to body mass decreases as overall size increases. This means that large animals such as cows are at a disadvantage in losing excess body heat. They are also at greater risk of becoming overheated. Calves, on the other hand, have a greater amount of surface area relative to body mass and, therefore, are much better at dissipating heat than a mature cow.

Avenues for the dissipation of heat in cows include both non-evaporative and evaporative cooling mechanisms. Between the temperatures of −17.8 and 10°C (0–50°F), 75 per cent or more of heat loss from the body occurs by non-evaporative cooling (i.e. conduction, convection and radiation). However, at temperatures of 29.5°C (85°F) and above, nearly 80 per cent of heat is dissipated by evaporative cooling (i.e. the evaporation of water from the skin and respiratory tract). In general, whenever temperatures exceed 21°C (70°F), evaporative cooling becomes the predominant mechanism of heat loss in cattle.

Bos indicus (Zebu) cattle have larger and a greater number of sweat glands than *Bos taurus* cattle, but actual sweating rates are only slightly higher. The evaporation of water from the cow's skin is a very effective cooling mechanism. It is enhanced by conditions which provide air movement which moves water vapour away from the skin thereby increasing the vapour-pressure gradient in the immediate air space surrounding the animal.

The primary obstacle to evaporative cooling is high relative humidity. Humid air is more saturated with water vapour. Thus, the vapour-pressure gradient is reduced. In some environments this is exacerbated still further by limited air movement. This results in very low water evaporation rates and consequently minimal cooling. In hot and humid environments this condition may be overcome by a combination of sprinkling the skin with water and forced air movement with fans. Fanning cools wetted cows by accelerating the water vaporization rate.

Effects of heat stress on performance

Prepartum heat stress

Elevated environmental temperatures during the last trimester of gestation alter blood flow to the uterus and maternal–fetal hormone concentrations. The result is lower calf birthweight and reduced milk yield in the subsequent lactation. Approximately 60 per cent of fetal growth occurs during the last 90 days of gestation. Chronic heat stress during late gestation leads to reduced blood flow to the uterus which retards placental and fetal growth. As a consequence, placental mass is reduced and calf birthweights are lowered by as much as 6 to 8 per cent. Studies have also shown that milk yield is related to calf birthweight and lower calf birthweights are associated with reduced milk production. Although the precise reasons for reduced milk yield are unknown, most researchers believe that hyperthermia in late gestation interferes with normal hormonal regulation of mammary development, lactogenesis and milk yield.

Peripartum heat stress

Cows calving during daylight hours in hot climates with direct exposure to solar radiation are particularly subject to hyperthermia and heat stroke (p. 935). This is particularly true for cows experiencing hypocalcaemia at calving, when control of body temperature by natural mechanisms is greatly diminished. Therefore close monitoring of calving cows is essential in hot climates.

Heat stress at parturition also creates significant consequences for calves. Once delivered, calves born in stressful conditions are weaker and slower to suck colostrum. Indeed, passive transfer of immunoglobulins has a seasonal pattern in calves. Calves born during the hotter summer months have higher rates of failure of passive transfer whereas calves born during the more moderate times of the year tend to have better rates of passive transfer. At least one study suggests that an increase in serum corticosteroids in heat stressed neonates reduces permeability of the intestine to immunoglobulin absorption. Thus, it would appear that both physical and physiological mechanisms are responsible for high rates of failure of passive transfer in calves.

Postpartum heat stress

Reduced feed intake is a primary strategy for lowering body heat production. The consequence is a reduction in milk production of as much as 10 to 20 per cent or more. Similar effects on constituent (milk fat and protein) yield are observed. Milk quality parameters are also affected whereby somatic cell and bacterial counts tend to increase during periods of hot and humid weather. Although specific data are limited, the observed increase in somatic cell counts suggests a greater susceptibility to infection due to decreased host resistance or increased exposure to pathogens created by an environment more favourable for their propagation.

Improper ration formulation, intermittent feeding behaviour, a lack of cud chewing, elevated respiratory rates, excessive losses of saliva from drooling and an overall reduction in the buffering capacity may interfere with the normal buffering of rumen contents. This is believed to be a significant contributor to rumen acidosis (see p. 829), laminitis (see p. 420) and other lameness conditions (see Chapter 31) that seem to be particularly prevalent during periods of hot weather. Feeding the lactating cow is particularly challenging during periods of intense heat. The objective is to maintain some level of performance and homeostasis yet not add to the internal heat load or tendency toward rumen acidosis.

Heat stress has a major impact on reproductive performance. It lowers conception rates, reduces the length of the oestrous period and oestrous intensity, modifies endocrine function, alters the oviductal and uterine environment and increases early embryonic death by interrupting embryo development. The seasonal depression in reproductive performance that results is one of the most serious problems for the dairy and livestock industry of subtropical and tropical regions throughout the entire world.

Methods to reduce heat stress (p. 975)

Successful abatement of heat stress generally requires environmental modification. Critical components include shade, water in the form of a fog, mist or sprinkling and air flow – either natural or by forced air movement with fans. The primary objectives are to reduce direct solar radiation, lower air temperature, improve or assist air movement or in some cases increase the natural evaporative cooling from skin surfaces.

Natural shade

Trees are an excellent source of shade. They are not only effective blockers of solar radiation but the evaporation of moisture from leaf surfaces cools the surrounding air without appreciably interfering with air circulation. In addition, animals acquire very little radiant heat load from the shade of a tree compared with a metal roof. Therefore, trees are a highly desirable natural resource in the environment of the dairy cow. However, trees have a short life span in operations where they are not protected. In fact, most last only about one to two summers after the onset of cow exposure where stocking rates are high. As cows congregate to seek protection from the summer sun they quickly develop mud holes at the base of trees. This soon leads to death of the tree and loss of this natural shade source. In order to take advantage of natural shade, some effort must be made to ensure that trees are protected from damage by cows.

Artificial shade

Solar radiation is a major factor in heat stress and increases heat gain by direct as well as indirect means. Blocking its effects through the use of properly constructed shade structures alone increased milk production by 10–19 per cent in studies conducted in Florida. Options include permanent or portable shade structures. In the following sections consideration will be given to design and maintenance factors.

Permanent shade structures

Major design parameters for permanent shade structures include:

- Orientation
- Floor space
- Height
- Ventilation
- Roof construction
- Feeding and water facilities
- Waste management system.

The preferred orientation of a shade structure depends upon whether or not cows are confined to the structure. Alignment of the long axis in an east–west direction achieves the maximum amount of shade under the structure and is therefore the preferred orientation for confined animals. On the other hand, where cows are free to move with the shadow of the structure a north–south orientation is better because this orientation will allow sunlight to dry out as much as 35–50 per cent of the area beneath the shade structure during both the morning and afternoon hours. This is particularly important for shade structures with earthen floors.

Some prefer concrete slab floors. A reinforced concrete slab at least 10 cm (4 inches) thick, with a smooth finish and grooved for good footing, is recommended. If a flush system is to be used the floor should be sloped 1.5–2 per cent. Water availability, space and environmental concerns are currently of interest in floor scraping and removal of manure solids from the premises. Various other waste handling facilities incorporate settling basins, liquid/solid separators, pumping and gravity-flow systems.

Guidelines regarding the size of shade structures vary according to climatic conditions. Some recommend 1.75–2.5 m^2 (19–27 square feet) of floor space per cow. However, for hot and humid environments, some would recommend a floor space equivalent to 5.5–6.0 m^2 (60–65 square feet) per cow. Space requirements are doubled for hot and humid climates to provide an additional open area for improved air movement.

Natural air movement under a shade structure is affected by its height and width, the slope of the roof and the presence of, or size of, the ridge opening. Air movement may occur naturally as breezes through the open sides of structures or by thermal buoyancy, in which air warmed by the presence of animals and thermal radiation through the roof creates air flow toward the ridge opening. A steady flow of air through a shade structure requires the following design specifications:

- Shade structures of 12 m (40 feet) or less in width require a minimum eave height of 3.7 m (12 feet).

Structures wider than 12 m (40 feet) should have eave heights of at least 5 m (16 feet) or more.
- There should be at least 15 m (50 feet) of clearance between adjacent buildings or other obstructions.
- Gable roofs should have at least a 4:12 slope (6:12 is acceptable but difficult to work on) and a continuous open ridge. Ridge caps if desired should have a minimum of 0.3 m (1 foot) of clearance between the cap and the roof peak.
- Ridge openings should be a minimum of 0.3 m (1 foot) wide plus 5 cm (2 inches) for each 3 m (10 feet) of structure width over 6 m (20 feet).
- Painting metal roofs white and adding insulation directly beneath the roofing will reflect and insulate from effects of solar radiation and will reduce thermal radiation on cows.

Thermal radiation from the roof of shade structures can add significant heat load to cattle, particularly in low structures without a ridge opening. In these types of structures thermal radiation can be reduced by cooling the roof with water, adding insulation or painting the roof with a reflective type of paint. However, it should be remembered that these additions to the structure do not cool air, reduce humidity or augment the natural evaporative cooling mechanisms of cows beneath the shade structure. Furthermore, proper design of the shade structure (adequate eave height and an open ridge) will naturally limit thermal radiation effects. When faced with the need to retrofit cooling into an ill-designed existing structure, the priorities should be directed to cooling the cows rather than the roof. Roof cooling (beyond painting with a reflective paint), while beneficial, is a secondary consideration.

Portable shade structures

Portable shades offer some advantages over permanent structures in their ability to be moved as required to cleaner and drier locations. However, protection from solar radiation is less than that achieved in permanent structures. Shade cloth patterns come in various weaves providing 30–90 per cent shade. One of the more common types is a woven polypropylene fabric which provides 80 per cent shade. While longevity is considerably less than that expected of permanent structures, shade cloth if properly maintained (kept tight) can last 5 years or longer.

Cooling by reducing ambient air temperature

As temperatures rise above the upper critical temperature threshold of 25.5°C (78°F) the dairy cow begins to increase heat loss via the respiratory tract and skin surface. However, despite the remarkable efficiency of these thermoregulatory responses to dissipate heat, as temperatures continue to rise these natural mechanisms are overwhelmed, leading to hyperthermia and reduced performance. In these circumstances efforts to minimize additional heat gain and supplement cooling become necessary. Water and air movement become the agents by which the micro-environment is cooled and evaporative cooling by the cow is augmented.

Evaporative cooling pads and fans

Air temperatures can be lowered by air conditioning or refrigeration, but the expense of such types of mechanical air cooling makes these impractical for cooling dairy cows. A more economically feasible method to cool the micro-environment is the evaporative cooling pad (corrugated cardboard or similar material) and fan system which uses the energy from air to evaporate water. This process cools the air and raises its relative humidity. Although these systems are most effective in arid climates, they have been observed to reduce air temperature in humid climates as well.

High pressure foggers (see also Chapter 71)

In recent years interest in high pressure foggers has grown. These systems offer effective cooling but with lower water use. Foggers disperse very fine droplets of water which quickly evaporate, cooling the surrounding air and raising the relative humidity in the process. The typical design incorporates a ring of fogger nozzles attached to the exhaust side of a fan. As fog droplets are emitted (200 psi) they are immediately dispersed into the fan's air stream where they soon evaporate. The temperature of the animals is reduced as they inspire the cooled air and it is blown over their bodies. Fogger systems are most effective in areas of low humidity. However, even where humidity is normally quite high, daytime humidity is still low enough to allow effective cooling with fogger systems. In areas where relative humidity increases to nearly 90 or 100 per cent in the overnight hours foggers must be turned off. Once the air is saturated with moisture evaporation is reduced and cooling stops. High pressure foggers should be designed to operate during the less humid hours of the day. Finally, they should be used only in open-sided, ridge-vented, tall (greater than 3.7 m (12 feet)) barns. Low barns with side walls restrict air flow and fog droplet evaporation. This reduces cooling and makes for excessively wet conditions in the barn.

High pressure foggers are advantageous in the fact that they use far less water (13.5–23 litres (3–5 gallons)/cow per day) compared with sprinkler systems (135–230 litres (30–50 gallons)/cow per day). The primary disadvantage is that they require more maintenance. In-line water filters must be cleaned or checked daily to prevent clogging of fogger nozzles.

Misters

A mist droplet is larger than a fog droplet but cools air by the same principle. These systems do not work well in windy conditions or in combination with fans in humid environments. In warm humid environments mist droplets are too large to evaporate fully before settling to the ground. The consequence is wet bedding and wet feed. A further complication with misters is the formation of an insulating layer of air between the droplets of water on hair shafts and the cow's skin. When this occurs it impedes natural evaporative heat loss from the skin and can result in body heat build-up.

Enhancing the cow's natural mechanisms of heat loss

Protecting the cow from solar radiation with shades and reducing ambient air temperatures through the process of water vaporization and controlled ventilation are important considerations in cooling dairy cattle. Various combinations of these techniques have proven to be particularly useful in arid climates. Cooling in hot and humid climates, on the other hand, can be more challenging. Instead of trying to lower ambient air temperature, another technique is to provide shade, wet the skin and move air to enhance the cow's primary mechanism for the dissipation of heat – evaporative cooling from the skin.

Sprinklers and fans

Sprinkling systems utilize a larger size water droplet that is able to wet the hair coat to the skin. Cooling is accomplished as water evaporates from the hair and skin. In combination with forced air, sprinkling substantially increases the loss of body heat over that possible by sweating alone. Several studies have demonstrated upper body sprinkling followed by forced-air ventilation to be an effective means to reduce body temperature, increase feed intake and boost milk yield. This combination has been applied to holding areas outside milking areas, shade structures, feed barns and free-stall barns with a high degree of success.

Sprinkler and fan systems require a properly sloped concrete floor with facilities to handle water run-off at rates of somewhere between 230 and 450 litres (50 and 100 gallons) of water per animal per day depending upon sprinkling rates. In early Florida studies water use amounted to 455 litres (120 gallons)/cow per day (sprinkling for 30 seconds every 5 minutes when ambient air temperatures exceeded 26.5°C (80°F)). Later work has shown that rates of 230 litres (50 gallons)/cow per day or less will provide effective cooling. Consequently, in addition to plans for water run-off and containment, some determination of the water supply is advised.

Sprinklers should be located above the cows, with nozzles directed such that they wet the cows but not the feed. The type of nozzle chosen depends upon the volume of water and sprinkling rate desired. Generally, low pressure (10 psi), 180° spray nozzles, capable of delivering the equivalent of 1.25 mm (0.05 inches) of rainfall per sprinkling cycle, are used. This sprinkling rate assures that the cows will be wetted to the skin. Nozzles are spaced approximately every 2.5 m (8 feet) or as far apart as necessary to provide overlapping coverage.

Fans (0.5–1.0 hp) capable of air flow rates of 11 000 cfm or greater are recommended. Ninety centimetre (36 inch) fans rated as such can be hung above the sprinklers every 9 m (30 feet) (every 1.2 m (40 feet) for 120 cm (48 inch) fans). They should be tilted downward at a 20–30° angle (from vertical) to direct the flow of air on to the cows. An air velocity of 120–185 m (400–600 feet) per minute over the cow is desired. The system combines fans and sprinkling, with cows being sprinkled for 1–2 minutes at 15-minute intervals. Fans should be run continuously. The entire system should be thermostatically controlled to operate automatically when ambient air temperatures reach or exceed 26.5°C (80°F).

Sprayers in parlour exit lanes

Exit lane sprayers are available commercially and designed to automatically spray water on to cows as they pass through. Fan nozzles and timing of the spray are designed to spray only on to the cow's back and sides. Fan spray nozzles must have a flow rate of at least 36 litres (8 gallons) per minute at 40 psi. These systems would seem to have greatest appeal in operations where cows travel some distance from the milking parlour to feed and in loafing areas. A less complex system can be made by simply locating an ordinary shower nozzle above cows in the parlour exit lane. Cows can be showered as they leave the parlour.

Cooling ponds

Tradition has held that it is better to limit or exclude access of cows to streams and farm ponds, and with good reason. Experience has shown that free access to streams and ponds may predispose to a number of infectious diseases and some toxicities in dairy cattle. Most notable of these are leptospirosis (see pp. 734–7) and mastitis (see Chapter 23) caused by a variety of organisms, particularly *Protheca* species (achlorophyllic algae). As a result, most advise that cows be fenced away from streams and ponds. Cooling ponds, therefore, represent a controversial method for the management of heat stress. However, studies in the USA have found that cooling ponds not only effectively reduce body temperature, but have no apparent adverse effect on udder health.

The primary mode of heat loss in cooling ponds is conduction, with a small amount lost by evaporative cooling during the 5–10 minutes after exiting the pond. Water temperature of the cooling ponds studied in the USA generally ranged from 24 to 30°C (75 to 86°F), or occasionally higher. At this temperature there was a favourable heat transfer gradient between the cow's body and the pond water.

Major questions remain as to how cooling ponds should be designed or maintained. Some operations that rely on ponds for cooling cows maintain them by providing a constant inflow of water, with an overflow at one end of the pond. They also drain, dredge and fill them with new sand every 1 to 2 years. Although total bacterial content does not appear to be appreciably affected there is less build-up of organic material. There is some evidence that allowing cows access to stagnant or natural ponds may negatively affect milk quality and the incidence of mastitis. Cows from herds with man-made ponds, which are maintained regularly, produce milk with lower bacteria and somatic cell counts compared with cows from herds which have no ponds or natural ponds. Thus, one would conclude that the use of ponds for heat stress management should be accompanied by plans for pond maintenance.

Further reading

Beede, D.K. & Shearer, J.K. (1991) Heat stress, part IV: nutritional management of dairy cattle during hot weather. *Agri-Practice*, **12**, 5–13.

Beede, D.K., Bray, D.R., Bucklin, R.A., Elvinger, F. & Shearer, J.K. (1987) Integration of cooling methods for environmental management systems in hot humid environments. *Proceedings of the 24th Annual Florida Dairy Production Conference*, pp. 68–93.

Bray, D.R. (1986) Housing systems for dairy cattle in Florida. *Southeastern Dairy Review*, **25**, 12–13.

Bray, D.R., Beede, D.K. & DeLorenzo, M.A. *et al.* (1991) Environmental modification update. *Proceedings of the 28th Annual Florida Dairy Production Conference*, pp. 134–40.

Bray, D.R., DeLorenzo, M.A. & Elvinger, F.C. *et al.* (1989) Cooling ponds and milk quality. *Proceedings of the 26th Annual Florida Dairy Production Conference*, pp. 63–72.

Bray, D.R. & Shearer, J.K. (1988) Environmental modifications on Florida dairies. *Proceedings of the 25th Annual Florida Dairy Production Conference*, pp. 52–9.

Bucklin, R.A., Bray, D.R. & Beede, D.K. (1988) Methods to relieve heat stress for Florida dairies. *Florida Cooperative Extension Service Circular 782.*

Bucklin, R.A., Turner, L.W., Beede, D.K., Bray, D.R. & Heurleen, R.W. (1991) Methods to relieve heat stress for dairy cows in hot, humid climates. *Applied Engineering in Agriculture*, **7**, 241–7.

Buffington, D.E., Collier, R.J. & Canton, R.H. (1983) Shade management systems to reduce heat stress for dairy cows. *Transactions of the ASAE*, **26**, 1798–802.

Collier, R.J. & Buffington, D.E. (1979) Common Florida shade management systems to reduce heat stress. *Proceedings of the 16th Annual Florida Dairy Production Conference*, pp. 36–45.

Collier, R.J., Doelger, S.G., Head, H.H., Thatcher, W.W. & Wilcox, C.J. (1982) Effects of heat stress during pregnancy on maternal hormone concentration, calf birth weight, and postpartum milk yield of Holstein cows. *Journal of Animal Science*, **54**, 309–19.

Collier, R.J., Eley, R.M., Sharma, A.K., Pereira, R.M. & Buffington, D.E. (1981) Shade management in a subtropical environment for milk yield and composition in Holstein and Jersey cows. *Journal of Dairy Science*, **64**, 844–9.

Collier, R.J., Simerl, N.A. & Wilcox, C.J. (1980) Effect of month of calving on birth weight, milk yield, and birth weight–milk yield interrelationships. *Journal of Dairy Science*, **63**(Suppl 1), 90.

Erdman, R.A. (1988) Dietary buffering requirements of the lactating dairy cow: a review. *Journal of Dairy Science*, **71**, 3246–66.

Flamenbaum, I.D., Wolfenson, D., Mamen, M. & Berman, A. (1986) Cooling dairy cattle by a combination of sprinkling and forced ventilation and its implementation in the shelter system. *Journal of Dairy Science*, **69**, 3140–7.

Hahn, G.L. (1985) Management and housing of farm animals in hot environments. In *Stress Physiology in Livestock, Volume II, Ungulates* (ed. by M.K. Yousef), pp. 151–74. CRC Press, Boca Raton.

Igono, M.O., Johnson, H.D., Steevens, B.J., Krause, G.F. & Shanklin, M.D. (1987) Physiological productive and economic benefits of shade, spray and fan systems versus shade for Holstein cows during summer heat. *Journal of Dairy Science*, **70**, 1069–79.

Ingraham, R.G., Gillette, D.D. & Wagner, W.D. (1974) Relationship of temperature and humidity to conception rate of Holstein cows in a subtropical climate. *Journal of Dairy Science*, **57**, 476–81.

Roman-Ponce, H., Thatcher, W.W., Buffington, D.E., Wilcox, C.J. & Van Horn, H.H. (1977) Physiological and production responses of dairy cattle to a shade structure in a subtropical environment. *Journal of Dairy Science*, **60**, 424–30.

Schneider, P.L., Beede, D.K., Wilcox, C.J. & Collier, R.J. (1984) Influence of dietary sodium and potassium bicarbonate and total potassium on heat stressed lactating dairy cows. *Journal of Dairy Science*, **67**, 2546–53.

Shearer, J.K. & Beede, D.K. (1990a) Heat stress, part I: thermoregulation and physiological responses of dairy cattle in hot weather. *Agri-Practice*, **11**, 5–18.

Shearer, J.K. & Beede, D.K. (1990b) Heat stress, part II: effects of high environmental temperature on production, reproduction, and health of dairy cattle. *Agri-Practice*, **11**, 6–18.

Shearer, J.K., Beede, D.K., Bucklin, R.A. & Bray, D.R. (1991) Heat stress, part III: environmental modifications to reduce heat stress in dairy cattle. *Agri-Practice*, **12**, 7–18.

Shearer, J.K., Bray, D.R., Elvinger, F.C. & Reed, P.A. (1987) The incidence of clinical mastitis in cows exposed to cooling ponds for heat stress management. *Proceedings of the 26th Annual Meeting, National Mastitis Council*, pp. 66–70.

Strickland, J.T., Bucklin, R.A., Nordstedt, R.A., Beede, D.K. & Bray, D.R. (1989) Sprinkler and fan cooling system for dairy cows in hot, humid climates. *Applied Engineering in Agriculture*, **5**, 231–6.

Taylor, S.E. (1985) *Evaluating the potential benefits of using an evaporative cooling system for Florida dairy cattle.* Masters thesis, University of Florida.

Thatcher, W.W. & Collier, R.J. (1985) Effects of climate on bovine reproduction. *Current Therapy in Theriogenology*, pp. 301–9.

Thatcher, W.W., Gwazdavskas, F.C. & Wilcox, C.J. *et al.* (1974) Milking performance and reproductive efficiency of dairy cows in an environmentally controlled structure. *Journal of Dairy Science*, **57**, 304–7.

Turner, L.W., Chastain, J.P., Hemken, R.W., Gates, R.S. & Crist, W.L. (1989) Reducing heat stress in dairy cows through sprinkler and fan cooling. *Transactions of the American Society of Agricultural Engineers, Paper No 89-4025.* St Joseph, MI.

Wiersma, F. & Armstrong, D.V. (1988) Evaporative cooling dry cows for improved performance. *Transactions of the American Society of Agricultural Engineers*, Paper No 88-4053. St Joseph, MI.

Wolfenson, D., Flamenbaum, I. & Berman, A. (1988) Dry period heat stress relief effects on prepartum progesterone, calf birth weight, and milk production. *Journal of Dairy Science*, **71**, 809–18.

Chapter 9
Nutrition

J.M. Wilkinson

Introduction	95
Fermentation in the rumen	96
Saliva	98
The actions of micro-organisms	98
Fermentation of different types of feed	98
Actual and potential digestion	99
Optimizing digestion in the rumen	99
Feed intake	100
Is feed intake under control?	100
Concentrates	100
Roughages	101
Rumen capacity	101
Digestibility of forages	101
Speed of digestion	101
Grazed pasture	101
Probable levels of intake	102
Energy requirements	103
Requirements and allowances	103
Partition of feed energy	104
Efficiency of use of metabolizable energy	104
Energy requirements of growing cattle	104
Energy requirements of lactating cattle	105
Protein requirements	106
Microbial protein synthesis	107
Metabolizable protein	108
Requirements for metabolizable protein	110
Composition of feeds	111
Cellulosic and non-cellulosic feeds	111
Energy and protein in feeds	112
Physical form	113
Feed preservation	114
Drying	114
Ensiling	114
Primary and secondary fermentations	115
Typical analytical composition of silage	116
Additives for silage	116
Additives for hay and moist grain	117
Feed processing	117
Physical processing of roughages	117
Chemical processing of roughages	117
Processing of cereals	118
Feeding management	118
The importance of selective eating	118
Targets for sward surface height at pasture	118
Buffer feeding	119
Frequency of feeding and ruminal acidosis	119
Out-of-parlour feeders	119
Flat-rate feeding	120
Total mixed rations or complete diets	120
Diet formulation	120
Condition score	121
Feed budgeting	122

Introduction

The bovine animal, along with the other ruminants, depends very heavily on its symbiotic relationship with the microbial population of the rumen. Thus any consideration of the nutrition of the bovine must be focused on the rumen as the most important part of the bovine digestive system. The fermentation in the rumen is dominated by the degradation of plant cell walls, of which the most abundant constituent is cellulose. This adaptation to plant cell wall digestion, in addition to cell content degradation places the bovine in an important strategic position relative to other animals.

Van Soest (1994) classified cattle feeding habit as being one of grazing fresh grass, rather than browsing trees and shrubs. Cattle have a greater need for water than other ruminants, possibly because they retain fibre for relatively long periods in the rumen. A high free-water content, typically around 90 per cent, is essential for optimal bacterial activity. In addition, there is less absorption of water in the large intestine and a higher water content in the faeces than with sheep and goats.

The bovine is a relatively unselective eater compared with the other ruminants. This may be a disadvantage when tree and shrub leaves are abundant at a time when pasture supply is scarce because of drought. But the bovine can and does browse. In situations of excess food supply over consumption, selective eating occurs.

In temperate regions of the world, a constant supply of feed throughout the year is achieved by preserving excess herbage growth as hay or as silage. This activity, coupled with the production of root crops specifically for use when grass growth is slow or non-existent, has transformed the annual cycle of production from one totally dependent on grass growth to one which is not. Thus beef cattle, for example, no longer lose weight in the winter when grass is scarce, but are able to maintain or even increase in weight on a winter diet of hay, silage or stored root crops. The development of the human food and drink industry has released a wide range of by-products, such as bran from the milling of grain for flour, and spent grains from the brewing of beer and the production of spirits. These by-products, which are not edible by the human population, play a vital role in the nutrition of the bovine when grazed pasture grass is in short supply.

A remaining challenge in bovine nutrition is to achieve a similar constancy of feed supply to that of the temperate regions of the world, to bovine populations in regions where drought is common, and where the technology of feed preservation and by-product utilization is less well developed.

In this chapter, the fermentation in the rumen is described, with particular emphasis on the kinetics of the process and its interaction with feed intake. Requirements for energy and protein are then considered. The composition of feeds is outlined, together with technologies for feed preservation and feed processing. Finally, the management of the feeding of the bovine is outlined in relation to maintaining stability in the rumen, maximizing intake and meeting requirements for high levels of productivity.

Fermentation in the rumen

The rumen accounts for more than half the total volume of the digestive tract of cattle. The animal relies very heavily on the reactions that occur in the rumen for its supply of major nutrients. Thus on a sole diet of grazed grass some 90 per cent of the animal's total energy and protein supply is derived directly from the rumen micro-organisms and the end-products of their metabolism. Therefore, the importance of maintaining optimal conditions for fermentation cannot be overstressed.

The symbiotic relationship between the micro-organisms of the rumen and the host animal has been crucial to the survival of the bovine, since the animal itself does not produce the enzymes to degrade the cellulose and hemicellulose in plant cell wall material. This task is undertaken by the microbial population of the rumen.

In the wild, surrounded by foliage and limited supplies of feeds containing starch or sugar, the bovine's fermentation of plant cell wall material secured not only the supply of energy, but also a vital supply of microbial protein. The ruminant has evolved a nutritional niche whereby it is independent of external sources of amino acids and B vitamins – a considerable advantage when grass is the only feed available.

Fermentation in the rumen is the anaerobic process of microbial activity, which also occurs in the lower digestive tract of animals and in the preservation of crops by ensilage. Essentially, dietary carbohydrates, proteins and some fats are reduced to short-chain fatty acids with the production of carbon dioxide, methane and ATP.

The short-chain fatty acids produced in the digestive tract are principally acetic, propionic and butyric acids, although occasionally lactic acid is also produced.

The most important bacteria involved in fermentation in the rumen are the cell-wall digesting or cellulolytic micro-organisms. The concentration of bacteria in rumen fluid is about 10^{10} to 10^{11} bacteria/ml, with most being attached to particles of food. The predominant species of bacteria varies with the type of fermentation, which depends on the principal substrates in the diet. Thus the major species of bacteria in the rumen of animals given a diet of grass are those which digest cellulose and hemicellulose, such as *Ruminococcus albus*, *Ruminococcus flavefasciens* and *Bacteriodes succinogenes* (see Table 9.1).

Other species, such as *Streptococcus bovis*, ferment starch to acetic acid and ethanol. This species, along with other streptococci, can produce lactic acid and are more tolerant of acid conditions than other species of rumen bacteria. Acidosis can occur if the diet of the animal is changed abruptly from cellulose to starch or sucrose. The population of bacteria in the rumen changes from cellulolytic to amylolytic as the pH falls. Lactic acid accumulates and accelerates the fall in pH. Even a small fall in the pH of the rumen from pH 7 to pH 6 is reflected in a reduction in cellulose digestion and a change in the population of the bacteria towards the more acid tolerant species.

Proteins are degraded to a varying extent during the fermentation to their constituent amino acids. Some amino acids are used directly by bacteria and protozoa, but most are used as a source of energy and are broken down further to ammonia and volatile fatty acids. Ammonia is used as a substrate for the production of microbial protein, with the excess being absorbed into the animal's portal blood and converted to urea in the liver. The extent to which proteins are degraded during the fermentation in the rumen depends on their solubility, which is generally relatively high. However, solubility is lower in feeds which have been subjected to heat treatment during processing. Thus the degradation of protein in brewer's grains is only about 0.6, compared to 0.9 for fresh herbage. Protein degradation also depends on the time the material spends in the rumen, and is lower for diets which pass rapidly through the rumen (concentrates and feeds of small particle size) than for long forages which are digested slowly.

Protozoa and fungi are also involved in the fermentation process. These organisms can digest cellulose, starch, sugars and fats to produce acetic acid, butyric acid, lactic acid, hydrogen and carbon dioxide.

Table 9.1 Common types of rumen micro-organisms and their action.

Species	Energy source	Fermentation products	Requirements
Bacteria			
Bacteroides			
amylophilus	Starch	F, A, S	CO_2, NH_3, BrVFA
succinogenes	Cellulose	F, A, S	CO_2, NH_3, BrVFA, SVFA, Vit.
Ruminococcus			
albus	Cellulose, xylan	F, A, E, H_2, CO_2	BrVFA, CO_2, NH_3, Vit.(A)
flavefaciens	Cellulose, xylan	F, A, S, H_2	
Butyrivibrio			
fibrosolvens	Xylan, starch	F, A, B, L, H_2, CO_2	BrVFA, A, CO_2, NH_3, Vit.(A)
Lachnospira			
multiparus	Pectin	F, A, L, E, H_2, CO_2, A, Vit.	
Selenomonas			
ruminantium	Lactate, starch	A, P, L, CO_2, H_2	A(CO_2)
Methanobacterium			
ruminantium	Formate, H_2	Methane	A, BrVFA, Haem, CO_2, NH_3
Protozoa			
Holotrichs			
Isotricha	Starch and sugars	A, B, L, H_2	
Dasytricha	Starch and sugars	A, B, L, H_2	
Entodiniomorphs			
Entodinia	Starch	F, A, P, B, (L)	
Epidinium	Starch, hemicell.	A, B, H_2, (F, P, L)	
Ophryoscolex	Starch	A, B, H_2, (P)	
Diplodinium			
Eudiplodinium		H_2, fatty acids	
Polyplastron			

Symbols: F, formate; A, acetate; P, propionate; B, butyrate; BrVFA, branched-chain VFA; E, ethanol; L, lactate; S, succinate; SVFA, straight-chain VFA; Vit., B vitamins.

The predominance of the weak acids acetic, propionic and butyric in the end-products of fermentations in the digestive tract highlights the importance of buffering agents to maintain the pH of the environment close to neutrality. Saliva, containing sodium and potassium bicarbonate and urea, is the most important buffering agent in the rumen, and the amount of saliva produced during eating and rumination is therefore crucial to the neutralization of the fermentation acids (see below). Long fibre is often included as a supplement to diets high in concentrates to stimulate chewing and rumination.

The constant flow of saliva (p. 98) into and outflow of digesta from the rumen, and the absorption of digested nutrients into the portal blood, ensure that in most nutri- tional circumstances the environment for fermentation remains relatively constant. However, digestive disor- ders can arise to disrupt the equilibrium. Toxins, pro- duced by undesirable bacteria and from moulds present in foods, can damage the sensitive lining of the wall of the rumen and reduce the absorption of nutrients. Sudden changes in diet can change the microbial population and result in the production of lactic acid in the rumen, as in the fermentation of crop material in the silo, with a con- sequent reduction in rumen pH. If the pH of the rumen falls below pH 5 and remains at a low level, there is a risk of rumen stasis which can result in bloat because the animal can no longer eructate the gases produced by the fermentation.

Methane loss from the rumen is estimated to account for about 8 per cent of the total gross energy eaten by the animal. Apart from the rumen fermentation, methane is also lost to the environment from hind gut fermentations and together these fermentations constitute a significant contribution of methane to the global environment. Ways of reducing methanogenesis include chemical food additives (ionophores), and changing the pattern of fermentation to increase the proportion of propionate and to reduce the proportion of acetate.

Saliva

Feeds are chewed during eating and also regurgitated during rumination to allow very thorough mastication. Throughout these activities large quantities of saliva are mixed with food. The effect of saliva is to buffer the acids that are produced in the rumen as a result of the fermentation. This buffering is vital to the maintenance of the correct type of fermentation, and can even prevent the collapse of normal rumen function in extreme situations.

The principal buffering constituent of saliva is bicarbonate. It has been estimated that a dairy cow may produce up to 3.5 kg of bicarbonate per day. Clearly, the need for adequate buffering is more important if the diet is rapidly fermented than if it is only slowly fermented. Further, if the diet is acidic, as in the case of silage, it is essential that salivary secretion is sufficient to prevent a build-up of excessive acidity in the rumen or in blood.

It follows that feeds which stimulate rumination are more useful to the maintenance of optimal conditions for fermentation in the rumen than those which do not. Unfortunately many constituents of high-energy concentrates, such as molasses and ground cereal grains, are fermented rapidly in the rumen and do not stimulate rumination. At the other extreme, hay and straw are chewed extensively to break down the fibre and their rate of digestion is also relatively slow. Hence a compromise with respect to saliva production is required; fibre is required together with concentrated feed sources in order that saliva output is maintained.

The actions of micro-organisms

The major organisms responsible for digestion in the rumen are anaerobic bacteria and protozoa, although anaerobic fungi are thought to be responsible for much of the initial colonization of feed particles in the rumen. The cellulolytic bacteria adhere to particles of fibrous feeds and secrete enzymes that gradually erode out the digestible material. Their enzymes break down hemi-cellulose and cellulose to glucose and fructose. Starch and pectins are also similarly degraded (Fig. 9.1). In the case of plant cell wall material, this erosion continues until lignified tissue is encountered. Lignin, which is cross-linked to hemicellulose and cellulose, provides structural strength to the plant and is also very resistant to bacterial enzymic attack.

The protozoa in the rumen mainly ferment starch and sugar, but they also consume bacteria. The protozoa are thought to be active in assisting the bacterial population in adapting to new feeds.

The end-products of bacterial digestion are short-chain acids acetic, propionic and butyric (the volatile fatty acids, VFA), microbial cells (and their constituent protein), and the gases methane and carbon dioxide. Methane comprises the major gaseous energy loss as a result of fermentation. Gas is lost by eructation whilst the VFA are mainly absorbed through the rumen wall.

Some common types of rumen micro-organisms and their actions are summarized in Table 9.1.

Fermentation of different types of feed

The fermentation of plant cell walls is optimal at relatively high rumen pH (around pH 7.0) because the bacteria responsible are sensitive to excess acidity. Their growth is depressed if rumen pH falls below about pH 6.2. The principal end-product of cellulose fermentation is acetate, an important precursor of milk fat.

Starch and sugar are fermented to give propionic and butyric acids as the main end-products. The micro-organisms responsible for their fermentation are more tolerant of acidity than those which ferment cell wall. Some species of starch-digesting bacteria (e.g. *Streptococcus bovis*, *Selenomonas ruminantium*) produce lactic acid, a stronger acid than the VFA. Large amounts of lactic acid can predispose the animal to rumen stasis and to acidosis (see p. 829).

Protein is fermented to yield ammonia and VFA from the carbon skeletons of amino acids. The ammonia may be used by bacteria to synthesize new protein in their cells, but since bacterial growth is generally limited by the energy available from carbohydrate digestion, rather than from protein digestion, ammonia in excess of microbial requirements can easily be produced, especially on high-protein diets. Excess ammonia is converted, at an energy cost, to urea in the liver and excreted in urine. A deficit of ammonia in the rumen slows down bacterial growth, reduces rate of digestion and depresses feed intake. Thus the rate of release of ammonia should match as closely as possible the release of energy (see Fig. 9.2).

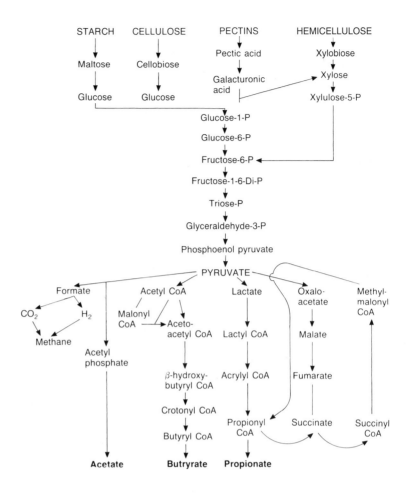

Fig. 9.1 Chemistry of rumen fermentation.

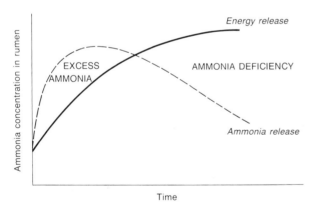

Fig. 9.2 Typical patterns for the rates of release in the rumen of ammonia from the breakdown of protein, and of energy, following a meal. The rate of ammonia release should match as closely as possible that of energy, either by reducing the amount of quickly degraded protein in the diet, or by increasing the quantity of readily-fermentable energy (e.g. starch or sugar) in the diet.

Actual and potential digestion

Fibre that has been reduced to a small enough particle size at which it can pass out of the rumen, and which has also resisted being digested by microbial activity, is liable to pass on down the tract and out in the faeces. The rate of passage out of the rumen can influence the extent to which fibrous particles are actually digested. The faster the rate of passage, the lower the actual, relative to the potential, digestibility.

The same concept applies to protein, especially that fraction which is available for microbial fermentation in the rumen. A high-yielding dairy cow, given a high-quality diet with a fast rate of passage of feed through the rumen, will have a relatively lower fibre digestibility than a dry cow given less of the same diet, or a diet of lower energy content. However, the protein in the diet of the high-yielding cow will have a lower digestibility in the rumen, yield less ammonia and provide more undegraded protein to the abomasum than that in the dry cow's diet (see Table 9.13). Paradoxically, the lower the actual, relative to potential, digestibility in the rumen, the worse off the animal is with respect to energy, but the better off it is likely to be with respect to protein.

Optimizing digestion in the rumen

It follows from the above discussion that the following principles need to be adopted in order to optimize the fermentation in the rumen:

- Cell wall is the principal source of digestible energy in the diet of the bovine, and conditions in the rumen should be optimal for its digestion.
- Sufficient saliva must be produced to maintain rumen pH above pH 6.5, otherwise cell wall digestion will be reduced.
- Adequate degradable protein must be supplied to meet the requirements for microbial protein synthesis (see section on protein requirements, p. 106).
- Supplementary energy in the form of starch or sugar must not interfere with the maintenance of the above conditions in the rumen (see section on feeding management, p. 118).

When cell wall digestion is optimized, then feed intake is likely to be maximal, at least with respect to fibrous feeds (see below).

Feed intake

Most diets for cattle are offered in excess of the amount the animal actually consumes, although there are situations where the amount of feed offered each day is restricted intentionally. Two such situations are readily apparent: the dry cow and the suckler cow in late lactation. Both situations require that the animal does not overeat and become excessively fat.

The concept of voluntary feed intake is discussed in this section, that is, the amount of feed the animal will eat when offered an excess supply so that about 10 to 15 per cent of the daily amount offered is refused.

Is feed intake under control?

The fact that cattle can become overfat suggests that feed intake is under relatively imprecise control. Equally, sparse availability of range pastures or the provision of very low quality roughages as the sole feeds can lead to inadequate levels of feed intake and chronic undernutrition. The animal can suffer from deprivation because it is unable to ingest, or digest, enough nutrients daily to meet its requirements for maintenance of body weight. Nevertheless, there is evidence that cattle eat to satisfy their demand for energy to maintain weight and produce tissue growth or milk. The generalized relationships between the energy content of the diet and dry matter intake (Figs 9.3 and 9.4) suggest that signals received by the brain when the animal's energy needs are met in turn elicit the response to cease eating. Perhaps cattle eat as much as possible whilst at the same time attempting to minimize the total discomfort which may be caused physically or metabolically. Signals to commence eating may be metabolic (for example, the concentration of a metabo-

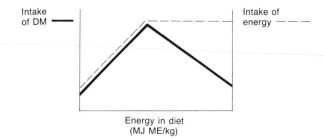

Fig. 9.3 Simplified relationship between the energy content of the diet and feed intake. As the energy content of the diet increases, dry matter intake will increase until it reaches a maximum. If energy content increases further, dry matter intake is reduced because metabolic factors, rather than the bulk, or 'fill', of the diet now control intake.

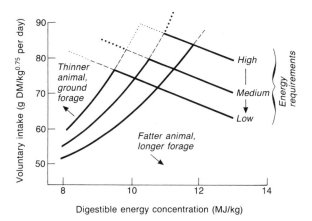

Fig. 9.4 Composite diagram of the relationships between intake and animal and feed factors in ruminants. At any given energy content, intake is higher for cows that have a greater requirement for energy (or potential milk production). Also, intake of dry matter is greater the thinner the cow, and the smaller the particle size of the feed. Source: Forbes (1983), reproduced with permission of CABI International.

lite such as acetate in blood), but the signals to cease eating may be physical (bulkiness of the food or restriction of rumen capacity by the fatness of the animal) or metabolic (concentrations of absorbed nutrients in blood), depending on the type of food. These concepts are discussed in more detail below.

Concentrates

With concentrates, satiety occurs long before the capacity of the rumen is reached. Intake is determined by the animal's capacity to metabolize the nutrients absorbed following digestion. Enhanced rate of metabolism, for example following the administration of somatotrophin, is reflected in increased feed consumption of high-energy diets where physical limitations do not apply (see below).

Roughages

With roughage feeds the volume of the rumen usually restricts intake. Thus intake is proportional to the volume of the rumen – the larger the rumen, the more feed is consumed. Larger animals eat more than smaller animals because their rumen volumes are greater.

Rumen capacity

Animals with large rumen capacities relative to their total body weight eat more roughage than those with relatively smaller rumen volumes. The implications are that calves should be reared on diets that encourage rumen development, and cattle should be selected for large rumen capacities. Channel Island cattle (Jersey, Guernsey) typically eat more food relative to their body weight than Holstein cattle because, although they weigh much less, their rumen capacities are relatively greater. Thinner cattle tend to eat relatively more than fatter cattle (Fig. 9.4).

Digestibility of forages

Digestibility or energy concentration of forage feeds exerts a large influence on feed intake (Fig. 9.5). However, the relationship between intake and digestibility is much less evident for silages than for dried forages, where the pattern of fermentation in the silo, particularly the presence or absence of residual sugar and the pH value of the silage, can have an overriding influence on intake. Thus at the same digestibility drier silages of higher pH value and higher residual sugar concentrations tend to be eaten in greater amounts than more extensively fermented silages, possibly because they provide more readily available nutrients to the rumen microbial population.

Speed of digestion

Speed of digestion also has an important influence on intake, since it determines the length of time the feed remains in the rumen. Legumes are digested at a faster rate than grasses of the same overall digestibility, partly because they contain less cell wall than grasses (Fig. 9.5). Also, the structure of the cell walls of legumes enables bacteria to gain access more rapidly than with grasses.

The cell contents of forages are fermented very quickly in the rumen, provided they are released by eating and by rumination. For example, young grass may contain up to 40 per cent of its dry matter in the

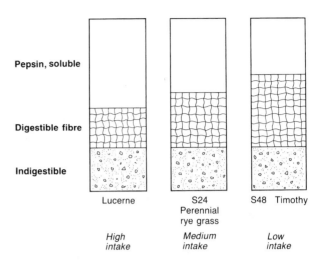

Fig. 9.5 Variations in the ratio of material soluble in acid pepsin (cell contents) to digestible fibre (cell wall) in three forages of the same digestibility, but differing in intake. Source: Osbourn (1967), reproduced with permission of the British Grassland Society.

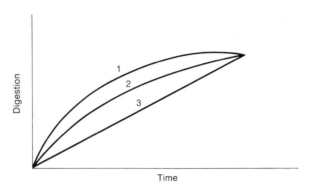

Fig. 9.6 Three feeds with the same potential digestibility but different speeds of digestion. The animal will eat most of feed 1 and least of feed 3. Reproduced from Orskov (1998) with permission of Chalcombe Publications.

form of cell contents, principally sugars and proteins, and in this regard it is nearer to a concentrate in terms of its speed of digestion in the rumen.

Cell walls are generally fermented at a slower rate than cell contents. The actual rate of cell wall digestion depends on initial particle size, the extent to which it is broken down by rumination, and the extent to which it may be lignified. Three feeds with the same potential digestibility but different speeds of digestion are represented in Fig. 9.6. The feed with the fastest speed of digestion will be eaten in the greatest amount by the animal.

Grazed pasture

Unlike indoor feeding, grazing animals select what they eat to a considerable extent, particularly when the

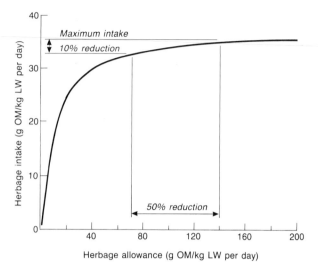

Fig. 9.7 Relationship between daily herbage allowance and herbage intake in grazing lambs. Source: Hodgson (1975), reproduced with permission of the British Grassland Society.

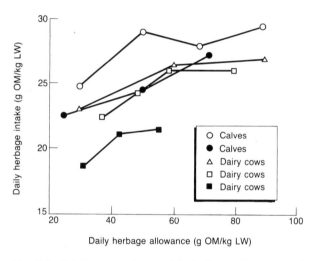

Fig. 9.8 Relationship between daily herbage allowance and herbage intake in cattle. (Data from different studies.) Source: Hodgson (1975), reproduced with permission of the British Grassland Society.

herbage on offer is heterogeneous and is offered in excess of consumption. Thus a measure of the digestibility of the herbage on offer is of little use as an indicator of intake, since the animals are usually able to select material of higher digestibility than the average of that on offer.

Herbage intake under grazing is predominantly influenced by the amount on offer. To achieve maximum intake, the amount on offer should exceed that actually consumed by three to four times (Figs 9.7 and 9.8).

Intake is usually expressed relative to liveweight, and it follows that the amount of herbage on offer should

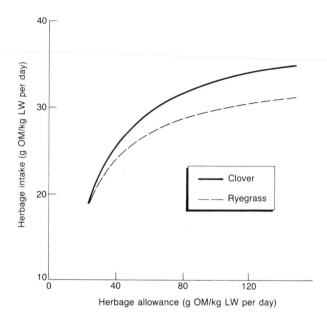

Fig. 9.9 Herbage intake of lambs grazing perennial ryegrass and red clover. Source: Gibb & Treacher (1978), reproduced with permission of Cambridge University Press.

be expressed per kilogramme liveweight rather than per hectare. It follows that stocking rate, a commonly used but empirical and inflexible way of describing herbage allowance, should not be expressed as number of animals per hectare, but as kilogrammes of liveweight per hectare (see section on feeding management, p. 118).

The relationship between herbage allowance and intake holds for animals in different physiological states, and for legumes as well as grasses (Fig. 9.9).

Studies of grazing behaviour and herbage intake by animals grazed on adjacent monocultures of grass and clover demonstrated that the grazing bovine has a strong preference for clover. Clover comprised 70% of total dry matter intake, and this preference was greater earlier in the day than during evening grazing, suggesting that some discomfort may have been induced following large meals of clover which the animal attempted to attenuate by preferentially eating grass in subsequent grazing meals.

Probable levels of intake

Estimated levels of voluntary dry matter intake for growing and lactating cattle are shown in Tables 9.2 and 9.3. The relative intake of cows given the same diet throughout lactation, expressed as a percentage of the mean for the whole lactation, is shown in Table 9.4. The important feature in Table 9.4 is the relatively low intake in the first month of lactation, when the demand for nutrients for milk production is at its highest, and

Table 9.2 Estimated feed intake of growing cattle (kg DM/day). Reproduced from Allen (2001) with permission of Chalcombe Publications.

	Well-preserved grass silage	Poorly-preserved grass silage	Big bale silage	Maize silage	Hay	Barley straw	Concentrate
Metabolizable energy (MJ/kg DM)	11.0	10.0	10.5	11.0	9.0	6.5	12.5
Liveweight (kg)	Forage intake (kg DM/day)						
200	4.3	3.6	3.9	4.5	3.6	2.4	6.0
300	5.8	4.8	5.2	6.1	4.8	3.2	8.0
400	7.2	6.0	6.5	7.6	6.0	4.0	9.0
500	8.5	7.1	7.7	9.0	7.1	4.8	9.5
600	9.7	8.1	8.8	10.3	8.1	5.5	10.0
Reduction of forage DM intake/kg concentrate DM fed							
	0.5	0.4	0.5	0.6	0.3	0.2	–

Table 9.3 Probable dry matter intake of cows in mid and late lactation (kg/day). From Ministry of Agriculture, Fisheries and Food (MAFF, 1984).

Liveweight (W) (kg)	Milk yield (Y) (kg/day)							
	5	10	15	20	25	30	35	40
350	9.3	9.8	10.3	10.8	11.3	11.8		
400	10.5	11.0	11.5	12.0	12.5	13.0		
450	11.8	12.3	12.8	13.3	13.8	14.3	14.8	
500	13.0	13.5	14.0	14.5	15.0	15.5	16.0	
550	14.3	14.8	15.3	15.8	16.3	16.8	17.3	17.8
600	15.5	16.0	16.5	17.0	17.5	18.0	18.5	19.0
650	16.8	17.3	17.8	18.3	18.8	19.3	19.8	20.3
700	18.0	18.5	19.0	19.5	20.0	20.5	21.0	21.5

Note: In the first 6 weeks of lactation, reduce these values by 2–3 kg DMI/day.

Based on DMI (kg/day) = $0.025W + 0.1Y$.

Table 9.4 Relative intake of dairy cows fed on the same diet throughout lactation (daily intake per cent of mean intake for complete lactation). From ARC (1980), reproduced with permission of CABI International.

Month	Relative intake	Month	Relative intake
1	81	6	108
2	98	7	101
3	107	8	99
4	108	9	97
5	109	10	93

the consequent deficiency in intake of nutrients which results in the mobilization of nutrients from body tissues.

Energy requirements

Requirements and allowances

The notion of requirements takes no account of the variation between animals when kept in groups. Hence, if a group is given enough feed to meet the mean requirement for a given performance, a proportion of the group will be underfed and a proportion will be

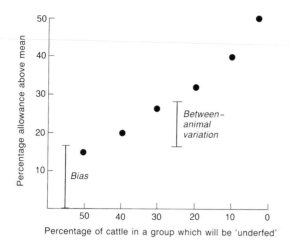

Fig. 9.10 Estimated allowances above mean requirements (ARC, 1980) required to meet the ME needs of a defined proportion of beef cattle in a group. Additional allowance due to bias in the estimate of requirements is shown separately from that due to estimated between-animal variation. Source: *Energy Group Report* (1988) Inter-Departmental Working Party.

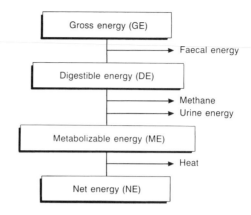

Fig. 9.11 Partition of energy.

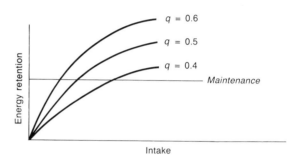

Fig. 9.12 Efficiency of use of ME for maintenance (k_m) is relatively high at 0.7. At twice the maintenance energy intake (common level for growing animals) efficiency of use of ME for growth (k_g) = 0.3 to 0.5 for diets ranging from $q = 0.4$ to $q = 0.6$; k_g declines further at higher levels of energy intake and correction must be made for the curvilinear decline.

overfed. Since underfeeding is considered to be the more serious failure of the system, allowances are made so that only a small proportion of the group remains underfed. If, as is the case with beef cattle, the metabolizable energy system of assessing requirement over-predicts performance, an additional increment (15 per cent) is added on to account for this inaccuracy. The result (Fig. 9.10) is that allowances may exceed requirements by some 30 per cent. 'Requirements' in practical feeding systems include a safety margin, although in most cases this margin is only 5 per cent and is arbitrary.

Partition of feed energy

The proportion of the gross energy (GE) of a feed that is absorbed by the animal depends on its digestibility. The amount remaining for metabolism (metabolizable energy, ME) is the digested energy less energy lost as methane or in urine. Further heat losses occur as a result of metabolism and the remaining energy (the net energy) is that which is available to the animal for maintenance of body weight, for weight gain or for milk production. The partitioning is shown diagrammatically in Fig. 9.11.

In calculating energy requirements, the term 'metabolizability' (q) is used. This is an expression of ME/GE, where GE is usually about 18.4 MJ/kg dry matter (DM) for conventional feeds. The greater the work of digestion, the higher the heat lost as a result of this work and the lower the q value of a feed. Thus q is generally

lowest for feeds of low digestibility, such as straws, and highest for concentrates.

Efficiency of use of metabolizable energy

The proportion of ME used for maintenance and productive functions, such as growth or lactation, depends on the efficiency with which it is utilized by the animal (k). This depends on q, the level of feeding above maintenance and on the productive purpose for which the energy is to be used. Thus for growing cattle, k for maintenance (k_m) varies as shown in Fig. 9.12.

Energy requirements of growing cattle

For growing cattle, a variable net energy system has been adopted to take account of the fact that k_m varies with q. The system involves assessing the animal production level (APL), which depends on the weight of the animal and the desired level of weight gain, the net energy allowance for the particular animal and level of

Table 9.5 Net energy allowances for maintenance and production NE_{mp} in growing beef cattle (MJ/day). From MAFF (1975).

Liveweight (kg)	Liveweight gain (kg/day)					
	0.25	0.50	0.75	1.00	1.25	1.50
100	14.7	17.4	20.7	24.6		
200	21.6	25.0	29.0	33.9	39.9	
300	28.6	32.6	37.3	43.1	50.2	
400	35.5	40.1	45.6	52.3	65.8	77.0
500	42.4	47.7	53.9	61.5	70.9	82.9

Table 9.6 Values for animal production level (APL) in growing beef cattle. From MAFF (1975).

Liveweight (kg)	Liveweight gain (kg/day)					
	APL					
	0.25	0.50	0.75	1.00	1.25	1.50
100	1.19	1.40	1.66	1.98		
200	1.15	1.33	1.54	1.79	2.11	
300	1.13	1.29	1.47	1.70	1.97	2.33
400	1.12	1.26	1.43	1.64	1.90	2.22
500	1.11	1.25	1.41	1.60	1.84	2.15

Table 9.7 Net energy values of feeds for maintenance and production in growing beef cattle. From MAFF (1975).

APL	Energy concentration in feed (MJ ME/kg DM)						
	8	9	10	11	12	13	14
	Net energy value (NE/kg DM)						
1.00	5.8	6.5	7.2	7.9	8.6	9.4	10.1
1.10	5.2	6.0	6.8	7.6	8.3	9.1	9.9
1.15	5.1	5.8	6.6	7.4	8.2	9.0	9.8
1.20	4.9	5.7	6.5	7.3	8.1	8.9	9.8
1.30	4.6	5.4	6.3	7.1	7.9	8.8	9.7
1.40	4.4	5.2	6.1	6.9	7.9	8.8	9.7
1.50	4.2	5.1	5.9	6.8	7.7	8.6	9.5
1.75	3.9	4.8	5.6	6.5	7.4	8.4	9.3
2.00	3.8	4.6	5.4	6.3	7.3	8.2	9.2
2.25	3.6	4.4	5.3	6.2	7.1	8.1	9.1

Table 9.8 Example of feed requirements for a 300 kg steer growing at 0.75 kg/day on silage (ME 10) and barley (ME 13).

1. Dry matter intake (DMI) (simplified), $0.02\,W = 6$ kg/day
2. Net energy for M + LWG (NE_{mp}) (from Table 9.5), 37.3 MJ/day
3. Animal production level (from Tables 9.6), 1.46
4. Net energy values of feeds (from $\dfrac{NE_m + NE_p}{ME_{mp}}$ or Table 9.7)
   Silage ME 10 = 5.9 MJ/kg
   Barley ME 13 = 8.6 MJ/kg
5. Energy concentration in ration,
   $NE_{mp}/DMI = \dfrac{37.3}{6} = 6.2$ MJ/kg
6. Pearson Square to calculate ration:
   Barley 8.6 ⟍ 0.3 $0.3/2.7 \times 6 = 0.67$ kg barley DM
               6.2
   Silage 5.9 ⟋ 2.4 $2.4/2.7 \times 6 = 5.33$ kg silage DM
                2.7
7. Divide by DM, $0.67/0.85 = 0.8$ kg fresh barley
   $5.33/0.25 = 21.3$ kg fresh silage

gain, and the net energy value of a feed, which depends on its ME content and the particular APL. The relevant information is shown in Tables 9.5, 9.6 and 9.7. For two ingredient rations, a Pearson square is used to solve the simultaneous equations to derive the amount of each feed required in the diet (see example in Table 9.8).

Energy requirements of lactating cattle

As with growing cattle, the main determinant of the ME requirement for maintenance is liveweight, but the ME system for lactating cattle also recognizes that k_m varies with q (Fig. 9.13). A further important consideration is the composition of the milk produced by the cow. The higher the fat and protein concentration, the higher the milk energy concentration and the greater the requirement for ME for milk production at any given dietary q value. However, in most practical feeding situations the q of diets for lactating dairy cows is unlikely to vary significantly from about 0.7, because of the need to include high-energy forages and concentrates to meet the total energy requirement. The values for ME required for milk production in Table 9.9 relate to a q value of 0.7 for simplicity. If the diet has a q value lower than 0.7, then the requirement should be increased accordingly (Table 9.9).

The requirement for ME to support the growth of the fetus during pregnancy increases progressively with the duration of gestation. For the first half of gestation the requirement is negligible, and in practice the energy requirement of the fetus only assumes significance in the last two months of pregnancy, i.e. in the dry period. The requirement for ME for pregnancy (Fig. 9.14) assumes a 40 kg calf at term. The requirement for heavier calves, such as Charolais × Holstein, is increased by direct linear scaling.

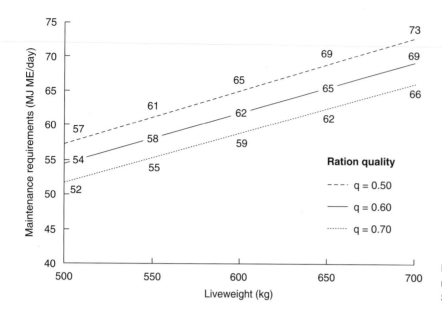

Fig. 9.13 Metabolizable energy requirement for maintenance in lactating cattle. Source: AFRC (1992).

Table 9.9 Metabolizable energy requirement (MJ/litre) for milk production. Reproduced from Chamberlain & Wilkinson, 1996 with permission of Chalcombe Publications.

Milk fat (% per litre)	Milk protein (% per litre)			
	3.00	3.20	3.40	3.60
q = 0.6				
3.00	4.39	4.47	4.54	4.62
3.50	4.71	4.79	4.86	4.94
4.00	5.03	5.11	5.18	5.26
4.50	5.35	5.43	5.50	5.58
5.00	5.67	5.75	5.82	5.90
q = 0.7				
3.00	4.16	4.23	4.30	4.37
3.50	4.47	4.54	4.61	4.68
4.00	4.77	4.84	4.91	4.98
4.50	5.07	5.14	5.21	5.28
5.00	5.38	5.45	5.52	5.59

q = gross energy/metabolizable energy.

The net energy value of weight change is assumed to be relatively constant in the case of adult cattle, but the impact of weight loss on the ME requirement varies according to the presumed utilization of the body tissue catabolized – milk production in early lactation and growth of the fetus in the dry period. The ME value of weight change also varies with the *q* value of the diet (Table 9.10).

The energy requirement of the cow is also influenced by the amount of activity, especially walking, that the animal undertakes daily. In most temperate areas of the world the energy expended in activity is considered to be moderate and the above requirements relate to that situation. However, cattle are sometimes subjected to extensive foraging under range and semi-arid conditions, and account should be taken of the increased energy required for activity when assessing requirements.

The total ME required is calculated as the sum of the above factors, but the overall efficiency of energy utilization of the lactating animal declines with increasing level of production, partly because of the faster rate of passage of food through the digestive tract at higher levels of voluntary intake and partly because the processes of absorption and metabolism are less efficient at higher levels of output. The correction for ME required depends on the animal production level (APL), defined here as the total ME required divided by the ME required for maintenance. Correction factors for level of production are in Table 9.11.

Protein requirements

Traditionally, protein requirements were expressed as digestible crude protein (DCP), that is, the proportion of the crude protein (CP or total nitrogen multiplied by 6.25) that is apparently digestible and therefore available to the animal. It is now recognized that DCP is totally inadequate as a system for assessing the protein requirements of ruminants.

The concept of digestible crude protein ignored the fact that a proportion of the digestible protein is degraded to ammonia by the action of the rumen microorganisms. Some of this ammonia is synthesized into

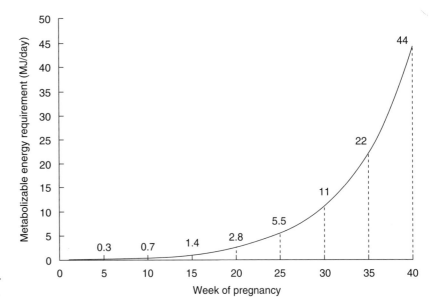

Fig. 9.14 Metabolizable energy requirement for pregnancy. Source: AFRC (1992).

Table 9.10 Metabolizable energy value (MJ ME) of weight changes in dairy cows given diets of different qualities (*q*). Reproduced from Chamberlain & Wilkinson, 1996 with permission of Chalcombe Publications.

	Live weight change (kg/day)			
q	−1.00	−0.50	0.50	1.00
Lactating cows				
0.5	−23.3	−11.6	19.4	38.8
0.6	−22.0	−11.0	18.3	36.7
0.7	−20.8	−10.4	17.4	34.7
Dry, pregnant cows				
0.4	−24.8	−12.4	34.5	69.0
0.5	−24.8	−12.4	27.7	55.4

q = gross energy/metabolizable energy.

Table 9.11 Correction factors for metabolizable energy requirement according to the animal production level (APL). Reproduced from Chamberlain & Wilkinson, 1996 with permission of Chalcombe Publications.

APL	Correction factor
0.7	0.99
1.0	1.00
2.0	1.02
3.0	1.04
4.0	1.05
5.0	1.07

APL = total ME/ME$_{maint}$

microbial protein in the rumen; the rest is absorbed into the bloodstream, converted to urea in the liver and excreted in the urine.

There are many situations where the animal's requirements can be met entirely by microbial protein. However, in some situations, particularly with high-yielding dairy cows, the animal requires more protein than that supplied by the microbial cells and it is necessary to supply additional dietary protein to the abomasum that has not been broken down *en route* through the rumen.

Microbial protein synthesis

Microbial protein is of high value to the ruminant in that its balance of essential amino acids is very close to

the animal's requirement (Table 9.12). Most classes of ruminant livestock can fulfil their total requirement for metabolizable protein (MP) from the supply of microbial true protein (MTP) alone. The exception is the high-yielding dairy cow, where supplementary digestible undegraded feed protein is required to meet the animal's total requirement for metabolizable protein (see below). In this situation, there may also be a requirement for supplementary essential amino acids such as methionine and lysine.

Much of the dietary protein eaten by the animal is degraded in the rumen to ammonia by the microbial population and it is possible to include non-protein nitrogen, such as urea, in diets which are deficient in degradable protein. Such deficiencies might arise in situations where the dietary ingredients, such as straw or maize silage, are low in total protein, or where the degradability of the feed protein is relatively low, as a result of heat-treatment during processing.

Table 9.12 Amino acid composition of bacterial protein and animal proteins (g amino acid/100g protein). From Van Soest (1994).

Amino acid	Microbial protein	Milk	Beef
Isoleucine	5.8	5.6	5.1
Leucine	8.0	10.2	8.0
Lysine	9.2	8.2	9.1
Methionine	2.5	2.9	2.7
Cysteine	1.4	1.0	1.3
Phenylalanine	5.3	5.4	4.5
Tyrosine	4.9	4.5	3.8
Threonine	5.7	5.0	4.6
Tryptophan	1.5	1.4	1.3
Valine	5.8	7.4	5.3
Arginine	5.3	4.0	6.7
Histidine	2.1	3.0	3.7
Alanine	6.8	3.8	6.4
Aspartic acid	11.9	8.5	9.6
Glutamic acid	12.4	23.0	17.3
Glycine	5.4	2.2	5.6
Proline	3.6	9.4	5.1
Serine	4.7	5.9	4.5

The production of microbial protein in the rumen depends on the supply of degradable protein and the supply of fermentable metabolizable energy (FME). The supply of degradable protein depends on the feed source and also on the time the feed spends in the rumen. Rumen outflow rate depends on the APL. The APL is therefore higher for high-producing animals than for low-producing animals. Degraded protein is not used with complete efficiency for microbial protein synthesis because some of the quickly degraded fraction is lost as ammonia through the rumen wall and is converted to urea in the liver. The proportion of quickly degraded protein (QDP) which is lost from the rumen is presumed to be 0.2, so that only 0.8 of the QDP is available to the rumen microbial population. All the slowly degraded protein (SDP) is potentially available to the micro-organisms and, together with 0.8 of the QDP, is the *effective* rumen degradable protein (ERDP) and is the amount of protein (or nitrogen) available for microbial growth and metabolism. However, the amount of ERDP which the microbial population can utilize depends on the amount of energy available, known as the fermentable metabolizable energy or FME. Some sources of energy in foods are considered to be of low value to the microbes, particularly those which yield low levels of ATP during their digestion in the rumen. Thus the energy in lipids and in silage acids is discounted, and the energy in undegraded protein should also be discounted (but is not) in the calculation of FME.

FME is therefore the total metabolizable energy minus the gross energy content of the lipids and (in the case of fermented feeds like silages) the content of fermentation acids. The yield of microbial crude protein (MCP) per MJ of FME, known as Y, depends on the APL because at lower APL the outflow rate from the rumen is reduced and at the lower outflow rate bacteria and protozoa die before passing out of the rumen and are digested by other rumen microbes. Their protein is recycled to produce new microbial protein. However, this process requires energy so additional FME is utilized with no net increase in yield of microbial protein.

The limit to the total yield of MCP is either the supply of ERDP (g per day) from the diet itself, in which case MCP production equals the supply of ERDP. Or, when the limit to the total yield of MCP is FME, the total amount of MCP produced is equal to the yield of MCP per MJ of FME (Y, which ranges from 8 g MCP/MJ FME at an APL of 1.0 to 11.5 at an APL of 4.0) multiplied by the total supply of FME in MJ per day. The *lesser* of the two values is taken as the production of MCP in the rumen.

It is unusual to find a situation where the two limiting factors to the production of MCP – ERDP and FME – are equal and where the calculation of MCP production by the two methods gives the same result. For example, most grass silages contain an excess of ERDP and a deficit of FME, whilst maize silage has a deficit of ERDP relative to FME. The skill in formulating diets is to achieve the correct overall balance between the total supply of ERDP, the total supply of FME (see Figs 9.16 and 9.17 for examples of the ERDP and FME contents of different feeds) and their respective rates of digestion in the rumen.

Having calculated the production of MCP, this value is then reduced to take account of the fact that about 0.75 of MCP is true protein and that it is absorbed into the blood with an efficiency of about 0.85 (Fig. 9.15). Thus microbial true protein supply is only about 0.64 of the MCP produced.

Metabolizable protein

The digestion and metabolism of dietary protein are shown in simplified form in Fig. 9.15. Dietary crude protein (CP) (Total N × 6.25) contains true protein, polypeptides, peptides and non-protein nitrogenous compounds (NPN) such as amino acids, amines, amides and ammonia. Urea, recycled to the rumen in saliva, is produced in the liver from ammonia which is in excess to that used by the microbial population of the rumen to synthesize microbial protein (see above). The amino acid content of microbial true protein is very constant,

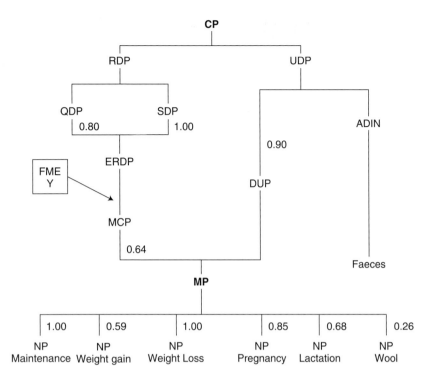

Fig. 9.15 The metabolizable protein system. Reproduced from Chamberlain & Wilkinson (1996) with permission of Chalcombe Publications.

and similar to the amino acid composition of tissue protein (beef) and also of milk (Table 9.12).

The degradable fraction, or ERDP, which yields microbial protein, is only part of the total supply of protein to the animal (Fig. 9.15). The protein which is not degraded in the rumen is termed undegraded dietary protein, of which a proportion, insoluble in acid detergent (ADIP or ADIN × 6.25), is indigestible. The remainder is known as the digestible undegraded protein or DUP.

The extent of degradation depends not only on the inherent characteristics of the protein source, but also on the time the material is exposed to degradation in the rumen, i.e. on outflow rate from the rumen. Thus the same protein may have quite different values when given to different types of cattle (Table 9.13).

The supply of MP to the animal has two components (Fig. 9.15): MTP derived from the growth of bacteria and protozoa in the rumen (see the section on microbial protein above) and digested undegraded feed protein (DUP), which has passed intact through the rumen and has been digested in the abomasum together with the microbial protein. The rate of production of microbial protein in the rumen depends on the supply of ERDP, the supply of FME to the rumen microbes and the speed of flow of digesta out of the rumen. The supply of undegraded feed protein is also affected by the speed of flow of digesta through the rumen (Table 9.13). The speed with which feed particles pass through the rumen depends mainly on the APL of the animal.

Table 9.13 Example of differences in the proportion of degraded and undegraded soyabean meal protein according to class of livestock. Reproduced from Orskov, 1998 with permission of Chalcombe Publications.

Dairy cows		Growing cattle		Suckler cows	
ERDP	DUP	ERDP	DUP	ERDP	DUP
0.50	0.50	0.65	0.35	0.85	0.15

ERDP = effective rumen degradable protein.
DUP = digestible undegraded protein.

The higher the APL, the faster the rate of passage of feed through the rumen. Thus MP supply depends not only on the feed itself but also on the type of animal to which the feed is being given. The requirement of the animal for MP depends on its level of productivity. The major requirement for MP in adult female ruminants is for the production of milk during lactation (see below), but the animal also requires MP for maintenance and growth, including the growth of the fetus during pregnancy, and for the production of wool. MP is released from the breakdown of muscle tissue during periods of body weight loss. MP is presumed to be utilized with variable efficiencies (net protein, NP) depending on its use (Fig. 9.15), with an efficiency of 1.0 for maintenance and with variable efficiencies for pregnancy (0.85), lactation (0.68), growth (0.6) and wool (0.26).

Table 9.14 Metabolizable protein (MP) requirement for maintenance. Reproduced from Chamberlain & Wilkinson, 1996 with permission of Chalcombe Publications.

Live weight (kg)	MP requirement for maintenance (g/day)
400	216
450	236
500	256
550	275
600	293
650	312
700	329
750	347

Table 9.15 Metabolizable protein (MP) requirement for milk production. Reproduced from Chamberlain & Wilkinson, 1996 with permission of Chalcombe Publications.

Milk yield (litres/day)	Milk protein (% per litre)			
	3.00	3.20	3.40	3.60
	MP requirement (g/day)			
10	427	456	484	513
20	855	912	969	1026
30	1282	1368	1453	1539
40	1710	1823	1937	2051
50	2137	2279	2422	2564

Table 9.16 Metabolizable protein (MP) requirement for pregnancy. Reproduced from Chamberlain & Wilkinson, 1996 with permission of Chalcombe Publications.

Week of gestation	MP requirement (g/day)
5	1
10	3
15	8
20	17
25	34
30	64
35	114
40	191

Table 9.17 Metabolizable protein (MP) allowances for weight change in dairy cows. Reproduced from Chamberlain & Wilkinson, 1996 with permission of Chalcombe Publications.

Live weight change (kg/day)	MP requirement (g/day)
−1.0	−131
−0.5	−66
0	0
0.5	122
1.0	245

Requirements for metabolizable protein

The requirement of the animal for MP depends on the amount of protein produced in tissue growth or in milk. The young calf has a high rate of lean tissue growth relative to its feed intake. Hence the concentration of protein in its diet needs to be relatively high. The cow yields more milk and eats less feed in early lactation than in mid-lactation. At this time the energy output in the milk is higher than that consumed in the feed because the cow is using stored reserves, mostly body fat. However, fat from body reserves yields no metabolizable protein and as a result she requires more protein per unit of feed in early lactation than later on.

If sufficient energy is provided to maintain the animal, then microbial protein produced from ERDP is likely to be sufficient to meet the maintenance requirement for MP. On the other hand, if the animal is restricted to a submaintenance level of feeding, then it will lose not only body fat but also protein from muscle tissue.

The protein requirement of the bovine animal is generally considered in terms of the main activities of the body – the maintenance of essential functions, lactation, pregnancy and weight change. The requirements of cattle of different liveweights for metabolizable protein for maintenance are shown in Table 9.14.

The requirement for MP for lactation is quantitatively the most important and varies with milk yield and also, though to a much lesser degree, with the protein concentration in the milk. Values for the requirement for MP for milk production are shown in Table 9.15.

The requirement for MP to support fetal growth in pregnancy is very low in the early stages and only becomes of significance in the final two months of gestation (Table 9.16). Allowances for MP for weight loss and the requirement for weight gain are shown in Table 9.17.

The total requirement for MP is calculated as the sum of the requirements for the appropriate bodily functions. Thus, for a dairy cow weighing 600 kg liveweight, yielding 20 litres of milk of 3.2% protein, in her fifteenth week of pregnancy and gaining 0.5 kg liveweight/day the total requirement is 293 g for maintenance (Table 9.14) + 912 g for milk production (Table 9.15) + 8 g for pregnancy (Table 9.16) + 122 g for weight gain (Table 9.17) = 1335 g MP/day.

In some situations the total protein requirement is expressed as a recommended concentration of crude

Table 9.18 Recommended concentrations of crude protein in diets for cattle.

Dairy cows		Beef suckler cows		Growing beef cattle		
Milk yield (litres/day)	Dietary crude protein (g/kg dry matter)	Milk yield (litres/day)	Dietary crude protein (g/kg dry matter)	Liveweight (kg)	Dietary crude protein (g/kg dry matter) ME of total diet (MJ/kg DM)	
					11.0	12.0
0	135–145	0	120	100	180	210
10	145–155	5	150	200	140	150
20	155–165	10	150	>200	130	140
30	165–175					
40	175–180					
50	180–190					

protein in the total diet dry matter. This may appear to be an oversimplification, but where the degradability characteristics of the protein in some dietary ingredients are not known, or where there is uncertainty about the actual animal production level, then diets should be formulated according to the recommended concentrations of crude protein in Table 9.18.

Tests of the MP system with dairy cows have revealed that the system works reasonably well at low to medium levels of milk yield (20 to 30 litres/day), but that at higher levels of production the MP required is underestimated. This implies that the efficiency of utilization of MP for milk production is not constant at 0.68 (see section on metabolizable protein), but that it decreases at increased levels of output. The values for MP requirement for lactation in Table 9.15 have been adjusted upwards to take account of the decrease in efficiency of utilization of MP for milk production above a milk yield of 25 litres/day. Other systems of assessing protein supply and requirements, for example the French PDI system, also take account of the relatively greater requirement for MP of the high-yielding cow.

Composition of feeds

Cellulosic and non-cellulosic feeds

Feeds for cattle are best described in terms of the major components that undergo fermentation in the rumen. In other words, the conventional division into concentrates and roughages is only a crude way of distinguishing between feeds that contain mainly non-cellulosic (starch, sugar and protein) or cellulosic (plant cell wall) material.

The division into cellulosic and non-cellulosic feeds is relevant because the two fractions are fermented by

Table 9.19 Classification of feeds. From MAFF (1986b) and Lonsdale (1989).

Mainly cellulosic (NDF >500 g/kg DM)	Mainly non-cellulosic (NDF <500 g/kg DM)
Straw	Kale
Hay	Very young grass
Grass (except very young grass)	Maize silage
Silage (except maize)	Fodder beet, root crops
Brewers' grains	Cereal grains
Malt distillers' draff	Molasses
Pectin-extracted fruit	Molassed sugar beet pulp
Coffee grounds	Maize gluten feed
Unmolassed sugar beet pulp	Soyabean meal
Bran	Fat
Wheat feed	Cottonseed cake
	Distillers' dark grains
	Citrus pulp
	Legume seeds

different types of bacteria and at different rates (see section on fermentation in the rumen, p. 96). Cellulosic feeds are fermented at a slower rate, occupy more space in the rumen and are usually eaten in smaller quantities (i.e. at a slower rate) than non-cellulosic feeds.

When formulating diets it is useful to recognize the different fermentation patterns of the two types of feed and their different rates of intake by the animal. With productive cattle it is important to avoid too much of one type, or intake may be depressed – by acidosis if too much non-cellulosic material is eaten, or by a slow fermentation in the rumen and slow outflow rate if too much cellulosic material is eaten.

Feeds are classified into those which are mainly cellulosic and those which are mainly non-cellulosic, as

Table 9.20 Classification of raw materials according to their energy and protein contents. The degradability of the protein is also indicated*. Reproduced from Lonsdale (1989) with permission of Chalcombe Publications.

Protein content (g/kg DM)	Metabolizable energy content (MJ/kg DM)		
	High >12.0	Medium 9.0–12.0	Low <9.0
High **>200**	Maize gluten meal (prairie meal) (B) Groundnut cake (A) Soyabean meal (B) Sesame meal (B) Soya beans (whole processed) (C) Condensed corn steep liquor Lupins (sweet) (B) Pot ale syrup (A) Linseed meal (B) Spent wash syrups (A) US corn distillers' dark grains (C) Beans (field) (C) Wheat distillers' dark grains (C) Malt distillers' dark grains (C) Peas (B) Delactosed whey syrup (A) Copra expeller (B) Maize gluten feed (B)	Rapeseed meal (B) Sunflower seed meal (B) Cottonseed cake (B) Safflower meal (A) Malt culms (B) Brussels sprout packhouse waste (A) Malt residual pellets (B) Brewers' grains (B) Palm kernel meal (extr.) (B)	Cotton cake (undec.) (B) Sunflower seed meal (undec.) (B) Safflower meal expeller (A)
Medium **120–200**	Maize germ meal (B) Whey (A) Triticale (A) Wheat (A)	Wheat bran (B) Dried forages (grass, lucerne) (B) Wheatfeed (A)	Rice bran (C) Shea nut meal (D) Rape meal (D)
Low **<120**	Barley (A) Oats (A) Sugar beet pulp (molassed, dried, pressed, ensiled) (B) Potatoes (A) Maize grain (B) Carrots (A) Citrus pulp (B) Molasses (A) Manioc (B)	Pectin extracted fruit (B) Apple pomace (B)	Oatfeed (C)

* Degradability: category A = 0.71–0.90, B = 0.51–0.70, C = 0.31–0.50, D = <0.31.

shown in Table 9.19. Some forage feeds, which would at first sight be considered cellulosic, are not. High-quality grass, for example, typically contains less than half of the DM as cell wall or neutral detergent fibre (NDF) (MAFF, 1992); maize silage also contains less cell wall than cell contents, because of its high grain content; typically 250 to 300g of the DM of maize silage is starch. Fodder beet contains 650g sugar per kg DM, but it is contained within cell walls and is released in the rumen for fermentation at a slower rate than, say, the sugar from molasses.

Energy and protein in feeds

The two most important nutrients are energy and protein. Other nutrients, particularly minerals, can limit efficiency of feed use, but in practice if a wide range of feeds is included in the diet the risk of mineral imbalance is low. Most farmers add proprietary mineral supplements to the diets of their cattle. However, particular deficiency situations do arise due to inadequate management, for example hypomagnesaemia (see Chapter 46).

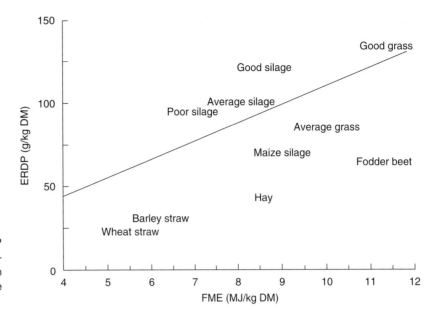

Fig. 9.16 Typical concentrations of ERDP and FME in selected forage crops. Reproduced from Chamberlain & Wilkinson (1996) with permission of Chalcombe Publications.

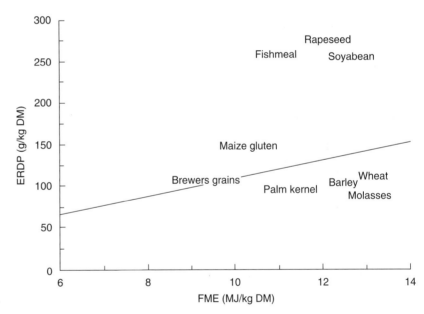

Fig. 9.17 Typical concentrations of ERDP and FME in selected concentrates. Reproduced from Chamberlain & Wilkinson (1996) with permission of Chalcombe Publications.

A simple classification of feeds is one which takes into account the concentrations of ME, FME, ERDP and DUP (see sections above for definitions of terms), as in Table 9.20. A fuller description of the composition of feeds is given in the UK Ministry of Agriculture, Fisheries and Food's book *Feed Composition* (MAFF, 1992).

An alternative way of considering feed sources is in terms of the balance between ERDP and FME, shown in Figs 9.16 and 9.17 for selected forages and concentrates, respectively. Maize silage, fodder beet, hay, straw, molasses and cereal grains are typically deficient in

ERDP relative to FME, whilst fishmeal, rapeseed meal, soyabean meal and maize gluten feed typically contain an excess of ERDP relative to their concentrations of FME.

Physical form

There are three easily recognizable categories for the physical form of feeds: (i) liquids, (ii) moist solids and (iii) dry solids. Examples of each category are shown in Table 9.21.

Table 9.21 Examples of the physical forms of raw material feeds. Reproduced from Stark & Lonsdale (1989) with permission of Chalcombe Publications.

Liquid	Moist solid	Dry solid
Condensed corn steep liquor	Apple pomace	Bran (wheat and rice)
Delactosed whey syrup	Brewers' grains	Cereal grains
Fresh whey	Brussels sprout	Citrus pulp
Molasses	packhouse waste	Distillers' dark grains
Pot ale syrup	Carrot rejects	Dried grass and lucerne
	Maize gluten feed*	Legume seeds
	Pectin-extracted fruit	Maize germ meal
	Potatoes	Maize gluten feed*
	Sugar beet pulp*	Maize gluten meal
		Malt culms
		Malt residual pellets
		Oatfeed
		Oilseed residues
		Sugar beet pulp*
		Wheatfeed
		Whole oilseeds

* Available as either a moist or dry solid.

Liquids range from very low DM materials such as whey, which has handling characteristics similar to water, to viscous liquids such as molasses, which has a typical DM content of 750 g/kg fresh weight. With the exception of whey, most liquid feeds have been condensed prior to shipment, in an attempt to reduce haulage costs.

Moist solids comprise those which contain fermentable sugars (e.g. fresh grass, molassed sugar beet pulp) and are usually stored as silage (see section on feed preservation, see below), and those which are low in fermentable components (e.g. apple pomace), and which benefit from the addition of a preservative.

Dry solids are a common form of feed and include cereal grains and by-products from the flour milling industry, hay, straw and residues from oil seed extraction. The DM content of dry solids is usually in the range 830 to 930 g/kg fresh weight. Higher moisture contents increase the risk of spoilage during storage and for this reason most manufacturers of dry feeds aim to approach 900 g DM/kg fresh weight if possible. Hay is usually stored at an initial DM content of around 800 g/kg, but final DM content is typically 850 g/kg fresh weight.

Feed preservation

The principle of preservation is to prevent the development of spoilage organisms such as the putrefying bacteria and moulds. These organisms prefer warm temperatures, low levels of acidity (pH 6 to 8), oxygen and water. Hence preservation may be achieved by cooling (preferably freezing), by acidification, by exclusion or removal of oxygen, or by drying.

Drying

Drying is the most effective form of feed preservation. It is also the most costly and therefore tends to be used with the more valuable feeds (e.g. cereals) and with feeds that are prone to deterioration (e.g. citrus pulp).

The DM content of cereals is normally increased by drying to 850 to 870 g/kg prior to storage. Hay is dried in the field to about 800 g DM/kg fresh weight, unless it is to be dried artificially in the barn, when it may be harvested in a moist state at between 650 and 750 g DM/kg. Drying in the barn proceeds until the safe DM content, more than 800 g/kg, has been reached and the crop shows little sign of heating and moulding.

Ensiling

The process of ensilage involves the fermentation of plant water-soluble carbohydrate (WSC) monomers (simple sugars, mainly fructose and glucose) to organic acids, principally lactic acid. The acidity thus produced effectively 'pickles' the crop or feed in a stable state in the absence of air.

Fermentation is an anaerobic process. The crop must be completely sealed from the air to facilitate the growth

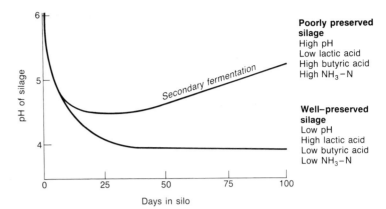

Poorly preserved silage
High pH
Low lactic acid
High butyric acid
High NH₃−N

Well−preserved silage
Low pH
High lactic acid
Low butyric acid
Low NH₃−N

Fig. 9.18 Patterns of fermentation and changes in the pH value of silage as a result of secondary fermentation.

of the desirable anaerobic bacteria that are present on the crop in the field in relatively small numbers. As much air as possible should be removed from the crop at the time of ensiling, so that residual oxygen is exhausted as rapidly as possible. This is achieved by first chopping the crop as it is harvested from the field, by consolidating it once the crop is in the silo and finally by sealing it completely using a plastic sheet.

Primary and secondary fermentations

It is important to distinguish between primary and secondary fermentations, and to recognize that both are quite distinct from the process of aerobic spoilage that occurs on exposure of silage to the air at the time of feed-out.

Primary fermentation essentially comprises the conversion of sugars or WSC, mainly fructose and glucose, to lactic and other acids as the result of the metabolism of bacteria. This process can be rapid and completed in a few days.

Secondary fermentation, which sometimes follows the primary fermentation, involves the degradation of lactic and other acids, with the formation of evil-smelling acids like butyric acid. The process can also be accompanied by the complete degradation of nitrogenous compounds to ammonia. The main organisms involved in secondary fermentation are the obligate anaerobic clostridial bacteria.

At the point of entry to the silo the pH of the fresh crop is usually about 6.0. The crop is still alive, but it is consuming the products of photosynthesis (sugars) by respiration and producing carbon dioxide, water and heat. In addition, aerobic bacteria such as the Enterobacteriaceae (coliforms) consume sugars to produce acetic acid and degrade protein to ammonia.

As the supply of oxygen is exhausted, the primary fermentation dominates, with lactic acid the predomi-

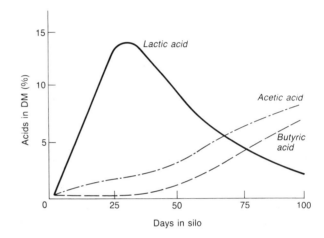

Fig. 9.19 Typical changes in the content of fermentation acids in silage as a result of secondary fermentation.

nant product. Acidity increases as the conversion of sugars to acids continues.

Primary fermentation proceeds until either the supply of fermentable substrate is exhausted or the amount of free water (i.e. that not associated with products of fermentation) is reduced to a sufficiently low level to restrict bacterial activity. A stable low pH is reached. The silage contains lactic acid as the main fermentation acid and the amount of protein completely degraded to ammonia is small (see Fig. 9.18). However, if the supply of sugar in the crop is low, or its resistance to acidification or buffering capacity is relatively high, secondary fermentation may occur during the storage period. In this situation the silage is unstable. Wet crops of low sugar content are particularly prone to secondary fermentation. Typical changes in the content of fermentation acids in silage as a result of secondary fermentation are shown in Fig. 9.19.

Table 9.22 Crops ranked in order of their 'ensilability'. Reproduced from Wilkinson (1990) with permission of Chalcombe Publications.

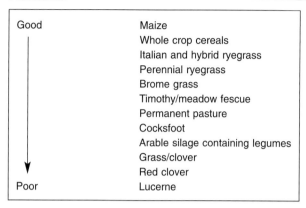

Good	Maize
	Whole crop cereals
	Italian and hybrid ryegrass
	Perennial ryegrass
	Brome grass
	Timothy/meadow fescue
	Permanent pasture
	Cocksfoot
	Arable silage containing legumes
	Grass/clover
	Red clover
Poor	Lucerne

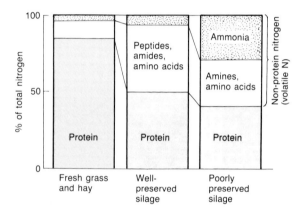

Fig. 9.20 The nitrogenous components of fresh grass, well-preserved silage and poorly preserved silage. Source: Wilkinson (1985).

Some crops, because they have a relatively low content of WSC or have relatively high buffering capacities, are more prone than others to secondary fermentations – their 'ensilability' is relatively low. Crops are ranked in order of their ensilability in Table 9.22. Maize combines adequate WSC with low buffering capacity, whilst the converse is true for the legumes, lucerne in particular.

Wilting in good weather prior to harvest has the effect of concentrating the sugars in the crop, and this is beneficial in terms of reducing the risk of secondary fermentation.

Silages that have undergone secondary fermentation are poorly preserved, but paradoxically they tend to be relatively stable on exposure to air. A major consequence of clostridial activity is an increase in the proportion of nitrogen present as ammonia in the silage (Fig. 9.20). Digestibility and energy value are also reduced due to secondary fermentation; hence losses of nutrients are elevated in poorly preserved silages.

Typical analytical composition of silage

Typical values for the composition of grass and maize silages made in bunker silos under European conditions are shown in Table 9.23. The most notable differences between grass and maize silage are in crude protein and NDF, which are higher for grass than maize, and in starch which is very low in grass silage. Poorly-preserved grass silages normally contain elevated levels of ash, fibre, acetic acid, butyric acid and ammonia–N, whilst energy values are depressed compared to well-preserved material. Amino acid–N is reduced as a proportion of the total non-protein nitrogen, indicating greater degradation to amines, amides and ammonia. Wilted grass silages generally undergo less extensive fermentations and consequently have higher pH values than wetter silages, residual (i.e. unfermented) WSC, lower concentrations of fermentation acids and less ammonia–N (Table 9.23).

Additives for silage

The main objective in applying an additive at the time of harvest is to prevent the multiplication of clostridia. The lactic acid bacteria are more tolerant of acid conditions than are the clostridia, so traditionally their growth has been inhibited by direct acidification of the crop with an organic acid such as formic, or an inorganic acid such as sulphuric. The former is relatively more expensive, but it does have a specific antimicrobial action against clostridia, whilst sulphuric acid acts solely through its effect in reducing pH. Some products comprise mixtures of acids and synergistic properties are claimed for them.

If the pH of the crop can be reduced from 6.0 to about 4.5 by acidification at the time of harvest then the risk of clostridial growth is greatly reduced.

An alternative approach is to accelerate the production of lactic acid by the direct inoculation of the crop at harvest. Provided sufficient live bacteria are added (ideally l million colony forming units/g fresh crop) and provided the content of fermentable sugar in the crop is sufficient for their growth then good preservation quality should be assured. Problems can arise with inoculants if there is insufficient sugar, either because the crop itself is deficient or because the crop is too wet at the time of ensiling. The most common species of bacteria in inoculants is *Lactobacillus plantarum*.

Enzyme additives, containing hemicellulase and cellulase, are another type of additive; the object in this case is to generate extra sugar from cell wall components to ensure sufficient acidification during primary fermentation so that clostridia are inhibited.

Products are now available which contain both lactic acid bacteria and enzymes. It is essential, however, to

Table 9.23 Typical composition of grass and maize silage stored in bunker silos.

| | Grass silage | | | Maize silage |
| | Direct-cut | | Wilted | |
	Poorly preserved	Well preserved		
pH	5.5	3.8	4.5	4.0
DM (g/kg fresh weight)	160	180	360	300
Ash (g/kg DM)	110	80	90	55
Crude protein (g/kg DM)	160	160	150	90
NDF (g/kg DM)	650	550	550	450
WSC (g/kg DM)	0	0	50	85
Starch (g/kg DM)	0	0	0	250
Lactic acid (g/kg DM)	50	150	65	100
Acetic acid (g/kg DM)	25	20	35	45
Butyric acid (g/kg DM)	35	0	0	0
DOMD (g/kg DM)	675	700	700	720
ME (MJ/kg DM)	10.8	11.2	11.2	11.5
NH_3-N (g/kg total N)	300	75	40	30
Amino acid–N (g/kg total soluble N)	405	700	750	650

establish that the active ingredients in these biological additives really are active, and have not been destroyed by processing, packaging or storage.

Additives for hay and moist grain

The risk of development of moulds and mycotoxins in moist hay and moist grain may be reduced by adding an effective preservative at the time of storage. Propionic acid and salts of propionic acid such as ammonium bis-propanoate, added at 15kg active ingredient per tonne of fresh crop at the time of harvest, are effective in reducing mould development in both hay and grain and also in big bale silage, where moulding due to incomplete sealing is a common problem.

Feed processing

Physical processing of roughages

Traditionally, feeds like hays and straws were chopped or ground prior to feeding. There is now increasing evidence to indicate that although these procedures may be convenient for the processor, they are less than ideal from the point of view of the nutrition of the animal.

With fibrous feeds such as straw, intake is often limited by the speed with which long particles are reduced in size by chewing so that they can pass out of the rumen. Grinding removes this restriction to intake, but a consequence is that particles pass out of the rumen before they are fully digested. The net result is that although dry matter intake is increased, digestibility is reduced and nutrient intake is little changed.

Chopping long forages also reduces the opportunity for the animal to select the best quality material on offer. However, if straw is to be used in a complete diet, coarse chopping is a useful way of incorporating the feed uniformly into the total mixture.

Long fibre with an average particle length of at least 150mm is essential for milk fat synthesis and for the maintenance of rumen function on high-concentrate diets. It is therefore important to bear in mind that physical processing of roughages can diminish their value with respect to milk quality and the health status of the rumen.

Chemical processing of roughages

The use of alkalis, such as sodium hydroxide, for upgrading straw is not new, but recently additional benefits from the use of the technique have been recognized.

Essentially, the technique involves adding sodium hydroxide to straw at about 50 kg per tonne fresh weight. The alkali degrades and swells the plant cell wall material, with a consequent increase in digestibility and intake. The benefits are valuable where straw is plentiful and where it comprises a high proportion of the total diet, for example in the case of beef suckler cows.

The residual alkalinity in straw treated with sodium hydroxide can help to reduce the risk of ruminal acidosis in high-yielding dairy cows given diets containing large proportions of concentrates and/or highly acid silages. In these situations, where fibre is needed to maintain milk fat content but the overall energy content is required to be high at the same time, the provision of a source of long fibre of enhanced digestibility is also valuable.

Ammonia (usually added in aqueous form at 30 kg NH_3 per tonne fresh weight) is a useful alternative alkali to sodium hydroxide. It has the advantage of also contributing nitrogen, a valuable feature if the diet is deficient in rumen degradable nitrogen, but a disadvantage if silage of high protein content is the major forage in the diet.

Urea may also be used to upgrade straw, but both the moisture content of the straw and ambient temperature need to be relatively high for the technique to be successful.

The effect of an increase in digestibility of straw on intake can be considerable. Thus a 10 per cent improvement in digestibility can lead to a 50 per cent increase in dry matter intake. Since the feed consumed is more digestible, the increase in ME intake is even greater.

Processing of cereals

Grinding of cereals was traditionally considered essential to achieve complete digestion by cattle. A trade-off was accepted between rapid digestion in the rumen and possible acidosis on the one hand and poor digestibility with undigested grains appearing in the faeces on the other. It is now accepted that the passage of a few undigested grains has no measurable effect on digestibility, but that forage digestibility can be reduced when grain is overprocessed.

The need for cereal processing depends on the size of the reticulo-omasal orifice. In the case of sheep and calves less than 150 kg liveweight, it is difficult for whole barley and whole oat grains to pass through the orifice, whilst it is easy in larger cattle. Thus whole grains may be given to young calves, but some processing is necessary for older cattle. If possible, the extent of process-

ing should be as small as possible: it is sufficient to crack the seed coat. Crimping is better than rolling, but treatment with sodium hydroxide, which has the effect of breaking the seed coat by swelling it, is probably the best method from the animal's point of view. In addition to slowing down the rate of digestion of the starch in the grain, the residual alkali buffers acidity in the rumen.

Feeding management

Successful nutrition of the bovine not only requires an understanding of the principles of nutrient requirement, nutrient supply and animal response; it also involves appropriate management of feed resources. This includes presenting the correct amount of feed to the animal for the appropriate period of time, formulating diets from available resources that meet requirements, taking into account the condition of the animal and the desired direction and rate of change in weight and condition and budgeting ahead so that rapid changes in diet are avoided and performance targets are achieved.

The importance of selective eating

The need to maintain stability in the rumen has led to the presentation of feeds to the animal over a large proportion of the day. This is particularly so with forages and straws, where rate of intake is relatively slow. It is also important that the animal has access to feed for most if not all the time when selectivity is desirable.

At pasture, maximum intake is only achieved when herbage is offered in substantial excess (Figs 9.7 to 9.9). In general, the amount of herbage on offer should be three to four times the amount eaten in order to achieve maximum potential voluntary intake (see section on grazed pasture, p. 101).

Targets for sward surface height at pasture

A simple guide to the amount of herbage on offer is the sward surface height of the grazed pasture. Regular measurement of sward height or sward mass is a useful tactical aid to pasture management. Targets for sward height for growing, lactating and dry cows are shown in Table 9.24.

It is important to measure sward height in grazed areas, since herbage that is rejected due to contamination by faeces, urine or treading is unlikely to be eaten until the height of herbage in grazed areas is well below that at which intake is restricted below maximum.

Table 9.24 Target sward surface heights (cm) for rotational and continuous grazing.

	Spring	Early summer	Late summer	Autumn
Lactating cows and growing cattle				
Rotational grazing				
Pregrazing	10–15	12–16	14–18	10–15
Postgrazing	6–7	7–8	8–9	6–7
Continuous grazing	6–7	7–8	8–9	6–7
Dry cows[a]	4–5	4–5	4–5	4–5

[a] Postgrazing, rotational and continuous grazing.

Buffer feeding

The concept of buffer feeding was developed as a way of reducing losses in output from grazed pasture, especially when herbage allowance was apparently adequate but intake less than maximal due to poor weather, inadequate grass growth, short day length or reduced time of access to pasture.

The buffer feed should be less acceptable than the herbage on offer at pasture, otherwise the buffer acts as a substitute rather than a supplement for grazed grass. Typically, silage or hay are used as buffer feeds, offered *ad libitum* at the farm buildings to dairy cows after each milking or placed in the grazing field for other classes of stock.

Frequency of feeding and ruminal acidosis

It is significant that when cereal concentrates are offered *ad libitum* the animal eats a little at a time. Thus the general practice in feedlots, and in areas of the world where milk is produced from high-concentrate diets, is to allow the animals 24-hour access to all feeds (both concentrate and roughage) to avoid ruminal acidosis, otherwise known as 'feedlot bloat'. This condition is caused by the rapid fermentation of starches and sugars, and can occur as the result of infrequent ingestion of large feeds of concentrates. It can also occur as the result of inadequate long fibre to maintain rumination and saliva production. Essentially, the condition is due to the dominance in the rumen fermentation of lactic acid producing bacteria (p. 829). Ruminal stasis can occur at low rumen pH (less than pH 5.5) and the inability of the animal to eructate leads to the accumulation of gas and the resultant bloat (p. 832).

Cattle given concentrates *ad libitum* should therefore also be allowed access to long forage or a source of roughage such as straw, at about 15 per cent of the total diet dry matter.

Traditionally, dairy cows were given concentrates, usually in the form of milled compounded feeds, in the parlour at milking and forages *ad libitum* for the rest of the day. With ever-increasing milk yields per cow, the pressure on the available time in the parlour meant that the cow had difficulty consuming a large feed of compounds during the milking period. Further, the rapid fermentation of the two relatively large meals (sometimes as much as 5 kg/meal) meant that rumen pH decreased, fibre digestion slowed down and forage intake was reduced as a result (see Fig. 9.21). Accordingly, a mid-day feed of compounds or of by-products such as dried sugar beet pulp was introduced to reduce the quantity of compound to be fed through the parlour.

Sodium bicarbonate may be a suitable ingredient of the diet when the cow is suffering from acidosis. However, the problem with bicarbonate is that it is relatively unpalatable and large quantities are required to have a significant effect. Thus the addition of 100 to 150 g/cow per day is insignificant by comparison with the 3 kilogrammes of bicarbonate produced in saliva daily. It is better therefore to include feeds, like hay or straw, to stimulate rumination and salivation.

Out-of-parlour feeders

The advent of computerized cow identification has enabled cows to be rationed accurately in the parlour according to yield, and it was a relatively logical step to introduce out-of-parlour feeders to allow the higher-yielding individuals to eat compounds and concentrates during the rest of the day. The nutritional advantages were that higher levels of compounds could be given to those cows that 'deserved' to receive them, and in a relatively large number of meals per day. Feeders could be programmed to deliver equal proportions of the total day's allocation in up to 12 feeds per day; cows not

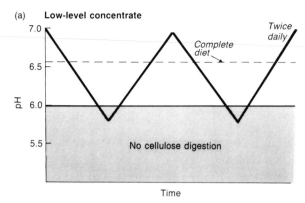

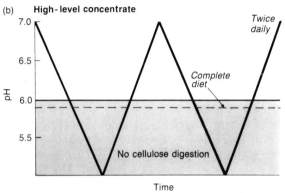

Fig. 9.21 It is important to prevent the pH of the rumen from falling below 6.0 for long periods of time, otherwise cellulose digestion will be greatly reduced. The problem is less at low levels of concentrate feeding (a) than at high levels (b). Reproduced from Orskov (1998) with permission of Chalcombe Publications.

taking their feeds were readily identifiable and could be checked for disease immediately.

Flat-rate feeding

The introduction in Europe of milk quotas placed a limit on output, and the emphasis switched to simplifying the day-to-day feeding management of the dairy herd, especially in those herds where the input of concentrate was moderate and where the supply of grassland for grazing and silage was adequate and reliable throughout the growing season.

The principle of flat-rate feeding is that all cows receive the same amount of concentrate, irrespective of their actual or potential milk production, together with silage *ad libitum*. The system works best when there is a compact calving pattern, with most cows at the same stage of lactation, and when the input of concentrates is relatively low. Silage quality should be relatively high and if necessary the level of concentrate should be reduced when the herd is in late lactation to prevent cows becoming overfat.

In practice, higher-yielding cows in the herd eat more silage and it is important that the silage is on offer *ad libitum* otherwise these animals are underfed. Peak lactation yields tend to be lower than in herds given concentrates to yield, but the rate of decline in yield post-peak tends also to be slower than in herds fed to yield, giving a flatter lactation curve for flat-rate feeding.

Total mixed rations or complete diets

The main principle of complete diet feeding is that the animal receives an intimate mix of slowly and rapidly fermented feeds, thus balancing the inflow to the rumen of feeds with widely differing rates of fermentation and (it is hoped) thereby maintaining stable conditions in the rumen.

However, with high proportions of concentrates in the mix, the level of acidity in the rumen may be so high that fibre digestion is permanently depressed (Fig. 9.21). In this situation, the proportion of propionate in the rumen volatile fatty acids is elevated and as a result cows tend to gain in weight and produce milk of relatively low fat content. Overfat cows with fatty livers were a feature of early mismanagement of herds given complete diets.

Thus, provided cows in late lactation and dry cows are not given the same high-energy mix as higher-yielding animals, complete diets offer a logical approach to feeding management. By-products can be incorporated into complete diets with greater ease than in other feeding systems. Higher voluntary feed intakes are usually achieved than with separate feeding, and milk compositional quality is often improved as a result of the higher energy status of the animal and improved fibre digestion in the rumen. On the other hand, the investment in mixer-wagons can be considerable and there is little evidence of improved overall efficiency of feed utilization by animals given total mixed rations compared to the same diet in separate feeds of forages and concentrates.

Diet formulation

Diets are formulated to meet calculated requirements for major nutrients (see sections on energy and protein requirements, pages 103, 106), taking account also of the needs of the animal for macro- and microelements. Recent research in the USA indicates that formulations for lactation should also take account of dry matter content and the content of NDF (cell wall) in the total diet. The dry matter content of the whole diet should be between 500 and 650 g/kg fresh weight for maximum intake, whilst the content of NDF should be between 350 and 450 g/kg DM for maximal output of milk

Table 9.25 Target condition scores for beef suckler cows. Reproduced from Fuller (1988) with permission of Chalcombe Publications.

Stage of reproductive cycle	Target condition score	
	Autumn-calving cows	Spring-calving cows
At calving	3	2.5
At mating	2.5	2
Mid-pregnancy	2	3

Table 9.26 Feed budget for a dairy herd of 100 cows, average milk yield 6500 l/cow, calving September to November.

Feed	Budget
Grazing	
Spring	5 cows per hectare
Early summer	3.5 cows per hectare
Late summer and autumn	2.5 cows per hectare
Silage	10 tonnes fresh weight per cow at 10.5 MJ ME/kg DM
Concentrates	
When cows are housed	1.4 tonnes per cow
When cows are grazing	0.1 tonnes per cow

Table 9.27 Feed budget for suckler cows (t fresh weight/cow and calf per annum). Silage and other feeds 25 per cent DM.

Grazing
Hill pastures and semi-arid lowlands: 0.5–1.0 cows/ha
Upland pastures: 1.2–1.8 cows/ha
Lowland temperate pastures: 1.5–2.1 cows/ha

Winter feeding

	Autumn calving	Spring calving
Lowland herds		
Concentrates	0.4	0.2
Silage	3.5	2.5
Straw	1.0	0.8
Other feeds (wet byproducts)	0.3	0.4
Upland herds		
Concentrates	0.4	0.2
Silage	4.7	4.5
Straw	0.6	0.5
Other feeds	0.2	0.4

Hill herds: as for upland herds except silage 5.5 t/head to allow for longer winter period

Table 9.28 Feed budgets for growing beef cattle.

Grazing
Target liveweight (t/ha) at 250 kg N/ha

May	2.2
June	2.0
July	1.7
August	1.6
September	1.4
October	1.4
Average	1.7

Increase by 4 kg for each extra kg of N

Silage and concentrates (t/head)

	Silage (25% DM, 10.5 ME)	Concentrates
Overwintered store cattle and finishing suckled calves	3	0.3
18-month beef	5	0.9
Silage beef (15–16 months)	6	0.8
Cereal beef (11–12 months)	*	1.6

* 0.2 t straw/head to maintain rumen function.

fat. Constraints in diet formulation programmes now include dry matter and NDF in addition to conventional prediction equations for voluntary intake and nutrient requirements.

Condition score

Condition scoring cows is relatively easy; there is no fleece to hide the animal's fatness (or thinness). The essential areas for physical examination are: (i) the transverse processes of the lumbar vertebrae at the top of the loin, halfway between the last rib, (ii) the hip bone and (iii) the tail head (see Chapter 2, Fig. 2.1).

Scoring should ideally be carried out by feeling the extent of subcutaneous fat cover at the tail head and at the lumbar area. With practice, visual scoring is possible taking into account the visibility of the ribs and the amount of fat at the tail head. Cows in condition score 1 have no fat at the tail head and their ribs are prominent. The ribs are visible in condition score 2 but not in condition score 3 and above. As condition score rises above 2, the amount of fat visible at the tail head increases.

Target condition scores for cows at different stages of the production cycle are shown in Table 9.25.

Regular condition scoring helps to identify overthin cows that require preferential treatment (extra feed) and overfat cows, especially those in late pregnancy, that are at risk of dystokia at calving. Scoring in early lactation to monitor the effectiveness of nutrient inputs to achieve weight gain at mating is an essential part of successful rebreeding. Economies may also be made in high-energy feeds at times when the whole herd is scored as being slightly overfat.

Feed budgeting

Feed budgeting is the extension of daily diet formulation to annual feed planning. Future levels of output are set and a feeding policy is developed which takes into account the home-produced feeds available, or likely to become available during the year, and the type and quantity of purchased feeds required to meet the target level of output. A buying strategy is developed to meet the projected requirements.

Simplified examples of feed budgets for grazing and winter feeding are shown in Tables 9.26 to 9.28 for dairy cows, suckler cows and growing beef cattle, respectively.

References and further reading

Agricultural Research Council (1980) *The Nutrient Requirements of Ruminant Livestock*. Commonwealth Agricultural Bureaux, Farnham Royal, Bucks, CABI Publishing, Wallingford, pp. 1–347.

Agricultural Research Council (1984*) The Nutrient Requirements of Ruminant Livestock, Supplement No. 1*. Commonwealth Agricultural Bureaux, Farnham Royal, Bucks, pp. 1–45.

Agricultural and Food Research Council (1992) Technical Committee on Responses to Nutrients, Report No. 9, Nutritive Requirements of Ruminant Animals: Protein. *Nutrition Abstracts and Reviews, Series B: Livestock Feeds and Feeding*, **62**, 787.

Allen D.M. (2001) *Rationing Beef Cattle*, 2nd end. Chalcombe Publications, Lincoln, pp. 1–89.

Chamberlain, A.T. & Wilkinson, J.M. (1996) *Feeding the Dairy Cow*. Chalcombe Publications, Lincoln, pp. 1–241.

Forbes, J.M. (1983) *The Voluntary Food Intake of Farm Animals*. CABI Publishing, Wallingford, pp. 1–206.

Fuller, R. (1998) *Suckled Calf Production*, 2nd edn. Chalcombe Publications, Lincoln, pp. 1–105.

Gibb, M.J. & Treacher, T.T. (1978) The effect of herbage allowance on herbage intake and performance of ewes and their twin lambs grazing perennial ryegrass. *Journal of Agricultural Science, Cambridge*, **90**, 139–47.

Hodgson, J. (1975) The influence of grazing pressure and stocking rate on herbage intake and performance. In *Pasture Utilisation by the Grazing Animal* (ed. by J. Hodgson & D.K. Jackson), Occasional Symposium No. 8, British Grassland Society, pp. 93–103.

Lonsdale, C.R. (1989) *Straights: Raw Materials for Animal Feed Compounders and Farmers*. Chalcombe Publications, Lincoln, pp. 1–87.

Ministry of Agriculture, Fisheries and Food (1975) *Energy Allowances and Feeding Systems for Ruminants*. Technical Bulletin 33. HMSO, London, pp. 1–79.

Ministry of Agriculture, Fisheries and Food (1984) *Energy Allowances and Feeding Systems for Ruminants*. Technical Bulletin 433. HMSO, London, pp. 1–85.

Ministry of Agriculture, Fisheries and Food (1986a) *Nutrient Allowances for Cattle and Sheep*. P2087. HMSO, London, pp. 1–6.

Ministry of Agriculture, Fisheries and Food (1986b) *Feed Composition*. Chalcombe Publications, Marlow Bottom, Bucks, pp. 1–69.

Ministry of Agriculture, Fisheries and Food (1992) *Feed Composition, UK Tables of Feed Composition and Nutritive Value for Ruminants*, 2nd edn. Chalcombe Publications, Canterbury, Kent, pp. 1–99.

Orskov, E.R. (1998) *The Feeding of Ruminants: Principles and Practice*, 2nd edn. Chalcombe Publications, Lincoln, pp. 1–90.

Osbourn, D.F. (1967) The intake of conserved forages. In *Fodder Conservation* (ed. by R.J. Wilkins), Occasional Symposium No. 3, British Grassland Society, pp. 20–28.

Stark, B.A. and Lonsdale, C.R. (1989) Straights for compounders and farmers In: *Ruminant Feed Evaluation and Utilisation* (ed. by B.A. Stark, J.M. Wilkinson & D.I. Givens), Chalcombe Publications, Lincoln.

Van Soest, P.J. (1994) *Nutritional Ecology of the Ruminant*, 2nd edn. Cornell University Press, New York, pp. 1–476.

Wilkinson, J.M. (1985) *Beef Production from Silage and Other Conserved Forages*. Longman, London, pp. 1–140.

Wilkinson, J.M. (1990) *Silage UK*, 6th edn. Chalcombe Publications, Lincoln, pp. 1–185.

Chapter 10
Alternative Forages

M. Tame and the late P.S. Jarvis

Introduction	123
Forage maize (corn)	123
Fodder beet	124
Swedes	125
Stubble turnips (leaves and roots)	125
Kale	125
Forage rape	126
Lucerne	126
Red clover	127
White clover	128
Peas	129
Sainfoin	129
Lupins	129
Rye	129
Triticale	130
Whole crop silage: whole wheat	130
Whole crop cereal with peas	130
Wet byproducts used in dairy cow rations	131

Introduction

The main forage crops in the UK and many other countries for cattle are conserved grass in the form of hay or silage, otherwise straw. Economic and nutritional considerations have led to a quest for alternative forages.

Feeding dairy cows, dairy heifers, suckler cows and beef animals is a mixture of science and art. Any ration needs to be balanced for energy, protein, minerals, vitamins and water, to meet the required production objectives. Energy sources will include starches, sugars and digestible fibre, whilst protein will be of rumen degradable and digestible undegradable protein and will contain a wide range of amino acids. The ration must be palatable, digestible, appetizing and free from dirt, stones, harmful bacteria and moulds. Some feeds are enhancers of dry matter intake (DMI), whilst others substitute for existing ingredients in the ration. Thus brewers' grains, sodium hydroxide-treated straw, maize, etc., are enhancers of DMI whereas, for example, barley and wheat substitute for each other.

The UK Ministry of Agriculture, Fisheries and Food and the Agricultural and Food Research Council have published standards for energy, protein and the major minerals for maintenance and production for lactating and fattening animals. Knowledge is incomplete, and the art of feeding stock relates to adjusting feeds, introducing different ingredients and measuring and observing the results.

The figures shown in Table 10.1 act as a starting point in the compilation of dairy cow rations, particularly as feeds can vary in analysis. Alternative forages will need to fit the criteria laid down for each animal's production. However some forages, such as maize and lucerne, are DMI enhancers and so they can be perfectly satisfactory at lower energy densities in winter rations.

Dairy heifers, calving at two years old, need to grow at 0.7–0.8 kg/head daily to attain a satisfactory calving weight, and beef animals in the final stages of fattening require growth rates in excess of 1 kg/head daily.

Total farm profitability determines whether or not alternative forages feature in a farming system. Factors to be considered include soil type, labour availability, working and fixed capital requirements, value for money, yield variability, rotational considerations and feeding facilities. The majority feature in winter rations, but kale and stubble turnips are often grazed in the summer and early autumn, while lucerne and red clover are versatile protein sources in the summer. They can be grazed (with caution because of bloat) or conserved as silage. Red clover is usually in a grass ley mixture, but lucerne is generally grown as a pure stand.

A brief description will be given of some of the crops available together with their use and integration into cattle rations.

Forage maize (corn)

The typical analysis of forage maize silage per kg dry matter (DM) is:

DM = 28 per cent, metabolizable energy (ME) = 10.8 MJ, digestible crude protein (DCP) = 70 g, neutral detergent fibre (NDF) = 360 g, modified acid detergent fibre (MADF) = 215 g

Minerals: Ca = 3.9 g, P = 1.8 g, Na = 0.2 g, Mg = 2.4 g

Yield on National Institute of Agricultural Botany (NIAB) plots = 12.0 t DM/ha

Table 10.1 Winter ration criteria for Friesian/Holstein dairy cows.

	Milk yield (kg/day)			
	35	**25**	**18**	**Dry**
Minimum DM (%)	38	33	26	22
Energy density	12.0	11.4	10.8	9.5
Minimum MADF fibre (%)	15	18	22	25
Approximate DMI	20.9	17.1	14.7	9.3

Note: protein guidelines are 400 g DCP for maintenance and 60–65 g DCP/kg milk, with sufficient undegradable as well as degradable protein in the ration.

For Jersey cows with milk yields of 25, 18, 13 and 9 kg respectively, the protein requirements are 350 g DCP for maintenance and 70–75 g DCP/kg of milk.

Maize silage is best stored in long, narrow clamps to limit the amount of heating and hence spoilage when the clamp is opened. Most maize is grown in the southern counties of Britain but as more early-maturing varieties are being bred, the frontiers are being pushed further north.

The true value of maize (corn) is often underestimated by conventional equations. Maize silage costs less to produce than grass silage, and is complementary to it. In a dull, wet summer, the ME can be under 10 but is still as good as most grass silages made in similar weather. Generally, it is a high-energy, low-protein conserved forage that has limited fibre and is low in minerals, particularly calcium, phosphorus, sodium, copper, zinc, iodine and manganese. The greater the proportion of maize in the ration, the more deficiencies need to be corrected.

A typical ration for a dairy cow yielding 25 kg milk might include 32 kg grass silage, 14 kg maize silage, 1 kg soya bean meal, 5.5 kg maize gluten and 0.15 kg high phosphorus minerals. Research work, particularly by Phipps (pers. comm.), has shown that by including at least 25 per cent of the silage as maize increases forage DMI, lowers the cost and increases milk production and hence the weight of fat and protein. The response is greater with 63 per cent digestibility ('D' value) silage compared with 68 D grass silage. With a ration based on 40:60 grass:maize silage and 6 kg concentrates, DMI and milk yield were increased by 2.8 and 2.9 kg respectively compared with grass silage and 6 kg concentrates. Maize silage combines well with lucerne silage, but needs an addition of 1–2 kg straw to provide fibre.

Maize silage can be used as the sole source of forage for dairy cows. An example ration for a cow producing 25 kg milk would be 27 kg maize silage, 3.5 kg caustic treated straw, 2 kg molasses, 2 kg sugar beet pulp, 3 kg maize gluten, 2.5 kg rapeseed meal, 1.5 kg soya bean meal and 0.3 kg mineral/vitamin supplement. As the DM of maize silage increases, so does the DMI.

Maize silage can be introduced to young cattle at under three months old, but additional protein, vitamins and minerals are necessary. Typically, a 300 kg heifer growing at 0.65 kg/day requires 5.1 kg DM of maize silage, 0.2 kg 50 per cent vegetable protein and one per cent non-protein nitrogen (urea) added to maize silage; 1 kg of a 34 per cent protein/mineral/vitamin supplement would also be suitable.

Bull beef animals have higher intakes of maize than grass silage. A beast weighing 300 kg needs 6 kg DM of maize silage plus 1.5 kg of a 34 per cent protein/mineral/vitamin concentrate supplement to gain 1 kg/day. This quantity of supplement is kept constant over a range of weights so that the crude protein of the complete ration declines as the animal matures.

Maize fits well into a grass silage system and can be self-fed or forage-box fed. It can be fed as a green crop prior to harvest, and used as a buffer feed in spring for cows at pasture.

Fodder beet

The typical analysis of fodder beet per kg DM is:

DM = 18.3 per cent, ME = 11.9 MJ, DCP = 34 g,
   NDF = 127 g, MADF = 83 g
Minerals: Ca = 3.9 g, P = 1.8 g, Na = 2.4 g, Mg = 1.4 g
Yield on NIAB plots = 14.2 t DM/ha (excluding the
   value of fodder beet tops (leaves), which can add up
   to 30 per cent to the DM)

Ensiled tops are higher in protein minerals (especially phosphorus) and fibre and can complement the diet, but are difficult to harvest and utilize efficiently. Fresh tops can contain harmful oxalic acid and lead to calcium problems but the problem is reduced with wilting. Thus they can cause scouring and milk fever in freshly calved cows.

Fodder beet is used primarily as a low-cost concentrate replacer for dairy cows, at a maximum of 4–4.5 kg DM (22–25 kg fresh weight). As a high-energy source, it will need to be balanced by additional degradable and undegradable protein. In limited cases, it can be used as part of the maintenance ration but additional protein, fibre (as hay or straw) and minerals will be required.

For a dairy cow yielding 25 kg milk, with 40 kg grass silage producing more than maintenance, 15 kg of fodder beet, 4 kg maize gluten and 2.25 kg of a proprietary 20 per cent protein, high-energy concentrate complete the ration. A mix of other dry concentrates such as barley and soya bean meal can replace maize gluten.

Harvested fodder beet can be fed from a hopper or behind an electric fence provided that sufficient feed space is available to avoid uneven intakes between cows in the herd. It is more commonly fed as part of a complete diet in a forage wagon, but the beet must be free from dirt and preferably finely chopped or shredded to integrate in the ration.

Strip-grazing beet in the field produces a multitude of problems: poisoning from tops (even when topped this can be via secondary growth in the spring), waste of feed and foot troubles (see Chapter 31).

When used as a concentrate replacer, fodder beet enhances the butterfat and protein percentages in the milk, but observations suggest that it depletes the compositional quality when used as part of the maintenance ration.

A combination of fodder beet and soya bean meal can add to DMI and hence milk yield and quality, particularly replacing a 10.8 ME grass silage. The grass silage uptake has been shown to decrease from 9.6 to 7.0 kg DM/cow per day. When fodder beet was added to a poorer silage and with no soyabean meal, compositional quality was not improved. As well as lowering the ration cost, fodder beet partially acts as a concentrate replacer.

Fodder beet should be finely chopped or shredded in the rations for dairy heifers over one year old when they are changing their teeth. For these animals average grass silage up to 2 kg DM (11 kg fresh weight) of fodder beet can be fed in place of sugar beet pulp to ensure good growth rates and conception. Using a straw-based ration, a 300 kg heifer growing at 0.8 kg/day could receive 3 kg straw, 14 kg fodder beet, 1.2 kg barley and 1 kg soya bean meal. If ammonia or urea-treated straw is used, 11 kg fodder beet and 1 kg barley could produce the desired results. Alternatively, 2 kg DM from both fodder beet and brewers' grains with *ad libitum* straw should produce a palatable and productive ration. Amounts will, of course, be increased as the animals grow.

Gleadthorpe Experimental Husbandry Farm (1984, 1985) developed a fodder beet system that utilised its low cost when compared with concentrates for Friesian × Hereford heifers and steers. Crushed beet was introduced when the animals weighed 200 kg. Both fishmeal and soyabean meal have been used as the protein sources with minerals and straw also added if necessary.

In many cases, fodder beet requires much additional capital for sowing, harvesting, storing, cleaning and chopping the beet, but it can be grown in most areas of the UK and other temperate areas. In a wet autumn on heavy soils, harvesting can be difficult, but it is a relatively cheap source of energy. Mangels, which have a DM of 10–15 per cent, are in the main similar to fodder beet for feeding but crop yield is less.

Swedes

The typical analysis of swedes per kg DM is:

DM = 10.5 per cent, ME = 13.1 MJ, DCP = 64 g,
NDF = 140 g, MADF = 114 g
Minerals: Ca = 3.5 g, P = 2.6 g, Na = 1.5 g, Mg = 1.1 g
Yield on NIAB plots = 7 t DM/ha

The crop is generally grown in the cooler west and north of Britain. Fungal problems such as powdery mildew and club-root can limit crop yields.

Swedes have a low protein and high energy content, but a relatively low yield of DM. They are used primarily for beef and sheep as well as for human consumption.

Swedes could be utilized by dairy cows on a similar DM basis to fodder beet, but are more costly to produce. Despite their low DM (10.5 per cent) they are likely to be DMI enhancers. Similarly, they can be fed to dairy heifers by incorporation in straw-based rations. The low DM of swedes could assist consumption, but chopping or slicing is advantageous. Swedes may be grazed *in situ*, especially by sheep.

Stubble turnips (leaves and roots)

The typical analysis of stubble turnips per kg DM is:

DM = 8.0 per cent, ME = 11.6 MJ, DCP = 130 g
Figures for fibre levels and minerals are not available
Yield on NIAB plots = 3.8 DM/ha (relates to the tops and that portion of the root that is above ground)

These quick-growing turnips are a very useful catch crop being sown in the spring as a prelude to a grass reseed in the autumn or after winter barley in July as a break crop.

Stubble turnips are grazed by dairy cows *in situ* behind an electric fence in midsummer and autumn, particularly where grass production is limited. In the summer, stubble turnips and *ad libitum* ammonia-treated straw complement grass, while in the early autumn the same combination can substitute for a limited amount of silage on free-draining soils. Stubble turnips can also be fed to sheep and suckler cows, but are little used for dairy heifers and beef animals because they are unlikely to be constrained by an electric fence. The cost per unit of energy is similar to grazed grass. Fungal problems such as powdery mildew and alternaria leaf spot can limit crop yields.

Kale

The typical analysis for kale per kg DM is:

DM = 13.6 per cent, ME = 12.6 MJ, DCP = 119 g,
 NDF = 208 g, MADF = 161 g
Minerals: Ca = 12.1 g, P = 3.5 g, Na = 1.2 g, Mg = 1.4 g
 (varieties differ in analysis)
Yield on NIAB plots = 8.6 t DM/ha

Kale can be grown in most areas of the UK but yields can be adversely affected by dry weather.

Protein and minerals are contained in the leaves and carbohydrates and fibre occur in the stem. Thus, the proportion of leaf to stem influences the feed value of kale.

Kale is a low DM, high-protein feed that is high in calcium, but low in phosphorus, copper, manganese and iodine. Goitrogens can interfere with iodine use in the dairy cow (see pp. 257, 586). Excessive amounts of kale can lead to haemolytic anaemia (see p. 941).

In the past, kale was strip-grazed in the autumn and up to midwinter and, together with hay, provided the maintenance portion of the dairy cows' ration. The practice has been largely curtailed as herds moved towards autumn calving, and a continuity of feed during the winter season became necessary. In addition, foot troubles were very common and udders needed additional washing. Currently, kale is grazed *in situ* in the summer and early autumn in a similar fashion to stubble turnips with ammonia-treated straw. It tends to be fed to mid- and late-lactation cows and should not exceed 30 per cent of the ration. In practice, 3–4 kg DM/head per day are consumed together with 1–2 kg of ammonia-treated straw. Kale can be cut and carted to all classes of stock, and may be strip-grazed by sheep in winter.

Forage rape

The typical analysis of forage rape per kg DM is:

DM = 14 per cent, ME = 9.5 MJ, DCP = 144 g
 (no fibre figures are available)
Minerals: Ca = 9.3 g, P = 4.2 g, Na = 2.3 g, Mg = 2.1 g
Yield on NIAB plots = 5.4 t DM/ha

Rape can be grown in most areas of the UK. Forage rape can be used as a catch crop like stubble turnips and kale but is lower yielding than the latter and higher yielding than the former. The principles of feeding and the reservations on use of forage rape are similar to kale. Forage rape can cause taints in milk and should be introduced into the ration slowly. It can be grazed *in situ* from July to December, or be zero-grazed.

Lucerne

The typical analysis of lucerne silage per kg DM is:

DM = 29 per cent, ME = 9.5 MJ, DCP = 134 g,
 NDF = 464 g, MADF = 357 g
Minerals: it is claimed to be high in minerals, except sodium, and to have good buffering capacity in the rumen. Ca = 17.6 g, P = 3.0 g, Mg = 1.8 g
Yield on NIAB plots = 14.7 t DM /ha

Lucerne (alfalfa) is now the most important forage crop on a worldwide basis. While some 1 million ha are suitable for the crop in the UK, only around 22 000 ha are cultivated. The crop grows best in areas where the night temperature remains above 10°C and where daytime temperature is in the range 15–25°C. It is an erect, deep-rooting and hence very drought tolerant crop which is well suited to cutting. The exceptionally deep rooting habit requires a well-fissured alkaline subsoil. The soils also need to be free draining as the plant is not tolerant of a high water table. Top soil pH should be maintained at 6.2 or higher, preferably above 6.5 as root nodulation does not occur at pH levels below 6.2. Lucerne is not a competitive crop (Sheldrick *et al.*, 1995).

The advantages of lucerne are its reduced fertilizer requirement (it fixes very high levels of nitrogen); its persistence (it will stand regular cutting for up to 5 years); its drought resistance; its high protein level (up to 24% protein at tight bud stage); its high digestibility; the slow fall in D value; its low level of lignification and its high levels of calcium and vitamins A and E (Koivisto, 1999, pers. comm.).

Its disadvantages are that in the small seedling stage it is frost susceptible. It is not tolerant of wet conditions requiring a free draining soil. It is susceptible to stem eelworm and sitona weevil and some varieties are susceptible to verticillium wilt. In some conditions downy mildew and various leaf spots may occur.

All seed should be checked to ensure that it has been fumigated against stem eelworm and all seed should be inoculated with *Rhizobium meliloti* in areas where it has not been grown in the last few years. A seed rate of 20–25 kg/ha is recommended, except in particularly favourable areas where the rate may be reduced to 15–20 kg/ha. The target seedling density should be 425 plants per square metre, although a mature stand may only have 120–150 plants per square metre. The crop should be sown between late April and the first week in August. Lucerne should not be sown with grass as the latter is too competitive.

Another disadvantage is its low yield in the establishment year, although this can be overcome by undersowing it into a spring cereal crop or a semi-leafless pea crop. After establishing the nurse crop and controlling weeds the lucerne should be broadcast and either rolled or raked in. Alternatively the two crops can be drilled at the same time, although this makes weed control more difficult. If there is adequate late summer/early autumn rainfall the crop can be established in late summer, no later than mid-August, after a winter cereal crop.

Decaying lucerne roots exude chemicals known as medicarpins which inhibit germination of lucerne so it is not possible to 'stitch in' seed to fill areas where the crop has died out.

Fertilizer requirements are relatively low as there is no requirement for nitrogen after establishment. The main requirements are for phosphate and particularly potash.

Lucerne is ideally suited to a cutting regime. The crop should be allowed to flower before the first cut and should then be cut at intervals of 35–40 days, with the last cut being made in September to allow at least 6 weeks for recovery before the first frost. After the first frosts the crop will normally stop growing, at which time it is safe either to cut or lightly graze the crop. The ideal cutting time is mid-bud stage.

Dry matter yields from a well-established crop of lucerne under ideal conditions could be as high as 14 tonnes dry matter/ha, although average yields will be 10–12 tonnes dry matter/ha. The first cut is normally expected to contribute about 35 per cent of the total, with the second, third and fourth cuts contributing 35, 20 and 10 per cent, respectively.

Ensiling lucerne is more difficult than grass silage as the sugar levels are much lower and for ensiling to be successful it is strongly recommended that the crop is wilted to 30 per cent dry matter. If the dry matter prior to ensiling is much higher than this there is a very real danger that losses will be high as a result of leaf shatter.

Lucerne is not usually grazed because of the risk of bloat, although there are instances where it has been grazed successfully. This requires a slow introduction and all the usual precautions to avoid tympany.

Because of its ability to fix large amounts of nitrogen and its very deep and extensive root system lucerne is well suited to organic systems, although its inclusion in a rotation will extend it considerably.

Red clover

The typical analysis for red clover silage per kg DM is:

DM = 22 per cent, ME = 9.8 MJ, DCP = 135 g

Figures are not available for the fibre levels and mineral content, but like lucerne, red clover has high intake characteristics and the ME is likely to be close to 10 MJ/kg DM

Yield on NIAB plots = 13.5 t DM for first harvest year, and 11.1 t/ha for the second harvest year

The use of red clover declined dramatically to the late 1990s. However, the recent interest in organic farming has spearheaded a revival of interest in the last five years.

Red clover yields well on a range of soils with a pH of 6 or higher and adequate soil moisture. Summer rainfall is also a prerequisite for good yields. Water-logged soils, on the other hand, should be avoided and heavy soils subject to structural damage from smearing and the use of heavy machinery will shorten the life of the crop. Unlike white clover, red clover does not produce stolons (runners) and has a single crown to the plant that is susceptible to damage.

As a general rule red clover is sown with Italian rye grass and with the more modern varieties a fairly aggressive rye grass is required as the clover tends to take over in the second year. Seed rates are usually around 3 kg/ha with a target plant density of 200/m^2. It is important that the red clover seed is fumigated against stem eelworm. Modern varieties will usually give two heavy cuts, with a third lighter cut over the first two years. There is a significant decline in productivity in year three, although the new variety Milvus is claimed to give good production over a three-year period. Growing red clover with Italian rye grass will not only give a heavier crop, by up to 30 per cent annually, but also raise overall digestibility. Annual yields of dry matter are usually in the range 9–12 tonnes/ha for pure stands and 11–13 tonnes/ha when grown with companion grasses. Yields in organic systems will be almost, if not as high as in conventional systems because of the high levels of nitrogen fixed. Red clover can fix up to 245 kg nitrogen/ha (Lampkin, 1990).

Red clover is sensitive to soil potash levels as large amounts are removed from the field under cutting. Potash level can be improved by the appropriate use of slurries to which it responds well. If high protein levels are to be achieved in the first cut the use of some artificial nitrogen may be necessary as nitrogen fixation by clovers is temperature dependent and in cold and wet seasons little nitrogen may be fixed before the first cut is made. The protein level in the first cut material is often very low in organic systems where the use of artificial nitrogen is not permitted. However, it has usually increased to around 18–20 per cent by the time the second cut is made.

The low levels of sugar in clover can lead to poor fermentation in ensiled crops of pure red clover. Ensiling grass/red clover is often more successful because of the sugar contributed from the grass. The quality of the fermentation is also likely to be improved by wilting the crop to approximately 30 per cent dry matter whenever possible, but care should be taken not to exceed this as leaf loss due to shattering occurs above this level. If the material has to be ensiled at a significantly lower dry matter the use of an inoculant is recommended.

Weed control can be a problem as red clover is sensitive to many of the herbicides currently available. Control of weeds in organic systems is often achieved by undersowing into a spring cereal nurse crop, a technique which could also be used in conventional systems.

A gap of at least four and preferably five years should be allowed between red clover crops to reduce the risk of pests and diseases, particularly stem eelworm and *Verticillium*.

The risk of bloat in cattle is reputedly higher with red clover swards than white clover swards and as a result red clover is grazed less frequently (p. 833). However, with careful management it can be avoided. The red clover should be introduced slowly and once introduced it should be a consistent component of the diet. The risk is highest in cold wet weather and when the animals are particularly hungry. Lambs in particular grow very well on grass/red clover swards and increased growth rates can also be achieved with young stock and beef cattle (Thomas *et al.*, 1982).

Because of its ability to fix large amounts of nitrogen, red clover is an important part of the fertility building cycle in organic systems.

White clover

In the last few years interest in white clover has increased significantly and it is increasingly being used in grazing swards. Again, interest has been fuelled by the increasing interest in organic husbandry.

Varieties tend to be classified according to leaf size, with the smaller leafed varieties being more suited to sheep grazing and the larger leafed varieties being more suited to cattle grazing and/or conservation. More recently, varieties have been introduced which are more cold tolerant, resulting in earlier growth and nitrogen fixation. Soil pH should again be 6 or higher for good germination and growth, and on some soils this may mean the regular application of lime to maintain this pH.

White clover is much longer-lived than red clover and will typically be expected to survive for six years or more under good management. Typical seed mixtures will contain between 1 and 2 kg/ha in a total mix of 12 kg/ha (the total seed rate may need to be higher in adverse conditions, e.g. low rainfall and light soils). White clover seed is very small and germinates more successfully if broadcast on to the surface rather than being drilled into the seedbed. Grass varieties need to be chosen with care to avoid either the grass or the clover becoming the dominant species. Work in this area has been done by the Kingshay Trust, from whom recommendations are available to its members.

Production levels from grass/white clover swards are lower than from grass/red clover swards and are likely to be of the order of 6 tonnes of dry matter/ha with no artificial nitrogen input to 7.6 tonnes/ha with 200 kg artificial nitrogen/ha. However, at this level the clover content of the second cut will be suppressed (Sheldrick *et al.*, 1995). These same authors state that under ideal conditions herbage yields equivalent to those from grass swards receiving in excess of 300 kg nitrogen/ha have been recorded. It is recommended that no more than 50 kg of nitrogen/ha is used. In organic systems where the use of artificial nitrogen is not permitted it should be noted that the protein content of the first cut is often very low, particularly in cold and wet seasons when it is typically between 10 and 12 per cent (Weller & Cooper, 2001; Tame, pers. obs.).

The proportion of grass to clover can be managed to some extent by alternating cutting with grazing. The growth of the white clover is light sensitive; allowing the sward to grow will mean that eventually the clover will be shaded out as the grass grows taller. This is particularly so in autumn and early spring when the temperatures are low enough to suppress clover growth but not grass growth. The clover content can be increased by an intensive grazing and/or cutting regime, although the proportion of clover increases naturally through the season (Weller & Cooper, 2001). Ensiling grass/white clover is less difficult than grass/red clover because of the generally lower clover content and higher sugar level contributed by the grass, but even so wilting to around 30 per cent dry matter is again recommended. At dry matter levels much higher than this leaf shatter will be a problem.

Weed control can be a problem in newly established swards, particularly with annual weeds such as chickweed. This can be controlled by the careful use of an appropriate herbicide, although most will have some adverse effect on the clover. In organic systems successful control is achieved by the use of mechanical control or by undersowing into a nurse crop of spring cereals.

Grass/white clover swards are used principally for grazing and it is worth noting that milk production will be 1–1.5 litres/cow higher from a grass/clover sward than from an all-grass sward.

Care needs to be taken in the autumn to ensure that late grazing by sheep does not damage the stolons of the clover as such damage may result in a loss of clover in the following spring.

White clover also plays an important part in soil fertility building in organic systems because of its ability to fix nitrogen even though it fixes less than red clover, 150 kg/ha under good conditions (Lampkin, 1990).

Peas

The typical analysis for pea silage per kg DM is:

DM = 25.9 per cent, ME = 8.8 MJ, DCP = 146 g,
   NDF = 517 g, MADF = 384 g
Minerals: Ca = 12.7 g, P = 4.4 g, Na = 0.4 g, Mg = 2.0 g
Yield (estimated) = 7 t DM/ha

Pea silage can be a byproduct from the production of vining peas and may be more like straw. Peas can also be grown on their own, but need some physical support and are usually sown in conjunction with spring barley on the basis of 40:60 peas:barley by seed weight. Newman & Luffman (1984) have produced the arable silage mixture (barley was cut at the cheesy stage) with a DM of 43.2 per cent, ME of 10.2 MJ and DCP of 147 g. They observed that the silage yield at 10 t DM/ha was very palatable. Depending on the stage of lactation, when fed to 200 dairy cows in Somerset, it produced rises in DMI between 10 and 20 per cent over grass silage. (Dry matter intake of grass silage tends to be in the range of 7–10 kg depending on the quality and quantity of the silage.) The arable silage mixture can also be fed to dairy heifers and beef animals. Peas are not an easy crop to establish and whole crop cereal silage may be preferred.

Sainfoin

A typical analysis for sainfoin silage per kg DM is:

DM = 24 per cent, ME = 8.4 MJ, DCP = 124 g
Figures for fibre and minerals are not available
Yield (estimated) = 7.5 t DM/ha

Sanfoin is a little grown crop although there has been some revival of interest in the last few years. A research programme is currently under way at the Royal Agricultural College at Cirencester (Lane & Koivisto, 1999). In most aspects the requirements, establishment and management of sanfoin are very similar to those for lucerne.

The main differences are that the most commonly available varieties of sanfoin are significantly less productive than lucerne with fewer cuts. However, some recent varieties that will soon be available from Eastern Europe, notably Hungary, may well be almost as productive as lucerne. Another difference which has significant practical and nutritional implications is that sanfoin has a relatively high tannin level which means that there is no risk of bloat from grazing it. Indeed, very high growth rates have been achieved in lambs grazing sanfoin (Koivisto, pers. comm.). It is also likely that the tannin content of sanfoin may have the effect of reducing the rate of protein breakdown in the rumen.

Again sanfoin is well suited to organic systems although, like lucerne, its inclusion in a rotation will extend the length of the rotation considerably.

Lupins

Interest in this crop has been growing in recent years particularly as large areas are grown in continental Europe, 60 000 ha in northern Germany alone, and particularly in Australia, 1 million ha. While the crop is normally grown as a grain crop it can also be harvested as a forage crop. When cut at ten to twelve weeks post-emergence it gives a high yield of good quality forage. Crude protein levels may be as high as 20 per cent, with a good energy level and up to 20–25 per cent starch.

Recommended types are the white, apically dominant varieties or the yellow branched varieties. The crop is tolerant of a wide range of soil types provided that the pH is within the range 5–7. The crop should be sown from mid-March to mid-April. The seed rate will depend on type and the seed should be inoculated. Weeds need to be controlled in the early stages of the crop. Yields as high as 10 tonnes of dry matter/ha have been reported, although it is too early to know whether this is typical under UK conditions.

Lupins seem to be particularly well suited to organic systems because of the high level of nitrogen fixation and the fact that the crop is in the ground for such a short time means it fits well into rotations.

Rye

The typical analysis for grazed rye per kg DM is:

DM = 23 per cent, ME = 9.5 MJ, DCP = 88 g
Figures are not yet available for fibre and mineral
   content
Yield (estimated) = 7.7 t DM/ha

Rye is grown on its own or in a mixture with Italian ryegrass to produce an early bite in the spring on light land with a low pH. It is usually strip-grazed by dairy cows once daily and its feed value often decreases rapidly. Zero-grazing is possible. Any surplus can be conserved as big bale silage and used for any class of stock. In some areas it is followed by forage maize and could be drilled after an early maturing variety of maize in the autumn. Many dairy farmers prefer buffer feeding of silage in late spring or other combinations of feed as an alternative to growing small areas of rye.

Triticale

Feed analysis figures are not available for triticale, which is a hybrid of wheat and rye. Triticale can perform a similar function to rye, and is said to have lower DM yields than rye in the earlier part of the season, but its digestibility stays at a higher level than rye as the crop matures. Feeding value is likely to be similar to whole crop silage. If cut in mid June, it can have a DM of 25 per cent and an ME of 9.6 MJ. Both sugar and fibre levels are higher than grass.

Whole crop silage: whole wheat

A typical analysis for whole wheat silage (Newman, pers. comm.) per kg DM is:

DM = 50 per cent, ME = 10.7 MJ,
   crude protein = 9 per cent, NDF = 400 g, pH = 8
Yield (estimated range) = 7–10 t DM/ha

There has been a considerable increase in interest in whole crop cereal silage over the last decade both in fermented and in urea-treated form.

The addition of whole crop cereal silage to the diets of both cattle and dairy cows results in a significant increase in dry matter intake, particularly with the urea-treated form. However, there are some very significant differences between the two forms.

The fermented form of whole crop has the advantage that it has a much higher digestibility and results in a larger increase in milk output and a small increase in milk quality, mainly in butterfat. The disadvantage is that it is lower in protein and is aerobically unstable, although this latter disadvantage can be overcome to some extent by adequate chopping, good consolidation and good clamp management.

Urea-treated whole crop has the advantages that there is a large increase in dry matter intake, it is aerobically stable and the added urea results in a higher nitrogen content. However, the disadvantage is that the digestibility, particularly of the starch, appears to be much lower and the large increase in dry matter intake is reflected in only a small increase in milk output and quality (Sutton *et al.*, 1997). As a result urea treatment of whole crop cereal silage is not recommended.

The objective should be to grow the crop as for a good grain yield with winter wheat being sown at a rate of 150–200 kg/ha and spring wheat at up to 240 kg/ha. If a spring crop is to be undersown the seed rate should be roughly half the figure just given. There will of course be a yield penalty with the lower sowing rate. Winter wheat should be harvested at between five and six weeks after ear emergence and at a dry matter of 35–40 per cent (Kristensen, 1995). Winter barley should be harvested slightly earlier at four to five weeks post ear emergence and at a dry matter of 30–35 per cent. However, in the UK the suggestion is that winter wheat can be harvested at up to 45 per cent dry matter (MDC, 1995). Yields for winter wheat are 10–12 tonnes dry matter/ha with conventional systems and 6–10 tonnes in organic systems depending on where it is placed in the rotation and whether it is undersown with grass/clover. If the dry matter is much higher than 50 per cent it is likely that grain will be excreted, undigested, the amount increasing with higher dry matter.

Whole crop cereal is well suited to use as a buffer feed to supplement grazing in the summer, particularly in organic systems where its starch and low protein content can be used to balance the very high levels of degradable protein in the grass/clover swards from mid-summer onwards. Indeed, whole crop cereal silages fit very well into organic systems as a whole as the early harvest allows a grass/clover ley to be established in August. It also allows a degree of flexibility in the system as it can be taken either for grain or for forage depending on the season.

Whole crop cereal with peas

The major disadvantage with whole crop cereal silages is that they are low in protein. This can be overcome to a greater or lesser extent by growing whole crop cereals as a bi-crop with peas. The target should be for at least 40 per cent peas in the crop. The peas should be a short-strawed, coloured, flowered variety. Sowing rate will depend on the proportion of peas required, but with a 50:50 mix the seed rates would be around 125 kg/ha wheat and 270 kg/ha peas depending on variety and seed size.

The crop should be harvested at 14–15 weeks post sowing when the cereal grain is at the doughy stage and the pea seed is at the yellow wrinkled stage. The protein and starch are optimized at this stage (Adesogan, pers. comm.). When harvested at this stage the silage should have a crude protein content of 16–18 per cent, with 40 per cent peas in the mix. If higher crude protein levels are required the proportion of peas should be increased. In the same study digestibility is reported to be higher than grass silage when fed to sheep. A further trial showed that the total intake, milk yield and milk composition of cows fed whole crop/pea silage was higher than or comparable with cows fed first-cut/ryegrass silage and 4 kg more concentrate. As with fermented whole crop, the silage needs to be very well consolidated in the clamp and clamp management at feed-out must be very good.

Table 10.2 Analysis of byproducts fed to dairy cattle.

Food	DM (%)	ME (MJ)	DCP (g)	NDF (g)	MADF (g)	Ca (g)	P (g)	Na (g)	Mg (g)
Brewers' grains	22.0	11.7	189	572	219	3.3	4.1	0.1	1.5
Cabbage	10.6	13.7	181	586	140	7.2	4.5	1.2	1.5
Carrots	13.0	12.8	62	–[a]	–	5.9	3.4	0.8	1.8
Parsnips	15.0	13.3	67	–	–	–	–	–	–
Potatoes	20.4	13.3	80	73	39	0.4	2.0	0.2	1.0
Pressed sugar beet pulp	25.4	12.3	60	557	259	9.0	1.1	0.6	2.0
Apples	13.6	12.2	–	111	101	0.5	0.9	0.1	0.3
Apple pomace	23.0	8.7	–	503	375	1.7	1.4	0.2	0.6

[a] –, no reliable information available.

Yields under a conventional system should be around 11–12 tonnes dry matter/ha, while under organic management it should be 7–10 tonnes of dry matter/ha.

Wet byproducts used in dairy cow rations

The products shown in Table 10.2 can be incorporated in winter rations for dairy cows and other stock. They are likely to be fed with straw and other ingredients for other cattle, and to supplement grass silage and act as a concentrate replacer for dairy cows.

Vegetable waste, e.g. Brussels sprouts, cabbages and cauliflowers from vegetable processing plants, could have a similar feed value to kale. Potato waste, pressed sugar beet, peas and beans are occasionally available. Good storage facilities and the avoidance of waste are necessary for the above products. They will all need to fit in with the ration criteria for the appropriate class of stock.

References

Gleadthorpe Experimental Husbandry Farm (1984) In *Gleadthorpe Experimental Husbandry Farm Annual Review*, pp. 15–17.

Gleadthorpe Experimental Husbandry Farm (1985) In *Gleadthorpe Experimental Husbandry Farm Annual Review*, pp. 38–40.

Kristensen, V.F. (1995) The production and feeding of whole crop cereals in Denmark. In *Whole-Crop Cereals* (ed. by B.A. Stark & J.M. Wilkinson). Chalcombe Publications, Lincoln, pp. 21–38.

Lampkin, N. (1990) Crop nutrition. In *Organic Farming*. Farming Press, p. 84.

Milk Development Council (MDC) (1995) *Making the Most of Whole Crop Cereals*. MDC.

Newman, G. & Luffman, B.J. (1984) Lucerne, red clover and forge peas: management, utilization and incorporation into feed systems. In *Occasional Symposium of the British Grassland Society* (ed. by D.S. Thompson), pp. 147–51.

Sheldrick, R.D., Newman, G. & Roberts, D.J. (1995) White clover. In *Legumes for Milk and Meat*. Chalcombe Publications, Lincoln, p. 27.

Sutton, D.J., Abdalla, A.L., Phipps, R.H., Cammell, S.B. & Humphries, D.J. (1997) The effect of replacement of grass silage by increasing proportions of urea treated whole crop wheat on food intake and apparent digestibility of milk products by dairy lows. *Animal Science*, **65**, 343.

Thomas, C., Aston, K., Daley, S.R. & Hughes, P.M. (1982) A comparison of red clover with grass silage for milk production. *British Society of Animal Production Winter Meeting, Harrogate*.

Thomas, C., Aston, K. & Daley, S.R. (1985) Milk production from silage, 3. A comparison of red clover and grass silage. *Animal Production* **41**, 23–31.

Weller, R.F. & Cooper, A. (2001) Seasonal changes in the crude protein concentration of mixed swards of white clover/perennial ryegrass grown without fertilizer N in an organic farming system in the United Kingdom. *Grass and Forage Science*, **56**, 92.

Wilkinson, J.M. & Stark, B.A. (1990) *Whole Crop Cereals – Making and Feeding Cereal Silage*. Chalcombe Publications, pp. 1–86.

Part 2
DISEASE

Chapter 11
Diagnosis and Differential Diagnosis in the Cow

R.G. Eddy and P.J.N. Pinsent

The clinical attitude	135
The clinician's approach to the clinical case	136
The clinical examination	136
The main presenting syndromes	138
Drooling at the mouth (kiddling, slobbering)	138
Vomiting	139
Acute abdominal pain (colic)	139
Acute abdominal distension	140
Anterior abdominal/posterior thoracic pain	142
Chronic bloat (chronic and subacute ruminal tympany)	146
The liver	147
Constipation	148
Diarrhoea	149
Tenesmus (straining)	150
The unthrifty or emaciated cow	150
The 'downer' cow	151
The cow ill during or after calving	151
Pyrexia of unknown origin (PUO)	151
Sudden death	152
Jugular stasis (cording)	153
'Redwater' (blood or blood pigments in urine)	154
Cows breathing badly (hyperpnoea and dyspnoea)	155
Acute nervous and convulsive syndromes	155

The clinical attitude

Veterinary clinicians must develop certain special attributes in relation to their environment. They must be inquisitive, questioning, curious and observant. They must notice everything around them, and, if possible, explain it. They must always be critical in the true sense of the word. They spend their lives diagnosing disease and must understand quite clearly that, as health is normality, then disease is simply deviation from normality. From this, it follows that veterinary surgeons will never be able to detect and recognize disease, i.e. deviation from the normal, until they know the normal. They must learn the normal in all domestic species in many different circumstances. For normality is relative, not absolute. It is relative to breed, age, nutrition, the stage of lactation or pregnancy, management and many other factors.

Thus normality is relative to environment. The veterinarian, therefore, must consider the environment as critically as he does the patient. Is it suitable? Does it predispose to, or even cause, the abnormality present in the patient? Does it cause stress? Remember that the environment can only be appreciated if one considers the animal's viewpoint: for example, if it is thought that the ventilation in a calf house is suspect, it may well be advisable to get your head down among the calves!

If it is accepted that disease is often related to environment, nutrition or management, then it follows that in an adverse environment other animals in the group may also be affected. In such circumstances, it is always well worthwhile looking carefully at the rest of the group, if necessary, animal by animal. It may well be that others are showing the same signs albeit to a lesser extent. Such an observation may be very helpful not only in diagnosis, but also from the viewpoints of treatment and prevention.

The veterinarians of today must concern themselves with the health of the herd as well as the individual and it is almost negligent to omit from the examination of the individual cow, a look, however brief, at the other stock in the group.

The other side of the coin is that, in unusual environmental conditions, when you are not certain whether the cow's response is normal or not, it is often very helpful to look at the rest of the group. If they are all showing the same response, then either they are all abnormal, which is unlikely, or they represent normality, in which case, the patient is also normal.

It should be remembered that the owner and his staff are an important part of the patient's environment, and can play a large part in the disease process and progress. They, equally with, or perhaps even more than, other environmental factors, merit critical assessment. Are they competent? Are they humane? Are they interested? Are they truthful? Have they contributed to the disease process? They merit critical study, for the staff are inextricably involved with their animals and the one cannot be considered without the other.

The important diagnostic principles that should always be followed are shown below.

(1) Be systematic.
(2) Adopt a routine that is found suitable and stick to it.
(3) Take nothing on trust.
(4) Apply continual critical assessment to oneself and monitor one's own attitudes and techniques.
(5) Consider all the time:
  (a) Is there a problem?
  (b) If so, then define it.
  (c) Having defined it, what is best done about it?

The clinician's approach to the clinical case

There is nothing magical about clinical work. It depends upon care, patience, thoroughness, method and logical routine; a routine of examination that covers all the likely eventualities. Once having evolved such a procedure, there should be no short cuts without good reason, and, however cursory some sections of the examination, for various reasons, sometimes have to be, nothing should be omitted without due consideration.

The clinical examination

The owner's message

The owner's message (usually termed the owner's complaint) should include name and full address, and may reach the clinician by direct word of mouth, by telephone or by mobile or radio telephone direct to his car. The owner's complaint will also include the type of animal and the main presenting syndrome, e.g. a scouring cow, a downer cow, a convulsing cow or a bloated cow. It is important to distinguish between the owner's complaint and his diagnosis. The owner's message will often be in the form of a diagnosis and the clinician must be aware that this will frequently be wrong. For example, a farmer may assume that a recumbent cow and recently calved will be suffering from milk fever. However, a full clinical examination may reveal acute mastitis or calving paralysis.

There are a limited number of main presenting syndromes, and the clinician should learn differential lists for each of them, to include only the major differential conditions, not the rarities. It should be remembered when considering the differential lists that the common things occur commonly; that is why they are common!

The clinician should know the main presenting syndrome and its differential list, and during the journey to the farm should consider the following points.

(1) The time of year. Many diseases are seasonal, e.g. the coughing calf indoors in November probably has a viral or bacterial based pneumonia, but the coughing calf at grass in August probably has husk.
(2) The part of the country. Each type of country has its own disease problems, e.g. in the hills one meets malignant catarrhal fever, bracken poisoning and piroplasmosis, while in intensive lowland dairying areas one meets coliform mastitis, milk fever and hypomagnesaemia.
(3) The individual farm. The clinician will often know that a specific farm has a particular disease problem, e.g. a parasitic problem among the young stock, because they are overcrowded and underfed.
(4) The type of management. For example, heavily stocked cubicle yards with straw bedding often lead to environmental mastitis.

Such patterns of disease become second nature to veterinary surgeons, and always hold good for the part of the country in which they work, although revision might be necessary in a practice 400 miles away.

The clinician will, therefore, arrive at the farm with a diagnosis already half formed. It will be adaptable, not dogmatic, a *working hypothesis*, to be confirmed or refuted; however, it is quite remarkable how often this hypothesis stands up to the test of full clinical examination, and, more importantly, refutes the presence of any other disease process.

Thus, if the clinician knows that the cow to be visited is showing convulsive signs at pasture, that it is early May, that it is an intensive dairy area in Britain the chances that the disease condition is anything other than hypomagnesaemia are too remote to be significant. Nevertheless, a clinical examination is always necessary.

History

History is all important and the foundation of diagnosis.

(1) Immediate history is the story of the present illness.
(2) Past history is anything in the animal's earlier life that may be relevant, e.g. calving and service dates, something similar at the same point in a previous lactation, and so on.
(3) Herd or group history is important when adverse nutritional or management factors may be relevant to the present illness.

History taking is an art – it does not come naturally, but must be learnt and practised. After a few pleasant introductory words, questioning can begin while walking to the animal, which may be approached, but should not, if at all possible, be disturbed. First, look. Check the owner's statements mentally by reference to the animal and the surroundings. Do not hurry the owner at first: let him or her talk, then ask your own questions, checking each statement and following a routine that suits you. You are not wasting time for you are, meanwhile, carrying out the next two parts of the clinical routine.

Do not ask leading questions in the hope of saving time, or in the hope of confirming one's half formed diagnosis, for they often produce inaccurate or misleading answers. Human nature being what it is, owners may either agree with you because they think they ought to, or disagree because they are contra-suggestive.

Study the owner or stockworkers. Are they reliable? Are they telling the truth? Are they covering up errors in management? Are they guessing? Every clinician must be interested in the human animal; after all, it is the owner whom you serve, advise, encourage or console. In a way, the owner is as much your patient as the cow. Admittedly, owners seldom deliberately falsify their story, but it is wise to beware the guilty one, the bombastic one, the one who knows it all or the one involved in the sale or purchase of the affected animal.

Description

A formal description is more relevant to the examination of a horse, but it is often very useful for the clinician to classify the animal under observation mentally while the history is unfolding, e.g. a young Friesian cow, recently calved and heavily in milk. It is always dangerous to be uncertain as to the exact type of animal under examination as it may lead to loss of face in discussion of the case and, occasionally, even to serious error.

Preliminary inspection/observation

Like the description, this inspection, *note* inspection not examination, takes practically no time, and is carried out during history taking. The clinician observes the behaviour of the animal or group of animals and makes a mental note of the conditions in the animal's environment.

At this stage, do not touch, do not disturb. Stand well back and observe from a distance, looking over the pen wall or gate. Put the picture in its frame. One is looking for the deviations from normality that constitute disease, so:

(1) One must know the normal.
(2) If the animal is frightened, pushed about or even handled, abnormalities may appear due to annoyance and fear. The minutiae that might have given a diagnostic lead will be masked. Condition, vigour, demeanour, respiratory pattern, appetite, rumination, faecal passage and type, and response to environment should all be noted.

Preliminary examination

The animal may now be touched but it is essential to proceed quietly, with as little fuss as possible. This stage of the examination includes the rate and character of the pulse, the temperature and a check on skin, eye, membranes, udder and ruminal movement. Although pulse character and rate are very important, it is frequently quite impossible to examine the pulse properly in a modern dairy cow that has been separated from the others, driven into a crush and clamped by the neck. It is usually not possible to do more than check the heart and heart rate with a stethoscope.

The clinician may well have arrived at a diagnosis at this stage, but if not is probably aware of the system of the body involved. In this case, he may only need to confirm his views, by examination of that system and by checking out the other systems quickly, even mentally.

Nevertheless, the position may still be far from clear, and the clinician will then have to embark upon a systematic examination. The procedure so far described will have taken no more than a few minutes, but if a full systematic examination becomes necessary, the case becomes much more time consuming.

Systematic examination

This includes all the manual and instrumental techniques necessary as part of such an examination, even including surgical intervention in some cases. The clinician, according to training and inclination, may interpret the word systematic as meaning (i) thorough, starting at the nose and finishing at the tail or (ii) system by system, in which case a mental list of the systems or sections that should be examined can be ticked off mentally when satisfied.

There is merit in adopting the second routine. It enables one to examine first the system or disease section that seems most likely to be affected from the preliminary evidence. Should the provisional diagnosis be confirmed, then a great deal of time will be saved, for it will only be necessary to check the remaining systems briefly, even, in some cases, mentally, to make sure that there is no other disease or lesion present. If there is no provisional diagnosis in mind, then it is reasonable to begin the systematic examination with the digestive system. In cows, this is the most likely cause of illness in obscure cases. Subsequently, the less important systems and sections can be examined as necessary.

A logical list of systems and disease groups for examination is as follows:

- Digestive system
- Respiratory system
- Circulatory system
- Urinary system
- Genital system
- Locomotory system
- Nervous system
- Skin
- Sense organs
- Lymphatic system
- Liver
- Udder
- Parasite problems
- Metabolic disease
- Allergies.

The last five headings on this list are, of course, not systems: nevertheless, they are very important disease sites (liver and udder) or disease groups that are logically considered as entities on the clinician's list.

A rectal examination is an important and useful aid to diagnosis and must always be included if the presenting signs are not conclusive. The bladder, uterus and ovaries, kidney and rumen are easily palpable, as are the caecum and small intestines if dilated.

Laboratory and special examinations

These are very important today, although increasing costs and the decline of dairying have unfortunately decreed that most laboratory work, apart from statutory Ministry investigations, or that done in the practice, is limited to the diagnosis of herd problems, rather than individual cow disease.

It is important that the clinician should never become a slave to the laboratory. The laboratory investigation is intended to confirm or refute the provisional diagnosis (working hypothesis) already in your mind.

Clinical examination comes first. Laboratory results can be inaccurate, irrelevant and confusing as well as expensive, but if used logically and critically they can be of great help.

Laboratory investigations include: haematology, biochemistry, bacteriology, virology, parasitology, serology, biopsy (histology) of tissues or fluids and, finally, necropsy.

Even after full examination, one may not have a complete diagnosis. However, there should be sufficient evidence to make a provisional diagnosis, which will allow

a logical course of treatment and, where relevant, prevention. The clinician must be prepared to think, form a working programme even on insufficient evidence, have enough confidence to convince the owner and enough adaptability to modify the programme tactfully if, and when, new evidence appears.

Owners, of course, are only partly interested in diagnosis. Prognosis is much more important to them. Will the cow get better? Will she be fully productive again? Is she worth treating? And today, unfortunately, another factor enters the equation. Will it be inconvenient to treat the cow; will she need nursing or extra care? If so, she is likely to be slaughtered, provided that she has antibiotic clearance and is likely to pass meat inspection.

The main presenting syndromes

It is not intended to discuss here the detailed techniques of the clinical examination of the various body systems. Every clinician has learnt these techniques as part of basic training, and there is excellent coverage in many textbooks, e.g. Boddie's *Diagnostic Methods in Veterinary Medicine* (1970). Instead, this chapter sets out to consider the differential diagnosis of some, although by no means all, of the main presenting syndromes that occur from day to day in the dairy cow.

Drooling at the mouth (kiddling, slobbering)

This is due to factors causing excess salivation, or factors preventing normal swallowing or combinations of both.

Bacterial or viral lesions in mouth

In countries where foot-and-mouth disease (FMD) has not occurred for a number of years, the possibility of infection must always be considered (see Chapter 43c). Thus the UK outbreak of 2001 shows how important it is that the disease is always remembered in differential diagnosis. Its occurrence was 33 years after the last major outbreak. The consequences of failure to recognize this disease are quite terrifying. Any salivating bovine animal, whether lame or not, whether pyrexic or not, must be treated as a possible case of foot-and-mouth disease until the clinician is satisfied that it is not. Other pyrexic diseases with oral lesions may give cause for concern, particularly bovine virus diarrhoea (BVD)/mucosal disease (see p. 853), infectious bovine rhinotracheitis (IBR) (see p. 289) and occasional cases of malignant catarrhal fever (see p. 935), but, fortunately, the mouth lesions and signs caused by these three diseases are usually relatively superficial and mild.

Actinobacillosis causes mechanical difficulty in tongue movement. The lesion is obvious, but painless even when ulcerated (see p. 824).

Calf diphtheria is limited to the young animal, causes pain as well as difficulty in mastication or suckling and produces inflammatory swelling with necrosis of the mucous membrane of the cheek (see pp. 250, 822, 825).

Foreign bodies

These are rare in the mouths of cattle, but the lids of cans occasionally become wedged between the lower molars and the cheek. Rarely, a stick becomes impacted between the rows of lower molars, or a molar itself loosens (see p. 825).

Interference with swallowing

This may be due to paralysis of the fifth or seventh cranial nerves which, in turn, may be due to listeriosis, meningeal abscesses or, particularly in the case of the seventh nerve, to trauma to the side of the head or face.

Fifth nerve paralysis makes the cow unable to close her mouth completely. The lips are in apposition but the teeth are not, a fact which is easily checked by flicking the lower jaw upwards, when the clicking together of upper and lower molars may be heard. Fifth nerve paralysis may often lead to accumulation of partly masticated food or cud in the pharynx, producing marked discomfort and gagging.

Seventh nerve paralysis causes unilateral or bilateral paralysis of the lips and cheek, and if of central origin, as in listeriosis (see p. 904), also causes flaccidity of the eyelids, with resultant keratitis and drooping of the ear on the affected side. This condition also leads to dropping of the cud bolus out of the mouth on the affected side and thus, ultimately, to loss of condition.

Oesophageal choke, particularly in the high oesophageal position, causes anxiety, even distress, with arching of the neck and profuse salivation. Choke may also cause varying degrees of ruminal tympany (see p. 826).

Dilatation and diverticulum of the oesophagus, particularly in the low cervical position, may produce similar, though milder, signs, as accumulation of food in the diverticulum may eventually lead to blocking of the oesophageal lumen, with resultant accumulation of food and saliva above the lesion.

Actinobacillosis of the oesophageal groove may lead not only to low-grade ruminal tympany but also to reflux of ruminal and reticular fluid into the mouth, so that in shippen-housed (i.e. tied) cows, a pool of such fluid may be found in the manger in the morning (see p. 823).

Excess salivation of CNS origin

This may be seen in lead poisoning, for the toxin affects the salivary nucleus. Blindness and aimless wandering in the cow, abdominal pain and convulsions with bellowing in the calf, should help the diagnosis.

In the 'licking mania' ketotic complication of milk fever or in 'nervous acetonaemia' (see p. 794) excess salivation is due to the compulsive chewing so characteristic of the disease.

Rhododendron poisoning

This may cause profuse salivation, and even vomiting, as well as diarrhoea (see p. 943).

Organophosphorus compounds

These may also cause salivation and diarrhoea (see p. 940).

Acute photosensitization syndromes

These may well cause profuse salivation, as well as lacrimation, jaundice and, later, the onset of necrosis of the non-pigmented skin areas (see p. 884).

Acute dyspnoea

This condition, as in very severe pneumonia, may cause obvious salivation as a result of mouth breathing.

Acute anaphylactic shock

This often causes profuse drooling of saliva as well as tachypnoea, subnormal temperature, cold extremities, oedema, and a very rapid heart (see p. 927).

Vomiting (see p. 825)

Vomiting is very rare in the cow and, to all intents and purposes, only occurs in *laurel* and *rhododendron poisoning* (see p. 943). Very occasionally a peptic ulcer of the abomasum will cause problems (see p. 844). Regurgitation of rumen fluid or content (false vomiting) may occur in cases of acute bloat (see p. 852), acidosis (see p. 829) or where there are lesions in the oesophageal groove (see p. 147), e.g. actinobacillosis or a foreign body ('wire') (see p. 837).

Occasionally, cases of oesophageal dilatation and diverticulation may accumulate material above the obstruction until it overflows into and out of the mouth.

Acute abdominal pain (colic)

It is interesting that acute colic pain of the type seen in the horse is relatively rare in cattle, and several of the syndromes that cause the most acute pain are not, in fact, obstructive gut lesions, as one would expect, and may not even involve the alimentary tract at all.

Acute gut obstruction

This may be due to the following causes:

- Abomasal torsion (see p. 842);
- Torsion of caecum, colon, or ileum or common mesentery (see p. 847);
- Strangulated mesenteric hernia (see p. 1113);
- Strangulated scrotal hernia (see p. 1113);
- Gut tie: the entrapment of gut in peritoneal tears at the edge of the internal inguinal ring due to castration by traction in the slightly older animal (see p. 1113);
- Intussusception (see p. 847);
- Obstruction of ileum by the stalk of a lipoma (see p. 849).

Abomasal or large gut torsion produces a degree, sometimes very considerable, of right-sided abdominal distension, not normally seen in small gut obstructions. In gut tie, there may be considerable distension in the inguinal region, whilst scrotal hernia obviously produces distension of the scrotum on the affected side. It is, however, very easy for the clinician to overlook scrotal or inguinal swelling unless aware of the possibility. These acute obstructive conditions cause the most acute colicky abdominal pain in the very early stages, but such pain is often very transient and by the time the case is presented to the veterinary surgeon, temperature is falling, pulse rate is rising, body surfaces are becoming cold and even clammy, and a dull toxaemic and shocked appearance develops as circulatory obstruction, necrosis and gangrene of the obstructed gut supervenes. Intussusception is sometimes an exception in that many cases of bovine intussusception, particularly if large gut is involved, show little more than depression and dullness even in the early stages. Rectal examination is a useful diagnostic procedure.

Acute enteritis (Chapters 14, 15, p. 850)

Acute enteritis, particularly salmonellosis (see Chapter 15), is similar to acute cereal overeating, e.g. barley poisoning, in that some cases show spectacularly acute abdominal pain, often with some degree of tympany, which remains noticeable for a considerable time, often several hours, before the characteristic profuse diarrhoea begins. Laparotomies have been performed on a number of occasions at this stage of the disease in the belief that the condition was one of acute gut obstruction. Once diarrhoea appears, temperature falls often to normal or below, while signs of dehydration, electrolyte imbalance and shock appear.

Acute fermentative colic

This condition, involving the caecum and colon and producing right flank tympany, may occur on rich pasture, particularly in wet weather, and may be difficult to differentiate from acute obstructive conditions. Fortunately, these conditions generally respond to analgesics and antispasmodics before serious diagnostic errors occur (p. 847).

The passage of a calculus down the ureter

This may produce the most spectacular colicky pain, which fortunately is usually relatively transient. Diagnosis is obviously extremely difficult (see p. 263).

Photosensitization involving teats

Acute photosensitization (see p. 884) in cattle, e.g. Ayrshires with sparingly pigmented teats and udders, can produce an inflammatory exudative lesion of teats and skin of the udder that is so painful that the cow behaves exactly as if suffering from an acute abdominal catastrophe. Diagnostic error will only be avoided if the clinician remembers the invariable rule that whatever may seem to be affecting a cow, the udder and teats must always be examined.

Acute abdominal distension

This is one of the important and relatively common presenting syndromes in the cow. All causes of abdominal distension in the cow are covered by the memory rhyme (the seven Fs), which runs as follows: fat, fetus, fluid, flatus, faeces, food or foreign body. Severe abdominal distension may originate at several sites.

Ruminal

Dietary ruminal impaction: This occurs in housed fattening cattle on store diet, hay or straw, with limited water (see p. 236). The massive ruminal impaction, absence of ruminal movement, raised temperature and pulse rate, painful frequent abdominal grunt, and hard scanty faeces produce a syndrome requiring differentiation from *acute traumatic reticuloperitonitis* ('wire') (see p. 837) in its very early stages, although the impactive mass in the 'wired' rumen is never so great.

A similar condition, although much less severe, may occur in dairy cows tied in shippens during the winter should the water bowl cease to function, a mishap that frequently escapes the attendant's notice, and is always worth checking. Modern systems of building and management have markedly decreased the incidence of these two conditions.

Impaction of the rumen with grain (see p. 829) occurs in cows that have broken into a food store and eaten greedily, but even when the attendant is unaware of this, or will not admit it, the nature of the case generally becomes apparent in two to three days when profuse diarrhoea, staggering, recumbency, subnormal temperature, rapid pulse rate and other evidence of toxic effects occur in severe cases. In cases seen soon after ingestion of large quantities of grain, palpation of the left sublumbar fossa may produce the same sensation as handling a sack of grain. If, as is generally the case in Britain, the grain is barley, the interim period of impaction, with arched back, grunt, depression and moderate tympany is usually transient, and within a few hours the profuse diarrhoea so characteristic of barley poisoning appears.

Vagus indigestion (see p. 855): This condition is usually a complication of 'wire' that has produced adhesions, involving the medial wall of the reticulum and the cranial sac of the rumen, interfering with the function of the vagus nerve receptors in their walls. The atonic rumen, gradually filling with water and saliva, eventually produces a massive left-sided fluid distension in a cow steadily losing body condition.

Acute ruminal tympany (see p. 832): Acute ruminal tympany presents relatively little diagnostic difficulty. The condition includes clover and kale bloat and oesophageal obstruction (choke). The history, environmental circumstances, season of the year and the gagging, retching and salivating associated with most cases of choke are generally reasonably conclusive, although in very acute cases, of course, it pays to relieve the tympany via the left sublumbar fossa before worrying too much about the aetiology.

It is worth remembering that a thirsty cow, housed overnight in old-fashioned accommodation and released to drink its fill of very cold water, may easily become, transiently, quite alarmingly tympanitic, due presumably to the chilling effect of the frosty water on the rumen musculature.

The acute ruminal tympany of a cow that, for one reason or another, e.g. milk fever, has collapsed into lateral recumbency should not require mention. It is, however, surprising that it is still quite commonplace to find that such a cow has not been supported in sternal recumbency, as the condition demands.

Peritoneal

Acute diffuse peritonitis (see p. 849): This condition occurs when the special ability of the bovine peritoneum to withstand and localize peritoneal infection fails for various reasons, allowing a virulent diffuse exudative process to spread across the peritoneal cavity. Usually, the condition stems from the breakdown of the defensive mechanisms isolating 'wire' in reticular diaphragmatic adhesions, but the leakage or rupture of a superficial liver abscess may produce the same result.

The peritoneal cavity fills with thin evil smelling pus of *Arcanobacterium (Actinomyces; Corynebacterium) pyogenes*: there are widespread adhesions, temperature falls, pulse rate rises, scanty diarrhoea develops, body condition falls away and the cow is toxic and in pain. The fluid wave is very obvious and confirmation by paracentesis is easy. The condition most likely to cause confusion is the massive milky ascites that may follow extensive liver damage and obstruction to the portal circulation. Inspection and examination of peritoneal fluid provides straightforward differentiation.

Peritoneal tympany: A gas-filled abdominal cavity may occur following perforation of an abomasal ulcer at a point free of attached omentum, causing acute pain over much of the anterior abdomen, particularly on the right side. Grunting, tooth grinding, falling temperature and rising pulse rate are followed by progressive peritoneal tympany due to leakage of gas from the abomasal lumen into the abdominal cavity.

Abomasal

Dilatation and/or torsion of abomasum (see p. 842): Dilatation and/or torsion of the abomasum on the right produces right-sided distension, very marked in cases of torsion, which also causes acute and even colicky pain.

Acute left abomasal displacement (see p. 839): This condition produces significant abdominal distension of the left flank, but such cases are exceptional. All abomasal cases are amenable to diagnosis by normal auscultation methods.

Intestinal

Acute tympanitic fermentative intestinal colic: This condition, which usually resolves without too much difficulty, can produce massive right-sided distension.

Torsion of caecum and colon on the common mesentery (see p. 847): This serious and usually fatal complication of fermentation and atony also produces massive right-sided distension. Differentiation depends upon demeanour, rectal examination, pulse rate and upon progress of the case following initial medication.

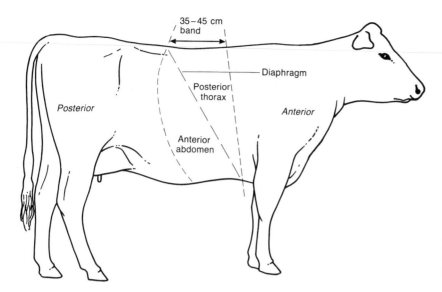

Fig. 11.1 Lateral view of cow showing anterior abdominal/posterior thoracic area.

Uterine

Hydrops amnion and allantois (see p. 1119): These conditions produce very marked abdominal distension. Diagnosis is helped by rectal examination. Uterine rupture producing extra-uterine pregnancy in the last third of pregnancy is marked by the formation of much fibrinous exudate in an abdomen filled with free uterine fluid and containing fetus and membranes. Such an abdomen is distended and shows a fluid wave which, on rectal examination, appears to be unassociated with the uterus. There is abdominal pain, rapid pulse and often severe illness. Diagnosis depends upon an accurate history and the ballottement of a fetus in the lower abdomen, even though rectal examination reveals a partially involuted uterus.

Anterior abdominal/posterior thoracic pain

The organs and structures enclosed within a 35–45 cm band encircling the cow immediately behind the withers provide a group of diseases of great importance to the bovine clinician. Viewed from a lateral position, the diaphragm divides this area into the posterior thorax anteriorly and dorsally, and the anterior abdomen ventrally and posteriorly (Fig. 11.1).

The band described encircles lungs, mediastinum, heart, pleural cavity and great vessels in front of the diaphragm, and rumen, reticulum, omasum, abomasum, liver, gall-bladder, spleen and the anterior part of the peritoneal cavity posteriorly with much of the greater and lesser omental sheets. Differential diagnosis is often difficult and is not helped by the fact that both thoracic and abdominal lesions occur within this imaginary belt.

Traumatic reticulo-peritonitis

The classical and traditional condition affecting this area is traumatic reticulo-peritonitis ('wire') (see p. 837) and it is very convenient to use this condition, less common nowadays, but well known and recognized, as a yard-stick with which to compare the numerous other conditions of the posterior thorax and anterior abdomen.

The possibility of overlooking a penetrating foreign body, a serious mistake for both patient and clinician, is always at the back of one's mind when examining a bovine abdomen. It is always a considerable relief if one can eliminate the possibility of a foreign body and its complications, and such a process is, of course, very important to the surgeon when considering the site of a possible exploratory laparotomy. Nevertheless, neither the confirmation nor the refutation of a provisional diagnosis of traumatic reticulitis is easy without exploratory laparotomy. Thus, the clinical syndrome presents such wide variations in both the extent and intensity of signs that it is probably true to say that the only constant clinical sign is the presence of some degree of pain in the anterior abdomen. The range of differential diagnoses is therefore wide and includes several groups of clinical conditions, each capable of confusion by virtue of exhibiting one or more of the signs associated with reticulitis.

The acute clinical syndrome not infrequently encountered at the onset of the condition includes complete inappetence, and ruminal and reticular atony, resulting in ruminal impaction and slight tympany, with absence of ruminal movement and cudding. Constipation may also be a feature. Temperature may be 40–40.5°C (104–105°F) with a pulse rate of 80–90/minute. There is a marked drop in milk yield. The painful focus in the anterior abdomen results in general rigidity with arched back and protruding neck, disinclination to lie down and spontaneous grunting accentuated by movement, defaecation and micturition, and very marked on pinching the withers or applying upward pressure to the xiphisternal region.

This acute syndrome is by no means constant, even at the onset of reticulitis, and when present usually abates in 24–36 hours as the intensity of pain lessens and varying degrees of ruminal and reticular motility return. Temperature tends to fall into the 39–39.5°C (102–103°F) range, pulse rate may be in the normal range or slightly raised, appetite, although poor, is not completely absent, ruminal impaction and tympany largely disappear and faeces regain normal consistency. The painful rigid stance relaxes and although the back remains somewhat stiff and arched, pain may require elicitation by the clinician rather than being obviously spontaneous. Rumination, however, nearly always remains absent, or irregular and occasional.

In some cases the only clinical signs are slightly depressed appetite and rumination, subnormal milk yield and indications of pain so slight that they amount to no more than unwillingness to depress the back, so that even mild and painless diseases such as acetonaemia have to be considered in differential diagnosis.

Localized peritonitis

The acute and subacute syndromes described above are, of course, essentially those of localized peritonitis, and pictures similar in broad outline will result from other causes of localized peritonitis, although the veterinarian may be able to differentiate the focus of pain.

(1) Penetration of the involuted uterus or the vaginal fornix by a catheter or damage to the anterior vagina at service may produce a picture similar, save for considerably less interference with alimentary motility and for pain response on pressure over the posterior abdomen or on rectal examination. Such injuries frequently evoke straining, indicating the need for vaginal examination.

(2) Postoperative peritonitis may well provide a syndrome similar to that of moderately acute traumatic reticulitis, but the fact of recent operation and the possibility of peritonitis resulting therefrom will be obvious to the clinician, particularly after procedures such as trocharization for the relief of bloat.

(3) Perforation of an abomasal ulcer (see p. 844) may present a picture broadly similar to that of acute traumatic reticulitis if seen in the early stages before diffuse peritonitis, collapse and death occur. However, there is likely to be acute pain over a much wider area of the anterior abdomen, particularly on the right side, than is the case in reticulitis. Any temperature rise is likely to be transient only, but the pulse rate will be considerably in excess of that expected in reticulitis and may exceed 100/minute. There will be grinding of the teeth and loud groaning as well as grunting of a similar type to that seen in acute reticulitis. The cow will not eat, is greatly depressed and remains largely recumbent. In a proportion of cases, though by no means all, the abdomen becomes distended with gas, presumably by leakage through the perforation, and a state of true peritoneal tympany develops. This syndrome must also be considered in the differential diagnosis of acute abdominal distension.

(4) A peritonitis syndrome varying from a very acute picture associated with shock to a subacute picture sometimes associated with straining is occasionally met with as the result of penetration of the rectum by a foreign body, usually a broom or pitchfork handle, introduced through the anus by a person with sadistic tendencies. Such a lesion is always detectable by rectal examination.

(5) The more acute lesions of tubercular peritonitis (see p. 863), as seen in the breakdown forms of the disease, occasionally produce an abdominal syndrome similar to that of traumatic reticulitis. Unless there are obvious coincidental signs of tuberculosis, diagnosis is made only on opening the abdomen with the intention of performing rumenotomy when the blood-streaked, caseating and even exudative lesions of the acute disease may be only too obvious. This syndrome is now rare in more developed countries but might occur should the disease again break out.

Having considered the differentiation of traumatic reticulitis from other causes of peritonitis, one must now be prepared to differentiate moderately severe forms of the disease from conditions which, although not involving peritonitis, cause pain in the anterior abdomen or posterior thorax. This question of pain in the anterior abdomen or posterior thorax is, of course, very important in the diagnosis of reticulitis. One must remember that the reticulum, diaphragm, liver, abomasum, omasum, heart, pleurae, oesophagus and the posterior lung areas all lie approximately along the vertical line between the point at which one pinches the withers and the point at which one applies the bar.

Bacterial endocarditis (see p. 726)

Classically described and reviewed by Rees Evans (1957), bacterial endocarditis obviously requires differentiation from other cardiac diseases, but it is not generally realized that, in its earlier stages, before signs of venous congestion and circulatory stasis supervene, endocarditis can easily be confused with traumatic reticulitis. Pain, often intermittent in nature, and causing rigidity of stance with abduction of the left, or both, elbows, and discomfort when pressure is applied to the withers, xiphisternum and left ventral aspect of the chest, is probably due to infarction of the lungs or myocardium. This is not unlike that due to a foreign body penetrating the reticulum. Once venous congestion is clinically obvious, the fact that the heart is diseased becomes apparent and from this point the clinician must eliminate other cardiac diseases, particularly traumatic pericarditis.

Previous to the development of venous congestion, accelerated respirations with dyspnoea and coughing on exercise, the peculiar 'shifting' lameness of endocarditis, the tendency towards a markedly high pulse rate even when temperature is responding to antibiotics and the presence, in some cases, of recognizable abnormality of heart sounds may all help in differentiating endocarditis from reticulitis. The author is cautious on the subject of heart sounds, for although he has frequently been assured by skilled cardiologists that a murmur will always be audible in this disease, he has frequently failed to detect one in cases with a right-sided lesion. It is noticeable that endocarditis cases tend to retain a relatively bright demeanour and reasonable appetite until the late stages of the disease. The white cell picture is of limited value as many cases present total and differential counts similar to those produced by a penetrating foreign body, although there is a tendency for both total white cell count and neutrophil percentage to be higher than in that disease.

Certain cases of pneumonia and pleurisy (see Chapter 49a,b)

These conditions, particularly the latter, exhibit signs of posterior thoracic pain that may simulate reticulitis and careful auscultation of the chest is necessary in an attempt to confirm the presence of abnormal thoracic sounds. Pleurisy is very painful in the early dry stages, but becomes painless as effusion develops. Respirations are rapid and shallow, but as effusion builds up, they become deep and swinging.

Impaction of the abomasum (see p. 844)

Impaction of the abomasum, involving primarily the pyloric outlet with large quantities of fibrous foodstuffs,

sand or gravel, may occur very occasionally. There is a slow diminution in appetite and milk yield and progressive ruminal impaction comprising solid food material with, occasionally, a little gas. Rumination ceases and constipation occurs. Temperature is never more than slightly raised, but pulse rate may eventually exceed 100/minute. At first, there is slight anterior abdominal pain only, but as the disease progresses, pinching of the withers and pressure over the xiphisternum are resented markedly. Pain may, in contradistinction to the case in reticulitis, be evoked by pressure over the anterior part of the right flank. The white cell picture may be in the normal range or similar to that of 'wire'. Although the patient becomes much weaker and more depressed than is the case in reticulitis, it is doubtful whether differentiation will be made before exploratory laparotomy reveals the distended doughy abomasum.

The author believes that true abomasal impaction is very rare, and that most of the cases described as abomasal impaction in the past have shown distension of the fundic portion of the abomasum with material like dry rumen contents and an accumulation of fluid within the rumen, which suggest very strongly that they are, in fact, cases of 'vagus indigestion' (p. 855). Lymphosarcoma can cause the problem (p. 693).

Painful conditions of the liver (see p. 147)

These obviously present a problem in differentiation within the group of diseases causing pain in the anterior abdomen or posterior thorax. The liver is a very difficult organ from the clinician's viewpoint. It is anatomically inaccessible and, in spite of the considerable volume of work carried out in recent years, there are still no entirely satisfactory tests of liver function in the bovine species.

The cow has large reserves of liver tissue, and very considerable damage may occur without the production of a clear-cut syndrome. Liver biopsy is of limited value in that the portion of liver obtained may be quite unrepresentative of the whole. The author prefers to make an incision behind the last rib, in the right sublumbar fossa, sufficiently large to allow a manual examination of the liver and even, using a small torch, limited visual examination. A biopsy specimen can, if required, be obtained through such an incision with the minimum of risk.

Pyelonephritis (see p. 725)

In its more severe forms pyelonephritis produces pain that, although not sited in the anterior abdomen, can easily lead to confusion with traumatic reticulitis, particularly as the white cell count is also usually raised. It may be said that, in spite of the raised temperature and pulse rate, the arched back and the grunt not infrequently present, urine examination leaves the diagnosis beyond doubt. Nevertheless, failure to observe the urine may easily lead to error. Rectal palpation will reveal an enlarged kidney or differentiate cystitis from pyelonephritis (p. 725).

Impaction of the omasum

Another confusing condition, which is practically impossible to diagnose in life, is impaction of the omasum. The disease, which is fortunately very rare, produces slow weight loss, inappetence, low-grade anterior abdominal pain and general dullness. Ulceration and necrosis of the abomasal leaves are found at post-mortem examination.

Diaphragmatic hernia (see p. 848)

In cattle diaphragmatic hernia produces signs much more suggestive of anterior abdominal pain, particularly reticulitis, than of any thoracic involvement. It is, in fact, probable that many cases arise due to weakening of the diaphragmatic muscle by previous foreign body ('wire') damage. The hernial ring is usually small, involving parts of the reticulum and sometimes the omasum. The resulting low-grade pain may actually be due to areas of peritonitis caused by the original 'wire'. The interference with reticulum and omasum, due to the constriction of the hernial ring and the development of adhesions, sometimes leads to 'vagus indigestion' (p. 855).

Uterine torsion (see p. 1118)

It is worth remembering that the occasional cow which develops uterine torsion very early in parturition may show subacute or chronic abdominal pain with progressive inappetence and constipation. Such a case may show little or no further signs of developing labour.

Cases of acute traumatic reticulitis (see p. 837) *with ruminal impaction requiring differentiation from other conditions presenting this feature*

These conditions are discussed in the section on ruminal impaction and include dietary ruminal impaction in yarded cows on fibrous feeds, e.g. hay or straw, with limited access to water. A less spectacular ruminal impaction may occur in dairy cows tied in shippens during the winter should the water bowl cease to function or in groups when the water supply is reduced or ceases, e.g. freezing, bursts in piping, etc.

Impaction of the rumen with grain shows varying degrees of ruminal distension and discomfort for varying periods before diarrhoea supervenes (p. 829).

Subacute and chronic ruminal tympany (see p. 832): These do occur in traumatic reticulitis, particularly in the early stages, and often superimposed on a degree of ruminal impaction. A number of other conditions also result in slight ruminal tympany, which forms a differential group in its own right (see chronic bloat, p. 832).

Cases of traumatic reticulitis (see p. 837) *requiring differentiation from other causes of anterior abdominal pain and conditions causing stiffness and rigidity of stance*

Tetanus (see p. 733): This is not infrequently misdiagnosed as reticulitis in the first instance. Not only is there subacute tympany, but the arched back, stiff unbending stance and marked constipation of tetanus can be quite confusing.

Bilateral solar ulcer (see p. 417), *laminitis* (see p. 420) *and other hind foot lesions* (see Chapter 31): Similarly, but with less justification, cases of bilateral solar ulcer, laminitis (coriosis) and other painful bilateral hind foot lesions may cause similar confusion.

Injury to lower cervical vertebrae: Occasionally, cows suffer injury to the lower cervical vertebrae, resulting in pain, stiffness and reluctance to bend the lower neck or back, and such cases have sometimes been diagnosed as traumatic reticulitis.

Complications of, and sequelae to, traumatic reticulitis (see p. 837) *causing confusion in diagnosis of anterior abdominal/posterior thoracic pain*

(1) Cases are encountered where a piece of wire loose in the reticulum, by reason of its shape, repeatedly pricks the reticular wall and is then dislodged, producing minor episodes of pain and localized peritonitis that rapidly resolve. By the time operation has been decided upon, the animal is substantially normal and surgery is withheld, only for the syndrome to be repeated after varying intervals of time. It is possible that such 'pricks' should be included with transient phases of abomasal displacement as the reason for many of the 'nonspecific inappetence' cases so well known to every bovine clinician.

(2) A difficult problem is the case where traumatic reticulitis is strongly suspected and rumenotomy carried out, only to find that in spite of the presence of definite reticular adhesions, no foreign body can be found. There are three possibilities. Firstly, the adhesions may be longstanding and bear no relation to the present illness, i.e. the diagnosis is

incorrect. This possibility can be checked by applying digital pressure to the adhesions – if pain is provoked, they are probably pertinent to the present ill health. Secondly, the foreign body may have become dislodged and passed down the gut, or even regurgitated, in which case prognosis is good. Thirdly, the foreign body may have passed completely through the reticular wall and be buried in adhesions and reactionary tissue beyond. Here the prognosis is obviously grave.

One can only advise a wait-and-see policy, but such cases do present difficulties in the management of clients who expect the production of a foreign body and, in its absence, are frequently inclined to doubt the diagnosis and regard the operation as an error on the part of the clinician.

(3) An occasional, but nevertheless difficult, case is the cow from whose reticulum a foreign body has previously been removed and which now, weeks or months later, is showing a clinical syndrome suggestive of 'wire'. Has there, in fact, been a penetration by a further foreign body or are the signs due to further infection or abscess formation in the old adhesions? In cases that do not respond promptly to antibiotic therapy it is always wise to re-operate, for even if no further foreign body is involved, an abscess may be found that can be drained into the reticulum.

(4) A further group of conditions occurs where a foreign body penetrating the reticulum has since penetrated another organ. Signs, in these cases, are usually related largely to this secondary occurrence and the signs, all-important prognostically, of the primary foreign body aetiology tend to be masked. The classical example of this type of condition is traumatic pericarditis, producing a syndrome very well recognized, but presenting considerable difficulty at times in differentiation from endocarditis.

Penetration of the thoracic cavity to produce suppurative pneumonia or pleurisy also occurs, tending to produce a subacute thoracic syndrome with progressive loss of condition. It is of considerable importance prognostically to know whether such a condition is due to a penetrating foreign body or not and it is often extremely difficult, in the presence of pain in the posterior thorax, to decide whether pain exists in the anterior abdomen as well. The white cell picture will not help, and exploratory laparotomy may be necessary as a diagnostic aid.

Similarly, foreign body penetration of the liver may occur causing a large area of suppuration, which may produce a clinical picture similar to the acute liver fluke syndrome previously mentioned, but with reticuloruminal interference as well. Extensive liver lesions of this type occasionally interfere sufficiently with the bile ducts to cause jaundice.

(5) Occasionally, traumatic reticulitis leads to acute diffuse peritonitis, the abdomen filling with pus and producing abdominal distension, toxaemia, depression, weakness and diarrhoea, leading to death (see abdominal distension, p. 140).

(6) Vagus indigestion is also a complication of traumatic reticulitis (see abdominal distension, p. 855).

Chronic bloat (chronic and subacute ruminal tympany) (see p. 852)

All conditions producing low-grade ruminal tympany must fall into one or other of two main groups: (i) those affecting normal rumino-reticular tone and motility and (ii) those causing partial obstruction to the escape of gas from the rumen, motility and tone remaining normal.

Conditions affecting normal rumino-reticular tone and motility

Chronic inflammatory lesions of the mucous membrane and wall of the reticulum and the oesophageal groove: Actinobacillosis of these sites is the most important condition of this group (see p. 823). The smooth painless fibrous plaque of this disease interferes with both eructation and rumination, producing a mild tympany most obvious after feeding. If the oesophageal groove is badly affected there is often a prolonged retching gurgling noise as the cow makes laboured attempts to bring up the first bolus of a new period of rumination. There may be drooling from the mouth.

Therapeutic response is normally rapid enough to be considered diagnostic.

Occasionally, inflammatory thickening and *A. pyogenes* abscessation of the area resulting from foreign body lacerations and partial penetrations may occur, also affecting eructation and rumination. Chronic ruminal atony can occur in calves with oesophageal groove problems.

Inflammatory changes (peritonitis): Inflammatory changes involving the serous lining of rumen, reticulum or even abomasum are more important, leading to poor motility and even atony of the rumen-reticulum. The classic syndrome in this group, as already mentioned, is *traumatic reticulo-peritonitis* ('wire', p. 837). Even in longstanding cases, where some degree of rumen movement has returned, there may well be chronic ruminal tympany often superimposed on low-grade ruminal impaction.

A *peptic abomasal ulcer* (see p. 844) sufficiently advanced to involve the peritoneal lining may well form omental adhesions, and may even perforate among these adhesions, so that there is no leakage into the peritoneal cavity itself. Such a cow, instead of dying within 24–36 hours of acute diffuse peritonitis, toxaemia and shock with massive peritoneal tympany, as described under abdominal distension, will pass into a state of intermittent low-grade pain, abnormal or negligible rumino-reticular movement with slight and intermittent ruminal tympany. There will be lethargy, weight loss and intermittent diarrhoea.

Acidosis (see p. 829): This shows its classical features in barley poisoning, but many recently calved high-yielding cows on a high-energy diet develop mild acidosis after each feed. The slight ruminal tympany plus near-diarrhoeic faeces in a lethargic cow with sub-optimal appetite and milk yield is familiar in intensive dairy herds.

Vagus indigestion (see p. 835): Occasional cases of vagus indigestion (see complications of traumatic reticulitis, p. 837, and abdominal distension, p. 140) show an accumulation of ruminal gas forming a marked, but chronic, tympany that may even mask the fluid present.

Tetanus (see p. 733): Tetanus frequently produces a moderate tympany (see rigidity of stance and gait, p. 145).

Cold water: Under ruminal distension, the effect of cold water on the ruminal musculature is mentioned. In some herds, in which all the cows drink water from troughs in the yard, the whole herd may show a degree of post-drinking tympany.

Botulism (see p. 721): With its generalized muscle weakness, botulism shows subacute tympany as a minor part of a fatal progressive disease.

Conditions causing partial obstruction to the escape of gas from the reticulo-rumen

Motility and tone being normal, these conditions will cause low-grade tympany.

Oesophageal wall lesions (see p. 825): Usually traumatic in origin, these include oesophageal stricture, oesophageal wall abscesses, oesophageal dilatation and oesophageal papillomata, which are usually sited at the cardia.

Lesions causing external pressure on the oesophagus (see p. 832): These lesions will also produce chronic tympany. They include thymic lymphosarcoma in young cattle (p. 698) and enlarged posterior mediastinal lymph nodes in the adult. Such enlargement is an important cause of chronic tympany and is usually due to one of three infective organisms: *A. pyogenes*, *Actinobacillus ligneresi* and, occasionally, *Mycobacterium bovis*.

Diaphragmatic hernia (see p. 848): This condition also not infrequently leads to chronic tympany.

Diagnosis of chronic and subacute ruminal tympany

Diagnosis depends firstly upon a careful clinical examination to decide whether the tympany is related to a specific alimentary condition or whether it is due to loss of gastric tone as a result of a more general disease. If the condition is primarily alimentary, and one believes there is no oesophageal obstruction, then auscultation should be carried out to check that the left flank tympany is ruminal and not abomasal (i.e. left displacement). Auscultation should leave one in no doubt, although it is not always easy to distinguish between a gas-filled abomasum, early vagus indigestion (p. 855) and reticular actinobacillosis (p. 823).

The liver

The liver is practically impossible to examine clinically by normal methods. It is unfortunately true that unless one adheres to a strict routine, it is only too easy to examine a cow without even thinking about the liver. The liver has many functions and failure, therefore, may produce a variety of signs.

Signs include lethargy, slow weight loss, anaemia, low-grade or acute abdominal pain, massive abdominal haemorrhage, ascites, abdominal distension, chronic venous congestion, ataxia, ventral oedema, photosensitization, endocarditis, encephalopathy, dyspnoea with pulmonary thrombosis, massive nasal haemorrhage and, occasionally, jaundice. All these conditions may originate in hepatic disease. Also, one must consider the diverse problems of the high-yielding cow calving down with a very fat liver predisposing to metritis, coliform mastitis, ketosis, low solids, milk fever and even infertility.

The liver, it seems, not only is the site of specific disease conditions in its own right, but also may be a background factor predisposing to disease in other organs and systems. In the face of this diversity of signs, all one can suggest is that the clinician should always consider the possibility of liver disease when examining a cow. He/she is then unlikely to miss liver pathology when it occurs.

Laboratory tests, e.g. haematology, serum proteins, serum enzymes (aspartate aminotransferase (AST), serum alkaline phosphatase (SAP) and particularly gamma-glutamyl transferase (γGT)), may be helpful, though by no means conclusive. Paracentesis may occasionally help in the presence of ascites, while liver biopsy is at least theoretically useful. Unfortunately, these techniques are expensive and the farmer of today is very unwilling to authorize them in any but the most valuable of individual cows.

So consideration of the liver must be as rigid a rule as checking the udder, and a mental list of the syndromes involved in hepatic disease can be a great help.

Abscessation (see p. 830)

This is usually due to *A. pyogenes* or *Fusobacterium necrophorum en route* from the rumen, and is probably only clinically significant when extensive. Obviously, cereal overeating and other conditions likely to damage the rumen wall will predispose to liver abscesses. Bacteraemias also come from navel infections and pyaemias.

Complications of hepatic abscessation may be very serious:

● Rupture into the abdominal cavity leading to an acute diffuse peritonitis.
● Rupture into a major vessel, leading to major haemorrhage, shock and sudden death.
● Vena cava thrombosis, usually where the vena cava passes through the diaphragm. This produce hepatic portal obstruction leading to abdominal distension and ascites; however, it may produce pulmonary thromboembolism leading to pulmonary abscessation. There will be a painful cough, and dyspnoea, with rupture of abscesses into blood vessels producing severe and often recurrent haemorrhage via the nose and mouth (see p. 867).

Hepatic necrosis

Hepatic necrosis due to *Fusobacterium* invasion causes pyrexia, inappetence, lethargy, rapid pulse, weight loss, ataxia and occasionally signs of anterior abdominal pain. The presence of jaundice is variable, but is diagnostically helpful when it occurs.

Cholecystitis

This condition is rare and difficult to diagnose. Such cases show ataxia, anterior abdominal discomfort and jaundice, with lowered appetite and milk yield. Temperature may be raised.

It is interesting that jaundice is much more likely to occur in obstructive hepatic conditions than in parenchymatous change.

Cirrhosis

Cirrhosis in cattle, for all practical purposes, means liver fluke infestation (p. 276). This condition must never be forgotten. It occurs in adults as well as young stock, in herds as well as individuals, and although wasting, submaxillary oedema and anaemia may well be present, the disease may merely cause chronic unthriftiness and suboptimal yield during the winter months, thus needing differentiation from a nutritional energy deficit. In fact, both problems may occur in the same herd, particularly between parturition and peak yield.

It is worth remembering that in severe fluke infestation, constipation is more likely than diarrhoea, and that during the migratory stage of the young flukes, a low-grade abdominal pain syndrome may occur that requires differentiation from 'wire'.

Liver fluke infestation (see p. 276) has far-reaching effects. It may lead to infertility, presumably due to weight loss, to low milk solids and to salmonellosis, or to endocarditis due to bacteria passing to the liver and then into the circulation.

Cirrhosis also results from ragwort poisoning (p. 945), causing weight loss, ataxia, encephalopathy, occasional jaundice and terminal tenesmus in the affected animal. The encephalopathy produces blindness, head pressing and dragging of the hind fetlocks reminiscent of lead poisoning in the adult cow. Ragwort poisoning during the grazing period may well trigger photosensitization.

Other syndromes involved in liver disease

Tuberculosis (see p. 862) and *neoplasia* of the liver are relatively rare. Neoplasia includes lymphosarcoma and adenocarcinoma and is, to all intents and purposes, impossible to diagnose in life, while fatty livers may follow bacterial or chemical toxicity, but are much more common as the result of overfeeding or inappropriate feeding.

The fatty liver syndrome (see p. 801), resulting from excessive weight gain pre partum, has gained prominence in recent years, but is probably less common today. The syndrome may be involved in many diseases in early lactation.

Constipation

Quite apart from the acute gut obstruction syndromes, constipation may occur in diverse circumstances in cattle.

(1) Unsuitable fibrous diet, e.g. straw, may produce ruminal impaction.
(2) Insufficient water intake may produce ruminal impaction.
(3) External pressure on the gut, e.g. fat necrosis (see p. 849), lymphosarcoma (see p. 693), adhesions.

(4) Pain:
- (a) Postoperative pain.
- (b) Injured back – faeces dry out in rectum.
- (c) Injured anus and rectum – painful bladder.

(5) Weakness or paresis: milk fever, broken back. Constipation is, of course, a very useful differential sign of milk fever (p. 781).

(6) Some poisons, e.g. lead (see p. 944) and ragwort (p. 945).

(7) Pyrexia.

(8) Anaemia. e.g. fluke (see p. 276), piroplasmosis (see p. 748). In both these diseases, constipation becomes very marked in long-standing cases.

(9) Ketosis: mild constipation is a frequent clinical sign (see p. 793).

(10) Hypocalcaemia (see p. 781).

(11) Peritonitis (see p. 849).

Constipation is, of course, rare in dairy cattle and if faeces are completely absent, acute gut obstruction (p. 1113) caused by intussusception (p. 847), caecal or intestinal torsion (pp. 846, 847) will be the most likely reason.

Diarrhoea

Varying degrees of diarrhoea are normal today in intensive dairy herds feeding concentrates and silage.

Not all conditions causing diarrhoea originate primarily in the digestive tract, but from the viewpoint of differential diagnosis, it is best to consider all conditions causing diarrhoea together.

Acute diarrhoea

(1) Most toxaemic conditions produce diarrhoea, e.g. diffuse peritonitis (p. 849), acute mastitis (staphylococcal, coliform or *A. pyogenes* (Chapters 23, 24)), acute septic metritis (p. 519), traumatic pericarditis. These conditions all involve damage by bacterial toxins, and the diarrhoeic faeces tend to be relatively scanty, but dark and sticky with a fetid odour.

(2) Several acute septicaemic diseases are associated with acute enteritis and diarrhoea, e.g. anthrax (see p. 717), transit fever (see p. 286) and other forms of acute pasteurellosis (see p. 728), and, of course, salmonellosis (see Chapter 15).

(3) Some virus diseases, e.g. malignant catarrhal fever (see p. 935) or the BVD/mucosal disease complex (see p. 853).

(4) Several plant poisons, e.g. solanin from green potatoes (see p. 943), water dropwort (see p. 943), and rhododendron (see p. 943).

(5) Several chemical poisons, e.g. arsenic (see p. 941) and certain organophosphorus compounds (see p. 940).

Chronic diarrhoea

(1) Johne's disease (see p. 857): the classical form of chronic diarrhoea with loss of weight, particularly from the hindquarters, ventral and submaxillary oedema and anaemia.

(2) Tuberculosis of the intestine (see p. 862), very rare today, is always secondary to pulmonary lesions, and is similar, clinically, to Johne's disease.

(3) Ulceration of the abomasum (see p. 844) produces scanty and intermittent diarrhoea in a cow losing weight, becoming anaemic and showing signs of low-grade anterior abdominal pain. Erosion of such an ulcer into a blood vessel in the abomasal wall produces more profuse, tarry faeces and may cause death.

(4) Amyloidosis is very rare indeed (see p. 928).

(5) Lymphosarcoma of the large gut is also very rare in cattle (see p. 693).

Herd diarrhoea

(1) Winter scours, or winter dysentery, has long been recognized as an acute, pyrexic and occasionally slightly dysenteric condition, which races through a housed dairy herd in winter conditions and then dies out with minimal long-term damage. There has been discussion as to the aetiological organism, various viruses and *Campylobacter* spp. having been incriminated (see p. 852).

(2) Various nutritional diarrhoeas:
- (a) Spring grass.
- (b) Frosted roots or kale.
- (c) Fodder beet poisoning, the leaves of which causes a hypocalcaemia-like syndrome and diarrhoea.
- (d) Acidosis (see p. 829), whether due to excessive root feeding or more commonly due to excessive cereal overload. The classical acidosis syndrome is that of barley poisoning with its acute abdominal pain and low-grade tympany, followed by profuse diarrhoea (see p. 830).

(3) Mineral deficiencies, e.g. copper (see pp. 254, 298) and cobalt (see p. 295) deficiency, producing chronic diarrhoea with weight loss and anaemia.

(4) Parasitic diarrhoea, e.g. parasitic gastroenteritis (see p. 267) and coccidiosis (see p. 282), largely affecting young stock.

(5) Toxicity, e.g. antibiotic contamination of the feed.

There is no easy way to diagnose the diarrhoeic animal. It is necessary to consider all environmental factors, including nutrition, stage of lactation, season of year, housing or pasture; whether the condition is an individual animal or herd problem and whether it is acute or chronic in nature.

Other signs besides diarrhoea may indicate whether the faecal changes are due to a primary gut problem or are secondary to a systemic disease.

Finally, one must utilize whatever laboratory tests for bacteria, parasites, viruses or minerals are available under the circumstances. Even so, there will be one-off conditions, rarely met with in one's practice area, which will, from time to time, elude the diagnostic net!

Tenesmus (straining) (see p. 838)

This condition occasionally occurs in cattle. *Coccidiosis* (see p. 282) in calves is an excellent example due to painful inflammatory changes in the hindgut. The *BVD/mucosal disease* (see p. 853) complex in young stock may have the same effect. Straining is also seen in the late stages of *ragwort poisoning* (see p. 945), in occasional cases of *terminal intussusception* (see p. 847) and sometimes in *urolithiasis in the male* (see p. 263).

It may also follow *sadistic human behaviour*, when sticks or broom handles have been forced into the rectum, frequently penetrating the wall of the hind gut some 30–45 cm (12–18 inches) proximal to the anus.

Occasionally, there will be sufficient straining to pass hard dry faeces in the cow with milk fever of some hours duration, to produce transient doubt in the attendant's mind as to the possibility of there being a further calf *in utero*. Obviously, the most frequent causes of straining in the cow are obstetrical, e.g. parturition, dystokia (p. 1115) or vaginal injury (p. 519).

Rectal examination may make things much worse if tenesmus is marked, but a look at the mucous membrane just within the anus with a pencil torch may be very helpful. In coccidiosis, cryptosporidosis and the BVD complex, particularly, the acutely inflamed nature of the hindgut often spreads right to the anus itself.

The unthrifty or emaciated cow

Starvation

Even in developed countries today, starvation can still be seen in poorer areas as a primary condition, but much more frequently appears as a relative energy deficit in high-yielding cows near peak yield. In the period from parturition to peak yield, it is frequently associated with ketosis.

Ketosis (see p. 793)

Ketosis is nothing more nor less than energy deficit and may if untreated produce very severe weight loss.

Liver fluke infestation (see p. 276)

Liver fluke infestation, reaching its most dangerous in terms of liver damage in the late autumn and winter months when autumn-calved cows are at peak yield and possibly in energy deficit, accentuates the whole picture of energy deficit and ketosis.

Chronic hypomagnesaemia (see p. 787)

In cold windy weather in late winter, heavily pregnant cattle develop a state of chronic hypomagnesaemia as a result of low food intake and cold, becoming thinner and poorer until some additional stress triggers off the acute convulsive phase.

These four conditions, interconnected to varying degrees, account for much of the unthriftiness found in dairy herds. A further condition, which may also be involved, is copper deficiency (p. 298).

Copper deficiency (see p. 298)

Copper deficiency may be either in its own right or resulting from molybdenum excess. In the latter case, there will be diarrhoea, but many herds exist in a low-grade copper deficiency, particularly at the beginning of the grazing season when the rapid grass growth dilutes the copper uptake, with weight loss and infertility the only signs.

Other conditions leading to weight loss

On an individual animal basis, Johne's disease (p. 857), which does not always cause diarrhoea in the early stages, and, historically, tubercular emaciation (p. 862) are important causes of weight loss, as are abomasal disorders such as left displacement (p. 839) and ulceration (p. 844). Chronic liver disorders, e.g. ragwort toxicity (p. 943) or multiple abscessation (p. 829), may also result in poor thriving to the point of emaciation before clear-cut aetiological pointers appear.

A number of other conditions lead to weight loss and suboptimal yield, but reasonable and sensible clinical examination should produce a definitive diagnosis without real problems. These conditions include the following.

- Lameness (laminitis, solar ulcer and white line lesions) (Chapter 31), often ignored by farmers who completely fail to realize the serious nature of the long-term effects.
- Chronic pyelonephritis (see p. 725), which should be obvious provided the clinician remembers to examine the urine.
- Actinobacillosis of the tongue or oesophageal groove area, already discussed on pp. 823–6.
- Paralysis of the fifth or seventh cranial nerve.
- The long-term toxic and depressing effects of mastitis, metritis, or postoperative peritonitis with adhesions and peritoneal abscessation.

The 'downer' cow (see pp. 439, 797)

A 'downer' cow used to be defined as a cow that remained recumbent after treatment for milk fever due to a continuing hypophosphataemia (p. 791). But, by general usage, the term has come to mean any cow recumbent at, or near, parturition, and thus there is a large differential list.

Preparturient

- Liver fluke (see p. 276) and/or starvation (see p. 796). These cows may have cirrhotic livers. They are thin, weak and lethargic, but not ketotic.
- The fat cow syndrome (see p. 796). Occasionally, grossly fat preparturient cows with pathologically fatty livers may become recumbent.

Parturient

(1) Prolonged dystokia may lead to exhaustion.
(2) Rupture of cervix or uterus leads to recumbency through shock and is quickly fatal.
(3) Traction injuries.
  (a) Sacroiliac disarticulation (see p. 448).
  (b) Sciatic nerve paralysis (see p. 439).
  (c) Torn adductor muscles (see pp. 439, 459).
  (d) Fractured pelvis (see p. 446).
  (e) Fractured femur (see pp. 441, 444).
  (f) Peroneal paralysis, which is much more likely to occur after milk fever than after parturition, because it is secondary to muscle atony in recumbency (see p. 438).

Parturient and postparturient

- Complications of milk fever (see p. 781)
- Fractures, dislocation and muscle injuries (see Chapter 32).
- Ruptured gastrocnemius (see p. 451).
- Peroneal paralysis (see p. 438).
- Sciatic nerve paralysis (sensory and motor) (see p. 439).
- Pressure ischaemia of hindleg or legs, which may lead to ischaemic muscle degeneration, particularly the semimembranosus and semitendinosis muscles. Serum AST and creatine phosphokinase levels rise markedly (see p. 439).
- Ketosis and licking mania (see p. 793).
- The cows seems bright and well, but stays down. Never attempt to make a cow with milk fever get up before it is entirely ready to do so (see p. 797).

Notice that the following conditions are all important in the differential diagnosis of the 'downer' cow (see pp. 439, 797).

- Acute staphylococcal (see p. 332) or coliform (see p. 334) mastitis.
- Acute septic metritis (see p. 519).
- Hypomagnesaemia (see p. 787).
- Cereal over-eating: acidosis (see p. 829).
- Fodder beet poisoning (see p. 149).
- Botulism: a condition increasing in frequency and associated with the feeding of big bale silage. Diagnosis is aided by a normal temperature, slow pulse rate and slowly progressive generalized muscular weakness affecting both voluntary and involuntary muscle (see p. 721).
- Internal haemorrhage, with fast pounding heart, white membranes, rapid respirations and often a subnormal temperature.

Diagnosis of the 'downer' cow is never easy, unless there is an obvious major fracture.

It is important that every 'downer' cow should be given full doses of calcium and phosphorus, and possibly also magnesium. It may be very logical to argue that a particular cow cannot possibly be a case of hypocalcaemia, but it is easy to be wrong. It is much safer to treat, just in case. With reasonable care no harm can be done.

Once satisfied that metabolic possibilities have been covered, a careful examination of the available parts of the skeleton should be carried out, but may not be very fruitful. It is not easy to assess injuries to the legs of a 'downer' cow deep in sludge or slurry!

It is vital that the udder and the uterus should be properly checked and, as far as the udder is concerned, every quarter must be examined however difficult access may be.

The cow ill during or after calving

There is no excuse in cases of periparturient illness for the taking of any form of short cut. The clinician must be satisfied that the cow has not developed any form of milk fever, and even when satisfied, it may be wise to give calcium/magnesium mixture subcutaneously as a precautionary measure.

The uterus must be examined to make sure that it is not infected and not damaged and, above all else, that there are no more calves within. Even after removing the third calf, the uterus should be checked for the fourth!

It is essential that the udder is properly examined. A parturient dairy cow may be very ill and dangerously toxaemic before the udder shows more than a small crepitating area just above the teat, and that may be all that is noticeable in some cases.

Pyrexia of unknown origin (PUO)

Obviously, many conditions may cause a marked rise of temperature in a cow, but a lethargic cow with a temperature of 40.5–41°C (105–106°F) is more likely to be a case of incipient mastitis (Chapter 23) than anything else, and should always be treated as such in the absence of other signs.

The next possibility is an active pulmonary hyperaemia as an early stage of pneumonia, while an acute septicaemic condition, such as salmonellosis (Chapter 15), may show pyrexia and little else for some 8–12 hours before diarrhoea supervenes. A rectal examination may discover diarrhoea in the early stages that will not have been seen by the stockman. During this period, the total white cell count may be as low as 1500–2000 per mm³, with a neutrophil percentage of less than 10 per cent.

One should remember that *anthrax* (see p. 717) is also an acute septicaemic condition, and there have been many cases of early anthrax where lethargy and a temperature of 41–42°C (106–108°F) are the only signs present. In young stock, severe diarrhoea, often bloodstained, with injected membranes, may supervene within a few hours to be followed by ataxia, collapse and death. In the adult cow, it is not infrequent for the hyperpyrexic early anthrax picture to be followed by collapse, subnormal temperature, clammy skin, cyanotic mucous membranes, restlessness and anxiety, followed quickly by coma and death. The clinician must beware of a stage in this process when the cold recumbent cow is easily mistaken for a severe milk fever case. Realization will come when it is seen that injection sites are trickling dark blood, while spreading haematomata appear where a vaginal examination has been performed, the teats have been handled or the stockworker has gripped the cow's nose.

Sudden death

This is a dangerously misleading heading. Very many cows that the owner regards as cases of sudden death are in fact cows found dead, which is quite a different matter. A cow found dead may well have taken 12 hours or more to die, depending on the diligence of the stockworker and when the cow was last seen.

If one can assume that sudden death means that a cow has collapsed and died, if not immediately then within the hour, then the differential diagnosis is fairly clear-cut.

Acute infections

- Anthrax: every case of sudden death is anthrax until proved otherwise (see p. 717).
- Blackleg (see p. 723): usually young stock but may occur in young adults. The lesion is usually obvious at post mortem. The causal organism is *Clostridium*

chauvoei and bruising of muscle groups predisposes to the problem (see p. 723).
- Wound gas gangrene infections: other clostridial organisms involved in wound infections, usually obvious at post mortem (see p. 724).

Occasional cases of acute coliform (see p. 334) infections, salmonellosis (see Chapter 15), pasteurellosis (see pp. 281, 728) and RSV pneumonia may produce a very rapid, sudden and unexpected death.

Acute pasture conditions

- Bloat: classical signs and environment, with a reasonably clear post-mortem picture, provided that the carcass is examined within an hour or so of death (see p. 832).
- Hypomagnesaemia: classical convulsive syndrome on spring grass. The carcass is often covered with debris, sweat and mud, with signs of convulsive movement in the grass for a considerable distance around (see p. 787).
- Fog fever: occurs in late summer or early autumn. As it is a herd problem there are usually other animals with signs. The lungs show a fairly characteristic post-mortem picture (see p. 866).

Electrocution and lightning strike (see p. 930)

There may be no signs whatsoever on the carcass, particularly in electrocution cases. The behaviour of neighbouring cows, if there is any witness, may help in electrocution, while it goes without saying that if a cow is to be struck by lightning, there must be a thunderstorm.

Accident or catastrophe

Road traffic accidents do occur but strangulation and asphyxiation as a result of faulty yokes and feed trough fittings are probably more common.

Catastrophes also include such events as a wire in the reticular wall being forced in one movement into the heart. The perforated abomasal ulcer leading to shock, peritoneal tympany and toxaemia is also included in this grouping.

Acute haemorrhage

This may result from the following:

- Wire penetration into a great vessel.
- Mammary vein rupture following injury.
- Teat vessel haemorrhage following injury.
- The rupture of a coronary vessel.
- The erosion of an abomasal ulcer into an artery in the abomasal wall.

- Damage to uterine or vaginal vessels after forced traction in dystokia cases.
- The erosion of a hepatic abscess into a major vessel.
- A thromboembolic pulmonary lesion originating from liver (see p. 867).
- A superficial haemangioma, often sited dorsally in the lumbar sacral area.
- Occasional acute cases of the pyrexia, pruritis and haemorrhage syndrome (see p. 884) bleed from the gut, and all other tissues. They also show raised temperature, severe general pruritis and aggressive behaviour before collapse and death.

It should be noted that all these haemorrhagic syndromes, with the exception of rupture of a coronary vessel, may not necessarily produce immediate death, but may instead produce a cold, staggering and severely anaemic animal with rapid pulse rate, rapid respirations, loudly beating heart and subnormal temperature. Early anthrax, peracute salmonellosis, acute babesiosis and acute bracken poisoning may produce the same collapsed and anaemic syndrome.

Acute anaphylactic reactions (see p. 927)

There may be much saliva around the mouth with oedema of the larynx, pharynx, eyelids, skin of face and head, etc. On the other hand, the only lesions may be pulmonary.

Poisons (see Chapter 54)

Theoretically, a number of poisons may cause sudden death in the cow but, practically, sudden death by poisoning will be due to one of the following:

- Yew (see p. 947);
- Water dropwort (see p. 943);
- Bracken: acutely haemorrhagic (see p. 946);
- Strychnine: rarely found today in Britain;
- Arsenic: rarely found today (see p. 941);
- Lead: may cause sudden death in calves, but not usually in cows (see pp. 906, 944);
- Copper (see p. 948).

Jugular stasis (cording)

Care must be taken in the interpretation of jugular stasis. There is often confusion between jugular stasis and jugular pulsation, and it must be emphasized that jugular pulsation may occur in perfectly normal cows, especially if the head is held low as while grazing.

Jugular stasis may occur in conditions involving space-occupying lesions in the anterior mediastinum, e.g. thymic lymphosarcomata in young stock, mediastinal lymphosarcomata in the adult (p. 693) or large mediastinal abscesses.

Nevertheless, the more common causes of jugular stasis (distension) stem from the heart itself.

Traumatic pericarditis (see p. 731)

Previously the most common form of cardiac disease in the cow, this condition has now become relatively rare in Great Britain.

Chronic vegetative endocarditis (see p. 726)

This condition has become much more frequent. It is probable that, 30 years ago, many cases of endocarditis were missed completely for the clinician was so used to 'wire' and pericarditis that all cases of congestive heart failure were diagnosed as pericarditis and sent to the knacker's yard after the most superficial examination.

There are a number of important clinical differences. The pericarditis case is much more toxaemic and therefore more depressed. Transition from relative health to acute illness is much more sudden, although there may, of course, have been low-grade reticulitis signs at some previous stage. Pain is more marked and very readily elicited by wither pinching. Cardiac sounds start with slight friction sounds synchronous with the heart beat, which is usually more than 100/minute. Within a day or so, the tinkling splashing sounds indicative of gas/fluid production within the pericardium can be heard, and in a further day or so the sac is grossly distended with pus, and splashing and tinkling have ceased. The heart sounds are now muffled and may, in fact, be louder on the right side because the pressure of the distended pericardium against the left thoracic wall tends to extend the whole structure across to the right.

Gross jugular and mammary engorgement and dependent oedema will now be present at jaw, neck, brisket and lower abdomen. Pulse rate may well reach 140/minute.

Endocarditis, on the other hand, runs a more gradual course. For some time, the picture may be one of low-grade anterior abdominal pain, plus a temperature rise to 40–41°C (104–106°F). Pain is felt over a much wider area of the chest. The pulse rate is not generally very greatly raised at first. The cow is often relatively bright and may even eat a little, but exercise tolerance is very poor. Heart sounds, at first, are no more than loud, and even later in the disease it is not always possible for ordinary mortals to hear the cardiac murmur that is stated to be invariably present in this disease. The reason for this seems to be that, in most cases, the lesion is right-sided.

At first, therefore, and for several days at least, vegetative endocarditis falls within the anterior abdominal/posterior thoracic pain grouping and is easily mistaken for 'wire'. There may even be a wire, for although most cases derive the valvular infection from the rumen via the liver, from the udder, uterus, pharynx or feet, occasional cases are met in which the primary pyogenic focus is a penetrating reticular foreign body. It is interesting that, in most cases of vegetative endocarditis, the white cell count and the temperature fall during antibiotic treatment, but the pulse rate is unaffected.

Eventually, jugular congestion, shifting lameness, dependent oedema, pulmonary signs, and even haematuria may all appear.

In right-sided cases, pulmonary thromboembolism may cause marked thoracic pain, whilst ascites and engorged mammary and jugular veins are very noticeable. In left-sided cases, pulmonary congestion causes dyspnoea and coughing with less pain, but haematuria due to renal infarction is more likely.

Myocardial abscesses

Myocardial abscesses of considerable size may sometimes occur, producing a clinical picture similar to that of endocarditis, but with lower temperature rises and a slower course.

Other causes of jugular stasis

Fatty degeneration of the heart, and tubercular pericarditis, are usually masked by more obvious systemic signs of the respective diseases.

'Redwater' (blood or blood pigments in urine)

With very few exceptions, disease of the urinary tract in cattle produces significant urinary haemorrhage, and the differential diagnosis obviously includes the numerous haemolytic conditions producing urinary haemoglobin.

Obviously, therefore, when presented with a 'redwater' case, the first stage in diagnosis is to decide whether the case is one of haematuria or haemoglobinuria. Microscopical examination or centrifuging the urine will supply the answer, but usually the simple expedient of standing some urine in a container for a few minutes, while clinical examination is proceeding, will give a satisfactory answer. The clinician must remember that many cows with redwater are not presented as such, for stockworkers rarely notice or even see a cow urinate, except by chance. If asked whether the urine is normal, the invariable answer is that it must be or it would have been noticed. This is wishful thinking, upon which no reliance can be placed.

Once differentiation between blood and blood pigment has been made, diagnosis becomes much easier.

Haematuria

- Chronic cystic haematuria (enzootic haematuria (see p. 947) or chronic bracken poisoning (see p. 946));
- Pyelonephritis (see p. 725);
- Calculi (see p. 263);
- Neoplasia other than is involved in the first list point.

These four conditions show primary lesions within the urinary tract.

Enzootic haematuria (see p. 946) has a regional incidence dependent upon the prevalence of bracken. It tends to occur in older home reared cows and the blood in the urine, slight at first and slowly increasing, contains very little pus or exudative material.

Pyelonephritis (see p. 725) is much more likely to be encountered in dairy herds, but is, for some reason, a rare disease today in Britain compared with its incidence in the 1950s and 1960s.

There are systemic signs varying from very acute to very mild, but diagnosis is greatly assisted by the presence of pus, debris and renal casts, as well as blood, in the urine. Rectal examination may help and the presence of pain is another differential point, for enzootic haematuria is painless and afebrile. Bacteriology on the urine of pyelonephritis may, in fairly early cases, produce a culture of *Corynebacterium renale*, which is the primary causal organism. Remember that the pain, the temperature and the arched back invite confusion with 'wire' unless the clinician keeps pyelonephritis in mind in such cases, particularly in the first third of lactation, and insists on inspecting a urine sample.

Urolithiasis (see p. 263) occurs largely in the young male, and other signs such as straining, the absence of significant amounts of urine and, eventually, 'water belly' overshadow the presence of blood spots in the urine.

Neoplasia of the urinary tract, other than that due to chronic bracken poisoning, is very rare.

A number of conditions occur in which haematuria is but one of a number of fairly obvious systemic signs, so that the urinary blood, when present, is not important in diagnosis:

- Vegetative endocarditis (see p. 726).
- Septicaemic conditions, e.g. anthrax (see p. 717) and acute pasteurellosis (see pp. 286, 728).
- Acute bracken poisoning: a disease with markedly raised temperatures and generalized haemorrhages, which behaves like an acute septicaemia and probably is one (p. 946).

It is worth remembering that very high doses of sulphonamides may theoretically produce crystalluria and haematuria, but sulphapyridine, the sulphonamide that most frequently produced these signs, is no longer used.

Haemoglobinuria

Piroplasmosis is an acute, pyrexic, and acutely haemolytic tick-borne disease of certain areas of Britain and other countries caused by *Babesia divergens*. The clinical signs include profuse diarrhoea, followed by stubborn constipation in a non-premune cow, progressive anaemia, with very rapid pulse rate, loudly pounding heart, and deep port wine coloured urine (see p. 748).

Bacillary haemoglobinuria is a peracute and rapidly fatal pyrexic disease due to *Clostridium haemolyticum* (now renamed *Cl. oedematiens* type II). It affects young stock in certain rough hill areas, but is of relatively little importance overall (see p. 719).

Postparturient haemoglobinuria is seen during the weeks following parturition in cows in certain parts of eastern Scotland and occasionally in England. It is non-febrile, but progressive and frequently fatal due to very severe anaemia, and is possibly associated with root and straw feeding and abnormalities in phosphorus metabolism. It is too rare today to be of real significance (see p. 792).

Kale and rape poisoning are too well known to merit detailed consideration. Large quantities are required and wilted kale is much less likely to cause problems. It is worth remembering that rape in excess may also produce abdominal pain, nervous signs and/or dyspnoea (see p. 941).

Leptospira icterohaemorrhagiae produces haemoglobinuria in the calf, but this is most unlikely to occur in the adult (see p. 735).

Very cold water, thirstily drunk, may cause haemoglobinuria in the calf, but not in the adult.

Copper toxicity, increasing in the UK, may apparently produce haemoglobinuria (see p. 948).

Cows breathing badly (hyperpnoea and dyspnoea)

The clinician must not assume that rapid respirations in cattle necessarily indicate the presence of pneumonia. Cattle 'blow' for many reasons.

Physiological

Cattle breathe more rapidly when full after feeding, after exercise, in hot and humid weather and when they are nervous or frightened. A herd coming in for milking on a hot summer afternoon after a mile walk from lush grazing may all appear dyspnoeic! When asked to comment on a cow's respiratory pattern, it is always worth comparing it with that of neighbouring cows.

Pathological

Respiratory rates:

(1) Increase markedly in many diseases due to pyrexia.
(2) Increase and become jerky in acutely painful conditions, e.g. septic feet, acute laminitis (see p. 417).
(3) Increase in acute toxaemic conditions, e.g. summer mastitis (Chapter 24), coliform mastitis (see p. 334) and acute septic metritis (see p. 519).
(4) Increase in metabolic disease, e.g. hypomagnesaemia (see p. 787) or acidosis (see p. 829).
(5) Increase markedly with a much shallower thoracic excursion in conditions that prevent full pulmonary expansion, e.g. ruminal tympany, ruminal impaction and pleural effusion.
(6) Increase in conditions in which the upper respiratory tract is blocked at least in part, e.g. malignant catarrhal fever, IBR (see p. 289) and pharyngitis.
(7) Increase and become shallow in conditions that interfere with the function of the respiratory muscles, e.g. tetanus (see p. 733).
(8) Increase very markedly in severe anaemic conditions, e.g. piroplasmosis (see p. 748) and haemorrhage.
(9) Increase and become laboured in conditions that, for various reasons, decrease the amount of active lung tissue, for example:
  (a) active pulmonary congestion prior to pneumonia (see p. 860);
  (b) chronic venous congestion, e.g. vegetative endocarditis (see p. 726);
  (c) acute anaphylactic conditions (see p. 927);
  (d) 'fog fever' (acute pulmonary oedema and emphysema) (see p. 866); and
  (e) pneumonia (see p. 864).

Acute nervous and convulsive syndromes

Nervous signs occur relatively frequently in cattle of all ages, and vary from mild signs of ataxia and head pressing on the one hand to hyperaesthesia, circling, muscular tremors, aggression, collapse and convulsions, on the other.

Acute hypomagnesaemia (see p. 787)

This condition occurs in dairy cattle on heavily fertilized high-protein pasture at turn-out in spring, and again in the autumn. It also occurs in winter and early spring in beef cattle on exposed pasture. Hyperaesthesia, with muscular tremors of face, eyelids, ears and muscles of the head and neck, is followed by strabismus, generalized muscular tremors and collapse in generalized clonic convulsions.

Transit tetany

This occurs during transport, largely in preparturient cattle under stressful conditions. Signs are similar to those of hypomagnesaemia, but blood may be low both in magnesium and calcium.

Bovine spongiform encephalopathy (BSE) (see p. 909)

This shows more slowly developing hyperaesthesia with ataxia and behavioural changes prior to collapse. These changes include apprehension occasionally amounting to panic, obsessive licking of nose and lips, semaphoring of ears, refusal to pass through doorways, kicking off the milking clusters in the parlour, reflex kicking at other times and muscular tremors of neck and shoulders.

Hepatic encephalopathy

Hepatic encephalopathy, occurring as a complication of certain forms of liver disease, e.g. ragwort (see p. 945) or other forms of plant poisoning, is due to the effect upon the brain of ammonia released from the damaged liver. Signs are ataxia, dullness, slow circling, head pressing and collapse. Occasional periods of excitement are seen.

Tubercular meningitis (see pp. 251, 862)

Not to be forgotten in these days when bovine tuberculosis is on the increase, tubercular meningitis may be seen in half-grown cattle as a sequel to congenital tuberculosis or the consumption of milk from cows with mammary tuberculosis. Ataxia, stumbling, bellowing and an inco-ordinate aggression with head pressing followed by collapse were frequently seen in this condition. In the days of horned cattle, fracture of one or both horns often occurred as a result of head pressing. Blindness in one or both eyes might also occur.

Lead poisoning (see p. 944)

In the adult lead poisoning produces blindness and aimless wandering, often complicated by trauma due to collisions with walls, trees, etc. Bellowing frequently occurs.

Rape poisoning (see p. 941)

Rape poisoning may produce excitement, aggression, blindness and bellowing, a nervous syndrome, which may be complicated by dyspnoea, haemoglobinuria and constipation.

Listeriosis (listerellosis) (see pp. 251, 904)

Listeriosis occasionally occurs in silage-fed cattle, producing an initial pyrexia followed by hyperaesthesia, a tendency to aggression, circling, head pressing, facial paralysis with drooping of one or both upper eyelids and a dry keratitis. One or both ears may also be involved, and occasionally the fifth cranial nerve as well as the seventh is affected so that chewing and swallowing are impaired and food becomes impacted in the pharynx and mouth.

Ketosis (acetonaemia) (see p. 795)

Ketosis is normally a sign of energy deficit in high-yielding dairy cattle between two and six weeks after calving. The condition may well be subclinical, doing no more than reducing yield. At its worst, it produces inappetence for concentrates, lethargy and constipation, with a normal or subnormal temperature and pulse rate.

Occasionally, a nervous form occurs producing ataxia and excitement, with marked head signs, the patient licking itself and anything within reach in an obsessive fashion, holding the bars of the shippen or parlour in its teeth and chewing to such an extent that tongue and lips may bleed forming a bloodstained froth. Ketone bodies are present at high levels in blood, milk and urine.

Occasionally, this licking frenzy may occur as a complication of milk fever. It is known as 'licking mania' and is believed to be ketotic in origin.

Acute inflammatory, exudative and/or haemorrhagic lesions in the brain

Acute inflammatory, exudative, and/or haemorrhagic lesions within the brain may cause marked excitement bordering on mania before collapse occurs. This picture may occur in anthrax (see p. 717), in which case diagnosis will be helped by generalized haemorrhage and oedema, and is also sometimes seen in malignant catarrhal fever accompanied by marked nasal and ocular discharge, with heat and pain over the sinuses of the head. Horns, if present, feel hot and in cattle with white horns they become very reddened and may, in fact, become loose. There is usually profuse diarrhoea.

Convulsive syndromes that are relatively frequent among calves

Lead poisoning (see pp. 906, 944): This is still common, causing abdominal pain, blindness, salivation and con-

vulsions, with marked bellowing and leading rapidly to death.

Magnesium tetany (see p. 255): In beef calves fed dam's milk alone without supplement magnesium tetany appears at 12–16 weeks of age, producing star gazing, stilted gait, muscular tremors and hyperaesthesia leading to convulsions and death. Abdominal pain, blindness and bellowing are not features of magnesium tetany.

Gammexane (gamma BHC) poisoning (see p. 942): This condition is due to feeding milk in buckets contaminated with gammexane, after mixing insecticides, and causes very severe clonic convulsions and death.

Linseed poisoning (see p. 941): The acute dyspnoeic picture with gasping and muscular spasm that follows the feeding of warm wet linseed to calves may look much like a convulsive picture unless one is aware of the signs of prussic acid poisoning.

Muscular dystrophy (see pp. 258, 302): Calves dying of heart failure due to the cardiac form of muscular dystrophy will normally be housed calves fed only on dam's milk. Vitamin E intake may therefore be low, and at two to three months of age any sudden excitement, such as the arrival of the dam at feeding time, may trigger off a cardiac failure episode with cyanosis and anoxia which, nevertheless, may superficially resemble a convulsive syndrome.

Cerebrocortical necrosis (see p. 261): Cerebrocortical necrosis (CCN) occurring in housed or yarded calves may produce star gazing, hyperaesthesia and ataxia but, occasionally, leads to a severe convulsive picture.

References

Boddie, G.F. (1970) *Diagnostic Methods in Veterinary Medicine*, 6th edn. Oliver and Boyd, Edinburgh.
Rees Evans, E.T. (1957) Bacterial endocarditis of cattle. *Veterinary Record*, **69**, 1190–202.

The Calf

Chapter 12
Outline of Clinical Genetics

G.B. Young

Introduction	161
Deleterious major genes	161
Genes and disease in different species	162
Genetic epidemiology	162
Economic loss	162
Modes of inheritance	162
Dominant genes	162
Semidominant genes	162
Recessive genes	163
Sex-limited and sex-linked genes	163
Multiple alleles	163
Irregular inheritance	163
Genetic polymorphism	163
Chromosomal abnormalities	163
Epidemiology and control	164
Controlling dominants	164
Controlling recessives	164
Controlling an irregularly inherited defect	164
Genes exhibiting good and bad effects	164
Assessing controls	165
Investigating genetic diseases	165
Pedigree analysis	165
DNA analysis	165
Differentiating genetic and infectious diseases	165
Genetic counselling	166
Genetic defects and artificial insemination	166
Genetic defects and egg transplanting	166
Polygenic deleterious genes	166
Sterility and infertility genes	167
Calving difficulties	167
Susceptibility and resistance genes	167
Metabolic disease genetics	168
Disease genetics and cattle improvement schemes	168
Inbreeding depression	168
Intensive single-character selection	169
Balanced selection	169
Positive selection for health	169
Selection and longevity in dairy cows	169
Bull mothers	169
Crossbreeding	169
Health recording schemes	169
Recent advance	169
Cloning	170
The genomics revolution	170
Conclusions	171

Introduction

Genetics in hereditary diseases corresponds to the microbiology of infections. Before Pasteur's contribution to bacteriology, infections were crudely controlled by isolation, but his work greatly improved preventive measures. Similarly, genetics greatly improves the precision in controlling hereditary diseases.

Many genetic problems are complex and exhibit a spectrum from being entirely genetic to entirely environmental. The genetic component may be divided into major gene and polygenic effects. Polygenes each have a small effect and produce continuous variation. Most disease due to major genes is, however, also influenced by minor genes and many diseases currently considered polygenic may in reality be affected by relatively few major genes.

Observations and experimentation indicate that, like the well-studied *Drosophila*, cattle carry a genetic load of deleterious major genes producing gross abnormality and of deleterious polygenes producing subfertility, increased disease susceptibility and poor physique. With current knowledge many polygenic constitutional defects can only be studied biometrically, but the final aim is to recognize individually every gene and its location on specific chromosomes. Recombinant DNA technology now makes this theoretically feasible.

Deleterious major genes

Every body system is subject to abnormal inheritance. Indeed, if, as the embryo unfolds, a defect occurs early, several subsequent systems may be involved, producing a syndrome. Environmental disturbances, or other genes sometimes inherited differently but affecting the same developmental pathway, can produce identical diseases or syndromes.

Genetic diseases affect all ages from conception to senility. Congenital malformations, observed at birth, may be genetic or due to maternal effects such as infections, nutritional deficiencies or drugs. Genes control the synthesis of proteins and, when defective, generally result in an enzyme reduction or deficiency.

Molecular genetics has developed the concept of control genes, influencing structural genes, but most genetic diseases are still thought of in terms of structural or chromosomal mutations.

Genes and disease in different species

The basic genetic physical structure of all species from worms and fruit flies to humans is similar. For example, the control homeobox genes, the molecular architects organizing other genes and switching them on and off at the correct time, are universally responsible for the division into head, thorax and abdomen. The gene that controls eye development in humans, when inserted into a fly, produces normal fly development. This common, genetic, evolutionary heritage implies that genetic malformations present in one species will often also be present in others. The luxate gene in mice, humans and Galloway cattle is an example. Further genes can be transferred from one species to another. Using transgenics, most known human genetic diseases have been transferred to mice.

Mammalian species probably have around thirty thousand genes and yet only three hundred are thought to separate mice from men. Different species are therefore likely to suffer from similar infections and infestations. Tuberculosis and the influenzas illustrate the point. Studying genetic disease similarities and dissimilarities between species constitutes comparative genomics.

Genetic epidemiology

All cattle breeds possess several genetic diseases, some common to many breeds, others specific to individual breeds. Several hundred have been described and many more are known.

Most persist at a low frequency. Some appear almost sporadically in many different herds over the years. Others are concentrated in a few herds in sudden outbreaks. Occasionally, a defect increases until individual or collective action reduces its frequency. If breeders relax, its frequency increases again, producing a cyclical pattern.

Economic loss

Calf loss may reach 20 per cent within a herd for several years, as in Galloway tibial hemimelia (p. 176). Maternal mortality may be high as in prolonged gestations in many breeds (p. 183). Difficult parturitions reduce yield and late abortions result in long dry periods. In later developing defects, e.g. hip dysplasia (p. 453), only cull value is obtained. The bull has to be replaced, the breeding programme is disrupted and pedigree sales drop. Counterselection substantially reduces economic selection.

Few breeders escape genetic disease at some time. Economic data are not available on either the direct loss due to major deleterious genes or the greater indirect loss from counterselection. Genes capable of producing defects are, however, abundant and most cattle probably carry several. Only fear of inbreeding and continual selection against defects prevents more frequent outbreaks.

Modes of inheritance

Inheritance is duplicate: each individual has two genes (units of inheritance) for a particular character or function at each locus on the chromosomes. A parent passes one on a random basis to an offspring, the other coming from the second parent. Chemically, genes are deoxyribose nucleic acid (DNA) and the fine structure of the gene has been elucidated, but for most clinical purposes the gene may still be regarded as the unit of inheritance.

Dominant genes

In regular dominance every carrier is affected. The disease is generally inherited from one parent and half its offspring are affected. A new dominant gene producing a severe effect tends to be lethal and produces single isolated effects. Surviving dominants produce relatively minor defects, e.g. notched ears in Ayrshires.

Irregular rather than regular dominants are more common in cattle. An individual may carry the gene but not manifest it due to intangible environmental effects or modifying genes (incomplete penetrance). Half of its offspring also carry the abnormal gene but a proportion similarly do not manifest it, producing irregular segregation ratios.

Hereditary ataxia (p. 178) in Aberdeen Angus illustrates this inheritance. Transmitting bulls mated to noncarrier cows leave around 25–40 per cent of calves affected instead of the expected 50 per cent, so penetrance is from 50 to 80 per cent.

Some late-developing defects, such as arthritic conditions in bulls (p. 176), could, in theory, be due to dominants. The bull would not exhibit the disease until old, and bred from, and because of culling, the relationship and ratios between bull and offspring might not be easily noticeable.

Semidominant genes

These are quite common in cattle. A single gene produces a defect but a double dose increases its severity. In the single dose, the abnormal gene converts a Kerry into the small, more desirable, Dexter, but a double dose produces monsters. Matings of Dexters produce on average 25 per cent Kerry types, 50 per cent Dexter types and 25 per cent bulldog monsters (see p. 175).

Many dwarves exhibit this inheritance. Often, as in snorter dwarves in Herefords, the carrier conformation is only slightly different from normal and slightly better (heterozygote advantage). Selection for carriers then spreads the disease. At the limits, one-quarter of the calves are defective.

Recessive genes

A single gene does not show in a carrier because of the normal dominant gene. The defect only appears with a double dose. Neither parent is affected yet the defect has come from both parents.

In carrier matings one in four of the offspring are normal (RR), two are carriers (Rr), and one will be affected (rr). This is true on average but not for individual or small groups of matings. Moreover, pure recessives giving exact ratios are rare, even with the traditional genetic model of *Drosophila*.

The abnormal gene is usually considered neutral in carriers but in some cases, probably more than is currently understood, it may be detected biochemically. Carrier recognition is a major field of genetics and should always be sought in major recessive outbreaks in cattle.

Recessive defects may also have reduced penetrance. Since the frequency of recessive homozygotes is generally low, if further reduced by incomplete penetrance, inheritance is best described simply as irregular, and calculating the penetrance of a recessive is generally unprofitable.

Recessive defects often appear following line breeding. A breeder obtaining good daughters from one bull is often tempted to use related bulls on these. These related males may carry the same recessive gene derived from a common ancestor. Some second matings are thus between carriers, and defects appear. The pedigrees of affected animals often reveal common ancestors within a few generations.

Sex-limited and sex-linked genes

Many cattle diseases are limited to one sex, for example, testicular hypoplasia (p. 182). The other sex, however, plays an equal role in inheritance and the defective genes are in the non-sex autosomes. This inheritance must be distinguished from sex-linked recessive inheritance where the abnormal gene is carried on the X chromosome and a carrier cow transmits the disease to half her bull calves, and leaves half her heifer calves as carriers; a cow with a double dose of the harmful gene would show the disease. Since sex-linked recessives are not transmitted by unaffected bulls, they are rare in cattle.

Multiple alleles

Each locus on the chromosome may have not just two but several genes present. Various combinations of these genes may produce a gradation of severity of a condition. For example, a series of multiple alleles reducing melanism successively dilutes coat colour from normal agouti to albinism. Multiple alleles may contribute to the variation in clinical expression of many diseases. They are also a common form of inheritance in many disease-related biochemical variants.

Irregular inheritance

Many, indeed most, genetic diseases of cattle are inherited irregularly. They do not provide simple genetic ratios and are characterized by sporadic incidence and occasional concentration within families. Arthrogryposis in Charolais characterized by calves with twisted limbs (see p. 177), cleft palates and a twisted spine, illustrates the problem. More than half of all artificial insemination (AI) bulls produce a few defective calves but a few (about 5 per cent) leave around five per cent of affected calves.

Cryptorchids provide another example of non-Mendelian inheritance. Cryptorchidism is frequently sporadic (p. 182). Most extensively used sires leave some cryptorchids. Many cryptorchids leave mainly normal offspring and most cryptorchids have normal parents. Occasionally, however, affected or normal bulls sire a higher proportion of affected offspring than average. Their incidence also increases markedly on inbreeding. Cryptorchidism thus has a genetic component and probably both male and female contribute to its occurrence.

Such defects result from unknown environmental factors and genetic susceptibility, either recessives or dominants, exhibiting a very sensitive threshold of manifestation.

Genetic polymorphism

This is a discontinuous variation which persists in a population apparently more or less at random. Cattle blood groups are an obvious example. Their relative proportions are not maintained by a balance between mutation increasing the defect and selection removing genes in affected animals. Most, however, will probably be ultimately shown to affect fitness. Many may be relics of resistance mechanisms to much earlier plagues.

Chromosomal abnormalities

Structural chromosomal mutations, such as duplications, deficiencies, inversions, translocations (p. 184) and alterations in chromosomal number, are not uncommon in cattle. Large chromosomal breakages produce complete sterility and small breakages subfertility. Both are inherited like irregular dominants. Bulls with low conception rates due to minor chromosomal abnormalities pass the defect directly to their sons.

Many chromosomal defects, often difficult to detect, are probably present in early embryos, and account for a considerable proportion of early embryonic mortality and some reduction in conception rate. The uterus, however, acts as a clearing house for such defects and few progress to birth.

Epidemiology and control

Breeds are generally organized hierarchically. A few top herds supply bulls to less influential breeders who in turn supply commercial producers. If a harmful gene spreads in the top strata these bulls spread carriers through the breed. Similarly, if the defect is eliminated from the top herds then sires free from the defective gene slowly reduce the defect in the other herds. The origin and increase of a harmful mutant in the top herds is probably due to mutation and genetic drift.

Control is the sum of the control efforts of individual breeders. Affected herds select against the gene, and breeders soon learn from which herds to reduce their purchases. The distribution of non-carrier bulls reduces the incidence.

The desirability of control will vary with the severity and frequency of the defect. A defect causing dystokia justifies considerable counterselection, but a minor defect such as colobomata very little. Strong selection against a defect may also relax selection for important economic characters.

Controlling dominants

A regular dominant spreads directly down through a breed but such direct transmission is rare in cattle except for minor defects such as some forms of polydactyly. If required, culling all affected animals eliminates the defective gene.

Dominants exhibiting incomplete penetrance, however, commonly spread directly. The lower the penetrance, the greater the likelihood of this occurring. If penetrance is high a few offspring will pinpoint a carrier parent and transmitters can be culled. If penetrance is low, control is more difficult, since many offspring are required to detect carriers.

Controlling recessives

At breed level, epidemiology and control of recessive genes will depend on the gene frequency. This is simply the proportion of genes of a particular type in the population. Since each animal has two of these genes, the proportion of carriers is approximately twice the gene frequency, and the incidence of affected individuals is the square of the gene frequency. Thus, if the incidence of a recessive defect is 1 per cent, the gene frequency is 10 per cent and the proportion of carriers about 20 per cent. Even a low incidence of defects thus implies large numbers of carriers.

Moreover, this gene frequency will be the average for the whole breed and much higher frequencies will occur in farms that have used carrier males recently. Thus the outbreaks and frequencies will be patchy with some farms heavily affected and others with few or no defects. This often renders measurement of the incidence of a defect in a breed difficult. A useful guide is that a defect attracts notice when around 1 per cent of calves are affected in the breed so that about 18–20 per cent of animals are carriers.

Reduction in frequency can be rapid if the initial frequency is high but is slower as the frequency decreases or if the initial frequency is low. Thus breeders can rapidly reduce a recessive defect at high levels but eliminating it completely is very difficult.

The main difficulty in selecting against a recessive is the large number of carriers that cannot be recognized on visual inspection. However, if all bulls and cows producing defects are culled, experience shows the incidence of the defect soon drops to acceptable levels.

Controlling an irregularly inherited defect

In a disease such as arthrogryposis (p. 177) all bulls leaving defects cannot be culled but only bulls transmitting most frequently. Similarly, in defects such as cryptorchidism, control is based on not using affected animals or close relatives and this is effective in maintaining a low frequency.

Irregular defects such as cryptorchidism (p. 182) would only increase if affected animals were continuously used. Why they persist at a low level despite generations of natural and artificial selection is unknown although carrier advantage may be suspected.

Genes exhibiting good and bad effects

Some pleiotropic genes or closely linked gene complexes produce both desirable and undesirable effects and selection for the good effects may spread the gene. For example, some genes producing desirable coat colours also cause infertility. Selection for the coat colour may thus spread infertility or maintain it at a low level, as in white heifer disease (p. 183).

A gene may be beneficial when single but harmful in a double dose as in selection for the desirable conformation in American beef breeds resulting in unconscious selection for carriers.

Inheritance involving advantageous and disadvantageous effects may be much more common in cattle than suspected.

Assessing controls

Excessive controls, such as compulsory recording of all abnormalities, are sometimes advocated. Controls are essential, particularly where a defect has become a problem, but they should be kept in proportion. They should be kept to the minimum level necessary, so that selection for efficient production can proceed as rapidly as possible.

Investigating genetic diseases

Inheritance may be suspected when other factors are excluded, the defect runs in families and previous reports implicate genetics. Since environmental defects may simulate genetic conditions and similar clinical defects have different genetic causes inheritance in the affected herd should be investigated.

Inheritance exists when one bull has sired all the defects and another contemporary bull has left none when mated to similar females in a similar environment. However, such controls are often not available and a properly designed experiment may be necessary.

If line breeding is being practised a new defect is probably genetic. If recessive, both sexes are affected equally and the incidence within a herd seldom rises above 15–20 per cent. The disease may disappear as unaffected males are brought in. Since environmental changes are often made simultaneously confusion may arise.

Simple recessive defects resemble each other fairly closely – one dropsical calf tends to be similar to another. Where considerable variation in clinical appearance or age of onset is present a simple recessive is unlikely.

In cattle, and especially in a small herd, establishing the exact inheritance may be difficult. Often all that can be said is that the disease runs in families and comes from either one parent only or, alternatively, the genetic factors are present in both parents.

Breed differences are also suggestive of genetic disease but not conclusive because of possible confounding between breed and environment. This is particularly true where infections or mineral deficiencies are involved.

Pedigree analysis

A few generations intensively studied are better than long pedigrees. A list of normal and affected animals born during and immediately prior to the outbreak, their sex, sire, dam and maternal grandsire is generally adequate. This list will indicate if simple genetic ratios exist.

With recessives one out of four offspring of carriers are affected, but in practice the common ratio obtained is one in eight. This occurs when two carrier males are used successively. The first carrier leaves on average half of his daughters carriers (as well as half his sons). In mating the second carrier bull to the carrier daughters, one out of the four offspring are defective. About one in two × one in four, i.e. one in eight of the second bull's offspring are defective.

Care has to be taken with pedigrees since as many as 10 per cent may be inaccurate. Few pedigree investigations fail to produce anomalous cases.

DNA analysis

Almost weekly a new gene for a human disease, located by deciphering the genome, is recorded and some breast cancers are already subject to routine screening, particularly in patients with a family history. Although mapping the genome in cattle is being pursued in some laboratories, financial restraints limit progress. Moreover, reliable results require great technical skill to narrow down the suspected DNA sequences, which may involve several hundred genes, to the required gene and to assure the specific gene is involved. Until more progress is made reliance for diagnosis and control in livestock has to be placed on the more standard but still relevant procedures such as pedigree analysis outlined previously.

Predicting future diseases seems to cause substantial ethical and insurance problems in humans, but in livestock, while similar problems will arise, they are relatively trivial. In contrast, predicting future diseases in livestock is one major way ahead in reducing disease incidence.

Differentiating genetic and infectious diseases

Genetic and infectious diseases may, on occasion, be confused. Their epidemiology can be similar, with deleterious genes or infectious agents radiating out from heavily diseased foci. Moreover, many infectious diseases through close contact are familial and genetic resistance may be present, enhancing the familial aspects. Pathology may even be similar, since an invading organism can affect the same developmental pathway as a deleterious gene. The crucial distinctions are the isolation of an infectious agent and experimental transmission of the disease or the establishment of fairly clearcut genetic ratios, perferably the former.

Genetic counselling

In the event of a genetic disease a breeder should be advised to change the bull immediately, thus eliminating the appearance of the defect and reducing the carrier incidence in offspring. Continuous use of non-carrier bulls gradually reduces the number of carriers.

If a carrier male has had only restricted use all his daughters should be culled. However, where the herd has many carrier females, culling should be gradual to avoid decimating the herd. Known carriers and low-producing females should be culled first. Where the abnormal gene occurs in a particularly good strain its frequency should be reduced rather slowly so as to preserve the strain intact, i.e. some defects should be suffered to maintain production qualities.

In a serious outbreak a breeder might test a male on about 20 of its daughters or half sisters, or on 10 known carrier females. Generally, however, test mating is expensive and best avoided.

Control of defects inherited as irregular dominants or in a non-Mendelian fashion, follows the same principles. The bull should be changed and transmitting females culled.

When a defect rises in frequency, the breed society should seek veterinary advice. After ensuring that the disease is recognizable, both clinically and pathologically, its mode of inheritance and methods of control are then explained to breeders so they can counterselect most effectively. Prenatal diagnosis and selective abortion, although feasible, should only have limited application in valuable animals in cattle practice.

Genetic defects and artificial insemination (see Chapter 39)

Artificial insemination centres seldom suffer outbreaks of genetic disease because they avoid inbreeding, particularly in the larger units, and rapidly withdraw bulls transmitting defects. Although most bulls carry several defective genes, few leave many defects in their progeny since their cow population is unlikely to have a high gene frequency for the same defect. While a carrier bull leaves half his daughters carriers, each time a non-carrier is used on the succeeding daughter's generations, the carrier incidence is halved.

Automatically eliminating bulls leaving three or so affected offspring is rather rigid. Selection against bulls leaving calves causing maternal mortality, late developing defects, or leaving three affected calves in their first 100 offspring should be more intense than against bulls producing unimportant defects, or producing a few abnormalities among several thousand normal calves. Again, a few defects among several thousand normal calves is tolerable from a bull transmitting efficient production.

When an undesirable gene is increasing, an AI centre should buy bulls from sources thought to be incidence free. Even with limited numbers of offspring and a low gene frequency, carrier bulls should soon be detected. For a serious condition, bulls might be progeny tested on known carrier females.

Testing all bulls on their daughters would test for any deleterious gene. Since most bulls probably carry several such genes, the bulls available would be limited. Where older bulls are being used, the test might be of some value, although low production in the inbred daughters would be a disadvantage.

Generally, AI, because of its scientific basis and monitoring procedures, is an agent for reducing rather than increasing defects.

Genetic defects and egg transplanting

Routine egg transfer permits intense selection among females and potentially concentrates even further the genetic base. It thus enhances the risk of spreading genetic defects. Provided proper surveillance is instituted and donors transmitting defects rapidly withdrawn, like AI, it should however decrease rather than increase genetic disease.

Polygenic deleterious genes

There is very marked individual variation in fertility, in susceptibility to infections and metabolic diseases and in conformation and physique. The genetic part of continuous variation is considered to be due to many additive genes, each with a small effect. They produce a bell-shaped distribution whose mean can be shifted by selection.

Multifactorial inheritance, particularly from field data, is measured by a heritability estimate – the ratio of genetic influences to all influences (genetic and environmental). Heritability estimates tend to vary widely according to the method of calculation and the particular field data chosen and are commonly averaged to obtain a generalized more reliable estimate. Individual estimates have to be treated with great caution, especially when used to predict rates of progress under selection. Strictly speaking they apply only to the population from which they are obtained and their predictive value is limited to a few generations at most.

Sterility and infertility genes

Infertility genetics is little understood. Although there is substantial automatic natural selection present for fertility, the marked decline in fertility with inbreeding and its restoration on crossbreeding demonstrates the existence of many infertility and subfertility genes.

Difficulties and inaccuracies in statistically measuring fertility, and the different indices used, have produced very different estimates of its heritability. Most studies suggest the heritability of pregnancy rate in cattle is low, almost zero. Some based on sire/son comparisons, however, suggest figures as high as 40 per cent.

Intense selection for yield is thought by some workers to lower fertility. It can be argued that a few per cent decrease in pregnancy rate might be overestimated in comparison with high yield. Lengthening calving intervals, however, markedly reduce profitability and selection for fertility should remain a high priority with some culling of sons of bulls with low pregnancy rate.

Semen volumes and sperm numbers, concentration, motility and morphology show marked age, breed, weight and individual variation (see p. 604). Semen characteristics are considered to be moderately heritable (15–20 per cent) and should respond to selection to improve semen quality but progress would be slow. The correlation between sperm characteristics and fertility is, however, not entirely clear and some semen standards may be unnecessarily high, leading to reduced selection for other characters. Specific sperm defects which are common, e.g. knobbed sperm, are often due to single genes and should be strongly selected against. Testicular size and conformation are also influenced considerably by genes. The difference in libido between beef and dairy bulls is sufficient to indicate the strong genetic influence in libido.

At the herd level most infertility problems are transient and non-genetic. Similarly, repeat breeding in individual cows is usually of environmental or management origins. Oestrous expression, however, plus time of onset of post partum cyclicity, probably has a considerable genetic component associated with hormonal differences.

Calving difficulties

Genetic selection for yield and growth rate increases body size and larger cows inevitably have increased calving problems. Friesians, for example, have more difficulties than Jerseys or Ayrshires. At the extreme limit in pure, large, continental breeds cows can only produce a few calves before becoming sterile. Counterselection is impossible as long as growth rate is given priority and the only remedy is Caesarean section.

Susceptibility and resistance genes

Susceptibility and resistance genes are widespread and genetic variation in disease resistance has always been demonstrated when adequately sought. Animals relatively resistant to one disease are often susceptible to another. Resistance is sometimes polygenic but, with increasing research, it has often been found to be dependent on relatively few genes.

In natural epidemics an invading organism frequently spreads rapidly causing heavy mortality. Some genetically resistant animals almost invariably survive and subsequently multiply. After initial oscillations, host and parasite settle down to coexist. Initially acute diseases tend to become chronic as genetic immunity develops.

Before control, selection for resistance genes must have been intense. This effect is still obvious in tropical countries, for example, where Zebus are markedly more resistant to local disease than exotic breeds. In grading up by crossbreeding, a proportion of Zebu genes has to be retained and indeed in high-disease areas improvement of indigenous cattle may be preferable. For many large countries resistance genes dictate a stratified breeding programme from pure exotics to pure indigenous cattle. In tropical countries genotype–environment interactions are of prime significance.

In European cattle the most obvious example of genetic resistance is in mastitis. There are marked breed differences. Heritability estimates vary enormously but are probably around 10–15 per cent. Daughters of infected dams are more susceptible and some bulls transmit substantially more mastitis than others. In one extensive survey most mastitis cases were daughters of relatively few AI sires.

Selection to raise the frequency of mastitis-resistance genes, even with AI, although feasible, would be difficult. Many daughters, perhaps 250, would be required to classify the bull. Currently sires' daughters are classified mainly on first lactation yield when mastitis is less frequent and the effect of AI on mastitis incidence is probably neutral. It is dangerous to assume that selection for high heifer yield automatically implies selection for health, as many diseases occur in later lactations.

Calf scours and pneumonia also have a genetic component, associated with colostral antibody. This varies genetically, as does the vitality of the calf, influencing its suckling ability.

BSE is another infectious disease where mouse research published and some unpublished research on scrapie and BSE's epidemiology suggest there are strong genetic and familial factors operating. Research has been hindered by the need to prevent its spread to humans. Since safety in humans can only be guaranteed by its elimination in cattle, the genetic factors involved justify much further research.

There are marked species and individual differences in the severity of foot-and-mouth disease and selection could probably enforce this resistance, but vaccination would seem the best approach in such an infectious, rapidly spreading disease involving many viral strains. Isolating the experimental animals could also prove a major, although not insuperable, problem.

Parasitic infections, however, are emerging as a very possible candidate for scientific counterselection. They tend to be chronic, natural selection resistance already exists and regular treatment is expensive. This field is likely to develop, perhaps particularly in tropical livestock development centres (LDCs).

The greatest progress in artificially selecting for disease resistance depends on detecting biochemically resistant and susceptible animals. Considerable progress is being made on this front, centring around immune response genes. These control the ability of the animal to produce antibody against certain specific antigens. The *Ir* genes are on the part of the chromosome that contains the genes controlling the acceptance of tissue grafts, the histocompatibility genes. These latter can be detected serologically and both *Ir* genes and histocompatability genes form a multiple allelic series.

As knowledge of this gene complex increases and the genetic basis of immunity is understood in finer detail, positive selection for resistance to disease may become more feasible. Artificial insemination, egg transplanting and, ultimately, gene transfer are the obvious instruments.

Selection for disease resistance is likely to be profitable, however, only where vaccines are not available, although in some cases genetically more resistant animals respond more effectively to vaccines. Both approaches may in some circumstances be complementary.

Metabolic disease genetics

Individual variation in susceptibility to metabolic disease is well demonstrated by milk fever. It has a heritability estimate of around 20–25 per cent and a repeatability of about 20 per cent, indicating how sus-

ceptible cows can be. There are also breed variations, Channel Island breeds being particularly liable. Breed variation in hypomagnesaemia and acetonaemia also exists.

The anaemia common in high-yielding cows provides one of the best experimental examples of the strength of biochemical individuality. In one unpublished twin study, despite marked prolonged nutritional and weight differences, haemoglobin, red blood cells, packed cell volumes and mean haemoglobin concentrations were all so highly determined by individuality that pair members closely resembled each other in blood pattern, despite the nutritional differences within and between pairs. Individual differences overshadowed the nutritional effect.

Such individual differences indicate the need for caution in interpreting disease status from blood analysis in individuals. Because of individual variation normality is difficult to define. A single animal with a low haemoglobin may not be anaemic but merely exhibiting a normally determined low value. Blood tests are generally most valuable at the herd level in preventive medicine.

Selection for increasing yields is putting dairy cows under increasing stress and metabolic diseases are steadily increasing in developed countries. Both milk fever and acetonaemia are basically diseases of high yielders and almost unknown in less-developed countries.

Disease genetics and cattle improvement schemes

These are essentially interwoven. Improvement schemes carry risks as well as rewards. Those based on AI and egg transplants steadily to improve rates of progress involve the risk of inbreeding depression.

Inbreeding depression

Since relatively few males are required to avoid inbreeding, in theory it presents little problem in improvement schemes.

As technology reduces bull numbers and AI sires are followed by their sons more care will be necessary. Using a few score bulls for several million cows should not cause serious inbreeding provided sons are not chosen repeatedly from only the very best sires, causing an undue concentration on very few sires. However, after many decades, such a system could cause a serious accumulation of inbreeding effects. Remedies would include importations, using stored semen or splitting the breed into small units and exchanging bulls. Similarly, with egg transplanting overconcentration on a few mothers has to be avoided.

In practice, however, more inbreeding may be occurring than is generally suspected and with inadequate recording the risks may be being underestimated.

Intense single-character selection

Single-character intense selection in all species reduces fertility and frequently produces other undesirable correlated responses. The balanced homeostasis of the animal is upset. At the extreme it often uncovers major defects, e.g. pygmies in downward selection for weight.

Intense selection for yield in dairy cattle increases mastitis, udder oedema and metabolic diseases. The genetic, early, high-peak yields in dairy cows, much higher than in any other species, induces stress. High yielders also suffer increased digestive disorders, foot problems and calving difficulties. High yielders, although more profitable, thus require expensive health care, particularly to maintain mammary function.

The genetic reduction in fertility associated with high yield is probably sufficiently serious to reassess current selection programmes in dairy cattle. Increased efficiency of production, rather than yield alone, should be the objective.

Balanced selection

In future, greater emphasis is likely to be placed on balanced selection. Factors such as growth rate and mature size, body conformation and composition, food intake and efficiency and perinatal mortality and disease resistance are likely to be built into selection indices. Selection will probably also occur under controlled conditions as well as using field data. The aim will be better balanced and healthier animals and hence more profitable dairy cattle.

Positive selection for health

Selection and longevity in dairy cows

The very short lifespan of dairy cows (and bulls) is probably due to poor management and particularly inadequate fertility control. Genetic selection for health and longevity could, however, contribute substantially to better health. In livestock, positive eugenics is possible.

Longevity has a considerable genetic component independent of yield. The heritability of survival to the sixth lactation may be around 20 per cent. Theoretically,

selection for longevity at the end of the first lactation is possible but would require too many daughters and measurements to be economically feasible. As biochemical individuality is explored in greater depth it may become possible.

Bull mothers

A simple approach to improving health, and longevity is to place a much greater emphasis on older bull mothers, cows that have successfully over five or six lactations resisted mastitis, metabolic disease and infertility. This approach is now being implemented.

Crossbreeding

Crossbreeding schemes, even those where the primary objective is blending different maternal and paternal characters, greatly improve health and vigour.

The simplest explanation of hybrid vigour is that the load of recessive deleterious genes, which can be exposed on inbreeding, are covered up by normal alleles on crossbreeding. Crossbreeding is extensively used in beef production, particularly where hardiness is vital, as in exposed hill areas.

Systematic crossbreeding schemes are being used in some Scandinavian, eastern European and tropical countries but generally have been little developed in western Europe.

The best schemes of cattle improvement, maximizing both health and efficiency, are probably based on combining crossbreeding and selection and using selection indices. Dairy cattle improvement is only in its infancy and with increasing research and development such schemes are likely to develop in the West.

Health recording schemes

Another approach to genetically improving health is a greater emphasis on health recording schemes. Currently, the most effective of these are devoted to improving fertility control, particularly regular calving and improved heat detection and, to a lesser extent, early detection of metabolic breakdown. With improved design, however, they are likely to detect bulls transmitting undesirable qualities such as mastitis susceptibility and poor heat expression.

Recent advances

The full significance and utility of the two fundamental genetic achievements of the last decade, the human genome project and cloning, are only now being explored, but the genetic revolution will have a major impact.

Cloning

Livestock cloning, when a relatively reliable success rate is achieved, should greatly advance medical science, enabling the rapid build-up of flocks and herds containing specific genes for generating pharmaceutical products, as in various Roslin Institute research projects. Investigation of the current reproductive and malformation difficulties should also enhance our understanding of cell differentiation, and cell multiplication and division, with implications for genetic diseases and even ageing and cancer.

Commercial cloning to achieve rapid once and for all improvement may require greater caution. Widespread use of identical animals could leave them exposed to new, rapidly spreading, emerging diseases and without biological diversity, whole populations could be affected. The Irish potato famine was basically caused by cloned potatoes. Moreover, the aim is to improve animals every generation rather than stabilize current populations with prize-winning livestock. In certain circumstances, however, where scientifically improved animals have been developed, limited commercial cloning could prove worthwhile. Cloning valuable animals before they succumb to infertility or disease could be regarded as dysgenic.

One underestimated benefit would lie in exploring nature and nurture. Currently, field heritability studies tend to produce lower values than twin studies, and the problems of nature and nurture are far from being satisfactorily resolved. In twin research the existence of only two identical twins reduces replication and requires very complex experimental designs. Clones would greatly simplify this. In field studies the introduction of clones into different herds and environments would also greatly improve the measure of genetic variation. Apart from specific genetic studies, readily available clones would improve nutritional and disease research, raising the whole standard of cattle research, as pure lines have done in mice.

The genomics revolution

The most significant result from the human genome project is a reduction in the gene count from an estimated hundred thousand or so to nearer thirty to forty thousand. Since there are probably hundreds of thousands of proteins, the one gene, one enzyme hypothesis

is, therefore, untenable and each gene must encode for several proteins – estimates vary from the tens to several hundreds.

This conclusion leads to a switch in emphasis from genomics to proteomics as the fundamental key to understanding the body and attempts are now being made to produce a comprehensive catalogue and map of all the proteins. This will be very difficult since proteins are complex, may interact with other proteins, once created may be modified and can be transient.

This changing emphasis is having a major effect on drug development and therapy. Although in a fluid state, the new concepts are already tending to emphasize the importance of individual drug treatment, and helping to explain why different drugs act differently in different patients and the occasional side-effects in block busters and vaccines. The key seems to lie in genetic individuality producing genetic variation in individual proteins and hence different responses to different drugs. Medicine, at present, could be regarded as a diverse collection of symptoms and empirical treatments, but is slowly being converted into a science. The day when each valuable animal has its own genetic profile and can be treated accordingly, however, is a very long way off, but that is the direction in which genomics and proteomics seem to be leading pharmacogenetics.

Not only some mammals but many infectious agents, such as the cholera bacterium, have been successfully sequenced, work which should lead to more effective vaccines. Likewise sequencing biting insects such as the mosquito should ultimately lead to better insecticides. With infectious agents and parasites evolving rapidly to overcome current therapies, sequencing should provide a better understanding of the resistance mechanisms they are developing (they are fairly well understood in bacteria already) and this in turn should help provide better control systems.

In evolutionary terms the reduction in gene numbers seems to imply that the vast variation in life forms, including the domestic species and their parasites, may be due more to control genes, switching genes on and off, rather than a large number of genes producing different proteins.

In animal breeding terms it is difficult to overestimate the significance of genomics and proteomics. Currently improvement is largely based on biometrics, particularly heritabilities. In the future this is likely to be supplemented and possibly finally replaced by screening the DNA and looking for genes, particularly major genes, which influence production and disease. In the even longer term such genes are likely to be inserted into the genotype – after all, all genes in different species can be regarded as part of one vast network – and the future of livestock improvement lies in genetic engineering.

Perhaps after a long latent period, during which the immense successes of microbiology has dominated medicine, the old-fashioned subject of medical diathesis or constitutional medicine, rejuvenated by Mendelism, is now reasserting itself.

Conclusions

Thus in cattle improvement, the future is likely to see a greater emphasis on selection for survival and efficiency as well as production, and genetics will become a core subject in cattle preventive medicine. With gene transfer enabling resistance genes to be built in to cattle, a new Pasteurian age is developing and the prospects seem limitless.

Further reading

Brock, D.J.H. & Mayo, O. (eds) (1972) *The Biochemical Genetics of Man*. Academic Press, London and New York, pp. 1–725.

Emery, A.E.H. (1983) *Elements of Medical Genetics*. Churchill Livingstone, Edinburgh, London, Melbourne, New York. pp. 1–283.

Hamori, D. (1983) *Constitutional Disorders and Hereditary Diseases in Domestic Animals*. Elsevier Scientific Publishing Company, Amsterdam, Oxford, New York. pp. 1–728.

Lerner, I.M. (1954) *Genetic Homeostasis*. Wiley, New York, pp. 1–134.

Nicholas, F.W. (1987) *Veterinary Genetics*. Oxford University Press, Oxford, UK, pp. 1–580.

Pirchner, F. (1983) *Population Genetics in Animal Breeding*. 2nd edn. Plenum Press, New York and London, pp. 1–414.

Chapter 13
Congenital Conditions

A.H. Andrews

Introduction	173	Nervous system defects	178
Cardiovascular system	173	Hydrocephalus	178
Ectopia cordis	173	Cerebellar hypoplasia	178
Ventricular septal defects	173	Inherited cerebellar ataxia	178
Multiple cardiac lesions	174	Cerebellar abiotrophy (premature ageing)	178
Patent foramen ovale	174	Congenital spasms	178
Patent ductus arteriosus	174	Familial ataxia and convulsions	178
Aortic stenosis	174	Progressive ataxia	179
Persistence of the right-sided aortic arch	174	Bovine progressive degenerative myeloencephalopathy	
Persistent truncus arteriosus	174	(Weaver syndrome)	179
Abnormal origin of the carotid arteries	174	Inherited neurodegenerative disease (shaker calf	
Aortic coarctation	174	syndrome)	179
Cardiomyopathy	174	Idiopathic epilepsy	179
Blood disorders	175	Lysosomal storage diseases	179
Factor XI deficiency	175	Mannosidosis	179
Bovine leucocyte adhesion deficiency (BLAD)	175	Spastic paresis	179
Simmental hereditary thrombopathy	175	Neonatal spasticity	180
Skeletal defects	175	Periodic spasticity	180
Achondroplastic calves (bulldog calves,		Inherited congenital myoclonus	180
chondrodystrophia fetalis)	175	Maple syrup urine disease (branched-chain ketoacid	
Complex vertebral malformation (CVM)	175	decarboxylase deficiency, BCKAD)	180
Congenital joint laxity and dwarfism syndrome (CJLD)	175	Congenital pastern paralysis	180
Osteopetrosis (metaphyseal dysplasia)	176	Perosomus elumbis	180
Atlanto-occipital fusion	176	Ocular defects	180
Mandible and face abnormalities	176	Exophthalmus with strabismus	181
Vertebral column defects	176	Colobomata	181
Defects of the limbs and claws	176	Congenital cataract	181
Osteoarthritis	176	Persistent hyaloid vessels	181
Arachnomelia	177	Skin defects	181
Displaced cheek teeth	177	Symmetrical alopecia	181
Lymphatic system	177	Congenital hypotrichosis	181
Inherited lymphatic obstruction	177	Epitheliogenesis imperfecta	181
Alimentary tract defects	177	Keratogenesis imperfecta (baldy calves)	181
Cleft palate (palatoschiasis)	177	Inherited parakeratosis (lethal trait A46)	181
Harelip	177	Interdigital hyperplasia	182
Smooth tongue (epitheliogenesis imperfecta linguae		Albinism	182
bovis)	177	Familial acantholysis	182
Atresia ilei	177	Congenital ichthyosis	182
Atresia coli	177	Body cavity defects	182
Atresia ani	177	Umbilical herniae (navel ruptures)	182
Muscular system defects	177	Inguinal herniae	182
Congenital flexure of the pastern joints	177	Scrotal herniae	182
Arthrogryposis ('curled calf disease')	177	Schistosoma reflexus	182
Muscular hypertrophy (double muscling, muscular		Diaphragm defects	182
hyperplasia, culard)	178	Reproductive system defects	182
Multiple tendon contracture	178	Testicular hypoplasia	182
Joint hypermobility	178	Cryptorchidism	182
Achondroplastic deviation	178	Wolffian duct aplasia	183

Ovarian aplasia	183
Ovarian hypoplasia	183
Müllerian duct aplasia	183
Duplication of the reproductive tracts	183
White heifer disease	183
Prolonged gestation	183
Hermaphroditism	183
Freemartinism	183
Urinary system defects	184
Pervious urachus	184
Other defects	184
Congenital porphyria	184
Familial polycythaemia	184
Congenital goitre	184
Anomalous twins	184
Chromosomal translocations	184

Introduction

Most farmers will, at times, have calves that show defects of a varying degree at birth. Such defects, although congenital, may be due to genetic or environmental factors or their interaction. The overall level of incidence of congenital defects ranges considerably in surveys from 0.2 to 3.0 per cent. It should be remembered that genetic defects are not always apparent at birth. The incidence of all specific defects is very small, but detailed investigation of any anatomical system will often show slight deviations from the norm. Genetic causes can be inherited on a dominant, recessive or additive basis and often they are influenced by the environment. In many cases all that can be said about a particular condition is that it is familial. Factors connected with the environment are many-fold. Other problems are the result of bacterial or viral infections, nutritional deficiencies, chemical poisoning and physical insults. If the condition occurs in the early stages following fertilization (i.e. up to day 14 after fertilization), death of the embryo occurs and it is resorbed. During the embryo and organogenesis stage (15–44 days after fertilization) the effect is variable. In many cases there is death of the embryo with resorption or abortion, whereas in others the embryo remains viable and there is congenital absence, deficiency or disturbance in function. Once the fetus stage is reached (day 45 to birth) then again death can occur resulting, if early, in resorption, otherwise mummification or abortion and, if later, in stillbirth. In other cases the fetus survives and may be normal or suffer growth retardation, reduction in size or organic function, or the animal may become weak.

It is often difficult to diagnose the problem and to decide whether a congenital condition is inherited or not, and if it is, whether control of the condition is necessary. Often it is hard to ascertain the frequency of a problem, as farmers are reluctant to admit its presence and also how frequently it is occurring. In many cases with large herds and limited labour, abortions or deformities are often missed. When the condition is present in the offspring of bulls used in artificial insemination the frequency may again be hard to determine because of the disinclination of farmers to report the problem. An indication as to whether or not a problem is of genetic origin may be obtained from the type of defect apparent and the knowledge already available about the condition. Other evidence may be a sudden outbreak of a defect following the use of a new sire and which only affects calves of his parentage. In some cases there is evidence of a gradually increasing number of similar abnormalities that occur over a number of years. Following an investigation, it may be shown that a defect is confined to a particular family within a herd or to the progeny of certain dams.

In most cases the history will show a much lower incidence of any inherited defect in crossbred animals than in pedigree ones. Some genetic problems are noted as being very common in certain breeds or families within the breed and this aids a tentative diagnosis of the condition, e.g. hip dysplasia in Herefords (see p. 453). The history should be indicative of a relationship between the condition and mating systems rather than the time of year, disease incidents, etc. The reuse of the same bull in repeat sire–dam matings may also indicate the inherited nature of the condition and its mode of inheritance, as also can sire–daughter or sire–half-sister matings, but these involve a considerable period of time before any mode of inheritance can be suggested or confirmed.

Some of the more common conditions are described under generalized headings of the systems involved.

Cardiovascular system

Ectopia cordis

This is an uncommon congenital abnormality where the heart is present outside the thoracic cavity. The cause is unknown. The heart is usually positioned in the region of the lower neck and can be seen pulsating when some distance from the calf. Some cases are displaced into the abdominal cavity.

Ventricular septal defects

These are the most common form of congenital heart lesion in calves. They vary in their size, which determines the severity of the signs and their location, but they are often high on the septum. In some cases the animal survives for many years with nothing untoward being suspected. The defects can be single or combined with abnormalities of the blood vessels. The defect allows blood to pass from the left to the right ventricle.

The signs mainly depend on the size of the defect. If it is small the animal may grow normally, have a normal exercise tolerance and a normal life expectancy. Such cases are usually only detected when the animal is examined for some other reason. Occasionally, calves will suddenly drop dead with no premonitory signs at a few weeks to several months of age. In severe cases there will be some stunting in growth, decreased exercise tolerance and a varying degree of listlessness. Other calves will remain recumbent at birth and die soon afterwards. In the uncomplicated case there is no cyanosis, but on auscultation all animals have a systolic murmur that is very obvious and can be heard on both sides over a wide area of the chest. At necropsy there is an interventricular defect and this is often just ventral to the aorta. In some cases there may be an enlarged liver.

Multiple cardiac lesions

There are many of these but all tend to be uncommon. In most cases the animal is born dead, weak or stunted. Often other congenital defects are also exhibited. Tetralogy of Fallot is probably the most common and involves a ventricular septal defect with pulmonary stenosis, a dextroposed aorta and a secondary ventricular hypertrophy. Eisenmenger's syndrome is relatively similar to tetralogy of Fallot with a ventricular septal defect, a dextroposed aorta but there is no pulmonary stenosis. Other multiple cardiac lesions include a double aortic arch and a double outlet to the right ventricle.

The affected animals usually die. Those that survive show a very poor growth rate, severe dyspnoea when exercised, and lassitude. Cyanosis is present in many cases, particularly after exercise, although in Eisenmenger's syndrome, cyanosis may not develop until late. Auscultation of the heart will reveal a murmur.

Patent foramen ovale

This normally takes about seven to ten days to close completely in the normal calf. Patency is relatively common. In many cases there is little blood transport, but if it does occur it is usually from left to right and so there is normally no cyanosis. Hypertrophy of the right ventricle may sometimes arise. There are usually no signs unless other defects are present. Cyanosis is absent unless there is subsequent right ventricular hypertrophy.

Patent ductus arteriosus

Although patent during intra-uterine life, the ductus arteriosus closes within a day of birth and at least by five days old. The condition is relatively common and the cause is unknown. Blood passes from the aorta to the pulmonary artery. Signs are often limited other than poor exercise tolerance and lassitude. There is no cyanosis, but there is a continuous murmur often known as a machinery murmur as it increases and decreases with each cardiac cycle. The condition can be corrected surgically.

Aortic stenosis

This is very uncommon and is just below or at the aortic semilunar valves' attachments. Some animals show few signs, others show dyspnoea. There is a systolic murmur. Death can occur suddenly with respiratory distress.

Persistence of the right-sided aortic arch

This is rare, but when it occurs the oesophagus is encircled by blood vessels, causing constriction. There is usually regurgitation of milk after feeding and this normally starts at birth or soon afterwards.

Persistent truncus arteriosus

This condition occurs very rarely.

Abnormal origin of the carotid arteries

This may affect one or both arteries, which may derive from the pulmonary artery instead of the aorta. This results in weakness of the myocardium in the ventricle of the affected side due to anoxia, and leads to congestive heart failure.

Aortic coarctation

This is a constriction at the site of entry of the ductus arteriosus and results in a systolic murmur and poor pulse.

Cardiomyopathy

A condition often with polydipsia, hyperpnoea and dyspnoea for one to seven days before death has been described in Australian Poll Hereford calves with a tight curly hair coat. At post-mortem examination there is vascular congestion of the liver, spleen and lung with diffuse streaking of the entire myocardium. It appears to be a genetic condition, possibly associated with a simple autosomal recessive mode of inheritance.

Blood disorders

Factor XI deficiency

The main congenital coagulation deficiency reported in cattle involves factor XI (plasma thromboplastin antecedent). It has been reported in North America and recently in Britain. It has been shown to be present in some Holstein–Friesian breed lines and is transmitted as an autosomal recessive trait. Factor XI protein is concerned at an early stage of the contact or intrinsic activation pathway of blood coagulation. This pathway converges with the extrinsic one due to tissue damage, resulting in the activation of factor X. Following activation the factor converts prothrombin to thrombin, which in turn changes soluble fibrinogen to an insoluble fibrin clot. Bleeding problems can vary from minor to profuse with haematuria and post-injection haemorrhage.

Bovine leucocyte adhesion deficiency (BLAD)

This is a genetic problem caused by an autosomal recessive gene type of inheritance in Holstein cattle which came into prominence in the 1990s. It is characterized by a deficiency in the Mac-1 (CD11b/CD1S) cell surface receptor of the integrin family. The lack of adhesion results in an inability to combat disease effectively. The problem is seem in certain genetic lines of Holstein bulls, some of which have been very widely used by AI for their increased milk production characteristics.

Animals involved are not easy to detect initially as they are more susceptible to infections and so suffer more enteric and respiratory problems and growth rates are poor. There is usually oral ulceration, which is recurrent, and on post-mortem examination some have peritonitis. Most animals die between two and about seven months old, although some have survived longer. Many of the signs are similar to BVD infection, BIV, mineral deficiencies and parasitic problems including coccidiosis, cryptosporidiosis and parasitic gastroenteritis. Diagnosis is often difficult, but if BVD is eliminated and the animal has a marked leucocytosis it is likely to be the cause. This can be confirmed by laboratory examination of blood to show the presence of the genetic defect and looking at the pedigree to determine the presence of certain affected bulls. Many reputable cattle semen companies will indicate the presence of the BLAD factor within their bulls. Treatment has been successfully undertaken by bone marrow transplant but is not recommended as it is helping to perpetuate a genetic defect. If a mating does produce an affected calf

then it should not be repeated and bulls should be used which do not carry the BLAD gene.

Simmental hereditary thrombopathy

A bleeding disorder resulting from impaired aggregation of platelets has been diagnosed in Simmental-sired cattle. The signs may not be manifested early in life, although later it causes a prolonged bleeding time after even minor trauma. These animals become severely debilitated or die. The problem has mainly been recorded in Canada, where it is recorded sporadically in the cattle population. The data available suggest that the inheritance is the result of the inheritance of at least two genes rather than a simple Medelian recessive.

Skeletal defects

Achondroplastic calves (bulldog calves, chondrodystrophia fetalis)

Although it has been associated with the Dexter breed, it can also occur in the Friesian, Hereford, Jersey and Guernsey. It is basically a defect of interstitial growth. The condition is mainly a recessive gene except that it is dominant in the Jersey. When Dexters are mated together 25 per cent of the offspring are bulldogs, 50 per cent are Dexters and 25 per cent are Kerry-type Dexters with long legs. Most calves are aborted at about seven months' gestation. The calves usually have very short limbs, flattened skulls with a foreshortened face and short nose. There are often abdominal hernias and anasarca. In many animals there is hydrocephalus due to the deformed cranium.

Complex vertebral malformation (CVM)

A problem recently discovered by Danish scientists. It involves the Holstein breed and appears to have a genetic basis, possibly with a recessive-type inheritance pattern. It appears to have been carried by some bulls widely used for AI across the world. The problem is of malformed calves which appear visually to have a foreshortened neck and thorax; the spinal cord may be twisted, with deformed carpal and metacarpal joints. It appears that there can also be an increase in abortions, heart and lung abnormalities and low birthweight. Control is obtained by ensuring dams are not mated to known carrier bulls or other bulls descended from the same bloodlines.

Congenital joint laxity and dwarfism syndrome (CJLD)

The condition is also known as long bone deformity/chondrodystrophy syndrome and in Canada 'acorn calf syndrome', as it occurs at a time when acorns are around. The condition is seen mainly in the calves of suckler cows and very occasionally dairy heifers. The calves are mainly born in the spring from dams which have usually been fed only pit or clamp silage or rarely big bale silage with no other feeds. Various causes have been suggested but it appears to be nutritional in origin, directly or indirectly, as the addition of another feed such as straw, hay, cereals, etc. to the diet usually prevents or greatly reduces its occurrence.

There are various forms of the condition which have been grouped together and may be variations on the same problem or different problems. In the dwarfism syndrome animals are born at full gestation but have long bone shortening. Other signs can include increased (laxity) or decreased joint movement (chondrodystrophy) and some of these can improve. The fetlocks are often involved. The head may be domed or the face dished, there may be superior brachygnathia. The fore limbs may show lateral bowing or the hind can be sickle hocked. Severely affected calves are unable to rise and my have kyphosis. Post-mortem reveals the skeletal abnormalities; there may also be hepatic fibrosis.

The cause is unknown although silage feeding is critical. There appears to be an interference in normal bone metabolism: it may be a calcium/phosphorus imbalance, or vitamin D, A or copper deficiency. Manganese problems have been suggested but supplementation does not improve the problem. There appears to be no genetic link.

Osteopetrosis (metaphyseal dysplasia)

This has been recorded in black and red Aberdeen Angus and Hereford calves. It is thought to be due to an autosomal recessive gene. The calf may be born prematurely. At birth it is small and of low weight, with brachygnathia inferior (shortened mandible), protrusion of the tongue, impaction of the molar teeth, misshapen coronoid and condyloid processes, open fontanelle, thickened cranial bones, shortening of the long bones and a lack of bone marrow. Radiographs show the homogeneous bone shaft.

Atlanto-occipital fusion

This is rare and is due to a failure of the first cervical vertebra to separate from the occipit and thereby form a joint. It need not necessarily be apparent at birth. The main signs are ataxia with inability to coordinate limb movements. There are then abnormal flexures of the cervical region and recumbency.

Mandible and face abnormalities

The terms 'overshot' and 'undershot' are often used for these conditions, but they have variable definitions. Abnormal length of the upper and lower jaws is better termed superior or inferior prognathia and shortening of the upper or lower jaw is superior or inferior brachygnathia respectively. Most newborn calves show a degree of inferior prognathia, but this condition resolves. However, persistent inferior prognathia is more common than inferior brachygnathia (parrot mouth). The conditions are thought to be inherited. Problems can arise from impaction or non-apposition of the molar teeth. Extreme hypoplasia or agnathia are rare. Lateral deviation of the face with normal development of the mandible (campylognathia) is occasionally seen.

Vertebral column defects

Various abnormalities have been reported including spirabifida, lordosis (ventral deviation), kyphosis (dorsal deviation) and scoliosis (lateral deviation). Occasionally, there is partial or total agenesis of the posterior part of the spinal column; screwtails are reported in Red Polls and wrytails in Jerseys and Holsteins. Ankylosis of the intervertebral joints has been recorded.

Defects of the limbs and claws

Occasionally, duplication of all or part of the limb occurs and in other animals the whole or various bones of the limb are absent. One problem recently described is tibial hemimelia in Galloway cattle. Polydactyly or extra digits have occasionally been seen. A quite frequent abnormality is the partial or complete fusion of the digits (syndactyly or mule foot). The condition is reported in the Holstein, Aberdeen Angus, Hereford and Chianina. It occurs more commonly in the front than the hind legs and the right limbs are more often affected. It can be inherited as a simple autosomal recessive trait. Duplication of the whole limb (polymelia) is very rare. It can be attached to the thigh of the normal limb by soft tissue and a pseudoarthrosis may develop between the femoral head and the pelvis.

Osteoarthritis

Although it can be nutritional in origin, it can also be inherited in Jersey and Holstein Friesian cattle. There are two main conditions, namely degenerative arthropathy, which mainly involves the hips, and degenerative osteoarthritis, which primarily affects the stifle joints. The latter condition develops in older cattle over a period of one or two years. The stifle shows crepitation and the limb is not raised much off the ground when walking. The articular cartilages show degeneration.

Arachnomelia

This condition involves the limbs having very long, thin distal extremities like a spider and the bones are brittle. It has been recorded in the Simmental breed. Often there is spinal curvature and inferior brachygnathia, which often affects other body systems.

Displaced cheek teeth

The lower mandible tends to be shorter and narrower than normal with abnormal eruption or impaction of the cheek teeth.

Lymphatic system

Inherited lymphatic obstruction

This has been reported in Ayrshire calves and is caused by the autosomal recessive condition. The lymph nodes tend to be small and the lymphatic vessels are large and tortuous. The condition results in oedema, which varies from slight to severe. The calves may be born dead. The oedema may be so gross as to cause dystokia. Oedema can be of the head, neck, ears, tail and legs. In slight cases there is oedema of the legs and these animals may survive. Accessory lobes may be present at the base of the ears.

Alimentary tract defects

Cleft palate (palatoschiasis)

This can occur as an individual condition but is normally associated with other conditions, particularly arthrogryposis.

Harelip

This has been recorded in cattle but its mode of inheritance is not known. Occasionally, ingestion of lupin (*Lupinus sericeus*) can result in the condition.

Smooth tongue (epitheliogenesis imperfecta linguae bovis)

This is seen in the Holstein–Friesian and Brown Swiss. It is the result of an autosomal recessive gene and leads to the filiform lingual papillae being small. The animals tend to be in poor condition with a poor coat and increased salivation.

Atresia ilei

This condition has occasionally been reported and there is disruption of patency. The signs are of a distended abdomen and this may lead to dystokia. Some cases are due to a recessive gene.

Atresia coli

This has been recorded in Aberdeen Angus and other breeds. The calves survive only a few days.

Atresia ani

This may be inherited and is seen in several breeds including the Friesian. The animal is usually born bright, but will usually die within a week unless surgical relief is provided.

Muscular system defects

Congenital flexure of the pastern joints

This is common and present in most breeds. In the Jersey it is considered to be caused by an autosomal recessive gene. The calves show knuckling over on one or both front fetlocks, and occasionally the hind limbs are also affected. The condition is usually reversible and most calves recover within about six weeks. In some cases it may be necessary to splint the limbs. Manganese deficiency in the dam can also lead to the condition as can locoweed or poison vetch (*Astragalus* and *Oxytronis* spp).

Arthrogryposis ('curled calf disease')
(see pp. 451, 925)

By definition this is a permanent joint contraction. The condition is normally bilaterally symmetrical and the forelimbs are affected more than the hind limbs. The muscles show marked atrophy, they are pale in colour and there is replacement of many muscle fibres with fat. Cleft palate is often also present. The condition is common in the Charolais breed where it is a recessive gene. The gene is probably more prevalent than it should be because carrier dams appear to have advantages in improved longevity and fertility. Infection of the fetal calf by akabane virus can result in the condition, as can lupin (*Lupinus sericeus*) ingestion.

Muscular hypertrophy (double muscling, muscular hyperplasia, culard)

This is a characteristic with some production potential in that some muscles have increased numbers of muscle fibres. The condition is seen in the South Devon, Limousin, Charolais and Belgian Blue and the degree of skeletal muscle involvement varies. It occurs most commonly in the hind limbs with a rounding of the hindquarters. The muscles affected have deep grooves along the intermuscular septa and this may be seen in the muscles of the shoulder, back, rump and hindquarters. Many of the animals tend to stand in a stretched position. The calves tend to be less viable at birth and because of the increased muscle size dystokia is common. In the Belgian Blue dystokia results partly from a narrowing of the dam's pelvis.

Multiple tendon contracture

This has been recorded in Shorthorn cattle and results in dystokia due to the calf's limbs being fixed in extension or flexion. There is a lack of mobility of the limbs and often positioning is abnormal. The problem involves the tendons and there is limb muscle atrophy. The calves are born dead or are destroyed because they are unable to stand. The condition is thought to be inherited by a single recessive gene.

Joint hypermobility

The cause of the condition is unknown but in Jersey calves it is a single autosomal recessive gene. The joints are very mobile and can be bent into very abnormal positions with overextension and flexion of all or most of the upper fore and hind limb joints.

Achondroplastic deviation

Most cases appear to be inherited as a single recessive characteristic and involve the Aberdeen Angus and Hereford breeds but cases have been reported in the Holstein and Shorthorn. The calves have short legs, a wide, short head and the mandible protrudes far in front of the dental pad. The eyes bulge and the tongue protrudes. Breathing is stertorous with the forehead protruding and the maxilla distorted.

Nervous system defects (see Chapter 51)

Hydrocephalus

This is uncommon in calves and can be inherited or congenital. It is often associated with other deformities. e.g. congenital achondroplasia. The condition is seen in the Holstein and Hereford and is in-herited. Infection of the fetus with akabane virus can produce the problem and it is thought vitamin A deficiency can contribute to the condition. It can result from obstruction to the drainage of cerebrospinal fluid from the ventricles or cranial malformation. In both conditions the animals are born dead or die in a few days. There are usually ocular defects.

Cerebellar hypoplasia

This is also known as Hereford disease, but is seen in the Holstein and Shorthorn and appears to be genetic. During pregnancy, infection with BVD or *Neospora* can produce the condition (see p. 900). The cerebellum tends to be small, tough and leathery or even absent. Most calves are obviously affected at birth; there is swaying of the neck, with inability to stand and blindness occurring in severely affected animals. Less badly affected calves have exaggerated and incoordinated limb movements. The animals are conscious and able to drink. Some will survive for several months.

Inherited cerebellar ataxia (see p. 893)

This condition is described as being due to a single autosomal recessive gene. It is seen in the Holstein, Jersey and Shorthorn and the signs are similar to cerebellar hypoplasia, although they are not apparent at birth. The gross lesions are minimal and consist of a wet glistening appearance to the cerebellar white matter, which appears on histology to be reticulate.

Cerebellar abiotrophy (premature ageing)

This condition is seen in Hereford and Simmental calves and appears when four to eight months old. There is the sudden onset of ataxia, which then progresses slowly. The animals are not blind. Calves remain strong but become recumbent or decline slowly into a spastic ataxia. Histologically, there is ageing or degeneration of the cerebellar neurones (see p. 893).

Congenital spasms

The condition has only been reported in the Jersey and there is a continual tremor of the head, neck and limbs. The animal cannot walk and it may die in a few weeks.

Familial ataxia and convulsions (see p. 893)

These have been reported in Aberdeen Angus calves and appear to be an incomplete dominance. The signs are seen within a few hours of birth but can occur when two or three months old with the sudden onset of tetanic spasms, which last for three to twelve hours. In mild cases there is a stiff, exaggerated movement but in the severe form there may be convulsions with recumbency, opisthotonus and paddling of the forelimbs. Following the initial signs there is a residual ataxia with a goose-stepping action, which lasts weeks or months. Necropsy shows lesions of degeneration of the cerebellar cortex Purkinje cells. Diagnosis depends on age, signs and their remission.

Progressive ataxia (see p. 894)

This has been recorded in the Charolais in Britain and subsequently in France. The signs do not develop until the animal is about a year old and they are seen as a progressive ataxia. The animal has increasing difficulty in rising until it may become permanently recumbent. Histologically, there is a myelin degeneration of the white matter of the cerebellum and internal capsule.

Bovine progressive degenerative myeloencephalopathy (Weaver syndrome)

The condition is inherited, appears to be linked with high milk production and occurs in the Brown Swiss breed, although a similar condition has been described in the Murray Grey. Signs usually develop between five months and two years, with the occasional one starting after that time. The problem is one of a progressive (it often stretches over one to one and a half years) bilateral hind limb weakness with the animal showing an increasingly broad-based stance when standing, ataxia and dysmetria. Thus the animal gradually has increasing difficulty in rising, a weaving action and often goose stepping of the fore limbs while starting to drag its hind legs. Although there are proprioceptive deficits, limb reflexes are normal. The animal is bright and alert throughout the condition. At post-mortem examination there are lesions in the white matter of the cerebellum and at all levels within the spinal cord. The lesions include axonal degeneration and vacuolation of the white matter due to large intercellular spaces and axonal spheroidal degeneration. There may be muscular wasting but without muscular dystrophy. Chromosomal examination confirms the defect.

Inherited neurodegenerative disease (shaker calf syndrome)

This syndrome, which has been described in Canadian horned Hereford cattle, is evidenced by a severe muscular tremor and shaking of the head, body and tail. The animal has difficulty in rising, a wobbly spastic gait and

an inability to bellow. Histological examination reveals accumulations of neurofilaments within the neurones of the central, peripheral and autonomic nervous systems.

A similar clinical syndrome has been recorded in Holstein male calvers and is probably caused by a sex-linked recessive mutation. On histology, there are spinal cord changes with spongiform lesions with cavitation.

Idiopathic epilepsy

This condition occurs when the calves are a few months old and mainly involves the Brown Swiss. It is inherited as a dominant characteristic. The convulsions are epileptiform and are seen when the calf is stimulated. They disappear once the animal is one to two years old.

Lysosomal storage diseases (see p. 892)

There is a generalized glycogen storage problem in beef Shorthorns with muscle weakness, incoordination of gait and eventual recumbency. In the Friesian there is a GM_1 gangliosidosis where there is an accumulation of ganglioside (GM_1) in the nervous tissue due to reduced activity of the enzyme β-galactosidase. At about three months old the animal begins to grow more slowly, is blind and has a staring coat.

Mannosidosis

The condition has been recorded in Aberdeen Angus and Murray Grey cattle in New Zealand, Australia and recently in Britain (see p. 892). It is inherited as an autosomal recessive trait and is a deficiency of a specific lysosomal hydrolase enzyme, α-mannosidase, and this causes the accumulation of mannose and glucosamine in secondary lysosomes. The signs develop from one to fifteen months old and most animals die by one year. There is, at first, slight hind leg ataxia, then a fine lateral head tremor, slow vertical head nodding, aggression and loss of condition. Diagnosis is based on reduced tissue and plasma levels of α-mannosidase. Histologically, accumulations of mannose and glucosamine are seen in the nerve cells, fixed macrophages and epithelial cells of the viscera. Tissue and plasma levels of α-mannosidase are about half the normal level in heterozygous animals and can thus be detected.

Spastic paresis (see p. 458)

There is an extension of the stifle and tarsal joints of one or both hind limbs. The condition is seen in the Friesian, but other breeds can be affected. Signs are not usually present until the animal is several weeks or months old, when they start to progress. Contraction of the Achilles tendon, gastrocnemius and superficial flexor tendons overstraighten the hock joint, so that the os calcis is moved cranially towards the tibia. Usually, one leg is more affected than the other and this limb may appear shorter. In the later stages of the severe cases, the leg may swing backwards and forwards like a pendulum. The condition is considered to be inherited. However, the genetic influence is considered to be small, and it is thought that the phenotypic expression as a probably multifactorial recessive genotype depends on mostly unknown environmental factors. Where only small numbers of an AI bull's offspring are affected and the animal is of high genetic merit, it has been suggested that it should still be used as a sire (see p. 166). Surgery can relieve the condition but the animals should not be used for breeding. Recently, analysis of cerebrospinal fluid concentrations of homovanillic acid, the main metabolite of dopamine, has shown levels to be lower in spastic paresis calves than normal contemporaries. The possibility of a disorder in dopamine metabolism has therefore been suggested as a possible cause of the condition.

Neonatal spasticity

This condition involves a single recessive characteristic in the Jersey and Hereford. The animal is born normal but within the first week it develops convulsions of the head, neck and limbs, preceded by neck deviation and bulging eyes.

Periodic spasticity

This has been recorded in the Guernsey and Holstein breeds. It appears to be a single recessive character with incomplete penetrance and is often not noticed until the animals are adult. Early signs involve the hind end, with difficulty in rising; the hind limbs are stretched backwards and the back depressed. The back muscle may fasciculate and the condition progresses from a few seconds duration to last up to 30 minutes. The animal cannot walk during the attack.

Inherited congenital myoclonus

The condition does not involve oedema of the central nervous system and is therefore described as inherited congenital myoclonus (see p. 893). It is inherited as an autosomal recessive gene and is seen in America, New Zealand and Australia to affect Hereford and polled Hereford-cross calves. It has also been reported in Britain in the Hereford, Jersey and South Devon. Animals are usually produced after a shorter than normal gestation period. They are bright and alert but

recumbent, often in lateral recumbency and some are unable to move their head. There is extension and crossing of the hind limbs with hypersensitivity to noise and touch. Often when animals are encouraged to stand there are myoclonic spasms with the body becoming rigid. At necropsy there is usually damage to the hip joints, probably secondary to myoclonic contractions. There is no oedema of the central nervous system. The main differential diagnosis is maple syrup urine disease. No treatment is possible and the same mating pattern should not be used again.

Maple syrup urine disease (branched-chain ketoacid decarboxylase deficiency, BCKAD)

This condition is possibly inherited as an autosomal recessive gene. It is very uncommon but may be seen in polled Hereford calves (see p. 893). There are higher than normal concentrations of branched-chain amino acids in plasma and/or serum, urine, cerebrospinal fluid and formalin-fixed cerebral tissue. It has been suggested that the condition is analogous to branched-chain ketoacid decarboxylase deficiency or maple syrup urine disease. There is dullness, opisthotonus and recumbency and a poor response to touch or auditory stimuli. At post mortem there is severe stratus spongiosus. The main differential diagnosis is inherited congenital myoclonus.

Congenital pastern paralysis

The defect is lethal due to prolonged recumbency and in Red Danish cattle at birth can take the form of opisthotonus–muscle tremor with spastic extension of the limbs and exaggerated tendon reflexes. There is neuronal degeneration in many parts of the brain and spinal cord. In the Norwegian Red Poll a similar condition is seen but only involving opisthotonus and muscle tremors.

Perosomus elumbis

This occurs very occasionally in ruminants. There is aplasia or hypoplasia of the spinal cord caudal to the thoracic area. This results in rigidity of the hind limbs, there is muscle atrophy and no joint movement. Most cases are born dead.

Ocular defects (see p. 914 onwards)

Reports of ocular defects in cattle are few. Anophthalmia and microphthalmia occur infrequently. Entropion is also very rare. Dermoids can occur on the eyelids, conjunctiva and cornea, but they are commonest on the third eyelid.

Exophthalmus with strabismus (see p. 918)

This has been recorded in the Hereford and Holstein is combined with strabismus in Shorthorns and their crosses in Britain and Jerseys in America. The signs, particularly in the Shorthorn, are usually delayed until a year old, although occasionally young calves are affected. The condition is progressive and defective vision is observed first, followed by protrusion and deviation of both eyeballs medially with difficulty in focusing. The condition is considered to be inherited as a recessive gene, but some occur in cases of cerebellar hypoplasia or mucosal disease.

Colobomata (see pp. 923, 924)

These problems appear to have a high prevalence in the Charolais. There is an absence of part of one or more of the structures of the eye. The condition occurs during early gestation, when the eye is developing. Although always bilateral, it may not be symmetrical and it is usually found associated with the optic disc and the tapetum nigrum below the disc. The retina is involved and in some animals the choroid and sclera are also affected. The condition is present at birth and does not progress. The mode of inheritance has been debated, but a dominant gene with incomplete penetrance, autosomal recessive or polygenic inheritance have all been suggested. Signs are not usually apparent although an ophthalmoscopic examination will reveal the lesion. The very severely affected animal can be blind, and a few others are considered to be hyperexcitable due to the defective vision.

Congenital cataract (see p. 923)

Lens opacity is present from birth. The condition has been recorded in the Friesian, Hereford, Jersey and Shorthorn. Some cases in the Holstein and Jersey are considered to be due to an autosomal recessive gene or infections. A form of nuclear cataract in Friesian and Friesian-cross calves appears to be more common in calves born in the summer months and is considered to be of environmental origin. The condition is bilateral and not progressive. In most animals the degree of involvement of each eye is similar. In severe cases blindness is apparent. It is not always possible to examine the fundus of the eye, but in most affected calves there is no abnormality of the retina or optic disc (see p. 923).

Persistent hyaloid vessels

These are quite common and are the vestige of the earlier development of the eye. They have no practical significance.

Skin defects

Symmetrical alopecia

This is apparently inherited as a single autosomal recessive characteristic in Holstein cattle. It involves animals born with a normal hair coat but which is then lost in a symmetrical pattern over the body. It occurs between six weeks and six months of age and affects both pigmented and non-pigmented areas.

Congenital hypotrichosis

Several forms are recorded that vary both in inheritance and degree. There may be partial or complete loss of hair and the condition is present at birth. In some instances the animals will grow satisfactorily provided there is sufficient shelter.

Epitheliogenesis imperfecta

This condition can occur in either sex and reports include Holstein, Ayrshire and Jersey calves. Most animals die within a few days of birth. It is considered to be caused by an autosomal recessive gene. There are normally areas of varying size devoid of skin or mucous membrane. The defects are often distal to the tarsal and carpal joints. Lesions may also occur on the muzzle, tongue, hard palate, cheeks and nostrils.

Keratogenesis imperfecta (baldy calves)

The condition appears a few months after birth and is lethal. It has been observed in the Friesian and is due to an autosomal recessive gene. The skin tends to develop alopecia, there is a loss of body condition and the horns do not grow. The skin then becomes scaly, thickened and folded, particularly on the neck and shoulders. There is alopecia and raw areas may develop, particularly on the knees, hocks, elbows, axillae and flanks. The joints tend to be stiff and there is overgrowth of the hooves.

Inherited parakeratosis (lethal trait A46)

This is possibly an autosomal recessive condition. It is seen in Friesian cattle and is thought to be due to an increased zinc requirement. The signs are usually seen about four to eight months after birth with alopecia and parakeratosis of the limbs, muzzle and under the jaw. The animal becomes stunted and, if untreated, it dies in about four months. At necropsy there is thickened skin with thick crusts over the skin lesions. The spleen shows hypoplasia. Diagnosis depends on low serum zinc levels (normal 12–27 μmol/l; 80–120 mg/100 ml) and history of parakeratosis. Therapy must continue for the rest of the animal's life and as a calf about 0.5 g zinc oxide or 1 g zinc sulphate daily is required. The dose should be increased as the animal grows older (see p. 260).

Interdigital hyperplasia (see p. 429)

This condition is particularly seen in the Hereford and it is considered to have a genetic predisposition. The condition tends to be present in the older animal and can be surgically removed, but has a tendency to recur.

Albinism

Varying types occur. In partial albinism the coat colour is normal for the breed or a dilute colour, but the iris is blue and white centrally, with a brown border. Incomplete albinism is characterized by a white or mainly white coat and the iris may be blue, grey or white. The condition is inherited by an autosomal dominant gene. In complete albinism the coat is pure white and the iris white or pink. The condition is inherited as a simple autosomal recessive trait.

Familial acantholysis

This has been recorded in Aberdeen Angus calves. There is a loss of skin at the carpal and metacarpal joints and coronet, where there is horn separation. The defect is one of defective collagen in the basal and prickle layers.

Congenital ichthyosis

This is also known as fish scale disease in that there is alopecia and the presence of a horny epidermis.

Body cavity defects

Umbilical herniae (navel ruptures)

These are found with a low frequency in several breeds, but especially the Friesian and Holstein. It would appear in some cases to be due to the environment, following infection, to a dominant gene with incomplete penetrance, or autosomal recessive genes. In one study of the progeny of Holstein bulls, more cases occurred in the female than the male offspring. In the male many

umbilical herniae are missed unless a conscious effort is made to look for the defect. This is due to the hernia occurring just anterior to the prepucial orifice. If the hernia is small it may not need to be treated. Larger hernias may need surgical repair (see p. 1122) by suturing across the hole or surgical webbing may need to be introduced. Many cases are inherited and the animal should be recorded as often the hernia is hard to detect in the adult. Do not breed from affected cattle.

Inguinal herniae

These occur far less commonly than umbilical herniae. Little is known about aetiology.

Scrotal herniae

Like inguinal herniae, these are rarely seen but can occur in the Sussex and Friesian breeds. Little is known about the aetiology, but there is a familial trait.

Schistosoma reflexus

This is a group of conditions in which there is longitudinal fissure in the body wall. The cause is unknown, but it may be due to the failure of the somatopleure of the blastodermic vesicle to close. At birth the vertebral column is angulated with the head and tail showing approximation dorsally. The abdominal and thoracic organs lie free in the dam's uterine cavity.

Diaphragm defects

These occur occasionally and, depending on size and position, they may or may not involve abdominal organ herniation.

Reproductive system defects

Testicular hypoplasia (see p. 618)

This occurs sporadically in all breeds of bull. The problem can be bilateral or unilateral as well as being partial or complete. The left side is more commonly affected. Work on gonadal hypoplasia in Swedish Highland cattle showed an inherited origin and this is probably also the case in British breeds.

Cryptorchidism (see p. 482)

There is incomplete descent of the testicles into the scrotum and this may be unilateral or bilateral, although the former is more common. Bilateral cryptorchidism usually produces a sterile animal. The condition occurs in most breeds including the Friesian and Hereford. Although studies of aetiology are few, it is considered to have an inherited basis.

Wolffian duct aplasia

This is normally seen in the area of the epididymal head.

Ovarian aplasia

This occurs occasionally with or without other reproductive abnormalities.

Ovarian hypoplasia

As with testicular hypoplasia, this has mainly been recorded in the Swedish Highland breed where it is inherited.

Müllerian duct aplasia

Various forms can occur and all are uncommon, but the main form is uterus unicorni.

Duplication of the reproductive tracts

This can occur as a deficient union or exaggerated union of the Müllerian ducts. They can result in a partial or complete duplication of the cervix or uterine body or vaginal septa.

White heifer disease

The condition used to be common in the white Shorthorn with up to 10 per cent of them being affected. It is now rare, but can be found in other breeds. There are varying degrees of involvement. In all cases there is partial or complete persistence of the hymen. This may be the only abnormality, but in other animals there are abnormalities cranial to the hymen. These defects may include the absence of the cranial vaginal cervix, uterine body or horns. The ovaries are functional and in most cases there is a distension of the normal organs due to the accumulation of the products of secretion.

Prolonged gestation

This has been recorded in most dairy breeds and in some cases it has an inherited origin. There are two main forms of the condition.
(1) Prolonged gestation with fetal giantism. In these animals the fetus continues to grow *in utero* before parturition 21 to 100 days late. The cow usually calves with no udder development or ligament relaxation and usually first stage labour is minimal, necessitating a Caesarean section. The calves tend to be heavy, have well-erupted teeth and a good coat growth. The adrenals of the calves are hypoplastic and following delivery most are weak and die in hypoglycaemic crisis. The condition is the result of an autosomal recessive gene.
(2) Prolonged gestation with adrenohypophyseal hypoplasia. This is due to a recessive gene and it is mainly recorded in the Channel Island breeds. The gestation length is increased by weeks or months and parturition occurs about seven to fourteen days after the calf's death. There is again no udder development and few signs of parturition. The calf in this case is small and ceases to grow after the seventh month of gestation, so it can often be delivered by manual traction. It may show disproportionate dwarfism, craniofacial defects that may cause hydrocephalus, alopecia and abdominal distension. There is no or only partial development of the adenohypophysis.

It should be remembered that the gestation period of some of the larger beef breeds such as the Charolais, Simmental and Limousin is longer than for the Friesian or most British beef breeds.

Hermaphroditism

Both true and pseudohermaphrodites occur. In the true form there are gonads of both sexes, although they may be combined into an ovo-testis. In the pseudohermaphrodite, cattle are genetically female with female gonads but they have partial masculinization of the external genitalia. The animals usually exhibit normal oestrous behaviour and on investigation have normal ovaries. However, the vulvar orifice is usually small and displaced ventrally.

Freemartinism

This is seen in twins where a female is developing with a male and this affects about 11 out of 12 such twins. The calf contains both normal 60 XX chromosomes and a few 60 XY (male) chromosomes. Occasionally, a female calf will be born singly with this abnormality and this is due to the death of the other twin. Freemartins are usually sterile.

The external genitalia resemble a female, but the vulva is smaller than normal. Later a tuft of hair develops at the vulva and in many cases an over-sized clitoris is found. Internally, there is a varying amount of agenesis or hypoplasia of the Müllerian system and stimulation of the Wolffian system. The ovaries tend to be hypoplastic and the vagina is usually non-patent, which allows diagnosis of the condition in the calf by the passage of a probe. However, occasionally the vagina is tubular and terminates at the normal position of the cervix, which is absent. The uterus tends to be two thick cords and there are two thin ducts that extend from the gonads to the intrapelvic urethra. There are often seminal vesicles present and sometimes testicles.

Urinary system defects

Pervious urachus

The defect occurs occasionally in calves. However, it may go undetected for weeks or even months, particularly in the male. Urine is discharged in a dribble from the urachus. All urine may be passed via the urachus although in some cases passage is also via the urethra. The condition may lead to cystitis and, as the umbilicus does not heal, there is often omphalophlebitis, septicaemia and polyarthritis. Surgical correction of the condition is possible and can be successful.

Other defects

Congenital porphyria

This is very rare. It is mainly seen in the Friesian and Holstein. It is caused by a simple recessive gene and occurs more frequently in the female than the male. There is increased porphyria in the blood and urine leading to the accumulation of the product in the tissues. The teeth tend to be pink or brown in colour and this can be seen in the newborn. The urine is red or purple and animals will develop cutaneous photosensitization and anaemia. There are high levels of uroporphyrins and coproporphyrins in the blood.

Familial polycythaemia

The condition is seen in the Jersey and is inherited as a simple autosomal recessive trait. There are early deaths. Those alive have poor growth, congestion of the mucosae and dyspnoea. There is a reduced erythrocyte count, packed cell volume and haemoglobin concentration.

Congenital goitre

This is an inherited condition but animals can be kept alive although mortality is high. Goitre also occurs when iodine deficiency affects the gestating dam (see pp. 257, 301)

Anomalous twins

There is faulty division in monozygotic twinning and this results in various abnormalities. There are varying degrees of conjunction, but double-headed monsters are most often seen. Others have a single head and the posterior part of the body is divided. In some cases the separation of the vertebral column may be almost complete, resulting in Siamese twins. Occasionally, small amorphous monsters called amorphous globosus or acardiac twins occur. They are related to double monsters and identical twins. They are found attached to the fetal membranes of the other calves and comprise an outer skin enclosing adipose tissue.

Chromosomal translocations

There are always 60 chromosomes present in the normal bovine. Translocation is the fusion of two morphologically distinct chromosomes. The most common is 1/29 translocation where there is fusion between number 1 and 29 pairs; it is also referred to as the Robertsonian translocation. It has been recorded in the Swedish Red and White breed, Charolais, Red Poll, British White and other breeds. The condition appears to be of importance in that there is reduced fertility in such animals due to early embryonic death.

Further reading

Blowey, R.W. & Weaver, A.D. (2003) Congenital disorders. In *Colour Atlas of Diseases and Disorders in Cattle*, 2nd edn. Mosby, Edinburgh, pp. 1–9.

Chapter 14
Calf Diarrhoea

P.R. Scott, G.A. Hall, P.W. Jones and J.H. Morgan

Introduction	185
Causative mechanisms in diarrhoea	185
Altered ion transport	185
Passive malabsorption	187
Intestinal motility	187
Osmotic effects	187
Tissue hydrostatic pressure and increased permeability	188
Types of diarrhoea	188
Role of the large intestine	189
Effects of diarrhoea and their clinical signs	189
Metabolic and hormonal changes	191
Infectious agents	191
Bovine rotavirus	191
Bovine coronavirus	199
Calici-like virus (Newbury agent)	200
Astrovirus	200
Breda virus	201
Escherichia coli	201
Campylobacter spp.	204
Cryptosporidium parvum	204
Investigating an outbreak of calf diarrhoea	206
Epidemiology	206
Mixed infections	207
Management of diarrhoea	209
Rehydration	209
Nutrition	210
Drugs	210
Environment	210
Microbial environment	210
Immunological environment	210
Nutritional environment	212
Physical environment	212
Necrotic enteritis	213

Introduction

Diarrhoea in the neonatal calf is a serious welfare problem and a cause of economic loss due to mortality, treatment costs and poor growth. Calf diarrhoea is an example of a complex or multifactorial disease, resulting as it does from an interaction between the calf, its environment and nutrition and infectious agents (Fig. 14.1). Successful control of an outbreak will depend on recognition of the important factors in that outbreak and correction of the problems. Identification of the infectious agents involved is important because it permits a logical approach to disease control. Appropriate advice on nutrition, colostrum feeding, vaccination, hygiene and the use of antibiotics can only be given if it is clear which infectious agents are present and what their contribution to the disease process might be.

Causative mechanisms in diarrhoea

The digestive tract may be regarded as a high fluid flow system in which 80 per cent of the fluid contained within it is secreted into it and 20 per cent is ingested. Secreted fluid originates from salivary glands, gastric mucosa, pancreas, liver and small and large intestinal mucosa. Of the water that enters the digestive tract, 95 per cent is absorbed. Diarrhoea may be defined as an increase in faecal water loss due to increased faecal water content or to increased volume of faeces excreted or to a combination of both. The occurrence of diarrhoea indicates an imbalance between absorption and secretion of water and electrolytes. Only a slight imbalance in the equilibrium between secretion and absorption, in favour of secretion, may lead to severe diarrhoea because very large volumes of fluid are fluxing in both directions. There are several possible causes of imbalance.

Altered ion transport

Diarrhoea due to altered ion transport is caused by reduced absorption of sodium ions by villous enterocytes (Fig. 14.2), by increased secretion of chloride ions by crypt cells (Fig. 14.3) or by both mechanisms acting together. These changes are stimulated in calf diarrhoea by bacterial enterotoxins produced by enterotoxigenic *Escherichia coli* (Fig. 14.4). These bacteria, held on the gut surface by fimbrial adhesins, release enterotoxins. The subunit A of the heat-labile toxin activates adenylate cyclase located on the basolateral membrane which, in turn, raises the production of intracellular cyclic adenosine monophosphate (cyclic-AMP). Increased production of cyclic-AMP reduces sodium ion absorption by villous cells (Fig. 14.5) and

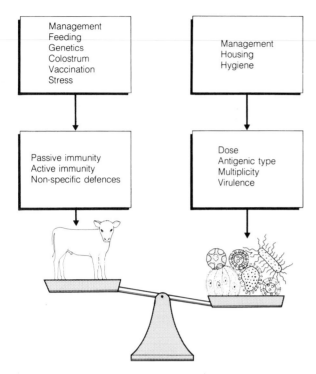

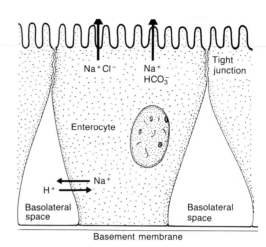

Fig. 14.3 Line drawing illustrating some mechanisms of sodium secretion by crypt enterocytes. Sodium ions are secreted through the luminal surface and chloride and bicarbonate ions and water are transported within sodium ions.

Fig. 14.1 Interactions between management, the calf and enteric agents. Reproduced from Morgan (1990).

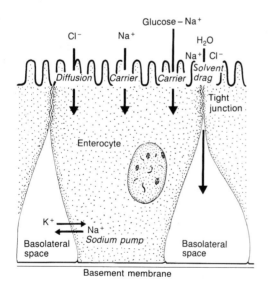

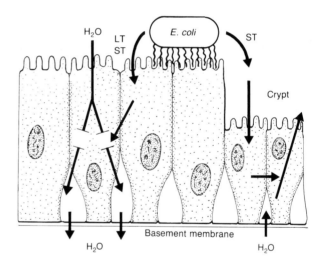

Fig. 14.4 Line drawing illustrating the mechanisms by which enterotoxigenic *E. coli* cause diarrhoea. Bacteria are attached to the enterocyte surface by fimbriae and secrete heat-labile enterotoxin (LT) or heat-stable toxin (ST), which act on metabolic pathways in villous enterocytes to block water absorption and on metabolic pathways in crypt enterocytes to stimulate water secretion.

Fig. 14.2 Line drawing illustrating some mechanisms of movement of sodium and chloride ions and water from the intestinal lumen into basolateral spaces. The sodium pump expels sodium ions from the villous enterocyte into the basolateral space. Sodium ions diffuse along the electrochemical gradient created by the sodium pump, through the enterocyte luminal surface membrane, where passage is assisted by glucose-dependent and glucose-independent carrier systems. Chloride ions and water follow the movement of sodium ions.

consequently water absorption is reduced. At the same time secretion of chloride ions, and therefore water, is stimulated in crypt cells (Fig. 14.6). The heat-stable enterotoxin activates guanylate cyclase, stimulating intracellular synthesis of cyclic guanosine monophosphate (cyclic-GMP), which probably stimulates secretion and reduces absorption, although the precise mechanisms are not known (Fig. 14.5).

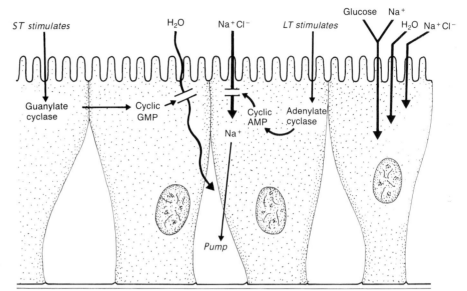

Fig. 14.5 Line drawing illustrating the effects of heat-stable entero-toxin (ST) and heat-labile entero-toxin (LT) on movement of water through villous enterocytes into basolateral spaces. ST inhibits water absorption via cyclic-GMP and LT, acting via cyclic-AMP, blocks absorption of sodium ions and water along the glucose-independent carrier system. The glucose-dependent carrier system is not affected by either toxin.

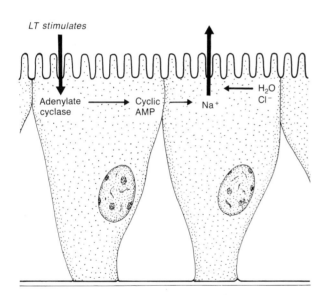

Fig. 14.6 Line drawing illustrating the effects of heat-labile enterotoxin (LT) on the secretion of sodium ions by crypt ente-rocytes. LT increases production of intracellular cyclic-AMP and this stimulates secretion of sodium ions, which carry with them chloride ions and water.

Passive malabsorption

Diarrhoea may be the consequence of water mal-absorption (Fig. 14.7). If malabsorption occurs then normal secretory processes and fluid loss due to tissue hydrostatic pressure will continue and will cause diar-rhoea. Water malabsorption will follow a direct reduc-tion of active uptake of sodium ions from the intestinal

lumen. Malabsorption also occurs when morphological changes reduce the absorbing surface area. The best example of such morphological change is villus stunt-ing produced by viral enteritis. The mature villous enterocytes can be regarded as the functional compart-ment of the small intestine, with absorption as one of the principal functions. A substantial reduction in the number of villous enterocytes causes a corresponding loss of function. Furthermore, crypt hyperplasia occurs in viral infections and immature secretory cells migrate onto the villus, increasing secretory capacity. In addi-tion to loss of absorptive capacity there is also loss of digestive capacity, therefore maldigestion occurs, which can lead to an osmotically induced diarrhoea.

Intestinal motility

Increased intestinal motility may contribute to the development of diarrhoea, resulting in decreased transit time and insufficient time for normal absorption. The role of motility is now considered to be less important than was thought previously.

Osmotic effects

Lactose, the major sugar in cows' milk, is split into glucose and galactose by the enzyme galactosidase (lactase), which is located on microvilli of jejunal ente-rocytes. These monosaccharides are rapidly absorbed and therefore have little osmotic effect. Viral enteropathogens destroy mature enterocytes, thus creating a transient deficiency of galactosidase. Conse-quently, lactose passes undigested to the colon together

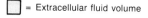
= Extracellular fluid volume

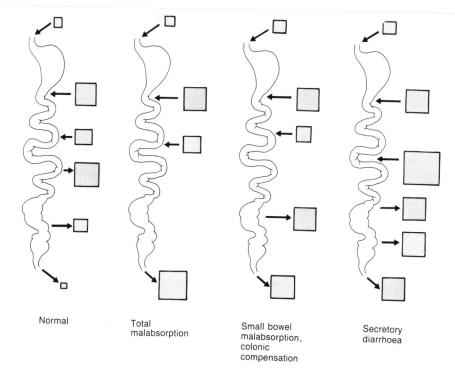

Fig. 14.7 Fluid fluxes in normal growing pigs (40 kg) and pigs with diarrhoea. Volumes of fluid entering and leaving the intestines are drawn in proportional size to the extracellular fluid volume shown at the top. Most water is absorbed by the distal small intestine and colon in pigs of this age and colonic compensation is likely to be much less in neonatal pigs. Source: Argenzio (1984).

Normal

Total malabsorption

Small bowel malabsorption, colonic compensation

Secretory diarrhoea

with an osmotic equivalent of water. It may be inferred from studies of pigs, goats and horses that the consequence of increased lactose in the colon depends on the balance between input of lactose and the fermentative capacity of the colonic microbial flora. If the calf possesses a well-developed colon and colonic microbial flora and the amount of lactose entering is not excessive because of restricted dietary intake and/or slight intestinal damage, then the lactose will be fermented to short-chain fatty acids. These will be absorbed through the colonic mucosa, a process that facilitates the absorption of sodium ions and water by the colonic mucosa. These processes are 'anti-diarrhoeal' (Fig. 14.8). In a young animal, with a poorly developed colon and colonic microflora, there may be little fermentation of lactose that remains in the lumen, holding water and contributing to the diarrhoea (Fig. 14.8). In an animal with a well-developed colonic microflora, dumping of large amounts of lactose into the colon as a result of *ad libitum* feeding and severe intestinal damage results in hyperfermentation and the production of lactic acid rather than short-chain fatty acids. Lactate is poorly absorbed and draws water into the colon by osmosis, exacerbating the diarrhoea. These mechanisms explain why withholding milk from calves with rotavirus scour reduces the severity of the diarrhoea (Fig. 14.8).

Tissue hydrostatic pressure and increased permeability

Tissue hydrostatic pressure results in a continual seepage of water from the mucosa into the lumen and this can contribute to the pathogenesis of diarrhoea if malabsorption is present. Seepage may be increased by inflammation of the mucosa, which allows greater leakage of fluid between enterocytes. In very severe inflammatory conditions, for example acute salmonellosis, the epithelium may be so extensively damaged as to allow erythrocytes to leak from capillaries, through the epithelium into the lumen; clearly other blood constituents will be lost also.

Types of diarrhoea

Having examined the various pathophysiological processes that can give rise to diarrhoea, two general types of diarrhoea can be recognized.

Secretory diarrhoea

A diarrhoea resulting from net movement of fluid into the gut lumen despite fasting. Faeces are

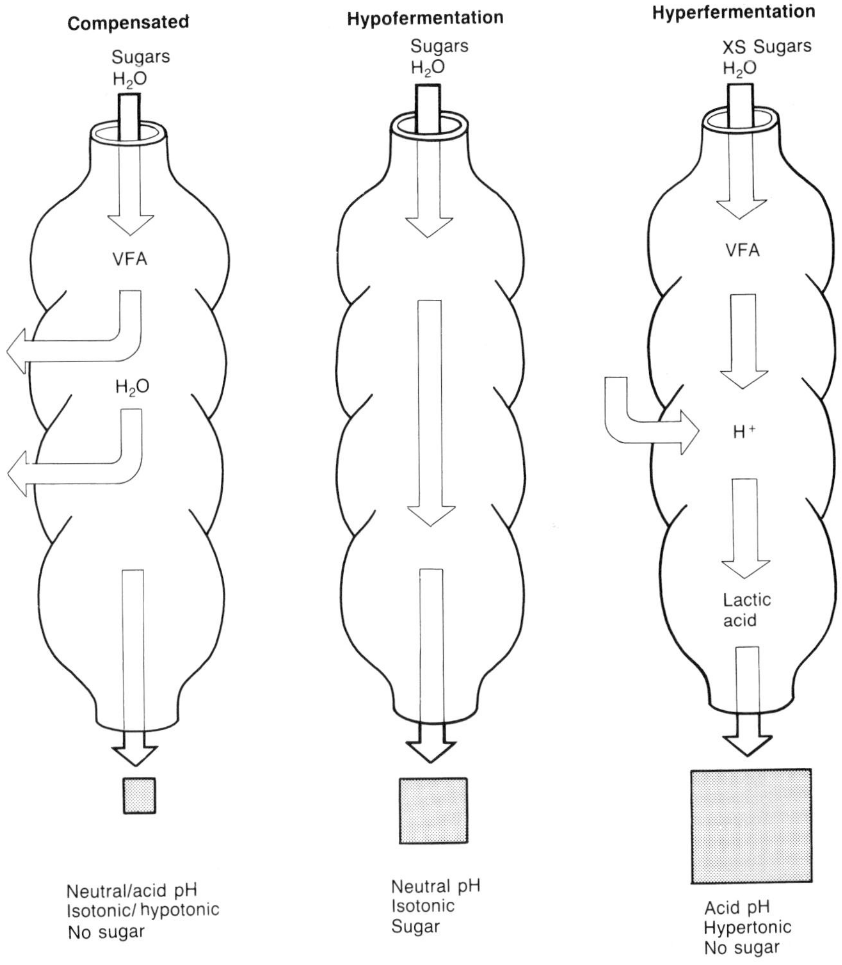

Compensated
Sugars
H_2O

VFA

H_2O

Neutral/acid pH
Isotonic/ hypotonic
No sugar

Hypofermentation
Sugars
H_2O

Neutral pH
Isotonic
Sugar

Hyperfermentation
XS Sugars
H_2O

VFA

H^+

Lactic
acid

Acid pH
Hypertonic
No sugar

Fig. 14.8 Three alternative consequences of a small intestinal maldigestion and malabsorption, as seen in rotavirus infection. In the 'compensated' situation, the colonic flora is well developed and microbial fermentation of the moderate amounts of malabsorbed carbohydrate yields volatile fatty acids (VFA). These are rapidly absorbed, stimulating water absorption and promoting colonic compensation so that diarrhoea does not occur. If the colon and colonic flora are poorly developed there is hypofermentation and consequently no compensation, and diarrhoea occurs. If the colonic flora is well developed and is overloaded with sugar, hyperfermentation occurs and lactic acid is produced that promotes osmotic diarrhoea. Source: Argenzio (1984).

characteristically isotonic with plasma, watery and alkaline, and the volumes produced are usually large. The faeces are alkaline because sodium and bicarbonate ions are secreted by the ileum. In compensation, the colon may be exchanging potassium ions for sodium ions. Acute secretory diarrhoea is always caused by a bacterial infection.

Osmotic diarrhoea

A diarrhoea where the faeces may have high osmolality due to unabsorbed molecules with osmotic activity, usually of dietary origin. Faeces may contain undigested lactose and faecal pH will vary, depending on the amount of lactose fermented to short-chain fatty acids or lactic acid. Osmotic diarrhoea may also be thought of as a diarrhoea caused by malabsorption and maldigestion. Faecal volume is smaller than in secretory diarrhoea and the diarrhoea is reduced or abolished by fasting. Viruses are one cause of this.

Role of the large intestine

Most diarrhoea in the calf originates in the small intestine and as a result small intestinal function has received most study. It is evident that the large intestine, particularly the colon, is a very important site of water absorption and consequently may contribute to the development of diarrhoea if its functional capacity is overwhelmed or impaired by the fermentative mechanisms described above. Similarly, its function may be impaired by infection with *Cryptosporidium*, coronavirus or enterohaemorrhagic *E. coli*. Ingesta entering the colon from the small intestine may be damaging.

Effects of diarrhoea and their clinical signs

The systemic effects of diarrhoea, which eventually culminate in death, are precipitated by a single event, the

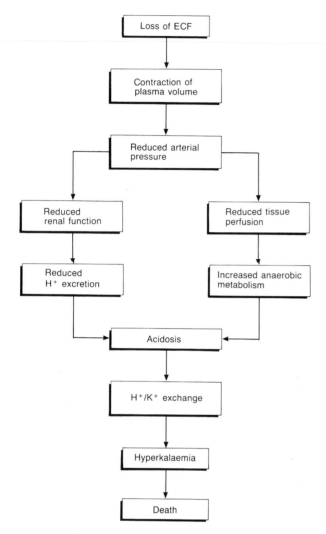

Fig. 14.9 The systemic consequences of diarrhoea. Reduction of extracellular fluid volume leads to acidosis, an exchange of extracellular H⁺ for intracellular K⁺ leading to hyperkalaemia causing cardiac failure. Source: Argenzio (1984).

loss of extracellular fluid. Endogenous secretion into the gastrointestinal tract in 24 hours may equal the extracellular fluid volume. Loss of 7 per cent of the extracellular fluid volume leads to clinical signs and loss of 30 per cent results in death.

Diarrhoea causes changes in plasma constituents that are similar regardless of the cause of the diarrhoea (Fig. 14.9). When neonatal colostrum-fed calves were experimentally inoculated with coronavirus, the water and electrolyte losses were severe (Lewis & Philips, 1978). Faecal water loss increased 28-fold, faecal volume increased 22-fold and faecal water content increased from 73 to 94 per cent. Renal water loss was reduced to 30 per cent of normal and there were severe losses of

sodium and chloride ions and considerable losses of bicarbonate and potassium ions. There was loss of body weight, 12.7 per cent between onset of diarrhoea and death. Plasma volume decreased by 40 per cent leading to a 39 per cent increase in haematocrit and a 33 per cent increase in plasma protein concentration. The increase in plasma protein concentration was lower, possibly because of protein loss by catabolism or by leakage into the intestinal lumen. Both these values vary widely between individuals and are of little value in assessing severity of fluid loss.

Contraction of plasma volume gives rise to the clinical signs of sunken eyes and 'tenting' of skin folds; it leads to a fall in arterial blood pressure, which stimulates peripheral vasoconstriction. Peripheral vasoconstriction, in its turn, leads to poor tissue perfusion with blood, localized ischaemia and lower metabolic activity so that the temperature of peripheral tissues falls, approaching ambient temperature prior to death; the extremities, the ears and mouth, feel cold. Rectal temperature increases until near to death when it falls rapidly to below normal.

Acidosis is an important consequence of diarrhoea and a number of factors contribute to its development. A major factor is loss of bicarbonate ions in faeces and, additionally, there may be absorption of acids produced by microbial fermentation of lactose in the large intestine. Loss of extracellular fluid (dehydration) causes decreased perfusion of the kidney with blood, causing reduced renal function, which leads to decreased excretion of hydrogen ions by the kidney. Finally, lactic acidosis may develop because of increased production of lactate following peripheral hypoxia, and decreased utilization of lactate due to decreased delivery of lactate to the liver. The ability of the liver to use lactate for gluconeogenesis may be impaired because of increased intracellular concentration of hydrogen ions. Indeed, the liver may become a lactate producer rather than a lactate utilizer. The calf attempts to reduce metabolic acidosis by panting to increase exhalation of carbon dioxide. Intracellular acidosis occurs in parallel with the fall in the blood pH. Intracellular production of hydrogen ions increases and hydrogen ions move into cells. This movement of hydrogen ions into cells forces potassium and sodium ions to be lost and hyperkalaemia develops. However, potassium is also lost in the faeces, so that the plasma concentration may, theoretically, be increased, normal or decreased depending on the rate of loss from plasma into faeces, and from cells into plasma. In general it is increased. The loss of potassium ions from cells into the interstitial fluid causes levels of intracellular potassium to fall and levels in interstitial fluid and plasma to rise and, consequently, adjacent to cells, the ratio of extracellular potassium : intracellular potassium is reduced. This redistribution of potassium causes a reduction in the resting potential of cell membranes, which has serious and eventually lethal effects on cardiac muscle function. As the concentration of potassium ions in plasma rises, heart rate falls and there is a decreased amplitude, or loss of the P wave. The activity in plasma of the myocardial enzymes lactate dehydrogenase isoenzyme 1, creatinine phosphokinase 1 and aldolase is raised indicating cardiac damage. Thus death from acute severe diarrhoea in the calf appears to be due to potassium cardiotoxicosis.

Metabolic and hormonal changes

Hypoglycaemia frequently occurs in acute severe diarrhoea of calves, especially young calves near death. Anorexia, decreased absorption of nutrients, minimal glycogen reserves, inhibited gluconeogenesis, increased glycolysis due to reduced tissue perfusion and anoxia and insulin-like effect of bacterial endotoxins on liver may contribute to the hypoglycaemia. Signs of hypoglycaemia are weakness, lethargy, convulsions and coma. Hypoglycaemia stimulates corticoid secretion; plasma concentration of corticosterone and hydrocortisone are elevated in calves with diarrhoea and are higher in calves that die. Theoretically, corticosteroids help counter hypoglycaemia by stimulating gluconeogenesis but their effects may be blocked. Plasma aldosterone concentrations are increased in calves with diarrhoea probably due to acidosis, hypovolaemia, hyperkalaemia and hyponatraemia. The actions of aldosterone are helpful in that sodium and water retention is increased as is excretion of potassium and hydrogen ions. There is, however, decreased renal function, which limits the helpful actions of aldosterone.

Infectious agents

The elucidation of the infectious causes of calf diarrhoea has been a major area of progress over the last 30 years. For many years, salmonellas were the only known cause, but in 1967 it became clear that a small number of strains of *E. coli* caused a watery diarrhoea and subsequently these came to be known as enterotoxigenic *E. coli* (ETEC). Rotavirus was the first viral enteropathogen to be recognized, followed by coronavirus, and more recently Breda virus. Approximately 20 years ago, *Cryptosporidium parvum* was found to cause diarrhoea in calves. Most recently, *E. coli* have been identified that cause diarrhoea without producing enterotoxins; these include strains that infect the large intestine and cause mild dysentery, the enterohaemorrhagic *E. coli* (EHEC), and strains comparable to human enteropathogenic *E. coli* (EPEC).

Bovine rotavirus

The agent

Rotavirus is a new genus within the family Reoviridae. The virus contains double-stranded RNA in 11 segments. Particles have a wheel-like appearance; a wide hub formed by the core, spokes formed by 20 outer capsomers and an often ill-defined outer rim (Fig. 14.10). Incomplete particles lacking the outer capsid layer are frequently seen in faeces. Almost all bovine rotaviruses share a common antigen and have been classified as group A rotaviruses.

Epidemiology

Bovine rotavirus is universally present in all cattle herds but is a more significant problem in single-suckled beef calves than dairy calves because of the much greater risk from cross-contamination between calves, the seasonal nature of the calving pattern and financial restrictions leading to lower nutritional inputs during late gestation.

The incubation period varies from 15 hours to five days and is followed by virus excretion which commences in the second week of life. Many infections are subclinical but a proportion results in severe diarrhoea and even death if not treated promptly. The peak incidence of diarrhoea occurs at about 10 to 14 days of age. Initially, calves are dull and reluctant to suck. The dam's udder becomes distended with milk and may be the first indication to the diligent stockperson that the calf is unwell. Diarrhoea develops which is pale yellow or white and may contain mucus; dehydration and metabolic acidosis develop in more severely affected calves

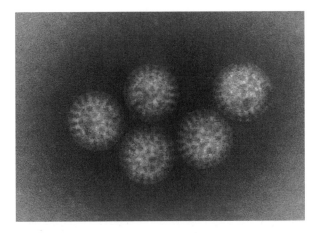

Fig. 14.10 Transmission electron micrograph of a cluster of five bovine rotavirus particles. Visible are the wide hub, spokes formed by the capsomeres, and the outer rim. (Courtesy of Dr J.C. Bridger, Royal Veterinary College, University of London.)

and may be fatal. At this stage the calf may have abdominal distension due to fluid sequestration in the small intestine. Excretion of copious amounts of yoghurt-like faeces is typical of rotavirus infections that are uncomplicated by other enteropathogens and the faeces are thought to have this appearance because they represent the passage of partially digested or undigested milk.

Occurrence of pyrexia is variable, but when it occurs it is usually mild (<39.5°C) and may be more suggestive of a focal bacterial infection such as omphalophlebitis or polyarthritis.

Pathogenesis

Rotaviruses infect mature enterocytes, located on the surface of villi. Particles are detected in the cytoplasm, usually in dilated cisternae of the endoplasmic reticulum. Masses of granular or finely fibrillar virus precursor (viroplasm) containing virus cores are present outside the cisternae. Particles released from viroplasm pass into the cisternae; some bud through the membrane of the endoplasmic reticulum and acquire an envelope. Viral multiplication within the cells initiates degenerative changes, the cell exfoliates and the rapid loss of large numbers of cells leads to fusion and stunting of villi. The columnar epithelium is replaced by enterocytes that are cuboidal or squamous and the epithelium contains increased numbers of immature cells from the crypts (Fig. 14.11). In very severe cases the villi may be obliterated leading to a totally flat epithelium. The pathogenic process may commence in the upper jejunum and progress along the small intestine to the ileum, producing a wave of damage (Mebus

et al., 1971). There is variation in pathogenicity between strains; whilst some strains may only damage a limited length of upper jejunum, others may damage the entire length of the small intestine. Some poorly virulent strains are able to infect enterocytes, replicate within them and cause enterocyte loss, but not at a sufficiently rapid rate to outpace repair mechanisms and cause lesions and diarrhoea. The existence of strains of low virulence has implications for accurate diagnosis of rotavirus diarrhoea because it may be assumed that such strains could be excreted by calves with diarrhoea caused by other enteropathogens. To be confident in a diagnosis of rotavirus diarrhoea, it is necessary to identify rotavirus in the faeces of significantly more diarrhoeic calves than in age-matched, clinically normal calves on the same farm. On the basis of present knowledge, groups of four affected and four normal calves are adequate.

The changes in intestinal structure affect its function. Loss of mature enterocytes with their lactase, and their replacement with immature enterocytes containing less lactase, results in a reduced capacity of the mucosa to digest lactose, especially in the jejunum. Because the surface area of the small intestine is reduced, there is reduced ability to absorb the glucose and galactose that is produced from the digestion of lactose. Thus lactose accumulates in the large intestine, where by virtue of its hypertonicity it prevents absorption of water from faeces and contributes to the development of water loss and dehydration. Bacterial fermentation of the lactose may increase the osmotic effects. As a result of enterocyte loss, the population of enterocytes on the villi changes from mature cells with digestive and absorptive function to predominantly immature cells with

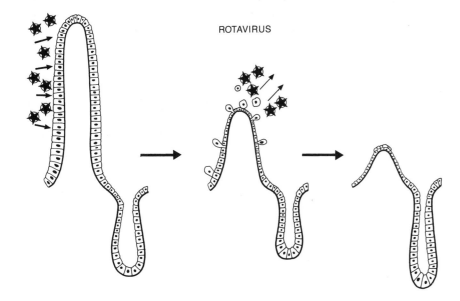

ROTAVIRUS

Fig. 14.11 Line drawing illustrating the development of the small intestinal lesion in rotavirus infection. Mature enterocytes are infected and virus replication causes enterocyte death and sloughing. Villi stunt and the surviving enterocytes are cuboidal or squamous. Mitosis increases in the crypts, which elongate. The star within a circle represents a virus particle.

secretory function. The number of cells in the crypts (secretory cells) also increases. Thus the functional balance may change from absorption to secretion.

Prevention

Virtually all calves that have sucked colostrum will have serum antibody to rotavirus, which can be detected by a number of tests. These antibodies, however, do not protect against infection and disease because for protective purposes neutralizing antibody is required in the gut lumen. This is because the entire disease process occurs on the mucosal surface and if antibodies are to interfere with the pathogenic process they must be present in the gut contents that bathe the mucosal surface; luminal antibodies neutralize virus and prevent initial infection and spread of infection from enterocyte to enterocyte. There is recent evidence, however, suggesting that serum antibodies, which originated from the colostrum of hyperimmune cows, can be transferred to the gut where they are protective.

Following natural infection, calves are immune to disease; this is thought to be the result of an active mucosal immunity provided by IgA and cell-mediated mechanisms. Repeated episodes of reinfection without signs occur throughout life, maintaining herd immunity and the virus in the population and environment.

Colostrum contains antibodies to rotavirus that help protect the calf against infection and disease. The concentration of antibody in colostrum and early milk from unvaccinated cows declines rapidly, reaching levels that are thought to be non-protective three to four days after parturition (Fig. 14.12).

Under farm conditions where rotavirus is always present, feeding colostrum only immediately after birth delays, rather than prevents, rotavirus excretion and calves are susceptible to infection and disease in the second week of life. Protection of the calf has been achieved by providing enhanced passive protection to calves by vaccinating dams with commercial combined inactivated vaccines containing rotavirus, coronavirus and *E. coli* K99 one to three months before the anticipated calving date. Because rotavirus is endemic in herds, cows have antibodies to rotavirus in their serum and parenteral administration of a single dose of inactivated virus absorbed onto aluminium hydroxide gel, and the whole emulsified in a light mineral oil, boosts these pre-existing serum antibodies. Consequently, the concentration of antibody in colostrum and milk is increased and antibody is present in milk for longer than in unvaccinated animals. Thus, dam vaccination is essential on those farms which have experienced losses due to viral diarrhoea in young calves. This system is suitable for both suckled calves, and for artificially reared calves where hyperimmune colostrum is saved from the first six to eight milkings and stored in a cool place and ideally fed at a rate of 2.5 to 3.5 litres per day for the first two weeks of life.

It is essential that all calves ingest sufficient good quality colostrum within the first six hours after birth with values equivalent to between 7 and 10 per cent of bodyweight commonly quoted. Factors that may reduce the level of specific antibody accumulation in the colostrum differ between beef and dairy cows because of the lower nutritional and management inputs in beef herds and the higher prevalence of metabolic disease in high-yielding dairy cows.

Problems with sufficient colostrum accumulation in the udder of beef cows include debility of the dam, poor nutritional status during late gestation, intercurrent disease such as fascioliasis and chronic mastitis caused by *Arcanobacterium pyogenes* (summer mastitis) (Chapter 24). Dystokia is more common in beef calves leading to extended intervals to standing and sucking. As a general rule, those calves born following an assisted calving should receive 2 litres of colostrum within the first two hours of life and be closely supervised to ensure normal sucking behaviour.

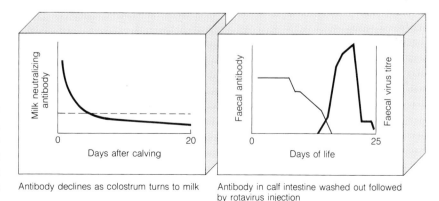

Fig. 14.12 Graphical illustration of changes that occur in neutralizing antibody to rotavirus in cows' milk after calving and faecal antibody to rotavirus and faecal virus in the early days of a calf's life. Reproduced from Morgan (1990).

Antibody declines as colostrum turns to milk

Antibody in calf intestine washed out followed by rotavirus injection

Recumbency resulting from hypocalcaemia, over-crowding of the calving accommodation, slippery underfoot conditions and poor mothering ability, especially in dairy heifers, may delay the ingestion of sufficient colostrum by the newborn dairy calf.

Dam vaccination may not prevent all episodes and rotavirus diarrhoea may follow stressful events such as housing and disbudding if undertaken before the calves are six weeks old.

Diagnosis

Rotavirus infection produces the complete range of clinical signs from no observed abnormality through to severe diarrhoea and dehydration with high mortality even in treated calves. The incubation period is one to three days depending upon the level of viral challenge. Isolation of rotavirus from faecal samples does not necessarily indicate a diagnosis of rotavirus diarrhoea because rotavirus can be isolated from a high proportion of normal healthy calves without signs of diarrhoea. Comparison of faeces samples collected from healthy and diarrhoeic populations of calves may be necessary to determine the precise aetiology but such sampling will prove cost-prohibitive in most farm situations. Determination of the age of affected calves, and vaccination status of their dams against infectious causes of neonatal diarrhoea, will assist in determining the aetiology of the disease outbreak, noting that mixed infections are common. For example, *Cryptosporidium* spp. often exacerbate the severity of diarrhoea caused by rotavirus infection.

Calves with rotavirus infection during the early stages of disease typically show signs of mild depression and salivation, reluctance to stand and suck and profuse diarrhoea when eight to fourteen days old. Disease rapidly spreads among young calves present on the farm when clinical signs may be seen from six days of age. There is extensive faecal staining of the perineum and tail. The faeces are yellow and fluid but without blood or mucosal casts. The rectal temperature is usually within normal limits during the early stages unless there is evidence of focal bacterial infection. Without oral rehydration therapy the affected calf becomes dehydrated, hypothermic and weak, and remains in sternal recumbency. The eyes are sunken and the skin becomes tight and inelastic, consistent with 8 to 10 per cent dehydration within 48 hours, unless treated appropriately. As hypovalaemic shock develops, peripheral vasoconstriction causes the calf's extremities to feel cold. At this stage the calf is often hypothermic (<38.0°C). Without treatment, death may ensue within 72 hours of the onset of diarrhoea.

In most situations diarrhoeic calves have been treated by farm staff with oral rehydration solutions which alter the clinical presentation, whereby profound acidosis is the main presenting feature rather than severe dehydration. The abdomen appears distended and the abomasum and intestines are distended with fluid and 'slosh' when succussed.

Calves treated with oral rehydration solutions by the farmer using an oesophageal feeder often have normal hydration status but become severely acidotic, causing profound weakness and depression extending to stupor. There is no relationship between the degree of dehydration and the severity of the acidosis. The eyes are not sunken and the skin tent duration is normal. Fluid distension of the abdomen is obvious. The respiratory rate is increased above 40 breaths per minute with increased depth of expiration. The heart rate is often less than 90 beats per minute.

A thorough clinical examination is essential in all young calves with diarrhoea because of the likelihood of other focal infections such as early bacterial meningoencephalitis, respiratory disease, omphalophlebitis and possible associated peritonitis, hypopyon and polyarthritis. Indeed, the diarrhoea reported by the client may be the agonal stage of a septicaemia, although such peracute infections usually occur in calves less than six days old.

In normal calves more than two days old the umbilical remnant is dry and shrivelled, hastened by its immersion in strong veterinary iodine solution immediately after birth and again six to 12 hours later. Omphalophlebitis manifests as a swollen (>3 cm diameter), wet and painful umbilicus which may discharge pus under digital pressure (see p. 249). Localized peritonitis associated with omphalophlebitis may result in the formation of fibrinous adhesions and associated ileus which proves difficult to detect on clinical examination alone. Abdominocentesis is difficult to perform on such recumbent calves because of the fluid-distended intestines and the scant fibrinous nature of the adhesions. Similarly, abdominal ultrasonography fails to identify such early adhesions. Calves with peritonitis fail to respond to standard fluid therapy and antibiotic therapy regimens, with the adhesions identified at post-mortem examination.

Polyarthritis manifests as hot, distended and painful joints, typically the fetlock, hock and carpal joints, resulting in the tendency for calves to adopt lateral recumbency rather than sternal recumbency associated with weakness (see pp. 249, 455).

Laboratory diagnosis of rotavirus

Enzyme-linked immunosorbent assays (ELISA) have been developed for rotavirus and a plate ELISA is used by many diagnostic laboratories. Some diagnostic laboratories use the polyacrylamide gel electrophoresis method, which has proved to be equally satisfactory. The diagnostic kits available to practice laboratories in the UK are a dot ELISA, a latex method and a plate ELISA system. The plate ELISA system requires a minimum of equipment and also tests for bovine coronavirus and K99[+] *Escherichia coli*; a modification to the system has permitted the detection of *Cryptosporidium* spp.

The identification of rotavirus particles or antigen in the faeces of calves with diarrhoea does not automatically lead to a diagnosis of rotavirus disease in the outbreak. Rotavirus antigen was detected in 50 per cent of faeces from healthy calves aged one to two weeks in a study in which an ELISA test was used. Thus, in order to reach a sound diagnosis, and using that test to identify excretors, it was necessary to show that significantly more than 50 per cent of diarrhoeic calves were excreting rotavirus. This was achieved by examining faeces from four calves with diarrhoea and four matching normal calves on the farm. The number of calf faeces that will need to be examined in an investigation of an outbreak will depend on the ability of the diagnostic test in use to detect excretion by normal calves.

Treatment (see p. 209)

Veterinary treatment of calf diarrhoea is generally limited to collapsed animals which have failed to respond to oral rehydration solutions. Administration of oral rehydration solutions is frequently made by the farmer using an oesophageal feeder. While this procedure has considerable time savings, it is frequently used for weak recumbent calves without a strong suck reflex which serves to further delay veterinary involvement to the stage where calves are profoundly acidotic when presented. In veterinary practice therefore, treatment of calf diarrhoea involves the correction of acidosis rather than simple correction of hydration status, although both problems may have to be tackled at the same time.

Basic animal husbandry is frequently overlooked in many modern beef production systems. The diarrhoeic calf should be isolated in a warm, dry and well-bedded pen. In beef herds, the dam should be separated from the calf by a gate which allows visual contact. Hypothermic calves should be warmed and this is best achieved with convector heaters rather than heat lamps.

Intravenous fluids are essential because most severely affected diarrhoeic calves are profoundly acidotic (see example below), with variable degrees of dehydration depending upon previous oral rehydration therapy.

Example: treatment of diarrhoeic calf under field situations

The objectives of intravenous fluid therapy include the correction of extracellular fluid volume, plasma pH, blood glucose concentration and plasma concentrations of sodium and potassium, restoration of cellular potassium and the provision of nutrients.

A 10 day-old, 45 kg single suckled beef calf is presented with profuse diarrhoea with faecal staining of the tail, perineum and hind legs. The calf is weak, unable to rise or remain standing when lifted. It is markedly depressed with cold extremities. The skin tent is about three seconds. The eyes do not appear sunken but the scleral vasculature is pale. The heart rate is 85 beats/minute and the respiratory rate is 45 breaths/minute. Two litres of an oral rehyration solution have been administered by oesophageal feeder twice daily for the past two days.

Typical laboratory values: Typical laboratory values are listed below for this calf but such analyses are rarely possible under field situations. Excellent clinical recovery rates for such cases are achieved in general practice using estimations of the base deficit based upon the clinical examination

Packed cell volume = 31%	Arterial blood gas analysis:
Total plasma protein = 68.0 g/l	pH = 6.9
Sodium = 128 mmol/l	pCO_2 = 46 mmHg
Potassium = 7.2 mmol/l	HCO_3 = 7 mmol/l
Chloride = 105 mmol/l	Base deficit = 20 mmol/l

The calf is estimated to be only 5 per cent dehydrated. The serum potassium concentration is elevated because intracellular K^+ ions exchange with H^+ and pass into the extracellular fluid. However, the intracellular (and total body) K^+ ion concentrations will be lowered, but this deficit is more safely replaced by the oral rehydration solution rather than the intravenous fluid. Diarrhoeic calves are not markedly hypoglycaemic and nutrients are better supplied in the oral rehydration solution, and then milk, than in the intravenous fluids.

Intravenous fluid therapy: The fluid requirements are calculated as:

45 kg × 0.05 = 2 litres

The daily requirement of 75–150 ml/kg should be added to this deficit. The fluids should be warmed to body temperature before administration and insulated if left suspended in a cold environment.

Base deficit: The base deficit is estimated from the clinical findings whereby profoundly weak and depressed/stuporous calves, in the absence of septicaemia or bacterial meningoencephalitis, have a base deficit in the region of 20 mmol/l. As an alternative practical guideline, calves able to maintain sternal recumbency are reported to have a base deficit of 15 mmol/l, whilst those in lateral recumbeny have a deficit of 20 mmol/l (Naylor, 1996). However, such distinction is not necessary to achieve excellent results, even under less than ideal practice situations.

The total base deficit (or negative base excess) can be calculated as:

$$\text{base deficit} \times \text{bicarbonate space} \times \text{dehydrated calf} \\ \text{weight} = 20 \times (0.3 \text{ to } 0.6) \times 45 = 270 \text{ to } 540 \text{ mmol} \\ \text{bicarbonate}$$

There is considerable debate as to which value should be employed for the bicarbonate space because this value is higher in neonates than adults. In practice situations, where blood gas analysis is rarely available, an estimate of 20 mmol/l for base deficit in recumbent stuporous calves is commonly used in conjunction with an estimate of 0.5 to 0.6 for the bicarbonate space. While it is accepted that there will be errors in such a simplified approach, this regimen has proved very reliable in general practice where the rapid response to intravenous fluid therapy spiked with bicarbonate is the most valuable indicator of success of the fluid therapy regimen.

Typically, stuporous calves should be much improved after three to four hours, and be able to stand six to eight hours after the start of intravenous fluid therapy. A thorough initial clinical examination will eliminate focal and septicaemic infections from the list of differential diagnoses. Re-evaluation of the diagnosis and/or treatment is necessary if the calf's condition has not markedly improved within six hours of commencing intravenous fluid therapy. The two most common reasons why the calf's condition has not improved are: the extent of the base deficit has been underestimated and insufficient bicarbonate has been infused or, less commonly, that the calf has bacterial meningoencephalitits (see pp. 251, 901).

Some practice laboratories use a Harleco apparatus to determine total CO_2, which is a useful index of the severity of the metabolic acidosis. However, determination of metabolic acidosis using either the Harleco or blood gas analysis necessitates hospitalization of the calf with the attendant risks of contaminating the facilities with a range of enteropathogens, some of which are serious zoonoses. While blood samples can be transported to the practice laboratory for blood gas analysis, such retrospective information may not be so helpful because financial considerations frequently preclude a second veterinary visit to correct any estimations based upon clinical findings. Alternatively, with accurate information on the precise severity of the acidosis, the farmer can be instructed to spike the intravenous fluid with materials left on the farm.

Treatment regimen: Under practical conditions on farm a 14 gauge (or 16 gauge) catheter should be stitched into a jugular vein as this makes fluid administration much easier because the calf can be left unattended. A 5 cm by 5 cm area of skin overlying a jugular vein is shaved and aseptically prepared. A stab incision through the skin overlying the jugular vein using a 15T blade greatly facilitates catheter placement. If the calf is severely dehydrated and cannot be catheterized easily, either the first litre of fluid can be administered through a 16 gauge hypodermic needle or the calf is suspended by its hind legs to distend the jugular veins, thereby facilitating catheterization.

A typical treatment regime for a recumbent acidotic calf would commence with 1 litre of isotonic saline spiked with 200 mmol bicarbonate (16 g sodium bicarbonate) administered intravenously over 20 to 30 minutes. This solution can be administered while the veterinary surgeon remains on the farm suturing the catheter in position, securing the fluid administration set, and possibly attending further calves with diarrhoea or collecting faecal samples as appropriate.

A further 3 litres of isotonic saline solution containing the balance of the estimated bicarbonate deficit (approximately 400 mmol) should then be administered over the next four to six hours, by which time the calf's demeanour will be much improved. The calf should be able to stand and suck a teat enthusiastically at this stage. An oesophageal feeder should be used only as a last resort to administer oral fluids because the calf's demeanour and willingness to suck are valuable indicators of the calf's recovery. Indeed, early cases of bacterial meningoencephalitis may be difficult to differentiate from profound acidosis, but acidotic calves should respond well within six hours to spiked intravenous fluid therapy and suck, whereas those with meningoencephalitis will not and may progress to opisthotonus with spontaneous nystagmus. Alternatively, in cases where meningoencephalitis is suspected during the veterinary examination, lumbar CSF can be collected under local anaesthesia and inspected visually for turbidity caused by white cell infiltration.

This approach to fluid therapy of collapsed acidotic calves described above has been employed in many farm animal practices because the calf remains on the farm and is visited by the veterinary surgeon, thereby removing the risk of introducing enteropathogens, including *Salmonella* spp., into the practice hospital facilities with the potential for disastrous consequences. Often only one veterinary visit is possible for each diarrhoeic calf because of cost limitations, but this system of intravenous fluid administration works well in practice.

Most diarrhoeic calves are not profoundly hypoglycaemic and the addition of glucose to the intravenous solutions is generally not undertaken. Energy supply is better given as a component of the oral rehydration solution therapy (high energy rehydration solution), which often commences within six to eight hours of the start of intravenous fluid administration. Recently-introduced oral rehydration solutions have a high energy content designed to counter the energy deficit state caused by witholding milk from the calf's diet. As soon as the suck reflex returns, the calf should be offered either one litre of oral rehydration solution or milk at alternate feeds every two hours.

Other intravenous fluids: Clinical evaluation of the alkalinizing effect of various bases in diarrhoeic calves suffering from severe dehydration and acidosis (Kasari & Naylor, 1986) clearly demonstrated the advantages in both speed and extent of administering isotonic saline solutions containing bicarbonate compared to those solutions containing either lactate or acetate.

Lactated Ringer's solution should not be used to treat severe acidosis because it contains only 30 mmol/l of lactate, which would necessitate in excess of 15 litres to counter severe acidosis in a calf. Furthermore, lactate must be metabolized to yield bicarbonate but the young calf cannot fully utilize D lactate in the racemic mixture. Hypertonic (7.2%) saline solutions are not indicated in the treatment of acidotic calves because of their lack of alkalinizing effect, although successful treatment of mild acidosis in experimental calves has been reported using a hypertonic saline solution containing sodium bicarbonate (Dupe *et al.*, 1993).

The administration of sterile isotonic saline solutions spiked with bicarbonate described above has obvious advantages over non-sterile fluids made using tap water; however, solutions prepared using small water purification plants are reported to work well under practice conditions. A typical mixture of salts available in the UK (Electrolyte ED; Vetoquinol Ltd) added to 5 litres of water yields 141 mmol/l sodium, 4 mmol/l potassium, and 35 mmol/l bicarbonate, which can then be spiked with additional sodium bicarbonate. Extra bicarbonate can be administered either as a 1.3 per cent isotonic solution (65 g sodium bicarbonate to 5 litres, yielding 150 mmol/l bicarbonate) or by adding 35 g sodium bicarbonate to yield 400 mmol in addition to the 175 mmol already present in the 5 litre solution (Grove-White, 2000).

Oral rehydration solutions: There are a large number of oral rehydration solutions available but all utilize the active glucose/sodium-linked gut transport system whereby sodium is transported across the gut wall into the extracellular fluid and water follows along the osmotic gradient. Other molecules, including acetate, propionate, glycine and glutamine, also play an important role in sodium transport.

The original World Health Organization (WHO) oral rehydration solution was an equimolar solution containing approximately 100 mmol/l sodium and glucose and was the basis of the first generation oral rehydration solutions introduced into veterinary practice during the 1970s. Potassium was present to assist in restoring any deficits. These solutions contain no bicarbonate or precursor and are therefore unable to correct a significant acidosis, but are effective in many cases of calf diarrhoea associated with dehydration. Viral causes of neonatal diarrhoea were not reported in the United Kingdom until the mid-1980s (Snodgrass *et al.*, 1986), and these oral rehydration solutions proved effective in the treatment of bacterial and nutritional causes of calf diarrhoea which were not usually associated with severe metabolic acidosis.

The widespread occurrence of rotavirus-induced diarrhoea and associated metabolic acidosis led to the development of oral rehydration solutions containing 80 to 120 mmol/l bicarbonate as a precursor, whether lactate, propionate or citrate. These solutions have been referred to as 'second generation' oral rehydration solutions. While these solutions are very effective in meeting the primary objectives of correcting hypovolaemia, moderate metabolic acidosis (and associated hyperkalaemia) and hyponatraemia, they fail to provide sufficient calorific support and treated calves lose considerable body condition during treatment when milk is withheld from the diet.

'Third generation' oral rehydration solutions contain much higher concentrations of glucose (up to 375 mmol/l) and sodium (up to 133 mmol/l) to counter the energy deficit which results when milk is withheld from the calf's diet. Such hypertonic solutions do not worsen diarrhoea due to osmosis or produce hypernatraemia and, when compared to standard oral rehydration solutions, these 'third generation' solutions have reduced the liveweight loss which results from calf diarrhoea.

Further developments in oral fluid therapy ('fourth generation') include the addition of the amino acid glutamine to promote enteric sodium uptake and sustain villus form and function. A high-calorie oral rehydration solution with glutamine was more effective in correcting plasma, extracellular fluid and blood volume than solutions without (one WHO-type solution and two high-glucose but glutamine-free solutions) using an *Escherichia coli* model (Brooks *et al.*, 1997).

In summary, an oral rehydration solution should be judged on the composition of the solution in mmol/l and not on a dry matter percentage basis. The sodium concentration should not exceed 130 mmol/l. The bicarbonate concentration (usually as a precursor such as citrate, acetate or propionate) should be in the region of 80 to 120 mmol/l. The role of glycine may be overstated with respect to sodium transport but it aids palatibility. High-energy-containing oral rehydration solutions, with glucose concentrations up to 375 mmol/l, limit liveweight loss during diarrhoea and should be considered if milk is withheld for more than two days. The addition of glutamine to the oral rehydration solution appears to offer numerous advantages over other solutions (Brooks *et al.*, 1997).

Treatment with oral rehydration solutions: As detailed above, there is an almost bewildering list of oral rehydration solutions which can be used to treat diarrhoeic calves, each supported by its own experimental and clinical database. For veterinary practitioners presented with a recumbent calf with severe metabolic acidosis, the most critical treatment is appropriate intravenous fluid therapy. No oral rehydration solution will correct the moderate to severe base deficit in these profoundly weak and recumbent calves. Within six to eight hours of the start of intravenous fluid therapy the calf should be much improved, with return of the suck reflex. This clinical improvement indicates that the acidosis has been largely corrected, but to counter ongoing losses 1 litre of a high-calorie oral rehydration solution with a high alkalinizing ability should be offered eight times daily (note: this may be twice the recommended rate detailed in the product data sheets). The presence of a vigorous suck reflex is the best indicator that the calf is recovering and is a more important factor than the continued production of fluid faeces.

The calf should be returned to a milk diet as soon as possible, and this should be a complete change. The milk must not be diluted with an oral rehydration solution. Typically, when milk is added to the diet, the calf will continue to have profuse diarrhoea for a few days but it will possess a strong suck reflex, be bright and alert with no signs of weakness. Assessment of the calf's recovery based upon demeanour, activity and appetite is more important than the negative aspect of the continued production of fluid faeces.

Traditionally, milk was withheld from diarrhoeic calves until solid faeces were passed, which often did not occur until after four or more days of administration of only oral rehydration solutions. This calorific deprivation led to considerable body condition loss and a protracted convalescence. Some clinicians recommend that milk and an oral rehydration solution are alternated every two to four hours during the early convalescent phase, thereby largely overcoming the calorie deficit but still retaining the benefits of the oral rehydration solution. Oral rehydration solutions with an increased glucose content as energy source should be chosen if the calf is fed only oral rehydration solution for more than 24 hours (third or fourth generation oral rehydration solutions).

Antibiotics: Antibiotics are frequently employed in the treatment of diarrhoeic calves despite the fact that significant bacterial causes are limited to age-specific periods within the first four days (enterotoxigenic *E. coli*) and at over three weeks old (*Salmonella* spp.). Unsupervised widespread use of antibiotics prescribed by veterinary surgeons for the treatment of calf diarrhoea has been claimed to result in an increased prevalence of muliple resistant enteropathogens in humans, which cautions against their use except for specific bacterial causes (see also p. 210).

Enterotoxigenic *E. coli* do not display a high degree of antibiotic resistance and the commonly used antibiotics such as trimethoprim-sulpha are effective. Such calves do not develop a bacteraemia and oral antibiotic administration is preferable. Many *Salmonella* spp. infections result in bacteraemia with localization in the lungs, joints and growth plates. Antibiotic selection should be guided by bacterial isolation and antibiotic sensitivity testing. Improved biosecurity and hygiene, and possibly dam vaccination, should all be considered to control salmonellosis in neonatal calves, thereby reducing the need for antibiotic therapy. The use of fluoroquinolone antibiotics to treat salmonellosis in calves should be carefully considered and employed only where there is no alternative antibiotic.

The use of antibiotics in rotavirus diarrhoea is not indicated, but care must be taken not to overlook focal bacterial infections. Indeed, it is possible to overlook early cases of bacterial polyarthritis and meningoencephalitis, but such infections generally appear in calves less than six days old whereas rotavirus infection causing recumbency and stupor occurs in calves more than eight days old with a history of diarrhoea for the past two days or more.

Following intravenous fluid therapy it is important that the catheter is removed within 24 hours to reduce the risk of thrombophlebitis; parenteral antibiotics should not be necessary simply because the jugular vein has been catheterized.

Non-steroidal anti-inflammatory drugs: Non-steroidal anti-inflammatory drugs (NSAIDs) such as flunixin meglumine and ketoprofen have been recommended for diarrhoeic calves but have not been fully evaluated as a supportive treatment. Some reports refer to reduced severity of scouring following flunixin injection while other clinicians comment that dehydrated calves must not be given NSAIDs.

Protectants: Protectants, e.g. kaolin and pectin mixtures, are used as an adjunct to treatment but their value in serious cases is doubtful.

Convalescence

Convalescence from rotavirus-induced diarrhoea is often protracted because of physical loss of absorptive capacity of the small intestine. The villus epithelial cells are lost, resulting in stunted villi (Fig. 14.11). These lining cells are intially replaced with undifferentiated squamous and cuboidal cells, and only later replaced by specialized aborptive columnar cells. Extended oral administration of certain antimicrobials may prolong this delay to normal absorptive capacity.

Management

The management of an outbreak of rotavirus diarrhoea, once it has been diagnosed, should be based on the twin concepts of reducing exposure to infection and enhancing resistance to infection by ensuring passive transfer of specific antibody induced by timely vaccination of the dam (see p. 1006). Good hygiene will not be successful in controlling spread of infection because rotavirus is endemic and highly infectious, but it will help to reduce the build-up of infection throughout the calving period and thus reduce the infectious challenge to which calves are exposed; several studies have recorded beneficial results from good hygiene.

Unlike dairy herds, most beef cattle have a seasonal calving pattern with over 90 per cent of the cows calving during a nine week period, which presents problems with stocking levels in farm buildings and calving accommodation. Beef cattle should calve outdoors wherever possible. Newly-calved cows and their calves should be moved to clean pastures as soon as possible after birth. The stocking density on these pastures should be kept as low as practicable to prevent environmental contamination and build-up of infection. Problems with rotavirus diarrhoea usually appear during the second half of the calving period and are often associated with adverse weather conditions during early spring or late autumn, when young calves are crowded in sheltered areas of the field facilitating build-up of infection. Infection builds up rapidly in housed beef herds where poor building design and lack of sufficient straw bedding material aggravate overstocked conditions. The provision of a dry, well-bedded creep area for calves may reduce the level of challenge but is not suffcient to prevent disease.

To assist good hygiene, calving accommodation and calf pens on dairy farms should be designed for ease of cleaning and with adequate drainage. An 'all-in, all-out' policy should be adopted where possible, especially in units rearing purchased calves. Pens should be cleaned between batches, steamed, disinfected and allowed to dry.

Disinfectants that have been reported to be effective against rotavirus are 0.25 per cent formaldehyde, 2 per cent phenol, 1 per cent sodium hypochlorite, 0.25 per cent propiolactone, quaternary ammonium compounds and iodophores. Mixing calves of different ages should be avoided and stress should be limited by staggering management interference such as castration, disbudding and changing of accommodation.

Bovine coronavirus

The agent

Bovine coronavirus (BCV) is a member of a group of viruses with a characteristic morphology seen in the electron microscope (Fig. 14.13). The virions, which contain single-stranded polyadenylated RNA, are pleomorphic spherical particles 70 to 220 nm in diameter with a corona of widely spaced club-shaped surface projections (peplomers), which are 20 nm long. Bovine coronavirus has two types of peplomer of different length. There is only one serotype of bovine coronavirus.

Signs

Calves usually become infected with coronavirus when they are between one and three weeks old, although disease may occur in calves up to three months of age. Transmission of infection is by the faecal–oral route. Calves develop diarrhoea in a manner virtually

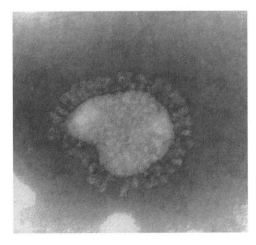

Fig. 14.13 Transmission electron micrograph of a single particle of bovine coronavirus. The particle has an irregular shape and is covered by a corona of peplomers. (Courtesy of Dr J.C. Bridger, Royal Veterinary College, University of London.)

identical to rotavirus; studies of experimental inoculations suggest that the incubation period is 20 to 30 hours. Generally, coronavirus diarrhoea is more watery and of greater severity than rotavirus diarrhoea, leading more rapidly to dehydration and acidosis. The severe diarrhoea also leads to substantial losses of sodium, potassium, chloride and bicarbonate ions. Fluid yellow faeces are passed at first and these turn to a yellow liquid containing milk clots and mucus.

Pathogenesis

Bovine coronavirus infects mature enterocytes located on the surface of villi and epithelial cells of the upper respiratory tract. The small intestine is severely damaged due to sloughing of infected cells, especially the ileum, and cells on the surface and in the crypts of the large intestine are also killed. Infection of the upper respiratory tract does not appear to cause lesions. Virus particles are assembled in the cytoplasm by a budding process through the rough endoplasmic reticulum. They are subsequently transported through and accumulate in the Golgi complex and are released from the cell by lysis. The range of lesions seen in the small intestine is identical to those produced by rotavirus and repair can occur rapidly because small intestinal crypt cells are largely unaffected. Virus damage to colonic crypt cells results in atrophy of the mucosal ridges and dilated crypts containing dead exfoliated cells. The mechanisms by which the intestinal damage caused by bovine coronavirus results in diarrhoea are thought to be the same as described for rotavirus. The presence of severe lesions in the ileum, caecum and colon, areas of the small and large intestine that absorb water, may account for the more watery nature of the diarrhoea seen in BCV infections. It is not clear whether or not strains of BCV vary in virulence, as is seen in bovine rotaviruses.

Prevention

There are two inactivated vaccines available in the UK which combines coronavirus, rotavirus and E. coli K99 to provide protective antibody in colostrum and early milk. The vaccines are administerd 12 to 13 weeks before the anticipated calving date.

Diagnosis

Bovine coronavirus is universally present on all cattle farms, as indicated by the presence of antibodies in all adults. Diagnosis of coronavirus disease, like that of rotavirus disease, is based on the detection of virus or virus antigen in intestinal tissue or faeces. Assays using ELISA have been developed for detection of bovine coronavirus and are used by diagnostic laboratories. The existence of bovine coronavirus excretion by clinically normal calves is recorded, although it is not seen as commonly as is rotavirus.

Management

An outbreak of BCV diarrhoea should be managed in the same way as an outbreak of rotavirus diarrhoea; that is, aim to reduce exposure to infection and enhance resistance to infection by vaccination of the dam and ensuring adequate passive antibody transfer (see p. 1006).

Sick calves should be moved to isolation facilities to help prevent a build-up of infection and to facilitate the provision of rehydration therapy. Diarrhoea induced by BCV is often more watery than that caused by rotavirus, possibly because the colon is less able to absorb water because it is damaged by the infection. The watery diarrhoea is likely to lead to severe dehydration and rehydration therapy as outlined for rotavirus is indicated (see pp. 195–6).

Calici-like virus (Newbury agent)

Particles of calf calici-like virus measure approximately 33 nm in diameter and have an indefinite feathery outline with dark hollows on the surface. Some particles have a 10-spiked sphere morphology. The virus was first detected in faeces of calves with diarrhoea and the pathogenic process has been studied in gnotobiotic calves. As far as is known, the disease is confined to the unweaned calf, although a gnotobiotic calf aged 60 days was susceptible to infection and disease. In gnotobiotic calves, clinical signs of enteric disease are identical to those seen in rotavirus infections and the lesions are comparable to those produced by rotavirus and BCV.

Two antigenically distinct isolates of Newbury agent have been identified and infection with either virus did not protect against clinical illness following infection with the other virus three weeks later. There are no specific diagnostic tests for the calf calici-like viruses, other than electron microscopic examination of faeces concentrated and purified by ultracentrifugation. They might be suspected as the aetiological agent in cases that appeared clinically similar to rotavirus, but are negative for rotavirus and other enteropathogens. Calves with diarrhoea caused by a calici-like virus may be managed as though they were infected with rotavirus.

Astrovirus

Astrovirus is a descriptive name for viruses with a star-like pattern on their surface in the electron microscope. They have a diameter of 28–30 nm and contain single-stranded RNA. Astroviruses have also been detected in faeces of lambs with diarrhoea where the virus infected enterocytes causing mild villus stunting in the mid small intestine. Astroviruses have been detected in calf faeces in association with diarrhoea but experimental infection of gnotobiotic calves with astrovirus did not cause diarrhoea. Nevertheless, antibodies to astrovirus are widespread in cattle sera, having been found in 11 out of 22 herds in the UK and in 30 per cent of cattle sera examined in the USA. Recently, astroviruses were shown to infect and damage the specialized epithelium of the dome villi (Fig. 14.14) in the Peyer's patches of calves. These calves did not develop diarrhoea, but severe diarrhoea occurred in mixed infections of astrovirus and rotavirus or astrovirus and Breda agent. It is probable that astrovirus are not pathogenic on their own, but may increase the severity of the disease produced by other enteropathogenic viruses. There are no routine tests to detect astroviruses in faeces, but in the research laboratory they can be identified by electron microscopic examination of faeces concentrated by centrifugation.

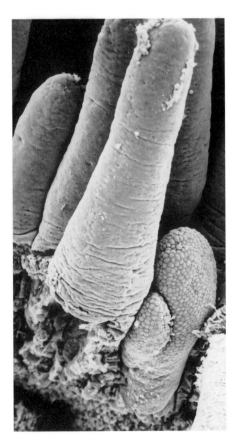

Fig. 14.14 Scanning electron micrograph of calf small intestine illustrating absorptive villi and a dome villus covered by a characteristic epithelium, which is thought to be specialized for antigen uptake and which has been shown to be susceptible to infection and damage by bovine astroviruses.

Breda virus

This virus was first described as causing calf diarrhoea in the USA in 1982. Lesions were similar to those produced by coronavirus. Jejunal and ileal villi were stunted and there were crypt abscesses in the small intestine and particularly in the colon. There were areas of necrosis of the surface epithelium of the colon.

There are no tests available commercially which detect Breda virus in faeces. Electron microscopy of faeces and thin sections through ultracentrifuge pellets may be used in the research laboratory and, because all isolates of Breda virus possess common antigens, antibodies to these can be used in an immunofluorescent test of intestinal sections and in an ELISA test. Examination by ELISA of over 200 faeces from UK calves with diarrhoea failed to detect Breda virus. However, in a separate study, antibodies to Breda virus were detected in 55 per cent of cattle sera.

Escherichia coli

Three groups of *E. coli* have been identified that appear to cause diarrhoea in calves. Strains that elaborate a heat-labile enterotoxin or a heat-stable enterotoxin are called the enterotoxigenic *E. coli* (ETEC). A second collection of strains exists that colonize the small intestinal mucosa and cause diarrhoea, but do not elaborate enterotoxins. Characteristically, these strains attach closely to the luminal surface of enterocytes, often in cup-shaped depressions or on cytoplasmic protrusions, described as 'pedestals'. This attachment of bacteria to the enterocyte surface usually results in the microvilli being effaced and the lesion has been named the 'attaching and effacing' (AE) lesion (Fig. 14.15). Comparable strains cause diarrhoea in children and are called enteropathogenic *E. coli* (EPEC). It is appropriate to use this term for equivalent calf strains, but care is required because the term enteropathogenic *E. coli* has been used in the veterinary literature for many years to describe strains associated with diarrhoea, regardless of their pathogenic mechanism.

A third group of strains colonizes the surface of the large intestine and causes a mild dysentery. These strains also cause AE lesions but because they cause blood to be lost into the lumen of the large intestine, they are called enterohaemorrhagic *E. coli* (EHEC); once again comparable strains cause a similar disease in children. Some EPEC and EHEC, but not all, produce a toxin that kills Vero cells *in vitro* and is called Verocytotoxin (VT) or Shiga-like toxin (SLT). This toxin does not cause AE lesions, but is probably involved in the pathogenic process. *Escherichia coli* that produce VT are referred to as VT+ *E. coli* or VTEC. VTEC have been isolated from calves with diarrhoea,

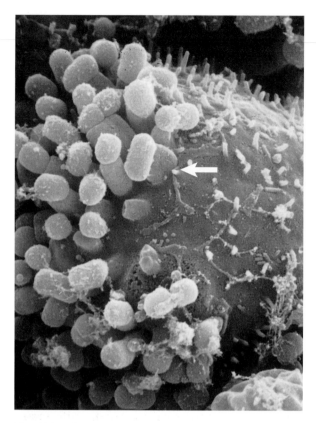

Fig. 14.15 Scanning electron micrograph of an enterocyte in the colonic mucosa of a gnotobiotic calf inoculated experimentally with an enterohaemorrhagic *E. coli* (strain S102–9). Bacteria are attached closely to the surface of the enterocyte, often on 'pedestals' (arrow) and the microvilli have been effaced.

but they may also be present in the faeces of healthy calves. In an epidemiological study, they were found to be as common in the faeces of healthy calves as in the faeces of calves with diarrhoea. Therefore, designation of an *E. coli* as a VTEC may not necessarily define it as an isolate capable of causing diarrhoea and demonstration of a VTEC in the faeces of a calf or calves with diarrhoea does not constitute a diagnosis of the cause of the diarrhoea.

Enterotoxigenic E. coli

Enterotoxigenic *E. coli* most commonly cause diarrhoea in calves under four days old. In experimentally infected newborn calves the incubation period is 12 to 18 hours. Calves are depressed and anorexic and rapidly dehydrate and die. In calves ETEC diarrhoea can be diagnosed clinically because it causes disease in very young calves and because it produces a very profuse and much more watery diarrhoea than any other of the calf enteropathogens.

Enterotoxigenic *E. coli* possess two virulence attributes (determinants) that distinguish them from non-pathogenic strains: ability to adhere to the mucosal surface of enterocytes and, as mentioned previously, ability to produce enterotoxins (see Fig. 14.4).

Adhesion is mediated by filamentous protein structures called fimbriae, sometimes called pili or adhesins, which bind to specific receptors on the enterocyte cell membrane. Adhesion mediated by fimbriae does not bring the bacterium in close contact with the enterocyte luminal surface as is the case of EPEC and EHEC. The microvilli are unaltered and 'cups' and 'pedestals' are not seen. The presence of receptors is affected by age, and susceptibility to infection is greatest in the newborn calf when expression of receptors is greatest. These fimbriae are antigenic and so many of them are known by their antigenic name (e.g. K99, F41). Their adhesive ability allows ETEC to overcome the peristalsis of the small intestine by sticking to the mucosal surface. The adhesion antigens commonly found in ETEC of calves are K99 and F41; they often occur together but may be present independently. K99⁺ strains are also capable of inducing diarrhoea in pigs, foals, lambs, goats and possibly other ruminants. Adhesion of the bacterium to the enterocyte surface confers another advantage to the bacterium because enterotoxins are released close to their receptor sites. The ability of ETEC to produce fimbriae and enterotoxins is determined by genes that are usually carried on a single plasmid and thus occur together. It is adequate, therefore, to diagnose ETEC infection by detecting either the enterotoxin or the adhesin.

Detection of adhesins forms the basis of the diagnostic tests for ETEC because they are easier to detect than enterotoxins. Special culture media may be required to encourage ETEC to express adhesins because, in general, K99 and F41 are poorly produced by bacteria *in vitro*, although they are readily produced by bacteria growing in the gut. Once expressed they can be detected using specific antisera in agglutination, haemagglutination or ELISA tests.

It is helpful to understand the mechanisms of absorption and secretion in the small intestine before considering how the enterotoxins produced by ETEC cause diarrhoea. Absorption occurs through the activity of the mature villus enterocyte. Sodium ions are transported out of enterocytes through the basolateral cell membranes into the basolateral spaces by an energy-dependent mechanism, the sodium pump. This creates a concentration gradient extending from the lumen into the enterocyte. Sodium ions, followed by chloride ions, diffuse along the concentration gradient from the lumen through the microvillous surface, assisted by a brush border carrier system. The osmolality in the basolateral spaces increases and water passes from the lumen along the osmotic gradient (see Fig. 14.2). There are several carrier systems that assist the entry of sodium ions; one system does not utilize the products of digestion, another utilizes glucose, which is specifically absorbed through the luminal surface of enterocytes and each molecule of glucose carries with it a molecule of sodium. Chloride ions and water follow and this flow of water traps additional sodium and chloride ions by solvent drag (Fig. 14.2). Carrier systems for amino acids and citrate also transport sodium ions and water through the intestinal mucosa. These carrier systems, particularly the glucose carrier system, are particularly important in oral rehydration therapy. Secretion occurs from crypt cells; sodium passes into the intestinal lumen taking chloride and bicarbonate ions and water with it (Fig. 14.3). Cyclic-AMP stimulates this secretory activity.

The heat-stable enterotoxin (ST) is the enterotoxin usually produced by ETEC strains from calves. Two forms of ST occur (ST_A, and ST_B), but only ST_A occurs in calves. Both forms stimulate guanylate cyclase activity within enterocytes, causing increased levels of intracellular cyclic-GMP, which inhibits absorption by villous enterocytes but has no effect on secretion.

The heat-labile enterotoxin (LT), rarely produced by calf ETEC strains, is made up of two subunits. Subunit A stimulates adenylate cyclase activity within enterocytes. Subunit B assists entry of subunit A into enterocytes. Adenylate cyclase raises the levels of cyclic-AMP in mature villous enterocytes and crypt cells. In mature villous enterocytes, cyclic-AMP inhibits the independent pathway for the absorption of sodium ions and therefore of chloride and water (see Fig. 14.5). In crypt cells, it stimulates sodium secretion, which takes with it chloride and water (see Fig. 14.6).

Although the main mechanism for the pathogenesis of diarrhoea is attributed to enterotoxins, which do not cause visible damage to the gut, experimental infections of gnotobiotic and conventional calves, both colostrum fed and colostrum deprived, have revealed a pathology associated with ETEC infections that probably contributes to the development of diarrhoea. Villi become stunted and fused together and the enterocytes change shape from columnar to cuboidal. These cells are probably immature enterocytes and these changes indicate an increased rate of enterocyte loss.

Immunoprophylaxis against ETEC-induced diarrhoea is based on the use of immune colostrum. Dam vaccination is used to stimulate high levels of antibody in the colostrum and this approach is particularly successful because calves are susceptible to this disease for only the first few days of life when colostrum is fed. Vaccines containing the K99 fimbriae, or dead bacteria with the K99 antigen expressed on the surface, are used because adhesion is an important component of the pathogenic process.

It is possible to recognize clinically an outbreak of calf diarrhoea caused by ETEC because of the severity and age group of calves affected. An outbreak characterized by the rapid onset of severe, very watery diarrhoea, which quickly causes dehydration and collapse and which is frequently fatal and occurs in calves that are less than 96 hours old, is likely to he caused by ETEC. In some circumstances, calves may die before there is evidence of profuse diarrhoea. There is rapid and severe dehydration. The calf quickly becomes recumbent. Sequestration of fluid in the abomasum and intestines gives the abdomen a bloated appearance which 'sloshes' on succussion. The rectal temperature may be elevated in the early stages but rapidly falls to subnormal. Affected calves are rarely acidotic. Faecal bacteriology will confirm the diagnosis. ETEC diarrhoea is not common in the UK (less than one per cent of calf diarrhoea outbreaks), but outbreaks have been associated with poor housing and management at calving.

There are a number of possible causes of recumbency in neonatal calves which must be excluded from the differential diagnosis list, including congenital heart defects, rupture of liver/spleen following dystokia and bilateral femoral nerve paralysis. Atresia coli/ani cases present with increasing abdominal distension, progressive weakness and dehydration leading to recumbency. Septicaemia and bacterial meningoencephalitis are also commonly encountered in calves less than four days old. Congenital neosporosis has also recently been reported as a cause of recumbency in neonatal calves.

The immediate response must be rapid isolation and treatment of sick calves by rehydration with an electrolyte solution. Acidosis is not a feature of diarrhoea in calves less than six days old and spiking intravenous fluids with bicarbonate is not indicated in calves with enterotoxigenic E. coli infections. Rehydration may be given by intravenous infusion if the calf is unable to feed; intravenous infusions may be changed to oral administration as the calf recovers strength. Less severely dehydrated calves may be treated only by oral rehydration. The biochemistry of oral rehydration has been discussed earlier (pp. 197–8). Oral antibiotics should be administered to all calves at birth in the face of an outbreak until the vaccine administered to all remaining pregnant cattle can provide protective immunoglobulins in the colostrum. Antibiotic resistance is not a problem in such outbreaks thus antibiotic selection is not critical to a successful outcome. Fluid therapy is the first priority because calves may die of dehydration before any beneficial effects are obtained from antibiotic therapy.

Following immediate management of an outbreak with fluid therapy and antibiotics, it is essential to introduce dam vaccination (see p. 1006). It should be possible to eliminate the infection from the herd with the use of antibiotics, dam vaccination and good hygiene. ETEC with the K99 antigen are absent from most farms and disease prevention should concentrate on exclusion of the infection by good herd biosecurity.

Enteropathogenic E. coli, *enterohaemorrhagic* E. coli *and verocytotoxin-producing* E. coli

There are no specific clinical signs of diarrhoea caused by EPEC and VTEC although a yellow watery diarrhoea has been reported. The mean age of calves with diarrhoea caused by EHEC was 15 days. Calves maintained a normal appetite and did not develop pyrexia, but a mild diarrhoea containing blood was seen. In prolonged cases there was dullness, signs of abdominal pain, dehydration and weight loss.

Although the EPEC, EHEC and VTEC are capable of causing diarrhoea in calves and have been associated with outbreaks of disease, it is difficult to diagnose their specific involvement. Presence of frank blood in the faeces is suggestive of EHEC, especially if salmonellas and cryptosporidia are not isolated from faeces. The presence of these enteropathogens will be suggested by the failure to find other agents and possibly by the finding of *E. coli* in association with the mucosa of the small or large intestine.

Clinical signs of septicaemia

In many situations it can prove difficult to differentiate the cause of the calf's depression, lethargy and weakness between profound acidosis or early septicaemia/bacterial meningoencephalitis. Most septicaemic calves are less than six days old and this age prevalence differs from the typical occurrence of viral-induced diarrhoea and acidosis (more than eight days old). Septicaemic calves usually present with episcleral injection, toxic mucous membranes and evidence of multi-organ system involvement such as joints, respiratory tract and eyes. Pyrexia above 39.5°C is not a consistent finding in septicaemic calves while diarrhoea is often only present during the terminal stage of illness.

Lumbar cerebrospinal fluid (CSF) collection and visual inspection of the turbid sample on farm enables immediate diagnosis of bacterial meningoencephalitis and appropriate aggressive antimicrobial therapy (Scott & Penny, 1993). This sampling procedure is recommended in those cases where the clinician is unsure of the diagnosis. On-farm collection of lumbar CSF in depressed calves is a simple procedure which only requires a knowledge of the bony landmarks and an appropriate length hyopdermic needle without stylette (see p. 896). With appropriate aseptic precautions, there is little risk of spinal meningitis. Selection of a narrow gauge hypodermic needle, and removal of only 1 to 2 ml of CSF, will greatly reduce any risks associated with sudden release of CSF pressure.

Campylobacter *spp.* (see p. 852)

The related campylobacters, *Campylobacter jejuni* and *C. coli*, have been recognized recently as important enteric pathogens in humans. They are the most common cause of diarrhoea in developed countries and they are one of the three most common causes of human diarrhoea in developing countries; *E. coli* and rotavirus are the other two enteropathogens of major importance. Recognition of the importance of campylobacters followed marked improvements in culture techniques that improved isolation and identification from faeces. They have been isolated from healthy and diseased domestic animals and poultry for many years and, not unexpectedly, the most common sources of infection in human outbreaks are fresh poultry, minced meat and unpasteurized milk.

The recognition of animal products as the source of human infection has prompted a reassessment of the importance of *C. jejuni* and *C. coli* in causing enteric disease of farm animals. Since the 1930s, campylobacters have been thought of as the cause of an enteric disease of housed adult cattle in the winter–syndromes referred to as 'winter dysentery', 'winter scours', 'vibrionic enteritis'. The above association has, however, been questioned and more recently a coronavirus has been implicated as the cause of winter dysentery (see p. 852). The association of campylobacters with calf diarrhoea has been examined in experimental infections and in case-control studies of field outbreaks. The results have shown that *C. jejuni* is present on all farms and most case-control studies have failed to demonstrate an association between excretion of this organism and calf diarrhoea. In the majority of experimental studies, inoculation of calves with *C. jejuni*, even using high doses, resulted in colonization without diarrhoea. *Campylobacter jejuni* may be detected in up to 80 per cent of weaned calves, indicating that isolation of this organism from calves with diarrhoea does not constitute a diagnosis. *Campylobacter coli* is less commonly isolated from cattle and experimental inoculations and case-control studies indicate clearly that it is non-pathogenic. *Campylobacter fetus* subsp. *fetus* and *C. hyointestinalis* are also commonly isolated from cattle of all ages, but most evidence suggests that they are not a cause of intestinal disease.

Cryptosporidium parvum (see p. 286)

Cryptosporidium parvum is an enteric coccidia recognized commonly in calves and lambs and is a zoonosis.

The organisms are spherical or ovoid parasites that adhere to the microvilli of enterocytes, particularly in the ileum, but also in the large intestine. Cryptosporidia exhibit three important differences from other enteric coccidia: excreted oocysts are directly infective to new hosts, cryptosporidia are not host specific so that infection can spread between mammalian species, including man, and finally they are unaffected by most existing anticoccidial drugs (see pp. 206, 1029).

The life cycle commences with the ingestion of oocysts containing sporozoites, which become trophozoites. In the asexual phase of the life cycle the trophozoites mature to schizonts containing eight merozoites, which are liberated and infect new enterocytes to form a second generation of merozoites. In the sexual phase, macrogametes fuse with microgametes and give rise to zygotes, which form oocysts. Sporozoites form within oocysts in the intestinal lumen or whilst they are still attached to the surface of enterocytes so that oocysts excreted in the faeces are directly infective to new hosts without an obligatory period of maturation outside the host body. Consequently, infection can spread rapidly within a group of calves and the pattern of spread is similar to that seen with rotavirus and not similar to that seen in *Eimeria* spp.

Cryptosporidiosis is seen in neonatal calves, usually when they are aged one to two weeks (peak 11 days old), at about the same time as they develop rotavirus diarrhoea. Most calves appear to become infected, but not all develop diarrhoea. Subclinical infections are not thought to be the result of passive protection by colostral antibodies because experiments have shown that antibodies that are fed are not protective; subclinical infections remain unexplained. Experimental infections indicate an incubation period of two to five days and close association between occurrence of diarrhoea and excretion of oocysts. Depression and anorexia accompany the profuse watery green diarrhoea, which contains mucus and occasionally blood. Diarrhoea may be intermittent and lasts two to 14 days (usually about seven) and causes dehydration which often requires treatment with oral rehydration solutions. Morbidity is usually high and mortality low, although some outbreaks have been associated with high mortality.

Infected mucosae (Fig. 14.16) are congested and villi are stunted in the ileum. Enterocytes in the small and

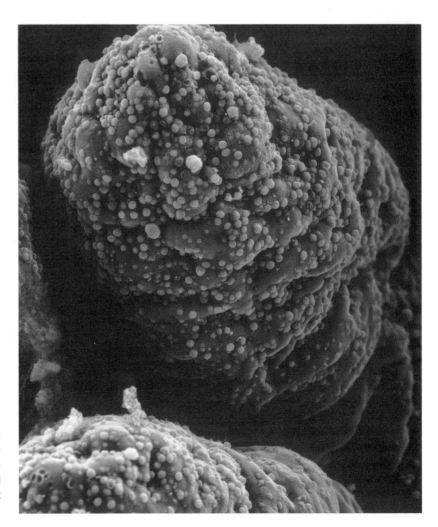

Fig. 14.16 Scanning electron micrograph of the ileal mucosa of a calf naturally infected with *Cryptospordium parvum*. The surface of the villi is heavily infected and partially exfoliated enterocytes are present at the tip of the villus.

large intestines become cuboidal or squamous and crypts may become dilated and filled with exfoliated cells and neutrophils. The lamina may become infiltrated with mononuclear inflammatory cells, neutrophils and eosinophils. Cryptosporidia appear to cause diarrhoea by destroying mature enterocytes, but by an unknown mechanism. The population of mature enterocytes is reduced in size and numbers of immature cells are increased. Mucosal lactase activity is markedly depressed and there is reduced ability to digest and absorb food. Intestinal secretion may be enhanced due to the increased numbers of secretory cells in the mucosa. The self-limiting nature of natural and experimental infections and the widespread detection of antibodies indicate that immune responses occur that are protective. No further information is available on immunity.

Cryptosporidiosis can be diagnosed by detection of oocysts in faecal smears but more reliable results are obtained from stained gut sections. However, such material is rarely available due to the low mortality. Several staining methods are available, of which the Giemsa stain, the modified acid fast method and auramine are the most widely used. Alternatively, mucosal smears of ileum may be stained with Giemsa or histological sections of ileum stained by haematoxylin and eosin. The histological method is of little value if autolysis is advanced because the enterocytes will have sloughed from the mucosal surface. The most reliable method is to make and stain smears of oocysts concentrated from faeces using flotation techniques.

Management of an outbreak presents problems; although a large number of chemotherapeutic agents have been tested for efficacy against *Cryptosporidium*, only halufiginone has been found to be effective. Most workers recommend high levels of hygiene as the best approach to control, but oocysts are extremely resistant to a variety of disinfectants, including iodophor, cresylic acid, sodium hypochlorite, benzylkonium chloride, sodium hydroxide and aldehyde-based disinfectants. Ammonia and formalin are effective disinfectants. The organism is susceptible to freezing and thawing and to temperatures over 50°C. Steam cleaning is strongly recommended.

Investigating an outbreak of calf diarrhoea

The investigation should start with a farm visit to examine the calves clinically and establish a picture of calf husbandry and of the outbreak. Enterotoxigenic *E. coli* diarrhoea can be suspected on the basis of age of affected calves. Faeces, not rectal swabs, should be collected as soon as possible after the onset of diarrhoea

and before treatment commences and should be examined for rotavirus, coronavirus, *Cryptosporidium* and *Salmonella* spp. Samples from very young calves with watery diarrhoea should be tested for K99$^+$ *E. coli*. Faeces should be collected from affected calves and age-matched healthy calves on the farm, a minimum of four calves in each category. Faecal collection should continue if the outbreak persists to monitor for changes in enteropathogens being excreted.

Where a problem persists, or no diagnosis has been reached, samples may be sent to a research laboratory for examination by electron microscopy or for the detection of EPEC, EHEC and VTEC. A post-mortem examination of a calf submitted alive to a laboratory may help to elucidate the significance of results of faecal examination and indicate the presence of other agents not detected by faecal examination. Laboratories are frequently asked to assist in the diagnosis of the aetiology of calf diarrhoea outbreaks on the basis of samples submitted from one or two calves only. Clearly this is pointless, because diagnosis of disease caused by an endemic agent is based on the detection of the agent in a higher percentage of the faeces of calves with diarrhoea than in healthy calves on the same farm. Where data are not available from healthy calves on the same farm, results from other studies may be considered. Rotavirus and cryptosporidia have rarely been found in more than 50 per cent of randomly selected healthy calves and coronavirus is usually detected in less than 25 per cent. Figures above these values may be taken as a tentative diagnosis.

Salmonellas, which may be suspected clinically, are often only detected qualitatively. Merely isolating these bacteria is relatively meaningless; quantitative bacteriological techniques should be used to demonstrate excretion of large numbers of bacteria from calves with diarrhoea. It is only worth looking for K99 adhesins where the outbreak is suggestive of ETEC, i.e. if calves under four days of age are affected and there is severe watery diarrhoea.

Epidemiology

On a farm basis, the infectious agents that have been associated with neonatal calf diarrhoea can be divided into three groups: those infections that are usually absent but may be introduced and cause an outbreak of disease (ETEC, *Salmonella* spp.); the ubiquitous agents (rotavirus, coronavirus, and cryptosporidium) that are invariably present on every farm; and those agents for which inadequate epidemiological data are available (Breda virus and VTEC). Although there is evidence to support the view that all the above infectious agents are able to cause diarrhoea in calves, it is clear that their

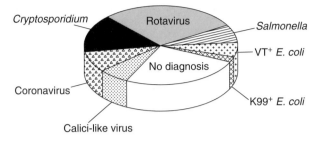

Fig. 14.17 Prevalence of pathogenic agents in calf diarrhoea.

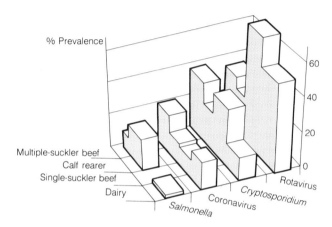

Fig. 14.18 Correlation of farm type with prevalence of pathogens in calf diarrhoea. Reproduced from Morgan (1990).

presence in the intestinal tract does not inevitably lead to disease and they are not all equally important in the aetiology of calf diarrhoea.

The prevalence of these agents in calves with diarrhoea in southern Britain, as determined from 45 outbreaks of calf diarrhoea, is shown in Fig. 14.17 (Reynolds *et al.*, 1986); another survey examined outbreaks in northern England and southern Scotland (Snodgrass *et al.*, 1986). Rotavirus was associated most frequently with calf diarrhoea and was most common on dairy farms and single-suckler beef units (Fig. 14.18). Cryptosporidia oocysts were associated with calf diarrhoea slightly less often than rotavirus and were more common in beef suckler units than in dairy farms. In southern England, salmonellas occurred in 25 per cent of outbreaks and were most often a problem for rearers of calves bought in from markets. Enteropathogens were not detected in 31 per cent of faeces of calves with diarrhoea. Rotavirus and cryptosporidia were excreted by up to 50 per cent of normal calves, and on the basis of this evidence an outbreak of rotavirus-induced or cryptosporidia-induced diarrhoea should only be diagnosed if more than 50 per cent of calves with diarrhoea are excreting either enteropathogen. Coronavirus was

detected rarely in clinically normal calves and it was invariably associated with disease, usually in outbreaks with high mortality. Results of two surveys show that diarrhoea caused by ETEC was uncommon in the UK at that time; this may still be the situation. Intermittent excretion of ETEC may occur throughout life, often unassociated with diarrhoea, making interpretation of diagnostic findings difficult and emphasizing the need for quantitative bacteriology.

These survey data have been reproduced by numerous monitoring organizations over the past 15 years which clearly indicates the important role of rotavirus and coronavirus in neonatal enteritis. Vaccination is highly effective against these viral causes of diarrhoea but the need for annual vaccination and perceived high cost have resulted in many beef calves remaining unprotected.

Mixed infections

With the recognition of enteropathogenic agents and the development of diagnostic tests, it has been possible to look at outbreaks of diarrhoea and at individual animals to assess the importance of mixed infections. Results of surveys of faeces of calves with diarrhoea indicate that although single infections may result in diarrhoea, the likelihood of diarrhoea occurring increases with the number of enteropathogens present. When 21 moribund calves with diarrhoea were examined in detail by necropsy, two or more enteropathogens were detected in 19 calves (Hall *et al.*, 1988). The most common combination of enteropathogens revealed by these studies has been rotavirus and cryptosporidia and the way in which these infections can overlap in rearing pens is illustrated in Figs 14.19 and 14.20. Studies of distribution of infection of the gut mucosa with these two agents and the severity of the lesions have shown that either agent, as a single infection, might not cause sufficient intestinal damage to cause diarrhoea, but together they could. A study of the intestinal pathology of normal calves that were excreting rotavirus showed that there were severe lesions in the anterior small intestine and mild lesions in the mid small intestine, but the lower small intestine and large intestine were normal (Reynolds *et al.*, 1985).

Cryptosporidia, however, infect and damage the lower small intestine and the large intestine, so that in a combined infection the cumulative damage would be sufficient to cause diarrhoea (Fig. 14.21). Similarly, if simultaneous infection with coronavirus and either rotavirus or calici-like virus occurred there would be cumulative damage because the former infects and damages the lower small intestine and large intestine, whilst the latter infects and damages the upper small

208 • Chapter 14

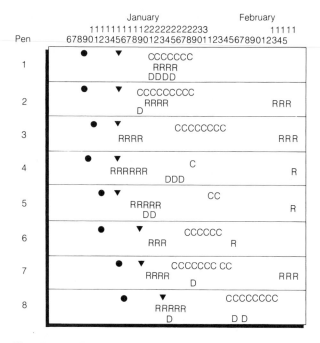

Fig. 14.19 The spread of rotavirus and *Cryptosporidium* between calves in adjacent pens. (●) Day of birth, (▼) day of move to rearing pens. C, *Cryptosporidium* excretion; R, rotavirus excretion; D, day of diarrhoea. Reproduced from Morgan (1990).

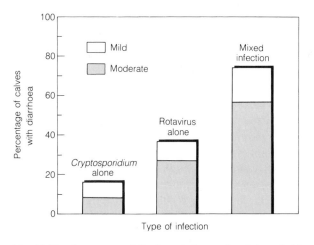

Fig. 14.20 Occurrence of diarrhoea in farm calves infected with either rotavirus or *Cryptosporidium* and in mixed infections.

intestine. The concept that mixed infections involving rotavirus, cryptosporidia, and coronavirus cause cumulative damage in the small and large intestines is based on information presently available concerning the predilection sites of these pathogens. There is, however, evidence that different strains of rotavirus and coronavirus may have different predilection sites within the small intestine and this could affect the development of cumulative damage.

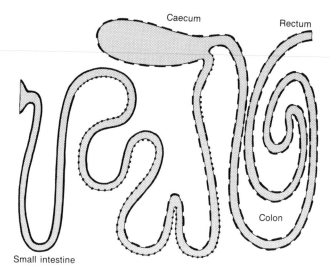

Fig. 14.21 Line drawing illustrating the small and large intestines of the calf and indication of those parts susceptible to infection by rotavirus (· · ·) and those susceptible to infection by *Cryptosporidium* spp. (---). Reproduced from Hall (1989).

Many of the recognized enteropathogens infect and damage the small intestine and coronavirus, Breda virus, EHEC and cryptosporidia also damage the large intestine. However, assuming that diarrhoea is more likely to occur when both the small and large intestines are damaged, there is a need to study the infectious agents that damage the large intestine. Diarrhoea was often associated with infections and lesions throughout the small and large intestines in a study of the pathology of 21 calves with diarrhoea in southern Britain (Hall *et al.*, 1988); coronavirus and bacteria adherent to the mucosal surface were associated with the lesions in the large intestine. The results indicate that these bacteria, some of which were EHEC, were contributing to the development of diarrhoea. Evidence from field studies also suggests that mixed infections are important in the development of diarrhoea. In a longitudinal study of calves, from birth to weaning, only 15 per cent of calves that excreted *Cryptosporidium* sp. and 37 per cent of calves that excreted rotavirus experienced diarrhoea, but in calves in which the two infections occurred together, 75 per cent developed diarrhoea (Fig. 14.20).

Rotavirus and ETEC were the infectious agents first identified as able to cause diarrhoea in calves and, as a result, combined inoculations with these agents were studied by several groups. The interaction between these two agents was studied despite the fact that ETEC cause diarrhoea in calves that are less than 48 hours old, whereas the mean age of calves with rotavirus diarrhoea is ten days. The conclusions reached from these studies were that combined infections were more severe, although it was unclear whether this was due to additive effects or synergism.

Management of diarrhoea

The first priority is to treat fluid depletion, i.e. restore extracellular fluid volume so as to counter shock and acidosis.

Rehydration (see also p. 195)

Oral fluids are very satisfactory in the less severely affected animals. They are usually isotonic with plasma and contain sufficient K^+ and HCO_3^- to replace faecal losses and Na^+ and glucose in equimolar amounts. Such preparations are formulated to utilize the pathways of absorption of glucose, amino acids and citrate, which carry water with them. These formulations have been improved by inclusion of 80 to 100 mmol/l bicarbonate as a precursor, usually citrate, which is catabolized to give bicarbonate ions which helps to counter metabolic acidosis. Energy is supplied as glucose and citrate. More recently, oral rehydration solutions have been introduced which contain up to 375 mmol/l glucose in an attempt to counteract the energy deficit when milk is removed from the calf's diet. An oral rehydration solu-tion containing glutamine, a simple amino acid and high levels of glucose has also recently been introduced with the claim that this combination will have a beneficial effect on mucosal architecture by reducing the severity of villous atrophy and promoting repair. Commercially prepared oral rehydration solutions are sophisticated formulations and should always be used.

As a rule of thumb, if the calf is weak and presents in lateral recumbency, use intravenous therapy; if it can lift its head but has no suck reflex, use intravenous therapy. If the calf can drink, offer electrolyte solution by teat and bottle as reluctance to suck may be the first indicator of septicaemia/bacterial meningoencephalitis. The calf should be fed every two to four hours and care-fully monitored; loss of an active suck reflex indicates deterioration of the calf's condition and veterinary attendance is necessary without further delay.

The efficacy of oral rehydration varies with the type of diarrhoea. In secretory diarrhoea, the sodium glucose absorption system is unaffected by bacterial enterotoxins and glucose/electrolyte solutions are very effective in rehydrating the animal. Nevertheless, the diarrhoea continues and this should be stressed to the client (Fig. 14.22). The small intestine may be so

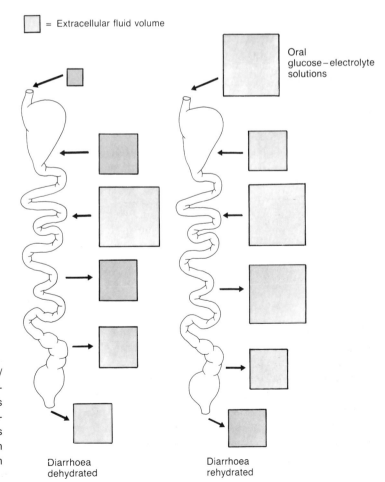

Fig. 14.22 Effect of orally administered glucose/electrolyte solution of fluid fluxes in secretory diarrhoea in the pig. Where glucose/electrolyte solution is not given, there is a net loss of water and dehydration develops. Where glucose/electrolyte solution is given, the diarrhoea continues but there is a net gain of fluid by intestinal absorption and rehydration occurs. Source: Argenzio (1984).

severely damaged in very severe viral infections that oral electrolyte solutions are ineffective. In less severe viral infections, for example many rotavirus infections of calves, sufficient functional surface may remain for oral electrolytes to be effective.

Nutrition

The energy requirements of a newborn calf are approximately 2500 kcal/day, equivalent to 600 g of glucose. The glucose content of 10 litres of an oral glucose/electrolyte solution containing 80 mmol glucose is 144 g, which does not supply sufficient energy but this can be largely overcome by feeding an oral rehydration solution containing 375 mmol/l. A rational approach is to feed electrolyte solution alone for one to two days and subsequently alternate feeds of milk and electrolyte solution. While mixing electrolyte solution and milk does not appear to interfere with clotting of milk in the abomasum, this method is to be avoided if possible. With suckled calves, separate the calf and the cow, feed electrolyte and then allow the calf to suck the cow for approximately five minutes.

Drugs (pp. 189, 229)

In severe dehydration, rehydration must be the first priority. There are two situations where the use of antibiotics is indicated: infections with *Salmonella* spp. or with pathogenic *E. coli* (ETEC, EHEC and VTEC). Broad-spectrum antibiotics and antimicrobials have been used widely as a primary form of treatment of calves with neonatal diarrhoea, without sound reason in many cases. Most therapeutic trials for treatment of diarrhoeal calves with antibiotics have been uncontrolled or used small numbers of animals and have not, therefore, been convincing.

The disadvantages of using antibiotics are that some directly damage the intestinal mucosa, delaying repair, and may contribute to the development of diarrhoea. Antibiotics add significantly to production costs, they may contribute to the problem of resistance factors in the enterobacteria, they may result in residues in meat and antibiotic use may result in the carrier state in *Salmonella* infections.

Environment

The impact of environment on the pathogenesis of calf diarrhoea may be discussed under the following headings: microbial environment, immunological environment, nutritional environment and physical environment.

Microbial environment

The enteropathogens that have been discussed are all excreted in faeces in very large numbers by clinically sick calves. It is clear, therefore, that once an outbreak is established the major source of infection is faecal contamination of the environment by clinically affected calves. Other animal sources or reservoirs of infection have been described; rotavirus and coronavirus are excreted by calves and cows with subclinical infections and similar situations could be expected for the other enteropathogens, which have been investigated less well. Studies of dairy systems (Greene, 1983; McNulty & Logan, 1983) have shown the value of cleansing, disinfection and use of the 'all-in all-out' system in the control of diagnosed and undiagnosed calf diarrhoea. Calving accommodation and calf pens should be designed for ease of cleaning, steaming and disinfection and with adequate drainage. Pens should be well ventilated, but draught free. Pens and utensils should be kept clean, and pens kept dry with adequate straw.

The same principles apply in beef systems (Radostits & Acres, 1980). Firstly, it is important to remove the source of infection from the calves' environment, or minimize it. Measures that can be adopted include the following.

- Avoid confining the herd, especially at calving. Avoid using calving paddocks in which mud and faeces soon predominate and where animal density is high.
- Regularly change the pastures that the herd grazes.
- Do not calve cows and heifers on the pasture on which they have been held during winter; move them to clean areas just before calving.
- Do not calve on the same area year after year. Avoid calving in barns and sheds where infection builds up rapidly, and ventilation and sunlight are restricted, encouraging survival of infection.
- Choose a calving ground that is sheltered and well drained. Avoid creating local areas within calving grounds where animals congregate and infection builds up, i.e. restricted feeding or watering areas.
- Calving areas should be cleaned up and left vacant during summer.
- Isolate calves, as far as is possible, from the contaminated environment by removing calves from areas contaminated by diarrhoeic calves. Reduce crowding of calves by dividing the calving herd into small subgroups and dispersing newborn calves with their mothers soon after birth.

Immunological environment

Neonatal calves are more resistant to enteric infections when suckled than when fed artificial feeds, regardless of whether or not there is absorption of colostral immunoglobulins. This suggests that components of colostrum and milk that are not absorbed have an intestinal role in protecting the neonate. The other quite distinct protective function provided by the immune components of mammary secretions is their absorption to provide passive circulating antibody, which prevents invasion of micro-organisms.

Specific protective systems in colostrum and milk
(see p. 1002)

Immunoglobulins are concentrated from the cow's serum into colostrum from five weeks prepartum. The classes of immunoglobulins that are present in colostrum and milk are IgA, IgG_1, IgG_2 and IgM. IgA and IgG_2 each comprises 5 per cent of colostral immunoglobulins and IgM comprises approximately 7 per cent. The majority of colostral immunoglobulins (80 to 90 per cent) are IgG_1 and the concentration of IgG_1 in colostrum is three to twelve times that of maternal serum, because of selective secretion by the acinar epithelial cells of the mammary gland.

Colostral proteins are absorbed very rapidly and efficiently by the small intestine of the newborn calf. The small intestinal villi are covered by highly vacuolated enterocytes, which are specialized in the uptake of macromolecules by pinocytosis. The ability to absorb macromolecules may persist for up to 24 hours after birth and its disappearance is known as 'closure of the gut'. Although the gut may remain 'open' for up to 24 hours, closure occurs rapidly after ingestion of the first feed. If the first feed is colostrum, all is well, but if the first feed is milk, the gut will 'close' and colostrum fed subsequently will not be absorbed. Thus, IgG_1 is absorbed into the blood of the calf in large amounts during the first 24 hours of life. All macromolecules presented are absorbed but IgG_1 is predominant and therefore it is absorbed in greatest amounts. IgA in milk provides a passive intestinal humoral immunity in other species. In ruminants the predominance of IgG_1 in milk suggests that it has a similar function. Determination of passive antibody transfer can be easily achieved by measuring total plasma protein concentration using a refractometer where values greater than 65g/l are considered optimum and concentration below 50g/l inadequate.

The immune components of mammary secretions have two functions. Firstly, colostral antibodies absorbed into the circulation of the neonate provide passive circulating antibody, which prevents invasion of micro-organisms (e.g. septicaemic *E. coli*). Secondly, colostral antibodies that are not absorbed due to gut closure, and milk antibodies, act within the gut lumen, providing passive local immunity. Milk antibody has

been shown to protect calves from ETEC, probably by anti-adhesive activity. Absorbed colostral antibody may also influence enteric infections because IgA is absorbed along with IgG_1 and some is resecreted onto mucosal surfaces.

Studies of the concentration of immunoglobulins in the blood of diseased calves showed that calves with the lowest levels of immunoglobulin had highest mortality; colisepticaemia was the major killer, either rapidly or via abscesses in the umbilicus, liver and joints. Calves with low levels of immunoglobulins may also show a greater incidence of diarrhoea.

Colostral antibodies, if they are to be absorbed effectively or if they are to have a protective function in the gut lumen, must resist rapid degradation. The mechanisms that protect colostrum from degradation in the gastrointestinal tract are the low activity of pancreatic protease in the neonatal calf, the presence of a trypsin inhibitor in colostrum, the high buffering capacity of colostrum, the reduced secretion of acid in the abomasum in the first three days of life and the resistance of IgG_1 to proteolysis by chymotrypsin. The enterocytes of the newborn calf are specialized for non-selective macromolecule absorption by pinocytosis and vesicle transport. This process results in rapid and effective uptake of antibodies (IgG_1) because these are the major macromolecules in colostrum.

There are, in addition to protective immunoglobulins, non-specific protective systems in colostrum and milk (Reiter, 1978; see also Chapter 58). Lactoferrin, an iron-binding protein present in colostrum and milk, inhibits bacterial growth, possibly by reducing availability of iron to bacteria. There are appreciable amounts in bovine colostrum but little in bovine milk. Citrate, also present in colostrum, competes for iron, making it available for bacteria. Therefore, normal colostrum is not bacteriostatic for *E. coli*, but once the citrate is removed colostrum is bacteriostatic. Conditions in the calf small intestine apparently favour the action of lactoferrin because citrate is rapidly absorbed from the calf small intestine and bicarbonate, which assists binding of iron and lactoferrin, is secreted into the small intestine. The antibacterial action of lactoferrin is enhanced by specific antibodies in colostrum. The lactoperoxidase/thiocyanate/hydrogen peroxidase system is inhibitory or lethal to bacteria via the production of an oxidation product. Lactoperoxidase is synthesized by the mammary gland, thiocyanate ions are present in milk and are secreted into the calf stomach and cow's milk contains glucose and glucose oxidase, which provide hydrogen peroxide; hydrogen peroxide is also produced by lactobacilli, which are the predominant bacteria in the flora of the stomach and small intestines of newborn calves. Thus, all the components of this protective system are present in the calf *in vivo*.

The absorption of colostral immunoglobulins is influenced by several factors and 20 to 50 per cent of calves attain inadequate serum IgG levels. The time of the first colostrum meal is an important determinant of serum immunoglobulin concentration; late feeding leads to lower levels. Also, first-milk colostrum has the highest concentration of immunoglobulins, therefore preparturient leaking or milking leads to poorer quality postparturient colostrum. Colostrum is secreted prepartum and once removed is not replaced. The amount of immunoglobulin absorbed varies with its concentration in the colostrum and this is more important than the quantity of colostrum consumed.

Maternal nutrition may affect colostrum production. Poor nutrition does not, apparently, influence the concentration of immunoglobulin in colostrum but decreases the amount of colostrum produced, therefore sucking calves achieve lower levels of serum immunoglobulin; heifers produce less colostrum than cows. A second feed of colostrum increases the absorption of immunoglobulin from the first feed, presumably because the second feed displaces colostrum from the upper gastrointestinal tract into the jejunum.

The presence of the dam improves the efficiency of absorption of immunoglobulins by the calf by up to 80 per cent. Lower serum levels are obtained if the calf and dam are separated at birth and colostrum is fed by bucket. The dam licks and cleans the newborn calf in the order: thorax, back, abdomen, head, neck and perineum. The placenta is then eaten. Suckling does not occur unless the licking process occurs. An easy parturition leads to early licking. Beef cows mother better than dairy cows; they lick longer and stand better to be sucked. The speed at which calves stand is important because they then start to seek the teats. If cows have calved standing then sucking is likely to start earlier. Field-born calves have higher levels of serum immunoglobulins than box-born calves. The cow is likely to be the primary object of teat-seeking attention but in a box the walls may confuse the calf. Low pendulous udders delay successful sucking.

Farmers should be encouraged to ensure that all calves receive a minimum of 2 litres of colostrum soon after birth, certainly within 4 to 6 hours. Practical recommendations to enhance colostrum uptake include the following:

- Do not separate dam and calf until 24 hours postpartum.
- Provide bedding to allow the calf to stand easily.
- Encourage early feeding, which is very beneficial. The calf may need assistance to ensure this.
- Keep a supply of frozen colostrum for use after prepartum leakage.

- Encourage outdoor calving in warm weather; it is more likely to lead to higher levels of serum immunoglobulins.

Methods of measuring the concentration of immunoglobulins in calf serum include the following:

- Single radial immunodiffusion: convenient, accurate and capable of measuring IgG_1, IgG_2 and IgA.
- Zinc sulphate turbidity test: depends on the selective precipitation of immunoglobulin by zinc sulphate; there is good correlation between zinc sulphate turbidity and total immunoglobulin content of serum.
- Sodium sulphite precipitation method.
- Refractometry: measures total protein.

The immunoglobulin content of colostrum can be assessed simply and accurately with a hydrometer (Fleenor & Stott, 1980) and one designed specifically for the purpose is available in the UK.

Nutritional environment

Skim milk powders, which have been severely heat treated, and some non-milk proteins (e.g. soya) do not coagulate well in the abomasum. This may result in gastric stasis and reduced secretion of gastric acid and enzymes, which causes increased escape of undigested protein into the duodenum and reduced secretion of pancreatic enzymes. These events result in diarrhoea. Soya initiates immune-mediated intestinal damage in some calves and heated soya may contain substances that are directly damaging to the intestinal mucosa. Some feeding methods may upset the balance between the calf and the infectious agents to which it is exposed, thus precipitating diarrhoea. These include feeding cold milk, bucket feeding, high-fat diets and skim milk. Alternatively, feeding methods that are said to alleviate diarrhoea include use of acidified milk and fermented colostrum, even though it is less well absorbed than fresh colostrum.

Physical environment

Hypogammaglobinaemia is more common in single-suckled beef herds where the stocking density is high, presumably due to poor mothering and supervision. Calf mortality is less if the person who looks after the calves is the farmer, or a member of his or her family.

Single penning helps reduce the spread of infection, as do solid walls between pens. Aspects of the physical environment that contribute to the development of diarrhoea by stressing calves are inclement weather, particularly snow and rain, cold wet bedding and overcrowding.

Necrotic enteritis (See p. 238)

Necrotic or necrotizing enteritis is the term used to describe a distinct clinicopathological syndrome characterized by severe diarrhoea, pyrexia and neutropaenia in two to three month-old beef calves (Penny *et al.*, 1994). The disease has been reported to occur in the same beef herd for four consecutive years, affecting approximately 5 per cent of calves when seven to 12 weeks-old (Penny *et al.*, 1994). Despite intensive supportive and antibiotic therapy approximately 25 per cent of affected calves died after five to 10 days of illness. The clinical presentation of necrotic enteritis is not dissimilar to coccidiosis but the morbidity is much lower and the findings more severe in nature.

Affected calves are dull and depressed and do not suck. These calves are moderately (5 to 7 per cent) to severely (8 to 10 per cent) dehydrated, and pyrexic (39.5 to 42.0°C) with pale mucous and oral membranes. Sudden onset profuse dark green diarrhoea containing fresh blood is a consistent feature. Tenesmus is also a common feature and becomes more prominent during the latter stages of the disease and may cause temporary rectal prolapse. There is rapid loss of body condition and affected calves have a gaunt appearance with a tucked-up abdomen. This syndrome has many clinical features of mucosal disease but oral erosions and ulceration are observed in less than 50 per cent of calves, and there are no interdigital lesions.

Muco-purulent ocular and nasal discharges, commonly seen in mucosal disease, are not observed in necrotic enteritis. The age-specific occurrence of necrotic enteritis differs from mucosal disease which more commonly affects yearling cattle although BVD/MD persistently affected cattle may die of intercurrent disease, especially bacterial pneumonia, from two months old. BVD antigen has not been detected in blood samples from affected calves nor from fresh tissue samples. No recognized enteropathogen has been isolated from faecal examinations. There is mild to severe anaemia and profound leucopaenia caused predominantly by a severe non-regenerative neutropaenia.

The administration of oral and/or systemic antibiotics has no effect on the outcome of necrotic enteritis. Supportive therapy comprising oral and intravenous fluids, and flunixin meglumine, may effect a temporary improvement but does not alter the prognosis.

Erosion or ulceration of the hard palate is common but no oesophageal ulceration has been recorded. Consistent findings are necrotizing lesions in the abomasum and small and large intestine, particularly involving the terminal ileum and colon. Abomasal lesions range from discrete 1 to 3 cm diameter oval ulcers to large confluent areas of ulceration and necrosis in the pyloric region. Haemorrhagic or necrotic lesions overlying gut-associated lymphoid tissue (Peyer's patches) are common.

References

Argenzio, R.A. (1984) Pathophysiology of neonatal diarrhoea. *Agri-Practice*, **9**, 25–32.

Brooks, H.W., White, D.G., Wagstaff, A.J. & Michell, A.R. (1997) Evaluation of a glutamine-containing oral rehydration solution for the treatment of calf diarrhoea using an *Escherichia coli* model. *The Veterinary Journal*, **153**, 163–70.

Dupe, R., Bywater, R.J. & Goddard, M. (1993) A hypertonic infusion in the treatment of experimental shock in calves and clinical shock in dogs and cats. *Veterinary Record*, **133**, 585–90.

Fleenor, W.A. & Stott, G.H. (1980) Hydrometer test for estimation of immunoglobulin concentration in bovine colostrum. *Journal of Dairy Science*, **63**, 973–7.

Greene, H.J. (1983) Minimise calf diarrhoea by good husbandry: treat sick calves by fluid therapy. *Annales de Recherches Vétérinaires*, **14**, 548–55.

Grove-White, D. (2000) Intravenous fluid therapy in the diarrhoeic calf. *UK Vet*, **5**, 56–61.

Hall, G.A. (1989) Mechanisms of mucosal injury: animal study. In: *Viruses and the Gut, Proceedings of the Ninth BSG: SK&F International Workshop*, 27–29.

Hall, G.A., Reynolds, D.J., Parsons, K.R., Bland, A.P. & Morgan, J.H. (1988) Pathology of calves with diarrhoea in southern Britain. *Research in Veterinary Science*, **45**, 240–50.

Kasari, T.R. & Naylor, J.M. (1986) Clinical evaluation of sodium bicarbonate, sodium lactate and sodium acetate for the treatment of acidosis in diarrhoeic calves. *Journal of the American Veterinary Medical Association*, **187**, 392–7.

Lewis, L.D. & Philips, R.W. (1978) Pathophysiologic changes due to coronavirus-induced diarrhoea in the calf. *Journal of the American Veterinary Medical Association*, **173**, 636–42.

McNulty, M.S. & Logan, E.F. (1983) Longitudinal survey of rotavirus infection in calves. *Veterinary Record*, **113**, 333–5.

Mebus, C.A., Stair, E.L., Underdahl, N.R. & Twiehaus, M.J. (1971) Pathology of neonatal calf diarrhoea induced by a reo-like virus. *Veterinary Pathology*, **8**, 490–505.

Morgan, J.H. (1990) Epidemiology, diagnosis and control of undifferentiated calf diarrhoea. *In Practice*, **12**, 17–20.

Naylor, J.M. (1996) Neonatal ruminant diarrhoea. In *Large Animal Internal Medicine* (ed. by B.P. Smith), 2nd edn. Mosby, St Louis, p. 404.

Penny, C.D., Scott, P.R., Watt, N.J. & Greig, A. (1994) Necrotic enteritis of unknown aetiology in young beef calves at pasture. *Veterinary Record*, **134**, 296–9.

Radostits, O.M. & Acres, S.D. (1980) The prevention of epidemics of acute undifferentiated diarrhoea of beef calves in western Canada. *Canadian Veterinary Journal*, **21**, 243–9.

Reiter, B. (1978) Review of the progress of dairy science: antimicrobial systems in milk. *Journal of Dairy Research*, **45**, 131–47.

Reynolds, D.J., Hall, G.A., Debney, T.G. & Parsons, K.R. (1985) Pathology of natural rotavirus infection in clinically normal calves. *Research in Veterinary Science*, **38**, 264–9.

Reynolds, D.J., Morgan, J.H., Chanter, N., Jones, P.W., Bridget, J.C., Debney, T.G. & Bunch, K.J. (1986) Microbiology of calf diarrhoea in southern Britain. *Veterinary Record*, **119**, 34–9.

Scott, P.R. & Penny, C.D. (1993) A field study of meningo-encephalitis in calves with particular reference to cerebrospinal fluid analysis. *Veterinary Record*, **133**, 119–21.

Snodgrass, D.R., Terzdo, H.R., Sherwood, D., Campbell, L, Menzies, J.D. & Synge, B. (1986) Aetiology of diarrhoea in young calves. *Veterinary Record*, **119**, 31–4.

Further reading

Acres, S.D. (1985) Enterotoxigenic. *Escherichia coli* infections in newborn calves: a review. *Journal of Dairy Science*, **68**, 229–56.

Angus, K. (1987) Update: Cryptosporidiosis in domestic animals and humans. *In Practice*, **9**, 47–9.

Grimshaw, W.T.R. (1987) Efficacy of sublactam-ampicillin in the treatment of neonatal calf diarrhoea. *Veterinary Record*, **121**, 162–6.

Michell, A.R., Bywater, R.J., Clarke, K.W., Hall, L.W. & Waterman, A.E. (eds) (1989) *Veterinary Fluid Therapy*. Blackwell Scientific Publications, Oxford.

Moerman, A., de Leeuw, P.W., van Zijderveld, F.G., Baanvinger, T. & Tiessink, J.W.A. (1982) Prevalence and significance of viral enteritis in Dutch dairy cattle. In *Proceedings XIIth World Congress on Diseases of Cattle, Amsterdam*. Vol. 1. pp. 228–36.

Pearson, G.R. & Logan, E.F. (1986) Pathological and immunological aspects of neonatal enteritis of calves. *Veterinary Annual*, **26**, 68–75.

Roy, J.H.B. (1990) The Calf. In *The Management of Health*, Vol. 1, 5th edn. Butterworths, London.

Saif, L.J. & Smith, K.L. (1985) Enteric viral infections of calves and passive immunity. *Journal of Dairy Science*, **68**, 206–8.

Snodgrass, D. (1986) Prevention of calf diarrhoea by vaccination. *In Practice*, **8**, 239–40.

Chapter 15
Salmonellosis

P.W. Jones, P.R. Watson and T.S. Wallis

Introduction	215
Classification	216
Resistance to antibiotics	217
Epidemiology of salmonellosis in cattle	218
The carrier state	219
Pathogenesis	220
Initiation of infection	220
Interaction with the intestines	221
Systemic spread and persistence	224
Signs of disease	225
Adults	225
Calves	226
Diagnosis of salmonellosis	226
Control measures and vaccination	227
Vaccination	228
Antibiotic therapy	229
Summary	230

Introduction

Salmonellosis is a collective description of a group of diseases caused by bacteria of the genus *Salmonella* with signs that vary from severe enteric fever to mild food poisoning. One of the characteristics of *Salmonella* is that different serotypes vary in the range of animals that they can infect and cause disease. For example, *S. typhimurium* and *S. enteritidis* have a very broad host range and infections with these serotypes have been associated with virtually all warm-blooded animals. In contrast, other serotypes have a more limited host range and this has been interchangeably referred to as host specificity, restriction or adaptation. The highly host-specific serotypes infect only phylogenetically closely-related host species; for example *S. typhi* infects only human beings, *S. abortusovis* infects only sheep and goats and *S. gallinarum* infects only poultry. Other serotypes are predominately associated with disease in one species but may also infect a limited number of other host species. For example, *S. dublin* is usually associated with cattle, but natural infection by this serotype may occur in other animals, including human beings and sheep.

Salmonellosis as a disease of human beings, cattle, sheep, pigs and poultry is manifested clinically by one of three major syndromes: a peracute systemic infection, an acute enteritis or a chronic enteritis. In humans, this ranges from the generalized typhoid infection, through the less severe paratyphoid infections to a mild gastroenteritis. The majority of serotypes produce a mild to severe gastroenteritis that only rarely becomes generalized and severe infections are most often encountered in very young, old or immunologically-compromised patients. It is generally accepted that *Salmonella* gastroenteritis is a zoonotic disease, mainly contracted by consuming large numbers of salmonellas in food of animal origin or foods contaminated with animal products in which the salmonellas have proliferated. There is, however, convincing evidence not only that infection can be a sequel to the consumption of small doses but that direct person-to-person contact is involved in many outbreaks.

The disease in cattle differs from the disease in humans, where the majority of cases in the developed world represent self-limiting intestinal infections, but which occasionally have a high mortality even when treated.

Until recently salmonellosis in animals in the UK was characterized by the large proportion of infections caused by the 'host-specific' and 'host-restricted' serotypes: *S. choleraesuis* in pigs, *S. abortusovis* in sheep, *S. pullorum* and *S. gallinarum* in poultry, and *S. dublin* in cattle. Recently, apart from the latter, these serotypes have virtually disappeared in the UK although they remain important in other parts of the world. Salmonellas may be carried by animals in the absence of clinical signs and this is probably the normal situation in pigs and poultry, although *S. enteritidis* (phagetype 4) became associated with clinical disease in the latter.

The cycle of infection between man and farm animals is often called the '*Salmonella* cycle', which is shown in Fig. 15.1. Some of the links in the cycle are tentative and the main source of infection for humans is animal products and the principal sources of infection for domestic animals are other animals of the same species and contaminated feed.

Whilst it is accepted that infections in the human population are usually associated with the consumption of animal products such as eggs, meats and milk, it is

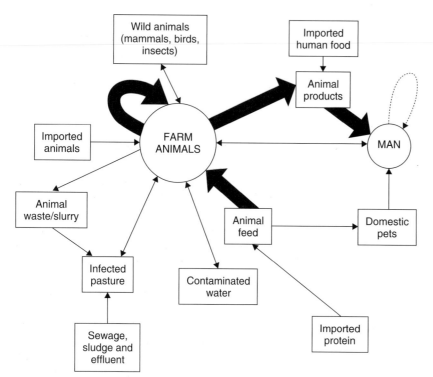

Fig. 15.1 The 'Salmonella cycle'.

not always realized that it is possible for the farm animal population to become infected by direct contact with man or the waste products of man such as sewage and sewage-polluted waters. It is further complicated by the possibility of the spread of disease by wild animals such as rodents, birds and insects and by the recycling of animal products and wastes from one animal species to another. Thus an understanding of salmonellosis and the eventual solution of the current disease problems may only arise from an interrelated study of the disease in all groups of animals and of the manner in which the bacteria responsible contaminate the environment and pass from one animal to another.

Classification

Strains of the genus *Salmonella* obey the definition of the family *Enterobacteriaceae*: they are straight rods, usually motile with peritrichous flagella (*S. pullorum/gallinarum* which cause disease in poultry are the non-motile exceptions), facultatively anaerobic, ferment glucose usually with the production of gas (*S. typhi* and some strains of *S. dublin* are the exceptions) and reduce nitrate to nitrite. Most are prototrophic (grow in artificial media with glucose as the sole source of carbon and energy and ammonium ions as a nitrogen source). Most host-specific and host-restricted

strains are auxotrophic, e.g. *S. typhi* requires tryptophan for growth, *S. dublin* requires nicotinic acid and *S. choleraesuis* requires cysteine.

The genus is subdivided into serotypes (or serovars), which in some classifications are grouped into subgenera on the basis of their biochemical reactions. Subgenus I contains the 'typical' salmonellas isolated mainly from warm-blooded animals, and these are the bacteria which normally cause disease in cattle. The serotypes (or serovars) within a subgenus cannot, with rare exceptions, be distinguished biochemically and differentiation is on the basis of the possession of somatic (O) antigens and diphasic flagellar (H) antigens in the Kauffmann–White scheme. The antigenic formula consists of three parts delimiting the O antigens and the H antigens which may occur in two phases. O antigens have arabic numbers and H antigens have letters in phase 1 and letters and numerals in phase 2, since the same antigens may occasionally occur as phase 1 or phase 2 in different serotypes. Thus the common cattle pathogen *S. dublin* has the antigenic formula 1,9,12:gp:-; this denotes that it is distinguished by the presence of O antigens 1, 9 and 12 and H antigens g and p. It does not have a second phase. The other common cattle pathogen *S. typhimurium*, which is diphasic, has the formula 1,4,5,12:i:1,2. When initiated the scheme comprised 44 serotypes and varieties organized in five O groups (A–E), but it has since expanded to include

Table 15.1 The antigenic formulae (Kauffmann–White scheme) of *Salmonella* serotypes commonly isolated from cattle in the UK.

Serotype	Antigens		
	Somatic	Flagella	
		Phase 1	Phase 2
S. saintpaul	1,4,[5],12	e,h	1,2
S. derby	1,4,[5],12	f,g	–
S. agona	1,4,12	f,g,s	–
S. typhimurium	1,4,[5],12	i	1,2
S. agama	4,12	i	1,6
S. bredeny	1,4,12,27	l,v	1,7
S. heidelberg	1,4,[5],12	r	1,2
S. indiana	1,4,12	z	1,7
S. stanleyville	1,4,[5],12,27	z_4,z_{23}	[1,2]
S. montevideo	6,7,14	g,m,[p],s	[1,2,7]
S. virchow	6,7	r	1,2
S. infantis	6,7,14	r	1,5
S. mbandaka	6,7,14	z_{10}	e,n,z_{15}
S. newport	6,8	e,h	1,2
S. enteritidis	1,9,12	g,m	[1,7]
S. dublin	1,9,12,[Vi]	g,p	–
S. panama	1,9,12	l,v	1,5
S. anatum	3,10	e,h	1,6
S. give	3,10	l,v	1,7
S. havana	1,13,23	f,g,[s]	–

–, flagella antigens occur in first phase only.
[], not always present.
1,14,27, phage-determined, not always present.

over 2400 serotypes organized in 48 O groups. The antigenic formulae of serotypes commonly involved in disease in cattle are shown in Table 15.1.

The names given to the serotypes do not follow the usual rules of nomenclature. The first serotypes to be identified, such as *S. typhi*, *S. choleraesuis*, *S. abortusovis* and *S. typhimurium*, were given names that indicated the disease with which they were associated or their common animal host, and these names, which have become accepted by clinical microbiologists, continue in common use. Serotypes isolated subsequently are named after the town or region in which they were first isolated, such as *S. dublin*, *S. liverpool*, *S. crossness* and *S. bareilly*, or are designated solely by their antigenic formulae. As an aid to epidemiological studies many of the commonest serotypes have been further subdivided into phagetypes, biotypes, plasmid types, etc.

In alternative classifications which are increasingly being used *Salmonella* is considered as one or two species (with subspecies *S. enterica* subsp. *enterica*, *S. enterica* subsp. *salamae*, *S. enterica* subsp. *arizonae*, *S. enterica* subsp. *diarizonae*, *S. enterica* subsp. *houtenae*

and *S. enterica* subsp. *indica*). The names of serotypes are not considered as species names and are not printed in italics. The species name is usually *S. enterica* and the serotypes are written, for example, as *S. enterica* (sometimes subsp. *enterica*) serovar typhimurium or *S. enterica* serovar dublin.

Resistance to antibiotics (see p. 1038)

A feature of salmonellosis in cattle during the last four decades has been the development of strains resistant to one or more antibiotics. This has occurred most commonly in a relatively small number of phagetypes of *S. typhimurium* and has been the subject of considerable debate on the use of antibiotics prophylactically, therapeutically and as growth promoters in calves. It is, however, generally accepted that resistance is developing under the selective pressure of the indiscriminate use of antibiotics. This is thought to be particularly true both of the use of mixtures of antimicrobials for therapy without diagnosis and antimicrobials mixed into animal feeds. The problem was first recognized in the 1960s when the number of antibiotic-resistant strains isolated from cattle rose from less than 3% at the beginning of the decade to more than 60% by 1965 and most of the isolates belonged to one phagetype (DT29). This phagetype disappeared at the end of the decade and the proportion of antibiotic-resistant isolates declined, but by the end of the next decade the proportion had again risen to approximately 60%. This was due to the emergence of two closely related types (DT193 and DT204) and was associated with the development of chloramphenicol resistance. Although these two phagetypes also subsequently declined, they were replaced during the 1980s by the closely related phagetype DT204c. This phagetype became endemic, particularly amongst market-purchased calves and in the calf-rearing trade. It subsequently declined and was replaced by phagetype DT104. This multiply-resistant phagetype also became established in sheep and pigs.

Strains of *S. dublin* isolated in the UK, unlike *S. typhimurium*, have remained comparatively sensitive to antibiotics. In contrast, strains isolated in Holland, Belgium, Germany and the USA are usually resistant to a number of antibiotics. The reason for the difference between British isolates and those from North America and Europe has not been explained satisfactorily but is usually attributed to the selection pressure of antibiotics in animal feed. Presumably the same pressure is exerted in the UK as elsewhere and is equally applied on *S. dublin* as on *S. typhimurium*. Multiply-antibiotic-resistant strains of *S. dublin* resistant to chloramphenicol began to be reported in the UK from 1979 and the chloramphenicol resistance was transmissible, although located on R plasmids distinct from those carrying the same resistance genes in *S. typhimurium*.

Epidemiology of salmonellosis in cattle

In cattle the disease, which has been recognized for two centuries, has a world-wide distribution and has been associated primarily with *S. dublin* and *S. typhimurium*. Other serotypes infect cattle more sporadically and these 'exotic' serotypes have become more common in the UK during the past 50 years, although during the last 20 years approximately 100 serotypes other than *S. dublin* and *S. typhimurium* have accounted for only about 10 per cent of incidents. The number of outbreaks caused by the 'exotic' serotypes has declined in the last few years. There was a dramatic rise in the incidence of salmonellosis in cattle between 1960 and 1969 due to an increase in isolations of *S. dublin*. This was followed by an equally dramatic decline in both *S. dublin* and total incidents and a slight rise in *S. typhimurium*. Over the last 20 years the incidence has remained about the same and at present *S. dublin* and *S. typhimurium* are isolated at about the same frequency, with the former being more common in adults and the latter more common in calves.

Recent estimates would suggest that approximately 20 per cent of UK cattle herds may be infected with salmonellas at any one time, although obvious disease is a much rarer event. Serological surveys have suggested a history of infection in up to 75 per cent of UK dairy herds. In the UK approximately 400 to 500 incidents (outbreaks in a single herd) of salmonellosis in cattle are reported annually. This is almost certainly an underestimate since disease outbreaks often are not reported and carriage in the absence of disease is common.

The distribution of salmonellas in cattle in other parts of the world is similar to the UK. *S. dublin* is endemic in northern Europe and western North America and *S. dublin* and *S. typhimurium* tend to be present in most advanced dairying areas and intensive cattle rearing regions. In the rest of the world occurrence is more sporadic and serotypes other than *S. dublin* and *S. typhimurium* are commonly involved.

A feature of *Salmonella* infections in all species, however, is a continual fluctuation in the proportions of the serotypes involved. It is common for a serotype to be introduced to the country and to establish in one or more species, possibly as the predominant serotype, and then to decline without any apparent reason or without the intervention of public health or veterinary authorities. The predominance of *S. hadar* in poultry and the human population in the 1970s to 1980s is a good example and it may possibly be predicted that the

epidemic of *S. enteritidis* phagetype 4, which replaced *S. typhimurium* as the predominant serotype in poultry and the human population in the 1980s and 1990s, will follow the same course. It is always possible, therefore, for the relative importance of *S. typhimurium* and *S. dublin* to change and the relative importance of these two serotypes in cattle should not be judged on the basis of isolations over only a few years.

Salmonellosis occurs in calves in all months of the year but there is a peak of disease associated with all serotypes between October and December, with a low incidence in June and July. This is associated with calving patterns rather than a true seasonal increase and reflects the distribution of calvings in dairy herds and may change. Similarly, since the source of calves sold through markets to fattening units is bull calves from dairy herds and surplus cross-bred heifer calves from dairy and beef units, there is also a seasonal incidence in fattening units since most outbreaks in calves occur within a few weeks of purchase from markets.

The importance of salmonellosis as a disease of calves was demonstrated by a survey carried out by researchers at the Institute for Animal Health, Compton, and is described in detail later in this chapter (p. 219). In this survey samples of faeces from diarrhoeic calves on 45 farms in the south of England were examined for the presence of a variety of putative enteropathogens including salmonellas, rotavirus, calici-like viruses, coronavirus, *E. coli*, cryptosporidia and campylobacters. Salmonellas were isolated from 12 per cent of diarrhoeic calves in 24 per cent of diarrhoea outbreaks. In 37 of the outbreaks, samples were taken from normal calves of similar age to the calves with diarrhoea and a comparison between isolation rates from healthy and diarrhoeic calves was prepared. Salmonellas were isolated from 12 per cent of diarrhoeic calves compared with only 3 per cent of normal calves, thus showing a clear association of the organism with disease. Salmonellas were associated with an outbreak of severe dysentery on six farms while single cases of typical salmonellosis occurred in three outbreaks, and salmonellas were detected with other agents as part of a diarrhoea problem in two outbreaks where dysentery and pyrexia were not recorded. This highlighted the problem of arriving at a diagnosis in an outbreak of enteritis when several organisms may be involved as part of a disease syndrome. Since salmonellas may be carried by apparently healthy animals, isolation of the organism, unless it is present in large numbers ($>10^5$ per gramme of faeces), is not proof of the cause of disease. There was a correlation between the type of farm and the isolation of salmonellas from diarrhoeic calves. Diarrhoea was more likely to be associated with salmonellas in units (calf-rearer, multiple-suckler) where large numbers of calves were purchased from markets, although a large number of isolations were also made from calves on dairy farms.

The source of most outbreaks is probably animal-to-animal contact, although there are distinct differences in the epidemiology of the disease in adults and calves, and between serotypes. The main sources of infection for cattle herds are probably bought-in cattle, contaminated feed, contaminated animal wastes spread on pasture, human sewage sludge spread on pasture, contaminated water courses, birds, particularly gulls, rodents, insects and human contact. Infected cattle may excrete up to 10^8 salmonella/g of faeces and contamination of the environment in the proximity of other cattle by excreting animals will obviously be a potent source of infection. In an outbreak of *S. saintpaul* infection in two large dairy herds, infection rapidly spread from cows to their calves, presumably by contact with the contaminated environment of calving barns, and all calves that eventually became infected were excreting salmonellas within 72 hours of birth. Dairy calves may thus become infected by contact with their dam, other calves or the contaminated environment. The collection of calves for intensive rearing, which involves transport to markets and dealers' premises, produces an ideal environment for dissemination. When salmonellosis gains a foothold in calves subjected to this treatment it spreads so rapidly that entire herds in rearing premises may become infected.

There have been several reports that demonstrate the importance of salmonellas in market-purchased calves and in rearing units. One of these was a survey of almost 600 market-purchased calves supplied to 11 rearing units. Frequent swabbing of the calves indicated that less than 1 per cent were infected when they arrived at the rearing units but within the next six weeks over half the calves became infected. The calf units examined in this survey were cleaned and disinfected between batches of calves and yet salmonellas could still be isolated from the environment after cleaning in over half of the units. In a similar study of a calf unit in Berkshire, UK, which bought calves from local markets, 250 calves were examined over a two-year period and 51 were shown to be infected with one of four different phagetypes of *S. typhimurium*. Phagetype DT204c, which was multiply-antibiotic-resistant, was isolated at the beginning of the survey. This was eventually removed by destocking and a rigid hygiene programme. The calf units were steam-cleaned, after which *S. typhimurium* DT204c was still isolated from environmental samples. Following further steam-cleaning and washing with disinfectant the organism was no longer detectable in the environment but was detectable from the next batch of calves introduced to the units. Although it is not certain that this was the result of environmental contamination the organism was not isolated from the calves on arrival. Subsequent batches of calves (20 or 30 per batch) were examined on arrival and three further serotypes, *S. typhimurium*, *S. agama* and *S. binza*, were isolated. Salmonellas were subsequently isolated from 20 per cent of calves that developed diarrhoea on the farm.

Both of these surveys amply demonstrate that infection in a limited number of calves can spread rapidly in young, susceptible animals subjected to the stress of the marketing and rearing systems and once established it may be difficult to remove the organism from an infected environment. It may also be possible that salmonellas, which cannot be recovered on normal bacteriological media may, although non-recoverable, remain viable and infective for animals.

The manner in which animals in previously uninfected dairy herds become infected is more problematical, and the source of infection may vary from serotype to serotype. Most outbreaks are probably associated with the introduction of infected stock or contaminated feed but polluted water supplies, the spreading of contaminated animal manures and human sewage sludge on pasture, and contamination of pasture or feed by scavenging birds may also be involved. Outbreaks have also been described where the probable source of infection was direct human contact. Insects may also be involved in mechanical transmission since it is difficult to contain salmonellosis outbreaks when animals are kept in units that are not insect-proofed and similar difficulties have been described in rearing *Salmonella*-free pigs unless fattening units were rendered fly-proof.

The epidemiology of *S. dublin* in dairy herds differs from that of other serotypes. *Salmonella dublin* has a precise geographical distribution. The organism has remained established in adult cattle in Wales and in southwest and northwest England. It is thought that this distribution may, in part, be due to an association between *S. dublin* and *Fasciola hepatica*, although this may be fortuitous and merely indicate that both are influenced by similar climates and survive better in wet conditions. *Salmonella dublin* probably persists on farms in these areas because recovered animals remain infected and excrete the bacteria in their faeces, either continuously or intermittently. Elsewhere in the UK the disease is predominantly one of calves in calf-rearing units rather than adults and it is introduced to the units with the introduction of infected animals.

The carrier state

Animals which excrete salmonellas continuously ('active carriers'), usually in concentrations of greater than 10^5/g of faeces, can be detected by bacteriological examination which will also detect 'passive carriers', animals that ingest salmonellas in their feed and pass them in their faeces without actual infection of the intestine or the mesenteric lymph nodes. When removed from an infected environment these latter animals stop excreting. Active excretion is usually a sequel to clinical enteritis or septicaemia and infected animals may excrete for many years and perhaps for life. It may also develop in animals that have not shown clinical signs, although this probably occurs only in cases of concurrent fascioliasis. In such cattle, *S. dublin* is characteristically present in the gall-bladder and alimentary contents without necessarily colonizing the rest of the animal. However, although active (persistent) excretors are an obvious source of infection for other cattle, and although the source of calf infection is assumed to be adult cattle, field studies have shown that the majority of calves infected with *S. dublin* are home-bred on farms where there is no clinical evidence of adult salmonellosis. This is characteristic of the disease and has led to a search for other sources of infection.

Many of the infections occur in closed herds; other sources of infection such as feed are not appropriate to a 'host-restricted' serotype such as *S. dublin* and although contaminated streams may be implicated, this gap in the epidemiology is usually explained by the existence of 'latent carriers'. These are animals that have salmonellas somewhere in their tissues or alimentary tract but only rarely excrete the organisms in their faeces. It has been suggested that infection with *S. dublin* is mainly latent, but is activated by stress, particularly at parturition, and the birth of congenitally infected calves to latent carriers or to cows that excrete *S. dublin* would only intermittently explain the occurrence of disease in calves on farms where searches for active carriers are unsuccessful. It is possible to detect greater numbers of excretors by bacteriological examination of faeces taken at calving and surveys have revealed animals which, although found to be infected with *S. dublin* at necropsy, were not detected as carriers by previous faecal sampling. It has not proved possible, however, to create such animals experimentally and serological tests for their detection have been singularly unsuccessful.

Serum agglutination tests (SAT) may detect a proportion of actively infected animals but they do not detect latent carriers and so far other immunological tests are equally unsuccessful, although they may be useful in detecting active carriers and infected herds. Delayed hypersensitivity skin tests can distinguish systemically infected animals but they may, unfortunately, also detect convalescent and recovered animals. It is possible that many unexplained outbreaks may be the result of human contact or extended survival of the organism in the environment, although most evidence, particularly from field studies, would favour the latent carrier hypothesis.

In contrast to *S. dublin*, infection with other serotypes does not appear to result in active or latent carriers. Adult cattle usually excrete for a maximum of a few weeks following infection and excretion that is detected for longer periods probably reflects recontamination from the environment, although the establishment of some 'exotic' serotypes such as *S. saintpaul* for up to a year has been reported. Similarly, *S. saintpaul* has been shown to be retained in the tissues of calves for up to eight weeks after excretion had apparently ceased.

Pathogenesis

An overview of the main stages involved in *Salmonella* pathogenesis is presented in Fig. 15.2.

Initiation of infection

Cattle are probably infected with salmonellas by the oral route, although respiratory and conjunctival infection may also occur. The dose required to initiate infection is thought to be high and will be dependent on the age, immunity and dietary status of the animal and virulence of the infecting strain. However, it is probable that animals are infected naturally by much smaller doses since factors such as concurrent parasitism (particularly fascioliosis), ketosis, metritis, mastitis, cystitis, pneumonia, viral infection, dietary changes, pregnancy, food and water deprivation and other stress factors such as freezing, wet weather or worming may lead to increased susceptibility. In calves, colostrum, whether normal or immune, is particularly important and animals that have either not received colostrum or have received insufficient amounts are particularly susceptible. Natural infections have been described where animals may have been infected with very small doses, particularly from infected feed. In one such outbreak dairy cattle were infected from a component of feed containing less than three *S. mbandaka*/g and the infection spread to their calves. The experimental infectious oral dose for calves has been variously estimated as between 10^5 and 10^{11} organisms, although doses in excess of 10^8 are normally required. The dose for adult cattle is approximately 10^{11} orally and greater than 10^8 intravenously.

Gastric acidity is responsible for eliminating a large proportion of ingested organisms in both monogastric animals and ruminants. In ruminants, survival of salmonellas is further reduced by the high concentration of short-chain fatty acids in rumen fluid and consequently salmonellas disappear rapidly from the rumen of regularly fed cattle. Factors which alter the acidity and composition of rumen fluid, such as starvation and

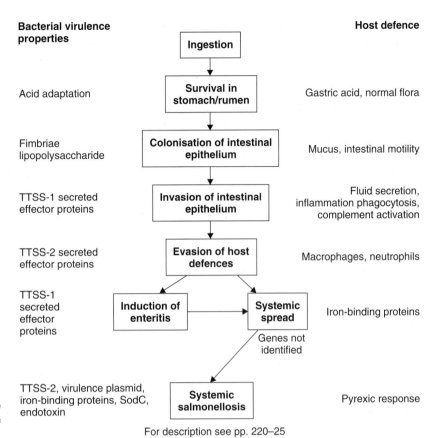

**Bacterial virulence
properties**

Acid adaptation

Fimbriae
lipopolysaccharide

TTSS-1 secreted
effector proteins

TTSS-2 secreted
effector proteins

TTSS-1
secreted
effector
proteins

TTSS-2, virulence plasmid,
iron-binding proteins, SodC,
endotoxin

Host defence

Gastric acid, normal flora

Mucus, intestinal motility

Fluid secretion,
inflammation phagocytosis,
complement activation

Macrophages, neutrophils

Iron-binding proteins

Pyrexic response

Ingestion

Survival in
stomach/rumen

Colonisation of intestinal
epithelium

Invasion of intestinal
epithelium

Evasion of host
defences

Induction of
enteritis

Systemic
spread

Genes not
identified

Systemic
salmonellosis

For description see pp. 220–25

Fig. 15.2 A tentative overview of the pathogenesis of salmonellosis. TTSS = type three protein secretory system.

refeeding, achlorhydria or administration of antacid, increase susceptibility to infection. Salmonellas that survive passage through the stomach(s) will probably be phenotypically altered. Experiments *in vitro* have shown that exposure to low pH and/or short-chain fatty acids results in the induction of expression of up to 50 proteins. This correlates to increased bacterial resistance to further exposure to low pH. Several bacterial genetic loci have been shown to regulate this acid-adaptation response. Three of these genetic loci, *rpoS*, *fur* and *phoP/phoQ*, have previously been implicated in regulating virulence in the mouse model of systemic salmonellosis and mutation of several of the other genes has also suggested a link between acid adaptation, survival within murine macrophages and virulence in mice. To date, there have been no studies on the effect of acid adaptation on pathogenesis in bovine salmonellosis.

Interaction with the intestines

After passage through the stomach(s), surviving salmonellas must be able to resist several host innate defences, including lysozyme and lactoferrin, and to prevent their removal from the intestines in the normal movement of food by peristalsis. The bacterial flora of the intestines may also be inhibitory to infection and the absence of a fully developed intestinal flora may in part account for the comparative lack of resistance of young animals to salmonellosis. Despite these host defences, salmonellas are able to associate rapidly with the intestinal epithelial monolayer. Bacterial motility and chemotaxis may aid this process by allowing the bacteria to move more freely within the intestinal lumen, to sense the presence of the epithelial mono-layer and to penetrate the overlying mucus layer.

The interaction between salmonellas and the intestinal mucosa is highly dynamic. Salmonellas are rapidly able to mediate their own uptake into epithelial cells and this is associated with a dramatic, but temporary, 'ruffling' of the apical membrane of the epithelial cell at the site of bacterial entry (Figs 15.3 and 15.4). The main initial site of entry is probably the distal ileum. This may be because the intestinal contents are held within the distal ileum for some time before entry into the caecum and it may also be partly due to the relatively high number of M cells (specialized epithelial cells overlying the Peyer's patches) in the distal ileum. In mice M cells are interspersed between enterocytes and salmonellas can clearly be seen preferentially interacting with the M cells. In calves, M cells form a

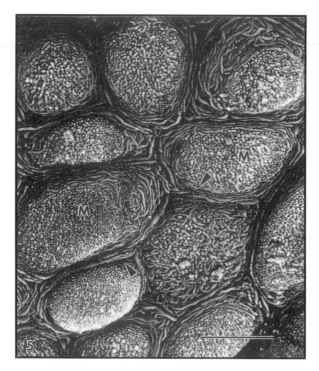

Fig. 15.3 Scanning electron micrograph of uninfected bovine ileum showing a group of typical M cells (M) on a domed villus. The cells have characteristic microfolds with a central area of short microvilli.

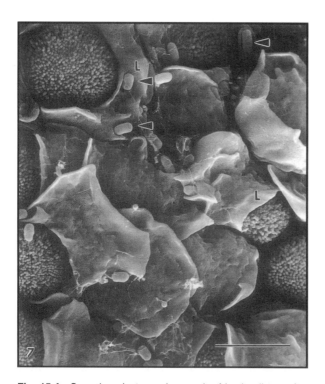

Fig. 15.4 Scanning electron micrograph of bovine ileum after infection with *S. typhimurium*. The peripheral microfolds of the M cells are ruffled and bacteria (arrowheads) are being engulfed by the membrane ruffles.

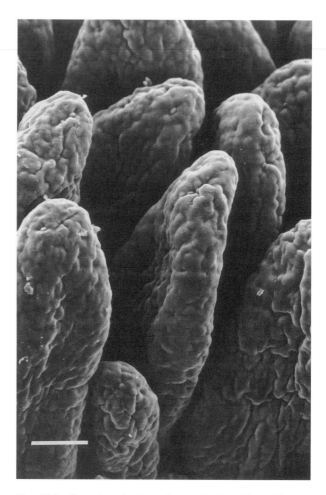

Fig. 15.5 Scanning electron micrograph of uninfected bovine ileum showing the normal morphology of villi.

homogeneous monolayer over the dome villi (villi associated with the Peyer's patches) and so the relative interaction of salmonellas with M cells and enterocytes is more difficult to assess. It appears, however, that salmonellas will initially interact with the M cells (within 10 minutes of direct inoculation into the distal ileum) and are not taken up by the enterocytes until slightly later (approximately 20 minutes after inoculation).

The mechanism of *Salmonella* invasion has been extensively studied. The bacterial genes involved in invasion are clustered together at one site on the chromosome, which has been named *Salmonella* pathogenicity island 1 (SPI-1). SPI-1 encodes a type 3 protein secretion system (TTSS-1: so called after comparison to two previously described secretion systems), regulatory genes and several effector proteins which are secreted by TTSS-1. TTSS-1 can be viewed as a proteinaceous microsyringe that spans the bacterial inner and outer membranes. The main function of TTSS-1 is the

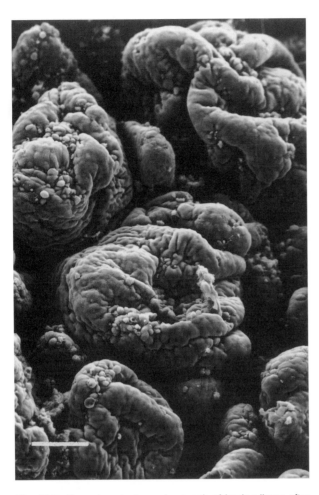

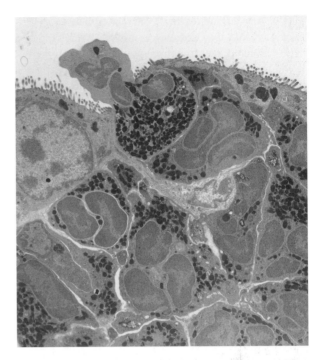

Fig. 15.7 Transmission electron micrograph of dome villus after infection with *S. typhimurium*. There are a large number of PMN leucocytes, one of which appears to be crossing the epithelial monolayer.

Fig. 15.6 Scanning electron micrograph of bovine ileum after infection with *S. typhimurium*. The villi are shortened and there is an abnormal extrusion of enterocytes.

co-ordinated secretion of specific bacterial proteins, not only out of the bacterial cell, but also directly into the target epithelial cell. The translocated proteins interfere with specific components of the host cell signalling pathways and cytoskeleton, resulting in bacterial uptake and potentially influencing the subsequent induction of enteropathogenic responses.

Infection of the intestines by *Salmonella* may result in several pathological changes (Figs 15.5–15.7). These can be studied using the calf ligated ileal loop model, which has been developed by researchers at the Institute for Animal Health, Compton. Results from this model correlate well with those from orally-inoculated animals. Short sections of the ileum are sealed *in situ* by surgical silk to form individual loops and each loop is directly inoculated with up to 10^9 salmonellas. This is an appropriate inoculum size, since faeces from infected calves may contain up to 10^8 salmonellas/g. The main advantage of this model is that pathological responses

to several strains can be quantified in a single animal, thus dramatically reducing the number of animals required for such experiments. In infected ileal loops there is an increase in the rate of epithelial cell shedding, which could be viewed either as a bacterial cytotoxic activity, allowing further invasion, or as a host defence mechanism to eliminate infected cells rapidly.

An inflammatory response is initiated in the intestines by the production of cytokines and other pro-inflammatory mediators by infected host cells. It is unclear whether this is a generalized host response to invading bacteria, which will release pro-inflammatory molecules such as endotoxin, or if it is the result of the direct action of specific bacterial proteins acting on epithelial cells without necessarily requiring bacterial invasion. It results in a large influx of inflammatory cells, particularly polymorphonuclear (PMN) leucocytes, into the intestinal mucosa and lumen. However, salmonellas are relatively resistant to the bactericidal activity of PMN leucocytes and their influx may cause considerable damage to the mucosa by disrupting cellular junctions and releasing the contents of their granules extracellularly. The most striking pathological change is the increase in net fluid secretion by infected mucosa. By 12 hours after inoculation with either *S. typhimurium* or *S. dublin*, as much as 30 to 40 ml of fluid may have accumulated in a 6 cm ligated ileal loop. This fluid secretion may initiate the physiological response of the infected host to eliminate infecting bacteria, but it will also be advantageous to the bacteria, because it mediates their dispersal into the environment.

This characteristic secretory response has led many investigators to look for enterotoxin activity associated with salmonellas. Despite numerous reports of enterotoxic activity in various extracts from salmonellas and using various enterotoxin assays, there is no conclusive evidence that *Salmonella* produce a classical enterotoxin. A *Salmonella* gene has been cloned on the basis of its homology to the cholera toxin gene from *Vibrio cholerae*. However, mutation of this gene in either *S. typhimurium* or *S. dublin* did not reduce fluid secretion into infected ligated ileal loops in calves. Despite the lack of evidence that *Salmonellae* produce a classical enterotoxin, there is growing evidence that they do produce proteins with enterotoxin activity, but which lack a receptor-binding domain and therefore require viable bacteria to translocate them into target host cells. The best characterized of these proteins is called SopB, and it is dependent on TTSS-1 for translocation into epithelial cells. SopB affects inositol phosphate eukaryotic cell signalling, which may lead to interference with chloride channel function and hence affect movement of electrolytes and water. Mutation of SopB in *S. dublin* significantly reduces fluid secretion and the influx of PMN leucocytes in calf ligated ileal loops. SopB is located within a small *Salmonella* pathogenicity island called SPI-5 and mutation of the other genes within SPI-5 also reduces enteropathogenic responses in bovine ligated ileal loops, although the biochemical basis of this is not known.

Elucidation of bacterial factors involved in the interaction of *Salmonella* with the intestines is advancing rapidly, but there is still a lack of knowledge as to how *Salmonella* induces enteritis. In addition to the intimate interaction with epithelial cells, bacteria also spread rapidly to the lamina propria and mesenteric lymph nodes, as well as being returned to the gut lumen by extrusion of infected epithelial cells. A significant proportion of luminal bacteria appear not to invade during the initial stages of infection. The presence of high numbers of luminal bacteria may extend the symptoms of enteritis by providing a continual source of bacteria to interact with epithelial cells. In addition, many of them will be expelled in the copious diarrhoea associated with disease, and are therefore vital to bacterial spread between animals. Salmonellas that have invaded the lamina propria and beyond may also contribute to enteritis. For example, *S. dublin* carrying mutations in TTSS-2, a second TTSS which is not required for invasion of bovine intestines but is required for subsequent intracellular persistence, are highly attenuated

in orally inoculated calves. The mechanisms of bacterial spread from the epithelial monolayer and the way in which intracellular persistence contributes to enteritis are not known. Several of the host responses to invasive bacteria may contribute to enteritis. For example, loss of epithelial cells will reduce the absorptive capacity of the intestines; the associated increase in crypt cell mitosis will alter electrolyte balance, and hence water movements, and the PMN leucocyte influx and associated vasodilation and mucosal damage may alter absorptive function, as well as allowing further bacterial spread. The relative importance of these host responses compared to the direct action of bacterial proteins, such as SopB, on epithelial cell function is not known.

Systemic spread and persistence

Salmonellas are able to spread rapidly to systemic sites, particularly the liver, lungs and spleen. In experimentally infected calves this may occur within 6 hours after oral inoculation. The most probable route of spread is via mesenteric lymph nodes, the efferent lymph draining these nodes, and subsequent entry into the general circulation via the thoracic duct. Cannulation of efferent lymphatic vessels draining bovine mesenteric lymph nodes has demonstrated that *S. dublin* leaves the nodes in efferent lymph. In general, the growth of *S. typhimurium* and *S. dublin* in the bovine liver and spleen appears to be relatively well controlled and in calves infected experimentally it is unusual to recover more than 10^5 bacteria/g of tissue, even at the peak of disease. However, the bovine infection model most commonly used (four-week-old Friesian calves) usually results in a predominantly enteric disease and may not be an appropriate model for the systemic disease occurring in some very young calves or adult cattle. The pathogenesis of systemic disease has been mainly studied in mice and the results extrapolated to other animal species. Natural resistance of mice to infection with *Salmonella* is controlled by a genetic locus called *Nramp*1, which affects the ability of macrophages to control intracellular bacterial growth in the reticuloendothelial organs during the early stages of infection. Resistance to salmonellosis in cattle may also be under genetic control and several researchers have commented on the variations in susceptibility to salmonellosis amongst breeds of cattle. For example, Friesian calves are thought to be less susceptible than Channel Island calves, although the genetic basis of this is not known. A homologue of *Nramp*1 has been identified in cattle, but its contribution to susceptibility to salmonellosis is not yet clear.

Several bacterial factors involved in systemic spread and/or persistence have been identified. A variety of

Salmonella mutants that are unable to persist within murine macrophages *in vitro* have reduced virulence in mice and several bacterial genetic loci influencing persistence, including those encoding TTSS-2 and the two component transcription regulators PhoP/PhoQ have been identified. Mutation of one such gene, *slyA*, is highly attenuating in mice but only slightly attenuating in calves, which highlights the differences in pathogenesis between these infection models. In contrast, the *spv* (*Salmonella* plasmid virulence) genetic locus is required for systemic virulence in both mice and cattle. This locus is located on a high molecular weight plasmid, called the virulence plasmid, which is present in many *Salmonella* serotypes. The existence of large molecular weight plasmids in many of the more important serotypes of *Salmonella*, including *S. typhimurium*, *S. dublin*, *S. choleraesuis* and *S. enteritidis* (but interestingly not in *S. typhi* which causes the severe disease typhoid fever in humans), has been described for more than 20 years. The plasmid harboured is characteristic of the serotype and they were originally called 'serotype-specific plasmids'. Naturally-occurring plasmid-free strains and strains from which the plasmid has been removed are avirulent in the mouse model of salmonellosis. In calves infected experimentally, plasmid-containing strains cause enteritis and a generalized systemic infection while plasmid-free strains induce enteritis in the absence of the generalized infection. It thus appears that plasmid genes are involved in the ability of salmonellas to proliferate within the host and that in cattle both plasmid and chromosomal genes are essential for the full expression of the disease. The virulence plasmid may not be carried by all isolates of a given serotype, particularly *S. typhimurium*, and this may explain, in part, the variation in the degree of severity of salmonellosis observed in the field where some outbreaks involve enteritis only whilst in others this develops into systemic infection.

The mechanism by which the *spv* genes contribute to systemic virulence is not known, although one study suggests the locus promotes bacterial replication *in vivo*. The virulence plasmid does not contribute to persistence within macrophages *in vitro* and although carriage of the virulence plasmid increases the lysis of macrophages during *Salmonella* infection *in vitro*, this is not attributable to the *spv* locus. The lysis of macrophages during *Salmonella* infections *in vivo* has received little study and the relative contributions of macrophage persistence and lysis to pathogenesis need to be assessed. The TTSS-2-dependent secreted effector proteins are thought to promote bacterial net growth *in vivo* by two distinct mechanisms: firstly by promoting bacterial replication rates; and secondly by preventing killing of bacteria by macrophages.

Systemic spread and persistence may have several pathological consequences. Release of endotoxin in systemic organs may result in haemorrhages, leucopenia, leucocytosis, hypotension, hypoglycaemia and shock. Mutation of endotoxin to make it less inflammatory reduces the mortality in mice infected with *S. typhimurium* without affecting the net rate of bacterial growth in the liver and spleen. This suggests that fatal systemic infection, at least in mice, is due to the inflammatory response of the host to endotoxin. Bacterial spread to systemic sites may prolong enteritis by allowing continual reinfection of the intestines via the biliary system and may also lead to systemic complications such as pneumonia or abortion. Abortion may occur before, during, after or even in the absence of enteric symptoms. The placenta becomes infected and the subsequent rapid bacterial multiplication results in a pyrexic response, severe damage to the placenta and possible infection and death of the fetus *in utero* or the birth of infected calves. Systemic spread may also lead to the development of the carrier state, characterized by the continual faecal excretion of salmonellas.

Signs of disease

Adults

The disease in adult cattle is usually sporadic, although *S. dublin* has become endemic in some areas of the country and acute and subacute forms are recognized. In the characteristically severe form of the disease produced by *S. dublin* in adult cattle the onset is usually sudden. Fever, dullness, anorexia and abruptly depressed milk yield at first associated with firm faeces, which may contain blood, are rapidly followed by severe diarrhoea. The faeces often become watery and contain large numbers of salmonellas (up to 10^8/g). The fever usually persists for several days, then animals rapidly become cold and recumbent and death, which may be preceded by abortion, occurs in approximately 75 per cent of untreated animals between four and seven days from the onset of clinical signs. In some animals the disease is more protracted and cattle may become emaciated and dehydrated and show signs of abdominal pain. A milder disease, characterized by diarrhoea and abortion, or abortion in the absence of other clinical signs, from which animals usually recover, also occurs. A similar disease is produced by other serotypes including *S. typhimurium*, although in these cases abortion is a less frequent event. Survivors of *S. dublin* infections often remain as carriers, possibly for life, while infection with other serotypes seldom results in the carrier state although excretion of types such as *S. saintpaul* for up to two years after infection has been reported.

Calves

In calves, disease usually occurs between two and six weeks after birth. Characteristically, calves become dull and anorexic and develop a fever. Diarrhoea follows, which in young calves involves the excretion of faeces with the colour and consistency of putty. This may be bloodstained and may contain fibrin and mucus. Eventually, the faeces become dark brown and watery with an offensive odour. More rarely the faeces are heavily bloodstained, become stringy due to the presence of undigested milk and pseudomembrane formation and may contain shreds of necrotic intestinal mucosae. In older calves the faeces are usually watery, dark brown and offensive. The calves become very weak and dehydrated and death usually occurs after five to seven days of illness in untreated individuals.

The disease is very variable; in some calves, especially those two to three days old, bacteraemia and septicaemia occur and the animals collapse and die without diarrhoea. In other animals the disease may be so mild as to pass unnoticed or may be associated with diarrhoea in the absence of systemic disease. Diarrhoea may be prolonged in some calves, which may eventually die as a result of dehydration, electrolyte loss and acid–base imbalance. In both calves and adults systemic infection may lead to complications such as pneumonia, meningitis and osteitis; polyarthritis and gangrene may occur when the disease has been prolonged. Mortality from acute salmonellosis may be as high as 70 per cent and all calves in a herd may become infected. Recovered calves do not normally appear to become carriers of either *S. dublin*, *S. typhimurium* or the exotic serotypes and consequently infected calves do not grow into infected adults. However, the disease is often slow to resolve and salmonellas have been isolated from calves up to six months after their initial infection. The disease produced by different serotypes in calves is usually similar, although the peak incidence of disease and mortality with *S. dublin* is at four weeks of age compared with three weeks for *S. typhimurium*. Calves from dams infected with *S. dublin* may be infected from birth and these are particularly likely to succumb to septicaemia rather than enteritis.

Diagnosis of salmonellosis

It will be apparent from the description above that diagnosis of salmonellosis presents several difficulties. The clinical signs and findings at post-mortem examination are not unique to salmonellosis and although a tentative diagnosis may be made this should be confirmed in diseased animals or at necropsy by isolation of the organism. Diseased animals showing signs of enteritis usually excrete large numbers of organisms in their faeces and determination of viable counts, rather than enrichment cultures, should be used (see below). For this reason faecal samples rather than swabs should be taken and these should obviously be obtained before administration of antibiotics. It may also be possible to isolate the organism from oral secretions and by blood culture, although these are less reliable than faeces cultures and must be taken with care to avoid contamination. Animals that have died of salmonellosis usually have large numbers of salmonellas distributed throughout their tissues and samples of spleen, liver, hepatic, mediastinal and bronchial lymph nodes may yield counts in excess of 10^6 organisms/g. Similar concentrations may also be present in the wall and contents of the ileum, caecum, colon and associated lymph nodes. Samples should be taken from the gut and internal organs in order to distinguish animals that have died of enteritis without septicaemia. Samples of fetal fluids, vaginal mucus and cotyledons should be taken from animals that have aborted. Counts will again give a more reliable result since the cotyledons from animals that have aborted due to *S. dublin* infection will usually contain between 10^8 and 10^{10} organisms/g.

Identification of carriers by bacteriological examination is more difficult and an attempt must be made to distinguish 'active carriers' (persistent excretors) from 'passive' carriers and 'latent carriers' (intermittent excretors). Faeces samples are more reliable than swabs and should distinguish persistent excretors whose faeces usually contain in excess of 10^5 salmonellas/g. Animals should not be assumed to be excretors on the basis of one isolation, nor should they be considered to be free of infection unless at least three negative faecal samples have been obtained. Even in this latter case 'latent carriers' and animals that will eventually clear the infection, and yet are still harbouring salmonellas, will be missed. There may be an advantage in taking samples from adults at calving although care must still be observed to distinguish 'passive carriers'. Traditionally, samples of gall-bladder or bile have been taken to identify carriers at slaughter. Unfortunately, these may not always contain salmonellas unless animals are infested concurrently with *F. hepatica* and a variety of tissues including alimentary contents and superficial lymph nodes need to be examined. It may be possible to isolate salmonellas from the walls of the omasum, abomasum and rumen or from lymph nodes such as the bronchial node, prescapular node and retropharyngeal node when all other tissues are negative. Similarly, salmonellas have only very rarely been isolated from the tonsil although this has been the preferred site for some investigators. Identification of infected herds may be achieved by faecal samples but this may present similar difficulties to identifying individual infected animals, particularly in the case of *S. dublin*. A simple, less expensive and probably more reliable method is to take samples of slurry where this is available.

A variety of enrichment techniques and isolation media are available for the cultivation of salmonellas. They rely on promoting the selective growth of salmonellas, whilst inhibiting the growth of contaminants, and identification on the basis of colony morphology and biochemical reactions. The choice of media depends upon the environment from which the organism must be isolated and often depends upon the subjective choice of bacteriologists who specialize in *Salmonella* isolation. In general, a range of liquid enrichment media and the use of at least two types of solid isolation media are necessary to guarantee the isolation of the majority of serotypes. Enrichment media depend upon allowing salmonellas to grow, albeit sometimes in an inhibited manner, whilst suppressing other bacteria through the action of chemicals, dyes, antibiotics and enhanced incubation temperature. In common use are media containing sodium selenite or tetrathionate and dyes such as brilliant green or malachite green to which salmonellas are relatively resistant.

After enrichment in liquid culture, colonies of *Salmonella* are isolated on solid selective agars such as MacConkey, Brilliant Green, Deoxycholate citrate, EF-18, Rambach, Hektoen, Bismuth sulphite and Salmonella–Shigella. These rely on the resistance of salmonellas to a variety of antibiotics, bile salts and dyes, which inhibit other bacteria, and lack of fermentation of sugars such as lactose and sucrose to differentiate colonies of *Salmonella* from other bacteria which grow on the media despite the presence of inhibitors. More recent techniques include the use of immuno-magnetic separation (IMS) and PCR (polymerase chain reaction) or fluorescence PCR, but the use of these is usually confined to research laboratories. Once isolated, the identification of salmonellas to genus level is carried out on the basis of biochemical reactions for which a variety of rapid kits are available. Further identification is carried out by slide and tube agglutination tests, which define the serotypes according to the Kauffmann–White scheme. Since a large number of differential sera are required this is usually the province of dedicated laboratories.

Important serotypes such as *S. typhimurium* and *S. enteritidis* may be further subdivided by phagetyping (there are more than 200 phagetypes of *S. typhimurium* but one or two phagetypes predominate in the UK at any one time, although 20 to 30 are usually present), plasmid analysis or a variety of molecular techniques including ribotyping (rRNA gene restriction patterns), PFGE (pulse-field gel electrophoresis), IS200 typing (a method of comparing restriction patterns of DNA after hybridization to a probe to a unique (IS200) *Salmonella* insertion sequence), DNA fingerprinting (RFLP: restriction fragment length polymorphism) and AFLP (amplified fragment length polymorphism where DNA fragments are amplified by PCR). Although used for research purposes, a phagetyping scheme for *S. dublin* is not available in the UK (recent studies identified 26 groups of *S. dublin* by phagetyping but more than 50 per cent belonged to one group) and this serotype is subdivided into biotypes. Unfortunately, although seven distinct, stable biotypes have been identified, the majority (approximately 75 per cent) of strains isolated in the UK belong to the same biotype and the scheme is of little use in epidemiological investigations.

A number of serological techniques are also used in an attempt to identify *Salmonella*-infected animals. Unfortunately, no single test has proved useful in distinguishing all infected animals, some of which do not mount an antibody response, and all suffer from an inability to distinguish infected animals from others which, although previously infected, no longer harbour the organism. Various techniques such as ELISA have been developed but they are usually no more successful than more traditional methods and are not in routine use.

Control measures and vaccination

Attempts to control salmonellosis in cattle have involved the use of strict hygiene measures, antibiotics and vaccination, either singly or in combination. Most of the control measures are obvious from the discussion presented above and the role of antibiotics and vaccination is described below. To prevent the introduction of salmonellosis to herds it is necessary to provide animals with uncontaminated feed and water, to control ingress of rodents and birds and limit human contact. When adult stock have to be 'bought in' these should be quarantined and examined bacteriologically. Exacerbating factors such as ketosis and liver fluke infestation should be controlled and particular care should be taken in maintaining the health and hygiene of animals at calving. This should include the use of individual calving boxes and thorough cleaning between animals. Calves should be encouraged to absorb sufficient colostrum. To prevent acquisition of infection in calf-rearing units only good quality calves from herds of known health history should be purchased and strict hygiene should be observed during feeding and cleaning. Units should be run on an all-in, all-out basis and calf houses should be thoroughly cleaned (preferably by steam-cleaning, disinfection or fumigation) between batches. In the event of a disease outbreak, affected animals should be quarantined and restrictions should be placed on the movement of susceptible stock.

Human contact with infected animals should be restricted and strict hygiene should be observed when moving between groups. During the course of an extensive outbreak of salmonellosis due to *S. saintpaul* in two large dairy herds many methods to control infections and reduce mortality were attempted. These included the use of an emergency vaccine, which had no effect on mortality but reduced the duration of faecal excretion, and treatment with oxytetracycline and ampicillin, which reduced mortality and the number of persistent excretors. Other measures included restriction of movement of stock and personnel, the use of impermeable clothing and disinfectant sprays, removal of predisposing factors such as dietary imbalance, reduction of stocking densities, segregation of susceptible animals, prompt antibiotic treatment of sick animals and removal of 'persistent excretors'. These measures were designed to reduce the level of environmental contamination. This is primarily due to contamination with the faeces of diarrhoeic animals and 'persistent excretors' from which calves may be infected either at birth, particularly when communal calving facilities are used, or when housed in the same buildings as adults. Once infected, calves may excrete such large numbers of organisms that less than 0.1 g of faeces may contain a lethal dose for other calves. Thus any measure that reduces environmental contamination may help to break the cycle of infection. Methods that appeared successful in this particular outbreak were prompt antibiotic treatment of sick calves, removal of adult carriers, reduction in stocking densities and segregation of susceptible animals.

Salmonellosis may be spread from farm to farm and amongst cattle on infected premises by the disposal or use of animal wastes on pastures as a fertilizer. The number of organisms contained in such materials is usually low and the risk can be reduced to an acceptable level if sensible restrictions are observed. The following code of practice designed to reduce the number of salmonellas should be followed:

(1) When possible, slurry should be spread on arable land or land used for conservation. Salmonellas do not survive for long enough on grass to be a danger in hay, nor do they survive efficient silage making.
(2) Composted waste may safely be spread on pasture to be grazed by animals but slurry should be stored for at least one month prior to spreading.
(3) Pasture treated with stored slurry should not be grazed for at least one month after spreading. If the slurry cannot be stored, this interval between spreading and grazing should be extended. In addition, since young animals may be more susceptible to salmonellosis they should not be allowed to graze pasture dressed with slurry for at least six months after spreading.
(4) The principal danger to cattle occurs when fresh unstored slurry, particularly pig slurry or poultry manure, must be applied to pasture. This danger can be reduced by using low application rates and by leaving pasture as long as possible before grazing.
(5) Consideration should be given to mechanical separation of slurry. This produces a solid fraction that readily composts and a liquid fraction in which salmonellas die off rapidly.
(6) Slurry should not be spread by equipment which involves the production of spray.

These recommendations were designed to reduce the risk of infections from animal wastes but they may be applied, with minor modifications, to the disposal of human sewage sludge on agricultural land. However, water authorities disposing of sewage sludge produce their own codes of practice that should be followed.

Vaccination (see p. 1006)

Prevention of salmonellosis by vaccination has been attempted since the late nineteenth century. There has been considerable scientific debate on the relative importance of humoral and cell-mediated immunity, but it is now generally agreed that solid immunity probably depends on both humoral and cellular responses. Although the humoral response is not totally protective it plays an important role in the suppression of infection in its early stages. However, a cellular response is probably required for complete elimination of the organism. In consequence, both live and killed vaccines have been used for the prevention of salmonellosis in cattle and attempts have been made to protect calves actively and passively by transfer of maternal antibody in colostrum. In the UK only an inactivated vaccine is available. The inactivated vaccine, which is licensed for use in both adults and calves, is a formalin-killed preparation of *S. dublin* and *S. typhimurium*. This vaccine has been the subject of recent field and experimental tests and has been shown to be effective when used to induce antibodies in adults, which could be transferred to calves in colostrum.

The majority of recent attempts at developing new vaccines have utilized live, attenuated *Salmonella* strains. These have either been naturally occurring avirulent strains, laboratory-derived strains, spontaneous undefined mutants or, more recently, genetically-manipulated strains. Amongst the first of these, originally produced in the USA, were strains in which mutations were introduced into genes encoding enzymes in aromatic amino acid biosynthesis pathways known as Aro deletants or Aro strains. Such strains are unable to synthesize chorismate from which *p*-aminobenzoic acid, a precursor of folate, and dihydroxybenzoate, a precursor of the iron-binding protein enterochelin, are produced. In the absence of *p*-aminobenzoic acid and dihydroxybenzoate, which are not found in mammalian tissues, they will not grow. Aro strains of *S. dublin* and *S. typhimurium* have been produced and tested experimentally in calves. They induce good protection when administered orally or parenterally, are claimed to cross-protect against challenge with heterologous serotypes and are claimed to be safe. They do not establish in the host, do not cause side-effects and are genetically stable. Their only disadvantages are that not all constructs are equally protective and that they may not be able to protect calves less than three weeks of age. More recently, constructs deficient in more than one enzyme or constructs with auxotrophic and other mutations have also been produced. These strains, which because they have two or more independent mutations are thought to be safer than strains with a single mutation, have also been shown to be effective vaccines for calves and may even be able to protect animals within the first month of life. As yet none of these strains are available commercially for use in the UK.

It is also probable that such strains are not able to protect against infection with a variety of serotypes. No study to date has shown good cross-protection between different serotypes for any significant period of time after vaccination. In one recent study wild-type *S. typhimurium* and *S. dublin* strains were used to infect ligated loops of calves previously immunized with either serotype. Although protection against bacterial invasion and induction of enteropathogenic responses was demonstrated it was clearly serotype-specific, despite the two serotypes being closely related and sharing common virulence mechanisms. It is difficult to imagine how effective cross-protection between serotypes may be obtained in future. It may be possible to include more than one serotype in a live vaccine. Recent evidence suggests, however, that distinct vaccine strains can interfere with each other when used in combination. Such interference could compromise efficacy.

Another problem with live vaccines that depend for attenuation on metabolic defects is that they are still equipped with a full battery of virulence mechanisms and may in some circumstances still be able to cause disease such as diarrhoea either in vaccinated animals, animals in contact or, in the case of food animals, in the human population who later consume their meat. A common problem with live vaccines has been mild diarrhoea and excretion of the vaccine strain in the faeces of vaccinated animals. Recent research on the mechanisms by which salmonellas induce enteritis may alleviate this problem. *Salmonella* type III protein secretion systems are responsible for the delivery of effector proteins into host cells, which influence *Salmonella* intestinal invasion, induction of inflammation, fluid secretion, bacterial replication and avoidance of host defence mechanisms (*vide infra*). Targeted mutagenesis in *Salmonella* that results in the disruption of genes influencing *Salmonella*-induced inflammatory responses and net bacterial growth, but not invasion, can optimise the phenotype of vaccine strains such that they remain invasive, and thus immunogenic, but not virulent.

Since calves may become infected within the first few days after birth and the peak of mortality occurs between three and four weeks of age, passive protection by vaccination of adult animals would appear to be the ideal way of protecting calves. Unfortunately, attempts at passive protection have met with conflicting results. However, an experimental vaccination regimen based on dam vaccination and prolonged colostrum feeding has been described. Cows were vaccinated with formalin-inactivated *S. typhimurium* approximately seven weeks and two weeks preparturition. Calves were given the opportunity to suck from their dam for 48 hours following parturition and were then fed cold, stored colostrum from their own dam for a further eight days. These calves were resistant to a normally lethal challenge of *S. typhimurium* or *S. dublin* given five days after birth and excreted salmonellas in their faeces for only a short period after infection. Mortality was also reduced in calves that sucked from a vaccinated dam and were then fed on normal colostrum and in calves born to unvaccinated cows and later fed on 'immune' colostrum. In cases of outbreaks with exotic serotypes the use of emergency vaccines for control has been successful.

Vaccines may have an important role to play in the prophylaxis of bovine salmonellosis, but until improved vaccines become available they will not be a substitute for good husbandry and hygiene.

Antibiotic therapy

It is not intended to discuss treatment of animals infected with salmonellosis in detail here since this is based on the use of antibiotics and fluid replacement therapy as described earlier (p. 195). Although antibiotics are not used in the treatment of gastroenteritis in humans their use is justified for bovine salmonellosis, which can become a systemic disease with a high mortality in the absence of treatment.

The concern with the use of antibiotics is that they have the potential of predisposing to colonization with salmonellas, increasing levels and duration of excretion by carriers and of selecting for antibiotic-resistant strains (see p. 210). The effect of antibiotics on an animal and its resident micro-organisms will depend upon the dose level, duration of administration and antimicrobial spectrum of the antibiotic. The effects of antibiotics to which salmonellas are sensitive at therapeutic doses must be distinguished from the effects of the same antibiotic at subtherapeutic concentrations and the effects at either concentration of antibiotics to which salmonellas are insensitive. Similarly, since the antibiotic may have an effect upon the salmonellas or the normal flora or both, the age of the animal host is important since age is often the principal factor in determining the composition of the normal flora. An antibiotic to which salmonellas are sensitive, used at the correct therapeutic dose, may be predicted to reduce excretion. The same antibiotic at a subtherapeutic dose may lead to increased multiplication of salmonellas due to a suppressive effect on the activity of growth-suppressing normal flora. Similarly, the use of an antibiotic to which salmonellas are resistant, but the normal flora sensitive, may be expected to result in increased multiplication and excretion.

Antibiotic therapy in uncomplicated *Salmonella* gastroenteritis in humans has not been recommended for more than 40 years. Therapy apparently does not shorten or otherwise alter the clinical course of infection and has frequently been shown to prolong postconvalescent excretion. However, antibiotics have been used extensively to treat salmonellosis in cattle without undue complications. It should be clear from the remarks above that the antibiotic sensitivity of the organism should be determined and the information used to choose the preferred antibiotic. The use of antibiotics for prophylaxis is more controversial and most authorities have reported that medication with antibiotics has no part to play in the prevention of salmonellosis. The use of antibiotics in the treatment of an outbreak of *S. saintpaul* infection has been described above. In the same outbreak antibiotics were successfully used prophylactically and have also been used to effect a bacteriological cure in adult carriers and calves.

Summary

- Salmonellosis is a disease which ranges in man and animals from severe enteric fever, through severe enteritis (with complications) to mild food poisoning.
- The disease has a worldwide distribution.
- Salmonellosis is caused by bacteria of the genus *Salmonella*, of which over 2400 types (serotypes) have been identified.
- The disease is characterized by host specificity. Some types cause disease only, or primarily in one animal species, whilst others are ubiquitous and cause disease in many species.
- The disease in animals in the UK is most severe in cattle and particularly calves, and can result in high morbidity and mortality. The principal serotypes involved are *S. dublin* and *S. typhimurium*. The former is endemic in dairy herds, particularly in the west of the UK, and may be maintained in herds by 'carriers'. The disease is also frequently mild or characterized by carriage of salmonellas in the absence of disease.
- The disease is controlled in cattle by vaccination and the application of strict hygiene.
- Some serotypes, and particularly *S. typhimurium*, have developed resistance to a number of antibiotics and multiple antibiotic resistance may be transferred between strains.

Further reading

Wallis, T.S. & Galyov, E.E. (2000) Molecular basis of Salmonella-induced enteritis. *Molecular Microbiology*, **36**, 997–1005.

Wray, C. & Wray, A. (2000) *Salmonella in Domestic Animals*. CAB International, Wallingford, Oxon.

Chapter 16
Digestive Disorders of Calves

R.W. Blowey

Introduction   231
Abomasal milk clot failure and milk scour   231
Problems with milk substitutes   232
Oesophageal groove dysfunction   233
Ruminal bloat   234
  Signs   235
  Treatment   235
Rumen impaction and 'pot-bellied' calves   236
Abomasal ulceration   236
  Signs   236
  Treatment   237
Abomasal dilatation   237
Chronic peri-weaning diarrhoea   237
Colic   238
Necrotic enteritis   238

Introduction

The young calf is particularly susceptible to digestive disorders, with the major presenting clinical sign of scouring (diarrhoea) being a significant cause of economic loss due to ill-thrift and death. Immediately after birth the calf is exposed to a wide range of infectious agents, to which it must develop an immunity. Many calves are hand-reared and consequently within a few days their diet may change from whole milk to milk substitute. Later they must learn to eat solid food, to be weaned at six to eight weeks old. Such rapid changes of feed and feeding systems, in combination with a changing immune status, render the calf susceptible to a wide variety of infectious diseases and nutritional disorders. Infectious conditions are described elsewhere in this book (see Chapters 14, 15). This chapter discusses the common nutritional disorders.

Abomasal milk clot failure and milk scour

Abomasal volume in the newborn calf is 1.0–1.5 litres. It has a neutral pH, thus allowing the first feed of colostrum to pass through unclotted, so that immunoglobulin molecules can be absorbed whole through the intestinal epithelium. Initially, renin coagulates milk (optimally at pH 6.5), with clot formation within minutes of ingestion. The clot contracts, expressing the whey proteins (albumin and globulin), minerals and lactose in liquid whey, which begins its passage into the duodenum 5–10 minutes later. After two to three days the number of parietal cells in the abomasal epithelium increases and they begin to secrete hydrochloric acid. Abomasal pH falls. This converts pepsinogen secreted by chief cells into the active form of pepsin. Both pepsin and renin are capable of clotting milk and both can digest the milk protein casein, but pepsin is most effective at pH 5.2 and, additionally, can digest a wider range of proteins. The pepsin digestion system is not fully developed until approximately seven to ten days old and until that stage calves should, ideally, receive either whole milk or a substitute consisting of whole milk. Similarly, the very young calf has an immature intestinal digestive system. Pancreatic proteases can cope with whey proteins, pancreatic lipases with fat and intestinal lactase degrades the milk sugar lactose into glucose and galactose. The ability to digest starch does not develop until the calf is at least seven days old and full activity of maltase, sucrase and amylase systems, allowing the calf to digest non-milk carbohydrate, is not complete until three weeks old.

Figure 16.1 is a flow diagram of digestion in the young calf. Complete digestion of the abomasal milk clot (or 'curd') by lipases and proteases may take 6–8 hours and hence calves fed twice daily are without nutrients for only a short period. Calves left with their dams may suckle seven to ten times each day and any remaining curd forms a nucleus for the next milk clot.

If abomasal milk clot formation is poor, then whole milk spills over into the duodenum, where casein cannot be digested. In addition to altering the osmotic balance, this provides an excellent medium for bacterial fermentation in the lower intestine and scouring results. Similarly, if excessive quantities of milk are provided (greater than 1.5l for the young calf), or if a hungry calf is allowed to gorge itself, then abomasal digestive processes become overloaded and whole milk spills into the duodenum. This can also be a problem with suckler calves, especially if the dam is a 'milky' Friesian or Holstein crossbred animal. Although the calf may suckle every few hours, overloading and

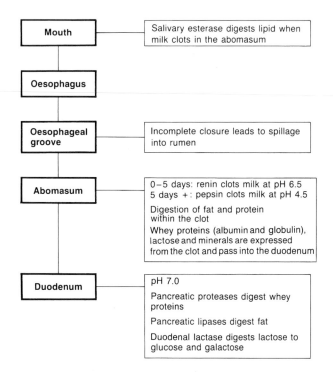

Fig. 16.1 Flow diagram of digestion in the young calf.

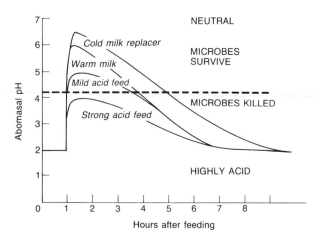

Fig. 16.2 The effect of type of milk and milk substitute on abomasal pH (Webster, 1984).

dietary scouring can still occur. This is particularly common if cows are put with the calves only twice daily.

On bucket-rearing systems a variety of management factors can lead to poor abomasal milk clot formation. These include:

• Nervous or stressed calves, for example feeding immediately after arrival from market, dehorning or some other stressful procedure.
• Irregular feeding times.
• Milk substitute fed at the wrong temperature or incorrect strength (see p. 233).
• Inflammation of the abomasum (see p. 237).

Many enzyme systems are induced, that is, enzyme activity develops following exposure to substrate. Calves should therefore be reared on a single type of milk substitute and, preferably, from a single batch purchased to cover the whole rearing period. A sudden change in the ingredients of the milk substitute could lead to incomplete digestion of protein, fat or carbohydrates, which later undergo putrefactive fermentation in the lower intestine, resulting in malabsorption, a fetid diarrhoea and weight loss. Such calves are more susceptible to colonization by pathogenic *Escherichia coli* and salmonellae.

Irregular feeding and its influence on abomasal pH can also have an effect on the susceptibility of a calf to infection. Most ingested enteric infections are killed at an abomasal pH below 4.5. The very young calf, which

for the first few days of life has an abomasal pH of 6.5, is particularly susceptible to infection therefore. However, this is counteracted by surface-active antibodies contained in whole milk and colostrum. In the older calf, the acidity of the empty abomasum, i.e. after complete digestion of the curd 6–8 hours after the previous feed, may fall to as low as pH 2.0. Following a feed of milk, pH rapidly rises towards neutrality (e.g. pH 6.5), the extent and persistence of this rise depending on the volume and nature of the liquid milk ingested. With warm whole milk, abomasal pH falls to below 4.2 within three hours of a meal and bacterial killing once again becomes effective. Figure 16.2 indicates the periods required for other feeds.

Clearly, calves that develop a poor abomasal milk clot, or that have other abomasal disorders (e.g. abomasal dilation, p. 237), resulting in increased pH values, will be more susceptible to infection. In addition, improperly digested fats passed in the faeces produce steatorrhoea, with subsequent hair loss over the legs and perineal region (Plate 16.1). Affected calves will be unthrifty and in poor condition, due to poor absorption of nutrients.

Treatment with oral electrolytes for two to three days and dietary correction is normally effective.

Problems with milk substitutes

A full review of liquid feeds and feeding systems is beyond the scope of this book. Those interested should consult more authoritative texts such as Webster (1984). Because of the immaturity of the pepsin–HCl system, calves should receive colostrum and whole milk for the first three to four days of life. Most conventional milk substitutes are based on skim milk powder (SMP), to which is added lipids and fats from a variety of sources, all highly emulsified to ensure even suspension throughout the milk when it is reconstituted. These SMP substitutes should clot in the abomasum. Addition of weak organic acids (e.g. citric or fumaric) reduces the pH to 5.7 and thus improves keeping quality. Fully acidified milk powders, with a pH of approximately 4.2, have an even better keeping quality. As casein would clot at this low pH it cannot be used and strong acid powders primarily consist of whey proteins (albumin and globulin) with added fat. Without casein they do not clot in the abomasum, but this does not seem to produce any increase in digestive problems. Such 'zero' replacers (so-called because they contain no skim milk powder) are commonly used in *ad libitum* calf feeding systems.

If skim milk powder is overheated during manufacture, casein is denatured, abomasal milk clot formation is poor, undigested casein passes into the small intestine and scouring may result from putrefactive bacterial fermentation. Most proprietary milk substitutes are carefully monitored and the majority of problems associated with their feeding are managerial in origin. The first golden rule must be *to read the manufacturer's instructions*. To achieve even dispersal of the product, and especially of the fat, many manufacturers recommend that milk is mixed at a higher temperature (45–50°C) and then cooled to just above blood heat (42°C) before feeding. A thermometer is needed to do this. The temperature cannot be judged manually. On a hot day milk will feel cool and consequently may be fed too hot. On a cold day the temperature may be overestimated and the milk substitute consequently fed too cold. Milk substitute mixed below the optimum temperature produces an inferior product. Added protein and minerals sediment to the bottom of the bucket and are wasted. In addition, poorly dispersed fats remain as a layer on the surface of the milk, forming a ring around the calf's muzzle after feeding, which produces secondary alopecia (Plate 16.2). If a long row of calves is fed from a single container, the milk for the last calf may be appreciably cooler. Again fat will rise to the surface and alopecia may develop on the muzzle. A fall of only 6°C in the temperature of the milk fed will *double* the time taken to form the abomasal clot. Undigested milk may then leak from the abomasum, thus reducing its nutritive value and possibly inducing diarrhoea. Conversely, however, if milk is fed too hot calves simply will not drink it, but no adverse effects have been observed. It is interesting to compare this with our own liking for hot drinks.

Milk fed at the wrong strength can cause problems. Powder is normally added at 125 g/l for twice-daily feeding and 150 g/l on once-daily systems. Abomasal milk clot will be optimal at these concentrations. If too dilute, clot formation is poor. Milk should not, therefore, be fed 'half strength' for scouring calves, as this may retard clot formation. Although some proprietary electrolyte preparations state that they can be used with whole milk and improve clotting time, there is some evidence that the clot thus formed is less stable. In general, therefore, it is best to avoid diluting milk substitutes and if electrolytes are to be given, they should be fed separately. Similarly, calves should not be allowed to drink large volumes of water immediately after milk, as this will have the effect of diluting the milk.

Probably the biggest problem with milk substitutes comes from careless mixing. Stirring with the hand is simply not adequate: a whisk, whether manual or mechanical, is essential. Carelessly mixed powders leave lumps and a sediment of protein in the bottom of the bucket and poorly dispersed fat rises to the top. Trials have shown that up to 60 per cent of the oils in a replacer may be wasted in this way, producing poor growth, stunted calves and possibly scouring due to inadequate abomasal clot formation.

Oesophageal groove dysfunction

From as early as two weeks of age the young calf begins picking at hay, grass or other solid foods. Bacteria ingested with this food, initially *E. coli* and lactobacilli, initiate ruminal fermentation. With increasing age, the rumen becomes progressively more anaerobic and an adult ruminal flora eliminates the early organisms. The inability of *E. coli* and salmonellae to survive for significant periods in the rumen is one reason for encouraging early ruminal development. However, at this age rumen fermentation alone would be unable to provide adequate nutrients for the rapidly growing calf and milk needs to continue 'monogastric' digestion in the abomasum. Milk entering the rumen is both wasteful and dangerous and hence it should bypass the rumen and reticulum to enter the abomasum direct. This is achieved via the oesophageal groove. In the anterior wall of the dorsal sac of the rumen there is a muscular channel that runs from the distal end of the oesophagus into the rumino-omasal orifice, as shown in Fig. 16.3. A reflex action from suckling results in muscular closure of this groove, to form an enclosed pipe, and milk is then transferred directly into the abomasum. As the calf gets older, the thought of being fed and the sight, sounds and stimuli associated with the arrival of its milk will be sufficient to evoke closure. It is most important that closure occurs prior to feeding and hence the establishment of a standardized feeding regimen is vital. The calf needs to know that it is about to be fed, that a pleasurable event is forthcoming. Ideally the calves should be able to both see and hear the feed being prepared, as this will induce a state of

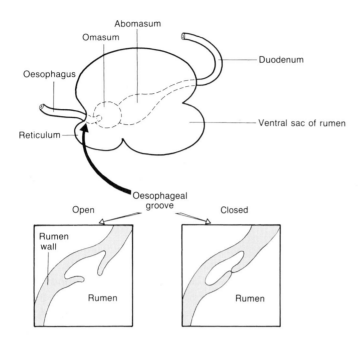

Fig. 16.3 The oesophageal groove.

expectation and stimulate oesophageal groove closure. Feeding times should be consistent each day. Milk should be provided at the correct and consistent temperature, in the same amount at each feed and of a similar taste and consistency. Calves with wagging tails and calves which butt the bucket (or udder, or teat) are enjoying their food and the oesophageal groove is well closed.

Calves on a teat need to work reasonably hard to get their milk – a pile of saliva beside the teat is a good sign. Conversely, if milk flow is too rapid, for example a badly damaged teat with an open orifice, the calf will almost choke with the rate of flow and milk could spill into the rumen. A sawn-off milking machine liner fitted onto a bottle and used by some farmers as a teat produces a much too rapid flow rate. Stressed calves, for example those that have just arrived from market, may not achieve groove closure and should therefore be given electrolyte solutions for their first feed. Similarly, calves should not be moved, handled, dehorned, etc. immediately before feeding. Slow drinkers present a problem. While the milk is warm, oesophageal groove closure may be adequate. However, if the bucket is left in front of the calf it may drink later, with possible milk spillage into the rumen. Some calves fail to learn to drink adequately and must be finger or teat suckled until weaning, although this is preferable to reluctant drinking with inadequate groove closure. Bucket height and teat position are important. The bottom of the bucket must be at least 30 cm above the floor of the pen, which means that it must be raised as straw bedding accumu-

lates. Unfortunately, it is all too common to see calves on their knees trying to drink from a bucket some way below pen level. Teats for milk substitute should be positioned such that the calf has sufficient space to stand back to suckle and at a height that allows its nose to be tilted upwards and the oesophagus at least horizontal.

Milk spilt into the rumen undergoes rapid fermentation. This may produce an acute and sometimes fatal bloat and colic, within 15–30 minutes of feeding. In more chronic cases, ruminal development is retarded and abnormal products of digestion pass into the intestine, producing scour. Chronic pain restricts food intake and therefore growth and development. The Charolais calf in Plate 16.3 has a typically distended left flank caused by ruminal bloat. The superficial haemorrhage resulted from trocarization with a needle. A pasty scour is evident on the tail.

Treatment of oesophageal groove closure is, in effect, treatment of chronic bloat and is discussed in the next section.

Ruminal bloat (see also p. 832)

The development of normal rumen function is a complex process and any interference can produce bloat. Organisms ingested with feed from approximately two weeks onwards eventually establish an anaerobic fermentation. It is the ingestion and subsequent fermentation of solid feed that stimulates the rapid expansion in size of the rumen, although full development is not complete until 12 weeks old, when the rumen comprises approximately 80 per cent of the total volume of the four stomachs. During this period, development of the rumen papillae is affected by the type of food offered. Inadequate long fibre and fermentation of a high-concentrate diet leads to low ruminal pH and acidosis. This can restrict development of papillae to such an extent that inflammation and ulceration of the ruminal wall permits bacterial 'leakage' and subsequent hepatic abscessation. The addition of 10–15 per cent chopped straw to concentrates, especially high-starch products, will improve rumen fermentation, thereby increasing the overall digestibility of the ration and promoting increased dry matter intake, since high acidity depresses the activity of cellulolytic bacteria. Calves that do not have hay on offer should therefore be bedded freshly each day, with ample palatable straw. Long fibre encourages rumination and subsequent saliva production, which in turn both neutralizes and dilutes ruminal acidity. Long fibre essentially acts as a 'scratch factor' and stimulates rumen motility. Silage or other forages may be used, but it seems critical that the fibre length is 5.0 cm or above. The rate of ruminal contractions and subsequent eructation and gas release varies with the physical presentation of the diet, as shown in Table 16.1, and with dietary constituents. High-forage diets produce greater ruminal activity than high concentrate. It has been suggested that concentrate intakes in heifer calves being reared for dairy replacements should be restricted, as this will encourage greater consumption of forage and the development of a larger rumen, capable of sustaining greater intakes later in life.

Irregularities at any stage of rumen development can lead to bloat, but the two most common causes are oesophageal groove failure, with subsequent fermentation of milk in the rumen, and acidosis caused by high-level feeding of improperly formulated concentrates. In both cases the bloat is caused by ruminal atony.

Table 16.1 Effect of the physical form of diet on ruminating behaviour of calves 6–9 weeks old (from Webster 1984, adapted from Hodgson, 1971).

	Grass pellets	Long or chopped grass
Eating (min/24 h)	132	276
Ruminating (min/24 h)	138	459
Eating (min/kg DM)	85	320
Ruminating (min/kg DM)	70	535
Dry matter intake (g/24 h)	1553	862

Signs

Typically, bloat is seen 15–30 minutes after a feed of milk or concentrate. Mild cases may deflate spontaneously over 3–4 hours, as ruminal contractions recommence. More protracted cases may remain bloated until the next feed, because bloat depresses feed intake and is therefore, to an extent, a self-perpetuating phenomenon. Affected calves are uncomfortable, with bouts of colic, often leading to kicking at their abdomen. Many develop a chronic scour (see colour plate 16.3), leading to general poor growth and unthriftiness. Death frequently occurs with acute cases.

Treatment

The syndrome may develop in both preweaned and postweaned calves and treatment is similar, the method used depending on the severity of the condition. Acute bloat must be deflated, either using a large bore needle through the rumen wall or, preferably, by stomach tube. Oral antibiotic will depress gas production. Penicillin may be the drug of choice, since lactobacilli proliferate in both concentrate overload acidosis and milk fermentation. Withdrawal of food and feeding electrolyte solutions for two to three days helps to remove the fermenting substrate. Calves should then be returned to a liquid milk diet for two to three weeks and eventually reintroduced to solid food. Even then, a proportion of cases recur and in many instances this protracted treatment is, for a variety of reasons, impractical. In such cases the construction of a permanent ruminal fistula in the triangle between the most caudal point of the last rib and the lumbar transverse processes is indicated. Under local anaesthesia, the rumen wall is sutured to the skin and a fistula is created. Although rumen contents may spill onto the flank, this does not appear to upset the calf and in many animals the improvement in growth and general condition following surgery is dramatic. A proportion of fistulae seal spontaneously after six to twelve months. Others require surgical correction, although this is not normally performed for beef animals.

On farms where bloat is a common problem, feeding and management systems should be examined, especially in relation to the encouragement of early ruminal development. Highly nutritious concentrates should be offered from two to three weeks old onwards, preferably in small amounts each day, to ensure freshness and palatability. Water should be freely available, especially on once-daily milk feeding. Inadequate access to water restricts concentrate intake and occasionally a long drink by a thirsty calf with a dry rumen leads to rapid fermentation of concentrates and subsequent bloat. In this respect the placing of buckets is important. Water should always be freely available, but the calf must be 'programmed' to regard it as a drink, namely without stimulating the oesophageal groove closure reflex. However, milk is a food and as soon as the calf has finished, replace the milk bucket with another containing concentrate. (Many farmers leave the milk bucket *in situ* – to avoid the transfer of infection – and simply add the concentrate bucket.) The calf immediately puts its head in and starts to eat, thus encouraging concentrate intake and, at the same time, discouraging excessive water drinking. Even so, occasional calves will still drink to excess, looking bloated and uncomfortable when they do so. In such cases, water is best withheld until 2–3 hours after the feed of milk, accepting the risk of bloat following rapid fermentation of dry ingested concentrates.

Rumen impaction and 'pot-bellied' calves

Postweaning feeding is a critical stage of the calf's development. The rumen is not fully mature, being more acid (i.e. lower pH) than the adult and unable to synthesize sufficient microbial protein, relative to energy, to meet the calf's high requirements for growth. Preweaning, milk has passed directly into the abomasum and this source of undegradable protein must be replaced by high-quality undegradable foods, e.g. fishmeal or linseed meal, after weaning. The higher the growth rate required, the higher will be the requirement for additional undegradable protein. As feed conversion is much more efficient at a younger age (Table 16.2), it is still cost-effective to feed expensive, nutritious diets to freshly weaned calves.

If the diet largely consists of poor-quality forages, the calf's growth will be stunted, and the rumen will be distended with slowly fermenting foods. If concentrate intakes are inadequate, hungry calves may consume large amounts of forage. Fermentation rates will decrease and rumen distension is exacerbated. Affected calves have a 'pot-bellied' appearance, i.e. the lower abdomen is distended, often on the right as well

Table 16.2 The effect of age on feed conversion (Blowey, 1999).

Body weight (kg)	Feed conversion ratio
50	2:1
100	3:1
300	5.5:1
500	8.5:1

as the left flank, but overall body condition, in terms of fat and muscle cover, will be poor. Ruminal contractions may be slow and the rumen feels 'doughy' on palpation. In an extreme case, where poorly grown calves left without food for many hours were allowed unlimited access to palatable straw, the author has seen severe illness and even death due to ruminal impaction. However, this is rare. Rumen impaction is almost the reverse of bloat, in that it is associated with overconsumption of dry, fibrous and relatively indigestible foods, sometimes compounded by inadequate access to water. It may be a group problem of poor dietary management, or the result of inadequate trough space, when the smaller members of the group get pushed out and have to exist on forage alone.

Abomasal ulceration

Abomasal ulceration is common in artificially reared calves, the majority of cases being asymptomatic and seen only at post mortem (for example in veal calves). Surprisingly, perhaps, the incidence is higher in those veal calves that have had access to forage. Many clinical cases are seen at two to three weeks old, when they first start eating solid food, or in animals that have developed pica, often as a result of chronic illness. These points suggest that ulcers may result from large, inadequately digested particles of hay or straw, passing from the rumen to the abomasum. There is undoubtedly an increase in ulceration in calves with trichobezoars (hair balls), but whether the hair balls lead to ulceration, or whether chronic ulceration stimulates the calf to lick and eat hair (in the same way as chronic ruminitis) is uncertain. Ulceration occurs in association with abomasal dilation (see p. 237) and may also result from ruminal acidosis and starch overload, allowing undigested starch to spill over into the abomasum. Fungal hyphae are visible microscopically in a proportion of ulcers and may be involved in the pathogenesis.

Signs

The majority of ulcers in calves are subclinical although some may haemorrhage, producing melaena and anaemia, which is occasionally fatal. Others produce a localized peritonitis of the abomasal serosa, whilst perforating ulcers lead to acute peritonitis and death. The three-week-old Friesian calf in Plate 16.4 was recumbent, in considerable pain, with a subnormal temperature (37.5°C) and sunken eyes. Regurgitated rumen contents are visible at the mouth. Death followed within two hours, despite abomasal drainage, lavage and parenteral metoclopramide. On post mortem (Plate 16.5) two large ulcers, one perforated with a white diphtheritic lining, were present, typically on the greater curvature of the abomasum.

Treatment

The treatment of abomasal ulcers is largely symptomatic. Valuable calves with extensive haemorrhage may be given a blood transfusion, but bleeding ulcers are less common in calves than in adult cattle. Kaolin has been used, but probably antacids such as magnesium oxide or magnesium silicate give a better response. Metoclopramide at 0.5–1.0 mg/kg body weight has been used to alleviate abomasal atony (Biggs *et al.*, 1989). Drainage and lavage may be indicated in concurrent abomasal dilation and ulceration. Antibiotics are indicated when peritonitis is suspected.

Abomasal dilatation

Also known as abomasal bloat, this condition of unknown aetiology produces a shock syndrome in calves, typically at two to three weeks old, when they first start eating solid food. Many cases are fatal. Affected calves are very dull, with sunken eyes and subnormal temperature, and are often reluctant or unable to stand. Enteritis may occur, but it is not a consistent feature. The enlarged abomasum, distended by excess fluid and occasionally with gas to produce tympany, can be ballotted on the lower right flank. The accumulated fluid has a much higher pH (range 5–7) than a normal calf with an empty abomasum (pH 2–3), thus allowing the bacterial count to increase to 10^5–10^9 ml, with coliforms predominating. A normal calf has an abomasal pH range 2–4 and a bacterial count of 50000/ml, with mainly staphylococci and *Bacillus* species and very low numbers of *E. coli*. This has led to the proposal that abomasal dilation is an enterotoxaemia, similar to 'watery mouth' in young lambs (Price, 1989).

Abomasal drainage may be achieved by deep insertion of a stomach tube. With the calf in lateral recumbency on a straw bale and its head hanging down, the excess fluid is discharged under gravity. The abomasum can then be flushed two to three times with electrolyte solutions and, if the calves are treated symptomatically for shock and acidosis and fed electrolytes for 24–48 hours, recovery rates are acceptable. Metoclopramide at 0.5–1.0 mg/kg body weight has been reported useful to overcome abomasal atony (Biggs *et al.*, 1989), but the current author has met with very limited success.

In those cases that reach post mortem, a degree of abomasal ulceration, sometimes with fungal hyphae, is often present.

Acute abomasal bloat may also occur in milk substitute-fed calves within 20 to 30 minutes or less after feeding. Affected animals are seen in severe distress, kicking at the distended abdomen or rolling on the floor. Some cases are fatal, others respond to relaxant therapy, for example pethidine or mepramizole. On post mortem the milk has often failed to clot, but no other lesions are seen and the cause remains unknown. It has been suggested that it is more common with infrequent and irregular feeding times.

Chronic peri-weaning diarrhoea

A well-recognized syndrome of a chronic persistent grey/brown scour occurs in calves 4–10 weeks old, i.e. before or after weaning (Blowey, 1988, 1994, 2000; Bidewell *et al.*, 1999) and when consuming concentrates. Morbidity is usually high but mortality is low and the few detailed post mortems reported have not shown consistent findings. There may be fibrous impaction of the rumen and a distended colon. Many cases of mild 'looseness' often pass unreported, but if the condition progresses, appetite falls and marked weight loss occurs. The diarrhoea may be unusually persistent, with many cases continuing for 4–6 weeks, leading to marked weight loss and stunting. The condition can be a major problem for feed companies because it often becomes apparent following (but not necessarily associated with) a delivery of food.

A range of treatments have been used, but none is particularly effective and most calves seem to eventually self-cure. Faecal examinations of affected calves reveal a range of organisms including *Giardia*, cryptosporidia, coccidiosis, *Campylobacter* species and rotavirus. Motile protozoa are commonly seen in fresh faecal smears and although calves can excrete giardial cysts asymptomatically, *Giardia duodenalis* has been reported to cause chronic diarrhoea in calves in the USA (O'Handley *et al.*, 1999). Although faecal coccidial oocyst levels are often low, the author has examined an outbreak where intestinal histopathology was typical of coccidiosis and there was an apparent improvement in the remaining calves following the use of in-feed decoquinate at 1.67 kg/t if *ad libitum* or 2.22 kg/t if feed was restricted to 375 g/50 kg body weight of calf. It has been suggested that the syndrome is similar to colitis in pigs, where a primary dietary imbalance leads to proliferation of intestinal parasites. The rate at which the syndrome passes through several groups of calves would suggest that an infectious cause is also involved (Plate 16.6).

Management factors have been implicated, particularly those relating to digestive upsets. The syndrome is seen more commonly (but not exclusively) with calf pellets rather than coarse mix, presumably because calves eat coarse mix more slowly, chew it more thoroughly and saliva production is therefore increased.

Feeding rancid food, digestive upsets associated with poor abomasal groove closure and use of 'milking cow' concentrates and maize gluten, both of which are unsuitable for calves with an improperly developed rumen, have all been suggested as causes. Hygiene seems to be important and a thorough cleaning of the affected area helps. The syndrome is more common in group housed/fed calves rather than in animals penned singly and keeping calves individually penned until one to two weeks postweaning will help (Blowey, 2000).

Treatment is largely symptomatic and includes antimicrobials, anticoccidials and vitamins. Macrolides, for example tilimicosin, have been used and sulphonamides and other anticoccidial agents. Badly affected calves should be returned to a whole milk diet, without access to solid food, and possibly fed three to four times daily. One severe outbreak dealt with by the author appeared to improve through the use of in-feed decoquinate. Lasalocid could also be used. There is an urgent need for more epidemiological information on predisposing factors.

Colic (see also p. 845)

Colic is commonly seen in young calves. It occurs in association with many of the syndromes described earlier in this chapter, namely oesophageal groove dysfunction, acidosis, ruminal bloat, ruminal impaction, abomasal ulceration and abomasal dilatation. True intestinal spasmodic colic occurs and may precede enteritis and subsequent diarrhoea. Colic may also be a sign of a more serious abdominal disorder, for example torsion of the root of the mesentery, intussusception, acute peritonitis, cystitis with urethral obstruction or atresia ani/coli. The latter condition is seen within 24–48 hours of birth.

The treatment of colic therefore depends on the diagnosis and is discussed in the relevant section.

Necrotic enteritis (see also p. 213)

This syndrome, first reported in the UK in 1991, affects spring-born suckler calves at 2–4 months old, when they are at pasture. Morbidity is low but mortality is high (Penny, 1999). Clinical signs are a sudden onset of profuse haemorrhagic diarrhoea, which later becomes scant and mucoid with tenesmus. Coccidiosis is therefore an important differential. Pyrexia is common and the animal becomes progressively more depressed, anaemic and dehydrated, with death following in 7–10

days. There may be additional respiratory signs, with a muco-purulent occulo-nasal discharge originating from ulceration of the mouth and pharynx and in some cases crusting lesions of the nostrils are seen. On post mortem the characteristic findings are erosive ulcers throughout the gastro-intestinal tract, with some being sufficiently deep to produce areas of localized peritonitis. The ileum, caecum and colon are the organs most commonly affected. Kidneys may be pale and swollen, with infarcts, and there may be lesions of inhalation pneumonia as a consequence of the pharyngeal ulceration (Penny, 1999).

Typical haematological findings reflect the pathology and include anaemia, leucopenia, neutropenia and raised urea values. Treatment is symptomatic and includes antibiotics, NSAIDs and fluid therapy. The aetiology is unknown. Although the pathology is strongly suggestive of BVD (p. 853), the virus is rarely isolated from affected calves.

References

Bidewell, C.A., David, G.P., Gonning, R.F., Harwood, D.G., Higgiov, R.J., Jones, J.R. & Laren, R.D. (1999) Persistent periweaning calf diarrhoea. *UK Vet*, **4**, 35–8.

Biggs, A.M., Dainton, J.T. & Tucker, M.E. (1989) Metoclopramide for preventing watery mouth. *Veterinary Record*, **124**, 312.

Blowey, R.W. (1988) *A Veterinary Book for Dairy Farmers*, 2nd edn. Farming Press, Ipswich, p. 54.

Blowey, R.W. (1994) Calf feeding practices in relation to health. *Cattle Practice*, **2**, 375–82.

Blowey, R.W. (1999) *A Veterinary Book for Dairy Farmers*, 3rd edn. Old Pond Publishing, Ipswich, pp. 21–66.

Blowey, R.W. (2000) Chronic peri-wearing diarrhoea – the clinical syndrome. *Cattle Practice*, **8**, 89–90.

Blowey, R.W. & Weaver, A.D. (1991). *A Colour Atlas of Diseases of Cattle*. Wolfe Publications, London.

O'Handley, R.M., Cockwill, C., McAllister, T.A., Jelinski, M., Morck, D.W. & Olsen, M.E. (1999) Duration of naturally acquired giardiosis and cryptosporidiosis in dairy calves and their association with diarrhoea. *Journal of the American Veterinary Medical Association*, **214**, 391–6.

Orskov, R. (1987) *The Feeding of Ruminants*. Chalcombe Publications, Marlow, Bucks, pp. 1–90.

Penny, C.D. (1999) Necrotising enteritis in beef suckler calves. *UK Vet*, **4**, 24–8.

Price, T.P. (1989) A treatment of calf enterotoxaemia. In *Proceedings of British Cattle Veterinary Association 1988–1989*, pp. 185–93.

Webster, J. (1984) *Calf Husbandry Health and Welfare*. Granada Technical Books, pp. 1–202.

Chapter 17
Calf Respiratory Disease

A.H. Andrews

Introduction   239
Enzootic and cuffing pneumonias   239
   Epidemiology   239
   Aetiology   240
   The environment   240
   Management   242
   The calf   242

Introduction

Bovine respiratory disease (BRD) in calves in the developed world occurs under two main management systems. The *first* involves young, housed calves, usually dairy bred and either reared for beef or as dairy replacements. These are weaned from their dams within a few days of birth and then fed milk substitute or milk until weaned, usually between five and eight weeks of age. Under such conditions these calves can succumb to one of two different respiratory syndromes. Often one will lead into the other. The first is a problem of slow, insidious onset known as chronic or cuffing pneumonia, whereas the second is more sudden and acute in occurrence and is given a variety of names, the most common being calf pneumonia, acute pneumonia or enzootic pneumonia.

Fewer problems occur with calves suckling their mothers in the beef herd until weaning. However, on occasion similar types of acute and chronic pneumonia occur while the animals are housed, Unusually, outbreaks occur in suckler calves whilst with their dams at grass. These outbreaks are often precipitated by a stress such as a management change or marked alteration in the weather. However some of these are less obvious in their precipitating factors. Investigation of these problems often shows *M. haemolytica* to be present. However, *Haemophilus somnus*, infectious bovine rhinotracheitis (IBR), bovine respiratory syncytial virus (RSV) and parainfluenza III virus (PI3) have all been detected in various outbreaks. It must also be remembered that calves can pick up lungworm infection and this, when in low concentrations, will still cause lung damage. This on its own can create clinical signs or activate organisms present within the respiratory tract.

The *second problem* is in a management system involving weaned suckled calves, usually six months to two years old and mainly reared outside. This disease occurs following transport and housing and results in a condition best described as transit fever or shipping fever (see Chapter 20). All the syndromes are best defined by the circumstances in which they occur because their aetiology is complex and mainly multifactorial in nature. This involves the susceptibility of the animal, the environment in which it is kept, the management of the animal as well as the various disease agents to which it is subjected. In many BRD problems the causal agents will be similar in each of the syndromes and it is only the management conditions that will be different.

Enzootic and cuffing pneumonias

The aetiology of pneumonia in young calves is extremely complex in both the acute and the chronic form. It is fair to suggest that the disease is multifactorial. It is usually seen in calves reared indoors, particularly when they are reared for beef production and so have moved farms at an early age. Most cases occur between two and five months and usually following weaning from a milk-substitute diet. The causes of the problem are partly infectious agents, the environment, management and the animals themselves.

Epidemiology

Chronic

It is very difficult to determine the incidence of chronic or cuffing pneumonia as most affected calves are not treated and they do not die. In addition, by the time animals reach slaughter weight or are culled the residual damage is minimal. However, in a survey of dairy-bred animals reared on a farm it was found that 11 per cent had significant pneumonic lesions and it was estimated that this resulted in a 7.2 per cent reduction in liveweight gain (Thomas *et al.*, 1978).

Acute

Very few studies have been undertaken into the incidence of this condition. However, Thomas (1978) obtained health records for 12 beef farms in 11 British counties. The records covered 11050 animals between 1970 and 1977. Mortality of bought-in calves is variable according to the rearing system used. However, a figure of 5.5 per cent is usual and it can be suggested that about half these deaths are due to enzootic pneumonia. This was seen in the Thomas study, which showed a death rate of 2.7 per cent from pneumonia out of a total mortality of 5.9 per cent. The overall number of animals treated for pneumonia was 32.6 per cent although the levels on individual farms varied from 3.1 to 52 per cent. Recent routine studies of individual outbreaks produced an overall incidence of signs of 68.4 per cent (range 41.7–90.5 per cent) (Andrews, 2000). It should also be remembered that some calves require more than one treatment for pneumonia. Again, there are few records for this but a level of retreatment of 10 per cent of all susceptible animals is probably not unrealistic. The recorded level was 8.9 per cent being treated on more than one occasion over a five-year period (Thomas, 1978) in a group of 2040 animals of which 22 per cent became ill initially. Another problem is that besides mortality, calves may become chronically affected and fail to thrive. Culling probably doubles the mortality due to disease and a level of 3.6 per cent was found in the study by Thomas. The reduction in liveweight gain in animals treated for pneumonia but which were not culled or died, compared with those untreated, was found to be 2.6 per cent (Thomas *et al.*, 1978). A study of eight outbreaks on dairy herds in 1997–99 showed an average cost per ill animal of £43 and a cost per animal within the group of £30. Veterinary and medicine costs amounted to only 40 per cent of the total costs of the outbreak (Andrews, 2000).

Aetiology

A large number of different infectious agents have been isolated and suggested to be involved in the aetiology of both chronic and acute calf pneumonia. Often the enzootic form is called 'viral pneumonia'. However, it is generally considered this term is a misnomer as it presupposes the aetiology and in most cases, even when viral agents are present, they only form part of the disease complex. It is usually considered that the most important agents involved in the chronic or cuffing form are mycoplasmal. They include *Mycoplasma dispar* and *Ureaplasma* spp. When it comes to the acute form there is a very long list of pathogens. Many have been seen in the disease but may not necessarily have produced the problem experimentally (see Table 17.1). However, certain agents do seem to be more commonly

involved. Thus the three main mycoplasmal agents are *M. bovis*, *M. dispar* and *Ureaplasma* spp., although *M. canis* is increasing. In the case of viruses, those most commonly implicated are bovine respiratory syncytial virus (BRSV), parainfluenza III (PI$_3$) virus, infectious bovine rhinotracheitis (IBR) and bovine viral diarrhoea (BVDV) virus.

The bacterial pathogens involved form a very long list and one or more tends to be isolated from most cases of disease. It is often postulated that these may be secondary invaders after primary damage by mycoplasma or viruses. The most commonly isolated organisms are *Mannheimia haemolytica*, *Pasteurella multocida* and *Haemophilus* spp., especially *Haemophilus somnus*. In addition, cases that involve toxaemia often include *Arcanobacterium* (formerly *Actinomyces*, *Corynebacterium*) *pyogenes* and *Fusobacterium necrophorum*. *M. haemolytica* serotype A1 is the most common serotype isolated, although serotype A6 is becoming increasingly common. The organism has also been involved in pleuropneumonia problems. The involvement of bacteria in this complex condition of enzootic pneumonia is also enforced by the fact that in most naturally occurring outbreaks of disease there is some clinical response following the use of antibiotics.

The environment

Various factors in the environment tend to be considered to be important. There is a popular belief that the disease is often associated with low environmental temperatures and a high humidity (see p. 974). Often a respiratory problem is associated with a sudden drop in temperature 24 to 72 hours previously. It is thought that the cold may allow infection to flare up partly by affecting the respiratory defence mechanisms and it also allows disease spread by encouraging calves to huddle together. It appears that the alveolar macrophages, ciliated and mucus-secreting cells are susceptible to the environment and cold stress inhibits clearance from the lungs. In the cold, animals reduce heat loss by slowing down their respiratory rate and by a partial reduction in the pulmonary ventilation rate (Webster, 1981b). This causes a reduced pulmonary oxygen tension and it has been shown that hypoxia reduces the clearance rate of some organisms in mice (Green & Kass, 1965), and there is a reduction in mucociliary rate and alveolar phagocytic activity (Thomson & Gilka, 1974). The probable role of hypoxia in respiratory infection is indicated by the fact that most lung consolidation occurs in the ventral parts of the apical and cardiac lobes and these tend to be the areas of lowest oxygen tension and the slowest rate of clearance of pathogens (Veit *et al.*, 1978).

At times, outbreaks of disease occur with a high temperature and a low humidity. Thus rearing at a temper-

Table 17.1 Infectious causes of enzootic pneumonia. The cause is often multifactorial, probably often mycoplasmal infection followed by viral and bacterial causes.

Viruses	Mycoplasmas	Bacteria
Respiratory syncytial virus (BRSV)[a]	*Mycoplasma bovirhinis*	*Mannheimia (Pasteurella) haemolytica*[a]
Parainfluenza virus II	*M. dispar*[a]	*P. multocida*[a]
Parainfluenza virus III (PI₃)[a]	*M. mycoides* subsp. *mycoides*	*Arcanobacterium (Actinomyces, Corynebacterium)*
Reovirus types 1,2,3 (Reo)	(little importance in Europe)	*pyogenes*[a]
Bovine viral diarrhoea virus (BVDV)[a]	*M. alkalescens*	*Streptococcus pneumoniae*
Adenovirus types 1,2,3,4	*M. arginini*	*Staphylococcus aureus*
Enterovirus	*M. bovis*[a]	*Strep. bovis*
Rhinovirus type 1 (RV)	*M. canis*	*Staph. epidermidis*
Infectious bovine rhinotracheitis	*M. bovigenitalium*	*Strep. mitis*
(IBR)[a]	*Acholeplasma laidlawii*	*Strep. faecalis*
Respiratory bovine coronavirus	*A. modicum*	*Aerococcus viridans*
	A. axanthum	*Acinetobacter* spp.
	Ureaplasma spp.[a]	*Micrococcus luteus*
	Ureaplasma diversum	*Staphylococcus* spp.
	Leach's group 7 mycoplasmas	*Neisseria* spp.
		Chlamydiales spp.
		Actinobacillus lignieresii
		Klebsiella spp.
		Corynebacterium bovis
		C. xerosis
		Streptococcus spp.
		Aerococcus spp.
		Haemophilus spp.
		Haemophilus somnus[a]
		Aeromonas spp.
		Bacillus spp.
		Alcaligenes faecalis
		Micrococcus roseus
		Micrococcus spp.
		Escherichia coli
		Fusobacterium necrophorum[a]

[a] Thought to be the most important causes.

ature of 21°C (70°F) and 47 per cent relative humidity (RH) predisposed Friesian and Jersey calves to respiratory disease compared with those kept at a temperature of 14°C (60°F) and 36 per cent RH (Roy *et al.*, 1971). It does seem that a high relative humidity may be beneficial at a high environmental temperature as it increases the sedimentation rate of airborne particles and thereby reduces the bacterial count of the environment. These factors have formed the basis for the establishment of the sweat box system for pigs (Gordon, 1963) and this is why water drips are often used in buildings for veal production.

Although it is generally recognized that respiratory disease commonly occurs at certain times of the year, and under certain weather conditions, it is only recently that attempts have been made to determine why. In housed dairy-bred calves on one farm two peak levels of enzootic pneumonia occurred; the first was between

October and December and the second from February to May (Thomas, 1978). A study of a veal-calf unit over a 14-month period showed extensive outbreaks of disease in October, April and early June (Miller *et al.*, 1980).

The relationship between season and respiratory disease is probably partly due to management influences, particularly the housing of animals in close proximity, thereby assisting in the build-up and transfer of infection. However, the correlation between weather and disease is harder to prove, and in a disease outbreak involving veal calves no relationship was found (Miller *et al.*, 1980). A sudden drop in environmental temperature is often followed one to three days later by an outbreak of respiratory disease in housed, dairy-bred calves or housed single-suckler calves (Wiseman, 1978). Pneumonia in Irish calves housed in naturally ventilated buildings also tended to be precipitated by change in weather, such as frost, rain and wind or damp, humid conditions (Bryson *et al.*, 1978).

Body temperature regulation in cattle is well developed, so they can tolerate both heat and cold (Webster, 1981a). However, draughts in buildings can result in chilling, which increases the metabolic rate and perhaps reduces resistance to infection (Webster, 1981b), but high relative humidity on its own does not chill cattle (Webster, 1979). Webster (1981b) therefore postulated that the main effect of weather was compounded by the building itself. Thus a badly constructed building with poor ventilation would reduce ventilation rate, and the water-carrying capacity of the air would be detrimentally affected by bad ventilation and possibly poor drainage. Such conditions could lead to the relative humidity remaining at more than 90 per cent for several days, and this in turn would increase the survival and spread of pathogenic organisms. Some support for this view has been obtained by work showing an increased survival of small airborne bacteria at high relative humidities (Jones & Webster, 1981). There is thus an increase in the number of infective particles that are not removed in the nasal passages and these are deposited further down the respiratory tract, possibly causing disease.

Management

The time of weaning appears to be important in that more lung lesions are found in calves weaned at five weeks than those on an *ad libitum* milk substitute diet until 14 weeks old (Roy *et al.*, 1971). The reason for this is not clear but it might be due to the lower levels of energy intake, or lower availability of a micronutrient (Roy *et al.*, 1971); or perhaps inhaled dust or fungal spores, which are more prevalent when dry feed is eaten, exacerbate the problem (Lacey, 1968); or due to weaning being less stressful or the calf more resistant to respiratory disease at an older age.

There is a relationship between colostral antibody levels and respiratory disease (Thomas & Swann, 1973). This apparent resistance to disease might be due to the ingestion of increased levels of specific antibody or due to an indirect effect resulting from a reduced amount of enteric disease, or possibly the gradual reduction in passive immunity allowing a more orderly exposure of the calf to respiratory pathogens. When colostral antibodies are low there is a relatively fast loss of antibody, which may then allow the invasion of many pathogens (Williams *et al.*, 1975).

The purchase of a large number of calves from different sources for dairy and beef production and keeping them in the same housing allows the easy spread of potential respiratory pathogens to other animals in close proximity. It is considered by many

authors (Wiseman, 1978) that it is the collection of a large number of young calves of a similar age and putting them into the same air space that is the main reason for the problem of pneumonia in intensively reared calf systems. It is not always accepted that the number of calves in a single air space is more important than the air space or floor area per calf. However, overcrowding is a major factor in allowing disease development and spread. Other factors involved in increasing disease levels are the inadequate cleaning and disinfection of the building between batches, as well as not allowing the accommodation sufficient rest between calf intakes. In some cases younger animals are mixed with an older group, thereby allowing transmission of micro-organisms from the old, apparently clinically normal animals. Economic considerations may also influence the picture if there is a reluctance to employ preventive measures such as vaccination, etc. Several management procedures such as castration, disbudding and weaning all appear to have an effect on the level of disease. The importance of microbial agents is indirectly indicated by the importance of adequate uptake of colostrum (Phillips, 1975; Thomas, 1979).

The calf

There appear to be some breed differences in susceptibility to respiratory disease and Friesian and Jersey calves are more likely to be infected than Ayrshire or Hereford × Friesians (Roy, 1980). It has been postulated that this may be due to an increased skin thickness in some breeds, which provides better insulation.

Signs

Chronic: The condition is one of gradual onset. There is generally no illness and so the calf is bright, eats well, but it may have a slight mucoid or mucopurulent oculo-nasal discharge. The temperature is normal or slightly raised at 38.5–39.5°C (101–103°F); the respiratory rate may be at any level from normal to 100 per minute with a normal pulse. There is a dry, explosive cough that is usually produced singly. On chest auscultation there are noises of whistling, wheezing or squeaking and these are more commonly heard at expiration, although often they occur at both inspiration and expiration. The sounds are most common in the anterior and ventral parts of the chest.

Acute: Although one calf may be seen to be ill to begin with, several animals will usually become sick within the next 24–48 hours. There is normally a reduction in feed intake of the group and widespread coughing will be apparent. The affected animals appear dull and the head tends to be carried lower than normal. There is inappetance, pyrexia (40–40°C, 104–107°F) and a dull, sweaty coat. Other signs including a mucoid or mucopurulent oculo-nasal discharge, tachypnoea (respirations are usually over 40 per minute), dyspnoea and hyperpnoea are normally present. In all but very severely ill calves there tends to be an increase in the amount of coughing; the cough itself may be of a harsh, dry, hacking type, but in others it will be moist. Pinching the upper trachea often elicits a cough. On auscultation of the thorax there are usually loud, harsh sounds or whistling, wheezing or squeaking. These sounds may be present at inspiration or expiration, but more commonly they are heard at the latter and in some cases there are fluid sounds such as bubbling or gurgling, which will be audible in the cranio-ventral parts of the lungs. In some bacterial infections, where there is marked lung consolidation, few sounds are present.

Necropsy

Chronic: Lesions tend to be confined to the ventral parts of the lung lobes and involve, in decreasing severity, the apical, cardiac and cranial parts of the caudal lobes. The area involved may be 5–40 per cent of the lung tissue and it tends to be red or purple in colour and to be indurated. Histologically, there are accumulations of lymphocytes in the peribronchiolar tissue and it is this that produces a cuff; macroscopically it is seen as a mottling of the lesion's cut surface. When accumulation is great, then the lymphocytes can cause a narrowing of the bronchiolar lumen and cause the surrounding alveoli to be compressed. Resolution of the lesions occurs over several months provided that they are uncomplicated. The bronchial and mediastinal lymph nodes are usually enlarged and there is often a fibrinous pneumonia.

Acute: Within the clinical entity of acute pneumonia there are three types of pathological entity that can be recognized involving the lungs (Pirie, 1979).

Type 1. There is localized consolidation particularly of the cranial lobes and the tissue is dark red, friable and there is no gross evidence of necrosis. Interstitial emphysema may be present. Histologically, there is an absence of peribronchiolar cuffing, but there is necrosis of the bronchiolar epithelium. The changes are often suggestive of a viral infection, but in many cases the presence of a virus cannot be proven because of the absence of inclusion bodies or positive immunofluorescence. PI3 infection can be suspected when there is alveolar and bronchiolar epithelium proliferation and eosinophilic intracytoplasmic inclusion bodies are present. RSV infection can result in alveolar epithelium hyperplasia and large multinucleate syncytial cells. Bronchial collapse occurs with adenovirus infection due

to bronchiolar necrosis; there are basophilic and eosinophilic intranuclear inclusion bodies in epithelial and other cells. Intranuclear inclusion bodies, particularly in the epithelial cells of the trachea and bronchi, are seen in IBR.

Type 2. There is often marked consolidation of the cranial lobes with red or red/grey hepatization with widespread tissue necrosis and in many cases suppuration and this may involve up to 70–80 per cent of the lung. This type of lesion is often characteristic of bacterial infection. Extensive consolidation and suppuration are particularly seen in *A. pyogenes* and *F. necrophorum* infections.

Type 3. This is characteristic of calves that suddenly develop respiratory distress. The syndrome is often called atypical interstitial pneumonia. At post-mortem examination there is interstitial emphysema, pulmonary oedema and congestion, with alveolar epithelial hyperplasia and hyaline membrane formation.

Besides the lungs, there is usually gross enlargement and congestion of the mediastinal and bronchial lymph nodes. In some cases there is fibrinous pleurisy and the heart may be enlarged with epicardial and endocardial haemorrhages. Sero-sanguinous fluid may be present in the thorax and pericardial sac (Thomas, 1979).

Lesions of pleuropneumonia result in a thickened pleura with the lung showing thickened interlobular septa with variable amounts of lung consolidation showing dark red to grey hepatization.

Diagnosis

Chronic: Several animals are affected and are usually indoors. The problem is gradual in onset and although the animals show respiratory signs they are bright and eat well. The respiratory signs include single, dry coughing.

Acute: Again this affects a group of calves. Respiratory signs are present and the animals are usually obviously ill. Nasopharyngeal swabs or broncho-alveolar lavage can be undertaken to examine for bacterial, viral or mycoplasmal presence. The last two groups require placement in a transport medium. Fluorescent antibody tests are available for most of the more important viral causes. Even when a potential pathogen is recovered it does not always mean that it is the same agent as is causing trouble in the lungs. Paired serum samples can be taken two weeks apart. This may indicate the cause but is only of value if control measures can then be implemented for the future. Post-mortem material can be cheeked for the presence of organisms and for histology to indicate the type of pathogen which might be involved.

Differential diagnosis

Chronic: This needs to be differentiated form acute pneumonia but in the latter case the animal is ill. Inhalation pneumonia is likely only to involve a single animal, which again is ill, and there is usually a related history. Tuberculosis may cause problems but usually there is a herd history and the dam may be showing signs. Muscular dystrophy (see p. 258) can produce respiratory signs but usually such animals have a fast pulse rate and raised serum creatine kinase, and aspartate and aminotransferase levels. Congenital heart defects (see pp. 173–4) will usually only involve one animal and there is a heart murmur, possibly with signs of cyanosis. Salmonellosis can result in signs but the calf is noticeably ill with diarrhoea (see p. 226).

Acute. Chronic pneumonia is a major differential diagnosis but the animals are not really ill in such cases. Uncomplicated IBR infection (see p. 289) could cause difficulties but there are mainly upper respiratory signs and a noticeable conjunctivitis. Salmonellosis (Chapter 15) will usually present with enteric signs. Although mucosal disease (see p. 853) can give rise to respiratory signs, there is usually also diarrhoea and, in some cases, mouth ulceration. Inhalation pneumonia mainly involves a single animal and there is an appropriate history. Tuberculosis will be detected by a history of disease in the herd. Congenital heart defects (see pp. 173–4) involve a single animal and there is usually a heart murmur. Calf diphtheria (see p. 251) results in stertor and is again a single animal problem. Malignant catarrhal fever (see p. 935) affects single animals and there is lymph node enlargement, corneal opacity and often nervous signs present. Acidosis (p. 829) can mimic pneumonia.

Treatment

Chronic: Therapy is usually not necessary unless the calf is showing severe coughing. Several antibiotics are of use, including tylosin at 4–10 mg/kg (2–5 mg/lb) body weight, oxytetracycline at 10 mg/kg (5 mg/lb) body weight, spiramycin at a dose of 20 mg/kg (10 mg/lb) body weight of spectinomycin at 20–30 mg/kg (10–15 mg/lb) body weight. The macrolide antibiotics (tilosin, erythromycin, spiramycin) are all concentrated in the lungs and have good efficacy against mycoplasmal infections. The fluorquinolones have activity against mycoplasma but probably cannot be recommended for this purpose due to human health implications.

Acute:

(1) Antimicrobials. If more than 30 per cent of the animals are affected at one time and need treatment it is probable that many others are incubating the condi-tion, so that it is often a good policy to persuade the farmer to treat all the cattle in the group, ideally using a different antibiotic. As with most disease, the earlier treatment is started, the less the mortality and the fewer the animals that have to be culled because of chronic disease. The drugs commonly used are given in Table 17.2. The therapeutic agent administered should have a broad spectrum of activity and ideally it should be bactericidal. The choice will most probably have to be based on previous successful usage on that farm or elsewhere. It is best not to use long-acting preparations because if there is no response to treatment it will make the initiation of subsequent therapy very difficult. If an animal dies then culture of swabs from the lung, bronchial and mediastinal lymph nodes and the subsequent antibiotic sensitivity of the isolates may be of use. The ideal is to culture swabs from material in carcasses that have not been treated. The culture of nasal or pharyngeal swabs from live infected calves is of less value as it cannot be certain that the organism cultured will be the same as the one causing disease in the lungs. However, it does indicate possible pathogens.

Therapy should be continued for three to five days, depending on the drug used and the response to treatment. In acute cases the choice of antimicrobial agent is normally dictated by those that can be given intravenously. Intratracheal administration of antibiotics has been advocated by some practitioners and in such cases those in aqueous solution are preferable to those in organic solvent. No antibiotic is at present licensed in Britain for this route of administration. Those compounds most commonly used have included erythromycin, trimethoprim and sulphadoxine.

(2) Corticosteroids. Some of the compounds available are shown in Table 17.3. The drugs commonly in use today include betamethasone, dexamethasone, prednisolone, flumethasone and triamcinolone. These compounds provide symptomatic relief only and do not cure the condition. Many people consider them to be overused (Pirie, 1979), but often an animal will show little or no improvement on antibiotic therapy alone, only to recover rapidly once corticosteroids are added to the treatment regimen. Their action is to suppress all stages of inflammation regardless of whether the cause is physical, chemical or immunological in origin. Thus in the acute stage, corticosteroids reduce vasodilation, oedema formation and leucocyte infiltration (Eyre, 1978). The drugs also have a 'euphoric' effect on the dull animal and this may allow the calf to eat and otherwise speed its recovery (Pirie, 1979).

The main problem with corticosteroids is the unselective suppression of inflammation that therefore includes those parts of the inflammatory and immune response, such as macrophage infiltration, which are

Table 17.2 Some of the antimicrobial compounds used in calf pneumonia therapy.

Antimicrobial compounds	Bactericidal (C) or bacteriostatic (S)	Route of administration	Dosage	
			(mg/kg)	(mg/lb)
Amoxycillin	C	i.v., s.c., i.m., oral	7 (15 LA)	3.5 (7 LA)
Amoxycillin and	C	i.m., s.c.	8.75 (am)	4.38 (am)
clavulanic acid			1.75 (cl)	0.88 (cl)
Ampicillin	C	i.v., s.c., i.m., oral	2–7	1–3.75 (7.5 LA)
Baquiloprim and	C	oral	4–8 (baquil)	2–4 (baquil)
sulphamidine			36–72 (sulpha)	18–36 (sulpha)
Ceftiofur	C	i.m.	1	0.5
Chloramphenicol (some countries)	S	i.v., s.c., i.m., oral	4–10	2–5
Danofloxacin	C	i.m.	1.25	0.6
Enrofloxacin	C	s.c.	2.5 or 7.5	1.25 or 3.75
Erythromycin	S	i.m.	2.5–5	1.25–2.5
Florfenicol	S	s.c., i.m.	40 (s.c.), 20 (i.m.)	20 (s.c.), 10 (i.m.)
Marbofloxacin	C	i.v., s.c., i.m.	2	1
Oxytetracycline	S	i.v., s.c., i.m., oral	10 (20 LA)	5 (10 LA)
Penicillin plus			10–15 (pen)	5–7.5 (pen)
streptomycin	C	s.c., i.m.	10–20 (strep)	5–10 (strep)
Spectinomycin	C	i.m.	12.5–30	6.25–15
Spiramycin	S	i.m., oral	20	10
Sulphadimidine	S	i.v., s.c., oral		
initial			200	100
maintenance			100	50
Sulphamethoxypyridazine	S	s.c., i.m.	22	11
Sulphapyrazole	S	i.v., s.c., i.m.	30–100	15–50
Tilmicosin	S	s.c.	10	5
Trimethoprim and sulphadiazine	C	i.m., oral	15–22.5 (active)	7.5–12 (active)
Trimethoprim and				
sulphadoxine	C	i.m.	15 (active)	7.5 (active)
Tylosin	S	i.m., oral	4–10	2–5

LA, long-acting; am, amoxycillin; cl, clavulanic acid; baquil, baquiloprim; sulpha, sulphadimidine; pen, penicillin; strep, streptomycin; active, active ingredients.

Table 17.3 Corticosteroids used in respiratory disease in calves.

Drug	Dose per animal (mg)
Betamethasone	2–10
Cortisone	up to 500
Dexamethasone	2–5
Flumethasone	0.5
Hydrocortisone	up to 300
Prednisolone	up to 20
Triamcinolone	up to 5

concerned with the control and removal of infectious organisms. In such an environment an organism can multiply and spread within the animal. This may be the agent that caused the pneumonia or an opportunist organism that enters the body. The reduction in the immune response can also increase the ability of the same organisms to reinfect the animal following recovery. It is therefore essential that antibiotic therapy is administered concurrently with corticosteroid therapy and in most circumstances it is probable that a bactericidal drug is indicated rather than a bacteriostatic drug. Adequate therapeutic doses of the antibiotic should be given and maintained for sufficient time. Another problem with the prolonged use of corticosteroids is that there is a risk of inducing permanent adrenal insufficiency, but this has produced little worry in cattle.

(3) Non-steroidal anti-inflammatory drugs (NSAIDs) (see Chapter 62). These drugs are salicylate-like compounds and although many are not registered for use in cattle, they do help reduce inflammatory reactions by blocking the synthesis of prostaglandins and inhibiting kinin formation (see p. 1050). They also antagonize the actions of some of the chemical

Table 17.4 Some non-steroidal anti-inflammatory drugs.

	Route of administration	Dose[a]
Acetyl salicylic acid	Oral	1.0–4.0 g/animal
Carprofen	Injection (i.v., s.c.)	1.4 mg/kg (0.7 mg/lb)
Flunixin meglumine	Injection (i.v.)	2.2 mg/kg (1.0 mg/lb)
Ketoprofen	Injection (i.v., i.m.)	3 mg/kg (1.5 mg/lb)
Meclofenamic acid	Oral	2.2 mg/kg (1.1 mg/lb)
Meloxicam	Injection (i.v., s.c.)	500 µg/kg (250 µg/lb)
Naproxen	Oral	10 mg/kg (5 mg/lb)
Phenylbutazone	Oral/injection	4.4 mg/kg (2.2 mg/lb)
Sodium meclophenamate		

[a] Doses are only guidelines. Note that many of the drugs are not registered for use in cattle in some countries.

mediators in the lungs such as 5-hydroxytryptamine (5-HT) and histamine, which are mainly released from mast cells in response to antibody–antigen reactions (Pirie, 1979). Besides an anti-inflammatory action, NSAIDs have two properties that corticosteroids do not possess, namely they are anti-pyretic and analgesic. Until the availability of flunixin these compounds were little used in Britain although they are frequently prescribed in Holland where corticosteroids are not allowed to be used for respiratory diseases in calves. Some of the main drugs available are shown in Table 17.4. The drugs most commonly used in Britain are carprofen, flunixin meglumine, ketoprofen and meloxicam.

(4) Antihistamines (see Chapter 62). These drugs have been used in the past but most clinicians have found them to be of little use in calf pneumonia. This is probably because the main chemical mediator of cattle is not histamine but 5-HT. The histamine that is released occurs very quickly following the antibody–antigen reaction so that antihistamines can only be of use in the early stages of the inflammatory response (Pirie, 1979).

(5) Sympathomimetics. These drugs are all adrenaline-like and their actions to a varying degree are similar to it.

Although both adrenaline and isoprenaline are of some use in relieving respiratory signs, they are little used because of their stimulatory effects on the heart. This is because adrenaline acts on many types of receptors that are designated α and β, those of the heart and lung being β_1 and β_2 receptors, respectively. Recent work has produced compounds that will act on only one type of receptor and not on the others. For various reasons including some of their other potential properties their use has been curtailed in many countries.

(6) Xanthine derivatives. Those commonly in use are etamiphylline camsylate and diprophylline, but others are available and are given. Their actions are relatively similar to those of adrenaline. There is stimulation of the central nervous system where caffeine is the most powerful, myocardial stimulation where aminophylline and diprophylline are strongest, bronchodilation and diuresis. Their main uses in respiratory disease are bronchodilation and, to a secondary extent, fluid removal. The mild action of these drugs compared with substances such as adrenaline means that they are all relatively safe.

(7) Expectorants. One drug used at present as a spasmolytic is bromhexine hydrochloride, which can be given orally or by intramuscular injection at a dose of about 0.5 mg/kg body weight for five to seven days. Its action is mainly to reduce the viscosity of mucus and thereby help in its expulsion, resulting in improved respiratory function. Other expectorants have often been used in chronic cases of coughing. These include a mixture of strychnine hydroxide, arsenic trioxide and ferric ammonium citrate given at a dose of about 5 ml orally twice daily, or diphenhydramine hydrochloride, ammonium chloride, sodium citrate and menthol at 5–10 ml orally two or three times daily. There is limited benefit form the antihistaminic action of diphenhydramine hydrochloride in cases of calf pneumonia.

(8) Antisera. Several antisera are available in some countries that have been produced either in cattle or horses against *P. multocida*, the septicaemic and pneumonic strains of *M. haemolytica* and, in some cases, diplococci. Little experimental work is available to demonstrate their efficacy or lack of it and so their use is speculative (Thomas, 1979). As has already been indicated there are numerous organisms involved in the aetiology of calf pneumonia and it would be only right to expect benefit in some cases where the organisms in the anti-sera are a major factor in the disease process.

(9) Supportive therapy. During the disease phase many animals become partially or completely anorexic

and it has been suggested that multivitamin injections, particularly of the vitamin B group, may be of use in overcoming any temporary deficiencies that might occur as the result of the low storage of vitamins (Thomas, 1979). As vitamin A is of use in epithelial repair it may be advantageous to inject this compound to ensure speedy respiratory mucosal regeneration.

(10) Nursing. As with many other diseases, although nursing is important, it is often neglected. Affected animals should be removed from the in-contact group partly to reduce spread of infection and also to allow access to feed and water away from competition. Feed supplied should be highly palatable and non-dusty to encourage uptake. The environment of the convalescent calf should include plenty of bedding, and draughts must be avoided. The provision of oxygen by means of a mask and reducing valve has been used in animals at indoor agricultural and fatstock shows.

(11) Vaccination. It is possible to obtain rapid confirmation as to the aetiology of outbreaks of calf pneumonia. If the cause is viral it is possible to use live vaccines and to vaccinate in the face of an outbreak. This can be very effective provided it is undertaken in the early stages of disease among the group. It appears to produce non-specific interferon followed by good specific immunity to the virus vaccinated against. To be effective a live vaccine needs to be used and it must be administered intranasally.

Prevention (see pp. 1007–11)

As the disease is multifactorial, preventive measures include attention to management as well as possible vaccination. Thus ensuring there are no more than 30 calves in any one air space as well as making sure that different age groups are not mixed is helpful. If disease tends to follow particular patterns it is best to alter the time of undertaking stressful procedures such as weaning, castration and disbudding. Often ensuring castration and disbudding are undertaken more than two weeks before weaning can be helpful. Increasing the duration of feeding milk substitute can also be useful, as well as ensuring weaning is not undertaken at a time when this is likely to result in pneumonia. Gradual weaning is often helpful, particularly when cattle are fed in groups on a milk dispensing machine that will provide feed throughout the 24 hours.

When calves are home-reared, it should be ensured that they receive adequate amounts of colostrum. All calves should be given adequate good quality feed. If calves are bought-in they should be examined at entry and any which show purulent ocular or nasal discharge rejected. Calves should not receive dusty or overmilled feed. As disease occurs on the same farms year after year, the time when disease starts should be noted and checked to see if it can be associated with any changes in management, etc. Calves bought as batches should be kept together and not mixed with other batches. An all-in all-out policy for rearing calves is best advocated. Ideally, calves should be reared before and after weaning in the same building for at least a month and preferably longer.

There are various vaccines available and, as might be expected with a disease of such complex aetiology, the results experienced by different farmers and veterinary surgeons are extremely variable (see p. 1007). In some cases this may be due to the type of vaccine used. It is thought that the age incidence of enzootic pneumonia may well coincide with the decline in colostral immunity. Thus peak onset of pneumonia in housed calves is often at two to four months old when concentrations of serum IgG_1, IgG_2 and IgA are at their lowest (Corbeil et al., 1984). It must also be remembered that several of the pathogens involved in the disease complex are immunosuppressive. These organisms include M. dispar, ureaplasmas and M. bovis as well as BRSV. In consequence, vaccination of calves where the organisms are already present in the animals is likely to reduce the immune response.

Dead vaccines are used to provide immunity against P. multocida and septicaemic and pneumonic strains of M. haemolytica. Following successful experiments (Gilmour et al., 1979) several M. haemolytica vaccines for serotypes 1 and 6 are now available in Britain. Killed polyvalent vaccines are used in some countries, and contain artigens such as RSV, PI_3, IBR and BVDV. They are usually administered parenterally and usually require two injections to produce immunity. Recent developments have included combined live and dead viral components of the four main antigens which are injected intramuscularly. When live vaccines are used, the integrity of the vaccine must ensure absence of other potential contaminants, both viral and other pathogens. Subsequently, modified live intranasal vaccines have been available. A study of the live IBR vaccine in the absence of disease showed virus could be isolated from most animals (10/11) and there was sero-conversion in 7/11 (Lucas et al., 1982). Although good immunity was conferred to animals by modified live vaccination, it was shown that some cattle became carriers after exposure to field strains of IBR (Nettleton & Sharp, 1980).

A dead vaccine has been produced against M. bovis, but it has had only limited success experimentally. There are several live vaccines used in Europe including ones against respiratory syncytial virus and parainfluenza III virus. A vaccine for PI_3 has been licensed and it is possible others will eventually be available in Britain and elsewhere.

From experience, the vaccines themselves do appear to have variable results on individual farms. This is probably due to the type of vaccine used, i.e. live or dead, other underlying pathogens, the level of infective dose and whether or not the particular pathogens present in the vaccine are responsible for disease on that farm. Before embarking on a vaccination programme it is important to ensure that the pathogens on the farm are correctly identified so that the programme can be introduced correctly. Such regimens will usually work well on farms housing just home produced cattle. However, there is a particular problem for farmers who continually buy in batches of calves as the pathogens introduced with each group are likely to be different. Thus it is very difficult to create a suitable vaccination policy to prevent pneumonia, unless several vaccines are used to cover most of the major pathogens. Such a policy is obviously costly and at times very wasteful as it will result in immunization for diseases that are not present. This has led to the suggestion that in such units it is best to make a diagnosis as to the likely cause of enzootic pneumonia in the first animal(s) to be affected. If the agent is primarily viral then the calves can be vaccinated in the face of an outbreak.

References

Andrews, A.H. (2000) Calf pneumonia costs! *Cattle Practice*, **8**, 109–14.

Bryson, D.G., McFerran, J.B., Ball, H.J. & Neill, S.D. (1978) Observations on outbreaks of respiratory disease in housed calves. I: Epidemiology, clinical and microbiological findings. *Veterinary Record*, **103**, 485–9.

Corbeil, L.B., Watt, B., Corbeil, R.R., Betzen, T.G., Brownson, R.K. & Morrill, J.L. (1984) Immunoglobulin concentrations in serum and nasal secretions of calves at the onset of pneumonia. *American Journal of Veterinary Research*, **45**, 773–8.

Eyre, P. (1978) Pharmacological considerations of current methods of therapy. In *Respiratory Diseases in Cattle. Current Topics in Veterinary Medicine Volume 3* (ed. by W.B. Martin), pp. 409–16. Martinus Nijhoff, The Hague.

Gilmour, N.J.L., Martin, W.B., Sharp, J.M., Thompson, D.A. & Wells, P.W. (1979) The development of vaccines against pneumonic pasteurellosis in sheep. *Veterinary Record*, **104**, 15.

Gordon, W.A.M. (1963) Environmental studies in pig housing. IV. The bacterial content of air in piggeries and its influence on disease incidence. *British Veterinary Journal*, **119**, 263–73.

Green, G.M. & Kass, E.H. (1965) The influence of bacterial species on pulmonary resistance to infection in mice subjected to hypoxia, cold stress and ethanol intoxication. *British Journal of Experimental Pathology*, **46**, 360–6.

Jones, C.R. & Webster, A.J.F. (1981) Weather-induced changes in airborne bacteria within a calf house. *Veterinary Record*, **109**, 493–4.

Lacey, J.C. (1968) The microflora of fodders associated with bovine respiratory disease. *Journal of General Microbiology*, **51**, 173–7.

Lucas, M.H., Roberts, D.H., Sands, J.J. & Westcott, D.V.E. (1982) The use of infectious bovine rhinotracheitis vaccine in a commercial veal unit: antibody response and spread of virus. *British Veterinary Journal*, **138**, 23–8.

Miller, W.M., Harkness, J.W., Richards, M.S. & Pritchard, D.G. (1980) Epidemiological studies of calf respiratory disease in a large commercial veal unit. *Research in Veterinary Science*, **28**, 267–74.

Nettleton, P.F. & Sharp, J.M. (1980) Infectious bovine rhinotracheitis virus excretion after vaccination. *Veterinary Record*, **107**, 379.

Phillips, J.I.H. (1975) Bovine respiratory disease. In *Veterinary Annual*, 15th issue (ed. by C.S.G. Grunsell & F.W.G. Hill), pp. 13–15. Wright, Bristol.

Pirie, H.M. (1979) *Respiratory Diseases of Animals*, pp. 68–70. Notes for a Postgraduate Course, Glasgow Veterinary School.

Roy, J.H.B. (1980) *The Calf*, 4th edn. Butterworth, London.

Roy, J.H.B., Stobo, J.F., Gaston, H.J.G., Anderton, P., Shotton, J.M. & Ostler, D.C. (1971) The effect of environmental temperature on the performance and health of the preruminant and ruminant calf. *British Journal of Nutrition*, **26**, 363–81.

Thomas, L.H. (1978) Disease incidence and epidemics – the situation in the UK. In *Respiratory Diseases of Cattle. Current Topics in Veterinary Medicine, Volume 3* (ed. by W.B. Martin), pp. 57–65. Martinus Nijhoff, The Hague.

Thomas, L.H. (1979) *Respiratory Disease in Housed Calves*, pp. 1–22. Booklet 2181. MAFF Publications, Middlesex.

Thomas, L.H. & Swann, R.C. (1973) Influence of colostrum on the incidence of calf pneumonia. *Veterinary Record*, **92**, 454–5.

Thomas, L.H., Wood, R.D.P. & Longland, J.M. (1978) The influence of disease on the performance of beef cattle. *British Veterinary Journal*, **134**, 152–61.

Thomson, R.G. & Gilka, F. (1974) A brief review of pulmonary clearance of bacterial aerosols emphasizing aspects of particular relevance to veterinary medicine. *Canadian Veterinary Journal*, **15**, 99–107.

Veit, H.P., Farrell, R.T. & Troutt, H.F. (1978) Pulmonary clearance of *Serratia marcescens* in calves. *American Journal of Veterinary Research*, **39**, 1646–50.

Webster, A.J.F. (1979) Housing and husbandry of the veal calf. In *Veterinary Annual*, 19th issue (ed. by C.S.G. Grunsell & F.W.G. Hill), pp. 49–53. Scientechnica, Bristol.

Webster, A.J.F. (1981a) Optimal housing criteria for ruminants. In: *Environmental Aspects of Housing for Animal Production. Proceedings of 31st Easter School*, University of Nottingham School of Agriculture (ed. by J.A. Clark), pp. 217–32. Butterworths, Sevenoaks.

Webster, A.J.F. (1981b) Weather and infectious disease in cattle. *Veterinary Record*, **108**, 83–7.

Williams, M.R., Spooner, R.P.L. & Thomas, L.H. (1975) Quantitative studies on bovine immunogobulins. *Veterinary Record*, **96**, 81–4.

Wiseman, A. (1978) Influence of environment on respiratory disease. In *Respiratory Diseases of Cattle. Current Topics in Veterinary Medicine, Volume 3* (ed. by W.B. Martin), pp. 149–57. Martinus Nijhoff, The Hague.

Chapter 18
Other Calf Problems

A.H. Andrews

Stillbirth/perinatal weak calf syndrome 249
Joint ill or navel ill 249
Oral and laryngeal necrobacillosis 250
   Oral form 250
   Laryngeal form 251
Meningitis 251
Otitis 252
Bovine papular stomatitis (BPS) 252
Calcium, phosphorus and vitamin D deficiency 253
Copper deficiency 254
Hypomagnesaemic tetany of calves 255
Vitamin A deficiency 256
Iodine deficiency 257
Iron deficiency 258
Selenium/vitamin E deficiency 258
Zinc deficiency 260
Furazolidone poisoning 260
Iodism 261
Cerebrocortical necrosis (CCN, polioencephalomalacia) 261
Urolithiasis 263

Stillbirth/perinatal weak calf syndrome

This is an important cause of losses in the young calf and has considerable economic consequences to the farmer. Very few studies have been undertaken to determine the factors involved. However work done in Northern Ireland (McCoy *et al.*, 1997) showed that nearly half (46 per cent) of the animals examined had non-inflated lungs and so were true stillbirths and another 22.7 per cent had severe trauma (mainly rib or spinal fractures) from calving. Otherwise the largest number of weak calves (36.7 per cent) had thyroid abnormalities and within the study 20 per cent had low thyroid iodine levels. Other problems were of an infectious nature including leptospirosis (13.4 per cent), pneumonia (9.1 per cent) and bacterial isolation (9 per cent); virus isolation was low.

Iodine deficiency is more common than recognized in suckler herds and dairy and suckler heifers who receive limited feed supplementation. The problem normally arises from increased calf mortality as abortion, still-births, weak calves and neonatal mortality. The calves have enlarged thyroids (greater than 14 g is suspect), parturition is slow and often there are retained placentae. Poor fertility may be seen with suboestrus and delayed ovulation, lowered milk yield, lowered libido in bulls, ill thrift in cattle and lowered herd immunity.

Joint ill or navel ill (see p. 455)

Joint or navel ill is a common problem in the calf. At birth there is a sudden change from the fetal circulation to that of the newborn calf. The blood vessels in the umbilical cord rapidly lose most of the blood within them but still remain patent, thereby allowing the introduction of infection. Infection can be caused by a single organism or a mixture. A wide variety can be involved including *Streptococcus* spp., *Escherichia coli*, *Erysipelothrix insidiosa*, *Pasteurella multocida*, *Arcanobacterium (Actinomyces, Corynebacterium) pyogenes* and *Fusobacterium necrophorum*. The problem normally arises from calving taking place in conditions with poor hygiene. Often the calf will not have had sufficient intake of colostrum and usually the navel will not have been treated. Many infections also enter via the tonsils.

Infection entering the umbilicus may result in a local reaction at the point of entry into the body, between the muscle layers or in the peritoneum. In other cases entry is via the urachus and can lead to local infection. Otherwise the bacteria may pass via the umbilical vein to the liver and then in the blood to the body. When infection is present in the blood it may cause a septicaemia or eventually result in chronic illness due to localization in organs such as the heart, brain, eye and most often the joints, leading to joint ill.

Signs

The signs vary and can be restricted to local inflammation of the navel or the abdominal wall muscles. In such cases the navel is swollen, soft and usually painful. The umbilical blood vessels are swollen at their base. Localized peritonitis may be difficult to detect. Where there is septicaemia, the calf rapidly becomes ill with depression, pyrexia (40.5°C, 105°F) and accelerated respiratory and pulse rates. The mucous membranes become reddened and there are often petechial haemorrhages. There may be a varying degree of dehydration, followed later by acidosis, recumbency and death.

In cases of bacteraemia that localize, the signs are often missed for several weeks or even months. In some animals there is inappetance, dullness and an intermittent slightly raised temperature (39–40°C, 103–104°F). Other signs depend on the organs affected. When there is local infection of the urachus the animal will become unthrifty and slightly slow to move. There may be a slightly raised tail with micturition. In animals with localization in the heart valves, endocarditis results with a heart murmur. If the eye is involved there is panophthalmitis with hypopyon. In the case of meningitis there is likely to be nystagmus, hyperaesthesia and tonic–clonic convulsions. The most common form is joint ill and one or more joints may be involved. In many cases there is bilateral involvement with pain and swelling, commonly of the carpal joints. Aspiration of the affected joints usually reveals thick pus. The animal tends to become lame and to have an altered stance.

Necropsy

Post-mortem examination may reveal the presence of infection in the umbilical vessels, which are swollen and contain blood. There may be localized peritonitis. In the septicaemic form petechial and ecchymotic haemorrhages are evident on the subserosa and submucosa of various organs. In the more chronic form various organs will show inflammation and abscessation.

Diagnosis

Diagnosis is aided by the presence of a swollen navel as well as by the signs. There may be a neutrophilia and blood culture may be helpful. The main difficulty is in differentiating the condition from other forms of enteritis, septicaemia and locomotor problems such as muscular dystrophy (see p. 258). If surgery is contemplated it is best to X-ray the joint lesions first.

Treatment and control

Treatment of the septicaemia will usually involve the use of antimicrobials, which in the main should be given intravenously. Appropriate antibiotics include amoxycillin, ampicillin, oxytetracycline, sulphonamides or potentiated sulphonamides. Chloramphenicol can be of use in some countries and florfenicol has been used successfully although not licensed for the purpose. In less severe cases other treatments such as penicillin and streptomycin may be given by the parenteral routes. The duration of therapy should be at least five days. If the animals are dehydrated, parenteral or oral electrolyte solutions will be required. In the more localized forms involving the navel or urachus, the infected material should be removed. There are problems in the treatment of localized chronic infection such as joint ill. In some cases the use of potentiated sulphonamides or lincomycin by injection has given good results. Surgical opening of the joints with removal of pus and affected tissue and joint flushing can be useful. Slow release gentamicin polymethylmethacrylate (PMMA) beads have been used in cases of septic arthritis with evidence of concurrent osteomyelitis. The beads are inserted after debridement of osteomyelitic bone via an arthrotomy incision or with arthroscopic examination. Success rates in early cases have been good (Butson, 1994).

Control is dependent on whether the calves are on their farm of origin or have been bought-in. If the former, then all navels should be dipped immediately after birth in an appropriate disinfectant. Tincture of iodine or iodine teat washes are useful for this purpose. Generally they allow the navel to be sterilized and help to cause desiccation. Antibiotic aerosols are used but it is often difficult to ensure the whole navel is completely covered. In purchased animals the navels should be examined, and calves with enlarged navels rejected. The joints of the animals should also be inspected. The navels should be dipped in an appropriate disinfectant solution on arrival at the farm.

Oral and laryngeal necrobacillosis

This is also known as calf diphtheria and there are two forms: oral which is most common, and laryngeal. The condition is caused by *Fusobacterium necrophorum*.

Oral form (see also p. 822)

This is quite common and is usually sporadic in occurrence although there may be outbreaks where hygiene is poor. In such cases it is probably spread by dirty milk pails, machine teats or feeding containers. Individual cases sometimes occur where fibrous and coarse food is offered. Although mainly seen in housed calves, it can also occur at pasture. Affected calves are usually up to three months old and often have intercurrent disease, nutritional deficiency or their teeth are erupting. The incubation period is about four days.

Signs

The major sign is a swelling of the cheek, particularly in the region of the first cheek teeth. The calf is often bright and active with a normal temperature. Opening the mouth reveals a necrotic swelling in the cheek, in which may be impacted food material, and there may be a foul smell. The animal may salivate a little. In a few cases there is also involvement of the tongue, which may become swollen and protrude from the mouth. Neglected cases may extend to the nasal cavity, pharynx, lungs, abomasum and coronets of the legs.

Necropsy

On post-mortem oral lesions are usually well circumscribed with an area of oedema and a necrotic centre. If the necrotic area is lost, an ulcer is seen.

Diagnosis

The main differential diagnoses are foreign bodies in the mouth, papular stomatitis, mouth and jaw injuries and BVD/mucosal disease. All are quite easy to eliminate by thorough oral examination.

Laryngeal form

This form is less common and is sporadic in occurrence. It has been seen in animals up to and over a year old.

Signs

These cattle tend to be dull with inappetance or anorexia. Often there is pyrexia (40.5°C, 105°F) and there may be stertor. Usually respirations are dyspnoeic to a varying degree. There may be a cough that is moist and painful. Palpation of the larynx is resented and can elicit the cough. The mouth may be foul smelling. Many of these animals do not respond well to treatment and the diphtheritic area may become detached resulting in sudden asphyxiation or lung infection.

Necropsy

The lesion in the larynx is normally well embedded into the laryngeal cartilage. When lung lesions occur there are necrotic areas present surrounded by a catarrhal pneumonia.

Diagnosis

The main differential diagnoses are laryngeal oedema, laryngitis, necrotic enteritis and vocal cord paralysis. These may be hard to eliminate unless an endoscopic examination is undertaken or an exploratory laryngotomy is performed.

Treatment

In either case the animal should be isolated from the others. It should have its own feed and water buckets.

In the oral form, parenteral or oral therapy is usually successful. Suitable antibacterial agents include oxytetracycline, potentiated sulphonamides, streptomycin, sulphonamides orally or parenterally or penicillin parenterally. Therapy for three to five days is usually sufficient in the oral form. When the animal is inappetant it should be encouraged to eat. In the laryngeal form, therapy needs to be continued for longer (e.g. 2–3 weeks) and should be parenteral. If breathing is very laboured then it may be necessary to undertake a tracheotomy and insert a tracheal tube. In some cases success is only achieved by surgical removal of the necrotic area and then using an intratracheal tube until the laryngeal oedema has reduced.

Control

If more than a single case occurs, hygiene should be improved. The calves should be fed with their own buckets and quality feed should be used. The milk and water buckets should be cleaned and disinfected after each feed and the feed bucket disinfected at least twice a week. Occasionally, it is necessary to give oral antibiotics as a prophylactic measure. Suitable agents include chlortetracycline and oxytetracycline.

Meningitis (see p. 901)

This is an inflammation of the meninges. The condition is uncommon and most often occurs following a pre-existing disease such as septicaemia. The organisms that can be involved are usually bacteria and include *Listeria monocytogenes*, *Escherichia coli*, *Pasteurella multocida* and *Haemophilus somnus*. A secondary meningitis can follow infection with *Mycobacterium bovis*. Although most cases are haematogenous in origin, a few result from spread of local infection or can follow disbudding, skull injuries, otitis media or frontal sinusitis. In most instances meningitis is the result of central infection causing local swelling and inflammation around the nerve trunks. Spinal meningitis will often lead to hyperaesthesia of the body, muscular tremors in the limbs and neck and an arched back.

Signs

The condition usually starts with a sudden onset of pyrexia and in many cases toxaemia. There is hyperaesthesia to any cutaneous sensation and muscular tremors of the neck and head with opisthotonus and paddling movements of the limbs. There may be ocular lesions with hypopyon and ophthalmitis. The animal may appear blind and the pupillary reflex may be sluggish.

Ophthalmoscopic examination may show the retinal irises to be engorged with oedema of the optic disc.

Necropsy

On post-mortem examination the meninges are thickened and opaque, especially ventrally, and there is engorgement of the meningeal vessels with haemorrhaging. The cerebrospinal fluid (CSF) is often cloudy.

Diagnosis

This is difficult in the live animal but the nervous signs are an indication and there is a leucocytosis. Confirmation can only be obtained by examination of the CSF, showing it to be cloudy with a high white cell count and possibly bacteria present. The differential diagnosis includes coccidiosis (see p. 282), septicaemia (see p. 204), vitamin A deficiency (see p. 256), hypomagnesaemia (see p. 255) and poisoning with various substances (see Chapter 54)

Treatment and control

Treatment involves the use of a broad-spectrum antimicrobial that will penetrate the blood–brain barrier. The potentiated sulphonamides or chloramphenicol in countries where available are probably most useful. Florfenicol has also been used although it is not licensed for this use. These preparations are able to diffuse into the CSF. Results of therapy are generally disappointing. Prevention is difficult but should involve the rapid treatment of all septicaemias, otitis or local injuries. Disbudding should always be undertaken with care.

Otitis (see also p. 903)

Otitis media and externa both occur. The condition has recently been more frequently diagnosed in calf-rearing units in America and Britain. The cause is unknown but most outbreaks have been preceded by enzootic pneumonia and it is thus possible that an ascending infection occurs along the Eustachian tube. In some outbreaks up to 30 per cent of calves have been involved. In individual cases of otitis media there may be extension from an otitis externa or from navel infection via the haematogenous route. The organisms involved vary but vitamin A deficiencies have been reported in some outbreaks. The external ear form is such that there are often streptococci and staphylococci present. When there is middle ear infection these two species may be present, or *M. haemolytica*, *Haemophilus* spp. or *Neisseria catarrhalis*.

Signs

In otitis externa the animal is well and has a normal temperature but the ear tends to be droopy with a foul-smelling purulent discharge. In middle ear infection, unless bilateral, the head is rotated and there is a degree of incoordination. The animal is often dull and there is inappetance. Radiography may show rarefaction of the tympanic bulla.

Diagnosis

This condition is differentiated from brain or spinal abscesses or injury by the rotation of the head.

Treatment and control

Treatment of the external form is relatively simple and involves the local application of antibiotics, in practice often from intramammary tubes. Suitable antibiotics include cloxacillin, chlortetracycline and penicillin and streptomycin. Otitis media is much less satisfactory to treat and involves puncturing the tympanic mucosa, irrigation with antiseptic solutions and local and parenteral antibiotics. Prevention is difficult as the cause is often unclear but it should involve adequate treatment of all cases of calf pneumonia.

Bovine papular stomatitis (BPS)

This is caused by a virus of the genus parapoxvirus. The condition is very common throughout the world. Lesions can occur in any age of animal and both sexes. However, most lesions are seen in young cattle. The virus causes pseudocowpox in cows (see p. 364). The organism has a high morbidity and is found in the saliva and nasal secretions. Spread is by contact. The disease is usually of little importance except in the differential diagnosis of other oral lesions, although occasionally it can be of financial significance. The condition found is variable but can be seen in calves of seven days old or more. It can be transferred to others, particularly following a bite, cut or scratch. Most lesions are local but may take many weeks to heal. Occasionally, systemic signs occur (see p. 822).

Signs

The lesions vary in severity. The mild form is the most common with the animal remaining healthy, eating well with no evidence of pyrexia, diarrhoea or respiratory distress. The lesions tend to be ring-like and pathognomonic. The periphery of the lesion is a thin red zone, within which is a white, slightly raised area of hyperplasia, with a yellow or brown centre due to tissue necrosis. Lesions heal from the middle outwards. Most involve the rhinarium and mouth and are often found near erupting teeth. Occasionally, a second type of lesion is a brownish-purple colour and usually the size of the ring lesions. It heals from the middle outwards producing a horseshoe shape lasting from four days to about two weeks. However, areas of lesions may last several months overall.

The severe form is less common and often associated with other intercurrent disease, e.g. parasitism. Lesions are slightly raised, diffuse and roughened, and are yellow or grey in colour. They are seen in any part of the mouth and can involve marked sloughing of the mucosae. As the more diffuse lesions heal, an underlying circular form often remains. In some cases saliva is held in the mouth making the lips wet.

Necropsy

Death from BPS is rare. Most lesions are in the mouth or rhinarium but may occasionally be seen in the oesophagus, rumen, reticulum and abomasum. Typically, there are no vesicles and on histology there is a ballooning degeneration of the stratum spinosum cells, which may contain eosinophilic intracytoplasmic inclusion bodies.

Diagnosis

Diagnosis is dependent on examining the lesions, the animal remaining healthy, viral isolation, histopathology and use of an electron microscope. Immunity can be measured by the serum neutralization test but levels are usually low. The main conditions to be differentiated are foot-and-mouth disease, mucosal disease, malignant catarrhal fever, rinderpest, vesicular stomatitis, BIV, BLAD and mycotic stomatitis.

Treatment

Treatment is not justified but in severe cases concurrent infections can be treated. Antibiotic therapy is recommended to resolve secondary infections. Prevention is not practical at present but the condition is less severe in healthy herds so good nutrition and freedom from parasites are important.

Calcium, phosphorus and vitamin D deficiency (see p. 462, 791)

These conditions are all closely related and it is best to consider them together. All three compounds can lead to primary and secondary deficiency, but conditions relating to their lack are very rare in calves. The diseases of the skeleton that do occur are usually associated with faulty mineral supply rather than vitamin D problems.

Calcium is well absorbed in the calf's small intestine. Therefore, primary deficiency is extremely unlikely, as is secondary deficiency, which could possibly occur if very high levels of cereals were fed without additives or high phosphorus levels were used. The daily calcium requirement of calves is 10–30 g ($\frac{1}{3}$–1 oz) depending on size and growth rate.

Phosphorus is very efficiently absorbed from milk, but less so from dry feeds. Primary deficiencies may resemble rickets. Secondary problems resulting from low vitamin D levels, high calcium or high vitamin A are rare. Phosphorus deficiency is widespread due to the types of soil present in an area. Leaching by rain or constant removal by cropping can lead to phosphorus-deficient soil. Excessive calcium, iron or aluminium can also result in the problem. The optimum calcium : phosphorus ratio is 2 : 1.

Vitamin D is usually provided by good quality hay and exposure to sunlight. Present feeding systems include supplementation of milk substitutes and so do not normally predispose to the problem, although lush green feeds contain much carotene and other substances that have anti-vitamin D properties. The optimal daily intake is 7–12 iu/kg body weight (3.5–6 iu/lb).

Signs

The signs are usually only seen in the best-growing calves. There is some degree of lameness, particularly of the forelimbs, which are bent forwards or laterally. The limb joints and costochondral junctions are swollen. In some calves the back will be arched and in severe cases the tail is elevated. There may be a marked tendency to lie down.

Necropsy

On death the animal is in poor condition. The ribs are easily cut and the limb bones are soft with thin, compact bone and they are easily fractured. The joints tend to be enlarged with thickened epiphyseal cartilage.

Diagnosis

Diagnosis is usually on clinical signs. The alkaline phosphatase level will be raised. The levels of serum calcium and phosphorus will depend on the cause of the condition but phosphorus will be low if it is due either to vitamin D or phosphorus deficiency. Radiographic examination shows the bones to lack density and the ends have a diffuse appearance. The epiphyses tend to be widened and irregular. The ash content of the bone is reduced from 60 per cent to 45 per cent and the ash:organic matter ratio will be reduced from the normal 3:2. The main problems to be differentiated are copper deficiency (but the plasma and/or liver copper concentrations will be low), arthritis and epiphysitis.

Treatment and prevention

Treatment varies according to the cause. In minor Ca:P imbalances sufficient vitamin D is all that is necessary. Where the skeletal deformities are pronounced, treatment will have only limited effect. Otherwise in calcium deficiency check there is no excess phosphorus present. Calcium should be provided but not to excess as this may cause other deficiencies. If phosphorus is deficient, dicalcium phosphorus or disodium phosphate should be used. The ratio of calcium:phosphorus of 2:1 should be provided by the diet. A vitamin D injection of 3000–5000iu/kg body weight will provide adequate levels for one to three months. Response to treatment is usually slow. Prevention requires ensuring adequate levels of minerals and vitamin D in the diet. Bone meal and dicalcium phosphate are ideal sources of both calcium and phosphorus but they are expensive and cannot be used in many countries. Ground limestone is a useful cheap method of ensuring adequate calcium in the diet, but its overuse can result in other mineral deficiencies.

Copper deficiency (see Chapter 21)

This is either primary due to a lack of copper in the diet or secondary when the dietary level is adequate but there is a failure in digestion, absorption or metabolism of the copper. In calves, deficiency can be seen at a few weeks old although it is much more common when three or four months old. This is because copper is stored in the liver and there is preferential absorption from the dam. Milk contains little copper although levels are high in colostrum. In the milk-fed animal absorption in the small intestine is high (up to 80 per cent) but this falls as the animal becomes a ruminant (2–10 per cent). Milk substitutes tend to be supplemented with copper and so most cases arise in calves sucking their dams or at grass. Problems often occur in the spring or summer when the mineral content tends to be lower.

Primary deficiency depends on the soil type and is common on sandy soil, particularly where there is much rain and leaching, and on peat. Secondary deficiencies are probably more numerous than primary. They can be due to high molybdenum levels and this effect is increased by the presence of sulphur, which may be in the form of protein. High levels of iron, zinc, lead, cadmium and calcium carbonate also reduce copper absorption.

Copper is concerned with the formation of cytochrome oxidase, which regulates oxidation processes and electron transfer in tissues. It is also part of the enzyme lysyl oxidase, which is used for elastin or collagen synthesis and deficiency results in skeletal defects and blood vessel fragility. Copper is also present in caeruloplasmin, which releases iron from stores into plasma for erythropoiesis and deficiency results in anaemia.

Signs

The signs of *primary deficiency* are that the calves have a reduced growth rate; sometimes there is a scour but not usually as pronounced as in secondary deficiency. There may be a stilted gait with some ataxia developing after exercise, but recovery occurs after rest. Ribs and limb bones may develop spontaneous fractures, the shaft thickness may be reduced and there is osteoporosis. Thickened epiphyses, particularly in the fetlock region, may be noted, and stiffness of the joints.

Secondary deficiency is usually seen in calves sucking the dam or grazing. There is again a stiff gait and unthriftiness. Molybdenosis is characterized by severe scours. Some calves become very lame with epiphyses that are painful to palpate and usually the distal ends of the metapodial bones are enlarged. On radiography there is a thickened irregular epiphyseal plate, and the metaphyses are thickened. In some animals depigmentation of the hair occurs.

Necropsy

On post mortem there is usually emaciation with anaemia seen as thin, watery blood and pale tissues. Where copper levels are low there are deposits of haemosiderin in the liver, kidney and spleen. The limb bones may show evidence of rarefaction and fracture. A thickening of the epiphyseal plates, particularly of the metapodial bones, may be present. In the small intestine there may be villous atrophy. Histologically, the bones show osteoporosis.

Diagnosis

In practice the majority of cases are diagnosed because of the area where the animals have lived, and most calves will be sucking a cow or at pasture. The signs give an indication of the condition and it usually affects several animals. Examination can involve looking for anaemia with a reduced erythrocyte count ($2–4 \times 10^{12}$/l;

normal, $5–10 \times 10^{12}$/l) and low blood haemoglobin (5–8 g/100 ml; normal, 8–15 g/100 ml). Plasma copper levels are low (normal, >15 μmol/l; deficient, <0.9 μmol/l) as are liver levels (normal, 100–200 ppm dry matter (DM); deficient, <50 ppm DM). Cytochrome oxidase (normal, >7.0 μmol/g wet liver) and caeruloplasmin levels are low. Copper can also be estimated in the diet, pasture and soil. Often response to copper therapy gives an indication.

Treatment

When therapy is undertaken it is important to confirm the presence of copper deficiency, as overdosing is toxic. Oral administration of 1.5 g copper sulphate weekly is very useful, but requires constant handling of the calves. Parenteral administration of copper can overcome the problem. Copper sulphate has been used at a dose level of 200 mg/calf. A methionine copper complex can be administered as a deep intramuscular injection at a dose of 40 mg/calf, as can diethylamine copper oxyquinoline sulphonate at a rate of 0.24 mg/kg body weight by subcutaneous injection and copper edetate as a subcutaneous injection of 50 mg. Experiments in sheep have shown high doses of copper methionine subcutaneously to be safer than calcium copper edetate and diethylamine copper oxyquinoline (Mahmoud & Ford, 1981) but it was considered that this might have been the result of the rapidity of absorption depending on the route of injection. A comparison of the efficacy of copper preparations in cattle showed copper edetate to be best with copper diethylamine oxyquinoline sulphonate 19 per cent worse, aqueous copper methionate 36–48 per cent worse, and cupric sulphate producing the second-best result. The injections also cause a local reaction, with copper diethylamine oxyquinoline sulphonate giving least damage, copper edetate producing an intermediate reaction and copper methionate causing most swelling (Suttle, 1981a).

Prevention

Prevention is to ensure that the level of copper in the diet of dams and calves is at least 10 mg/kg dry matter of feed. When deficiency has been determined it may be necessary routinely to inject or drench the cattle. However, no such programme should be undertaken unless a sample of the animals has been checked to ensure blood copper levels are low. The timing of the first injection (in severely affected herds) is at about six weeks old, but subsequent injections need to be based on further blood sampling. Copper sulphate can be used as a drench at a level of 1.5 g weekly. Cupric oxide needles have been used to alleviate hypocupraemia in heifers (Suttle, 1981b). A form of soluble glass has been used to release copper slowly from an intraruminal bolus. The use of pasture dressing annually with 5.6 kg/ha (5 lb/acre) copper sulphate is effective. As there is a possibility of poisoning, animals should not graze the pasture until after heavy rain or three weeks after application. The copper supplementation of water has been advocated (Farmer *et al.*, 1982). Salt licks containing 0.5 per cent copper sulphate are safe in use but are not permitted in all countries.

Hypomagnesaemic tetany of calves (see p. 787)

The condition occurs most commonly in calves on high-milk or milk-substitute intakes that are receiving little other feed. It results from a hypomagnesaemia that may be associated with hypocalcaemia. The young calf has a serum magnesium level similar to the dam and receives extra magnesium in its colostrum. However, milk is deficient in this element and if it constitutes most of the feed then there will be a gradual fall in circulating magnesium levels. This is partly allayed by the absorption of magnesium from bones. The calf is also able to absorb magnesium very efficiently from the small and large intestine in early life but this capacity reduces so that by three months old it becomes poor. The problem is often seen in veal or suckler calves after two months of age. Occasionally, hypomagnesaemia is seen in the young calf about two weeks old and this is due to poor absorption, which can occur with diarrhoea, the feeding of liquid paraffin or the use of fibrous feed, which increases salivation and thereby causes the body to lose magnesium. A calf requires 1–5 g daily, according to size and growth rate.

Signs

In the early stages there is hyperexcitability to stimuli with increased ear movements, interspersed with the ears being held back. There tends to be opisthotonus, ataxia and head shaking. The animal may have trouble drinking from a bucket on the ground. The temperature is normal and the pulse rate rapid. Later on there are muscular fasciculations with jaw champing, frothing at the mouth and a spastic gait. Convulsions may occur starting with the calf stamping its feet, pricking its ears, retracting its eyelids and the head being held up. The animal may fall and show tonic–clonic movements of the legs with uncontrolled passage of urine and faeces, a fast pulse over 200/minute with heart sounds audible away from the chest and respirations ceasing. The temperature is often raised to 40.5°C (105°F) due to muscular exertion. If the convulsions are severe the pulse is often imperceptible, cyanosis develops and the animal dies within about 30 minutes. In some cases there are periods of relative normality between bouts of convulsions.

Necropsy

On post-mortem examination there is usually extensive haemorrhage and congestion of the organs including the aorta, mesentery, pericardium, gall-bladder and intercostal walls.

Diagnosis

Diagnosis depends on the history of the feeding regimen used or presence of diarrhoea as well as the signs present and serum magnesium levels (normal, 0.9–1.4 mmol/l, 2.2–3.4 mg/100 ml). Clinical signs may occur at 0.12–0.33 mmol/l (0.3–0.8 mg/100 ml). In animals that die the Ca:Mg ratio in the caudal vertebrae or rib bone is increased from a normal of 70:1 often to over 90:1. The aspartate aminotransferase and creatine kinase levels also tend to be raised because of the increased muscular activity. The main differential diagnoses involve conditions resulting in clonic convulsions. These include tetanus (but the course is usually longer) (see p. 733), arsenic, lead or mercury poisoning (but in all these there is colic and diarrhoea and with lead there is blindness). Strychnine poisoning can occur and results in a stiff gait. Hypovitaminosis A may well result in night blindness. Encephalitis (which may be viral or bacterial in origin) or meningitis may be difficult to determine. *Clostridium perfringens* (*welchii*) type D produces apparent blindness and a raised blood glucose level (normal, 2.5 mmol/l, 45 mg/100 ml).

Treatment and prevention

Treatment should include the use of magnesium sulphate (50 ml of 25 per cent solution) subcutaneously and possibly calcium borogluconate intravenously. Magnesium given intravenously can lead to medullary depression and cardiac embarrassment. If necessary the animal should be sedated with acepromazine or xylazine. When the problem is the result of diarrhoea then this should be rectified. The condition in the older calf is prolonged and there will be greatly reduced magnesium levels in bone, etc. Thus these animals will need to be supplemented with 2–4 g magnesium oxide or 4–8 g magnesium carbonate daily.

Prevention involves the provision of roughage, usually as good quality hay, from ten days of age. This is difficult in suckler calves but can be overcome by feeding the cows with magnesium oxide (calcined magnesite) at a level of 60 g daily. Magnesium can also be given to calves in the form of magnesium boluses or in molassed creep feed.

Vitamin A deficiency

The condition results from a deficiency of the fat-soluble vitamin A or its dietary precursor carotene. Secondary deficiency can arise where there is sufficient vitamin A/carotene in the diet but it does not reach a normal tissue level due to a failure in digestion, absorption or metabolism. In calves the condition may result in skeletal changes, which can affect the brain or spinal cord. The condition can be congenital or postnatal and is often partly due to the nutritional status of the dam. Usually, a diet of green food will provide sufficient of the precursor carotene and hence vitamin A. Thus problems do not occur at pasture until there are periods of prolonged drought, which can cause deficiency in the calves of affected dams or beef calves about six months old.

The condition is more common in housed animals fed diets likely to be deficient in vitamin A such as straw, cereals or sugar beet pulp. The dam's nutrition is important in that carotene in green food does not pass across the placental barrier until it is converted to vitamin A. It can then be taken up by the fetus and stored in the liver, as also can the vitamin A in water-soluble injections or fish oils. Colostrum is a major source of vitamin A for the calf and the introduction of extra carotene or vitamin A to the dam's diet precalving can be useful. The vitamin A requirement for a pregnant cow is about 80 iu/kg body weight daily and that for a calf is about 40 iu/kg.

Calves that are fast-growing, stressed or in a high environmental temperature require more vitamin A. Many factors that influence the vitamin A and carotene contents of feeds can lead to secondary deficiencies. Vitamins C and E help to prevent vitamin A loss, and the uptake of the vitamin is inversely proportional to the phosphate present in the diet. The vitamin is not very stable and so pelleting of the rations, storage at high temperatures and rancidity all decrease the content of the diet. Wood preservatives such as chlorinated naphthalenes inhibit carotene conversion to vitamin A and prolonged oral use of liquid paraffin or other mineral oils can produce a deficiency. Vitamin A is used to produce visual purple for the retina, normal epithelium and bone, and for normal CSF absorption.

Signs (see p. 925)

Congenital: Calves are born blind due to impingement of bone on the optic nerve. Other signs are due to increased CSF resulting in syncope with the calves showing tonic–clonic convulsions, ventral flexion of the head and neck, retraction of the eyeballs and tetanic closure of the eyelids. The calves are not blind. They may die during convulsions. In some outbreaks the affected calves develop severe diarrhoea and occasionally otitis media.

Postnatal: One of the most common lesions is the presence of large amounts of brown, bran-like scales in the coat and this is particularly seen in fast-growing animals. A reduction in growth rate may occur but is usually also the result of other deficiencies combining with that of vitamin A. Classical xenophthalmia with thickening and whitening of the cornea is unusual. When it does occur, it may be accompanied by serous ocular discharge. Nervous signs usually start with ataxia and weakness of the hind limbs and then the forelimbs. Increase in CSF pressure results in nerve compression and can lead to fainting with animals showing tonic–clonic convulsions for up to half a minute. The signs are similar to those for congenitally affected animals. Night blindness is more likely to be seen in yearling cattle.

Necropsy

Following death it may be possible to see the constrictions of the optic nerve, or the cranial cavity or vertebral cord may be reduced in size leading to injury to the spinal nerve roots. Histologically, there is squamous metaplasia of the interlobular ducts of the parotid salivary gland that is pathognomonic. The epithelium of the prepuce, reticulum and rumen shows hyperkeratosis. The liver may show focal necrotic areas.

Diagnosis

Diagnosis depends on post-mortem findings, plus a history of a lack of green feed and the signs. The deficiency can be confirmed by determining plasma vitamin A levels (normal, 25 μg/100 ml; deficient, <10 μg/100 ml) and CSF pressure (normal, <100 mm H_2O).

The condition needs to be differentiated from hypomagnesaemia where the animal is not blind, lead poisoning where there is abdominal pain, tetanus where there is no blindness and *Clostridium perfringens* (*welchii*) type D where there are high blood glucose levels. Bacterial and viral encephalitis and meningitis (see p. 251) usually result in pyrexia.

Treatment and prevention

Treatment involves the parenteral administration of aqueous vitamin A at a rate of 400 iu/kg body weight. The animals often respond quickly to treatment even where convulsions are occurring. Subsequently, an adequate level of vitamin A should be present in the diet to provide 40 iu/kg body weight. Often in practice daily allowances are doubled. Green feed or early-cut hay, good quality silage or dried grass should be given. However, very high daily levels of vitamin A supplementation in the diet can lead to exostoses on the digits and loss of epiphyseal cartilage. This produces lameness, ataxia and poor hoof development. Where it is difficult to supplement the diet, injections of vitamin A can be used every two months at 5000 iu/kg body weight, but dietary supplementation should be the primary aim.

Iodine deficiency (see p. 301, 586)

This can be the result of a primary lack of iodine. Secondary deficiency is recorded following high intakes of brassicas, high calcium ingestion, heavy bacterial contamination of feed or water, a low level intake of linseed meal or other plants containing cyanogenetic glycosides. Iodine deficiency occurs in most parts of the world where there is a high rainfall and there is little exposure to oceanic iodine. Soils with a high calcium content are likely to be deficient. The condition is mainly seen in the newborn calf of a deficient dam, usually in suckler herds. Iodine forms part of the hormone thyroxine, and a deficiency will result in the pituitary increasing the production of thyrotrophic hormone. This in turn leads to goitre. Calves born alive are prone to die if chilled, etc.

Signs

Many of the affected calves are aborted or stillborn and usually there is evidence of thyroid enlargement (goitre). If the animal is born alive it will be weak and disinclined to suck. Occasionally, the gland will be felt to pulsate. Very rarely areas of alopecia are apparent. The cow is often slow in calving.

Necropsy

The thyroid glands are enlarged and heavier than usual (normal fresh weight 6.5 g; a weight greater than 14 g is suspect). Histologically, there is thyroid hyperplasia.

Diagnosis

Diagnosis depends on the area or a diet containing goitrogenic plants. There is thyroid enlargement in the calves and several heifers or cows abort or produce stillborn or weak calves. Plasma protein-bound iodine levels are low (normal, 24–140 μg/l). The plasma inorganic iodine can be used (optimum 100–300 μg/l;

marginal 50–100 μg/l; low 20–50 μg/l; very low <20 μg/l). Most (90 per cent) of circulating iodine is bound as thyroxine and normal values are 36–89 μg/l (80–160 nmol/l). The thyroid weight is increased and the iodine content of the gland is low (normal, 15.6–39.0 mmol/kg DM; deficient, 9.5 mmol/kg DM). Differential diagnosis is mainly to eliminate other causes of abortion (see Chapter 37).

Treatment and prevention

Treatment is to ensure that the calf sucks and is kept in a warm, draught-free environment. Thyroid extract can be used at a dose of 1–2 mg/kg body weight (0.5–1 mg/lb). Intravenous sodium iodide can be used at a dose of 5–7 g for the young calf, but it is not without risk; potassium iodide can be used orally at about 3 g per calf. Iodism (iodine poisoning) can sometimes develop (see p. 261).

Prevention involves allowing the dams adequate iodine in the diet. A recommended level is 0.8 mg/kg DM for pregnant and lactating cows. The level for calves should be 0.12 mg/kg DM. Pouring on to the coat 7 ml of 5 per cent tincture of iodine weekly can be helpful. One millilitre of tincture of iodine per cow per day in the water or 800 mg potassium iodide per cow every two weeks by drench or added to the drinking water can work. Injections of iodized poppy seed oil can assist. A bolus of 3400 mg iodine with selenium and cobalt can release iodine for five to six months. Some fertilizers are high in iodine and seaweed meal can be given in the feed and typically contains 50–100 mg/kg DM iodine.

Iron deficiency

Iron deficiency is not common in cattle and the primary condition is mainly seen in veal calves without access to roughage. The secondary condition usually follows heavy infestation with sucking lice such as *Haematopinus eurysternus* and *Linognathus vituli* or after haemorrhage. The primary condition can occur in veal calves or others fed predominantly raw milk or unsupplemented milk substitute. The calf has only sufficient iron for about three weeks after birth and milk is a poor source of iron. In the case of veal calves there is an attempt to maintain iron levels low to keep the meat white. Over half the iron in the body is in the form of haemoglobin with small amounts present in myoglobin and in enzymes used for oxygen utilization. The normal blood haemoglobin values for adult cattle are 8.0–15.0 g/100 ml. However, the value in a calf at birth is 12.9 g/100 ml, dropping to 10.4 g/100 ml on a diet of milk and solid feed (Holman, 1956). The calf's daily iron requirement is 50 g and as only about 2–4 g are received

from the cow's milk there is a need to supplement with hay, straw and cereals. The only source of iron for veal calves on slats without roughage is the milk substitute and this needs to be supplemented. Levels less than 19 mg soluble iron/kg DM of feed are likely to result in problems.

Signs

The main sign is a reduction in appetite followed by reduced weight gain. The mucous membranes tend to become pale, but death is extremely rare.

Necropsy

Necropsy findings are of pale muscles with the blood thin and watery and clotting slowly. The liver tends to be enlarged and there is moderate anaemia. Diagnosis depends on the history of the diet and signs. It can be confirmed by haematological examination demonstrating a reduced erythrocyte count and low haemoglobin value. The serum iron level is low (normally 30 mol/l, 167 μg/100 ml when born, reducing to 12 μmol/l, 67 μg/100 ml at three weeks). The main differential diagnoses are those of copper and cobalt deficiency but signs additional to the anaemia will be present.

Treatment and prevention

Treatment usually involves the injection of 1 g of iron weekly to each calf as iron dextran or 0.5–1.0 g iron as ferric polygalactofuranose. Vitamin B$_{12}$ is also often used at levels of 5–10 μg/kg body weight. Prevention is by supplying milk substitute containing an iron concentration of 25–30 mg/kg DM. This will ensure that the animal has a normal appetite and growth and it will help to produce pale meat suitable for veal (Bremner *et al.*, 1976). This is because the level is sufficient to give an acceptable blood haemoglobin without there being enough to produce much myoglobin. Most milk substitutes for calf rearing contain considerably more iron.

Selenium/vitamin E deficiency

(see p. 302)

Vitamin E and/or selenium can be deficient and result in muscular dystrophy, also known as white muscle or fish flesh disease. It can be seen at any age after birth. Selenium deficiency is mainly dependent on the area where crops are produced. Soils derived from granite or pumice are deficient. Alkaline soils encourage selenium absorption by plants. The condition appears to be becoming increasingly important, probably due to the increased cost of bought-in feeds causing farmers to use more home-produced crops for their animals. The accepted level of selenium in feeds is 0.1 mg/kg DM. Selenium is mainly used by the body in the production of the enzyme glutathione peroxidase.

Vitamin E deficiency is much more dependent on the type of crop grown and its storage, etc. Vitamin E levels tend to be high in green pasture, silage, dried grass or kale. Adequate levels of the vitamin are also present in cereal grains, well-cured fresh hay, maize silage and brewers' grains, but deficiencies can occur on poor quality hay, straw or root crops unless there is a suitable supplement provided. Vitamin E tends to deplete with storage. Calf diets high in unsaturated fatty acids, as can occur where cod liver oil, fishmeal, soya bean meal or linseed oil are fed, may become deficient due to their oxidation, resulting in rancidity and the destruction of vitamin E. Storage of grains when wet or with propionic acid can also reduce the vitamin E level. Normal levels for growing cattle are considered to be 150 mg of α-tocopherol, and for the calf, milk substitutes should contain antioxidants and 300 iu/kg DM α-tocopherol.

The condition affects muscles, particularly cardiac, skeletal and diaphragmatic. Deficiency can occur in suckler calves sucking mothers with low selenium or vitamin E levels or in artificially reared calves on deficient diets. The condition results from unsaturated fatty acids entering the muscle cells where they accumulate. They are oxidized to lipid peroxides, which result in degeneration and calcification. It is believed vitamin E helps prevent lipid peroxide formation within the muscle cells whereas selenium compounds with many unsaturated points are known as polyunsaturated fatty acids and these are particularly common in vegetable oils, which therefore predispose to peroxide formation.

Signs

The signs vary in degree and in the sudden death syndrome the calf appears perfectly healthy but while drinking or normally within 30 minutes of feeding the animal will suddenly collapse. Death is usually within a minute of collapse. Mortality is 100 per cent.

Acute muscular dystrophy is again sudden in origin. The animal becomes dull and lies in lateral recumbency. There is respiratory distress, a heart rate often elevated to 150–200 beats/minute and irregular. The rectal temperature is normal, the calf is fully conscious and has normal eye reflexes. Most calves die within 6–18 hours and the mortality approaches 100 per cent.

The most common form seen is subacute muscular dystrophy and the morbidity is variable between about 10 and 40 per cent of calves. The signs depend on the muscles affected. The animal may stand stiffly; it is reluctant to move and when it does it may have a stiff gait. The calf is often weak and will not stand for long.

However, it is fully conscious with normal appetite, normal temperature and usually normal respiratory rate, but the heart rate may be raised. In many cases the gait is abnormal and it moves by rotation of the hocks. In some cases the affected muscles are swollen and firm on palpation. It has been shown that there is increased susceptibility to infectious diseases such as calf pneumonia due to delayed lymphocytic response.

Necropsy

On necropsy of calves with the sudden death syndrome there are often no macroscopic lesions. Other cases may show congestion of the liver and lungs. The heart shows a slight pallor of the myocardium. Histologically, lesions not otherwise apparent can be detected with a haematoxylin basic fuchsin–picric acid method and these are considered to be peracute myocardial degeneration. In acute muscular dystrophy there are localized streaks in the diaphragm and skeletal muscles. In the latter they tend to be bilaterally symmetrical white or grey areas in the muscles. In the heart there may be cardiac hypertrophy and myocardial degeneration with pulmonary congestion and oedema. Histologically, there is no inflammation but changes vary and include hyaline degeneration and coagulative necrosis. In subacute muscular dystrophy there is usually no cardiac involvement but the skeletal muscles show bilateral grey or white areas.

Diagnosis

Diagnosis depends on the area and diet provided as well as the signs. Decreased glutathione peroxidase levels occur (normal >23 iu/ml RBC) and the normal level of selenium in the blood is 0.63 µmol/l. There are raised plasma creatine phosphokinase and aspartate transaminase levels. The blood vitamin E level normal range is 3.0 to 18.0 µmol/l and it will be low in deficiency. Otherwise liver and kidney levels of selenium can be examined (normal, 3 and 30 µmol/kg DM). Response to treatment can be determined as a means of diagnosis.

Treatment

Therapy can involve the use of vitamin E and/or selenium depending on the cause of deficiency. The dose of DL₂-α-tocopherol acetate is about 6 iu/kg body weight. Selenium can be injected as 0.1–0.15 mg/kg sodium selenite. Long-acting selenium injections are obtainable. The combined injections have become available and produce acceptable results. Selenium can also be given in the form of reticular bullets or in soluble glass. The diet should provide sufficient vitamin E and selenium. Cows with calves at foot or in late pregnancy can be given a combined vitamin E/selenium injection to supplement their calves.

Prevention

For prevention, growing calves should be given a supplement at the rate 0.1 p.p.m. selenium of the total ration and 150mg/head of α-tocopherol daily. Cows should receive a supplement of vitamin E during the last two months of pregnancy. Injections of selenium and vitamin E can be used; selenium bullets or soluble glass intraruminal boluses are also of value. Pastures can be top-dressed with fertilizer containing sodium selenite 75–150g/ha (1–2oz/acre) or foliage dusting or spraying can be undertaken at 17.5g/ha (¼oz/acre). Analysis of pasture should be undertaken to determine that toxic levels of selenium are not produced; this can occur at levels of 0.5mg/kg. Selenium can be added to the drinking water.

Zinc deficiency

This can be either primary due to a lack of zinc, or secondary due to impaired uptake. It is usually seen in calves from six to ten weeks old, particularly in the period after weaning, and most commonly they are housed. Usually, calves do not show signs on diets containing 40 ppm zinc, but it is probable that calcium and highly fibrous diets reduce zinc availability and perhaps low copper levels reduce uptake. A congenital skin condition occurs in Friesian calves resulting in an increase in requirement (see p. 181).

Signs

Signs usually occur about two weeks after the deficient diet is introduced. The main signs are of poor growth with possible stunting. There is alopecia and parakeratosis often affecting the limbs, muzzle, vulva, anus and tail head. There are fewer lesions on the main part of the body. In some cases any wounds or abrasions will take longer to heal. Most animals do not die but skin biopsies show increased thickness of all skin components and the stratum corneum contains nucleated epidermal cells.

Diagnosis

Diagnosis is partly on the lesions and a biopsy shows parakeratosis. Normal plasma zinc levels are 9–18µmol/l (80–120µg/100ml). Serum alkaline phosphatase, albumin and amylase levels fall whereas serum globulin levels rise. The calves usually start to respond to therapy in about a week.

Treatment and prevention

Treatment involves oral medication with zinc sulphate at a level of 2g weekly, or 1g weekly by injection is useful. Any calcium oversupplementation should be corrected and fibrous roughage should be reduced. A diet containing 50 p.p.m. zinc should prevent the condition. Weekly oral medication with 0.5g zinc sulphate can be helpful. Long-term control can be obtained with zinc-containing fertilizer.

Furazolidone poisoning (see p. 941)

Furazolidone was a common form of prophylactic medication in calves, which can result in problems of toxicity. However, its use is now banned in many countries. There are two syndromes, one of which (the acute) involves overdosing at levels of 20–30mg/kg body weight and the classic condition results from long-term feeding of low levels, often 2mg/kg. Both are usually the result of poor mixing, which allows some animals in a group to receive more than the others. Mortality in both cases is high and the chronic form may be seen several days after furazolidone feeding ceases.

Signs

In the acute form there are nervous signs with hyperexcitability, including muscle tremors, arched back and possibly circling, convulsions and death normally within a few days. When the chronic condition occurs there tend to be necrotic lesions and haemorrhages in the mouth and lower gut. This results in melaena or dysentery.

Necropsy

After death few lesions are seen in the acute condition but when chronic there are haemorrhages and necrosis in the alimentary tract. Haemorrhages are present on the peritoneal and pleural surfaces and there is decreased myelopoiesis in the bone marrow.

Diagnosis

Diagnosis depends on the signs and feeding the compound and can be confused with bracken poisoning (see p. 946) or anthrax (see p. 717).

Treatment and prevention

Little therapy can be given in either case but in the acute form furazolidone feeding should be stopped at once. Noise should be kept to a minimum and excitement should be avoided. Sedatives such as acepromazine, xylazine or magnesium sulphate can be helpful. In the chronic form little can be done, except perhaps to give blood transfusions. Prevention, where allowed, involves the correct dosage of furazolidone being offered to calves and it should be thoroughly mixed. If given with milk substitute from a bulk container the milk must be constantly agitated. Furazolidone in the micronized form or combined with diethyl sulphoxide or other nitrofurans will reduce the risk. Therapy with furazolidone in those countries where still allowed, whether medicinal or prophylactic, should not be repeated.

Iodism (see pp. 302, 823)

The overuse of sodium or potassium iodide in therapy for conditions such as actinobacillosis, iodine deficiency or ringworm can lead to iodism. The signs depend partly on the form of administration. If intravenous the animal can show considerable discomfort with dyspnoea, staggering and tachycardia. When given subcutaneously there may be swelling following injection for about two days and local discomfort for about two hours after administration. In the oral form the coat becomes stary, with a scaly skin and often a fine, white dandruff. There is excessive lacrimation and nasal discharge with, in some cases, a degree of inappetance. If problems arise in treatment from the intravenous route then the iodine should be given subcutaneously or orally. When signs occur following oral administration, treatment should be discontinued.

Cerebrocortical necrosis (CCN, polioencephalomalacia)

Aetiology

It is a deficiency of thiamine caused by endogenous thiaminase. Thiaminase has been found to be produced by *Clostridium sporongenes* and certain *Bacillus* spp. which can be found in cases of CCN. However, this does not mean they are the only factors (see p. 903).

Occurrence

It is a sporadic condition which can occasionally occur as outbreaks. Most animals affected are fast-growing, well-nourished animals between 6 and 18 months old. It can occur following deprivation of food followed by good grazing or feeding with concentrate.

Similar syndromes can be produced experimentally by feeding large amounts of bracken or horsetail which contain high levels of thiaminase. Amprolium is also a specific thiamine antagonist and has also been used experimentally. Molasses toxicity results in a similar problem due to a fall in the proprionate levels. Thiamine is naturally synthesized in the rumen. It forms an essential component of several enzymes used in glucolysis in the brain. Deficiency in thiamine results in increased blood pyruvate levels and a decrease in the lactate : pyruvate ratio as well as a depression of the erythrocyte transketolase level. This causes an interference with normal carbohydrate metabolism and the cerebral cortex in particular requires the oxidative metabolism of glucose.

It is possible that thiamine deficiency might have a direct metabolic effect on the neurones, particularly in the calf which is very dependent on the pentose pathway of metabolism in which the transketolase enzyme limits the rate of activity. Thiamine pyrophosphate is a coenzyme for several carbohydrate metabolic reactions and it is associated with transketolase in the pentose pathway of glucose oxidation. There tend to be marked cerebral oedema and cerebral necrosis and the signs are mainly the result of an increase in intracranial pressure.

The morbidity is usually low but occasionally up to 25 per cent. However, mortality can be 25 to 50 per cent if not treated early, with higher levels in young cattle (six to nine months) than older ones.

Signs

In acute cases there is a sudden onset of nervous signs including blindness, muscle tremors, particularly of the head and neck, head pressing, jaw champing and frothy salivation. Animals tend to be hard to handle and in the early stages signs may be intermittent. Although the animal appears blind, and the menace reflex is absent, the palpebral and pupillary reflexes are present. The convulsive signs soon become continuous with the animal becoming recumbent. The signs are then of opisthotonus, nystagmus, optic disc oedema, often strabismus and clonic–tonic convulsions which become worse when the animal is stimulated. The temperature is normal, the ruminal movements are normal but the heart rate is variable. Calves often die in one to two days although older animals show signs for a longer period. Recovery following therapy may well take two to four days or longer.

The signs of the subacute form last for a few hours to several days and include blindness, head pressing and standing. The condition will resolve in some cases. However, in an outbreak of CCN some of the animals show anorexia, partial impairment of eyesight and a mild depression. Almost all of the subacute animals recover within 24 hours of therapy.

Although recovery may occur, some animals may still remain blind. The longer the time between onset of signs and therapy, the less favourable the prognosis. When cattle remain dull and anorexic after three days' treatment they are unlikely to recover and should be slaughtered.

Necropsy

Most of the animals do not show any gross changes in the body other than the brain. There is usually increased intracranial pressure with a yellowing and compression of the dorsal cortical gyri. The cerebellum tends to be compressed into the foramen magnum and recovered animals show decortication of the motor area and occipital lobes. Histologically there is bilateral necrosis of the dorsal occipital and parietal cerebral cortex and also, occasionally, the thalamus, basal ganglia, lateral geniculate bodies and mesencephalic nuclei. Cerebellar lesions also occur.

Diagnosis

Diagnosis can be made from the following:

(1) History – age of animals, a change in feeding and the condition of the animal.
(2) Signs – blindness, normal palpebral and pupillary reflexes; normal ruminal movements, normal temperature but otherwise many nervous signs.
(3) Blood pyruvate and lactate levels are increased.
(4) Urine pyruvate levels increased.
(5) Erythrocyte transketolase activity reduced (Table 18.1).
(6) Pyruvate kinase levels are much increased.
(7) Thiamine levels in erythrocytes, blood and plasma may be in the normal range.
(8) Blood creatine phosphokinase (CPK) levels may occur.
(9) Thiaminase levels increased in rumen liquor and in faeces.

(10) Haematology virtually normal although total and differential counts may show a mild stress reaction.
(11) Increased cerebrospinal fluid pressure, 200–350 mm saline (normal 120–160 mm saline).
(12) Histology – bilateral necrosis in cerebral cortex (bisect brain longitudinally, put one half in buffered formalin, the other is deep-frozen).
(13) Green fluorescence of brain when exposed to long-wave ultraviolet light.

Differential diagnoses are shown in Table 18.2.

Treatment

Thiamine hydrochloride should be administered intravenously at a dose of 10 mg/kg (5 mg/lb) BW, and the dosage should be repeated every three hours or so for five treatments. A response will occur in 24 hours if animals are caught in the early stages, otherwise recovery is slowly progressive over several days. Multivitamin injections are often used but although they are suitable for follow-up therapy, in the initial stages insufficient thiamine will be administered unless very large doses are given.

Nursing is important and the cattle should be presented with wholesome food including at least 50 per cent good quality roughage. Rumen liquor from cattle on predominantly roughage diets may be helpful. The use of dried brewers' grains can help the conditions as they contain high levels of thiamine and others of the

Table 18.1 Differences in thiamine levels within certain tissues of the body in animals with or without cerebrocortical necrosis. (After Edwin *et al.*, 1979.) TPP = total plasma protein.

	CCN (±SEM)	Not CCN (±SEM)
Liver dry (µg/g)	2.5 ± 0.43	11.1 ± 2.11
Heart dry (µg/g)	2.5 ± 0.56	13.2 ± 2.12
Brain dry (µg/g)	1.8 ± 0.37	7.7 ± 1.52
Erythrocyte transketolase (% TPP effect)	172	15

Table 18.2 Differential diagnoses.

Disease	Differential diagnoses
Listeriosis	Unilateral facial paralysis, pyrexia
Lead poisoning	Abdominal pain, diarrhoea, no pupillary reflex, no ruminal movements
Coenuriasis	Slow onset, circling
Molasses poisoning	Similar to cerebrocortical necrosis but history of feeding large quantities and also glucose levels fall whereas thiamine levels remain normal
Amprolium poisoning	Similar to cerebrocortical necrosis but history of feeding it
Bracken or horsetail poisoning	Similar to cerebrocortical necrosis but highly unlikely to cause such a manifestation other than experimentally
Haemophilus somnus	Infection, but usually pyrexia and neutrophilia

B vitamin group. Levels of 0.5–1.0 kg/300 kg BW (1–2 lb/6 cwt) have been suggested.

Control

The precipitating factors for CCN are still not known, which makes it difficult to recommend preventive measures. As the condition is the result of endogenous thiamine activity, provision of extra thiamine is of limited value. Most natural feeds contain thiamine at a level of 2 ppm and this, plus the vitamin synthesized in the rumen, is normally sufficient. Provision of adequate amounts of roughage should prevent the condition and a level of 1.5 kg roughage per 100 kg BW is suggested.

Urolithiasis

Urinary calculi are either organic or inorganic. The organic type are less common and form casts or urinary deposits. The inorganic ones tend to be crystalline and are more common. The condition is usually seen in calves that are housed, with milk substitute as their main source of feed or in weaned growing animals fed high levels of concentrates. Some pastures are problem areas, which can be due to high plant oestrogen, oxalate or silica levels. Most calculi in housed animals contain calcium or magnesium ammonium phosphate although struvite and oxalate deposits occur at times. At pasture, carbonates of calcium, magnesium and phosphorus are most common. Vitamin A deficiency has been suggested as a precipitating factor both indoors and when cattle are grazing. The urinary pH has an influence and phosphate and carbonate calculi form more readily in an alkaline than an acid urine (adult ruminant urine is alkaline with a pH of 7 to 9). Binding of the calculi occurs with mucoprotein in the urine and this is seen more frequently when oestrogens from plants or growth promoters are present, or the ration is pelleted.

Urolithiasis can occur in all animals fed a predisposing diet regardless of sex; however, the condition is mainly seen in the male because signs are not normally observed unless some form of urethral blockage occurs. More cases are found in castrated than entire animals. Calculi can lodge anywhere in the urethra but occur most commonly at the sigmoid flexure of the penis with the region of the ischial arch being the second most common site.

Signs

Most of the signs are associated with partial or complete blockage of the urethra. This is seen as frequent attempts to urinate, which may be accompanied by the passage of small amounts of urine, often blood-tinged, or the attempts are unproductive. Calculi may be present on the prepucial orifice hairs. There is usually evidence of mild to severe colic with kicking at the belly, paddling movements and tail swishing. In most untreated cases with complete urethral obstruction, there will be perforation of the urethra or bladder rupture. When either takes place there is usually a period of relief from abdominal pain. When bladder rupture has occurred the urine enters the abdomen, which becomes distended and there is a fluid thrill present on percussion. In those with urethral perforation, urine tends to dribble under the skin, causing ventral abdominal distension, which will start to progress anteriorly. In most cases there is some toxaemia and possibly uraemia and this is seen as inappetance, with increasing dullness of the animal, which will ultimately become comatosed and die.

Necropsy

At necropsy there is usually some degree of cystitis, often with urinary deposits present in the bladder. When the bladder ruptures there is much fluid in the abdomen and in those cases of urethral perforation there will be erosion in the area of the calculus and urine, possibly with cellulitis, present subcutaneously. The position of the calculus can be ascertained by the passage of a catheter.

Diagnosis

The diagnosis depends on the history, particularly of the area and feeding as well as the sex of the animal and signs. If there is bladder rupture then the fluid can be aspirated from the abdominal cavity. It is often difficult to determine that urine is present without its odour and appearance. Urinary crystals may be present on prepucial hairs and these should be analysed. The main differential diagnoses are ascites, intussusception and constipation.

Treatment

Treatment of the condition is primarily by surgery. If the animal is nearing slaughter and there is no bladder rupture or urethral perforation then casualty slaughter is best. Otherwise, treatment is usually only successful in the early stages and all treated animals and others in the group must be carefully examined for several days subsequently. It may be possible to perform a urethrotomy and remove the calculi. Provided the stones are distal to the ischial arch then the provision of a urethrotomy in the perineal region may overcome the problem and, if it proves impossible to remove the calculi, the opening can be made permanent. Medical treatment can include hyoscine butylbromide injected intravenously or intramuscularly at a dose of 20–40 mg/animal, or 5–10 ml of protein-free pancreatic extract possibly repeated once or twice. Acetylpromazine can give useful results acting as a smooth muscle relaxant. Withdrawal of concentrates may assist the condition and the provision of salt water following relief of the blockage is useful.

Prevention

Prevention is partly dependent on feed alteration, and precipitation of phosphate can be avoided by having a correct ratio of calcium to phosphorus, which should be at least 1.2:1, but levels up to 2.5:1 have been suggested. The concentration of magnesium in the diet should be kept low and this means that the maximum amount of magnesium oxide that should be added to the diet is 200 g/t ($\frac{1}{2}$ lb/ton) of feed. In the concentrates, up to 3 per cent salt has been recommended and it is thought to have an ionic effect rather than just causing diuresis. Such diets should only be used where there is always free access to water. The addition to feed of urinary acidifiers such as ammonium chloride or phosphoric acid can be helpful. In animals at pasture the use of salt in the water can reduce the concentration of silicic acid in the urine, thereby preventing silica calculi formation. Adequate water supplies must always be available at pasture and areas likely to produce urolithiasis are best grazed by female cattle.

References

Bremner, J., Brockway, J.M., Donnelly, H.T. & Webster, A.J.F. (1976) Anaemia and veal calf production. *Veterinary Record*, **99**, 203–5.

Butson, R.J. (1994) Bovine septic arthritis: a review of current and future treatment regimes. *Cattle Practice*, **2**, 315–21.

Edwin, E.E., Markson, L.M., Shreeve, J., Jackman, R. & Carroll, P.J. (1979) *Veterinary Record*, **104**, 4–8.

Farmer, P.E., Adams, T.E. & Humphries, W.R. (1982) Copper supplementation of drinking water for cattle grazing molybdenum-rich pastures. *Veterinary Record*, **111**, 193–5.

Holman, H.H. (1956) Changes associated with age in the blood picture of calves and heifers. *British Veterinary Journal*, **112**, 91–104.

McCoy, M.A., Smyth, J.A., Ellis, W.A. & Kennedy, D.G. (1997) Stillbirth/perinatal weak calf syndrome. *Cattle Practice*, **5**, 31–4.

Mahmoud, D.H. & Ford, B.J.H. (1981) Injection of sheep with inorganic injections of copper. *Veterinary Record*, **108**, 114–17.

Suttle, N.F. (1981a) Comparison between parenterally administered copper complexes of their ability to alleviate hypocupraemia in sheep and cattle. *Veterinary Record*, **109**, 304–7.

Suttle, N.F. (1981b) Effectiveness of orally administered cupric oxide needles in alleviating hypocupraemia in sheep and cattle. *Veterinary Record*, **108**, 417–20.

Growing Cattle

Chapter 19
Endoparasites

S.M. Taylor and A.H. Andrews

Introduction 267
Nematodes 267
Parasitic gastroenteritis (PGE) 267
Parasitic bronchitis (husk, hoose) 272
Stephanurosis (kidney worm) 274
Bunostomosis 275
Haemonchosis 275
Trematodes 276
Fasciolosis 276
Paramphistomosis (stomach fluke disease, intestinal
amphistomiosis) 279
Schistosomosis (bilharziosis) 279
Cestodes 280
Taenia saginata 280
Echinococcus granulosus and hydatid cysts 281
Protozoa 282
Coccidiosis 282
Neosporosis 283
Toxoplasmosis 284
Sarcosporidiosis (sarcocystosis) 284

Introduction

Although cattle of all ages may become infected with many species of parasites, clinical disease caused by parasitism is mainly observed in groups of animals under 18 months of age, especially when two preconditions coincide:

(1) The availability of large numbers of the infective stages of the parasite (a variable that is usually dependent on the relationship between the bionomics of the parasite and suitable maturation conditions).
(2) The presence of susceptible cattle grazing on the contaminated area.

When these two conditions are fulfilled, the resultant simultaneous maturation of large numbers of parasites in a specific host organ produces severe tissue disruption and the consequent signs associated with the parasite involved. The gastrointestinal tract, lungs and liver are the organs most commonly affected. It is prudent, therefore, when considering the diagnosis and treatment of parasitic disease, to inquire whether the two preconditions have existed and to involve their separation as part of the therapeutic and prophylactic advice given.

Nematodes

Parasitic gastroenteritis (PGE)

The term itself is currently specifically associated with the presence of large numbers of nematodes in the abomasum and intestines rather than any other endoparasites. The nematodes in the abomasum are generally considered to be the primary pathogens, with those in the intestines playing a lesser but synergistic role.

In temperate areas the predominant worms in the abomasum are those of the genus *Ostertagia*, with *O. ostertagi* the most important and numerous. In the small intestine *Cooperia oncophora* and *Nematodirus helvetianus* are commonest.

There are two common forms of ostertagiosis, type I and type II, and since they are the result of different manifestations of the bionomics of *O. ostertagi* they will be described separately.

TYPE I OSTERTAGIOSIS

This form of the disease is characterized by a profuse watery diarrhoea in calves at grass. The faeces, because of the grass diet, is usually green. There is rapid loss of weight in severe cases, coupled with a slight hypoalbuminaemia due to protein loss and in chronic cases this can eventually result in submandibular oedema. It is most common in late summer and autumn in northern temperate areas.

Aetiology and epidemiology

The direct cause is the ingestion over a relatively short period of large numbers of the infective larvae of *O. ostertagi*. The presence of such large numbers of larvae is a result of several epidemiological interactions, a

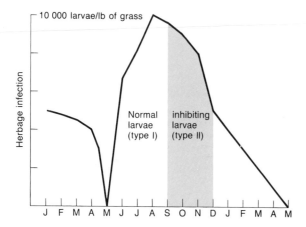

Fig. 19.1 Normal annual pattern of worm larvae on pasture in northern temperate countries.

working knowledge of which is necessary if the best advice on treatment and prophylaxis is to be offered.

The annual pattern of fluctuations of infective larval numbers on calf grazing was described by Michel (1969), and can be seen in Fig. 19.1, which shows that the number of infective larvae in northern temperate areas is lowest in May and June but rises to a peak in late August and September. Summarized, the pattern arises from the following sequence of events. Calves put out to graze in April or May, on grazing that has been used for cattle (and especially calves) during the preceding year, ingest some of the infective larvae remaining on the pasture from the contamination produced in the previous summer. These infective larvae develop into adults in approximately three weeks and egg-laying commences. The rate of hatching of these eggs is influenced by temperature and availability of moisture, and providing the latter is present increases as the temperature rises, reaching a peak in midsummer. The larvae thus hatched in May, June and July migrate or are washed out of faecal pats on to surrounding herbage to await ingestion by the eventual host. Their numbers are maximal in late July, August or early September, the precise timing depending on the climate in the area involved during the year in question. In normal climatic years in the British Isles the maximum number of infective larvae is found in southern England in late July, and in the west of Scotland and Northern Ireland in mid to late August. Wet summers produce an earlier peak but numbers of infective larvae decrease more quickly than normal due to more rapid depletion of the numbers in faecal pats and to dilution due to the more abundant grass growth under these conditions. Conversely, in dry summers the build-up is delayed; release of larvae from faecal pats does not take place under the autumn rainfall and the larval contamination is maximal thereafter.

Parasitic gastroenteritis normally occurs when calves or non-immune older cattle are grazed on pastures on which a large number of infective larvae are present. Typical cases occur in dairy herds where autumn-borne replacement calves are put out to graze for the first time in April or May. The pastures used are frequently close to the farmhouse to enable both ease of inspection and rehousing should weather conditions deteriorate. For these reasons the same fields frequently have the same use each year. The calves remain on the fields until midsummer, excreting eggs that initiate the midsummer larval increase. At that point, when grass in such paddocks requires resting, the farmer has aftergrass available after conservation for silage or hay. The calves are transferred to the aftergrass with or without anthelmintic treatment. Shortly afterwards, by which time the grass in the original fields has recovered slightly, spring-born calves are put out on to it. If no prophylactic measures are taken, the inevitable result of severe type I ostertagiosis ensues a few weeks later in the latter calves, caused by ingestion of massive numbers of infective larvae by fully susceptible cattle over a relatively short period of time.

Pathogenesis

Ingested infective larvae of *O. ostertagi* develop in the gastric glands in the abomasal mucosa, emerging 18–21 days later as adults. Whilst in the mucosa their presence produces distension of the parasitized acini, which in turn causes several pathological and biochemical lesions. Firstly, the hydrochloric acid-producing parietal cells in the acini are destroyed and replaced by rapidly dividing undifferentiated cells that do not produce acid. If the infection is severe and lesions extensive a thickened hyperplastic gastric mucosa results, little acid is produced and the pH of the abomasum rises from pH 2 to pH 7, and the intercellular junctions are disrupted. The change in pH has several major consequences. Above pH 4.5 pepsin ceases to be active in protein digestion; at pH 6 and above pepsinogen is not converted to pepsin and remains unaltered in excess and is reabsorbed into the bloodstream via the ruptured intercellular connections, raising the blood pepsinogen concentration. At the same time blood proteins such as albumin can leak outwards into the lumen. As a result of the rise in pH the abomasal contents become less bacteriostatic and bacterial overgrowth of the damaged wall results.

Signs

When all the above events occur the intestinal metabolism is also affected and the classical signs of acute diarrhoea, inappetance and weight loss commence.

TYPE II OSTERTAGIOSIS

This form of the disease is usually found in yearlings in the late winter or spring following their first season of grazing. Affected cattle can be housed or outwintered.

Aetiology and epidemiology

As with type I disease the direct cause is the simultaneous maturation of large numbers of *O. ostertagi*. The circumstances surrounding the event require some additional explanation, since the normal time of the disease is not when infective larvae on the pasture are most abundant.

Infective larvae present on pasture after September and ingested from that time until the following spring undergo a change in their normal parasitic development, which results in a period of delayed development at the early fourth larval stage while within the abomasal wall. The behavioural change has been shown to be more common in some strains of *O. ostertagi* than others and to be brought about by either cold or desiccation in their preparasitic exposure (Armour *et al.*, 1969). In the late autumn, calves that have not had adequate prophylactic treatment may harbour many thousands of such larvae but relatively few normally developing larvae or adult worms. Type II ostertagiosis results when these inhibited larvae resume their development in the late winter or spring, the emerging larvae producing the same lesions as those causing type I disease.

ATYPICAL FORMS OF PARASITIC GASTROENTERITIS

Parasitic gastroenteritis in beef herds

This is not usually a problem in spring-calving herds, since most of the infective larvae are consumed by the adult cows, which normally have enough immunity to prevent a high percentage of worms establishing and producing eggs. The calves that might transmit the infection are too young to consume much grass in the early part of the season. As a result the peak of infective larval numbers does not develop until September or October when most calves are weaned, treated and housed. Conversely, in autumn-calving herds in which calves are weaned in the following spring and grazed in the same manner as dairy replacements, the same epidemiological picture can result, i.e. type I ostertagiosis will occur in the absence of preventative measures.

Early-season type I ostertagiosis

In areas where climatic conditions allow autumn-born calves to be put out in March or early April, the number of infective larvae remaining on pasture can be sufficiently high to cause normal type I disease from 4 to 6 weeks after going to grass.

Nematodirosis in calves

Parasitic gastroenteritis due to large infections of the nematode *Nematodirus battus* has recently been observed. Normally recognized as a parasite of sheep, it has recently been observed to be able to be transmitted by cattle, both on farms where annual alternation of sheep and cattle has taken place and even where cattle only are kept, and has caused severe outbreaks of diarrhoea in calves.

Cooperiosis in calves

In the last decade, as a result of the widespread use of suppressive regimes with avermectins and moxidectin that are more effective against *Ostertagia* than *Cooperia* species, the prevalence of *Cooperia oncophora*, the commonest of that genus in northern Europe, has increased in comparison to *Ostertagia* species. In faeces samples taken during the first two-thirds of the grazing season on farms where intermittently applied avermectins have been routinely used for prophylaxis, *Cooperia* species eggs can form up to 90 per cent of the eggs excreted, with *Ostertagia* species forming the majority of the remainder. In such circumstances large *Cooperia oncophora* worm burdens can accumulate in a short time when hatching conditions are favourable. These can result in outbreaks of acute diarrhoea and loss of condition, and are rather similar to *Nematodirus battus* infections in lambs in spring, although in calves they usually occur in July or early August. If left untreated calves normally recover after a few weeks and become immune to *Cooperia oncophora*, but the loss of condition can be prevented by prompt treatment.

Parasitic gastroenteritis in adult cattle

Although uncommon, since most cattle acquire immunity by the age of 18 months, occasional individual cases can occur. Bulls that are grazed on calf paddocks and cows, which due to debilitating intercurrent diseases such as fascioliosis may have some of their normal immune reactions depressed, can both suffer from type II ostertagiosis.

Diagnosis

Affected animals invariably present with diarrhoea, which may be present to a greater or lesser degree in all members of the group. Younger animals are fre-

Table 19.1 Differentiation between type I and type II ostertagiosis.

	Type I	Type II
Seasonal incidence	Predominantly July–November; occasionally April–May	February–May
History	Usually in calves at grass for the first time, heavily stocked (8–10/ha). Occasionally in beef yearlings during the second year's grazing, and in individual cows and bulls transferred from hill herds to more intensive systems	*Always* in calves that grazed on heavily stocked pasture during the previous autumn, usually in younger members of group. Can also occur in bulls grazing calf paddocks. Occurs usually when housed or within 3 weeks of being put to grass
Clinical signs	Profuse green diarrhoea; will only usually recur once approx. 10 days after treatment. Rapid loss of body weight. Morbidity high, mortality low	Intermittent profuse diarrhoea. Recurs every 2 weeks until supply of inhibited fourth stages is exhausted. Morbidity low, mortality high
Laboratory findings[a]	Not usually anaemic PCV > 0.3 RBC > 7×10^6/mm^3 Hb > 10 g/100 ml Plasma pepsinogen 2–5 iu	Mild anaemia PCV 0.22–0.26 RBC 5.6 ± 10^6/mm^3 Hb 8.4 ± 0.5 g/100 ml Plasma pepsinogen 2–8 iu
Post mortem	pH abomasal contents >5.0 >50 000 adult *O. ostertagi* Severe abomasal reaction	pH abomasal contents >5.0 >50 000 adult *O. ostertagi* plus large numbers of immature fourth stages Severe abomasal reaction

[a] PCV, packed cell volume; RBC, red blood cell; Hb, haemoglobin.

quently the most severely affected. There will be a history that indicates grazing on potentially infected pasture during the preceding four to eight weeks in the case of type I ostertagiosis or during the previous late summer and autumn for type II ostertagiosis.

Specific diagnosis (see Table 19.1) can be assisted by the following tests.

(1) Faecal egg counts. Despite the dilution of faeces caused by diarrhoea, the nematode egg counts will be in excess of 1000 eggs/g. Counts may be higher in less severely affected calves that have not yet become severely diarrhoeic. In older animals and in some individuals in type II cases the faecal egg counts may be low enough to be misleading, and if suspected the results of other tests should be borne in mind.

(2) Plasma pepsinogen. In healthy calves the normal level of plasma pepsinogen is less than 1 international unit (iu) of tyrosine. In affected calves the level will normally be greater than 3 iu, and in very severely diseased individuals up to 4.5 iu. It should be pointed out that in adult cattle the normal pepsinogen level can be 1.5–2 iu, almost that found in calves in the prepatent period of type II ostertagiasis. Plasma pepsinogen levels in adults therefore should be carefully evaluated.

(3) Plasma gastrin. The plasma concentration of the hormone gastrin has been shown to rise at the time of patency in experimental infections and to peak at levels between 500 and 1000 pg/ml. Although still under investigation it may be used as a substitute for plasma pepsinogen in the future.

(4) Post mortem findings. In both type I and type II ostertagiasis the abomasum (providing the animal has remained untreated) will contain large numbers of adult *O. ostertagi*. The number can vary from 50 000 to 1 000 000 in extreme cases. In type II disease pepsin digest of the abomasal mucosa or incubation in lukewarm normal saline will reveal large numbers of inhibited fourth stage worms. The pH of the abomasal contents will be raised to pH 4.5.

Treatment (see Chapter 60)

Type I disease can be treated with almost any of the anthelmintics currently available such as levamisole, benzimidazoles or avermectins. Type II disease requires the use of some of the modern longer acting benzimidazoles or pro-benzimidazoles or avermectins such as ivermectin, doramectin, abamectin, eprinomectin or moxidectin. The avermectins and moxidectin are much the most effective in removing both adult and inhibited fourth stage parasites as a result of their persistence and slow excretion. Levamisole is much less effective for type II disease, as it has a poor efficiency against inhibited worms due to its rapid excretion (see p. 1021), and the benzimidazoles can vary in efficacy depending on the time of treatment in relation to the onset of inhibition of the worms, i.e. in the early and late stages of inhibition the larvae are thought to have a more active metabolism, and therefore absorb more anthelmintic; in the middle of the inhibition period they absorb less, and it is then that the benzimidazoles do not have the persistence necessary to kill the worms.

Prevention

As for most parasitic diseases, prevention is more cost-effective than treatment. Since there are no vaccines yet available for gastrointestinal nematodes, numerous schemes that combine grazing management and anthelmintic therapy have been developed. The methods fall into three types: (i) evasive; (ii) suppressive; and (iii) dilution.

Evasive strategies: The basis of this category (also called the 'Weybridge' system) was first enunciated by Michel (1968) at the laboratory of the same name. Using the knowledge of the epidemiology of parasitic gastroenteritis that had then become available, Michel pointed out that if susceptible cattle were removed from infected to uninfected grazing just before the summer increase in infective larval numbers, serious parasitism could be avoided. When combined with anthelmintic treatment at the time of movement the system reduces the level of nematode worm egg contamination on the clean grazing. In essence, therefore, the system involves taking no prophylactic action until early July. At that time, pasture which has not been previously used for cattle grazing that year is available, after grass has been taken for silage making or some other form of conservation.

The calves are given anthelmintic treatment before being moved to it. The timing of the treatment can vary with the pharmacokinetics of the anthelmintic used and its effect on nematode eggs if contamination of the aftergrass is to be avoided. For instance, the longer acting benzimidazole anthelmintics (e.g. oxfendazole, albendazole, fenbendazole) are ovicidal within a few hours after treatment and their slow rate of excretion means that cattle are protected from infection with susceptible parasites for approximately 30 hours after treatment. They can therefore be put back safely onto the contaminated grazing for 24 hours after treatment before transfer to the aftergrass. The same technique can be applied with avermectins and moxidectin, which

although not ovicidal have an even longer half-life and will inhibit further infections for at least two weeks. On the other hand, levamisole has a rapid excretion rate and is also not ovicidal. If reduction of contamination as well as nematode removal is intended, cattle treated with levamisole require to be yarded after treatment at least overnight, if not for 24 hours. After this first treatment in early to mid July, and depending on the availability of grass and its previous grazing history, the calves may require no further treatment until housed in late autumn, although in practice many are treated four to six weeks after the first movement. Although highly effective and the most economical method of prophylaxis when carried out carefully, it should be pointed out that although excellent for control of gastrointestinal nematodes it is not completely effective in the prevention of lungworm infection caused by *Dictyocaulus viviparus*.

Suppressive strategies: These have been introduced gradually since the mid 1970s and are also based on knowledge of the epidemiology of the infections. Unlike the evasive systems, which allow natural infection and pasture contamination to take place in spring and early summer, the basis of these methods is to suppress egg production during that period (Fig. 19.2). If pasture contamination is prevented or reduced, the summer increase of infective larvae is of such proportions as to cause a negligible risk of severe parasitism. Suppression is carried out by two different methods: (i) repeated anthelmintic treatments with standard preparations, the interval between which is determined by the pharmacokinetic properties of the chemical used; currently most of the anthelmintics used are avermectins or moxidectin: or (ii) the use of a device, usually an intraruminal bolus, which has a continuous slow release of the active anthelmintic for periods from 60 to 140 days. Such boluses are usually administered by balling-

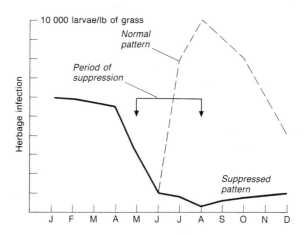

Fig. 19.2 Rationale for anthelmintic suppression.

gun at or just before susceptible calves are put out to grass in the spring, although recent experiments have shown that they can also be effective when given in midsummer to prevent infection in calves grazing previously contaminated fields. The length of prophylactic activity varies between different climatic areas and nematode species, e.g. in south-eastern areas of the UK suppression for eight weeks after being put to pasture in spring may be sufficient, but in wetter western areas it may require to be prolonged for a further five weeks and if lungworm infections are present on the farm for up to 15 weeks.

Dilution strategies: Originally described in New Zealand as the Ruakura method (McMeekin, 1954) and further amended by Leaver (1970), the methods consist of the grazing of paddocks in relays by groups of calves followed by groups of older cattle. The basis of the technique is that the greater consumption of infective larvae by the immune or partially immune adults will delay and reduce the build-up of infective larvae on the paddocks. Initially, no anthelmintic treatments were given, but in modern practice the method is frequently combined with either of the evasive or suppressive techniques.

The advantages and disadvantages of each of the three preventive methods are summarized in Table 19.2.

Parasitic bronchitis (husk, hoose)

Dictyocaulus viviparus is almost the sole cause of severe pulmonary helminth infections in cattle. Occasionally other parasites are found, but rarely in numbers sufficiently large to cause disease. In general, calves at grass from midsummer to autumn are those most frequently clinically affected, but heavy infections in animals of any age previously uninfected will produce signs. It is most prevalent in dairy-type calves, but is also common in weaned beef calves. The range of signs can vary from occasional coughing to severe respiratory distress, and is a reflection of the number of infective larvae ingested during a relatively short period.

Aetiology and epidemiology

The immediate cause of clinical symptoms is the ingestion two to four weeks previously of large numbers of infective larvae of *D. viviparus* by non-immune cattle. Experimentally, severe infections can be induced by a single administration of larvae at a rate of between 25 and 50 larvae/kg body weight. Typically, an affected calf weighing 300 kg will have ingested between 7500 and 15 000 L3 (third stage larvae). This is a much smaller infection than is required to cause parasitic gastroenteritis by *O. ostertagi*, and is an indication of lesser margin for error involved in ensuring adequate prophylaxis.

The epidemiology is more complex and infections are also much less predictable than are those of gastrointestinal nematodes, principally because at present not all details of larval survival and transmission are known. Infections are more prevalent in wetter areas, especially those in the west of the British Isles. One of the major differences between *D. viviparus* and gastrointestinal nematodes that has an influence on the unpredictability of infections is that the female worm produces eggs

Table 19.2 Advantages and disadvantages of the prophylactic methods for gastrointestinal parasites.

Method	Advantages	Disadvantages
Evasive	Low labour cost Low anthelmintic cost Not likely to lead to anthelmintic resistance in nematodes	Does not protect against lungworm Reduces the flexibility of pasture usage in the late summer
Suppressive	If carried out for long enough will reduce the chances of lungworm infection More likely to lead to anthelmintic resistance in target nematodes	Higher labour or anthelmintic costs especially in the case of slow-release boluses Allows more flexible use of grazing
Dilution	Lower anthelmintic costs	Requires excellent fencing and high labour costs and is generally used only in well organized dairy farms Is not effective for prevention of lungworm infection

containing fully developed larvae, which are passed in the faeces. These become infective within a much shorter time than the eggs of *Ostertagia* species and hence in optimal conditions can produce a rapid increase in their numbers. In addition to rapidity of maturation to infectivity, larvae are also dispersed from faecal pats by some of the following means: (i) ascending the common faecal fungus *Pilobolus* and being propelled into the air on discharge of the sporangium, to be carried by wind to adjacent areas; (ii) although unverified, there is evidence that earthworms or coprophagous beetles may act as transport hosts; (iii) also unverified, it has been reported that the European hare (*Lepus europaeus*) can be infected, although experiments have shown that the smaller blue hare (*L. timidus*), common in Ireland, is refractory to infection. In addition to these means of dispersal it has been shown that infective larvae can remain viable in soil as well as on pasture over the winter, and that small numbers of adult worms and hypobiotic larvae can survive and overwinter in infected animals despite their hosts having some immunity to further infection, only to mature and propagate larvae during the following spring.

Pathogenesis

After ingestion, infective larvae penetrate the intestinal mucosa, moult to the L4 stage of their life cycle and migrate via bloodstream and lymphatic channels to the lungs. This takes place approximately one week after being consumed, and up to this point no clinical effects are observed in the host. After that period, larvae break out of blood vessels into alveoli and small bronchioles, after which they moult to become young adults, and as they increase in size they ascend the bronchiolar tree towards the large bronchioles and bronchi. Larvae are first found in faeces from the 25th day after infection.

Signs

Clinical signs appear during the second week after infection and their severity depends on the number of developing worms. The signs range from occasional to repeated coughing, with a noticeably increased respiration rate in the worst affected. By the third week, severely affected cattle do little else except stand in a characteristic head extended position with rapid shallow breathing and frequent coughing.

Although most calves, if not severely affected, will recover after treatment, a small percentage will suffer a relapse of clinical signs in the absence of fresh infection. The precise aetiology of this is uncertain, but autopsy reveals an oedematous rubbery lung with alveolar epithelialization observed microscopically.

Necropsy

The pathological progression during maturation progresses from alveolitis and bronchiolitis to bronchitis and severe emphysema, sometimes with superimposition of a secondary bacterial pneumonia. If left untreated after patency even moderate infections can progress in severity due to aspiration of eggs and hatched larvae back into previously unaffected alveoli and smaller bronchioles, resulting in bronchitis and pneumonia.

Diagnosis

Affected cattle invariably present with varying degrees of respiratory abnormality, and since similar signs can occur as a result of infection by a variety of pathogens, careful differential diagnosis is advisable. The grazing history and time of the year in northern temperate areas invariably involve cattle grazing established pasture previously used by other cattle plus the appearance of clinical signs between July and October. Since the caudal lobes of the lung are more frequently affected, adventitious lung sounds are usually more apparent from these areas, in contrast to those from viral pneumonias, which usually affect the cranial and medial lobes. Confirmation of the diagnosis by identification of larvae in faeces or sputum samples can only take place after patency, which takes place approximately 25 days after infection, although it should be noted that in adults that are suffering from a re-infection the infection usually does not reach patency.

Treatment (see p. 1027)

In order to kill the worms and larvae present in the lung tissues, anthelmintic treatment is essential. The most effective are the avermectins and moxidectin; levamisole and some of the more recently developed benzimidazoles or pro-benzimidazoles, such as oxfendazole, fenbendazole, albendazole and netobimin, are also effective, but the incidence of alveolar epithelialization is more common after their use, since they have little persistent efficacy and reinfection can occur if the same grazing is used before and after treatment. Severely affected animals may also require antibiotic therapy to control secondary bacterial pneumonia, and if anorexia has been present rehydration with electrolytes may also be helpful. In most outbreaks a range of severity is observed and it is frequently advisable to house the worst affected cattle, especially if climatic conditions would be stressful even to healthy calves. In addition, because treatment of severe cases can exacerbate signs farmers should be warned of the possibility. In outbreaks involving adult dairy cows care should be taken that the anthelmintic used does not prevent sale of milk products for a prolonged period until a withholding time long enough to allow excretion of the drug has passed. The most appropriate drug currently available is eprinomectin, the use of which requires no period of milk withdrawal from sale.

Prevention

There are two major methods available, the first relying on inducing immunity and the second on suppression of infections.

Vaccination (see p. 1011): Immunity can be stimulated by the use of a live vaccine, which takes the form of two doses of 1000 infective larvae irradiated by gamma irradiation. Calves should be two months old before vaccination and the doses separated by four weeks and preferably both doses given before going to grass in the spring or before the time of earliest challenge in outdoor calves. Although the vaccine induces excellent protection against clinical disease it does not completely prevent all worms from natural infections completing their life cycle, so that the parasite can be maintained at a very low level on pasture grazed by vaccinated cattle. If the farmer neglects to vaccinate, parasite numbers can quickly increase sufficiently, if weather conditions are favourable, to affect non-immune cattle within their first grazing season.

Suppression: On farms where calves have suffered lung damage due to viral pneumonia, vaccination may be inadvisable because of the possibility of exacerbation of the existing lesions. Under these circumstances it has been found that regular anthelmintic treatments throughout the grazing season can suppress infection sufficiently to minimize the danger of clinical disease and at the same time allow some immunity to be induced by the natural ingestion of infective larvae from pasture which are subsequently killed before completion of their life cycle (see p. 1027). The method has also been successfully applied to normal healthy calves, but it requires to be carried out and monitored carefully, since there are potential problems in its use. Firstly, the length of time during which anthelmintic suppression is required may vary between areas with different climatic patterns and farming practices. In general in the British Isles it is necessary to provide anthelmintic cover until mid August. The methods of application require that the anthelmintic must be extremely effective against all stages of the parasitic life cycle of the nematode. Those anthelmintics used fairly successfully have been avermectins, either as injections or pour-ons administered at intervals after going to grass that are dependent on the particular pharmacokinetics of the drug used and the

time of turn-out to grass, and intraruminal boluses designed to release anthelmintic either intermittently or continuously for periods up to 140 days. The level of immunity stimulated depends on the number of larvae ingested from pasture and, since this can be highly variable, some cattle in a group may have inadequate resistance to future infection should they be exposed to it. As a result, careful monitoring is necessary after cessation of anthelmintic treatment and some thought required to plan cattle husbandry during the subsequent year and then as adults.

Stephanurosis (kidney worm)

Aetiology and epidemiology

This is mainly an infestation of pigs but it can infect calves and is due to *Stephanurus dentatus*. The adult is up to 45 mm in length.

The condition is found in the tropical and subtropical countries of Africa, East and West Indies, Brazil, Hawaii, Philippines, Australia and southern Europe where pigs are kept, but in calves adult worms do not develop. The larvae cause damage to the liver parenchyma during migration and produce thrombosis of the abdominal blood vessels, which may be fatal. Aberrant larvae can encapsulate anywhere in the host but the majority are found in all parts of the kidney. The eggs produced in the pig form hatch to produce first stage larvae. These develop to third stage infective larvae if there is warmth and moisture. The larvae are often ingested by earthworms and these act as a vector for infection. The infective larvae are otherwise susceptible to cold or drying. Transmission is either by ingestion, which may include earthworms, or by skin penetration. In the host they pass to the liver where they remain for a considerable time before going to other parts of the body.

Signs

They are mostly of anaemia, ill thrift and ascites. Many infestations are without signs.

Necropsy

Necrotic lesions with thrombosis in the mesenteric blood vessels and hypertrophy of the mesenteric lymph nodes are likely to be found. In a few cases there may be haemorrhages and abscesses in the lungs and kidneys.

Diagnosis

This will depend on the presence of calves grazing areas with infected pigs. An immunodiffusion test can be used. There is a marked eosinophilia.

Treatment and control

Fenbendazole at high doses may be effective. Calves should not graze pastures recently used by pigs.

Bunostomosis

Bunostomosis in cattle is caused by the hookworm *Bunostomum phlebotomum*. It mainly affects cattle up to one year old and causes a range of signs from unrest and mild abdominal pain to diarrhoea and eventually anaemia depending on the stage of the infection and the number of worms present. It is more prevalent in subtropical and tropical regions than in temperate; this distribution has become especially marked during the last decade as the worm, which does not occur in large numbers, seems especially sensitive to some of the modern anthelmintics and may now be absent from those areas where frequent suppressive anthelmintic treatments have been applied.

Aetiology and epidemiology

Bunostomum phlebotomum parasitizes the small intestine of cattle. Adults can reach 3.0 cm in length and are characterized by a large buccal capsule with lateral cutting teeth and a tooth-like structure in its base, which is the duct of an oesophageal gland. The worms suck blood, which can induce anaemia and in large numbers cause diarrhoea.

The eggs from adult females pass out with faeces. Depending on climatic conditions, a parasitic infective larva, which is susceptible to desiccation, will develop under optimal conditions of adequate moisture and warmth within one week. The infective larvae can infect susceptible cattle in either of two ways.

- By penetration of the skin after which it enters the bloodstream and passes to the lung, emerging into the alveoli and after further moulting up the bronchial tree to the pharynx, where it is then swallowed and passes to the intestine to mature.
- By direct ingestion after which it burrows into the intestinal wall during development to emerge as an adult.

The prepatent period is eight weeks. The worm flourishes in conditions of adequate moisture and warmth and thus is generally a subtropical problem, but disease has been recorded in countries as far north as Scotland, where it has been seen in cattle maintained indoors on damp straw bedding.

Signs

Heavy percutaneous larval infections cause restlessness, stamping and itching. Once in the intestine adults suck blood and cause haemorrhagic anaemia and hypoalbuminaemia, and small numbers (about 2000) in comparison to other gastrointestinal nematodes, other than *Haemonchus placei*, will cause very severe disease and death.

Diagnosis

It is difficult to diagnose when prepatent and mild anaemia is the main sign. When patent it should be differentiated from other parasites that cause haemorrhagic anaemia, e.g. *H. placei* and *F. hepatica*, and those deficiencies such as cobalt or copper (Chapter 21) that adversely affect erythropoiesis.

Treatment and control

The parasite is sensitive to modern anthelmintics and can be controlled by their suppressive or strategic use. Other measures in housed cattle should be the provision of dry bedding and its replacement when soiled. Once infected and treated, cattle normally develop a strong immunity to the parasite.

Haemonchosis

Haemonchosis is manifested by haemorrhagic anaemia and diarrhoea, and is caused by the presence in the abomasum of *Haemonchus placei* (synonym *H. similis*). As with bunostomosis it is mainly pathogenic in immature cattle, since infection in the first three years of life usually produces a strong immunity to reinfection. It also has a similar distribution, being commonest in subtropical and tropical countries, but present in most temperate countries and able to cause disease during any unusually warm periods of weather.

Aetiology and epidemiology

Adults of *H. placei* suck blood from the surface of the abomasum. They are fairly large in comparison to other abomasal nematodes and measure 3 cm in length when fully grown. In the female the ovaries and intestine are spirally intertwined to give the worm its 'barber-pole' appearance and nickname. The male has large barbed spicules, and both sexes a small lancet in the buccal capsule.

Female *H. placei* are very prolific egg producers and can lay up to 10000 eggs daily. The eggs are passed in faeces and undergo a typical trichostrongyline development to infective larvae. The time taken to reach this stage varies considerably between temperate and subtropical climatic areas. In the former, it may take several weeks in contrast to four days under suitable conditions. The conditions for development of

Haemonchus spp. have been studied in some detail, and it has been concluded that they require a temperature in excess of 18°C and rainfall of 5.3 cm/month for maximum translation, but can develop provided the mean minimum temperature is not less than 10°C. As a result of the combination of fecundity and rapid infective development in favourable conditions, pasture can become quickly contaminated with huge numbers of infective larvae. In the subtropics acute infections can therefore be found in susceptible young cattle, whereas in temperate areas infections are more likely to be chronic. Under adverse conditions in the tropics, e.g. dry seasons, infective larvae can undergo hypobiosis in a similar manner to *Ostertagia* spp., and resume development shortly before the rainy season commences.

Once ingested, larvae undergo two moults before becoming adult in 26–28 days, when infections become patent. After the first moult, the L4 larvae and subsequent adults suck blood, leaving haemorrhagic spots on the abomasal epithelium, and the resultant blood loss is the major pathogenic sequelae. However, in large infections the pH of the abomasal contents may be increased in the same way as in ostertagiosis, with the resultant digestive disturbance, raised plasma pepsinogen, possible bacterial overgrowth and diarrhoea. Once patent, peak egg production from females is normally reached between six and seven weeks after infection and may continue for a further six to eight weeks. Cattle, unlike sheep, develop resistance to the worm and unless immunologically compromised by intercurrent illness or malnutrition the population decreases rapidly thereafter and the animal remains fairly resistant for the remainder of its life.

Signs

There are two types of clinical picture. The first occurs in severe primary infections and presents severely anaemic, weak and sometimes diarrhoeic young cattle. The second is found in chronic lesser infections and typically causes weakness, lethargy, weight loss, a less acute anaemia, hypoproteinaemia, submandibular oedema and anasarca.

Diagnosis

Diagnosis can be confirmed if the infection is patent by the examination of faeces samples, which may reveal very high faecal egg counts. The plasma pepsinogen level may be raised. The grazing and past parasitic history may be helpful in differentiating from other causes of anaemia or diarrhoea such as fasciolosis, bunostomosis, copper or cobalt deficiencies, babesiosis, coccidiosis, bacillary haemoglobinuria and malnutrition.

Treatment and control

Anthelmintic treatment is the primary consideration and *H. placei* is susceptible to levamisole, avermectins, moxidectin and modern benzimidazoles as well as the flukicides rafoxanide, clorsulon and nitroxynil. This should be coupled with movement to uninfected pasture. Prevention can be achieved using similar methods as those described for ostertagiosis.

Trematodes

Fasciolosis

Fasciolosis in cattle is a chronic wasting disease caused by the presence in the liver and bile ducts respectively of immature and adult trematodes of the genus *Fasciola*. The disease is found in vast areas of the world, with the smaller *F. hepatica* (3.5 × 1 cm) in temperate countries and the larger *F. gigantica* (7.5 × 1 cm) in tropical regions the commonest species. Calves and yearlings are most commonly affected but any age of animal may be susceptible. Although it may take place at any time of the year, infection is most prevalent during autumn in temperate areas, with the resultant effects of disease becoming apparent in winter and spring.

Aetiology and epidemiology

F. hepatica: Multiplication of the parasite is partially climatically regulated, since its life cycle involves an intermediate host that requires adequate moisture and a suitable ambient temperature. The intermediate hosts are various species of snail of the genus *Lymnaea*, which are found on wet mud surfaces. In the British Isles, *L. truncatula* is the species involved. It prefers a neutral or slightly alkaline habitat, but can survive in fairly acid conditions such as peaty hills, although under such conditions individual snails remain small and the population low. At its maximum it can have a shell length of 1 cm. The snail population fluctuates, being least in winter and greatest in June and July, especially in years when late spring rainfall has been above average, when large numbers accumulate and are therefore available for transmission of *F. hepatica*.

Briefly summarized the life cycle of *F. hepatica* is as follows. The adult parasite in the bile ducts is a hermaphrodite and can be self- or cross-fertilized. Large numbers of eggs are produced by each parasite, which pass from the ducts to the gall-bladder and are subsequently passed into the intestine on contraction of that organ. Eggs are then passed in the faeces, but will not hatch unless moist and until an ambient temperature of 10°C is reached. Hatching at temperatures between 22 and 26°C takes nine days, but under normal temperatures in the months of May and June in the British Isles, it can take four weeks. On hatching, the released miracidium must locate and penetrate the foot of *L. truncatula* within three hours. Once in the snail, the parasite undergoes multiplication through stages of sporocyst and rediae and reaches the cercarial stage after a minimum of two months, although in colder temperatures it may take up to 16 weeks or should winter intervene complete development may cease until the following spring. Under natural conditions within the British Isles, cercariae from summer infections are released from snails between late August and October, and in some areas from overwintered infections in April or May. On release from the snail, which must take place in conditions of wetness, the cercariae swim to the nearest plant, encyst on its leaves and become the infective stage, termed metacercariae, several hundred of which can arise from one miracidium. Metacercariae on herbage can survive for several months and therefore maintain the infection from one year to the next.

Cattle become infected by ingestion of grass on which metacercariae are encysted. The metacercariae excyst in the small intestine, the wall of which they penetrate to reach the peritoneal cavity where they move to the liver and invade its capsule. At this point the flukes are very small (about 1 mm) but as they burrow through the liver parenchyma they gradually increase in size and in primary infections in cattle will reach the bile ducts after six to eight weeks, when they mature and become egg-laying adults 10–12 weeks after ingestion. In response to the presence of fluke in the liver parenchyma, the liver of cattle produces a more intense fibrous reaction than that of sheep, and the resultant cirrhosis is much more severe and is longer lasting. The liver cells of cattle do not regenerate as do those of sheep, and the result of even moderate infection in cattle is a more fibrous liver parenchyma than in most other species.

Within the bile ducts, the adult flukes suck blood and the spines on their cuticle cause multiple small haemorrhagic lesions. In cattle, the resultant fibrous reaction within the bile ducts is also more severe than in sheep and the bile duct walls thicken and become gradually calcified thereafter (Fig. 19.3). The result of the fibrous reaction during a primary infection in both bile ducts and parenchyma of cattle shortens the life span of adult flukes in the ducts to a maximum of 1.5 years and reduces the chances of flukes from subsequent infections being able to complete their life cycle. Cattle therefore become largely resistant to further infections, most of which do not become patent, and the few flukes that do so may take much longer than normal to reach patency and survive in bile ducts for a relatively short time.

F. gigantica: Although similar in many respects to *F. hepatica* it is not found in western Europe, but is widespread within tropical and subtropical climatic regions. The intermediate hosts are also snails of the genus *Lymnaea*, but the species are more aquatic than those transmitting *F. hepatica* and thrive in swamps, drainage channels and artificially flooded areas. As a result the epidemiology is closely tied to the periods of maximum rainfall, the snails being infected and development in the snail completed within these periods. Cercariae are shed towards the end of the wet season and encyst on herbage and even on the water surface at the start of the dry season.

The parasitic life cycle is similar to that of *F. hepatica* but each phase takes slightly longer with the result that patency of primary infections take three or four weeks longer than *F. hepatica*, eggs being found in faeces from 13 to 16 weeks after ingestion of metacercariae.

Signs

In severe infections there is a progressive loss of weight with anaemia and occasionally oedema. Subclinical infections cause a reduction in milk yield and reduction in the growth rate of young cattle.

Diagnosis: The disease is characterized by a gradual loss of condition that is exacerbated if the quantity and quality of feeding are suboptimal. A chronic anaemia develops and the packed cell volume (PCV) drops to approximately 20 per cent. Erythrocytes are hypochromic but normocytic, and while the leucocyte count may be slightly raised, the percentage of eosinophils in a differential count is greatly increased and may consist of up to 20 per cent of the total white cell count. In cows the total milk yield and the non-fat solids proportions may be reduced.

Diagnosis can be confirmed by the presence of fluke eggs in faeces samples, but detection is not always as simple as in sheep, especially in adults, since even in patent infections excretion of eggs is intermittent. Examination of plasma shows a hypoalbuminaemia, and during the migration phase the plasma glutamate dehydrogenase (GLDH) is raised. Once the epithelium of the bile duct walls becomes diseased, the plasma concentration of gamma-glutamyl transpeptidase (GT) rises and this is a useful diagnostic indicator.

Treatment (see pp. 1026, 1028)

Affected cattle are treated by administration of a fasciolicide. Of those currently used for cattle the commonest are triclabendazole, oxyclozanide, rafoxanide,

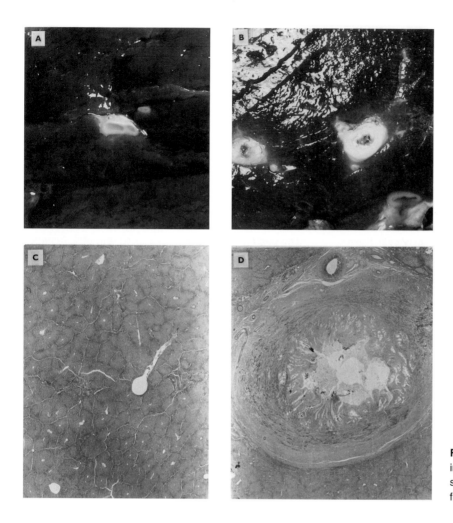

Fig. 19.3 (A) Normal and (B) liver fluke infected bovine liver. (C, D) Microscopic sections of the same stained to show fibrous tissue.

nitroxynil, albendazole, netobimin and clorsulon. All will remove more than 90 per cent of adult flukes from the bile ducts, but they have variable efficiencies against the immature stages migrating through the liver. The most effective is triclabendazole, which will remove developing flukes from a few days after ingestion. Rafoxanide, nitroxynil and clorsulon are effective against six-week-old flukes at normal dose rates and at increased dose levels affect those four weeks old. Albendazole, netobimin and oxyclozanide at normal dose rates remove only adult flukes from the bile ducts and are ineffective against immature flukes. All require withholding of meat and milk for human consumption for variable periods dependent on their pharmacokinetics (see p. 1026).

Prevention

There are four methods available that are used individually in suitable circumstances or can be combined in an attempt to give a more rapid reduction in the prevalence of the parasite.

• Prophylactic use of anthelmintics to reduce both the number of flukes in cattle and the number of eggs excreted. This is by far the commonest practice and involves treatment of cattle once or twice annually. In the British Isles such treatments take place in the autumn and late spring.
• If the areas of snail habitat are delineated and small and they can be drained. This is usually not cost-effective for fluke control alone if the sites are extensive.
• Small snail habitats can be fenced off during the time of greatest infection.
• Snail habitats can be treated with molluscicide. There can be environmental objections since many which were formerly in use were toxic to many species in addition to snails. The most satisfactory is *N*-tritylmorpholine, which although not available in the UK is used in many tropical countries.

Paramphistomosis (stomach fluke disease, intestinal amphistomiosis)

Aetiology and epidemiology

The cause of acute paramphistomosis in Africa is *Paramphistomum microbothrium*. Other *Paramphistomum* spp. and *Cotylophoron* spp. are found in ruminants in Africa and tropical and subtropical regions. In Asia, *Calicophoron* spp. are found and one species occurs in Africa. *Carmyerius* spp. are seen in Africa, India, Pakistan and the Middle East.

It has been recorded in a severe form in Australia, India and the USA. The life cycle is indirect and similar to that of *Fasciola*. It involves aquatic snails that are adapted to a variety of locations. Disease occurs only where there is a massive concentration of the infected planorbid snails. The metacercariae are ingested and the immature flukes develop in the duodenum, where they may be seen in the mucosa. The flukes are 3–4 mm long and 1–2 mm wide. They also develop in the abomasum but are less common. They then migrate through the abomasum to the rumen and reticulum, where again few are found. The prepatent period is very variable, being between one and a half to four months. Most outbreaks occur in the late summer, autumn or early winter when pastures are being contaminated with cercariae. Although all ages of cattle are susceptible, infestation is most commonly seen in yearlings. Fewer infestations occur in the adult, suggesting some degree of immunity.

Signs

Acute paramphistomosis is due to a massive infestation in calves. There is a persistent fetid diarrhoea without blood or mucus, anorexia, weakness, marked loss of condition and then recumbency. In some cases there is submaxillary oedema and a pallor of the mucosa. Death occurs in about one to two weeks after signs develop.

Chronic: In heavy infestations of adult flukes there is a chronic loss of weight, a dry coat and anaemia.

Necropsy

In the acute case there is severe inflammation of the duodenum and abomasum as the parasite penetrates deeply into the mucosa and sometimes the muscularis layer, and there is haemorrhage. There is muscular atrophy, subcutaneous oedema and fluid accumulation in the body cavities. Large numbers of small, immature, flesh-coloured flukes are present in the lumen. In less acute cases the duodenum is thickened and congested. There is fluid in the abdominal cavity.

Diagnosis

Most disease occurs with immature flukes and so it is not easy to detect in the live animal but it can be missed at post mortem. Often other parasitic infestations are present, which again causes paramphistomiosis to be overlooked. However, the history and area where the cattle are grazing can give some indications. There is a reduction in the red and white blood cells and a hypoalbuminaemia. Differential diagnoses include copper and cobalt deficiencies, liver fluke, parasitic gastroenteritis, Johne's disease in the adult and poisoning.

Treatment (see p. 1028)

Few of the modern trematocides have been found to be effective against paramphistomosis. Oxyclozanide at 18.7 mg/kg has variable efficacy from approximately 50 to 90 per cent. Niclosamide at 100 mg/kg is highly effective against intestinal paramphistomes but ineffective for adults. Brotianide at 55 mg/kg is effective against adult flukes but less so against the immature stages.

Control

Drainage of low-lying areas and destruction of the soil will considerably reduce infestation. The most susceptible animals, i.e. calves and immature cattle, should be kept away from likely snail habitats. Routine treatment against *Paramphistomum* before they mature and can infect snails is of use.

Schistosomosis (bilharziosis)

Aetiology and epidemiology

There are several parasites in the genus *Schistosoma*. *Schistosoma bovis* is found in African, Asian and southern European cattle. *Schistosoma mattheei* occurs in cattle in central and southern Africa and can infect man. *Schistosoma indicum* is found in India and Pakistan as is also *S. spindale*, which can also occur in south-east Asia and Indonesia. *Schistosoma japonicum* occurs in the Far East. *Schistosoma nasale* is again found in India and Pakistan and is unusual in that the adult occurs in the mucosal veins of the nose. Several minor species occur involving *S. curassoni*.

Various species of the parasite are widespread and the adults live in veins. Unlike most flukes, *Schistosoma* spp. are not hermaphroditic and the longer male carries the long slender female, which is up to 25 mm long, in a gyroectoplasmic canal. Infection can be via the skin or gut. After penetrating the skin the schistosomulae (young flukes) pass via the lymphatic system to the right side of the heart. They then go via the lungs into the circulation and then to the liver. They mature in the portal

Table 19.3 Intermediate snail hosts of *Schistosoma* spp.

Species	Intermediate snail host genus
S. bovis	*Bulinus* and *Physopsis*
S. indicum	*Indoplanorbis*
S. japonicum	*Oncomelonia*
S. mattheei	*Bulinus*
S. nasale	*Lymnaea* and *Indoplanorbis*

veins before migrating to their final area, usually the mesenteric veins, but they are also found in the urinary bladder veins in the case of *S. mattheei* and in the nasal mucosal veins in *S. nasale*. When infection is oral the gut is penetrated and the immature stages pass to the liver via the blood.

Once mature, eggs are produced that can hatch within minutes if conditions are right. The free-swimming miracidiae penetrate snail hosts producing sporocysts, daughter sporocyst and cercariae but there are no redia. The cercariae must infect the final host within one or two days or they die off as there is no metacercarial stage. There are various genera of snails involved depending on the species of *Schistosoma* (Table 19.3). All the snails like mud except for *Oncomelonia* spp., which are aquatic.

In many areas of Africa most of the cattle are infected but there are very few signs. Young cattle are more likely to be ill.

Signs

The main signs are of diarrhoea, which may contain blood and mucus and is intermittent. There is a loss of condition and reduced resistance to other diseases. Death occasionally occurs. Infestation with *S. nasale* causes a mucopurulent nasal discharge with dyspnoea. Chronic cases develop nasal granuloma.

Necropsy

In severe infestation there are small grey-white granules in the gastrointestinal tract with petechial haemorrhages and ecchymosis. The ileocaecal body may be enlarged and haemorrhagic. Granulomas may also be scattered through the liver parenchyma as well as the lungs and bladder. In *S. nasale* infestation there may be nasal granulomas.

Diagnosis

The signs and grazing history help but it is difficult to diagnose unless faeces are taken or nasal discharge if *S. nasale* is present. The eggs are large and characteristi-cally spiral. As the eggs hatch quickly they need to be fixed in 10 per cent formalin.

Differential diagnosis involves coccidiosis, try-panosomosis, poisoning and Johne's disease.

Treatment (see p. 1028)

Trichlorophan, an organophosphorus compound, can be used parenterally, or niridazole or thioxanthane derivatives such as becanthane or hycanthane may be used. Treatment must be performed carefully otherwise a large number of dead schistosomes will produce emboli and lead to hepatic infarction or portal occlusion.

Control

Immunity to the disease occurs but varies with the *Schistosoma* species. Control involves keeping cattle away from areas frequented by the intermediate host. Molluscicides can be of some benefit. Some vaccines are under development, e.g. a recombinant glutathione *S*-transferase derived from *Schistosoma bovis* has been shown to reduce both egg output and parasitic estab-lishment. Such vaccines can be expected to be available in the next year or two.

Cestodes

Taenia saginata

Taenia saginata is a cyclophyllidean tapeworm, for which man is the final host. It is transmitted to man by the ingestion of the intermediate larval stage in under-cooked beef. Although the larval stage can be found in any age of cattle, viable cysts are found mainly in cattle up to two years of age. The presence of the parasite in the muscles of cattle does not cause clinical signs unless the animal is very heavily infected and the myocardium is involved, but because it is a zoonotic infection its pres-ence can cause significant losses to the beef industry, especially in developing countries. In countries where sanitation standards are high it is a decreasing problem that on average is found in 0.5 per cent of bovine car-casses, with occasional heavy infections occurring under unusual circumstances. In those areas of Africa, Asia and parts of Latin America where human sanitation methods are poor or non-existent and local customs favour ingestion of raw or undercooked beef, the preva-lence may be up to 20 per cent.

Epidemiology

The adult tapeworm inhabits the intestines of man. Its scolex has no hooks, and apparently moves up or down the intestine depending on whether the host has eaten recently or not. When the host's stomach is empty the scolex moves back up the intestine towards the duodenum, and these movements produce hunger pains and vague intestinal discomfort. Fully grown the tapeworm may reach a length of 8 m. Mature egg-filled (about 25 000) proglottids are shed from its posterior end and are passed in faeces or wriggle out of the host's anus nocturnally. Anal pruritis and occasional diarrhoea are usually the only signs apart from the aesthetic and hygienic conditions involved.

The eggs are resistant to external conditions. They are inactivated within two weeks if desiccated, but are known to survive for 16 days in raw sewage, 71 days in liquid manure, 159 days on pasture and 200 days in sewage sludge. No normal method of handling sewage can inactivate them other than total incineration or extensive heat treatment. Extended periods of sludge digestion with or without heat may affect viability but technical proof is lacking. Chemical disinfectants other than some containing copper at very high pH (11.5) are not ovicidal.

Two-thirds of outbreaks in developed countries have been shown to be associated with the spreading of sewage sludge on agricultural land. The remainder have been presumed to be caused by spread of seagulls feeding at sewage plants and passing viable eggs through them on to grazing land, or by accidental flooding of pasture by contaminated effluent streams from sewage plants. Migrant labour from less developed countries and infected stockmen have been implicated in some isolated local multiple infections.

Once ingested, the egg hatches and the liberated oncosphere travels via the bloodstream to striated muscular tissue, including the myocardium. It develops in the muscle and reaches infectivity three months after ingestion, when it is recognizable as a whitish fluid-filled cyst with a diameter of approximately 1 cm, known as a cysticercus. It becomes enclosed in a thin fibrous capsule. Cellular immune reaction around it gradually increases and the capsule becomes thickened, eventually leading to the death of a high proportion of the cysticerci within 18 months and resistance to further infection, although some may survive for several years. After death the contents of the cysts become caseous and finally calcified. The masseter, tongue and heart muscles were generally considered preferential sites and are still examined carefully during meat inspection at abattoirs, in preference to damaging more expensive cuts of meat by the multiple incisions that would otherwise be necessary.

Control (see p. 1028)

There are no drugs suitable for ante-mortem treatment. Carcasses that are found to be infected are normally treated in one of two ways:

- If lightly infected they are frozen to a temperature of −10° for a minimum of 10 days, after which any previously viable cysticerci will have been killed.
- Heavily infected carcasses are usually condemned as unfit for human consumption and rendered after heat treatment into animal feedstuffs in some countries. The thermal death-point of cysticerci is 57°C and meat for human consumption should be raised to at least that temperature if the possibility of infection is to be avoided.

Echinococcus granulosus and hydatid cysts

There are two species of the taeniid tapeworm *E. granulosus*. The first is *E. granulosus granulosus*: the adult is found worldwide in the intestine of dogs and many wild Canidae but not the red fox. The intermediate form, the hydatid cyst, is found in domestic and wild ruminants, man and pigs, but not horses and donkeys. The second is *E. granulosus equinus*, which is almost exclusively found in Europe: adults parasitize the dog and the red fox, and horses and donkeys are the exclusive intermediate hosts.

Cattle therefore are affected by hydatid cysts of *E. granulosus granulosus*. The majority of hydatid cysts cause little apparent disease as they are situated in the liver or lung, their presence only becoming disclosed at abattoirs. Occasionally, they develop in sites where their gradually increasing size causes pressure on vital organs., the resultant disease being dependent on the organ and system affected.

Aetiology and epidemiology

The adult worms parasitize the small intestine of the dog. They are small worms, consisting of four segments of length 0.6 mm. Large numbers may be present in infected animals, each releasing one gravid segment daily containing many eggs, which are resistant to normal external climatic conditions and remain infective for up to two years. After ingestion by cattle or other hosts the oncosphere penetrates the wall of the intestine and is carried via the bloodstream to the liver or other organs where it lodges and starts to grow to become a hydatid cyst. Growth is relatively slow and may take at least one year to reach a diameter of 20 cm. In restricted sites the cyst assumes the shape of the space available, and daughter cysts may be formed and spread to other organs. If growth takes place in the omentum or mesentery, cysts can become very large. There is usually little cellular reaction around cysts in cattle. Since most cattle in developed countries are slaughtered in abattoirs there is little chance of further spread unless casualties are fed to farm dogs or packs of hounds. In underdeveloped countries or where carcasses are not disposed of, wild Canidae ingesting the offal become infected; the brood capsules from within the hydatid cyst evaginate, the scolex attaches to the intestinal wall and reaches adulthood and patency some six weeks later. Infection in dogs is usually symptomless.

Treatment and control (see p. 1028)

Affected cattle are not treated specifically for hydatidosis, principally because of the difficulty of diagnosis, but also because anthelmintics are only now becoming available for treatment of infected human beings. Activity against larval forms has been claimed for praziquantel and albendazole, although most cysts are excised.

Prevention is directed to ensuring that dogs do not become infected, either by regular treatment, the most effective anthelmintic being praziquantel, or by preventing the ingestion of infected offal.

Protozoa

Coccidiosis

Bovine coccidiosis almost invariably affects groups of cattle less than one year old, although it does occasionally occur in older animals. It is manifested by enteritis, diarrhoea and in severe cases dysentery. Not all members of the group are equally affected and light infections are self-limiting; severe infections can be fatal if untreated. The disease is caused by the ingestion over a short period of large numbers of oocysts of *Eimeria* species by non-immune cattle; the greater the infective dose, the more severe the signs produced. *Eimeria* are species-specific, and although 13 species have been isolated from cattle, *E. zuernii*, *E. bovis* and *E. alabamensis* are much the commonest and most pathogenic. They are found everywhere in the world where cattle are farmed. Cryposporidiosis is mentioned on pp. 204 and 286.

Aetiology and epidemiology

The presence of large enough accumulations of oocysts to cause disease is the result of farming practices that allow groups of cattle, which frequently have been stressed by transport and by mixing with others, to ingest food or water contaminated by faeces. It can happen either indoors on straw bedding, which is both damp and contaminated with faeces, or outdoors around drinking or feeding troughs. It can take place at any time of the year so long as conditions prevail that produce adequate moisture and temperature for

oocysts to survive and become infective, but frequently occurs three or four weeks after groups of purchased calves are mixed. In North America it has also been associated with the sudden stress of extreme temperature reductions in midwinter.

After ingestion, the oocyst is disrupted, releasing eight sporozoites each of which penetrates an intestinal epithelial cell and develops into a trophozoite. Multiple fission within the trophozoite produces a schizont, which after a few days ruptures the cell to release a large number of merozoites, which in turn invade other epithelial cells. There are up to four generations of schizogony depending on the species involved. The location of the cells invaded is important for the pathogenicity of the species, e.g. *E. zuernii* and *E. bovis* both invade cells in the lower ileum and later schizogony and gametogony (the term used to describe the sexual stages) take place in the epithelial cells of the caecum and colon. The gametocytes are formed deep in the epithelium and their rupture causes severe disruption of the lining of the caecum with resultant haemorrhage into the lumen. After gametogony, oocysts are formed that subsequently are passed in faeces. They are not immediately infective but require to undergo sporulation, in which the sporocyts and sporozoites are formed ready for further infection. The last process requires adequate moisture and warmth and takes 24–72 hours. The total life cycle from ingestion to patency occupies 15–17 days for *E. zuernii* and 15–20 days for *E. bovis*. Oocyst production during infection with a single species lasts for five to twelve days, but may be prolonged in multiple species infections. The oocysts are very resistant to external conditions and will survive for up to two years in suitable environments with adequate moisture. They can resist moderate frosts down to –8°C for two months, but are susceptible to drought, high temperatures and the chemical action of ammonia.

Signs

The presenting signs of diarrhoea or dysentery accompanied sometimes with severe straining in a group of calves leads to suspicion of coccidiosis.

Diagnosis

Examination of faeces samples for the presence of large numbers of oocysts can confirm the diagnosis. Care should be taken in interpretation of oocyst counts since small numbers are present in the faeces of many normal calves, and in severely affected diarrhoeic calves the main oocyst production phase may have passed or their numbers be misjudged due to the dilution factor of liquid faeces. Occasionally, calves may exhibit nervous signs, the reasons for which are as yet obscure, and viral diseases that have cerebral affects should be considered.

Treatment (see p. 1029)

Two considerations need to be borne in mind. Firstly, severely affected calves will require individual treatment with an anticoccidial and, if deemed advisable, fluid therapy with electrolytes and injections of antibiotics to control secondary bacterial infections. Anticoccidial treatments include injections of sulpha drugs or the oral administration of sulphadimidine at 140 mg/kg body weight daily for three days, or amprolium at 10 mg/kg for four or five days. Amprolium has been withdrawn from sale in many countries because of possible carcinogenesis, and it should be remembered that overdose with amprolium, which is a thiamine antagonist, has also been associated with production of cerebrocortical necrosis (CCN), so care should be taken to give the correct dose in those areas where it is available.

Secondly, prophylactic treatment for other calves in the group should be assessed, depending on the numbers involved. Lasalocid at 1 mg/kg body weight per day, monensin included in the diet at 16.5 ppm of the diet or decoquinate at 100 ppm, either continuously to suppress all infection or for two cycles of medication for a week separated by a week when it is removed, can protect from the infection and allow sufficient immunity to be stimulated. A long-acting intraruminal bolus consisting of 1.6 g baquiloprim plus 14.4 g sulphadimidine is also effective, and sulphadimidine itself can also be used prophylactically at 35 mg/kg, but it should be borne in mind that as light infections are self-limiting such treatments may not be cost-effective.

Other measures should be taken to reduce the chances of infection, i.e. removal of food contaminated with faeces and better siting of feeding and water troughs so that faecal deposition on food and in water is made less likely. If the problem is a recurring event with each batch of calves, thought should be given to a short period of anticoccidial treatment after two weeks of exposure to possible infection so that incipient infections are disrupted but sufficient stimulation of immunity has been allowed to take place. A potent anticoccidial of a novel chemical type, toltrazuril, has been used experimentally in this manner with great success and may constitute a significant future advance in the prophylaxis of the disease.

Neosporosis (see p. 584)

Aetiology

The cause is *Neospora caninum*, a coccidial protozoan discovered within the last decade, and now recognized as a ubiquitous parasite of cattle and dogs that also affects many other species of animals. Although it is the type species, recently, another species, *N. hughesi*, has been isolated from horses. Currently little is known of its development in animals that are naturally infected. The dog is the intermediate host, and is also a final host in prenatal infections. Infection can be both vertically transmitted from dam to calf *in utero* and lactogenically, naturally by ingestion of food and water contaminated with dog faeces containing *Neospora caninum* oocysts, or from cow to cow. The mechanisms of repeat congenital transmission are unknown at present.

Signs

It is a major cause of abortion in both dairy and beef cattle, and has been observed in almost all countries in the world. Cows of any age can abort from three months of gestation to full term, although most abortions occur at 5–6 months. Foetuses can be born alive or may die *in utero* and be mummified or reabsorbed. Calves that are infected may be born underweight and with neurologic symptoms such as ataxia, decreased reflexes and exophthalmia.

Necropsy

Tachyzoites and tissue cysts are found intracellularly in affected cattle. Tachyzoites measure 6 × 2 microns. Tissue cysts are oval, 102 microns long, and are found in the central nervous system and retina. Although infection can be found in many organs, the commonest site is the brain. The characteristic lesion is a focal encephalitis with necrosis and non-suppurative inflammation. Hepatitis can also be found in epidemic abortions.

Diagnosis

Ante-mortem diagnosis is by serologic methods. Several methods of assay of serum antibody are available, e.g. ELISA and indirect fluorescent antibody. A PCR (polymerase chain reaction) diagnosis of antigens is under development.

Treatment and control

At present treatments are largely experimental. Sulphonamides, pyrimethamine and clindamycin have been used in infected dogs, and decoquinate has been shown to kill *N. caninum* tachyzoites in cultures. Dogs should not be allowed to eat aborted fetuses or fetal membranes, and their faeces should be prevented from contaminating bovine feedstuffs.

Toxoplasmosis

Toxoplasmosis is a protozoan zoonosis that can infect any species of vertebrate. It is mainly recognized as being most pathogenic for sheep, however it occasionally causes human illness, and it can cause significant disease in cattle, although abortion is not as common a result as in sheep (see p. 895).

Aetiology and epidemiology

The parasite involved is *Toxoplasma gondii*. It has a two-host life cycle with both sexual and asexual stages. The definitive hosts are cats, both domestic and wild, which become infected by eating raw infected meat from the intermediate host, which can be any other species of vertebrate but is frequently a rodent. Once ingested the infective cysts are digested, each releasing large numbers of bradyzoites. They penetrate intestinal epithelial cells and undergo a coccidia-like series of schizogonies and finally gametogony in the small intestine to produce oocysts in faeces within one and a half weeks after ingestion of cysts. The cat then excretes oocysts for approximately two weeks. Oocysts remain viable for 17 months on pasture and if they contaminate animal feed any animal consuming it becomes infected.

Within the intermediate host, development is asexual. The oocyst wall is disrupted, releasing eight sporozoites which reach the lymph and blood vessels after penetrating the intestinal epithelium. The tachyzoites, as they are now called, are spread throughout the body to muscles, heart, lungs, liver, uterus and central nervous system, where they penetrate cells and multiply asexually. It is during this phase that the intermediate host becomes ill. After each multiplication the infected cells rupture, releasing 8–16 tachyzoites for further spread. After some days of such divisions the host develops some resistance to the organism and the spread of tachyzoites ceases, but is replaced by the formation of slow-growing cysts, each of which eventually contains large numbers of bradyzoites. Normally these remain until ingested, but should the host's immunity be reduced by other disease the invasive process can recommence. The tissue cysts are susceptible to freezing and cooking to 70°C for 30 seconds and therefore consumption of adequately cooked infected meat is harmless.

The organism is ubiquitous. Blewett (1983) reviewed the serological surveys that have been carried out in domestic animals and came to the estimate that antibody was present in 6.5 per cent of horses, 12.5 per cent of cattle, 23.5 per cent of pigs, 30 per cent of sheep and 40 per cent of cats. He also postulated that different animals vary in susceptibility to infection and in the rate of loss of antibody, and concluded that cattle return to a seronegative status much more rapidly than do sheep, which are as a result a more reliable indicator of the actual prevalence of the infection.

Diagnosis

At autopsy or in abattoirs the most common findings are multiple necrotic granulomatous foci in internal organs. Histopathological examination is necessary for confirmation. *In vivo*, cattle are presented with vague pyrexic disorders sometimes affecting the central nervous system. If pregnant cows are affected, stillborn or weak calves that die within a few days of birth may result. Such calves frequently manifest nervous signs such as tremors of the head or neck, teeth grinding or convulsions.

Serological diagnosis can be made using a variety of tests such as indirect immunofluorescence or enzyme-linked immunosorbent assay (ELISA), or the Sabin-Feldman dye test. Because of its ease of use, an ELISA using both anti-IgM and anti-IgG for detection of both acute and chronic infection is currently being developed.

Treatment and control

Treatment of acutely infected animals can be attempted by the use of pyrimethamine and sulpha compounds such as sulphadiazine or sulphadimidine. Results in animals have been disappointing compared with those in mice and humans. These drugs affect tachyzoites but not bradyzoites so that total elimination of the parasite is not possible. Recent experiments with the ionophore monensin have shown prophylactic activity in sheep, but there are no reports of its use in cattle (Buxton *et al.*, 1987). Other preventative measures include prevention of cat faecal contamination of animal food and adequate destruction of infected carcasses.

Sarcosporidiosis (sarcocystosis)

Aetiology

The cause is *Sarcocystis*, a coccidial protozoan that has a predator–prey life cycle. The indirect hosts are dogs, cats and man and each may contain several species of sarcocyst, each one specific for a different intermediate host. *Sarcocystis hirsuta* is present in the ox and cat species, *S. cruzi* in the ox and dog and *S. hominis* in the ox and man. In the final host the *Sarcocystis* spp. undergo an enteric cycle with oocysts in the cells producing sporocysts in the faeces. On entry to some intermediate hosts those infected via the dog undergo schizogamy in blood vessel endothelial cells before passing to the muscle. Those of the cat are not pathogenic and are found in the oesophagus, and throughout the tissues of the intermediate host produce microscopic cysts. If cattle are grazing and ingesting a few oocysts this probably results in a strong immunity. Signs develop about 26 days after infection (see p. 895).

Signs

Usually no signs occur but, following ingestion of massive doses, calves may develop anorexia, fever, emaciation and anaemia. Adults can suffer pyrexia, emaciation and abortion.

Necropsy

There are usually petechial and ecchymotic haemorrhages throughout the body, especially in the heart, brain, liver, lungs, kidneys and muscle. Some animals show emaciation, lymphadenopathy, anaemia and ascites. Death is usually due to necrotizing endocarditis. Histologically, schizonts can be found in the endothelium throughout the body and haemorrhages, lymphatic infiltration and oedema occur in the tissues and organs.

Diagnosis

This is usually based on post-mortem findings.

Treatment

Pyrimethamine at 1 μg/ml and trimethoprim at 5.0 μg/ml alone or in combination with sulphonamides have been shown to inhibit the development of *S. neurona* in cell cultures. Sulphonamides alone were ineffective. The difficulty with any treatment is the maintenance of sufficient concentrations of the drugs in the cerebrospinal fluid, and relapses are usually ascribed to failure to do so.

Control

This is difficult but involves keeping carnivores away from cattle. Infection in dogs and cats can be avoided by feeding them cooked meat.

References

Armour, J., Jennings, F.W. & Urquhart, G.M. (1969) Inhibition of *Ostertagia ostertagi* at the early fourth larval stage. II. The influence of environment on host or parasite. *Research in Veterinary Science*, **10**, 238–44.

Blewett, D.A. (1983) The epidemiology of ovine toxoplasmosis. I. The interpretation of data for the prevalence of antibody in sheep and other host species. *British Veterinary Journal*, **139**, 537–45.

Buxton, D., Donald, K.M. & Finlayson, J. (1987) Monensin and the control of experimental ovine toxoplasmosis: a systemic effect. *Veterinary Record*, **120**, 618–19.

Leaver, J.D. (1970) A comparison of grazing systems for dairy herd replacements. *Journal of Agricultural Science, Cambridge*, **75**, 265–72.

McMeekin, C.P. (1954) Good rearing of dairy stock. Bulletin, Department of Agriculture, New Zealand, No. 228.

Michel, J.F. (1968) The control of stomach worm infections in young cattle. *Journal of British Grassland Society*, **23**, 165–73.

Michel, J.F. (1969) The epidemiology and control of some nematode infections. *Advances in Parasitology*, **7**, 211–82.

Urquhart, G.M., Armour, J., Duncan, J.L., Dunn, A.N. & Jennings, F.W. (1987) *Veterinary Parasitology*. Longman Scientific, Harlow, pp. 1–286.

Chapter 20
Respiratory Diseases

A.H. Andrews

Shipping fever (transit fever, pasteurellosis)   286
Infectious bovine rhinotracheitis (IBR)   289

Shipping fever (transit fever, pasteurellosis)

Epidemiology

The condition is an important respiratory problem in groups of weaned suckled calves that have been sold, often via a market, hence the terms transit fever or shipping fever. They are usually over six months old and under two years. During part of the sale transactions they will probably have been mixed and grouped with other batches of animals of similar age during transport, at the market or following arrival at the finishing farm. Most cases occur within the first month of their entry to the fattening unit and most cases are seen at least 10 days after arrival (Andrews *et al.*, 1981). The disease is characterized by an illness of sudden onset with dullness, pyrexia and anorexia. It is an acute exudative bronchopneumonia with toxaemia as well as much fibrin present in the exudate and often accompanied by fibrinous pleurisy (Blood & Radostits, 1989). The condition is common in North America, Europe and Britain. It is particularly prevalent in the American cattle feedlot industry and is the largest cause of mortality in that system. In a Colorado survey 75 per cent of all clinical disease in yearling cattle and 64 per cent of all post-mortem diagnoses were due to respiratory disease (Jensen *et al.*, 1976). The morbidity and mortality rates vary considerably but a level of up to 35 per cent and a mortality of 5–10 per cent of those affected or 0.75–1 per cent of the susceptible population is often quoted (Blood & Radostits, 1989). More recently in Britain, morbidity rates of 73–100 per cent with a mortality of 0–8 per cent of those affected and an average mortality of 4 per cent have been reported (Andrews, 2000).

Aetiology

The aetiology of the condition is still open to disagreement. It is considered to be stress or management induced with the participation of infectious agents. The infection has been thought to be primarily viral, mainly due either to parainfluenza III (PI$_3$) virus or infectious bovine rhinotracheitis (IBR) virus, followed by secondary infection with either *Pasteurella multocida* or *Mannheimia haemolytica* (Pirie, 1979). *Mannheimia haemolytica* biotype A serotype 1 is considered to be the most common isolate although biotype T strains have also been found. *Mannheimia haemolytica* biotype A produces a heat-labile cytotoxin that is ruminant-specific destroying leucocytes (Sherwen & Wilkie, 1982). *Pasteurella multocida* infection is only isolated occasionally. Recently, it has been proved experimentally that *M. haemolytica* biotype A1 can produce the disease as a primary agent in non-immune calves (Shoo, 1989). Disease does depend on administering the organisms into the lungs either intratracheally (Friend *et al.*, 1977; Gibbs *et al.*, 1983) or intrathoracically (Houghton & Gourlay, 1984; Panciera & Corstvet, 1984). However, the exact mechanism by which the organisms enter the lung and result in lesions is not yet known. Other evidence of *M. haemolytica* involvement is that calves previously exposed naturally to the infection are much more resistant to experimental and natural pneumonic pasteurellosis (Confer *et al.*, 1984).

Although *M. haemolytica* can be isolated from the nasal passages it is only in small numbers when calves are healthy and unstressed. The organisms can be present in low numbers in the tracheal air but are not considered to be normal inhabitants of the lungs (Grey & Thomson, 1971). However, as the calves are transported, move to market and then enter the feedlot, the number of *M. haemolytica* biotype A1 increases in the nasal tract, the tracheal air and then the lungs, where bronchopneumonia can result (Frank & Smith, 1983). Thus management factors are important. The effects of stress are extremely difficult to quantify and have not been successfully undertaken experimentally to produce transit fever. However, transportation of yearling cattle does result in a rise in plasma fibrinogen levels, which is indicative of stress (Phillips, 1984). Increased fibrinogen levels also occur following confinement in unfamiliar surroundings and deprivation of food and water. In addition, it seems that cattle suddenly introduced to a diet consisting of large amounts of cereal are more prone to respiratory problems (Wilson *et al.*, 1985).

The environment tends to be important in that disease seems to be related to the season of the year (Andrews, 1978), fluctuations in daily ambient temperature and increased concentration of airborne particles 2.0–3.3 μm in diameter (MacVean *et al.*, 1986). Calves kept at a constant temperature of 16°C (60°F) showed minimum levels of nasopharyngeal bacteria at a relative humidity between 65 and 75 per cent. However, bacterial counts tend to rise at humidities on either side of this range (Jones & Webster, 1981).

The interrelationship of different micro-organisms and transit fever still needs further elucidation. However, cattle entering feedlots with low serological titres to IBR, bovine respiratory syncytial virus (RSV) and *Mycoplasma dispar* were at greater risk of being treated for BRD (Rosendal & Martin, 1986). It has also been shown that IBR, PI$_3$, bovine virus diarrhoea (BVD) and RSV are all associated with acute respiratory disease (Martin & Bohaz, 1986).

In many outbreaks of transit fever it is likely that the stress of movement plus mixing with other calves, the introduction to housing and a new diet are sufficient to initiate disease. The main organism involved is usually a *Mannheimia* species, especially *M. haemolytica* biotype A1. Spread of infection is optimized by crowded conditions in transport and markets. It is also probable that as animals go down with disease and pass on the infection, the organism increases in virulence. This can be seen in some outbreaks in which disease can be traced from individual animals to other members of the same group and then to other groups (Andrews, 1976).

Signs (see p. 921)

The peracute form is unusual but results in sudden death with no premonitory signs.

In the acute form the animals are dull and inactive with excessive oculo-nasal discharges, which may be mucupurulent. There is usually anorexia although the cattle still drink, and a marked fever (40–41°C, 104–106°F). There is rapid (40+/minute), shallow breathing and a soft, productive cough, which tends to increase with exercise. On auscultation there are bronchial sounds over the anterior and ventral parts of the lungs, which become louder as the condition continues. In some cases squeaks and high-pitched sounds are heard, together with a pleuritic rub. Later signs can include dyspnoea with marked abdominal breathing and an expiratory grunt. Diarrhoea occurs in a few animals. There is usually a favourable response to therapy.

Necropsy

Death is usually the result of anoxia and toxaemia although occasionally in young cattle there is septicaemia. Usually, over one-third of the lung shows marked consolidation and the ventral parts of the apical and cardiac lobes are most involved. Initially, there is lung congestion and then hepatitis with exudate and, in some animals, emphysema. Bronchitis and bronchiolitis are usually catarrhal, often with serofibrinous pleurisy and a fibrinous pericarditis. There is usually much pleural effusion.

Diagnosis

This depends on the history of age, recent movement, weaning or housing. The signs also help with severe respiratory signs involving the anteroventral parts of the lungs and pyrexia. Post-mortem findings of lung consolidation and pleurisy are present, and impression smears show bipolar staining organisms with methylene blue. *Mannheimia haemolytica* or *P. multocida* may be isolated from nasal swabs in live animals or lungs at post-mortem and their antibiotic sensitivity determined. Serology for antibody rise can be undertaken, as also can haematology but often the findings are variable.

Differential diagnosis

Differential diagnosis includes enzootic pneumonia (see p. 242) but this usually occurs in younger calves with a different history. Infectious bovine rhinotracheitis (see p. 289) usually shows mainly upper respiratory signs and a conjunctivitis. Fog fever (see p. 866) is mainly apparent in older cattle at grass after a pasture move in the autumn. Parasitic bronchitis (see p. 272) is present in cattle following grazing. Acute bronchopneumonia would be almost identical except for bacteriological isolation. Contagious bovine pleuropneumonia is severe in all age groups of cattle and the affected animals suffer severe pain and toxaemia with a high mortality (see p. 868).

Treatment

Therapy for shipping fever is given in Table 20.1. Treatment should begin early. Most cattle will usually show some improvement within one to three days of initiating treatment. Complete recovery may take four to seven days. Where severe outbreaks occur it may occasionally be necessary to use mass medication by water as most ill cattle still drink well. Anti-inflammatory agents are often useful in promoting a speedy recovery.

Prevention and control

Although the disease of transit fever is sporadic, many of the conditions that predispose to the problem can be defined. This should mean that methods of prevention should be relatively easy to institute. Ideally, the calves would be weaned at least two weeks prior to leaving the farm of birth (Andrews, 1976). They would be introduced to the type of feed to be provided on the rearing farm. In addition, they would be batched in groups that would go direct from the farm of birth to the rearing farm. In reality this does not happen as the farmer pro-ducing the calves hopes that by selling them at market he will obtain a better price than by selling direct. In addition, the first farmer will be little concerned about the subsequent disease status of his calves once they have left his farm for sale. This makes the possibility of vaccination prior to movement difficult.

As cattle go through markets, disease prevention tends not to be practised because many of the factors enhancing the likelihood of a disease outbreak are outside the control of the purchasing beef rearers. Thus they cannot control the time before moving, the trans-port of the animals from the farm of origin, their mixing

Table 20.1 Therapy for shipping fever.

Drug	Method of administration	Dose (mg/kg)	Dose (mg/lb)	Duration
Amoxycillin trihydrate	s.c., i.m.	7	3	Daily for 3–5 days
Ampicillin trihydrate	s.c., i.m.	5–10	2.5–5	Daily for 3 days
Baquiloprim and	oral	4–8	2–4	Once or repeat
sulphadimidine		36–72	18–36	after 48 hours
Cefquinome	i.m.	1	0.5	Daily for 3–5 days
Ceftiofur	i.m.	1.1	0.5	Daily for 3–5 days
Chloramphenicol (some countries)	i.m.	10	5	3–4 times daily for 3 days
Danofloxacin	i.v., i.m.	1.25	0.6	Daily for 3–5 days
Enrofloxacin	s.c.	2.5	1.25	Daily for 3 days
	s.c.	7.5	3.75	Once
Erythromycin	i.v., i.m.	5	2.5	Daily for 3 days
Florfenicol	i.m.	20	10	2 (48 hours apart)
	s.c.	40	20	Once
Marbofloxacin	i.v., s.c., i.m.	2	1	Daily for 3–5 days
Oxytetracycline	i.v., s.c., i.m.	10	5	Daily for 3 days
Oxytetracycline (long-acting)	i.m.	20	10	Usually once
Penicillin/dihydrostreptomycin	i.m.	(20–30 000 iu/kg)	(10–15 000 iu/lb)	Daily for 3 days
		20	10	
Penicillin (long-acting)				
benzathine	i.m.	5	2.5	Usually once
procaine	i.m.	6	3	Daily for 3–5 days
Spectinomycin	i.v., i.m.	10–20	5–10	Daily for 3–4 days
Spiramycin	i.m.	20	10	Daily for 2–3 days
Sulphadimidine	i.v., s.c., oral	150	75	Daily for 3 days
Tilmicosin	s.c.	10	5	Usually once
Trimethoprim and sulphadiazine	i.m.	4	2	Daily for 3–5 days
		20	10	
Trimethoprim and sulphadoxine	i.v., i.m.	3	1.5	Daily for 3–5 days
		12.5	6	
Tylosin	i.m.	4–10	2–5	Daily for 3–5 days
Mass medication				
Oxytetracycline	oral	5	2.5	Daily for 5 days
Sulphamidine	oral	100	50	Daily for 5–7 days
Trimethoprim and sulphadiazine	oral	25	12.5	Daily for 5–7 days
Tylosin	oral			Daily for 5 days

All animals should be provided with good-quality feed and adequate ventilation. Corticosteroids, e.g. betamethasone, dexamethasone, are often found to help in reducing the level of exudation. NSAIDs may be useful in reducing inflammation, and *Mannheimia* antisera may also be helpful.

with other cattle or the conditions present at market. Likewise they will probably have little direct say as to how the animals are transported or their mixing with other groups before their entry to the rearing farm. It is only once the cattle reach the rearers that control measures can be undertaken. Obviously, they can ensure that the animals are kept in as satisfactory an environment as possible and are only lightly stocked. This is best done by having the animals outside but this is resisted by most farmers because of the inconvenience and extra labour required. The new ration for the cattle can also be introduced slowly.

The problem is worse in North America where calves often travel vast distances. Here various preconditioning programmes are undertaken. It is advised that calves should be fed prior to weaning and kept in the same place once the dams are removed. Following weaning, regular checking of the calves several times a day should be practised. When animals are travelling they should be given adequate periods of rest and offered feed and water. They should also be well bedded during transit. Some farmers inject multivitamin preparations before moving and vaccines can be used, including those against *Mannheimia* and PI_3 virus.

In many countries antibiotics are used following the move. These have given variable results mainly due to predicting when injections should be undertaken. This is because most problems occur about seven to ten days after entry to the feedlot or farm. When used, it is probably best to give long-acting preparations and initiate therapy when the first animals show disease. Use of antibiotic medication in the feed or water is a common practice in North America and while it appears to reduce mortality it has no effect on morbidity.

Vaccination

If it is considered that *M. haemolytica* and at times *P. multocida* form an important part of the disease syndrome of transit fever then it might be possible to obtain some protection by vaccination. Various vaccines are present in Europe but currently only three are available in Britain.

In North America various *Pasteurella* bacterins and viral vaccines have been used to assist with the control of transit fever. Their efficacy appears to be low and literature reviews suggest that at present there is little evidence to show the efficacy of such vaccines under feedlot conditions (Myers, 1984).

Recently in North America several new vaccines have become available. One of these is a *M. haemolytica* vaccine/bacterial extract. This has been shown to be effective to controlled challenge provided two doses of vaccine have been administered prior to challenge (Sherwen & Wilkie, 1988). Response in a field trial has however shown only a slight decrease in morbidity of disease, with slight improvement in relapse rates and response to treatment (Bateman, 1988; Jim *et al.*, 1988).

Infectious bovine rhinotracheitis (IBR)

Aetiology

Infectious bovine rhinotracheitis (IBR) is a highly infectious and contagious disease of cattle. It is caused by a virus known as bovine herpes virus 1 (BHV 1). It is generally considered that there are several strains of the virus, although often the differences between the strains are not easily shown in the laboratory. The disease is seen in North America, Europe and Africa. It is considered that the outbreak of severe respiratory disease that occurred in Great Britain in the mid-1970s was due to a new strain being imported. Several European countries are undertaking eradication campaigns, many of which are progressing satisfactorily. They often involve initial vaccination with marker vaccines and then blood testing, and movement restrictions until the disease is no larger present.

While the disease is primarily one of cattle, it can also infect deer, goats and pigs. The main sources of infection between animals are nasal discharge (or eye discharge), when it is affecting the respiratory system, and vaginal or preputial discharges, semen, or the fluids and tissues of the fetus when the infection involves the reproductive tract (see p. 579).

Epidemiology

In most cases of respiratory infection disease is spread by aerosol. The genital form of the disease is contracted venereally. As respiratory infection is spread via the air, it can spread by direct contact between the animals or where the cattle are in the same air space, i.e. there is air contact. This can only be avoided by ensuring the walls extend from floor to ceiling and there is no contact with other animals either at the front of the pens or with other groups on either side. However, generally there is a need for close sustained contact between groups. This is why disease is often slow to spread within and between groups. It often takes two to five weeks to spread in a group. However, unexplained outbreaks of IBR do occur on isolated farms.

Latent infection: There is a problem with BHV 1 in that it is able to become a latent infection. Thus once an animal is infected with a strain of the virus or vaccinated with a live viral vaccine, the virus may remain in the animal for the rest of its life without it showing any signs of illness. The site of latency is arguable but the virus can be found in the trigeminal nerve of clinically normal cattle. However, if the animal is stressed at all, such as when moved or calving, or becomes ill, the virus may be shed. Shedding can also occur in bulls when mating. This shedding may be, but is often not, accompanied by any signs of disease. Corticosteroid injections may promote virus shedding. The level of this latent infection is variable but can be up to 10 per cent of clinically normal animals. In addition, while most of these cattle will show antibody levels to the BHV 1 virus, some do not. Thus all cattle in herds where disease occurs have the capacity to spread disease even when there are no clinical signs of disease present in the herd. The only way of knowing whether or not disease is present is to look at the results of milk or blood tests. If a blood test shows an antibody titre (positive response) to BHV 1 in cattle other than calves it means that the animal(s) have been exposed to infection and could possibly be carriers. If a blood test from an animal is negative it generally means that the animal is unlikely to have been exposed to infection, but it does not completely rule out the possibility that the animal is a latent carrier of disease. Thus tests on individual animals are of limited significance; however, on a herd basis repeated negative tests indicate that it is highly unlikely infection is present. When tests show several animals with antibody levels in the herd then infection is present. The calf that receives colostrum from its infected mother will also show a positive antibody level to the test although not necessarily being infected. The antibody provided from the colostrum will usually remain for one to six months, depending on the amount received from the mother.

Incubation period: The incubation period for the disease is very variable. Experimentally, it usually takes three to seven days. However, in most beef units disease occurs about 10–20 days after introduction of infected or susceptible animals. Longer incubation periods do occur. This is quite likely when it is considered that latent carriers may not be shedding virus at a particular time.

Signs

Respiratory disease: This disease is the most common form. It is usually seen in cattle over six months old but can occur at a younger age. The signs vary considerably but typically they tend to be worst in animals from about six months to two years old.

(1)   Mild disease. This is just a conjunctivitis, i.e. slight reddening to the lining of the eye and eyelids with some discharge, usually watery and clear (see p. 921). This often occurs when the disease strain is mild or degree of infection is low, or the animal is resistant.

(2)   Subacute disease. This is commonly seen in adult cattle and often is of only short duration. There is a marked rise in temperature lasting only a day or two (40°C, 104°F). Often there is a marked drop in milk yield. Again the lining of the eyes is reddened with discharge and this also involves reddening of the lining of the nose with nasal discharge. The animals will salivate and there may be a short, expressive cough. Breathing is rapid and shallow. The animals recover in 10 to 14 days.

(3)   Acute disease. The signs are as in the subacute form but the temperature tends to be higher (40–41°C, 104–106°F). These signs are particularly present in growing cattle between six months and two years old. The respiratory signs are more likely to include a cough and there is some respiratory distress. The discharge from eyes and nose tends to become profuse, yellow, thick and purulent. The lining of the nose may show grey areas, which consist of dead tissues that smell and are shed. The signs tend to last a lot longer before recovery occurs.

(4)   Peracute disease. The animals develop very high temperatures (42°C, 108°F) with eye and nasal discharge, respiratory distress, cough and then death in about 24 hours.

Some cattle may die owing to complications and this is particularly so in the six month to two year age group. Here mortality may reach 10 per cent or more. However, it is usually only about 1 per cent. Some cattle keep a stertor (snoring breathing) for many months. Some become 'puffers' with bouts of respiratory signs including distress when breathing, loss of appetite and cough. These usually have a secondary bronchopneumonia and die in weeks or months after losing condition. Often they become recumbent before death.

Characteristically, there is a sudden outbreak of disease involving the respiratory tract. This will initially involve the group of cattle to which infection has been introduced. It will then tend to spread round all the other groups and ages of cattle. This can often take a few weeks or many months, dependent on the strain of virus, the level of infection and the degree of exposure to infection of each group. Characteristically, an outbreak in a group reaches a peak at about two or three weeks after its start and is over between the fourth and sixth week.

Reproductive form: In most cases the reproductive and respiratory forms are not seen together.

(1)   Infectious pustular vulvovaginitis. This is an infection of the vulva and vagina often lasting several weeks. It results in the discharge of pus from the vulva, usually in small quantities. There is reddening of the lining and

pustule presence. In some cases infection causes irritation in the vagina resulting in frequent urination and possibly increased straining (see p. 628).

(2) Infectious bovine penoposthitis. Bulls show a small amount of purulent discharge from the prepuce. The surface of the penis and prepuce may be reddened with haemorrhages and small necrotic areas.

(3) Endometritis. Infection of the uterus, with discharge, poor conception rates and short returns to oestrus, can occur if semen is infected.

(4) Abortion (see p. 579). This is becoming increasingly common and occurs some weeks or months after the animal is infected. Abortion is usually at six to eight months of pregnancy and often the placenta is retained following abortion. In some cases of infection calves are born weak at the normal time.

Generalized/alimentary form: This is seen in young newborn calves and is recorded mainly in America. It occurs when calves receive little or no immunity in the colostrum and are then subjected to infection. The animals show a severe temperature reaction, they do not eat and they salivate. The lining of the nose is red. The eyes may show a conjunctivitis. In addition, the lining of the mouth and the soft palate (at the back of the throat) are reddened with mucus present. The opening to the trachea, i.e. the pharynx, is also reddened with much discharge present. There is usually severe respiratory distress with a bronchopneumonia. Some calves show severe diarrhoea and dehydration.

Central nervous system/encephalitic form: This is seen in calves under six months old and involves brain signs. The animals show incoordination with bouts of excitement and depression. In other cases there are convulsions, bellowing and blindness with salivation. This nervous form is rare.

Other infections: Reports of infections of the udder and intestinal tract have been made. However, these are rarely the only systems affected.

Necropsy

Respiratory form: In uncomplicated cases, lesions are restricted to the upper respiratory tract terminating at the upper bronchi. Inflammation of the muzzle and the nasal cavities varies from some congestion and petechiation with mucoid exudate, to a fibrinopurulent exudate with necrosis of the nasal mucous membranes. The submandibular and retropharyngeal lymph nodes tend to be swollen and oedematous. There is a laryngotracheobronchitis, which varies from a mild congestion of the mucous membranes with a mucoid discharge to large areas being covered by a necrotic layer of exudate (Pirie, 1979). In some cases there is pulmonary emphysema and secondary exudative bronchopneumonia, which may be purulent or necrotizing. Histologically, the mucous membranes show acute catarrhal inflammation and in some cases the epithelium and larynx tend to be infiltrated with neutrophils, lymphocytes, plasma cells and macrophages. In naturally occurring infections, inclusion bodies appear to be absent.

Abortion: Aborted fetuses often show marked autolysis and focal necrotic hepatitis.

Alimentary form: Epithelial necrosis of the turbinates, oesophagus, rumen and abomasum. Inclusion bodies are often evident in the surviving epithelium.

Nervous form: A non-suppurative encephalitis occurs particularly affecting the cerebral cortex and internal capsule.

Diagnosis

This will depend on the type but in the alimentary form it will depend on a history of IBR in the herd with virus present in the faeces or nasal swabs and possible necrotic areas on the turbinates. The nervous form is difficult to differentiate except that there is probably an IBR outbreak in the herd. At post-mortem examination the turbinates may show necrotic lesions.

In the respiratory form the history is that a new animal or group has entered the herd. In most cases several animals will be affected and besides varying degrees of respiratory signs there will usually be a conjunctivitis with copious, initially serous, ocular discharge. There may be necrosis of the nasal mucosa but this is absent in the mouth. The virus can be isolated in upper nasal or ocular swabs and is detected by fluorescent antibody staining. Otherwise paired blood samples will show a rise in titre to the enzyme-linked immunosorbent assay (ELISA) test. Other tests used include the serum neutralization test, indirect haemagglutination test, complement fixation test and virus neutralization test. Bulk milk testing will indicate the status of a dairy herd.

Treatment

There is a considerable divergence of opinion as to whether or not to use antibiotic treatment. If the disease appears to be uncomplicated, and this is unusual, then there would appear to be little point in therapy. If, however, as in most cases, there is secondary lung involvement, then therapy is justified. At the start of an outbreak all cases should be isolated as soon as possible because although it may not stop spread of the disease, the first animals are often clinically the worst affected. If antimicrobial agents are to be used, all ill calves should be treated for three to five days with any one of a number of drugs, including penicillin and streptomycin, oxytetracycline, ampicillin, trimethoprim and sulphadiazine, sulphadimidine, sulphamethoxypyridazine and sulphapyrazole. The animal should be given good, wholesome feed and it should be encouraged to eat and drink. Some farmers have vaccinated their calves with live vaccine after the start of an outbreak, with good results, but to be successful infection must not have become established. It should be remembered that for effective protection, vaccines should be introduced before the onset of infection. Several compounds have been found that are active against herpes viruses. However, many are toxic, but one drug, acyclovir, has been shown to be safe and may in the future be tried in animals.

Control

Management: It is best to keep a closed herd. However, in America, and also Britain, infection has been found in closed herds. Any new animal entering a known uninfected herd should be blood tested prior to entry. If the test is negative the animal should be isolated for a month and then retested. The use of corticosteroids may allow detection of virus in swabs of carrier animals. If the tests are all negative the animal can be allowed to enter the herd. The risks then of the introduction of infection are small. If the animal suffers a respiratory problem while in isolation the second test should not be until two or three weeks after the end of the episode. Some farmers may need to go to these lengths to keep their pedigree herds free from disease, because many European countries will not accept exports unless they are shown to have a negative titre for IBR. The same conditions at present govern the entry of bulls to some artificial insemination (AI) centres.

Vaccination (see p. 1010): An inactivated multicomponent vaccine has been available for a long time. The vaccine could be given as doses two to four weeks apart with a third injection at 10–12 weeks old. Its efficacy has at times been questioned. Subsequently, live IBR vaccines have become available. They are given by intranasal inoculation or injection and should be administered 24–48 hours after entry to the farm. Ideally, calves should be vaccinated 10 days prior to any movement. A gene-depleted live vaccine is available in some countries and allows control of disease. The immunity produced allows differentiation from that produced by the wild strain. This means the vaccination

can be used in an IBR eradication campaign. Live vaccines, as other vaccines, can present a possible danger if contaminated with other pathogens, such as BVDV.

Beef calves can be vaccinated about two weeks or so before they are weaned. One vaccine is temperature sensitive and so only replicates in the upper parts of the respiratory tract. However, the vaccine can still produce circulating antibody levels in some cattle, which will preclude their export or their sale to AI centres. Another vaccine does replicate in organs other than the lungs and produces a good systemic immunity. The vaccines provide effective immunity but they do allow the replication and re-excretion of the IBR virus, which can thus spread infection to non-vaccinated animals.

Several countries within the EU have successfully eradicated BHVI (IBR), including Denmark, Finland and Sweden. An EU-approved national compulsory eradication scheme is being undertaken in Austria. Control programmes are being pursued in the Netherlands, Belgium, France and Germany. A programme for the monitoring, screening, eradication and accreditation of freedom from IBR in being undertaken in the UK by Cattle Health Certification Standards (CHeCS).

References

Andrews, A.H. (1976) Factors affecting the incidence of pneumonia in growing bulls. *Veterinary Record*, **98**, 52–5.

Andrews, A.H. (1978) Some factors influencing respiratory disease in growing bulls and the effect of treatment on liveweight. In *Respiratory Diseases in Cattle*. Seminar in CEC Programme of Coordination of Research in Beef Production, Edinburgh, 8–10 November 1977 (ed. by W.B. Martin), pp. 169–80. Martinus Nijhoff, The Hague.

Andrews, A.H. (2000) Calf pneumonia costs! *Cattle Practice*, **8**, 109–14.

Andrews, A.H., Cook, G.L., Pritchard, D.G., Morzaria, S.P. & Gilmour, N.J.L. (1981) Observations on a respiratory disease outbreak in weaned suckled calves. *Veterinary Record*, **108**, 139–42.

Bateman, K.G. (1988) Efficacy of *Pasteurella haemolytica* vaccine/bacterial extract in the prevention of bovine respiratory disease in recently shipped feedlot calves. *Canadian Veterinary Journal*, **29**, 838–9.

Blood, D.C. & Radostits, O.M. (1989) Pneumonic pasteurellosis of cattle (shipping fever pneumonia). In *Veterinary Medicine*, 7th edn, pp. 663–73. Ballière Tindall, London.

Confer, A.W., Panciera, R.J. & Fulton, R.W. (1984) Effect of prior exposure to *Pasteurella haemolytica* antiserum on experimental pneumonic pasteurellosis. *American Journal of Veterinary Research*, **45**, 2622–4.

Frank, G.H. & Smith, P.C. (1983) Prevalence of *Pasteurella haemolytica* in transported calves. *American Journal of Veterinary Research*, **44**, 981–5.

Friend, S.C., Thomson, R.G. & Wilkie, B.N. (1977) Pulmonary lesions induced by *Pasteurella haemolytica* in cattle. *Canadian Journal of Comparative Medicine*, **41**, 219–23.

Gibbs, H.A., Allan, E.M., Selman, I.E. & Wiseman, A. (1983) Experimental bovine pneumonic pasteurellosis. *Veterinary Record*, **113**, 144.

Grey, C.L. & Thomson, R.G. (1971) *Pasteurella haemolytica* in the tracheal air of calves. *Canadian Journal of Comparative Medicine*, **35**, 121–8.

Houghton, S.B. & Gourlay, R.N. (1984) Bacteria associated with calf pneumonia and their effect on gnotobiotic calves. *Research in Veterinary Science*, **37**, 194–8.

Jensen, R., Pierson, R.E., Braddy, R.M., Saari, D.A., Lauerman, L.H., England, J.J., Keyvan, F.A.R., Collier, I.J.R., Horton, D.P., McChesney, A.E., Benitez, A. & Christie, R.M. (1976) Shipping fever pneumonia in yearling feedlot cattle. *Journal of the American Veterinary Medical Association*, **169**, 500–506.

Jim, K., Guichon, T. & Shaw, G. (1988) Protecting feedlot calves from pneumonic pasteurellosis. *Veterinary Medicine*, **83**, 1084–7.

Jones, C.R. & Webster, A.J.F. (1981) Weather induced changes in airborne bacteria within a calf house. *Veterinary Record*, **109**, 493–4.

MacVean, D., Franzen, D.K., Keefe, T.J. & Bennett, B.W. (1986) Airborne particle concentration and meteorological conditions associated with pneumonia incidence in feedlot calves. *American Journal of Veterinary Research*, **47**, 2676–82.

Martin, S.W. & Bohaz, J.G. (1986) The association between serological titres in infectious bovine rhinotracheitis virus, bovine viral diarrhoea virus, parainfluenza III virus, respiratory syncytial virus and treatment for respiratory disease in Ontario feedlot cattle. *Canadian Journal of Veterinary Research*, **50**, 351–8.

Myers, L.C. (1984) Questions on the efficacy of cattle vaccines. *Journal of the American Veterinary Association*, **184**, 5–7.

Panciera, R.J. & Corstvet, R.E. (1984) Bovine pneumonic pasteurellosis: model for *Pasteurella haemolytica* and *Pasteurella multocida*-induced pneumonia in cattle. *American Journal of Veterinary Research*, **45**, 2532–7.

Phillips, W.A. (1984) The effect of assembling and transit stresses on plasma fibrinogen concentration of beef calves. *Canadian Journal of Comparative Medicine*, **48**, 35–41.

Pirie, H.M. (1979) *Respiratory Diseases of Animals*, pp. 68–70, 71–4. Notes for a Postgraduate Course, Glasgow Veterinary School.

Rosendal, S. & Martin, S.W. (1986) The association between serological evidence of *Mycoplasma* infection and respiratory disease in feedlot cattle. *Canadian Journal of Veterinary Research*, **50**, 179–83.

Sherwen, P.E. & Wilkie, B.W. (1982) Cytotoxin of *Pasteurella haemolytica* acting on bovine leucocytes. *Infection and Immunity*, **35**, 91–4.

Sherwen, P.E. & Wilkie, B.W. (1988) Vaccination of calves with leukotoxic culture supernatant from *Pasteurella haemolytica*. *Canadian Journal of Veterinary Research*, **52**, 30–6.

Shoo, M.K. (1989) Experimental bovine pneumonic pasteurellosis: A review. *Veterinary Record*, **124**, 141–4.

Wilson, S.H., Church, T.L. & Acres, S.D. (1985) The influence of feedlot management on an outbreak of bovine respiratory disease. *Canadian Veterinary Journal*, **26**, 335–41.

Chapter 21
Trace Element Disorders

N.F. Suttle

Introduction	294
Differential diagnosis	294
Definitions	294
Cobalt disorders	295
Copper disorders	298
Iodine disorders	301
Selenium disorders	302
Manganese and zinc disorders	305

Introduction

The full impact that trace element disorders can have on the health of cattle was seen when Europeans attempted to carry their methods of animal production to the New World and to the Antipodes. The geologically young soils bordering Australia, and forming the Florida peninsula and the interior of New Zealand's North Island, were a graveyard for many an animal until the therapeutic effect of newly discovered essential trace elements became known. Crop and pasture growth was also limited by some of the deficiencies but these were the more easily diagnosed because they produced characteristic foliar abnormalities. The animal's needs were more difficult to delineate because they lacked clinical definition and persisted where the more modest needs of the plant had been met. Since those pioneering days, trace element disorders have been described in many areas of the world and they continue to appear when new methods of production are introduced, but it is important to keep them in perspective.

Differential diagnosis

Trace element disorders carry more than their fair share of blame for poor cattle performance, due to the non-specificity of most clinical signs, the pressures on practitioners to offer a quick diagnosis and the alacrity with which clients accept a diagnosis that may seem to exonerate them from blame. Figure 21.1 presents a scheme for differential diagnosis of some common problems. Of the three main lines of investigation shown, trace elements are only *part* of the *least probable* explanation, the

most common being malnutrition, which is likely to be a whole herd problem. A preliminary check must be made of the quantity and quality of available feeds (Sinclair & Suttle, 2001). Trace element disorders usually afflict only a minority of the herd but a preliminary 'audit' of the likely mineral inputs and needs may narrow the range of possible culprits (Suttle & Sinclair, 2000). Responses to a broad mix of micronutrients would confirm this line of investigation. Depending on the history of the farm or area, it may be beneficial to attempt an earlier definitive diagnosis by using a specific trace element supplement, but proof of responsiveness amongst an affected minority may require unconventional statistical techniques which take into account initial variation in performance (Suttle, 2000). There may be cross-over between lines of investigation: correction of a gut parasite problem might improve trace element status, while improving the major nutrient supply of a herd (by improving ration digestibility) may lower status and increase the risk of trace element disorders. Seasonal and annual variations in incidence mean that it will always be necessary to review the need for any trace element intervention from time to time. Overall, following such a scheme should improve the precision of diagnoses.

Definitions

Four terms will occur frequently in descriptions of the sequence of events that occur when cattle are deprived of essential trace elements, and these require definition:

- *Depletion*: the reduction of body stores of the element.
- *Deficiency*: the presence of subnormal concentrations of the element in blood or tissues.
- *Disorder*: the malfunction of trace element-dependent body processes (subclinical disorder).
- *Disease*: the presence of visible, clinical abnormalities.

They are particularly useful when describing the trace element status of cattle biochemically, and avoid the confusion caused by using the one word 'deficiency' to describe all four stages, and as a 'tag' for interpret-

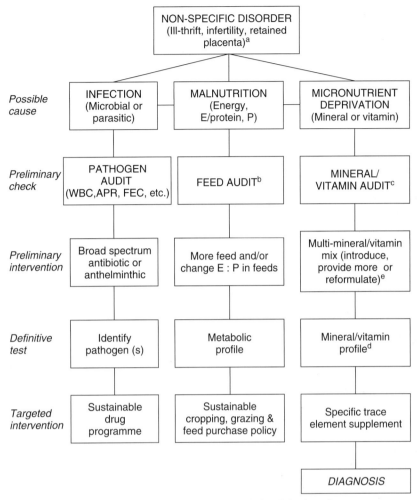

Fig. 21.1 Scheme for the differential diagnosis of trace element disorders with non-specific signs; proceed vertically with a given line of investigation only while test results are positive. WBC = white blood cell count; APR = acute phase proteins; FEC = faecal egg count.

[a] Firstly, rule out 'exotic' (e.g. plant, agrochemical or industrial poisons) or common (poor oestrous detection, large calf) factors.
[b] See Suttle (2002) for fuller details.
[c] See Suttle & Sinclair (2000) for fuller details.
[d] See Table 21.1 for best indices of trace element status.
[e] Some untreated animals must be left to prove effecacy and allow specific follow-up tests to be made.

ing indices of mineral status which rarely reflect onset of disorder or disease. Throughout this chapter, use will be made of 'marginal bands' for diagnostic criteria (Table 21.1), which reflect the uncertainty of detecting the onset of health-limiting conditions. The following descriptions of specific disorders concentrate on the more commonly encountered deficiencies of cobalt (Co), copper (Cu), iodine (I) and selenium (Se).

Cobalt disorders

Aetiology

The only known functions of Co arise from its place at the centre of the corrin ring of two cobalamin (Cbl)

molecules, methyl-(Me) and adenosyl-(Ado) Cbl, which have contrasting functions in the body. MeCbl acts as a coenzyme to methionine synthetase and is linked to folate metabolism, through the use of methyltetrahydrofolate as the methyl group donor. Deficiencies of this coenzyme can theoretically impair methionine synthesis and the bioavailability of folate and cause formiminoglutamic acid (FIGLU) to appear in urine. AdoCbl enables propionate to be used for gluconeogenesis via succinate and the tricarboxylic acid (TCA) cycle, acting as coenzyme to methylmalonyl-CoA isomerase: insufficiency causes methylmalonic acid (MMA) to accumulate.

The anorexia and anaemia that are successive debilitating consequences of deprivation may reflect the *dysfunction* of AdoCbl and/or MeCbl (Underwood

Table 21.1 Marginal bands for commonly used biochemical indices of micronutrient status in the diet, serum or tissues of cattle: mean values falling within bands indicate a possibility of benefit from trace element supplementation; the more extreme the value and the more parameters affected, the greater the possibility becomes; values below (above for Fe:Cu and thyroid weight) bands indicate a probable benefit.

	Cu	Co or vit B_{12}	I	Mn	Se	Zn
Diet[a] (mg/kg DM)	5–15	0.04–0.06	0.08–0.3	10–15	0.03–0.06	10–20
Serum[b] (μmol/l)	3–8	$0.25–0.5 \times 10^{-3\mathrm{M}}$	0.08–0.20	0.09–0.11	0.13–0.26[B]	6–9
Tissue[c] (μmol/kg DM)	150–300[nL]	0.2–0.4[L]	$9.5–15.8 \times 10^{3\mathrm{T}}$	11–13[H]	0.6–1.3[nL]	765–1070[R]

[a] Higher values are appropriate for: antagonist-containing diets (for Cu, Cu:Mo < 1–3, Fe:Cu > 50–100; Cu:sulphur < 0.0025); for I, with high goitrogen intake); for low agonist intake (e.g. for Se, low vitamin E intakes); for all elements when the digestibility of the ration is high.

[b] The ranges are for adults; newborns often have different norms (e.g. 3–9 μmol/l then being adequate for serum Cu).

[c] Superscript letters indicate sample origin: B = whole blood, H = heart, L = liver, M = milk, R = rib, T = thyroid; for the latter, an organ weight range of 0.3–0.8 g FW/kg LW is marginal; for the newborn (n), ranges may again differ, L Se being up to 3× that in the adult and L Cu 7–10× higher. Divide values by 3.3 (L) or 4.0 (H,T) for approximate fresh weight basis.

Conversion from μmolar to μg units requires multiplication by: 63.5 for Cu, 58.9 for Co, 126.9 for I, 54.9 for Mn, 79.0 for Se, 65.4 for Zn and 1355 for B_{12}; division by these factors converts mg to mmol units.

& Suttle, 1999). Loss of appetite was initially linked to Adocbl dysfunction and increased blood propionate concentrations, but disturbances of rumen fermentation (McDonald & Suttle, 1986; Kennedy *et al.*, 1991) and the accumulation of other metabolites (e.g. MMA, Rice *et al.*, 1989; succinate, Kennedy *et al.*, 1991; homocysteine, Stangl *et al.*, 2000) may also affect appetite. Loss of appetite would compound the effect of a diminishing supply of the glucose precursor, propionate. The anaemia of Co deficiency may reflect the role of MeCbl in DNA synthesis and red cell maturation.

The basic cause of cobalt-responsive disorders is a simple nutritional deficit that can be traced to impoverished soils in which crops or pastures have grown. Interactions can occur in the soil that leave most of the Co adsorbed in unavailable forms onto manganese oxides, particularly at alkaline soil pH with soil Mn >1 g/kg (Suttle, 2000). If extraction with 0.43 M acetic acid yields <0.3 mg Co/kg air-dry soil, deficiencies may develop. The diet should contain >0.05 mg Co/kg dry matter (DM) (Underwood & Suttle, 1999). Interactions in the animal have been postulated because Co can be incorporated into various analogues of B_{12} by the rumen microbes. There is thus competition for Co in the rumen between different forms of the vitamin. Cobalamins are selectively absorbed in association with intrinsic factor but if analogues find their way into the bloodstream or tissues, they might complicate the assessment of vitamin B_{12} status and compromise functions of the vitamin. However, protective mechanisms would probably have evolved, if they are needed, against analogues so copiously produced in the rumen.

Clinical signs

All ruminants require a dietary supply of Co for the synthesis of the essential vitamin B_{12} by rumen microorganisms. Cattle are less susceptible to a lack of Co than sheep, but when they succumb, they develop essentially the same clinical abnormalities in the same order: anorexia, loss of body condition, muscular wasting and finally an anaemia that is both normochromic and normocytic. In the early stages of the disease, the hair coat can become rough and discoloured (Judson *et al.*, 1982) and may be repeatedly licked. Appetite may become depraved (pica). Eventually, the skin becomes thin and fragile and the mucous membranes pallid. The clinical picture is thus one of a 'pining' or 'wasting' disease, indistinguishable from many other causes of ill-thrift. Cobalt-deprived cattle may be more susceptible to infections than normal cattle (MacPherson *et al.*, 1987a).

There is a neurological disease that affects cattle in Australia when they graze *Phalaris tuberosa* pastures called 'Phalaris staggers'; it can be prevented by Co dosage but not by administration of vitamin B_{12} and is, therefore, not a classical 'deficiency' syndrome. The response to Co may arise through the neutralization of fungal neurotoxins by the element (Underwood & Suttle, 1999).

Necropsy

At necropsy, cattle suffering from Co deprivation show the hallmarks of starvation. There is little body fat except occasionally in the liver, which may be pale and friable due to fatty infiltration; this condition is, however, far less common in cattle than in lambs or goat kids. In severely affected, anaemic individuals, bone marrow hypoplasia and splenic haemosiderosis will be found.

Diagnosis

Cobalt-responsive *disorders* are best diagnosed through responses in growth or health to Co or B_{12} supplementation in controlled trials (e.g. Duncan *et al.*, 1986). Biochemical confirmation of subclinical or clinical *disease* from the assay of plasma B_{12} is more difficult in cattle than in sheep. Plasma B_{12} concentrations appear to respond feebly to Co supplementation in cattle. Oral doses of Co ten times higher on a body weight basis than those that increase plasma B_{12} in sheep were apparently ineffective in cattle (N.F. Suttle & J. Brebner, unpublished data). High plasma B_{12} concentrations (>500 ng/l) are rarely found in cattle yet they are commonplace in sheep and values have often fallen to exceedingly low levels (<100 ng/l, e.g. Reid & McQueen, 1985) before cattle failed to thrive, though there are exceptions (e.g. Duncan *et al.*, 1986). The assay of B_{12} by the more favoured radioisotope dilution (RID) method is susceptible to interference from non-specific binders (Millar *et al.*, 1984; Schulz, 1987a, b); these include the transport proteins for B_{12} in bovine plasma (transcobalamins), which show quantitative differences from man (Schulz, 1987a) as well as seasonal anomalies (Millar *et al.*, 1984). Since binding affects the recovery of B_{12} after deproteinization of plasma or serum, it can impair assay by both microbiological and RID methods. The results of assays of B_{12} in bovine plasma can vary substantially between laboratories (Schulz, 1987b) and assays of the analogue component by difference, using specific and non-specific binders, are particularly prone to error. Extraction of the vitamin at alkaline pH overcomes the problem and modified assay kits are now available (Stangl *et al.*, 2000).

Assays of vitamin B_{12} in skimmed milk and liver are far more reliable than those in plasma and values for milk and liver from the same individual correlate reasonably well with each other, particularly at low levels that have diagnostic significance; milk B_{12} < 0.5 nmol (678 ng/l) indicates a possibility of ill health (Judson *et al.*, 1997b) (Table 21.1). By contrast, the relationship between plasma and liver B_{12} values is poor, particularly at low levels (Judson *et al.*, 1997a). Diagnostic thresholds for liver B_{12} in sheep have long been extrapolated to cattle; thus values <0.10 mg/kg fresh liver have been taken to indicate moderate to severe *deficiency* and values >0.19 mg (>140 pmol)/kg have been regarded as normal. There is a curvilinear relationship between Co and vitamin B_{12} concentrations in bovine liver which

shows better fit at low than at high levels (Mitsioulis *et al.*, 1995; Suttle, 1995); values between 0.06 and 0.08 mg Co/kg DM can be regarded as 'marginal' (Underwood & Suttle, 1999).

The diagnosis of Co disorders from the presence of abnormal metabolites in the blood and urine was developed in sheep and non-ruminants and extended to cattle. Quirk & Norton (1988) found that heifers grazing pastures low in Co (0.036 mg/kg DM) remained healthy and excreted no MMA or FIGLU in urine, despite low plasma B_{12} concentrations (96 pg/ml). After calving, milk yield was unaffected but very low B_{12} concentrations in the milk (42–86 ng or 31–63 pmol/l) caused depletion of plasma B_{12} in their calves (59–74 ng/l) and growth retardation, which was accompanied by increased urinary excretion of FIGLU. They concluded that MMA was less reliable than FIGLU as an index of *dysfunction* but their method for MMA was relatively insensitive (30 μmol/l). Assay of plasma MMA has been advanced as a measure of functional B_{12} status in sheep, with concentrations >5 μmol/l taken to be abnormal (Rice *et al.*, 1987): as yet plasma MMA has not been tested for the confirmation of Co dysfunction in cattle but a marginal band of 5–15 μmol/l may well prove useful. Increases in plasma homocysteine are found after prolonged Co deprivation (Stangl *et al.*, 2000).

Treatment or prevention

Although there are clearly differences in B_{12} metabolism between cattle and sheep, there is no evidence that these affect the methods of treating and preventing disorders. The injection of B_{12} as cyano- or hydroxycobalamin, 2–6 mg/50 kg liveweight, provides protection for several weeks, even though responses in plasma B_{12} soon dissipate. Slow-release, injectable preparations of B_{12} are being developed in the Antipodes.

Heavy cobalt oxide pellets given orally, in pairs or singly with a 'grinder', improve the B_{12} status of growing and adult cattle for several months (Judson *et al.*, 1981; Quirk & Norton, 1988), even when a change in formulation halves their Co content (Judson *et al.*, 1997b); the soluble glass bolus can also give sustained protection (Allen *et al.*, 1985). The effectiveness of infrequent oral doses of Co in anthelmintics has not been tested but weekly doses of 35–70 mg Co without anthelmintic are said to be effective (Underwood & Suttle, 1999). Cobalt supplementation via the drinking water can be practised where there is a piped water supply (MacPherson, 1983). Use of 'protected' or chelated forms for oral use is contraindicated because Co must be given in forms which can be rapidly incorporated into vitamin B_{12} by rumen microbes. Evidence that volatile fatty acid (VFA) production by rumen microbes is influenced by

Co deficiency (McDonald & Suttle, 1986; Rice *et al.*, 1989; Kennedy *et al.*, 1991) suggests a possible advantage for the oral route over the injection route, since only the former meets the needs of the microbes for B$_{12}$. Comparisons between methods have rarely been conducted but one at least showed no advantage in calf growth for oral Co versus injected B$_{12}$ (Judson *et al.*, 1981).

Administration of Co on a group basis via licks containing 0.1 per cent Co or mineral mixes containing up to 0.4 per cent Co may provide an inexpensive means of prevention but could not be guaranteed to protect all individuals. The best long-term strategy on certain soil types will be to apply Co salts, such as hydrated CoSO$_4$, at 2–3kg/ha, every three to four years. Responses may, however, be short-lived on sandy soils and negligible on calcareous or recently limed soils containing >1g Mn/kg DM because most of the Co becomes 'fixed' in the soil.

There is virtually no risk of overdosing with cobalt, but this should not be used as an excuse to overfeed Co to animals whose capacity to synthesize and absorb B$_{12}$ is strictly limited.

Copper disorders (see also Chapter 18)

Aetiology (see p. 254)

Most Cu-responsive disorders in cattle are induced: they are induced in the rumen where the anaerobic degradation of sulphur(S)-rich, fibrous feeds leaves little of the ingested Cu in a soluble form. After weaning, less than 10 per cent of the total Cu input is absorbed during passage down the gastrointestinal tract and the percentage can be reduced to as little as 1–2 per cent by small increments in dietary Mo (Underwood & Suttle, 1999). Again it is transformations in the rumen that are pivotal: extrapolating from sheep, it appears that the progressive substitution of S^{2-} for O^{2-} in molybdate creates thiomolybdates, which complex Cu and bind it to the solid phase. Surplus trithiomolybdate (MoOS$_3$) is absorbable and capable of changing the distribution of Cu in the blood and tissues (Underwood & Suttle, 1999). Just how important the systemic effects of thiomolybdates are under normal grazing conditions has yet to be determined. The 'tell-tale' appearance of abnormal plasma fractions, such as TCA-insoluble Cu, has been restricted to experimental situations, involving high levels of dietary Mo (35mg/kg DM; Wang *et al.*, 1988), and they may serve as slow release pools of Cu in the long term (Underwood & Suttle, 1999).

Most cases of Cu-responsive growth retardation in cattle are associated with abnormally low ratios of Cu:Mo in the herbage (<3.0; Phillippo, 1983) and it has

been suggested that they may reflect direct effects of Mo on the central control of appetite (Phillippo *et al.*, 1987b). It is, however, premature to discount the role of Cu (Suttle, 1988; Underwood & Suttle, 1999) and other factors that influence Cu status should not be ignored. Copper absorption in cattle is as sensitive to Mo inhibition as it is in sheep and the equations derived for grazing sheep to predict Cu absorption (Suttle, 1983b) should give an approximate weighting for cattle. High S intakes from the diet (Suttle, 1983a) or drinking water (Smart *et al.*, 1986) also suppress Cu absorption. Poor Cu absorption, and hence disorders, will therefore be more common on lush, immature, S-rich swards than on brown, mature swards and in wet than in dry seasons. Copper is also absorbed better from hay than from fresh grass of similar S content (Suttle, 1983b). Ensiled grass is a good source of absorbable Cu while S concentrations are low (about 2g/kg DM), but availability probably falls rapidly as concentrations rise to 3g/kg DM if cattle share the characteristics of sheep (Suttle, 1983a). High iron (Fe) concentrations also lower Cu status in cattle (Bremner *et al.*, 1987; Phillippo *et al.*, 1987b; Gengelbach *et al.*, 1997), are often raised in spring and autumn pastures and have been implicated in incidents of hypocuprosis (Jarvis & Austin, 1983; McFarlane *et al.*, 1990). There is debate over whether or not the Fe × Cu antagonism requires the presence of moderate amounts of dietary S (Suttle, 1988).

The principal determinants of hypocuprosis in grazing cattle are therefore raised soil Mo, alkaline soil pH (which encourages Mo uptake), sward immaturity, high rainfall (or irrigation), heavy fertilizer N use and high soil ingestion, rather than the Cu content of the soil or herbage, on all but the most impoverished, sandy soils.

Shortage of absorbable Cu leads to (i) rapid *depletion* of liver stores, (ii) a lowering of caeruloplasmin synthesis and a drop in plasma Cu (i.e. *deficiency*) and (iii) a reduction in cuproenzyme activities in the erythrocyte and tissues (*dysfuntion*). Although cytochrome oxidase and superoxide dismutase have been the most studied, others such as lysyl oxidase and dopamine hydroxylase will almost certainly follow the non-ruminant pattern in showing disorder (Suttle, 1988). Effects on growth, cardiac function and bone development cannot be attributed to a particular enzyme deficiency with certainty. Even the depigmentation once attributed to diminished tyrosinase activity must be open to other explanations now that it is known to be produced by Co as well as Cu deprivation (Judson *et al.*, 1982). Connective tissue defects, including those in the ligamentum nuchae, are probably due to lysyl oxidase deficiency leading to defective cross-links in elastin. Digestive disturbances may result from disruption of mitochondrial respiration and villous atrophy, but enhanced inflammatory reactions to gut parasites cannot be ruled out in grazing animals (Underwood & Suttle, 1999).

Clinical signs

The sequence and severity of signs associated with a lack of dietary Cu in cattle (hypocuprosis) depend upon the rate and stage of development at which it occurs. There are no definitive reports of teratogenic or neurological effects, comparable with swayback in sheep (cf. Richards & Edwards, 1986). In the growing calf, loss of hair colour, growth retardation and changes in metatarsal conformation are the earliest signs of abnormality followed by diarrhoea and finally anaemia. Black hair usually turns grey and red/brown hair becomes light brown. The 'foxy brown' discoloration of the Friesian is not attributable to copper deprivation (Mee, 1991). Cardiac hypertrophy has been reported in experimentally depleted calves and this may be an early manifestation of the myocardial degeneration that can cause sudden death after prolonged deficiency in the field (Suttle, 1988). Addition of small amounts of the Cu antagonist, molybdenum (Mo), to the diet (2 mg/kg DM) accelerates rather than changes these clinical manifestations of disorder. At much higher Mo concentrations (>10 mg/kg DM), animals may develop diarrhoea immediately upon exposure to the antagonist (Suttle, 1988).

Infertility has long been associated with Cu deprivation in cattle but there is little published evidence that deficiency leads to impaired reproduction unless Mo is involved (Phillippo *et al.*, 1982, 1987a). Molybdenum-induced deficiency is associated with delays in the onset of oestrus, impaired conception rate and anoestrus: these abnormalities have yet to be induced experimentally by other antagonists of Cu, such as Fe (Phillippo *et al.*, 1987a). Copper-responsive infertility in cattle given Mo, therefore, may result from the direct or indirect suppression of the release of luteinizing hormone (Phillippo *et al.*, 1987a).

Anaemia is a late sign of Cu dysfunction in growing calves (Suttle, 1988) and may be associated with Heinz body formation in the periparturient cow (Black, 1981). The *in vitro* viability and/or function of neutrophils from Cu-deficient cattle is poorer than that of cells from normal cattle (Suttle, 1988) but exposure to Mo can increase leucocyte counts (Gengelbach *et al.*, 1997); there is no evidence yet for impaired resistance to infections *in vivo* (Arthington *et al.*, 1996).

Necropsy

The pathology of bovine hypocuprosis is largely unhelpful because the histological changes underlying the clinical signs, like the signs themselves, are non-specific. The earliest and most dramatic lesions are likely to be those affecting the epiphyseal growth plates in the costochondral junctions and metatarsal/metacarpal bones. These can become overgrown to the point that they spill over to leave islets of collagen distal to the plate in various states of irregular calcification and fibrotic replacement (Suttle, 1988). Gross degenerative changes are also seen in connective tissues such as the ligamentum nuchae. In severe cases showing diarrhoea, villous atrophy in the duodenal and jejunal regions is likely to be seen (Suttle, 1988) but is indistinguishable from that caused by gut parasites.

The anaemia of Cu deficiency in the bovine is similar to that of Fe deficiency, i.e. macrocytic and hypochromic. Cardiac lesions including fibrosis of the myocardium have been reported in natural outbreaks only once, over 40 years ago, in Australia. While cardiac hypertrophy was seen in some experimentally depleted calves, which took a long time to develop clinical signs; it was not present in others that were depleted more rapidly (Suttle, 1988).

Attention switched from the lesions that underlie the expected and familiar clinical signs to those which, though less spectacular, occur earlier and may underlie the debilitating effects of the disorder. Fell and his associates (Fell *et al.*, 1985; Fell, 1987) found basement membrane defects in the pancreatic acinar cell, the duodenal enterocyte and kidney tubule, pointing to perhaps a common early failure of proteoglycan organization.

It remains to be seen whether Mo can cause distinctive histological or ultrastructural changes at central sites such as the pineal body which may be crucial to the development of disorder (Phillippo *et al.*, 1987a) and whether or not these are Cu-dependent.

Diagnosis

Since none of the clinical signs of Cu deprivation given above is specific, diagnosis must be supported by biochemical tests showing subnormal tissue Cu status. Because availability has such a major effect on Cu uptake, herbage or dietary Cu concentrations alone are almost worthless and should be accompanied by measures of Mo and S and predictions of available Cu (Suttle, 1983a). In green swards, which contain enough sulphur to potentiate the Mo antagonism, Cu:Mo ratios <3.0 indicate a risk of hypocuprosis. Even then, other factors such as initial Cu reserves, other dietary antagonists (Fe and ingested soil) and the rate of animal production may determine the outcome of events. Genetic variation in bovine Cu metabolism is far less pronounced than that found in sheep (Underwood & Suttle, 1999). Fe:Cu ratios in the range 50–100 indicate the possibility of a Cu-responsive disorder; these and other guidelines for the biochemical assessment of risk are summarized in Table 21.1.

The conventional criteria of Cu status in the animal, i.e. liver and blood Cu concentrations, are most dependable when herbage Mo concentrations are low (<5 mg/kg DM). Under these circumstances the ranges 150–300 μmol (10–20 mg) Cu/kg DM for liver and 3–9 μmol (0.2–0.6 mg) Cu/l for plasma can be regarded as 'marginal', except for the newborn (Table 21.1): as group means, they indicate that some individuals are likely to benefit from Cu supplementation and that cheap measures to improve Cu status would be prudent. Newborn calves require *higher* marginal ranges for liver (790–3150 μmol Cu/kg DM) and *lower* ranges for plasma (3.0–4.5 μmol Cu/l). At very high dietary Mo concentrations (35 mg/kg DM), changes in the distribution of Cu in the plasma and liver may complicate the assessment of Cu status (Wang *et al.*, 1988). With less extreme though still unusual Mo concentrations (>5 mg/kg DM) in pasture, 'teart'-like conditions may operate for critical periods, with animals responding to Cu while normocupraemic. Low caeruloplasmin : Cu ratios in plasma have been claimed to indicate the antagonistic influence of Mo, but they can be low when the antagonist is Fe (Gengelbach *et al.*, 1997). The relationship between caeruloplasmin and total Cu in bovine plasma is not perturbed in molybdeniferous areas of Scotland (N.F. Suttle & J. Small, unpublished data). It remains to be seen whether supplements that achieve normocupraemia invariably provide a sufficient defence against Mo-induced infertility and whether other parameters such as plasma Mo or plasma Fe concentrations have merit for diagnosing Mo-induced ill health (Phillippo *et al.*, 1987a, b). In establishing Cu as a limiting factor to production in a new area, a response to a specific Cu treatment affords the best assessment, though not necessarily showing Cu deprivation to be the primary cause (see p. 254).

Treatment or prevention

The treatment of Cu deficiency is achieved readily by single oral doses of Cu or parenteral injections of the element. In animals close to market weight the use of chelates of Cu with ethylene diamine, tetra-acetic acid (EDTA), glycine or methionine may result in unacceptable, 'cold' abscesses at the injection site, whether given subcutaneously or intramuscularly. Use of water-soluble complexes such as the hydroxyquinoline sulphonate and heptonate will avoid abscess formation but increase risks of acute toxicity (e.g. Suttle, 1981).

Prevention of deficiency and disorder can be achieved to varying degrees of precision and duration with oral and parenteral supplements. Copper oxide particles are more effective than serial injections, pro-viding protection for several months (Judson *et al.*, 1985; Rogers & Poole, 1988). Soluble glass boluses are likely in time to give equally sustained protection and are particularly suited to the extensive grazing situation (Allen *et al.*, 1985; Judson *et al.*, 1985; Givens *et al.*, 1988). During periods of supplementary feeding or housing, the use of Cu salts as forage additives or cereal supplements commends itself. Where food supplements are not given, a free-access mineral mixture containing >500 mg Cu/kg is likely to afford protection to the majority of the individuals that take to it in a given herd. If Cu proves to be useful as an antidote to Mo rather than an essential nutrient in some situations by rendering toxic thiomolybdates less available, the provision of Cu by slow rumenal release or steady dietary supplementation may have advantages over other forms of supplementation. The use of chelated forms of copper, such as 'proteinates' or copper lysine, as dietary supplements has given no consistent advantage over simple, cheap inorganic forms and cannot be relied upon to 'protect' copper from molybdenum or other antagonists (Underwood & Suttle, 1999).

Toxicity (see p. 948)

Copper poisoning rarely occurs through the ingestion of excess Cu in weaned cattle because of poor absorption and a well-developed capacity to excrete surplus Cu via the bile. Tolerance of diets containing >250 mg Cu/kg DM for several months has been reported in Friesian steers (Felsman *et al.*, 1973). Much higher absorptive efficiencies prior to weaning mean that calves reared on milk substitutes are relatively vulnerable, but they can tolerate up to 500 mg Cu/kg DM for brief periods (6 weeks; Jenkins & Hidiroglou, 1989). Oral drenching with $CuSO_4$ solutions can cause haemolytic crises similar to those found in the more vulnerable sheep, but slower rates of exposure via the diet may sometimes cause or contribute to hepatic crises. Rapidly growing bull calves can die suddenly and show biochemical evidence of liver injury, in the form of raised AST activities, and Cu overload, in the form of raised kidney Cu levels, without evidence of haemolysis (no jaundice or increase in kidney iron) and only marginally raised liver Cu (C. Low, pers. comm.). Diagnosis of toxicity becomes possible when 'liver enzyme' values in serum are raised and values for indices of copper status enter the following 'marginal' ranges: serum, 0.018–0.020 mmol Cu/l; liver 6.4–16.0, kidney 0.6–0.8 and diet 1.57–3.14 mmol Cu/kg DM (multiply by 63.5 to obtain mg or ppm units). False 'highs' for plasma Cu during acute infections will be accompanied by Cu : Zn ratios >3–4. Acute Cu poisoning can be caused by overdosage via the parenteral route (Mylrea & Byrne, 1974) and is characterized by haemolytic crises and jaundice.

Iodine disorders (see pp. 257, 586)

Aetiology

Iodine has only one function in the body, as a constituent of the hormone tri-iodothyronine (T_3), which regulates basal metabolic rate. The hormone is formed by the removal of iodine (deiodination) from thyroxine (tetra-iodothyronine, T_4), the physiologically inactive form synthesized in the thyroid gland. Disorders can arise either from a simple lack of iodine in the diet or from the impairment of iodine metabolism by ingested goitrogens. Simple iodine deprivation rarely occurs in coastal regions or on small islands because of the large atmospheric inputs of iodine of marine origin. Diets containing <0.1 mg I/kg DM are inadequate, those with 0.1–0.2 mg/kg DM marginal; levels are usually much higher in spring than in summer pasture (Underwood & Suttle, 1999). In areas where winter temperatures are low, iodine requirements probably increase in proportion to energy expenditure/kg LW, making the newborn particularly vulnerable. Selenium deprivation may increase the risk of iodine disorders through its role as an activator of several deiodinase enzymes (see 'Selenium disorders' on p. 302).

Ingestion of inorganic, cyanogenetic goitrogens in certain grasses (e.g. *Paspalum* spp., *Cynodon aethiopicus*), legumes (e.g. *Trifolium repens*, *Medicago sativa*), brassicas (e.g. *B. oleracea*) and by-products (e.g. cassava meal) leads to the formation of thiocyanate in the rumen which impairs iodine uptake by the thyroid. Organic, thiouracil-type goitrogens (e.g. in *B. campestris*, *Leucena leucophela* and rapeseed meals) can impair iodine incorporation into T_4 in the thyroid and its conversion to T_3 in the tissues. Exposure to both types of goitrogen increases risk of disorder and only the former type can be countered by providing more iodine.

Clinical signs

Iodine deprivation is no longer synonymous with goitre. While goitre in the newborn remains the commonest manifestation, lack of iodine also has a specific effect on brain development and non-specific effects on growth, fertility, milk yield and on the skin and its appendages (Underwood & Suttle, 1999).

Necropsy

Thyroid enlargement occurs as an adaptive response to iodine deprivation and undoubtedly provides a simple first measure of the *possibility* of iodine deficiency. In clinically significant, chronic pre- or postnatal iodine deprivation, enlargement of the thyroid is gross and there is no need to weigh the gland. Problems of interpretation arise when the degree of iodine deprivation and associated changes are less pronounced. In the UK, the limit of normality for thyroid weight was 0.33 g FW/kg LW, but recent work in Northern Ireland has shown that a higher margin is necessary. Iodine deprivation can cause thyroid weights to reach 0.79 g/kg LW without causing stillbirths (McCoy *et al.*, 1997) and iodine supplementation of beef cows significantly reduced thyroid weight *without* reducing calf mortality or stillbirths (Smyth *et al.*, 1992). Sound interpretation requires a marginal band of 0.3–0.8 g/kg LW (Table 21.1). Spurious increases in thyroid weight may occur during the trauma of a difficult calving as part of a generalized oedema.

Diagnosis

Biochemical and histological criteria can contribute to diagnosis in cases of marginal deprivation, but the most commonly used criteria present the greatest problems of interpretation.

Thyroxine: T_4 is transported in plasma bound to proteins, but concentrations in the blood are a poor and unreliable index of *functional* iodine status. Proper assessment of iodine *dysfunction* requires measurements of T_3, T_3:T_4 ratios and thyroid-stimulating hormone (TSH), the hormone secreted by the pituitary in response to iodine deprivation. The detection of raised TSH concentrations in the bloodstream indicates that an animal needs more T_3 and is prompting the thyroid gland to increase hormone synthesis. A recent experiment (McCoy *et al.*, 1997) confirms the unreliability of T_4 assays. Pregnant heifers were fed a diet sufficiently low in iodine to cause a 2.5-fold increase in thyroid weight of their newborn calves when compared with an iodine supplemented control group. No significant differences in plasma T_4 concentrations were found between the two groups in either mother or offspring and mean values (60–202 nmol/l) were in the normal range. There is also a spontaneous fall in plasma T_4 during early lactation to values that are subnormal for other stages (20–40 nmol/l).

Serum iodine: The element has been measured *in toto* and in protein-precipitable and butanol-extractable forms in serum, but rarely in proven clinical or subclinical cases of iodine deprivation, and diagnostic limits can only provisionally be set. Each parameter is a better measure of the degree of excess than of inadequate iodine supply (Table 21.1).

Thyroid iodine: Thyroid iodine concentrations largely reflect the amount of iodine in thyroglobulin which is lying in store. Since iodine stores can be depleted before cellular changes occur and cellular changes increase the size of the thyroid, tissue iodine concentration alone will be of limited value in determining the total amount of iodine present in the gland. Many authorities use the yardstick proposed in the 1930s that clinical goitre is associated with thyroid $I_2 < 1.2$ g/kg DM and $1.2–2.0$ g I_2/kg DM becomes a marginal range (Puls, 1994; Table 21.1).

Milk iodine: Concentrations of iodine in bovine milk are linearly related to iodine intake (Underwood & Suttle, 1999) and have proven diagnostic value in the ewe. Puls (1994) suggests that values <25 μg I/l indicate 'deficiency' in cows, much lower than the corresponding value for ewes (<80), yet this probably overlaps the 'marginal' range.

Histological criteria: A sequence of microscopic cellular changes occur in the thyroid as the organ responds to the stimulus from TSH. Firstly, stores of surplus thyroxine in colloidal form are removed – some pathologists call this 'colloidal goitre', but this does not mean that the abnormality has reached a clinical or life-threatening stage, rather that *depletion* is complete. With stores of thyroglobulin denuded, the epithelial cells which produce thyroxine increase first in number (hyperplasia: 'hyperplastic goitre') and then in size (hypertrophy); it is the latter process which lies behind visible, clinically significant goitre. Hyperplasia can occur in calves which are normal at birth (McCoy *et al.*, 1997) and may be caused by the stress of a prolonged calving. Undue diagnostic significance should not be attached to thyroid abnormalities, although these may be the only post-mortem 'abnormality' to be recorded.

Treatment and prevention

Congenital goitre must be prevented because there is no response to treatment and only the chronic forms of iodine disorders in older animals are amenable to treatment. Simple and thiocyanate-induced deprivation can be prevented by providing inorganic iodine supplements in iodized salt licks or mineral mixes containing *c.* 0.1 g I/kg. Substantial losses can occur by volatilization in hot climates and the use of less volatile forms such as periodates is then indicated. Slow-release boluses are being developed and a long-lasting form for parenteral administration (iodized poppyseed oil) has long been used, although it is no longer obtainable in some countries due to a failure to update product licences. Problems induced by organic goitrogens can be avoided by using cultivars selected for low glucosinolate content and by-products of such crops (e.g. canola rapeseed meals). Manipulation of the rumen

microflora in isolated populations can limit endogenous goitrogen synthesis from mimosine-containing shrubs such as *L. leucophela* (Jones & Meggarity, 1983).

Toxicity (see pp. 261, 823)

Iodine is a cumulative poison which eventually suppresses thyroid activity. Tolerable exposure is therefore a multiple of daily intake × length of exposure, rather than a set dietary concentration. The marginally tolerable concentration over three to four months' exposure is 25–50 mg I/kg DM (Newton *et al.*, 1974) and is rarely encountered under farm conditions unless there is access to seaweed (4–6 g I/kg DM). Iodosis is characterized by poor growth and respiratory disorder in calves (Newton *et al.*, 1974) and by perinatal mortality in offspring of the adult cow (Fish & Swanson, 1983). Once lactation has begun, the cow herself becomes less vulnerable because she is able to secrete much of any excess dietary or therapeutic iodine in milk. Use of iodine in the form of ethylene diamine dihyroiodide (EDDI) for treating foot rot and 'lumpy jaw' in the USA has resulted in many cases of iodosis (see page 261 and Underwood & Suttle, 1999, for further details).

Selenium disorders (see p. 258)

Aetiology

The principal function of Se in animals relates to its intracellular presence in the glutathione peroxidases, a family of antioxidant enzymes (once GSHPx, now GPXn with n ≥ 6), which use various potentially dangerous peroxides as substrates. Selenium has been linked with iodine metabolism in ways that indicate a separate function, independent of GPX (Arthur *et al.*, 1988). While the basic cause of Se disorders is obviously a shortage of the element in the diet, which in turn can be traced to soil formations also deficient in Se (Underwood & Suttle, 1999), other factors are probably involved in field outbreaks of Se-responsive disease. Calves fed experimental diets of exceedingly low Se content (0.01–0.02 mg/kg DM) indoors can be depleted of Se to the point that they have undetectable activities of GPX1 in their blood and yet do not develop myopathy (Arthur, 1988; Reffett *et al.*, 1988). In one study (Arthur, 1988), the failure to induce myopathy was the more surprising because the diet was also low in vitamin E, which also contributes to antioxidant defence in the tissues.

The importance of dietary sources of oxidant stress was demonstrated by workers in Belfast (Rice & McMurray, 1982), who showed that the addition of polyunsaturated fatty acids (PUFA, progenitors of lipid peroxides) to diets deficient in vitamin E and Se, simulating the composition of PUFA-rich spring grass, will precipitate myopathy. Other stressors may yet be required to induce myopathy because Arthur (1988) has shown that feeding of PUFA-rich grass indoors to calves deficient in Se and vitamin E did not precipitate the disorder, whereas grazing the same grass produced acute myopathy. He suggested that exercise or some other component of the environmental change at turnout contributed to the development of muscle damage. The excitable behaviour of the calf will of course result in increased activity of muscles involved in locomotion, circulation and respiration: muscular exercise is known to induce oxidant stress and exacerbate the effects of vitamin E deficiency (Jackson, 1987). It is highly likely that the intense and sometimes prolonged muscular activity of the uterus at parturition makes it particularly vulnerable to Se (and vitamin E) deficiency. Adverse weather conditions have been implicated in outbreaks of acute myopathy and the cause of Se-responsive disorders is thus multifactorial (Underwood & Suttle, 1999).

Clinical signs

Selenium deprivation in cattle can impair development throughout life. The suckling calf can develop chronic skeletal and cardiac myopathy if the dam's diet is low in Se (Hidiroglou et al., 1985), while the calf on pastures deficient in Se can suffer growth retardation before (Morris et al., 1984) and after weaning (Gleed et al., 1983). In spring, calves can develop acute myopathy with myoglobinuria when turned out to graze. Selenium supplementation has improved conception rate in cows (McClure et al., 1986) and heifers (MacPherson et al., 1987b). At parturition, cows of low Se status are more likely to retain the placenta than Se-supplemented cows and they are the more susceptible to metritis and cystic ovaries (Harrison et al., 1984). Selenium deprivation also affects the circulatory system: the growing calf can develop a Heinz-body anaemia (Morris et al., 1984) and when calving coincides with turnout, the cow which is both Cu and Se deficient may be vulnerable to haemolysis and haemoglobinuria (Black, 1981).

Despite the variety of clinical signs caused by a lack of Se, it is rare for more than one sign to appear in a single herd. Problems of muscular dystrophy have not been reported in the many studies of retained placenta, which is probably the commonest Se-responsive condition in cattle. Similarly, growth retardation and muscular dystrophy have not been reported in the same outbreak of disorder. Selenium deficiency in cattle has been associated with impaired phagocyte function in vitro, prompting speculation that Se deficiency would lead to decreased resistance to disease, but these suggestions have not always been confirmed in experimental studies (Reffett et al., 1988). There are several reports of inverse relationships between blood Se or glutathione peroxidane (GPX) activity with somatic cell counts in bovine milk (e.g. Erskine et al., 1989) and experimental evidence that addition of Se to diets of marginal Se concentration decreases the duration of clinical mastitis (Smith et al., 1984). Similar responses can be obtained with supplements of vitamin E (Weiss et al., 1997), making interpretation of responses to Se combined with vitamin E (the commonest approach) either difficult or impossible. Improvements in calf survival in herds on diets of marginal Se concentration (0.03–0.05 kg Se/kg DM) have been reported, but vitamin E as well as Se was given and the role of Se alone is again unclear (Spears et al., 1986).

Diagnosis

The differential diagnosis of Se-responsive disorders is complicated by the non-specific clinical signs of disease: most can also be attributed to vitamin E deficiency while others, such as retained placenta and growth retardation, have many possible causes of both nutritional and non-nutritional origin. The tolerance of low plasma and blood Se (or GPX1) concentrations in the absence of exacerbative factors confirms that measures of Se (or GPX) alone cannot confirm a selenium disorder. Neither is there likely to be a simple relationship between dietary Se concentration and incidence of disease.

In monitoring Se status, the assay of GPX once largely replaced that of whole blood Se because it was easier to assay, yet highly correlated with blood Se concentration. Enzyme activities were converted to blood Se equivalents for comparative purposes. Interpretation of blood GPX activities is, however, complicated by many factors. The measurement of GPX activity is subject to wider interlaboratory variation than most analyses in the clinical context: Blanchflower et al. (1986) identified some important variables. The use of an assay kit helped to standardize results, but differences can still arise and each laboratory should determine and quote its own Se equivalence for GPX activity. Results are variously reported per ml blood, per g haemoglobin and per ml cells: while these will be highly correlated with each other within laboratories, the use of common conversion factors for comparative purposes may introduce errors. The slow turnover of erythrocytes ensures that blood GPX activity reflects past rather than present Se supply. The data of Hidiroglou et al. (1985) indicate that it may take four months for blood GPX (and Se) fully to reflect an improved Se supply and just as long to reflect a waning supply. It should be noted that the GPX in blood is now regarded as a dispensable, storage form of the element and indicative of *depletion* rather than *dysfunction*. Plasma Se responds immediately to changes in dietary supply and is a useful adjunct to blood GPX in assessing Se status concentrations of 100–120 nmol (8–10 µg/l being 'marginal' and suggesting possible benefits from Se supplementation (Underwood & Suttle, 1999).

Very small differences in Se status may determine vulnerability. In the study of Hidiroglou *et al.* (1985) for example, myopathy occurred in calves in one year when blood GPX1 declined from 29 to 19 iu/g haemoglobin (Hb) and plasma Se from 11 to 6 µg/l, but not in the next when the respective falls were 51 to 28 iu/g Hb and 16 to 13 µg/l. Pasture Se was consistently low at 0.02–0.04 mg/kg DM. In a survey of the Se status of cattle in north-east Scotland (Arthur *et al.*, 1979), 85 per cent of herds had a blood Se status 50 µg/l, a threshold below which a risk of clinical disease was once suggested, but only 10 per cent had a recent history of myopathy; the winter diets mostly contained <0.05 mg Se/kg DM. In New South Wales, herds of growing cattle with blood Se concentrations usually <20 µg (0.25 µmol)/l rarely benefited from Se supplementation and those that did were not distinguishable from their blood Se levels (Langlands *et al.*, 1981). Studies in New Zealand with dairy cows indicated a critical blood Se concentration as low as 12 µg/l below which milk fat yield fell (Fraser *et al.*, 1987). The latter studies both involved grazing animals with plentiful supplies of vitamin E.

The clinically significant thresholds for dietary and blood Se concentrations probably vary with the Se-responsive condition and the dietary supply of vitamin E. Incidence of retained placenta can be reduced in cows receiving diets of higher Se content (0.04–0.05 mg/kg DM) than those giving freedom from myopathy. Higher thresholds for blood GPX activities and Se concentrations of 50 µg/l may sometimes be needed for normal reproduction (McClure *et al.*, 1986; Underwood & Suttle, 1999), but studies with grazing heifers in New Zealand show possible tolerance of much lower values (Wichtel *et al.*, 1996). Marginal bands must therefore be used (Table 21.1).

The greatest limitation of blood GPX for monitoring disorder is that the target tissue in Se deficiency is often muscle not blood. Furthermore, there are wide variations between muscles in their GPX content and in the lipid composition of their membranes (Rice & Kennedy, 1988). Measurement of blood GPX alone is unlikely to reflect the risk of lipid peroxidation and hence myopathy in crucial muscles. Guidelines for the interpretation of selected indices of Se status are given in Table 21.1. The assay of a peroxidation product in accessible membranes (e.g. malondialdehyde in erythrocytes) may provide an integrated measure of net oxidative stress but has yet to be tested in ruminants and would not be a specific test for Se (Suttle, 2000). As with other trace elements, the surest diagnosis is often provided by responsiveness to effective Se supplements. By plotting a measure of final performance against performance prior to supplementation (e.g. LWG), it is sometimes possible to identify a small minority of a population which would benefit from additional Se, while mean performance remains unchanged (Suttle, 2000).

Treatment or prevention

The many different methods for administering Se orally and parenterally have been reviewed (Allen, 1983; MacPherson, 1983) and three were compared by MacPherson and Chalmers (1984). Long-term supplementation can be achieved by both routes. By administering heavy metal (iron oxide) (e.g. Hidiroglou *et al.*, 1985; McClure *et al.*, 1986) or soluble glass boluses (Judson *et al.*, 1985) orally and by injecting a relatively insoluble Se salt, barium selenate, in an oily base (MacPherson & Chalmers, 1984; MacPherson *et al.*, 1987b), blood Se concentrations have been increased for at least five months. Supplementing the drinking water (MacPherson & Chalmers, 1984), the pasture (by slow-release fertilizer application; Sanson, 1990; Whelan *et al.*, 1994) or the winter diet (Stowe *et al.*, 1988) with Se can also provide long-term protection. Stowe *et al.* (1988) concluded that a supplement of 2 mg Se/day upon an estimated basal intake of 0.51 mg/day was not sufficient to raise plasma Se in the periparturient cow to 'acceptable levels' (>60 µg/l); nevertheless retained placenta and metritis was only half as prevalent in treated as in untreated cows. Oral supplementation prior to calving (13–45.5 mg/day for 15 days) can raise the Se status of offspring substantially and for several months (Enjalbert *et al.*, 1999). Use of organic forms of selenium such as yeasts or selenomethionine can change the partition of the supplement in weaned or adult cattle and increase the transfer of selenium to milk when compared to inorganic sources but is unlikely have any therapeutic, nutritional or economic advantage in the treated animal (Underwood & Suttle, 1999).

It is questionable whether long-term Se supplementation is the most cost-effective way of treating what are usually short-term problems. The Se-responsive diseases associated with parturition and turnout are acute conditions that can be effectively treated or prevented by single injections of Se as selenite or selenate (e.g. Eger *et al.*, 1985; McMurray & McEldowney, 1977). There is considerable variation in dosage practice. For example, for the prevention of retained placenta, Se doses have varied from 2.3 to 50 mg: the highest dose rate, equivalent to 0.1 mg/kg liveweight, is the most commonly used.

Selenium has generally been given with vitamin E and it is impossible to assess retrospectively whether there was invariably a need for both nutrients. The limited studies in which only one nutrient was given to some animals show that the benefit of providing vitamin E with Se varies from farm to farm. The need for dual supplementation may also depend on the nature of the clinical problem. A combination of oral vitamin E with parenteral Se reduced the incidence of retained placenta in one instance in which the separate treatments were ineffective, but Se alone reduced the prevalence of metritis and cystic ovaries (Harrison *et al.*, 1984). In the treatment of acute myopathy at turnout, McMurray and McEldowney (1977) found that vitamin E (2.8 mg/kg liveweight) was less effective than Se (0.0625 mg/kg liveweight) and added nothing when given with Se. In this situation cattle of low vitamin E status were turned onto grass of naturally high vitamin E concentration. The variable responses to vitamin E given with Se will be due largely to the wide variations found in the vitamin E status of housed cattle.

Selenium toxicity (see p. 943)

Disorders occur naturally either when pastures contain plant species (e.g. *Astragalus*) which accumulate selenium avidly from normal soils ('Blind staggers') or when a combination of selenium-rich soil and high pH allows high levels of selenium to accumulate in normal plant species ('Alkali disease') (O'Toole & Raisbeck, 1995). Accidental toxicity can be caused by errors in adding the small amounts of selenium needed to supplement feeds, exposure to multiple supplementary sources and multiple doses (e.g. Se-supplemented anthelmintics) and failure to scale oral drenches or parenteral injections carefully to liveweight. Because selenium is well absorbed, the oral route poses almost as big a threat as the parenteral route. Selenium is a cumulative poison and tolerable daily intakes and dietary concentrations decrease as duration of exposure increases. Lesions occur principally in the hoof, which overgrows to the point where it may be shed, causing a severe, debilitating lameness. The disorder can be distinguished from laminitis (see p. 420) by the fact that the lesions are epidermal rather than dermal (O'Toole & Raisbeck, 1995). The marginal ranges for indices of selenium status within which toxicosis becomes a possible diagnosis are as follows: diet, 50–75; liver, 30–50; hoof, 25–63 and hair 63–126 µmol Se/kg DM (Underwood & Suttle, 1999; multiply by 79 to obtain values in µg): the corresponding range for blood is 25–30 µmol Se/l (McLaughlin *et al.*, 1989). Preventive measures include the removal of 'Se-accumulator'

species from pastures, treatment of soils with fertilizers which lower selenium uptake (ammonium and calcium sulphates) by plants, rotational grazing with less susceptible species such as sheep and improved soil drainage. Oral administration of sulphate-rich mixtures may prevent or alleviate signs (Arora *et al.*, 1975)

Manganese and zinc disorders

(see p. 260)

Cattle deprived of elements such as Mn and Zn under experimental conditions develop diverse clinical symptoms, but the diets used contained far less Mn and Zn than the levels provided by the vast majority of natural diets (Underwood & Suttle, 1999). Field cases of Mn and Zn deprivation would require either an abundance of dietary antagonists which impair the utilization of the element or other factors which massively increase animal needs for Mn and Zn. There is a possibility that 'protection' of protein sources from rumen degradation might allow phytate to escape and lower absorption of both elements and that fine grinding of cereals might have a similar end result (Suttle, 2000). In the field, soil ingestion provides a rich adventitious source of manganese while access to galvanized feed and drinking troughs provides additional Zn, further reducing the risk of disorders. Little attention has therefore been given to reliable assessment of Mn and Zn status in the animal. Serum Mn and Zn concentrations are probably reasonable indices of deficiency (Table 21.1), but marginal concentrations cannot yet be set with certainty for the former; liver values are poor indicators of status for both Mn and Zn (Underwood & Suttle, 1999). Assessment of hypozincaemia is complicated by the fall in values which accompanies the acute phase of microbial infections; this complication can be ruled out by discarding results for samples with raised haptoglobin or fibrinogen levels or high Cu:Zn ratios (>3–4). Intervention with Mn and Zn supplements is rarely necessary and use of expensive chelated sources is unlikely to improve animal status or performance any more than inorganic Mn or Zn sources (Olson *et al.*, 1999; Underwood & Suttle, 1999). Toxicities of Mn or Zn rarely occur.

References

Allen, W.M. (1983) Parenteral methods of trace element supplementation. British Society of Animal Production Occasional Publication No. 7, pp. 87–92.

Allen, W.M., Drake, C.F. & Tripp, M. (1985) Use of controlled release systems for supplementation during trace element deficiency – the administration of boluses of controlled release glass to cattle and sheep. In *Proceedings of Fifth International Symposium on Trace Element Metabolism in Man and Animals* (ed. by C.F. Mills, I. Bremner & J.K. Chesters), pp. 719–22. Commonwealth Agricultural Bureaux, Farnham Royal.

Arora, S.P., Parvinder, K., Khirwar, S.S., Copra, R.C. & Ludri, R.S. (1975) Selenium levels in fodders and its relationship with Degnala disease. *Indian Journal of Dairy Science*, **28**, 249.

Arthington, J.D., Corah, L.R. & Blecha, F. (1996) The effect of molybdenum induced copper deficiency on acute phase protein concentrations, superoxide dismutase activity, leucocyte numbers and lymphocyte proliferation in beef heifers inoculated with bovine herpesvirus-1. *Journal of Animal Science*, **74**, 211–17.

Arthur, J.R. (1988) Effects of selenium and vitamin E status on plasma creatine kinase activity in calves. *Journal of Nutrition*, **118**, 747–55.

Arthur, J.R., Morrice, P.C. & Beckett, G.J. (1988) Thyroid hormone concentrations in selenium-deficient and selenium sufficient cattle. *Research in Veterinary Science*, **45**, 122–3.

Arthur, J.R., Price, J. & Mills, C.F. (1979) Observations on the selenium status of cattle in the north-east of Scotland. *Veterinary Record*, **104**, 340–1.

Black, H. (1981) Post-parturient haemoglobinuria in Northland. *Proceedings of the Sheep and Beef Cattle Society of New Zealand Veterinary Association's 11th Seminar*, Massey University, Palmerston North, pp. 11–14.

Blanchflower, W.J., Rice, D.A. & Davidson, W.B. (1986) Blood glutathione peroxidase: a method for measurement and the influence of storage, cyanide and Drabkin's reagent on enzyme activity. *Biological Trace Element Research*, **11**, 89–100.

Bremner, I., Humphries, W.R., Phillippo, M., Walker, M.J. & Morrice, P.C. (1987) Iron-induced copper deficiency in calves: dose–response relationships and interactions with molybdenum and sulphur. *Animal Production*, **45**, 403–14.

Duncan, I.F., Greentree, P.L. & Ellis, K.J. (1986) Cobalt deficiency in cattle. *Australian Veterinary Journal*, **3**, 127–8.

Eger, S., Drori, D., Kadoori, I, Miller, N. & Schindler, H. (1985) Effects of selenium and vitamin E on incidence of retained placenta. *Journal of Dairy Science*, **68**, 2119–22.

Enjalbert, F., Lebreton, P., Salat, O. & Schelcher, F. (1999) Effects of pre- or post-partum selenium supplementation on selenium status in beef cows and their calves. *Journal of Animal Science*, **77**, 223–9.

Erskine, R.J. Eberhart, R.J. & Hutchinson, L.J. (1989) Blood selenium concentrations and glutathione peroxidase activities in dairy herds with high and low somatic cell counts. *Journal of American Veterinary Medical Association*, **190**, 1417–21.

Fell, B.F. (1987) The pathology of copper deficiency in animals. In *Copper in Animals and Man* (ed. by J. McC. Howell & J.M. Gawthorne), pp. 1–28. CRC Press Ltd, Boca Raton, Florida.

Fell, B.F., Farmer, L.J., Farquharson, C., Bremner, I. & Graca, D.S. (1985) Observations on the pancreas of cattle deficient in copper. *Journal of Comparative Pathology*, **95**, 573–90.

Felsman, R.J., Wise, M.B., Harvey, R.W. & Barrick, E.R. (1973) Effect of graded levels of copper sulphate and antibiotic on performance and certain blood constituents of calves. *Journal of Animal Science*, **36**, 157–60.

Fish, R.E. & Swanson, E.W. (1983) Effects of excessive iodide administered in the dry period on thyroid function and health of dairy cows and their calves in the peri-parturient period. *Journal of Animal Science*, **56**, 162–72.

Fraser, A.J., Ryan, T.J., Sproule, R., Clark, R.G., Anderson, D. & Pederson, E.O. (1987) The effect of selenium on milk production in dairy cattle. *Proceedings of the New Zealand Society of Animal Production*, **47**, 61–4.

Gengelbach, G.P., Ward, J.D., Spears, J.W. & Brown, T.T. (1997) Effects of copper deficiency coupled with high dietary iron or molybdenum on phagocytic function and response of calves to a respiratory disease challenge. *Journal of Animal Science*, **75**, 1112–18.

Givens, D.I., Zervas, G., Simpson, V.R. & Telfer, S.B. (1988) Use of soluble glass rumen boluses to provide a supplement of copper for suckled calves. *Journal of Agricultural Science, Cambridge*, **110**, 119–204.

Gleed, P.T., Allen, W.M., Mallinson, C.B., Rowlands, G.J., Sansom, B.F., Vagg, M.J. & Caswell, R.D. (1983) Effects of selenium and copper supplementation on the growth of beef steers. *Veterinary Record*, **113**, 388–92.

Harrison, J.H., Hancock, D.D. & Conrad, H.R. (1984) Vitamin E and selenium for reproduction in the dairy cow. *Journal of Dairy Science*, **67**, 123–32.

Hidiroglou, M., Proulx, J. & Jolette, J. (1985) Intraruminal selenium for control of nutritional muscular dystrophy in cattle. *Journal of Dairy Science*, **68**, 57–66.

Jackson, M. (1987) Muscle damage during exercise; possible role of free radicals and the protective effect of vitamin E. *Proceedings of the Nutrition Society*, **46**, 77–80.

Jarvis, S.C. & Austin, A.R. (1983) Soil and plant factors limiting the availability of copper to a beef suckler herd. *Journal of Agricultural Science*, **101**, 39–46.

Jenkins, K.J. & Hidiroglou, M. (1989) Tolerance of the calf for excess copper in milk replacer. *Journal of Dairy Science*, **72**, 150–6.

Jones, R.J. & Meggarity, R.G. (1983) Comparative responses of goats fed on *Leucena leucephala* in Australia and Hawaii. *Australian Journal of Agricultural Research*, **34**, 781–90.

Judson, G.L., Koh, T.-S., McFarlane, J.D., Turnbull, R.K. & Kempe, B.R. (1985) Copper and selenium supplements for cattle: evaluation of the selenium bullet, copper oxide and the soluble glass bullet. In *Proceedings of the Fifth International Symposium on Trace Element Metabolism in Man and Animals* (ed. by C.F. Mills, I. Bremner & J.K. Chesters), pp. 725–8. Commonwealth Agricultural Bureaux, Farnham Royal.

Judson, J.G., McFarlane, J.D., Baumgurtel, K.L., Mitsioulis, A., Nicolson, R.E. & Zviedrans, P. (1997a) Indicators of vitamin B$_{12}$ status in cattle. In *Trace Elements in Man and Animals – 9: Proceedings of the Ninth International Symposium* (ed. by P.W.F. Fischer, M.R. Abbe, K.A. Cockell & R.S. Gibson), pp. 310–11. NRC Research Press, Ottawa, Canada,

Judson, J.G., McFarlane, J.D., Mitsioulis, A. & Zviedrans, P. (1997b) Vitamin B$_{12}$ responses to cobalt pellets in beef cows. *Australian Veterinary Journal*, **75**, 660–2.

Judson, G.J., McFarlane, J.D., Riley, M.J., Milne, M.L. & Horne, A.C. (1981) Treatment of cobalt deficiency in calves. In *Pro-*

ceedings of the Fourth International Symposium on Trace Element Metabolism in Man and Animals (ed. by J. McC. Howell, J.M. Gawthorne & C.L. White), pp. 191–4. Australian Academy of Science, Canberra.

Judson, G.L., McFarlane, J.D., Riley, M.J., Milne, M.L. & Horne, A.C. (1982) Vitamin B$_{12}$ and copper supplementation in beef calves. *Australian Veterinary Journal*, **58**, 249–52.

Kennedy, D.G., Young, P.B., McCaughey, W.J., Kennedy, S. & Blanchflower, W.J. (1991) Rumen succinate production may ameliorate the effects of cobalt-vitamin B$_{12}$ deficiency on methylmalonyl CoA mutase in sheep. *Journal of Nutrition*, **121**, 1236–42.

Langlands, J.P., Wilkins, R.F., Bowles, J.E., Smith, A.J. & Webb, R.F. (1981) Selenium concentration in the blood of ruminants grazing in northern New South Wales. I. Analysis of samples collected in the National Brucellosis Scheme. *Australian Journal of Agricultural Research*, **32**, 511–21.

McClure, T.J., Eamens, G.J. & Healy, P.J. (1986) Improved fertility in dairy cows after treatment with selenium pellets. *Australian Veterinary Journal*, **63**, 144–6.

McCoy, M.A., Smyth, J.A., Ellis, W.A., Arthur, J.R. & Kennedy, D.G. (1997) Experimental reproduction of iodine deficiency in cattle. *Veterinary Record*, **141**, 544–7.

McCoy, M.A., Smyth, J.A., Ellis, W.A. & Kennedy, D.G. (1995) Parenteral iodine and selenium supplementation in stillbirth perinatal/weak calf syndrome. *Veterinary Record*, **136**, 124–6.

McDonald, P. & Suttle, N.F. (1986) Abnormal fermentations in continuous culture of rumen microorganisms given cobalt-deficient hay or barley as food substrates. *British Journal of Nutrition*, **56**, 369–78.

McFarlane, J.D., Judson, J.D. & Gouzos, J. (1990) Copper deficiency in ruminants in the South East of Australia. *Australian Journal of Experimental Agriculture*, **30**, 187–93.

McLaughlin, J.G., Cullen, J. & Forristal, T. (1989) Blood selenium concentrations in cattle on seleniferous pastures. *Veterinary Record*, **124**, 426–7.

McMurray, C.H. & McEldowney, P.K. (1977) A possible prophylaxis and model for nutritional degenerative myopathy in young cattle. *British Veterinary Journal*, **133**, 535–42.

MacPherson, A. (1983) Oral treatment of trace element deficiencies in ruminant livestock. British Society of Animal Production Occasional Publication No. 7, pp. 93–106.

MacPherson, A. & Chalmers, J.S. (1984) Methods of selenium supplementation of ruminants. *Veterinary Record*, **115**, 544–6.

MacPherson, A., Gray, D., Mitchell, D.B.B. & Taylor, C.N. (1987a) *Ostertagia* infection and neutrophil function in cobalt-deficient and cobalt-supplemented cattle. *British Veterinary Journal*, **143**, 348–53.

MacPherson, A., Kelly, E.F., Chalmers, J.S. & Roberts, D.J. (1987b) The effect of selenium deficiency on fertility in heifers. In *Proceedings of 21st Annual Conference on Trace Substances in Environmental Health* (ed. by D.D. Hemphill), pp. 551–5. University of Missouri.

Mee, J.F. (1991) Coat colour and copper deficiency in cattle. *Veterinary Record*, **129**, 536.

Mee, J.F., Rogers, P.A.M. & O'Farrell, K.J. (1995) Effect of feeding a mineral–vitamin supplement before calving on the calving performance of a trace element deficient dairy herd. *Veterinary Record*, **137**, 508–12.

Millar, K.R., Albyt, A.T. & Bond, G.C. (1984) Measurement of vitamin B$_{12}$ in the livers and sera of sheep and cattle and an investigation of factors influencing serum vitamin B$_{12}$ levels in sheep. *New Zealand Veterinary Journal*, **32**, 65–70.

Mitsioulis, A., Bansemer, P.C. & Koh, T.-S. (1995) Relationship between vitamin B$_{12}$ and cobalt concentrations in bovine liver. *Australian Veterinary Journal*, **72**, 70.

Morris, J.G., Chapman, H.L., Walker, D.F., Armstrong, J.B., Alexander, J.D., Miranda, R., Sanchez, A., Sanchez, B., Blair-West, J.R. & Denton, D.A. (1984) Selenium deficiency in cattle associated with Heinz body anaemia. *Science*, **223**, 291–3.

Mylrea, P.J. & Byrne, D.T. (1974) An outbreak of acute copper poisoning in cattle. *Australian Veterinary Journal*, **50**, 169–72.

Newton, G.L., Barrick, E.R., Harvey, R.W. & Wise, M.B. (1974) Iodine toxicity, physiological effects of elevated dietary iodine on calves. *Journal of Animal Science*, **38**, 449–55.

Olson, P.A., Brink, D.R., Hickok, D.T., Carlson, M.P., Schneider, N.R., Deutscher, G.H., Adams, D.C., Colburn, D.J. & Johnson, A.B. (1999) Effects of supplementation of organic and inorganic combinations of copper, cobalt, manganese and zinc above nutrient requirement levels on post partum two-year-old cows. *Journal of Animal Science*, **77**, 522–32.

O'Toole, D. & Raisbeck, M.F. (1995) Pathology of experimentally induced chronic selenosis (alkali disease) in yearling cattle. *Journal of Veterinary Diagnostic Investigation*, **7**, 364–73.

Phillippo, M. (1983) The role of dose–response trials in predicting trace element deficiency disorders. British Society of Animal Production Occasional Publication No. 7, pp. 51–60.

Phillippo, M., Humphries, W.R., Atkinson, T., Henderson, G.D. & Garthwaite, P.H. (1987a) The effect of dietary molybdenum and iron on copper status, puberty, fertility and oestrous cycles in cattle. *Journal of Agricultural Science, Cambridge*, **109**, 321–36.

Phillippo, M., Humphries, W.R. & Garthwaite, P.H. (1987b) The effect of dietary molybdenum and iron on copper status and growth in cattle. *Journal of Agricultural Science, Cambridge*, **109**, 315–20.

Phillippo, M., Humphries, W.R., Lawrence, C.B. & Price, J. (1982) Investigation of the effects of copper status and therapy on fertility in beef suckler herds. *Journal of Agricultural Science, Cambridge*, **99**, 359–64.

Puls, R. (1994) *Mineral Levels in Animal Health*, 2nd edn, p. 120. Diagnostic data, Sherpa International, Clearbrook BC.

Quirk, M.F. & Norton, B.W. (1988) Detection of cobalt deficiency in lactating heifers and their calves. *Journal of Agricultural Science, Cambridge*, **110**, 465–70.

Reffett, J.K., Spears, J.W. & Brown, T.T. (1988) Effect of dietary selenium on the primary and secondary immune response in calves challenged with infectious bovine rhinotracheitis virus. *Journal of Nutrition*, **118**, 229.

Reid, T.C. & McQueen, T.P. (1985) Cobalt supplementation for beef cattle. In *Proceedings of Fifth International Symposium on Trace Element Metabolism in Man and Animals* (ed. by C.F. Mills, I. Bremner & J.K. Chesters), pp. 739–41. Commonwealth Agricultural Bureaux, Furnham Royal.

Rice, D.A. & Kennedy, S. (1988) Vitamin E: functions and effects of deficiency. *British Veterinary Journal*, **144**, 482–96.

Rice, D.A., O'Harte, F.P.M., Blanchflower, W.J. & Kennedy, D.G. (1989) Methylmalonic acid in the rumen of cobalt-deficient sheep and its effects on plasma methylmalonic acid. *Proceedings of Nutrition Society*, **48**, 141A.

Rice, D.A., McLoughlin, M., Blanchflower, W.J., Goodall, E.A. & McMurray, C.H. (1987) Methylmalonic acid as an indicator of vitamin B$_{12}$ deficiency in grazing sheep. *Veterinary Record*, **121**, 472–3.

Rice, D.A. & McMurray, C.H. (1982) Recent information on vitamin E and selenium problems in ruminants. Roche Symposium, Basle, Hoffman La Roche, pp. 1–19.

Richards, R.B. & Edwards, J.R. (1986) A progressive spinal myelinopathy in beef cattle. *Veterinary Pathology*, **23**, 35–41.

Rogers, P.A.M. & Poole, D.B.R. (1988) Copper oxide needles for cattle: a comparison with parenteral treatment. *Veterinary Record*, **123**, 147–51.

Sanson, R.L. (1990) Selenium supplementation of sheep by topdressing pastures under high rainfall conditions. *New Zealand Veterinary Journal*, **38**, 1–3.

Schulz, W. (1987a) Unsaturated vitamin B$_{12}$ binding capacity in human and ruminant serum – a comparison of techniques including a new technique by high performance liquid chromatography. *Veterinary Clinical Pathology*, **16**, 67–72.

Schulz, W. (1987b) A comparison of commercial kit methods for assay of vitamin B$_{12}$ in ruminant blood. *Veterinary Clinical Pathology*, **16**, 102–106.

Smart, M.E., Cohen, R., Christensen, D.A. & Williams, C.M. (1986) The effects of sulphate removal from the drinking water on liver copper and zinc concentrations of beef cows and their calves. *Canadian Journal of Animal Science*, **66**, 669–80.

Smith, K.L., Harrison, J.H. & Hancock, D.D. (1984) Effect of vitamin E and selenium supplementation on incidence of clinical mastitis and duration of symptoms. *Journal of Dairy Science*, **67**, 1293–300.

Smyth, J.A., McNamee, P.T., Kennedy, D.G., McCullough, S.J., Logan, E.F. & Ellis, W.A. (1992) Stillbirth/perinatal weak calf syndrome: preliminary pathological, microbiological and biochemical findings. *Veterinary Record*, **130**, 237–40.

Spears, J.W., Harvey, R.W. & Segerson, E.C. (1986) Effects of marginal selenium deficiency and winter protein supplementation on growth, reproduction and selenium status of beef cattle. *Journal of Animal Science*, **63**, 586–94.

Stangl, G.I., Schwarz, F.J., Jahn, B. & Kirchgessner, M. (2000) Cobalt-deficiency-induced hyperhomocysteinaemia and oxidative status of cattle. *British Journal of Nutrition*, **83**, 3–6.

Stowe, H.D., Thomas, J.W., Johnson, T., Martenuik, J.V., Morrow, D.A. & Ullrey, D.E. (1988) Responses of dairy cattle to long-term and short-term supplementation with oral selenium and vitamin E. *Journal of Dairy Science*, **71**, 1830–9.

Suttle, N.F. (1981) Comparison between parenterally administered copper complexes of their ability to alleviate hypocupraemia in sheep and cattle. *Veterinary Record*, **109**, 304–307.

Suttle, N.F. (1983a) Assessment of the mineral and trace element status of feeds. In *Proceedings of the Second Symposium of the International Network of Feed Information Centres* (ed. by G.E. Robards & R.G. Packham), p. 211. Commonwealth Agricultural Bureaux, Farnham Royal.

Suttle, N.F. (1983b) Effect of molybdenum concentration in fresh herbage, hay and semi-purified diets on the copper metabolism of sheep. *Journal of Agricultural Science, Cambridge*, **100**, 651–6.

Suttle, N.F. (1988) The role of comparative pathology in the studies of copper and cobalt deficiencies in ruminants. *Journal of Comparative Pathology*, **99**, 242–57.

Suttle, N.F. (1995) Relationship between vitamin B$_{12}$ and cobalt concentrations in bovine liver. *Australian Veterinary Journal*, **72**, 278.

Suttle, N.F. (2000) Minerals in livestock production. In *Proceedings of the Ninth Congress of The Asian–Australasian Association of Animal Production Societies* (ed by G. Stone) Suppl. C, pp. 1–9.

Suttle, N.F. (In press) Differential diagnosis of micronutrient–responsive disorders in beef suckler herds. *Cattle Practice*.

Suttle, N.F. & Sinclair, K. (2000) Suckler cow nutrition 2. Minerals and vitamins. *Cattle Practice*, **8**, 193–9.

Underwood, E.J. & Suttle, N.F. (1999) *The Mineral Nutrition of Livestock*, 3rd edn. CABI International, Wallingford.

Wang, Z.Y., Poole, D.B.R. & Mason, J. (1988) The effects of supplementation of the diet of young steers with Mo and S on the intracellular distribution of copper in liver and on copper fractions in blood. *British Veterinary Journal*, **114**, 543–51.

Weiss, W.P., Hogan, J.S., Todhunter, D.A. & Smith, K.L. (1997) Effect of vitamin E suplementation in diets with a low concentration of selenium on mammary gland health of dairy cows. *Journal of Dairy Science*, **80**, 1728–37.

Whelan, B.B., Barrow, N.J. & Peter, D.W. (1994) Selenium fertilizers for pastures grazed by sheep. I. Selenium concentrations in whole blood and plasma. *Australian Journal of Agricultural Research*, **45**, 863–75.

Wichtel, J.J., Craigie, A.L., Freeman, D.A., Varela-Alvarez, H. & Williamson, N.B. (1996) The effect of selenium and iodine supplementation on growth rate and on thyroid and somatotropic function in dairy calves at pasture. *Journal of Dairy Science*, **79**, 1865–72.

Adult Cattle
Mastitis and Teat Conditions

Chapter 22

Anatomy, Physiology and Immunology of the Udder

K.G. Hibbitt, N. Craven and E.H. Batten

Anatomy of the udder   311
  Introduction   311
  Early development of the udder   311
  The adult bovine mammary gland   313
The physiology of lactation   316
  Introduction   316
  Mammogenesis   316
  Lactogenesis   317
  Milk synthesis and secretion   318
  Milk ejection   319
  Galactopoiesis   320
  Manipulation of lactation   321
Immunology of the udder and teat   321
  Non-specific immunity   321
  The teat canal as a mechanical barrier   322
  Antimicrobial substances within the teat canal   322
  Antimicrobial substances in mammary secretions   322
  Specific immunity: lymphocytes   323
  Immunoglobulins in mammary secretions   323
  Phagocytic cell mobilization in the mammary gland
  and phagocytosis   324

Anatomy of the udder

Introduction

The mammary gland is essentially a skin gland. It is believed to have evolved by modification of a sweat gland and retains two common features: development by ingrowth of ectoderm; and a bilayered epithelium of inner secretory cells and outer myoepithelial cells, which by contracting promote flow of milk from the peripheral alveoli into the major ducts. Assuming the new function of catering for the immune welfare and nutrition of the neonate, the mammary gland has evolved into a highly branched compound structure with enormous numbers of dilated alveoli. This pattern allows for both synthesis and storage of milk on a large scale. Yet neither function is possible until the cow becomes pregnant, when the rudimentary and inactive gland undergoes massive growth to definitive structure and only then begins to synthesize secretion.

Early development of the udder

The first trace of mammary development appears in bovine embryos of 1.5 cm length as two short lines in the ectoderm running from the umbilicus caudally into the groin. Each line is several cells thick, but intense proliferation of cells in the basal layer at focal points produces an ingrowth, the mammary hillock (Fig. 22.1a). This soon enlarges into an ovoid mammary bud (Fig. 22.1b) invested by a condensation of inductive mesenchymal cells. As the rudiment of the duct system each mammary bud determines the site where a gland will form. By the seventh week of gestation in fetuses 9 cm long, four primary mammary buds are usually present, two on each side, defining the future quarters of the udder. Extra buds occasionally form and develop into supernumerary teats. Active proliferation of mesenchymal cells around the mammary bud lifts the epidermis into a rudimentary teat by the 8-cm stage. Simultaneously, vigorous proliferation of cells near the inner end changes the mammary bud into a solid cellular column, which elongates vertically into the mesenchyme (Fig. 22.1c) as the rudiment of the duct system, the future single galactophore. Meanwhile, division among the epidermal cells below the original bud produces an epidermal cone at the base of the duct primordium.

By the 19-cm stage the growing duct primordium is longer than the teat and slightly swollen at the inner end. Here a cavity or lumen appears and soon spreads proximally towards the teat apex. On reaching the epidermal cone the split remains narrow as the lumen of the future teat canal. Later this will open on the teat apex and both teat canal and superficial epidermis will be lined by a common, thick, stratified squamous, keratinizing epithelium.

By the 35-cm stage (Fig. 22.2) the growing duct rudiment has differentiated into three distinct regions:

(1) An upper spheroid chamber distended with fluid represents the future gland sinus or milk reservoir.
(2) A slightly longer mid-portion forms the more slender teat sinus.
(3) A narrow teat canal within the epidermal cone, but still closed from the exterior by a plug of horny cells.

(a) **Mammary hillock: 2.5 cm fetus**

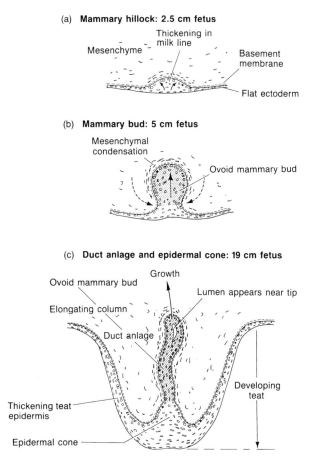

(b) **Mammary bud: 5 cm fetus**

(c) **Duct anlage and epidermal cone: 19 cm fetus**

Fig. 22.1 (a) Transverse section of a mammary line at the level of a localized cellular proliferation, which forms a mammary hillock and determines where a gland will develop. (b) Later stage showing an ovoid mammary bud with cells more basophilic (stippled) than in the epidermis. A condensation of mesenchymal cells surrounds the bud. Curved broken arrows indicate growth of mesenchyme, which elevates a rudimentary teat. (c) Sustained proliferation (upper arrow) near the tip converts the mammary bud into a columnar vertical ingrowth, the precursor of the axial duct and storage sinuses. Meanwhile, division among the subjacent epidermal cells produces a cone, which later splits to form the lumen of the teat canal (from Turner, 1952).

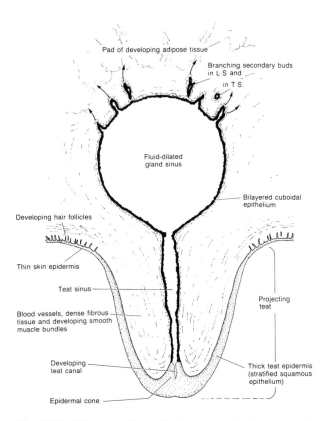

Fig. 22.2 Diagrammatic vertical section of the teat and mammary rudiment in a 35-cm fetus. Stratified epithelium is shown dotted. It appears distinctly thicker in the epidermal cone, where the teat canal lumen is forming, and over the surface of the teat rather than above it where hairy skin is differentiating. Derivatives of the original mammary bud are lined by double cuboidal epithelium (black) and comprise the narrow teat sinus leading from the fluid-distended gland sinus. Up to 10 short secondary buds project from the dome of the sinus and later will branch to form major ducts as they grow into the overlying cushion of fat. LS, longitudinal section; TS, transverse section (from Turner, 1952).

From the domed roof of the gland sinus several short solid epithelial cords, the secondary sprouts, project dorsally into the overlying pad of differentiating adipose tissue. When canalized these secondary sprouts represent the bases of the 10 or more major lactiferous ducts, which in the adult deliver milk into the gland sinus for storage. The teat sinus, gland sinus and duct bases are lined by a bilayered cuboidal epithelium. As also in the terminal alveoli, which differentiate later in pregnancy, the inner cells are potentially secretory, while the outer differentiate into myoepithelial elements. In contrast the lowest and narrowest part of the axial lumen, forming the teat canal, is lined by thick,

stratified squamous epithelium continuous with and identical to the glabrous epidermis of the teat. The latter is distinctly thicker, even in the fetus, than the epidermis above the teat where hair follicles differentiate from solid cellular ingrowths. The mesenchyme around and between the rudimentary epithelial ducts differentiates to provide blood vessels, lymphatics, small amounts of smooth muscle and an extensive fibroelastic stroma. Tracts of denser white fibrous and elastic tissue form the suspensory ligaments and dorsally numerous lobules form in the pad of adipose tissue.

Just before birth tertiary sprouts develop as short side branches from the secondary ducts, but thereafter the gland remains in an arrested state of development until puberty. Some extension to the ducts occurs during oestrous cycles, but full structural differentiation of the mammary gland is completed only during pregnancy under the influence of progesterone from the corpus luteum and other hormones. During the first half of pregnancy, intense cell proliferation at the blind ends elongates the ducts, which branch repeatedly establishing an extensive tree. At the peripheral tips of the large number of fine ducts thus formed narrow tubular prospective alveoli then differentiate. In the second half of pregnancy, protein secretion and lipid droplets slowly accumulate, dilating the alveoli into saccular chambers 120 µm across and filled with stored colostrum awaiting release in the first sucking after birth.

The adult bovine mammary gland

The cow's udder comprises four quarters, each an individual gland drained by a teat. The four secretory glands are structurally separate and function independently, without flow of milk between them. Receiving a large flow of blood and laden with stored milk, the lactating udder often weights 50–60 kg. Support for this massive weight is provided by dense fibrous suspensory ligaments that insert into the pelvis and tendons of the abdominal wall. The ligaments spread laterally and ventrally over the udder, then coverge inwards to join paired median ligaments. These form a double vertical partition separating glands on the left from those on the right. Septa of interlobular connective tissue span between the lateral and medial ligaments and support the heavy lobules of parenchyma. As the medial ligaments contain relatively more elastin than the predominantly collagenous lateral ligaments the full udder drops in the midline and the teats become splayed outwards.

Blood supply

During the production of 20 kg of milk each day 9000 kg of blood circulate through the udder of the cow. Most of this rich supply arrives through the inguinal canal in the external pudendal arteries derived from the external iliac trunks. The udder also receives a subsidiary supply, cranially through the subcutaneous abdominal artery and caudally via the perineal artery. Numerous small veins leaving the parenchyma anastomose and converge around the base of the udder into a circular vessel that is drained by three trunks: the large subcutaneous abdominal vein, which passes cranially and penetrates the abdominal wall near the xiphoid cartilage; the external pudendal vein, which departs through the inguinal canal; and the perineal vein.

Innervation

The principal nerve supply derives from branches of the third and fourth lumbar nerves, which traverse the inguinal canal. Contributions from the first and second lumbar nerves supply the cranial, and from the perineal nerves the caudal regions respectively. These are mainly sensory nerves, but they carry from the caudal mesenteric plexus sympathetic fibres, which modulate blood flow by direct action on the arterioles. Whereas the skin and particularly the teats receive a rich sensory supply, nerves are sparser in the glandular parenchyma and chiefly, if not entirely, vasomotor: the secretory alveoli lack a nerve supply. After the skin is anaesthetized the deeper mammary tissue may be incised without apparent sensation.

Mammary gland: histological organization

Histologically classified, the lactating udder is a large, lobulated, compound exocrine gland with dilated alveoli storing milk. Each alveolus is a single or bifid sac, slightly longer than wide and distended to an internal diameter of 120–150 µm by milk (Fig. 22.3). The lining epithelium is bilayered. The inner secretory or alveolar cells vary from tall cuboidal (8 µm) in the partially empty gland to stretched squamous (3 µm) in full distension state. Synthesis and release of milk constituents (fluid, casein, lactose and lipid) is continuous, until temporarily arrested by negative feedback. The outer contractile myoepithelial cells are indistinct in routine sections, but staining for alkaline phosphatase reveals their spider shape, with branching processes embracing the curved contour of the alveolar wall (Fig. 22.4). Towards term and during lactation the large alveoli have a rich capillary supply and are packed closely together into polyhedral lobules about 2 mm across. The alveoli drain into intralobular ducts which, unlike those in salivary or lacrimal glands, are indistinct, since they resemble the alveoli in size, milk content and secretory lining. The heavy lobules are enclosed and bound together by thin septa of supportive connective tissue. This also carries distributing arteries and veins, lymphatics and the larger interlobular ducts, which converge and unite into major ducts opening into the gland cistern.

The teat

Each teat has a single narrow teat canal, which dorsally opens into a wider teat cistern lined by bilayered epithelium. Normally, the teat canal is kept closed by sphincter action of the surrounding smooth muscle and elastic tissues. Thus in section the lumen is a narrow

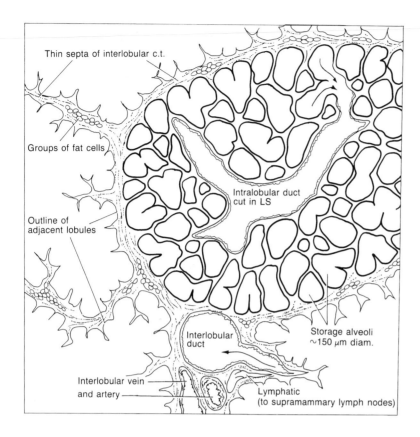

Fig. 22.3 Histological features of the lactating udder, showing large polyhedral lobules supported by thin septa of connective tissue carrying the distributing service vessels: interlobular ducts emerging (at lower right) from lobules, arteries supplying and veins draining the dense networks of perialveolar capillaries. Nearby collecting lymphatics carry a considerable flow of afferent lymph rich in lymphoeytes, neutrophils and macrophages and during infections, e.g. mastitis, carrying antigens that induce immune responses in the supramammary lymph nodes.

In each lobule the alveoli tend to be similar in size, but are generally smaller, averaging 60 μm across, with a tall cobbled epithelium in lobules that released milk at the previous lactation. When fully distended with milk, as shown, alveoli approach 150 μm in diameter and have a thin stretched lining. Smaller profiles represent alveoli slices in oblique to tangential planes. Intralobular ducts drain milk from alveoli (curved arrows), but unless fortuitously sliced in longitudinal section are almost indistinguishable from the alveoli, being comparable in width and lined by identical secretory epithelium. c.t., connective tissue; LS, longitudinal section (diagram by E.H. Batten).

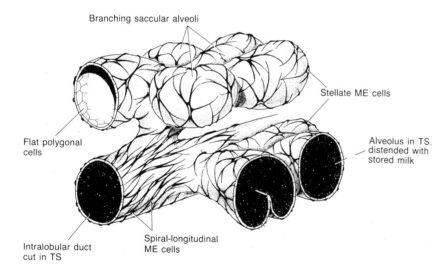

Fig. 22.4 Diagram showing several branching milk-distended alveoli of the lactating udder draining into a relatively wide intralobular duct. In the sectioned profiles fat droplets in the milk are shown white against a black background. Contraction of the network of stellate myoepithelial cells (cytoplasm black, nuclei white) expels milk from the alveoli into the intralobular ducts. In turn these become shortened and compressed by the contraction of the spirally aligned myoepithelial cells, which propel milk towards the larger interlobular ducts. ME, myoepithelial cells; TS, transverse section (after Linzell, 1961).

stellate crevice, with the lining of thick, keratinizing, stratified squamous epithelium thrown into several longitudinal folds that almost meet centrally (Fig. 22.5). The teat is robustly constructed and well adapted to tolerate the shear stresses generated by a suckling calf or milking machine.

Structurally the teat wall comprises five distinct tissue layers: superficial epidermis, then dermis, intermediate layer, fibrous lamina propria and internally the epithe-

lium of the teat canal. The teat is covered by thick, stratified squamous, keratinizing epidermis with neither hair follicles nor sweat and sebaceous glands. Whereas the thinner skin over the udder is relatively loosely attached and can freely be moved over the underlying glandular lobules, the teat skin is immobile and tightly anchored to the deeper fibromuscular core. This firm surface is well suited to withstand mechanical shear forces set up by suckling, hand or machine milking. In

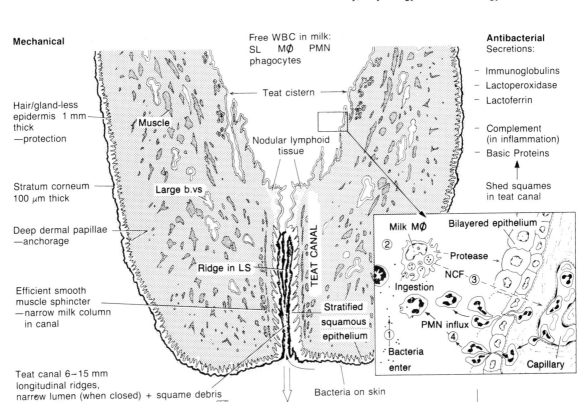

Fig. 22.5 Diagram of a vertical section of a cow's teat, showing on the left factors that protect against mechanical trauma during suckling or milking, and on the right defences against ascending infection by bacteria from the skin surface (curved arrow) entering the teat canal.

Milk normally contains shed epithelial cells, from both alveoli and ducts, squames from the teat canal, small lymphocytes (SL), macrophages (MØ) and neutrophils (PMN). As phagocytes the last two cell types often contain small droplets of fat ingested from the milk. Subepithelial plasma cells occur near the ring of nodular lymphoid tissue that surrounds the rosette or inner end of the teat canal, where the stratified, keratinizing lining gives way to a bilayered cuboidal epithelium of the teat cistern. Insert right summarizes the early response to mastitis-forming bacteria experimentally introduced into the teat canal. Bacteria (1) are ingested by milk macrophages (2), which release enzymes that damage and loosen the inner layer of the epithelium and neutrophil chemotactic factor (NCF), which induces (3) within 4 hours the emigration of large numbers of PMN from the subepithelial capillaries and venules. After insinuating through the cisternal epithelium the PMN (4) join with the macrophages in the ingestion and killing of bacteria. WBC, white blood cells; b.vs, blood vessels; LS, longitudinal section (diagram by E.H. Batten).

the lactating cow the teat epidermis is remarkable for three features.

(1) In thickness about 1 mm, it is comparable with muzzle epidermis and some 12 times deeper than epidermis of hair skin (75 µm in frozen sections, which preserve the 30 layers of horny squames only 1 µm thick).

(2) The protective stratum corneum is a compact layer, 100 µm deep and comprising as many overlapping layers of dead horny squames.

(3) The underside is deeply papillated: epidermal pegs interdigitate with narrow, deep intrusions of dermal connective tissue.

Over this interface the area of adhesive basement membrane is fivefold greater than in the flat underside of hairy epidermis. This interlocking pattern binds epidermis securely and inseparably into the dermis and dissipates shear stresses from the surface through the deeper tissues. The dermal fibrous mat continues into the dense fibromuscular layer, without the intervening loose superficial fascia typical of thin skin.

Beneath the epidermis the dermis carries a rich capillary network and numerous fine bundles of sensory fibres derived from lumbar nerves 2–4. Despite its thickness as a protection against wear, teat epidermis is highly sensitive, since the penetrating dermal papillae carry sensory nerves and endings to within 200 µm or less of the surface. This rich innervation receives tactile stimuli and relays to the central nervous system impulses that lead to the release of oxytocin from the pars nervosa into the blood. In turn, circulating oxytocin induces contraction of myoepithelial cells, promoting flow from the terminal alveoli and along the ducts during milk let-down. The deeper regions of the dermis contain dense collagenous tissue surrounding bundles of smooth muscle arranged mainly longitudinally.

The third or intermediate layer contributes much of the strength of the teat wall, as it contains numerous bundles of smooth muscle set in coarse fibroelastic tissue. These muscle bundles are aligned in longitudinal, circular and oblique planes. Major blood vessels are present, including distributing arteries, a complex plexus of anastomosing veins and numerous collecting lymphatics, which drain to the supramammary nodes.

The lamina propria resembles the dermis in its fibroelastic components, but carries more microvessels catering for the nutrition of the adjoining epithelium of the teat canal. During ascending infections with pathogenic bacteria, increased emigration from the local venules creates leucocytic infiltrations beneath regions where epithelial cells have been damaged, as explained in Fig. 22.5.

Both the teat cistern and the gland cistern dorsal to it are lined by a common bilayered cuboidal epithelium. Under scanning electron microscopy the superficial cells fit closely in hexagonal profiles densely covered with microvilli (Fig. 22.6). In the junctional region

around the inner opening of the teat canal (earlier termed Furstenberg's rosette from the mucosal creases) the surface cells are more rounded and protruding, with sparser microvilli. In this region just beyond the barrier epithelium of the teat canal the lining may be a lymphoepithelium important in the uptake or penetration of invading antigens. Intraepithelial lymphocytes are profuse and both diffuse and nodular lymphoid tissue are present in the lamina propria. The accumulations of plasma cells and germinal centres (Fig. 22.7) often present there provide evidence of local humoral immune responses.

The physiology of lactation

Introduction

The secretion of milk by specialized mammary glands in the female for the nourishment of the newborn is the essential characteristic that distinguishes mammals from other animals. This feature is epitomized in the dairy cow which, as a result of intensive selection, has a disproportionately high output of energy in milk in relation to body size. Continuing improvements in milk yield and feed efficiency are the result of refinement of the genetic make-up of stock and improvements in management and nutritional practices. This focusing of effort on increasing milk production has prompted the facetious comment that the modern dairy cow should perhaps be regarded as an appendage of the udder rather than vice versa! Indeed, the readjustment of physiological processes that occurs in order to meet the extra metabolic demands of lactation involves not just differentiation and activation of mammary tissue but extends to changes throughout the body. Not the least of these is the hormonal regulation of nutrient utilization and partitioning between the mammary gland and other organs.

Milk is a complex secretion and its production is under complex control. By understanding the underlying physiology, the relevance of correct nutritional and husbandry practices in maintaining health and optimizing performance may be better appreciated.

Mammogenesis

Mammogenesis may be defined as the growth and differentiation of the mammary gland to the stage prior to active secretion. Since milk yield is ultimately dependent on the number of secretory cells and their activity, factors that influence the former during mammogenesis can have lasting implications for subsequent milk production.

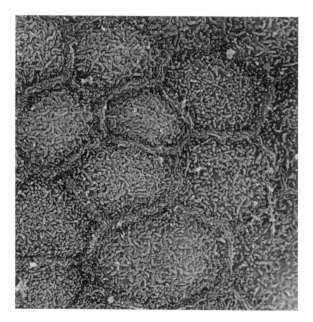

Fig. 22.6 Characteristic outline of teat epithelial cells covered with irregular microvilli (×9000). From Collins *et al.* (1986).

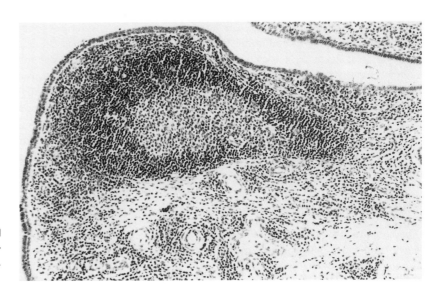

Fig. 22.7 A lymphoid nodule with germinal centre beneath the double cuboidal epithelium lining Furstenberg's rosette (HE × 32). From Collins *et al.*, 1986.

From birth to puberty mammary growth is isometric, i.e. in balance with the growth rate of the whole body, but just prior to the onset of ovarian activity mammary growth becomes allometric (i.e. exceeds that of the body surface). Only during the first pregnancy does marked branching of the duct system and lobulo-alveolar development occur, with expanding parenchyma displacing adipose tissue within the mammary fat pad. Lobulo-alveolar proliferation accelerates as pregnancy advances with division of secretory cells continuing at least until the onset of lactation. Balanced mammary development exhibits a crucial dependence on hormonal stimulation. The hormones principally implicated include steroids (oestrogens, progesterone and adrenal corticoids) and protein hormones (prolactin, somatotropin and placental lactogen). Thyroid hormones are possibly also involved. Many of these hormones interact synergistically to promote the different stages of mammogenesis. Oestrogens and somatotropin are responsible for ductal development whereas progesterone and prolactin appear to regulate lobulo-alveolar proliferation. The additional presence of adrenal corticoids maximizes this growth. Placental lactogen may, in some species, also stimulate alveolar formation but in the cow relatively little enters the maternal circulation.

During the period of allometric growth just prior to puberty the administration of exogenous somatotropin to heifers appears to promote an increase in mammary parenchyma. It is known that excess energy consumption during the period of allometric growth in heifers offered a high plane of nutrition results in lower mammary secretory tissue weight and is also associated with low milk production during subsequent lactation. It has been suggested that these effects of overfeeding during this critical phase of mammary development may in fact be caused by a decrease in endogenous levels of somatotropin, as has been observed during high plane feeding. Thus the interplay between nutritional management and hormonal balance during mammogenesis may have important consequences for subsequent production.

Mammary development is partly reversed during advancing lactation when gradual involution occurs. These effects become more pronounced during the dry period. A period of non-lactation between successive lactations is an essential prerequisite for maximal milk production. Milk yields in the next lactation are definitely impaired if cows are dry for less than six weeks. On the other hand there is little or no advantage to be gained in terms of an increase in subsequent lactation yield by extending the dry period to more than eight weeks.

Lactogenesis

The initiation of milk secretion (lactogenesis) in all mammals is closely coordinated with parturition. Parturition itself involves a complex interplay of endocrine controls with marked differences between species. There are two general concepts as to what constitutes the main lactogenic trigger, the positive stimulus of lactation-promoting hormones and the release from the inhibitory effects of progesterone. A peak in blood prolactin levels coincides with, but is not essential for, parturition. Suppression of prolactin release in cows inhibits the final stages of secretory cell differentiation and results in reduced milk yield. Thus elevation of prolactin (together with adequate amounts of adrenal corticoids) and the permissive effect of progesterone withdrawal, appear to provide the main lactogenic stimulus in the cow. An additional feature may be the removal near term of a locally produced inhibitory factor (possibly prostaglandin $F_{2\alpha}$).

Lactogenesis requires the preferential supply and uptake of nutrients by mammary tissue. Nutrient availability is enhanced by the disconnection of the fetal supply at parturition and increases in mammary blood flow and local selective nutrient uptake become evident.

Milk synthesis and secretion

The constituents of milk are synthesized mainly from small molecules absorbed from the blood, specific carrier systems probably assisting their entry into secretory cells. The blood supply provides not only precursors for milk synthesis but also adequate energy-yielding substrates to drive the synthetic processes.

Lactose (milk sugar) is a disaccharide composed of one molecule of glucose and one of galactose. In bovine milk its concentration, at about 4.8 per cent, is the most consistent of any constituent due largely to its influence in maintaining the osmolality of milk. Blood glucose is the main precursor of lactose but small amounts may also be formed from amino acids, glycerol and acetate. The final enzyme-catalysed step in lactose synthesis from glucose involves an enzyme, 'lactose synthetase', which is unique to mammary tissue. This is composed of two protein components and the availability of the second component, α-lactalbumin (a milk protein), determines the rate of synthesis of lactose, which occurs in the Golgi membranes of secretory cells.

Milk protein synthesis involves the assembly of different amino acids in a specific order along a chain. It takes place in the ribosomes of the rough endoplasmic reticulum (RER in Fig. 22.8) of secretory cells, proteins destined for secretion being released into the lumina of the endoplasmic reticulum. Total amino acid nitrogen uptake by mammary tissue entirely accounts for the output of nitrogen in milk protein. However, the proportions of different amino acids absorbed by the glands are at variance with their appearance in milk

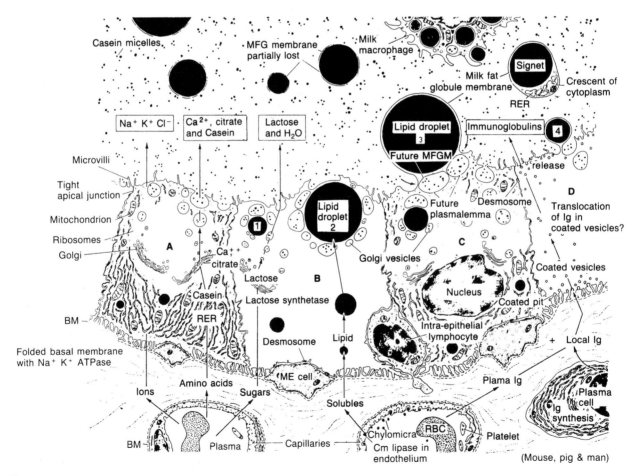

Fig. 22.8 Mammary alveolus secretory pathways. RBC, red blood cell; Ig, immunoglobulin; RER, rough endoplasmic reticulum; BM, basement membrane; MFG, milk fat globule; MFGM, milk fat globule membrane (diagram by E.H. Batten).

protein, indicating that some are metabolized while others are synthesized by mammary tissue. The majority of milk proteins are synthesized locally and are unique to milk (e.g. caseins). However, certain blood proteins and similar proteins synthesized by plasma cells adjacent to secretory epithelia are also transferred into lacteal secretions – in large amounts in colostrum (*see below*).

The fat content of bovine milk varies widely between and within breeds and is influenced by diet and environmental factors. The majority of milk fat is in the form of triglycerides, which are assembled in or near the endoplasmic reticulum of secretory cells using fatty acids and glycerol synthesized in the cytosol. Approximately half of the fatty acids in milk are derived directly from the blood – chiefly those greater than 14 carbons in length. *De novo* synthesis of fatty acids utilizes volatile fatty acids arising from rumen fermentation, fatty acid synthesis from glucose being negligible in ruminants. Acetate and β-hydroxybutyrate are important precursors and contribute mainly to the synthesis of shorter-chain fatty acids. The glycerol required for milk triglycerides is partly derived from hydrolysis of blood lipids and partly by synthesis from glucose. Esterification of fatty acids with glycerol is followed by aggregation of triglycerides to form the characteristic fat droplets of secretory cells.

The mechanisms for cellular release of secretion differ for the various components of milk. Instead of combining into a large exocrine granule typical of zymogenic and serous cells, milk protein remains separate as multiple small granules. These are visible only ultrastructurally and present a large surface area, which facilitates rapid digestion. Non-immune protein, such as casein, is delivered from the rough endoplasmic reticulum to the Golgi complex, where through the agency of lactose synthetase, lactose is added. This causes the vesicles leaving the Golgi to swell osmotically. As they rise through the supranuclear cytoplasm the vesicles become tightly clustered around the sides of the lipid droplets, which lie free in the cytoplasm and may be up to 5 μm in diameter. Subsequently, membranes of the more superficial vesicles fuse with the apical plasma membrane and their content of protein, lactose, calcium and fluid is emptied into the alveolar lumen by conventional exocytosis. As the vesicles successively discharge, their inner walls remain over the surface of the protruding lipid as the milk fat droplet membrane. Ultimately undercut by the fusion of membranes between the lowest vesicles, the milk fat droplet is liberated into the lumen without damage to the cell and in a manner reminiscent of the shedding from an erythroblast of a pyknotic nucleus of comparable size.

The process of milk fat release is best termed micro-apocrine, since it does involve some loss of cell components – the membrane investing the lipid and beneath it usually a thin veil of cytoplasm, as illustrated in Fig. 22.8. About 5 per cent of droplets are signet-shaped, with a crescentic fragment of cytoplasm containing a few mitochondria or short profiles of rough ER. Immune proteins, such as various immunoglobulins arriving via the blood or derived from local plasma cells, are taken into the cell base by receptor-mediated endocytosis into coated vesicles, translocated through the cytoplasm and released at the apical membrane.

Mature milk is characterized by a high concentration of potassium and a relatively low sodium concentration similar to the situation within the secretory cells. Milk is 86 per cent water. The amount of water (and hence milk volume) is determined largely by the rate of lactose secretion since lactose is not reabsorbed across epithelial cell membranes and it exerts an important osmotic 'draw' within the milk duct system.

Milk ejection

In the interval between milkings, milk continues to be synthesized and secreted at a more or less constant rate into the alveolar lumina and thence to the large collecting ducts and sinuses. The resistance of the teat sphincter retains the milk in the sinuses but much of the milk remains within alveoli and will not flow out passively even when the teat sphincter is patent. Forcible expulsion is, therefore, required to remove this alveolar milk from the gland. Milk ejection is under neuroendocrine control.

The milk ejection reflex involves stimulation of nerve receptors in the skin of the teat. Mechanical stimulation triggers an impulse in afferent mammary nerves. This impulse is transmitted via the spinal cord and ultimately arrives in the posterior hypothalamus. Specialized neurones in this region synthesize oxytocin (a peptide hormone) and a carrier protein. In addition to receiving the afferent excitatory stimulus originating from the teat, the neurones also receive facilitatory and inhibitory impulses that arise in other parts of the brain. If the net result of these impulses is stimulatory, neurosecretory granules are released into blood capillaries from axons that terminate in the posterior pituitary. Thus following mechanical stimulation of the teats of cows, oxytocin increases rapidly in the blood, reaching a peak within 2 minutes.

In mammary tissue, contractile myoepithelial cells form a basketwork surrounding the alveoli. Oxytocin in mammary blood binds with high affinity to receptor sites on myoepithelial cells (Fig. 22.4), resulting in contraction of the cells and expulsion of the milk from the alveoli.

Although sucking and milking are the most potent and natural stimuli to elicit the milk ejection reflex, udder washing and even visual and auditory cues associated with milking routines can substitute, as the reflex becomes conditioned by experience. Stressful stimuli which involve the release of catecholamines and activity of the sympathetic nervous system can have negative influences on oxytocin release, mammary blood flow and oxytocin binding to myoepithelial cells, thereby inhibiting milk ejection. Myoepithelial cells also contract to an extent in response to direct mechanical stimuli, independently of oxytocin release. Palpation of the udder (or butting by calves) may trigger this local so-called 'tap reflex'.

Galactopoiesis

Frequent milk let-down and its removal from alveolar lumina assists in the maintenance of milk production (galactopoiesis) by preventing 'end product inhibition'. Nevertheless, the continued secretion of milk also depends on a continued hormonal drive, which induces and maintains the synthetic enzyme complement of secretory cells and also ensures an adequate supply of substrates. The chief hormones implicated in the maintenance of lactation are different from those responsible for lactogenesis.

The essential role of the pituitary gland in the maintenance of lactation in all mammals has long been recognized. The roles of the various pituitary hormones have been revealed by studies on hypophysectomized animals with hormonal supplementation or by the use of specific antagonists. In most species (i.e. rabbits, pigs, dogs, humans) prolactin has been identified as the key galactopoietic hormone and suppression of prolactin secretion by bromocriptine has a rapid effect in inhibiting milk secretion. In ruminants, however, suppression of prolactin secretion has only a partial (sheep) or no inhibitory effect (cows, goats) on lactation. In these species, somatotropin (pituitary growth hormone) provides the main galactopoietic stimulus. The dose-dependent stimulation of milk yield in dairy cows that follows administration of somatotropin has been known for many years. With the advent of recombinant DNA technology, commercial exploitation of this effect is now practicable and our knowledge of the role of somatotropin has increased as a result of the considerable recent research on this topic.

The release of somatotropin into circulation from the anterior pituitary is under the influence of various hypothalamic peptides that arrive in the hypophyseal portal blood supply; these include a specific somatotropin releasing hormone and an inhibitory peptide, somatostatin. Thyroid hormone releasing hormone also enhances somatotropin release and synergizes with the

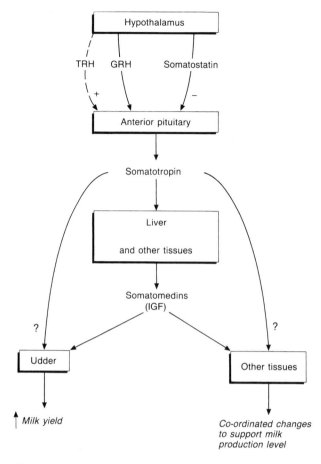

Fig. 22.9 Regulation of somatotropin release and its effects on milk production. TRH, thyroid hormone releasing hormone; GRH, growth hormone releasing hormone; IGF = insulin-like growth factor.

action of the specific releasing hormone. A direct effect of increased levels of somatotropin is the induction in the liver and other organs of the synthesis of other peptides known as somatomedins or insulin-like growth factors (IGFs). IGFs in turn appear responsible for mediating many of the effects attributed to somatotropin (Fig. 22.9).

It seems likely that somatotropin does not exert its galactopoietic effect by direct stimulation of the udder. Rather it acts by partitioning available energy away from body tissues and towards milk production but the increased yield is not merely a passive response to an increased nutrient supply. There is also an increased synthetic activity per secretory cell. Administration of somatotropin also elevates cardiac output and mammary blood flow. It is considered that this increase in blood flow is, at least in part, a consequence rather than a cause of the increased activity of mammary tissue.

The metabolic effects of administering supplementary somatotropin to dairy cows are well documented.

In early short-term studies, acute responses of hyperglycaemia ('diabetogenesis') and elevation of circulating free fatty acids ('lipolysis') were reported. In contrast, there is now substantial evidence from studies where somatotropin has been administered for long periods which indicates that the significant increases in milk yield are perfectly balanced by increased voluntary feed intakes and alterations in metabolism of body tissues such that steady-state concentrations of blood metabolites are maintained. These coordinated changes are consistent with the role of somatotropin as a homeorhetic control, allowing a substantial shift in the partitioning of nutrients to the mammary gland.

The key role of somatotropin in milk production is underscored by the evidence that cows selected for high genetic merit for yield show higher endogenous levels (basal and after stimulation) of somatotropin than low yielders. Furthermore, somatotropin levels decline with advancing lactation in line with milk production. Somatotropin levels are also influenced by nutritional status independently of these genetic effects. Underfed cows have generally higher somatotropin levels than those that are well fed, although this may be offset by a lower somatotropin responsiveness of the underfed animals.

Other hormones with a suggested role in galactopoiesis include adrenal corticoids and thyroid hormones. In most species adrenal corticoids are essential for lactation but there is little evidence that plasma levels are a limiting factor. Thyroxine and triiodothyronine may have a stimulatory effect on milk yield via effects on metabolic rate.

Immediate increases in milk yield can be obtained by commencing three times a day milking, which indicates that the secretory capacity of mammary cells can be increased. Frequency of milking does not appear to affect endogenous somatotropin levels. The mechanisms are not fully understood but may involve the removal of inhibitors.

Manipulation of lactation

The continuing steady increase in annual average milk yields of dairy cows is the result of judicious genetic selection and improvements in management, especially nutritional management. Experts expect these trends to continue for some years to come. However, a growing understanding of the physiological processes of lactation, together with advances in biotechnology, now make possible a variety of new ways to control and manipulate lactation.

Administration of somatotropin to prepubertal heifers has been shown to increase mammary parenchyma but whether this translates into increased milk yields is not yet clear. Nevertheless, optimal nutritional management during this period is clearly of practical relevance in influencing mammogenesis and subsequent yield.

The hormonal manipulation of galactopoiesis has considerable commercial potential, both in a free market for milk products and for efficient quota management under a milk quota system. Biotechnology-derived somatotropin in prolonged-release formulations is already available for commercial use in some countries (see p. 1073). Endogenous somatotropin production may also be enhanced by administering releasing factors or by immunization of animals against their natural inhibitory peptide, somatostatin. Research into such approaches is under way.

Developments in direct genetic transfers between mammalian cells make possible the insertion of extra somatotropin genes which, if expressed, will enable cows to produce high endogenous levels of somatotropin. The genes might be triggered by an external stimulus such as a dietary factor. Such transgenic 'super cows' could be propagated rapidly using modern reproductive techniques. Transgenic techniques might also be employed to modify the characteristics of the milk constituents produced.

There are also opportunities for optimizing milking procedures to exploit physiological controls of lactation more fully. Further automation of the milking process culminating in robotic milking may permit milking several times a day and, with some sophistication, optimal prestimulation, stripping and individual quarter milking.

Immunology of the udder and teat

Immunity in the mammary gland may be divided into two systems (see Chapter 29). Firstly, a non-specific system that offers a first line of defence when a pathogen invades, and frequently is able to resist the invasion of a number of potentially infectious agents. Secondly, if the non-specific system fails, the tissues of the mammary gland can adapt and produce a specific defence against each infectious agent. Frequently this system, once developed, remembers the invading pathogen, which can be resisted by the specific defence system on a later occasion.

Non-specific immunity

Most infections of the mammary gland of the dairy cow enter through the teat canal so the teat provides a very important barrier to infection, particularly since its exterior surface is frequently exposed to a most contaminated environment. The defences of the mammary gland may be considered under several headings.

The teat canal as a mechanical barrier

The length of the teat canal has no effect on the susceptibility of cows to mastitis but it has been reported in the literature that teat ducts from quarters susceptible to infection had a larger diameter than those from resistant quarters. Differences in teat duct patency might be expected to correlate positively with ease of milking but a relationship between milking characteristics and the incidence of intramammary infection is not universally accepted. Teat ducts with a temporary patency, such that a continuous unbroken column of milk is maintained for some time after milking, may offer a means of entry for micro-organisms and a way in which they may be transported upwards through the duct. In capillary columns of milk at 37°C, micro-organisms are capable of rising rapidly in association with ascending milk fat globules. Any mechanism, therefore, that is likely to break the fat-rich milk column and prevent an upward passage of bacteria is likely to increase the mammary gland defences. Various suggestions have been made on how the teat duct closes, e.g. it may close in a spiral fashion 'wringing out' the last drops of milk, but as the streak canal has ridges arranged longitudinally a spiral wringing would not be effective. Teat canal keratin is a white wax-like material derived from the surface cells of the stratified squamous epithelium and which forms a network in the lumen of the canal, thereby trapping invading bacteria and disrupting the milk column. Another simple mechanical method of preventing organisms from penetrating the teat canal is the flushing action during milking. Organisms not adhering to the teat canal wall or the keratin mesh at the beginning of milking are soon flushed out. The higher infection rate of quarters at drying off has been attributed to the cessation of milking and the consequent failure to flush out pathogens. Later in the dry period, there is an increase in the antimicrobial properties of the canal, which may restrict bacterial multiplication.

Antimicrobial substances within the teat canal

Antimicrobial substances in the teat canal may contribute to the defence of the mammary gland. The antimicrobial role of esterified and non-esterified fatty acids, particularly myristic acid, palmitoleic acid and linoleic acid has been described. These fatty acids are present in the teat canal keratin and it was suggested that the unsaturated fatty acids were the most inhibitory.

Some proteins isolated from the teat canal also play an important role in the defence of the mammary gland. At physiological pH they carry a positive charge and bind electrostatically to the mastitis pathogens which, at the same pH, carry a negative charge. The inhibiting effect of the various concentrations of these proteins has been demonstrated *in vitro* on the growth of staphylococci and streptococci. This antimicrobial activity of these proteins was not seen when micro-organisms were incubated with whole keratin under *in vitro* conditions. The cationic protein under these conditions would have already bound to other negatively charged molecules in the keratin. In the living animal continuous synthesis of these cationic proteins would overcome such binding. Despite the antimicrobial environment within the teat canal, local colonization by Gram-positive cocci has been reported, but the growth is very feeble with a low percentage viability.

Antimicrobial substances in mammary secretions

Non-specific antimicrobial substances in mammary secretions also contribute to the defences of the mammary gland. Lactoferrin is an iron-chelating protein which, in the presence of bicarbonate, inhibits the growth of micro-organisms having a high iron requirement. The activity of this protein is inhibited by the presence of citrate. Lactoferrin is thought to exert its most protective effects in the mammary secretions during the dry period when its levels are high compared with those in full lactation. These higher concentrations of lactoferrin may also influence the defences of the dry gland through the modulation of leucocyte functions.

Another antibacterial system present in milk involves the enzyme lactoperoxidase. This enzyme, in the presence of thiocyanate and hydrogen peroxide, can produce a short-lived highly oxidative system that is bacteriostatic for Gram-positive and bacteriocidal for Gram-negative organisms. Thiocyanate is present in milk, particularly in animals fed on diets containing legumes or brassicas. Doubt has been expressed in the past over the source of hydrogen peroxide (H_2O_2). Phagocytosing neutrophils are likely to be one source of H_2O_2 and some can be produced by the metabolism of catalase-negative organisms such as streptococci. Another enzyme present in milk, xanthine oxidase, may also contribute by generating H_2O_2. Recent research has demonstrated that xanthine oxidase is present in the teat duct and secretory tissue of the bovine mammary gland. The action of xanthine oxidase on its substrate leads to a release of hydrogen peroxide, which is then available to the lactoperoxidase system.

In addition to the above, antimicrobial systems that operate locally within the teat canal are likely also to be operative in the milk itself and in deeper parts of the mammary gland. The role of lysozyme in bovine body fluids, including milk, is equivocal. Some authors doubt its existence and, if present, the concentration would be extremely low, but possibly increasing in mastitis. As yet no defensive role has been ascribed to lysozyme in bovine tissues.

Antimicrobial cationic proteins, as found in the teat canal, may also be present in milk during mild inflammation. These proteins possess similar properties to the cationic proteins in the milk cells and are thought to have left the cells by a process of reverse pinocytosis.

Earlier methods used by many workers attempting to demonstrate haemolytic complement were too insensitive, but more recently a sensitive microassay revealed that low levels of haemolytic complement are present in milk throughout lactation, albeit usually masked by the anticomplement activity of the milk. Complement levels are highest in colostrum, in inflamed glands and in late lactation. A high correlation between the levels of serum albumin and the third component of complement during an inflammatory response suggests that complement components are passively transferred into the milk but this relationship is not seen in normal milk. Although the defensive role of the classical complement pathway remains in doubt it has been established that complement-sensitive organisms, such as some strains of *Escherichia coli*, are killed by the alternative complement pathway. *In vitro* tests, however, do not support this since serum-sensitive strains of *E. coli* can be grown in milk drawn from the udder. It is possible, however, that *in vivo* a very mild inflammatory response is needed to elevate slightly the serum-derived complement in milk.

Specific immunity: lymphocytes (see Chapter 29)

Lymphocytes are present in cows' milk at all stages of lactation and constitute 1–2 per cent of the milk cell population, which is low compared with that of human milk. Lymphocytes consist of T and B cells together with a population of lymphoid cells, which do not consistently carry markers of either T or B cells, the so-called null cells. The ratio of these cells (T:B:null) is similar to that in peripheral blood, but the percentage of B cells is slightly increased in dry gland secretions. Lymphocytes in mammary secretions are functionally competent, responding to mitogens and antigens. However, some responses of the T cells from mammary secretions to mitogens are lower than those of T cells from the systemic circulation. The precise reason for this difference in responsiveness is not clear, although it is known that mammary secretions contain soluble immunosuppressive factors that may be responsible. In addition, the T cell population in the mammary secretion may contain a greater proportion of suppressor cells which would inhibit responses.

Differences in the functional activity of T lymphocytes in blood and those in mammary secretions are evident as differing responses to specific antigens. Much of this work has been carried out using human mammary secretions and supports the view that lymphocytes in the mammary secretion form a distinct subpopulation. They belong to a mucosal immune system in which lymphocytes migrate from secretory surfaces of the body, e.g. the gut, to the mammary gland, but this is not the case in ruminants.

A similar migration occurs with B cells, but in the cow it has been suggested that following intestinal immunization there is a migration of antigen-stimulated IgG lymphoblasts and perhaps of antigen to the spleen and peripheral lymph nodes. This would be consistent with the appearance of serum-derived IgG antibodies in the colostrum and milk. When antigen is infused directly into the udder all classes of antibody, but particularly IgA and IgG$_1$, are produced locally from antibody-forming cells in the glandular stroma and in the regional supramammary lymph nodes.

Tissues in the terminal inner portion of the teat contain a high proportion of plasma cells, lymphocytes and macrophages, which may be involved in local immunity, and antibody-containing cells have been demonstrated in germinal centres in the distal Furstenberg's rosettes of the teat cistern (Fig. 22.7). Of the plasma cells in this region 88 per cent synthesize IgG$_1$, 10 per cent IgM while only a few synthesize IgA. The distribution of these cells does not change in relation to the mammary secretory activity.

Although the homing of lymphocytes to the mammary gland appears to be well established in some species, not all migrate into the secretions; in the rat mammary gland some remain in the alveolar and ductal epithelium. These intraepithelial lymphocytes are likely to be the predominating cell types infiltrating bovine mammary tissues and remain in association with the epithelia after a *Staphylococcus aureus* infection. Information from other species may reveal the precise identity and function of these cells. In humans a substantial proportion are T cells. Intraepithelial lymphocytes may form an important defence against infection at mucosal surfaces. Currently, there is a paucity of information on the role or even existence of natural killer (NK) and killer (K) cells in the bovine mammary gland; nevertheless, there is some evidence to suggest that lymphocyte activity in bovine mammary tissues may differ from that of other species.

Immunoglobulins in mammary secretions (see p. 380)

Milk contains most immunoglobulin classes in differing amounts that vary during lactation. IgG$_1$ is present in

Table 22.1 Immunoglobulin (mg/100 ml) to the blood and mammary secretions of the cow (from Lascelles, 1979).

	IgG$_1$	IgG$_2$	IgA	IgM
Blood serum	1400	1300	39	380
Colostral whey	1000–9000	250	470	540
Milk whey	40	6	11	9

the largest concentrations and it passes from the blood to the milk by a process of selective transfer. During inflammation of the udder, IgG$_2$ and other proteins are transferred from the blood. Some immunoglobulins such as IgM and IgA are locally produced and they arise from cells of the lymphoblast-plasma cell series that are located close to glandular epithelium in various parts of the mammary gland. The distribution of immunoglobulin classes in blood, colostrum and milk is shown in Table 22.1.

It will be noted from Table 22.1 that colostrum has a markedly higher concentration of IgG$_1$ than serum. This concentration is associated with the presence of specific receptor sites for this immunoglobulin on the membranes of bovine mammary epithelial cells. There are suggestions in the literature that the levels of IgA in milk and colostrum have probably been underestimated because much of the IgA is associated with milk fat globule membranes, and some IgM may also be globule bound. The precise origin of IgG$_2$ and IgA in the mammary gland of the cow remains in doubt. A local synthesis of IgG$_2$ has been reported in the cow but this was not confirmed in the ewe. There appears to be less disagreement concerning the origin of IgM and IgA, which are thought to be largely derived from local synthesis in the mammary gland of the cow, but in the ewe the synthesis of these immunoglobulins appears to be confined to the period of mammary involution whereas in early and mid-lactation large amounts are transferred from the blood.

Inflammation of the mammary gland leads to a rapid increase in levels of immunoglobulin and other serum proteins, including complement, within the first few hours. In this situation IgM and IgG$_1$, together with serum-derived complement, control the growth of serum-sensitive coliform organisms. Phagocytosis by neutrophils is more efficient if they are coated with specific IgG$_2$ antibodies.

The precise role of IgA in the mammary gland of the cow remains in doubt. Some workers believe that it may block IgG- or IgM-mediated complement fixation, in which case it would have detrimental effects on the protection of the mammary gland in early infection. On the other hand, it may activate complement, but this may not be of great importance due to the low levels of com-

plement in milk. There have been some reports that IgA antibodies assist the binding of bacteria to fat-globule membranes. This would hinder the mammary defence system by making the bacteria more difficult to phagocytose.

Phagocytic cell mobilization in the mammary gland and phagocytosis

The most effective system of udder defence against invading pathogens is the phagocytic activity of neutrophils. Normally, these cells are present in milk in very low numbers, the predominating leucocytes in the milk of healthy cows being macrophages and lymphocytes. Neutrophil numbers, however, rapidly increase in the very earliest stages of infection. The value of neutrophils in early infection was seen when unrestricted growth of bacteria occurred in the mammary gland of cows rendered neutropenic by the administration of anti-bovine leucocyte serum.

Neutrophil recruitment within the mammary gland is likely to be triggered by the presence of bacteria and bacterial products, which stimulate the formation of endogenous inflammatory mediators. These mediators lead to a margination of neutrophils in capillary vessels, cause a relaxation of endothelial cell junctions and allow a diapedesis of the neutrophils into the surrounding subepithelial connective tissues. The neutrophils in turn may release other inflammatory agents, further accelerating the process of neutrophil mobilization. The identity of the inflammatory mediators, which has been studied by a number of workers, includes prostaglandins produced by the cyclo-oxygenase pathway, and leukotrienes produced by lipo-oxygenation and interleukins. Prostaglandins have been measured in bovine milk and shown to increase in concentration from 4 hours after the administration of intramammary endotoxin. Prostaglandins are synthesized in bovine mammary tissue and may also be generated by neutrophils.

Pathogens entering the mammary gland and causing mastitis are rarely invasive. Therefore, if an antimicrobial environment is to be produced in the mammary gland neutrophils must be present in the teat and lactiferous sinus regions, the ducts and in the alveolar lumen. Milk collects in the teat and lactiferous sinus regions and it is thought that neutrophils are attracted as far as the luminal surface of the two-cell-thick epithelium by a concentration gradient of chemotactic factors originating from the lumen of the gland. Under these conditions, the neutrophils pass through the basement membrane and between the epithelial cells (Fig. 22.5). In severe staphylococcal infections the surface cells suffer toxic damage and in some cases this leads to large areas of epithelial erosion. Infections with *E. coli* frequently lead to more localized toxin-induced epithelial lesions and it is from these regions that the neutrophils migrate into the lumen.

A rapid neutrophil migration is essential for the efficient defence of the mammary gland following *E. coli* invasion, but particularly if the response occurs before the bacterial count in the milk exceeds 10^4/ml. Some cows, however, particularly if recently calved, fail to recruit neutrophils into their milk, and this leads to an unrestricted bacterial growth and severe damage within the mammary gland tissues. This situation may not be observed clinically since there may be a complete lack of inflammatory reaction. Nevertheless, these animals soon become severely ill and death may follow. Frequently, cows respond with a neutrophil recruitment but there is often a delay such that bacterial numbers may increase to a high level. Bacteria and neutrophils may then coexist in the mammary gland resulting in a protracted mastitis.

A rapid neutrophil response is also beneficial for controlling the growth of *Staphylococcus aureus* in mammary tissues, thereby preventing severe disease. A complete elimination of these organisms, however, rarely occurs and frequently a chronic subclinical disease remains in which small numbers of organisms are present in the milk, which has a permanently elevated cell count. These chronic infections may not be immediately obvious to the herdsman due to the very low grade inflammatory response in the tissues.

In any consideration of the immunology of the bovine mammary gland, availability of opsonins to permit the efficient phagocytosis of invading pathogens must be considered. The effector mechanisms of the phagocytes in the mammary gland may be activated by the Fc region of one or more classes of immune globulin and/or by fragments of the complement system bound to particles. Phagocytic cells have receptors for opsonins, where the opsonin is recognized and binds. This is linked with an effector unit that triggers the cell function. Different species of animals have different specificities for their receptors for different classes of immune globulin. Non-ruminant neutrophils have not been shown to bind to cytophilic antibody but cytophilic IgG_2 is active for ovine neutrophils and increases the bacteriocidal activity against *Staphylococcus aureus*. IgG_2 from immune bovine serum or milk whey will opsonize *E. coli*. Furthermore, the major opsonin for neutrophil phagocytosis of mammary gland pathogens using decomplemented non-immune bovine serum is IgM.

References

Collins, R.A., Parsons, K.R. & Bland, A.P. (1986) Antibody containing cells and specialised epithelial cells in the bovine teat. *Research in Veterinary Science*, **41**, 50–5.

Lascelles, A.K. (1979) The immune system of the ruminant mammary gland and its role in the control of mastitis. *Journal of Dairy Science*, **62**, 156–60.

Linzell, J.L. (1961) Recent advances in the physiology of the udder. In *Veterinary Annual* (ed. W.A. Pool). John Wright and Sons, Bristol, 44–53.

Turner, C.W. (1952) The Mammary Gland. In *The Anatomy of the Udder of Cattle and Domestic Animals*. Lucas Brothers Publishers, Columbia, 176–83, 203–7.

Further reading

Butler, J.E. (1974) Immunoglobulins of the mammary secretions. In *Lactation: a Comprehensive Treatise*, Vol. III (ed. by B.L. Larson & V.R. Smith), p. 217. Academic Press, New York.

Cowie, A.T. (1977) Anatomy and physiology of the udder. In *Milking Machine* (ed. by C.C. Thiel & F.H. Dodd), pp. 156–78. National Institute for Research in Dairying, Reading.

Craven, N. & Williams, M.R. (1985) Defences of the bovine mammary gland against infection and prospects for their enhancement. *Veterinary Immunology and Immunopathology*, **10**, 71–127.

Hibbitt, K.G., Cole, C.B. & Reiter, B. (1969) Antimicrobial proteins isolated from the teat canal of the cow. *Journal of General Microbiology*, **56**, 365–71.

Larson, B.L. (ed.) (1985) *Lactation*. Iowa State University Press, Ames, Iowa.

Mepham, T.B. (ed.) (1983) *Biochemistry of Lactation*. Elsevier, Amsterdam, New York.

Peel, C.J. & Bauman, D.E. (1987) Somatotropin and lactation. *Journal of Dairy Science*, **70**, 474–86.

Poutrel, B. (1982) Susceptibility to mastitis: a review of factors related to the cow. *Annales de Recherches Veterinaires*, **13**, 85–99.

Weber, A.F., Kitchell, R.L. & Sautter, J.H. (1955) Mammary gland studies. 1. The identity and characterisation of the smallest lobule unit in the udder of the dairy cow. *American Journal of Veterinary Science*, **16**, 255–63.

Chapter 23
Mastitis

P.W. Edmondson and A.J. Bramley

Introduction   326
Dynamics of herd infection   326
Effects of lactation age and stage   327
Teat canal   327
Transmission, sources and control of udder pathogens   328
Diagnosis of clinical mastitis   328
Diagnosis of subclinical mastitis   329
   Cytological examination   329
   Bacteriological examination   329
   Biochemical and other tests   330
Use of individual cow or quarter sampling in herd
    investigations   330
Cattle housing and mastitis   331
Machine milking and mastitis   331
   Milking hygiene   332
Aetiology of mastitis   332
   Staphylococcus aureus   332
   Streptococcus agalactiae   333
   Streptococcus dysgalactiae   333
   Streptococcus uberis and other aesculin-hydrolysing
    streptococci   333
   Coliforms   334
Arcanobacterium (Actinomyces, Corynebacterium)
    pyogenes   334
   Mycoplasmas   334
   Leptospira infection   335
   Coagulase-negative staphylococci and
    Corynebacterium bovis   335
Recommendations for control of mastitis   335

Introduction

Mastitis is the most prevalent infectious disease of adult dairy cattle. Several species of bacteria, fungi, mycoplasmas and algae have been isolated from the natural disease or have been shown to reproduce it experimentally. The predominant species are listed in Table 23.1. Furthermore, many clinical cases of mastitis that are due to infection are negative on bacteriological culture of the mammary gland secretion (Dairy Federation 1987a).

The inflammation, characteristic of mastitis, may be undetectable without the use of diagnostic tests applied to the milk or secretion. This is termed subclinical mastitis. Subclinical mastitis results in raised somatic cell counts in affected animals. This can result in a raised somatic herd cell count. It is essential to maintain a low cell count in order to comply with statutory milk quality requirements, e.g. the EU requires all milk to be under 400000 cells/ml, and to ensure that there is no penalty to milk price. In the UK, many farmers with cell counts over 150000/ml are penalized.

The subclinical stage may be prolonged or proceed rapidly to clinical mastitis in which external signs of disease such as swelling and hardness of the affected gland(s) or clots or discoloration of the secretion are present. Nevertheless, the subclinically infected quarter has a lowered milk yield, altered milk composition and excretes the infecting organism. Subclinical mastitis is a major element in the worldwide economic loss associated with mastitis, which exceeds £$^1/_2$ billion annually.

Dynamics of herd infection

Figure 23.1 illustrates the dynamics of udder disease within the herd. The mammary glands can be placed in one of three categories: uninfected, subclinically infected or clinically infected. The relative proportions of animals in these categories vary between herds. Pathogen type also influences the dynamics. For example, coliform infections tend to become rapidly clinical while *Staphylococcus aureus* infections often persist as subclinical infections for weeks or months. Clinical mastitis will usually be treated with antibiotic therapy and the clinical cure rates are variable and will depend on the pathogen. Bacteriological cure rates vary from 90 per cent for most coliform infections to as low as 25 per cent with *Staphylococcus aureus* in older cows.

The mammary gland has a range of defence mechanisms of which phagocytosis of invading organisms by polymorphonuclear leucocytes is probably the most important. Spontaneous elimination of infection by these mechanisms will occur. The rates of spontaneous elimination are low for staphylococcal infections (<20 per cent), high for *Escherichia coli* (>70 per cent) and intermediate for streptococcal infections.

Table 23.1 Species of micro-organism frequently isolated from clinical bovine mastitis.

Staphylococcus aureus	Escherichia coli
Streptococcus agalactiae	Klebsiella pneumoniae
Streptococcus dysgalactiae	Enterobacter sp.
Streptococcus uberis	Proteus sp.
Arcanobacterium	Pseudomonas aeruginosa
(Actinomyces;	Citrobacter sp.
Corynebacterium)	
pyogenes	
Bacillus cereus	
Mycoplasma bovis	Prototheca
Mycoplasma californicum	Aspergillus sp.
Mycoplasma canadense	Fungi

Table 23.2 Distribution of clinical coliform mastitis cases with stage of lactation when first found.

Lactation stage when found (weeks)	Number of coliform cases	Percentage
0–1[a]	86	20.8
2–5[b]	94	22.9
6–10	48	11.6
11–20	58	14.1
21–30	51	12.4
31–40	33	8.0
>40	41	10.0

[a] Uninfected at drying-off.
[b] Uninfected at calving.

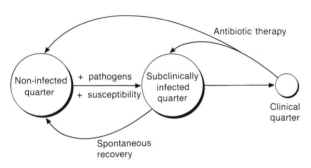

Fig. 23.1 Pattern of intramammary infection and clinical mastitis in a dairy herd.

Effects of lactation age and stage

Udder infection may develop when the cow is lactating or dry. Infection rates are highest in the early dry period although these infections may not persist or develop into clinical mastitis until the next lactation. Clinical mastitis is most common at calving and in the first three months of lactation. The incidence of clinical disease and new infection may increase with lactation number. An example for coliform mastitis incidence by stage of lactation is shown in Table 23.2.

The precise reasons for these effects of age and stage are not known. The high incidence of mastitis around calving is largely a consequence of high new infection rate in the dry period and a periparturient suppression of host defences. Increasing disease with age is probably not due to increased intramammary susceptibility but to increasing ease of penetration of the teat duct by pathogens and accumulated previous infections.

Teat canal

The teat canal is the primary defence mechanism between the semisterile udder and the outside environment. The bovine teat canal varies in length from 4 to 18 mm, with a median of 12 mm. It has a heavily keratinized surface and the keratin lining is crucial to the maintenance of its barrier function (Plate 23.1). Keratin traps bacteria as they try to penetrate the teat canal. Excess keratin is removed by shear forces during the milking process and this is a normal event. If there are poor shear forces, excess keratin and bacteria are not removed and may grow up and invade the udder. The barrier function has both physical and chemical elements. Antibacterial lipids and basic proteins have been identified within the keratin lining of the teat duct (Williams & Mein, 1985).

The diameter of the canal and the depth of the keratin layer have been shown to be positively and negatively correlated with infection respectively. Certain defects in machine milking operation can adversely affect the defensive properties of the teat duct, increasing mastitis incidence (see section on machine milking, p. 331 and Chapter 26). Any damage to the teat end or teat canal is likely to increase the likelihood of new infections. This will occur due to a weakened physical barrier and also the increased bacterial colonization on the damaged teat canal.

Colonization or infection of the streak canal, particularly adjacent to the teat orifice, is common with pathogens such as Staph. aureus or Streptococcus dysgalactiae. Such colonizations may persist for long periods in the absence of intramammary infection but are largely prevented or eliminated by postmilking teat disinfection. Other organisms are often present within the teat duct including Corynebacterium bovis and coagulase-negative staphylococci and there are reports of the isolation of anaerobes. The environmental organisms, such as coliforms and Strep. uberis rarely colonize the teat duct and this difference is important in the pathogenesis of infection.

Transmission, sources and control of udder pathogens

Broadly, the micro-organisms causing bovine mastitis can be partly classified into two groups: contagious and environmental.

Contagious mastitis: The udder and teats are the reservoir of infection. Transmission occurs *during* the milking process or udder preparation by contaminated hands, udder cloths and liners. Infection establishes on the surface of the teat and teat canal. Bacteria may then penetrate the mammary gland. Most infections are subclinical and result in raised cell counts. Control measures include postmilking teat disinfection, dry cow therapy and culling. Contagious bacteria include *Staphylococcus aureus*, coagulase negative *Staphs*, *Streptococcus agalactiae* and *Strep. dysgalactiae*. If a herd somatic cell count is over 200 000/ml then this indicates that there is a problem with contagious mastitis. Careful application of control measures based upon teat disinfection and dry-cow antibiotic therapy will eradicate *Strep. agalactiae* over the course of one to two years provided infected animals are not introduced into the herd. *Strep. agalactiae* can also be eliminated through the use of 'blitz' intramammary treatment during lactation and these bacteria are very sensitive to any of the penicillin antibiotics. Levels of *Staph. aureus* and *Strep. dysgalactiae* will also fall to low levels. In some herds, poor elimination rates of staphylococcal infection by therapy will require the heavy culling of chronically infected animals to achieve rapid progress.

Environmental mastitis: The environment is a reservoir of infection. Infections are transmitted onto teats *between* milkings or during udder preparation. Organisms are forced up through the teat canal during the milking process or after milking if cows are allowed to lie down immediately following milking. Most infections cause clinical mastitis. Sub-clinical infections are less common with *E coli*, but frequently occur with *Strep uberis*. Environmental mastitis is controlled by provision of a clean environment, adequate accommodation for cows, milking through correctly functioning machine, good udder preparation and pre-milking teat disinfection. Environmental organisms include *E coli*, *Streptococcus uberis* (straw bedding), *Klebsiella* spp. (sawdust and shavings) and *Bacillus* spp. Although there is potential for interquarter transfer at milking time it appears not to be the predominant infection mechanism. Postmilking teat disinfection does not prevent infection. Antibiotic therapy has some beneficial effects on coliform mastitis prevention but does reduce the rate of new dry-period infection with *Strep. uberis*.

Environmental mastitis is controlled through good environmental management, a good milking routine, an efficient milking machine, vaccination against coliform mastitis and premilking teat disinfection.

Diagnosis of clinical mastitis

The detection of clinical mastitis depends upon the examination of the mammary gland and its secretion. The affected gland may show swelling, heat, pain and/or hardness. The secretion may be clotted, serous or, occasionally, bloodstained (Plate 23.2a,b). In acute cases systemic signs of disease may also be present including pyrexia, anorexia and occasionally recumbency in toxic *E. coli* and *Staph. aureus* infections. Examples are shown of the clinical changes in Plate 23.2 (c,d).

Clinical disease is most commonly seen in lactating animals, particularly in early lactation, but may develop in the non-lactating gland also. Because the dry animal is rarely closely scrutinized some of these cases remain undetected until calving. 'Summer mastitis' is an acute disease of the non-lactating mammary gland and may affect cows, heifers or young calves. Characteristically, it is caused by mixed infection with *Arcanobacterium pyogenes* and anaerobic bacteria, commonly *Peptococcus indolicus*.

It is important (and in many countries statutory) that dairy cows are examined before each milking for signs of clinical mastitis. This allows abnormal milk to be discarded and the affected animal to be given therapy as rapidly as possible, thereby reducing tissue damage and giving higher cure rates, and minimizing the risks of infection transfer. Discarding mastitic milk also helps to protect the herd somatic cell count and bactoscan or TBC. An alternative to examination of the foremilk for abnormalities during preparation for milking is to use in-line filters, installed in the long milk tube to screen the total milk produced. Disadvantages of this approach are that (i) not all cases of clinical mastitis result in the formation of clots that are trapped in the filters; (ii) the affected quarter(s) have to be identified by an additional examination of the strippings milk; (iii) the abnormal milk may have passed to the bulk supply prior to detection, particularly in direct-to-pipeline milking systems and (iv) many milkers fail to check the filters. Palpation of the udder after milking also aids clinical mastitis detection but the increase in cows milked per person hour and the provision of automatic cluster removers have precluded this process in many parlour operations. Some milking equipment contains sensors to aid the detection of abnormal milk and this is likely to become more common.

Diagnosis of subclinical mastitis

A range of tests can be applied to milk to detect subclinical mastitis (Schultze, 1985). These tests generally measure the somatic cell count or detect the presence of infecting organisms. These changes are both cytological and biochemical. Most tests are laboratory based although the California Mastitis Test (CMT) and electrical conductivity measurements can be used at the cow side. Tests can be placed in three categories and applied either alone or in combination.

Cytological examination (see p. 323; Chapter 25)

Milk from a healthy, uninfected bovine mammary gland contains somatic cells comprising macrophages, neutrophils and lymphocytes. The number of these is usually <50000 cells/ml milk. When mastitis is present the cell count increases, primarily as a consequence of neutrophil infiltration. Subclinically infected quarters have cell counts in excess of 20000 cells/ml but, because of the dynamic nature of the disease, this value can vary considerably and will sometimes fall below this threshold (Table 23.3).

During clinical episodes the cell count will be elevated, counts in excess of 5000000 cells/ml being commonplace. The cell count is detectable by a microscopic count or by electronic means. Detailed descriptions of the methods employed are available (Dairy Federation, 1984). An indirect estimate of cell counts can be made

Table 23.3 Variation in the cell count of a quarter infected with *Staph. aureus* compared to an uninfected quarter in a Friesian heifer.

Milking No.	Somatic cell count C × 1000 cells/ml	
	Control quarter	Infected quarter
1	13	424
2	80	3943
3	64	528
4	84	4046
5	44	797
6	91	4540
7	107	1471
8	61	1446
9	64	528
10	84	4046

using a variety of tests such as the CMT or Whiteside test. These tests are based upon a gelling reaction between the nucleic acid of the cells and a reagent, either a detergent (CMT) or sodium hydroxide (Whiteside). The reactions are categorized from 0 to 4. Reactions of 3 and 4 have a high probability of infection being present. The advantage of the count is that the results are available immediately, are repeatable, cheap and give an individual quarter result. Many countries employ cell counting of herd bulk milk as an estimate of herd mastitis levels. Individual cow milk cell count services are available in many countries as an intermittent or regular service (e.g. National Milk Records in England and Wales and the Dairy Herd Improvement Association in the USA). A consistently high bulk milk cell count is characteristic of a high level of subclinical infection in the herd. Herds with counts <200000 cells/ml generally have little economic loss associated with subclinical disease. Such herds may however still suffer significant costs due to a high incidence of clinical mastitis, associated with short-duration infections such as coliforms.

Bacteriological examination

The secretion from a normal mammary gland is sterile although it may acquire bacteria from a colonized teat duct during collection. Therefore, the detection of a pathogen in an aseptically collected milk sample is indicative of infection. The number of organisms excreted per millilitre of milk from an infected gland fluctuates widely; hence the recovery of even low numbers of bacteria can be regarded as meaningful if the sample has been taken with adequate care and is not contaminated. Bacteriological examinations have the advantage of being positive or negative, whereas most other tests require the imposition of a threshold value which varies between animals and herds (Dairy Federation, 1987a).

A suitable sample is required for bacteriological examination obtained by an aseptic technique. Samples can be frozen (−20°C) prior to examination although this reduces pathogen numbers (particularly Gram-negatives) and precludes cytological and some biochemical examinations. The bacteria most commonly causing bovine mastitis will grow aerobically on blood agar. The more unusual causes of mastitis such as anaerobes, *Mycoplasma* spp. and *Leptospira* spp. require more specialized techniques not appropriate to the practice laboratory. The inclusion of 0.1 per cent aesculin in the blood agar is useful in the differentiation of *Strep. uberis* from other streptococci. A volume of milk is spread over the surface of the agar plate, which should be incubated for 24–48 hours at 37°C. An advantage of a bacteriological examination is that the causative organism can be identified and provides a possibility for antimicrobial sensitivity testing. Some organisms such as *Staph. aureus* may be shed intermittently and in small numbers in milk. With these infections, a negative result may indicate that the bacteria have not been isolated due to a dilution effect. Repeat sampling may be necessary in order to confirm a negative result. Disadvantages include cost, complexity and time delay. Detailed methods for the collection and bacteriological examination of milk samples for infection are available (Dairy Federation, 1981).

Biochemical and other tests

Inflammation of the mammary gland leads to a variety of compositional changes in milk either because of local effects or because of an increase of serum components entering the milk. Some of these changes can be used to screen for subclinical mastitis.

Significant changes in ionic composition occur with both Na$^+$ and Cl$^-$ levels increasing, K$^+$ decreasing. The individual ions can be directly determined but more commonly the net change in ionic composition is used, measured as an increase in electrical conductivity. Both laboratory and farm-based meters exist and milking equipment incorporating electrodes to measure milk conductivity during milking is marketed in some countries. There are a variety of other factors which may affect electrical conductivity such as oestrus. The majority of electrical conductivity meters work on pooled milk from all quarters and are unlikely to be very accurate due to a dilution effect. However, as for the majority of the milk parameters, the conductivity values of normal and infected quarters overlap and conductivity values vary between herds. These facts make the application of threshold values for diagnosis inaccurate. A fall in lactose concentration is also usual and has been employed diagnostically but has poor discrimination.

Enzymatic changes also occur. Some of the enzyme changes are associated with the increase in cell count (e.g. catalase), others with secretory cell damage (e.g. part of *N*-acetylglucosaminidase (NAG) increase) or with increased permeability (plasmin). The use of NAG has been widely tested and found to correlate well with cell count and infection and offers promise as a cow-side test.

As serum components leak into the mastitic gland they can be employed as indicators of inflammation. The most studied have been antitrypsin and bovine serum albumin (BSA). Automated methods for the detection of antitrypsin have been developed and the test is more sensitive than BSA. Table 23.4 summarizes the major compositional changes in milk due to udder infection and inflammation. For more detail of these

Table 23.4 Changes in milk composition associated with mastitis (examples of 'typical values').

	Somatic cells (1000)	
	Normal <20 to 75	Mastitic 100 to >10000
Sodium (mg/100 ml)	57	104
Chloride (mg/100 ml)	100	200
Potassium (mg/100 ml)	170	150
Conductivity (mM NaCl)	<50	>56
Lactose (mg/ml)	48	44
Catalase		increased 20-fold
NAG		increased 6-fold
BSA (mg/ml)	0.25	>0.6

NAG, *N*-acetyl glucosaminidase; BSA, bovine serum albumin.

tests and their application the reader is referred to Schultze (1985).

Use of individual cow or quarter sampling in herd investigations

Mastitis control relies upon the application of effective control measures to the herd rather than identification or special treatment of individual animals. It is essential to identify the organisms responsible for the problem and in high cell count herds, the proportion of cows infected. This requires bacteriology and individual cow cell count data which will help to identify the nature of a herd problem or individual animals for segregation or culling. As payment of milk on the basis of cell count becomes more common then the emphasis placed on these systems tends to increase.

If the aetiology of clinical mastitis is to be determined then a microbiological analysis is needed. Such analyses provide information on the patterns of the disease within a herd since there will be delay between sampling and diagnosis during which therapy will usually have begun. Often a broad-spectrum antibiotic is employed to cover the range of possibilities. However, the pattern of disease may be helpful in determining the attention needed to remedy the herd problem. The isolation of *Strep. agalactiae* indicates either that teat disinfection and dry-cow therapy are not being employed effectively or infected animals have been introduced. A pattern of high herd cell count, repeated clinical cases and the frequent isolation of *Staph. aureus* would be typical of poor elimination of infection by lactation or dry-period therapy. This might prompt the use of bacteriological analysis of samples taken after treatment or at drying-off and calving.

Individual cow cell count or other diagnostic tests can be used to identify chronically infected animals for culling, treatment during lactation and other options, although such animals might be identifiable via an examination of clinical records. In the majority of herds the records are unfortunately inadequate for such a purpose. When using individual cow cell counts or other indirect tests the variation in inflammation should be remembered. Confident diagnosis on a single sample is not possible. The changes in these measures due to lactation stage and yield are also relevant. Cell counts in colostrum and in dry-cow secretion are naturally elevated and diagnostically unreliable. As lactation declines and yield falls cell count and electrical conductivity increase slightly. Milk composition and cell count may remain permanently altered or elevated in glands that have suffered severe secretory tissue damage, even if the causative organism has been successfully eliminated (see Chapter 25).

Cattle housing and mastitis

In many countries climatic conditions require that cattle are housed for at least part of the year with consequences for mastitis. In some countries cows are housed all year round. Housing increases the risk of mastitis because the confinement of the animals and the multiplication of micro-organisms in various litters elevate teat challenge, and consequently mastitis. Prominent among these bacteria are the coliforms, *Strep. uberis* and faecal streptococci.

The relationship between housing and mastitis is most clearly established for coliform mastitis. Coliform bacteria have been shown to multiply readily in organic litters, particularly sawdust, reaching counts of >100 million/g. These numbers often exceed those found in bovine faeces and impose a risk of infection. Sawdust has been shown to act as a source of *Klebsiella pneumoniae*, particularly if not kiln-dried, and can lead to severe mastitis problems. Some outbreaks have been controlled by switching from sawdust to sand, which tends to harbour lower numbers of coliforms and reduces the risk of disease.

Streptococcus uberis colonizes the bovine gut and is excreted in faeces and consequently contaminates cattle litter. In straw, multiplication of the organism often occurs leading to high levels of teat challenge and increased infection rates (Bramley, 1982). Since *Strep. uberis* is particularly infectious for the non-lactating or parturient udder this can be a particular problem if dry-cow or calving accommodation is not adequately cleaned and bedded.

Since multiplication in the litter is a crucial factor in increasing challenge to the teat surface, regular removal

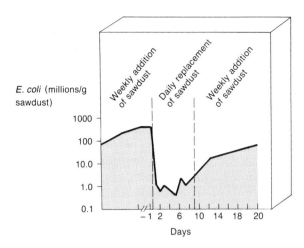

Fig. 23.2 Controlling coliform contamination of sawdust in cubicles by daily removal and replacement.

and replacement of bedding offers the soundest basis for reducing it (Fig. 23.2; Dodd *et al.*, 1984). Herds which house cattle in straw yards should clean these out every 4 to 6 weeks. In mild weather, this may need to be reduced to every 3 to 4 weeks.

The climate within cattle housing is also important since high humidity favours the survival and multiplication of micro-organisms. It has been found that cattle litter generally appearing to be clean and dry can harbour high numbers of micro-organisms and this can pose significant problems when giving advice over herd mastitis problems.

The design and size of yards and cubicles influence cow cleanliness and thus milk bacteriological quality and mastitis. Cubicles that are too short will leave cows' udders lying in the alleyway while those which are too long will lead to dunging on the cubicle surface itself. Obviously, the correct dimensions vary depending upon breed and age. There should be 5 to 10 per cent more cubicles than cows. In loose housing, a lying area of 6 m² for a Holstein cow should be allowed. Overcrowding in loose yards will lead to an increase in environmental infections, in particular *Strep. uberis*. Improper placement of access gates and water troughs in yards will lead to excessively dirty lying areas. Use of dung channels and grids can increase the incidence of damaged teats, etc.

These and other ways in which the environment influences mastitis are the subject of a review by the International Dairy Federation (Dairy Federation, 1987b). Detailed information on suitable dimensions and designs for cattle housing are also available (pp. 42–4).

Machine milking and mastitis

There is unequivocal evidence that the events occurring at milking time influence the incidence of mastitis.

These influences may be via the hygiene practised at milking time or because of effects of the milking machine *per se*. For details on how the milking machine can affect mastitis see Chapter 26.

Milking hygiene

The milk secreted by infected cows contains varying numbers of pathogenic micro-organisms. Herd milking provides opportunities for the transmission of these bacteria between udder quarters and cows via the milking machine itself, the milker's hands or cloths.

Various techniques can be employed at milking time to reduce transmission including:

(1) Using disinfected water for teat washing.
(2) Employing individual paper towels or cloths for teat drying.
(3) Wearing clean rubber gloves.
(4) Applying a suitable disinfectant to the teat surface after milking.
(5) Disinfecting or heat treating the cluster between milking cows.
(6) Premilking teat disinfection.

In addition, segregation of infected animals from the healthy herd can be used although it is impractical in most herds and requires the use of individual cow cell counts or a similar test. The use of measures such as those described above can reduce infection rates by about 50 per cent, effects being greatest against *Staph. aureus*, *Strep. agalactiae* and *Strep. dysgalactiae* (Fig. 23.3). The measures are less effective against coliforms and *Strep. uberis* infection because of their wider distribution in the environment.

Of the various measures to prevent new intramammary infections among milking cows, postmilking teat disinfection is the most valuable. Various disinfectants are used, most commonly iodophors, chlorhexidine and hypochlorite. Emollients are often added to promote good skin condition and rapid healing of lesions. These disinfectants will rapidly destroy bacteria reaching the teat surface during milking and will prevent colonization of the teat duct and the infection of teat lesions. The speed of kill of the postmilking teat disinfectant is not important provided that it is effective. This is contrary to the action of premilking disinfectants which must have a rapid speed of kill. This fast action is required to avoid slowing down the milking procedure.

The importance of premilking hygiene in the production of milk of high bacteriological quality should be emphasized. Data show that effective washing of the teat followed by drying significantly reduces the bacterial content of bulk milk. Washing without drying will result in bacteria being put in suspension. This solution will be sucked in with the milk and increase the bac-

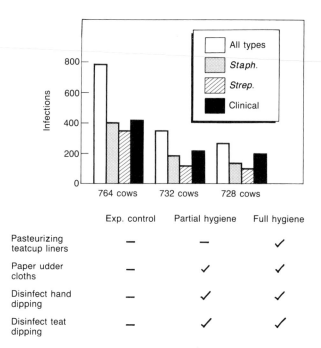

	Exp. control	Partial hygiene	Full hygiene
	764 cows	732 cows	728 cows
Pasteurizing teatcup liners	—	—	✓
Paper udder cloths	—	✓	✓
Disinfect hand dipping	—	✓	✓
Disinfect teat dipping	—	✓	✓

Fig. 23.3 Effect of milking time hygiene on new udder infections.

toscan or TBC. There will be an increased risk of liner slip and impact forces at the teat end. These factors will increase the risk of environmental infections. Ideally, a suitable concentration of an approved disinfectant (usually iodine or chlorine) should be included in the wash water supply. There have been examples of coliform and *Pseudomonas* mastitis problems associated with contaminated udder wash water supplies. These are unlikely where mains water is in use although uncovered water storage tanks may become contaminated with faeces or carcasses of small animals and provide a source of infection. For a review of this subject see Bramley & McKinnon (1990)

Aetiology of mastitis

It has already been stated that mastitis is a consequence of intramammary infection with one or more microorganisms of many different genera. The following section provides information on the most common or important of the different mammary infections.

Staphylococcus aureus (see p. 385)

In many countries this organism is the predominant cause of subclinical mastitis but is also isolated from clinical disease. The important sources of infection are infected udders, teat ducts or teat lesions. Extramammary sources do exist, notably the vagina and tonsils but do not appear important in the pathogenesis of infection. It has proved possible to eradicate *Staph. aureus* mastitis from individual herds by the application of hygiene at milking time and culling. The major limitation to more effective control of *Staph. aureus* mastitis remains its poor response to antibiotic therapy. Cure rates are highest in first and second lactation animals. In older cows cure rates during lactation may be as low as 25 per cent following intramammary antibiotic therapy. Even following the use of dry-cow therapy, cure rates of 33 per cent in older cows are common. There are a variety of reasons for this of which antibiotic resistance plays only a minor role. *In vitro* demonstration of sensitivity of *Staph. aureus* to an antibiotic is no guarantee of therapeutic success. The ability of the bacteria to survive inside polymorphonucleocytes (PMN), macrophages and epithelial cells, protected from antibiotic action, may significantly contribute to their therapy resistance. Additionally, the pathological changes, notably granulomata and fibrosis, induced in chronic *Staph. aureus* infections renders chronically infected cows essentially incurable. Most commonly *Staph. aureus* udder infection is chronic, acute mastitis being less common than with other bacteria. However, acute gangrenous *Staph. aureus* infections can arise in which uncontrolled growth of the organism occurs elaborating large quantities of α toxin. Such infections are probably not due to strains of increased virulence but rather to a failure by the host to mount an effective defence. Workers in California showed the critical role of the PMN in this defence since subclinically infected cows, made neutropenic, rapidly developed acute gangrenous *Staph. aureus* mastitis (Schalm *et al.*, 1976) (for therapy see p. 396)

Streptococcus agalactiae (see p. 387)

The sources of *Strep. agalactiae* are similar to those of *Staph. aureus*, namely the teats and udder. Consequently, milking time hygiene is an effective means of preventing infection during lactation. The presence of *Strep. agalactiae* in a herd suggests that there are defects in milking hygiene, postmilking teat disinfection and/or dry-cow therapy. Since *Strep. agalactiae* is easily eliminated by intramammary antibiotic therapy it is eliminated from herds employing teat disinfection and dry-cow therapy effectively and routinely. It is possible to include the elimination of infection by blitz therapy during lactation. Blitz therapy is where all quarters of infected cows are treated with intramammary antibiotics. The whole herd may be treated or selected animals. The level of infection relates well to individual cow cell counts. It is important to confirm that *Strep. agalactiae* is the cause of the high cell count before embarking on blitz therapy. The disease may exist as an acute clinical mastitis or persist as a subclinical infec-

tion. The duration of infection is shorter than staphylococci, primarily because of the better response to therapy. More rapid elimination of *Strep. agalactiae* can be achieved by diagnosis and treatment of infected animals although the economic basis for this is doubtful (for therapy see p. 396).

Streptococcus dysgalactiae (see p. 387)

This organism has both contagious and environmental characteristics often associated with poor teat skin condition. Very good control of lactation infections can be achieved by teat disinfection indicating that cow-to-cow transfer is an important mechanism. However, infection in the dry period and in heifers is commonplace, particularly among animals not protected by dry-cow therapy. Outbreaks of clinical mastitis with *Strep. dysgalactiae* frequently follow a breakdown in herd hygiene practices or increases in teat lesions. The incidence of teat lesions can increase rapidly following failures in pulsation, excessive milking vacuum or adverse housing or climatic conditions. In such outbreaks the machine should be given a thorough examination by an expert and the teats closely inspected for damage. The inclusion of a high level of a suitable emollient in the teat dip can promote rapid healing of lesions and prevent their colonization.

Clinical *Strep. dysgalactiae* mastitis can be acute with anorexia and pyrexia in addition to the local signs. However, the response to therapy is usually rapid and elimination rates with penicillins are similarly high to *Strep. agalactiae*. *Streptococcus dysgalactiae* is also encountered in mixed culture with other organisms, notably *A. pyogenes* and *P. indolicus* in summer mastitis. The bacteria can be isolated from bovine tonsils and the bovine genital tract and these sources, allied to the ability of the organism to infect and colonize lesions, may be important in the pathogenesis of dry-period infections.

Streptococcus uberis *and other aesculin-hydrolysing streptococci* (see p. 387)

These organisms are an important cause of bovine mastitis and, in some herds, are the major cause of clinical disease. Several species can be involved but the predominant one (>70 per cent) is *Strep. uberis*. Others include *Strep. bovis*, *Strep. faecalis* and *Strep. faecium*. Infection with these organisms is not controlled by postmilking teat disinfection although dry-cow antibiotic therapy reduces infection rates by about 50 per cent. However, *Strep. uberis* remains the commonest cause of infection in the dry period and susceptibility to infection has been shown to increase following drying-off (Marshall *et al.*, 1986). In untreated dry cows the highest rates of infection occur in the initial two weeks following drying-off while in animals given antibiotic therapy at drying-off infection tends to be periparturient. The high infection rates in the dry period and the failure of post milking teat disinfection to control disease emphasize the independence of milking and transmission. The bacteria are widely disseminated on the cow, are present in low numbers in cattle faeces and multiply in bedding materials, particularly straw, to reach high levels. Deep straw yards for housing dry cows seem to pose a particular risk factor. Not all strains are virulent for the lactating gland and a capsular layer is often elaborated conferring resistance to phagocytosis. Susceptibility of the lactating gland to infection may be influenced by the lactoperoxidase system, which in turn can be affected by feeding regimens altering milk thiocyanate levels. Although *Strep. uberis* is sensitive *in vitro* to a range of antibiotics, intramammary therapy often is ineffective and chronic infections are common in some herds. Under these circumstances cow-to-cow transmission may become more important (for therapy see p. 396)

Coliforms (see pp. 383, 1016)

The coliform species most commonly implicated in mastitis are *E. coli*, although other species including *Enterobacter aerogenes*, *Pseudomonas aeruginosa*, *Ent. oxytoca*, *K. pneumoniae* and *Citrobacter* spp. are also encountered. Infection is more common among housed cows and occurs particularly around calving. Subclinical infection is less common and peracute mastitis occurs frequently around calving. About 50 per cent of these peracute infections die. Treatment involves frequent stripping to remove endotoxin, antibiotic, supportive therapy including hypertonic saline and oxytocin, etc. The use of anti-inflammatory drugs, particularly non-steroidal anti-inflammatories, may also be helpful. Many new *E. coli* infections occur during the dry period but do not manifest as a clinical disease until into the next lactation. The incidence of coliform mastitis has increased despite the adoption of the National Institute for Research in Dairying (NIRD) five-point plan, improved milking machines and better hygiene. Transmission between cows is unimportant in pathogenesis and the use of postmilking teat disinfection and dry-cow therapy does not reduce infection rates. The primary source of infection is bovine faeces although secondary multiplication of the bacteria to high numbers in cattle litter is often a factor (see section on cattle housing and mastitis, p. 331).

Infection with coliform bacteria leads to a rapid development of inflammation and often the influx of neutrophils eliminates the infection (Hill *et al.*, 1979). In some animals, particularly in early lactation and in

high-yielding cows, this is not effective, possibly because the rate of neutrophil diapedesis is poor. Recent research indicates that low levels of selenium may be implicated in the process (Erskine *et al.*, 1989) (for therapy see p. 396)

Arcanobacterium (Actinomyces, Corynebacterium) pyogenes (see Chapter 24)

This bacterium is often involved in suppurative conditions in cattle, including mastitis. It is most frequently encountered as one of the mixture of pathogens responsible for 'summer mastitis' in northern Europe. This acute clinical disease of the non-lactating animal has been described in the section on diagnosis (see p. 328). *Arcanobacterium pyogenes* may also infect the lactating cow, or infection may be carried over from the dry period. Infection in the lactating cow is usually associated with teat damage.

The epidemiology of summer mastitis has been much studied because of its epidemic and destructive nature. The disease has been associated with fly-borne transmission and the sheep head fly *Hydrotaea irritans* has been shown able to carry *A. pyogenes*, *Strep. dysgalactiae* and the anaerobic peptococci responsible for the disease. With one exception transmission experiments with infected flies have proved unsuccessful but data do reveal that the use of insecticides or barriers (surgical tape, Stockholm tar, etc.) reduces the disease incidence. The most effective control measure is the prophylactic use of dry-cow therapy. A review of the epidemiology, transmission and pathogenesis has been published (Thomas *et al.*, 1987).

Mycoplasmas (see p. 385)

In recent years several species of *Mycoplasma* have been recognized as important causes of bovine mastitis. The most common cause is *Mycoplasma bovis* but other species implicated include *M. bovigenitalium*, *M. canadense*, *M. californicum* and *M. alkalescens*.

Characteristically, infection with *Mycoplasma* spp. leads to a mastitis, often involving multiple quarters, which is refractory to antibiotic treatment. The secretion may remain normal at the onset although a granular or flaky deposit is recognized on standing. In the later stages a purulent or thick secretion, without offensive smell is often reported. Swelling and firmness is common but after a few days the mammary gland may reduce in size. Milk secretion is severely reduced. Swelling of the supramammary lymph nodes occurs and there may be pyrexia, transient malaise and arthritis. Secretion of mycoplasmas in the milk frequently lasts for two months and often for longer. Intermittent shedding is common. Clearly, such cows constitute an infection risk for the herd. Most reports relate to infection in lactating cows but outbreaks among dry cows, notably with *M. californicum*, do occur (Jasper, 1982).

Diagnosis requires the application of specific microbiological and serological tests in specialist veterinary diagnostic laboratories. These involve culture from milk onto selective media and a range of serological tests, often growth inhibition, to identify the species.

The most severe problems with this disease have occurred in large dairy herds in California and Florida. It should be considered as highly infectious and affected animals either removed or isolated within the herd. Examination of bulk milk has proved a useful screening method for affected herds. If a herd is suspected of having a problem with *Mycoplasma* mastitis then specialist advice should be rapidly sought. For further information the reader is referred to detailed reviews (Boughton, 1979; Jasper, 1982) (for therapy see p. 396)

Leptospira *infection* (see also p. 737)

Increasing concern has arisen over leptospirosis for a variety of reasons. Most importantly organisms of the hebdomadis subgroup are pathogenic for man. The organism most involved is *Leptospira hardjo* and this is responsible for the so-called 'milk drop syndrome' and is also associated with abortion in affected herds. The characteristic milk drop appears initially as a mastitis, usually with the milk yield of all four quarters falling to zero within 24 hours. Pyrexia is common and the udder secretion is thickened or clotted and occasionally bloody. The udder remains flaccid and the condition usually resolves within seven to fourteen days. Cases may be restricted to a few animals or up to 50 per cent of animals may become affected over a period of two to three months (Jackson & Bramley, 1983). Antibiotic therapy with tetracyclines or streptomycin may aid the resolution of the clinical phase and reduce carriers although immunity develops following infection. A vaccine is available, which requires an annual booster to ensure adequate protection. Infection of human beings may occur via infected urine droplets, particularly in herringbone milking parlours and leads to a febrile illness characterized by severe headaches. In a proportion of cases this can lead to complications including meningitis and encephalitis.

Coagulase-negative staphylococci and Corynebacterium bovis

The incidence of coagulase-negative staphylococci has increased as herd cell counts have decreased. Several species of coagulase-negative staphylococci are commonly isolated from aseptically collected milk samples.

These include *Staph. epidermidis*, *Staph. simulans* and *Staph. xylosus*. Most of these organisms are of low virulence although some isolations are associated with clinical disease. These organisms generally produce a slight elevation of somatic cell count, which may increase resistance to infection with major pathogens.

Similarly, *Corynebacterium bovis* is not usually associated with clinical disease and primarily colonizes the distal teat duct. It is associated with suboptimal teat disinfection. It is rapidly eliminated by antibiotic therapy and its spread is prevented by effective teat disinfection. In the absence of such measures it may be isolated from >70 per cent of aseptically collected milk samples. Growth on blood agar may require incubation for 48 hours, preferably at 30°C, and stimulation by fatty acids supplied either by the milk or by additions to the media such as Tween 80.

Recommendations for control of mastitis

In the USA, UK and Australasia and many other parts of the world there is a recommended mastitis control scheme based upon the '5-point plan'. The elements in the scheme are as follows:

(1) Apply an approved teat disinfectant after every milking.
(2) Treat clinical cases of mastitis.
(3) Infuse long-acting antibiotic into all quarters at drying-off.
(4) An annual milking machine test and appropriate maintenance.
(5) Cull cows showing repeated cases of clinical mastitis.

These measures were the basis of controlled experimentation in many countries and have been widely employed since the 1970s. Teat disinfection is to reduce

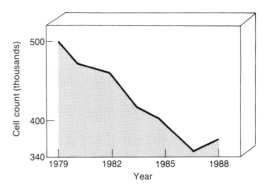

Fig. 23.4 Reduction in bulk milk cell count in England and Wales between 1979 and 1988.

rates of new infection during lactation; the dry-cow therapy serves to eliminate a high proportion of sub-clinical infections present at the end of lactation and to prevent many new dry-period infections. Treatment of clinical mastitis assists the elimination of infection and in the resolution of clinical signs of disease and culling is employed to remove chronically affected cows. Finally, the milking machine maintenance is intended to ensure efficient milking and prevent machine-induced infections as described above (therapy for mastitis is dealt with in Chapter 30).

A review of the progress in mastitis control following the introduction of these techniques has been described by Booth (1988). This shows major reductions in clinical mastitis incidence and in the reduction of bulk milk cell count (Fig. 23.4). The present status of improving mammary gland immunity is described in Chapter 29.

References

Booth, J.M. (1988) 1. Control measures in England and Wales. How have they influenced incidence and aetiology? *British Veterinary Journal*, **144**, 316–22.

Boughton, E. (1979) *Mycoplasma bovis* mastitis. *Veterinary Bulletin*, **49**, 377–87.

Bramley, A.J. (1982) Sources of *Streptococcus uberis* in the dairy herd. I. Isolation from bovine faeces and from straw bedding of cattle. *Journal of Dairy Research*, **49**, 369–73.

Bramley, A.J. & McKinnon, C.H. (1990) The microbiology of raw milk. In *Dairy Microbiology*, Vol. 1 (ed. by R.K. Robinson). Academic Press, New York.

Dairy Federation (1981) Laboratory methods for use in mastitis work. International Dairy Federation Bulletin 132, Brussels.

Dairy Federation (1984) Recommended methods for somatic cell counting in milk. International Dairy Federation Document 168, Brussels.

Dairy Federation (1987a) Bovine mastitis. Definition and guidelines for diagnosis. International Dairy Federation Bulletin 211, Brussels.

Dairy Federation (1987b) Environmental influences on mastitis. International Dairy Federation Bulletin 217, Brussels.

Dodd, F.H., Higgs, T.M. & Bramley, A.J. (1984) Cubicle management and coliform mastitis. *Veterinary Record*, **114**, 522–3.

Erskine, R.J., Eberhart, R.J., Grasso, P.J. & Scholz, R.W. (1989) Induction of *Escherichia coli* mastitis in cows fed selenium-deficient or selenium-supplemented diets. *American Journal of Veterinary Research*, **50**, 2093–2100.

Hill, A.W., Shears, A.L. & Hibbitt, K. (1979) The pathogenesis of experimental *Escherichia coli* mastitis in newly calved dairy cows. *Research in Veterinary Science*, **26**, 97–101.

Jackson, E.R. & Bramley, A.J. (1983) Coliform mastitis. *Veterinary Record* (In Practice Suppl., Vol. 5, No. 4) 135–46.

Jasper, D.E. (1982) The role of *Mycoplasma* in bovine mastitis. *Journal of the American Veterinary Medical Association*, **181**, 158–73.

Marshall, V.M.E., Cole, W.M. & Bramley, A.J. (1986) Influence of the lactoperoxidase system on susceptibility of the udder to *Streptococcus uberis* infection. *Journal of Dairy Research*, **53**, 507–14.

Schalm, O.W., Lasmanis, J. & Jain, N.C. (1976) Conversion of chronic staphylococcal mastitis to acute mastitis after neutropenia in blood and bone marrow produced by an equine anti-bovine leukocyte serum. *American Journal of Veterinary Research*, **37**, 885–94.

Schultze, W.D. (1985) Development in the identification of diseased udder quarters or cows. Proceedings International Dairy Federation Seminar *Progress in the Control of Bovine Mastitis. Kieler Milchwirtschaftliche Forschungsberichte*, **37**, 319–28.

Thomas, G., Over, H.J., Vecht, U. & Nansen, P. (eds) (1987) *Summer Mastitis*. Martinus Nijhoff, the Netherlands, 1–224.

Williams, D.M. & Mein, G.A. (1985) The role of machine milking in the invasion of mastitis organisms and implications for maintaining low infection rates. Proceedings International Dairy Federation Seminar *Progress in the Control of Bovine Mastitis. Kieler Milchwirtschafiliche Forschungsberichte*, **37**, 415–25.

Further reading

Blowey, R.W. & Edmondson, P.W. (1995) *Mastitis Control in Dairy Herds*. Miller Freeman, Ipswich, UK, pp. 1–196.

Bramley, A.J. & Dodd, F.H. (1984) Mastitis control–progress and prospects. *Journal of Dairy Research*, **51**, 481–512.

Schalm, O.W., Carroll. E.J. & Jain, N.C. (1971) *Bovine Mastitis*. Lea & Febiger, Philadelphia, pp. 1–360.

Chapter 24
Summer Mastitis

J.E. Hillerton

Aetiology   337
Epidemiology   337
Transmission   337
Pathogenesis   338
Clinical disease   338
Treatment   339
Control   339

Summer mastitis is an acute or peracute multifactorial infection of the non-lactating bovine mammary gland although clinical signs are often not obvious until parturition. The disease is reported from all four continents where dairy cattle are herded. It is, however, most prevalent in northern Europe and particularly common in some European cattle such as the Friesian/Holstein breeds, being rare in the Zebu.

Aetiology (see p. 334)

Bateriological analysis of summer mastitis secretion shows a complex infection. Usually *Arcanobacterium* (*Corynebacterium*) *pyogenes* predominates and the severity of the infection is related to toxin production from synergistic growth with other bacteria that are anaerobic (see p. 338). *Peptococcus indolicus* is the most common anaerobe but *Bacteriodes melaninogenicus* and *Fusobacterium necrophorum* are often found. An undescribed microaerophilic coccus, the Stuart–Schwann coccus is also found. It rarely grows in pure subculture. *Streptococcus dysgalactiae* is also common and believed by some to be a primary agent predisposing to *A. pyogenes* infection.

Much of the reported variation in bacterial culture, and especially isolation of anaerobes, probably results from suboptimal collection and transport of samples, allowing anaerobes to die out.

Epidemiology

Summer mastitis is considered to be epidemiologically most severe in northern Europe. It is also prevalent in Japan, and parts of the USA, as well as being reported from Greece, Australia, Zimbabwe and Brazil. The incidence varies greatly from country to country, as does the severity of the infection. Most cases in North America are recognized when heifers calve with a non-functional quarter from which the causative bacteria can be recovered, whilst in Japan systemic illness is more common.

The incidence of summer mastitis varies locally. It is greater in the more intensive dairy areas but does not just depend on the density of cattle. It is only in the dairy industry that the importance of the disease is well recognized. It can be prevalent in beef cattle but loss of function of one-quarter is not so important economically in the suckler cow. The Dutch, Germans and Danes believe that summer mastitis is associated with sandy soils, but these correlate well with the best grassland. The high humus content, open structure and free-draining of sandy soils are particularly suitable for foraging, soil-dwelling insect larvae.

The disease is most common in summer and early autumn but can also occur in spring. As well as season, it is particularly associated with calving pattern. In Ireland, with many spring-calving herds, the spring incidence is marked. The black and white dairy breeds seem most susceptible and in the absence of preventive measures the incidence is greatest in older cows.

Transmission

It is a long and widely held belief that flies are involved in the transmission of summer mastitis.

The peak incidence of disease in northern Europe occurs in July, August and September when flies are most abundant on cattle. The sheep headfly (or plantation fly), *Hydrotaea irritans*, is the most frequent visitor to the teats of dry cows and heifers. Flies around pastured cattle have been shown to carry the summer mastitis pathogens even in the absence of disease in the herd. The disease prevalence is coincident with the geographical distribution of the fly in most of Europe. Control of flies on cattle reduces the incidence of summer mastitis. Some 60 per cent of infections occur in the front quarters, which, it has been suggested, flies can reach more easily.

Various studies using *Hydrotaea irritans* to transmit summer mastitis have given incomplete results. The flies have been shown to carry the various bacteria and to be able to regurgitate the bacteria on to teat skin several days after a previous meal. Contaminated teats have been demonstrated to be one precursor to disease. Recently a study in Sweden confirmed a much earlier, anecdotal, UK report that contaminated *H. irritans* could transmit summer mastitis experimentally.

Summer mastitis also occurs frequently outside the fly season and in areas where the sheep headfly is not found. No other obvious vectors have been suggested in these situations. Cases of clinical mastitis, especially in newly calved cows, involving the same complex of bacteria, have been reported throughout the year. There are likely to be several risk factors to these infections including appropriate exposure to the bacteria and teat damage.

Initial cases of summer mastitis in an outbreak probably occur by chance. Increased incidence will depend on the density of animals at risk; hence there is a peak incidence in late summer-calving herds simply because more animals are challenged when they are most susceptible. Probably the role of the fly is to increase the challenge. It therefore is involved in secondary transmission. The fly may also contribute by stressing animals. Fly pestering can reduce milk yields by inducing gross behavioural changes. Susceptibility to infection during late gestation when there are other environmental and husbandry stressors, especially poor forage and heat, may increase with fly challenge.

Pathogenesis

Damage to secretory tissue is caused primarily by a toxin from *A. pyogenes*, with other virulence factors including a haemolysin, a coagulase and a hyaluronidase. The activity and quantity of these appears to be enhanced in mixed culture with *P. indolicus*.

The route of invasion of the udder by a mixture of bacteria is unknown but it seems unlikely that simultaneous invasion by up to five species of bacteria occurs. It is possible to isolate one or more of these pathogens from the udder of the lactating or dry cow in the absence of overt clinical signs so it is likely that some predisposing factor(s) is needed to cause clinical disease.

Evidence for the teat route of invasion in natural infections comes from the frequency of summer mastitis following teat-end damage. It has been possible to produce infections following surface contamination of

the teat with *A. pyogenes* alone. There is, however, no unequivocally accepted mechanism. Possibilities, each with proponents, include colonization of the teat skin or orifice spreading through the teat duct into the gland, bacteria entering the gland by draining via a supra-mammary lymph node from another site and invasion by haematogenous spread. All of the pathogens are ubiquitous on cattle, easily recoverable from mucous membranes and various lesions, and so a number of routes of invasion may occur naturally.

Clinical disease

Diagnosis of the later pathogenic stages of summer mastitis is relatively easy and requires little experience. Early stages are more difficult to distinguish from other infections.

The infection is most probably ascending so the primary sites are in the teat or in lactiferous tissue near the base of the teat. Initially, there is local inflammation and oedema. Expression of udder secretion may reveal a foul smell indicative of anaerobic bacteria. In summer months the teat may be attractive to flies and if the animal is housed the hind legs attract biting flies. Slightly later, behavioural changes in the animal related to toxaemia become apparent. The animal may be lethargic, inappetant, stop cudding and will become detached from the herd. These signs are easy to recognize at pasture. In newly calved and housed animals the first signs are often tenderness in the quarter, which can be confused with excessive intramammary pressure, and local temperature. The secretion will be discoloured, thick and creamy, rather than colostral, perhaps very clotted in a serous fluid, and frequently foul smelling.

In addition to the extreme mastitis, in later stages pyrexia and lethargy develop. If the infection remains local there may be rupture of mammary abscesses to the exterior. More commonly, the animal becomes systemically ill with progressive lameness from the hind legs, swelling of joints and an elevated temperature. The bacteraemia/toxaemia may be fatal in a few per cent of cases; similarly there may be abortion. Perinatal death is substantially increased and many calves, often born prematurely, fail to thrive.

The infection develops rapidly after the initial recognizable signs so confirmation of summer mastitis by bacteriology is rarely quick enough. Attempts have been made to develop cow-side diagnosis of anaerobic involvement based on specific metabolites but no practical technique is available. The time delay for confirmation is impractical. Evidence shows that 80 per cent of preliminary diagnoses of summer mastitis are correct (Hillerton *et al.*, 1987). The other infections would also respond readily to the same therapy so unless drastic action, such as teat amputation or immediate culling, is indicated misdiagnosis in favour of summer mastitis has no economic or welfare disadvantages.

Treatment

A number of different approaches to treatment can be taken. The one selected should depend on the anticipated outcome of the case, which in turn depends on the clinical severity of the infection. In a small number of cases the only recommendation is for immediate culling. Less drastic is to treat the infection purely as an abscess; to amputate the teat and drain. This is practised commonly in northern Europe with non-pregnant younger animals, which are often then reared for beef.

In cows and heifers near to or at parturition the prognosis depends on the speed of diagnosis. In most cases in dry cows the infection is sufficiently well developed that destruction of secretory function is virtually complete. A clinical cure can sometimes be achieved but rarely a bacteriological cure. The prognosis is much better if the infection is diagnosed early, and therapy started immediately.

The pathogens are susceptible to a wide range of antibiotics including penicillin/streptomycin preparations. However, there is a poor cure rate when the only therapy is infusion into the udder. This is because the tissue destruction is extensive locally and so diffusion of the antibiotic is limited. A greater success has been claimed for erythromycin, which diffuses more readily. Success has also been claimed for anti-anaerobe preparations containing metronidazole. Chlortetracycline can be useful in the lactating animal but should not be used in the dry gland as all secretory funtion will be destroyed.

Claims have been made for a variety of other preparations including proteolytic enzymes mixed with antibiotics but controlled studies are rare. Usually, the most successful outcome follows a coordinated effort: frequent stripping of the quarter combined with parenteral intramuscular antibiotics and an intramammary infusion. This conventional approach, although labour intensive, affords the best prognosis for the udder. If systemic involvement is established then treatment of clinical signs to secure the health of the animal is all that can be achieved as the function of the infected quarter has been lost.

The patient should be quarantined as it is a source of further infection.

Control

Summer mastitis is so destructive and expensive that considerable investment in time and materials to control the disease is made by the 40–45 per cent of farmers who regularly experience losses. Preventive measures are neither simple nor foolproof and usually are damage-limiting rather than totally preventive. The basic aims are to limit exposure to infection from the herd, to prevent colonization of lesions and to prevent spread of bacteria to the mammary tissue.

Assuming that summer mastitis infections will arise anyway it is important to recognize these early and segregate an infected animal to limit direct transfer of bacteria via, for example, bedding systems and indirect transfer by flies. *Hydrotaea irritans* do not pester housed cattle, so separate housing of infected animals is good practice.

The epidemiological spread of infection is related to the density of susceptible animals and the abundance of vectors. Reducing the density of late gestation cattle by spreading the calving pattern and completely avoiding the fly season of July, August and September in northern Europe are likely to be highly effective strategies.

Considerable effort is spent on fly control but this is the least effective method of disease control as persistent presence of insecticide on teats is hard to achieve. The synthetic pyrethroids now in common use are applied in ear-tags or as pour-ons to the back and probably spread by diffusion in sebum. However, the teats lack hair and sebaceous glands are sebum deficient, so limiting spread. Effective fly control on teats is only achieved by direct application or frequent reapplication of insecticide, or by the use of two ear-tags per animal.

There has been a gradual decline in the proportion of dry cows suffering summer mastitis, and in the number of herds affected, in England and Wales since 1988. This has been coincident with the control of flies by use of ear tags and later by pour-on formulations.

Frequently, summer mastitis follows infected lesions on or near the teats. These can be prevented or limited by use of surgical tapes, ensuring that the teats are cleaned first and not bandaged too tightly, or by frequent application of teat disinfectant. Many farmers teat-dip dry cows and heifers daily. This allows frequent inspection, trains the heifers to the milking parlour and ensures good teat condition. Prevention of teat lesions may reduce greatly the attractiveness for flies.

The best tested and most effective means of reducing the incidence of summer mastitis is the general application of prophylactic antibiotic infused into the teat at drying-off. Following administration of synthetic penicillins in a long-acting base, summer mastitis rarely occurs within three weeks. Longer effects are achievable with some preparations. Where the incidence of disease warrants extra investment it is advisable to repeat the application of antibiotic after three weeks. The main problem is avoiding milk contamination after an early calving. All the evidence available shows a significant reduction of summer mastitis following use of dry-cow therapy. It can also be applied to heifers if the antibiotic is introduced gently into the teat duct.

Attempts to produce a vaccine against summer mastitis have met with little success. This remains a long-term goal and will become more likely as multi-valent vaccines are developed.

Reference

Hillerton, J.E., Bramley, J.A. & Watson, C.A. (1987) The epidemiology of summer mastitis: a survey of clinical cases. *British Veterinary Journal* **142**, 520–30.

Chapter 25
Bulk Milk Testing and Mastitis Monitoring

D.J. O'Rourke and R.W. Blowey

Cell counts	341
What is a somatic cell count?	341
Factors affecting the somatic cell count	341
Determination of the cell content of milk	342
Interpretation of somatic cell counts	343
Total bacterial counts	345
Sources of bacteria	346
Bulk tank analysis	346
Mastitis monitoring	348
Introduction	348
Recording systems	348
Analysis of information	349
Target figures	350
Uses of mastitis monitoring	350

Cell counts

What is a somatic cell count?

The majority of somatic cells found in milk are white blood cells, with the remainder mainly epithelial cells shed by the secretory tissue of the udder. White blood cells are found throughout the body and their main function is to protect against disease. When large numbers accumulate they are visible as pus. The measurement of the number of somatic cells in milk is known as a somatic cell count.

Factors affecting the somatic cell count

Mastitis

Inflammation in the udder is in no way different from inflammation in other tissues. The cardinal signs of inflammation, namely swelling, redness, heat, pain and loss of function may not always be of recognizable intensity in mastitis. Signs of clinical mastitis are grossly visible but subclinical mastitis may go unnoticed. The majority of mastitis cases are bacterial in origin. One of the basic host responses to a bacterial infection is the infiltration of white blood cells from the blood into the udder. This is accomplished through the processes of diapedesis and chemotaxis. The degree and nature of the cellular response are likely to be proportional to the severity of the infection. In addition to bacterial infections, there are certain other factors, some of which are physiological, that affect the cellular content of milk.

Stage of lactation

The somatic cell count is high during the first week of lactation, then soon decreases and remains low for several weeks after which a gradual increase occurs until the end of lactation. As the milk volume decreases in the latter part of lactation, an apparent increase in cell numbers occurs from mere concentration of cells in a smaller volume of milk. The presence of high cell numbers in colostrum may be due to an excessive desquamation of epithelial cells in a small volume of milk in a gland resuming functional activity after a dormant period (Schalm *et al.*, 1971).

Lactation age

The somatic cell count increases with the lactation age of the cow (Fig. 25.1) (Blackburn, 1966). On the basis of histopathological examination of the udders, the increase in the average number of polymorphonuclear leucocytes with advancing lactation age was attributed to an increase in the extent of subacute inflammation of the ducts as well as an increase in the severity of lobular lesions.

Stress

A sudden upset in the cows' routine, for example a herd blood test or coming indoors in the autumn, can cause a raised cell count for a day or two.

Oestrus

Bulling cows tend to have increased cell counts that are probably stress related.

Milking interval

Irregular milking intervals will influence the somatic cell counts in milk. Comparisons of somatic cell counts in milk have generally shown higher counts for shorter

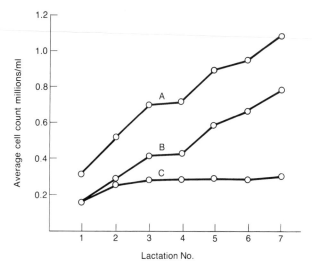

Fig. 25.1 Average cell count for each of seven lactations. A, total cell count; B, polymorphonuclear leucocyte count; C, count of cells other than polymorphonuclear leucocytes. Source: Blackburn (1966), reproduced with permission of Cambridge University Press.

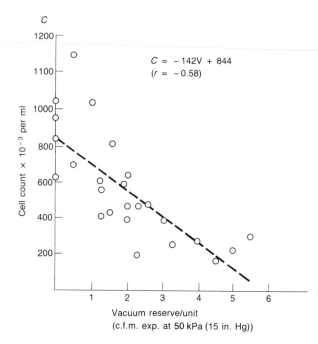

Fig. 25.2 Relationship between mean cell count of herd bulk milk (C) and vacuum reserve per unit (V). Source: Nyhan & Cowhig (1967).

milking intervals. This variation in cell numbers is explained on the basis of total volume of milk secreted leading to a greater dilution of somatic cells during the longer milking interval (Schalm *et al.*, 1971).

Milking machine

A significant correlation between cell counts and milking machine reserve air was observed by Nyhan and Cowhig (1967) in a survey of milking machine efficiency and mastitis in a random sample of 26 dairy farms (Fig. 25.2). Six of the herds were milked with machines that had a vacuum reserve of more than 0.11 m^3/min free air (4 ft^3/min free air) and these were the only herds with a mean bulk milk cell count of <300 000 cells/ml. However, later work in Australia (Olney *et al.*, 1983) concluded that in the absence of mastitis infections vacuum fluctuations, vacuum level, overmilking or varying pulsator rates will not cause stress or irritation that will lead to an increase in somatic cell counts.

Determination of the cell content of milk

Reference method: microscopic counting (Heeschen, 1975)

The method of microscopic counting of cells in a dry stained smear has been available for many years now although it has some possible errors. The optical and manual operations involved are tedious, especially in the case of serial tests, and the following sources of error must not be overlooked.

(1) Distribution of cells in the smears may not be homogeneous. The decision as to whether the stained structures observed are actually cells may be difficult in some cases and must be made subjectively.
(2) To estimate the cell content every microscopic field examined must be multiplied by a relatively large factor, and this can be a source of considerable error.

Consequently, the primary object of microscopic counting is the screening of other counting techniques.

Electronic particle counting

This can be carried out by the following methods.

Coulter counter (International Dairy Federation (IDF, 1981)): With the aid of the Coulter counter it is possible to determine rapidly and accurately the number of particles over a certain size in a suspension. Prior to the determination of the number of cells, the milk is treated as follows.

(1) Cells are stabilized to make them resistant to further treatments.
(2) The milk to be examined is diluted with an electrolyte.
(3) The fat globules are dispersed to well below the Coulter counter threshold.

The treated milk is passed through a 100μm aperture located between two electrodes. When a particle passes through the aperture, a small quantity of highly conductive liquid in the circuit is displaced by a particle of lower conductivity. The increased resistance raises the voltage, producing a voltage pulse proportional to the volume of the particle. The number of pulses indicates the number of particles passing through the aperture. The pulses are fed into a threshold circuit so that only those exceeding a particular threshold value (T) are counted.

Fossamatic (IDF, 1981): This instrument is an automatic microscope for counting cells in liquids. Cells are stained with ethidium bromide and are then excited with a high-energy lamp, causing them to emit light at a characteristic wavelength. The emitted light energy is detected electronically, the result being displayed and printed out for each successive sample.

Accuracy of these methods

The precision obtained in the Fossamatic instrument is comparatively high. However, it is not essentially different from that obtained in the Coulter counter. In practical operation, the Fossamatic instrument has proved to be superior to other methods tested. This applies to the rate of samples as well as the handling of the instrument (Heeschen, 1975).

In an International Dairy Federation (IDF) questionnaire in 1983 on the cell counting methods 20 countries indicated they used Fossamatic, 17 used Coulter counter and two used the microscope method.

Interpretation of somatic cell counts

Somatic cell counts can be carried out both on herd bulk milk and individual cow's milk.

Herd bulk milk

Monthly cell counting has been shown to provide a fair estimate of the subclinical mastitis status of a herd; furthermore, the annual mean can be updated on a rolling basis by substituting the current month's count of the same month of the previous year (Booth, 1985).

A herd of cows with physiologically normal quarters could expect a bulk milk cell count (BMCC) of <200000 thousand cells/ml. Herds with cell counts below this figure do exist (26 per cent of herds in England & Wales; Booth, 1997) but evidence shows that even in these herds there is some subclinical infection (Tables 25.1 and 25.2). A BMCC of 200000 cells/ml is considered to be a realistic upper limit for herds with mastitis under control (Table 25.3).

Table 25.1 Distribution of cow and quarter infections shown against cell count ranges. Source: Pearson & Greer (1974).

Cell count ranges (×10³ cells/ml)	No. of herds	Infections	
		In quarters (%)	In cows (%)
219–490	12	9.61	25.8
535–789	12	17.76	42
1005–1700	5	29.54	54.4

Table 25.2 Estimated infection prevalence and losses in milk production associated with elevated BMCC. Source: Eberhart *et al.* (1982), reproduced with permission of the International Association for Food Protection.

BMCC (×10³ cells/ml)	Quarters infected (%)	Production loss[a] (%)
200	6	0
500	16	6
1000	32	18
1500	48	29

[a] Production loss calculated as a percentage of production expected at 200000 cells/ml.

Table 25.3 Guidelines for interpretation of bulk milk cell counts.

Bulk milk cell count (×10³ cells/ml)	Estimate of mastitis problem
<200	Slight
200–400	Average
400–700	Bad
>700	Very bad

The prevalence of quarters infected clinically, and perhaps more importantly subclinically, with major pathogens such as *Staphylococcus aureus* or *Streptococcus agalactiae* and *Strep. uberis*, and to a lesser extent *Strep. dysgalactiae*, is the most important factor affecting the BMCC. Fenlon *et al.* (1995) confirmed this in a survey of 30 dairy herds, where they found a good correlation between the number of mastitis streptococci (*Strep. agalactiae*, *Strep. dysgalactiae* and *Strep. uberis*) found in bulk tank milk and BMCC. Gram-negative organisms such as *Escherichia coli* are usually rapidly eliminated from the udder and do not tend to cause many subclinical infections. Unless milk from clinical cases reaches the bulk tank, infections of this type do not tend to influence the BMCC significantly; BMCC,

FractionBox

therefore, is a poor indicator of Gram-negative infections (David & Jackson, 1984).

Both monthly and annual rolling mean figures must be examined to detect trends over a period of time rather than figures for a single month. Where subclinical infections with major pathogens like *Staph. aureus* are not well controlled it is possible to see a gradual increase in BMCC over a period of time, rather than a sudden explosive increase. A sudden spectacular rise in the BMCC where the levels have been consistently <250 000 cells/ml could indicate an outbreak, with mastitic milk reaching the bulk milk supply due to faulty detection.

Fifteen countries reported a decrease in national mean cell in an IDF survey (Booth, 1995) (Table 25.4).

Table 25.4 National mean cell counts in 1990 and 1993. Source: Booth (1995). Reproduced with permission of the International Dairy Federation.

Country	Cell count (× 10^6/ml)		Change (%) 1990–93	Mean[a]
	1990	1993		
Austria	379	313	−66 (17)	A
Belgium	307	265	−42 (14)	G
Denmark	368	309	−59 (16)	A
Finland	282	186	−96 (34)	A
Germany	274	237	−37 (14)	G
Hungary	419	351	−68 (16)	A
Iceland	471	408	−63 (13)	A
Italy	434	426	−8 (2)	A
Japan	260	280	+20 (8)	A
Netherlands	320	280	−40 (13)	A
New Zealand	345	255	−90 (26)	W
Norway	206	194	−12 (6)	A
Sweden	230	231	+1 (0)	G
Switzerland	117	104	−13 (11)	A
UK	329	277	−52 (16)	G

[a] A, arithmetic; G, geometric; W, weighted.

Can the BMCC be too low? There is a perception that too low a cell count can lead to an increase in susceptibility to mastitis. However, BMCC is not a measure of resistance to mastitis. Resistance against mastitis depends on the teat barrier being intact and the ability of the cow to mobilize large numbers of efficient neutrophils in a short period of time. Timms (1990) confirmed this when he showed that cows with a low somatic cell count (SCC) were not at greater risk of mastitis infections when compared to cows with a high SCC. In a survey of 125 herds with a low BMCC (<150 000 cells/ml) in the Netherlands the rate of clinical mastitis was significantly related to certain variables that increased the exposure of environmental micoorganisms: poor cubicle cleanliness, rubber mats in cubicles and drinking water from sources other than public water all increased the rate of clinical mastitis (Schukken *et al.*, 1990). Berry (1992) found that it is possible to have a low cell count and achieve a low incidence of mastitis in a survey of 35 herds in England and Wales with a BMCC of less than 70 000 cells/ml.

Why is the BMCC important? Within the dairy industry, BMCC has become the single most important test used to measure milk quality, to regulate whether milk can be sold and to determine the price paid for raw milk (Bennett, 1993; Wells & Ott, 1995; Leslie *et al.*, 1996). Reasons to include BMCC as a pricing component include: (i) domestic consumer demands for quality, (ii) processor need for high-quality raw milk for further processing, (iii) to help improve udder health and (iv) pressure from international markets for documented high-quality dairy products (Wells & Ott, 1995). EC Directive 92/46 states that all milk (liquid milk or milk for manufacture) must have a BMCC of less than 400 000 cells/ml.

Buyers are offering incentives for low BMCCs (Table 25.5), but some may question whether they, the buyers, need low cell counts in milk. Badinand (1994) indicates that the quality of milk is reduced once the number of cells is greater than 70 000 to 100 000/ml. Inflammatory

Table 25.5 Incentives to reduce cell counts. Source: Milk Marketing Board and Milk Marque (UK).

Cell count (×10^3)	Apr 1994	Apr 1995	Oct 1995	Apr 1996	Cell count (×10^3)	Apr 1997
					0–150	+0.2 p/l
<250	−	+0.2 p/l	+0.2 p/l	−	151–250	−
251–400	−	−	−	−0.2 p/l	251–400	−0.5 p/l
401–500	−0.5 p/l	−0.5 p/l	−1.0 p/l	−2.0 p/l	>400	−6.0 p/l
500–1000	−1.0 p/l	−3.0 p/l	−4.0 p/l	−6.0 p/l		
>1000	−2.0 p/l					

p/l, pence/litre.

Table 25.6 Effects of mastitis on milk and milk products. Source: Munro *et al.* (1984), reproduced with permission of the Australian Journal of Dairy Technology.

Substrate	Alterations
Raw milk	Development of a rancid flavour; lower heat stability of whey proteins
Pasteurized milk	Reduction of flavour and quality
Recombined concentrated milk	Less stable proteins
Cheese	Reduced starter activity; changed clotting time; reduction of curd firmness; losses of fat and casein with the whey; lower yield
Butter	Impairment of flavour; less flavour; oxidative taste; longer churning time; inhibition of diacetyl production

changes in the mammary gland influence the process of milk synthesis both quantitatively and qualitatively. The changes in constituents of milk affect the major components (lactose, fat and proteins) as well as fatty acids, protein fractions, caesins, whey proteins, anions and cations, conductivity enzymes, etc. With increasing numbers of somatic cells the growth of starter cultures in milk may be adversely influenced (Table 25.6). Rennetting time and heat stability of the milk can be impaired (Heeschen & Reichmuth, 1995).

Individual cow's milk

The normal somatic cell count in milk in various parts of the same udder varies widely from near zero in uninfected areas to something in the order of three hundred million cells per litre in the worst infected areas. A cow can have <200 000 somatic cells/ml with some small area of the gland badly infected.

Many farmers have monthly somatic cell counts (SCC) carried out on the milk samples taken from cows for milk recording purposes. These can provide a rather more detailed monitor of the herd mastitis situation than that provided by the monthly BMCC. The cost of monthly SCC testing for one year is very low and can be recovered in mid-sized herds by preventing one or two clinical cases of mastitis. The recovery of the cost is many times the out-of-pocket expense because of the many uses of SCC data and the number of cows at risk in a year's time. SCC reach the highest level in milk within the first several hours after milking and reach a low point just prior to milking (Schalm *et al.*, 1971). Anything less than a daily composite has reduced reliability and repeatability. Repeated samples over days or months add perspective to the cow's udder health history and improve the interpretation of SCC. Monthly SCC data accumulated over a year for a cow or herd describe more completely the mastitis history of the herd for the previous year. Greater confidence is gained as more samples are represented.

Table 25.7 Interpretation of individual cow milk cell count.

Count (thousand cells/ml)	Interpretation
Less than 200	Probably uninfected
200 to 500	Suspicious: possibly infected in one quarter
Over 500	Infected in at least one quarter

Individual cow cell counts (Table 25.7) can be of value to farmers and their veterinary surgeons for the following reasons:

- To estimate the proportion of cows in a herd that are infected;
- To screen the herd in order to identify cows for bacteriological examination;
- To identify cows for possible culling (at least two samples at monthly intervals are required);
- As a guide to the effectiveness of dry-cow therapy;
- In a herd with a high total bacterial count (TBC) where the equipment has already been checked, as the first step in identifying the cows that may be the cause of the high TBCs.

Stage of lactation can have some effect; counts are high in the first week after calving and tend to rise slightly in the last few weeks of lactation. First calvers that have never been infected will normally have counts of 100 000 cells/ml or less.

Total bacterial counts

Although by no means a new technique, there has been a recent increase in interest in the use of quantitative and semi-quantitative bacterial counts in bulk milk as an aid in the monitoring and investigation of mastitis and milk hygiene problems. The majority of samples submitted are for the investigation of herd problems with milk hygiene, rising cell counts and/or a high incidence of clinical mastitis. With the majority of countries now basing payment on both the cell count and bacterial count of milk, the results also have economic importance. It is vital that any sample taken is kept refrigerated during transit from the bulk milk tank to the processing laboratory, and this can produce practical difficulties.

EC Directive 92/46 states that all milk (liquid milk or milk for manufacture) must have a total bacterial count (TBC) of less than 100000 bacteria/ml. Consequently, milk supplies are subject to testing for TBC as a measure of milk quality and bonus/penalty payments are applied according to the level. The bacterial count obtained refers to all bacteria which includes sapro-phytic bacteria, faecal organisms such as *E. coli* as well as other major udder pathogens.

Sources of bacteria

Bacteria in milk comes from three main sources:

- From within the udder
- External contamination of cows' teats
- The milking plant

If there is a problem with cooling and refrigeration of milk all three sources may contribute to an increased TBC.

From within the udder

The milk from a healthy uninfected quarter contains virtually no bacteria. Neave (1975) found counts of up to 28 million bacteria/ml in a quarter with subclinical *Strep. uberis* infection. However, the majority of quarters with subclinical infections (*Staph. aureus, Strep. dysgalactiae* and *Strep. uberis*) had counts of around 10000 bacteria/ml. Bacterial counts from quarters with coliform infections were slightly lower.

Milk from cows with clinical mastitis should always be withheld. Neave (1975) found counts of up to 680 million bacteria/ml, and several quarters with counts greater than 100 million bacteria/ml (although 10^5 or 10^6/ml is more usual). Two litres of such mastitic milk added to 2000 litres of bulk milk may raise the TBC by 100000 bacteria/ml (Cousins, 1978).

Herds with satisfactory average TBC sometimes experience occasional wild fluctuations. This may indicate that mastitis cases are not being detected promptly and mastitic milk is entering the bulk tank. It is therefore essential for mastitis detection to be as thorough as possible especially where milking is direct to pipeline (David & Jackson, 1984).

TBC levels can provide some information regarding the mastitis situation in a herd. However, it must be borne in mind that a considerable number of bacteria come from other sources, such as soiling on teats and the milking apparatus (Bramley *et al.*, 1984).

External contamination of cows' teats

Attention to udder hygiene and housing, especially cubicle beds and passage ways, is important in reducing contamination from the udder skin. The handling of cows' teats before milking must always result in the risk of transfer of bacteria between teats and from one cow to another. Herds where teats were dry wiped with paper towels had the lowest BMCC and TBC in both the summer and winter period, followed by those herds where only dirty teats were washed and dried with paper towels (O'Rourke, 1987).

Contamination from the milking equipment

Contamination of the milking equipment is generally found to be the most frequent cause of high bacterial counts. Probably the two major causes are cracked and perished rubberware and inefficient cleaning of the plant (see Blowey & Edmondson, 2000a).

Bulk tank analysis

The organisms counted and the standards currently in use by one processing laboratory (Blowey & Edmondson, 2000a) are shown in Table 25.8. Other laboratories may use different criteria. In addition, a semi-quantitative screen is carried out for all other bacteria isolated from that sample. The target values have been reduced in line with the increasingly strict standards being imposed by the milk purchasing companies (Blowey *et al.*, 2000).

TBC vs Bactoscan

Typically TBC is the number of viable bacteria per ml of milk when cultured on milk agar medium at 37°C for

Table 25.8 Target values for different bacterial types in bulk milk. LPC, laboratory pasteurised count.

Organism	Target value (cfu/ml)
Thermoduric/LPC	<175
Coliforms	<20
Pseudomonas	<500
Total staphylococci	<200
Staph. aureus	<10
Strep. uberis	<2200
Total bacteria count	<5000

48 hours. It therefore measures the number of bacteria which grow at a specific temperature on a specific culture medium. Most bacterial counts are now measured automatically by Bactoscan. This counts all viable organisms, irrespective of their favoured growth temperature or cultural requirements. Bactoscan levels are therefore higher than TBCs, by a factor of approximately four- to five-fold. However, there is no direct relationship between the two, as this will depend on the type of bacteria present in any particular sample (Blowey & Edmondson, 2000b).

Thermoduric count

The number of thermoduric organisms present in the sample (i.e. organisms which are not killed by heating to 64°C for 35 minutes) is taken as an indicator of poor milking plant cleaning. This may be caused by inadequate quantities of hot water (less than 18 litres per cluster), inadequate water temperatures, a lack of swirling and jetting during the washing routine, inadequate amounts of dairy chemical used or particularly hard water leading to inactivation of the circulation cleaner. Many farms are now able to achieve a thermoduric count of 10 cfu/ml or lower, although with problem herds the count may rise to above 600 cfu/ml.

Coliform count

Coliform counts or, more precisely, enterobacteriacae, are taken as an indication of the amount of faecal contamination on teats. This could therefore indicate a problem with poor housing, or poor premilking teat preparation or both. High coliform counts could also arise from cows clinically or subclinically affected by *E. coli* mastitis, with the milk entering the bulk tank. This could occur, for example, where foremilking is not practised and where mastitis detection is poor. Fluctuating cell count and Bactoscan values are often associated with increased levels of clinical mastitis, especially *E. coli*, *Strep. agalactiae* and *Strep. uberis*.

Pseudomonas count

Pseudomonads are non-enteric coliforms, sometimes referred to as non-lactose-fermenting coliforms or NLFs. An increasing number of NLFs were found in milk samples from clinical samples and high cell count cows (Blowey *et al.*, 2000), and subsequent testing showed that these were primarily *Pseudomonas* species. The pseudomonad count is taken as an indicator of non-enteric, non-faecal environmental contamination, and raised levels are likely to be found in herds with poor premilking teat preparation and/or poor environmental hygiene.

Staphylococcus aureus count

High *Staph. aureus* counts are commonly found in herds with high cell counts and indicate that additional attention to hygiene is needed during the milking process and careful postmilking teat disinfection, to prevent the spread of infection. Spread of infection is by hands, teat wipes and especially the teat liners (inflations). In a proportion of herds the *Staph. aureus* levels in bulk milk are quite high and yet cell counts are acceptable. Advice given in these circumstances is that the herd is at risk from a rising cell count, and that there are probably a number of carrier cows present in the herd.

Total staphylococcal count

The total staphylococcal count was introduced because, with the elimination of *Staph. aureus*, there has been an increasing number of herds with high cell counts caused by coagulase negative staphylococci (CNS). This range of organisms includes *Staph. epidermidis* and *Staph. haemolyticus*.

Differential screen

The differential screen is a semi-quantitative assessment of other bacteria present in the milk sample. The bacteria commonly found include:

- *Streptococcus uberis*. Herds with high levels of *Strep. uberis* in bulk milk samples tend to have more clinical mastitis and may have widely fluctuating Bactoscans. *Strep. uberis* can sometimes be associated with somatic cell count problems, even when staphylococcal levels are low.
- *Streptococcus dysgalactiae* has been associated with poor teat skin condition, particularly in heifers. High levels of total staphylococci or *Staph. aureus* may also be present, as both organisms are associated with poor teat skin condition.
- *Streptococcus agalactiae* is sometimes identified from herds that did not even know that the cows were infected. *Strep. agalactiae* can be the cause of increased bulk milk tank somatic cell counts and high and fluctuating Bactoscans.
- *Corynebacterium bovis* has been associated with suboptimal postmilking teat disinfection. If staphylococcal levels are rising and *C. bovis* is identified in significant numbers in bulk milk samples, then it would suggest that additional attention needs to be paid to postmilking teat disinfection.
- Other organisms include *Strep. faecalis*, *Bacillus* species, yeasts and moulds. The presence of a wide range of these environmental organisms is often associated with high coliform and *Pseudomonas*

counts and with an increased incidence of clinical environmental mastitis. Poor housing and/or poor premilking teat preparation could be involved.

Mastitis monitoring

Introduction

There are few conditions in dairy cows that lend themselves to such a detailed objective numerical monitoring as mastitis. Mastitis is still a significant problem in dairy herds in all countries and many of the factors leading to a high incidence are associated with hygiene and husbandry, i.e. they are under the direct control of the farmer or stockman. It is therefore vital that there is a constant monitoring to ensure that all parties involved are made aware immediately a problem starts to develop.

One of the largest British surveys, starting with 45 000 cows in 378 herds, was completed in 1983 (Wilesmith *et al.*, 1986). Defining a 'case' of mastitis as one quarter affected and with a separate case commencing if seven days had elapsed since the disappearance of clinical signs, they found an incidence of 54.6 cases per 100 cows in 1980, declining to 41.2 cases per 100 cows by 1982. This is in broad agreement with the data of Blowey (1986), reporting a much smaller survey of 22 herds monitored by a veterinary practice, where the incidence of mastitis fell from 51.0 cases in 1979 to 31.8 cases per 100 cows in 1985 (Table 25.9). More recently Kossaibati *et al.* (1998), in a study of 144 well-recorded

Holstein/Friesian herds in England (average herd size 132 cows) over three years, recorded an incidence of 43.4 quarter cases per 100 cows per year. The disease affected 25.9 per cent of the cows in the herd each year, with 1.6 quarter cases per affected cow, giving an overall recurrence rate of 19.4 per cent. This would suggest that some cows are more susceptible to clinical mastitis than others. Although there has been little improvement over the past 10 to 15 years, these figures represent a marked reduction in incidence compared with the 1960s, when Kingwell *et al.* (1970) recorded an incidence of 120 cases per 100 cows per year. The marked reduction in incidence since this period has been associated with the implementation of the 'five-point plan', and the control of contagious infections. There has been little decrease in environmental infections however, possibly because the doubling of teat end milk flow rates (from 0.8 to 1.6 kg/Q/min) that has been associated with increased yields has led to a 12-fold increase in susceptibility to new infections (Grindal & Hillerton, 1991).

Recording systems

The precise system used by the farmer to keep mastitis records is not particularly important, provided:

- It is used accurately and kept up to date;
- All information is recorded, namely date, cow identity, quarter affected, treatment used, withdrawal period and results of bacteriological samples (if taken);

Table 25.9 The average performance of the 22 herds monitored (Blowey, 1986).

Period of records	Number of herds being recorded	Herd size	Rolling mean herd milk cell count (×10³/ml)	Annual milk sales (l)	Percentage cows affected	Mastitis cases/ 100 cows	Intramammary tubes used per cow	Intramammary tubes used per case treated	Percentage cases which recurred
Oct. 1979– Sept. 1980	22	91.7	346	6011	26.5	51.0	2.6	5.1	25.0
Sept. 1980– Aug. 1981	24	105	302	5820	25.4	49.6	2.7	5.8	16.3
March 1981– Feb. 1982	22	101	310	5921	25.8	459	2.4	5.6	14.9
April 1982– March 1983	16	123.7	302	5949	27.2	493	2.5	5.0	16.1
April 1983– March 1984	16	123.8	255	5651	23.6	42.7	1.9	4.2	13.1
April 1984– March 1985	23	111.5	243	5479	19.6	31.7	2.1	7.1	10.3

- The records are in a form that is acceptable and usable for the person compiling them;
- They are easily accessible and regularly reviewed by both the farmer and his veterinary adviser and any necessary action is taken following this review.

An analysis of data needs to be carried out at least every six months. Intervals longer than this would fail to achieve the aims of the monitoring (detailed later in this section, p. 350). It is also important to be seen to be using the data, thereby maintaining the interest and enthusiasm of the herdsman for continuing with the recording. Wall charts are the simplest method of recording; computers may be used, while others use a specific mastitis recording booklet, with a page for each cow (Fig. 25.3; Blowey, 1983). This has the advantage

COW No: _____

Date	Quarter	Tubes	Sample

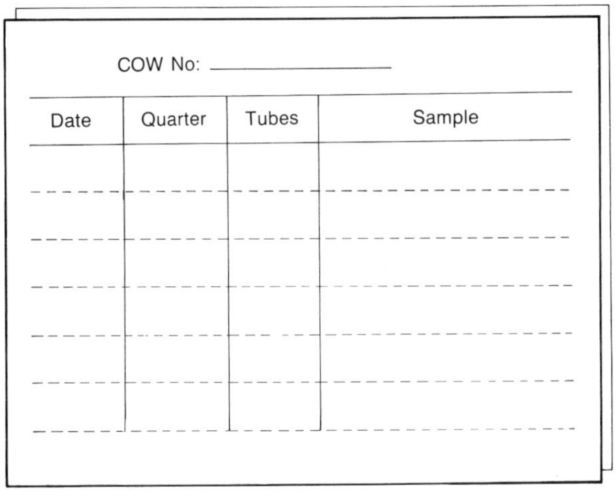

Fig. 25.3 A page from a herdsman's mastitis recording book. This is kept during the life of the cow.

that a cow's lifetime mastitis history is readily available. Whatever system is used, it must be capable of producing information on previous disease, to assist with decisions on culling.

Analysis of information

Regular checks must be carried out by analysing the recorded information in order to:

- Assess the incidence of mastitis on each farm and hence the efficacy of the control procedures in use;
- Compare the performance of the farm with 'standard targets' or with the herds of other members of the group being monitored.

The wide variety of criteria that can be used to monitor mastitis are shown in Table 25.10, which is part of a 'league table' taken from a herd recording programme (Blowey, 1984). Bulk milk cell count is clearly the traditionally used parameter, but this is mainly a reflection of subclinical *Staph. aureus*, *Strep.uberis* or *Strep. agalactiae* contagious mastitis. It provides relatively little information on the incidence of environmental mastitis. The percentage of cows affected gives the proportion of cows in the herd that have been clinically affected by mastitis during a 12-month recording period. Any one of these cows may have had mastitis in one or more quarters and any one quarter may have had two, three or more mastitis incidents over a 12-month period. Defining a case as one quarter affected once, and a remission of clinical signs for six days or more being needed before a new case commences, then the case incidence of mastitis can be calculated. As far as the farmer is concerned, this will be a more accurate reflection of the 'amount of mastitis' occurring in the

Table 25.10 A 'league table' derived from mastitis data analysis.

Herd number	Number of cows	Rolling mean cell count ($\times 10^3$)	Mean herd yield (annual sales) (l)	Percentage cows affected	For whole herd			For mastitic cows		
					Cases per 100 cows	Tubes used per cow	Tubes used per case	Average number of cases	Recurrence (%)	Quarters per cow
1	65	321	5800	38	60	3.5	5.7	1.6	15	1.4
2	81	745	6000	21	30	0.9	2.9	1.5	12	1.3
3	46	275	5850	19	40	4.1	9.4	2.2	45	1.2
4	134	267	5178	21	30	1.2	4.6	1.2		1.2
6	95	346		29	70	9.8	13.5	2.5	33	1.6
7	110	333	6500	27	70	2.7	3.8	2.6	40	1.6
8	132	272	6036	28	60	1.8	2.9	2.2	29	1.6
9	50	441		30	70	2.1	3.1	2.2	36	1.4
10	60	210		18	60	1.7	2.8	3.4	35	2.2

herd. If a herd has a low percentage of cows affected, but a high number of cases per 100 cows (for example herd 7, Table 25.10), then that herd has a problem with either (i) a large number of down-calving cases, with maybe all four quarters affected at the same time or (ii) a proportion of 'chronics' in the herd, which have had repeated attacks of mastitis in one or more quarters over the lactation. This can be expressed as the proportion of treated cases that recurred and is clearly very high for herd 7.

These two situations can be separated by monitoring the percentage that recurred, namely the proportion of treated quarters that required a second or subsequent treatment during a 12-month recording period. Additional information can be obtained by calculating indices for the cows affected, namely for 'mastitic cows' (Blowey, 1984). For example, in this category (i) 'cases per mastitic cow' gives an indication of the average frequency with which a cow gets mastitis during a 12-month period and (ii) 'quarters per mastitic cow' then gives a further indication of whether it is one quarter being regularly affected, or all four quarters affected at once.

In many instances, intramammary antibiotic tube usage is obtained from different sources, e.g. the veterinary practice or other sales invoices. This has the advantage in that it provides a check on the accuracy of the data being supplied by the farmer. For example, if it is calculated that 10 tubes are used for each case treated, there are several possible explanations:

(1) The cases treated are very slow to respond, either because the wrong antibiotic is being used, or because there is an unusually resistant organism or because treatment is not instigated until the case is quite well advanced.
(2) Tubes are being used at a rate well in excess of the manufacturer's recommendations.
(3) Tubes are being used for purposes other than the treatment of mastitis.
(4) Not all cases of mastitis are being recorded. This is the most likely cause of an extremely high tube usage per case.

The mean tube usage per cow in the herd and per case treated as recorded by Wilesmith et al. (1986) was slightly higher than that recorded by Blowey (1986) (Table 25.9). However, on individual farms Wilesmith et al. (1986) found that average tube usage over a 12-month recording period varied from 0.9 to 53.5 tubes per case treated (Table 25.11). It was for this reason that they concluded that tube usage was not a reliable indicator of mastitis incidence within a herd. However, coincident with a decrease in mastitis incidence from 54.6 to 41.2 cases per 100 cows per annum, there was a decline from 280 to 259 tubes used per 100 cows.

Table 25.11 Case incidence and tube usage over a 3-year recording period. Source: Wilesmith et al. (1986).

	1980	1981	1982
Cases/100 cows	54.6	49.8	41.2
Tubes used/100 cows	280	273	259
	(33–1032)	(23–1112)	(19–1003)
Tubes used/clinical case	6.1	6.1	5.8
	(1.1–29.4)	(0.9–53.5)	(0.9–19.5)

Table 25.12 Targets for herd mastitis incidence. Source: Blowey & Edmondson (2000a).

	Target	Interference level
Percentage cows affected per annum	20	25
Cases/100 cows per annum ('mastitis rate')	30	40
Milking cow antibiotic tubes/ cow in herd per annum	1.4	2.5
Milking cow tubes used per case	4.5	6.0
Percentage cases requiring a repeat treatment during a 12-month period	10	20
Percentage dry cows affected per annum	1.0	2.5

Similarly, in the data of Blowey (1986) (Table 25.9), tube usage fell from 260 to 210 tubes used per 100 cows in a period when mastitis incidence declined from 51.0 to 31.7 cases per 100 cows per annum. Tube usage would therefore appear to give some indication of mastitis incidence, although it is not a figure that should be used in isolation.

Target figures

Targets for mastitis incidence have been suggested by some authors and are shown in Table 25.12. These can be used by an individual farmer to assess the progress of a control scheme.

Uses of mastitis monitoring

Most points have been referred to already, but an appraisal of the uses of recording makes a useful summary of the subject.

- To monitor the progress of an individual cow. Any cow that has had four or more cases in one quarter during a 12-month period should be considered for culling, or at least for special treatment.
- To monitor herd status. Is mastitis incidence acceptable or should more effort be put into control? The surveys of both Blowey (1986) and Wilesmith *et al.* (1986) showed a marked decrease in mastitis incidence over the recording period and it is likely that the simple discipline of recording, leading to an increased awareness of the problem, will lead to improvements.
- A recording system provides an opportunity for greater veterinary involvement in on-farm advice and discussion. Recording in itself often provides the herdsman with greater motivation in mastitis control, and this is particularly the case if league tables are supplied, indicating how well a specific herd compares with the others being monitored.
- If problems occur, an analysis of the records can sometimes indicate the likely epidemiology of the organisms involved and hence the control measures required. For example, a herd with a high percentage of cases requiring repeat treatments is likely to be affected by staphylococcal or streptococcal cow-to-cow transmitted mastitis. Alternatively, because a heavily contaminated environment tends to expose all cows to the same level of infection, a high incidence of environmental mastitis would be seen in the records as a high percentage of cows affected, almost an equal number of cases per 100 cows, but only low numbers of cases per mastitic cow and a low percentage of cases recurring. For herds with environmental mastitis, clinical case incidence will commonly be high but the cell count remains low.

References

Badinand, F. (1994) Maitrise du taux cellulaire du lait. *Recueil de Médecine Vétérinaire*, **170**, 6–7, 419–27.

Bennett, R. (1993) Lead, follow or get out of the way: the new PMO SCC policy. *Dairy Food & Environmental Sanitation*, **13**, 74–9.

Berry, E.A. (1992) Mastitis incidence in low cell count herds. *Veterinary Record*, **130**, 479–80.

Blackburn, P.S. (1966) The variation in the cell count of cow's milk throughout lactation from one lactation to the next. *Journal of Dairy Research*, **33**, 193–8.

Blowey, R.W. (1983) Data recording and analysis in dairy herds. In *Proceedings of the Society of Epidemiology and Preventive Medicine*, pp. 19–28.

Blowey, R.W. (1984) Mastitis monitoring in general practice. *Veterinary Record*, **114**, 259–61.

Blowey, R.W. (1986) An assessment of the economic bene-fits of a mastitis control scheme. *Veterinary Record*, **119**, 551–3.

Blowey, R.W., Davis, J.R. & Edmondson, P.W. (2000) Bulk milk analysis – an opportunity for greater on-farm involvement. *UK Vet*, **3**, 26–30.

Blowey, R.W. & Edmondson, P.W. (2000a) In *Mastitis Control in Dairy Herds*. Farming Press, Miller Freeman, Ipswich, UK, p. 142.

Blowey, R.W. & Edmondson, P.W. (2000b) In *Mastitis Control in Dairy Herds*. Farming Press, Ipswich, UK, p. 133.

Booth, J.M. (1985) Bulk milk somatic cell counting: methods in use and a proposal for the standard presentation of data. In *Proceedings of the International Dairy Federation Seminar Progress in the Control of Mastitis*, Kiel, Germany, pp. 274–81.

Booth, J.M. (1995) Progress in the control of mastitis. In *Proceedings of the International Dairy Federation Seminar Progress in the Control of Mastitis*, Tel Aviv, Israel, **4**, 3–10.

Booth, J.M. (1997) Progress in mastitis control – an evolving problem. *Proceedings of British Mastitis Conference*, 3–8.

Bramley, A.J., McKinnon, C.H., Staker, R.T. & Simpkin, D.L. (1984) The effect of udder infection on the bacterial flora of the bulk milk of ten dairy herds. *Journal of Applied Bacteriology*, **57**, 317–23.

Cousins, C.M. (1978) Milking techniques and the microbial flora of milk. In *Proceedings XXth International Dairy Congress*, Paris.

David, G.P. & Jackson, G. (1984) The collection and interpretation of herd mastitis data. *British Veterinary Journal*, **140**, 107–14.

Eberhart, R.J., Hutchinson, L.J. & Spencer, S.B. (1982) Relationship of bulk tank somatic cell counts to prevalence of intramammary infection and to indices of herd production. *Journal of Food Protection*, **45**, 1125–8.

Fenlon, D.R., Logue, D.N., Gunn, J. & Wilson, J. (1995) A study of mastitis bacteria and herd management practices to identify their relationship to high somatic cell counts in bulk tank milk. *British Veterinary Journal*, **151**, 17–25.

Grindal, R.J. & Hillerton, J.E. (1991) Influence of milk flow rate on new intramammary infection dairy cows. *Journal of Dairy Research*, **58**, 263–8.

Heeschen, W. (1975) Determination of somatic cells in milk technical aspects of counting. In *Proceedings of the International Dairy Federation Seminar on Mastitis Control*, Reading, England, pp. 79–92.

Heeschen, W. & Reichmuth, J. (1995) Mastitis: influence on qualitative and hygienic properties of milk. In *Proceedings of the International Dairy Federation Seminar Progress in the Control of Mastitis*, Tel Aviv, Israel, **3**, 3–13.

International Dairy Federation (IDF) (1981) Recommended methods for somatic cell counting in milk. Document 132, pp. 5–16.

Kingwell, R.G., Neave, F.K., Dodd, F.H., Griffin, T.H., Westgarth, D.R. & Wilson, C.D. (1970) The effect of a mastitis control system on levels of subclinical and clinical mastitis in two years. *Veterinary Record*, **87**, 94–100.

Kossaibati, M.E., Hovi, M. & Esslemont, R.J. (1998) Incidence of clinical mastitis in dairy herds in England. *Veterinary Record*, **143**, 649–53.

Leslie, K.E., Godkin, M.A. & Schukken, Y.H. (1996) Milk

quality and mastitis control in Canada: progress and outlook. In *Proceedings 35th Annual Meeting of National Mastitis Council*, pp. 19–30.

Milk Marketing Board of England & Wales (MMB) (1985) The use of mastitis cell counts on individual cow milk samples. Leaflet No. ICCCS/VS/885.

Munro, G.L., Grieve, P.A. & Kitchen, B.J. (1984) Effects of mastitis on milk yield, milk composition, processing properties and yield and quality of milk products. *Australian Journal of Dairy Technology*, **39**, 1, 7–16.

Neave, F.K. (1975) Diagnosis of mastitis by bacteriological methods alone. In *Proceedings of the International Dairy Federation Seminar on Mastitis Control*, Reading, UK, pp. 19–36.

Nyhan, J.F. & Cowhig, M.J. (1967) Inadequate milking machine vacuum reserve and mastitis. *Veterinary Record*, **81**, 122–4.

Olney, G.R., Scott, G.W. & Mitchell, R.K. (1983) Effect of milking machine factors on somatic cell count of milk from cows free of intramammary infection. *Journal of Dairy Research*, **50**, 135–52.

O'Rourke, D.J. (1987) To wash or to wipe – a survey of pre-milking teat preparation. In *Proceedings British Cattle Veterinary Association, 1987–88*, pp. 130–3.

Pearson, J.K.L. & Greer, D.O. (1974) Relationship between somatic cell counts and bacterial infections of the udder. *Veterinary Record*, **95**, 252–7.

Schalm, D.W., Carroll, E.J. & Jain, N.C. (1971) *Bovine Mastitis*. Lea & Febiger, Philadelphia.

Schukken, Y.H., Grommers, F.J., Geer, D. van de, Erb, H.N. & Brand, A. (1990) Risk factors for clinical mastitis in herds with a low bulk milk somatic cell count. 1. Data and risk factors for all cases. *Journal of Dairy Science*, **73**, 3463–71.

Timms, L.L. (1990) Can somatic cells get too low? *Dairy Food & Environmental Sanitation*, **10**, 494–7.

Wells, S.J. & Ott, S.L. (1995) Individual and bulk milk tank somatic cell count results: what is the quality of the US milk supply? In *Proceedings 34th Annual Meeting of National Mastitis Council*, pp. 11–22.

Wilesmith, J.W., Francis, P.G. & Wilson, C.D. (1986) Incidence of clinical mastitis in a cohort of British dairy herds. *Veterinary Record*, **118**, 199–203.

Chapter 26
The Milking Machine

D.J. O'Rourke

The equipment 353
Functions of main components of a milking machine 353
Milking machine testing 355
    Static test 355
    Dynamic test 356
Milking machines and mastitis 357
Developments in milking machine technology 357
    Shields 357
    Ball claw 358
    Hydraulic milking 358
    Automatic milking systems 358
    Automatic cluster removers 359
    Large-bore pipelines 359
    High- and low-line plants 359
    Liner design 359
    Backflushing 360
    Automatic teat disinfection 361
Control measures 361

The equipment

A milking machine installation consists of a pipework system linking various vessels and other components, which together provide the flow paths for air and milk. The forces necessary to move air and milk through the system arise from the fact that the system is maintained at a vacuum. Thus it is atmospheric pressure that forces air, intramammary pressure that forces milk, into the system and the combination of these forces causes flow.

A milking machine has five basic components and any machine, no matter how big, can be broken down into these components (Figs 26.1–26.3):

- Vacuum pump: to supply the vacuum
- Regulator: to control the vacuum level
- Pulsators: to open and close the liners
- Clusters: to attach to the cow
- Containers: to store the milk

Figure 26.1 shows diagrammatically the flow of air and milk through a bucket milking machine. Milk enters the teatcups and travels through the short milk tubes to the claw where air is admitted to break up the columns of milk and improve milk flow away from the claw. The milk and air travel along the long milk tube to the container (bucket). A pulsator is normally situated on the lid of the container and this admits air, which aids in the collapse of the liners during the closed phase of pulsation. Air is also admitted through the regulator, which is situated on the vacuum pipeline.

The flow pattern is similar in the milking pipeline machine except that the milk and air from each claw flow through the milk pipeline to a common receiver where air and milk are separated (Fig. 26.2). Depending on the type of milk pump used, air may be admitted when milk is released from the receiver and pumped to the bulk tank.

The flow pattern of the recorder type of machine is similar to the milking pipeline machine except that air admitted at the claw is separated from the milk at the recorder jar (Fig. 26.3). Air has to be admitted at this point through a special inlet or through the teatcups at the end of each milking operation to force the milk from the recorder jar to the receiver jar (which is under vacuum). Some air may pass along with the milk as the jar empties, especially if the controls are not very expertly handled. This air is separated from the milk at the receiver jar.

Functions of main components of a milking machine

Vacuum pump: To extract air and maintain the machine under vacuum.

Interceptor: To prevent the ingress of foreign matter into the vacuum pump.

Sanitary trap: To prevent milk vapour from entering the pulsators.

Vacuum regulator: To maintain a constant vacuum level. It limits the maximum level by admitting air into the plant when a predetermined vacuum level

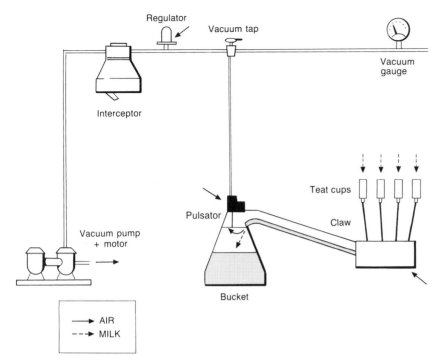

Fig. 26.1 Bucket milking machine.

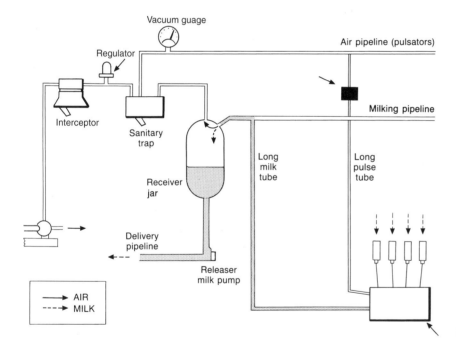

Fig. 26.2 Milking pipeline machine.

has been reached. When the vacuum level drops, the regulator closes; this stops admission of air and the vacuum level rises until the preset level of vacuum is reached, at which time the regulator opens again and admits air.

Pulsation: This causes the liner to open and close: when there is vacuum in the pulsation chamber the liner opens and milk flows; when air is admitted into the pul-

sation chamber the liner collapses, milk flow stops and the teat is massaged. In fact, milk generally flows when the liner is more than half open. The exact function of pulsation has not been established but is now thought to be relief of congestion around the teat orifice. Figure 26.4 shows a typical pulsation chamber waveform containing four phases: (i) a phase, liner opening; (ii) b phase, liner fully open; (iii) c phase, liner closing; and (iv) d phase, liner fully closed.

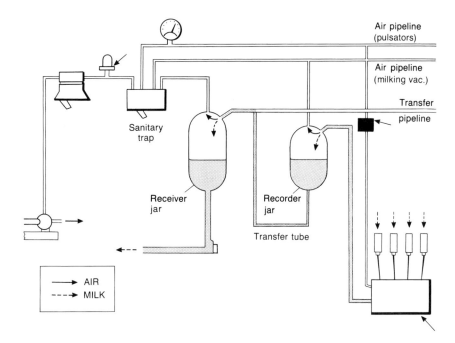

Fig. 26.3 Recorder milking machine.

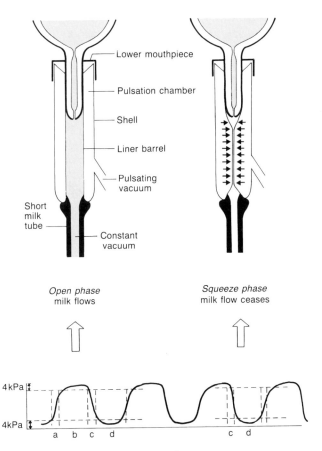

Fig. 26.4 Pulsation chamber waveform.

Liners: The performance of liners is related to various dimensions of liners and various other physical properties of the liner. The liner is the major determinant of milking characteristics (O'Shea, 1982).

Milking machine testing

Milking machines are tested to assess whether they are in good mechanical condition and conform to working standards as laid down by the standards institution of that country where used. Static and dynamic tests are used.

Static test

This type of test has been carried out for many years. It is basically an engineer's test to check for correct functioning of the components of the machine. The machine is set for milking and plastic bungs placed in the liner mouthpieces. No milk flows and, therefore, the test does not give an indication of how the machine will perform during milking.

There are three measurements to look for when interpreting a static test report:

(1) *Effective reserve.* Vacuum within the plant is created by the vacuum pump. Air is used by the pulsators, air holes in the claws and leaks in the plant, etc. The spare vacuum capacity left after compensating for these leakages is called the effective reserve. The effective reserve is used to compensate for additional leakages during cluster application and removal and cluster fall-off.

(2) *Pulsation.* Table 26.1 shows the recommendations for pulsation characteristics.

(3) *Leakages:* The static test will measure the air consumption of the major components in the machine

Table 26.1 Recommendations for pulsation characteristics. Source: O'Shea (1982), reproduced with permission.

Parameter	Acceptable range
Rate	53–63 c/min
Ratio (atb : ctd)	55–70%
d-value	Not less than 15%

and there is a set of standards for the maximum consumption allowed. It is worth checking that the results of the test are within the normal range.

Practical tips

As a veterinary surgeon in practice there are two simple ways of checking the effective reserve of a machine:

(1) Put plant in milking position with plastic bungs in the liners. For every five units, open one and let air in. If the effective reserve is sufficient the vacuum level, as read at the vacuum gauge, should not drop by more than 2 kPa (about ¾ inch Hg) (O'Shea, 1982).
(2) Again put plant in milking position with plastic bungs in the liners. By letting air in the plant, via the gate valve, drop vacuum to 33 kPa (10 inches Hg). Close off air leakage. The vacuum should return to 50 kPa (15 inches Hg) within 3 seconds (Mein, 1984).

Dynamic test

Dynamic testing was indicated in only 1 per cent of herds (O'Callaghan *et al.*, 1982) where there was a mastitis problem and the static test had revealed no faults. At that time, equipment was either very sophisticated and expensive (UV recorder) or crude (pulsation pen recorder). In recent years, with the advent of computer technology, new recording machines specially designed for dynamic testing have been developed.

In dynamic testing the vacuum level is measured at the clawpiece and other areas of the machine, e.g. the recorder jar, throughout the milking of a number of cows. This allows the determination of what is happening when milk and air are flowing in the machine and also assessment of the ability of the milker to use the machine properly.

There are three measurements to look for when interpreting a dynamic test reading:

● *Cyclic fluctuations*: generated within the claw as a result of pulsation (Fig. 26.5).

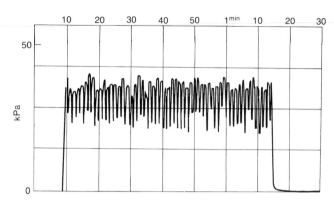

Fig. 26.5 Vacuum changes (cyclic fluctuations) at the teat end during milk flow.

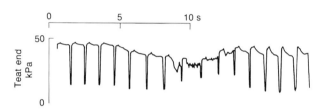

Fig. 26.6 Vacuum changes (irregular fluctuations) at the teat end during milk flow. Source: Nyhan (1968).

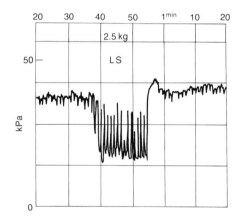

Fig. 26.7 Liner slip at the teat end during milk flow. LS, liner slip; 2.5 kg, flow rate of 2.5 kg/min.

● *Irregular fluctuations*: occur as a result of changes in airflow during milking, which leads to a drop in vacuum (Fig. 26.6).
● *Liner slip*: sudden air admission between the liner and the teat (Fig. 26.7). A problem exists if more than five slips or falls per 100 cows require correction by the milker(s) (Mein, 1984).

It should be noted that 50 per cent of the faults detected in a dynamic test are operator related.

Milking machines and mastitis

The milking machine can act as vector in three ways: (i) cow-to-cow transfer of bacteria via contaminated clusters; (ii) internal flow between clusters within the plant; and (iii) quarter-to-quarter transfer within the cow via the claw.

A farm survey in Ireland in 1967 showed a highly significant regression of bulk milk cell count on effective reserve of the miking plant, i.e. as effective reserve decreased cell count increased (Nyhan & Cowhig, 1967). Subsequent work showed that unstable vacuum (a combination of large irregular fluctuations and moderate cyclic fluctuations) caused higher new infection rates than stable vacuum.

Further work carried out at the National Institute for Research in Dairying (NIRD) at Reading in the early 1970s (Cousins, 1972; Cousins *et al.*, 1973; Thiel *et al.*, 1973) found that large irregular fluctuations or large cyclic fluctuations *per se* did not increase new infection rates. However, any combination of large irregular fluctuations with substantial cyclic fluctuations caused a large increase in new infections. The results also suggested that infections were most likely to be initiated towards the end of milking.

During the late 1970s research workers at Moorepark in Ireland (O'Callaghan *et al.*, 1976; O'Shea *et al.*, 1976, 1979, 1981; O'Shea & O'Callaghan, 1978, 1982) showed that plant vacuum stability *per se* had little effect on new infection rate. It was suggested that the effect of generalized vacuum instability is mediated via increased liner slip, i.e. sudden air admission between the liner and the teat. Liner slip, in turn, is largely a function of liner design and also of vacuum stability.

When slip occurred in one quarter, impacts of milk droplets were detected in other quarters connected by the claw to the teat in which the slip occurred and a higher number of new infections occurred in these impacted quarters.

This liner slip theory is compatible with many other results. Liner slips are more frequent at foreteats; infections are more often seen in hind quarters (Rabold & Picher, 1980). Slip frequency is most common at morning milkings and high flow rates and infections are most frequent in cows with high milk flow rate (O'Shea *et al.*, 1980).

Further work carried out on simulated liner slips at Moorepark in the early 1980s (O'Shea *et al.*, 1981) yielded the following results:

- There were equal numbers of new infections with inaudible and audible liner slips.
- Liner slips at start of milking or the end of milking only, or during the total milking caused almost equal numbers of new infections.
- Liner slips increased new infections when teats were heavily contaminated with environmental bacteria (*Escherichia coli* and *Streptococcus dysgalactiae*).

Liner slip is now considered to be the major mechanism of spread of mastitis at milking (O'Shea *et al.*, 1981).

Baxter *et al.* (1990) found that new intramammary infection rates (IMI/100 cow days) were 0.379 in cows milked with high-slip liners and 0.277 in those milked with low-slip liners ($p = 0.056$). Clinical cases per 100 cow days were 0.211 in the high-slip group and 0.158 in the low-slip group ($p > 0.05$). Rogers and Spencer (1991) found that variation between cows in machine liner slips, and manual milking machine adjustments within and across lactation number and days in milk can be partially explained by udder and teat morphology. Wider teats (distances between teats) were associated with increased liner slips and increased manual milking machine adjustments. More tilted udders (rear quarters lower than front quarters) were associated with increased liner slips and tended to be associated with increased manual adjustments. In addition, poor unit alignments, larger teat diameter and longer teats tended to be associated with increased liner slips.

Developments in milking machine technology

Shields

During the late 1970s research workers at Reading developed shields (deflector plates) in the teatcup chamber between the short milk tube and the teat end (Fig. 26.8). Trials on 15 herds in England and 16 herds

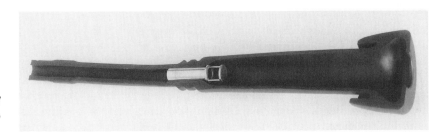

Fig. 26.8 Shielded liner. Photo courtesy of Institute of Animal Health (IAH), Compton.

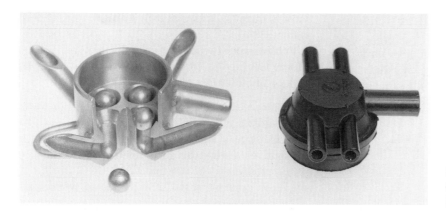

Fig. 26.9 Ball claw cluster. Photo courtesy of Institute of Animal Health (IAH), Compton.

in Australia showed that shields prevented about 10 per cent of quarters from becoming infected (Griffin *et al.*, 1980a).

Ball claw

In the early 1980s research workers at Reading developed a cluster to prevent the transfer of pathogens between teats during milking (Griffin *et al.*, 1980b). It was a simple practical modification of the clawpiece for each of the four short milk tube connectors (Fig. 26.9). Field trials showed an overall 14 per cent reduction in new infection rate due to the clawpiece (Griffin *et al.*, 1982). However, there was an unexpected larger reduction (17 per cent) in new infection rates from environmental sources of exposure (*Streptococcus uberis*, coliforms and others) than from those (8 per cent) transmitted mainly at milking time within the udder or on teat sores (*Staphylococcus aureus*, *Strep. agalactiae* and *Strep. dysgalactiae*).

Hydraulic milking

Following research on the ball claw, Griffin and Grindal carried out an experiment to ascertain the effects of blocking the air bleed on new infections. Initial results from a closely controlled small scale experiment in a research herd showed that teat end condition was improved and that it was at least equal in preventing mastitis to milking with the valve clawpiece with airbleeds (Griffin, 1985). This new method of milking was christened 'hydraulic milking'. Research at Compton on the ball claw under hydraulic milking conditions has shown that as the liner starts to open, high vacuum levels (up to 90 kPa) are generated beneath the teat (Grindal, 1987). Although high vacuum levels have been shown to increase teat damage during conventional milking (Smith & Peterson, 1946), further trials with hydraulic milking have not shown this to be a

problem. Grindal and Griffin (1989) carried out four trials comparing hydraulic milking with the valve clawpiece with airbleeds. Milk flow rate was increased by 20 per cent and milking time was decreased by 26 per cent with hydraulic milking. Quarter infection ratios were low in both groups with only two out of 88 quarters infected with challenges with *Streptococcus agalactiae* and *S. dysgalactiae* in each treatment group.

Automatic milking systems

About 100 automatic milking systems are currently in use on farms in Germany (Schon *et al.*, 1997). Milking robots are used at 200 Dutch dairy farms and it was forecast that >800 farms would be using them by 2000 (Ipema *et al.*, 1998). Data (1996–98) on milk quality were compared between 28 Dutch dairy farms using milking robots and those with machine milking three times/day (28 farms) and twice/day (49 farms). Parameters were somatic cell count, pH of milk fat, freezing point, clarity, fatty acids, milk fat and milk proteins. The use of a milking robot resulted in increased somatic cell counts and pH of milk fat, and decreased percentages of milk fat (from 4.43 to 4.37 per cent) and milk proteins (from 3.49 to 3.42 per cent). The main differences are due to the construction, design and cleaning of milking robots and cooling tanks (Klungel *et al.*, 1998).

Working and utilization of a milking robot were studied in a herd of 40 cows during the first 12 weeks of lactation (Pomies *et al.*, 1998). After a training period, cows had free access to the robot for 18 hours/day. During starting phase, frequency of breakdown of the robot was 1.4 times/week, the rate of automatic attachment of the cluster when a cow entered the robot was 80 per cent (70 per cent within the first two attempts) and manual attachment was 2.6 per cent. Five cows were removed from the robot due to problems on the front right quarter (reference for attachment of

Table 26.2 Recommendations for sizes of milking pipelines. Source: O'Callaghan *et al.* (1982).

Number of units	Minimum bore of milking pipeline (mm)
2–5	31
6–8	38
9–20	50

cluster). The number of daily milkings was 2.4 and the daily milk yield was 27.9 kg. Clinical mastitis and milk composition and quality were similar to normal values of the herd, except for butyric acid bacterial counts, which were three times higher in the robotic-milked cows.

Automatic cluster removers

Automatic cluster removers (ACRs) are an important development in eliminating overmilking and improving labour efficiency. Persistent and excessive overmilking can cause external damage to the teat, which may increase the susceptibility to udder infection (Shepherd, 1985). However, ACRs are not recommended in two stalls per unit herringbone parlours. Limited overmilking does not increase new infection rate. ACRs do not reduce the work routine time, unless operators have been spending time moving up and down the pit to remove clusters as soon as cows have stopped milking. ACRs improve throughput in rotary parlours, provided teat disinfection is automated; in this case one operator less is needed. ACRs which admit air blasts into the claw (to activate the automatic shut-off) at cluster removal should not be used (O'Shea *et al.*, 1984). Ramussen (1993) showed that early cluster removal (400 g/min), when compared to normal level for cluster removal (200 g/min), decreased machine-on time by 0.5 minutes, increased average milk flow rates slightly, improved teat condition significantly and reduced the change in teat end thickness during milking of first lactation cows. Early removal did not affect milk yield or composition or the incidence of subclinical mastitis.

Large-bore pipelines

These are used in the USA, where it is not uncommon to see milk lines of 75 mm (3 inches) in diameter. At present, standards for sizes of pipelines are recommended by the International Dairy Federation (Table 26.2). At a National Mastitis Council Meeting in the USA, it was stated that the American standards for 38 mm (1½ inches) and 50 mm (2 inches) pipes are rea-sonable, while the 62 mm (2½ inches) and 75 mm (3 inches) may not have been thoroughly evaluated (Spencer, 1981).

High- and low-line plants

Milking systems can be divided into two types depending on the level of the milking pipeline in relation to the cow's udder. Where the milking pipeline is above the udder it is called a high line and a low line if it is below the udder.

Midi-level pipelines (1.2 to 1.5 m above cow standing level) are recommended. Very high pipelines increase the level of cyclic fluctuations at the teat end (Thiel *et al.*, 1968). Low-level pipelines (under the cow standing level) decrease fluctuations and increase milking rates by 3 to 8 per cent (Phillips & Copeman, 1969). However, low-level plants are susceptible to contamination by urine and faeces. In herringbone parlours one unit must be used per stall, which is only 60 per cent as efficient as two stalls per unit (O'Callaghan *et al.*, 1982). In midi-level pipeline plants vacuum fluctuations are reduced by having air admission holes in the claw (Thiel *et al.*, 1968) but if these holes are not kept patent mastitis levels are likely to increase (Hopkirk *et al.*, 1943).

Liner design

Liner design can have a greater effect on milking characteristics than any other machine factor. Six-fold differences in strip yield, eight-fold differences in the incidence of liner slips and 33 per cent differences in milking times between liner types have been reported.

Machine-induced congestion and oedema is reduced by milking with a 'narrow-bore' liner with a soft mouthpiece. The internal diameter of a liner is usually measured at a point 75 mm below the mouthpiece. Liners should have a barrel diameter about 1–2 mm less than the average diameter of the teats after milk letdown (approximately 21–22 mm). Liners should be designed to fit teatcup shells. The mouthpiece should not be distorted by the shell, but the liner should be held firmly enough not to twist easily in the shell. Teatcup shells should all be the same length (within 2 mm) to ensure uniform liner tension and to distribute the cluster weight more evenly between the four quarters (National Mastitis Council, 1996).

In North America narrow liners with a supple mouth are preferred, as these are thought to reduce the risk of oedema of the teats. It is considered that the diameter of the liner should be 1–2 mm less than that of the teat after milking, thus providing sufficient friction between the liner and the teat. The liner should also be long enough to enclose the teat completely. The liner must be well aligned in the teatcup. Liners may be made from natural rubber, synthetic rubber, silicone or a mixture of these products; the material used will largely determine the lifetime of the liner (Levesque, 1998). Most manufacturers recommend that rubber liners are used for between 2000 and 2500 cow milkings and then changed. The recommended life of silicone liners is 5000 cow milkings or 5 months – whichever comes first. Theoretically they have a longer life than rubber liners as silicone does not absorb fat. However, in practice they are more susceptible to tearing and puncturing than rubber liners and are likely to split if cows step on them, as well as being three to four times more expensive.

Backflushing

Liners are a potent method of disseminating pathogens both within and between cows. The number of pathogens recoverable from liners after milking infected cows is related to the number of bacteria in milk from the infected cow. Consequently, it is recommended that clusters should be disinfected between the milking of infected cows. The most common practice is to dip the cluster in a disinfectant solution for a couple of seconds. Such a practice generally reduces the number of pathogens transferred from cow to cow. However, such practice has often been rendered ineffective because contamination of milk neutralized the disinfectant solution, air locks within the cluster prevented entry of the disinfectant or the milker failed to carry out the procedure correctly.

Results from studies carried out at NIRD (Neave, 1971) indicated that circulating water at 85°C through the cluster for at least 5 seconds is the best way to achieve near sterilization of liners between milkings, although a cold hypochlorite flush reduced numbers of bacteria to very low numbers (Table 26.3).

Laboratory experiments showed a large reduction in bacteria (about 99 per cent) after backflushing with cold water (Jasper & Bushnell, 1978) and an initial flushing with an iodine disinfectant appeared to give better results. The authors concluded that even though complete sterility may not be achieved, backflushing should be helpful in reducing cow-to-cow transfer of pathogens on liners. Around this time automatic backflushing systems using cold water rinses with or without a chemical disinfectant between cold rinses were developed.

Eriksen and Rasmussen (1994) carried out a 9-week experiment with 283 cows in two groups, a control and an experimental group. The teatcup liners of the experimental group were backflushed with the Airwash system between milking each cow. The liners were flushed with a combination of compressed air and lukewarm water through small inlet valves placed in the short milk tube. The flushing sequence was water for 4s and compressed air for 2s, repeated for 30–40s. Automatic backflushing of liners reduced the total bacteria count by 50 per cent, coliforms by 68 per cent and *Staphylococcus aureus* by 61 per cent without having any effect on udder health and somatic cell count.

Table 26.3 Disinfection of teatcup clusters after removal from cows with mastitis. Source: Neave (1971), reproduced with permission of The British Cattle Veterinary Association.

Treatment of cluster	Time	No. tested	% positive after disinfection	No. of *Staph. aureus* recovered per cluster
Cold water flush	5s	19	100	100 000–800 000
Cold hypochlorite circulation (0.03%)	3min	19	100	50–2000
Circulation of water at 66°C	3min	18	22	0–80
Circulation of water at 74°C	3min	85	0	0
Circulation of water at 85°C	5s	530	3	0–15

Table 26.4 A comparison of teat disinfection methods. Source: Anon (1983).

	Dipping	Hand spraying	Auto spraying
Time taken (min/cow)	0.08–0.10	0.04–0.08	Nil
Teat-end coverage (%)	95–100	79–97	96–99
Volume used (ml/cow)	5–10	10–13	30
Chemical type	Various	Iodophor	Dilute hypochlorite

Automatic teat disinfection

Several automatic teat disinfection systems are available. These are fitted to the exit race of the parlour and consist of a pressure spray unit fitted with a set of nozzles. The spray is activated by an electronic control unit, which detects the presence of the cow (Hunter, 1985). Table 26.4 shows that with automatic teat spraying it is possible to achieve as good coverage as dipping. Automatic spraying will use more chemical. However, as it is outside the parlour it is possible to use the much cheaper chemical hypochlorite.

Control measures

The milking machine is only one component that can be involved in mastitis. Mastitis control involves continued implementation of each of the recommendations in the five-point control programme. Changing some of the components in the milking machine may help in the short term, but only a concerted effort in carrying out the full programme will control mastitis in a herd in the long run.

The following points are recommendations that should help to reduce mastitis resulting from the milking machine:

- Maintain proper vacuum levels.
- Attach and remove clusters properly to minimize massive changes in vacuum and resulting from entry of air into the clawpiece.
- Make sure clusters are attached properly on each cow.
- Select liners with low slip characteristics. Replace rubber liners every 2500 milkings or every 6 months, whichever comes first, and siliconized at 5000 milkings or every 5 months, whichever comes first.
- Dry teats before attaching clusters in order to reduce the number of bacteria.
- Have the machine tested at least once a year.

References

Anon. (1983) Effectiveness of teat spraying. *Dairy Farmer*, **30**, 26.

Baxter, J.D., Eberhart, R.J., Spencer, S.B. & Rogers, G.W. (1990) Effect of milking machine liner slip on new intra-mammary infection. *Journal of Dairy Science*, **73**(Suppl. 1), 258.

Cousins, C.L. (1972) *The relationship between the milking machine and new intramammary infection*. PhD thesis, University of Reading.

Cousins, C.L., Thiel, C.C., Westgarth, D.R. & Higgs, T.M. (1973) Further short-term studies of the influence of the milking machine on the rate of new mastitis infections. *Journal of Dairy Research*, **40**, 289–92.

Eriksen, L. & Rasmussen, M.D. (1994) Automatic backflushing of teatcup liners by the Airwash system. [Danish] Effekten af afskylning af pattekopperne med Airwash-systemet pa bakterieforekomst og yversundhed. Forskningsrapport fra Statens Husdyrbrugsforsog. Statens Husdyrbrugsforsog, Tjele, Denmark: 1994. No. 25.

Griffin, T.K. (1985) The use of valve clawpieces in the control of mastitis. In *Proceedings of the International Dairy Federation Seminar Progress in the Control of Mastitis*, Kiel, Germany, p. 625.

Griffin, T.K., Bramley, A.J., & Dodd, F.H. (1980b) Milking machine modifications in the control of bovine mastitis. In *Proceedings of the International Workshop on Machine Milking and Mastitis*, Moorepark, pp. 19–29.

Griffin, T.K., Grindal, R.J., Staker, R.T., Shearn, M.F.H., Bramley, A.J., Simpkin, D.L., Higgs, T.M. & Westgarth, D.R. (1982) Development and evaluation of control techniques for bovine mastitis. Control of intramammary infection by modification of the design of the milking machine. Report of the National Institute for Research in Dairying, Reading, pp. 37–8.

Griffin, T.K., Mein, G.A., Westgarth, D.R., Neave, F.K., Thompson, W.H. & Maguire, P.D. (1980a) Effect of deflector shields fitted in the milking machine teat cup liner on bovine udder disease. *Journal of Dairy Research*, **47**, 1–9.

Grindal, R.J. (1987) Effect of ball-valve milking clusters on udder disease. *Veterinary Record*, **121**, 250–2.

Grindal, R.J. & Griffin, T.K. (1989) Effect of hydraulic milking on milking performance, teat condition and lipolysis. *Journal of Dairy Research*, **56**, 45–53.

Hopkirk, C.S.M., Palmer-Jones, T. & Whittlestone, W.G. (1943) The effect of closed air admission holes on the health of the udder of dairy cows. *New Zealand Journal of Agriculture*, **66**, 30–1.

Hunter, A.C. (1985) Milking Routine. In *Hygienic Milk Production*. The Scottish Milk Marketing Board, p. 42.

Ipema, B. Smits, D. & Jagtenberg, C. (1998) Practical experiences with milking robots. [Dutch] Praktijkervaringen met melkrobots. *Praktijkonderzoek Rundvee, Schapen en Paarden*, **11**, 37–9.

Jasper, D.E. & Bushnell, R.B. (1978) Influence of premilking sanitation on transfer of infection during milking. In *Proceedings of the International Symposium on Milking Machines and Mastitis*, 17th Annual Meeting of the National Mastitis Council, Louisville, Kentucky, pp. 231–41.

Klungel, G., Slaghuis, B. & Hogeveen, H. (1998) Milk quality after the use of milking robots requires attention. [Dutch] Melkkwaliteit bij automatisch melken verdient aandacht. *Praktijkonderzoek Rundvee, Schapen en Paarden*, **11**, 33–6.

Levesque, P. (1998) Teatcup liners. (French) Les manchons trayeurs. *Producteur de Lait Quebecois*, **18**, 34–6.

Mein, G.A. (1984) Simple 'on-farm' checks of a milking machine installation. Interpretation of machine test report forms. Seminar for Veterinarians on Milking Machines and Mastitis, Werribee, Australia.

National Mastitis Council (1996) Liner design influences milking characteristics. In *Udder Topics*, August 1996.

Neave, F.K. (1971) The control of mastitis by hygiene. In *The Control of Bovine Mastitis* (ed. by F.H. Dodd & E.R. Jackson). British Cattle Veterinary Association, Reading, p. 55.

Nyhan, J.F. (1968) The effect of vacuum fluctuations on udder disease. In *Proceedings of the Symposium on Machine Milking*, Reading, pp. 71–82.

Nyhan, J.F. & Cowhig, M.J. (1967) Inadequate milking machine vacuum reserve and mastitis. *Veterinary Record*, **81**, 122–5.

O'Callaghan, E., O'Shea, J., Kavanagh, A.J. & Doyle, H.J. (1982) Machine milking and milking facilities. *An Foras Taluntais*, p. 24.

O'Callaghan, E., O'Shea, J., Meaney, W.J. & Crowley, C. (1976) Effect of milking machine vacuum fluctuations and liner slip on bovine mastitis infectivity. *Irish Journal of Agricultural Research*, **15**, 401–17.

O'Shea, J. (1982) Milking machines – the function and performance of components. *Irish Veterinary Journal*, **36**, 78–87.

O'Shea, J. & O'Callaghan, E. (1978) Milking machine effects on new infection rate. In *Proceedings of the International Symposium on Milking Machines and Mastitis*, 17th Annual Meeting of the National Mastitis Council, Louisville, Kentucky, pp. 262–8.

O'Shea, J. & O'Callaghan, E. (1982) The effect of liner slip on mastitis infection rates. In *Proceedings of the Conference on Dairy Production from Pasture*, New Zealand Society of Animal Production, Hamilton, pp. 77–8.

O'Shea, J., O'Callaghan, E. & Leonard, R.O. (1980) Milking performances of commercial clusters with standard pulsation. In *Experiments on Milking Machine Components, Moorepark, 1976–1979*, pp. 40–64.

O'Shea, J., O'Callaghan, E. & Meaney, W.J. (1979) Relationship between milking machine and the incidence of mastitis in dairy cows. *Irish Journal of Agricultural Research*, **18**, 225–35.

O'Shea, J., O'Callaghan, E. & Meaney, W.J. (1981) Incidence of new infection rate in dairy cows subjected to solenoid-induced air blasts during milking. *Irish Journal of Agricultural Research*, **20**, 163–83.

O'Shea, J., O'Callaghan, E., Meaney, W.J. & Crowley, C. (1976) Effects of combinations of large and small irregular and cyclic vacuum fluctuations in the milking machine on the rate of new udder infection in dairy cows. *Irish Journal of Agricultural Research*, **15**, 377–99.

O'Shea, J., O'Callaghan, E. & Walsh, J.P. (1984) Machine Milking Research. In *Moorepark 25th Anniversary Publication, Part II: Animal Health and Machine Milking*, pp. 166–8.

Phillips, D.S.M. & Copeman, P.J.A. (1969) Some recent research on milking machine design. *Proceedings of the New Zealand Society of Animal Production*, **29**, 26–36.

Pomies, D., Vimal, T., Bony, J. & Coulon, J.B. (1998) Introduction of a milking robot on an experimental farm: first results obtained at INRA. [French] Mise en place d'un robot de traite dans une ferme experimentale: premiers resultats obtenus a l'INRA. *Rencontres Recherches Ruminants*, No. 5, 335–8.

Rabold, K. & Picher, D. (1980) Some environmental influences on mastitis of cows in South Germany. In *Proceedings of the International Workshop on Milking Machines and Mastitis*, Moorepark, pp. 121–7.

Rasmussen, M.D. (1993) Influence of switch level of automatic cluster removers on milking performance and udder health. *Journal of Dairy Research*, **60**, 287–97.

Rogers, G.W. & Spencer, S.B. (1991) Relationships among udder and teat morphology and milking characteristics. *Journal of Dairy Science*, **74**, 4189–94.

Schon, H., Wendl, G. & Liebler, J. (1997) Use of automatic milking systems in dairying. [German] Einsatz automatischer Melksysteme in der Milchviehhaltung. *Landtechnik*, **52**, 322–3.

Shepherd, H.M. (1985) Milking equipment. In *Hygienic Milk Production*. The Scottish Milk Marketing Board, p. 64.

Smith, V.R. & Peterson, W.E. (1946) The effect of increasing the negative pressure and widening the vacuum release ratio on the rate of removal of milk from the udder. *Journal of Dairy Research*, **29**, 45–53.

Spencer, S.B. (1981) Sizing milking systems – a review. Annual Meeting of the National Mastitis Council, pp. 141–6.

Spencer, S.B. (1991) Effect of vacuum and milking machine liners on liner slip. *Journal of Dairy Science*, **74**, 429–32.

Thiel, C.C., Clough, P.A., Westgarth, D.R. & Akam, D.M. (1968) Factors affecting vacuum within the teat-cup liner during milking. *Journal of Dairy Research*, **35**, 303–16.

Thiel, C.C., Cousins, C.L., Westgarth, D.R. & Neave, F.K. (1973) The incidence of some physical characteristics of the milking machine on the rate of new infection. *Journal of Dairy Research*, **40**, 117–29.

Chapter 27
Skin Infections of the Bovine Teat and Udder and Their Differential Diagnosis

J.K. Shearer, J.R. Townsend and E.P.J. Gibbs

Introduction	363
Infectious lesions of the teat	363
Bovine herpes mammillitis (BHM)	363
Pseudocowpox	364
Papillomatosis (teat warts)	365
Cowpox	365
Vesicular stomatitis	366
Laboratory diagnosis	366
Diagnostic techniques	366
Treatment	367
Prevention and control	367
Non-infectious lesions of the teat end	367
Introduction	367
Theleitis	368
Teat trauma	368
Chemical injury	369
Environmental injury	369
Milking-machine-induced teat lesions	370
Insect-induced teat lesions	370
Differential diagnosis of skin lesions of the bovine teat	370

Introduction

Teat lesions in milking cattle are due to a variety of causes, infectious and non-infectious. Viral skin infections of the bovine teat and udder are principally due to pseudocowpox virus, bovine herpesvirus 2 and papillomavirus, but, on occasions, teat lesions may occur in association with a generalized viral infection, such as foot-and-mouth disease, vesicular stomatitis, or mucosal disease. Although the vernacular use of 'cowpox' to describe any teat infection is common, cowpox (as caused by cowpox virus) is an unusual disease and has been recognized only in Europe. There are several bacterial and non-infectious skin conditions of the teats and udder that can be equally as troublesome as viral infections. Irrespective of cause, when teat infections occur in a milking herd they predispose cattle to secondary bacterial infection by *Staphylococcus aureus*, *Streptococcus dysgalactiae* and other bacteria. Cows, and particularly newly calved heifers, become difficult to milk and the milking time may be prolonged by as much as 50 per cent.

Currently, there are no vaccines in use to protect cattle from any of the viral teat diseases and treatment is palliative. Differentiation of the diseases affecting the teats and skin of the udder is important, however, for reasons of public health and exotic disease control; cowpox and pseudocowpox are zoonotic diseases causing skin infections that can affect milking personnel or herdspersons and any vesicular lesions on the teats should always raise suspicion of foot-and-mouth disease.

In this chapter, particular attention is given to bovine herpes mammillitis and pseudocowpox, the two diseases that cause greatest concern to dairy farmers in the industrial nations of the world.

Infectious lesions of the teat

(see Table 27.1)

Bovine herpes mammillitis (BHM)

Aetiology

Bovine herpes mammillitis (BHM) is caused by bovine herpesvirus 2 and is closely related, if not identical, to Allerton virus (p. 887), the causative agent of pseudolumpy skin disease; it is unrelated to bovine herpes virus 1, the aetiological agent of infectious bovine rhinotracheitis.

The genome is linear double-stranded DNA, 220 kbp. The virus produces intranuclear inclusions and syncytia in infected cells.

Epidemiology

Also known as bovine ulcerative mammillitis, BHM was first recognized in Scotland. The virus has since been isolated from affected cattle worldwide in countries such as the USA, Australia and Brazil.

In the northern hemisphere, BHM commonly occurs as a seasonal disease between August and December. In a completely susceptible herd, the disease spreads quickly with nearly all cows developing infection over one to two months. In other herds, only the newly calved heifers introduced into the milking herd for the first time are affected. Recrudescence of clinical disease

Table 27.1 Infectious conditions of the teat and udder skin of cattle.

Cowpox and vaccinia
Pseudocowpox
Bovine herpes mammillitis (BHM)
Bovine papillomatosis (warts)
As part of generalized disease, e.g.
foot-and-mouth disease
rinderpest
lumpy skin disease
mycotic dermatitis

is unusual, even though latent infections do occur. Whether latently infected older cattle are the reservoir of infection from which the newly calved heifers become infected is conjectural. It is thought that susceptible pregnant cows may become infected some time before parturition, but do not develop the lesions until calving.

The method of transmission of the virus between farms with closed herds is unknown, although biting flies have been incriminated as possible vectors.

Clinical signs and lesions

Bovine herpes mammillitis is a disease initially characterized by a painful oedematous teat swelling. The incubation period ranges from three to seven days. The disease is generally more severe than either cowpox or pseudocowpox and the lesions are ulcerative rather than proliferative. Newly calved heifers are usually the most severely affected, particularly if they have postparturient oedema of the udder. Initial lesions are followed by the development of an irregularly shaped vesicle (0.5–5.0 cm in diameter) (Plate 27.1). Within 24 hours, the vesicles rupture, leaving an ulcerated surface that exudes copious serum (Plate 27.2). Upon drying, this exudate forms a thick, dark reddish-brown scab (Plates 27.3 and 27.4). In the absence of secondary infection, healing is complete in three weeks by granulation and regrowth of the epithelium (Plates 27.5–27.8). Lesions on the udder may coalesce with those of the teat and may extend to the perineum resulting in vulvovaginitis as a sequel to infection of the skin of the mammary gland.

Differential diagnosis

Bovine herpes mammallitis usually occurs in summer and autumn. The oedema of teats, vesication and ulceration and extensive scab formation over most of the teat surface are strongly suggestive of BHM. Epidemics of BHM can occur in a region, which can lend support to the diagnosis.

Pseudocowpox

Aetiology

Initially confused with cowpox virus, it was not until 1963 that it was demonstrated in the USA that pseudocowpox virus was a member of the genus *Parapoxvirus*. Pseudocowpox virus is closely related to the virus of orf (contagious ecthyma, contagious pustular dermatitis) of sheep, and also to the bovine papular stomatitis virus.

The virus contains a linear double-stranded DNA, 130 kpb, and produces intracytoplasmic inclusions in infected cells.

Epidemiology

Referred to in the past as false cowpox, varicella, waterpox, udderpox and natural cowpox, pseudocowpox occurs in most countries of the world. It is the most common infectious cause of teat lesions in North America and the UK. Lesions of pseudocowpox may be seen in a herd during any season of the year. The immunity is short-lived, lasting four to six months; thus, pseudocowpox is commonly seen as a chronic problem in most herds. Although herd morbidity may reach 100 per cent, only 5–10 per cent of the herd may be infected at any one time. Nevertheless, it may occur as an acute herd problem, which spreads rapidly affecting a majority of the cows in the herd. Lesions in such primary outbreaks are frequently more extensive.

Clinical signs and lesions

The clinical presentation of pseudocowpox is variable. Usually no systemic illness is noted and vesicle formation may not be observed. After an incubation period of about six days, localized erythematous and oedematous areas appear on the teats. These lesions are painful, making cows difficult to milk. Within 38 hours, a small orange papule develops, followed by the formation of an elevated small dark red scab (2–3 mm) (Plate 27.9). In some cases, a vesicle will form in the centre of the papule, but this is rare with pseudocowpox in contrast to bovine herpes mammillitis. The progressive enlargement of the edges of the lesions (Plate 27.10) leads to umbilication of the central scab. Healing of the lesion is centrifugal and the primary scab is often shed after 10 to 12 days, leaving the classical raised 'horseshoe' or 'ring' lesion, which is pathognomonic for pseudocowpox (Plate 27.11). As adjacent lesions enlarge, they may coalesce to form linear scabs extending the entire length of the teat (Plate 27.12). Pseudocowpox lesions are primarily found on the teat; however, 5–10 per cent of affected animals develop lesions on the udder. Healing usually occurs within four to five weeks, leaving no scars.

In herds where 'teat chaps' are common, pseudocowpox virus can be detected in many of the lesions.

In humans, pseudocowpox virus causes localized infection on the fingers or hands, commonly called 'milker's nodule'. These nodules are painful and may extend to the entire arm of the person affected.

Differential diagnosis

In contrast to BHM, pseudocowpox is a chronic problem in most herds. Lesions are proliferative, progressing to small 'ring' or horseshoe' type lesions rather than ulcerative. Atypical lesions (Plates 27.13–16) may be observed and confused with warts or mild traumatic injuries to the teats and udder but, in general, a careful examination of the herd will allow the clinician to differentiate pseudocowpox from other diseases. It must be remembered that pseudocowpox is often present in herds where the major problem may be due to BHM or even cowpox.

Papillomatosis (teat warts) (see p. 882)

Aetiology

Bovine teat papillomatosis (teat warts) is a common finding of dairy cattle throughout the world. The causative agents of teat warts are several distinct strains of bovine papilloma virus (BPV). The strains most commonly implicated are BPV-1, BPV-5 and BPV-6. These strains of BPV are classified as members of one of two subgroups. Strains in subgroup-A, which include BPV-1 and BPV-5, produce warts with both dermal and epithelial components (fibropapillomas). Subgroup-B strains, of which BPV-6 is a member, produce warts with only epithelial proliferation (papillomas). The virus contains a closed, circular, double-stranded DNA approximately 8000 bp in size.

Epidemiology

The method of infection is thought to be similar to other bovine cutaneous warts in that transmission is by direct contact with infected animals or fomites. The virus needs cutaneous damage, such as abrasions, to gain entry into susceptible tissue. After infection occurs, incubation times of 1 to 6 months have been demonstrated under experimental conditions. Abattoir studies have shown that teats often have multiple warts and that prevalence increases with increasing parity.

Clinical signs and lesions

Because of the tendency of BPV strains to produce morphologically distinct warts, presumptive identification of the causative BPV strain of a teat wart may be possible through gross examination. BPV-1 has been demonstrated to be responsible for fibropapillomas of the penis and teats. The teat warts have a filamentous or frond-like appearance. These warts are normally seen on younger animals and will typically regress over a period of 1–12 months. BPV-5 produces small 'rice grain' fibropapillomas, so named because of their white and elongated appearance. These warts are seen in cattle of all ages, and, if natural regression occurs, it does so over periods of greater than a year. The warts produced by BPV-6 are papillomas that have a frond appearance and are considered the most common type of teat papilloma. These frond papillomas may regress, usually in a time frame of greater than a year.

Cowpox

Aetiology

Cowpox virus shares with Jenner a central role in the development of vaccines and the control of smallpox in man. The current use of vaccinia virus (the derivative virus used for protection of man from smallpox) in a new role as a recombinant vaccine vector for many diseases, maintains attention on cowpox. Few people realize that cowpox was considered an unusual disease even in Jenner's time. Occasional outbreaks of cowpox still occur in Europe, but from the perspective of the dairy industry they are of little importance.

The causative agent of the cowpox is an orthopoxvirus, very similar to, but distinguishable from, vaccinia virus by its biological properties in laboratory animals and its larger genome (220 kbp compared with 185 kbp for vaccinia virus). The virus produces intracytoplasmic inclusions in affected cells.

Epidemiology

The epidemiology of cowpox is unknown. Cowpox virus has been isolated from skin infections in man and carnivores in which no direct contact with cattle could be established. It is currently thought that rodents are reservoirs of the virus.

Once infection is present within a herd, however, the disease appears to spread by the milking machine and the hands of milkers. Between and within herds, biting insects may also be responsible for mechanical transmission. At present, the disease is confined to western Europe. In other areas of the world, outbreaks of teat lesions, clinically indistinguishable from cowpox but caused by vaccinia virus from an uncovered vaccination site in an attendant, have been reported. Since the eradication of smallpox in 1979, most countries have discontinued vaccination against smallpox, although military personnel and others are now vaccinated because of the threat of bioterrorism. Currently, there is little likelihood of vaccinia infections occurring naturally on the teats of cattle in most parts of the world, but if widespread use of vaccinia recombinants becomes popular, either in man or domestic animals, a resurgence in vaccinia mammillitis in cattle is conceivable.

Clinical signs and lesions

The incubation period is approximately five days, after which an irregular prodromal fever and tenderness of the teats is noticed. A roseolar erythema occurs at the site of future pock development: oedema may be localized to the area of the erythema or may involve the whole teat. A vesicle forms three to four days after the initial onset of signs (Plate 27.17) and rapidly progresses to a pustule, which subsequently ruptures and suppurates (Plate 27.18). The classical development of a thick red scab ranging in size from 1 to 2 cm in diameter and said to be pathognomonic for cowpox may now form (Plate 27.19), but more frequently an ulcerated surface is observed (Plate 27.20). Healing is centripetal and, in uncomplicated cases, takes place within three weeks. Immunity to reinfection is said to be lifelong.

Vesicular stomatitis (see p. 710)

Aetiology

Vesicular stomatitis (VS) is a sporadic disease of cattle in the US, but is endemic in other areas of the western hemisphere. VS is caused by a vesiculovirus of the family Rhabdoviridae. Vesicular stomatitis virus has a genome that consists of a single-stranded, negative-sense RNA approximately 11 kbp in length.

Epidemiology

The epidemiology of vesicular stomatitis virus is not completely understood at this time. The disease is seen most commonly in the form of sporadic outbreaks, but the inter-epidemic host is, as yet, unknown. Outbreaks are seen less frequently in more temperate climates and after the first frost of the year. The virus is probably transmitted by direct contact with contaminated milking equipment, ingestion of contaminated materials, and a number of different biting insects. The antibodies produced by natural infection seem to provide little protection from reinfection. Persistent viral infection has been theorized, but has not been clearly demonstrated.

Clinical signs and lesions

Following an incubation period of only 24–48 hours, fever and vesicle formation will be observed in cattle infected by vesicular stomatitis virus. The vesicles will develop into erosions on the mouth (especially the tongue), teats and, rarely, the coronary band. The oral lesions will lead to the clinical signs of excessive salivation and feed refusal. The teat lesions produced by VS are often indistinguishable from those produced by foot-and-mouth disease. For this reason, VS is considered of great regulatory importance.

Laboratory diagnosis

Sample collection

An accurate diagnosis of the cause of teat lesions may be possible with a thorough examination of both affected and apparently healthy cows within a herd (or group in larger herds). However, for a definitive diagnosis, laboratory confirmation is required. An accurate laboratory diagnosis requires adequate tissue samples to be submitted. For submitting good quality samples when a virus is suspected as the causative agent, the clinician should remember the following guidelines.

- During the early stages of the disease, the titre of the virus is highest at the affected sites.
- Viruses require living cells and may be inactivated by disinfectants, light exposure, pH extremes and desiccation.
- Secondary bacterial infection of skin samples is common in later stages of the diseases.
- Skin scrapings should come from animals with early lesions and be transported on cold packs.
- Samples for virus isolation should be collected into virus transport media and transported on cold packs.
- To avoid erroneous results, more than one animal and multiple lesions should be sampled.
- An area that will be collected as a skin scraping or biopsy should be washed with saline, not alcohol (alcohol will inactivate the viruses).
- Scrapings should extend to the periphery and base of a lesion.

A wide range of laboratory tests may be used for making the diagnosis of the viral agent responsible for a teat lesion. Brief descriptions of common diagnostic laboratory tests are included below.

Diagnostic techniques

Electron microscopy

Electron microscopy has emerged as a very accurate and useful test for practitioners. The advantages of electron microscopy include a rapid diagnosis and the ability to detect non-viable virus and combined viral infections.

Tissue culture

Virus isolation using tissue culture is an alternative if electron microscopy is not available. Acceptable samples may be derived from early scabs, vesicular fluid or scrapings of the raw surface of lesions. Some strains of pseudocowpox may fail to grow *in vitro*, but vaccinia virus can be distinguished from cowpox virus on tissue culture.

Histological identification

Collection of a biopsy of a teat lesion is seldom easy. If one is collected, the tissue should be preserved in 10 per cent formol saline or preferably Bouin's solution. Each of the infections discussed above has a characteristic histopathology if an early lesion is sampled. Combined with immunohistochemistry, this technique is useful for the differentiation of the specific causative strain of BPV responsible for teat warts. The disadvantage of this diagnostic technique is the difficulty in collecting a teat biopsy and the necessity of an early lesion of sampling.

Paired serum samples

Paired serum samples collected during the acute stage of the infection and 14 days later may provide a diagnosis. A diagnostic 4-fold rise in serum antibodies is observed in cowpox and BHM, but pseudocowpox generally does not elicit a serological response. A primary problem with this test is that the cow may already be past the acute stage of the illness by the time she is tested. This is especially true of BHM, for which acute stage serum samples must be taken within two days of the appearance of lesions. For practical purposes, however, a clinical diagnosis of BHM may be made by the detection of high BHV-2 antibody titres in a single sample.

Treatment

There are many differing opinions on the treatment of ulcerative teat lesions produced by viruses. However, all the treatments have the similar primary therapeutic objectives of promoting healing and limiting secondary bacterial infection. Many treatment protocols rely on the use of different combinations of astringents and topical antibiotics. Topical corticosteroids and anaes-

thetic ointments have also been recommended, but in large herd outbreaks this type of treatment may be difficult to justify financially. Large multiple-use containers of ointments should be avoided, as they may become contaminated with virus and serve as a source of new infections. Strict hygiene must be followed if applying ointments by hand, as the hands of treatment personnel may transfer the infection to uninfected teats. A commonly recommended alternative therapy is the spraying of a teat dip containing emollients (such as 10 per cent glycerin) to reduce bacterial and viral numbers and soothe damaged skin.

Teat warts, on the other hand, may often go ignored until an increase in size interferes with milking and requires treatment. Surgical removal of the warts, either by excision or cryosurgery, may be effective. Autogenous and commercial vaccines have also been used as treatments, with varying degrees of success. Vaccine failures in the past were possibly due to a combination of using one strain of BPV to treat a lesion caused by a different strain and a lack of cross-protection between strains. Vaccination has been reported to be effective for the prevention of warts caused by BPV-1 and BPV-6, but not for BPV-5. Autogenous vaccines probably provide the best potential for success.

Prevention and control

Although the treatment of individual cows suffering from teat lesions is necessary, it is also important to institute prevention and control strategies within the herd. Ideally, new herd additions should be quarantined for at least 14 days before their introduction into the herd. All infected cows should be isolated or, more reasonably, milked last. All milking equipment should be thoroughly disinfected after use on an infected cow. Milkers should wear gloves in the parlour and disinfect the gloves between cows. Concerted efforts should be made to reduce the fly and insect population. Teat skin condition must be preserved by removing sources of trauma, including improperly functioning milking equipment and poorly maintained housing. Finally, the use of autogenous vaccines (such as in the case of papillomatosis) may provide some protective benefit.

Non-infectious lesions of the teat end (see Table 27.2)

Introduction

In addition to infectious lesions of the bovine teat and udder are those caused by traumatic events, chemical injury, environmental conditions, insects and the

Table 27.2 Non-infectious conditions of the teat and udder skin of cattle.

Traumatic, e.g.
    barbed wire
    grazing kale
    mud
    'treads'
Irritant chemicals, e.g.
    incorrect strength disinfectants
    any corrosive agent
Photosensitization
Excessive postparturient oedema
Milking machine induced
Insect induced

milking machine. As discussed earlier, teat lesions, regardless of cause, are frequently colonized by staphylococci and *Strep. dysgalactiae*. Lesions occurring at the teat end increase the risk of mastitis. Consequently, high new infection rates and increased numbers of clinical cases of mastitis are common sequelae in herds where lesions involving the teat end are prevalent (Plate 27.21). Lesions of the teat barrel are less likely to cause mastitis directly, but do cause greater milking difficulty. The increased risk of mastitis occurs more as an indirect response to the pain experienced by the cow during milking, resulting in reduced milkout and milking speed.

Theleitis

This is a non-specific condition of the inner wall of the teat often associated with inflammation due to traumatic injury or infectious conditions of the teat and udder. Inflammation involving the teat results in a thickening and hardening of the wall of the teat cistern that in the most severe scenario could lead to partial or complete occlusion of the teat. Theleitis is believed to be a significant, if not primary, reason for the development of non-functional teats or 'blind quarters'. However, a Florida study suggests that many blind quarters are due to non-mastitis/theleitis related factors. Blind quarters are generally described as those with an absence of mammary tissue or those which lack a functional teat or teat sphincter. Duraes *et al.* (1982) studied the incidence of blind quarters in 1177 first parturitions in a Florida herd where all five major dairy breeds (Holstein, Guernsey, Jersey, Brown Swiss and Ayrshire) plus Holstein–Guernsey cross-breds were represented. A total of 38 (3.2 per cent) heifers had 48 (1 per cent) blind quarters at calving. The highest incidence occurred in Holsteins. The other breeds including the cross-breds did not differ in frequency of occurrence. Adjusting production figures for length of record, cows with one blind quarter produced only 59 kg (130 lb) (1.7 per cent) less milk for the lactation. Despite the seemingly insignificant impact on performance, records indicated that animals with blind quarters were culled an average of 57 days earlier than herd mates.

Teat trauma (see p. 1127)

Traumatic lesions of the teat are most commonly the result of the cow stepping on her teats or wire cuts. They are a troublesome problem for the veterinarian as well as the dairyman. Histologically, the teat wall contains an abundance of elastic connective tissue that provides for expansion and contraction of the teat as it fills and evacuates milk in the lactating cow. The near constant movement associated with these physical dynamics of the teat combined with milking preparation procedures and milk collection complicate the normal process of healing.

The dairyman's challenge is in getting cows with teat lesions milked. Because these lesions are generally painful and cows resist preparation and milking procedures they are difficult if not hazardous to milk.

A further complication is mastitis. Teat lesions are readily colonized by bacteria and thus serve as an important reservoir of infection. Udder preparation cloths, hands of the milker and milking machine components facilitate the transfer of infectious organisms between quarters of the same cow and can be responsible for cow-to-cow transmission as well. Emphasis on milking hygiene procedures becomes crucial in control of new infections whenever teat lesions are present.

Depending on severity and the period of time prior to discovery, teat lacerations may be repaired surgically. Fresh superficial lacerations of the teat skin (within 12 hours of occurrence) in which the vascular supply has not been significantly damaged have the best prognosis. These are generally amenable to surgical closure. If, on the other hand, such lesions go unnoticed for a couple of days and become heavily contaminated, cleansing in mild disinfectant solution and removal of the skin flap tissue is likely to be the best therapeutic approach.

Teat lacerations (see Chapter 66) that extend into the teat cistern are of greater concern and generally carry a more guarded prognosis. Exposed edges of the teat cistern lining must be sutured using a suture pattern that will turn the edges inward creating an impervious seal. If this is not achieved healing cannot occur and draining fistulae will often develop. The teat wall muscle layers and skin may be closed separately. Most advise intramammary and/or systemic therapy for four to five days as a precaution against the development of mastitis. A protective bandage allowing access to the teat end for milking is recommended. Some suggest that milk be retrieved from the gland through the use of teat cannulas. Mastitis is a frequent secondary complication.

Pastured cattle have a lower incidence of teat trauma than confined cattle. Housing factors of primary importance are associated with the amount of space available to the cow for resting and rising. Further, individual cow characteristics and conformation increase the potential for teat trauma in some cows.

Chemical injury

Postmilking teat dipping is widely advocated for control and prevention of new mastitis infections. However, this practice has also increased the potential for chemical injury of teats and teat ends. The accidental or inadvertent use of concentrated udder wash or cleaning products in place of teat dip has been observed to cause serious teat lesions with a single application.

Teat lesions may also occur as a result of the application of an improperly mixed or defective teat-dip product. Iodophor-based teat dips, primarily because of their widespread use, are frequently the offenders. However, the problem has been observed with quaternary ammonium dips, chlorhexidine-based dips, dodecyl benzene sulfonic acid and hypochlorite teat dips. Lesions appear as dry, roughened, proliferative regions around the teat end that are usually discoloured by the teat dip. This discoloration may be present on 40–50 per cent of the teats in the affected herd. Changing to a dip with better conditioning properties will result in the rapid improvement of teat skin health.

In the case of the iodophor dips, problems have arisen secondary to freezing of the dip on farm or in transit. When these solutions freeze they separate, sending emollients to the bottom of the container while leaving excessive amounts of the active ingredients in a layer suspended above. The subsequent application of this concentrated iodine can cause teat irritation and lesions. Depending on the degree of insult these lesions can be quite severe.

Environmental injury

Teat chaps

Teat chapping is a common problem in the more temperate regions of the world where climatic conditions favouring dampness and cooler temperatures prevail. Activities associated with milking such as udder preparation, the milking process and postmilking teat dipping all exacerbate chapping problems. Chaps usually occur as horizontal cracks in the teat skin. Serum exudates from these cracks result in the formation of linear scabs (Plate 27.22). The surrounding teat skin may appear dry or leather-like and flake.

The primary significance of chaps is that they are readily colonized by staphylococci and *Strep. dysgalactiae* and thus constitute a threat to individual cows affected as well as the herd. Drying of the teats and udders before cows leave the milking parlour, particularly during inclement weather conditions, is an important preventive measure. Further, the use of teat-dip products containing hydroscopic skin softening agents such as glycerine or lanolin is helpful in controlling chapping problems.

Freezing or frost-bite

Initially, frozen teats will appear reddened or pale. If severe, the lesion progresses to the state where a scab forms over the distal half of the teat. In time, usually several days, this scab will loosen and fall off, exposing a raw, denuded teat end. As a second scab begins to develop the duct may become occluded. Milking becomes difficult and may require opening of the streak canal surgically.

In less severe cases, scab formation does not occur and cows become receptive to milking after only a few days. Cows immediately leaving the milking parlour with wet teats (from dip or milk) to areas with inadequate protection during cold weather may develop frost-bite on the teat ends. Freezing of the droplet on the teat end confines the lesion to the teat-end orifice area. The result is as described above for frozen teats.

Treatment consists of attempts at keeping the teat duct patent and preventing the development of mastitis. Severely affected cows may need to be culled. Drying of the teats and udder prior to exit from the milking parlour and provision of adequate wind breaks and shelter for milking cows is essential. The suspension of teat dipping procedures should be considered during extremely cold winters.

Sunburn

Severe reddening and drying of the teats and udder are observed in sunburn conditions, when blisters may form. Lesions are most severe on unpigmented skin or where the skin is devoid of hair. The application of moisturizers, ointments and salves to the affected areas is advised for treatment. For burns caused by fire see p. 934.

Photosensitization (see p. 884)

This condition occurs when photodynamic agents are eaten in their preformed state. Upon exposure to sunlight, the unpigmented skin areas develop an erythema and oedema, which results in severe lesions that most commonly appear on the lateral aspects of the teats and udder (Plate 27.23). Medial aspects of affected teats remain soft and cool. These lesions are highly susceptible to secondary bacterial infection.

Milking machine-induced teat lesions

The milking machine is assumed to be a major cause of teat lesions. However, most lesions associated with the milking machine are mild unless malfunction results in extremely high vacuum or pulsation failure. Damage may be by direct trauma to the teat or indirect, occurring over an extended period of time through the induction of degenerative changes in the teat. These changes in teat tissue health are primarily associated with circulatory disturbances, resulting in oedema and hyperkeratosis. Proper pulsation is essential for the circulation of blood and lymph in the teat. When normal circulation is disrupted teat-end health diminishes.

Direct damage to the teat may be caused by excessive milking vaccum, inadequate pulsation and careless use by the operator. Although rare, subcutaneous haemorrhages in the teat epithelium and prolapses of teat duct tissue are possible consequences with severe malfunctions of milking equipment or its use.

Calluses and hyperkeratosis of teat ends

Because of its appearance, hyperkeratosis of the teat end is often mistakenly diagnosed as a prolapsed sphincter. Hyperkeratosis of teat ends is a common finding in hand milked dairy cows as well as beef cattle. Histopathology of this material will confirm it to be excess keratin, which some refer to as callouses. These callouses may be rough or smooth and thus logically implicated as possible risk factors for mastitis. However, according to studies in the USA, the presence of hyperkeratatic lesions at the teat end had no effect on the prevalence of mastitis unless accompanied by erosions or scabs.

The exact cause of hyperkeratotic lesions in dairy cattle is unknown, but appears to be related to certain milking practices and milking-machine-related factors. For example, high levels of milk production and extended milking times, failure to apply appropriate premilking stimulation and overmilking increased the degree of lesions. Vacuum levels and pulsation ratios (within normal limits) had no effect on the degree of hyperkeratosis observed. On the other hand, a Wisconsin study indicated that hyperkeratosis of teat ends appeared to increase in relation to the compressive load of the milking machine liner.

Black spot

This condition is observed as a lesion of the tip of the teat commonly associated with excessive vacuum levels and overmilking. It is a particularly troublesome problem as the lesions are quite painful and frequently harbour mastitis pathogens, notably *Staphylococcus* sp. *Fusobacterium necrophorum* is also usually present in the lesions, but difficult to isolate. The specific location of this lesion at the tip of the teat end significantly increases the risk of mastitis in affected animals. Control of the condition requires correction of the predisposing cause and application of an effective teat dip containing emollients or other skin conditioning agents such as glycerol.

Insect-induced teat lesions

Summer mastitis is an acute suppurative disease of the non-lactating mammary gland (see Chapter 24). First described in Europe, it has been reported in the USA and other countries as well. It occurs sporadically throughout the year in Europe, with annual incidences in England and Wales estimated to be around 2 per cent of heifers and dry cows. In the USA, some estimate incidences of 5–6 per cent on certain farms during the summer months.

While some questions remain, in both the USA and Europe epidemics of summer mastitis have been coincident with periods of greatest fly challenge. Further, data indicate that effective fly control reduces disease incidence. These findings support the possibility of insect involvement. European data suggest that biting flies are responsible for the initial damage to the teat end and implicate the cattle fly, *Hydrotaea irritans*, as the infectious vector in summer mastitis (see Chapter 24).

Differential diagnosis of skin lesions of the bovine teat

The following is an aid to the diagnosis of lesions of the udder and teats in severely affected milking herds (see Table 27.3; Plates 27.1–32). With the exception of teat chapping and milking machine damage, the aetiology of which appears to be complex, most outbreaks of teat lesions in cows are due to three types of virus: (i) cowpox, (ii) pseudocowpox and (iii) BHM.

Table 27.3 The clinical appearance and diagnosis procedures for teat conditions (other than BHM, cowpox, bovine vaccinia mammillitis and pseudocowpox).

Condition	Clinical appearance	Confirmatory diagnostic procedure
Blackspot (Plate 27.27)	Scabby infection of teat orifice with *Fusobacterium necrophorum* but often other organisms	Isolation of *F. necrophorum* (often unsuccessful)
Chaps (teat) (see Plate 27.22)	Skin fissures often through dermis. Haemorrhage may occur with scab formation at the fissure edge. Often horizontal lesions	None. Parapox virus particles may be found but their importance unknown. Heavy bacterial contamination of lesion common
Folliculitis and impetigo	Pustule with surrounding erythema	Isolation of *Staphylococcus aureus*
Foot-and-mouth disease (see Plate 27.24)	Vesiculation of teat, buccal and interdigital mucosae. Pyrexia	Presence of virus. *Notifiable* in most countries
Mud abrasion (Plate 27.28)	Abrasions on lateral surface of the udder	
Photosensitization (see Plate 27.23)	Lesion progresses from erythema, oedema to serous exudation through skin. There is then necrosis, ulceration and scab formation. Pigmented areas of teat unaffected	
Ringworm (Plate 27.29)	Typical grey crusty lesions	Isolation of *Trichophyton verrucosum*
Theleitis and serous exudate from udder skin in peracute mastitis (Plate 27.30)	Teat swollen, painful with udder skin involved. Cow febrile and toxic	Isolation of bacteria
Vesicular stomatitis	Vesiculation of teat, buccal and interdigital mucosae	Virus isolation. As similar to foot-and-mouth may need to notify

Warts
  Filiform (Plate 27.31)
  White nodule (Plate 27.32)
	Pedunculated attachment to teat
	Broad attachment to teat. Variable in size. Some warts intermediate between filiform and nodule	

Accurate diagnosis is important for varius reasons. A major factor is the zoonotic potential of cowpox and pseudocowpox. Secondly, there is the need to differentiate foot-and-mouth disease as occasionally vesicles occur on the teats before their appearance in the mouth and foot (Plate 27.24).

When investigating an outbreak it is best to examine as many cattle as possible because the lesions in a single cow may not be typical. Often mixed disease occurs (Plates 27.25, 27.26) and an assessment of the development of lesions rather than just examination of the most severely affected cattle helps in the diagnosis.

On occasion the clinical appearance of the lesions can be modified by environmental factors, thereby making recognition of the condition difficult. Such factors include the teat cluster, mud or coloured teat dips. In these problems laboratory diagnosis becomes essential, although it is advisable in all disease investigations.

Reference

Duraes, M.C., Wilcox, C.J., Head, H.H. & Van Horn, H.H. (1982) Frequency and effects on production of blind quarters in first lactation dairy cows. *Journal of Dairy Science*, **65**, 1804–807.

Further reading

Farnsworth, R.L. (1996) Observations on teat lesions. In *Proceedings of the National Mastitis Council*, pp. 93–8.

Farnsworth, R.L. & Seiber, R.L. (1979) Relationship of teat end lesions to intramammary infections. In *Proceedings of the National Mastitis Council*, pp. 17–24.

Francis, P.G. (1984) Teat skin lesions and mastitis. *British Veterinary Journal*, **140**, 430–6.

Gibbs, E.P.J. (1984) Viral diseases of the skin of the bovine teat and udder. *Veterinary Clinics of North America. Large Animal Practice*, **6**, 187–202.

Gibbs, E.P.J., Johnson, R.H. & Osborne, A.D. (1970) The differential diagnosis of viral skin infections of the bovine teat. *Veterinary Record*, **87**, 602–609.

Gibbs, E.P.J. & Rweyemamu, M.M. (1977) Bovine herpesvirus, 1, 2 & 3. *Veterinary Bulletin*, **47**, 317–43, 411–25.

Sieber, R.L. & Farnsworth, R.J. (1978) The etiology of bovine teat lesions. In *Proceedings of the National Mastitis Council*, pp. 5–15.

Sieber, R.L. & Farnsworth, R.J. (1984) Differential diagnosis of bovine teat lesions. *Veterinary Clinics of North America. Large Animal Practice*, **6**, 313–21.

Chapter 28
Factors Affecting Milk Quality

R.W. Blowey and R.A. Laven

Introduction	373
Feeding and milk composition	373
Feeding before calving	373
Feed constituents	373
Dietary fat	375
Dietary protein	376
Feeding systems	376
Non-nutritional factors	377
Age of cow	377
Stage of lactation	377
Season of the year	377
Disease	377
Genetic variation	378
Management factors	378

Introduction

Most countries with a developed dairy industry now pay producers on the basis of both total volume sold and compositional quality, and with the slowly increasing move for a larger proportion of milk to be used for manufacturing, this trend is likely to continue. In addition, many countries also have a milk quota system and to maximize profitability, a farmer must produce a specified amount of milk of optimum quality. Much attention has therefore been paid to factors affecting milk quality, the most important aspects of which are reviewed in this chapter. The composition of average Friesian/Holstein milk is given in Fig. 28.1. Feeding has by far the greatest impact on milk quality and as such will be discussed first.

Feeding and milk composition

This is an extremely complex area to study, since it is often difficult to differentiate the separate effects of, for example, plane of nutrition, system of allocation of food, frequency of feeding and feed composition. Superimposed on this are effects of feeding before and after calving and the problem of differentiating between compositional values and overall yield. For example, in a high-yielding cow the milk fat content (g/kg milk) may be reduced, but the overall fat production (g/day) may be increased.

Feeding before calving

Severe underfeeding, leading to cows calving down in condition score 2 (overall scale 1–5, see p. 10) or less, will reduce milk yield, fat, protein and lactose and although these effects are greatest in early lactation, they will persist throughout it. The extent of the depression is approximately 20 g/kg (0.2 per cent) in milk fat and 10 g/kg in protein. Less severe underfeeding has little effect on milk protein, and provided that high quality diets are provided after calving, some of the effects on milk quality can be eliminated (Garnsworthy & Topps, 1982).

Feeding a high energy density diet (11.7 MJ/kg DM) precalving significantly increases milk fat concentration in early lactation; however, this effect does not persist and there is no significant effect on fat yield and no effect on protein concentration or yield.

Very fat cows have an increased fat content in their milk, and it has been estimated that milk fat increases by 2 g/kg for each 1.0 unit rise in condition score. This effect lasts for the first five to six weeks of lactation only, and is related to fat concentration only; indeed total fat *yield* is often depressed in very fat cows.

Feed constituents (see p. 112)

The greatest effect arises from the forage:concentrate ratio in the ration and its influence on milk fat content. Milk fat is synthesized from the fatty acids acetate and butyrate, products of the ruminal fermentation of forage and other feeds containing fibre. As the level of concentrates in the ration increases, the proportions of acetate and butyrate fall and that of propionate rises. There is also a decrease in ruminal pH and a depressed activity of cellulolytic degradation, which can eventually result in depressed dry matter (DM) intake. The extent of the depression varies with the materials being fed, but as an approximate guide, forage:concentrate ratios should not be allowed to fall below 60:40 (or 50:50 if fed as a total mixed ration). For example,

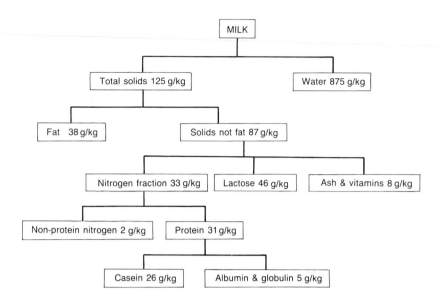

Fig. 28.1 The compositional quality of milk.

Table 28.1 Effect of proportion and type of concentrate in a mixed diet on milk production in early lactation. Source: Sutton *et al.* (1985).

	600 (g/kg diet)		700 (g/kg diet)	
	Starchy concentrate	Fibrous concentrate	Starchy concentrate	Fibrous concentrate
Consumed (kg air dry feed/day)				
Hay		7.2		3.5
Concentrates		10.8		14.0
Dietary ADF (g/kg DM)	192	231	136	180
Milk yield (kg/day)	26.3	26.5	32.0	25.5
Fat concentration (g/kg)	41.5	42.9	22.6	36.2
Fat yield (kg/day)	1.09	1.12	0.73	0.91

ADF, acid detergent fibre.

Sutton (1986) calculated that milk fat fell by 5 g/kg (0.05 per cent) for every 100 g/kg decrease in the proportion of hay in the diet, even when the overall energy content of the ration remained constant. However, there was a good deal of variation and probably a better way of estimating dietary effect is to express the overall fibre content of the diet on the basis of acid detergent fibre (ADF). Milk fat has been shown to fall when overall dietary ADF drops to below 200–250 g/kg DM. This is equivalent to approximately 450 g long forage/kg dietary DM, although on much higher forage diets, milk yield could be depressed.

The type of concentrate also has an effect. The energy fraction of a concentrate can be derived from four main sources, namely:

● Sugar, for example molasses.
● Starch, for example barley and maize.

● Digestible fibre, for example sugar-beet pulp, cotton seed, citrus pulp, etc.
● Fats and oils.

Table 28.1 (Sutton *et al.*, 1985) shows that concentrates containing a high level of digestible fibre cause less depression of milk fat and produce an overall higher fat yield (kg/day), even though total milk volume is reduced due to lack of starch. This was particularly noticeable at the higher levels of concentrate feeding. It is, of course, the amount of starch in the ration and its conversion into propionate and glucose that is one of the main determinants of the volume of milk produced. The energy in digestible fibre products such as sugar-beet pulp is derived from cellulose and hemicelluloses and is slowly fermented. Maize is also slowly fermented and as such causes less depression of milk fat, compared with other more rapidly fermented starch

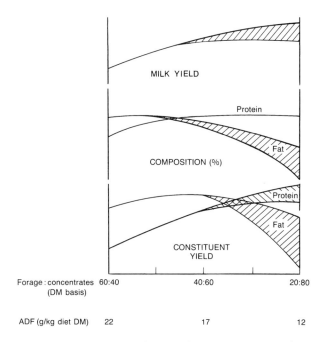

Fig. 28.2 The relationship between forage : concentrate ratio or acid detergent fibre (ADF) and milk yield and composition.

sources such as barley. Uncooked ground maize will, to a certain extent, pass through the rumen and into the small intestine. This possibly explains why maize-based concentrates give an overall lower level of yield than conventional barley products. Both features are particularly noticeable at higher concentrate intakes. Root crops, e.g. fodder beet, have most of their energy stored as the sugar sucrose. Generally, they produce better levels of fat, but lower yields than a comparable amount of starch.

The effect of diet on milk protein is different from that seen with milk fat. On high-forage diets, increasing the proportion of concentrate in the ration (especially high-starch concentrate) will increase milk protein, but only up to a level of 50–60 per cent of concentrate in the diet. Beyond this, milk yield may rise and milk fat concentration will fall, but protein levels will remain constant. The net effect is an overall rise in protein yield. These changes are represented diagrammatically in Fig. 28.2.

Increasing the intake of rumen bypass protein will also increase milk protein, even if requirements for metabolizable protein have been met. This effect is enhanced if the amount of rumen bypass starch is increased, suggesting that the mammary gland requires a balance of precursors and energy to produce higher levels of dietary protein.

Clearly, within a quota system there will be an optimal level for a farmer, both in terms of milk yield

and milk quality, but this will depend on the economic milk price : concentrate cost ratio prevailing at the time, and a full discussion is well outside the scope of this review.

Of course, low forage intakes may not occur intentionally. Poor quality fodder such as very wet, very acid or very butyric silages will depress intakes and thereby increase the concentrate : forage ratio. A more common problem is probably inadequate access. Self-feeding consolidated silage, particularly behind an electric wire, may depress intakes of even good quality material by as much as 5–10 per cent and could further exacerbate the problem.

There is no requirement for 'long fibre' in the basal ration to maintain milk quality, and diets containing long fibre length generally give the same milk quality as finely chopped silage (Thomas, 1984). However, there is some evidence that silage diets give better milk quality than rations of equal metabolizable energy intake based on hay. Fine grinding of forage will depress milk fat when used as the sole ration, but if used as a supplement to conventional forage it has no effect (Thomas, 1984).

Dietary fat

Manufacturers may increase the energy content of a concentrate by adding fat, either directly into the product or by fat-spraying the outside of the cubes. Fat 'prills' may also be added to the ration, e.g. a complete diet, as a separate constituent. Provided that saturated (or 'hard') fats such as tallow, coconut or palm kernel oil are used, and only to a maximum of 5–6 per cent, this will increase the fat content of the milk. However, milk protein content will be slightly depressed, but as milk yield is likely to increase, overall milk protein yield remains constant. Levels of fat above 7 per cent interfere with ruminal function, leading to a depression of both total milk yields and the fat and protein contents.

Increased levels of unsaturated ('soft') fats, such as maize, cotton seed, groundnut and especially fish oils, should not be used because they will coat the surface of fibre particles in the rumen, thereby depressing fibre digestion and leading to a fall in the milk fat content. However, if the fat can be protected from rumen degradation (such as with heating or formaldehyde treatment), the fat will bypass the rumen, resulting in no depression of fibre digestion. This will allow the long-chain fatty acids to be utilized more fully and overall milk fat will therefore rise. Protecting unsaturated fat also has a significant impact on the fatty acid composition of milk. As a result of hydrogenation of dietary fatty acids in the rumen, milk fatty acids are primarily (75 per cent) saturated fat. Protecting unsaturated fat can significantly increase the proportion of unsaturated fats in milk (and reduce the proportion of saturated fat). Mansbridge and Blake (1997) showed that inclusion of either full fat soybeans or partially oil-extracted rapeseed in the diet resulted in a significant reduction in the proportion of palmitic acid (the predominant saturated milk fatty acid) in milk. Additionally, feeding oil-extracted rapeseed significantly increased the concentration of oleic acid (a mono-unsaturated fatty acid) and linolenic acid (a polyunsaturated fatty acid), while feeding full fat soyabeans resulted in significant increases in linoleic and linolenic acid. Milk and milk products produced from cows fed protected diets could be a valuable aid in reducing saturated fat intake.

Dietary protein (see p. 106)

The effects of dietary protein on milk quality, including milk protein, are less well defined. It is the energy content of the ration that has the major effect on milk protein, particularly at high forage intakes. Severe dietary protein deficits will depress milk protein, although this may be partly because the requirements of the ruminal micro-organisms have not been met and as such total dry matter intake, and therefore the overall dietary energy intake, is inadequate.

Feeding systems

It is possible to overcome some of the effects of high concentrate, low forage diets by feeding the cows more frequently. In a series of experiments at the National Institute for Research in Dairying (Sutton, 1986), cows were given concentrate diets varying from 600 to 900 g/kg (namely 40 per cent to 10 per cent forage) fed either twice daily or up to six times daily. The results are given in Table 28.2 and show that for all levels of concentrate feeding, milk fat was higher with a greater frequency of daily feeds. As one might expect, the differential was greatest at the highest level of concentrate feeding, where twice daily feeding had produced a severe depression of milk fat. The concentrate used was a standard material containing high levels of starch. Had a highly digestible fibre product been used, it is unlikely that the depression of milk fat would have been so great – hence the response to more frequent feedings would also have been considerably less. It is generally assumed that diets leading to high propionate and low acetate in the rumen will reduce milk fat. However, increasing the frequency of feeding does not seem to depress propionate concentrations sufficiently to account for the full benefit to milk fat synthesis. It would appear that high plasma insulin concentrations are the main factor depressing milk fat and that the release of insulin is stimulated by peaks of propionate production, such as occurs after a large feed of concen-

Table 28.2 Effect of number of daily meals of starch-based concentrates on milk yield and composition. Source: Sutton (1986).

Concentrates				
(kg/day)	10.0	11.5	12.8	14.0
(g/kg diet)	600	700	800	900
ADF (g/kg diet DM)	192	162	124	99
Milk yield (kg/day)				
2 meals	19.3	19.7	20.6	23.0
6 meals	20.8	20.2	24.5	21.4
Milk fat (g/kg)				
2 meals	34.3	32.6	31.6	17.9
6 meals	36.2	39.2	35.3	29.7
Milk protein (g/kg)				
2 meals	31.4	33.2	31.7	32.0
6 meals	31.8	34.1	31.2	33.2

trate, rather than the steady supply of propionate that will be a feature of more frequent feeding. The effect of increased levels of insulin is to promote lipogenesis in adipose rather than mammary tissue.

Table 28.2 shows that milk protein is unaffected by frequency of feeding, or by the level of concentrate fed at these high levels of concentrate:forage ratio.

Complete diets (see p. 120) offer an opportunity for even feeds of concentrate throughout the day. When milk fat is low, due to depression by an excessive concentrate:forage ratio, feeding the same constituents in a complete diet will lead to an increase in the fat content. Milk protein may also increase on complete diets, but this is thought to be due to the effects of an increased dry matter intake, rather than any particular effect on frequency of feeding.

Since the introduction of milk quotas in the UK (see p. 24), there has been a greater tendency to feed forage, and concentrates have been fed on a 'flat-rate' basis, rather than the more traditional system of a basic allocation for maintenance and an increasing quantity of concentrate depending on yield. Provided that good quality forage is available *ad libitum* (and this is essential to the success of the system), there is no significant effect on milk quality throughout the lactation. Since high levels of 'starchy' concentrates promote high yields, cows calving onto a 'flat-rate' system tend to 'peak' at a lower level in early lactation and hence the 'dilution' effect of high yields depressing milk quality is not seen. Any reduction in milk quality on a flat-rate system is compensated for by slightly higher quality later in lactation. If access to forage is restricted, then clearly decreasing concentrate in early lactation will depress milk protein.

The depression of milk fat caused by high-concentrate diets can also be counteracted by the use of buffers. The most commonly used compound is sodium bicarbonate, fed at 12.5–15 kg/t, or 100–125 g/cow per day. The extent of the improvement depends on the original level of milk fat, the response being greatest in herds where butterfat is already low due to high levels of starchy concentrate being fed twice daily. Feeds such as sugar beet pulp also have a good buffering capacity (sometimes also known as the cationic exchange capacity), whereas others, such as maize gluten, can lead to a more acid fermentation. It is interesting to speculate on the effects of the use of sulphuric acid as a silage additive. This is a 'strong' acid, thus requiring a greater buffering, and could exacerbate milk fat problems in a way that formic or lactic acids would not.

Non-nutritional factors

Age of cow

Heifers generally have the highest milk quality, there being a fall of about 3 g/kg (0.3 per cent) in fat and 7 g/kg (0.7 per cent) in solids not fat (SNF) per lactation thereafter. The rate of decline continues until approximately the fifth lactation, after which it becomes more gradual. The decline in SNF is primarily due to a decline in lactose and mainly occurs during the first three lactations. Protein declines by only approximately 1 g/kg (0.1 per cent) per lactation over this period.

Stage of lactation

Milk quality is, of course, very high at calving (colostrum has at least double the dry matter content, i.e. 25 per cent, of normal milk, see p. 211), but then declines as yield increases, reaching a minimum at about 50–70 days after calving. Milk fat may drop by as much as 10 g/kg (1.0 per cent) and protein by 3 g/kg (0.3 per cent) over the period. This depression is partly due to a 'dilution' effect of high yields and partly to the inherent inability of the early lactation cow to consume sufficient energy to meet the demands of production. Feeding high levels of 'starchy' concentrates and, in so doing, boosting the volume of milk produced, can in some circumstances exacerbate the decline in milk quality. Both milk fat and protein tend to increase after 70 days, but milk protein only rises significantly if the cow becomes pregnant, and the rapid rise in both fat and protein that occurs in later lactation (e.g. six months after calving) is greater in the pregnant animal. Farms practising 'block calving', for example from August to October, often experience a marked fall in milk quality two to three months later (e.g. November

to February) due to the fact that a large number of cows are at peak yield and relatively few are pregnant.

Changes in lactose follow an opposite pattern. The lactose content of colostrum is low, but rises rapidly after calving to reach a peak by two weeks into lactation. This level is maintained until six weeks, but there is then a steady fall, the rate accelerating towards the end of lactation. Changes in lactose are therefore a mirror image of changes in fat and protein.

Season of the year

In the UK there is a sharp fall in milk fat at the end of winter, when cows are turned out to grazing. This can be partly offset by providing access to hay or straw, although intakes of such forages are often poor when highly palatable grass is available and, if only 1–2 kg are consumed, this will have little benefit. To overcome the situation (and to improve grassland management and conservation), a system of 'storage' or 'buffer' feeding has been introduced, whereby cows are kept in at night on silage. Experiments carried out at Crichton Royal Farm (Table 28.3) showed that this significantly improved butterfat and although yields were marginally lower, overall fat yield was increased. However, protein yields were lower.

Often there is also a fall in milk protein during the winter housing period (November to March in the UK), probably due to a lower energy content of the diet at this time of the year and also to a stage of lactation effect. Protein levels then rise rapidly in April and May, following turnout to spring grazing. There is very little seasonal change in lactose concentrations.

Disease

Liver fluke (see p. 276) can depress both milk fat and milk protein and this depression in milk quality may be

Table 28.3 The effect of silage feeding at grazing on milk quality. Source: Phillips & Leaver (1983).

	Grazing	Restricted grazing and silage
Milk yield (kg/day)	19.9	18.9
Milk composition		
Fat (g/kg)	35.6	39.4
Protein (g/kg)	35.1	34.8
Solids yield		
Fat (g/day)	708	745
Protein (g/day)	698	657

Table 28.4 Approximate breed variations in milk yield and quality. Source: MMB (1983).

	Milk yield (kg)	Milk fat (g/kg)	Protein (g/kg)
Ayrshire	4988	39.0	33.8
British Friesian	5610	37.8	32.6
British Holstein	6292	37.3	32.0
Guernsey	4017	46.4	36.3
Jersey	3876	51.9	38.5

seen in the absence of any other clinical signs of fluke. Heavy infestations of lice (see p. 741) and gastrointestinal worms (see p. 267) may also reduce milk quality, but these are unlikely in adult milking cows.

Mastitis (see Chapter 23) leads to a reduction in yield, lactose and butterfat. For example, a herd with a cell count of 750 000 cells/ml could be losing 750–900 l/cow per year, 50g/kg (0.5 per cent) lactose and a smaller amount (30g/kg, 0.3 per cent) of milk fat. Milk protein levels will increase slightly with mastitis, but the protein is of lower quality, with increased levels of globulin and decreased casein. High cell count milk is therefore of reduced value for manufacture.

Genetic variation

It is well known that Channel Island cattle such as the Jersey and Guernsey have higher milk quality than other breeds. Approximate breed values are given in Table 28.4. Of course there are large variations between individual animals within a breed, and this is the basis of genetic selection. The selection of animals on the basis of yield alone could lead to a decrease in fat and protein contents and care should be taken to ensure that bulls with a high improved contemporary comparison (ICC) for both fat and protein are selected. There is less genetic variation within breeds for protein and lactose than for fat and hence the greatest rate of genetic progress will be made by selecting for fat. For example, the range of fat content within a breed is over 20g/kg, whereas genetic variation for protein is only approximately 10g/kg (Crabtree, 1984). The genetic variation for lactose is even lower.

Management factors

Milking intervals would appear to have an effect on milk quality in that on twice-daily milking, the fat content is higher in the afternoon. This is entirely due to a 'carryover' effect (Dodd, 1984). At the end of milking, some 10–20 per cent of the milk present remains in the udder and cannot be removed. The fat content of this milk is very high, 150g/kg (15 per cent) or higher, and it is withdrawn at the next milking. If there is an uneven interval between milkings, milk produced after the shorter interval will have a higher fat content because of the reduced 'dilution' effect of the additional milk produced. The total daily fat production remains constant, irrespective of the variation in milking interval and therefore of fat content. Increasing the frequency of milking to three or even four times daily does not alter milk quality significantly, although yields may rise by 10–15 per cent.

References

Crabtree, R.M. (1984) Milk compositional ranges and trends. In *Milk Compositional Quality and its Importance in Future Markets* (ed. by M.E. Castle & R.G. Gunn), pp. 35–42. BSAP Occasional Publication No. 9, Edinburgh.

Dodd, F.H. (1984) Herd management effects on compositional quality. In *Milk Compositional Quality and its Importance in Future Markets* (ed. by M.E. Castle & R.G. Gunn), p. 77. BSAP Occasional Publication No. 9, Edinburgh.

Garnsworthy, P.C. & Topps, J.H. (1982) The effect of body condition of dairy cows at calving on their food intake and performance when given complete diets. *Animal Production*, **35**, 113–19.

Mansbridge, R.J. & Blake, J.S. (1997) Nutritional factors affecting the fatty acid composition of bovine milk *British Journal of Nutrition*, **78** (Suppl 1), S37–S47.

National Dairy Council (NDC) (1997) *United Kingdom Dairy Facts and Figures*, pp. 1–208. National Dairy Council, London.

Phillips, C.J.C. & Leaver, A.D. (1983) The effect of offering silage to set-stocked dairy cows. *Animal Production*, **36**, 507.

Sutton, J.D. (1986) In *Principles and Practice of Feeding Dairy Cows*, pp. 203–18. NIRD Technical Bulletin No. 8.

Sutton, J.D., Bines, J.A. & Napper, D.J. (1985) Composition of starchy and fibrous concentrates for lactating dairy cows. *Animal Production*, **40**, 533.

Thomas, C. (1984) Milk compositional quality and the role of forages. In *Milk Composition Quality and its Importance in Future Markets* (ed. by M.E. Castle & R.G. Gunn), pp. 69–76. BSAP Occasional Publication No. 9, Edinburgh.

Chapter 29

The Enhancement of Bovine Mammary Gland Immunity Through Vaccination

K.P. Kenny, T. Tollersrud and F.D. Bastida–Corcuera

Introduction	379
Anatomy of the bovine mammary gland	379
Defence mechanisms of the gland	379
Immunoglobulin in lacteal secretions	380
Biological activity of antibody	380
Complement	381
Cells of the mammary gland	381
Cytokines	382
Intramammary infection	382
Virulence factors and immune response to major pathogens	383
Escherichia coli	383
Klebsiella spp.	384
Mycoplasma spp.	385
The summer mastitis complex	385
Staphylococcus aureus	385
Streptococcus spp.	386
Mucosal immune system	388
Generation of immune response	388
Limitations of vaccination	389

Introduction

The examination of immunological methods to increase resistance of the dairy cow to pathogens which cause mastitis has been ongoing for almost a century. This is a controversial area of bovine immunity with the existence of two schools of thought on the role of immunological intervention in mastitis control programmes. The first believes it is not possible to generate protective immunity in the mammary gland and control measures should be based on management, therapeutic strategies and genetic selection (Mellenberger, 1977). The second opinion is vaccination has a role in a mastitis control programme (Colditz & Watson, 1985). The latter view, founded on an improved knowledge of the bovine immune system and the principal pathogens of the gland, is supported by reports which indicate heightened resistance to infection with certain pathogens. The success of coliform mastitis vaccines has spurred novel studies on *Streptococcus uberis* mastitis. Such vaccines will complement conventional control measures which are less effective against environmental pathogens.

Anatomy of the bovine mammary gland (see Chapter 22)

The bovine udder comprises four mammary glands. The main arterial supply is from the bilateral external pudendal arteries. The venous return is via the external pudendal veins and the subcutaneous abdominal veins. There are two lymph vascular systems: a superficial and a deep set. The superficial set drain the cutaneous area and the teat walls. The deep set is associated with the finer branches of the arteries and veins. The lymphatics drain into the superficial inguinal (supramammary) lymph nodes and the lymph passes to the deep inguinal node.

The mucosa of the teat or streak canal is arranged in longitudinal folds and is lined by stratified squamous epithelium which constantly undergoes keratinization. A slightly projecting fold marks the proximal end of the teat canal, the Furstenberg's rosette area. The teat cistern (sinus) is the cavity directly proximal to the teat canal, and this continues into the parenchyma of the udder as the gland cistern (lactiferous sinus), which possesses a two-layered columnar epithelium. The secretory tissue is divided into lobes which are composed of lobules and there is an extensive duct system. The epithelium of secretory alveoli is a single layer of cuboidal cells. The alveoli are surrounded by a stromal layer which is more pronounced in the non-lactating gland.

Defence mechanisms of the gland

Non-specific and specific defence mechanisms exist in the bovine mammary gland (Outteridge & Lee, 1988). Non-specific factors include teat and teat duct shape and structure, teat duct patency and teat duct keratin. Teat duct keratin owes its protective properties to fatty acids and basic proteins. During milking there is a mechanical flushing of the teat canal. The enzyme lysozyme can cleave certain bacterial cell walls, but is present at very low concentrations in bovine secretions. Lactoferrin can bind iron and reduce the availability of iron to micro-organisms, but citrate inhibits this protein. The lactoperoxidase/thiocyanate/hydrogen peroxide system has activity against micro-organisms. Complement can be activated by the lipopolysaccharide of Gram-negative organisms and cause lysis of these bacteria by the alternative pathway.

Four specific defence mechanisms operate in the gland. These are mediated by antibodies directed against epitopes of the pathogens or their toxins, in conjunction with phagocytic cells and complement. The mechanisms include prevention of bacterial adherence to epithelial cells, neutralization of bacterial toxins, opsonization of pathogens and direct lysis of pathogens. The key role of humoral immunity reflects the extracellular location of mastitis pathogens. A role for cellular immunity has not yet been established although laboratory studies have shown the ability of staphylococci and streptococci to achieve an intracellular location in cultured mammary epithelial cells.

Two methods can be employed to heighten resistance. One could increase non-specific protection which would be widely effective against all pathogens. The strategic use of cytokines at key points in the lactation cycle has yielded encouraging results. The administration of gamma-interferon lessens the severity and duration of experimental *Escherichia coli* infection, but there are no reports of field trials describing the effect of such administration on naturally occurring infections. An alternative approach is to stimulate specific immunity for each mastitis pathogen. The latter is difficult because there are many causative bacteria. The challenge is to characterize the virulence factors of the principal pathogens, identify their protective epitopes and then establish and maintain sufficient protective antibody in milk.

Immunoglobulin in lacteal secretions
(see p. 323)

Four classes of antibody have been described in the bovine (Butler, 1986): IgA, IgE, IgG and IgM. IgG_1 and IgG_2 are two subclasses of IgG. The half-life in serum of IgA, IgM, IgG_1 and IgG_2 is 3, 5, 17 and 22 days respectively. Serum IgA of cattle is probably synthesized by bronchial or gut associated lymphoid tissue, while IgM and IgG are most likely synthesized by the spleen and peripheral lymph nodes. Immunoglobulin concentrations in serum and colostral secretions are listed in Table 29.1.

Antibody present in lacteal secretions may be synthesized locally or derived from serum via selective transport or transudation. Inflammation of mammary epithelium causes an increase in the passage of antibodies from blood to lacteal secretions via transudation. IgA is the major immunoglobulin in most bovine

Table 29.1 The concentration of immunoglobulin in serum and colostral secretions. Values are expressed in mg/ml.

	IgA	IgM	IgG_1	IgG_2
Serum	0.37	3.0	11.2	9.2
Colostral whey	4.7	7.1	48.2	4.0
Milk whey	0.08	0.08	0.5	0.06

secretions, but not in milk. Around 50 to 100 per cent of milk IgA is produced locally. Plasma derived IgA is selectively transported into most mucosal secretions by vesicular transport following its binding to secretory component on epithelial cells. There are conflicting reports concerning the origin of milk IgM with some indicating it is entirely serum derived while others suggest that 75 per cent is locally synthesized. Most milk IgG_1 is serum derived. About 90 per cent of IgG_2 found in milk is locally produced. To increase specific IgG_1 in milk one must increase the serum level of specific IgG_1, whereas for IgA one must generate appropriate plasma cells in the lamina propria.

Biological activity of antibody
(see Chapter 22)

Antibody molecules can be considered as having two components. Firstly the two antigen binding sites recognize and bind antigen. Secondly, the Fc portion of the molecule is considered the effector part because it can fix complement components and interact with specific Fc receptors on phagocytic cells. For certain protective effector functions, antibody must not only be directed against a particular epitope but must be of the correct isotype.

Secretory IgA serves to protect mucosal surfaces from colonization and penetration by undesirable micro-organisms. It can augment the bacteriostatic effects of lactoferrin and can function as an opsonin. Lacteal IgA is largely associated with milk fat globules. IgG_1 and IgG_2 are efficient at fixation of complement and able to neutralize bacterial toxins. Cytophilic antibodies are capable of attaching to certain cells in such a way that these cells can subsequently adsorb specific antigen. It has been shown that IgG_2 is cytophilic for bovine blood neutrophils and for ovine mammary neutrophils. Bovine macrophages were found to be capable of binding both IgG_1 and IgG_2 *in vitro*. Live vaccines are believed to preferentially stimulate IgG_2. IgM is 10 to 20 times more effective than IgG in complement fixation. This ability to fix complement may explain why IgM is bactericidal for Gram-negative pathogens. In this manner it can also opsonize micro-organisms for uptake by phagocytic cells. IgM can also agglutinate bacteria and permit them to be flushed out at milking.

Table 29.2 The cellular composition of gland secretions (%).

	PMN[a]	Macrophage	Lymphocyte	Epithelial
Colostrum	62	35	4	0
Milk	3	79	16	2
Dry gland secretion	3	89	7	1

[a] PMN, polymorphonuclear neutrophil.

Complement (see Chapter 58)

The complement system consists of more than 29 distinct plasma and membrane proteins, several of which are enzymes. The system is activated either by antibody binding to the bacterium (classical pathway) or by carbohydrate structures on the surface of the organism (alternative pathway). Triggering of the system results in a sequence of biochemical reactions in which one component activates another component in a cascade fashion. Complement thus bridges the innate immune system based on recognition of foreign carbohydrates and the induced immune system based on specific antibody formation.

The terminal part of the reaction is the formation of a membrane attack complex which causes lytic lesions to form in the membrane of the invading microorganism. Resistance to complement (serum resistance) is the only virulence factor identified among strains of Gram-negative bacteria isolated from cases of bovine mastitis. Serum-sensitive bacteria are either killed or do not grow in normal milk, whereas serum-resistant organisms generally multiply, and only the latter are able to cause mastitis.

There are several effector mechanisms by which complement aids phagocytosis. When the complement cascade is activated, component C3b is deposited on the surface of the bacterium. This C3b coating promotes adherence to and ingestion by phagocytes, which possess surface receptors for C3b. Products of complement activation include C3a and C5a which are chemoattractant for neutrophils and C5a can activate neutrophils. The inflammatory mediators responsible for the influx of neutrophils into milk have not been conclusively identified. Infusion of activated complement induces inflammation in dry glands but not in lactating glands. Levels of complement in lacteal secretions are highest as lactation ends, in the dry period and in colostrum. In normal milk the concentration of C3 is 1–4 per cent of serum, but milk does contain anti-complementary activity. In mastitis there is an increase in complement components in milk due to transudation.

Table 29.3 Lymphocyte composition using flow cytometry.

	T cell	B cell	Null	Macrophage
Peripheral blood	48	20	10	22
Milk	52	14	9	25
Dry gland secretion	43	19	11	27

Cells of the mammary gland

In dry and lacteal secretions the predominant cell type is the macrophage while in colostrum the polymorphonuclear neutrophil (PMN) serves this role. The number of cells per millilitre in dry period secretion is greater than that of normal milk. The cellular composition of gland secretions is outlined in Table 29.2.

Identification of cells in milk and blood can be performed by microscopic examination of stained smears. Flow cytometry is a sensitive technique which allows further differentiation of the mononuclear cell population in blood and gland secretions (Table 29.3). It is unclear why these two techniques yield different results for the macrophage content of dry gland secretion.

Mammary *lymphocytes* can respond to mitogens and particulate and soluble antigens; however, these responses are lower than those of peripheral blood lymphocytes from the same animal. T lymphocytes can produce cytokines which effect recruitment and activation of other cell types. T cells may be further subdivided according to their accessory molecules (CD4 or CD8) or antigen receptors (alpha-beta or gamma-delta). The majority of T cells in milk express alpha-beta T cell receptors. The ratio of CD8+ to CD4+ cells in blood is 1.5, while in mammary secretions it is 0.85. Some activated CD8+ cells may suppress the proliferation of CD4+ cells in the course of *S. aureus* mastitis and this may adversely effect antibody production by B cells.

The mammary *macrophage* functions in phagocytosis and killing of bacteria, eliminates fat in the involuting gland and plays a role in local immunity through antigen processing and presentation. After they have phagocytosed bacteria, mammary macrophages generate chemoattractants for PMN, while after exposure to endotoxin they release cytokines. Although critical for phagocytosis of *Strep. uberis* they may provide an intracellular location for *Staph. aureus* and their phagocytic capacity is reduced by dry secretion. A considerable population of macrophages exists beneath the alveolar and ductal epithelium.

Milk from normal uninfected glands contains less than 300000 cells per millilitre and the predominant cell is the macrophage. Subclinically infected quarters contain around 750000 cells per millilitre, while the secretion of infected quarters contains millions of cells per millilitre and in both these instances the predominant cell is the polymorphonuclear *neutrophil* leukocyte (PMN). A pre-existing leukocytosis confers increased resistance to infection; however, increased amounts of serum factors in the milk typically accompany this leukocytosis. When intramammary devices increase cell counts to 900000 per millilitre in strippings, protection against a wide variety of mastitis pathogens is achieved. Such high cell counts are not desired by the dairy industry.

There is a large pool of mature neutrophils present to fight infection. The half life of the cell in the bloodstream is about nine hours, with a substantial number developing in the bone marrow. Upon infection of the gland, PMNs adhere to capillary endothelium via receptors and pass through it by diapedesis. They then migrate down chemotactic gradients and enter the lumen of the gland through the mammary epithelium. Antibody and complement promote contact and recognition of the pathogen, which is ingested and exposed to the microbiocidal system of the PMN. Both oxygen dependent and independent pathways exist within neutrophils to kill ingested microbes. Some bacteria such as *Staph. aureus* possess defence mechanisms against oxidative damage by neutrophils and may survive within the phagosome. PMNs are viable for 1–2 days in the mammary gland, then undergo apoptosis (programmed cell death) before ingestion by macrophages.

Phagocytosis by mammary PMNs is much less efficient than that by blood PMNs. PMN function in the mammary gland is impaired by milk fat globules, casein and the lower glycogen content of milk PMN compared to blood PMN. PMN function can also be impaired by bacterial toxins. Cows vary in both the ability of their PMN to phagocytose and in the capacity of their milk to support phagocytosis. Despite high levels of phagocytic cells in the gland during the dry period, the gland is very susceptible at this time to new infection. This may reflect the poor phagocytic efficiency of these cells or the unfavourable nature of the non-lactating gland for them. Fc receptor function is impaired by dry secretion and colostrum.

PMN function has limitations, as evidenced by chronic infections with some pathogens persisting in the face of a high SCC. To increase the efficacy of phagocytosis one could increase and maintain a high level of opsonin in milk through immunization, select for cows with superior phagocytic ability or decrease PMN mobilization time in response to pathogen invasion. Antigen-specific inflammatory responses can be established in the gland by parenteral immunization and one of the effector inputs of vaccination is the more rapid response of the PMN to infection. One could also increase and maintain a high PMN concentration in milk; however, this will adversely affect milk quality.

Cytokines

Cytokines are a group of regulatory proteins which act as intracellular communication signals and are secreted in very low amounts by a variety of cell types. Most cytokines possess multiple biological properties and regulate the activity of cells which participate in specific and non-specific immunity. Some can also alter physiological processes and cause pathological changes. The immunomodulatory capacity of these molecules is complex and interactions exist between cytokines – the cytokine network. Tumour necrosis factor (TNF), interleukin-1 (IL-1), interleukin 2 (IL-2), interleukin 6 (IL-6) and interleukin 8 (IL-8) have been detected in milk during inflammation. These and other cytokines have been shown to affect bovine mammary leukocytes *in vitro* and to a lesser extent *in vivo*. Their role as vaccine adjuvants and therapeutic agents is being evaluated.

Intramammary infection
(see also Chapter 23)

To induce mastitis a pathogen must pass the teat canal and enter the gland, survive the bacteriostatic and bactericidal mechanisms and use the available nutrients to replicate. Colonization of the gland reflects both the adherence capacity of the pathogen and its ability to utilize nutrients in lacteal secretion to multiply. *Strep. agalactiae* and *Staph. aureus* adhere readily to ductular epithelial cells, while *Escherichia coli*, *Klebsiella* spp. and *Arcanobacterium pyogenes* adhere poorly. If they are to maintain infection within the gland, bacteria must multiply at a rate which exceeds that at which they are eliminated. The outcome of infection depends on the rate of growth of the organism, the production, absorption and activity of toxins and the immune status of the host.

Virulence factors and immune response to major pathogens

Escherichia coli (see also Chapter 23)

Escherichia coli mastitis is an opportunist infection. When 290 *E. coli* isolates were examined, 82 per cent could be grouped into 63 O-serogroups, the remainder being untypable (Linton & Robinson, 1984). Mastitis isolates do not possess the virulence factors associated with invasive or enteropathogenic strains of *E. coli* and cannot be distinguished from faecal isolates. Serum resistance, which is the capacity to withstand killing by complement, is the key feature of mammary isolates. The contribution of a capsule is unclear because most unencapsulated strains are serum resistant. Serum-sensitive strains are killed rapidly, with over 90 per cent killed in 15 minutes by freshly collected 10 per cent normal bovine.

When serum-resistant strains gain access to the lactating gland they commence to multiply and lipopolysaccharide (LPS), also called endotoxin, is released from the bacterial cell wall. Endotoxin is found in 50–100 per cent of lacteal secretions and 15 per cent of blood samples of cows with coliform mastitis. The exaggerated response of the host to endotoxin is often responsible for the severity of this mastitis. Fever, disseminated intravascular coagulation, hypotension, shock, complement activation and death can occur. Macrophages are the principal method by which endotoxins are removed. In the presence of LPS macrophages become activated and secrete IL-1, IL-6 and TNF. These cytokines mediate endotoxic events and are responsible for many of the clinical signs associated with this condition.

E. coli does not adhere to mammary epithelial cells. The organisms grow in secretions and there is little tissue invasion. Mammary lesions in *E. coli* mastitis are confined to the superficial layer of the teat and lactiferous sinus where extensive sloughing and necrosis of epithelial cells is evident. Secretory tissue is not involved. The response of cows to *E. coli* infection of the gland may be a function of the physiological state of the gland. The dry gland is much less responsive to endotoxin than the lactating gland and mild histopathological changes are noted following infusion. *E. coli* is incapable of establishing itself permanently in the gland in the first half of the dry period and this may be due to lactoferrin (Bramley, 1976). One experiment revealed that in the 30 days before parturition bacteria maintained infection in 14 of 37 inoculated quarters and all of these quarters had peracute toxic mastitis after parturition.

Following infusion of 500 colony forming units (CFU) of *E. coli*, newly calved cows mobilize PMN slowly and appear to be refractory to the presence of irritants in the udder. This permits great bacterial replication and a large subsequent release of endotoxin which is often fatal (Hill, 1979). Killing of some *E. coli* strains within the udder requires a neutrophilia only, whereas for others up to 30 per cent serum products are required. For virulent strains a PMN response and opsonin are typically required. In decomplemented non-immune serum, colostrum and whey, the main opsonin for *E. coli* is IgM and there is no absolute requirement for complement in the opsonization of *E. coli* by the adult dairy cow. Later research found IgG_2 from immune bovine serum or whey opsonic for *E. coli*. Encapsulated isolates are more resistant to uptake by PMN and require greater amounts of opsonin than non-encapsulated isolates.

The Gram-negative cell wall consists of an inner cytoplasmic membrane and a cell wall which is composed of mucopolysaccharide–peptidoglycan, phospholipid protein and lipopolysaccharide. LPS is composed of three distinct subunits. The outermost O polysaccharide is linked to the core polysaccharide which is covalently bound to the lipid A. Free lipid A in soluble form expresses all the typical *in vivo* properties of endotoxin. Resistance to the bactericidal activity of normal serum is attributable to the O antigen of the LPS. When compared to serum-sensitive strains, LPS from serum-resistant strains is relatively enriched in long-chain O antigen subunits. These O polysaccharides may mask lipid A which could activate the alternative complement pathway. If the longer polysaccharide chains do bind C3b, the distance from the outer membrane of the bacteria is too far for insertion of the complement membrane attack complex.

The O polysaccharides are made up of a series of identical repeating oligosaccharide units containing three to five sugars each. The O polysaccharide is immunodominant and displays great diversity in length and sugar constituents whereas the core polysaccharide is conserved. Antibody to the O polysaccharide antigen or LPS affords protection against homologous challenge only. Because of the great diversity of the O polysaccharides of LPS, a search for shared epitopes on other parts of the molecule has been undertaken in an effort to find an antigen that could be used for active immunization. Gram-negative core antigens have immunological homology across bacterial species, but are typically masked by the immunodominant O polysaccharide.

In contrast to smooth organisms, rough mutants, called so because of their colonial morphology, have incomplete synthesis of O polysaccharide side chains and consequently varying amounts of the core glycolipid are exposed. The *E. coli* J5 strain is an Rc mutant of *E. coli* O11:B4 and has an LPS devoid of O antigen (see p. 1016). Animals immunized with killed J5 bacteria are able to make antibodies to the core region and are protected from challenge with heterologous live organisms. Antibody to J5 cross-reacts with LPS extracted from other Gram-negative bacteria which cause mastitis, in particular *Klebsiella* spp. The protective factor induced by vaccination is considered to be antibody to core glycolipid which binds to invading bacteria at a time when the core antigens are most exposed, that is, early in their growth phase. This antibody promotes opsonization of Gram-negative bacteria and may also be bactericidal or reduce growth of the organism. The protective ability of antibodies to core glycolipid may also reflect their ability to bind to released LPS, neutralize the toxic effects of lipid A and thereby diminish systemic signs. Such release would occur during bacterial growth or after antibiotic therapy, phagocytic destruction or complement mediated lysis.

Initial studies of IgG_1 antibody titres to the core antigens of J5 showed that titres of less than 1:240 were associated with 5.33 times the risk of clinical coliform mastitis (Tyler *et al.*, 1988). This vaccine has been the subject of several field trials. In one trial, 246 cows received three doses of J5 killed cells (7.5 billion bacteria per dose) in Freund's incomplete adjuvant, twice in the dry period and once after calving, while 240 unvaccinated cows served as controls. Six cases of clinical coliform mastitis occurred in vaccinates with 29 occurring in control cows (Gonzalez *et al.*, 1989). In a separate trial which lasted 30 months, cows received either vaccine or placebo at dry-off, 30 days later and at calving. There was no difference between groups in the percentage of quarters infected with Gram-negative bacteria at calving. In the control group, 67 per cent of these infections became clinical in the first 90 days of lactation compared to 20% in the vaccinated group (Hogan *et al.*, 1992a).

Cows directly challenged with coliform bacteria via the intramammary route have provided data which are less supportive of the efficacy of the J5 vaccine. One experiment found no difference between vaccinates and control cows subsequent to challenge with 150 CFU of a serum-resistant strain (Hill, 1991). Both groups displayed acute clinical mastitis with systemic signs, a decrease in milk production and large numbers of bacteria in the milk. In an American study, cows immunized at drying off, 30 days later and at calving were challenged with a virulent field strain 30 days into lactation (Hogan *et al.*, 1992b). Lower milk bacteria counts were observed in vaccinates but SCC and local clinical signs did not differ between groups. Milk yield

and dry matter intake was higher in vaccinates. In a separate trial of similar design, cows were challenged one month after calving with a field strain known to cause mild clinical mastitis. No differences in temperature, milk production and systemic signs were observed between groups, but vaccination reduced the duration of both infection and local clinical signs.

It is known that cows which succumb to natural clinical coliform mastitis are in a complex physiological state with alterations in neutrophil function, including receptor expression, rate of diapedesis and phagocytic capacity. Measurement of these parameters can predict which cows will suffer severe clinical mastitis in response to experimental challenge. These animals may receive greatest benefit from vaccination and field trials would more accurately reflect this benefit. For immunological prevention of Gram-negative infection to be a possibility three requirements must be met. A common antigenic structure must exist; this must function as an immunogen and the response to this immunogen must generate protective antibodies. Large field trials indicate that the J5 bacterin achieves this goal. Cows vaccinated in the dry period and at calving have a lower incidence of clinical coliform mastitis in early lactation. The vaccine does not reduce the incidence of intramammary infection with coliforms at calving, but reduces the number of infected quarters which display clinical signs. Two new areas of research include the use of a *Salmonella typhimurium* Re17 bacterin to prevent coliform mastitis and the effect on *E. coli* of antibodies specific for membrane proteins involved in iron transport.

Klebsiella *spp.* (see also Chapter 23)

Klebsiella pneumoniae (*K. pneumoniae*) and *K. oxytoca* are environmental pathogens and opportunist invaders of the bovine mammary gland. Within the genus *Klebsiella* there are over 70 capsular types and eight somatic types or O groups. Thirty-three capsular types of *K. pneumoniae* were isolated from cows belonging to 12 herds and within individual herds up to 13 types could be found. The primary feature of pathogenic strains is their ability to withstand the bactericidal effects of normal serum. Some are also adapted to grow in the secretion of non-lactating glands. Following infusion of small numbers of serum-resistant bacteria into normal mammary glands a severe mastitis is evident. This mastitis is prevented by a pre-existing leukocytosis or by the presence of specific antibody.

Cell wall O antigens are responsible for resistance to serum bactericidal activity. The capsule confers resistance to phagocytosis in the absence of specific antibody. Although type-specific protection can be achieved by vaccination with the homologous capsular polysaccharide, the numerous capsule types recovered from lacteal secretions preclude the use of a polyvalent capsular vaccine. Antibody specific for core glycolipid of *E. coli* J5 strain cross-reacts with endotoxin extracted from *K. pneumoniae*. This antibody is reputed to bind to these core antigens during the log phase of bacterial growth and in this manner afford protection.

Mycoplasma *spp.* (see also Chapter 23)

Mycoplasmas lack a cell wall and are surrounded by a membrane which is similar to the cytoplasmic membrane of bacteria. Several species of mycoplasma cause mastitis but *Mycoplasma bovis* (*M. bovis*) is most prevalent. Cows in all stages of lactation are susceptible but those in early lactation suffer more severely. Antibiotics have little success but after a prolonged time cows may recover. Resistance to killing by serum is a virulence determinant and a pre-existing leukocytosis does not prevent cows from challenge. Neutrophils are not capable of killing *M. bovis* unless specific antibody is present.

Udders with a quarter which had resolved infection were examined and it was found all quarters of the udder were resistant to challenge. Quarters recovered from infection were immune for up to six months, but over one year postinfection all quarters were susceptible to reinfection. Studies of the immune response to *M. bovis* have failed to differentiate between resistant and susceptible animals. Systemic antibody does not appear to protect from infection and the immunity may be based on locally produced IgA and IgG and the action of T lymphocytes. Immunization with protein extracts assists cows in eliminating infection. No attenuated strains have been identified.

The summer mastitis complex
(see also Chapter 24)

There are conflicting views on what are the causative organisms of summer mastitis and how these organisms spread and invade the gland. Summer mastitis typically affects the non-lactating gland of heifers or dry cows and involves mixed bacterial infections. *Arcanobacterium pyogenes* (*A. pyogenes*), *Peptostreptococcus indolicus* (*P. indolicus*), a microaerophilic coccus and *Streptococcus dysgalactiae* are the pathogens believed to have a role in this condition. *Fusobacterium necrophorum* and *Bacteroides melaninogenicus* have also been recovered from the secretion of affected glands. Sorensen (1972) could induce summer mastitis in heifers with *A. pyogenes* and *P. indolicus* or with these two organisms and a microaerophilic coccus. Cultures were more virulent if grown together and infused rather than grown separately and then mixed for infusion.

A. pyogenes does not adhere to mammary epithelial cells and this may explain why summer mastitis is typically associated with the non-lactating gland. This bacterium grows best in lacteal secretion when the pH is greater than 7, as in the dry gland, and secretes haemolysin and proteases. *P. indolicus* stimulates the growth and haemolysin production of *A. pyogenes*. High titres of protease antibodies are found in the serum of infected cows. *P. indolicus* and the microaerophilic coccus produce enzymes which can damage tissue.

Early vaccines were composed without regard to the complex nature of the aetiology, typically containing *A. pyogenes* with or without hemolysin, and the results were poor. Sorensen showed that *A. pyogenes* alone had no protective effect but that a triple bacterin preparation composed of *A. pyogenes*, *P. indolicus* and the microaerophilic coccus gave encouraging results and merited further study (Sorensen, 1972). There is a marked lack of data on the immune response of the cow to these pathogens and approaches to vaccination will remain empirical for some time.

Staphylococcus aureus (see also Chapter 23)

Staphylococcus aureus has been described as a persistent pathogen of the gland due to the failure of therapy during the lactating period to achieve bacteriological cures. It is a contagious pathogen and infusion of 10 CFU into the teat sinus can cause mastitis. Much research has been performed to ascertain the benefit of immunization with staphylococcal antigens. Early attempts at vaccination were unsuccessful and these failures can be explained to a degree by the low numbers of bacteria used and by the culture of these bacteria in conventional media which does not support the expression of certain surface polysaccharide virulence factors. Later work demonstrated limited protection against homologous strains, a reduction in the severity of clinical infection and a reduction in spread of *Staph. aureus* mastitis in vaccinated herds.

The cell wall is composed of peptidoglycan, teichoic acid and protein A. Protein A can bind to the Fc portion of IgG molecules. Peptidoglycan was once considered to be the key cell surface component involved in promoting opsonization of *Staph. aureus*. Most bovine mammary isolates of staphylococci produce additional surface polysaccharides which are located outside the peptidoglycan layer. These polysaccharides may block antibody binding to peptidoglycan or prevent bound antibody interacting with phagocytic receptors. Their precise composition remains obscure and they have been described as exopolysaccharides, pseudocapsules and slime. Their production is typically associated with growth in milk. Such growth increases the virulence of a strain, induces anti-phagocytic properties and increases adherence to epithelial cells. A typing scheme based on chemically characterized capsular polysaccharides has been described for staphylococci. Serotyping of bovine isolates for capsular polysaccharides 5 and 8 typically found 50 to 70 per cent of isolates possessed one of these microcapsules, though in some countries non-typeable isolates predominated.

Staphylococcus aureus produces around 30 extracellular proteins, some of which have been shown to be virulence factors (Sutra & Poutrel, 1994). Alpha-toxin is believed to be responsible for much of the tissue damage seen in staphylococcal mastitis and beta-toxin has been shown to cause inflammation of the gland. Following experimental infection ulcerative and erosive lesions in the epithelial layer are evident throughout the ductal system. Toxins can also damage PMNs whose role in defence against *Staph. aureus* became apparent when anti-bovine leukocyte serum converted a chronic staphylococcal mastitis to an acute gangrenous type. Neutralizing antibodies can be induced through vaccination and these lessen the damage to secretory tissue.

The surface of staphylococci contains proteins which can bind the host tissue proteins fibronectin, fibrinogen and collagen. Attachment to ductal epithelial cells is an important step in colonization and is thought to be mediated by fibronectin binding protein. Specific antibody has been shown to prevent this adherence. During infection toxins may expose subepithelial connective tissue components to which the organism can bind in a specific manner.

Staphylococcal enterotoxins were originally described for their ability to cause food poisoning or toxic shock syndrome in humans. There is variation between countries in the proportion of bovine *Staph. aureus* isolates secreting these molecules. Recent research suggests they may have a role to play in staphylococcal mastitis by causing immunosuppression. Enterotoxins may activate $CD8^+$ T lymphocytes and decrease the response of $CD4^+$ T lymphocytes to staphylococcal antigens. As superantigens, enterotoxins may also contribute to inflammation by activating cells in a non-specific manner and causing the release of inflammatory cytokines. Bovine mononuclear cells proliferate in response to enterotoxin and secrete IL-2, gamma-interferon and TNF. It is difficult to stimulate neutralizing antibodies to these molecules.

In a field trial with a staphylococcal bacterin–toxoid preparation, fewer new infections, less culling and lower somatic cell counts were evident in vaccinated cows as opposed to controls. Each dose of bacterin contained 10 billion CFU of each of two strains of *Staph. aureus*, whose exopolysaccharide cross-reacted with most field isolates. The toxoid component contained alpha- and beta-hemolysins. A second trial found fewer clinical and subclinical cases in vaccinates but this difference was not statistically significant (Nordhaug *et al.*, 1994). Isolated exopolysaccharide in liposomes afforded sheep protection from infection.

Studies performed in Australia found vaccination with live bacteria protected the gland from infection. The protection afforded by vaccination with live bacteria is due to the generation of specific IgG_2 which is cytophilic for PMN. The use of live bacteria has significant disadvantages and consequently bacteria grown in a medium containing milk whey and then killed have been used. Killed bacteria stimulate IgG_2 when administered with the adjuvant dextran sulphate. In normal glands there is a 24 hour lapse between entry of bacteria into the gland and the accumulation of 500 000 PMNs per millilitre and this delay allows infection to become established. Vaccination can decrease this lag period to 6 hours and PMNs may enter the gland, carrying IgG_2 on their membrane.

Australian workers developed a vaccine containing killed bacteria, alpha-toxoid and beta-toxoid, emulsified in an adjuvant of mineral oil and dextran. Experiments have been performed to establish the efficacy of this Australian vaccine (Watson *et al.*, 1996). In challenge studies in sheep the incidence of peracute gangrenous and acute clinical mastitis and the decrease in milk yield was lower in the vaccinates. Heifers which received the vaccine had lower SCC and greater milk production after challenge, compared to controls. A field trial conducted on seven herds and over 1800 cows found 45 clinical cases of *Staph. aureus* mastitis in vaccinates and 67 cases in controls. This difference was not statistically significant. One of the herds had a high incidence of *Staph. aureus* mastitis and in this herd clinical and subclinical cases of mastitis were significantly lower in vaccinates compared to controls.

A better understanding of *Staph. aureus* suggests that protection depends on antibodies being generated to several virulence factors. Vaccines should generate antibodies specific for matrix binding proteins to prevent adherence and to the surface polysaccharides to promote opsonization. Neutralizing antibodies specific for alpha- and beta-toxins would lessen clinical damage and protect the cellular defences of the gland. The results of trials with experimental vaccines based on these three components will clarify whether vaccination has a role in preventing staphylococcal mastitis. When attenuated strains are administered by the intramammary route, they replicate but are eliminated by the gland. The capacity of such strains to stimulate protective immunity is being examined.

Streptococcus spp.

There are no cross-reactive protective epitopes shared by the streptococci which cause mastitis.

Streptococcus agalactiae (see also Chapter 23)

Streptococcus agalactiae (*Strep. agalactiae*) is a Group B streptococcus and is an obligate parasite of the bovine mammary gland where it colonizes the milk ducts. It can be eliminated from a herd through culture and therapeutic means. This easy step should take precedence over the task of generating protective antibody. The group-specific polysaccharide is common to all strains and *Strep. agalactiae* can be divided into five distinct serotypes based on the presence of type-specific surface antigens. A protein antigen designated X is frequently associated with bovine mastitis isolates. Attachment to epithelia is a prerequisite for colonization and surface lipoteichoic acid may aid in this attachment. *Strep. agalactiae* produces CAMP factor which is lethal for mice and rabbits.

The bactericidal activity of neutrophils for *Strep. agalactiae* is dependent on antibody and complement. Most opsonizing antibody is directed to the weakly immunogenic, type-specific polysaccharide and such antibody is a more efficient opsonin when it binds complement. The sera of cows contain low levels of natural opsonin. Mackie *et al.* (1986) found heifers became hyperimmune following systemic vaccination by the subcutaneous and intravenous routes. Despite high titres there was little real difference between the hyperimmune and non-vaccinated heifers following challenge with around 40 million bacteria and it was concluded that locally produced antibody may be required for protection. Antibodies to protein X increase the ingestion of bacteria by PMNs but do not increase the number of bacteria killed by PMN.

Streptococcus uberis (see also Chapter 23)

Streptococcus uberis (*Strep. uberis*) has been examined serologically, biochemically and by molecular biological techniques. It does not fit into the Lancefield classification with 25 per cent of strains typing as group E and smaller numbers belonging to other serogroups. A similar percentage of strains is CAMP positive. Sensitive molecular typing methods indicate most isolates are genetically dissimilar. This organism can be recovered from several body sites of the cow and from manure and soil. It has become a significant cause of mastitis and as an environmental pathogen is less affected by conventional control methods.

The susceptibility of the dry mammary gland to infection with *Strep. uberis* increases with time and in the second half of the dry period all quarters are susceptible. This bacterium binds low amounts of fibronectin, fibrinogen and type II collagen. Adherence to mammary epithelial cells has been described *in vitro*, but in experimental infections most bacteria were found in the alveolar exudate with just a small number associated with damaged epithelial cells. After infection there are many neutrophils in gland secretions but few contain *Strep. uberis*. The role of this cell in defence against *Strep. uberis* is unclear because isolates possessing a hyaluronic acid capsule resist uptake by neutrophils and capsular material can damage PMNs. Macrophages may be the key defence cell since they can ingest isolates which have been opsonized by IgG_1 and IgG_2.

Quarters previously infected with *Strep. uberis* are significantly protected from subsequent infection by the same bacteria. Immunization with killed bacteria via the intramammary or subcutaneous route offered protection from challenge with the immunizing strain and a strong inflammatory reaction was present in the gland. The bacterin did not afford protection from infection with wild-type strains. When live bacteria were administered subcutaneously and bacterial extracts by the intramammary route, a degree of protection was again noted. This protection did not extend to strains not included in the vaccine. As there was only a mild inflammation in the gland it was proposed that live vaccine affected the ability of the organism to replicate and a neutrophil response was not critical for protection from infection (Leigh, 1999).

Streptococcus uberis is unable to produce certain amino acids and must find them in its environment. Studies using chemically defined media found all strains require eight amino acids for growth, with some requiring 13 amino acids. The organism is incapable of hydrolysing proteins directly, but is able to convert bovine plasminogen to plasmin, a protease which can break down casein into peptides. The plasminogen activator of *Strep. uberis* is a protein of 30 kD; it is secreted by almost all isolates and specific neutralizing antibodies are stimulated following immunization.

In an experimental challenge trial, vaccination with plasminogen activator gave a significant degree of protection from clinical disease and greatly reduced bacterial numbers in milk (Leigh, 1999). Both of these protection indices were achieved in the presence of a mild inflammatory response and protection was correlated with the titre of neutralizing antibody specific for plasminogen activator. The studies conducted with *Strep. uberis* could be highly relevant to other mastitis pathogens and have underlined the importance of *in vivo* rather than *in vitro* studies.

Streptococcus dysgalactiae (see also Chapter 23)

Streptococcus dysgalactiae (*Strep. dysgalactiae*) is a group C streptococcus and possesses a hyaluronic acid capsule. The group C antigen is a carbohydrate and three type-specific antigens have been identified. This bacterium is able to cause mastitis on its own and is one of a number of pathogens involved in the summer mastitis complex. Strains of highest infectivity are those which adhere well to mammary epithelial cells. *Strep. dysgalactiae* binds well to fibronectin, moderately to fibrinogen and poorly to collagen. Protein G is present in the cell walls of some *Strep. dysgalactiae* and can bind bovine IgG. Such non-specific binding of immunoglobulin may protect the bacteria from gland defences. Cows develop protective antibody following immunization and hyperimmunized cows showed a degree of resistance to challenge exposure of the homologous strain.

Mucosal immune system

The concept of a common mucosal immune system was proposed following the observation that subsequent to intestinal exposure to antigen, specific immunity was evident at distant mucosal sites. Immunocompetent cells (specific lymphocytes) can migrate from Peyer's patch or mesenteric lymph nodes to distant sites, become resident and respond to sensitizing antigen. This does not seem to be true for ruminants since there is no selective migration of lymphocytes between the mammary gland and the gut of the cow. There are two major groups of recirculating lymphocytes in the cow: a peripheral and an intestinal pool. Labelled lymphocytes from the supramammary lymph node recirculated to the prescapular and supramammary lymph node whereas labelled ileac mesenteric lymphocytes were recovered from intestinal mesenteric lymph nodes. Local administration of antigen to the mammary gland would stimulate lymphocytes in the lamina propria to expand clonally and some of these cells would traffic to the supramammary lymph node.

Generation of immune response

Immune responses designed to protect the bovine mammary gland from infection can be generated by administration of antigen by various routes. Systemic immunization performed by the intramuscular, subcutaneous or intravenous route generates serum antibody. When mammary epithelium becomes inflamed sizeable amounts of circulating antibody pass into the lacteal secretions from the serum by transudation. Antibody has its greatest effect when present in lacteal secretions before infection is established. Direct injection of antigens into the udder stimulates both a local and a systemic response.

The primary course of events for humoral immunity involves antigen processing by macrophages and pres-

entation to $CD4^+$ T cells and to B cells. These $CD4^+$ cells release cytokines that stimulate the B cells to divide and produce antibodies. A small proportion of B cells become memory cells and if subsequently presented with their specific antigen they will proliferate rapidly and produce large amounts of antibody. Macrophages, T cells and B cells are present in the mammary gland and administration of antigen to the dry gland stimulates local synthesis of IgA and IgG_1. Such production persists well into lactation and is associated with the development of plasma cells in periductal connective tissue and interalveolar areas. The response is much less when antigen is administered to the lactating gland.

Intraperitoneal administration of antigen followed by local infusion recruits cells from systemic lymphoid tissues which have been primed by intraperitoneal immunization. Vaccination in the region of the draining lymph node of the mammary gland stimulates serum antibody and promotes production of local antibody. This may be due to the trafficking of lymphocytes. The J5 coliform mastitis was efficacious when administered subcutaneously or in the area of the supramammary lymph node. The administration of antigen in the region of the draining lymph node accompanied by local infusion is likely to have the greatest impact on the generation of antibodies in lacteal secretions.

The time of vaccination is another important factor since most infections occur at drying off, during the dry period and in the periparturient period. Almost 100 per cent of clinical mastitis occurs during lactation, with 60 per cent taking place in the first 40 days. Vaccination should be designed to offer maximum protection at these times. If systemic immunization is carried out at drying off, a booster given shortly before parturition by the intramammary route allows the gland to give a heightened and prolonged response through the next lactation (Watson & Lascelles, 1975).

Two components of a successful vaccine are the antigen and the adjuvant. As knowledge of the protective antigens of mastitis causing bacteria has grown, it is now appreciated the amount of antigen in a vaccine dose is critical and that the numbers of bacteria used in early studies were too low. Growth of Gram-positive cocci on conventional laboratory media can result in decreased expression of key bacterial antigens which are expressed during *in vivo* replication. Adjuvants are substances which act in a non-specific manner to augment the immune response to an antigen. Mineral oil, saponin and aluminium hydroxide are examples of adjuvants employed in veterinary vaccines. They can affect the magnitude, duration and isotypic composition of the immune response. The mechanism of action of adjuvants is not fully understood but includes slow release of antigen from a depot, alteration of lymphocyte circulation and release of cytokines.

Limitations of vaccination

The scientific literature contains numerous reports documenting the failure of vaccination to protect against intramammary challenge with a pathogen. There are fewer reports of protective products. These studies account for the two opposing views concerning the role of vaccination in mastitis control programmes. Challenge studies often have consisted of placing thousands of bacteria into the teat sinus, which is not an accurate reflection of natural infections in which only a few organisms will traverse the teat duct and reach the cistern to multiply. A better method to establish the efficacy of a vaccine is to perform field trials in herds where natural exposure to the pathogen will occur, with one half of the herd receiving vaccine and the remaining half receiving placebo. The evaluation of infection, clinical inflammation, persistence of leukocytosis, bacterial shedding and the effect on milk production will help determine vaccine efficacy.

The dairy cow undergoes periods of severe stress in each lactation cycle and immune dysfunction occurs at certain times. Immunosuppression can occur during pregnancy, lactation and parturition. Much interest has been directed to the four-day period prior to and subsequent to parturition, the so-called periparturient immunosuppression. Secretion taken just after drying off and at parturition has an inhibitory effect on blastogenic responses to mitogens. Proliferative responses to mitogens by blood and milk lymphocytes are low for one week before parturition and lowest on the day before calving (Kehrli et al., 1989). This may relate to the high incidence of clinical mastitis and intramammary infection which occur at calving and up to 30 days past calving. Certain indices of neutrophil function increased two weeks before parturition and decreased dramatically by the first week after parturition.

Because the concentration of PMNs is used to assess milk quality and a major defence component of the gland involves a leukocytosis with specific antibody, some authors argue that protection afforded by such a leukocytosis is, by definition, mastitis. Such a protective response can be interpreted in this manner. There is mounting evidence indicating that for certain pathogens, appropriate immunization strategies can reduce the number of clinical cases, reduce the number of new infections, improve the response to therapy and decrease the severity of clinical mastitis. If this involves a transient leukocytosis, it is likely farmers will accept the benefits.

The mammary gland of the cow has limited defensive capabilities with regard to PMN function and level of opsonins. In North America, good dairy cows yield on average 30 litres of milk for each day of their lactation. To maintain levels of antibody in this volume of secretion requires an enormous synthetic rate. Immunization does not confer absolute protection and at best will complement good husbandry and other mastitis control procedures. Vaccines for coliform mastitis will continue to be used widely while products to prevent *Staph. aureus* and *Strep. uberis* should become available in the near future. For other mammary pathogens there is little prospect of vaccines becoming available.

References

Bramley, A.J. (1976) Variations in the susceptibility of lactating and non-lactating bovine udders to infections when infused with *Escherichia coli*. *Journal of Dairy Research*, **43**, 205–11.

Butler, J.E. (1986) Biochemistry and biology of ruminant immunoglobulins. *Progress in Veterinary Microbiology and Immunology*, **2**, 1–53.

Colditz, I.G. & Watson, D.L. (1985) Immunophysiological basis for vaccinating ruminants against mastitis. *Australian Veterinary Journal*, **62**, 145–52.

Gonzalez, R.N., Cullor, J.S., Jasper, D.E., Farver, T.B., Bushnell, R.B. & Oliver, M.N. (1989) Prevention of clinical coliform mastitis in dairy cattle by a mutant *Escherichia coli* vaccine. *Canadian Journal of Veterinary Research*, **53**, 301–305.

Hill, A.W. (1979) The pathogenesis of experimental *Escherichia coli* mastitis in newly calved dairy cows. *Research in Veterinary Science*, **26**, 97–101.

Hill, A.W. (1991) Vaccination of cows with rough *Escherichia coli* mutants fails to protect against experimental intramammary bacterial challenge. *Veterinary Research Communications*, **15**, 7–16.

Hogan, J.S., Smith, K.L., Todhunter, D.A. & Schoenberger, P.S. (1992a) Field trial to determine efficacy of an *Escherichia coli* J5 mastitis vaccine. *Journal of Dairy Science*, **75**, 78–84.

Hogan, J.S., Weiss, W.P., Todhunter, D.A., Smith, K.L. & Schoenberger, P.S. (1992b) Efficacy of an *Escherichia coli* J5 mastitis vaccine in an experimental challenge trial. *Journal of Dairy Science*, **75**, 415–22.

Kehrli, M.E., Nonnecke, B.J. & Roth, J.A. (1989) Alterations in bovine lymphocyte function during the periparturient period. *American Journal of Veterinary Research*, **50**, 215–20.

Leigh, J.A. (1999) *Streptococcus uberis*, a permanent barrier to the control of bovine mastitis? *The Veterinary Journal*, **157**, 225–38.

Linton, A.H. & Robinson, T.C. (1984) Studies on the association of *Escherichia coli* with bovine mastitis. *British Veterinary Journal*, **40**, 368–73.

Mackie, D.P., Meneely, P.J., Pollack, D.A. & Logan, E.F. (1986) The loss of opsonic activity of bovine milk whey following depletion of IgA. *Veterinary Immunology and Immunopathology* **11**, 193–8.

Mellenberger, R.W. (1977) Vaccination against mastitis. *Journal of Dairy Science*, **60**, 1016–21.

Nordhaug, M.L., Nesse, L.L., Norcross, N.L. & Gudding, R. (1994) A field trial with an experimental vaccine against *Staphylococcus aureus* mastitis in cattle. 1. Clinical parameters. *Journal of Dairy Science*, **77**, 1267–75.

Outteridge, P.M. & Lee, C.S. (1988) The defence mechanisms of the mammary gland of ruminants. *Progress in Veterinary Microbiology and Immunology*, **2**, 1–53.

Sorensen, G.H. (1972) Sommer mastitis. Den mulige beskyttende virkning af to forskellige vacciner overfor eksperimentelle infektioner. *Nordisk Veterinar Medecin*, **24**, 259–71.

Sutra, L. & Poutrel, B. (1994) Virulence factors involved in the pathogenesis of bovine intramammary infections due to *Staphylococcus aureus*. *Journal of Medical Microbiology*, **40**, 79–89.

Tyler, J.W., Cullor, J.S., Osburn, B.I., Bushnell, R.B. & Fenwick, B.W. (1988) Relationship between serologic recognition of *Escherichia coli* O111, B4 (J5) and clinical coliform mastitis in cattle. *American Journal of Veterinary Research*, **49**, 1950–4.

Watson, D.L. & Lascelles, A.K. (1975) The influence of systemic immunization during mammary involution on subsequent antibody production in the mammary gland. *Research in Veterinary Science*, **18**, 182–5.

Watson, D.L., McColl, M.L. & Davies, H.I. (1996) Field trial of a staphylococcal mastitis vaccine in dairy herds, clinical, subclinical and microbiological assessments. *Australian Veterinary Journal*, **74**, 447–50.

Chapter 30
Antimicrobial Therapy of Mastitis

D.J. O'Rourke and J.D. Baggot

General considerations   391
Antimicrobial resistance   391
Pharmacology of the mammary gland   392
Intramammary preparations   393
Parenteral preparations   395
Selection of antimicrobial agent   396
Response to therapy   397
Therapy of mastitis   397
  During lactation   397
  During the dry period   399
Benefits of antimicrobial therapy for mastitis   402
  Improved milk quality   402
  Increased milk production   402
  Effective microbiological cures, eliminating reservoirs
    of infection   403
Costs associated with antimicrobial therapy   403
  Drug and veterinary costs   403
  Discarded milk   403
  Slaughter withdrawal periods   403
  Risks of new infections/altered host defences   403

General considerations

Mastitis is the single most common disease of the adult dairy cow, accounting for 30 per cent of all morbidity (Gardner *et al.*, 1990) and 38 per cent of health costs (Kossaibati & Esslemont, 1997). Additionally, in herds where the average culling rate was 23.8 per cent, mastitis was cited as the reason for culling in 10.1 per cent of cases and was the most common cause of death (8.9 per cent) (Esslemont & Kossaibati, 1997). Failure to achieve expected lactation yield as a consequence of clinical mastitis (Lucey & Rowlands, 1984; Rajala-Schultz *et al.*, 1999) and a reduction in milk yield caused by subclinical mastitis are responsible for even greater economic losses (Hortet & Seegers, 1998; Hortet *et al.*, 1999). Efficacious, economical treatment of mastitis is therefore an important component of livestock medicine.

The most frequent causes of mastitis are *Staphylococcus aureus*, *Streptococcus agalactiae*, *Strep. uberis*, *Strep. dysgalactiae*, *Escherichia coli*, *Enterobacter* sp., *Pseudomonas* sp., *Klebsiella* sp., *Arcanobacterium (Actinomyces; Corynebacterium) pyogenes* and *Mycoplasma* sp. (see Chapters 23 and 24). Differences in climate, management and national or regional regulatory efforts result in patterns of disease that vary markedly. The arid south-western regions of North America have repeatedly identified prevalences of intramammary *Mycoplasma* sp. infection exceeding those observed in other parts of the world (Jasper *et al.*, 1966; Jasper, 1980). In a survey of 50 California dairy herds (23 138 cows) potential mastitis pathogens were isolated from 22 per cent of cows (Gonzalez *et al.*, 1988). *Staphylococcus aureus* was isolated from all 50 herds, *Strep. agalactiae* from 47 herds and *Mycoplasma* sp. from 24 herds. The prevalence of mastitis pathogens (per cent cows) was *Staph. aureus* (9.1 per cent), *Strep. agalactiae* (9.3 per cent), *Mycoplasma* sp. (0.9 per cent), coliform bacteria (1.2 per cent) and other streptococci (0.9 per cent).

Laboratory testing is an integral part of treatment and control programmes and identification of the causal agents will have a direct bearing on subsequent therapy decisions. Several handbooks (International Dairy Federation, 1981; National Mastitis Council, 1999) and articles (Higgs & Bramley, 1981; Buswell, 1995) are available to assist in the identification of mastitis pathogens.

Antimicrobial resistance

Although useful as a guideline for antimicrobial selection, antibiotic sensitivity testing does not guarantee the efficacy of an antibiotic. Generally, the major streptococcal pathogens of the bovine mammary gland are sensitive (>90 per cent) to penicillin, ampicillin and erythromycin (Prescott & Baggot, 1988). Actual cure rates vary with clinical and lactation status.

There appears to have been no significant increase in bacterial resistance of mastitis-causing bacteria in the UK over the past 25 years. Craven *et al.* (1986) found a high incidence (69.8 per cent) of β-lactamase production which was similar to that (66.1 per cent) reported by Jones and Heath (1985). These studies indicated little change from the 70.6 per cent of penicillin-resistant strains reported by Wilson (1961). Recent surveys have indicated little change (Buswell, pers. comm.). It should also be noted that no staphylococci of bovine origin that are resistant to cloxacillin have been identified (Jones, 2000), despite its widespread use in both lactating and dry-cow intramammary preparation syringes for over 30 years.

Sensitivity patterns for the two most common Gram-negative intramammary pathogens, *E. coli* and *Klebsiella* sp., are reported in Table 30.1 and may be used to guide the choice of antibiotic when treating peracute mastitis (Mackie *et al.*, 1988; Prescott & Baggot, 1988). One should be cautioned that sensitivity patterns will vary locally according to antibiotic use. Historical susceptibility information drawn from individual farms will likely prove more useful. Table 30.2 reports *in vitro* sensitivity (Mackie *et al.*, 1988) and *in vivo* cure rates (Le Loudec, 1978) with respect to *Staph. aureus* for several commonly used antimicrobial agents. It should be noted that the percentage of sensitive isolates consistently exceeds cure rates. The absence of *in vitro* activity indicates bacterial resistance while sensitivity infers, but does not guarantee, clinical efficacy.

Pharmacology of the mammary gland

Antimicrobial therapy is applied in the treatment of clinical mastitis during lactation and in treating subclinical mastitis at the end of lactation, while the implementation of preventive measures is essential for decreasing the incidence of infection in the dairy herd. Clinical mastitis is often treated systemically which entails the repeated parenteral administration of an antimicrobial agent to which the causative pathogenic micro-organisms are susceptible at the drug concentration attained at the site of infection in the udder. The administration of an intramammary preparation in conjunction with systemic therapy is highly desirable, but the effectiveness of an infused antimicrobial is limited

Table 30.1 Antibiotic sensitivities of selected Gram-negative bacteria isolated from cattle with clinical mastitis (reported as per cent of isolates sensitive).

Antibiotic	Prescott & Baggot (1988)[a]		Mackie et al. (1988)
	E. coli	Klebsiella	Coliforms
Amoxycillin	–	–	51–65
Ampicillin	35	0	3–41
Cephalothin	60–73	82–93	–
Erythromycin	39	25	–
Framycetin	–	–	83–97
Furazolidone	92–98	25–92	88–99
Gentamicin	99–100	100	–
Lincomycin	29	17	–
Neomycin	56–70	33–90	19–93
Penicillin	0	0	–
Polymyxin	100	100	–
Spectinomycin	–	–	30–59
Streptomycin	73	77	49–61
Tetracycline	23	42–54	54–88[b]
Trimeth-sulfa	81	100	62–95

[a] Compiled from several sources.
[b] Oxytetracycline.

Table 30.2 Antibiotic sensitivities and bacteriological cure rates following treatment for *Staphylococcus aureus* after intramammary treatment with various antibiotics (adapted from Mackie *et al.* (1988) & Le Loudec (1978).

Antibiotic	% sensitive	Staph. aureus		No. of reports
		Mean % cure	Range	
Penicillin	19–62	32	0–87	12
Cloxacillin	100	41	21–84	14
Cephalosporins	100	72		1
Neomycin	72–98	27	25–36	2
Tetracycline	84–92	54	17–96	8
Tylosin		55	48–59	1
Erythromycin	72–98	63	51–76	2
Spiramycin		70	45–82	2
Rifamycin		66	65–66	2
Penicillin-streptomycin		39	21–78	2
Penicillin-neomycin		96	95–100	2
Ampicillin-cloxacillin		27	27–29	1

by decreased ability of the drug to ascend partially occluded milk ducts and by frequent stripping of the infected quarter.

Antimicrobial agents, like other drugs, cross the blood–milk barrier, which is a somewhat restrictive functional rather than an anatomical barrier, mainly by passive diffusion. Both non-polar lipid-soluble compounds and polar substances with sufficient lipid solubility passively diffuse through the predominately lipoidal barrier (Baggot, 1977). At a moderate level of milk production the ratio of the volume of blood circulating through the mammary gland to the volume of milk produced has been estimated to be 670:1; this provides ample opportunity for drugs to passively diffuse from the general circulation into milk. The rate of transfer is directly proportional to the concentration gradient across the blood–milk barrier and the lipid solubility of the drug. The milk-to-plasma equilibrium concentration ratio of total (non-ionized plus ionized) drug is determined by (i) the degree of ionization of the drug, which is pK_a/pH-dependent, in blood and milk, (ii) the charge on the ionized moiety and (iii) the extent of binding of plasma proteins and milk macromolecules. It has been shown that only the lipid-soluble, non-ionized moiety of a weak organic acid or base that is free (not bound to proteins) in the plasma can diffuse through the cellular barriers and enter the milk (Rasmussen, 1966). In normal lactating cows (milk pH range 6.5–6.8), weak organic acids attain milk ultrafiltrate-to-plasma ultrafiltrate equilibrium concentration ratios less than 1; oxytetracycline and rifampin, amphoteric drug molecules with moderate and high lipid solubility, attain equilibrium concentration ratios of 0.75 and *ca* 1,

respectively; weak organic bases, apart from aminoglycosides, spectionmycin and polymyxin B (drugs with low solubility in lipid), attain milk ultrafiltrate-to-plasma ultrafiltrate equilibrium concentration ratios greater than 1 (Baggot, 2000). The high concentration ratios attained by lipophilic organic bases (macrolides, lincosamides and trimethoprim) are attributed to the ion-trapping effect in acidic milk. Enrofloxacin and its active metabolite ciprofloxacin, formed by *N*-de-ethylation (a microsomal-mediated oxidative reaction) in the liver, would be expected to attain concentrations in milk that would be effective against Gram-negative aerobic bacteria, in particular *Escherichia coli*.

In the presence of mastitis, the pH of milk increases to within the range 6.9 to 7.2. As a consequence the ion-trapping effect on lipophilic organic bases is reduced while the concentrations attained by weak organic acids are somewhat increased. The inflammatory reaction in udder tissues enhances the passage of penicillins into milk. The increased pH of milk does not affect the concentrations attained by amphoteric drugs (fluoroquinolones, tetracyclines, rifampicin), but antimicrobial activity of these drugs is lower in milk than in extracellular fluid or *in vitro* determination would predict.

Intramammary preparations (Table 30.3)

Intramammary preparations are used, often in conjunction with parenteral preparations (depending on severity of infection), to treat clinical mastitis and at the end of lactation to treat subclinical infection and

Table 30.3 Distribution of antibiotics throughout the udder after intramammary administration (adapted from Ziv, 1980).

Good	Moderate	Poor
Amoxycillin	Penicillin G	Bacitracin
Ampicillin	Cloxacillin	(Dihydro)streptomycin
Cephalexin	Cephalonium	Gentamicin
Erythromycin	Cephapirin	Neomycin
Novobiocin	Cephacetrile	Polymyxins
Penethamate	Cefquinome	Framycetin
Quinolones	Tetracyclines	
Spiramycin	Other sulphonamides	
Sulphanilamide		
Tylosin		
Trimethoprim		
Rifamycin		
Amoxycillin-clavulanic acid		
Lincomycin		
Pirlimycin		

prevent the establishment of new infections during the dry period. The various preparations differ in nature, content and release pattern of the active ingredient(s) and in the length of the withdrawal periods (slaughter and milk withholding) but all preparations must be reasonably non-irritating to the udder. Intramammary preparations are formulated either to provide quick release of the antimicrobial agent or slow release of the antimicrobial over an extended period. The former are used mainly in lactating cows while the latter are used at the end of lactation (after the last milking) and in non-lactating cows. While the formulation of an intramammary preparation determines the pattern of antimicrobial release and may influence the withdrawal periods, the chemical nature and physico-chemical properties (in particular lipid solubility) of the drug govern its uptake and distribution in mammary tissue and its absorption into the blood. Drug transfer from treated to untreated quarters of the udder takes place via the bloodstream.

Following intramammary infusion antimicrobials with high lipid solubility (macrolides, trimethoprim, fluroquinolones, rifampicin) are readily taken up by and distributed widely in mammary tissue. Oxytetracycline is moderately lipid-soluble and the fraction that is not chelated with calcium in milk enters mammary tissue and distributes evenly in a manner that is not subject to the pK_a/pH-dependent ion-trapping effect. However, the antimicrobial effect, which is exerted mainly on streptococcal spp. and coagulase-negative staphylococci, is bacteriostatic. The susceptibility of coagulase-positive *Staph. aureus*, *E. coli* and *Klebsiella* spp. to oxytetracycline is variable and unpredictable. The uptake and distribution of sulfadiazine (pK_a 6.4) and sulphamethoxazole (pK_a 6.0), which are moderately lipid-soluble organic acids, are influenced by the degree of ionization in their local environment. Since sulphonamides are combined with trimethoprim in intramammary preparations the broad-spectrum antibacterial effect produced is bactericidal. The beta-lactam antibiotics (penicillins and cephalosporins), although they exist mainly in an ionized form in milk, are taken up by mammary tissue and distribute reasonably well but do not readily enter epithelial cells or kill bacteria within phagocytic cells (neutrophils and macrophages). The uptake of hydrophilic antimicrobial agents (aminoglycosides and polymixin B) from milk is low and their distribution is very limited and uneven because of selective binding to mammary tissue components. Antimicrobials that avidly bind to mammary tissue (polymyxin B, neomycin, streptomycin, spiramycin) have long withdrawal periods.

The frequency of milking and the efficiency of milk-out greatly influence the concentration of antimicrobial that could be attained in the udder. Since frequent stripping of the infected quarter(s) is recommended in cows with clinical mastitis, it follows that only quick-release intramammary preparations are suitable for use in lactating cows.

Intramammary preparations for use in lactating cows should contain a readily available form, usually water-soluble salt, of an antimicrobial agent with a low degree of binding to milk and mammary tissue proteins. The vehicle used and viscosity of the formulation should allow rapid release of the drug and ensure that effective concentrations are maintained throughout the recommended dosage interval. Examples of intramammary preparations that are formulated as suspensions and have a recommended dosage interval of 12 hours include cloxacillin sodium, oxytetracycline hydrochloride, ampicillin sodium–cloxacillin sodium combination and trimethoprim–sulfadiazine combination. Cefuroxime sodium and cefoperazone sodium (second- and third-generation cephalosporins, respectively) are formulated as an oily paste and oily suspension, respectively. While a 12-hour dosage interval is recommended for cefuroxime, a single dose of the cefoperazone preparation is considered to be usually sufficient for treatment. Quick-release intramammary preparations have short withdrawal periods, typically slaughter times of 7 days and milk withholding times of 3.5 days, or either may be less depending on the preparation.

Slow-release intramammary preparations may contain an antimicrobial agent with a high degree of binding to the secretions and mammary tissue proteins. Either a poorly soluble salt of an antimicrobial agent may be used or the formulation of the preparation be such that the rate of antimicrobial release is relatively constant, approaching zero order (Baggot & Brown, 1998). The formulation of slow-release preparations determines the antimicrobial concentration–time profile in the mammary gland to a greater extent than quick-release preparations. Since only a single dose of a slow-release preparation is infused, the antimicrobial content is generally higher than in quick-release preparations. The antimicrobial must remain active (be stable) throughout the extended duration in the udder and the preparation must not cause irritation. Examples of slow-release intramammary preparations include cloxacillin (as benzathine salt) with aluminium monostearate (suspension), ampicillin (as trihydrate)–cloxacillin (as benzathine salt) formulated as an oily suspension, procaine benzlypenicillin (oily paste) and dihydrostreptomycin sulphate-procaine benzylpenicillin (oily paste). The long withdrawal periods for these preparations preclude their intramammary infusion in lactating cows.

Intramammary administration permits delivery of the antibiotic directly to the mammary gland. Penicillin derivatives have demonstrated efficacy in intramammary treatment of *Strep. agalactiae*. Intramammary preparations for infusion are available as single-use syringes for a course of treatment of one, two or three syringes at 12- or 24-hour intervals depending on the product. Lactating cow (quick-release) products are generally designed for rapid clearance and, consequently, have shorter milk withholding periods. Antibiotics with extensive tissue binding (polymixin B and aminoglycosides) have extended milk withholding periods (Baggot, 2000). Dry-cow formulations, for the treatment of subclinical mastitis, are designed to produce extended duration of effective drug concentrations. This is achieved by using a higher concentration of the active drug or the benzathine salt of the active drug in oil or a repository vehicle.

For antimicrobial therapy with either a parenteral or intramammary preparation, or the concurrent use of both types of preparation, to be effective an antimicrobial concentration exceeding the MIC for the causative pathogenic micro-organism must be maintained at the site of infection for an adequate duration. Provided the appropriate antimicrobial is selected, the intramammary infusion of a slow-release preparation at the end of lactation may adequately meet this requirement. However, in the case of *Staph. aureus* infection, the administration of a parenteral preparation in conjunction with a slow-release intramammary preparation containing an antimicrobial, which is active against all strains of the bacterium, increases the effectiveness of therapy and consequently the recovery rate.

Parenteral preparations

Severe mastitis is usually treated systemically, although intramammary therapy will often be used adjunctively. An 'ideal' antimicrobial for systemic therapy of mastitis should have the following properties (adapted from Ziv, 1980):

- Low minimum inhibitory concentration (MIC) for the majority of mastitis-causing pathogenic micro-organisms.
- High biovailability following intramuscular injection.
- Lipid-soluble and predominately non-ionized in the blood, and have a low degree of binding to plasma proteins.
- A long apparent half-life to ensure that concentrations above (preferably several-fold) the MIC are maintained at the site of infection throughout the dosage interval (12 or 24 hours).
- Minimal adverse effects in cows.
- Short withdrawal periods (milk withholding and slaughter).

Parenteral preparations with pharmacokinetic properties that meet most of these criteria include procaine benzylpencillin, amoxicillin trihydrate–clavulanate potassium combination, trimethoprim–sulfadiazine (or sulphamethoxazole) combination and enrofloxacin. In order to obtain effective concentrations in milk oxytetracycline hydrochloride (conventional preparation) should be administered by slow intravenous injection. Long-acting parenteral preparations of oxytetracycline are not indicated in the treatment of mastitis. Macrolide antibiotics have good tissue penetrative capacity and the ion-trapping effect favours the concentrations attained in milk. An undesirable feature of their distribution is diffusion from the systemic circulation into ruminal fluid (pH 5.5 to 6.5) where the ion-trapping effect also applies. Because of their wide distribution in tissues and passage into ruminal fluid, high doses are required to attain effective concentrations in milk. In the case of spiramycin, the persistence of tissue residues is a major disadvantage. Since parenteral preparations of erythromycin and spiramycin cause tissue irritation at intramuscular injection sites, slow intravenous injection is the preferred route of administration.

Drugs are transferred from the general circulation to the mammary gland by passive diffusion (Baggot, 1977; Ziv, 1980). Consequently, non-ionized lipid-soluble agents that are not extensively bound to plasma proteins more readily reach the mammary gland (Table 30.4). Because milk is weakly acidic (pH 6.5–6.8), drugs that are weak bases (trimethoprim, macrolides, lincosamides) are preferentially concentrated by ion trapping (Ziv, 1980; Baggot, 2000). Of the antimicrobials that distribute well in the mammary gland following parenteral administration, only fluoroquinolones have broad-spectrum activity against Gram-negative pathogens. Because of bacterial resistance concerns for humans, the use of this class of antimicrobial in dairy cows is not approved. The low degree of lipid solubility of aminoglycosides and polymyxin B limits their passage into milk.

Table 30.4 Distribution of antibiotics throughout the udder after parenteral administration (adapted from Ziv, 1980).

Good	Moderate	Poor
Erythromycin	Amoxycillin	(Dihydro)streptomycin
Spiramycin	Ampicillin	Gentamicin
Tylosin	Cephalosporins	Neomycin
Trimethoprim	Penicillin G	Polymyxins
Baquiloprim	Rifamycin	Spectinomycin
Fluoroquinolones	Sulphonamides	
	Tetracyclines	

In the presence of clinical mastitis, the pH of the milk increases (6.9–7.2), approaching that of plasma. Under these circumstances weak acids (sulphonamides, penicillins, amoxycillin–clavulanic acid, cephalosporins, rifampin), although typically not concentrated in milk, may reach effective concentrations (Ziv, 1980; Durnford, pers. comm.; Baggot, 2000). Lipophilic drugs of various pharmacological classes will also be concentrated in milk in spite of the decreased ion-trapping.

The site of infection within the udder varies with the causative pathogenic micro-organisms and, in addition to bacterial susceptibility, influences the choice of antimicrobial agent. Since streptococcal mastitis is usually an infection of the milk compartment of the udder, antimicrobial agents that have limited membrane penetrative capacity and produce a bactericidal effect, such as penicillins (benzylpenicillin), may be selected for therapy. Even though coliform mastitis is an infection of the milk compartment, the choice of antimicrobial for systemic therapy is largely limited to enrofloxacin or trimethoprim–sulphonamide since the long withdrawal period for aminoglycosides precludes their use. *Staphylococcal aureus*, the principal causative micro-organism of subclinical mastitis, may reside in the intracellular space and within epithelial and phagocytic cells (Pyorala, 1995). The treatment of staphylococcal mastitis requires the administration (parenteral and intramammary) of an antimicrobial agent which can penetrate epithelial cells and tissues of the udder and is active against staphylococcal beta-lactamase. Amoxicillin–clavulanic acid combination and macrolide antibiotics (erythromycin and spiramycin) meet these requirements. The bacteriostatic effect produced by macrolides and their reduced antibacterial activity in milk could be disadvantageous.

Selection of antimicrobial agent

There are several factors to consider when selecting an antimicrobial agent, and the preparations (parenteral, intramammary) to use, for the treatment of mastitis. They include the nature and severity of the infection, the stage of lactation, the causative pathogenic micro-organism and its susceptibility, the relative cost of the various antimicrobial preparations, the incidence of mastitis in the herd and the usage pattern of intramammary preparations. Early diagnosis and the prompt application of appropriate treatment will reduce the extent of mammary tissue damage and will increase the rate of recovery and the return of milk production to or approaching the original level. It is desirable to select an antimicrobial that produces a bactericidal effect and has a narrow spectrum of activity and essential that treatment should continue for an adequate duration in order to achieve a bacteriological cure. Apart from preparations containing fixed combinations (trimethoprim–sulphonamide, amoxillin–clavulanate), the use of combination preparations should generally be avoided.

Having made a (tentative) clinical diagnosis of the nature of the mastitis and established the history of infection in the affected cow and incidence of infection in the herd, a pretreatment milk sample for bacterial culture should be properly (aseptically) collected. Immediate examination of a milk sample is a particularly useful aid in selecting an antimicrobial for empirical treatment, which should commence at this time. A parenteral and quick-release intramammary preparation may be used concurrently. The latter should be infused after stripping milk and other products (cellular debris, pus) from the infected quarter(s). Oxytocin, 5 to 10 units of diluted solution (10 units/ml), can be administered by slow intravenous injection to facilitate the completeness of stripping. The half-life of oxytocin is approximately 2 minutes. In addition to antimicrobial administration, supportive therapy should be provided.

Results obtained from the microbiology laboratory, interpreted in conjunction with the tentative clinical diagnosis and knowledge of the distribution of antimicrobial agents in the udder, facilitate selection of the appropriate drug. Mastitis, with the exception of summer mastitis, is usually caused by a single bacterial species. When *Staph. aureus* is the causative pathogenic micro-organism, it can be rapidly determined whether the strain isolated produces beta-lactamase (70 per cent of strains), although it should be recognized that milk induces production of the enzyme. The susceptibility of streptococci can be predicted, but it is necessary to determine quantitative susceptibility, using the broth dilution method (which measures MIC), of coagulase-positive staphylococci and enteric bacteria (*E. coli*, *Klebsiella* spp.). Knowledge of the susceptibility (predicted or measured *in vitro*) of the causative bacterial pathogen and of the pharmacokinetic properties of the antimicrobial agent of choice provides the information required for calculating the dose and selecting the dosage interval for the parenteral preparation. Dosage calculations are based on MIC which is assumed to be related to the concentration attained at the site of infection in the udder. An intramammary preparation containing an antimicrobial that will reach the site of infection and complement the activity of the antimicrobial in the parenteral preparation should be chosen and administered by intramammary infusion (after stripping the inflamed quarter) at the recommended dosage interval, which is usually 12 or 24 hours, for preparations intended for use in lactating cows.

Response to therapy

A combination of methods, applied two to three weeks after the end of treatment, should be used to assess the effectiveness of antimicrobial therapy. They include clinical examination, bacterial culture of an aseptically collected milk sample, tests based on changes in somatic cell count, protein, enzyme and electrolyte contents of milk (indication of inflammation) and return to the expected level of milk production (Pyorala, 1995). Discrepancy between the expected and obtained response to therapy may be attributed to inadequacy of the host defence mechanisms, acquired bacterial resistance, altered pharmacokinetic behaviour of the antimicrobial in the diseased animal or poor distribution in the udder with limited access to the site of infection. In the case of infection caused by *Staph. aureus* bacteria located in microabscesses, macrophages and fibrotic tissue, the bacterial pathogen may be virtually inaccessible to antimicrobial agents or may be in a state of dormancy. The bacteriological cure rate of staphylococcal mastitis is low, particularly when treatment is applied during lactation, while the high self-cure rate of coliform mastitis greatly influences the validity of attributing bacteriological cure to antimicrobial therapy (Sandholm & Pyorala, 1995). A reasonably satisfactory response rate to treatment of staphylococcal mastitis is obtained only when appropriate therapy with a parenteral preparation and a slow-release intramammary preparation is applied at the end of lactation after the last milking. The longer the antimicrobial(s) persists in the udder, the greater the likelihood of at least a moderately favourable response to therapy. The bacteriological cure rate can vary widely.

Therapy of mastitis

During lactation

Factors to take into account when choosing an intramammary preparation include:

- Antibacterial spectrum
- Cost of the preparation for usual duration of treatment
- With/without steroid
- Previous treatment history
- Availability of injectable 'partner' (parenteral preparation)
- Milk withholding time
- Personal preference

Compound preparations containing one or more antimicrobial agents and a corticosteroid (hydrocortisone or prednisolone) are available for intramammary infusion mainly in lactating cows. Amoxycillin trihydrate–clavulanate potassium and prednisolone are combined in a compound intramammary preparation (oily suspension) which provides greatly enhanced activity of amoxycillin against beta-lactamase producing *Staph. aureus* and has short withdrawal periods.

Steroids (prednisolone) are present in low dose and their activity is of short duration. There has been no convincing evidence of depressed antibody production or cell-mediated responses as a result of the inclusion of prednisolone in an intramammary formulation. In fact, it could be argued that the inclusion of prednisolone is supportable on grounds of cow welfare. Farmers will claim that the inclusion of the steroid will lead to a reduction in size of the inflamed quarter. Trials carried out with an amoxycillin–clavulanic acid formulation containing prednisolone confirm this observation (O'Rourke, 1994) (Fig. 30.1).

Most compound preparations contain antimicrobial agents that are selected on the basis of broadening the spectrum of antimicrobial activity without extending the withdrawal period. These compound preparations (more than one antibiotic) are of doubtful value and are often not successful in eliminating infection. Moreover, the concentration achieved by any one antibiotic in such preparations is likely to be lower than the optimum required for treatment and could facilitate the development of resistance (Egan, 1984). Unless the antimicrobials in a combination preparation act synergistically (Table 30.5) the use of compound preparations should be avoided.

In recent years veterinary practitioners have been debating the concurrent use of an injectable and intramammary preparation in the treatment of mastitis.

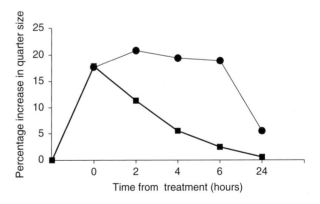

Fig. 30.1 Reduction in quarter size, experimentally infected with *Streptococcus uberis*, after treatment with amoxycillin and clavulanic acid formulations with and without prednisolone (O'Rourke, 1994). ■ = Lactating low formulation containing amoxycillin, clavulanic acid and prednisolone. ● = Same formulation without prednisolone.

There have been a number of studies indicating a beneficial effect in the treatment of *Staph. aureus* infections from the concurrent use of an intramammary and an injectable (Tables 30.6 and 30.7). However, the compatibility of the injectable and intramammary preparations should be taken into account whenever this form of treatment is being considered.

Peracute mastitis

Toxic mastitis is most commonly caused by the coliform organisms *E. coli*, *Klebsiella* spp., *Enterobacter* spp. and *Serratia* spp. Because of the severity of clinical signs the following therapeutic regimen is suggested:

(1) Frequent stripping of the affected quarter following the administration of oxytocin is probably the most important, yet most often neglected, component of therapy. Evacuation of the udder serves to remove both bacterial endotoxins and inflammatory host mediators, thus markedly reducing the severity of clinical signs.

(2) Antibacterial therapy: gentamicin, polymyxin B and potentiated sulphonamides have minimal inhibitory concentrations (MIC) and distribution properties suitable for the treatment of coliform mastitis.

(3) Intravenous fluids.

(4) Non-steroidal anti-inflammatory drugs.

The non-steroidal anti-inflammatory drugs have a more selective action than glucocorticoids in that they directly inhibit cyclo-oxygenase, although isoforms of the enzyme are inhibited to a varying degree depending on the drug. The consequence of cyclo-oxygenase inhibition is that the synthesis of prostaglandins

Table 30.5 Clinically useful antimicrobial drug combinations in veterinary medicine (adapted from Prescott & Walker, 2000).

Indication	Drug combination	Comment
Bovine *Staph. aureus* mastitis	Penicillin–streptomycin	Synergistic combination
	Amoxycillin–clavulanic acid	Potentiated combination

Table 30.6 Bacteriological cure rates for subclinical *Staphylococcus aureus* infections at 21 days post treatment with amoxycillin and penicillin G (Owens *et al.*, 1988). Reproduced with permission of the American Dairy Science Association.

Route	Regime	Bacteriological cure rate (%)
Intramammary (*n* = 40)	62.5 mg amoxycillin six times @ 12-hour intervals	25
Intramammary + injection (*n* = 35)	62.5 mg amoxycillin six times @ 12-hour intervals +9 000 000 iu procaine penicillin daily for 3 days	51.4

Table 30.7 Bacteriological cure rates for chronic *Staphylococcus aureus* infections at 20 days post treatment with spiramycin (Ziv, 1980).

Route	Regime	Bacteriological cure rate (%)
Injection (*n* = 18)	10 g spiramycin (IM) twice @ 72-hour intervals	16
Intramammary (*n* = 40)	500 mg spiramycin three times @ 24-hour intervals	40
Intramammary + injection (*n* = 35)	10 g spiramycin (IM) twice @ 72-hour intervals + 500 mg spiramycin three times @ 24-hour intervals	68

involved in central pyresis and pain perception as well as tissue inflammation is inhibited. Unlike glucocorticoids, the non-steroidal anti-inflammatory drugs do not produce immunosuppression. The rate of elimination (hepatic metabolism) of these drugs in cattle differs widely. The half-life of salicylate is 0.8 hours (3.5 hours when administered orally as aspirin, due to slow dissolution/absorption from ruminal fluid), ketoprofen (0.4 hours), flunixin (8.1 hours) and phenylbutazone (42–66 hours). They distribute to a similar extent, mainly in extracellular fluid, and enter milk by passive diffusion. Of these drugs, flunixin meglumine (2.2 mg/kg, administered by intravenous injection at 24-hour dosage intervals) may have a place in the treatment of acute *E. coli* (endotoxin) mastitis. The withdrawal period is slaughter 7 days, milk 12 hours. The antipyretic, anti-inflammatory and analgesic effects produced by the drug are largely dependent on the stage of the inflammatory process at which treatment is commenced. Early diagnosis of coliform mastitis would increase the beneficial effect produced by flunixin administration.

During the dry period

Routine dry-cow therapy provides the following advantages:

- Bacteriological cure of a higher proportion of *Staph. aureus* infections (Table 30.8).
- No loss of milk production.
- Prevention of new infections (including summer mastitis commonly due to *Arcanobacterium pyogenes*), especially in the early dry period.
- Treatment of infections caused by streptococci and other bacteria.

In herds with a high prevalence of contagious mastitis pathogens, the use of dry-cow therapy has been an efficacious and economically effective method of reducing the frequency of intramammary infections (Heald *et al.*, 1977). Berry *et al.* (1997) showed that cows treated with dry-cow therapy at the end of lactation produced 179 kg more milk during the first 120 days of the subsequent lactation when compared with control cows that received no therapy.

The efficacy of dry-cow therapy for subclinical mastitis is not invariably reliable, especially for chronic cases of mastitis caused by *Staph. aureus* (Table 30.9). There are, however, results indicating that an improved cure rate can be achieved when intramammary treatment is accompanied by systemic treatment (Table 30.10).

Strategies for dry period treatment

With consistent application of dry-cow therapy (DCT) in conjunction with other mastitis control measures the prevalence of contagious mastitis pathogens has declined to a low level in many herds (Kirk *et al.*, 1994), as is evidenced by bulk milk somatic cell counts (BMSCC) of <200 000 cells/ml. Some owners of herds with a low prevalence of contagious mastitis pathogens have stopped using dry-cow therapy and others are questioning the practice because of concerns about residues in the milk (Kirk *et al.*, 1994). Macmillian *et al.* (1983) indicated that in herds with low cell counts selective dry-cow therapy may be preferable to whole herd therapy.

A fact sheet entitled Dry Cow Therapy (Anderson & Cote, 1996) from the Ontario Ministry of Agriculture, Food and Rural Affairs recommends that selective dry-cow therapy should be used when the monthly bulk milk cell count (BMCC) is below 200 000 and the quarter infection rate is <15%. The following cows should be treated:

- Cows with peak somatic cell count (SCC) > 250 000/ml.
- Cows which have had a clinical case of mastitis.
- Cows from which a major mastitis pathogen(s) has been cultured.

In New Zealand the SAMM (seasonal approach to managing mastitis) plan was devised by the Dairy Research Corporation. It was adopted by the NZ Mastitis Advisory Committee and launched in 1993. The implementation of the plan contributed to a

Table 30.8 Bacteriological cure rates (percentages) for selected Gram-positive intramammary infections using cloxacillin (adapted from Griffin *et al.*, 1982).

Bacterium	Lactation		At drying off
	Clinical	Subclinical	
Streptococcus agalactiae	85	100	99
Staphylococcus aureus	26	52	61
Streptococcus dysgalactiae	90	98	96
Streptococcus uberis	77	82	87

Table 30.9 The responses of previously untreated or unsuccessfully treated staphylococcal infections to cloxacillin therapy given in lactation or at drying off (adapted from Griffin *et al.*, 1982).

	Previous lactation treatments			
Lactation therapy No previous drying-off treatments	0	1	2	>2
% response	46	21	17	12
1 or more previous drying-off treatments				
% response	25	15	13	7
Drying-off therapy	0	1	>1	
% response	61	46	24	
Previous drying-off treatments				
% response	60	24	10	

Table 30.10 Bacteriological cure rates for chronic subclinical *Staphylococcus aureus* infections at 15 days postcalving (Johansson *et al.*, 1995). Reproduced with permission of the International Dairy Federation.

Route	Regime	Bacteriological cure rate (%)
Intramammary (*n* = 42)	0.17 g penicillin benzathine +0.4 g dihydrostreptomycin in all 4 quarters	57
Intramammary + injection (*n* = 38)	20 mg/kg benzylpenicillin procaine for 5 days followed by 0.17 g penicillinbenzatin +0.4 g dihydrostreptomycin in all 4 quarters	79

substantial decline in somatic cell count levels in subsequent years (national average cell count is 178 000/ml). The criteria used for determining herd mastitis status and dry-cow therapy are show in Table 30.11.

The effects of three selection strategies for dry-cow therapy on prevention of new infections and rate of antibiotic usage were compared in a trial involving 1044 cows in 12 herds (Table 30.12) (Browning *et al.*, 1984). Selective cow treatment was identified as the preferred strategy. Blanket treatment resulted in increased antibiotic usage: 15.5 versus 6.4 tubes per infection eliminated with no additional benefit and selective quarter treatment resulted in a higher new infection rate (6.4 versus 3.9 per cent) during the dry period.

Berry *et al.* (1999) confirmed that this is still the case today in a study comparing dry-cow therapy versus no treatment. Dry-cow therapy resulted in a 10-fold reduc-

tion in clinical mastitis during the dry period and a 3-fold reduction in infected cows at calving and clinical mastitis in the first 21 days of lactation when compared to herds where there was no treatment (Table 30.13).

Hovi and Roderick (2000) found that the incidence of new infection during the dry period was three times higher in organic herds when compared to conventional herds (28.9 cases per 100 cows versus 9.2 cases per 100 cows). The authors point out that most organic dairy farmers felt that it was impossible to maintain low SCCs without using dry-cow therapy and culling healthy young cows.

Whilst we may implement selective dry-cow therapy, the key question is: are these untreated quarters more susceptible to infection during the dry period? The physiological process whereby the teat canal becomes closed through the formation of a keratin plug after drying off appears to be a major defence mechanism.

Table 30.11 Criteria used in the SAMM plan for determining herd mastitis status and dry-cow therapy strategy (Woolford *et al.*, 1995). DCT, dry-cow therapy. Reproduced with permission of the International Dairy Federation.

Criteria	Herd mastitis classification		
	High	Medium	Low
Average BMSCC, Jan–Mar (000/ml)	>400	150–400	<150
or			
% cows >150000/ml over Jan–Mar	>50%	20–50%	<20%
or			
% cows clinical in first month of lactation	>10%	3–10%	<3%
or			
15% cows clinical first 3 weeks of last dry period?	Yes	No	No
or			
Late season outbreak of clinical cases?	Yes	No	No
Recommended DCT strategy	*Total herd*	*Selective cow*	*Selective cow*

Table 30.12 Prevalence of infected quarters at drying off and calving plus the new infection rate during the dry period for three different dry-cow strategies (Browning *et al.*, 1984, reproduced with permission of Australian Veterinary Journal). DCT, dry-cow therapy.

Strategy	Drying off prevalence (%)	Calving prevalence (%)	New infection rate during dry period (%)
DCT	13.2	6.8	2.6
Selective cow	13.0	7.9	3.9
Selective quarter	13.1	10.0	6.4[a]

[a] $P \le 0.05$.

Table 30.13 Prevalence of clinical mastitis during the dry period, infected cows at calving plus clinical mastitis during the first 21 days of lactation (Berry *et al.*, 1999). DCT, dry-cow therapy.

Strategy	Clinical mastitis during the dry period (%)	Infections at calving (%)	Mastitis in first 21 days of lactation (%)
DCT	0.0	9.6	5.5
No treatment	10.5	32.8	16.4

Williamson *et al.* (1995), reporting on the observations of the dynamics of teat canal closure for a group of 657 quarters after drying off, noted that 50 per cent of teat canals were classified as 'closed' at 7 days after drying off. A further 45 per cent became closed over the following 50–60 days and 5 per cent remained 'open' at 90 days. During this study 83 per cent of all clinical infections during the dry period occurred within the first 21 days. Of the 52 clinical infections that were diagnosed

during the dry period, 97 per cent occurred in teats that had an 'open' canal.

The dilemma is how to protect quarters that are not treated with dry-cow therapy. In New Zealand a non-antibiotic preparation, Teatseal™, is available (Orbe-Seal™ in the UK). Teatseal is a dense, viscous material, which is infused hygienically into the teat as soon as possible after the last milking of lactation. It physically plugs the teat canal immediately after infusion thus

Table 30.14 Numbers of new intramammary infections (IMIs) over the dry period and at calving for the four treatment groups (Woolford *et al.*, 1998).

Experimental group	NC	PC	TS	TS + Ab
Total quarters allocated at drying off	528	528	505	505
New dry period clinical IMIs	18	2[a]	1[a]	2[a]
New IMIs at calving				
Streptococcus spp.	50	5[a]	4[a]	4[a]
Staphylococcus aureus	3	0	1	0
Coagulase-negative staphylococci	6	1	6	2
Coliforms	4	4	1	1
Other organisms	2	2	0	1
Clinical – no growth at culture	2	0	0	0
Total non-streptococcal IMIs	17	7[b]	8[c]	4[a]
Total new IMIs at calving	67	12[a]	12[a]	8[a]
Total new IMIs	85	14[a]	13[a]	10[a]
Overall incidence of new IMI rate (% quarters)	16.1	2.7[a]	2.6[a]	2.0[a]

Superscripts denote significant differences within rows between treatment groups and the negative control.
[a] $P < 0.01$; [b] $P \approx 0.05$; [c] $P < 0.1$
NC, negative control; PC, positive control (cephalonium); TS, Teatseal; TS + Ab, Teatseal + cloxacillin.

preventing bacteria from entering the teat. The teat canal then becomes closed from day one of the dry period and remains closed for the dry period.

A large-scale study has been carried (Woolford *et al.*, 1998) utilizing a total of 1200 cows across seven herds. Cows with late lactation SCCs of < 200000/ml were identified and sampled aseptically to establish the infection status of every quarter at drying off. At drying off uninfected quarters were randomly allocated to a treatment. The numbers of new intramammary infections (IMIs) during the dry period and at calving are shown in Table 30.14. In the 1998 study all three infused treatments (Teatseal, cephalonium (Cepravin DC), and Teatseal plus 600 mg cloxacillin (prior to infusion of the seal) showed about a 10-fold reduction in new clinical IMIs ($P < 0.01$) relative to the negative control (no treatment). The incidence of new IMI due to *Strep. uberis* at calving was 10-fold lower ($P < 0.01$) for prophylactic treatments compared to the negative control. It is also interesting to note that the prophylactic treatments reduced the incidence of postcalving clinical mastitis by approximately 50 per cent in the subsequent lactation compared to the negative control. This study indicated that use of Teatseal protects the gland against establishment of infection, by the presence of a physical barrier from day one of the dry period, which remains in place until calving.

Benefits of antimicrobial therapy for mastitis

Improved milk quality

Subclinical mastitis affects the quality of dairy products. Milk from infected cattle is less palatable, has a shorter shelf-life and produces lower yields of processed dairy products. Consequently, cooperatives, commercial concerns and regulatory agencies impose penalties, based on cell count and bacterial counts of bulk milk. The most severe penalty arises with milk that is deemed unfit for human consumption and discarded (BMCC > 400000 cells/ml in EU, see Chapter 25). Although treatment of clinical mastitis may not result in a microbiological cure, macroscopic milk quality will return to normal more quickly following treatment. The more rapid return to the production of saleable milk is an important benefit of treatment.

Increased milk production

The largest cost associated with mastitis is reduced milk yield as a result of clinical and subclinical infection. Lucey and Rowlands (1984) found that the mean reduction in milk yield where clinical mastitis occurred was 540 kg, the average lactation being 4830 kg. The reduction was greatest when infection occurred before peak yield, the proportional reduction being higher in higher-yielding cows. Where clinical mastitis occurred before peak yield, both peak yield and length of lactation were reduced, though the rate of decline from peak yield was unaltered. Where infection occurred between peak yield and 10 weeks after peak yield, lactation yield and length were both affected. Clinical mastitis occurring after peak yield appeared to have little effect on lactation yield. Results suggested that cows which contract mastitis are unlikely to achieve their full milk-yield potential in the following lactation. In a survey of just over 24000 dairy cows the daily loss in milk yield during the first 2 weeks after the occurrence of mastitis varied from 1.0 to 2.5 kg. Total loss over the entire lactation varied from 110 to 552 kg and depended on parity and the time of mastitis occurrence. Regardless of the time of occurrence during the lactation, mastitis had a long-lasting effect on milk yield; cows with mastitis did not reach their premastitis milk yields during the remainder of the lactation after the onset of the disease (Rajala-Schultz *et al.*, 1999).

Table 30.15 (a) Reduction in test day milk yield (kg)* in relation to somatic cell counts (SCCs) of Holstein cows without clinical mastitis, and (b) for SCCs of 200 000 cells/ml the reduction in test day milk yield (kg)* at days 50, 150 and 250 postpartum (Hortet *et al.*, 1999, reproduced with permission from Elsevier Science).

(a) Reduction in yield at various SCCs

	SCC (cells/ml)		
	100 000	200 000	600 000
Primiparous cows	0.30	0.61	1.09
Calving 2	0.32	0.63	1.13
Calving ≥3	0.30	0.60	1.07

(b) Reduction in yield at SCC of 200 000 cells/ml

	Day 50 postpartum	Day 150 postpartum	Day 250 postpartum
Calving 2	0.63	0.92	1.77
Calving ≥3	0.60	1.09	1.85

*Reduction in yield was calculated as the deviation from a reference value set at 50 000 cells/ml.

Reduction in milk yield is also associated with subclinical infection. Hortet and Seegers (1998) found in a review of 19 papers that there was an average loss of 80 kg of milk in primiparous and 120 kg in multiparous cows for each two-fold increase of the geometric mean of somatic cell count (SCC) > 50 000 cells/ml. The reduction in test day milk yield (kg) associated with SCC of less than or equal to 600 000 cells/ml in cows without clinical mastitis was assessed using monthly cow records collected for a one year period in 105 Holstein herds in France (Hortet *et al.*, 1999). Results indicated that for 100 000, 200 000 and 600 000 cells/ml the reduction in daily milk yield was approximately 0.30 kg, 0.60 kg and 1.10 kg, respectively (Table 30.15).

Effective microbiological cures, eliminating reservoirs of infection

A very real, but often overlooked, benefit of antimicrobial therapy relates more to the overall herd health status than the infected cow. This is because the infected cow is a reservoir of transmissible infection. Each infected cow may represent not only an individual with suboptimal health and production, but also a reservoir of infection. Each infected cow thus poses a threat to the productive capacity of non-infected cattle. *Strep. agalactiae* is an obligate parasite of the mammary gland. *Staphylococcus aureus* and *Mycoplasma* spp., although

not obligate parasites of the mammary gland, are transmitted from cow to cow (Bramley & Dodd, 1984). Identification followed by treatment, isolation or eradication can markedly reduce the numbers of new infections if coupled with appropriate hygienic measures.

Costs associated with antimicrobial therapy

Drug and veterinary costs

These costs will not be detailed, but should be considered when evaluating the costs associated with treatment.

Discarded milk

Available intramammary antibiotic preparations recommend milk withholding periods (discard times) that vary from 36 to 120 hours after the last treatment. Cattle with clinical mastitis are usually treated three times at 12 to 24 hour intervals. The antibiotic-contaminated, and hence discarded, milk may total as much as 420 litres in a high-producing cow. The decision to undertake treatment cannot be taken lightly. Dry-cow therapy is particularly cost-effective because it does not require milk discarding.

Slaughter withdrawal periods

Both systemic and local (intramammary) antibiotic preparations have slaughter withdrawal periods. Treated individuals cannot be marketed for salvage purposes, regardless of the success of treatment, until after the withdrawal period for the administrated preparation has ended.

Risks of new infections/altered host defences

Intramammary infusion of antibiotics is far from being an innocuous procedure. The infusion procedure may remove the keratin lining of the streak canal, an important barrier to intramammary infections (see pp. 313, 400). Strict hygiene must be practised to prevent accidental introduction of micro-organisms at the time of treatment. Only commercially available formulations of known efficacy and guaranteed safety are suitable for intramammary therapy. Special care must be exercised when large numbers of cattle are being treated on a single occasion. Explosive outbreaks of peracute and often fatal mastitis have been known to follow either poor hygiene during infusion of an intramammary product or use of a contaminated product.

References

Anderson, N.G. & Cote, J.F. (1996) Dry Cow Therapy. Factsheet 90-003. Ontario Ministry of Agriculture, Food & Rural Affairs.

Baggot, J.D. (1977) *Principles of Drug Disposition in Domestic Animals: The Basis of Veterinary Clinical Pharmacology.* W.B. Saunders, Philadelphia.

Baggot, J.D. (2000) Priniciples of antimicrobial drug bioavailability and disposition. In *Antimicrobial Therapy in Veterinary Medicine* (ed. by J.F. Prescott, J.D. Baggot & R.D. Walker), 3rd edn, pp. 50–87. Iowa State University Press, Ames, Iowa.

Baggot, J.D. & Brown, S.A. (1998) Basis for selection of the dosage form. In *Development and Formulation of Veterinary Dosage Forms* (ed. by G.E. Hardee & J.D. Baggot), 2nd edn, pp. 7–143. Marcel Dekker, New York.

Berry, E.A., Cocks, V. & Hillerton, J.E. (1999) Dry cow treatment strategies. In *British Mastitis Conference*, Stonleigh, p. 94.

Berry, S.L., Mass, J., Kirk, J.H., Reynolds, J.P., Gardner, I.A. & Ahmadi, A. (1997) Effects of antimicrobial treatment at the end of lactation on milk yield, somatic cell count, and incidence of clinical mastitis during the subsequent lactation in a herd with low prevalence of contagious mastitis. *Journal of the American Veterinary Medical Association*, **211**, 207–11.

Bramley, A.J. & Dodd, F.H. (1984) Reviews of the progress of dairy science: mastitis control – progress and prospects. *Journal of Dairy Research*, **51**, 481–512.

Browning, J.W., Mein, G.A., Brightling, P. Nicholls, T.J. & Barton, M. (1984) Strategies for mastitis control: dry cow therapy and culling. *Australian Veterinary Journal*, 71, 179–81.

Buswell, J. (1995) Simple mastitis bacteriology for the practice. *In Practice*, **17**, 426–32.

Craven, N., Anderson, J.C. & Jones, T.O. (1986) Antimicrobial drug susceptibility of *Staphylococcus aureus* isolated from bovine mastitis. *Veterinary Record*, **118**, 290–1.

Egan, J. (1984) Mastitis – a review. *Veterinary Update*, **1**, 5–11.

Esslemont, R.J. & Kossaibati, M.A. (1997) Culling in 50 dairy herds in England. *Veterinary Record*, **140**, 36–9.

Gardner, I.A., Hird, D.W., Utterback, W.W., Danaye-Elmi, C., Heron, B.R., Christiansen, K.H. & Sischo, W.M. (1990) Mortality, morbidity, case-fatality, and culling rates for California dairy cattle as evaluated by the National Animal Health Monitoring system, 1986–87. *Preventive Veterinary Medicine*, **8**, 157–70.

Gonzalez, R.N., Jasper, D.E., Farver, T.B. & Bushnell, R.B. (1988) Prevalence of udder infections and mastitis in 50 California dairy herds. *Journal of the American Veterinary Medical Association*, **193**, 323–7.

Griffin, T.K., Dodd, F.H. & Bramley, A.J. (1982) Antibiotic therapy in the control of mastitis. In *Proceedings of the British Cattle Veterinary Association 1981–82*, pp. 137–46.

Heald, C.W., Jones, G.M., Nickerson, S. & Bibb, T.L. (1977) Mastitis control by penicillin and novobiocin at drying-off. *Canadian Veterinary Journal*, **18**, 171–80.

Higgs, T.M. & Bramley, A.J. (1981) Laboratory techniques for the examination of milk samples. In *Mastitis Control & Herd Management* (ed. by A.J. Bramley, F.H. Dodd & T.K. Griffin), pp. 95–109. Technical Bulletin 4, NIRD, Reading.

Hortet, P., Beaudeau, F., Seegers, H. & Fourichon, C. (1999) Reduction in milk yield associated with somatic cell counts up to 600 000 cells/ml in French Holstein cows without clinical mastitis. *Livestock Production Science*, **61**, 33–42.

Hortet, P. & Seegers, H. (1998) Calculated production losses associated with elevated somatic cell counts in dairy cows: review and critical discussion. *Veterinary Research*, **6**, 497–510.

Hovi, M. & Roderick, S. (2000) Mastitis and mastitis control strategies in organic milk. *Cattle Practice*, **8**, 259–63.

International Dairy Federation (1981) Laboratory Methods for Use in Mastitis Work. Document No. 132. International Dairy Federation, Brussels, Belgium.

Jasper, D.E. (1980) Prevalance of *Mycoplasma* mastitis in Western states. *Californian Veterinarian*, **34**, 24–6.

Jasper, D.E., Jain, N.C. & Brazil, L.H. (1966) Clinical and laboratory observations on bovine mastitis due to *Mycoplasma. Journal of the American Veterinary Medical Association*, **148**, 1017–29.

Johansson, J., Fumke, H. & Emanuelson, U. (1995) Systemic treatment of chronic subclinical *Staphylococcus aureus* mastitis at drying off. In *Proceedings of the Third IDF International Mastitis Seminar*, Tel-Aviv, Israel (ed. by A. Saran & S. Soback), Book 2, pp. 54–7. National Mastitis Reference Center, Bet-Dagan.

Jones, T.O. (2000) Mastitis bacteriology: further problems, pitfalls and comments. *Cattle Practice*, **8**, 333–6.

Jones, T.O. & Heath, P.J. (1985) Beta-lactamase production in *Staphylococcus aureus* isolated from bovine mastitic milk. *Veterinary Record*, **117**, 340.

Kirk, J.H., DeGraves, F. & Tyler, J. (1994) Recent progress in treatment and control of mastitis in cattle. *Journal of the American Veterinary Medical Association*, **204**, 1152–8.

Kossaibati, M.A. & Esslemont, R.J. (1997) The costs of production diseases in dairy herds in England. *Veterinary Journal*, **154**, 41–51.

Le Loudec, C. (1978) Efficacites des antibiotiques contre les mammites bovines staphylococciques et streptococciques. *Annales de Recherches Vétérinaires*, **9**, 63.

Lucey, S. & Rowlands, G.J. (1984) The association between clinical mastitis and milk yield in dairy cows. *Animal Production*, **39**, 165–75.

Mackie, D.P., Logan, E.F., Pollock, D.A. & Rodgers, S.P. (1988) Antibiotic sensitivity of bovine staphylococcal and coliform mastitis isolates over four years. *Veterinary Record*, **123**, 515–17.

Macmillian, K.L., Duirs, G.F. & Duganzich, D.M. (1983) Associations between dry cow therapy, clinical mastitis and somatic cell count score with milk and fat production in ten New Zealand dairy herds. *Journal of Dairy Science*, **66**, 259–65.

National Mastitis Council (1999) *Laboratory Handbook on Bovine Mastitis.* National Mastitis Council, Washington, DC.

O'Rourke, D. (1994) Treatment of clinical mastitis in cattle. *Irish Veterinary News*, **48**, 54–9.

Owens, W.E., Watts, J.L., Boddie, R.L. & Nickerson, S.C.

(1988) Antibiotic treatment of mastitis: comparsion of intra-mammary and intramammary plus intramuscular therapies. *Journal of Dairy Science*, **71**, 3143–7.

Prescott, J.F. & Baggot, J.D. (1988) Bovine mastitis. In *Antimicrobial Therapy in Veterinary Medicine*, pp. 321–31. Blackwell Scientific Publications, Boston.

Prescott, J.F. & Walker, R.D. (2000) Principles of antimicrobial drug selection and use. In *Antimicrobial Therapy in Veterinary Medicine* (ed. by J.F. Prescott, J.D. Baggot & R.D. Walker), 3rd edn, pp. 88–104. Iowa State University Press, Ames, Iowa.

Pyorala, S. (1995) Staphylococcal and streptococcal mastitis. In *The Bovine Udder and Mastitis* (ed. by M. Sandholm, T. Honkanen-Buzalski, L. Kaartinen & S. Pyorala), pp. 143–8. University of Helsinki, Faculty of Veterinary Medicine, Helsinki.

Rajala-Schultz, P.J., Grohn, Y.T., McCulloch, C.E. & Guard, C.L. (1999) Effects of clinical mastitis on milk yield in dairy cows. *Journal of Dairy Science*, **82**, 1213–20.

Rasmussen, F. (1966) *Studies on the Mammary Excretion and Absorption of Drugs*. Carl Fr Mortensen, Copenhagen.

Sandholm, M. & Pyorala, S. (1995) Coliform mastitis. In *The Bovine Udder and Mastitis* (ed. by M. Sandholm, T. Honkanen-Buzalski, L. Kaartinen & S. Pyorala), pp. 148–60. University of Helsinki, Faculty of Veterinary Medicine, Helsinki.

Williamson, J.H., Woolford, M.W. & Day, A.M. (1995) The prophylactic effect of a dry-cow antibiotic against *Streptococcus uberis*. *New Zealand Veterinary Journal*, **43**, 228–34.

Wilson, C.D. (1961) The treatment of staphylococcal mastitis. *Veterinary Record*, **73**, 1019–24.

Woolford, M.W., Hook, I.S., Eden, M.T. & Joe, A.T. (1995) The 'SAMM PLAN' a seasonal approach to managing mastitis. *Proceedings of the Third IDF International Mastitis Seminar*, Tel-Aviv, Israel (ed. by A. Saran & S. Soback), pp. 59–63. National Mastitis Reference Center, Bet-Dagan.

Woolford, M.W., Williamson, J.H., Day, A.M. & Copeman, P.J.A. (1998) The prophylactic effect of a teat sealer on bovine mastitis during the dry period and the following lactation. *New Zealand Veterinary Journal*, **46**, 12–19.

Ziv, G. (1980) Drug selection and use in mastitis: systemic vs local therapy. *Journal of the American Veterinary Medical Association*, **176**, 1109–15.

Adult Cattle
Lameness

Chapter 31
Lameness in the Foot

R.W. Blowey

Introduction   409
Incidence and prevalence   409
Structure of the foot   411
  Hoof   411
  Corium   413
  Bone and associated structures   413
Weight bearing surfaces, hoof overgrowth and wear 413
  Hoof overgrowth   413
  Hoof trimming   415
Lesions causing lameness   417
  Sole ulcers and white line defects   417
  Sole ulcers   419
  Heel and toe ulcers   419
  White line defects   419
  Causes and control of coriosis (laminitis)   420
Other causes of foot lameness   425
Hoof disorders   425
  Foreign body penetration of the sole   425
  Slurry heel   425
  Vertical fissures (sandcracks)   425
  Hardship lines   426
  Horizontal fissures (sandcracks)   426
  Axial wall fissures   426
Skin disorders   426
  Interdigital necrobacillosis   426
  Digital dermatitis   427
  Interdigital dermatitis   429
Interdigital skin hyperplasia   429
  Mud fever   429
Bone and joint disorders   429
  Fracture of the pedal bone   429
  Apical necrosis of the pedal bone   429
  Deep pedal infections   430
General treatment and control of foot lameness   430
  Footbaths   430
  Nursing, dressings and footblocks   431

Introduction

Lameness remains a major problem for dairy herds worldwide. There are few other problems which produce as much pain and distress to the cow and very few other problems where the herdsman spends so much time and effort on routine prevention, namely hoof trimming. This chapter examines the incidence and costs of lameness, the anatomy of the digit, an approach to hoof trimming and the causes and control of lameness.

Incidence and prevalence

The incidence of lameness is defined as the number of cases recorded over a given period, usually a year. It is a longitudinal measure and is often expressed as the number of cases per 100 cows per annum. A single case of lameness is defined as one lesion in one claw. A repeat or new case can be a different lesion in the same, or another, claw, although it may be a recurrence of the same lesion after a period of time. Prevalence is the number of cases of lameness present at a single point in time, for example when the whole herd is examined on the same day, and is known as a cross-sectional measure.

A further distinction must be made between the incidence or prevalence of *lameness* and the incidence or prevalence of *lesions*, and care must be taken when comparing data. The majority of studies record the prevalence of lesions, as this produces a larger number of observations. Very few studies have examined the proportion of lesions that eventually translate into clinically detectable lameness, and yet this is an extremely important issue if we are to continue to use lesion prevalence studies to investigate the causes of lameness.

The results of studies of lameness incidence will depend on the person recording. Inevitably, studies by veterinary surgeons will give lower figures than those by farmers or stockmen, because rarely are all lame cows on a farm dealt with by a veterinarian. It is difficult to provide an average figure for the proportion of lame cows seen by veterinary practitioners. For example, the study of Clarkson *et al.* (1996) showed that 3 per cent of lame cows were examined by the veterinarian in Cheshire, 20.4 per cent in the Wirral, 21.7 per cent in Wales and 77.3 per cent in Somerset. An American study where observers went to each farm twice to record the number of lame cows showed that their recorded prevalence was 2.5 times higher than that estimated by the herd managers (Wells *et al.*, 1993).

Table 31.1 The incidence levels of lameness in several British Isles surveys.

Authors	Date	Recorders	Incidence (cases/100 cows per year)
Hedges *et al.*	2000	Veterinarians	68.9
Clarkson *et al.*	1996	Veterinarians and farmers	54.6
Esslemont & Spincer	1993	Veterinarians and farmers	36
Prentice & Neal	1972	Veterinarians	30
Booth	1989	Farmers	30
Arkins	1981	Farmers	28
Whitaker *et al.*	1983	Veterinarians and farmers	25
Esslemont & Kossaibati	1996	Veterinarians and farmers	24
Collick *et al.*	1989	Veterinarians	17
Bell & Miller	1977	Veterinarians	11
Eddy & Scott	1980	Veterinarians	7
Russell *et al.*	1982	Veterinarians	6
Leech *et al.*	1960	Veterinarians and farmers	4

Whitaker *et al.* (1983) estimated that in Britain veterinary surgeons saw only a quarter of the total lameness cases, the remainder being treated by the farmer. This was based on a study of 185 herds where the veterinary surgeon treated 25.2 per cent and the farmer 74.8 per cent of all lamenesses. As herds increase in size, the stockman becomes more competent and the number of lame cows seen routinely by the veterinary surgeon decreases.

The use of data produced by farmer recording produces problems of terminology and there will be errors in recording the causes of lameness. Hence many studies refer to 'under-run sole' or 'a foot abscess', when in fact the primary lesion was a white line disorder or a sole or heel ulcer. This produces further errors in our understanding of the incidence and causes of lameness. It is generally accepted that the incidence of lameness has increased over the past 40 years (Table 31.1) when a study provided by both veterinary surgeons and farmers gave an incidence of 3.88 per cent (Leech *et al.*, 1960). The last major British survey was in 1977 and involved 48 veterinary practices which recorded 7526 cases of lameness in 1821 dairy herds (Russell *et al.*, 1982). The average incidence amongst cattle was 5.5 per cent, although this varied between the veterinary practices from 1.8 to 11.8 per cent. Most lesions (88.3 per cent) occurred in the feet and 84 per cent of foot lesions were in the hind feet. The remaining 11.7 per cent of lameness occurred in the legs and trunk and the majority of these involved trauma (Russell *et al.*, 1982). A New Zealand farmer-recorded study of three herds in 1989/90 showed variations in lameness incidences of 38 per cent, 22 per cent and 2 per cent (Tranter & Morris, 1991).

An American study of 18 farms showed a median prevalence of 11.8 per cent of lactating dairy cows were clinically lame in the summer and 14.8 per cent in the winter (Wells *et al.*, 1995). No overall prevalence was provided because of the management differences.

A two-and-a-half-year UK study of 37 farms where both farmers and vets recorded lameness produced a mean annual incidence rate of 54.6 new lamenesses per 100 cows, varying on individual farms from 10.7 to 170.1 (Clarkson *et al.*, 1996). The mean incidence rates for the winter and summer were 31.7 and 22.9 respectively, with 78.7 per cent of the total in the outer claw. The mean prevalence rate was 20.6 per cent, ranging from 2.0 per cent to 53.9 per cent, with winter and summer rates being 25.0 per cent and 18.6 per cent, respectively (Clarkson *et al.*, 1996).

The trial reported by Hedges *et al.* (2000) was an 18-month intervention study involving only five farms in one area (Gloucestershire) of the UK. All lame cows were examined by veterinarians, so the study produced useful data on the incidence of lesions causing lameness. The incidence of lameness treated by both veterinary surgeons and farmers in 90 well-recorded UK dairy herds is shown in more detail in Table 31.2. The authors concluded that it should be a reasonable target for farmers to reduce lameness incidence to second quartile values, i.e. 11 per cent of the herd affected, giving a target of 14 cases/100 cows per annum. From other figures in Table 31.1 this would appear to be a rather optimistic target.

Although enormous research effort over the past 25 years has led to an increase in our understanding of lameness, the incidence has not declined significantly. One major reason for this is the advent of digital

Table 31.2 Incidence of lameness in 90 well recorded DAISY herds (Esslemont & Kossaibati, 1996).

	Weighted average values				
	Overall	Lowest quartile	Second quartile	Third quartile	Fourth quartile
Number of herds	90	22	23	23	23
% of herd affected by lameness	17.4	4.4	11.1	18.3	33.8
Cases per affected cow	1.4	1.0	1.2	1.4	1.8
Cases per 100 cows	24	4.7	14.1	24.6	47.4

dermatitis. First reported in the UK in the mid 1980s (Blowey & Sharp, 1988), digital dermatitis now accounts for around one third of all cases of lameness seen. In a UK study of five UK dairy herds involving over 1100 cow lactations over 18 months, where all lame cows were examined and recorded by a veterinarian, the incidence of digital dermatitis was 12.0 cases per 100 cows per annum, compared with sole ulcers at 13.9 cases/100 cows p.a. and white line disease at 12.7 cases/100 cows p.a. (Hedges *et al.*, 2000).

Several studies have attempted to record the frequency of lesions causing lameness, although results must be interpreted with care. Studies which rely on veterinary records of cases for which the farmer has requested attention for treatment will undoubtedly underestimate the incidence of conditions such as digital dermatitis and foul in the foot, as many farmers would treat these themselves. On the other hand, studies involving farmer recording may use vague terms such as 'under-run heel' or 'sole abscess', without defining the initial cause of the lesion (sole ulcer, white line, foreign body penetration, etc.), and these studies would lack accuracy. Table 31.3 summarizes five sets of data on lesions causing lameness.

Heel ulcers are a recently defined condition (Blowey *et al.*, 2000a) and may have been classified as under-run heel or foreign body penetration in other surveys. Axial wall fissures also appear to be of increasing importance worldwide (Vermunt, 1998) and may be a form of white line lesion as many follow the line of the axial groove.

Structure of the foot

The bovine claw consists of three main components, namely (Fig. 31.1):

- Hoof
- Corium
- Bone and associated structures

Hoof

The hoof, or horn capsule, is keratinized epidermis, similar to hair or finger nails. There are five distinct parts to the hoof, namely the periople, the wall, the sole, the white line and the heel. The wall, sole and heel consist of tubular horn, produced by the underlying papillary corium (or dermis). Keratinization of the epidermal cells is a physiological process involving a high rate of synthesis of keratin proteins inside the cell, plus the production of intercellular cementing substances. This must be carried out entirely by diffusion, because the epidermis is avascular. The strength, or quality, of the horn is determined by three main factors:

- The amount of keratin fibrils within the cell and the strength of their cross-linking disulphide bonds to form keratin masses.
- The amount and quality of the intercellular cementing substances which cement the keratinized cells together.
- The architecture of the horn itself, namely the ratio of tubular to non-tubular horn, which is effectively the density of the horn tubules.

Horn tubule density is approximately 80 tubules/mm^2 in the wall, decreasing to 20 tubules/mm^2 in the central sole area. There is no tubular horn in the white line. The wall is therefore the stronger part of the hoof, especially at the toe when it is more mature. As the number of horn tubules is fixed at birth, enlargement of the hoof, for example in older cows, is by an expansion of the intertubular cement. The very large flat foot of a cow is generally softer and weaker than the small compact foot of the heifer, because of its lower tubule density.

The *periople* is the hairless band of soft horn that separates the wall from the skin at the coronary band. It is continuous from one claw to the other and merges with the bulbs of the heel to give the smooth, waxy coating

Table 31.3 Types of lesion recorded as causing lameness.

	Study No.				
	1 % of lesions	2 % of lesions	3 % of lesions	4 % of lesions	5 Cases/100 cows per year
Sole ulcer	12.0			28	13.90
White line disease	18.0	39	16.8	22	12.70
Interdigital necrobacillosis	14.7		15.0	5	7.20
Foreign body penetration	12.3				3.10
Digital dermatitis				8	12.00
Interdigital dermatitis					
Interdigital skin hyperplasia	4.2			5	1.20
Interdigital foreign body	2.0		5.6	5	
Overworn sole/bruising	1.9	42		8	2.00
Vertical fissure (sandcrack)	1.1				0.54
Aseptic laminitis	4.7				
Under-run heel	7.7				
Deep sepsis	3.1		8.9		0.45
Heel ulcers					5.80
Axial wall fissures					1.07
Foot lesions	88.3		82.3		
Leg lesions	11.7				
Hind foot lesions			65.0		35.70

Key to study numbers:

(1) Russell *et al.* (1982), UK. Lameness reported by farmers and examined by veterinarians.

(2) Tranter & Morris (1991) New Zealand study of three dairy herds. All lame cows examined by veterinarians.

(3) McLennan (1988), Australia. Cases reported to veterinarians.

(4) Clarkson *et al.* (1996), UK. Lesions recorded by farmers and veterinarians

(5) Hedges *et al.* (2000), UK study of five dairy herds. All lame cows reported by farmers but examined by veterinarian.

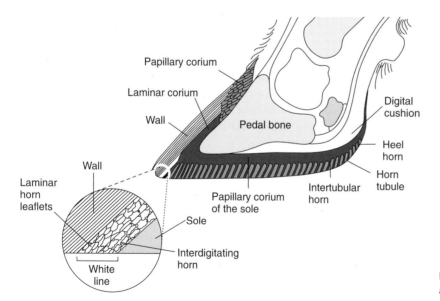

Fig. 31.1 The structure of the hoof wall and white line. (Diagram: Jane Upton.)

seen on good quality hooves. Its main function is to prevent dehydration of the horn. Deterioration with age or with hot, dry or windy conditions will predispose to vertical fissures.

The *wall*, produced by papillary corium beneath the coronary band (Plate 31.1), flows over the laminar corium at approximately 5 mm per month. As the length of the anterior wall, from the coronary band to the toe, is approximately 75 mm, new horn takes 15 months (75 ÷ 5 = 15) to come into wear at the toe.

The lamellae of the deeper layers of the epidermis (namely the hoof capsule) interdigitate with the laminae of the dermis (the corium). This produces a structure that is firmly attached to and protects the corium, but allows free movement for the horn wall and acts as a shock absorber during locomotion.

Sole horn is produced by the papillary corium of the sole and therefore consists of tubular horn and intertubular matrix (Fig. 31.1). The sole thickness varies from 10 to 15 mm and thus sole horn comes into wear two or three months after formation.

The *white line* is the cemented junction between the wall and the sole and runs from the heel, along the abaxial wall to the toe, caudally along the axial wall, then dorsally along the axial groove, to end in the interdigital cleft. The white line (Plate 31.2) consists of laminar horn leaflet cells and interdigitating horn cells. Both are produced from the adjacent corium at the toe, where the laminar corium of the wall joins the papillary corium of the sole. There is no tubular horn and hence white line horn is less mature and considerably weaker than the wall or the sole.

The *heel*, or bulb of the hoof, is a continuation of the perioplic layer, with horn tubules running obliquely in an anterior/ventral direction from the heel towards the sole. The softer heel horn can expand and contract during locomotion and, in conjunction with the underlying digital cushion, acts as both a shock absorber and vascular pump preventing venous stasis. Consequently heifers which remain stationary, standing for very long periods, may develop anoxia of the corium with subsequent poor horn production.

Corium

The corium is the modified dermis providing nerve and vascular supplies (and therefore nutrients) to the hoof horn externally and the bones and associated structures internally. Arteriovenous shunts across the top of the foot enable blood to bypass capillaries during weight bearing, although if the shunts remain open for too long, for example as a result of laminitis/coriosis, anoxia and consequently dyskeratotic horn formation result. The corium is structurally modified, enabling it to perform differing functions in various areas of the foot, namely:

● Papillae on the wall and sole extrude tubular horn.
● The laminar corium is a support structure where it interdigitates with lamellae on the hoof wall and in its distal extremities it produces white line cement.
● The digital cushion: within the heel and extending forwards to a point beneath the caudal edge of the pedal bone, the corium is impregnated with fat, fibrous and elastic tissue, to form a shock absorber and vascular pump. Trauma to the digital cushion results in a permanent replacement of fat and elastic tissue by scar tissue, with subsequent loss of function.
● On its internal aspect the corium provides nutrients and vascular support for the pedal and navicular bones. Arteriovenous shunts allow blood to bypass the foot during periods of weight bearing.

Bone and associated structures

The third phalangeal (pedal) bone, the distal sesamoid (navicular) and the distal interphalangeal (pedal) joint are all contained within the hoof capsule. The deep digital flexor tendon is attached to the flexor tuberosity of the pedal bone and within the heel is separated from the distal sesamoid by the navicular bursa. Small fibrous strands of tendinous structure, sometimes visible in the base of deep sole ulcers, are fragments of the deep flexor tendon. The suspensory apparatus of the pedal bone (Fig. 31.8) supports the caudal edge of the bone. It is firmly attached to the corium on the abaxial aspect and joins the suspensory ligaments of the leg axially.

Weight bearing surfaces, hoof overgrowth and wear

As the primary objective of hoof trimming is to restore the foot to its 'normal' shape, it is important to understand the correct weight bearing surfaces of the foot and the distortions that occur due to overgrowth. In a correctly shaped hoof, weight is taken on the heel, on the abaxial wall and, to a lesser extent, on the white line and 10–20 mm of adjacent sole, and on the axial wall running from the toe caudally along the first third of the axial space. The remainder of the axial surface of the claw should be non-weight bearing (Fig. 31.2). Other dimensions of the claw are given in Fig. 31.3.

Hoof overgrowth

The size and shape of the hoof at any one time will be a balance between the rate of growth and the rate of wear. As one might expect, there are a variety of factors that influence both processes. For example, horn growth is faster:

● In young animals
● With high concentrate feeding
● With more exercise
● On rough surfaces

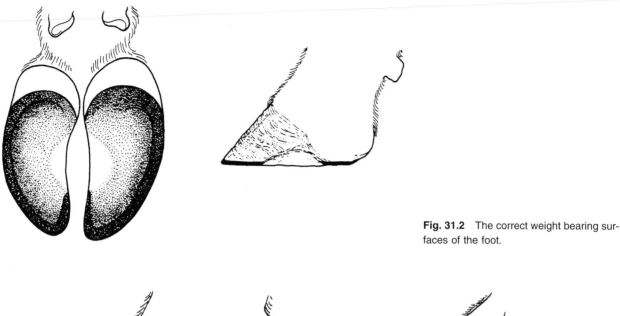

Fig. 31.2 The correct weight bearing surfaces of the foot.

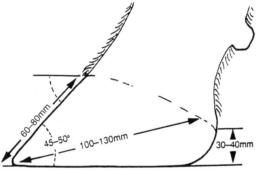

Fig. 31.3 Approximate dimensions and angles of a normal claw.

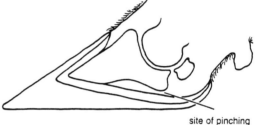

site of pinching

Fig. 31.4 Overgrowth at the toe leads to a caudal rotation of the pedal bone.

The rate of wear is increased by factors such as:

- Wet conditions underfoot, leading to softer horn which wears faster
- Excessive standing and walking
- Hard and/or abrasive floor surfaces

Overgrowth at the toe

The horn of the wall is generally harder than the horn of the heel, so although both may grow at the same rate, horn is worn away more slowly from the toe than from the heel. This results in overgrowth occurring *primarily at the toe*. The additional horn at the toe lifts the front of the foot and the front wall then forms a more shallow angle, decreasing from 45° to 30° or 20°, or even to the horizontal. In extreme cases the front wall becomes concave and the toe is lifted off the ground (Plate 31.3). These changes are shown in Fig. 31.4. Internally the pedal bone is rotated backwards, thereby putting even more pressure on its rear edge (the flexor tuberosity) and further increasing the risk of sole ulcers. However,

the pedal bone remains the same size, irrespective of the degree of overgrowth. In this respect the hoof is very different from the cow's horn, where the cornual bone lengthens with increasing length of the horn.

Overgrowth of the lateral wall

In some animals the wall of one claw grows faster than the other and starts to curl under the sole. This produces a corkscrew effect at the toe. Corkscrew claw may be a genetic trait or can be a result of coriosis/laminitis.

Overgrowth of the sole

A ledge of horn is commonly seen growing from the sole and extending into the axial space (Fig. 3.17, Plate 31.4). In some instances it may even overlap the adjacent claw, and may be so pronounced that it becomes the major weight bearing area of the foot. This has importance in the pathogenesis of sole ulcers, as the overgrowth of sole horn is immediately beneath the flexor tuberosity of the pedal bone and in an area where weight bearing should be minimized.

Disparity of claw size

The lateral claw of the hind foot is often considerably larger than the medial claw. There is no single reason for this and suggested causes include:

- The lateral claw is naturally slightly larger than the medial (Paulus & Nuss, 2002).
- Poorer suspension of the pedal bone within the lateral claw, leading to pinching of the corium and stimulating the growth of horn. The caudal edge of the pedal bone is suspended within a 'hammock', known as the pedal suspensory apparatus (fig. 31.8). This is connected to the laminae on the abaxial wall, and axially to the suspensory ligaments of the leg.
- A greater variation in load bearing on the lateral claw compared with the medial claw when the cow is walking (Toussaint-Raven, 1985).
- A leg conformation in which the hocks point inwards and the toes outwards.
- Excessive engorgement of the udder at calving, forcing the legs apart.
- The hind feet are the major propelling force of the cow during locomotion, pushing her forwards, whereas the front feet are the major weightbearing structures.

In the front feet the position is reversed: the medial claw is commonly larger than the lateral claw.

Negative net growth

At housing, and especially when housing and calving coincide, heifers invariably undergo a period of *negative net growth*. The rate of hoof horn growth is reduced but at the same time there is a rapid increase in wear, especially at the toe. This leads to a shortening and increased angle in the dorsal wall, plus a thinning of the sole. In some heifers the changes may be sufficiently extreme for the horn at the toe to become totally eroded, exposing the corium. Such heifers are said to have 'soft soles' or 'toe ulcers'. The syndrome is seen especially in heifers that have to walk long distances to and from pasture, for example in New Zealand and Uruguay, and also in young bulls introduced into a dairy herd. It may be occasionally seen in maiden heifers when they are housed at the end of their first grazing season.

Hardship lines

Temporary disruptions of hoof formation in the anterior wall lead to circumferential rings of variable thickness known an 'hardship lines'. When horn production is poor, a groove is formed and in extreme cases results in total cessation of horn formation, leading to a horizontal fissure. Because the dorsal wall is longer than the heel, the hardship lines often run from the sole surface of the abaxial wall, across the dorsal wall to the sole surface of the axial wall. 'Hardship lines' can be used to establish the chronology of previous episodes of coriosis/laminitis, and therefore the potential causes of current hoof problems.

Hoof trimming

A variety of methods have been described, but all have one common aim, namely to restore the foot to its correct shape and weight bearing surface. The manner in which this is achieved is less important and the following text simply describes one approach (Blowey, 1998), with emphasis being placed on the anatomical corrective stages, rather than the precise method used. Other approaches are described elsewhere (Toussaint-Raven, 1985). Although described as a four-stage process, in reality one part of the trimming process merges with the next.

Cut one

The overgrown toe should be cut to its correct length, which is approximately 75–80 mm from the coronary band to the toe, or one handspan. Most experienced hoof trimmers would simply estimate this distance but, when learning, it would be better to measure specifically. After cut one the cow is left with a 'square-ended toe'. In Plate 31.5 it can be seen that the white line now passes across the end of the toe and clearly the wall, which should be the correct weight bearing surface, is no longer weight bearing at this point. Although the anterior wall may now be the correct length, the toe is still too high and this means that the front angle of the anterior wall is too shallow. This is demonstrated in Fig. 31.5.

Cut two

The next stage is to remove the excess horn from the sole surface of the toe, thus dropping the toe relative to the heel and bringing the front wall back to a more

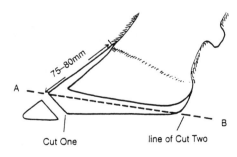

Fig. 31.5 Hoof trimming cuts one and two.

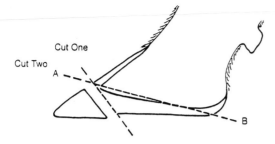

Fig. 31.6 Hoof trimming. Cut one should not be made too short.

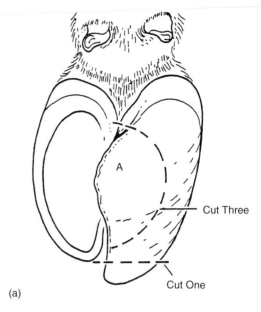

(a)

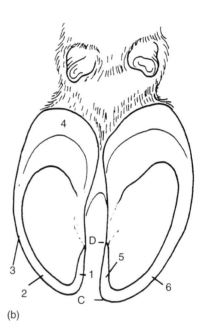

(b)

Fig. 31.7 Hoof trimming. Cut three and the finished foot.

upright position. The horn to be removed in cut two lies beneath the line AB (Fig. 31.5), which is a line joining cut one to the base of the heel. The first part of cut two can be performed by removing part of the wall using hoof clippers, but later stages should be carried out with a hoof knife, using thumb pressure to check this area of the sole regularly for signs of softening. A softening of the horn should not occur, but if it does then trimming must stop. There will only be a few millimetres of horn before the corium is penetrated and exposure of the corium in this area of the foot can lead to quite severe and protracted lameness.

If cut one was in the correct position it should be possible to remove horn from the sole surface of the toe until the white line and adjacent wall are once again clearly visible at the toe. The wall is now the weight bearing surface. It is important that this is achieved, otherwise the weaker white line structure would become weight bearing, with obvious adverse consequences.

It is vital that cut one does not make the hoof too short; this scenario is shown in Fig. 31.6. Because cut one was too short, a line drawn from the top of cut one to the bottom of the heel (AB in Fig. 31.6) would lead to exposure of the corium at the toe and this can produce severe lameness.

Cut three

Cut three consists of removing any axial overgrowth of the sole, followed by dishing the axial sole surface of both claws (Fig. 31.7a), so that weight bearing beneath the flexor tuberosity of the pedal bone is minimized. Cut three also slightly increases the space between the digits. This makes impaction by dirt and foreign bodies less likely, decreasing the incidence of diseases such as foul, interdigital dermatitis and interdigital skin hyperplasia ('corns').

Cut four

The final stage is to trim the two claws back to approximately the same size with the lateral claw 4–5 mm

longer. This usually means removing additional horn from the outer claw of hind feet and the inner claw of front feet, bringing the legs back to the upright position. This produces more even weight bearing.

General points

When trimming is complete, points 1, 2, 3 and 4 on Fig. 31.7b should all be on the same longitudinal horizontal plane, to provide adequate weight bearing. The two claws should also be of equal size and their two sole surfaces on the same transverse horizontal plane. Removal of the axial (inner) wall CD (Fig. 31.7b) is a common mistake made by some herdsmen who feel that the toes should not be touching once trimming is complete. This is a fallacy. If the wall CD was lowered the claw would be seriously destabilized, causing it to rotate inwards and allowing overgrowth of the lateral wall. In the worst case excessive removal of the axial wall might expose the corium, leading to severe lameness.

It is preferable not to remove any heel horn unless it is badly under-run, other than as part of cut four. If the heel is only slightly pitted, it is best left alone, since removal of the heel could lead to backwards rotation of the pedal bone and so predispose to sole ulcers.

One theory of hoof trimming recommends that it is advisable first to trim the medial claw to the correct shape and then use this as a template for trimming the lateral claw. Whilst this system may have its merits, it is the opinion of the current author that it is not always a correct course of action, and especially when dealing with lame cows. This is because it may be beneficial on welfare grounds to leave the medial claw slightly larger than normal in order to increase its weight bearing potential when there is a lesion in the lateral claw.

Timing of foot trimming

There is no one correct time to trim feet. Potential options include:

- When overgrowth occurs. Leaving a foot with overgrown horn not only makes walking uncomfortable but it also predisposes to the development of more serious lesions such as sole ulcers.
- When the cow is lame. Clearly all lame cows should have the affected foot lifted, trimmed and examined.
- At drying off. As many of the management and feeding 'insults' leading to lameness occur at the time of calving, it is ideal to have feet in optimum shape at this stage. In addition, at the end of lactation there may be a build up of horn from insults suffered in the previous lactation

Lesions causing lameness

The majority of the lesions causing lameness are in the foot. In this section these will be subdivided as follows:

- Sole ulcers and white line defects.
- Other hoof problems: foreign body penetration, horizontal and vertical fissures.

- Conditions of the skin: digital dermatitis, interdigital necrobacillosis, interdigital skin hyperplasia and mud fever.
- Disorders of the pedal and navicular bones.

Sole ulcers and white line defects

Pathogenesis

The horn of the white line and sole is produced by the corium. Damage or disruption of the corium will therefore be the primary change that later leads to the formation of poor quality horn, and this is eventually seen as defects such as sole ulcers and white line disorders. The syndrome is sometimes referred to as 'clawhorn disruption', although once again, as the primary defect is in the corium, then this is the area to which attention should be focused. Although the term 'laminitis' is often used, the majority of changes affect the whole corium, and particularly the papillary corium of the sole, where there are no laminae. Hence use of the term 'laminitis' in cattle is not particularly accurate. It is doubtful if laminitis occurs as a single entity in cattle, and the more general term of 'coriosis' is preferable.

Changes associated with the corium

Coriosis can occur as a result of trauma, infection, nutritional imbalance/excess and toxic states and commonly is a sequel to a combination of causes. The overall result will be the same, namely altered horn formation with the risk of lameness when the poor quality horn reaches the bearing surface of the sole.

Ossent (1995) describes three stages in the pathogenesis of sole ulcers and white line disease, all of which arise as a consequence of coriosis:

(1) Disruption of blood flow within the corium, leading to sludging, poor oxygenation of epidermal tissues and consequently poor keratin synthesis.
(2) The laminar suspension of the pedal bone within the hoof is disrupted and the bone sinks within the hoof.
(3) Compression of the corium, especially beneath the flexor tuberosity of the sinking pedal bone, leads to further ischaemic necrosis, disrupted horn formation and consequently the production of a sole ulcer.

The changes at the dermal–epidermal junction are still not fully understood. It is thought that they involve an initial release of vasoactive substances. Vasodilation in the corium leads to vascular stagnation and the opening of the arteriovenous shunts exacerbates this. The ensueing hypoxia leads to transudation, thrombosis and ischaemic necrosis, and consequently poor keratin synthesis and lamellar disruption.

Haemorrhage on the sole is often referred to as 'bruising'. This may be a correct term, although it should always be remembered that the 'bruise' was formed by an insult one or two months previously, when the horn now on the surface of the sole was being produced. As such, bruising of the sole cannot be implicated as a recent cause of lameness. The effect of mixing serum or blood with the horn can be likened to mixing sawdust with concrete – it weakens it considerably. This is particularly the case for the white line, which is an inherently weak structure, and at the sole ulcer site where there may be almost 'neat sawdust' because so much haemorrhage is present. The whole process is very similar to the changes which occur when a fingernail is bruised: the blood spot often starts at the corium of the skin–nail junction and then slowly grows to the distal extremity of the fingernail over the next few months.

Changes associated with the pedal bone

The ventro-axial border of the pedal bone is arched in shape. The pedal bone is suspended within the hoof by the laminae, with a much stronger attachment to the abaxial wall than to the axial wall (Fig. 31.8) of the hoof. When weight is transmitted down the leg the bone rotates slightly on the axial surface, putting increased weight on the flexor tuberosity. Increased weight bearing puts extra pressure on the corium and if it is already in a fragile state, then it is likely to become damaged. Pinching of the corium between the flexor tuberosity of the pedal bone above and the horn of the sole beneath leads to 'bruising' of the corium. This leads to defective horn formation and the changes will be seen on the bearing surface of the sole one or two

months later. The nature of the horn defects will depend on the severity of the initial corium damage, and are likely to appear as:

- Yellow discoloration – if serum only was released.
- Haemorrhage – if the blood vessels ruptured (Plate 31.6).
- A sole ulcer – if the damage to the corium was so severe that horn formation was totally disrupted (Plate 31.7).

If there is a generalized inflammation of the corium, then the suspension of the pedal bone within the foot is disrupted, allowing the bone to sink within the foot, as shown in Fig. 31.9. The corium is then displaced and the following changes occur:

- The 'sinking' bone puts further pressure on the corium, especially beneath the flexor tuberosity, the heel or the toe. Ulceration of the sole, heel or toe may result.
- Lateral displacement of the corium into the white line area leads to weakening and widening of the white line cement with increased risk of white line defects.

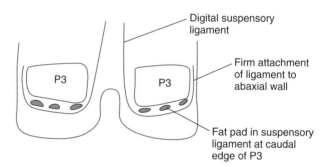

Fig. 31.8 Suspension of the pedal bone within the hoof.

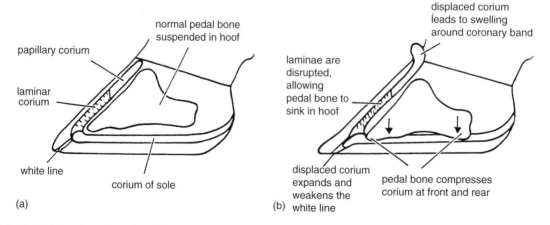

Fig. 31.9 Coriosis leads to disruption of the laminar suspension of the pedal bone.

- Dorsal displacement of the corium may produce a circumferential thickening above the coronary band.
- Anterio-ventral displacement of the pedal bone (i.e. movement towards the toe) may leave a horizontal depression or 'furrow' in the heel horn. This is a classic sign of disruption of the laminar suspension with subsequent movement of the pedal bone.

The poor laminar suspension on the axial wall compared with the abaxial wall (Fig. 31.8) leads to the axial aspect of the pedal bone, and especially its flexor tuberosity, having the greatest contact with the corium of the sole. This explains the typical site of the sole ulcer in zone 4 (mid sole) of the hoof. Once the pedal bone has dropped within the hoof it will never regain its original position. In addition, a corium that has been damaged by ischaemic necrosis heals by fibrosis and is therefore less able to produce good quality horn in the future. As a consequence, heifers affected by coriosis during their first lactation are more susceptible to lameness in later lactations. For example, in one study, heifers that developed lameness in their first lactation were almost three times as likely to go lame in their second lactation than their non-lame counterparts. Optimal management of the precalving and periparturient first lactation heifers is therefore vital as a long term lameness control measure.

Continual compression of the corium of the sole can lead to generalized poor horn formation, sometimes seen in older cows where a sole ulcer totally fails to heal. In such animals a layer of very poor quality 'horn', sometimes little more than a layer of fibrous tissue, may form over the ulcer site, and the tip of the flexor tuberosity of the pedal bone can sometimes be palpated as a hard lump immediately beneath.

Sole ulcers

A sole ulcer (Plate 31.7) is a physical condition, caused by trauma to a fragile corium, and treatment must therefore be aimed at minimizing this trauma. The main steps for treatment are:

- Dish the sole ulcer site so that weight bearing is minimized.
- Remove any under-run horn around the ulcer, to eliminate pockets of necrotic horn and infection, thus allowing the formation of new horn.
- Remove protruding granulation tissue.
- Reduce the size of the affected claw as much as possible, and maximize weight bearing on the sound claw. For more advanced cases, apply a block to the sound claw (e.g. Plates 31.7 and 31.20).

Note that no dressings are recommended: in fact many would consider them to be counterproductive. This is referred to later.

Heel and toe ulcers

Although sole ulcers are by far the most common, there can be areas of haemorrhage or even total perforation at other areas of the sole. Toe ulcers are thought to occur when the pedal bone sinks within the hoof 'bows first' – that is, the front of the pedal bone drops before the flexor tuberosity at the rear.

Heel ulcers are seen as small dark red/black marks (Plate 31.8) in the central sole area towards the heel (Blowey, et al., 2000a). Plate 31.8 shows a typical heel ulcer on the left claw and haemorrhage at the site of an early sole ulcer on the right claw. Some heel ulcers simply track down to the corium and fade to nothing. Others lead to under-running and abscessation of the sole at the sole–heel junction and can produce a marked lameness. Heel ulcers represent a significant cause of lameness (Table 31.3). They often occur in association with sole ulcers, although they are seen more commonly on the medial claw of hind feet. The cause of heel ulcers is not known, although one theory is that they are produced by pinching of the corium under the caudal edge of the pedal bone. At this point the bone is suspended in the pedal suspensory apparatus (Fig. 31.8), within which there are three fat pads acting as shock absorbers (Ossent & Lischer, 2000). The central fat pad has been shown to undergo cartilaginous change, and it may be the effect of this that leads to the formation of heel ulcers. Heel ulcers are hence in the *central* sole region at the junction of zones 4 and 6 (zone standardization from the Liverpool International Ruminant Digit Symposium 1990, cited by Greenough *et al.*, 1997). Sole ulcers typically occur in a more anterior and axial position on the *axial* aspect in the centre of zone 4, and toe ulcers are seen in zone 5 at the toe.

White line defects

Weakening of the white line, brought about by the inflammation associated with laminitis/coriosis, can result in a range of white line disorders. The most common of these are:

- Sterile abscessation.
- White line separation.
- White line penetration and abscess formation, with potential complications of infection tracking along the laminar corium towards the coronary band.

Sometimes the internal inflammation within the corium is so severe that pockets of necrotic tissue are formed. These can produce a sterile internal abscess and as there may be no obvious tracts running from the outside, they may be quite difficult to locate and treat. In severe forms of coriosis the whole sole becomes separated by an accumulation of inflammatory fluid. This is known as a *false sole*.

More commonly fissures develop vertically into the weakened white line, a process known as white line separation (Plate 31.9). This occurs especially if the cows are walking over rough or stony ground, or when they make sudden turning movements, as when escaping from an aggressive cow. Small stones may then become impacted and with continued walking these may eventually penetrate the corium. The most common point for white line separation and penetration is at zone 3, where the rigid abaxial hoof wall joins the flexible heel. During locomotion this is where there are the greatest sheer forces between the rigid hoof wall, the suspended pedal bone and the movements of the flexible heel horn. Once the corium has been penetrated, the invading foreign body (usually a stone or grit) introduces infection. For white line abscesses near to the heel, natural drainage is through the soft horn of the heel. White line abscesses close to the toe do not have such an easy escape route and often infection tracks upwards through the laminae, to discharge at the coronary band. This produces a more severe lameness because at the toe the pedal bone is tightly attached to the hoof, and there is therefore very little room for the pus to expand.

Whereas a sole ulcer results in damage to the underlying corium, the majority of white line lesions primarily produce separation of the horn from the underlying horn-forming corium. Uncomplicated white line lesions therefore normally heal much more quickly than sole ulcers. White line lesions in the axial groove are described on page 426.

The treatment of a white line abscess is very similar to that for a sole ulcer, namely:

- Remove all under-run horn, even if this means removing the wall from the sole to the coronary band, or the whole of an under-run sole. A few authors recommend leaving a bridge of hoof wall to prevent movement of each side of the bisected wall, but the danger of doing this is that the under-run infection will not be fully drained.
- Reduce the size of the affected claw, to minimize weight bearing, and leave the sound claw large.

Blocks and dressings are discussed on page 431.

When using a hoof knife to drain infection from the white line, it is important to remove the short section of adjoining hoof wall. Digging a deep pit into the white line with the curved point of the hoof knife has two disadvantages, namely:

- It leaves a pit which can easily become impacted with stones or dirt, thereby impeding drainage and predisposing to further white line impaction.
- By creating a pit, areas of under-run horn and pockets of infection are much more likely to be missed. If a small area of adjacent wall is removed, it is much easier to expose and drain the affected area.

Protruding granulation tissue is often an indication that there is adjacent under-run horn that needs to be removed, and use of a block on the sound claw to prevent weight bearing on the affected claw improves the rate of healing. A swollen, hot and painful coronary band is caused by infection tracking into deeper structures such as the navicular bursa or tendon sheaths, and in such instances antibiotic therapy and/or more radical treatment is indicated.

Causes and control of coriosis (laminitis)

Coriosis is clearly the primary factor responsible for defects in the horn capsule. In this section the aetiology, and consequently the control of coriosis, is described under the headings of parturition, excessive standing, nutrition and general management.

Parturition

Many authors have shown an association between parturition and increased incidence of lameness, with the peak incidence of white line lesions in first lactation heifers occurring nine weeks after calving, and sole ulcers at 14 weeks postpartum (Leach *et al.*, 1997). In cows the incidence peaks slightly later. Green *et al.* (2002) showed that lameness from all causes peaks in the second and third month after calving. The rings on a cow's horns, one for each calving (Plate 31.10), are said to be a reflection of the natural disruption in horn formation (Blowey, 1998) that occurs at calving. Livesey *et al.* (2000) suggested a decreased incorporation of amino acids into hoof horn at the time of parturition, presumably associated with a repartition of nutrients (sulphur amino acids) towards milk production. Hirst *et al.* (2000) showed that cows that develop lameness in their first lactation are more likely to become lame in subsequent lactations, and suggested yield as a contributory factor. Green *et al.* (2002), in an intervention study involving 1109 cow-years on trial, showed that high-yielding cows were more likely to become clinically lame than lower-yielding animals, but in the affected group, lame cows produced 396 litres per cow less milk than their non-lame counterparts.

The changes that occur in all periparturient cows appear to have a marked impact on the corium, horn strength and subsequent lameness. There is a decrease in the rate of rumination, and this leads to a 25–30 per cent decrease in dry matter intake, at a time when the cow's requirements (for the fetus and milk production) are rising rapidly. There is an increased risk of rumen acidosis and a marked immune suppression. Dietary change, namely moving from a low concentrate dry-cow ration to a high performance production diet, further increases the risk of rumen acidosis and coriosis.

Whatever the cause, the increased fragility of the corium during the periparturient period means that it is particularly susceptible to trauma. However, in most dairy systems this is when the greatest trauma to the corium occurs, due to excess periods of standing and aggressive interactive movements between cows as they become re-established in a different social group.

Even if they calve outside in a field, for a few days after calving cows, and especially heifers, will spend far more time standing and their lying times will be decreased. There is then more weight on the corium and a greater potential for bruising. It is not known whether the decreased lying times are due to inherent nursing behaviour (attending to the calf), discomfort from the perineum, an enlarged udder or to some other factor.

Diseases such as mastitis and metritis are more common immediately after calving. This also increases the fragility of the corium and in extreme cases will produce hooves with hardship lines and horizontal fissures. Heifers are likely to be worst affected, partly because they have often had no prior experience of the housing and milking system and partly because in many large dairies the heifers have been reared totally separate from the main herd. They are therefore additionally exposed to a whole range of new infections immediately postpartum, when immune suppression is at its maximum, and this further depresses horn formation. This leads to long periods of standing, producing increased hoof wear at a time when hoof growth is minimal. The 'negative net growth' which occurs around parturition and housing is referred to below and on page 415.

Excessive standing

Anything that leads to a decrease in lying times, especially in the immediate postcalving period when the corium is in its most fragile state, will increase the incidence of sole ulcers and white line disease.

One experiment (Leonard *et al.*, 1996) deliberately housed heifers in an overstocked cubicle building (17 cubicles for 35 heifers) immediately after calving.

Although the average lying time of the heifers was ten hours, some animals lay down for as little as five hours each day. This group showed the highest incidence of lameness and quite severe haemorrhage persisted in the sole horn for up to four months after calving. In most dairy systems heifers are forced to spend longer on their feet after calving. They will stand waiting to be milked, they spend longer standing to feed, because they are often last to feed, and need to eat more as lactation proceeds. They will have recently been mixed with the main herd and are now having to compete with older cows and fear may restrict their entry into a cubicle shed, especially if they are of low social dominance and have had no previous cubicle training.

Excessive standing may be bad for the immediate postpartum cow, but standing still is even worse. If the animal does not move, the vascular pumping mechanisms of the heel and digital cushion will be impaired. Vascular stasis predisposes to anoxia and damage to the corium, with resulting poor horn formation. It is essential that there are adequate loafing areas to allow the cows to walk around freely. Overcrowding should be avoided, even in collecting yards. Animals that are packed tightly together have little option but to stand still. Adequate loafing areas also help to improve oestrus expression and hence fertility.

The incidence of sole ulcers and white line disease will therefore be markedly reduced if animals are encouraged to maximize lying times in the immediate postcalving period, for example for the first two to six weeks after calving.

Post-calving comfort: Of all the above factors, cubicle comfort is probably the most important. Cubicles may make the management of cows easier, but they are not always ideal in terms of cow comfort and lameness. Several surveys have shown that the incidence of lameness in cows in straw yards is much lower than in those housed in cubicles. This must point to cubicles being less than ideal, especially for the immediate postcalving cow. A small but increasing proportion of farms are now housing their freshly calved cows in 'maternity' loose yards for the first two to six weeks after calving and then transferring them to cubicles. Experience from such systems suggests that in heifers especially, a postcalving period of loose housing leads to:

- Increased yields.
- A decreased incidence of lameness.
- Improved cubicle acceptance when the heifers are eventually transferred from the yard to the cubicles.

The third factor is perhaps the most surprising. One might have expected that cows and heifers that had got used to a straw yard would be very difficult to retrain to use cubicles. The fact that the reverse is true probably indicates that parturition is a stressful experience and that it is only when animals have fully recovered that they are able to withstand the rigours of the cubicle system. The major problem with straw yards is the increased incidence of environmental mastitis and hence perhaps the ideal situation would be a 'maternity group' housed in a low stocking density system of luxury cubicles.

Cubicle design: Cubicle comfort is obviously all-important. Ideally, cubicles should be long enough and wide enough (1.15 metres wide and 2.4 metres long) to accommodate the larger Holstein cows and with sufficient space at the front to allow the cow to lunge forward 1–1.5 metres as she stands up. If there are two facing rows of cubicles, a length of 2.2 metres is adequate. Cantilever-type divisions are ideal. Also recommended are a 100 mm fall from front to rear, a step of not more than 130 mm down into the dunging channel and a brisket rail at the front 1.75 m from the kerb, which prevents the cow from shuffling too far forwards, but at the same time provides ample space for lunging as she stands up.

When attempting to stand, the cow lunges forward 1 to 2 metres and lifts herself first onto her hind feet, then up onto her front feet. When she is lying down or half standing, therefore, much of her weight is taken on her knees. If the floor surface is hard, and particularly if it is also rough, cubicle acceptance will be low. The worst possible cubicle floor is a stone base, poorly compacted and with insufficient straw. In an attempt to get comfortable cows will shuffle forwards, until they are so close to the wall that they are unable to lunge to stand. If a proportion of the cows are too far forward in the cubicles, cubicle comfort should be re-examined.

Most cubicle bases are made of concrete. This is fine provided that it is deeply bedded, although it is often difficult to retain a well-matted straw bed. A variety of mats and mattresses are available and these are certainly much better than concrete alone. However, some bedding should be used, even with mats, otherwise hock sores will develop. A disadvantage of mats is that it is difficult to get large amounts of straw bedding to adhere to them, although the cows enjoy standing on rubber mats. Deep sand cubicles (for example 70 mm) also work well and reduce the incidence of mastitis, although sand may lead to problems with slurry disposal systems. Choosing the correct type of sand, which does not compact and consolidate, is essential.

The best cubicles are comfortable cubicles. While design and dimensions may be important, comfort is of even greater significance (see also pp. 40–42).

Nutrition

High starch/low fibre diets that lead to rumen acidosis undoubtedly predispose to coriosis and subsequent lameness, especially if fed both pre- and postpartum. Blowey *et al.* (2000b) used 48 multiparous cows to compare high starch (wheat-based) with equal energy high fibre (sugar beet pulp) rations fed pre- and postpartum. Sole haemorrhage scores at 24 weeks postpartum were significantly higher in the high starch group. Livesey and Flemming (1984) showed that 64 per cent of cows on a low fibre diet developed sole ulcers compared with only 8 per cent on the high fibre ration.

Concentrate intakes should be built up slowly after calving, to reach a peak at no less than two weeks post-calving for average yielding cows and probably three weeks for higher yielding animals, which peak later. Ideally no more than 4.5 kg of feed should be given in the parlour. The inclusion of 1–3 kg of long-chop straw, well mixed with the ration, helps to stimulate rumination, thereby promoting a good flow of saliva and decreasing acidosis. There is evidence that maintaining an ideal dietary cation–anion balance (DCAB) is beneficial (see p. 787). Acidosis can be recognized clinically by loose faeces, an increased incidence of digestive upsets, cud regurgitation and a sweaty coat.

Although high protein diets have occasionally been suggested as a cause of coriosis, most consider protein to be of less importance than other factors. High intakes of poorly fermented grass silage have also been implicated, although this could be due to toxic amines rather than high protein.

Even feeding during rearing influences the incidence of sole haemorrhage, with heifers fed high levels of concentrate being the worst affected. High fibre diets are now recommended for rearing dairy heifers.

Trace elements and vitamins: Many attempts have been made to improve hoof condition by mineral, vitamin and trace element supplementation. The use of zinc, particularly zinc methionine, is often promoted as a feed supplement having beneficial effects. If one of the reasons for the production of poor quality horn at calving is a temporary deficit of sulphur amino acids (see p. 419) then logic would suggest that supplementation with zinc methionine might be beneficial at this time, since methionine is a sulphur amino acid and zinc promotes healing.

Biotin has been shown to influence the differentiation of epidermal cells into hoof horn; it boosts the production of keratin and it stimulates the production of intracellular cementing substance (ICS). ICS is a vital component of non-tubular horn, such as is found in the white line, and this is perhaps why biotin supplementation has a major effect on white line disease. Although

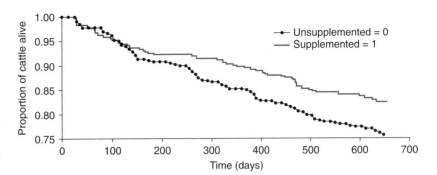

Fig. 31.10 Effect of biotin supplementation on white line lameness in dairy cows. No effect was seen until after 130 days of supplementation (Hedges *et al.*, 2001). Reproduced with permission of the American Dairy Science Association.

one might expect ruminal synthesis of biotin would meet the requirements of the cow, Da Costa Gomes *et al.* (1998) showed that with high concentrate diets producing rumen acidosis, *in vitro* biotin synthesis was reduced from 1.5 to 0.3 μg per day. Herds with significant problems associated with horn quality may benefit from biotin supplementation, although attention to dietary management would also be important.

In a study with 100 first lactation heifers, Midla *et al.* (1998) showed that supplementation with 20 mg biotin/day from calving produced a significant improvement in white line lesions at 100 days of lactation. In a more extensive split herd intervention study involving over 1100 cow lactations in five UK dairy herds, supplementation with 20 mg/day biotin significantly halved the incidence of lameness caused by white line lesions (Hedges *et al.*, 2001). Survival analysis demonstrated that supplementation needed to be given for 130 days before any difference in the two groups was seen (Fig. 31.10). In addition, only 28 per cent of supplemented animals required a repeat treatment in the same digit, compared with 72 per cent of unsupplemented controls (Blowey *et al.*, 2000c).

Hagemeister (1996) showed that animals receiving 10 mg biotin daily had significantly fewer sole ulcers and less heel erosion than unsupplemented controls, and Lischer *et al.* (1996) reported a correlation between biotin supplementation and the rate of healing of claw lesions. New horn formed more rapidly in those cows supplemented with 20 mg biotin/day. A two-year Canadian field study of 265 Hereford beef cows with a high prevalence of vertical fissures (sandcracks) demonstrated that supplementation with 20 mg biotin/ cow per day significantly reduced the prevalence of vertical fissures from 29.4 per cent to 14.3 per cent (*P* < 0.05; Campbell *et al.*, 1996).

General management

Many aspects of management have already been discussed in the housing and feeding sections. This section will cover a few miscellaneous points relating to lameness, placing particular emphasis on those factors which might damage the corium, especially in the early lactation animal.

Wet hoof: This is softer than dry hoof and therefore the sole is more likely to become penetrated or the corium bruised if the feet are damp. Cubicle passages should be scraped twice daily and the addition of small quantities of slaked lime to the cubicle beds once a week will help to dry the feet as well as control mastitis (see p. 391).

Floor surfaces: These should not be too rough, stony or have broken concrete, all of which could damage the corium. On the other hand, very slippery surfaces can lead to leg damage. An excellent demonstration that cows do not like walking on concrete is shown in Plate 31.11. A strip of second-hand rubber belting, approximately 1.5 metres wide, has been laid along the centre of a concrete track which runs from a dirt yard to the milking parlour at a dairy in California. Although the cows could walk anywhere they wished on the track, note how they all prefer to walk on the rubber belt. In the UK, if cows are allowed to amble out to a field at their own speed they will usually choose to do so by walking on the soft earth of a grass verge, rather than on stones (Plate 31.12). They even place their feet in exactly the same spot each time, making holes in the ground. This preference for a softer surface has led to the development of specific cow tracks. The ground is excavated to 0.3 cm deep and 1.0–1.5 metres wide and lined with a permeable geotextile road construction membrane which prevents sinkage of the track. A drainage pipe runs along the base, surrounded by a large aggregate, perhaps having fine stone on the top (Fig. 31.11). This is covered with a second special toughened membrane, which allows water to drain through but will not allow mud to rise up through it. Finally a layer of bark strippings, sometimes known as Cundy peelings, 100 mm (4 inches) deep, is placed on top of the upper membrane to provide a comfortable walking surface for the cows. Tractors and other vehicles must

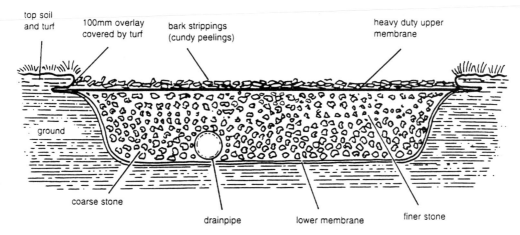

top soil and turf

100mm overlay covered by turf

bark strippings (cundy peelings)

heavy duty upper membrane

ground

coarse stone

drainpipe

lower membrane

finer stone

Fig. 31.11 Cross-section of a cow track.

not use the track. Similar tracks may be constructed in gateways, around water troughs and in other areas where the ground gets badly poached. On very well drained land some farmers have constructed a very simple track by scraping away the topsoil and then unrolling a large round straw bale onto the underlying stone. Wet bales, too badly soiled for straw yards, could be used. The straw needs replacing approximately every two or three weeks, depending on the weather, but it makes a good track and is certainly cheaper.

The influence of floor surface on white line disease is interesting. It is commonly stated that cows become lame because of a specific type of stone or gravel in a track, particularly if sharp flints are present. However, beef cattle could probably walk along the same track without stones penetrating their feet. This strongly suggests that it is the weakening of the white line which is the critical factor and not the sharpness of the stones.

Rough handling: This has also been shown to have an effect. A survey of farms showed that cows which were forcibly rushed along farm tracks by a herdsman, dog or tractor had a far higher incidence of lameness than farms where the cows were allowed to walk along at their own speed. This was presumably because in the latter case they chose their own footing, thus avoiding bruising to the sole and corium. Similarly, if heifers are introduced into a highly competitive situation where they are forced to make many sudden turning movements, this both increases hoof wear and forces the wall away from the sole, leading to an increase in white line defects. When walking, cows should be allowed to move at their own pace. Their heads will be down as they look at the ground surface in front of them for a safe and soft footing. If cows are being driven too fast, or if they are too crowded, then their heads will be high, they cannot see their footing and increased lameness may result.

Hoof wear: Both inadequate and excessive hoof wear can cause problems. Heifers reared and housed in totally bedded areas (straw, shavings or sand) may not receive sufficient hoof wear. The toes become overgrown, the foot rotates caudally and the corium may become damaged at the sole ulcer site. The provision of a lightly abrasive concrete feeding area is essential, both to keep the foot in shape and to stimulate sufficient horn production to produce the thick sole that is needed in the postpartum animal. At the other extreme, cows or heifers (and especially fresh calvers) that are made to walk long distances on gravel or even concrete roads can wear their soles so thin that they are easily compressed by thumb pressure. This syndrome is common in the grazing systems of Australia, New Zealand and Uruguay. Heifers reared on pasture are often introduced into the dairy herd immediately after calving and expected to walk long distances to and from grazing. This produces maximal wear at a time when hoof growth is minimal, and soft soles with subsequent bruising of the fragile postpartum corium leads to an increase in white line disease and toe ulcers (see 'negative net growth', p. 415). If heifers are exposed to concrete or some other hard surface for a few weeks before calving, this can stimulate an increased thickening of the sole and the severity of the syndrome is reduced.

A similar 'soft sole' syndrome is seen in young bulls introduced to work in a dairy herd, particularly if the bulls are large and do not use the cubicles. The soles of their hind feet, especially at the toe, can wear down to the corium. Ideally, bulls in cubicle systems should be rested in a straw yard, for example cubicles by day and a straw yard by night, or alternate weeks in cubicles and straw yards. On a daily basis bulls soon learn which is to be their period of lying and compensate for the cubicles by lying in the straw yards for long periods of time.

Conformation: Conformation affects the incidence of lameness, which is therefore influenced by genetics and breeding. Bulls should be chosen to give a good depth of heel and a good upright angle of the front wall, as in Fig. 31.3.

Foot trimming: The final management factor that influences the development of lameness is routine foot trimming. If parturition is a major stress period for the development of coriosis, then feet need to be in optimum shape at calving in order to minimize this effect. This is achieved by hoof trimming at drying off, and at any other time when they are overgrown.

Footbaths: The use of footbaths is discussed on p. 430.

Other causes of foot lameness

Hoof disorders:

- Foreign body penetration
- Slurry heel
- Vertical fissure (sandcracks)
- Hardship lines and laminitis
- Horizontal fissure
- Broken toe
- Axial wall fissures

Skin disorders:

- Interdigital necrobacillosis (foul of the foot or footrot)
- Digital dermatitis (hairy warts)
- Interdigital skin hyperplasia (corns, growths or tylomas)
- Mud fever

Bone and joint disorders:

- Pedal bone fracture
- Necrosis of the apex of the pedal bone
- Pedal arthritis

Hoof disorders

Foreign body penetration of the sole

Typical foreign bodies are stones (especially sharp flints), nails (particularly those with flat heads), fragments of wood, glass or tin and occasionally even the sharp root of a cast tooth will penetrate the sole. After removal of the foreign body it is essential to provide drainage by opening the sole at the point of entry and removing all under-run horn.

Slurry heel (heel horn erosion, heel necrosis)

In feet which have been exposed to slurry over a long period of time, the smooth, soft and pliable heel horn often becomes black and pitted and in more extreme cases totally eroded, especially in the axial area (Plate 31.13). Although perhaps not too serious externally, slurry heel causes important internal changes. Removal of weight bearing at the heel allows the foot to rotate backwards, thereby predisposing to sole ulcers. In advanced cases the flexor tuberosity no longer has adequate support and as a result penetrates the horn of the sole. The corium will be pinched as the cow walks and sole ulcers develop.

Deep slurry heel fissures may develop into an under-run sole, which may be further complicated by a secondary digital dermatitis. Erosion of the heel also predisposes to white line defects, and by predisposing to a caudal rotation of the claw, to sole ulcers.

There is no one single cause of heel horn erosion. As it is almost exclusively a condition of housed cattle, simple erosion by slurry seems to be the most probable factor. Others have suggested the involvement of specific bacterial infections such as *Dichelobacter nodosus* (Toussaint-Raven, 1985) or *Prevotella (Bacteroides)-melaninogenicus* (Greenough, 1987). Coriosis/laminitis may also be involved, leading to poorer quality heel horn, which is then more susceptible to the corrosive effects of slurry.

Treatment and control

Deep fissures may need to be investigated to eliminate (and correct) an under-run sole, but if the lesion is relatively superficial it is best left and treated topically. Removal of heel horn is commonly contraindicated, because to do so must inevitably lead to a caudal rotation of the claw and increase the risk of sole ulcers. Hygiene is the best control measure, maintaining the feet in a clean and dry environment, with regular footbaths. Lime, used in cubicles for mastitis control, also acts as a disinfectant and drying agent.

Vertical fissures (sandcracks)

Vertical fissures occur as a result of damage to a small area of the periople and underlying coronary band. Horn formation is disrupted at that point, although the adjacent horn continues to grow. This leaves a gap (the vertical fissure) running down the hoof wall from the point of disrupted production (Plate 31.14). In North America vertical fissures are commonly seen in both beef cattle and older dairy cows kept in sand lots where the combination of age, sand, wind and dry weather removes the protective periople. Vertical fissures can also be a result of a digital dermatitis infection on the coronary band. A two-year Canadian field study of 265 Hereford beef cows with a 37 per cent prevalence of sandcracks demonstrated that supplementation with 10 mg/day of biotin significantly reduced the incidence of sandcracks from 29.4 per cent to 14.3 per cent (Campbell et al., 1996).

For treatment, the full length of the fissure should be opened using the curved tip of the hoof knife. Even a small abscess can cause intense lameness. If the fissure is large, a block should be applied to the sound claw.

Hardship lines

Any disruption in horn formation may leave a groove, sometimes referred to as a 'hardship groove' (Greenough et al., 1997), encircling the hoof wall. These are the result of coriosis/laminitis. Inflammation of the laminae is said to lead to massive pressure under the hoof wall, causing the wall to push forward and the toe to lift. The eventual effect is a concave front wall with numerous hardship lines.

Horizontal fissures (sandcracks)

Animals severely ill, for example with mastitis, metritis or any toxic condition, may undergo a total cessation of horn formation. When horn production resumes, instead of a hardship groove, there may be a horizontal fissure encircling the hoof wall. Initially this may cause no problem, but as the defect moves distally towards the toe it loses its support and attachment at the heel. The protruding 'thimble' of horn is then able to rotate on the underlying corium, causing pinching, pain and lameness. Both claws of all four feet may be affected. The date of the illness can be calculated by measuring the distance from the coronary band to the fissure and dividing this by the rate of horn growth, namely 5 mm per month.

For treatment, the loose 'thimble' of horn is removed. If the corium is extensively exposed on one claw, a block should be applied to the other claw if it is sound. However, not all horizontal fissures lead to lameness. Some simply grow to the toe and are shed naturally. It is only necessary to trim the foot if the cow is lame. A cow with one long claw and one short, due to the horizontal fissure fragment having been shed from one claw only, is sometimes referred to as having a 'broken toe'.

Axial wall fissures

The white line junction runs along the abaxial wall from the heel to the toe, caudally along the axial wall at sole level and then passes obliquely in a proximal caudal direction along the axial wall to the coronary band in the interdigital space. White line lesions running obliquely along the axial wall are often referred to as axial wall fissures (Plate 31.15). Recently there has been an apparent increase in incidence (Vermunt, 1998). The cause is unknown, but wet conditions underfoot have been suggested. Due to their position in the interdigital space they are quite difficult to pare and lesions which damage the coronary band can lead to permanent vertical fissures. Digital dermatitis lesions affecting the coronary band in the interdigital space may be a further factor.

Skin disorders

Interdigital necrobacillosis
(foul of the foot, foot-rot)

This is a bacterial infection of the skin of the interdigital cleft. Two organisms are primarily involved, namely Prevotella (Bacteroides) melaninogenicus and Fusobacterium necrophorum. Cultural studies have suggested that P. melaninogenicus should be further subdivided into Porphyromonas asaccharolytica and Prevotella species (Berg & Weaver, 1994). Dichelobacter nodosus may also be involved. F. necrophorum is an obligate anerobic Gram-negative bacterium found in the intestinal tract of both cattle and sheep and it is widespread in the environment, surviving for up to ten months. The A and AB biotypes produce a potent exotoxin which causes a suppurative necrosis and depresses phagocytosis, and a degree of synergism may exist between B. melaninogenicus and F. necrophorum. Injury to the interdigital skin may be required to allow entry of infection. This is usually due to stones, stubble, kale stems, hardened dung in the interdigital area, sticks, very dry pasture, rough flooring, etc. Damage will be easier when the skin is soft due to continued wetting. In some instances the damage may be caused by penetration of spirochaete organisms. Reservoirs of infection may exist in wet, dirty areas such as the gateways to fields and around water and feed troughs. It is also possible that mild digital dermatitis or interdigital dermatitis might be the cause of the initial damage.

The condition has a worldwide distribution in both dairy and beef cattle. Usually only one or a few animals are affected at one time. However, the disease appears to be contagious with the incidence increasing in wet humid weather and interdigital skin damage. Epizootics can arise when cattle are moved to a new environment or mixed together. The most probable source of infection is discharge from the feet of infected animals. The same animal can be affected repeatedly and as susceptibility only changes slightly with age, acquired immunity to the bacteria appears to be poor.

Clinical signs

Typically 'foul' is seen as a sudden onset lameness, more commonly in the hind foot, and it is characterized by bilateral swelling above the coronary band of both claws, often with the digits forced apart. Pyrexia is common. Initial erythema of the interdigital skin progresses to a fissure and subsequent slough of the epidermis to expose the underlying necrotic dermis (Plate 31.16). Unless treated, lesions may progress to an infection of the navicular bursa, the flexor tendon sheath or even the distal interphalangeal joint. However, these complications are more commonly associated with the virulent condition known as 'superfoul'.

Treatment

A wide range of parenteral antibiotics including penicillin, oxytetracycline, sulphonamides, tylosin, tilmicosin, ceftiofur and cefquinome are all effective. The period of treatment required will vary with the severity of the initial lesion. The foot should always be lifted and examined to remove necrotic tissue and any predisposing foreign body and a topical antibiotic applied. Local treatment must improve the rate of healing and reduce the spread of infection into the environment.

Superfoul

This is a peracute form of interdigital necrobacillosis with a poor response to treatment unless aggressive therapy is instigated in the very early stages (David, 1993). Cultural examinations have indicated that the same organisms are present, although most cases are seen in herds concurrently infected with digital dermatitis. An 'invasive spirochaete', similar to both digital dermatitis and the spirochaete identified in peracute foot-rot in sheep, has been seen in lesions of superfoul. The main difference between foul and superfoul is the speed of onset and the severity of the lesions. Necrosis of the interdigital skin may be seen within 12 hours, with deep necrotic fissures into the dermis within 24 hours. Early and aggressive therapy is therefore essential. The treatments used are similar to conventional foul, but at a higher dose and for a longer period. Some benefit has been reported from the use of local anaerobic therapy such as clindamycin, spiramycin and metronidazole.

Prevention and control: Environmental hygiene and footbathing are the main control measures. If outbreaks occur, passages should be scraped with increased frequency, more bedding can be used, and if cattle are outside, they should be moved to a different paddock. Attention should be given to gateways, areas around water troughs and other gathering points to minimize

physical damage to the interdigital cleft. Frosted ground can also produce damage.

Disinfectant footbaths (formalin, copper sulphate, etc.) provide excellent control and are discussed on p. 432. Antibiotic footbaths have been used in the control of superfoul where digital dermatitis may be involved.

Digital dermatitis

This is a bacterial skin infection that primarily affects the epidermis. First reported in Italy (Cheli & Mortellaro, 1974), digital dermatitis now has a worldwide distribution. Figures of frequency of occurrence vary enormously depending on whether the incidence is recorded as a cause of lameness or whether prevalence of lesions is recorded. Many cows show low-grade lesions. For example, Laven (1999) found a lesion prevalence of 41 per cent in 1810 hind feet examined, although only a few of the cows were lame. Within the UK, digital dermatitis now represents approximately 30 per cent of all cases of lameness, which is probably why the overall incidence of lameness in cattle has not decreased since digital dermatitis was first reported in 1987 (Blowey & Sharp, 1988).

Aetiology

Histological studies were first to implicate spirochaetes (Blowey *et al.*, 1992; Read *et al.*, 1992). These had a predilection for keratinized cells and produced a toxin which is keratolytic. A possible association between *Borrelia burgdorferi* and other Treponemes has been suggested. Digital dermatitis-infected cows had a higher seropositivity to *B. burgdorferi* strain B31 and Treponemes 1-9185MED and 2-1498 than control cows (Demirkan *et al.*, 1999). Other workers have suggested the involvement of *Dichelobacter nodosus* and *Campylobacter faecalis*

While spirochaetes can often be found in large numbers at the junction of viable and necrotic tissue layers, they are often difficult to culture. However, successful culture techniques have been reported. Two different spirochaetes have now been demonstrated. One is a long, filamentous organism 12 μm long and 3 μm wide and the other a short spirochaete 5 to 6 μm long and 0.1 μm wide. They are also different on enzymatic analysis (Walker *et al.*, 1995). The most probable cause is an organism with characteristics most consistent with the genus *Treponema*. Potential isolates suggested are *T. phagedenis*, *T. vincentii* and *T. denticola*.

Epidemiology

There is considerable confusion in the literature between incidence of disease seen as lameness and prevalence of lesions, with few studies having examined large numbers of feet at a single point in time. Laven (1999) reported a 41 per cent lesion prevalence but did not relate this to lameness incidence. Hedges *et al.* (2000), in a study of over 1100 cow years in five UK dairy herds, found that digital dermatitis ranked approximately equal to sole ulcers and white line disease, and accounted for around 20 per cent of all cases of clinical lameness examined. Lesions are most commonly seen in housed cattle, especially dairy cows, but heifers and beef animals can also be affected. Lesions in hind feet are more common than in front feet and there would appear to be relatively little immunity, because affected cattle are more likely to have lesions on *both* hind feet (Laven, 1999) and reinfections occur in the same cows year on year, suggesting recrudescence of latent infections. Environmental hygiene is the main factor influencing disease, with the most severe outbreaks occurring in housed cattle in winter, although the increase in lesions and lameness seen in early lactation (Laven, 1999) could also be a reflection of periparturient immune suppression. The highest incidence of disease is seen in the early lactation period and this is associated with animals showing a high prevalence of lesions prepartum. Disease incidence is higher in lactating than dry cows. Suggested causes include lactating cows spending longer standing (for milking, moving and feeding), higher bacterial levels in slurry from higher concentrate diets, faeces are not as dry and stocking density is often higher.

Clinical signs

The earliest lesions of digital dermatitis are seen as a dry, painless, grey encrustation of hyperkeratotic material, often lining the caudal edge of the interdigital pouch. The pouch is most probably the major reservoir of infection in carrier animals, although similar encrustations can be seen along the junction of the heel horn and skin. More advanced lesions, and those sufficiently painful to cause lameness, are typically seen as a moist, light greyish-brown area of exudate, 10–20 mm in diameter, often with matted hairs and encircling the interdigital cleft (Plate 31.13). Cleaning the lesions reveals a red, raw area of epidermitis, very painful when touched and having a characteristic fetid odour and a granular 'strawberry' appearance. Advanced lesions create superficial epidermal erosions and irradiate across the heel bulbs, but ulceration into the dermis is rare: most lesions retain an epidermal covering. Longstanding, chronic lesions have a proliferative appearance, with marked epidermal hypertrophy and hyperplasia (Plate 31.17). These lesions are more prevalent in North America where they are referred to as papillomatous digital dermatitis (PDD) or 'hairy warts', although they are now becoming increasingly common in the UK.

Although the heel area is the most common site, lesions of digital dermatitis may also be seen in the interdigital space, on the sole following a sole ulcer, white line disease or some other lesion exposing the corium, adjacent to the accessory digits or at the anterior aspect of the interdigital space adjacent to the coronary band. Lesions at this point are particularly significant because they can damage the germinal layers of the hoof wall to produce a vertical fissure. In chronic cases granulation tissue may protrude from the fissure and because the corium is inflamed exostoses develop on the anterior wall of the pedal bone. Vertical fissures resulting from anterior digital dermatitis are currently a common indication for digit amputation.

Treatment

Most lesions regress following cleaning and topical application of antibiotics, although repeated treatments may be necessary. Lameness resolves but it is likely that lesions persist to recrudesce at a later date. A wide range of topical antibiotics have been used including lincomycin, combined lincomycin and spectinomycin, oxytetracycline, erythromycin, tylosin and tiamulin. Concurrent parenteral therapy is indicated for anterior lesions to reduce the risk of vertical fissure development. Frequency of application varies with lesion severity, but ideally the lesion should be cleaned and treated for at least two consecutive days. Severe lesions should be bandaged with topical antibiotics for 3–4 days.

Treatment of PDD (hairy warts) is more difficult because the organism is protected by 10–20 mm of keratinized epidermis. Ideally these lesions should be amputated at lower epidermal level, under local anaesthesia, and an antibiotic dressing applied for three to five days, although an antibiotic dressing alone may be sufficient. Single topical treatments and footbaths are not effective against PDD. Antibiotic and antiseptic footbaths are an important aspect of both treatment and control.

Prevention and control

Environmental hygiene is the most important control measure and factors which produce a cleaner and/or drier foot environment will lower disease incidence. Cubicle and feed passages should be scraped at least twice daily and accumulations of stale slurry such as may be found in cross passages and around water troughs should be avoided. Feet should be kept as dry as possible by good drainage, ample bedding and the use of lime in cubicle beds (which also helps in mastitis control). Footbaths are an important control measure, although antibiotics applied as a foot spray on a whole-herd basis have also been effective.

Interdigital dermatitis (IDD)

Considerable confusion exists in the literature over whether IDD is a separate entity or whether it is a combination of a chronic form of digital dermatitis confused with stages of slurry heel. Many of the lesions attributed to IDD contain the spirochaete of digital dermatitis. It is not generally considered to be a cause of lameness, but large numbers of cattle are said to be affected and this predisposes to other lesions such as digital dermatitis, foul, slurry heel and interdigital hyperplasia. *Dichelobacter nodosus* is said to be a common organism involved, but others dispute whether this organism ever causes problems in the feet of cattle.

Clinical signs

Many cases are mild, leading to irritation and hyperaemia of the interdigital skin, with lesions spreading onto the heel bulb. Fissures and necrosis of heel horn can result, with coronary band lesions said to disrupt hoof wall formation and lead to vertical fissures. The latter is also characteristic of anterior digital dermatitis

Control

Environmental hygiene and regular footbathing with copper sulphate or formalin are said to be effective in control.

Interdigital skin hyperplasia (see p. 182)

Also called corns, tylomas, fibromas and just 'growths', interdigital skin hyperplasia is an overgrowth of the natural skin fold adjacent to the axial hoof wall. There is a fold of interdigital skin adjacent to both the medial and lateral claw, and the hyperplasia may develop from either side. It is an overgrowth of skin with gross hypertrophy of the epidermis. The term 'fibroma' is therefore technically incorrect. The lesion is hereditary in certain heavier breeds of cows, especially beef breeds. In other cases it is secondary to chronic irritation of the interdigital skin, for example due to low-grade foul, digital dermatitis or simply impaction with dirt. Cows walking over rough surfaces, leading to excessive splaying of the claws, may show an increased incidence. Lameness occurs either when the lesion reaches such a size that it is compressed by the claws during locomotion or when it becomes secondarily infected, for example by digital dermatitis or foul.

Mild cases can be treated by removing excess horn from the axial wall and the axial surface of the sole. Many lesions regress spontaneously when they are no longer traumatized during locomotion, although low-grade digital dermatitis lesions are so common that it is always worth applying a topical antibiotic. Larger lesions require surgical amputation, although many recur. Regular footbathing through formalin is also said to resolve many lesions.

Mud fever

Mud fever occurs following exposure to cold, wet and muddy conditions. The lower leg becomes slightly swollen, with hard, dry and flaking skin. There may be hair loss and even bleeding if the skin cracks.

For treatment, the legs should be throughly washed and dried followed by application of a greasy antiseptic ointment or a teat spray which contains a high level of emollient. As the organism *Dermatophilus* may be involved, three days of injectable antibiotic (penicillin) may also help (see p. 886; Blowey & Weaver, 2003).

Bone and joint disorders

Fracture of the pedal bone

Bulling activity, with the mounting cow falling back heavily onto hard or rough concrete, is the most common cause of a fractured pedal bone. Bones weakened by age, fluorine poisoning or a foreign body penetrating the sole of the hoof may be at greater risk of fracture. Typically it is the inner claw of the front foot that is involved and by adopting a cross-legged stance the cow transfers her weight onto the sound lateral claw. However, the stance alone is not sufficient to diagnose fracture of the pedal bone. Cows with ulcers in both inner claws will adopt the same position. Most animals heal well if a block is applied to the sound claw.

Apical necrosis of the pedal bone

In a few cows, what initially appears to be a standard white line abscess at the toe sometimes fails to heal, even though it may have been treated thoroughly. At the second examination there will probably be a characteristic foul odour and even with further extensive removal of under-run tissues the toe fails to heal (Plate 31.18). In such cases the apex of the pedal bone has become infected (osteomyelitis). The negative net horn growth (p. 415) which occurs in the periparturient heifer, leading to erosion of toe horn, can be an exacerbating factor, especially if housing coincides with parturition. A similar condition is seen in weaned beef calves that continually run around the pen when introduced into feed lots.

Treatment must involve removal of all necrotic bone. Some clinicians report success with aggressive debridement of the bone, but this has not been this author's experience. Provided the coronary band remains intact, removal of the necrotic toe and the adjacent wall and sole with an embryotomy wire may result in full resolution. Ideally, a radiograph is needed to identify the extent of the necrosis, and as many pedal bones are already severely eroded (Plate 31.19), total amputation of the digit may be the best option (see p. 1119).

Deep pedal infections

Severe or neglected cases of sole ulcers, white line disease, interdigital necrobacillosis or foreign body penetration can lead to infection tracking into deeper tissues. Complications must be suspected when severe lameness follows treatment of an apparently standard lesion, when swelling appears above the coronary band of the affected digit or when pus can be expressed from a sinus when massaging the digit. In any of these instances it is the author's opinion that immediate and aggressive parenteral therapy should be instigated, for example oxytetracycline (2 g twice daily), tylosin or penicillin. If swelling of the coronary band was the only apparent lesion, this may be sufficient to effect resolution.

Deep infections may produce a retro-articular abscess (namely in the heel caudal to the deep flexor tendon), an infection of the navicular bursa, osteomyelitis of the navicular (distal sessamoid) bone or a purulent coronopedal arthritis. A range of treatment options is available, all of which involve aggressive antibiotic cover, and most will require a block applied to the sound claw, thus minimizing weightbearing on the affected claw (p. 432). The option chosen will depend on the severity of the lameness and the clinician's preference, and includes the following:

● Radical fenestration of the sole or wall to provide drainage, followed by regular flushing of the lesion to prevent overgrowth of granulation tissue which would impede drainage (Blowey, 1990).
● Insertion of a drainage tube, the upper end of which is strapped to the hock to allow ease of flushing at milking (Plate 31.20). The lower end is closed. A practical method of siting this tube is to use a trocar and cannula to follow the sinus tract into the foot and then exit above the coronary band.
● Permanent arthrodesis can be created by drilling through the pedal joint and curettage of the articular joint surfaces.
● A surgical approach, opening the joint from the heel, is also available.
● Digit amputation is relatively simple. It can be performed in the standing animal under regional intravenous anaesthesia and provided that there is no major ascending infection of the flexor tendon it

generally results in a good response. There is an additional requirement to redress the lesion regularly, however, and additional weightbearing on the remaining digit may lead to early culling. If amputation can be performed at drying off, then a single dressing change after two to three days may be sufficient, with the second dressing fully removed three to four days later. Most cases heal remarkably well (see also p. 1119).

General treatment and control of foot lameness

Footbaths

Footbaths are an excellent preventive measure for lameness and cows should be walked through once a week during the winter housing period. Solutions of 5–10 per cent formalin or 2.5 per cent copper sulphate or zinc sulphate have been used, as have a variety of other disinfectants. The main objective of a footbath is both to clean and disinfect the foot and in so doing it should help to reduce the incidence of conditions such as:

● Interdigital necrobacillosis
● Slurry heel and heel erosion
● Interdigital skin hyperplasia ('tylomas' or 'corns')
● Digital dermatitis

Formalin also has a drying action on the foot. However, it is unpleasant to handle and its use is not permitted in some countries. Similarly copper sulphate baths may not be permitted by some environmental authorities because of the risk of pollution. Often two baths are used, the first containing water to wash and clean the feet. There is then a raised concrete strip to drain off excess water before the cows walk into the second bath containing the active chemical, as shown in Fig. 31.12. The liquid in the bath needs to be only 80–100 mm deep, as only the claws need to be immersed. Overfilling, particularly with formalin, can lead to damaged skin on both feet and teats.

For best effects cows should have their heels cleaned by a water spray as they enter the milking parlour. Excess water then drains off during milking, after which the cows should exit through a footbath and into a clean environment, with the whole herd being bathed on the same day to avoid cross-contamination. If done carefully, a single passage through an antibiotic footbath will dramatically reduce the incidence of lameness due to digital dermatitis in as little as 24 hours. Unfortunately it does not eliminate infection from a herd.

A range of antibiotics have been used to treat and control digital dermatitis, and at varying concentrations. In most countries none are licensed for this use. The

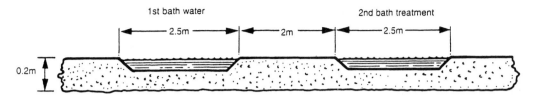

Fig. 31.12 Two footbaths in series.

following are the most common: oxytetracyclines at 4–6 g/litre, lincomycin at 1.0 g/litre, combined lincomycin/spectinomycin at 33 g lincomycin plus 66 g spectinomycin in 150 litres, erythromycin at 0.6 g/litre, tiamulin at 0.5 g/litre and tylosin at 1.3 g/litre. The dosage and frequency of bathing required depends on the severity of clinical signs, with a single or perhaps two passages through a fresh solution once every four weeks originally being the most common recommendation in the UK. (This was not effective on the hairy warts seen in North America, however.) Although this initially appeared reasonably effective, by the late 1990s all antibiotics appeared to be losing their effectiveness and revised concepts of footbathing were considered (Blowey, 2000). At that stage footbaths were instigated only when lameness appeared and usually when a small but significant proportion of the herd was lame. Clearly at this stage lesions have progressed to quite an advanced stage and a single treatment is likely to be less effective.

If footbaths were instigated at an earlier stage, before lesions appeared and especially if dry cows were treated on a preventive basis prior to calving, then it was likely to be more effective. A system of continual daily footbathings in 2.5–5 per cent formalin for periods of two to three weeks (Brizi, 1993; Blowey, 2000) was effective in reducing lesion severity, although even this does not totally eliminate infection from a herd and the treatment has to be repeated after intervals of three to four weeks. Some herds now use footbaths on a continual daily basis. Although formalin and other disinfectants do not penetrate the epidermis as well as antibiotic solutions, regular use eventually leads to drying and sloughing of superficial keratinized tissue. The black debris of hairy warts can be peeled off after two weeks of treatment, although in a proportion of cases characteristic granular areas of active dermatitis may still be visible beneath. Individual severely affected cows can be stood in formalin for 20–30 minutes and this also results in resolution of lesions. The system has also been effective against combined outbreaks of foul and digital dermatitis.

A variety of other footbath chemicals have been used including acidified ionized copper sulphate, hydrogen peroxide/peroxyacetic acid or quaternary ammonium disinfectants, a beta-ionine terpene compound and a triplex of copper, a peroxy compound and a cationic agent. The latter was found to be at least as effective as oxytetracycline.

Nursing, dressings and footblocks

Nursing

Lame cows obviously find walking difficult. They are much less able to compete with the rest of the herd, especially if they are at the lower end of the social dominance scale, which is commonly the case with lame heifers. In addition, they find it difficult to manoeuvre in and out of the cubicles. Cubicles are not easy to use at the best of times and if a cow is not fully mobile cubicles are even more difficult to negotiate. This results either in lame cows spending longer time standing, which exacerbates the digit lesion, or, when down, they spend a long time lying and do not feed sufficiently, resulting in marked weight loss. Ideally lame cows should be transferred into a straw yard, where it is easier for them to lie down and get up and where there is less competition for food. Many herdsmen have commented that moving lame cows from cubicles into straw yards results in an increase in yield in as little as 24 hours, especially in heifers.

Foot dressings

Opinions vary over the need to apply a bandage and dressing to an exposed corium, for example following the trimming of sole ulcers or white line lesions with under-run sole. There appears to be a minimal risk of infection from the environment penetrating the corium, even if cows with extensively under-run soles are allowed to walk out into the slurry, and it is surprising how quickly the exposed corium becomes covered by a layer of new horn. On the other hand, there are several potential disadvantages in applying a dressing, any of which may retard healing. These include the following:

- Unless changed almost daily, the dressing will absorb infection from the environment and impede drainage. Impeded drainage may allow infection to spread, producing further under-run horn.

- Dressings prevent exposure to air and air often promotes healing.
- The presence of a bulky dressing on the sole means that the affected sole becomes weightbearing. This could make sole ulcers worse and cannot be beneficial in the production of new horn.
- Astringents, sometimes used to reduce granulation tissue from a sole ulcer, may damage the corium and hence discourage the formation of the new horn, which is so badly needed to cover the sole.

Few clinicians now use dressings on uncomplicated sole ulcers or white line abscesses and most consider that this results in improved healing. Dressings are needed following amputation of a digit, amputation of large interdigital skin hyperplasia lesions, treatment of extensive digital dermatitis and occasionally to control haemorrhage.

Footblocks

The use of a block applied to the sound claw is an excellent practice as it both promotes healing and considerably improves the welfare of the cow. A variety of devices are available, for example:

- Tie-on shoes and boots
- Nail-on blocks
- Blocks and shoes which are glued on

Tie-on shoes are the least popular, because they are difficult to fix and by encasing the whole foot keep it damp and can retard healing. They also do not reduce weightbearing on the affected digit as effectively as other methods.

Nail-on blocks are used successfully in skilled hands, although the sole of the claw to be blocked needs to be flat. They are cheap and fast to apply, but they do not remain *in situ* for as long as the glue-on blocks: they may move slightly and occasionally create sole ulcers under the rear edge of the block. The nail holes must also weaken the sound claw.

Wooden blocks, rubber blocks and PVC shoes, all of which can be glued onto the sound hoof, are the most popular products. The PVC shoe (Plates 31.7 and 31.20) gives the best support because it is glued to both the wall and the sole, and weightbearing is therefore transferred to the wall, which is the correct weightbearing structure. The glue also sets more rapidly, thus facilitating ease of application, especially in colder climates. However, on cows with very large feet it may not be possible to push the shoe sufficiently far back towards the heel, and the foot can rotate caudally, leading to discomfort.

For all glue-on blocks, the sound claw should be scraped totally clean and dry with a hoof knife, avoiding even finger contact. Access to the inner wall can be improved by forcing the claws apart with a small roll of paper towel. With the PVC shoe the glue is mixed in the shoe until it forms a paste. When the paste is just starting to set the shoe should be pushed as far back towards the heel as possible. It is very important that the shoe or block supports the heel, otherwise the cow rotates backwards onto the sound claw, leading to discomfort and very rapid wearing of the block. Although some authors recommend removing blocks after two or three weeks to retrim the sound claw, most clinicians consider this unnecessary. On average, PVC shoes have been shown to remain in place for over two months, allowing ample time for the new sole to reform (Blowey *et al.*, 1999). The PVC shoes can easily be removed by clipping around their outer wall with hoof clippers.

References

Arkins, S. (1981) Lameness in dairy cows. Parts I and II. *Irish Veterinary Journal*, **35**, 135–40; 163–70.

Bell, E.M. & Miller, A.M. (1977) Lameness in cattle. Interim report, Edinburgh School of Agriculture.

Berg, J.N. & Weaver, A.D. (1994) Bacterial aetiology of diseases in the foot rot complex: recent research and nomenclature changes. In *Proceedings of the International Symposium on Disorders of the Ruminant Digit*, Banff, Canada, pp. 51–7.

Blowey, R.W. (1990) A simple treatment of deep foot infections in cattle. *Veterinary Record*, **127**, 515.

Blowey, R.W. (1998) In *Cattle Lameness and Hoofcare, An Illustrated Guide*. Old Pond Publishing, Ipswich.

Blowey, R.W. (2000) *Control of digital dermatitis. Veterinary Record*, **146**, 10.

Blowey, R., Girdler, C. & Thomas, C. (1999) Persistence of foot blocks used in the treatment of lame cows. *Veterinary Record*, **14**, 642–3.

Blowey, R.W., Hedges, V.J., Green, L.E. & Packington, A.J. (2000c) The effect of biotin supplementation on the treatment of white line lesions in dairy cows. In *Proceedings of the 11th International Symposium on Disorders of the Ruminant Digit*, Parma, Italy, September 2000.

Blowey, R.W., Ossent, P., Watson, C.L., Hedges, V.J., Green, L.E. & Packington, A.J. (2000a) Possible distinction between sole ulcers and heel ulcers as a cause of bovine lameness. *Veterinary Record*, **147**, 110–12.

Blowey, R.W., Phipps, R., Jones, A.K. & Barringer, A.J. (2000b) A comparison of the effects of high fibre and high starch diets on hoof lesion score in multiparous dairy cows. In *Proceedings of the 11th International Symposium on Disorders of the Ruminant Digit*, Parma, Italy, September 2000.

Blowey, R.W. & Sharp, M.W. (1988) Digital dermatitis in dairy cattle. *Veterinary Record*, **122**, 505–8.

Blowey, R.W. & Weaver, A.D. (2003) In *A Color Atlas of Diseases and Disorders of Cattle*. Mosby, London.

Blowey, R.W., Sharp, M.W. & Done, S.H. (1992) Digital dermatitis. *Veterinary Record*, **131**, 39.

Booth, J.M. (1989) Lameness and mastitis losses. *Veterinary Record*, **125**, 161.

Brizi, A. (1993) Bovine digital dermatitis. *The Bovine Practitioner*, **27**, 33–7.

Campbell, J., Greenough, P.R. & Petrie, L. (1996) The effects of biotin on sandcracks in beef cattle. In *Proceedings of the 9th International Symposium on Disorders of the Ruminant Digit*, Jerusalem, p. 29.

Cheli, R. & Mortellaro, C.M. (1974) La Dermatite digitale del bovino. In *Proceedings of the 8th International Meeting on Disorders of Cattle*, Milan, Italy, pp. 208–13.

Clarkson, M.J., Downham, D.Y., Faull, W.B., Hughes, J.W., Manson, F.J., Merritt, J.B., Murray, R.D., Sutherst, J.E. & Ward, W.R. (1996) Incidence and prevalence of lameness in dairy cattle. *Veterinary Record*, **138**, 563–7.

Collick, D.W., Ward, W.R. & Dobson, H. (1989) Association between type of lameness and fertility. *Veterinary Record*, **125**, 103–6.

Da Costa Gomez, C., Al Masri, M., Steinberg, W. & Abel, H.J. (1998) Effect of varying hay/barley proportions on microbial biotin metabolism in the rumen stimulating fermentor RUSITEC. In *Proceedings of the Society of Nutritional Physiologists*, No. 7, 14–28.

David, G.P. (1993) Severe foul-in-the-foot in dairy cattle. *Veterinary Record*, **132**, 567–8.

Demirkan, I., Walker, R.L., Murray, R.D., Blowey, R.W. & Carter, S.D. (1999) Serological evidence of spirochaetal infections associated with digital dermatitis in dairy cattle. *The Veterinary Journal*, **157**, 69–77.

Eddy, R.G. & Scott, C.P. (1980) Some observations on the incidence of lameness in dairy cows in Somerset. *Veterinary Record*, **106**, 140–4.

Esslemont, R.J. & Kossaibati, M.A. (1996) Incidence of production disease and other health problems in a group of dairy herds in England. *Veterinary Record*, **139**, 486–90.

Esslemont, R.J. & Spincer, I. (1993) Report No. 2. DAISY – The Dairy Information System. University of Reading.

Green, L.E., Hedges, V.J., Blowey, R.W., Packington, A.J. & Schukken, Y.H. (2002) The impact of clinical lameness on the milk yield of dairy cows. In *Proceedings of the 12th International Symposium on Disorders of the Ruminant Digit*, Florida.

Green, L.E., Hedges, V.J., O'Callaghan, C., Blowey, R.W. & Packington, A.J. (2000) Biotin supplementation to dairy cows – multivariate analysis of the prospective longitudinal study. In *Proceedings of the 11th International Symposium on Disorders of the Ruminant Digit*, Parma, Italy, September 2000, pp. 305–7.

Greenough, P.R. (1987) An illustrated compendium of bovine lameness, part two. *Modern Veterinary Practice*, February, 94–7.

Greenough, P.R., Weaver, A.D., Brom, D.M., Esslemont, R.J. & Galindo, F.A. (1997) Basic concepts of bovine lameness. In *Lameness in Cattle* (ed. by P.R. Greenough & A.D. Weaver), 3rd edn, p. 10. W.B. Saunders, Philadelphia.

Hagemeister (1996) Research Institute of Biology in Farm Animals, Rostock GDR, Research Report.

Hedges, V.J., Blowey, R.W., O'Callaghan, C., Packington, A.J. & Green, L.E. (2001) A longitudinal field trial of the effect of biotin on lameness in dairy cows. *Journal of Dairy Science*, **84**, 1969–74.

Hedges, V.J., Blowey, R.W., Packington, A.J. & Green, L.E. (2000) A longitudinal field study of the incidence and location of specific causes of lameness on claw health in dairy cows and the effect of biotin supplementation. ISVEE, Colorado, August 2000.

Hirst, W.M., French, N.P., Murray, R.D. & Ward, W.R. (2000) The importance of first lactation lameness as a risk factor for subsequent lameness. In *Proceedings of the 11th International Symposium on Disorders of the Ruminant Digit*, Parma, Italy, September 2000, pp. 149–51.

Laven, R. (1999) The environment and digital dermatitis. *Cattle Practice*, **7**, 349–56.

Leach, K.A., Logue, D.N., Kempson, S.A., Offer, J.A., Ternent, H.E. & Randall, J.M. (1997) Claw lesions in dairy cattle: development of sole and white line haemorrhages during the first lactation. *The Veterinary Journal*, **154**, 215–25.

Leech, F.B., Davies, M.E., Macrae, W.D. & Withers, F.W. (1960) *Disease, Wastage and Husbandry in the British Dairy Herd*. HMSO, London.

Leonard, N., O'Connell, J. & O'Farrell, K. (1996) Effect of overcrowding on claw health in first calved Friesian heifers. *Veterinary Journal*, **152**, 459–72.

Lischer, C., Hunkeler, A., Geyer, A. & Ossent, P. (1996) The effect of biotin in the treatment of uncomplicated claw lesions with exposed corium in dairy cows. In *Proceedings of the International Symposium on Disorders of the Ruminant Digit*, p. 31.

Livesey, C.T. & Flemming, F.L. (1984) Nutritional influences on laminitis, sole ulcer and bruised sole in Friesian cows. *Veterinary Record*, **114**, 510–12.

Livesey, C.T., Laven, R.A., Marsh, C. & Johnson, A.M. (2000) Changes in cysteine concentration in sole horn of Holstein cattle through pregnancy and lactation. In *Proceedings of the 11th International Symposium on Disorders of the Ruminant Digit*, Parma, September 2000, pp. 319–21.

McLennan, M.W. (1988) Incidence of lameness requiring veterinary treatment in Queensland. *Australian Veterinary Journal*, **65**, 144–7.

Midla, L.T., Hoblet, K.H., Weiss, W.P. & Moesschberger, M.L. (1998) Supplemental dietary biotin for prevention of lesions associated with aseptic subclinical laminitis (pododermatitis aseptica diffusa) in primiparous cows. *American Journal of Veterinary Research*, **59**, 733–8.

Ossent, P. (1995) The pathology of digital disease. *Cattle Practice*, **3**, 263.

Ossent, P. & Lischer, Ch. (2000) Sole ulcer, what's new about an old disease? In *Proceedings of the 11th International Symposium on Disorders of the Ruminant Digit*, Parma, Italy, September 2000, pp. 46–9.

Paulus, N. & Nuss, K. (2002) Claw measures at defined sole thicknesses. In *Proceedings of the 12th International Symposium on Lameness in Ruminants*, Florida, pp. 428–30.

Prentice, D.E. & Neal, P.A. (1972) Some observations of the incidence of lameness in dairy cattle in west Cheshire. *Veterinary Record*, **91**, 1–7.

Read, D.H., Walker, R.L., Castro, A.E., Sundberg, J.P. & Thurmond, M.C. (1992) An invasive spirochaete associated with interdigital papillomatosis of dairy cattle. *Veterinary Record*, **130**, 59–60.

Russell, A.M., Rowlands, G.J., Shaw, S.R. & Weaver, A.D. (1982) Survey of lameness in British cattle. *Veterinary Record*, **111**, 155–60.

Toussaint-Raven, E. (1985) *Cattle Footcare and Claw Trimming*. The Farmning Press, Miller Freeman, Ipswich.

Tranter, W.P. & Morris, R.S. (1991) A case study of lameness in three dairy herds. *New Zealand Veterinary Journal*, **39**, 88–96.

Vermunt, J.J. (1998) Axial wall cracks. In *Proceedings of the 10th International Symposium on Disorders of the Ruminant Digit*, Lucerne, Italy, September 1998, p. 141.

Walker, R.L., Read, D.H., Loretz, K.J. & Nordhausen, R.W. (1995) Spirochaetes isolated from dairy cattle with papillomatous digital dermatitis and interdigital dermatitis. *Veterinary Microbiology*, **47**, 343–55.

Wells, S.J., Trent, A.M., Marsh, W.E. & Robins, R.A. (1993) Prevalence and severity of lameness in lactating cows in a sample of Minnesota and Wisconsin herds. *Journal of the American Veterinary Medicine Association*, **202**, 78–82.

Wells, S.J., Trent, A.M., Marsh, W.E., Williams, N.B. & Robins, R.A. (1995) Some factors associated with clinical lameness in dairy herds in Minnesota and Wisconsin. *Veterinary Record*, **136**, 537–40.

Whitaker, D.A., Kelly, J.M. & Smith, E.J. (1983) Incidence of lameness in dairy cows. *Veterinary Record*, **113**, 60–2.

Chapter 32
Lameness Above the Foot

A.D. Weaver

Introduction	435
Nerve paralyses	436
Introduction	436
Suprascapular paralysis	436
Brachial plexus injuries	436
Radial paralysis	436
Femoral paralysis	437
Obturator paralysis	438
Tibial paralysis	438
Peroneal paralysis	438
Sciatic paralysis	439
Downer cow syndrome	439
Fractures	441
Introduction	441
First aid	442
Fracture repair	442
Long bone fractures: external fixation	442
Long bone fractures: internal fixation	444
Introduction	444
Humeral fractures	444
Femoral fractures	444
Tibial fractures	444
Growth plate and other injuries	444
Vertebral fractures	445
Pelvic fractures	446
Dislocations and subluxations	447
Hip joint	447
Sacroiliac luxation and subluxation	448
Stifle joint: femoropatellar	448
Stifle joint: femorotibial	449
Fetlock joint: metacarpophalangeal and metatarsophalangeal	450
Muscle and tendon injuries	451
Introduction	451
Specific muscles	451
Contracted flexor tendons	451
Traumatic flexor tendon injuries	452
Joint diseases	453
Osteochondrosis	453
Hip dysplasia	453
Degenerative arthritis	454
Infectious (septic) arthritis	455
Introduction	455
Septic arthritis: joint ill in neonate	455
Septic arthritis: older cattle	457
Miscellaneous neuromuscular diseases	458
Spastic paresis	458
Spastic syndrome	459

Diseases of skin and subcutis	460
Tarsal cellulitis	460
Carpal bursitis	461
Ankylosing spondylitis	462
Mineral imbalance-related lameness: rickets and osteomalacia	462
Osteomyelitis	463
Physeal dysplasia	464
Lameness of iatrogenic origin	465

Introduction

Lameness above the foot accounts for only 5–15 per cent of dairy cow lameness, and perhaps twice as great a proportion in beef cattle, for which data are lacking. Economic conditions in the UK and elsewhere in Western Europe have led to an increase in the size of the average dairy herd (see p. 23), but the labour force has been reduced. Additionally, only a minority of farmers have been financially secure enough to improve older dairy units, or to replace them with new accommodation. A personal survey of dairy cattle housing (Weaver, 1997) revealed their construction dates to be 1955 to 1994 ($n = 49$) mean 1976, i.e. over 20 years old. Seven units had undergone structural improvements 5 to 28 years (mean 19 years) later. In the period 1997 to 2000 two units were completely rebuilt, while six stopped operating as dairy farms. The result has been an apparent increase in both minor and more severe injuries in dairy cows. In the worst scenario a routine (herd fertility) visit to a dairy unit can reveal two downer cows, both needing urgent nursing care (see p. 440), while the labour – two or three experienced persons – is not always available immediately to move such cows to straw-bedded boxes.

Non-digital lameness problems due to poor accommodation arise from inadequate size and quality of cubicles, false economy of bedding requirements, overcrowding of cubicles and feeding areas, inappropriate mixing of first lactation heifers with mature cattle (leading to bullying, slipping and trampling of younger stock), and an increasing tendency to push cattle around rather than permit them to move at their own speed.

The results, discussed elsewhere in this chapter, include an increased incidence of skin and subcutaneous problems such as tarsal cellulitis (p. 460), carpal swelling (p. 460), traumatic tendon injuries (p. 451), pelvic damage (p. 446) and hip dislocation following falls (p. 447). Not one of these conditions is new. However, as housing systems in the present economic climate fail to satisfy two of the five freedoms – freedom from thermal and physical discomfort, freedom from fear and stress – there is a renewed obligation to recognize the deficiencies in specific dairy units and to advise on both economic and welfare grounds, the need for radical improvements. The introduction of herd health assurance schemes (p. 52) and increased welfare checks on many farms means that housing conditions for dairy herds are likely steadily to improve.

Economic conditions render many of the treatment and management modalities in this chapter hopelessly non-economic except in valuable predigree stock. It is therefore all the more important that early and accurate diagnosis (e.g. septic arthritis in neonate, p. 455, tibial fracture, p. 444) is sought and the options are discussed fully with the responsible person on the farm.

Nerve paralyses

Introduction

Nerve paralyses of the forelimb include the suprascapular, brachial plexus and radial. The main hindlimb involvement is with the femoral, obturator, tibial, peroneal and sciatic. The usual common aetiological component is trauma. The typical age of affected individuals varies from neonate to mature cow. The treatment in all forms involves careful nursing and supportive care (e.g. oral fluids), and management of the primary lesion (e.g. fracture). Sometimes multiple nerve injuries occur as in the downer cow syndrome, which is considered separately (p. 439).

Suprascapular paralysis

Aetiology and pathology

The suprascapular nerve originates from cervical 6 and 7 roots. It may be involved in brachial plexus injuries (see below). The nerve supplies the supraspinatus and infraspinatus muscles. It has no sensory component. It is occasionally injured by blunt trauma in calves butted by others at mangers and troughs when the vertical bar barrier bruises the scapular region. Associated injuries can include fractures of the scapular neck or acromium.

Clinical signs and diagnosis

Suprascapular paralysis causes few clinical signs initially. The shoulder joint may be slightly abducted and the forward phase of the stride shortened. After one week muscular atrophy causes increased prominence of the scapular spine ('sweeney').

Treatment

Treatment is purely palliative. Vitamin B complex may be given systemically. The prognosis is usually good.

Brachial plexus injuries

Aetiology

Trauma, as from sudden caudal and ventral displacement of the shoulder and entire forelimb, together with abduction can lead to separation of any group of the nerve roots C6 to T2. The nerves mainly affected are the radial, median and ulnar. Occasionally, the nerves are damaged by penetrating injury in the axilla with extensive additional damage to the vasculature. More frequently, the plexus is injured during traction in dystokia and severe abduction of the forelimb.

Pathology

The avulsion close to the spinal cord results in a complete loss of motor supply to the forelimb. Occasionally, the cranial segments of the network (supplying the suprascapular and axillary nerves) are spared.

Clinical signs and diagnosis

The forelimb is non-weightbearing and maintained in flaccid extension, with a tendency for the digits to be dragged. Sensation is absent from the level of the elbow distally. Muscular atrophy is evident after seven days.

Differential diagnosis includes radial paralysis (dropped elbow, more localized loss of skin sensation) and humeral shaft fracture with or without radial nerve injury (see p. 444), and forelimb dislocation.

Treatment and prevention

Since brachial plexus avulsion has a very poor prognosis, treatment is not usually justified. In calves with partial avulsion, anti-inflammatory drugs and limb support are suggested. Affected cattle should be confined to a well-bedded stall and care should be taken to avoid the development of decubital damage to the analgesic lower limb.

Radial paralysis

Aetiology and pathogenesis

The nerve (roots C7–T1) is damaged in its distal portion secondarily to humeral shaft fractures, which tend to be

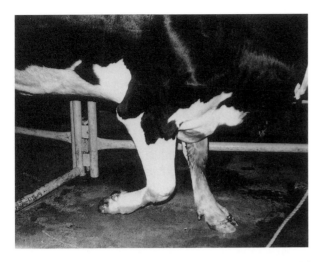

Fig. 32.1 Radial paralysis of right foreleg of six-year-old Friesian cow. Paralysis was present on standing following 120 minutes in right lateral recumbency for surgery of a septic parotiditis under general anaesthesia. Total recovery took 48 hours. The classical signs are present: dropped elbow, flexed carpus and inability to extend forelimb for weight bearing.

spiral, comminuted and to have sharp protruding spikes of bone. Radial nerve paresis frequently occurs following a long (one to two hour) period of general anaesthesia in lateral recumbency when the primary damage is a compressed vascular compartment. A dairy cow trapped under the lower horizontal bar of a cubicle division can also, on release, have radial paralysis. While partial paralysis is more common, complete radial paralysis can result from brachial plexus injuries or severe trauma. Cattle entering a crush fast and banging the shoulders against the yoke gate occasionally have a temporary partial radial paralysis.

Clinical signs and diagnosis

The main signs are a dropped elbow due to triceps paralysis, knuckled fetlock and an inability to advance the limb (Fig. 32.1). If the limb is placed in its usual position, the fetlock flexes as an attempt is made to bear weight. Sensory loss can be detected over the elbow and lateral aspect of the forearm.

Differential diagnosis includes humeral fracture with or without radial paralysis.

Treatment and prevention

The prognosis is good if the nerve has not been sectioned by humeral bone fragments. Treatment is supportive, keeping the animal on soft bedding and on non-slip surfaces. The fetlock should be bandaged to prevent iatrogenic trauma. Anti-inflammatory drugs and vitamin B complex may be given systemically.

Cattle maintained in lateral recumbency under general anaesthesia should have soft supporting surfaces and the down forelimb should be extended forwards to reduce the pressure on the vasculature to the lower parts of the limb. Also, the upper foreleg should not be roped tightly down against the table, whereby it would increase pressure on the lower leg.

Femoral paralysis

Aetiology and pathology

The femoral nerve (L4–6 spinal nerve roots) has a short course, ramifying in the iliopsoas and quadriceps muscles. It is liable to damage in the oversized fetus of large-framed breeds (Simmental, Charolais, Holstein) at delivery when presented in the 'hiplock' or 'stifle lock' position, which tends to cause femoral hyperextension as forced traction is exerted. The femoral nerve, usually unilaterally, is drawn against the pubic brim at the pelvic inlet. The injury can occur in either anterior or posterior presentation. The lesion is sometimes a rupture of the nerve, but more frequently involves very severe perineural haemorrhage and oedema. In other cases, the quadriceps femoris muscle is severely stretched and incurs damage to its vascular and nerve supply. The resulting quadriceps atrophy presents with typical clinical signs.

Clinical signs and diagnosis

The animal, usually a neonate, is unable to maintain the stifle in extension due to quadriceps dysfunction. The joint is flexed and the digit rests with minimal weight bearing. Usually, hock and digital joints are also flexed, though the toe is not dragged. A small area of loss of skin sensitivity may be detectable lateral and proximal to the stifle joint. Quadriceps atrophy within 10 to 14 days results in a triangular depression in the lateral cranial part of the thigh. Fibrosis of the remaining quadriceps muscle mass develops later. The stifle joint may become unusually prominent. Differential diagnosis involves dorsal or lateral patellar luxation, septic gonitis, femoral fracture or growth plate separation, hip dislocation and quadriceps rupture.

Treatment and prevention

The prognosis is guarded or poor. Recovery is unlikely in calves with femoral nerve rupture. The recovery time for regeneration was about four months in an experimental study when a 5 mm ($\frac{1}{4}$ inch) length of femoral nerve was resected surgically (Buchthal et al., 1984). Treatment is primarily careful supportive nursing care. Calves should receive colostrum by bottle within 6 hours of birth if the injury has prevented rising to suck.

Clean and dry bedding is essential. The calf should be frequently turned. Analgesics, anti-inflammatories, and vitamin E and selenium preparations should be given.

Obturator paralysis

Aetiology and pathology

Obturator paralysis classically involves unilateral or bilateral damage to the nerve, usually in heifers during dystokia due to fetal oversize or maternal immaturity, when the nerve (L4–L6 nerve roots) is damaged by fetal pressure on its course along the medial aspect of the ileum or along the pelvic floor. Experimental section of the nerve, which innervates the adductor muscles (gracilis, pectineus, adductor and external obturator), has caused mild abduction of one or both hind limbs but experimental animals have been able to rise without difficulty (Vaughan, 1964; Cox, 1981). A common synonym for obturator paralysis, 'calving paralysis', is considered a misnomer since the latter is usually associated with the 'downer cow' syndrome (Cox & Onapito, 1998) (see p. 439). Many clinical cases of so-called obturator paralysis have a more complex aetiology involving branches of the sciatic nerve or primary muscle damage.

Clinical signs and diagnosis

Abduction of the hindlimb (unilateral) or a straddled gait (bilateral) are the classical signs. Confusion clinically may result from the stance adopted by a heifer with an oedematous and overstocked udder and with pelvic fractures. Rectal and vaginal examination may reveal minor pelvic damage associated with the paralysis. Some cattle are recumbent and such recumbency is rarely due to simple unilateral obturator injury. Cattle are liable to slip with gross hindlimb abduction, giving rise to hip luxation. Skin sensation remains unimpaired. Diagnosis is based on the history of possible injury at parturition and on the characteristic stance and gait.

Treatment and prevention

The animal should be kept on non-slip surfaces to avoid possible hip luxation or femoral neck fracture. Sand on the concrete floor of a calving/isolation box, overlaid with plenty of straw, is ideal. The hocks and hind feet should be kept close together by a figure of eight pattern of rope above the hocks or fetlocks. The distance between these joints should not exceed 30 cm (12 inches), which permits the animal to rise. Supportive care should be continued for several days. Breeding management should be reviewed to avoid a high incidence of dystokia in heifers and to prevent damage during forced extraction of the fetus.

Tibial paralysis

Aetiology and pathology

Tibial paralysis is rare. It is associated with iatrogenic damage following deep infections in the caudal thigh musculature or lacerating injuries in the medial aspect of the hock with associated damage to related tendons.

Clinical signs and diagnosis

Tibial paralysis results in hock flexion from inability primarily to cause gastrocnemius contraction, which would result in hock extension. It also causes hyperextension of the digits in that the weight is borne more on the heels. Skin sensation is absent over the caudal aspect of the metatarsus and digits. Differential diagnosis includes peroneal paralysis and gastrocnemius and flexor tendon rupture.

Treatment and prevention

Treatment is symptomatic, involving confinement and vitamin B complex injections.

Peroneal paralysis

Aetiology and pathology

As with the tibial nerve, the peroneal nerve is a major branch of the sciatic nerve (L6–S2 nerve roots). Its common site of damage is over the lateral aspect of the stifle joint where the nerve lies relatively close to the skin surface. It is liable to injury following sudden (falls) or chronic pressure (prolonged recumbency).

Clinical signs and diagnosis

The hock is hyperextended, and fetlock and digits are flexed (knuckled over) (Fig. 32.2). The foot can be placed in its normal position. Skin sensation is lost dorsally from the fetlock distally to the coronary band. Diagnosis is easily made on the clinical signs and sensory loss. Differential diagnosis involves tibial paralysis and painful digital diseases.

Treatment and prevention

The prognosis is good with recovery usually evident in a few days. Self-induced trauma to the fetlock is minimized by application of a soft bandage or a light resin cast to the fetlock.

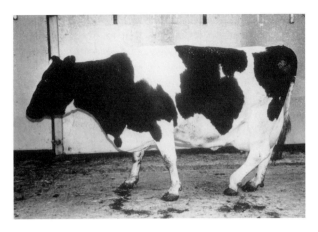

Fig. 32.2 Peroneal paralysis in six-year-old Friesian cow showing extended hock and knuckling of fetlock. Two days previously the digit had also been flexed. Some weight is now borne on claw normally. Total recovery took another three days.

Sciatic paralysis

Sciatic nerve paralysis involves the nerve that originates from three ventral roots (L6, S1–2). Damage to L6 root may be an important component of 'calving paralysis' or obturator paralysis (Cox, 1981) (see p. 438). The sciatic nerve is liable to damage unassociated directly with parturition but in prolonged unilateral recumbency. The site is usually close to the medial aspect of the femoral greater trochanter and may be associated with struggling. Such circumstances can involve partial recovery from milk fever or postparturient hypocalcaemia, as the cow struggles to rise on a slippery surface (e.g. concrete) (Cox & Onapito, 1998). Rarely, sciatic paralysis is secondary to femoral neck or pelvic fracture (pubis, ischium), or iatrogenic in origin from septic infection arising from intramuscular injections.

Clinical signs and diagnosis

The limb is entirely non-weightbearing. Sensation is lost from the limb distal to the stifle except for a strip on the medial aspect of the thigh distal to the mid-metatarsal region, which is supplied by the saphenous branch of the femoral nerve. Differential diagnosis should include femoral fracture, the signs of which will include crepitus, possibly swelling and abnormal mobility, and septic gonitis and tarsitis.

Treatment and prevention

The prognosis is usually hopeless. Many cases are presented as 'downer cows'. It is vital that this paralysis be recognized early, so that long-term nursing measures will not be instituted. Early slaughter is advisable.

Downer cow syndrome (see p. 797)

Defined as 'a cow down in sternal recumbency for unknown reasons', the syndrome usually affects high-yielding dairy cows in the first 48 hours postpartum. In the UK the incidence appears to be increasing as a result of overcrowding in cubicle houses (see p. 43). Veterinary attention may not be sought for 24 hours, as a response to calcium borogluconate therapy is awaited. The condition has a multiple aetiology including traumatic, metabolic, neurological and toxic infectious causes. The following are examples:

- Traumatic: sacroiliac luxation and subluxation, bilateral or unilateral coxofemoral luxation, rupture of gastrocnemius muscle, pelvic fracture, massive blood loss (profound anaemia).
- Metabolic: non-responsive hypocalcaemia, hypokalaemia.
- Neurological: lymphosarcoma infiltration into thoracic or lumbosacral spinal canal, bilateral peroneal paralysis, complications of obturator paralysis.
- Toxic infectious: septic metritis, acute coliform mastitis (pp. 334, 519).

The primary recumbency, whether due to dystokia (46 per cent of cases), milk fever (38 per cent), or other causes (16 per cent) (Chamberlain, 1987), is followed by secondary recumbency. The usual explanation for the development of a downer syndrome in a cow, which is unsuccessfully treated for clinical signs diagnostic of hypocalcaemic parturient paresis or milk fever, is that the hypocalcaemia has been treated too late and that unrecognized traumatic injury has already taken place. Half of all 'downer cows' develop within 24 hours of parturition. They tend to be high producers. The incidence is higher in winter. Survey data indicate a considerable range (3.8–28.2 per cent) in the incidence of downer cows as a percentage of cases of milk fever. One study revealed that 33 per cent of downer cows recovered, 23 per cent were slaughtered, and 44 per cent died or were euthanized.

Pressure damage causes ischaemia of muscles and nerves. Following a variable period of struggling, further skeletal injury such as gastrocnemius muscle rupture may occur. The differential diagnosis is often difficult since frequently a non-responsive milk fever cow does not appear to have any further specific abnormality.

The aetiology of this pressure damage involves effects resulting from the 'compartment syndrome' (Cox & Onapito, 1998). Increased pressure develops within an osteofascial compartment following external pressure or internal filling of the compartment with blood or oedematous fluid, or both. External pressure results in ischaemia, 'leaky' vessels, and a postcompression swelling. The effects of the crush syndrome, which refer to the systemic results or muscle damage, involve largely the absorption of muscle breakdown products.

One specific cause of the downer cow syndrome is pressure damage to the hindquarters following a period of prolonged recumbency (3–6 hours or more), resulting both in extensive muscle damage and reversible or irreversible changes in the sciatic nerve caudal to the proximal end of the femur and to the peroneal nerve.

Consideration of the aetiology and pathology of traumatic factors is reviewed in other sections (see Fractures, p. 441; Dislocations and subluxations, p. 447; Muscle and tendon injuries, p. 451).

Clinical signs and diagnosis

By definition the animal is recumbent. The cow is usually alert, eats, and can defecate and urinate. Affected cows make little or no attempt to rise in the hindlimbs. Some alert cows move around using the forelimbs and have been termed 'creeper cows'. Cows confined to a stanchion do not have facilities to demonstrate this movement, which may appear after the animal is transferred to a well-bedded stall or box. Dull or comatose and anorectic cows may be 'downers' due to systemic toxic factors (coliform mastitis, severe metritis). Occasionally, downer cows are hyperexcitable due to hypomagnesaemia or hypocalcaemia (see Chapter 46).

Rectal palpation is crucial to evaluate various traumatic aetiologies: sacroiliac (sub)luxation, pelvic fracture, severe, intrapelvic, soft tissue injury and coxofemoral luxation, as well as to check the state of the uterus (puerperium). External assessment includes palpation of the spine for abnormal angulation, swelling, or crepitus (fracture), musculature of the hindlimbs, especially the adductor group medially (muscle rupture), manipulation of the upper hindlimb and pelvis for evidence of fracture or dislocation, and determination of possible loss of skin sensation. The possibility of acute coliform mastitis should be investigated. The cow should be turned to the opposite side for similar examination of the other hindlimb. Cows usually prefer to lie with the more painful hindlimb uppermost.

Downer cows have variable changes in blood mineral levels, some showing a persistent hypocalcaemia, hypophosphataemia, and possible hypomagnesaemia. The role and significance of hypokalaemia is disputed. The release of potassium from damaged muscle cells does not necessarily cause hyperkalaemia because the usual coexisting hypocalcaemia has a tendency to cause hypokalaemia. All cases show an elevated creatine kinase (CK), which is specific for muscle injury. In one study (Chamberlain, 1986), CK peaked at 24 hours after onset of recumbency in cows that recovered to stand, and at 48 hours in cows that became permanent 'downers'. Plasma or serum CK values reflect the total mass of injured muscle, but CK half-life is such that it is of doubtful value as a prognostic indicator several days after initial recumbency, when little further active muscle damage may be occurring.

Plasma aspartate aminotransferase (AST) is elevated in animals with muscle damage. This enzyme is also released in cardiac myopathies, but postpartum increases in downer cows are almost invariably related to the muscle component.

In cows recumbent for over 48 hours (at the time of second clinical examination), clinical pathology can be reassessed. Urinalysis may now reveal proteinuria indicative of myoglobinuria (from muscle breakdown), ketonuria and bilirubinuria (from partial anorexia).

If the aetiology of the persistent recumbency remains in doubt, a repeat complete clinical examination should bear in mind less common causes (e.g. infiltration of lymphosarcoma into the spinal canal). A careful recheck of the history may aid diagnosis at this stage.

Treatment and prevention

The downer cow should be moved to a well-bedded loose box not later than 24 hours after the onset of recumbency. Ample food and water must be provided in low, wide-based containers.

The primary aim is to raise the cow. Any attempt should be made on a relatively non-slip surface. Personnel should be ready to assist with tail support following provocative stimulation (e.g. electric goad). Hip clamps, e.g. Bagshaw hoist, may be applied to the wings of the ilium for a maximum of 20 minutes. Usually, the ability of the cow to bear weight is obvious. While slung in this manner, the hindquarters should be checked for symmetry and the opportunity taken to flex and extend each hindlimb to check for fractures. Other devices for elevation include air cushions or bags, webbing slings and water flotation tanks (Smith et al., 1997). Some cows that can stand following hoisting require to be hobbled above the hocks or hind fetlocks to prevent abduction of the hindlimbs.

Hip clamps may be repeatedly applied for a few minutes of forced elevation of the hindquarters to improve circulation. When lowered, the cow should be placed with the previously dependent side uppermost.

The most important component of treatment is good nursing. The cow must be made comfortable. Owners should be observant for the possible development of a toxic (e.g. coliform) mastitis during recumbency. Rapid loss of weight, signs of systemic toxicity, and anorexia are grave prognostic indicators. Soft bedding is essential for effective nursing in all downer cows, which should be turned several times daily.

Fresh water should be available alongside a bucket containing a commercial electrolyte solution. Parenteral treatment includes repeated injection of solutions containing calcium–phosphorus–magnesium with glucose and potassium. Additional potassium should only be given by stomach tube (e.g. 50g KCl daily). Tripelennamine hydrochloride given as 12ml solution i.v. is an effective stimulant and antihistaminic that makes a downer cow appear more alert (Chamberlain, 1987). Analgesics such as phenylbutazone, flunixine meglumine and ketoprofen should be restricted to cows with obvious signs of pain.

The prognosis is good in well-nursed 'creeper cows' with some voluntary hindlimb movement and cows that are capable of a short period of weight bearing when hoisted or slung. The prognosis is poor in animals with no hindlimb movement. Proprioceptive reflexes should be repeatedly checked in such cows.

Generally, excellent nursing, a consistently good appetite, and some spontaneous movement should encourage owners to persist and practise patience.

Valuable prognostic indicators for survival in a limited British survey of 64 downer cows were as follows.

- On day 2 of recumbency: body condition score, quality of nursing care, absence of hypocalcaemia, relative hypomagnesaemia, and lower AST and CK enzyme levels.
- On day 4 of recumbency: survival was associated with little further rise of CK and with continued good nursing.

A US survey of 15 veterinarians' experience with slings used on 145 cows showed a recovery rate of 52 per cent.

Prevention depends primarily on the avoidance of parturient paresis associated with milk fever (see Chapter 46). Calving should take place in properly designed areas with good footing. Many farms will benefit from stalls with 30cm (12 inches) clean sand as bedding. On problem farms, successful reduction of the incidence of downer cows has been primarily attributed to improved observation for the initial signs of milk fever and its prompt treatment.

Periparturient cows should be placed onto a minimal slip surface and sand is excellent for this purpose if staw-bedded calving boxes are not available.

A high incidence of downer cows in first-calf heifers, where hypocalcaemia can be ruled out, may be due to dystokia. Breeding policies may require modification such as use of a smaller breed bull or later first service dates for heifers.

Prevention of the downer cow syndrome is particularly vital today since treatment is very labour-intensive and repeated veterinary involvement is too costly for the minimal profit margins of many dairy farms.

Fractures

Introduction

In the assessment of bovine fractures, several factors require consideration in each clinical situation.

Economics

With some exceptions, economic consideration is a vital factor. Many cattle not used for breeding, e.g. steers, are best slaughtered at once, since treatment would be costly. Young potentially valuable breeding stock fall into a different category, where slaughter value is negligible in comparison with the potential value following fracture healing.

Size, age and sex

Young cattle respond well to restrictions imposed during fracture immobilization. They tend to rise easily despite external fixation and to be less liable to develop decubital lesions. The soft thin cortices of long bones in calves make plate and screws generally an unsuitable means of internal fixation. Calves have a remarkable ability rapidly to produce a fibrous response at a fracture site and early callus formation.

Disposition

An advantage of fracture healing in cattle compared with horses is their tolerant disposition making handling easier.

Location and character

Generally, the more proximal the fracture, the more difficult is its anatomical reduction and rigid fixation. Thus humeral and femoral fractures have notoriously low recovery rates, while metatarsal and metacarpal fractures usually heal well. Fracture of the distal phalanx, in which displacement is minimal, is discussed elsewhere (see Fracture of distal phalanx, p. 429).

Comminuted fractures are the rule in cattle. Many fractures are closed initially but become open following inappropriate handling such as movement to a stall. The prognosis for open fractures, especially proximal fractures (humerus, tibia, femur), is guarded. Soft tissue damage is often limited to haematoma and oedema formation resulting from the original insult and movement of the fractured bone ends. In certain instances, significant nerve damage (e.g. to radial nerve in a spiral humeral shaft fracture) may be an important consideration in the prognosis.

Most fractures tend to be oblique or spiral in cattle. Maintenance of reduction while external or internal fixation is applied tends to be more difficult than with transverse fractures.

Duration of fracture

Unlike small animals and horses, the duration of a bovine fracture before presentation can often be 12–24 hours, a consequence of the relatively casual methods of husbandry practised on some farms. The result is invariably a greater degree of soft tissue injury than in a freshly presented fracture. One effect of a longer duration of movement at a fracture site is an open fracture.

First aid

Fractures should be immobilized on the farm premises as soon as possible. Suitable materials include padding with old towels or sheeting, and splinting with polyvinyl chloride tubing, or stiff rods such as broomsticks placed at 90° to each other (e.g. cranial and lateral surfaces of the forelimb to stabilize metacarpal fracture) and fixed in position with duct tape. The joints above and below the fracture should be immobilized. This technique is impossible in femoral, tibial and humeral fractures. In tibial fractures, a Robert Jones bandage comprising layers of cotton wool firmly bound by cotton bandage can achieve adequate immobility if sufficient bulk is applied.

Fracture repair

In certain fractures (e.g. rib) spontaneous healing is the rule. In others (e.g. external angle of ilium) repair usually takes place but a sequestrum may form. The sequestrum generally is only a cosmetic blemish but sometimes becomes infected and then requires removal.

Most fractures require treatment by methods of external or internal fixation, or both, if recovery is to take place.

Long bone fractures: external fixation

External fixation of fractures is usually satisfactory if the site is distal to the humerus or proximal tibial meta-

physis. A minimum of equipment is required, and extensive experience is unnecessary. External fixation is unsuitable for more proximal sites, in open fractures with gross contamination and fractures occurring in two limbs simultaneously. Young cattle develop osteomyelitis following open long bone fractures more frequently than older cattle. Careful examination of the fracture site, preferably after clipping of the skin, is essential to avoid missing an open fracture. External fixation alone may be contraindicated in very heavy animals.

Choice of materials and technique for external fixation

Immobilization techniques include the splint or cast, the modified Thomas splint, and both methods together.

Casting materials available today include plaster of Paris (one form of which is rapid-setting), thermoplastic polyester polymers (Hexcelite), and polyurethane resin incorporated into woven material of polyester (Cuttercast, Baycast) or fibreglass (Deltalite/Scotchcast). Casts should always be applied over a layer of padding. The depth of padding should be considerably greater if soft tissue swelling is anticipated at the fracture site and also should be generous over bone prominences. The padding should extend beyond the intended proximal point of the cast. The cast should immobilize the joints proximal and distal to the fracture site. Thus, in a one-month-old calf with a distal metacarpal shaft fracture, the cast should extend at least 8 cm (3 inches) proximal to the radiocarpal joint and similarly distal to the fetlock.

Positioning is very important in applying a cast. General anaesthesia is rarely necessary; xylazine is usually adequate for restraint and analgesia. The limb must be forcibly extended for fracture reduction and then maintained immobile until the cast has set. Traction on the distal part of the limb may be aided by inserting wire through holes drilled in the toes.

The advantages of a lightweight cast include increased comfort and ease of rising, and are achieved by fibreglass (e.g. Vetcast, Deltalite, Scotchcast), which has a strength five times greater than plaster of Paris. Weight reduction is also possible using several layers of plaster overlaid by fibreglass casting tape, once the plaster has hardened. Strength combined with lightness is the result.

Some fractures require radiography before reduction and immobilization to determine the extent and severity of bone damage. Fractures may also be radiographed two to three weeks after immobilization to assess the degree of healing. Removal of the cast at this time is often unnecessary. The radiolucency of cast materials varies, plaster of Paris being poor,

Deltalite/Scotchcast fair with some mottling, and Cuttercast/Baycast is excellent.

Extension bars have sometimes been incorporated into external casts. These U-shaped metal stirrups have the curved part of the U distal to the toes, so that weight is borne by the bar and transferred proximally to the cast, into which the two arms of the extension bar are buried during cast application. Such a device is only useful if there is a specific indication to avoid weight bearing by the digits. The effective increase in limb length makes standing up and ambulation more difficult. A modification is the hanging cast. This device comprises one or more intramedullary pins that are drilled through the proximal fracture fragment, and onto which a U-shaped bar is fitted after the usual external immobilization has been applied. When weight is borne, it is transferred proximally to load bearing by the proximal fracture site, so that the fracture site is not stressed.

Thomas extension splints may be put on either forelimb or hindlimb. Good padding is essential both at the points (axilla, inguinum) where maximal pressure will be applied, as well as at any contact points more distally. The Thomas extension splint must be 'made to measure' for the individual case (e.g. circumference of proximal and distal rings, length of cranial and caudal longitudinal bars). In growing stock the length should be slightly greater (e.g. 5 cm or 2 inches) than necessary, to permit growth. Some devices have expansion clamps or rings on the longitudinal bars to allow continual modification.

The bottom ring should be wired to the foot to maintain the leg in extension. Bandages and padding should be placed around the limb at potentially exposed areas before they are taped to the longitudinal bars. In the hindlimb, the metatarsus may be fixed to the caudal bar, the tibial (gaskin) area to the cranial bar. The extension splint should be checked carefully for fit and effective immobilization of the fracture site before release of the patient. Many cases will benefit from combination of an external cast (e.g. fibreglass) and a Thomas extension splint.

Cattle up to 350 kg (800 lb) will generally adapt well to Thomas splintage. Patients should be confined to a stall with relatively little straw bedding. Assistance to rise may be needed initially. The cast or splint should be checked daily for skin abrasions, cast fracture or slackness.

Neonatal and other calves less than a month old with simple fractures and rapid callus formation may require external support for two weeks only (Fig. 32.3). Other young cattle should be checked for progress at three weeks by removing the cast with an oscillating saw. Sometimes the same splint may be reapplied (e.g. with Deltalite, Cuttercast).

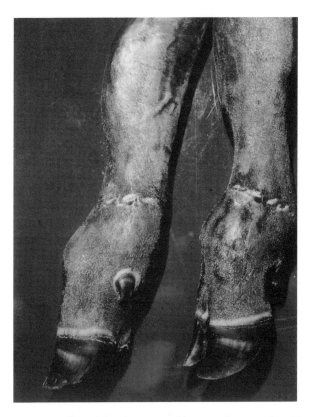

Fig. 32.3 Bilateral distal metacarpal fractures in a one-day-old Saler calf. Circular lesions result from pressure of obstetrical chains applied during forced extraction. In the absence of percutaneous infection (seen here) external immobilization from mid metacarpal to coronary level is indicated.

Humeral fractures in cattle aged two and a half months to three years can heal four to six weeks following Thomas splintage (Wintzer, 1961). In other cases, immobility has been unsatisfactory and nonunion has resulted despite massive callus formation.

Open fractures, at sites where external fixation is practical, require particular attention. The presence of skin perforation should carry the presumption of an open fracture even if bone cannot be seen or palpated through the injury. The wound is cleansed and carefully explored. Any free bone fragments should be removed. Larger wounds require debridement. It may be useful to take tissue samples or a blood clot for microbiological culture in the case of valuable cattle. Wounds should be copiously irrigated with a polyionic solution (isotonic balanced electrolyte with neutral pH). The value of adding a 0.1 per cent povidone-iodine solution (1:100 dilution of povidone-iodine 10 per cent solution) has not been established in cattle.

Antibiotics should be given parenterally in all open fractures in cattle. Natural and synthetic penicillins are the first choice. Systemic antibiotics should be continued for seven to ten days. Antibacterial sensitivity patterns may be checked via samples taken at an early stage and before antibiotics are given. Samples should preferably be taken from infected bone at surgery rather than from discharging sinus tracts where contamination with surface pathogens will complicate interpretation of laboratory results. Antibiotic therapy should be instituted as soon as possible following identification of an open fracture. Small wounds may be covered with a sterile protective dressing, but any external support of the fracture site should be removed after three to five days to permit quick assessment of the wound. Young cattle develop osteomyelitis following open fractures more frequently than adults. The reason may be a richer blood supply in the damaged area.

Long bone fractures: internal fixation

Introduction

Economic factors are often important in considering internal fixation of bovine long bone fractures. Expertise in the discipline is also essential for successful reduction and rigid support under aseptic surgical conditions.

Anatomical factors mean that long bone repair by internal fixation is most frequently required in humeral, femoral and tibial fractures. Young calves have very thin cortical bone and screws are liable to loosen or be stripped during insertion. Failure is the common result. Both access to the fracture site and reduction are much simpler in the calf than adult.

In adult cattle, where the cortex is thick and dense, the major problems are associated with general anaesthesia (e.g. regurgitation, rumen tympany, compromised ventilation), the soft tissue mass through which the fracture site is approached, and the initial difficulty of anatomical reduction, when muscle spasm compounds the degree of overriding of the fragment ends.

Specialist texts should be consulted for details of internal fixation of specific bovine fractures (Ferguson, 1997).

Humeral factures

Animals up to yearling size (e.g. 250 kg, 550 lb) are amenable to internal fixation unless the fracture is severely comminuted. Such fractures are usually midshaft oblique and spiral. The radial nerve is often involved (p. 436). There is often severe overriding, making reduction difficult. Intramedullary pinning (or stack-multiple-pinning) combined with cerclage wiring is often the technique of choice.

Humeral fractures are difficult to plate due to their short length and spiral configuration. Multiple bone fragments often necessitate the use of lag screws.

In older and heavier cattle, internal fixation is less successful due to greater mechanical forces. Often long-term Thomas splintage is adopted.

Femoral fractures

Femoral shaft fractures are relatively common in calves. Most have a history of forced extraction. The existence of concurrent disease should be evaluated (e.g. colostrum intake). No form of external immobilization is helpful. Internal pinning (Steinmann) rarely achieves sufficient immobility of the fracture site. The technique of choice is usually plate and screws, possibly double plating, with two plates placed at about 90° to each other (lateral and cranial).

Similar techniques may be attempted in older cattle. Reduction may present major problems. The huge mechanical force acting at femoral fracture sites makes bending of the plates or loss of screws common. Some femoral shaft fractures eventually heal with some months of stall rest alone.

Tibial fractures

Tibial shaft fractures are amenable to a variety of fixation techniques since exposure is relatively easy. Problems arise with severely comminuted or multiple fractures extending into the proximal and distal metaphyses. As alternatives to plate and screws, and additional support by a Thomas splint, some tibial fractures may be immobilized by cerclage wire with external support. Others best lend themselves to transfixation pinning. In this method two or three 6 mm Steinmann pins are placed through both cortices of both proximal and distal segments under strict asepsis, the protruding ends are cut to protrude about 2.5–5 cm (1–2 inches) from the skin, and a resin (methylmethacrylate) bridge is placed over these protrusions to immobilize the fracture site. The sites of skin puncture should be carefully covered with dressings to reduce the chance of infection tracking along the pins and causing osteomyelitis, which is the primary complication of this technique. Conservative treatment often fails to result in acceptable fracture resolution due to insufficient stabilization of the break. This often results in the development of severe lateral deformity of the limb with associated weight loss.

Growth plate and other injuries

Separation of the growth plate is a common complication of forced traction in dystokia. The usual site is the

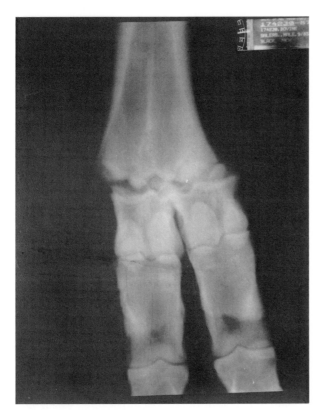

Fig. 32.4 Separation and displacement of distal metacarpal growth plate in 15-month-old Limousin bull. Complete recovery followed manipulation and traction reduction (over 1000 kg pull) and four weeks immobilization in resin cast.

distal metacarpus or metatarsus (Fig. 32.4). Non-weight bearing swelling and crepitus are major clinical signs. Cases must be distinguished from distal metacarpal/metatarsal shaft fractures and fetlock dislocation or subluxation. Most cases respond to manual reduction and some weeks' immobilization in a cast.

Other sites of growth plate separation include the distal femur, distal tibia and distal radius. Apart from external support, cross and Rush pinning are suitable methods of immobilization. The pins in the first method traverse the epiphysis obliquely to emerge through the opposite metaphysis. In Rush pinning, the pin is directed from the epiphysis to slide in a sledge-runner fashion proximally along the internal surface of the opposing diaphysis. Although such pins are liable to displace rather easily, healing is rapid and the success rate is high.

A specific and difficult orthopaedic problem is fracture of the femoral neck and separation of the proximal femoral epiphysis. Most cases result from dystokia. Diagnosis is difficult as precise localization of the fracture requires radiography. The differential diagnosis includes proximal femoral shaft fracture and pelvic fracture involving the acetabulum. The simplest method of treatment is confinement, which has a low success rate. Alternatively, the femoral head may be resected to permit development of a pseudoarthrosis, but lameness usually persists along with obvious muscle atrophy and compensatory conformational changes in the contralateral limb. Finally, internal fixation by Knowles pins or lag screws has been successful but requires intraoperative radiography to ensure the correct direction of insertion from the lateral aspect of the greater femoral trochanter.

Vertebral fractures

Aetiology and pathology

Elsewhere in this chapter, reference is made to long bone fractures and growth plate separation (p. 444) resulting from excessive traction during dystokia. But vertebral fractures due to forced traction, usually in an exotic beef breed such as Charolais, can lead to fracture and/or luxations in the caudal thoracic or cranial lumbar region (preferentially T12–L3). The common form is a fracture of the caudal physis of T13 (Schub & Killeen, 1988).

Postmortem changes include perirenal and perivertebral haemorrhage, fractured ribs, cord compression, severed cord, subdural haemorrhage, and myelomalacia.

Clinical signs and diagnosis

The calf is alive before traction is applied in dystokia, but following delivery the calf is weak, usually recumbent, with a swollen head, dyspnoea, and spinal deviation. These calves usually die within 24–48 hours from neurogenic shock (pain, trauma, hypoxia).

The normal rigidity of the spine in the affected thoracolumbar region invariably cannot tolerate the spinal curvature induced during typical traction on forelimbs of a fetus in anterior presentation when these dorsal structures become stretched and convex. When fetal hips lock on entering the maternal pelvis, the thoracolumbar region is approximately level with the maternal vulva. If the fetal body is then twisted and bent from side to side, acting as a pivot, a considerable risk of excessive shearing or traction forces can develop.

Treatment and prevention

The magnitude of traction forces in dystokia should be appreciated. Two men can exert a 350 kg pull for 30 seconds. A calf-puller device can produce over 500 kg traction. Adequate lubrication of the birth canal and an instinctive reluctance to use more than manual pressure are the two most important preventive measures, since treatment is useless. A greater willingness to adopt caesarean section in oversized viable fetuses will help prevent further accidental injuries (see p. 1115).

Pelvic fractures

Aetiology and pathology

Severe pelvic fractures are rare in cattle. Trauma is almost always involved. The most common pelvic fracture involves the tuber coxae, which is damaged during passage through a narrow doorway or in a sudden fall laterally onto hard ground (Fig. 32.5). Unlike other pelvic fractures, the tuber coxae fragment may be pulled ventrally by the fascia lata, becoming a sequestrum from an inadequate blood supply and may develop a septic draining tract to the exterior.

Another specific condition is separation of the pubic symphysis, resulting from excessive traction on a fetus in the pelvic canal of an immature heifer.

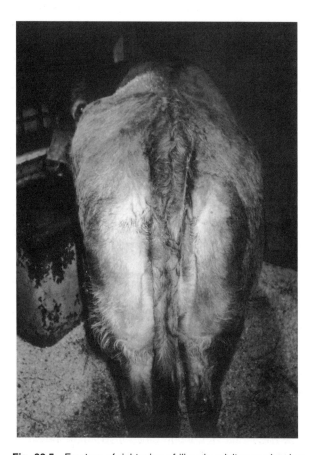

Fig. 32.5 Fracture of right wing of ilium in adult cow, showing asymmetry relative to the greater femoral trochanter and ischial tuberosity.

Osteoporosis is a predisposing factor to pelvic fracture in some high-yielding dairy herds.

Other pelvic fractures involve the wing or shaft of the ilium, tuber ischii, and the acetabular margin. The ilial fractures usually involve massive trauma, such as falls down cliffs. Tuber ischii damage may result from road traffic accidents in which the impact is caudal. Acetabular margin fracture chips often involve traumatic hip luxations.

Clinical signs and diagnosis

The degree of lameness varies considerably from nil (tuber coxae) to severe and even to recumbency (pubic and ilial shaft fractures). The external bony landmarks are frequently asymmetrical. Crepitus may be obvious as the animal walks. Rectal palpation will often permit localization of the crepitus and an appreciation of surrounding soft tissue injury. One useful technique is palpation during lateral rocking of the hindquarters. Fractures of the ilial shaft, pubis and cranial ischium can be appreciated on such rectal exploration. Vaginal palpation should be performed in mature cows and recently calved heifers.

Clinical diagnosis of acetabular fractures, which tend to involve the dorsal rim, is difficult as the localized crepitus must be distinguished from coxofemoral dislocation (in which the greater femoral trochanteric position is abnormal) and femoral neck or physeal fractures (which may be suspected from the increased mobility of the hip region in the affected limb). Radiography is essential for diagnosis in some cases, but, due to size and equipment constraints, is rarely feasible.

Other differential diagnoses include pelvic bruising leading to heamatoma formation and pelvic abscessation. Haematomas rarely cause lameness, while abscesses tend to have a more gradual onset and a protracted course. Several sites of pelvic fractures can lead to nerve trunk (sciatic, femoral, obturator) and blood vascular damage (middle uterine artery, internal pudendal, internal iliac arteries and veins).

Fractures of the bodies of the ischium and pubis invariably involve the obturator foramen, usually also the obturator nerve, and are serious in that marked pain and discomfort tend to cause prolonged periods of recumbency and a reluctance to stand. Commonly, both bones are fractured, making the pelvis unstable, and healing is then unlikely. In some cases, healing is liable to be accompanied by excessive callus formation. This sometimes extends to produce hip osteoarthritis and a persistent lameness.

Degenerative osteoarthritis of the hip in the older bulls and cows leads to considerable peripheral new bone formation. Sometimes, following minor trauma, small portions of the new acetabular dorsal rim are chipped off (pathological fractures), leading to a sudden increase in severity of the lameness. Often such fracture chips will heal by fibrous tissue, but lameness persists.

Treatment and prevention

Surgery is indicated in few cases of pelvic fracture, e.g. tuber coxae sequestrum. The only useful treatment is generally rest in a well-bedded stall. Use of hip clamps (e.g. Bagshaw hoist) to raise animals is contraindicated. Few cattle become acclimatized to slings, which may increase the discomfort caused by the fracture. Cases of pelvic fracture should be reassessed after three to four weeks of good nursing, and, in the absence of obvious improvement, most cases should be salvaged.

Dislocations and subluxations

Hip joint

Aetiology

Coxofemoral luxation is sporadic, occurring mostly in two to five-year-old cattle. It has an association with parturition and the early postpartum period. At this time, ligamentous relaxation is maximal and obturator or other nerve injury during dystokia may predispose cattle to abduct the hindlimbs and to slip the feet laterally resulting in a splayed-leg collapse.

Hip dislocation can occur in various directions, craniodorsal being most frequent (about 80 per cent of total), and cranioventral and caudoventral being less common.

Pathology

The gross pathological changes in luxation include rupture of the joint capsule and of the ligament of the femoral head (teres ligament), loss of articular cartilage and surrounding soft tissue, haemorrhage and oedema.

Clinical signs and diagnosis

A sudden onset of lameness is the only consistent sign. Other so-called typical signs refer only to the common craniodorsal luxation, when the leg is held rotated outwards, the hock medial, and stifle more lateral than normal. The leg may appear shortened and the greater femoral trochanters are asymmetrical, the affected side being relatively more dorsal. Movement of the limb is somewhat restricted and painful. Crepitus may be appreciated on limb abduction and flexion. Rectal palpation aids localization of crepitus to the hip. It will also help to differentiate the less common directions of luxation. In cranioventral luxation, abnormal movement may be appreciable cranial and lateral to the pelvic inlet when the cranial border of the pubis is followed. In caudoventral luxation into the region of the obturator foramen, movement may be noted as the leg is abducted, flexed and extended, released, taking the femoral head out of and back into the margin of the foramen.

Diagnosis may be confirmed in smaller cattle on ventrodorsal radiographs. Differential diagnosis includes femoral neck fractures, physeal separation, pelvic (acetabular) fractures, and greater femoral trochanteric fractures.

Treatment

Manipulative reduction should be attempted in all uncomplicated cases of craniodorsal luxation seen within 24 hours of the onset. The chance of successful manual reduction decreases markedly thereafter. Cases of caudoventral dislocation, which are often recumbent, perhaps due to additional obturator damage, have a poorer prognosis.

The common craniodorsal luxation is treated by careful positioning of the patient so that the body is fixed while the affected upper leg can be extended in various directions. Deep sedation (xylazine) is advisable. The leg is forcibly circumrotated in ever-increasing circles by an assistant to loosen up the periarticular soft tissues, which may be in spasm. A large, firm block is placed between the ground and the medial femoral region to act as a fulcrum when inward pressure is exerted on the stifle, tending to cause hip abduction. The limb is subject to controlled traction along the longitudinal axis of the limb. The veterinarian should concentrate on distal pressure on the greater trochanter. The amount of femoral head movement usually increases with time, and manipulation should not be quickly abandoned. Reduction is usually very obvious, and traction should be stopped at once, otherwise a caudoventral luxation may be produced. Once replaced, the limb is circumrotated slowly and carefully in an attempt to remove blood and other debris from the acetabulum. The animal should not be permitted to stand at once, since spontaneous reluxation is liable. The hindlimbs should be shackled above the hocks or fetlocks for 24–48 hours. A good non-slip surface should be beneath the cow when standing up and, if available, a hip hoist is a useful aid.

A high success rate has followed open surgery for reduction of hip dislocations (Tulleners et al., 1987). In this series few cases responded to manipulation. As experienced by others, caudoventral and cranioventral dislocations present special problems since limb traction cannot be exerted in the correct direction. The standard surgical approach is medial and cranial to the greater trochanter through the gluteal musculature. Care should be taken to avoid the sciatic nerve. The femoral head is mobilized and moved appropriately with a combination of manipulation by a non-sterile assistant handling the hock, which can be easily rotated slightly or, at will, abducted, and moved by appropriate instrumental leverage. Toggling through the femoral head and acetabulum to produce an artificial intra-articular ligament was unsuccessful in a long-term study.

Recumbency following hip dislocation and for a period after successful reduction necessitates a careful watch for the possible development of acute severe mastitis, since many cases have recently calved. Excellent nursing in good comfortable surroundings is essential for recovery.

Apart from a surgical series (Tulleners *et al.*, 1987) in which many animals were immature and, therefore, better surgical candidates, most cases have a guarded prognosis for craniodorsal dislocation and a poor prognosis for any other direction. Recumbency at presentation makes recovery less likely.

Hip dislocation is the clinical diagnosis in some 'downer cows' (see p. 439).

Sacroiliac luxation and subluxation

Aetiology

Sacroiliac displacement involves a partial or complete separation of the fibrocartilaginous joint surfaces. The aetiology usually involves excessive ligamentous flaccidity around parturition, when most cases occur. Some cases involve a degree of dystokia. A condition of sacroiliac distortion is recognized when there is no displacement, but excessive mobility of the joint surfaces is detectable. In true luxation considerable haemorrhage and soft tissue damage occurs in the joint space and peripherally (haematoma formation).

Clinical signs and diagnosis

Signs of sacroiliac luxation are characteristic. The lumbosacral spine is dropped relative to the sacral tuberosities of the ilium, which are correspondingly prominent. Cows initially prefer recumbency and show slight ataxia, hindquarter weakness, and some knuckling of the hind fetlocks. These signs are attributed to associated bruising of the ventral nerve roots of L5–S2. Crepitus can be easily elicited from the sacroiliac region. The dropped spine may develop over two to three days and be preceded by evidence of localized pain. Rectal palpation of luxation reveals the sacral promontory has been pushed caudally and depressed, so reducing the dorso-ventral diameter of the pelvic inlet. Very severe cases may be unable to stand as a result of spinal nerve trauma.

In cases of subluxation and distortion, the signs are relatively mild. Some hindlimb ataxia and weakness may appear. Crepitus may be noted during rectal palpation as the cow is walked forwards, and localized swelling over the ventral part of the joint is diagnostic when the history indicates a sudden onset.

Differential diagnosis includes coxofemoral osteoarthritis, pelvic fractures, obturator or other nerve damage, lumbar spondylitis and progressive hindlimb paralysis (spinal abscess, lymphoma).

Treatment and prevention

The prognosis is favourable for cases of distortion and subluxation that are confined to a well-bedded stall for a few days. More severe, recumbent cases of luxation or subluxation have a guarded or poor prognosis. A sacroiliac luxation never undergoes spontaneous reposition and manual reduction is impossible. However, some cows can survive for years with sacroiliac luxation despite the bizarre appearance of the hindquarters.

In nursing affected cows, no forcible attempt (hip clamp, electric goad) should be made to make them stand. Analgesics (phenylbutazone) every second day for one week may increase comfort.

Stifle joint: femoropatellar

Aetiology and pathology

Patellar luxation may occur dorsally, medially and laterally. Dorsal displacement (fixation) is seen in mature cattle as an intermittent condition, unassociated with any known trauma. Medial patellar displacement is rare and is usually congenital. Anatomical defects predisposing to medial luxation have not been clearly identified, though in newly calved heifers with large udders the abducted hindlimb posture may lead to temporary medial patellar luxation.

Lateral patellar luxation is occasionally seen as a specific entity in mature cattle and young calves. This luxation in calves may sometimes be secondary to quadriceps atrophy resulting from femoral paralysis (see p. 437). In calves that first show signs at three months (Weaver & Campbell, 1972) without a history of femoral paralysis, no predisposing factors have been identified.

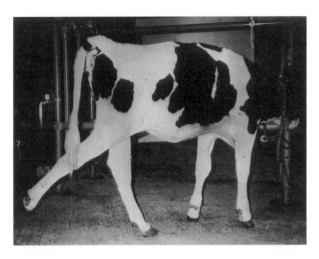

Fig. 32.6 Upward patellar fixation in 15-month-old Canadian Holstein heifer. The degree and duration of caudal extension were unusual. Heifer recovered following medial patellar desmotomy.

Clinical signs and diagnosis

In dorsal patellar luxation or fixation, the first sign may be initial hindlimb stiffness followed by a jerky action in which the limb remains extended caudally longer than usual, and is then pulled forwards and upwards in a movement resembling equine stringhalt (Fig. 32.6). This action may be intermittent and separated by several normal strides, or it may be repeated. If the animal is pushed backwards, the hindlimb may become fixed temporarily in extension. This extension may persist, whereby the foot is dragged along the ground (permanent upward fixation). Palpation reveals the patella to be more prominent and dorsal than usual, and the patellar ligaments are unusually easily felt. The patella is now resting partly in the supratrochlear fovea, while the medial patellar ligament is felt to be fixed around the medial trochlear ridge.

Both medial and lateral patellar fixation are associated with a characteristic posture. The stifle is markedly flexed, and the limb collapses on weight bearing, exactly as in femoral paralysis (p. 437). Bilaterally affected calves prefer recumbency. The patellar position is obvious visually and on palpation. It can usually be replaced on to the femoral trochlea but may immediately reluxate. Radiography can confirm the abnormal position but is a superfluous procedure. Differential diagnosis includes femoral nerve paralysis, quadricep muscle rupture, gonitis and distal femoral epiphyseal separation.

Treatment and prevention

Dorsal patellar luxation should be treated by medial patellar desmotomy if signs persist for more than a week. Surgery is preferably carried out in the standing case as an aseptic procedure following sedation and local analgesia. A large udder or a difficult temperament makes recumbency (affected side down) necessary in some cases. The surgical site is superficial to the most distal palpable point of the medial patellar ligament, close to its insertion into the tibial tuberosity. A 4 cm (1½ inch) long vertical skin incision is made cranial to the ligament. A tenotome is inserted just deep to the ligament with the blade in a vertical position. A Hey Groves knife, with a blunt rounded point, is ideal for this surgery. The conventional disposable scalpel blade and (Bard) handle are unsuitable since slight movement easily results in breakage and loss of the blade. The cutting edge is rotated through 90° towards the skin and the medial patellar ligament is sectioned without damaging or entering the joint cavity. A single non-absorbable skin suture achieves adequate wound apposition. The operated cow should walk normally at once. No deleterious long-term pathology has been reported in operated cattle.

Both medial and lateral patellar luxation are treated by a joint overlap procedure. In lateral luxation the femoropatellar joint is incised longitudinally about 1 cm (½ inch) medial to the patella, which is replaced in the trochlea. The capsule is closed by vertical mattress sutures in a joint capsular overlap procedure. Sometimes this technique fails to maintain the patella in position. The fascia of the thigh may then be split dorsally to permit replacement. Bilateral cases should be operated with a one week interval (Husband & Weaver, 1995). In medial patellar luxation, the overlap procedure is carried out lateral to the patella.

Stifle joint: femorotibial

Aetiology and pathology

Complete femorotibial luxation is rare and incurable. Subluxation is relatively common and is typically seen in the mature cow or bull as a result of primary cranial cruciate injury (see p. 455). Predisposing factors include heavy weight and sudden twists and falls as when mounting or being mounted by cows in oestrus. The cranial cruciate ligament is partially or completely ruptured (Fig. 32.7). Damage to the caudal cruciate is less likely. One or both tibial menisci are often torn and displaced at the time of rupture (Fig. 32.8). Secondary osteoarthritic changes quickly develop with initial loss of articular cartilage from the femoral condyles, followed by exposure and erosion of subchondral bone and peripheral osteophyte proliferation at the joint margins.

Detachment of the medial meniscus has been reported in young (1 month to 1 year) dairy cattle

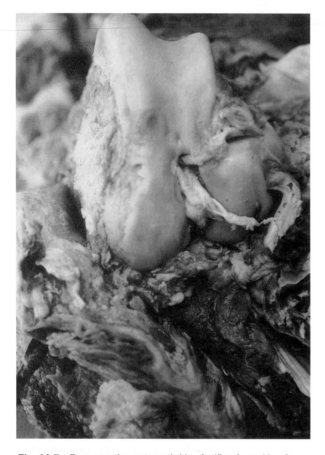

Fig. 32.7 Degenerative osteoarthritis of stifle of aged beef cow showing ruptured cranial cruciate ligament, massive osteophyte proliferation along margins of femoral trochlea and cartilaginous loss on femoral condyles.

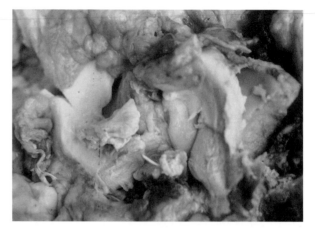

Fig. 32.8 Degenerative osteoarthritis of stifle joint of aged cow exposing damaged menisci and tibial condyles. Menisci are eroded and partially detached, allowing partial eburnation of the underlying tibial condyles. Surrounding musculature is pale due to extensive fibrosis.

following injury to the medial collateral ligament. Mounting activity has been postulated as a major aetiological factor (Nelson *et al.*, 1990).

Clinical signs and diagnosis

A sudden onset of a medium degree lameness is characteristic of femorotibial subluxation due to cruciate injury. There is generalized soft tissue swelling and crepitus may be spontaneous or may be induced by rotating the point of hock laterally and medially to produce some rotation of the tibial joint surfaces. The tibial tuberosity may be unusually pronounced and a 'drawer-forward' sign may be demonstrable initially. The animal, placed in lateral recumbency with the affected limb uppermost, has the stifle put into moderate extension. The clinician then attempts to move the proximal tibial region cranially, relative to the femoral condyles. Sometimes this movement is even appreciable as the animal walks. If not diagnostic on palpation,

and if radiographic facilities are available, lateral views of the stifle may demonstrate significant (approximately 2.5 cm (1 inch)) cranial displacement of the tibial plateau relative to the femoral condyles. In some cattle, arthrocentesis is advisable to rule out septic gonitis and to demonstrate the presence of cartilaginous debris and blood in the femorotibial joint. Other differential diagnoses include collateral ligamentous injuries, patellar fracture, and, in young cattle, proximal tibial epiphyseal separation.

Treatment and prevention

Radical surgery involving replacement of the ruptured cranial cruciate ligament by skin or synthetic material has occasionally been successful. These cases have either been experimental animals in which the ligament has been sectioned, or smaller animals in which surgery has been done very soon after the original injury. Most cases have lacked adequate long-term follow-up studies.

Fetlock joint: metacarpophalangeal and metatarsophalangeal

Aetiology and pathology

Dislocation is rare. It invariably involves rupture of both collateral ligaments as well as the intra-articular structures. Trauma is usually so severe that massive soft tissue injury exposes the joint surfaces. Subluxation either in a medial – lateral or cranial – caudal direction is seen sporadically.

Clinical signs and diagnosis

Clinical signs include a non-weight bearing stance, swelling, obvious gross displacement and crepitus on manipulation of the distal extremity. Diagnosis is usually easy. Differential diagnoses include epiphyseal separation in calves, and distal metacarpal, metatarsal and proximal phalangeal fractures. Subluxation presents with similar signs of gross swelling but crepitus may be hard to elicit. Subluxations can be successfully reduced following sedation and extension. A support bandage or cast should be applied subsequently.

Treatment and prevention

Treatment is usually hopeless. If the joint surfaces can be replaced to be congruent, a synthetic collateral ligament may be inserted by utilizing steel wire anchored to screws drilled into each epiphysis. Alternatively, the ligaments may be replaced with polypropylene material. It is usually impossible effectively to suture together the ruptured ends. In young calves the synthetic material may require later removal to permit normal growth of the epiphysis, otherwise the material is left *in situ*. Meniscopexy was successful in treatment of 20 out of 27 young cattle with medial collateral ligamentous and medial meniscal injury (Nelson *et al.*, 1990).

Muscle and tendon injuries

Introduction

The muscles most liable to rupture include the gastrocnemius, the adductor group and the cranial tibial (peroneus tertius). All three are particularly liable to damage when a heavy cow is struggling to rise postpartum (see Downer cow syndrome, p. 439).

Specific muscles

The gastrocnemius is particularly exposed to damage as a primary extensor of the hock. Prolonged recumbency, excessive weight, and possibly mineral imbalance leading to a degree of osteomalacia can predispose to gastrocnemius rupture.

The common site is the tendon–muscle junction. The rupture is usually complete and leads to considerable swelling due to extravasation of blood and the development of oedema. The hock is dropped and weight bearing is minimal. Diagnosis is rarely in doubt since the clinical picture is typical.

Gastrocnemius muscle rupture is treated by stall rest and maintenance of the hock in extension by means of a Thomas splint. In yearling animals, compression screws can be drilled from the caudal surface of the calcaneus into the distal portion of the tibial shaft to immobilize the tarsus for some weeks so that fibrous repair at the rupture site can take place.

Cranial tibial (peroneus tertius) rupture is also traumatic, resulting from falls or from excessive traction upwards of the hindlimb by ropes strung over an overhead beam and followed by severe struggling. The animal has a characteristic gait. While the hock is abnormally extended, the stifle remains flexed, in other words the reciprocal stifle–hock action is lost. When standing, any abnormality may be hard to detect, but the limb can be extended caudally so that the metatarsus and tibia form a straight line while the stifle remains flexed. The gastrocnemius tendon is then slack. The site of muscle rupture varies from its origin in the extensor fossa of the femur to the insertion and to the muscle belly itself. Some area of painful swelling is apparent and most cases respond to stall rest over a period of one to four weeks.

Adductor muscle damage has been briefly discussed under downer cow syndrome (see p. 439).

Ventral serrate rupture is spectacular due to loss of its normal anatomical function of supporting the chest in the form of a sling between the forelegs. The scapular cartilage projects above the level of the thoracic spine and is readily palpated subcutaneously. The prominence varies in degree, being more obvious when weight is borne and less obvious in the forward swing of the limb. Colloquially termed 'loose shoulder', Channel Island breeds, especially the Jersey, appear to be predisposed. This feature may reflect a smaller muscle mass relative to body weight. The aetiology in young cattle is possibly related to muscular dystrophy (vitamin E and Se deficiency; see page 258). Cases may be associated with turn-out to pasture. Pathological examination of chronic cases in adult cattle reveals severe muscle degeneration, fibrous tissue proliferation and serous infiltration. While mild cases may recover completely, complete rupture is incurable, but animals move around well, remain productive and emergency slaughter is rarely necessary.

Contracted flexor tendons

Aetiology and pathology

Contracted digital flexor tendons are the commonest congenital abnormality in cattle. The name 'contracted tendons' is a misnomer, as the primary abnormality is an arthrogryposis or articular rigidity, usually in flexion (Fig. 32.9). Most cases are mild and self-correcting as the calf moves around to an increasing extent. Some are more severe and sometimes associated with

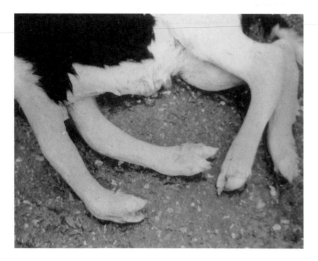

Fig. 32.9 Contracted flexor tendons (forelimb) and flexed hocks in a neonatal Holstein calf, which was unable to stand. Synonyms: arthrogryposis or articular rigidity.

other congenital defects such as cleft palate and arthrogryposis (see p. 177).

Contracted tendons usually affect both deep and superficial flexors, and sometimes the suspensory ligaments (see p. 178). The condition is bilaterally symmetrical in the forelimbs. The hindlimbs may have abnormal hock extensor rigidity and fetlock flexion.

Some breeds (e.g. Belgian Blue) have a very high incidence in which a relationship is suspected between relatively excessive fetal size and abnormal intrauterine posture. Dystokia is almost invariable in such cases. Akabane virus and the ingestion of various toxic plants (e.g. *Lupinus* species and locoweed) have been alleged in other high incidence outbreaks.

Clinical signs and diagnosis

Mild cases show about 10–20° excessive flexion of the carpus and fetlocks. Forced extension discloses the tautness in the flexor tendons and suspensory ligament. The abnormality is generally symmetrical. Some calves may have a split palate and arthrogryposis of the carpi and tarsi. Joints are not swollen and extension is not unduly painful. When moved, mild degrees of abnormal flexion will result in calves moving on the pastern, but, in severe cases, the calf is totally recumbent or will walk on the distal skin of the fetlock and rapidly develop abrasions and cellulitis, perhaps allowing secondary infection to establish itself and bring the risk of a septic arthritis.

Treatment and prevention

Some cases resolve but in others splinting of the leg is normally sufficient. A half-section of a 5 cm (2 inch) diameter polyvinyl drainpipe may be placed on a well-padded limb to immobilize the flexed joints in maximum extension. Such a splint in a neonatal calf must be checked by weekly removal and replacement. The toes should be left exposed to encourage weight bearing and walking. If the stance is not corrected in four weeks, surgery is indicated.

More severe cases will only respond to desmotomy, which should be undertaken at two to three weeks old, after the immediate neonatal stress period. Correction of carpal flexion is possible at the mediopalmar side of the carpus by an initial longitudinal incision through the retinaculum flexorum, exposure of the superficial part of the superficial flexor, and by complete transection of the retinaculum flexorum, which also involves section of the radial carpal flexor. If normal extension is not achievable, the deep flexor and deep part of the superficial flexor are transected, preserving carefully the neurovascular bundle of median artery, vein and nerves. Finally, the palmar carpal ligament may be sectioned. Exceptionally, with a radius–metacarpus angle <100°, it may be preferable to perform radiocarpal arthrodesis with resection of one or both carpal rows. The wound is closed by sutures and then bandaged and cast for five weeks.

Correction of fetlock flexion is similarly a multistep procedure. The skin incision is at the mediopalmar aspect of the metacarpus, and the superficial portion of the flexor tendon is transected. The deep flexor and deep part of the superficial tendon may be sectioned similarly for adequate extension. Small stab incisions may be made in the suspensory ligament. Bandaging and cast immobilization of the limb are again necessary.

Surgery is likely to be unsuccessful in very severe cases of contracted tendons where abnormal flexion creates an angle of <90° between radius and metacarpus.

Prevention of the primary aetiological stimulus is difficult as arthrogryposis leading to contracted tendons may result from infectious agents (bovine virus diarrhoea (BVDV), akabane virus) or toxic plant material.

Traumatic flexor tendon injuries

Sporadic traumatic injuries occasionally affect the flexor tendons and often result from contact with farm machinery. Adult cows may injure both deep and superficial flexor tendons in the metatarsal region, and an open infected wound results. Careful debridement under IVRA is indicated. A septic tenosynovitis necessitates pressure lavage with sterile isotonic saline b.i.d. for several days and systemic antibiotic cover. Selected cases of complete transection of both flexor tendons may heal following tenorrhaphy (e.g. carbon fibre or polyamide) and application of a limb cast. Despite prolonged convalescence most cases continue to be lame and the prognosis is guarded (Anderson *et al.*, 1996).

Joint diseases

Osteochondrosis

Aetiology and pathology

Osteochondrosis (OCD) is seen in young fast-growing beef cattle on a high calorie intake. Recently an American series of 29 cattle with osteochondrosis was dominated by dairy breeds, primarily mature males (Trostle *et al.*, 1997). Normal endochondral ossification is disturbed at the cartilaginous endplate of the epiphysis and at the metaphyseal growth plate, and is associated with a failure of vascular invasion. The thickness of articular cartilage increases as a result of continued growth and lack of wear, whereupon the failure of adequate nutrient diffusion causes a degeneration of the chondrocytes. The result is a characteristic cleft formation, producing cartilaginous flaps that undergo endochondral ossification (osteochondrosis dissecans). Another process is the formation of subchondral cyst-like lesions.

It is not yet known to what extent the changes are generalized, as most surveys have only examined specific joints (e.g. stifle, carpus or atlanto-occipital). Changes tend to be symmetrical. Sometimes the joint surfaces of several forelimb bones are normal, while significant changes occur in their physes. Osteochondrosis has been reported in the coxofemoral, femoropatellar, femorotibial and tibiotarsal joints of the hindlimbs, and in the scapulohumeral, humororadial, radiocarpal, and metacarpophalangeal joints of the forelimbs.

Clinical signs and diagnosis

Steers and young bulls are predominantly affected. Some lesions cause no clinical signs, while others produce a mild progressive lameness. Some lesions heal following production of fibrocartilage. This accounts for the larger percentage of lesions in autopsies than in clinical series of lame cattle. Other lesions progress to become a secondary degenerative osteoarthritis or degenerative joint disease (DJD). Exacerbations of a mild slight lameness have been attributed to additional joint trauma. If warranted, a doubtful case may be radiographed, but cartilaginous defects are unlikely to be demonstrated unless pneumoarthrography is performed. Suspicious evidence of osteochondrosis is the presence of a free calcified body within the joint ('joint mouse').

Treatment and prevention

Theoretically, as in the horse and dog, removal of the cartilaginous flap and curettage of the underlying bone is indicated. Surgical treatment has, however, not been adopted in cattle for economic and anatomical reasons. Management measures in high-incidence situations include a more restricted calorie intake and transfer to a softer bearing surface to reduce concussion. Lame steers should be confined. Osteochondrosis in a bull should stimulate consideration of its conformation as a possible predisposing factor.

Hip dysplasia

Aetiology and pathology

Hip dysplasia is seen in bulls of various fast-growing beef breeds, predominantly the Hereford and Aberdeen Angus, though isolated cases have been reported in numerous other breeds. In the Hereford breed, particular families have been alleged to have a high incidence. The condition is probably a sex-linked heritable characteristic. Although some cases are observed in the neonate, most develop in calves four to twelve months old with erosion of the acetabular cartilage close to the attachment of the accessory cartilage, which normally functions to extend the effective articulating surface (Fig. 32.10). The femoral articular cartilage usually undergoes a shallower but more extensive erosion.

Later changes include traumatic synovitis, fraying of the intra-articular ligament, and a tendency to subluxation. Secondary degenerative joint disease follows in a few weeks.

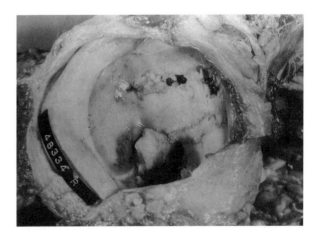

Fig. 32.10 Severe hip dysplasia seen in right acetabulum of nine-month-old Hereford bull. Severe fissuring and loss of cartilage and erosions in subchondral bone.

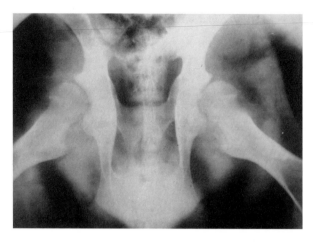

Fig. 32.11 Severe hip dysplasia evident in ventrodorsal radiograph of pelvis of five-month-old Angus bull that had experienced progressive hindlimb lameness for two months. Both femoral heads are subluxated and severe secondary osteoarthritis affects the acetabular rims.

Clinical signs and diagnosis

Lameness develops slowly and is preceded by a period in which abnormal lateral swinging of the hindquarters is seen. The bull calf spends increased periods in recumbency. Feed intake is reduced and hindquarter atrophy starts. Unilateral or bilateral crepitus is detectable in the hip region and may be localized more precisely if rectal palpation is feasible. The development of subluxation is recognizable from demonstration of the Ortolani sign: with the hand resting on the skin over the greater femoral trochanter, when weight is taken off the hind leg, a distinct 'plop' is felt as the femoral head drops into the acetabulum from its previous position on the dorsal acetabular rim.

In smaller calves, ventrodorsal pelvic radiographs may demonstrate secondary joint changes and a tendency to subluxàtion (Fig. 32.11). Any radiographic suggestion of shallowness of the acetabulum is usually the result of the secondary changes and not a primary anatomical feature.

Differential diagnosis is important in apparently unilateral cases. Stifle disease, acetabular and other pelvic fractures, hip luxation and slipped femoral epiphysis are all to be considered. A confirmed bilateral hip lameness in young bulls is usually diagnostic of hip dysplasia.

Treatment and prevention

No successful treatment has been reported. Affected bull calves and yearlings should be slaughtered. The hip joints should be retained for pathological confirmation of the clinical diagnosis.

Degenerative arthritis

Aetiology and pathology

Degenerative arthritis (degenerative joint disease, DJD) is attributed to a 'wear-and-tear' phenomenon. This chronic non-infectious disease involves primary degeneration of articular cartilage, generally accompanied by secondary sclerosis and eburnation of subchondral bone, peripheral osteophyte formation and surrounding soft tissue proliferation.

Though a common incidental finding at slaughter, its primary clinical significance is as a cause of progressive debilitating lameness involving major weight-bearing joints. In one study of the stifle and hip joints of cattle disease, atrophy frequently led to partial condemnation at slaughter (Weaver, 1977). A recent US study in 21 processing plants revealed that 11.9–16.5 per cent of beef and dairy cows and bulls had stifle arthritis ('stifled') or a broken leg. The stifle injury resulted in the loss of 17.9 kg tissue from trimming ($9.72 per carcase) (Roeber *et al.*, 2000). Other studies have shown the frequent involvement of the hock and carpal joints. Overweight and straightlegged cattle may be predisposed to early DJD but control studies are lacking. An inherited DJD of the stifles of Holstein cattle has been reported (Kendrick & Sittmann, 1966). Nutritional imbalance leading to osteochondrosis (see p. 453), which can lead to secondary DJD, is another aetiological possibility.

Subchondral bone cysts were the most frequent cause of stifle lameness in a Canadian survey (Ducharme *et al.*, 1985). The lateral tibial condyle was most frequently affected, followed by the opposing femoral condyle. The age range was six to eighteen months.

Early fibrillation of articular cartilage leads to necrotic and degenerative chondrocytes, which results in decreased proteoglycan production in the cartilaginous matrix. The cartilage becomes soft and somewhat yellowish. Chondrocyte destruction causes release of lysosomal enzymes, especially cathepsin D. Fibrillated cartilage withstands stress relatively poorly, and fissuring, thinning, or cartilaginous erosion follows.

Pain in DJD originates from the exposed subchondral bone and from the associated capsulitis and synovitis. Clinically, the joint enlarges as a result of the increased volume of synovia and soft tissue proliferation.

Clinical signs and diagnosis

A progressive lameness with gradual muscle atrophy and weight loss is commonly seen. The affected limb, usually hind, tends to be dragged as flexion of the affected joint is reduced. Movement of the stifle or hock results in palpable joint enlargement. In the stifle, proliferative changes (osteophyte formation, periarticular fibrosis) affect both femoropatellar and femorotibial compartments, and crepitus may be noted. Some cases of stifle DJD reflect a secondary response to cranial cruciate rupture or meniscal injury. In the hock, major changes are usually seen craniomedially, affecting the intertarsal and tarsometatarsal joint space (similar to equine 'spavin'). Relatively rarely do changes extend proximally to the tibiotarsal joint. Degenerative joint disease of the hip can be suspected in older cows when the more distal parts of the limb are normal clinically and where crepitus can be detected over the gluteal region and confirmed on rectal palpation.

Subchondral bone cysts can only be diagnosed on radiographic examination. Cases of DJD, ligamentous rupture and septic arthritis show ranging radiographic features. Degenerative joint disease of the stifle and hock shows the extent of the proliferative reaction. Lateral radiographs of the stifle in rupture of the cranial cruciate ligament have the 'drawer-forward' features seen in dogs. Septic arthritic cases on radiography demonstrate soft tissue swelling and distension of the joint capsule in early cases and, when more advanced, the radiographic changes include loss of subchondral bone.

Synovial fluid analysis is only justified when the differential diagnosis includes infectious arthritis or when fluid is withdrawn prior to injection of a local analgesic solution to assess whether lameness is lessened. Synovia in DJD is clear or slightly turbid, increased in volume, does not clot, has a low (<15 per cent) polymorphonuclear lymphocyte count, a normal protein (<2 g/dl), and a near-normal mucin precipitate (Weaver, 1997).

Differential diagnosis, apart from infectious forms of arthritis, includes fluorosis as a primary cause of DJD, osteoporosis, rickets and osteoarthritis deformans, all three of which occur in young growing animals, and osteomalacia. A sudden onset of lameness sometimes represents an exacerbation of a non-clinical DJD following a periarticular fracture (e.g. caudal surface of tibia in femorotibial DJD).

Treatment and prevention

Treatment is purely palliative. Affected cattle should be rested. Ketoprofen (10 per cent solution iv or im) has recently been shown to have analgesic properties in lame cattle. Phenylbutazone may be given (initially 5 mg/kg orally daily, then 5 mg/kg every second day) for its analgesic and anti-inflammatory properties. Aspirin (100 mg/kg orally b.i.d.) is an alternative regimen. Flunixin meglumine has few obvious advantages over either phenylbutazone or aspirin for arthritides and is considerably more expensive. Prolonged low-dosage therapy with phenylbutazone in cattle with painful arthritides has not led to any demonstrable deleterious effects such as gastrointestinal ulceration or renal papillary necrosis. Corticosteroids and dimethyl sulphoxide (DMSO) have also been advocated. The majority of young cattle with stifle lameness due to subchondral bone cysts formation recovered following conservative treatment (Ducharme *et al.*, 1985). Preventive measures include attention to the conformation of further breeding stock, especially bulls, to avoid a hindlimb conformation that is liable to lead to excessive concussive forces in progeny.

Infectious (septic) arthritis

Introduction

Infectious arthritis in this context is synonymous with septic arthritis. The rare primary septic arthritis develops from direct joint penetration by a contaminated foreign body. This section considers secondary septic arthritis resulting from spread of pathogens from an adjacent localized focus, and tertiary septic arthritis resulting from systemic or haematogenous spread from a focus elsewhere in the animal.

Septic arthritis: joint ill in neonate (see p. 249)

Aetiology and pathology

Joint ill in calves is classified as a tertiary septic arthritis. The primary infection is in the umbilicus, often as an umbilical abscess with extension along the umbilical veins towards the liver. Otherwise, spread is from a primary enteric infection. Common pathogens isolated are *Escherichia coli*, *Streptococcus* and *Staphylococcus* spp., *Arcanobacterium pyogenes*, *Erysipelothrix insidiosa* and *Salmonella* spp. Usually, more than one joint is affected, commonly the carpus, tarsus and femorotibial joints. The route of haematogenous spread is through metaphyseal or epiphyseal vessels or, alternatively, the synovial membrane. Establishment of foci of infection is naturally favoured by the slowed flow rate of blood through a network of venous sinusoids in the metaphyseal vessels.

Pathological changes start with an intense polymorphonuclear inflammatory response in the synovial membrane, the permeability of which is increased, permitting protein leakage into the synovial fluid. Later release of lysosomal and other enzymes into the synovia causes degeneration of the articular cartilage, which is weakened by defective nutrition due to an overlying fibrin deposit. The result is extensive loss of articular cartilage, acute synovitis, thickening of the

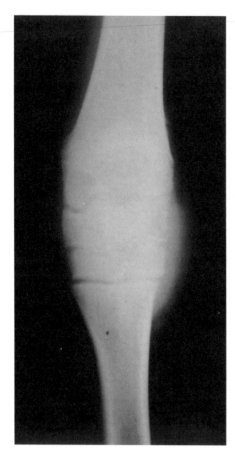

Fig. 32.12 Extensive soft tissue swelling of lateral aspect of left carpal region in a six-month-old Hereford calf. Bone lysis is evident in the distal part of the radial carpal and fused second and third carpal bones. Lysis resulted from transverse fracture of the proximal surface of the distal component of the joint. Recovery followed removal of the bone fragment, curettage and irrigation.

joint capsule, and sepsis in the growth plate and metaphysis (particularly associated with salmonella infection).

Clinical signs and diagnosis

The first sign is lameness. Later, joint swelling (Fig. 32.12) and pain are apparent. The joint capsule may be distended from an increased synovial volume. The presence and physical nature (serous, fibrinous or purulent) of such synovial effusions can be readily detected on ultrasonography (7.5 mHz linear transducer) in carpal, stifle and hock disorders (Kofler & Martinek, 2000). The polyarthritis is rarely symmetrical. Not all cases are associated with either gross umbilical sepsis or with severe enteritis. Calves that are immune depressed as a result of low gamma globulin levels (inadequate colostral intake) are at higher risk. Lameness becomes severe after a few days.

Radiology is not a great aid to diagnosis, as the only initial abnormality is the soft tissue swelling. After two to three weeks, changes suggestive of joint destruction are apparent.

Arthrocentesis is a more valuable aid to diagnosis in early cases. Apart from an increased volume, synovial fluid in a calf with joint ill is turbid, clots, and has a loose flaky character in the mucin precipitate. The protein content is >5 g/dl and a Giemsa smear reveals an almost pure (98 per cent) and massive population of polymorphonuclear lymphocytes. Taken aseptically, synovial fluid may be submitted for culture, but is often problematical with this particular material (see p. 457).

Differential diagnosis must be made from physeal and intra-articular fractures.

Treatment and prevention

Early and vigorous treatment is essential in joint ill. High therapeutic levels of systemic antibiotics should be given for two to three weeks. Intra-articular antibiotic medication is usually contraindicated, as the blood supply ensures adequate concentrations are obtained in synovia following systemic injection. Suitable antibiotics include penicillin, ampicillin and tetracyclines.

Joint lavage with a sterile polyionic solution or physiological saline is helpful. Generally, an in–out, through-and-through system using two 14 gauge needles is effective. Open arthrotomy with removal of the fibrin clots and purulent material along with curettage of the articular surfaces has been successful in some series. It appears more useful in less complex joints such as the stifle and fetlock rather than in carpus or tarsus.

Recently intra-articular therapy with gentamycin-impregnated polymethylmethacrylate beads has proved useful in neonatal septic arthritis with concurrent osteomyelitis. Such beads must be removed at a second surgery. Use of gentamicin-impregnated collagen sponges (Garamycin, Essex Chemie, Lucerne, Switzerland) which do not need later removal appear more promising, and further larger studies are awaited (Steiner & Zulauf, 2000).

Supportive care is important. Casting for three weeks of joint immobility (e.g. in fetlock) followed by bandaging for support reduces discomfort and so maintains the appetite. Low level oral dosage with phenylbutazone can improve the general attitude (p. 1050). Some calves also require management of the enteritis by fluid therapy (see pp. 195, 209) and others require drainage of an umbilical abscess. Inadequate levels of gamma globulins may, with difficulty due to the large volumes, be corrected by giving intravenous plasma.

Septic arthritis: older cattle

Aetiology and pathology

The main site of septic (infectious) arthritis in mature cattle is the distal interphalangeal joint resulting from secondary spread from a focus in the sensitive solar laminae or from complications of interdigital necrobacillosis (see pp. 420 and 426).

Septic digital arthritis is fully discussed elsewhere (p. 455). Other joints liable to be affected by septic arthritis include the fetlock, either by extension along the digital flexor sheath from a digital focus, or by direct trauma from a deep wound (Fig. 32.13). The major hindlimb weight-bearing joints, the tarsus, stifle and hip are occasionally involved as a result of haematogenous spread such as pyaemic vegetative endocarditis (e.g. from primary reticuloperitonitis) or in the tarsus from contiguous spread from an infected subcutaneous bursitis.

Organisms commonly recovered from septic arthritis in adult cattle include *A. pyogenes*, *E. coli*, *Staphylo-coccus* and *Streptococcus* spp. *Fusobacterium necrophorum* and *Bacteroides melaninogenicus* (anaerobe) have occasionally been reported. The major problem is *A. pyogenes*. Once infection is in the synovial fluid, joint destruction involves the same processes as described for DJD. The difference lies in the speed of destruction. The synovia is usually turbid or frankly purulent.

Some reports from the UK (Bracewell & Corbell, 1979; Wyn-Jones *et al.*, 1980) and USA (Madison *et al.*, 1989) noted an idiopathic, acute suppurative gonitis with severe lameness and synovitis. Articular erosions were evident radiographically on the lateral tibial plateau. Much evidence indicates the likelihood that *Brucella abortus* vaccination may have been the cause.

Clinical signs and diagnosis

Septic arthritis in a major weight-bearing joint causes a rapidly progressive disease with severe lameness, swelling and localized pain. In contrast to DJD, the animal may be anorexic and milk yield can drop abruptly in dairy cattle. Crepitus is not usually apparent. Arthrocentesis reveals a flocculent or purulent fluid that clots. It has a high leucocyte count of which over 90 per cent are polymorphs. The protein content often exceeds 8 g/dl and the mucin precipitate is abnormally flocculent.

A category 'suspect septic' refers to an early septic process associated with obvious lameness but apparently normal yellow synovia. The presence again of a high percentage of neutrophils in a dense leucocyte population is confirmation of early septic arthritis. Radiography in early (<10 days duration) septic arthritis is usually unhelpful. Ultrasound, on the other hand, can delineate the limits and physical nature of the fluid. From 14 days onwards, subchondral bone destruction and a peripheral periostitis are suggestive of joint sepsis.

Culture of synovial fluid is frequently negative in terms of isolation of pathogens, especially if antimicrobial therapy has already started. It is helpful if synovia is immediately inoculated into a diphasic culture bottle with sodium polyanetholsulphonate to enhance recovery of the organism. Culture of synovial biopsy material is usually more rewarding but is frequently impractical.

Treatment and prevention

The prognosis for septic arthritis is guarded or poor. Early aggressive treatment is essential. Parenteral antibiotic therapy should be initiated as soon as possible. Until sensitivity, based on synovial cultures, is available 48 hours after sampling, penicillin or

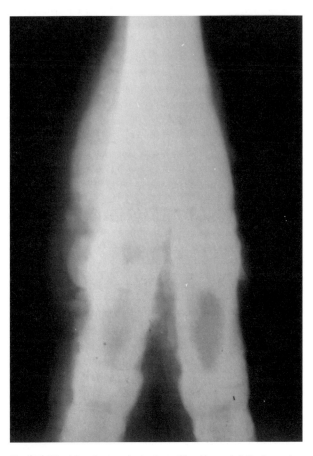

Fig. 32.13 Massive periosteal proliferation of fetlock region (metatarsophalangeal joint) of a four-year-old Holstein cow resulting from sepsis of the joint originating from an ascending septic tenosynovitis.

ampicillin is the drug of choice for most pathogens. Penicillin is most likely to be effective *in vivo* against all common pathogens except *Staphylococcus aureus* (where erythromycin, lincomycin, gentamicin, or cephalosporin may be better) and coliforms (gentamicin or trimethoprim–sulphadiazine).

The joint should be irrigated and drained (through-and-through lavage) through two wide-bore inflow–outflow portals produced by 14 gauge needles. Alternatively, small arthrotomy incisions may be made for the same purpose. Irrigation should be done with large volumes (>5l) of polyionic solutions, physiological saline, or with dilute (0.1 per cent) povidone-iodine solution.

Radical surgery also has a place if suitable facilities exist for the maintenance of asepsis and for general anaesthesia. Radical surgery comprises opening the joint following section of collateral ligaments and incision of joint capsule, evacuation of purulent material, curettage of infected cartilaginous surfaces, restoration of joint stability by suturing capsule and ligaments, and immobilization of the area, if in the distal limb, to prevent ankylosis. Such surgery appears more successful in the fetlock, carpus and tarsus than in the stifle, elbow, or shoulder joints.

Idiopathic gonitis (p. 1014) carries a good prognosis for recovery, regardless of the method of treatment. Heifers were treated successfully with a variety of antimicrobials, including procaine penicillin G, neomycin and ampicillin, and, in some cases, with through-and-through needle lavage with a polyionic solution. Lateral patellar arthrotomy with curettage of lytic areas on the lateral tibial plateau may be useful adjunct therapy.

There is no place for intra-articular antibiotics. Drainage of infective material from a poorly vascularized area is important, whereas systemic antibiotics adequately penetrate the well-vascularized joint capsule. Antibiotics should be given for at least two weeks. Preferred antibiotics are usually penicillin G, ampicillin, ceftiofur and gentamicin. Non-steroidal anti-inflammatory drugs should be given if pain is severe and persistent. The dosage is as for cases of DJD (see p. 455).

Miscellaneous neuromuscular diseases

Spastic paresis (see also p. 179)

Aetiology and pathology

Spastic paresis is a progressive condition of the hindlimbs of unknown origin. It is characterized by contraction of the gastrocnemius muscle and tendon and of other associated calcanean tendons and muscle bellies.

This spasm leads to severe extension of the hock. The condition has been observed in numerous breeds, but the highest incidence in dairy and beef cattle respectively is probably in the German and Dutch Friesian and the Aberdeen Angus.

It is hypothesized that an overactive stretch reflex is the major mechanism (De Ley & De Moor, 1977). Selective deafferentation of the gastrocnemius muscle by resection of the dorsal root fibres containing afferent nerve fibres (L5–6) abolished clinical signs. Plasma SGOT is reduced, and alkaline phosphatase is increased in affected calves, which also show a decreased P, Ca, and homovanillic acid concentration in CSF. The last-named effect indicates a lowered metabolic rate of CNS dopamine (De Ley & De Moor, 1975).

Gross and histopathological CNS lesions have generally been absent.

Clinical signs and diagnosis

The typical clinical signs are characteristic, and difficulty arises only in very early cases. Signs may start at six weeks to six months, rarely later. Cases encountered in adult cattle are best considered to be forms of progressive hindlimb paralysis, likely to involve spinal cord pressure resulting from vertebral exostoses.

The affected hindlimb is extended so that the hock angle is approximately 180° (normal is about 140°). The calf walks with a tendency to drag the toes. The limb may jerk intermittently at rest. It is advanced in a pendulum-like style. Later, less weight is taken and the calf may hop forward. Palpation reveals a very firm gastrocnemius muscle and tendon. The hock can be flexed manually without causing pain. On release the hock immediately adopts the original extended position (Fig. 32.14).

Lateral radiographs of the hock of calves affected for several weeks show several features indicative of the chronic overextension. The distal part of the tibial metaphysis is abnormally curved caudally; the distal tibial and tuber calcanei growth plates are widened; exostoses are present around the distal tibial growth plate, along with some osteoporosis. Often the most striking feature is a cranial curvature of the proximal part of the calcaneus.

In early cases, differential diagnosis includes dorsal patellar luxation, septic or non-infectious gonitis or tarsitis, fracture dislocation of the calcaneus, joint ill and luxation of the biceps femoris muscle.

Treatment and prevention

Since spastic paresis has a hereditary predisposition, breeding animals should be salvaged. Surgery can successfully alleviate the condition by either tenotomy or neurectomy.

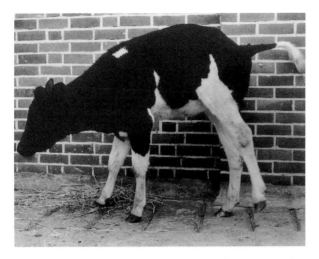

Fig. 32.14 Severe spastic paresis of left hindlimb of a four-month-old Friesian heifer, showing overextension of hock joint. Note spasm and elevation of the tail, and arched back as calf attempts to put more weight on the forelimbs.

Tenotomy has traditionally involved section of the gastrocnemius tendon and partial section of the superficial flexor tendon a little proximal to the point of the hock in the standing animal under local anaesthetic infiltration. A 6 cm (2½ inch) vertical skin incision is made caudally over the Achilles tendon to expose the two tendons. After section, the skin is sutured and the immediate surgical effect is usually pronounced hock flexion, with the joint initially close to the ground. Initial results have been consistently favourable, but a gradual recurrence of the abnormal posture is frequently seen, especially in older (six to ten-month-old) calves. Bilaterally affected calves should have the second leg operated four weeks following initial surgery.

It has been claimed that this classical operation ignores the fact that a second, deeply situated, tendon of insertion of the gastrocnemius muscle is left untouched. A modified operation, therefore, involves a lateral approach just cranial to the Achilles tendon, which is dissected to isolate the caudal component of the gastrocnemius tendon, from which a 2 cm (1 inch) length is resected. The superficial flexor tendon is left untouched. The cranial tendon of the gastrocnemius is identified and a similar tenectomy performed. In some cases, the dense fascia caudal to the distal end of the tibia is transected (Pavaux *et al.*, 1985).

Neurectomy of the tibial nerve or of its gastrocnemius branches is the alternative to tenotomy. Clinical results have been better than with tenotomy. Since identification of the multiple (seven or more) branches of the tibial nerve innervating the gastrocnemius

muscle is awkward, complete tibial neurectomy has been advocated (Boyd & Weaver, 1967). Surgery is performed under sedation and epidural block, or general anaesthesia. The site is the lateral thigh, between the two heads of the biceps femoris muscle. The tibial and peroneal nerves are identified by stimulation by forceps or by electrical means. Tibial nerve stimulation causes hock extension and fetlock and digital flexion. The tibial nerve should have a 2 cm (1 inch) portion removed at its most proximal point. Complications following this surgery are uncommon.

Spastic syndrome

Aetiology and pathogenesis

This chronic progressive disease, which is initially characterized by clonic–tonic spasms of the hindlimb musculature, is also known as 'crampy', 'stretches' or progressive hindlimb paralysis. The aetiology is unknown despite several attempts to find significant pathological lesions in the brain or spinal cord. Idiopathic muscular cramps is one current proposed explanation for the signs (Wells *et al.*, 1987).

The condition occurs in mature cattle of many breeds, both dairy (e.g. Holstein, Friesian and Guernsey) and beef (Hereford, Angus). The incidence in at least one breed (Danish Red) is significantly higher in bulls than cows. Many affected cattle have straight rear legs and poor hock conformation. Many bulls with spastic syndrome have spinal spondylosis. A single recessive gene with incomplete penetrance may be the mode of inheritance.

Clinical signs and diagnosis

Sudden episodic spasmodic contractions affect the muscles of both hindlegs, and sometimes also the back, neck and forelegs. The animal appears to be normal during recumbency. Signs are evident soon after rising.

The onset of the syndrome is slow, and signs may appear for a few months only to disappear for several weeks. The hindlimbs are hyperextended caudally in a fixed manner that may persist for several minutes. Spasms may extend forward to the forelimbs and neck muscles. The head is extended and the forefeet advanced with the back arched. If then forced to move, the gait is stiff and ungainly, and episodic lifting of the hindlimbs may also be seen during forward movement.

Animals generally spend considerable periods recumbent when the condition is advanced.

Other conditions that may confuse an initial diagnosis are relatively few but include bilateral DJD affecting the stifle or hock, and severe spinal spondylosis.

Treatment and prevention

The spastic syndrome is incurable. Palliative treatment has included vitamin D, bone meal (not available in many countries) and sedatives. Phenylbutazone has provided temporary relief in some cases. Affected bulls and apparently normal bulls that sire affected progeny should be culled from any breeding programme.

Diseases of skin and subcutis

Skin wounds are more liable around the limbs than the trunk and head. Their nature and treatment are adequately discussed in textbooks of general surgery. One unusual bovine problem is the constricting foreign body, usually rubber or wire, which slides over the foot to the level of pastern or metacarpus or metatarsus where it slowly becomes embedded in a mass of granulation tissue to present as a circumferential wound (Fig. 32.15). Such wounds require careful investigation because the band may be very deep and contacting bone.

Two specific disorders are discussed below. Generally, damage to skin and subcutis is more liable over pressure points such as the lateral aspect of the stifle, elbow and hock. Loss of the integument permits low-grade infection to become established. In a very contaminated environment such damage, arising from

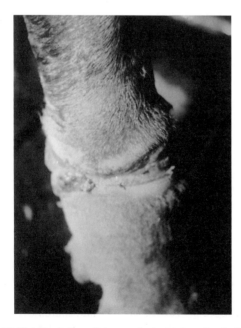

Fig. 32.15 Circumferential wound of metatarsal soft tissues. This two-year-old crossbred Hereford steer had a wire embedded deep to the soft tissues, resulting in mild lameness. Wound healed in four weeks following removal of foreign body.

pressure points and poor vascularity, may result in localized abscessation and pyaemic spread to the lungs, liver, kidneys and heart. The common organism is *A. pyogenes*.

Affected cattle should be put out on soft bedding, the wounds should be cleansed with chlorhexidine hydrochloride, and systemic antibiotics should be injected for five to seven days to prevent systemic spread. The prognosis for healing is good if appetite is maintained unless clinical signs of involvement of other organs (e.g. heart) are apparent, and suggestive of septicaemic spread.

Tarsal cellulitis

Aetiology and pathology

Almost all cases of hock enlargement result from repeated trauma against concrete surfaces in stanchions or loose housing. Typically, soft tissue swelling over the lateral aspect of the tarsus may be a false or acquired bursitis. Medial swelling of the joint is minimal unless the lateral enlargement is pronounced. Lameness is rare unless the fluid distension becomes massive, when mechanical restriction of joint flexion causes stiffness, or a low-grade infection arises. Radiographs have repeatedly shown the absence of bone changes.

The swelling is usually symmetrical. Hair loss and skin excoriation are evident. Usually the skin is not broken. Occasionally, a central area of skin sloughs, permitting a dirty red–brown material to escape. At this time, septic infection can supervene and a purulent discharge may be noted for several days before granulation tissue fills the cavity of the false bursa.

Clinical signs and diagnosis

The distribution of the swelling and absence of lameness are almost characteristic (Fig. 32.16). An infectious tarsitis causes a more diffuse swelling and obvious lameness, as will a tarsal bone fracture. Tarsal hydrarthrosis first causes synovial distension of the joint capsule cranially and medially, then both medial and lateral to the caudal border of the tibiotarsal bone, and cranial to the base of the calcaneus. Tarsal hydrarthrosis is a cosmetic blemish and causes no lameness.

Treatment and prevention

The seasonal occurrence of tarsal bursitis, becoming increasingly severe during the housed period and disappearing in the summer grazing months, is evidence that tarsal bursitis is related to the specific environment. Errors and deficiencies usually can be found in the lying-in areas of loose-housed herds. Some cows may

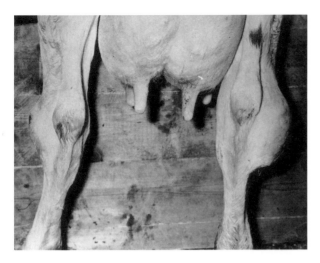

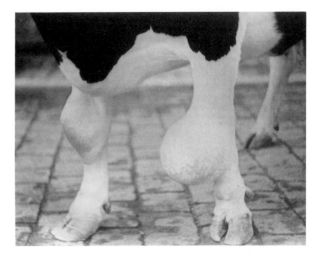

Fig. 32.16 Right tarsal bursitis in a five-year-old Holstein cow with digital problems resulting in prolonged recumbency. Left supratarsal skin shows evidence of previous injury.

Fig. 32.17 Severe bilateral carpal bursitis in an eight-year-old Friesian cow associated with *Br. abortus* infection (Czechoslovakia).

refuse to use cubicles and remain out on the slurry-covered concrete. They often have problems rising from the slippery surface, during which the wet skin of the lateral part of the hock is repeatedly abraded. Other cows suffer injury when they rise awkwardly in poorly designed or badly bedded cubicles. Standings that are up to 30 cm (12 inches) too short for the particular breed and neck rails placed 5 cm (2 inches) too low may force cows to stand with the hind feet in the passageway. Careful observation (e.g. during oestrous detection) will usually disclose the specific problem.

Treatment should be conservative and medical. It should never involve a long incision to drain fluid from the false bursa, neither should one attempt radically to dissect out this bursa. Most cases are best left untreated in the absence of lameness. If lameness eventually occurs as a result of a low-grade tarsal infection, systemic antibiotics (oxytetracyclines) rapidly reduce the size of the swelling. Corticosteroids are usually ineffective. Infected cases may be bandaged daily and be irrigated with warm water, but the response tends to be incomplete. A cluster of cases indicates a need to check the loafing areas and cubicles (Hughes, 2000).

Carpal bursitis

Aetiology and pathology

Carpal bursitis or carpal hygroma involves the skin, subcutaneous precarpal bursa and adjacent soft tissues. Very rarely does infection extend into the joint. Repeated contusion from contact points of the stanchions, stalls, or floor in housed cattle is the main predisposing factor. The condition is similar to tarsal cellulitis in that the swelling resolves in cattle when at pasture. Some cases have been associated with *Br. abortus* infection (Fig. 32.17; see also p. 580).

Clinical signs and diagnosis

A soft and painless swelling develops on the dorsal aspect of the carpus, usually with evidence of skin contusion. It tends to be symmetrical and no breed or age predilection is recognized. Minor swellings are merely a cosmetic blemish. The exceptional large grapefruit or melon-sized mass may cause slight mechanical lameness but is painless. The fluid appears to be synovia-like, yellow and clear, but less tenacious. It is produced by the bursal lining. The cavity tends to be multilocular. Differential diagnosis from a precarpal abscess or septic carpitis, both of which are painful and cause lameness, is simple.

Treatment and prevention

Surgical drainage is rarely necessary. Such drainage (as in tarsal bursitis, p. 460) is fraught with the risk of introducing infection into a sterile site. The skin is more liable to contamination every time the animal lies down. It is hard to protect the area with a bandage. Most cases respond if placed in a well-bedded straw yard (winter) or put to pasture (summer), i.e. into surroundings where predisposing trauma can be avoided.

Drainage is needed only when gait, feed intake and production are affected. The drainage should be done as an aseptic procedure. A mixture of antibiotic and corticosteroid solution should be instilled into various sections of the collapsed cavity and such injection should be repeated at weekly intervals.

Radical surgical removal of the bursa and excessive skin is possible, but is a haemorrhagic and time-consuming process despite the presence of a tourniquet proximal to the carpus. General anaesthesia is usually required as adequate local infiltration of the bursal wall is impractical.

Destruction of the bursal lining with an astringent (copper sulphate) or irritant disinfectant (tincture of iodine) is not advisable, as a severe local reaction is produced, and dissection, curettage and repeated irrigation of the wound are essential steps before secondary healing eventually occurs.

Prevention involves careful attention to the housing system for the existing herd. Problem cows should be put into straw yards before the swellings cause a clinical problem.

Ankylosing spondylitis

Aetiology and pathology

Generally confined to old bulls and defined as an acquired fusion of the ventral aspects of the bodies of the caudal thoracic and lumbar vertebrae, sufficient pressure may be exerted on the ventral and lateral spinal cord tracts or the ventral nerve roots to cause some hindlimb weakness, ataxia or paralysis. Exostoses first develop on the ligaments of the caudal 2–3 thoracic and cranial 2–3 lumbar spinal bodies (T11–L3). Degenerative changes in the intervertebral discs may predispose to exostosis formation. The new bone may extend into the spinal canal as 'replacement bone'. Sometimes, possibly resulting from a fall or a violent ejaculation, part of the exostosis may fracture, the fracture line extending through the vertebral body. Fluid exudate (blood, oedema) from the fracture may cause pressure on the spinal cord.

Clinical signs and diagnosis

An early sign may be a reluctance or difficulty in mounting cows, attributable to the mechanical effects of a relatively inflexible thoracolumbar spine. Usually there are no premonitory signs and the bull suddenly has difficulty in rising and may adopt a 'dog-sitting' position or may be completely paraplegic, dragging the digits caudally. Sometimes marked ataxia suddenly develops.

The site of trauma can rarely be accurately defined due to problems of size. Crepitus is rarely elicited. Swelling of the back musculature is not seen. On rectal examination, exostoses may be palpable dorsal to the aortic bifurcation, but such exostoses are a normal feature of mature and older bulls. In one extensive series of bulls followed to slaughter, severe signs of tail and hindlimb paralysis were only seen in two cases, though all bulls had varying degrees of ankylosing spondylitis.

Differential diagnosis includes other causes of spinal cord compression such as aberrant migrating larvae and infiltrating neoplasms such as lymphosarcoma as well as hindlimb degenerative joint disease.

Treatment and prevention

The prognosis depends on the degree and extent of nerve damage. In the progressive ataxic or paraplegic case, it is poor. Mild cases may improve following rest and use of corticosteroids and diuretics to reduce the oedema. Animals should be bedded on deep straw to prevent the development of decubital lesions. Many mild cases relapse following partial recovery. Slaughter on humane grounds is often the action of choice.

Mineral imbalance-related lameness: rickets, osteomalacia (see also p. 253)

Aetiology and pathology

Mineral, indeed nutrient, imbalance can result in lameness from calfhood through the growing yearling stage to maturity and old age. The pattern almost invariably involves an imbalance or deficiency of two or more factors.

During growth the important elements in normal development of healthy bone collagen, which is the framework for provisional calcification of the zone of hypertrophied cartilage, are vitamin D, copper, protein and energy. Mineralization of the cartilaginous matrix results in deposition of much calcium, phosphorus and carbonate, with lesser amounts of sodium, magnesium and fluoride. Vitamin D, calcium and phosphorus are essential to the formation of this bone mineral.

In the prenatal period, identified deficiency diseases resulting in abortion or the birth of progeny with skeletal defects include lupinosis (congenital arthrogryposis), manganese (contracted tendons), and zinc and vitamin A deficiencies (multiple defects).

Vitamin D deficiency in calves leads by a complex pathway involving the parathyroid gland, kidney and intestine to deficient calcification of long bones and of the cartilaginous matrix. The result in calves is rickets. The zone of provisional calcification is widened but the new osteoid is not mineralized. In adults, the same deficiency causes osteomalacia, which is rare except in northern Australia and South Africa. Usually a calcium: phosphorus imbalance is also involved. Vitamin

D-deficient diets may be identified on some farms where feed is home-mixed.

Clinical signs and diagnosis of rickets

Calves have enlarged metaphyses and growth plates of the long bones, especially the distal metatarsus and metacarpus, fetlock and pastern. The swellings are rather painful to pressure. The costochondral junction exhibits the classical 'rickety rosary' in calves. Radiographic changes include a widened area of radiolucency at the growth plate with flaring of the distal metaphyses, usually in the carpus, pastern and fetlock.

The diagnosis rests on the soft tissue swelling at characteristic sites, lameness, and in cases of doubt, feed analysis. Serum or plasma may reveal depressed levels of calcium, phosphorus and an elevated alkaline phosphatase.

Differential diagnosis includes physeal dysplasia and joint ill (polyarthritis).

Clinical signs and diagnosis of osteomalacia

The relative or absolute phosphorus deficiency, usually acquired from low phosphorus pastures, is classically associated with the development of pica and osteophagia, variable degrees of lameness including pathological fractures of long bones, weight loss, stiffness and recumbency. Deficiency tends to be exaggerated in cows due to the demands of pregnancy and lactation. Fertility may be severely reduced. Hypophosphataemia is accompanied by normal blood levels of calcium. The condition must be distinguished from DJD.

Vitamin D-deficient osteomalacia in grazing animals is seen in temperate climates with a shortage of sun-cured hay and affects cattle stressed by the demands of pregnancy and lactation. The clinical manifestation resembles the phosphorus-deficient form.

Treatment and prevention

In rickets, increased vitamin D in the ration along with restoration of a normal Ca:P ratio with adequate intake brings a rapid response.

Osteomalacia in adult cattle is treated by dietary supplementation with rations high in phosphorus.

Osteomyelitis

Aetiology and pathogenesis

Osteomyelitis of the limb bones in cattle occurs in two forms: one in growing cattle, the other in adults.

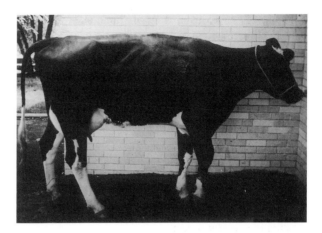

Fig. 32.18 Distal right radial septic physitis in two-year-old Holstein heifer. Weight bearing is minimal due to severe pain and soft tissue swelling. The aetiology, in the absence of penetration, was probably haematogenous.

A haematogenous form is seen in calves six to twelve months old as a result of *Salmonella* infection, which localizes in the metaphysis, physis and epiphysis of long bones such as the metacarpus as well as the upper limb where an embolic process may be responsible (Kersjes *et al.*, 1966; Gitter *et al.*, 1978). Blood flow through the metaphyseal sinusoids is slow, facilitating easy bacterial deposition and proliferation. Many clinical cases are multifocal and cause rapid destruction of bone. Other organisms in calves include *A. pyogenes* and *E. coli*. In older, growing cattle, less than two years old, a growth plate osteomyelitis may involve the distal metatarsus or distal tibia. Common bacterial isolates are *A. pyogenes* and *Salmonella* spp. (De Kessel *et al.*, 1982). Periarticular soft tissue swelling is prominent (Fig. 32.18). The radiographic extent of bone destruction is very variable and appears to be unrelated to the involvement of epiphysis and metaphysis, which are equally likely to be affected. Many cases have infected sequestra in the osteomyelitic focus.

In adult cattle, osteomyelitis of long bones is a sporadic isolated phenomenon. The aetiology may again involve haematogenous spread, or may arise following direct trauma. Open long bone fractures are an obvious example (see p. 441). Less obviously, saucer fractures of the diaphysis may lead to formation of a sequestrum. Sequestra in long bones of cattle are related to common sites of lacerating wounds, notably the proximal half of the dorsal aspect of the metatarsus (Firth, 1987). This author hypothesizes that severe contusion alone may produce sufficient subcutaneous soft tissue damage to render the area susceptible to infection and subsequent adjacent bone sequestration.

A chronic sequestrum in a long bone may develop a fistulous tract, which permits easier delineation of the bone by insertion of a positive contrast agent for a fistulogram.

A specific form of osteomyelitis is Brodie's abscess, which is a circumscribed abscess lined with a granular membrane surrounded by sclerotic bone. Synonyms are chronic fibrous osteomyelitis and chronic bone abscess. Though the lining is histologically a definite pyogenic membrane, bacteriological culture may be sterile. Both *F. necrophorum* and *A. pyogenes* have been involved in cases of Brodie's abscess in three and six-months-old calves (Weaver, 1972).

Clinical signs and diagnosis

Osteomyelitis usually causes severe, continuing pain with local swelling. These signs relate to the active process such as long bone infection following an open fracture when, if left untreated, purulent material, sometimes with bone spicules, is discharged to the exterior. Cellulitis may be severe and additional sinuses may form.

Osteomyelitis in calves where infection is within and surrounding the epiphysis presents differently. Localization of the lameness may be difficult due to the absence of local swelling but pain is usually evident.

Chronic osteomyelitis may not cause lameness when the infected focus is effectively walled off by dense sclerosed bone (involucrum). Sometimes, in such cases, lameness suddenly develops as infection flares up once more.

Osteomyelitis rarely extends to involve joints except in the digit and any resentment to joint flexion is usually due to extension from the diaphyseal or metaphyseal focus.

Systemic effects of osteomyelitis include lassitude, mild fever and a reduced appetite. Radiology is indicated in most cases to confirm the diagnosis, to determine the extent of the pathological process, and to assess the possibility of useful surgical intervention. Osteoporosis results from the loss of bone by erosion and its replacement by infected granulation tissue. Periosteal new bone is often evident and is variable in amount. Initially, the periosteum is elevated over an osteomyelitic focus with an underlying loss of cortical density. Later, in animals where a sequestrum forms, new subperiosteal bone is deposited while sclerosis is evident around the sequestrum.

Differential diagnosis of osteomyelitis with an open wound involves determining the primary lesion. Some cases of wounds may not involve the periosteum and lameness may reflect pain due to subcutaneous abscessation, septic myositis or extensive intramuscular abscessation. Open wounds should, therefore, be explored with a sterile probe.

Osteomyelitis of long bones without evidence of skin trauma must be differentiated from fissure fractures, subperiosteal haematoma, subcutaneous abscesses and rare bone tumours. In calves, haematogenous bacterial infection of metaphysis, growth plate and epiphysis must be distinguished from joint ill, epiphyseal separation and metaphyseal fractures.

Treatment and prognosis

Cattle with systemic involvement (pyrexia, anorexia) should be given parenteral antibiotics for three to five days. Many cases respond to this therapy. Non-responsive cases should be considered for surgery. This applies particularly to cases of Brodie's abscess and incision should be made over the metaphysis to attempt aspiration of the contents of the abscess if subperiosteal in position. In other cases a sinus tract through the cortex may be enlarged to evacuate the contents and to permit curettage of the adjacent necrotic bone and pyogenic membrane.

Cattle with open long bone fractures and osteomyelitis should have sequestra removed and check radiographic films taken. Treatment then depends on the type of fracture and extent of osteomyelitis. The options are discussed elsewhere (p. 442).

Calves with bacterial infection of the metaphysis sometimes respond to parenteral antibiotics alone, otherwise local debridement and irrigation of the focus is justified.

Physeal dysplasia

Aetiology and pathology

Physeal dysplasia, also loosely termed epiphysitis (though the epiphysis is not involved in an inflammatory process), is primarily a defective development of one or more growth plates, which later may become necrotic and inflammatory and later still may be purulent. The problem usually affects the lower limb, especially the carpal and fetlock joints. The pathogenesis apparently involves a reduced blood supply to the growth plate as a result of uneven or excessive mechanical pressure. The metaphyseal side, dependent on an adequate blood supply for calcification and ossification, is more affected than the epiphyseal surface. The pathological process has not been thoroughly investigated in cattle, but necrosis of the ground substance, resulting from folding of the cell columns and loss of continuity, has been noted histologically in housed fattening cattle. Poor-quality, uncomfortable floor surfaces predispose rapidly fattening cattle with limited exercise space to physeal dysplasia.

Gross pathology reveals some subcutaneous oedema and red or red–grey discoloration around the growth plate, which is either necrotic or, in severe cases, purulent. In its most severe form the growth plate undergoes separation.

Copper deficiency or a combined copper–molybdenum deficiency (see pp. 254, 298) has also been associated with physeal dysplasia as a result of defective collagen formation. The abnormal collagen does not permit normal mineralization. The result is stiffness and lameness in calves with a characteristic distal metatarsal swelling. Another result is an increased incidence of long bone fractures.

Clinical signs and diagnosis

The swellings are usually symmetrical, and hindlimbs are affected more often. The enlarged area in the lame calf or yearling is painful. Weight loss is rapid in beef cattle aged nine to eighteen months. Occasionally, several animals in a group of cattle are affected simultaneously following violent exercise, for example at turning out to pasture from confined housing. Isolated cases may result from trauma on slats.

In the copper-related form the limbs may be bowed either laterally or medially, the gait is stilted, and the swellings tend to be symmetrical. However, other signs of copper deficiency are present, including unthriftiness, a rough discoloured hair coat and diarrhoea.

Radiographic features include rarefying lesions with an increased width of the growth plate with irregularity and fragmentation, but with an absence of reactive change around the metaphyseal margin. The radiographic changes are more severe in cattle with physeal separation and secondary repair. Milder radiographic changes are evident in many cattle of the same group that do not show lameness.

The list of differential diagnoses includes rickets, traumatic separation of the growth plate, bacterial ostitis, septic arthritis and fractures. Radiography is necessary to permit this differentiation.

Treatment and prevention

Only the copper-related syndrome is responsive to treatment by an appropriate diet change. Mild non-copper-related cases respond to rest and external support by lightweight casting. Most cases of such

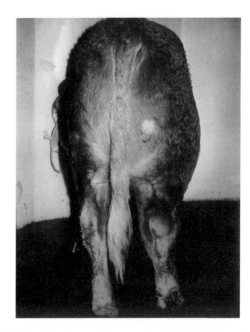

Fig. 32.19 Massive septic myositis in right hindquarters of two-year-old Saler bull. The light area (shaved) shows the site of exploratory needle puncture. Abscess cavity contained 12 litres of pus. *Actinomyces pyogenes* was recovered in pure culture. Severe oedema extends down to the hock. Recovery followed drainage and irrigation.

lameness should be salvaged before there is further weight loss.

Lameness of iatrogenic origin

Some forms of upper limb lameness may be the result of treatment for disease or injury. Various entities have been discussed elsewhere: radial paralysis from prolonged lateral recumbency during anaesthesia (p. 436), neonatal long bone fractures and physeal separations resulting from excessive traction in dystokia (p. 444), and traumatic injury and transection of the gastrocnemius tendon (p. 451). Another form of iatrogenic damage is that following intramuscular injections. Occasionally, particularly in calves, the sciatic nerve may be injured. More frequent is the development of an abscess following a subcutaneous injection, which rarely causes lameness but remains a cosmetic blemish. When a non-sterile preparation, or a dirty syringe and needle are used for an intramuscular injection, the results may be more serious. As a rule, infection is sealed off by fibrous tissue with no ill-effects. Sometimes the result is a massive abscess, which causes lameness and requires prompt surgical drainage and daily irrigation to prevent recurrence (Fig. 32.19).

References

Anderson, D.E., St.-Jean, G., Morin, D.E., Ducharme, N.G., Nelson, D.R. & Desrochers, A. (1996) Traumatic flexor tendon injuries in 27 cattle. *Veterinary Surgery*, **25**, 320–6.

Boyd, J.S. & Weaver, A.D. (1967) Spastic paresis in cattle. *Veterinary Record*, **80**, 529–30.

Bracewell, C.D. & Corbell, J. (1979) An association between arthritis and persistent serological reactions to *Brucella abortus* in cattle from apparently brucellosis-free herds. *Veterinary Record*, **106**, 99–101.

Buchtal, F., Rosenfalk, A. & Behse, F. (1984) Sensory potential of normal and diseased nerves. In *Peripheral Neuropathy* (ed. by P.J. Dyck), p. 995. W.B. Saunders, Philadelphia.

Chamberlain, A.T. (1986) Prognostic indicators in the downer cow. In *Proceedings of the British Cattle Veterinary Association*, pp. 57–68.

Chamberlain, A.T. (1987) The management and prevention of the downer cow syndrome. In *Proceedings of the British Cattle Veterinary Association*, 20–30.

Cox, V.S. (1981) Understanding the downer cow syndrome. *Compendium of Continuing Education for the Practising Veterinarian*, **3**, 45–53.

Cox, V.S. & Onapito, J.S. (1998) The many causes of downer cows. *AABP Bovine Proceedings*, **31**, 164–6.

Cox, V.S. & Farmsworth, R.J. (1998) Prevention and treatment of down cows: a continuum. *AABP Bovine Proceedings*, **31**, 167–9.

De Kessel, A., Verschooten, F., De Moor, A., Steenhaut, M. & Wouters, L. (1982) Bacteriele Osteitis–Osteomyelitis ter Hoogte van Groeiplaten bij het Rund. *Vlaams Diergeneesk. Tijdschr.*, **51**, 397–422.

De Ley, G. & De Moor, A. (1975) Bovine spastic paresis: cerebrospinal fluid concentrations of homovanillic acid and 5-hydroxyindolacetic acid in normal and spastic calves. *American Journal of Veterinary Research*, **36**, 227–8.

De Ley, G. & De Moor, A. (1977) Bovine spastic paresis: results of selective desafferation of the gastrocnemius muscle by means of spinal dorsal root resection. *American Journal of Veterinary Research*, **38**, 1899–1900.

Ducharme, N.G., Stanton, M.E. & Ducharme, G.R. (1985) Stifle lameness in cattle at two veterinary teaching hospitals (42 cases). *Canadian Veterinary Journal*, **26**, 212–17.

Ferguson, J.G. (1982) Management and repair of bovine fractures. *Compendium of Continuing Education for the Practicing Veterinarian*, **4**, S128–S136.

Ferguson, J.G. (1985) Special considerations in bovine orthopedics and lameness. *Veterinary Clinics of North America. Food Animal Practice*, **1**, 131–52.

Ferguson, J.G. (1997) Surgical conditions of the proximal limb. In *Lameness in Cattle*, 3rd edn (ed. by P.R. Greenough & A.D. Weaver), p. 262. W.B. Saunders, Philadelphia.

Firth, E.C. (1987) Bone sequestration in horses and cattle. *Australian Veterinary Journal*, **64**, 65–9.

Gitter, M., Gray, C., Richardson, C. & Pepper, R.T. (1978) Chronic salmonella infection in calves. *British Veterinary Journal*, **134**, 113–21.

Hickman, J., Houlton, J. & Edwards, B. (1997) *Atlas of Veterinary Surgery*, 3rd edn, pp. 261–2. Blackwell Science, Oxford.

Hughes, J. (2000) Cows and cubicles. *In Practice*, **22**, 231–9.

Kendrick, J.W. & Sittmann, K. (1966) Inherited osteoarthritis of dairy cattle. *Journal of the American Veterinary Medical Association*, **149**, 17–21.

Kersjes, A.W., Frik, Y.F. & Van de Watering, C.G. (1966) Bacteriele osteitis bij rundereen. *Tijd. Diergeneesk.*, **91**, 1537–47.

Kofler, J. & Martinek, B. (2000) Ultrasonographic imaging of disorders of the carpal region in 34 cattle – arthritis, tenoynovitis, carpal hygroma, periarticular abscess. *Proceedings of the International Symposium on Disorders of the Ruminant Digit*, Parma, Italy, September 2000, pp. 246–9.

Madison, J.B., Tulleners, E.P., Ducharme, N.G. *et al.* (1989) Idiopathic gonitis in heifers: 34 cases (1976–1986). *Journal of the American Veterinary Medical Association*, **194**, 273–7.

Nelson, D.R., Huhn, J.C. & Kneller, S.K. (1990) Peripheral detachment of the medial meniscus with injury to the medial collateral ligament in 50 cattle. *Veterinary Record*, **127**, 59–66.

Pavaux, C., Sautet, J. & Lignereux, J.Y. (1985) Anatomie du muscle gastrocnemien des bovins appliquée à la cure chirurgicale de la paresie spastique. *Vlaams Diergeneesk. Tijdschr.*, **54**, 296–312.

Roeber, D.L., Smith, G.C., Floyd, J.G. & Cowman, G.L. (2000) Lameness in breeding cattle in the United States: the National Market Cow and Bull Beef Quality Audit 1999. *Proceedings of the 11th International Symposium on Disorders of the Ruminant Digit*, Parma, Italy, September 2000, pp. 152–6.

Schub, J.C.L. & Killeen, J.R. (1988) A retrospective study of dystokia-related vertebral fractures in neonatal calves. *Canadian Veterinary Journal*, **29**, 830–3.

Smith, B.P., Angelos, J., George, L.W., Fecteau, G., Angelos, S., VanMetre, D., House, J.K. & Hullinger, P. (1997) Down cows: causes and treatments. *Proceedings of the American Association of Bovine Practitioners*, **30**, 43–5.

Steiner, A. & Zulauf, M. (2000) Fenestration of the abaxial hoof wall and implantation of gentamicin-impregnated collagen sponges for treatment of septic arthritis of the distal interphalangeal joint in 7 cattle. *Proceedings of the 11th International Symposium on Disorders of the Ruminant Digit*, Parma, Italy, September 2000, pp. 271–2.

Trostle, S.S., Nicoll, R.G., Forrest, L.J. & Markel, M.D. (1997) Clinical and radiographic findings, treatment, and outcome in cattle with osteochondrosis: 29 cases (1986–1996). *Journal of the American Veterinary Medical Association*, **211**, 1566–70.

Tulleners, E.P. (1986) Metacarpal and metatarsal fractures in dairy cattle: 33 cases (1979–1985). *Journal of the American Veterinary Medical Association*, **189**, 463–8.

Tulleners, E.P., Nunamaker, D.M. & Richardson, D.W. (1987) Coxofemoral luxations in cattle: 22 cases (1980–1985). *Journal of the American Veterinary Medical Association*, **191**, 569–74.

Vaughan, L.C. (1964) Peripheral nerve injuries: an experimental study in cattle. *Veterinary Record*, **76**, 1293–1301.

Weaver, A.D. (1972) Chronic localised osteomyelitis of the bovine limb. *British Veterinary Journal*, **128**, 470–6.

Weaver, A.D. (1977) An investigation into condemnations for hind limb disease in slaughtered cattle with particular reference to the stifle and hip joints. *Veterinary Record*, **100**, 172–5.

Weaver, A.D. (1997) Joint conditions. In *Lameness in Cattle*, 3rd edn, (ed. by P.R. Greenough & A.D. Weaver), p. 163. W.B. Saunders, Philadelphia.

Weaver, A.D. & Campbell, J.R. (1972) Surgical correction of medial and lateral patellar luxation in calves. *Veterinary Record*, **90**, 567–9.

Wells, G.A.H., Hawkins, S.A.C., O'Toole, D.T., Done, S.H., Duffell, S.J., Bradley, R. & Herbert, C.N. (1987) Spastic syndrome in a Holstein bull: a histologic study. *Veterinary Pathology*, **24**, 345–53.

Wintzer, H.J. (1961) A possible method of treating long bone fractures in cattle. *Dtsch. Tierarztl. Wschr.*, **68**, 226–8.

Wyn-Jones, G., Baker, J.R. & Johnson, P.M. (1980) A clinical and immunopathological study of *Brucella abortus* strain 19-induced arthritis in cattle. *Veterinary Record*, **107**, 5–9.

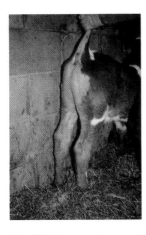

Plate 16.1 Hair loss over legs and perineum associated with steatorrhoea and diarrhoea (from Blowey & Weaver (1990) *A Colour Atlas of Diseases of Cattle*, Wolfe Publications Ltd, London) (p. 232).

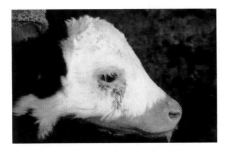

Plate 16.2 Alopecia on muzzle due to adherence of poorly dispersed fats from milk substitute (from Blowey & Weaver (1990) *A Colour Atlas of Diseases of Cattle*, Wolfe Publications Ltd, London) (p. 233).

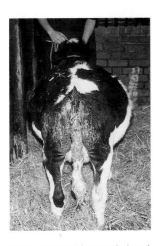

Plate 16.3 Rumen bloat and chronic scour caused by failure of the oesophageal groove to close (p. 234).

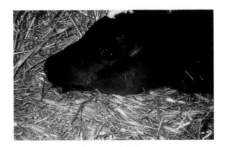

Plate 16.4 Perforated abomasal ulcer: calf *in extremis* (from Blowey & Weaver (1990) *A Colour Atlas of Diseases of Cattle*, Wolfe Publications Ltd, London) (p. 236).

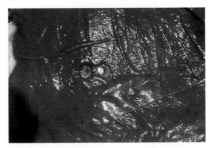

Plate 16.5 Perforated abomasal ulcer: abomasum at post mortem (from Blowey & Weaver (1990) *A Colour Atlas of Diseases of Cattle*, Wolfe Publications Ltd, London) (p. 236).

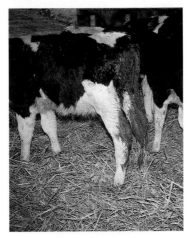

Plate 16.6 Chronic peri-weaning calf diarrhoea, a condition of uncertain aetiology (p. 237).

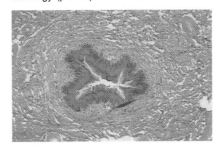

Plate 23.1 Transverse section of teat duct showing lumen and keratinized lining (p. 327). (×25)

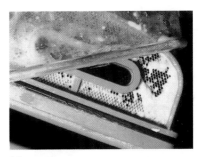

(a)

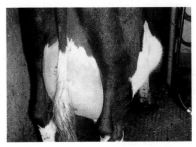

(b)

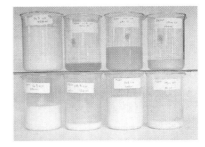

(c)

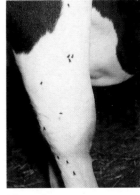

(d)

Plate 23.2 Signs of clinical mastitis. (a) Clotting of milk detected on a filter in the long milk tube. (b) Alterations to colour of milk due to mastitis. (c) Swelling and reddening of the rear quarters of a cow with acute coliform mastitis. (d) Oedema of leg of cow suffering summer mastitis. Note biting flies (p. 328).

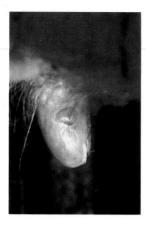

Plate 27.1 Early stage of bovine herpes mammillitis showing unilocular vesicle formation (p. 364).

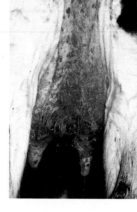

Plate 27.4 Bovine herpes mammillitis. In some cases, particularly in heifers, extensive scab formation can occur over the udder (p. 364).

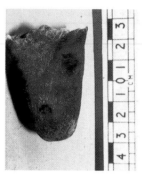

Plate 27.7 Bovine herpes mammillitis (two to three weeks). Necrotic tissue shed from cow (p. 364).

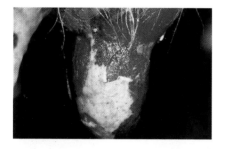

Plate 27.2 Bovine herpes mammillitis (two days). The vesicles have ruptured, producing a serous fluid and exposing a very congested dermis (p. 364).

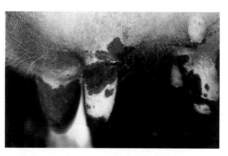

Plate 27.5 Bovine herpes mammillitis (about seven days). The initial oedema subsides and is followed by epithelial necrosis (p. 364).

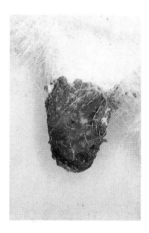

Plate 27.8 Bovine herpes mammillitis. The shedding of the necrotic tissue reveals a raw, granulated area, often becoming secondarily infected with bacteria (p. 364).

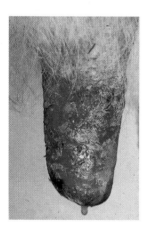

Plate 27.3 Bovine herpes mammillitis (four days). The exudate coagulates on the teat surface producing flat, smooth scabs. These darken to a red–brown colour (p. 364).

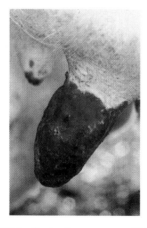

Plate 27.6 Bovine herpes mammillitis (about two weeks). An area of necrosis often involving most of the teat occurs as this is often shed as a whole (see Plate 25.7; p. 364).

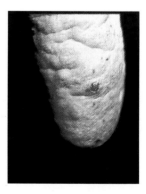

Plate 27.9 Pseudocowpox showing the formation of a small, dark-red elevated scab (p. 364).

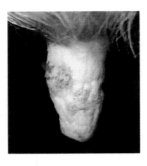

Plate 27.10 Pseudocowpox lesion (seven days), about 1 cm in diameter and somewhat resembling a mild cowpox lesion (p. 364).

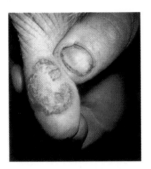

Plate 27.11 Pseudocowpox (10–12 days). A raised scab often known as a 'ring' or 'horseshoe' scab (p. 364).

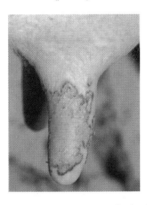

Plate 27.12 Pseudocowpox. Scabs have converged to form a single scab extending the teat length (p. 364).

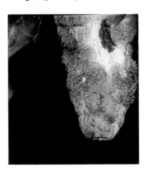

Plate 27.13 An atypical pseudocowpox lesion (p. 365).

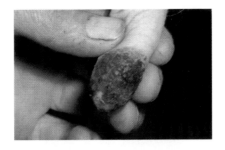

Plate 27.14 An atypical pseudocowpox lesion (p. 365).

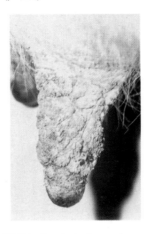

Plate 27.15 An atypical pseudocowpox lesion (p. 365).

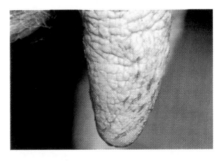

Plate 27.16 An atypical pseudocowpox lesion (p. 365).

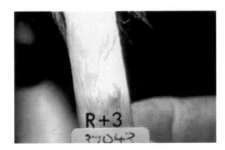

Plate 27.17 Cowpox showing development of a vesicle (p. 366).

Plate 27.21 (*right*) *Staphylococcus aureus* infection resulting in pustule formation surrounded by erythema (impetigo) (p. 368).

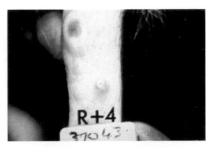

Plate 27.18 Cowpox following rupture of a vesicle (p. 366).

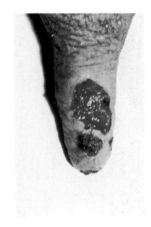

Plate 27.19 Cowpox with scab formation (p. 366).

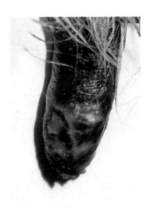

Plate 27.20 A severe cowpox involving most of the teat skin (p. 366).

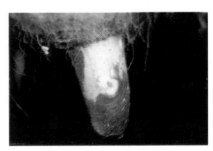

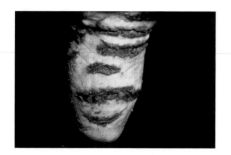

Plate 27.22 Teat chaps (p. 369).

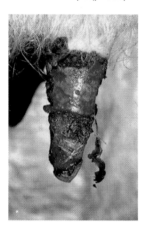

Plate 27.23 A teat with shedding of the skin following photosensitization (p. 370).

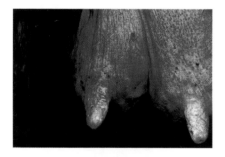

Plate 27.24 Foot and mouth disease. Vesiculation of the teat (p. 371).

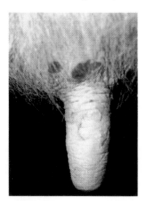

Plate 27.25 Pseudocowpox infection together with cowpox infection (p. 371).

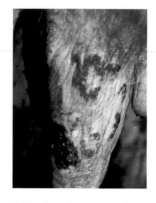

Plate 27.26 Pseudocowpox infection together with bovine herpes mammillitis (p. 371).

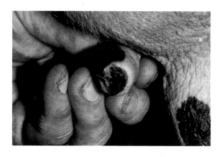

Plate 27.27 Blackspot of a teat orifice (p. 371).

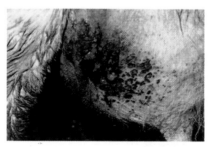

Plate 27.28 Mud abrasion of the lateral surface of the teat (p. 371).

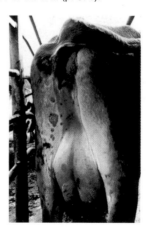

Plate 27.29 Ringworm lesions. Typical *Trichophyton verrucosum* lesions (courtesy of S. Smith, Hoechst Pharmaceuticals) (p. 371).

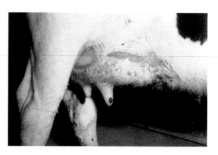

Plate 27.30 Thelitis and serous exudate of the udder skin in peracute mastitis (p. 371).

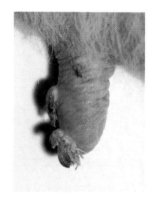

Plate 27.31 Filamentous papillomatosis of the teat (p. 371).

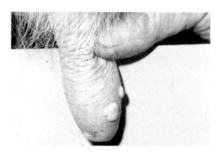

Plate 27.32 Nodular papillomatosis of the teat (p. 371).

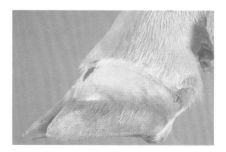

Plate 31.1 Hoof with corium removed (courtesy Dr P. Ossent) (p. 412).

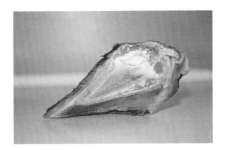

Plate 31.2 Cross-section of white line (p. 413).

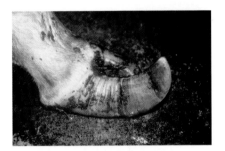

Plate 31.3 Gross claw overgrowth (p. 414).

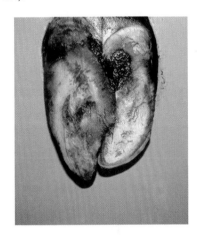

Plate 31.4 Overgrowth from the sole (p. 414).

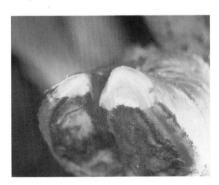

Plate 31.5 White line across a square-ended toe (p. 415).

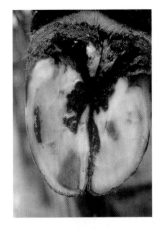

Plate 31.6 Haemorrhage at the sole ulcer site and in white line (p. 418).

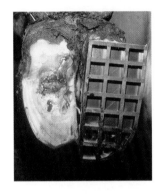

Plate 31.7 Typical sole ulcer (p. 418).

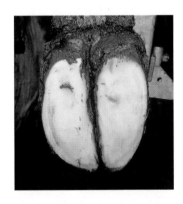

Plate 31.8 Heel ulcer on the left claw and an early sole ulcer haemorrhage on the right (p. 419).

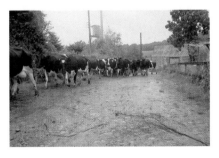

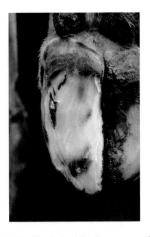

Plate 31.9 Typical white line separation with impacted stone at the abaxial wall (p. 420).

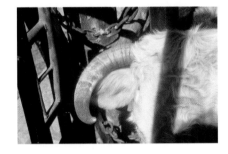

Plate 31.10 The rings on a cow's horns, one for each calving, demonstrates the disruption of horn formation in the periparturient animal (p. 420).

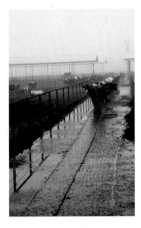

Plate 31.11 Cows prefer to walk on the soft surface of a rubber mat (courtesy Dr Karl Burgi) (p. 423).

Plate 31.12 (left) Cows walking along the grass verge to avoid the stony track (courtesy H. and D. Blanch) (p. 423).

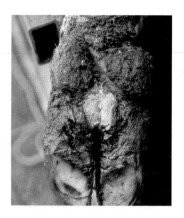

Plate 31.13 Digital dermatitis and slurry heel (p. 425).

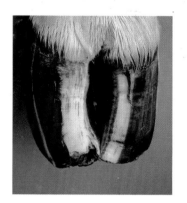

Plate 31.14 A vertical fissure (p. 425).

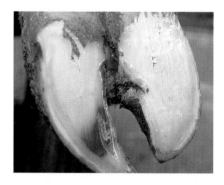

Plate 31.15 Axial wall fissure (p. 426).

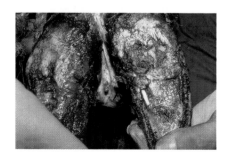

Plate 31.16 Interdigital necrobacillosis (p. 427).

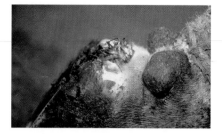

Plate 31.17 The chronic 'hairy wart' form of digital dermatitis (p. 428).

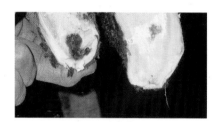

Plate 31.18 Necrosis of the apex of the pedal bone, viewed from the underside of the hoof (p. 429).

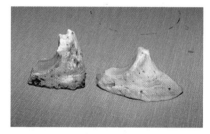

Plate 31.19 Necrosis of the apex of the pedal bone. Note the eroded bone on the left compared to the normal (p. 430).

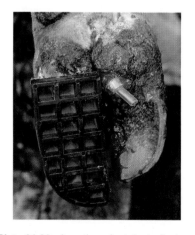

Plate 31.20 Insertion of a tube to flush and drain deep pedal infections (pp. 430, 432).

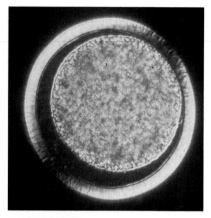

(a) Unfertilized ovum

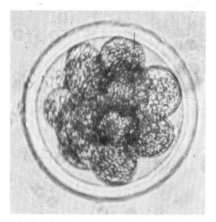

(b) 16-cell embryo (if at this stage on day 7 it will degenerate)

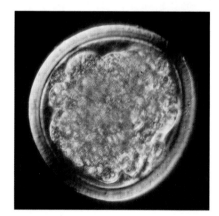

(c) Grade 1 morula

Plate 40.1 Classification and grading of embryos. Photographs courtesy of Colorado State University (p. 635).

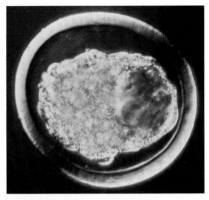

(d) Grade 1 early blastocyst

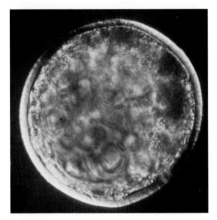

(e) Grade 1 blastocyst

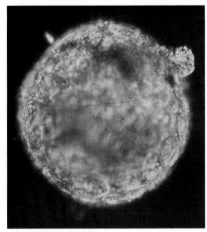

(f) Grade 1 hatched blastocyst

Plate 40.1 *Contd.*

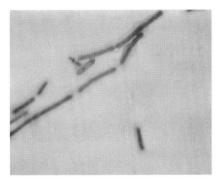

Plate 44.1 *Anthrax bacillium* with typical purple capsules in a smear from blood culture (×850) (courtesy of the Veterinary Investigation Centre, Aberystwyth) (p. 717).

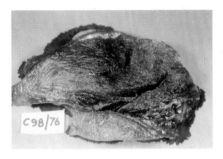

Plate 44.2 Blackleg due to *Clostridium chauveoi* in the thigh muscles of a calf showing the dark, dry and gangrenous lesion (courtesy of the Veterinary Investigation Centre, Carmarthen) (p. 723).

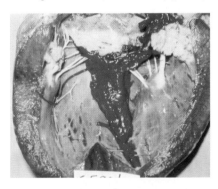

Plate 44.3 Endocarditis. Vegetative growth on the bicuspid valve (courtesy of the Veterinary Investigation Centre, Carmarthen) (p. 727).

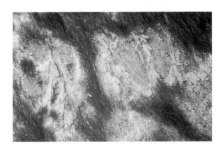

Plate 50.1 Generalized *Trichophyton verrucosum* infection of a Beef Shorthorn bull (p. 878).

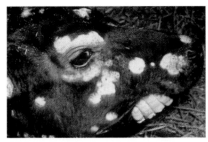

Plate 50.2 *Trichophyton verrucosum* infection of the head of a Friesian calf (p. 878).

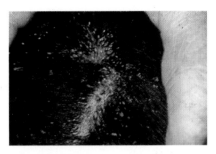

Plate 50.3 *Linognathus vituli* lice and ova (nits) on a calf (p. 880).

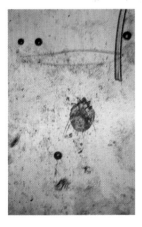

Plate 50.4 Wet preparation in potassium hydroxide solution of *Sarcoptes scabiei*. Mite 240 µm × 200 µm (p. 881).

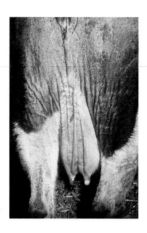

Plate 50.5 Friesian cow with generalized sarcoptic scabies (p. 881).

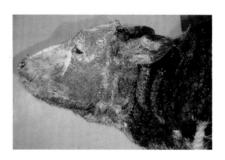

Plate 50.6 Hereford-cross calf with generalized sarcoptic scabies (p. 881).

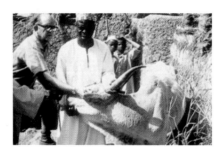

Plate 50.7 Cow with nodular lesions of demodicosis on the neck (northern Nigeria) (p. 882).

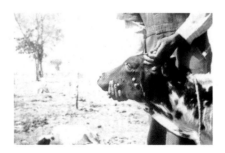

Plate 50.8 Viral papillomatosis. Calf with multiple lesions on the head and neck (p. 883).

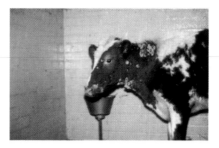

Plate 50.9 Viral papillomatosis. Ayrshire heifer with extensive cauliflower growths on the head and neck (p. 883).

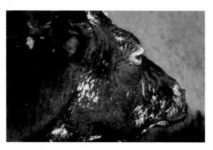

Plate 50.10 Pruritis/pyrexia/haemorrhagic syndrome. Head of a cow showing papule and exudative dermatitis (p. 884).

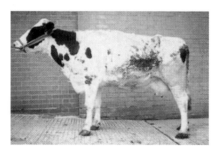

Plate 50.11 Friesian cow with severe photodermatitis (p. 885).

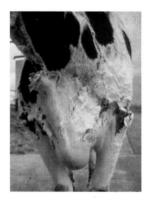

Plate 50.12 Friesian cow with severe photodermatitis. Note the non-affected densely melanotic skin (p. 885).

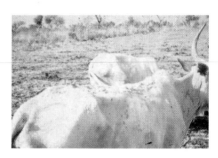

Plate 50.13 Dermatophilosis. Crusted lesions on the dorsum of a cow (northern Nigeria) (p. 886).

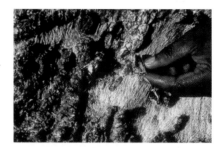

Plate 50.14 Dermatophilosis. Hyperkeratotic scab and crust (northern Nigeria) (p. 886).

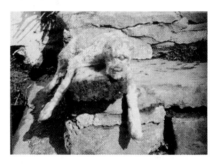

Plate 52.1 Cyclopia in a newly born Jersey calf (p. 918).

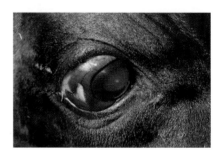

Plate 52.2 (a) Early esotropia (convergent squint) in a three-month-old Friesian calf (p. 918).

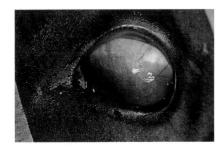

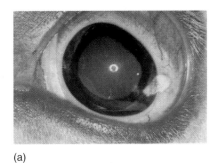

(a)

Plate 52.2 (b) Marked esotropia in an eight-month-old Friesian heifer. The globe has rotated medially to such an extent that mainly scleral tissue is visible within the palpebral fissure (p. 918).

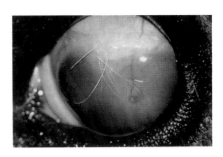

Plate 52.3 Epibulbar dermoid within the dorsal bulbar conjunctiva in a four-month-old Friesian calf; other ocular anomalies were also present (courtesy of S.M. Crispin) (p. 919).

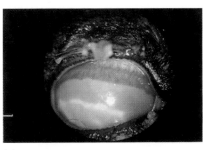

(a)

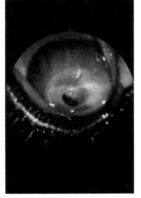

(b)

Plate 52.4 (*left*) Infectious bovine keratoconjunctivitis. (a) At eight days corneal vascularization has occurred. (b) Rupture of the cornea and staphyloma formation. Right eye in six-month-old Friesian (p. 920).

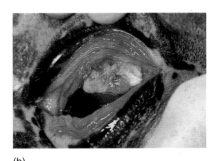

(b)

Plate 52.5 Squamous cell carcinoma. (a) Small precursor papilloma at the lateral limbus in a two-year-old Hereford cow, left eye (courtesy of S.M. Crispin). (b) Extensive involvement of the lateral bulbar conjunctiva, right eye (p. 922).

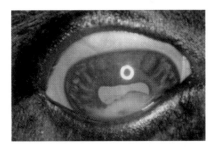

Plate 52.6 Anterior uveitis secondary to a septicaemia of undetermined aetiology. Right eye, two-year-old Friesian (courtesy of S.M Crispin) (p. 923).

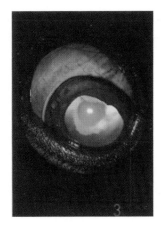

Plate 52.7 Congenital cataract in the right eye of a two-month-old Friesian (p. 923).

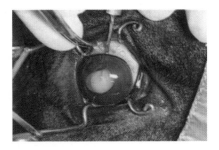

Plate 52.8 Lens discision for the treatment of congenital cataract. The Bowman's discision needle is used to break up the anterior capsule through a dilated pupil, and dislocate the cortical and cataractous lens material into the anterior chamber (p. 924).

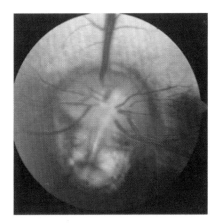

Plate 52.9 Typical papillary coloboma in a 12-month-old Charolais bull (courtesy of K. C. Barnett) (p. 924).

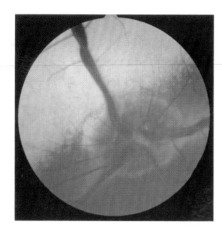

Plate 52.10 Normal bovine fundus with a remnant hyaloid tag over the centre of the optic papilla. Twelve-month-old Friesian (p. 924).

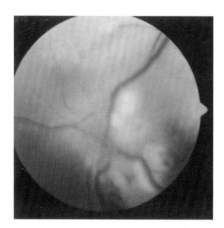

Plate 52.11 Severe papilloedema with disc haemorrhages in a seven-month-old vitamin A deficient calf (courtesy of K. C. Barnett) (p. 925).

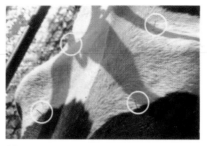

(a)

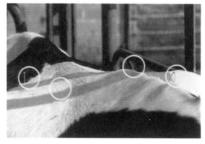

(b)

Plate 65.1 (a & b) Treatment for anoestrus. This comprises needles in Bladder 31 and Bladder 26. Each is bilaterally stimulated. Bladder 26 is antero-lateral to the sacro-iliac joint and Bladder 31 is posterior to this (p. 1098).

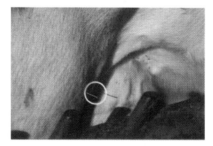

Plate 65.2 Stomach 36. This point is antero-lateral on the proximal end of the tibia in the depression lateral to the tibial crest. This is an important and commonly-used point with a wide variety of actions. This point is called Zusanli and is indicated in the treatment of melancholia, irritability, shyness, posterior paralysis, pain or swelling of the hindquarters, blood pressure defects, malfunction of genital organs and hormonal equilibrium. It is also useful in diseases affecting the skin (p. 1098).

Adult Cattle
Fertility

Chapter 33
Reproductive Physiology in Cattle

P.J. Hartigan

Introduction	471
The hypothalamus	471
The anterior pituitary gland	473
Neuroendocrine links	473
Feedback	474
Endocrine signals: generation and reception	476
Systemic constraints on reproduction	477
Puberty	479
Male physiology	481
Morphology of the testis	482
The spermatozoon	485
Neuroendocrine control	485
The epididymis	487
Seminal plasma	488
Female physiology	488
Oestrous cycle	488
Pregnancy	498
Physiology of the postpartum period	502
Take-home concepts for the clinician	505

Introduction

Reproductive efficiency in a cattle enterprise is a function of good management. Therefore, it is important that the help and advice provided to management by the veterinarian should be based upon a sound appreciation of the physiological mechanisms that control the principal reproductive events.

The essential numerical data on reproduction in cattle are well known: puberty in bulls and heifers at 10–15 months of age; normal oestrous cycles of 18–24 days (mean = 21 days); normal oestrus lasts 12–24 hours (mean = 18 hours); ovulation occurs about 24 hours after the LH peak at the beginning of oestrus; normal gestation lasts 278–293 days; the interval from parturition to first ovulation can be as short as 15 days. The physiological control of each of these events is exerted by a system of interdependent endocrine organs that form the hypothalamic–pituitary–gonadal (HPG) axis, an important limb of the neuroendocrine system.

The primary purpose of this chapter is to provide a succinct outline of the salient features of the neuroendocrine system as it affects reproduction. Why is it con-sidered necessary to do this in a text addressed primarily to clinicians? Essentially, because we believe that it will enhance the reader's understanding of the pathogenesis of many of the reproductive problems encountered in practice and, as a consequence, it will foster a more methodical and perceptive approach to diagnosis and treatment. Underpinning that belief is the knowledge that efficient reproductive performance in the female is dependent on an integrated and precisely timed sequence of hormonal changes that are regulated by the hypothalamus in response to changes in the external and internal environments. Of course, this means that the sequence and timing of the hormonal changes are vulnerable to a great variety of stressors and noxious agents. Many of these deleterious factors have been recognized – and will be mentioned later in the relevant sections – but it is likely that many more remain to be discovered, in particular subtle but significant stressors associated with modern developments in cattle husbandry. The individual best placed to identify 'new causes' of reproductive inefficiency is the informed clinician working with problem herds; however, such insights are less likely if the investigator is not fully alert to the central role of the neuroendocrine mechanisms and their sensitivity to the effects of dietary and metabolic factors, hormone imbalances, stressors, drugs, age and many other influences.

The hypothalamus

In the neuroendocrine system the dominant role is played by the hypothalamus, which acts as a relay station where neural and hormonal messages are decoded and translated into appropriate signals to ensure the cooperation of the endocrine system with the nervous system in regulatory activities. It is able to do so because it contains many neurones that are capable of forming and releasing peptide hormones (neurohormones) that regulate the functions of various organs, principally via the pituitary gland.

These regulatory peptides are synthesized and packaged into granules in the cell body of the neurone

471

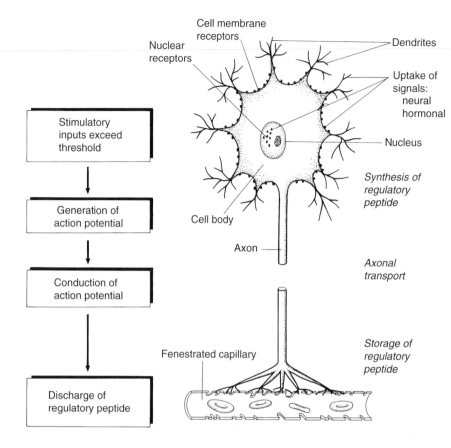

Fig. 33.1 This diagrammatic representation of a typical peptidergic
neurone depicts: (i) the uptake of
neural signals by dendrites; (ii) the
uptake of endocrine signals by specific
receptors located either in the cell
membrane (for water-soluble hormones: peptides, proteins) or in the
nucleus (for lipid-soluble hormones:
steroids, thyroid hormones); (iii) the
endocrine response to signals (synthesis, transport and storage of
regulatory peptide); (iv) the neural
response to signals (generation and
conduction of action potential, which is
responsible for the discharge of the
regulatory peptide).

before they are transported down the axon to the nerve terminals where they are stored pending release. The peptidergic neurones retain the electrophysiological properties of nervous tissue and they use their electrical activity to release the peptides.

A typical peptidergic neurone (Fig. 33.1) has many hundreds of synapses and through these it receives neural inputs (information) from most parts of the brain. (It also receives information from humoral inputs; we shall return to this topic later.) The neural and humoral inputs may be stimulatory or inhibitory; at any one moment the response of the peptidergic neurone will reflect its assessment of the current interplay between the synergistic and conflicting stimuli. When the stimulatory inputs exceed a critical threshold an action potential is generated, the nerve impulse passes down the axon and it causes the release of the (stored) peptide at the nerve terminals. Usually, the nerve terminals are in close apposition to capillaries with highly fenestrated walls that allow the peptide molecules to enter the vascular circulation promptly on release.

A simple example to illustrate the physiological phenomena just described is the milk ejection reflex (Fig. 33.2). This reflex depends on a suckling-induced release of oxytocin. Oxytocin is produced by peptidergic

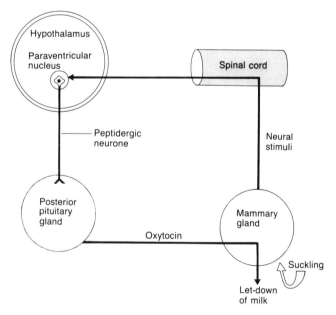

Fig. 33.2 Diagrammatic representation of the suckling reflex, in which neural stimuli elicit an endocrine response.

neurones whose cell bodies are located (principally) in the paired paraventricular nuclei in the hypothalamus and whose axons pass through the pituitary stalk into the posterior pituitary gland. Suckling evokes sensory impulses that travel via the spinal cord to the brain where they converge on the paraventricular nuclei and generate the impulses in the peptidergic neurones that lead to the release of oxytocin from the nerve endings in the posterior pituitary gland. The reflex is completed when the oxytocin in the blood perfusing the mammary gland induces 'let down' of milk. Conceptually, this is neuroendocrine regulation at its simplest: the neurone that 'reads' the afferent sensory message also produces and releases the effector hormone. This is possible only because the posterior pituitary gland, which arises as a downgrowth of neural tissue from the floor of the third ventricle, retains a direct neural link with the hypothalamus.

The anterior pituitary gland

The anterior pituitary gland (adenohypophysis) arises as an upgrowth from the roof of the primitive mouth and, therefore, it does not have a direct neural link with the hypothalamus. A vascular route has to be used to bring the regulatory peptides from the hypothalamus to the adenohypophysis. A specialized arrangement of the vasculature, the hypothalmo–hypophyseal portal system, has evolved for that purpose. In contrast to the normal sequence of arterioles, capillaries and venules, a portal system begins and ends with capillaries. In this instance, the superior hypophyseal artery gives rise to a plexus of capillaries (the primary plexus) in the region of the median eminence at the top of the pituitary stalk. From this the blood is drained by the hypophyseal portal veins, which pass down the pituitary stalk to end in a secondary plexus (the sinusoidal capillaries) within the anterior pituitary gland (Fig. 33.3). From there the blood returns to the general circulation via the anterior hypophyseal vein.

In contrast to the posterior pituitary gland, which does not produce the hormones it releases, the anterior lobe actually synthesizes the trophic hormones it releases into the circulation, including the gonadotrophins: follicle stimulating hormone (FSH) and luteinizing hormone (LH). However, the release of the trophic hormones is governed by stimulatory or inhibitory peptides produced in the hypothalamus. For instance, the secretion of FSH and LH is controlled by a gonadotrophin-releasing hormone (GnRH), which is synthesized by peptidergic neurones in the hypothalamus and is brought to the anterior pituitary gland via the hypothalamo–hypophyseal portal system. The axons of the neurones that produce GnRH end in the median eminence, in close apposition to the fenestrated capillaries of the primary plexus. When a nerve impulse induces a discharge of GnRH from the nerve terminals, this hypothalamic factor is transported via the primary

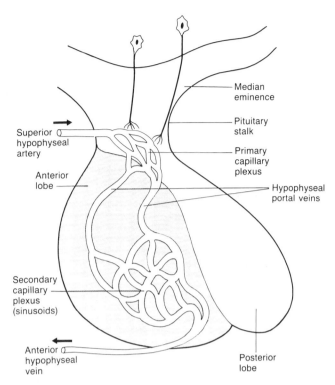

Fig. 33.3 The primary capillary plexus, the hypophyseal portal veins and the secondary capillary plexus form the hypothalamo–hypophyseal portal system that intervenes between the superior hypophyseal artery and the anterior hypophyseal vein. This is the route taken by GnRH which is synthesized by neurones whose cell bodies lie within the arcuate nucleus of the hypothalamus and whose axons abut onto the external walls of the capillaries in the primary plexus.

plexus, the hypophyseal portal veins and the secondary plexus to the secretory cells of the anterior lobe. It stimulates the release of the gonadotrophins, which enter the general circulation via the draining anterior hypophyseal vein. Other hypothalamic factors may exert inhibitory actions in the anterior pituitary gland, e.g. prolactin inhibitory factor (dopamine).

Neuroendocrine links

Since the peptidergic neurones form the functional links between the neural and endocrine systems, they need to be able to receive, decipher and react to signals generated by either system in response to changes in the internal and external environments. Neural signals from other regions of the brain converge on the hypothalamus bringing important cues from the special senses (sight, sound, smell), various exteroceptors (suckling, mating, pain), interoceptors (stimulation of

(a)

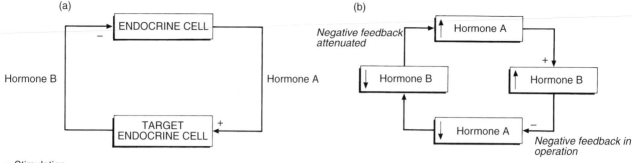

+ Stimulation
− Inhibition

Fig. 33.4 Negative feedback. Example: hormone A, FSH; hormone B, oestrogen. FSH stimulates the production of oestrogen by the granulosa cells of the ovarian follicle. The oestrogen exerts an inhibitory effect on the release of FSH by the pituitary gland. When the oestrogen declines the negative feedback is attenuated and secretion of FSH is increased.

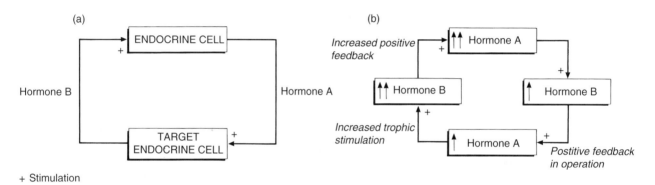

+ Stimulation

Fig. 33.5 Positive feedback. Example: the gonadotrophins FSH and LH (hormone A) stimulate the secretion of oestrogen (hormone B) by the granulosa cells of the preovulatory ovarian follicle (see Fig. 33.24). The rapidly rising concentration of oestrogen (the 'oestrogen surge') stimulates the hypothalamus and the pituitary gland to release a surge of gonadotrophins that is responsible for ovulation. Dilution abolishes the positive feedback at source.

the cervix and uterus) and stressors (physical, emotional, overcrowding). The peptidergic neurones also respond to humoral signals, especially to hormones acting through feedback loops. Again, the input may be stimulatory (positive feedback) or inhibitory (negative feedback). Although there are some important positive feedbacks, e.g. oestrogen prior to ovulation, the majority of feedback loops are negative.

Feedback

In its simplest form, a negative feedback loop (Fig. 33.4a) is a closed system in which hormone A stimulates the production and release of hormone B which, in turn, has an inhibitory effect on the cells that produce hormone A. Such a loop provides a very efficient mechanism by which circulating hormones are maintained

within stable normal limits while retaining their responsiveness to the immediate needs of the body. For instance, when the concentration of hormone B in the circulation rises towards its upper normal limit it exerts negative feedback on its trophic hormone. Thus, hormone A is prevented from exceeding its upper normal limit; the concentration of A in the circulation declines and, of course, so does the activity of its target cells. The resultant decline in hormone B attenuates the negative feedback inhibition (Fig. 33.4b) and the secretion of hormone A is enhanced before it falls below its lower normal limit.

In a positive feedback loop (Fig. 33.5a) hormone B stimulates rather than inhibits the production of more hormone A. This is an inherently unstable system in that it is liable to generate ever-increasing quantities of each of the hormones (Fig. 33.5b); in other words, it lacks the checks and balances of a negative feedback system. However, it is ideal for situations that call for

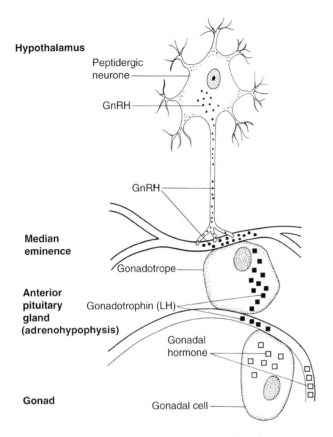

Fig. 33.6 Secretory cells in series: peptidergic neurone secretes GnRH; gonadotrope secretes LH, FSH; gonadal cell secretes testosterone, progesterone or oestrogen.

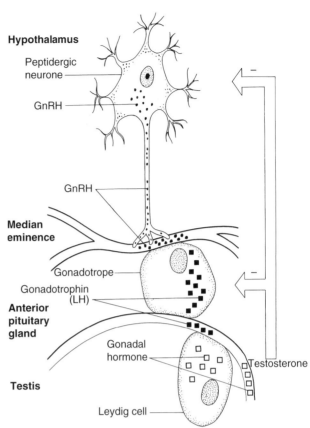

Fig. 33.7 Long loop negative feedback. LH induces Leydig cells to secrete testosterone; testosterone exerts so-called long loop feedback (i) on adrenohypophysis (suppressing secretion of LH) and (ii) on hypothalamus (suppressing secretion of GnRH).

short-term but self-limiting responses. The positive feedback loop may be a purely hormonal phenomenon; for example, the brief but highly significant period of positive feedback by oestrogen that elicits the preovulatory surge of LH. Other important positive feedback mechanisms are initiated by neural stimuli from exteroceptors, e.g. the suckling reflex, or interoceptors, e.g. stretch receptors in the cervix and vagina during the second stage of parturition, that induce reflex release of oxytocin. These two reflexes are excellent examples of self-limiting responses; removal of the physical stimulus terminates the reflex response almost at once.

The feedback mechanisms involved in the control of the reproductive tract are complex and involve several sets of secretory cells in series (Fig. 33.6). For descriptive purposes, three types of complex feedback loops are recognized:

- Long loop: for example, gonadal hormones acting at the level of the brain or pituitary gland (Fig. 33.7).

- Short loop: for example, pituitary gonadotrophins acting at the level of the hypothalamus (Fig. 33.8).
- Ultra-short loop: hypothalamic peptides acting at the level of the hypothalamus (Fig. 33.9).

The feedback effect of a particular hormone is not an intrinsic property of the molecule itself; for instance, although oestrogen is inhibitory (negative long loop feedback), during most of the oestrous cycle it exercises an essential stimulatory effect (positive long loop feedback) shortly before ovulation. Clearly, a single hormone can vary the message it conveys to the hypothalamus. This raises a crucial question: how do the gonadal steroids, the pituitary gonadotrophins and the hypothalamic peptides encode the signals that constitute the feedback messages? By definition, feedback depends on the ability of the target tissues to detect changes in hormone concentrations in the circulation, and to induce the appropriate readjustments (further changes). Hence, the system

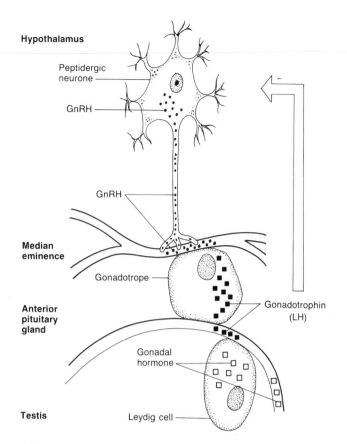

Fig. 33.8 Short loop negative feedback. GnRH induces the gonadotropes to secrete LH; LH exerts negative feedback on the release of GnRH by the hypothalamus.

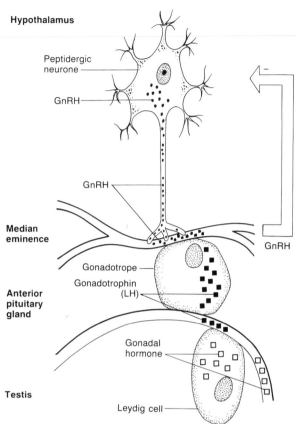

Fig. 33.9 Ultra-short loop negative feedback. The hypothalamic hormone (GnRH) regulates its own secretion.

depends on fluxes rather than constancy as the means of communication.

Endocrine signals: generation and reception

Two basic types of endocrine signals are used: pulses and surges (Fig. 33.10). A pulse of a particular hormone is a discrete burst of secretion of relatively short duration and modest amplitude. A surge occurs when a sequence of frequent pulses, often of high amplitude, produces a massive increase extending over a period of 12–24 hours.

Endocrine signals are detected only by cells that have specific receptors to which a particular hormone will bind. When the hormone interacts with the cells that produce it we refer to autocrine stimulation; when it interacts with another cell type located near the producer cell we call it paracrine stimulation; when it enters the blood stream and interacts with target cells elsewhere we call it endocrine stimulation. The recep-

tors may be located in the cell membrane or within the cell, mainly in the nucleus (see Figs 33.1 and 33.11). The polypeptide hormones, e.g. GnRH, and the glycoprotein hormones, e.g. LH, FSH, bind to receptors in the cell membrane (Fig. 33.11a), whereas the lipid-soluble gonadal steroids can diffuse through the cell membrane to react with intracellular receptors (Fig. 33.11b). The location of the specific receptors determines the mechanism by which the target cells express their characteristic responses to a hormone and, in turn, the different mechanisms determine the speed at which the final response is elicited.

When a gonadal hormone binds to its specific receptor in the nucleus of a target cell, it initiates a series of biochemical reactions that takes several hours to produce the new proteins that elicit the characteristic response to that hormone (Fig. 33.11b). By contrast, when a gonadotrophin binds to its receptor in the cell membrane, it elicits the final response much more rapidly because the resultant cascade of enzymatic activity utilizes enzymes that exist already within the cell. Binding of the hormone (the 'first messenger') to

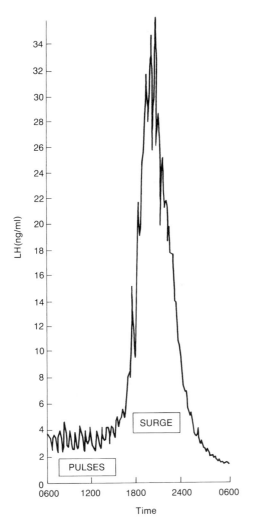

Fig. 33.10 Preovulatory surge of LH on day 18 of the oestrous cycle in a cow. (Redrawn from Rahe *et al.*, 1980).

the receptor activates an enzyme within the cell membrane that acts as a catalyst in a reaction that produces a 'second messenger', e.g. cyclic AMP, that, in turn, alters the activities of the enzymes that produce the final and characteristic response by the cell (Fig. 33.11a).

The sensitivity of a target tissue to a particular hormone will vary depending upon the number of specific receptors it has available for binding that hormone. At any time, the number of receptors depends on the balance between degradation and synthesis of receptors. A hormonal stimulus may increase the sensitivity of a target tissue by increasing the rate of synthesis of the specific receptors; a good example of this 'up regulation' is the increase in LH receptors induced in the granulosa cells of the preovulatory follicle by FSH

(see p. 492). Alternatively, the hormone stimulus may decrease the sensitivity of the target tissue because it increases the degradation and/or decreases the synthesis of receptors; for instance, GnRH can 'down regulate' its own receptors in the adenohypophysis, especially when the gonadotropes are subjected to constant stimulation rather than pulsatile stimulation by the releasing hormone (see p. 497).

The inherent mode of secretion of hormones in the neuroendocrine system is pulsatile and it is controlled by an oscillator or pulse generator in the hypothalamus. The activity of the pulse generator can be modulated both by neural inputs and by feedback signals from the median eminence, the pituitary gland and the gonads. In turn, the pulse generator will seek to ensure that the characteristics of the signals emanating from the pituitary gland and the gonads are altered so as to elicit the appropriate responses from target tissues in the reproductive tract. In that way the hypothalamus exercises fine tuning as well as gross control over reproductive events such as puberty, gametogenesis, oestrus, pregnancy, parturition and lactation.

Before we deal with the neuroendocrine regulation of those processes, it is appropriate to mention three systemic conditions that can constrain the reproductive system: energy balance, stress and neural–immune interactions.

Systemic constraints on reproduction

Energy balance

Although reproduction is critical for the survival of the species, processes that are of more immediate importance for the survival of the individual take top priority when an animal allocates available metabolic fuels among various energy-consuming activities (Fig. 33.12). Hence, changes in the availability of metabolic fuels affect reproductive functions, through actions at multiple sites in the central nervous system, pituitary gland, gonads and other peripheral organs (e.g. liver, skeletal muscles, adipose tissue). Negative energy balance leads to metabolic trade-off in which reproductive activity is curtailed, sometimes suspended. The suspension leaves the regulatory neuroendocrine apparatus intact; reproductive efforts can be resumed when the energy deficit has been repaired.

In many simple-stomach species the neural mechanisms that control the pulsatile release of GnRH (and, consequently, LH secretion and ovarian function) appear to respond to minute-by-minute changes in the availability of metabolic fuels (Bronson, 1989; Wade & Schneider, 1992). The response in ruminants may not be as immediate but it is significant, nonetheless. According to Roche *et al.* (2000), cattle are very sensitive to

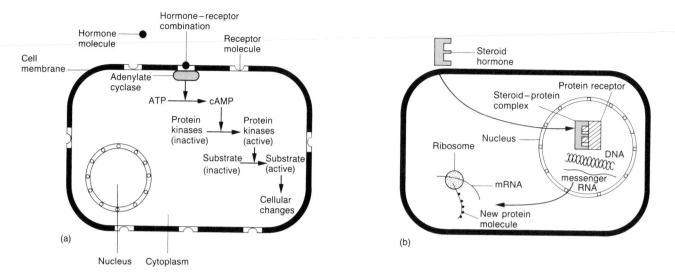

Fig. 33.11 Interaction of hormones with target cells. In (a) a glycoprotein (the 'first messenger') binds with receptors in the cell membrane and activates adenylate cyclase in the membrane. Adenylate cyclase converts ATP to cyclic AMP (the 'second messenger') which, in turn, activates various protein kinases. The resultant cascade of enzymatic activity produces the characteristic cell response to the endocrine signal. In (b) a steroid hormone enters the nucleus where it binds to its receptor. The receptor–hormone complex binds to a particular region of DNA and activates particular genes. The activated genes promote the synthesis of particular messenger RNA molecules that pass from the nucleus to the cytoplasm where they induce the synthesis of proteins (mainly enzymes) that are responsible for the characteristic actions of that hormone in that cell type.

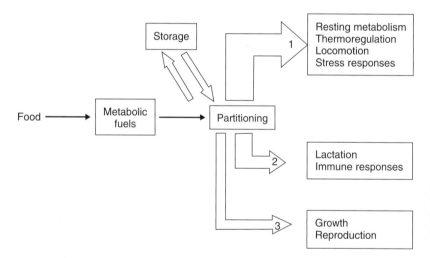

Fig. 33.12 Partitioning of energy by a lactating cow. The sizes of the arrows indicate the order of priorities rather than the quantities of metabolic fuels allocated to the different activities.

acute nutritional deprivation: after a lapse of three to five days, follicular growth is impeded and ovulatory ability is reduced. Chronic nutritional deprivation results in delayed puberty and, in adult females, it causes extended postpartum anoestrus and prolonged calving intervals.

Stress (see Chapter 67)

The effects of stress on reproductive functions are complex: during the stress response increased activity of the sympathetic nervous system induces catabolic responses that mobilize energy, promote its expenditure, and leave less available for use by the HPG axis; concurrently, cortisol released by the hypothalamic–pituitary–adrenal (HPA) axis acts as a counter-regulatory signal at all critical points in the HPG axis and at target tissues for the gonadal steroids (see Fig 67.6). Short-term acute stressors active at critical times in the reproductive cycle of a female can disrupt the orderly timed sequence of hormonal changes on which reproductive success is predicated. In such circumstances, failure to establish a pregnancy may be a 'one-off' eventuality without residual effects on the next attempt. On the other hand, stressors that generate allostatic load (see Chapter 67) may lead to attenuation or suspension of reproductive activities for periods of weeks or months until the counter-regulatory signals are quenched. In such cases, inhibition of the pulsatile release of GnRH may be the most significant action in the context of self-preservation of the organism, but inhibition at other critical points in the HPG axis may be responsible for more persistent carry-over effects during the recovery phase. Recovery of reproductive efficiency requires that the appropriate biochemical features (receptors, G-proteins, transcription factors, other signalling proteins, enzymes, metabolic cascades) be restored and functional at each of the critical points in the HPG axis. As happens at puberty and, again, in the early postpartum period, it may require more than one attempt to fully up-regulate the normal cascade of the HPG axis and reinstate the ability to reproduce.

Neuro-immune interactions

In recent years it has become increasingly evident that the interactions *between* behavioural, neural, endocrine and immune processes are as important to our understanding of homeostasis as are the interactions *within* each of the individual disciplines. In the present context, we focus on the bidirectional network through which the CNS and the immune system exert profound effects on each other. The nervous system impacts upon the immune system through several routes, systemic and local, including neuroendocrine pathways (e.g. the HPA axis), autonomic nerves and systemic nerves. In the reciprocal relationship, cytokines (see Box 33.1)

Box 33.1. Cytokines

Molecules, proteins or glycoproteins, produced by one or more cell types that regulate the activities of other cells. They bind to specific receptors on the cell membranes of target cells and, like hormones, they may act locally in autocrine or paracrine fashion, or they may be released into the bloodstream and interact with target cells elsewhere in the body. More than 100 cytokines have been identified; they are classified into several categories: interferons, insulin-like growth factors, interleukins, tumour necrosis factors, growth factors, transforming growth factors, and so on. Amongst a vast range of activities, they participate in haematopoiesis, cell proliferation, immune responses, inflammation, wound healing, modulation of cell metabolism. The nervous system can produce cytokines and it can respond to cytokines released peripherally; for instance, in fever, in sickness behaviour and in modulating neuroendocrine responses – which is the context in which we have introduced the term.

from activated immunocompetent cells can evoke a variety of neural, neuroendocrine, metabolic and behavioural responses regulated by the CNS; the effect is akin to activation of the central neural and hormonal components of the stress response (see Chapter 67): the main routes of communication are via the sympathetic nervous system and the HPA axis. The noradrenaline and glucocorticoids released by the counter-regulatory loops invoked by the cytokines can have profound biological effects in terms of the expenditure of energy, immunosuppression and interference with the functions of the HPG axis. Thus, for instance, the cross-talk between the brain and the immune system evoked by a severe bout of mastitis in early lactation can have a seriously negative impact on the restoration of cyclic ovarian activity and fertility.

Puberty (see also Chapter 5)

Puberty, the process by which animals become capable of producing offspring, is often given a very restricted definition. According to Short (1984), 'we generally refer to puberty as that moment at which the female first comes into oestrus and ovulates, or the male first produces spermatozoa in his ejaculate'. The trouble with this widely-held perception of puberty is that it concentrates exclusively on the apparent end-point of a protracted and complex physiological process and suggests that puberty is a discrete event that can be assigned to a particular day (or moment!). There is the additional problem that the apparent end-point (first release of the gametes) is not necessarily conclusive evidence that the animal has now reached the stage at which it can reproduce itself; for instance, it is clear that many heifers may not be capable of doing so until well after first ovulation.

In fact, the onset of puberty is a gradual process that is in train for several months during which there are significant morphological, physiological and behavioural responses to the progressive expression of both the steroidogenic and gametogenic activities of the gonads. The essential feature of the process is the maturation of the brain–hypothalamic–pituitary–gonadal axis, which culminates in the adult pattern of reproductive activity. The components of the hypothalamic–pituitary–gonadal axis are present before birth and, even at that stage, each component is capable of responding to appropriate hormonal signals. During gestation, steroid hormones released from the placenta have an inhibitory effect on the fetal hypothalamus that suppresses the activities of the axis. After birth the axis becomes an independent regulatory system that secretes increased amounts of gonadotrophins and gonadal steroids. However, the system is restricted to a relatively low level of activity (juvenile level); for instance, in the female the level of activity is well below that required for ovulation or cyclic ovarian activity. The restraint is due partly to fine sensitivity of the GnRH pulse generator to negative feedback by gonadal steroids and partly to inhibitory inputs from the neural circuits that modulate the activities of the hypothalamus.

The transition to sexual maturity is brought about by progressive changes in the neuroendocrine activities of the axis in response to a variety of internal and environmental factors. The 'gonadostat' hypothesis postulates that the essential change during the transition to sexual maturity is a progressive decrease in sensitivity of the hypothalamus to the negative feedback effects of gonadal steroids (Fig. 33.13) so that the frequency of GnRH pulses is increased progressively. This leads to an increase in the sensitivity of the pituitary

gonadotropes to GnRH and to an increase in the responsiveness of the gonads to the gonadotrophins (Fig. 33.14). Greater quantities of gonadotrophins are released from the pituitary gland and, in turn, greater quantities of steroids are released by the gonads. For instance, in the female the sensitivity of the hypothalamus to the negative feedback effect of oestrogen declines progressively and, as it does so, the increasing quantities of oestrogen from the ovaries can no longer hold the axis within the juvenile pattern of activity. There is a gradual movement of the regulatory system towards the adult pattern (Figs 33.13 and 33.14). Eventually, the ovaries produce a surge of oestrogen that exerts a positive feedback effect on the pulse generator in the hypothalamus (Fig. 33.14) and this induces a surge of LH that leads to ovulation.

As our knowledge of these changes expands, there is increasing evidence that sexual maturity is regulated to

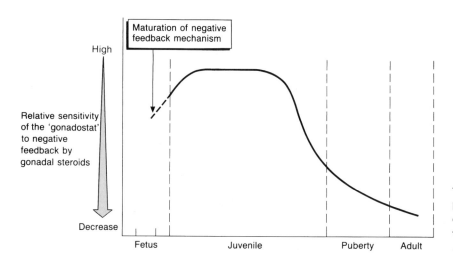

Fig. 33.13 Maturation of the negative feedback system and changes in set point of the hypothalamic gonadostat extending from fetal life through puberty to adulthood (modified from Grumbach *et al.*, 1974).

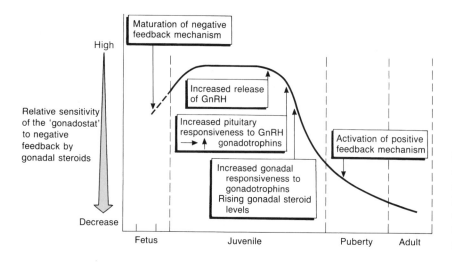

Fig. 33.14 The change in set point of the hypothalamic gonadostat (denoted by the dashed and solid lines) and the maturation of the negative and positive feedback mechanisms from fetal life to adulthood (from Grumbach *et al.*, 1974).

a considerable extent by changing patterns of neural control over the hypothalamus. These alterations in intrinsic neural activity do not appear to be dependent on gonadal hormones; however, they play a crucial role in that they gradually release the GnRH pulse generator from the restraints exercised by the central nervous system during the juvenile period, thus enabling it to respond to the gonadal steroids in the adult manner. It is evident that the classical 'gonadostat' hypothesis does not furnish an entirely satisfactory explanation of the onset of puberty in all its details. Nevertheless, it does provide a conceptual framework that is adequate for the purposes of this text.

The first ovulation is likely to be silent; it appears that the hormonal requirements for the expression of oestrus are small quantities of progesterone from a regressing corpus luteum followed by a surge of oestrogen from the preovulatory follicle – a sequence that is absent at the time of first ovulation. Thus, the first oestrus observed by the stockperson indicates that the process of puberty is well advanced but it does not provide a precise date for the 'moment' of puberty.

The earliest possible maturation of the individual components of the reproductive axis (and, therefore, of the axis itself) is determined by genes, i.e. there are inherent breed variations in the onset of puberty. However, in all breeds this process is subject to delays caused by a variety of endogenous and exogenous influences, some of which can be manipulated by the stockperson to ensure that the heifer is ready for breeding at the desired time. The principal environmental factors that influence the onset of puberty are: season of birth, level of nutrition, growth rate, photoperiod, high ambient temperatures, intercurrent diseases and presence of the male.

Specific reference to these factors will be made in the clinical segment of the text. For the moment, suffice it to say that, as a general guideline, the stockperson should devise a management strategy in the knowledge that the onset of puberty is a labile process that is conditioned by competition between the reproductive system and the other body systems of the growing animal for energy and specific nutrients. Reproduction, particularly in the female where it involves pregnancy followed by lactation, is an energy-consuming process to which Nature assigns a relatively low priority for the prepubertal animal. Evidence is accumulating from work on a number of species that inadequate intake of energy or nutrients can depress or abolish the activities of the GnRH pulse generator in the juvenile animal. This has been attributed, variously, to deficiencies in body weight, in rate of growth, in fat content or in fat:lean ratio. There is no agreement on the particular cue(s) that inhibit(s) the pulse generator but there is general acceptance of the thesis that the function of the generator is closely coupled with energy balance and that it is allowed to progress from the juvenile to the adult level of activity in the female only when the energetic status appears to be adequate to sustain pregnancy and lactation. It was anticipated that the hormone leptin, produced by adipose tissues, might prove to be the signal that triggers the onset of puberty: current evidence is that leptin is just one of many permissive metabolic factors that allow pubertal development to proceed; it may act as a permissive signal to increase GnRH secretion after the pulse generator has been sensitized to energy balance by other developmental or metabolic cues; it is not the trigger for the beginning of puberty (Urbanski, 2001; Smith et al., 2002).

Selective culling is an integral part of efficient management of the dairy herd. It can be practised successfully only when the stockperson has available an adequate number of high-quality heifers due to calve down at the appropriate time. This requires careful management of the prepubertal animal to ensure that the reactivation of the hypothalamic pulse generator is not delayed unduly by environmental influences, principally nutritional factors and subclinical diseases.

Similarly, young bulls intended for breeding purposes require careful management during the juvenile period because the onset of puberty in the male is also influenced by a variety of factors (including breed, season of birth, energy intake and liveweight gain) that affect the reactivation of the hypothalamic GnRH pulse generator.

Male physiology

In the male, puberty is associated with changes in the pattern of LH secretion, a gradual increase in the concentration of testosterone in the blood, rapid growth of the testes and the initiation of spermatogenesis. In essence, the adult pattern of GnRH release is attained and the testes proceed to fulfil two primary functions: the synthesis and release of androgens (steroidogenesis) and the production of spermatozoa (gametogenesis). In most male mammals, these functions are performed best at temperatures somewhat lower than body core temperature.

In the bull the testes are located in the pendulous scrotum, where they are attuned to function at 3–4°C below core temperature. The three principal mechanisms by which the scrotal temperature is reduced are as follows:

(1) Precooling of the arterial blood supply as it passes through the vascular cone in the spermatic cord. The vascular cone consists of a coiled segment of the spermatic artery that is surrounded by the

pampiniform plexus of the spermatic vein. Because of this anatomical arrangement the arterial blood and the venous blood are flowing in parallel but in opposite directions; this allows for an efficient countercurrent exchange of heat between the two vessels. The net result is that the arterial blood delivered to the testes is several degrees below body core temperature.

(2) Sweating from the many sweat glands in the scrotal skin.

(3) Physical contact with cold ground or other cold objects.

In very cold weather, the temperature at the base of the scrotum may be up to 7°C below core values but the bull can attempt to curtail the drop in temperature by drawing the scrotum closer to the (relatively) warm body wall by contracting the cremaster and dartos muscles.

The gametogenic function of the testes is much more heat sensitive than the steroidogenic function; for instance, a retained testicle in a cryptorchid animal ('rig') may secrete androgens but the seminiferous tubules will remain infantile in structure and they will not produce spermatozoa. The retained testicle has a propensity to develop neoplasms (see p. 182).

Morphology of the testis

The testis is surrounded by a thick fibrous capsule, the tunica albuginea, from which septa project inwards to divide the substance of the testis into lobules (Fig. 33.15). Each lobule contains one to four highly convoluted seminiferous tubules and interstitial tissue that fills the spaces between the convolutions.

The interstitial tissue contains blood vessels, lymphatic vessels, nerves and the steroid-secreting Leydig cells.

The seminiferous tubules are about 200μm in diameter and they may be up to 70cm long; they open at both ends into the rete testis (Fig. 33.15). The tubules contain two populations of cells: (i) a fixed population of non-proliferating somatic cells, the Sertoli cells, and (ii) a migratory population of proliferating, differentiating germ cells (Fig. 33.16).

Sertoli cells

The Sertoli cells have been described as the 'backbone' of the tubule. They are columnar cells that rest on the basement membrane and extend the full depth of the epithelial layer; they envelop the developing germ cells in deep recesses in their lateral walls and, ultimately, in their luminal surfaces. The Sertoli cells continually alter shape to accommodate the morphological changes in the germ cells during their migration from the base to the luminal surface. The plasma membranes of adjacent Sertoli cells form specialized interepithelial tight junctions that extend entirely around the circumference of each cell (Fig. 33.17). These junctions constitute the epithelial component of the blood–testis barrier that precludes the passage of many substances from the blood or interstitial fluid into the lumen of the seminiferous tubule. They also divide the intercellular spaces into two compartments: the basal compartment that contains the undifferentiated germ cells and the adluminal compartment that provides the appropriate microenvironment for the more differentiated germ cells (see below).

The basal surface of the Sertoli cell has specific receptors for FSH. The cells respond to the gonadotrophin by secreting (i) a nutrient fluid that sustains the germ cells in the intercellular spaces, (ii) androgen-binding protein that binds and transports testosterone to the epididymis and (iii) inhibin that modulates the secretion of FSH by negative feedback at the pituitary gland (Fig. 33.18). Sertoli cells also have receptors for androgens; it is known that testosterone can maintain the functional integrity of the Sertoli cell when FSH is withdrawn.

Sertoli cells are resistant to relatively high levels of heat, ionizing radiation and many toxins (e.g. cadmium, nitrofurans, cytotoxins) that destroy differentiating germ cells.

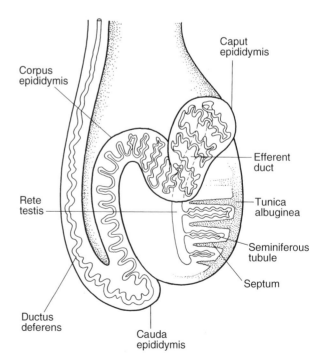

Fig. 33.15 Outline morphology of the testis.

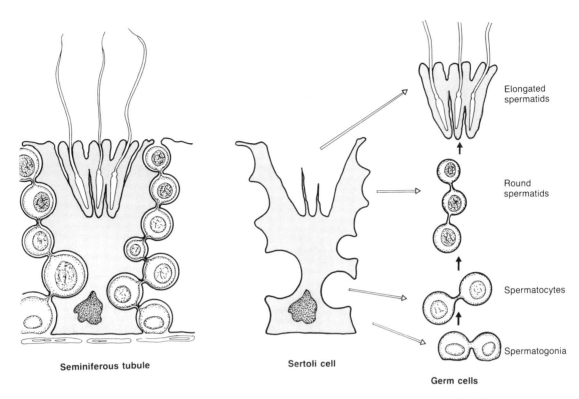

Fig. 33.16 The histology of the seminiferous tubule. The diagram depicts the Sertoli cell and the germ cells in intimate contact as they are *in vivo* and, also, separately to show the outlines of the individual cells. (Adapted from Fawcett, 1994.)

Germ cells

A detailed description of the process of spermatogenesis (see Table 33.1) is beyond the scope of this text. Suffice it to say that the spermatogonia are the stem cells and that they begin the process by undergoing a number of mitotic divisions in the basal compartment. These divisions produce a pool of cells that are joined to each other by intercellular bridges (Fig. 33.19).

Cohorts of spermatogonia from this pool are moved to the adluminal compartment while one spermatogonium from the group remains behind in the basal compartment. It enters a resting phase during which it is highly resistant to ionizing radiation and toxic agents. This will be the stem cell from which the next cycle of spermatogenesis will begin (two weeks later). In the meantime, the newly arrived cells at the base of the adluminal compartment proceed to undergo meiosis as primary spermatocytes (first meiotic division) and secondary spermatocytes (second meiotic division). The haploid secondary spermatocytes are still attached to each other by intercellular bridges and after a short period each of them divides to yield two spermatids. As the process of spermatogenesis proceeds the germ cells move progressively towards the lumen of the tubule,

still attached to the Sertoli cell; the final stages take place at the luminal surface. The conversion of the spermatid to the spermatozoon does not involve cell division, merely morphological reorganization (referred to as spermiogenesis). The principal changes are condensation of the nucleus and acquisition of the acrosome in the head region, reorganization of the mitochondria in the middle piece, development of the tail and loss of excess cytoplasm that moves caudally and is shed as the residual body, which is phagocytosed by the Sertoli cell. The intercellular bridges are lost with the residual bodies and each spermatozoon now is a separate cell, that soon escapes from the luminal surface of the Sertoli cell (spermiation). When the fully developed spermatozoon is released into the lumen of the seminiferous tubule it is non-motile. It is transported passively from the tubule into the rete testis and thence to the epididymis. Motility is acquired during passage through the epididymis.

In summary, during spermatogenesis the germ cells advance through three major processes:

(1) Proliferation of stem cells by mitosis in the basal compartment.
(2) Reduction of the chromosome number by meiosis in the adluminal compartment.

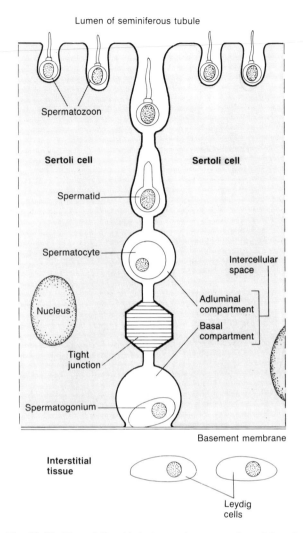

Fig. 33.17 The relationship between the germ cells and Sertoli cells during spermatogenesis.

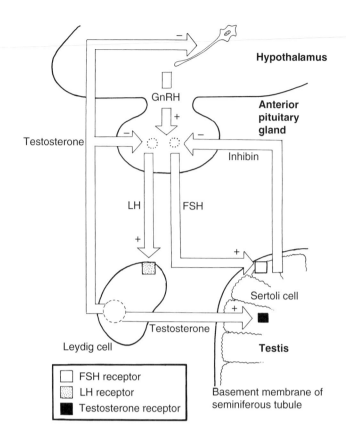

Fig. 33.18 Hormonal interactions in the hypothalamic–pituitary–testicular axis.

Table 33.1 Principal stages in the development of spermatozoa (spermatogenesis).

Cell type	Number of chromosomes
Spermatogonium	2n
Primary spermatocyte	2n
Secondary spermatocyte	n
Spermatid	n
Spermatozoon	n

(3) Morphological transformation of a conventional cell (the spermatid) into the very specialized structure of the spermatozoon (spermiogenesis) in the adluminal compartment.

This sequence of mitotic, meiotic and packaging events requires 56 days for completion in the bull. It is a very orderly sequence in which each of the component cells has a fixed lifespan so that cellular differentiation proceeds at a fixed rate. The spermatogonium that reverts to the resting phase remains quiescent in the basal compartment for 14 days (equivalent to 25 per cent of the entire cycle) before it enters mitosis and begins the next spermatogenic cycle. The cells derived from the new cycle advance in a similar orderly fashion behind the cells from the previous cycle as they move progressively towards the luminal surface. In fact, this arrangement means that four successive cycles of spermatogenesis

will be in train in the seminiferous epithelium at any moment. Furthermore, since both the intervals between the commencement of the cycles and the rates of progress of the cells through spermatogenesis are constant, a histological examination of a cross-section of a seminiferous tubule will reveal a characteristic set of cell associations at any one time. In most mammals the same set of cell associations is seen at all points in the circumference of the tubule (this represents the 'cycle of spermatogenesis'); however, adjacent segments of the tubule tend to have a different set of cell

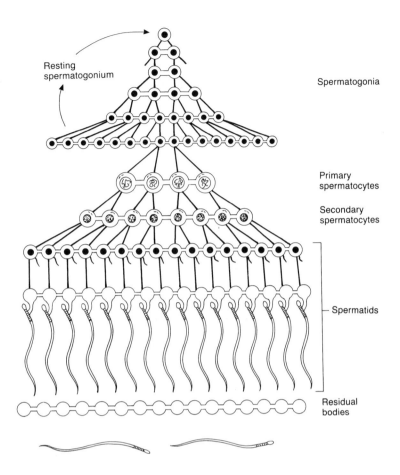

Fig. 33.19 The process of spermatogenesis. (Reproduced from Fawcett, 1994.)

associations, each either in advance of or behind its neighbours (this constitutes the 'wave of spermatogenesis').

Some of the progeny of the original spermatogonia do not complete the full course; large numbers (perhaps 20 per cent) of differentiating germ cells die without reaching maturity and these are removed by the Sertoli cells.

The spermatozoon

The essential features of the mammalian spermatozoon are depicted in Fig. 33.20. Only one structure warrants further comment at this juncture: the acrosome, an organelle that undergoes significant morphological change as an essential prelude to fertilization. The acrosome contains a number of lytic enzymes (particularly hyaluronidase, neuraminidase and acrosin); it has been described as a modified lysosome and, like all lysosomes, it has a bilaminar structure. The inner acrosomal membrane is adherent to the nuclear membrane, while the outer acrosomal membrane underlies the cell membrane. When the ejaculated spermatozoon undergoes the acrosome reaction in the female genital tract, the outer acrosomal membrane forms point fusions with the cell membrane creating a sequence of vesicles over

the head of the sperm and allowing the lytic enzymes to escape through the resultant pores (see p. 499).

Neuroendocrine control

The steroidogenic functions and the gametogenic functions are segregated anatomically: androgen synthesis by the Leydig cells in the interstitial spaces and spermatogenesis within the seminiferous tubules (Fig. 33.17). Both functions are controlled by the pituitary gland through the secretion of the gonadotrophins. Luteinizing hormone binds to specific receptors on the cell membranes of Leydig cells and they respond by secreting androgens (principally testosterone), which in turn inhibit LH secretion by negative feedback. When the concentration of testosterone in the blood declines sufficiently the 'brake' on LH secretion is released and the resultant rise in LH in the circulation induces the Leydig cells to secrete testosterone (Figs 33.18 and 33.21). The negative feedback effect of testosterone on LH secretion is exercised at the level of the hypothalamus (influencing the secretion of GnRH) and at the pituitary gland (modulating the responsiveness of the gonadotropes to GnRH). In this manner the hypothalamic–pituitary–Leydig cell axis maintains the

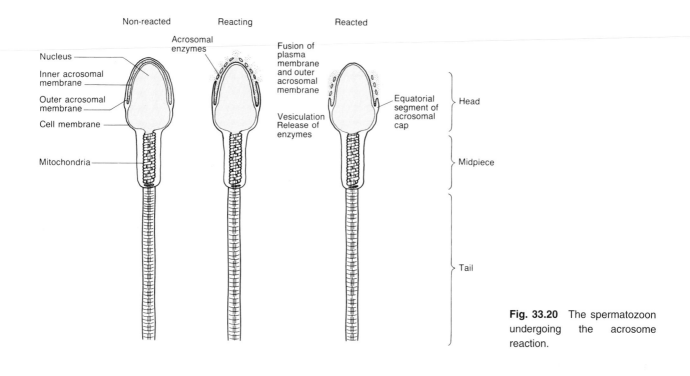

Fig. 33.20 The spermatozoon undergoing the acrosome reaction.

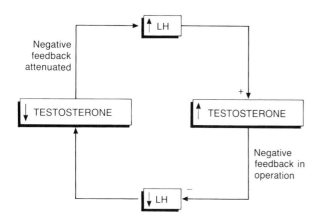

Fig. 33.21 The reciprocal relationship between the concentrations of testosterone and LH in the general circulation.

concentration of testosterone in the general circulation within normal limits.

Sertoli cells respond to FSH by secreting fluids and proteins that sustain the differentiating germ cells. Follicle stimulating hormone is absolutely essential for the initiation of spermatogenesis in immature animals but once the normal germinal epithelium has been established FSH does not appear to be essential for the start of each successive spermatogenic cycle. Another action of FSH is to stimulate the conversion of testosterone to oestradiol by the Sertoli cells. The Sertoli cells also secrete inhibin, a polypeptide that inhibits the release of FSH by the pituitary gland (Fig. 33.18).

There is no doubt that an intact hypothalamic–pituitary–testicular axis is essential for normal testicular function; however, apart from the fact that FSH is essential for the initiation of the process in immature animals, it is unclear what specific roles in the process of spermatogenesis are played by the individual hormones that constitute the axis. On the basis of information available in the literature, the following deductions have gained wide acceptance:

● Differentiating germ cells lack hormone receptors and, therefore, they are not affected directly by the hormones.
● Sertoli cells have specific receptors for FSH and for androgens but not for LH.
● Testosterone is required for the first mitotic division of the stem cell in the basal compartment.
● Testosterone is necessary for the reduction division of the primary spermatocyte.
● FSH is essential for the final steps in the maturation of the spermatids.
● There is controversy as to whether or not testosterone is required for the earlier steps in the maturation of the spermatids.
● It is likely that all the other steps in spermatogenesis can proceed without the specific intervention of a particular hormone.

Thus, FSH and testosterone exercise direct actions on the seminiferous tubules, while LH does so indirectly via the production of testosterone.

Histological–functional

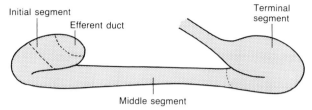

Anatomical

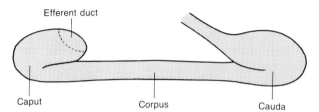

Fig. 33.22 The regions of the bovine epididymis.

It should be noted that even where specific hormonal stimulation is essential, the hormone serves to ensure that the event occurs but it does not alter the rate of progress of spermatogenesis, which is a feature that is determined by genes rather than by hormones.

The epididymis

When spermatozoa are transported from the rete testes through the efferent ducts to the initial segment of the epididymis they are neither motile nor capable of fertilization. They acquire these attributes during passage through the epididymis.

The epididymis is a highly convoluted tubule lined by specialized epithelium and surrounded by connective tissue, which incorporates concentric layers of smooth muscles that increase in thickness from the initial segment to the terminal segment. Anatomists describe the epididymis as consisting of three parts (Figs. 33.15, 33.22): the caput (head), the corpus (body) and the cauda (tail). A more recent histological–functional classification has designated at least eight regions in the epididymis of the bull, but for the purposes of this text it is sufficient to refer to the three principal segments used in that scheme: the initial segment, the middle segment and the terminal segment (Fig. 33.22). The efferent ducts empty into the initial segment, which is specialized for the bulk reabsorption of water and electrolytes. The middle segment, which includes most of the caput and corpus, is responsible for the sperm maturation. The terminal segment, largely the cauda, stores the mature spermatozoa pending ejaculation.

In many species the initial segment is the principal site for absorption of water from the luminal fluids. The

bull is an exception in that the bulk of the water has been absorbed by the efferent ducts before the contents reach the epididymis. The secretions from the epithelial cells of the initial and middle segments induce significant alterations in the functions and composition of most of the component parts of the spermatozoon. The principal functional changes are the acquisition of progressive motility and the ability to fertilize an egg. Fine structural changes have been observed in the plasma membrane, the acrosomal membranes, the nucleus and the tail. Changes in the composition of the plasma membrane appear to be central to the process of maturation of the spermatozoon as it passes through the epididymis; in particular, its protein composition is altered either by adsorption of components from the epididymal fluid or by modification or loss of existing components in response to enzymatic activity of the epididymal fluid. It is important to note that these biochemical changes are associated with the acquisition of the ability to fertilize but they do not complete the process of maturation – this will occur only after the ejaculated spermatozoa have been capacitated within the female genital tract (see p. 499).

Ejaculated spermatozoa have species-specific receptors that bind to the zona pellucida of the egg. The spermatozoa acquire these receptors in the epididymis, under the influence of testicular androgens.

The ability of the epididymis to facilitate maturation of the spermatozoa and to maintain the viability of the mature spermatozoa in the cauda is critically dependent on testicular androgens. Obviously, some of the testosterone reaches the epididymis in the arterial blood but it is probable that most of it comes via the efferent duct system bound to androgen-binding protein. The epithelial cells of the epididymis have androgen receptors and they rapidly convert the testosterone to dihydrotestosterone, which then regulates epididymal functions. It has been clearly established that the maturation of spermatozoa is regulated by dihydrotestosterone rather than by testosterone.

Movement of spermatozoa through the middle segment is by continuous peristaltic contractions of the smooth muscles that surround the epididymal tubule. The rate of transport in this segment is not influenced by ejaculation and in the bull it is estimated to take two to three days. It follows that the fertility of sperm should not be depressed even when the bull is ejaculating frequently. By contrast, the muscles surrounding the terminal segment are relatively inactive except when they are stimulated to contract during ejaculation; it follows that frequency of ejaculation can have a significant effect on the duration of storage of potentially fertile spermatozoa and on the numbers of fertile sperm available for ejaculation at a particular time.

Seminal plasma

The fluid portion of the ejaculate is called the seminal plasma. It consists of the testicular and epididymal secretions in which the spermatozoa are suspended when they pass from the cauda epididymis into the vas deferens plus the secretions from the various accessory glands, which are added as the spermatozoa are propelled along the vas deferens and the urethra during ejaculation. The seminal vesicles contribute fructose, the primary source of energy for the spermatozoa. Prostaglandins in the seminal fluid may assist transport of spermatozoa within the female tract by stimulating contraction of smooth muscle. The bull ejaculates 1–15 ml of semen containing 0.8–2.0×10^9 spermatozoa/ml. (Infertility in bulls is dealt with in Chapter 38 and some aspects of artificial insemination in Chapter 39.)

Female physiology

Oestrous cycle

By definition, the oestrous cycle is the interval between the onset of two successive periods of sexual receptivity (oestrus). Both the expression of oestrus and the duration of the cycle are the result of cyclic changes in the ovaries that involve two temporary endocrine structures (the ovarian follicles and corpora lutea) and their principal secretions (oestrogens and progesterone). For problems associated with the oestrous cycle see Chapter 35.

Oestrus

It has been shown that behavioural oestrus results from exposure of the anterior hypothalamus to both progesterone and oestrogen in physiological concentrations and in the proper temporal sequence. Progesterone on its own inhibits oestrus. Furthermore, in the absence of priming by progesterone, physiological concentrations of oestrogen fail to elicit the signs of oestrus; thus, in the pubertal heifer the first preovulatory follicle produces a surge of oestrogen that feeds back positively on the pulse generator and induces an effective ovulatory surge of LH, but it does not induce behavioural oestrus. In the adult cow the normal sequence is a high concentration of progesterone (P_4) for 10–14 days followed by a rapid decline in P_4 and an immediate increase in oestrogen from the growing preovulatory follicle (Fig. 33.23). This sequence results in behavioural oestrus that appears to be coupled with the preovulatory surge of LH so that ovulation occurs approximately 24 hours after the onset of oestrus.

The duration of oestrus may vary from 8 to 30 hours and the behavioural signs may recur frequently throughout the period or they may be evident during two shorter periods at the beginning and end with a quiescent period between them ('split oestrus').

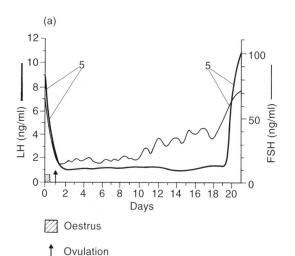

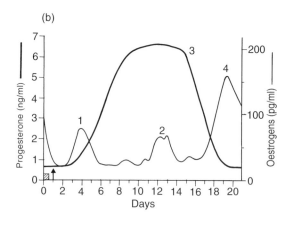

◫ Oestrus

↑ Ovulation

Fig. 33.23 Changes in concentrations of gonadotrophins (a) and ovarian steroids (b) in peripheral plasma during a 21-day oestrous cycle in the cow. During most of the cycle progesterone (P_4) secreted by the corpus luteum (CL) is the dominant hormone, exercising strong negative feedback on the hypothalamic–pituitary axis. However, the tonic concentrations of gonadotrophins released during the luteal phase induce two waves of follicles that are associated with small peaks of oestrogen (1, 2). When the CL regresses, the concentration of P_4 declines (3) and oestrogen concentration climbs to a peak, the oestrogen surge (4), which triggers a surge of gonadotrophins (5) that induces ovulation.

Length of the cycle

The cow is a polyoestrous animal and, if she is not pregnant, she will tend to return to oestrus repeatedly throughout the year at intervals of 18–24 days (mean = 21 days). By convention, the day of oestrus is designated day 0 and the length of the cycle is calculated from that baseline.

There can be considerable variation (within the normal range) in the length of the oestrous cycle: even successive cycles in the same cow may vary by several days. Most of this variation is due to differences in the duration of the luteal phase of the ovarian cycle, i.e. in the functional lifespan of the individual corpus luteum. Luteal regression may begin as early as day 15 or as late as day 19 of normal (20–24-day) cycles.

Regulation of the cycle

From a neuroendocrine perspective, the oestrous cycle is controlled by the secretory activities of three principal components: peptidergic neurones in the hypothalamus, gonadotropes in the adenohypophysis and steroid-secreting cells in the ovaries. It is clear that ultimate control is exercised by the hypothalamus through characteristic cyclic changes in the pattern of GnRH release, which are reflected in the circulating levels of FSH, LH, oestrogens and progesterone. Nevertheless, from the perspective of the practising veterinarian it would appear as if it is the ovary that times the events of the oestrous cycle. That perception will have been reinforced as a result of recent developments in ultrasound technology that have given the clinician visual access to the morphological changes in the female genital tract throughout the reproductive life of the cow; it is likely that it will be strengthened by this presentation, which emphasizes the central importance of the inherent rhythmicity with which cohorts of follicles emerge from the pool of resting follicles. In essence, the following text describes how the responses of the HPG axis determine the fate of the oocytes that are brought forward every seven to ten days in anticipation of being chosen to perpetuate the species.

Follicular development and its control during the oestrous cycle

Basic pattern: Each ovary has a large pool of oocytes, each contained within a follicle. The follicle is the basic functional unit of the female gonad; although it spends much of its lifespan in a dormant state, it does have a brief period of progressive growth and development that ends in either ovulation or degeneration (atresia). During this active phase it is an essential component of the hypothalamic–pituitary–gonadal (HPG) axis. It

Box 33.2. Some regulators of follicular growth.

From the pituitary gland
  Follicle stimulating hormone (FSH)
  Luteinizing hormone (LH)
  Prolactin (PRL)

Ovarian steroids
  Androgens
  Oestrogens
  Progesterone

Other regulatory factors[a]
  Inhibin
  Activin
  Insulin-like growth factor
  Insulin
  Follistatin
  Vascular endothelial growth factor
  Prostaglandins

[a] Chosen from among the scores of factors isolated from intrafollicular/extrafollicular sites. They have important extra-ovarian actions but are listed here in recognition of autocrine and paracrine activities during follicular growth.

responds to the gonadotrophins and it secretes a range of regulatory factors (Box 33.2), including steroid hormones (principally, oestradiol and progesterone) and the polypeptide inhibin; it also facilitates the maturation of the oocyte – but that is not a topic within the remit of this essay.

In its simplest form, the primordial stage, the follicle consists of an oocyte surrounded by squamous pregranulosa cells. The resting primordial follicles are thought to be under constant inhibitory influences to remain dormant. In due course, either due to a decrease in inhibitory influences or to positive stimuli by some paracrine or endocrine factors, growth is initiated in a cohort of primordial follicles. This process of *recruitment* begins long before puberty and is recurrent throughout reproductive life. The fate of a recruited follicle depends on whether or not the mutual interactions between the component parts of the HPG axis can shepherd it to ovulation. Those follicles that fall by the wayside on the long path to ovulation undergo atresia; obviously, that is the fate of all follicles recruited before puberty; it is also the fate of most of the follicles recruited after puberty.

In the adult ovary, most of the follicles progress slowly through several developmental stages to reach the antral stage after four months or so, at which point the follicle has acquired the histological features depicted in Figure 33.24. There is evidence that follicles can develop to the preantral stage in the complete absence of gonadotrophins; thereafter, they are

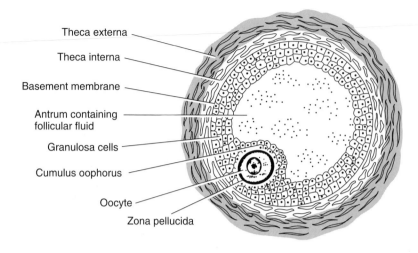

Fig. 33.24 The ovarian follicle has four distinct layers: the theca externa, the highly vascular theca interna, the basement membrane and the avascular granulosa cell layer. The basement membrane prevents direct access of capillaries to the granulosa cell layer.

Theca externa
Theca interna
Basement membrane
Antrum containing follicular fluid
Granulosa cells
Cumulus oophorus
Oocyte
Zona pellucida

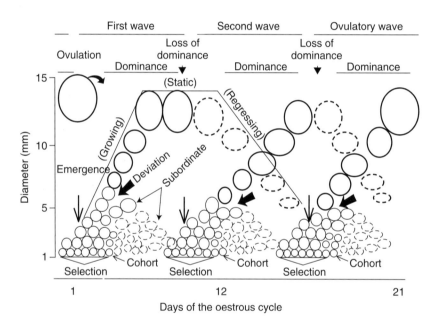

Fig. 33.25 A model explaining the terms associated with each wave of follicular development during the oestrous cycle of heifers. Based on ultrasound analysis, most heifers have one (first wave) or two waves (first wave, second wave) of follicular development during the luteal phase and a single wave of development (ovulatory wave) during the follicular phase. (From Ireland *et al.*, 2000, reproduced with permission of the American Dairy Science Association.)

gonadotrophin-dependent. FSH can stimulate growth of the follicle up to about 9 mm in diameter, while LH is required for further growth and for ovulation. In fact, the HPG axis provides the hormonal milieu that regulates the passage of the antral follicle through a complex sequence of processes known ('in the trade') as emergence, deviation, selection and dominance, and ovulation or atresia (Webb *et al.*, 1999; Ireland *et al.*, 2000).

The inherent pattern of follicular growth in cattle is wave-like (Fig. 33.25); it is set long before puberty and it persists during oestrous cycles, throughout most of pregnancy and during the early anoestrum of the postpartum period. In practice, the *emergence* of a wave is recorded as the first day on which a 4 mm or 5 mm follicle is detected by ultrasonography as the largest in a new cohort of growing follicles. Over the next two or three days all of the emergent follicles grow at a similar rate but then there is an abrupt divergence of individual growth rates (*deviation*; Fig. 33.26): growth continues unabated in one follicle, now grown to approximately 8 mm in diameter and destined to become dominant; in the subordinate follicles it comes to a halt and, soon, is followed by regression (Ginther *et al.*, 2001). About 8 hours before the beginning of deviation, the granulosa cells in the future dominant follicle acquire LH receptors. LH stimulates increased production of oestradiol and of insulin-like growth

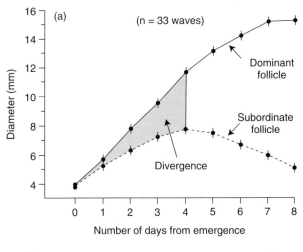

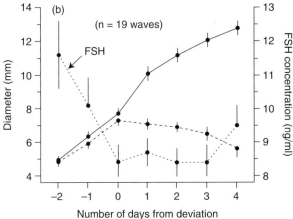

Fig. 33.26 Deviation. The patterns of growth in the dominant follicle and the largest subordinate follicle from the day of emergence. (a) The growth rates gradually diverge. (b) Before deviation, the growth rates did not differ significantly. The concentration of FSH reached a nadir on the day of deviation. (Reproduced from Ginther *et al.*, 1996 with permission of the Society for the Study of Reproduction.)

factor 1 (IGF-1). Systemically, the high levels of oestradiol and inhibin released by the dominant follicle suppress release of FSH from the pituitary gland; there is inadequate concentration of FSH to sustain the smaller follicles and they become atretic (Figs 33.26 and 33.27). Within the dominant follicle, oestradiol and IGF-1 increase the sensitivity of the granulosa cells to FSH, thus enabling that follicle to respond to (and thrive on) the low concentration that contributed to the onset of atresia in the subordinate follicles. If the largest follicle is ablated *before* deviation, the next largest follicle will proceed to dominance. Thus, the follicular wave has two phases (Fig. 33.28): the growth phase (initiated by FSH) and the dominance phase (initiated when FSH is close to its nadir; LH dependent).

Dominance is a consequence of *selection*, the process that results in the number of growing follicles being

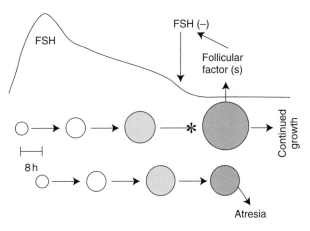

Fig. 33.27 Simplified model of deviation. The future dominant follicle emerges approximately 8 hours before the future largest subordinate follicle. Under the influence of FSH the two follicles grow at the same rate so that the larger follicle retains its initial advantage up to the point of deviation (marked by asterisk). As the follicles grow they secrete increasing quantities of oestradiol and inhibin, both of which diminish the secretion of FSH until there is insufficient to sustain the growth of subordinate follicles; they regress. However, changes in the dominant follicle, such as increased responsiveness to LH and the stimulatory activity of IGF-1, enable it to survive and enlarge in the presence of low concentrations of FSH. (After Wiltbank *et al.*, 2000.)

reduced to what is the 'species-specific ovulatory quota': in cattle, usually one follicle, occasionally two. The beginning of the selection phase cannot be identified by ultrasonography but the end of the phase is coincident with the onset of dominance, which can be identified.

Normally, each wave has a span of seven to ten days from emergence to ovulation or to the onset of atresia in the dominant follicle. The dominant follicle has the functional capacity to trigger the neuroendocrine cascade that culminates in ovulation but its fate is determined by the frequency of pulsatile LH secretion at the point of decision, essentially according to the phase of the cycle: the high frequency during the follicular phase enables it to ovulate; the low frequency during the luteal phase or during postpartum anoestrum results in atresia; an intermediate frequency (e.g. when there is suboptimal concentration of progesterone) is associated with extended dominance, which may have a deleterious effect on the competence of the oocyte. The next wave cannot emerge until after the dominant follicle has begun to regress.

Cyclic pattern: Usually, the bovine oestrous cycle has either two waves (modal days of emergence: days 0, 10) or three waves (modal days of emergence: days 0, 10, 16) of follicular growth, each emerging about a day after a transient peak in serum concentrations of FSH. During the luteal phase both progesterone from

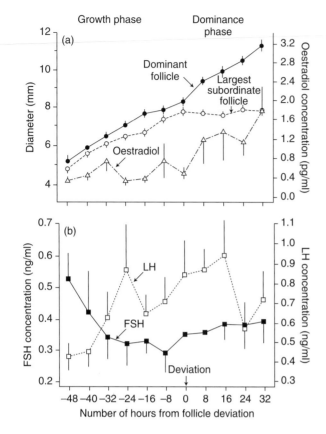

Growth phase   Dominance phase

Fig. 33.28 The follicular wave has a growth phase and a dominance phase. (a) Diameters of the dominant follicle and of the largest subordinate follicle before and after deviation; also, the contemporary concentrations of circulating oestradiol. (b) The contemporary concentrations of circulating FSH and LH. (Reproduced from Kulick *et al.*, 1999 with permission from Elsevier Science.)

the corpus luteum and oestrogen from the cohort of growing follicles (>5mm) restrain the hypothalamic–pituitary axis by negative feedback. The frequency of the pulse generator is reduced to one pulse of GnRH every 4–8 hours and the concentrations of gonadotrophins in the peripheral circulation are insufficient to induce ovulation. As a result, neither of the dominant follicles in the first two waves can ovulate; all of the follicles in the two waves undergo atresia. Luteolysis, which is required to remove this inhibition, occurs spontaneously when the uterus, under the trophic influence of progesterone followed by oestrogen and oxytocin, produces sufficient prostaglandin $F_{2\alpha}$ ($PGF_{2\alpha}$) to kill the corpus luteum (see p. 495). The resultant fall in progesterone concentrations releases the GnRH pulse generator, which increases its frequency to one pulse every hour (approximately). The concentrations of FSH and LH rise in the peripheral circulation, stimulating the cohort of follicles that initiates the follicular phase of the cycle and from within

which the new dominant follicle goes on to ovulate approximately three days later (Fig. 33.28), by which time it has grown to 16–20mm in diameter.

The phases of the oestrous cycle

Follicular phase: Each of the growing follicles has two populations of steroid-secreting cells: theca interna cells and granulosa cells (Fig. 33.29a). The cells of the theca interna have specific receptors for LH and they respond to this gonadotrophin by synthesizing androgens (androstenedione and testosterone) that diffuse across the basement membrane into the granulosa cell layer. During the early stages of folliculogenesis the granulosa cells have receptors for FSH and they respond to this gonadotrophin by converting the thecal androgens to oestrogen (Fig. 33.29b). As the follicles grow under the trophic influences of both FSH and oestrogen, the granulosa cells acquire increased numbers of FSH receptors and oestrogen receptors and they secrete increasing quantities of oestrogen-rich follicular fluid (Fig. 33.29c). Follicular oestrogen passes into the circulation and exerts negative feedback on the release of FSH from the pituitary gland: while the concentration of FSH is in decline, the dominant follicle is selected and the subordinate follicles regress (Figs 33.26, 33.27). The dominant follicle maintains FSH at low concentrations and becomes dependent on LH for continued growth and secretion of oestradiol (Fig. 33.30). LH stimulates the secretion of sufficient oestradiol to induce oestrus and to evoke the oestrogen surge that exerts a positive feedback on the hypothalamic–pituitary axis (Figs 33.30, 33.31). The frequency of the GnRH pulse generator increases, the sensitivity of the adenohypophysis to GnRH is increased by a self-priming action of the GnRH and the pituitary gland releases the preovulatory surge of LH. The response of the dominant follicle to LH is both morphological (growth, ovulation, formation of the corpus luteum) and secretory (oestrogen, progesterone).

Ovulation is critically dependent on the timing, frequency, and amplitude of the hormonal changes just described. For instance, an inappropriate pattern of LH secretion could lead to atresia or to undue persistence of the dominant follicle (with detrimental effects on the quality of the oocyte). The crucial hormonal event that initiates the ovulatory process is the switch from negative feedback by progesterone and oestrogen to positive feedback by oestrogen (Figs. 33.30, 33.31); again, the timing and rate of change of the oestrogen surge are critical: any significant deviation in either feature can result in delayed ovulation or anovulation.

Luteal phase: After ovulation, the basement membrane between the theca cells and the granulosa cells breaks down and the avascular granulosa cell layer is invaded

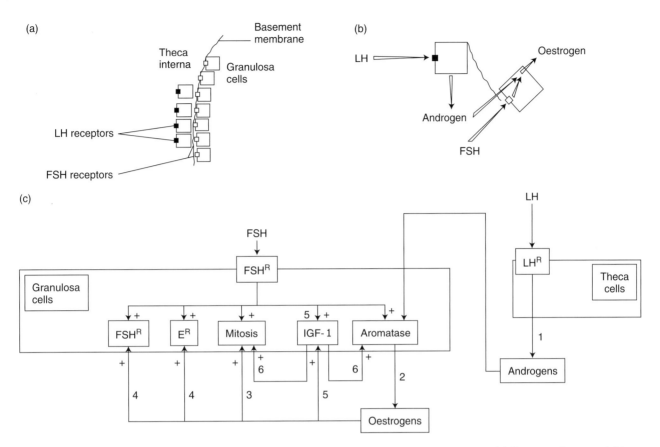

Fig. 33.29 Formation of oestrogen by ovarian follicles: (a) depicts the structure of the follicular wall; (b) illustrates the essential features of the production of oestrogen: LH stimulates the synthesis of androgens by the theca cells, FSH stimulates aromatases within the granulosa cells to convert the androgens to oestrogens; (c) depicts the biochemical events in the growing follicle between emergence and divergence: (1) LH stimulates theca cells to produce androgens; (2) FSH activates aromatase in granulosa cells to convert the androgens to oestrogen; In the granulosa cells, oestradiol (3) stimulates mitosis and (4) up-regulates receptors for FSH (FSH^R) and for oestradiol (E^R); (5) synthesis and secretion of IGF-1 by granulosa cells are stimulated by oestradiol and FSH; (6) IGF-1 further stimulates mitosis and aromatase activity in granulosa cells. Outcome: growth of the follicle and expansion of the antrum due to the combination of increased numbers of secretory granulosa cells with increased numbers of FSH and oestrogen receptors per cell.

by connective tissue septae that carry theca cells and blood vessels. The granulosa cells and the theca cells differentiate into luteal cells that secrete progesterone; they can also synthesize and secrete oestrogen, oxytocin and relaxin. The invading blood vessels undergo extensive branching and deliver a very large blood flow to support the very high metabolic rate of the mature corpus luteum; so rich does the vasculature become that endothelial cells comprise more than half of the constituent cells – in due course, these cells play a pivotal role in the process of luteolysis (see below).

Luteinizing hormone is the principal luteotrophin in the cow; under normal circumstances, tonic secretion of LH maintains the functional corpus luteum until PGF$_{2\alpha}$ from the uterus causes luteolysis at the end of the cycle. It is important to realize that 'normal circumstances' include the correct antecedent hormonal pattern:

specifically, serum progesterone at luteal phase concentrations for a few days before it subsides, followed by serum FSH at normal preovulatory concentrations. Failure of this sequence or inappropriate serum concentrations of either hormone seem to affect the lifespan of the corpus luteum (short luteal phase, prolonged luteal phase) and/or its capacity to secrete progesterone (inadequate luteal phase), phenomena that are common after the first ovulation at puberty or after calving. It is not known how the (prefollicular phase) progesterone exerts its influence on the activities of the next corpus luteum; it is possible that the FSH could do so through its role in the induction of LH receptors on the granulosa cells of the preovulatory follicle.

The corpus luteum grows progressively in size until days 16–18 of the oestrous cycle. Histologically, the mature corpus luteum is seen to contain two mor-

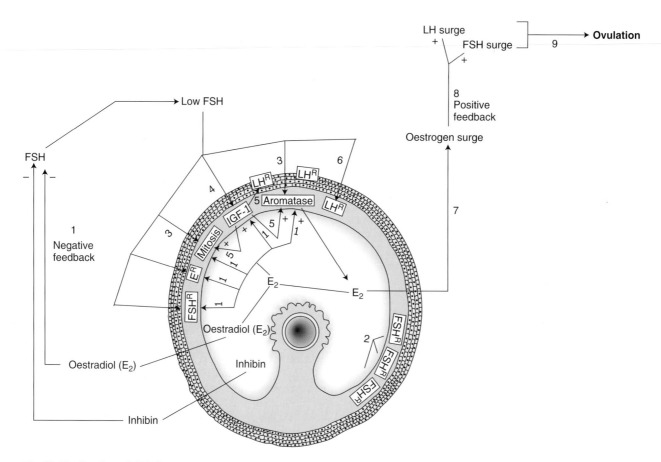

Fig. 33.30 Dominant follicle becomes the ovulatory follicle. When luteolysis occurs, the LH pulses attain the frequency that is required to progress the dominant follicle to ovulation. FSH induces mitosis and stimulates aromatase activity in granulosa cells and they secrete oestradiol and inhibin: within the follicle, oestradiol binds to receptors (E^R) in granulosa cells in which it (1) up-regulates E^R and receptors of FSH(FSH^R), stimulates aromatase activity, mitosis and secretion of IGF-1: systemically, both oestradiol and inhibin depress FSH secretion by the pituitary gland (negative feedback). (2) Granulosa cells have high number FSH^R [see (4) in Figure 30.29]. (3) The low levels of FSH continue to induce mitosis and to stimulate aromatase activity in granulosa cells (thus producing oestradiol and enlarging the antrum). FSH (4) and oestradiol (1) stimulate granulosa cells to secrete more IGF-1 – which, in turn, (5) enhances the steroidogenic and mitotic actions of FSH and oestradiol on granulosa cells, and enhances the steroidogenic action of LH on theca cells. FSH (6) in creases the number of LH receptors (LH^R) on granulosa cell. The cell division and the secretory activity accelerate the expansion of the dominant follicle: it may be 16 to 18 mm in diameter at the preovulatory stage. The rapid increase in secretion of oestrogen induced by the activities of LH, FSH and IGF-1 leads to a surge of oestrogen (7) which evokes, by positive feedback (8), coincident surges of the gonadotrophins (large surge of LH, smaller surge of FSH) and, consequently, ovulation (9).

phologically distinct populations of parenchymal cells: small luteal cells (10–20 µm) and large luteal cells (20–35 µm). All of the small cells are derived from thecal cells and, until the sixth day of the oestrous cycle, nearly all of the large cells are derived from the granulosa cells. After day six, some small luteal cells differentiate into large luteal cells, so that the large cells are of mixed origin and the proportion of large cells increases as the corpus luteum matures (from less than 2 per cent at days 3 to 5 to almost 5 per cent at days 10 to 18).

It is significant for the clinical management of the oestrous cycle to realize that the small luteal cells and the large luteal cells differ in their abilities to respond

to the recognized luteotrophin (LH) and luteolysin ($PGF_{2\alpha}$). Receptors for LH are numerous on the small cells but they are scanty or absent on the large cells. Therefore, LH stimulates the small cells to secrete progesterone but it has no such effect on the large cells. Despite this and the numerical predominance of small luteal cells throughout the luteal phase, it is generally agreed that most of the progesterone is secreted by the large luteal cells. Progesterone is secreted as pulses at a frequency that is different from that for LH. This does not diminish the importance of LH as the principal luteotrophin in the cow: LH does not have direct control over the quantities of progesterone secreted by the large cells but it does exert an important indirect

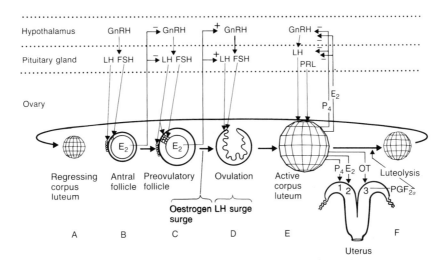

Fig. 33.31 Interrelationships between the hypothalamus, pituitary gland, ovary and uterus during the oestrous cycle. When the corpus luteum (CL) regresses at the end of a cycle (A), the hypothalamus and pituitary gland are released from the strong negative feedback exerted by progesterone (P_4) throughout the luteal phase of the cycle. FSH and LH stimulate the growth and secretory activity of a dominant ovarian follicle (B) that secretes increasing quantities of oestradiol (E_2). The initial low concentrations of E_2 have a negative feedback effect until the preovulatory follicle produces a surge of oestrogen (C) that exerts a positive feedback and results in a surge of LH that causes ovulation (D). A new CL develops under the trophic influence of both LH and, perhaps, prolactin (PRL). It secretes P_4 and E_2 that reassert a strong negative feedback effect on the hypothalamic–pituitary axis. In addition, the P_4 causes an accumulation of fatty acid precursors in the endometrium (1). After day 10, E_2 induces the synthesis of prostaglandin from the stored precursors (2). Finally, oxytocin (OT) causes the release of the $PGF_{2\alpha}$ (3), which is transferred from the uterus to the ipsilateral ovary by a counter-current mechanism (see Fig. 33.32) and induces luteolysis (F). (See Fig. 33.23 for changes in concentrations of the hormones in the peripheral plasma.)

control by regulating the differentiation of small cells into large luteal cells, a process during which the steroidogenic activities of the cells seem to be turned on fully and permanently. On the other hand, receptors for $PGF_{2\alpha}$ are numerous on large luteal cells but are absent from the small cells. Since the secretion of progestrone by the young corpus luteum (days 3 to 5) is invested almost entirely in the small cells, it is not surprising that it is refractory to the luteolytic action of $PGF_{2\alpha}$. The luteolysin becomes effective when the large luteal cells assume responsibility for most of the secretory activity.

It is well known that during the first four or six days of the oestrous cycle exogenous oxytocin can inhibit the growth of the corpus luteum and block its secretory activity. This is possible because the small luteal cells have specific receptors for oxytocin and interaction between the receptors and the peptide leads to inhibition of the LH-stimulated secretion of progesterone by the small cells. In the mature corpus luteum the large luteal cells synthesize oxytocin and it has been suggested that this peptide may play a significant role in local 'large-cell-to-small-cell communication' during prostaglandin-induced luteolysis.

Prostaglandin $F_{2\alpha}$ is formed in the endometrium. It leaves the uterus in the uterine vein and most of it is

transported in the venous blood to the lungs where approximately 65 per cent of it is degraded into its inactive metabolite, PGFM, in one passage. However, some $PGF_{2\alpha}$ is brought directly from the uterus to the adjacent ovary by means of a counter current mechanism (Fig. 33.32) that transfers the luteolytic agent from the uterine vein to the ovarian artery. Thus, in the cow, $PGF_{2\alpha}$ may act partly by the systemic route to augment the local counter-current transfer (McCracken et al., 1999).

Prostaglandin $F_{2\alpha}$ is released from the uterus in pulses and there is evidence that the minimum requirement for normal regression of the corpus luteum at the end of the oestrous cycle (i.e. effective luteolysis by endogenous $PGF_{2\alpha}$) is a pulse lasting one hour repeated about every six hours over a period of 24–30 hours. (By contrast, after day 5 of the oestrous cycle the corpus luteum can be removed by a single injection of exogenous luteolysin, in an appropriate dose.)

The timing and magnitude of $PGF_{2\alpha}$ release from the uterus is determined by the sequential interactions of progesterone, oestradiol and oxytocin. The central and peripheral actions of oestradiol are critical for luteolysis to occur (Binelli et al., 2001). During the early part of the oestrous cycle the endometrial cells have many receptors for progesterone and coupling of the steroid

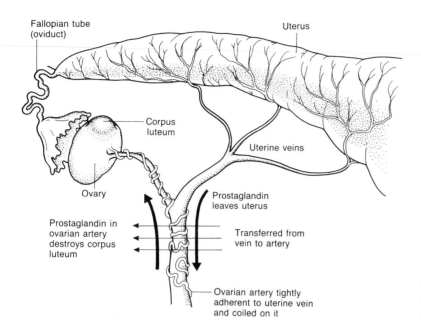

Fig. 33.32 The transfer of $PGF_{2\alpha}$ from the uterus to the ovary by a counter current mechanism.

with its receptors effectively blocks the production of $PGF_{2\alpha}$; however, it causes an accumulation of fatty acid precursors in the endometrium. After about 10 days the action of progesterone on the hypothalamus and on the endometrium begins to decline (possibly due to progesterone-induced loss of its own receptor: 'down regulation'), permitting oestrogen to effect changes both centrally and peripherally. Centrally, oestradiol from developing ovarian follicles appears to alter the frequency of the hypothalamic oxytocin pulse generator, which produces a series of intermittent episodes of oxytocin secretion; peripherally, it promotes the formation of endometrial receptors for oestradiol and oxytocin. In the endometrium, coupling of oestradiol with its receptors increases the synthesis of $PGF_{2\alpha}$ from the fatty acid precursors, while coupling of oxytocin (from the hypothalamus and from the corpus luteum) with its receptors leads to immediate pulsatile secretion of $PGF_{2\alpha}$ (McCracken *et al.*, 1999). It is probable that the duration of the pulses is determined by the rapid down regulation of oxytocin receptors (within one hour) and that the frequency of the pulses reflects the regeneration time of the oxytocin receptors in response to oestradiol (six hours).

$PGF_{2\alpha}$ causes a significant reduction in luteal blood flow and it couples with specific receptors on the large luteal cells. However, the other steroidogenic cells, the small luteal cells, do not have receptors for $PGF_{2\alpha}$ and it has to be assumed that some type of intercellular communication between the large cells and the small cells is involved in terminating the LH-induced secre-

tion of progesterone by the small luteal cells. Oxytocin, which is formed in the large luteal cells and has specific receptors on the small luteal cells, is an obvious candidate messenger. Recent studies (Meiden *et al.*, 1999) assign the pivotal role to endothelin 1 (ET-1), a peptide synthesized and released by the resident endothelial cells. The proposal is that $PGF_{2\alpha}$ elicits the release of ET-1 from the endothelial cells and of oxytocin from the large luteal cells; ET-1 acts on the steroidogenic cells to reduce their progesterone output; both $PGF_{2\alpha}$ and ET-1 induce vasoconstriction and consequent hypoxic conditions; ET-1 secretion is enhanced both by hypoxia and by oxytocin (Fig. 33.33). For structural regression it is envisaged that ET-1 initiates a cascade of events leading to recruitment and activation of phagocytic cells that release cytokines responsible for programmed cell death.

It is obvious that the functional corpus luteum plays a primary role in the control of the oestrous cycle, a fact that is central to all regimes that aim to control the cycle. In the past, the practice was to remove it manually *per rectum*, a procedure to be condemned. The mature corpus luteum (CL) is a very vascular organ; manual expression causes haemorrhage which will give rise to local adhesions, if it is not fatal. The CL can be removed by administration of exogenous luteolytic agents. It is insensitive to exogenous $PGF_{2\alpha}$ during the first four days of the cycle, but between day 5 and day 16 the administration of $PGF_{2\alpha}$ or an analogue will cause rapid luteolysis followed, within a few days, by oestrus and ovulation.

Messenger

Mechanisms by which luteal secretions are altered

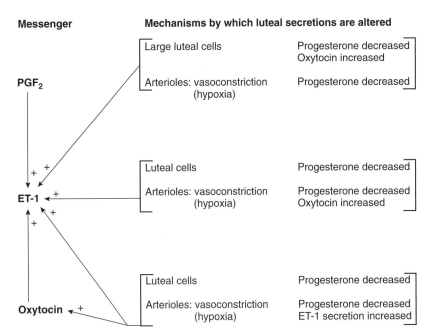

Fig. 33.33 Schematic representation of the putative role of endothelin-1 (ET-1) in functional luteolysis in cattle.

Pharmacological regulation of the oestrous cycle (see also Chapter 42)

The pharmaceutical industry has provided an array of natural and synthetic hormones – GnRH, gonadotrophins, steroids, prostaglandins – that can be used to regulate the oestrous cycle. The use of these agents for specific purposes will be described when we deal with the clinical conditions in which they have been found to be effective. Nevertheless, it is appropriate at this juncture to emphasize a few basic principles that should be borne in mind when the clinician is contemplating the use of reproductive hormones for therapeutic purposes.

The GnRH generator imposes a pulsatile mode of secretion on the hypothalamic–pituitary–ovarian axis. The component parts of the axis respond to hormonal signals that are encoded in the frequency and, to a lesser extent, the amplitude of the pulses. However, these target tissues may not be able to decode a hormonal stimulus that is either non-pulsatile or pulsatile at non-physiological frequencies. As an example, repeated small pulses of exogenous GnRH will induce pulsatile releases of gonadotrophins and these responses will be enhanced by the self-priming action of GnRH. On the other hand, continuous infusion of GnRH or intermittent infusions of GnRH at markedly non-physiological frequencies will soon lead to complete refractoriness of the pituitary gland to the continued stimulation (see p. 477). Therapeutic regimes should be planned with

due recognition of these observations. A single bolus of exogenous GnRH is likely to be effective only when a preovulatory follicle is present already.

During the luteal phase of the oestrous cycle the corpus luteum acts as an effective 'brake' on the pulse generator: pulse frequency is reduced so that circulating gonadotrophins are maintained at tonic concentrations and the dynamic surges required to cause ovulation cannot occur. Luteolysis removes the brake, the pulse frequency increases and ovulation occurs within four or five days. Hence, there are two methods by which control over the length of the cycle and ovulation can be achieved: the use of a luteolytic agent to kill the corpus luteum of the current cycle or the use of a progestogen to create an 'artificial' luteal phase, which will be followed by ovulation shortly after withdrawal of the progestogen. These methods can be used separately or in combination. Since prostaglandin does not kill the very young corpus luteum (less than five days after ovulation), the usual recommendation is to give two injections 11 days apart (see p. 682).

To date, neither of these methods has fully satisfied the requirements of the industry. Ideally, synchronization of oestrus should make it possible to achieve high rates of pregnancy to a single insemination at a predictable interval after treatment, without the need for detection of oestrus. Recent studies of the dynamics of follicular waves have revealed that the prime requirement is 'to have a recently selected dominant follicle of short duration dominance at the end of a progestagen or PGF$_{2\alpha}$ treatment regimen' (Roche *et al.*, 1999). Thus, the objective of current research efforts is to validate a regimen that will regulate both the luteal and follicular components of the periovulatory phase.

As mentioned, the response of the corpus luteum to an exogenous luteolysin depends on the stage of its development, and even when it is fully responsive the intervals from treatment to oestrus and ovulation can vary by some days depending on the stage of development of the dominant follicle at the time of treatment. For instance, if the current largest follicle is no longer functionally dominant, clinical response will be delayed until the dominant follicle of the next wave does the business up to a week later. Scientists have shown that it is possible to manipulate follicular waves to deliver ovulation within a time span that would satisfy the level of predictability required to make fixed-time insemination a viable proposition. However, the problem remains that some of the procedures that have been employed under 'laboratory conditions' do not lend themselves to ready application under field conditions. One such approach involved transvaginal ultrasound-guided ablation of all follicles greater than 5 mm (day 0) followed by PGF$_{2\alpha}$ (day 4) and LH or GnRH (day 5): all of 23 treated heifers ovulated within the same 24-hour period, 19 within the same 12-hour period (Bo *et al.*, 2002). Presumably, the next task is to replace surgical ablation by a pharmacological regimen that will selectively consign the current cohort of emerging follicles to immediate atresia, permitting the emergence of a new cohort, one of which then can be driven by exogenous hormones to ovulation within a predictable time span. It is known that the physiological activities of the follicle are modulated by a range of molecules produced locally within the follicle (growth factors, activins, inhibins, cytokines etc.: Box 33.2). The paracrine or autocrine actions of those molecules may hold the keys to precise manipulation of ovarian function.

Pregnancy

Transport of gametes in the female genital tract

Fertilization takes place in the oviduct, close to the junction of the isthmus and the ampulla (Fig. 33.34). Transport of the ovum from the ovary is achieved by muscular and ciliary activity and flow of fluids in the ovarian bursa and ampulla of the oviduct. After natural mating, spermatozoa have to traverse the cervix, the uterus and the uterotubal junction. Again, muscular activity and flow of fluids are largely responsible for the transport of the male gametes. The appropriate muscular activities, secretion and flow of fluids in the female genital tract are regulated by the ovarian hormones

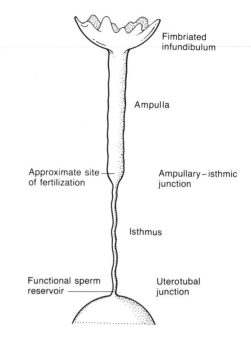

Fig. 33.34 Schematic diagram of the uterine tube (oviduct, Fallopian tube).

(oestrogens and progesterone) released in the correct concentrations and in the proper sequence. Therapeutic procedures that significantly alter the relative concentrations or sequence of the hormones can disrupt the transport mechanisms, which in some instances may cause the loss of gametes or of the conceptus.

The transport of spermatozoa is not an entirely passive process: the motility of the male gametes makes a significant contribution to the successful completion of the hazardous voyage from vagina to oviduct during which the vast majority of the spermatozoa are lost, partly as a result of phagocytosis but largely by expulsion to the exterior in cervical mucus. It appears from the literature that two distinct populations of spermatozoa arrive in the oviduct:

- Those that are transported rapidly but are incapable of fertilizing the ovum; and
- Those that are transported more slowly to the functional sperm reservoir, are viable and are capable of undergoing capacitation and the acrosome reaction, two processes that are essential if a spermatozoon is to acquire the capacity to fertilize an ovum.

Spermatozoa have been recovered from the ampulla of the oviduct within 3–5 minutes after mating. This rapid transport is due to muscular contractions in the female genital tract. During oestrus, the contractions begin at the cervix and move towards the oviduct; at the end of oestrus the direction of the contractions is reversed. Most of the spermatozoa that reach the oviduct during the initial rapid transport phase are damaged or dead and they do not include the sperm that fertilizes the ovum. It has been suggested that these non-viable spermatozoa may play a significant physiological role, by releasing products that elicit local muscular and secretory responses that facilitate transport and sustenance of the gametes.

According to Hunter and Wilmut (1984), viable spermatozoa are transported more slowly: heifers mated early in oestrus took 8–12 hours to establish an adequate population of viable spermatozoa in the oviduct. Then the gametes were sequestered, in a relatively quiescent state, in the caudal 2 cm of the isthmus for a further 18–20 hours before they began a progressive migration towards the site of fertilization. Thus, the caudal isthmus served as the functional sperm reservoir, the immediate source of viable spermatozoa at the time of ovulation. It is known that both the temperature and the oxygen tension are lower in that segment of the isthmus than they are in the ampulla and it is thought that these factors may be responsible for the depressed motility of the spermatozoa in the reservoir up to the time of ovulation. At ovulation, the temperature and oxygen tension are elevated in the lumen of the caudal isthmus, the sequestered spermatozoa begin to exhibit activated motility (hyperactivation) and they migrate to the site of fertilization. Hyperactivation is in response to the 'pick-up' of follicular fluid and the ovum by the oviduct.

Capacitation and the acrosome reaction

The spermatozoa deposited in the female reproductive tract are not immediately capable of fertilizing an ovum. During transport through the tract they undergo physiological changes that make them competent to penetrate the zona pellucida and fuse with the ovum, i.e. they undergo capacitation. It is thought that during capacitation the spermatozoon loses some proteins it has acquired, by adsorption or incorporation into the plasma membrane, during exposure to epididymal fluid or seminal plasma. This does not cause any visible change in the morphology of the spermatozoon but it does alter the physical and chemical properties of the plasma membrane, permitting an influx of calcium ions required for the induction of the hyperactivated form of motility and for the acrosome reaction. The hyperactivated motility endows the capacitated spermatozoa with strong thrusting power that facilitates migration from the isthmus to the ampulla and subsequent passage through the zona pellucida. The acrosome reaction is an essential prerequisite for fertilization – a spermatozoon with an intact acrosome cannot penetrate the ovum.

The acrosome reaction (Fig. 33.20) involves multiple point fusions between the plasma membrane and the outer acrosomal membrane over the front half of the sperm head. The fusions give rise to a series of small vesicles formed by fragments of both membranes. The vesicles are separated by small pores through which the acrosomal enzymes escape. There is controversy as to whether or not the escaping enzymes aid the passage of the spermatozoa through the cumulus oophorus in the cow. As the reaction proceeds, the pores enlarge at the expense of the vesicles so that the vesicles have been lost by the time the sperm penetrates the zona pellucida. When one of the advancing spermatozoa reaches the perivitelline space, it fuses with the plasma membrane of the ovum and its genetic material is incorporated into the conceptus at fertilization.

The fusion of the egg and the sperm triggers a series of reactions that prevent polyspermy by making both the zona pellucida and the plasma membrane of the ovum impenetrable to other spermatozoa.

It is often stated that capacitation requires a 6-hour sojourn in the female tract. However, it is unlikely that the processes would be synchronized to ensure that all the surviving spermatozoa would have been capacitated at a fixed minimum time after deposition in the female tract. Asynchrony in the time to capacitation would appear to be more advantageous in that it would allow for small populations of potential fertilizing spermatozoa to be available sequentially over a period spanning several hours before and after ovulation. Indeed, there is evidence that only 10–20 per cent of bovine spermatozoa have undergone capacitation and the acrosome reaction within three hours of insemination, while other spermatozoa do so several hours later. Again, the inappropriate use of exogenous hormones may hamper capacitation and the acrosome reaction.

Maternal recognition of pregnancy

Normally, the conceptus enters the uterus about 72 hours after ovulation, at the 8–16 cells stage. The cells (blastomeres) form a solid mass (morula) still contained within the zona pellucida. By day 7 or 8, fluid secreted by the blastomeres accumulates in a central cavity (blastocoele) and the zygote is now called a blastocyst. The cells have been arranged into two distinct populations (Fig. 33.35):

- The flattened trophoblast cells that form the wall of the blastocyst and ultimately will forms the chorion.
- A group of cells that forms the inner cell mass at one pole beneath the trophoblast cells and is destined to form the fetus.

The blastocyst hatches from the zona pellucida on days 9 to 11 and on day 13 it begins to elongate so that

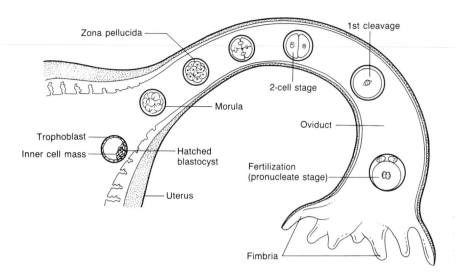

Fig. 33.35 Schematic diagram to illustrate the changes in the conceptus during transport down the uterine tube and into the uterine lumen (after McLaren, 1984).

during the third week it occupies most of the pregnant (ipsilateral) horn and a portion of the non-pregnant (contralateral) horn. The process of attachment begins at day 19 or 20 when there are definite areas of adhesion between the trophoblastic epithelium of the conceptus and the endometrial epithelium; implantation is completed between days 35 and 42. The conceptus plays an important role in prolonging the functional lifespan of the corpus luteum, an essential requirement for the maintenance of pregnancy. The critical period for the extension of the lifespan of the corpus luteum in the cow is between day 15 and day 17; if there is an elongated conceptus present at that time, the mother will 'recognize' that she is pregnant and the luteolytic pulsatile pattern of $PGF_{2\alpha}$ release from the endometrium will be attenuated or abolished.

Since maternal recognition of pregnancy precedes the physical attachment of the conceptus to the endometrium, it is evident that the utero-ovarian regulatory mechanisms that 'rescue' the corpus luteum are responding to a biochemical dialogue between the conceptus and the maternal tissue that is initiated by a variety of signal factors released into the uterine lumen by the preimplantation conceptus.

The bovine conceptus can synthesize a number of products (steroids, prostaglandins, peptides, proteins) that may interact with the maternal utero-ovarian axis. There is evidence to suggest that the conceptus releases different signal factors at different times and that the relative importance of each of these factors may change during these early days of pregnancy. A hypothesis consistent with current information is that the bovine conceptus initiates both antiluteolytic and luteotrophic activities. The main signal is the secretion of interferon-tau (IFN-τ) which reduces the secretion of $PGF_{2\alpha}$ by the

endometrium. The size of the blastodermic vesicle may be critical: a small conceptus may not secrete sufficient IFN-τ to prevent luteolysis. Putative luteotrophic factors include a lipid-like substance released by the conceptus between day 13 and day 18 of pregnancy and, possibly, PGE_2 from the endometrium.

Later in this text we shall pay serious attention to the effects of nutritional status on the resumption of normal ovarian and uterine functions after calving; therefore, it seems appropriate to mention at this juncture that the survival of the early conceptus may be put at jeopardy when the dam is fed excess protein in the diet. The resultant production of large quantities of ammonia in the rumen leads to elevated concentrations of urea in the blood which, in turn, so alters the ionic composition of uterine and tubal secretions that the pH is incompatible with the survival of the conceptus. Problems of embryonic loss are dealt with in Chapter 36.

Maintenance of pregnancy

Once the normal conceptus–endometrial–ovarian regulatory axis of pregnancy has been established, the uterus comes under long-term control by progesterone. In the cow, a fully functional corpus luteum is essential to maintain pregnancy up to day 235; thereafter, the adrenal glands seem to be able to secrete sufficient progesterone to maintain pregnancy in ovariectomized cows. The placenta contributes little to the circulating concentrations of progesterone at any time during pregnancy. The principal luteotrophin is LH; there is little evidence that prolactin plays any significant role (McCracken *et al.*, 1999). The corpus luteum maintains the plasma progesterone concentration above 10 ng/ml from the second week of gestation until term. Progesterone exercises a 'block' on the uterine muscle in that it depresses the amplitude of contractions, suppresses the reactivity to oxytocin and PGF$_{2\alpha}$ and prevents the development of synchronous coordinated contractions that might expel the fetus prematurely. It does not abolish the spontaneous contractility of the myometrial cells. Problems of fetal loss are dealt with in Chapter 37.

Parturition

Since parturition depends on coordinated rhythmic contractions of the myometrium as well as involuntary contractions of the abdominal muscles and 'softening' of the birth canal, the final preparation for delivery of the fetus must involve removal of the progesterone block. This is achieved by significant changes in the hormonal profile coupled with the acquisition of gap junctions by the myometrial cells.

The hormonal changes are initiated by the fetus, triggered by the recognition of 'stress' by the fetal hypothalamic–pituitary axis (Fig. 33.36). This results in the release of ACTH that stimulates the fetal adrenal to release increased amounts of cortisol. The cortisol induces the placenta to release increased quantities of oestrogens into the maternal circulation, and both the cortisol and the oestrogens act on the endometrium to increase the output of PGF$_{2\alpha}$, which causes luteolysis. Thus the oestrogen:progesterone ratio has been switched strongly in favour of oestrogen and the inhibitory effect of progesterone on the uterine muscle has been abolished. The oestrogens promote uterine contractility by stimulating the synthesis of contractile protein and of receptors for both oxytocin and PGF$_{2\alpha}$, and by facilitating the formation of gap junctions between adjacent myometrial cells. Gap junctions are intercellular structures that link cells and allow them to exchange ions and electrical impulses. In the parturient uterus they provide the routes through which electrical activity is propagated; in other words, they provide the structural basis for a functional syncytium that permits synchronization of myometrial contractions. Thus, the switch to oestrogen domination at full term enables the uterine muscle to develop spontaneous rhythmical contractions. The transition of the myometrium from a quiescent state to an active state has been termed

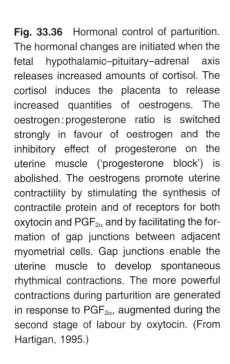

Fig. 33.36 Hormonal control of parturition. The hormonal changes are initiated when the fetal hypothalamic–pituitary–adrenal axis releases increased amounts of cortisol. The cortisol induces the placenta to release increased quantities of oestrogens. The oestrogen:progesterone ratio is switched strongly in favour of oestrogen and the inhibitory effect of progesterone on the uterine muscle ('progesterone block') is abolished. The oestrogens promote uterine contractility by stimulating the synthesis of contractile protein and of receptors for both oxytocin and PGF$_{2\alpha}$ and by facilitating the formation of gap junctions between adjacent myometrial cells. Gap junctions enable the uterine muscle to develop spontaneous rhythmical contractions. The more powerful contractions during parturition are generated in response to PGF$_{2\alpha}$, augmented during the second stage of labour by oxytocin. (From Hartigan, 1995.)

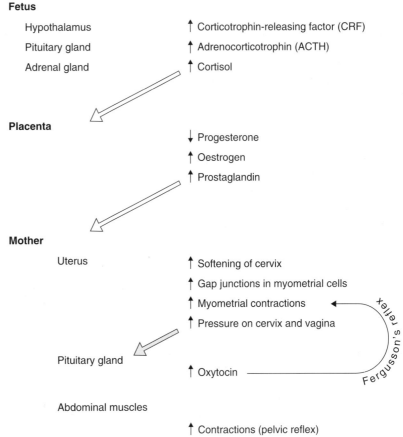

'activation'; the activated myometrium is capable of generating high-frequency, high-amplitude contractions in response to mechanical or biochemical stimuli. The more powerful contractions during parturition are generated in response to PGF$_{2\alpha}$, augmented during the second stage of labour by oxytocin. Both of these hormones influence smooth muscle activity by regulating the concentration of calcium ions in the myometrial cells. The concentration of free Ca^{2+} in myometrial cells increases about three-fold during contraction, through influx from extracellular sources and release from intracellular stores. A deficiency of calcium in a pregnant female at full term is associated with atony of the uterine muscle and a tendency to prolapse of the uterus.

Softening of the birth canal is achieved by the cascade of hormones: a rise in oestrogen concentrations followed by the activities of relaxin and PGF$_{2\alpha}$. Parturition can be induced after about day 255 of gestation by a single injection of a synthetic glucocorticoid that simulates the effects of fetal cortisol, or after 270 days by PGF$_{2\alpha}$. Retained placenta can be a problem with either method.

Tocolysis: Myometrial activity is inhibited by agents (such as β-adrenergic agonists and relaxin) that increase the intracellular levels of cAMP or cGMP, thus interfering with the interaction of free calcium ions with contractile protein.

Drugs that stimulate β$_2$-adrenoceptors of the myometrial cells have been used to relax the uterine muscle in non-pregnant cows undergoing embryo transfer and in pregnant cows at full term to delay parturition (tocolysis) or to facilitate obstetrical operations such as fetotomy, caesarean section or replacement of uterine prolapse. The duration of the tocolysis depends on the pharmacological effects of the agent and on the position of the fetus at the time of treatment. For instance, clenbuterol causes an outflow of calcium ions from the myometrial cells and that renders the cells unresponsive to oxytocin for some hours. When a single therapeutic dose of clenbuterol is given early in stage one of labour it can delay parturition for 5–8 hours, but if it is given in stage two after the cervix has been fully dilated the delay may be as short as an hour or two. It has been reported that when uterine contractility returns, the treated animal tends to have an 'easier' calving; it is suggested that this is due to greater widening and softening of the birth canal.

Physiology of the postpartum period

During pregnancy, the mechanisms for the synthesis and release of GnRH by the hypothalamus and those for the release of the gonadotrophins by the pituitary gland appear to remain intact and functional. The high concentrations of progesterone and oestrogen in the circulation exert a prolonged negative feedback on the maternal hypothalamic–pituitary–ovarian axis. The principal long-term effect of this inhibition is a progressive decline in the amount of LH in the pituitary gland, accompanied by a greatly diminished response of the pituitary gland to GnRH, a low concentration of LH in the circulation and relatively quiescent ovaries. The inherent wave-like pattern of follicular growth is not lost: it is in train within a few days after parturition, with the intrinsic periodicity of seven to ten days. However, the selected dominant follicle may not be able to trigger the neuroendocrine process that leads to oestrus and ovulation. Hence, immediately after calving, the cow has a period of anoestrum, the length of which can be influenced by age, season, nutritional status, dystokia, milk yield, suckling, uterine pathology or subclinical disease.

Re-activation of the hypothalamic–pituitary–ovarian axis

The primary objective of the neuroendocrine adjustments in the early postpartum period is to reinstate the ovaries as fully functional components of the hypothalamic–pituitary axis and to restore the pituitary stores of LH to their normal levels so that the pituitary gland can respond to pulses of GnRH by releasing pulses of LH of sufficient frequency and amplitude to stimulate follicular maturation; in general, this is achieved by day 10 postpartum. In addition, the cow has to cope with the myriad of endogenous and exogenous stressors that might interfere with her ability to progress the dominant follicle to its physiological destiny as a preovulatory follicle. The fate of the first-wave dominant follicle has a significant impact on the duration of the interval to first ovulation: for instance, Beam and Butler (1999) reported the interval as 20 days for those that ovulated (46 per cent of their cows), 51 days for those that regressed (31 per cent of cows) and 48 days for those that formed follicular cysts (23 per cent of cows).

Metabolic factors play key roles in the resumption of reproductive activity (Fig. 33.37). Following parturition, the high producing dairy cow is unable to increase dry matter intake as fast as is necessary to meet the increased nutrient demands for lactation; body reserves of fat and protein are mobilized to meet the deficit; in the circulation, the concentrations of non-esterified fatty acids and triglycerides are elevated, while the concentrations of glucose, insulin, and IGF-1 are diminished (Fig. 33.37) and the interval to first ovulation is extended. According to Beam and Butler (1999), the interval from calving to the nadir of negative energy balance has just as much significance for fertility as does

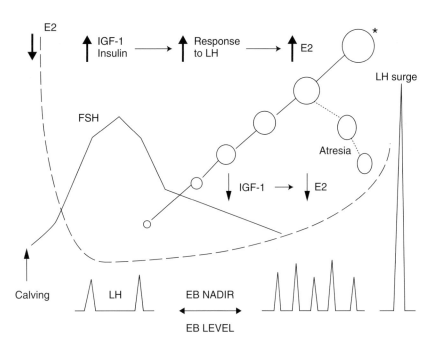

Fig. 33.37 A schematic model describing dominant follicle development (circles) and function in relation to changing metabolic and reproductive hormones, and energy balance (EB), during the first follicular wave postpartum in dairy cows. The first-wave follicle either ovulates (*) or undergoes atresia. LH pulse frequency is modulated by the day of the EB nadir and, to a lesser extent, the level of EB. The large upward arrows indicate increased insulin-like growth factor-1 (IGF-1) and insulin leading to improved responsiveness to LH and greater oestradiol (E_2) production by the dominant follicle. (From Beam & Butler, 1999, reproduced with permission of the Society for Reproduction and Fertility.)

the depth of the nadir. Available evidence seems to confirm that the modal interval to first ovulation has become longer in recent years.

It is suspected that the negative energy balance may be a factor in the pathogenesis of abnormal cycles (short luteal phase, prolonged luteal phase, follicular cysts) in cows that have returned to oestrus. The mechanisms by which the negative energy balance can inhibit ovarian activity are complex. For instance, there is some evidence that it may suppress LH pulse frequency; the low levels of insulin and IGF-1 may retard the growth of the dominant follicle; the steroidogenic activity of the dominant follicle may be so reduced that it is incapable of exerting the positive feedback on the hypothalamus and the pituitary gland that is required for ovulation; if the follicles that ovulate are small, they may form small corpora lutea that are incapable of secreting optimal concentrations of progesterone. It has been reported that cows that experienced deep negative energy balance over the first 10 days postpartum subsequently had subnormal progesterone concentrations in their third oestrous cycles.

Oestrous cycles in postpartum cows

The first ovulation may or may not be associated with oestrus; estimates of silent ovulation range from 40 to 70 per cent. Frequently, oestrus is not observed until the end of the first full-length interovulatory period. The first preovulatory surge of LH may be followed in some cows by a complete cycle with a normal luteal phase. However, other cows may have an initial cycle of normal duration but with reduced concentrations of progesterone. Another group that may constitute approximately 50 per cent of either the dairy herd or the beef herd has been reported to have a short luteal phase of five to ten days' duration during which the corpus luteum secretes reduced amounts of progesterone (Lamming *et al.*, 1981). These corpora lutea are not killed by the usual luteolytic process: their ability to synthesize progesterone is lost prematurely. The transient low levels of progesterone after the first ovulation may have a significant (but, as yet, unidentified) effect on hypothalamic function and they almost certainly play a role in ensuring that oestrus is expressed before the second ovulation.

As mentioned above, a variety of factors can delay the onset of oestrous cycles. Although the events leading to normal stores of LH in the pituitary gland are relatively independent of the suckling stimulus and environmental stressors, the events leading to an increased frequency of LH pulses are susceptible to inhibition by such factors.

In general, milked dairy cows ovulate earlier in the postpartum period than do suckling dairy cows or beef cows. For instance, Lamming's group at Nottingham has reported that milk progesterone profiles on 505 milked dairy cows indicated a mean calving-to-first-ovulation interval of 24 days compared with approximately 60 days for 365 suckled beef cows. Suckling depresses the frequency of LH pulses, probably because it induces a release of endogenous opioids that inhibit the normal pulsatility of the hypothalamic–pituitary axis. There are high concentrations of prolactin in the circulation of lactating cows but, according to Lamming *et al.* (1981), there is no evidence that hyperprolactinaemia plays a significant role in the suckling-induced inhibition of ovarian activity. The potency of the suckling stimulus declines with time after parturition. The duration of the period of inhibition can be influenced by other environmental factors, such as poor nutrition (e.g. when cows lose one unit or more in body condition score in early lactation) or season at calving (photoperiod?). For instance, cows that calved during January to June took significantly longer to resume ovarian activity than did those that calved during July to December (Lamming *et al.*, 1981).

Uterine involution

It should be emphasized that the uterus exercises some control over the activities of the ovaries by way of a local utero-ovarian axis and that uterine pathology can put a brake on the ovarian contribution to the larger neuroendocrine axis. Synthesis and metabolism of $PGF_{2\alpha}$ are elevated in the bovine uterus during the early postpartum period and this is reflected in the presence of a major metabolite (PGFM) in the blood at that time. There is accumulating evidence that ovarian function does not resume until the concentration of this metabolite has fallen below a critical threshold. There appears to be a significant negative correlation between the duration of elevated concentrations of PGFM after calving and the time required for completion of uterine involution (Lindell & Kindahl, 1983). Persistent uterine infections prolong the period of high concentrations of PGFM and the time to uterine involution. A problem may arise in the infected cow that ovulates very early in the postpartum period because these continuously elevated concentrations of prostaglandin are not sufficient to induce luteolysis and a mutual interdependence between the infection and the corpus luteum may be established, thus rendering the cow liable to develop pyometra. However, the majority of cows do not ovulate until after the microbial population of the uterus has been reduced to transient contaminants, a process that may be enhanced by the fluctuating levels of oestrogens released from the follicles that begin to grow in the ovaries as early as the first week postpartum and at intervals of seven to ten days thereafter.

During the second week after parturition the pool of antral follicles in the ovaries is increased both in dairy cows and in beef cows; the increase in numbers is largely due to the development of medium-size follicles (4–8 mm in diameter), particularly evident in the ovary contralateral to the previous pregnancy. This predominance of the contralateral ovary seems to persist for about four weeks, with the result that the majority of first ovulations are from the contralateral ovary. It has

been suggested that a very early ovulation from the ipsilateral ovary in an infected cow may increase the risk of development of pyometra (Hartigan *et al.*, 1974).

It is perfectly 'normal' for bacteria to invade the bovine uterus during the first few days after parturition. Bacteriological studies have revealed that a very wide range of micro-organisms, both pathogens and commensals, gain entry but repetitive sampling showed that when parturition was uncomplicated the contamination of the uterus was transient and that the isolates varied from one sample to the next. At the end of the fourth week postpartum only 30 per cent of the cows had bacteria in the uterus, mostly non-pathogens (Griffin *et al.*, 1974). Under optimal conditions, most cows have eliminated the pathogenic contaminants before cyclic ovarian activity begins. On the other hand, cows that experience dystokia, traumatic damage to the endometrium or retention of placental membranes are less efficient in dealing with pathogens. There is a significant reduction in the efficiency of phagocytic cells in the endometrium and uterine lumen and, as a result, potential pathogens may persist and induce endometritis or metritis. Again, in the majority of cows the endometritis tends to be short-lived; the combination of phagocytosis, local antibody production and myometrial contractions that are normal features of the involutionary period effect clearance of the micro-organisms and resolution of the endometritis. However, it is important to stress that infusion of irritants (antibiotics, iodine) that inhibit phagocytosis, extensive intra-uterine manipulation that damages the endometrium or an early ovulation that causes the onset of a precocious luteal phase may permit a pathogenic micro-organism to become established within the uterus, particularly if the concentration of PGFM is still high. In such circumstances the prostaglandin produced by the uterus is inadequate to cause luteolysis. The result is that the defence mechanisms of the host are depressed by the progesterone from the corpus luteum and the pathogens cause continuing damage to the endometrium, thus preventing the release of a luteolytic dose of prostaglandin. At this stage, the pathogen and the corpus luteum have established a mutual interdependence that predisposes to the development of pyometra. The vicious circle can be broken by exogenous prostaglandin. The important point is that inappropriate medication early in the postpartum period can interfere with the physiological progress of involution and induce long-term pathological consequences.

If a cow enters the second week postpartum without clinical evidence of an active inflammatory response, it is unnecessary – and it may be unwise – to resort to intrauterine antibacterial therapy: the drug may cause physical damage to the regenerating mucosa and – perhaps just as important – it may dampen the local immune response to micro-organisms that may challenge that system later, when the cow is inseminated.

If purulent endometritis/metritis develops it does not abolish ovarian activity immediately and totally. Initially, it causes prolonged cycles, usually with silent ovulations for some months before anoestrum supervenes. Obviously, the best prospects of full recovery to fertility will depend on diagnosis and treatment before the link between the hypothalamic–pituitary axis and the ovaries has been severed.

For problems seen in the postpartum period consult Chapter 34.

Uterine environment after resumption of cyclic ovarian activity

The quality of the luminal microenvironment of the female genital tract has a significant impact on fertility. The fluids secreted by the oviducts and by the uterus are the media in which the gametes are transported and sustained; the spermatozoa are capacitated, hyperactivated and acrosome-reacted, the ovum is fertilized and the conceptus is transported and sustained while it develops into the elongated blastodermic vesicle that implants in the uterus. The appropriate secretions, muscular activity and flow of fluids are governed by oestrogen and progesterone released from the ovaries in the correct concentrations, at the correct times and in a specific sequence. Therefore, any factor that alters the delicate balance of ovarian hormones during the oestrous cycle is a potential hazard to pregnancy, even when a normal fertile cow is bred to a highly fertile bull.

The composition of the tubal and uterine fluids changes on regional and temporal bases – specifically to meet the needs of the gametes and of the conceptus: in particular, the changing needs of the conceptus as it progresses from a single cell zygote to an elongated vesicle. It follows that the preimplantation conceptus is vulnerable to damage by anything that disrupts the hormonal balance or otherwise alters the secretions. However, it is not easy to disentangle the complex interrelationships between the various actions of the hormones, the secretory and muscular responses of the tubular tract, and the viability and developmental competence of the oocyte. For instance, there are several highly sensitive junctures at which short-term acute stress might interfere with the maturation of the oocyte, fertilization, embryogenesis or implantation; it would be virtually impossible to ascertain whether the pregnancy wastage was due primarily to low developmental competence of the zygote or to an inappropriate uterine microenvironment that was unable to sustain a fully competent conceptus. Frequently, it would be just as difficult to identify the cause of the acute stress. A similar cause-and-effect conundrum attaches to the

reports of long-term (up to the third cycle) deleterious effects on embryo survival in cows that experienced deep negative energy balance during the first 10 days after calving. Were the carry-over effects due to a loss of developmental competence that resulted in embryo mortality and suboptimal luteotrophic stimuli, or were they due primarily to deficient luteal function that made the uterine microenvironment suboptimal for the conceptus?

We have mentioned that ingestion of excess protein leads to elevated blood urea levels, lower pH of uterine fluids and lower fertility. The pregnancy wastage has been attributed to the deleterious effect of acidic uterine fluid on embryos (Butler, 2000) but O'Callaghan and Boland (1999) took a different view: on the basis of experiments involving reciprocal embryo transfers, they suggested that the effects on embryo quality are due to alterations in the tubal microenvironment or in the follicle rather than in the uterus.

The iatrogenic introduction of micro-organisms can seriously diminish the quality of the uterine microenvironment during the breeding season. The uterus has a higher degree of susceptibility to bacterial infection during the luteal phase than it has during oestrus. This is because the migration of neutrophils into and through the endometrium is inhibited by progesterone, which also depresses the phagocytic activity of the cells once they have arrived in the endometrium. Therefore, the clinician should exercise great care to avoid the introduction of contaminated or irritant material into the uterus during the luteal phase. For the same reason, cows should not be inseminated at mid-cycle or after conception. Persisting bacterial endometritis in a cyclic cow could induce embryo loss because (i) it damages the endometrium so that it is not possible to establish an efficient interface for the transfer of nutrients; (ii) it induces embryo mortality or retards expansion of the blastocyst which then fails to secrete enough IFN-τ to maintain the corpus luteum and/or (iii) it releases sufficient $PGF_{2\alpha}$ to induce premature luteolysis.

Problems of the postpartum period are dealt with in Chapter 34, with endometritis being discussed from p. 521.

Take-home concepts for the clinician

Readers must be aware that this overview of the basic elements of reproductive physiology in cattle is a simplified account of some highly complex phenomena; the aspiration has been to provide the broad concepts that ought to inform the diagnostic and therapeutic efforts of the clinician. So, what is the conceptual framework for the major themes presented here?

Overall control of reproductive activities is vested in the HPG axis, within which the dominant role is played by the hypothalamus, literally the nerve centre that coordinates and responds to the relevant neural, endocrine and immunological inputs. It exercises control through the actions of a pulse generator that is responsible for the pulsatile release of GnRH which, in turn, regulates the release of the gonadotrophins that determine the nature, intensity and timing of events in the genital tract. For instance, it is the frequency and, to a lesser extent, the amplitude of LH pulses that regulate the timing of ovulation. The *pulsatility* is modulated by *feedback*, by *energy balance* and by *stress*; to take a practical example, it is likely that ovulation will be suppressed when an animal is in negative energy balance and/or is stressed by other environmental challenges.

During the transition period the high-producing cow is exposed to a plethora of stressors (both intrinsic and extrinsic), is relatively immunosuppressed and, once lactation begins, is in significant negative energy balance; in such circumstances, reproduction has a relatively low priority in the *partitioning of energy* and it is likely that the resumption of cyclic ovarian activity will be delayed. Of course, the deleterious effect of the energy deficit on LH pulses is a major factor in the suppression of oestrus and ovulation, and in the low pregnancy rates to first service; however, the fact that approximately half of the mated cows calve to first service should convince us that there are other contributing factors that tip the balance away from a satisfactory level of herd fertility. Thus, management of the breeding programme demands attention to hygiene and the physical facilities, to body condition score, to feeding practices and to veterinary care throughout both the transition period and the breeding season. The prime objective is to minimize the *allostatic load* so that functions of HPG axis are not put at hazard by the coping strategies of an overburdened cow (see Chapter 67).

If there is a need to induce ovulation, the relevant conceptual framework derives from the inherent pattern of *follicular waves* that makes a cohort of newly recruited follicles available every seven to ten days. Treatment should be administered at the appropriate stage in a current wave or, as has been done by investigators pursuing the aspiration to eliminate the need for detection of oestrus after induced ovulation, in a new wave that has emerged after surgical ablation of the current wave (Bo *et al.*, 2002). The latter experiment is an exciting application of basic physiological information but it does prompt a rhetorical question: if an effective pharmacological regimen capable of chemical ablation of cohorts of recruited follicles is devised and is then used widely on a whole-herd basis, how is the consumer likely to respond to the news that milk on sale in the local store has been produced by cows that are 'hormone-laden'?

References

Beam, S.W. & Butler, W.R. (1999) Effects of energy balance on follicular development and first ovulation in postpartum dairy cows. *Journal of Reproduction and Fertility*, **Supplement 54**, 411–24.

Binelli, M., Thatcher, W.W., Mattos, R. & Baruselli, P.S. (2001) Antiluteolytic strategies to improve fertility in cattle. *Theriogenology*, **56**, 1451–63.

Bo, G.A., Baruselli, P.S., Moreno, D., Cutaia, L., Caccia, M., Tribulo, R., Tribulo, H. & Mapletoft, R.J. (2002) The control of follicular wave development for self-appointed embryo transfer programs in cattle. *Theriogenology*, **57**, 53–72.

Bronson, F.H. (1989) *Mammalian Reproductive Biology*. Chicago University Press, Chicago.

Butler, W.R. (2000) Nutritional interactions with reproductive performance in dairy cattle. *Animal Reproduction Science*, **60–1**, 449–57.

Fawcett, D.W. (1994) *A Textbook of Histology*. Chapman and Hall, London.

Ginther, O.J. (1996) Selection of the dominant follicle in cattle. *Biology of Reproduction*, **55**, 1187–94.

Ginther, O.J., Beg, M.A., Bergfelt, D.R., Donadeu, F.X. & Kot, K. (2001) Follicle selection in monovular species. *Biology of Reproduction*, **65**, 638–47.

Griffin, J.F.T., Hartigan, P.J. & Nunn, W.R. (1974) Non-specific uterine infection and bovine fertility I and II. *Theriogenology*, **1**, 91–106; 107–14.

Grumbach, M.M., Roth, J.C., Kaplen, J.L. & Kelch, R.P. (1974) In *Control of the onset of puberty* (ed. by M.M. Grumbach, G.D. Grove & F.E. Meyer), p. 158. Wiley, New York.

Hartigan, P.J. (1995) Cattle breeding and infertility. In *Animal Breeding and Infertility* (ed. by M.J. Meredith), pp. 86–186. Blackwell Science, Oxford.

Hartigan, P.J., Langley, O.H., Nunn, W.R. & Griffin, J.F.T. (1974) Some data on ovarian activity in post-parturient dairy cows in Ireland. *Irish Veterinary Journal*, **28**, 236–41.

Hunter, R.H.F. & Wilmut, I. (1984) Sperm transport in the cow: peri-ovulatory redistribution of viable cells. *Reproduction Nutrition Development*, **214**, 597–608.

Ireland, J.J., Mihm, M., Austin, E., Diskin, M.G. & Roche, J.F. (2000) Historical perspective of turnover of dominant follicles during the bovine estrous cycle: key concepts, studies, advancements, and terms. *Journal of Dairy Science*, **83**, 1648–58.

Kulick, L.J., Kot, K., Wiltbank, M.C. & Ginther, O.J. (1999) Follicular and hormonal dynamics during the first follicular wave in heifers. *Theriogenology*, **52**, 913–21.

Lamming, G.E., Wathes, D.C. & Peters, A.R. (1981) Endocrine patterns in the post-partum cow. *Journal of Reproduction and Fertility*, **Supplement 30**, 155–70.

Lindell, J.O. & Kindahl, H. (1983) Exogenous prostaglandin $F_{2\alpha}$ promotes uterine involution in the cow. *Acta Veterinaria Scandinavica*, **24**, 269–74.

McCracken, J.A., Custer, E.E. & Lamsa, J.C. (1999). Luteolysis: a neuroendocrine-mediated event. *Physiological Reviews*, **79**, 263–323.

McLaren, A. (1984) In *Reproduction in Mammals*, 2nd edn (ed. by C.R. Austin & R.V. Short), Book 2, p. 21. Cambridge University Press, Cambridge.

Meiden, R., Milvae, R.A., Weiss, S., Levy, N. & Friedman, A. (1999) Intra-ovarian regulation of luteolysis. *Journal of Reproduction and Fertility*, **Supplement 54**, 217–28.

O'Callaghan, D. & Boland, M.P. (1999) Nutritional effects on ovulation, embryo development and the establishment of pregnancy in ruminants. *Animal Science*, **68**, 299–314.

Rahe, C.H., Owens, R.E., Fleegen, J.L., Newton, A.J. & Harms, D.G. (1980) Patterns of plasma luteinizing hormone in the cyclic cow: dependence upon the period of the cycle. *Endocrinology*, **107**, 498–503.

Roche, J.F., Austin, E., Ryan, M., O'Rourke, M., Mihm, M. & Diskin, M.G. (1999) Regulation of follicle waves to maximize fertility in cattle. *Journal of Reproduction and Fertility*, **Supplement 54**, 61–71.

Roche, J.F., Mackey, D. & Diskin, M.G. (2000) Reproductive management of postpartum cows. *Animal Reproduction Science*, **60–1**, 703–12.

Short, R.V. (1984) In *Reproduction in Mammals*, 2nd edn (ed. by C.R. Austin & R.V. Short), Book 3, p. 139. Cambridge University Press, Cambridge.

Smith, G.D., Jackson, L.M. & Foster, D.L. (2002) Leptin regulation of reproductive function and fertility. *Theriogenology*, **57**, 73–86.

Urbanski, H.F. (2001) Leptin and puberty. *Trends in Endocrinology and Metabolism*, **12**, 428–9.

Wade, G.N. & Schneider, J.E. (1992) Metabolic fuels and reproduction in female mammals. *Neuroscience and Biobehavioral Reviews*, **16**, 235–72.

Webb, R., Gosden, R.G., Telfer, E.E. & Moor, R.M. (1999) Factors affecting folliculogenesis in ruminants. *Animal Science*, **68**, 257–84.

Wiltblank, M.C., Fricke, P.M., Sangsritavong, S., Sartori, R. & Ginther, O.J. (2000) Mechanisms that prevent and produce double ovulations in dairy cattle. *Journal of Dairy Science*, **83**, 2998–3007.

Wiltbank, M.C., Gumen, A. & Sartori, R. (2002) Physiological classifications of anovulatory conditions in cattle. *Theriogenology*, **57**, 21–52.

Chapter 34
The Postpartum Period

I.M. Sheldon, D.C. Barrett and H. Boyd

Introduction	508
Uterine involution	508
Regeneration of the uterine epithelium	509
Elimination of bacterial contamination	509
Return of ovarian cyclicity	509
Monitoring the postpartum period	511
Herd records	511
Individual clinical cases	511
History	511
Clinical examination	511
Principal factors affecting the postpartum period	512
Enhancement of the postpartum period	513
Postpartum lesions of the genital tract	513
Lacerations and haemorrhage	513
Uterine prolapse	514
Retained fetal membranes	515
Pneumovagina and urovagina	519
Vaginitis	519
Acute puerperal metritis	519
Endometritis	521
Pyometra	524
Postpartum anoestrus	525
Cystic ovarian disease	526
Prevention of postpartum disease problems	526
Breeding decisions and the management of the pregnant and periparturient cow	526
Therapy immediately postpartum	527
Conclusions	527

Introduction

The postpartum period is the time during which the genital tract recovers after parturition, and returns to a normal state ready for the next pregnancy. Despite a trend for extended lactation for higher genetic merit dairy cows producing high milk yields, the majority of farmers still select an earliest service date, or voluntary waiting period, between 40 and 60 days after calving. Similarly, in seasonally calved herds, a short period for recovery following pregnancy is often essential for those animals that calve during the later part of the season. Monitoring the uterus and ovaries in the postpartum period is important because delayed uterine involution, the presence of postpartum uterine infec-tion or abnormal ovarian function causes subfertility which results in substantial economic loss for the cattle industry. Retained fetal membranes, endometritis and cystic ovarian disease, for example, delayed conception by 25, 31 and 64 days, respectively compared with cows with a normal postpartum period (Borsberry & Dobson, 1989).

The events that comprise the postpartum period are uterine involution, regeneration of the endometrium, elimination of bacterial contamination of the uterus and the return of ovarian cyclical activity. The initial stimulus for these changes to occur is the expulsion of the fetus along with the associated membranes and fluids at calving.

Uterine involution

Uterine involution is the return of the genital tract after calving to normal non-pregnant dimensions. This involves physical shrinkage, necrosis and sloughing of caruncles, and the regeneration of the endometrium. There is considerable loss of tissue, with the mean weight of the uterus decreasing from about 13 kg before parturition to about 1 kg during a 30-day period (Kaidi *et al.*, 1991). The uterus and cervix contract rapidly immediately after calving and it is often difficult to insert a hand through the cervix 24 hours postpartum; the cervix only admits two fingers by 96 hours postpartum. Uterine involution occurs in a decreasing logarithmic scale with the greatest change during the first few days after parturition (Fig. 34.1). By 10 to 14 days postpartum the entire genital tract is palpable *per rectum* in normal animals, although the previously gravid horn can still be identified because it is longer and has a greater diameter than the con-tralateral horn. Although the time required for com-plete involution is 40 to 50 days, the changes in uterine diameter are almost imperceptible after 20 days post-partum. Involution is delayed by postpartum disease including milk fever, retained fetal membranes and uterine infection.

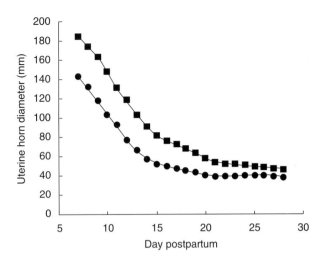

Fig. 34.1 The mean external diameter of the previously gravid (■) and non-gravid (●) uterine horns between 7 and 28 days postpartum.

Regeneration of the uterine epithelium

Following the loss of the allantochorion there is necrosis of the uterine caruncle and this has usually sloughed by day 12 postpartum. Sloughing of the uterine caruncles contributes significantly to the rapid reduction in weight of the involuting postpartum uterus because the caruncles account for over half of the weight of the uterus. The sloughed caruncles form the lochial discharge, along with the remains of fetal fluids and blood from the ruptured umbilicus. The lochia is usually a yellow to brown, viscous fluid without an unpleasant odour. The uterus of normal animals contains one to two litres of lochia immediately postpartum and the greatest discharge is in the first two to three days; it has virtually disappeared by 14 to 18 days after calving.

There is initially regeneration of the endometrium in the intercaruncular areas and then by centripetal growth of the cells over the caruncle. Epithelial regeneration is complete by about day 25 postpartum, but the deeper layers of tissues are not fully restored until 6 to 8 weeks postpartum. Whilst these epithelial changes are taking place the caruncles are shrinking. By 40 to 60 days postpartum the caruncles are only 4 to 8 mm diameter and 4 to 6 mm high, compared with 40 to 70 mm diameter and 25 mm high at calving.

Elimination of bacterial contamination

At calving, the vulva is relaxed and the cervix dilated, allowing bacteria to gain entry to the vagina and the uterus. The postpartum environment of the uterine lumen supports the growth of a variety of aerobic and anaerobic bacteria. Many of these bacteria are simple contaminants in the uterine lumen and are removed by a range of uterine defence mechanisms (Box 34.1). In one study, 93 per cent of the uteri obtained at an abattoir within 15 days of calving yielded bacteria on aerobic and anaerobic culture of lumenal swabs and endometrial tissue (Elliot *et al.*, 1968). The number of uteri from which bacteria were isolated had declined to 78 per cent by 16 to 30 days, 50 per cent at 31 to 45 days and 9 per cent by 46 to 60 days postpartum. In the live animal, there is a constantly fluctuating bacterial flora in the first 7 weeks postpartum due to spontaneous contamination, clearance and recontamination. However, uterine infection is commonly associated with *Escherichia coli*, *Arcanobacterium pyogenes*, *Fusobacterium necrophorum* and *Prevotella* (formerly *Bacteroides*) species. Indeed, *A. pyogenes*, *F. necrophorum* and *Prevotella* species have been shown to act synergistically to enhance the likelihood of uterine disease and increase the risk of clinical endometritis and its severity.

Box 34.1. Uterine defence mechanisms.

- Intrauterine neutrophils
- Physical barriers of the vulva and cervix
- Persistent uterine contractions and involution
- Caruncular sloughing (to expel adherent bacteria)
- Secretory immunoglobulins
- Cell mediated immunity
- Intrauterine pH (rises at oestrus to 7.0, from 6.4 during dioestrus, which reduces bacterial growth)
- Resident vaginal bacterial flora

Return of ovarian cyclicity

During the bovine oestrous cycle, ovarian follicular development occurs in a wave pattern starting with the emergence and recruitment of two to six follicles of 4 to 6 mm diameter (Savio *et al.*, 1988). One of these follicles is selected to continue to grow and become the dominant follicle, whilst the remaining follicles become atretic and regress (Fig. 34.2). Each follicular wave is preceded by an increase in circulating FSH concentration (Adams *et al.*, 1992). Selection of the dominant follicle results in oestradiol production, and negative feedback on FSH, with the follicle subsequently becoming LH dependent (Ginther *et al.*, 1996). Early luteal phase progesterone secretion, however, suppresses LH pulse frequency and the first dominant follicle under-

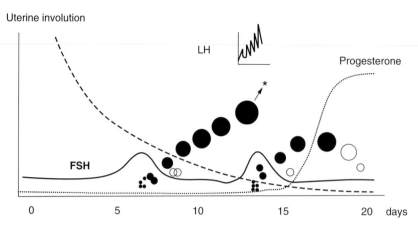

Fig. 34.2 Cartoon of resumption of ovarian cyclical activity in a dairy cow during the first 20 days postpartum. As uterine involution (--) progresses, there is a transient increase in plasma FSH concentration (——), followed by the emergence of several follicles > 4 mm diameter (•), with subsequent selection of a dominant follicle (●) and atresia of the subordinate follicles (○). The fate of the first dominant follicle is dependent on LH pulse frequency, which in the present case is sufficient to cause ovulation (*), and the subsequent formation of a corpus luteum secreting progesterone (...), heralding the return of ovarian cyclical activity.

goes atresia. Conversely, at the other end of the cycle, after luteolysis the LH pulse frequency increases, stimulating growth of another dominant follicle that increases plasma oestradiol concentrations, which subsequently stimulate an LH surge and ovulation.

Throughout pregnancy, regular periodic emergence of anovulatory follicular waves occurs in response to recurrent FSH surges, except for the last 21 days of pregnancy due to very high plasma progesterone and oestrogen concentrations. After parturition steroid hormone concentrations decrease to basal values, there is an increase in plasma FSH concentration within days of calving and that stimulates the emergence of the first postpartum follicular wave. Subsequently, the first dominant follicle is selected around day 10 to 12 postpartum (Savio *et al.*, 1990; Beam & Butler, 1997). These events occur in all postpartum cows irrespective of periparturient disease, environment or dietary deficiencies. However, the first dominant follicle has three possible fates: ovulation and formation of the first postpartum corpus luteum (return of ovarian cyclical activity), atresia with the emergence of one or more follicular waves without ovulation (anoestrus) or formation of an ovarian follicular cyst (Beam & Butler, 1997). In Europe, 70–80 per cent of first dominant follicles are ovulated in dairy cattle fed an appropriate diet whereas in the beef suckler cow ovulation of the early postpartum dominant follicles is less frequent (Roche & Boland, 1991). The prolonged interval to return of ovarian cyclicity in beef suckler cows is an expression of their failure to ovulate, rather than a failure to develop, dominant follicles. The principal factor determining the fate of the dominant follicles is LH pulse fre-

quency; ovulation generally occurs once the LH pulse frequency is one per hour. Therefore, factors that suppress LH pulse frequency in the postpartum period can delay the return of ovarian cyclical activity. Those factors causing anoestrus tend to be more common in the beef suckler cow, and include suckling or the maternal bond, low body condition score and inadequate nutrition. The principal factor causing anoestrus in dairy cattle is negative energy balance.

An interesting feature of ovarian follicular growth within 4 weeks of parturition is that there are fewer dominant follicles or corpora lutea in the ovary ipsilateral to the previously gravid uterine horn, compared with the contralateral ovary (Sheldon *et al.*, 2000). However, the presence of a dominant follicle in the ipsilateral ovary, although less frequent, is a positive marker of subsequent fertility.

Early return of cyclical ovarian activity is generally accepted to be beneficial for subsequent fertility (Darwash *et al.*, 1997); however, others have reported the converse (Smith & Wallace, 1998). Furthermore, it is suggested that an early postpartum first ovulation in the presence of uterine infection can lead to pyometra with persistence of a CL in the presence of pus within the uterine lumen (Olson *et al.*, 1984).

Farmers rarely observe oestrus at the time of the first postpartum ovulation in cattle, and in a significant number of animals the first luteal phase is relatively short. Using continuous observation, oestrus is detectable at the time of about 50 per cent of first and 95 per cent of second ovulations. It is suggested that a period of progesterone dominance prior to ovulation is important for oestrous expression.

Monitoring the postpartum period

Herd records

Recording the basic fertility parameters including the date of calving, dates of observed oestrus and service dates is invaluable for analysis to determine whether a herd is achieving its fertility targets (see also Chapter 41 (b)). The importance of efficient and accurate heat detection cannot be stressed too often to farmers. In addition, the recording of calving ease, the occurrence of retained fetal membranes, abnormal vulval discharge and other peripartum problems identify those herds, and animals within a herd, that warrant particular attention during the postpartum period.

Individual clinical cases

In many cows presented immediately after calving, diagnosis of postpartum problems is quite simple, for example retained fetal membranes or prolapse of the uterus. However, a cow that is acutely ill could be suffering from a variety of conditions and, therefore, a systematic approach to diagnosis is necessary both for differential diagnosis and to ascertain the severity of the condition. Investigation of the individual cow should include the history, a thorough physical examination and further investigations as indicated.

History

Questions should be asked to ascertain whether the cow was ill before calving and whether the illness was related to reproduction or was a condition that is obviously related, such as a pathological vaginal discharge. Information about previous feeding and management should be gathered, particularly relating to the transition period, with the object of determining whether the diet could have predisposed to metabolic diseases. Details of other postpartum problems in the herd in this and previous breeding seasons should also be obtained.

The place where the cow calved should be inspected to assess the level of environmental hygiene during calving. The farmer should be asked if the calving was assisted and, if so, how much and what help was given, by whom and what hygienic precautions were taken. It is also important to determine whether the client has given any treatment already.

Clinical examination

A thorough clinical examination must be undertaken, although the optimum time after calving for examination is debatable. Most often in outwardly healthy animals an examination is made three to five weeks postpartum to identify abnormalities of the puerperium that might lead to subsequent infertility. This may include the following procedures.

Physical examination

Body condition scoring of cows at drying-off, at calving, at routine postpartum examinations and at the time of insemination is an effective method to assess the adequacy of nutrition in a herd and to monitor energy balance. Indeed, changes in body condition score reflect the effect of negative energy balance on fertility as well as other markers of energy balance such as plasma concentrations of insulin-like growth factor 1 (IGF-1) and β-OH butyrate (BHB). In addition, the presence of ketosis can be established by analysis of urine, milk or serum, and is associated with postpartum uterine infection (Markusfeld, 1984). The use of milk analysis as a method of assessing the nutrition of dairy cattle and their metabolic status is discussed further in Chapter 47 (see p. 807).

Palpation *per rectum* of the genital tract is the predominant method of assessing uterine involution and the return of ovarian cyclicity. Uterine involution may be considered to be complete when the genital tract has contracted such that the uterine horns are of equal diameter and length and the uterus has returned to lie within the pelvic cavity. Return of ovarian cyclicity is usually determined by the palpation of a corpus luteum in the ovary; palpation of follicles in the ovary does not indicate return of ovarian cyclicity. Anoestrus cows may have ovarian follicles up to 18 mm diameter, but there is no corpus luteum. Palpation of ovarian structures more than 25 mm in diameter may indicate the presence of a follicular or luteal cyst. However, a substantial proportion of cystic structures identified before day 30 postpartum will spontaneously regress (Chapter 35).

Palpation *per rectum* alone is not sufficient to determine the adequacy of uterine involution and elimination of bacterial contamination. A vaginal examination is essential for the assessment of the presence or absence of postpartum uterine bacterial infection. Generally, a manual examination of the vagina is performed by inserting a lubricated, clean, gloved hand between clean vulval lips. During the examination, vaginal and cervical os lacerations and abnormalities are noted and a sample of vaginal mucus withdrawn and examined for character, volume and smell. The combination of a vaginal examination and a rectal palpation can be used to score the severity of endometritis, which is a prognostic indicator of the success rate of treatment for endometritis (Sheldon & Noakes, 1998). Observation of the vagina, vaginal mucus and the cervix with a speculum may provide additional information; sterile, disposable specula are available.

Ultrasonography

Real-time B-mode ultrasonography using a linear array transrectal probe has revolutionized the veterinarian's ability to monitor the return of ovarian cyclical activity and uterine involution. Visualization of the genital tract before day 10 postpartum is difficult, particularly in older animals, and a 5 MHz probe is more appropriate for examination of the enlarged uterus at this time. However, a 7.5 MHz probe is superior for examination of the ovaries. Ultrasonography is particularly useful for identifying ovarian follicles; a dominant follicle is usually defined as a follicle ≥9 mm diameter in the absence of other large growing follicles. However, caution has to be exerted when considering structure and function; the detection of a large follicle or follicular cyst alone does not indicate that it is endocrinologically active (Beam & Butler, 1997).

Use of the ultrasound machine's internal callipers allows measurement of the diameter of the uterus and ovarian structures and comparison with the expected normal values determined by sequential measurement of uterine horn diameter during the process of involution. In addition, abnormal contents of the uterine lumen are readily detected. The entire length of both uterine horns should be scanned, because often pus is localized within a limited section of the genital tract. However, the use of transrectal ultrasonography does not negate the value of performing a manual or specular examination of the vagina before examining the remainder of the genital tract.

Progesterone analysis

Estimation of plasma or milk progesterone by enzyme-linked immunosorbent assay (ELISA) or radioimmunoassay (RIA), collected two to three times per week after calving is adequate to determine the first postpartum luteal activity and abnormal patterns of ovarian activity. Milk samples are more practicable in the field because of the ease of collection. Samples of 10 ml of milk can be stored for at least a month in containers with a potassium dichromate tablet as a preservative (Lactab Mk III, Thompson & Capper, Runcorn) and refrigerated at 4°C.

Endometrial biopsy

Histological examination of endometrial biopsies has not been used as frequently in cattle as in mares. However, endometrial biopsies are valuable indicators of subsequent reproductive performance. Unfortu-

nately, the cost of collection and evaluation for the individual animal precludes the widespread use of the technique in cattle.

Bacterial culture

Guarded transcervical swabs can be used to collect samples of intrauterine fluid for bacterial culture and identification. It is essential that both anaerobic and aerobic cultures are used, which requires the use of a transport medium and specialized microbiological techniques. The predominant pathogens associated with endometritis are *A. pyogenes*, *E. coli*, *F. necrophorum* and *Prevotella melaninogenicus*. Sensitivity tests for selection of an appropriate antibiotic might be of value for herds with a high incidence of endometritis.

Principal factors affecting the postpartum period

There are a variety of factors than can influence the duration of the postpartum period. For convenience, we have already considered the various components of this period as separate entities; however, this does not reflect the normal situation. Uterine involution, bacterial infection and the return of ovarian cyclicity are all closely linked.

Abnormalities of the puerperium such as dystokia, retained fetal membranes, stillbirths, abortions and twins delay uterine involution and the return of ovarian cyclicity. In addition, these problems are associated with an increased risk of metritis and/or endometritis. Conversely, early postpartum ovulation prior to the elimination of bacterial contamination may predispose to pyometra if uterine infection persists in the presence of a corpus luteum.

Suckling has been widely reported to delay the return of ovarian cyclicity. It is interesting to compare studies using milk progesterone estimation to determine the mean time to postpartum resumption of ovarian cycles in dairy (Bulman & Lamming, 1978) and beef cows (Peters & Riley, 1982), which were 24.0 ± 0.6 and 59.9 ± 2.5 days, respectively. It would appear that this inhibitory influence, mediated by reduced LH secretion, is a function of the maternal bond attributable to the dam's own calf, rather than simply an effect of suckling or milk yield (Williams & Griffith, 1995). It has also been suggested that higher milk yields are associated with longer acyclic periods, although it is difficult to separate the effects of milk yield and confounding factors such as nutrition.

Inadequate nutrition, and particularly a diet deficient in energy, is the most important cause of postpartum anoestrus. Body condition score (BCS), particularly in beef suckler cattle, is an important factor affecting the resumption of ovarian cyclicity and cows with a body condition score less than 2.5 are likely to have a significant delay (see p. 10). In dairy cows, changes in BCS after calving are more important than BCS at calving.

Enhancement of the postpartum period

Shortening the postpartum period would increase the opportunity for rebreeding cattle after calving. Unfortunately, most practical attempts to advance uterine involution have been disappointing; a variety of therapeutic agents have been used in the early postpartum period with no significant effect.

A number of therapeutic agents have been used to try to induce ovulation in the early postpartum period and, therefore, shorten the interval to return of ovarian cyclicity; these agents include GnRH, progesterone and eCG (see p. 678). However, results are inconsistent and often of little long-term benefit to the fertility of the herd.

In the absence of consistently effective pharmacological methods of shortening the postpartum period, it is particularly important for the veterinary surgeon to be familiar with the management factors affecting this period and to give appropriate advice to clients to avoid their negative effects. For example, veterinarians should use condition score targets for key points in the management cycle such as at calving and drying off, in dairy cattle, or weaning, in beef suckler cows. In addition, it is important to ensure the cows are fed an appropriate diet, paying particular attention to the energy density of the ration.

Postpartum lesions of the genital tract

Traumatic injuries to the genital tract, bony pelvis and nerves of the pelvis sometimes occur during normal parturition. However, they are more common following dystokia. Postpartum problems include traumatic injuries such as penetrating wounds and tears of the uterus or vagina, tearing of the cervix or vulva, rectovaginal fistula formation, haemorrhage and haematoma, as well as other conditions such as retention of the fetal membranes and prolapse of the uterus (Noakes, 2001a).

Lacerations and haemorrhage

There is usually, but not always, a history of a protracted or particularly difficult *per vaginam* delivery of the calf.

The first action of the obstetrician after the delivery and resuscitation of a calf should always be to check the dam for trauma. If haemorrhage is apparent its severity should be assessed and appropriate action taken; severe haemorrhage involving a large artery can be rapidly fatal.

Traumatic and post-traumatic lesions are treated according to general principles of wound management. If the calf has been delivered without the use of epidural analgesia, but surgical intervention is required to control haemorrhage, then the use of an epidural should be considered. In order to prolong the duration of analgesia obtained by this method it may be advantageous to include xylazine in the epidural (Ko *et al.*, 1989; Holden, 1998). When a vaginal vessel is bleeding severely, an attempt must be made to clamp the traumatized vessel with artery forceps which can them be left in place for 24 hours. Ligation and the suturing of lacerations would also be indicated in some cases, although it is often impractical due to the inability to gain adequate access to the site. If bleeding vaginal vessels cannot be clamped or ligated the only other option is to apply pressure using materials such as clean towels or bedsheets or a pressure pad containing ice in an attempt to bring about constriction of the bleeding vessels and promote blood clotting.

Where haemorrhage is occurring from uterine lacerations, oxytocin may also be used to promote contraction of the uterus. In cases of uterine rupture, laparotomy and surgical repair may be the only alternative to emergency slaughter. Following severe haemorrhage a blood transfusion may be indicated as a life saving procedure.

In less severe cases the bleeding may stop spontaneously, although lacerations, severe bruising and tissue trauma may result in the later development of necrotic vaginitis. Where perivaginal fat prolapses through vaginal lacerations and becomes necrotic, this may have to be removed to allow closure of the vaginal tear. Infection with *F. necrophorum* or *Clostridium* species may result in a locally severe reaction and serious systemic illness or death.

In the case of necrotic vaginitis emollient fluids and antiseptics are applied locally along with an appropriate systemic antibiotic such as a cephalosporin or potentiated amoxycillin. Following any difficult parturition with associated trauma to the reproductive tract the cow is likely to benefit from the administration of systemic non-steroidal anti-inflammatory drugs (NSAIDs) (Chapter 62).

The response to treatment of many vaginal lesions is good and the clinical signs will disappear within about 10 days. In these cases there is no interference with future reproduction. In a few cases infection spreads and affects the uterus, with resultant poor prognosis for fertility. Scar tissue may cause narrowing of the birth canal and interference with the next calving.

For further information on nerve damage, the reader should consult Chapter 32.

Uterine prolapse

Uterine prolapse is a relatively common complication of third stage labour in the bovine, with the uterus prolapsing within hours of the calf being delivered and prior to the cervix contracting (Noakes, 2001b). The usual presentation is of a complete inversion of the gravid uterine horn. While prolapse of the uterus may follow a dystokia with a high degree of traction, it is also commonly seen as a sequel to a normal or unassisted second stage labour. Plenderleith (1986) reports that the condition is recorded in 0.5 per cent of assisted calvings and 0.3 per cent of all calvings, while Correa *et al.* (1992) report the condition in 0.6 per cent of calvings. The main predisposing factor in the aetiology of this condition is considered to be uterine inertia immediately postpartum. Hypocalcaemia (milk fever) (see p. 781), which results in a reduction of smooth muscle tone in the uterus, and elsewhere, has been shown to increase the risk of uterine prolapse threefold, while dystokia increased the risk fivefold (Correa *et al.*, 1992). The increased risk of hypocalcaemia in older cows may explain why multigravida are more commonly affected than primigravida. Factors that are considered to predispose to prolapse of the uterus are summarized in Box 34.2.

Box 34.2. Possible predisposing factors for uterine prolapse.

- Fetal oversize and maternal/fetal disproportion
- Prolonged dystokia
- Fetal traction
- Hypocalcaemia
- Retained fetal membranes
- Chronic disease, particularly cattle in very poor body condition

---

When notified of a case of uterine prolapse, the veterinarian should inform the client to wrap the prolapse in a clean sheet to prevent further trauma and contamination and reduce heat loss.

When faced with a case of uterine prolapse in a cow with overt clinical signs of hypocalcaemia, treatment of the hypocalcaemia should probably be carried out prior to replacing the uterus, in case regurgitation and aspiration of rumen contents occurs or the cow succumbs to the hypocalcaemia. However, a non-life-threatening hypocalcaemia which maintains a cow in recumbency

with reduced abdominal straining may actually aid replacement of the prolapsed organ if the procedure can be undertaken swiftly and treatment with calcium borogluconate is not delayed too long.

The replacement of the uterus is aided by the correct positioning of the cow. If the cow is standing the uterus may be lifted on a sheet with the aid of two assistants and replaced from that position. However, if the cow is recumbent she should be placed in sternal recumbence in the frog-leg position as described by Plenderleith (1986) (Fig. 34.3) and if possible positioned facing down hill. This positioning of the cow is achieved by rolling her onto one side and pulling the opposite leg straight back, before rolling her to the other side and repeating the process. If necessary, ropes can be used to hold the cow in this position until the uterus has been replaced. Replacement of the uterus is greatly aided by the administration of an epidural anaesthetic, possibly including xylazine (Ko *et al.*, 1989; Holden, 1998); this also reduces postoperative straining and improves pain relief for the cow. Before replacing the uterus it must be carefully checked for trauma and cleaned as much as possible using a warm, non-irritant, antiseptic solution or normal saline; lacerations of the uterus may require suturing. There is no absolute need to remove the placenta, but often the most effective way of cleaning the organ is to remove the heavily contaminated fetal membranes. However, if the placentomes are still intact and the fetal membranes are not removed easily they should be left in place.

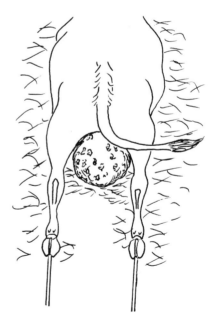

Fig. 34.3 Recumbent cow in the 'frog-leg' position for replacement of a uterine prolapse. Reproduced from Plenderleith (1986) with permission.

The weight of the uterus is best supported by an assistant on either side of the cow while the surgeon replaces the uterus little by little starting at the vulval lips. Gentle but continuous pressure is applied with a clenched fist or the open palm of the hand as portions of the uterus are pushed back into the vagina. Care must be taken to ensure that fingers are not pushed through the often friable uterine wall. Once the uterus begins to be replaced it is best to maintain momentum, as a single abdominal contraction from the cow while the uterus is not held can result in the entire uterus once again becoming prolapsed. As the uterus disappears within the vulval lips the veterinarian should continue to press it forward to the full length of his/her arm. It is important that the whole of the uterus passes through the cervix and that the total length of the uterine horn is fully replaced and any remaining inversion of the tip of the uterine horn reduced. This can be achieved using something to extend the veterinarian's reach such as a clean smooth-ended bottle. Alternatively a volume (5–10 litres) of warm clean water, normal saline or dilute antiseptic solution can be instilled into the uterus and then the majority can be siphoned back out. This has the added advantage that it also has a cleansing action, and any fluid remaining in the tip of the uterine horn may act to hold the uterus in place until the recurrence of normal uterine contractions results in its expulsion.

There is debate within the profession as to whether there is a need to suture the vulval lips closed after replacing a uterine prolapse. If suturing is considered necessary it is best to use Buhner's technique with obstetrical tape, although many other techniques are available (Hooper *et al.*, 1999). Following replacement of the uterus every effort must be made to restore uterine tone and promote involution and closure of the cervix. To this end hypocalcaemia must be treated and oxytocin may be administered; parenteral antibiotics and analgesics are also indicated. Some uterine prolapse cases prove fatal due to trauma and haemorrhage including rupture of the uterine and/or ovarian blood vessels, shock or the often concurrent hypocalcaemia. However, the prognosis depends largely on the following:

- The time lapse between the development of the prolapse occurring and professional treatments being undertaken.
- The degree of trauma that has taken place to the uterus.
- Associated periparturient conditions such us hypocalcaemia and haemorrhage.

There are few published reports looking at success rates for uterine prolapse cases. However, a study undertaken in New Zealand (Oakley, 1992) showed that 19 per cent of cows died within 24 hours of treatment and a further 16 per cent died or were lost to the study before the end of the next breeding season. Of those cows that were subsequently mated, 78 per cent were found to be pregnant, although 9 per cent subsequently aborted. This indicates that prompt attention to uterine prolapse gives a reasonable survival rate and acceptable subsequent conception rates. Possible complications following uterine prolapse are listed in Box 34.3.

Box 34.3. Possible complications of uterine prolapse.

- Hypocalcaemia
- Haemorrhage
- Metritis
- Endometritis
- Peritonitis
- Toxaemia/septicaemia
- Necrosis of devitalized tissue in longstanding cases
- Uterine rupture

Retained fetal membranes

Introduction

Retained fetal membranes (RFM) is a common condition that is defined as non-separation of the fetal membranes by 12 hours after calving (some authors extend this period to 24 hours before they consider the placental retention to be pathological). The incidence varies from study to study but tends to be about 5–10 per cent (Kossaibati & Esslemont, 1995; Parkinson, 2001); in a survey of >160 000 calvings in the Netherlands the average incidence was 6.6 per cent (Joosten *et al.*, 1988). In problem herds the incidence may be much higher. The year of calving, season of calving, parity of dam, calf mortality, calving difficulty and fetal presentation have all been shown to affect the incidence of RFM (Mee, 1991).

Diagnosis and consequences of retained fetal membranes

The diagnosis of RFM is self-apparent, the major variable being the effect of the condition on the cow's health. In many cases health is unaffected. However, the majority of cows have mild disturbances of appetite and body temperature. In a small number of cows, acute metritis develops causing severe illness, with typical signs of toxaemia and septicaemia. Without effective treatment this condition can be fatal. Some of the effects of RFM are summarized in Box 34.4. Economically, RFM represents one of the most significant postpartum abnormalities with each case reported to have a direct cost of approximately £85, mainly due to a reduction in milk yield and/or milk sales. When the effects on subsequent poor fertility are also considered

Box 34.4. Some of the effects of retained fetal membranes.

- Reduced dry matter intake
- Withholding of milk from the food chain and possibly a lowered milk production
- Increased incidence of postpartum metritis, endometritis and pyometra
- Increased time to first service
- Reduced conception rates/increased services per conception
- Increased days open
- Longer calving interval
- Predisposition of cows to other conditions such as left-displaced abomasum and laminitis
- Mortality

the cost is estimated to be around £300 per case (Kossaibati & Esslemont, 1997).

Aetiology

The specific pathogenesis of RFM still remains uncertain due in part to our poor understanding of normal placental separation in the bovine. However in simple terms there are considered to be two main ways in which fetal membrane retention occurs:

(1) Interference with the separation of the fetal villi from the maternal caruncles. This may be associated with the following:
  (a) Premature calving (induced or spontaneous) without the normal maturation of the placentome involving hormonal and structural changes in preparation for separation. This maturation involves changes in the molecular structure of collagen within the placentome and alteration in binucleate cell numbers in the trophectoderm. Spontaneous premature calvings will include many twin births as well as abortions.
  (b) Prolonged gestation may result in excessive growth of the dam's caruncles.
  (c) Trauma with oedema of the villi, which occurs after Caesarean section, torsion of the uterus and other dystokias.
  (d) Infectious conditions (with or without abortion) result in inflammatory changes that bind together the maternal and fetal tissue in the placentome.
  (e) Hyperaemia of the placentomes.
  (f) Necrosis of the villi.
(2) Observations on uterine contractions after calving suggest that in many cases of retained fetal membranes, their frequency and amplitude are greater

than in cows that released the membranes normally. However, on some occasions retention is associated with uterine atony: for instance, after overextension of the myometrium as in cases of hydrops allantois, or prolonged labour or in hypocalcaemic cows. It is unlikely, however, that uterine atony in the absence of some disturbance of the process of caruncle/cotyledon separation would result in RFM.

In addition to the above mechanisms, nutritional problems such as vitamin E/selenium, iodine and vitamin A deficiency have been reported to be associated with an increased incidence of RFM in some herds, although individual cows are not normally considered to develop RFM due to nutritional deficiencies.

Laven and Peters (1996) have reviewed the aetiology and pathogenesis of fetal membrane retention in detail.

Treatment

Over time the natural sloughing of the maternal caruncles and uterine involution contributes to the loss of the membranes. If left untreated, freeing of the fetal villi from the maternal caruncles eventually occurs as a result of bacterial putrefaction and autolysis over several days. The toxic products of this putrefaction accumulate within the uterus, causing a fetid odour that taints the milk making it unfit for human consumption.

Moller *et al.* (1967) describe a large clinical trial in which the results of a wide variety of treatments were studied. They pointed out that cows that are ill and cows with metritis must be treated, but they concluded that the evidence did not indicate a need to treat cases of uncomplicated placental retention. In fact it appeared that any type of drug therapy for this condition tended to depress subsequent pregnancy rates, whereas cows that were not treated (that is, membranes not removed, no drug therapy administered) had pregnancy rates that were not significantly different from those achieved by cows that passed the membranes at the proper time. In cows that remain healthy, treatment may therefore not be indicated. However, in a small proportion severe metritis and toxaemia may develop, which may be fatal if left untreated.

Manual removal of fetal membranes: Veterinarians have been arguing for decades over the need for manual removal of retained fetal membranes. It should be borne in mind that although the results of many field trials tend to favour non-removal, the arguments in favour of manual removal are said to include the following:

(1) It removes a major source of infection and putrefying protein.

(2) It removes the unpleasant smell, which can taint the milk, and physical presence of the retained membranes.

(3) The cow may be less likely to develop systemic illness.

(4) The cow may be less likely to have disturbed fertility later.

(5) The cow may be less likely to suffer from reduced milk yield.

(6) A small number of conservatively treated cows become very ill and require life-saving treatment.

These points are not necessarily sufficient justification for manual removal of RFM, as point 2 is a benefit to the farmer rather than the cow and points 3, 4 and 5 have been contradicted by many published trials. Points 1 and 6 are true, although there is little evidence that toxaemia occurs because the placenta has not been removed. Toxaemia can occur after removal of the placenta (Peters & Laven, 1996).

Those in favour of manual removal claim that the danger of reproductive or general disease is greatly reduced with gentle handling, a willingness to stop manual removal where the attachment is firm, and the concurrent use of local or systemic antibiotics. If manual removal is to be used this should not be attempted until a minimum of 96 hours after calving and in many cases it is necessary to leave for a longer time period than this. Manipulation should be confined to gentle traction on the membranes and not involve the manual breaking down of each individual placentome as this results in significant trauma to the endometrium.

The arguments used against manual removal of the retained fetal membranes include the following:

(1) Just after calving the cow is ready to deal with the large amount of infected material and decomposing necrotic caruncles that are sloughed off into the uterus in the normal course of events; the need to get rid of fetal membranes as well presents no insurmountable problem to most cows.

(2) Intrauterine manual intervention should be avoided because it interferes with the natural defence mechanism by reducing phagocytosis for several days.

(3) Manual removal of the membranes is never complete and numerous villi and remnants of placenta are left attached.

(4) Manual removal causes trauma and adds to the likelihood of local infection persisting.

(5) If the cow is ill, systemic treatment is sufficient to deal with the problem and manual removal may worsen the cow's condition.

Advocates of conservative treatment may intervene only if the animal develops signs of systemic disease, in which cases the treatment is systemic administration of a broad-spectrum antibiotic. Other veterinarians simply cut off the part of the membranes that is visible to reduce the smell and only apply other treatment in those (few) cases that become systemically ill.

It would seem that current practice in the field is often at odds with research findings regarding treatment of RFM. Laven (1995) undertook a survey of the methods used by British veterinarians for treating RFM and found that manual removal was used in some cases by at least 92.5 per cent of respondents. Ecbolic agents including prostaglandin $F_{2\alpha}$ (or analogues of $PGF_{2\alpha}$) and oxytocin were sometimes used by 84.2 per cent, with 15.7 per cent using oestradiol (no longer permitted in many countries) in an attempt to potentiate the effects of oxytocin. Most veterinarians reserved the use of antibiotics for cows that were systemically ill, but 18 per cent used them in animals with no overt illness. Only 1.6 per cent of respondents routinely left cases of RFM untreated.

At the present time it is difficult to say categorically that cows should or should not be treated by manual removal of the membranes, or which cows would benefit from manual removal rather than other medical or conservative treatment. However, it is in conditions such as RFM, where we need evidence-based medicine most, that treatment decisions of this type should be based on sound scientific and economic analysis to provide decision support rather than individual arbitrary decisions.

Ecbolic drugs: Prostaglandin $F_{2\alpha}$ or analogues have been administered systemically to encourage the removal of fetal membranes. Stevens *et al.* (1995) evaluated the use of an intrauterine infusion of oxytocin, subcutaneous injections of fenprostalene or a combination of both. They concluded that the interval from parturition to expulsion of the fetal membranes was unaffected by treatment, as was the frequency of subsequent displaced abomasum, ketosis and mastitis. However, Stocker and Waelchli (1993) found that the administration of $PGF_{2\alpha}$ after Caesarean section decreased the risk of retention of fetal membranes.

Similarly, oxytocin used up to 36 hours after calving may increase myometrial contractions and hasten expulsion of the membranes. Trial results have been variable regarding the use of oxytocin (Stevens & Dinsmore, 1997), however its administration may be of some benefit to counteract the effects of uterine relaxants used during obstetrical procedures or Caesarean sections. Oestrogen alone has also been used (but is probably contraindicated and is no longer available for use in food producing species in some countries). In short, ecbolic drugs are unlikely to be effective after a diagnosis of RFM has been made, but they may reduce the incidence of RFM in certain groups of cows if administered very soon after the delivery of the calf.

Collagenase: Eiler and Hopkins (1993) reported using collagenase as an infusion into the umbilical artery; a dose of 200 000 iu of collagenase was dissolved in 1 litre of saline and infused between 24 and 72 hours after parturition. The technique was reported to give an 85 per cent success rate in cases of spontaneous RFM. However, no further reports of this technique have appeared in the literature and it has not been accepted and taken up widely. This author has no personal experience of this technique and feels that there is a need for further research before it could be recommended.

Intrauterine medication: Various intrauterine medications have been advocated over the years including intrauterine infusions of oxytetracycline (Stevens *et al.,* 1995). Brooks (2001) compared two different intrauterine pessaries administered after manual removal of RFM, one containing penicillin, streptomycin and formosulphathiazole and another made up of 8 per cent iodoform in a vegetable gelatine base. He was unable to detect any difference in the efficacy of the two products as determined by subsequent fertility, but did not compare the treatment groups with negative controls.

Intrauterine antimicrobial and antiseptic treatments are probably best reserved for the treatment of the sequels of RFM, including endometritis (see p. 521), rather than being seen as a treatment for RFM itself. There is even a school of thought that advocates not suppressing bacterial putrefaction of the membranes by administering local intrauterine antimicrobials as this slows the release of the membranes. Some intrauterine medications may also interfere with the local immune response within the uterus.

Other treatments: Other treatments such as intravenous calcium borogluconate, corticosteriods, multivitamins (Laven, 1995) and oral calcium chloride gel (Hernandez *et al.,* 1999) are advocated by some. However, their use is controversial and like the more established treatment options there is a lack of evidence to support their use. In some cases these treatments may actually be detrimental and thus contraindicated.

It should perhaps also be borne in mind that other treatments administered to the postpartum cow such as NSAIDs (e.g. flunixin meglumine) may even induce RFM (Waelchli *et al.,* 1999).

In summary, there is little scientific evidence to support anything other than conservative treatment of

RFM, with close monitoring of the cow so that supportive therapy can be instigated rapidly in the small number of cases that develop systemic illness. Veterinary efforts should be concentrated on preventing the high incidence of RFM at the herd level and minimizing the reproductive and economic consequences of the condition.

Prevention of retained fetal membranes

General preventive measures for postpartum disease problems including RFM are discussed at the end of this chapter (p. 526). With specific reference to RFM, attempts at prevention by routine treatment of all cows at calving are generally ineffective and impractical because of the relatively low incidence and morbidity of the condition. However, incidence of retention is increased greatly when parturition is induced with corticosteroids and there is some evidence that $PGF_{2\alpha}$ can be an effective therapeutic agent in such cases. Gross *et al.* (1986) used dexamethasone to induce parturition in 66 cows; they injected $PGF_{2\alpha}$ into 40 cows within one hour of delivery and treated 26 cows with saline (controls). The incidence of retention in the $PGF_{2\alpha}$-treated cows was 8.8 per cent compared with 90.5 per cent in the controls. This approach to prevention is supported by findings that suggest that cows which subsequently develop RFM have lower levels of endogenous $PGF_{2\alpha}$ at the time of calving than those without RFM (Wischral *et al.,* 2001).

Effects of retained fetal membranes

The effect of retained fetal membranes on subsequent fertility depends on whether acute metritis, endometritis or pyometra develops or not. While there is argument about the best treatment at the time of retention, there is general agreement that it is important to monitor cases closely until the membranes are lost. They should also be examined again about 18–30 days after calving to identify and treat those cows that have developed endometritis or pyometra (see pp. 521, 524).

In an extensive field study with cows that retained the placenta for at least 48 hours, Leslie *et al.* (1984) reported that 14 per cent of the cows developed pyometra and 15 per cent developed chronic endometritis. In four herds in which a conservative approach to treatment was employed, metritis developed in 40 of 73 cases of retained fetal membranes (Sandals *et al.,*1979). From a study of days to service, days to conception and services per conception these authors concluded that the condition of retained fetal membranes alone has little effect on subsequent fertility. In a large field study (Halpern *et al.,* 1985) 45 per cent and 41 per cent of primiparous and pluriparous cows with retained fetal membranes developed metritis. In the heifers there was no significant adverse effect of retained fetal membranes on fertility. In adult cows with no subsequent metritis, retention for five or more days caused lower pregnancy rates than controls. Retention for more than seven days caused a long calving-to-service interval and low pregnancy rate. Borsberry and Dobson (1989), working in the UK, reported that RFM alone extended the calving interval by 25 days, but when it was associated with a subsequent endometritis this increased to 51 days. McDougall (2001) also reported that cows with RFM have lower pregnancy rates and take longer to conceive than unaffected herd-mates under New Zealand management systems. Rowlands and Lucey (1986) reported that the lactation yield following retained fetal membranes was 7 per cent lower than expected (Box 34.4).

Pneumovagina and urovagina

Pneumovagina may be caused by damage to the vulva during parturition or inadequate closure of an episiotomy incision. However, often there is no specific cause of pneumovagina or urovagina evident on presentation. Both conditions are often associated with a history of dystokia or delivery of a large calf; the affected cow frequently has a BCS < 2. Pneumovagina and urovagina may be unobserved until a genital tract examination or artificial insemination (AI) is performed. Occasionally, the herdsperson will observe a persistent dribble of urine from the vulva or hear air being sucked through the vulval lips.

The treatment of pneumovagina is to perform a Caslick's operation. Briefly, under epidural anaesthesia, the lips of the vulva are scarified along a 1 cm wide strip from the dorsal commissure to the level of the ischial arch, leaving 2.5–3.0 cm at the ventral commisure to permit urination. The lips of the vagina are sutured with a non-absorbable material. Concurrent vaginal and/or uterine infection is treated appropriately. Sutures are removed in 10 to 14 days and the animal artificially inseminated at the next oestrus.

There are a number of treatments for urovagina. Some cases will respond spontaneously, particularly those cases identified before 4 to 6 weeks postpartum and in animals that increase BCS. The return of ovarian cyclical activity, or possibly administration of $PGF_{2\alpha}$ to induce oestrus, may help resolution in some cases. The use of AI can be successful even in the presence of urovagina, in other cases. In severe or long-standing cases surgical intervention may be necessary. A caudal extension to the distal urethra can be constructed using the ventral vaginal wall or a transverse ventral shelf of tissue can be formed cranial to the urethral orifice.

Vaginitis

Vaginitis is often associated with a more extensive infection of the genital tract. However, inflammation may also be associated with pneumovagina, urovagina or following trauma during parturition. In addition, infectious causes of vaginitis are reported especially where natural service is practised. Infectious pustular vulvovaginitis caused by bovine herpes virus-1 (BHV-1) is probably the most common. However, other potential pathogens such as *Ureaplasma diversum*, *Mycoplasma bovigenitalium*, *Haemophilus somnus* and BHV-4 have also been implicated as causes of a mild granular vulvovaginitis (Cook, 1998).

The presenting sign of vaginitis is usually tenesmus; there may also be an abnormal vaginal or vulval discharge and changes in the mucosa, varying from hyperaemia through necrosis to gangrene in rare cases. Occasionally there is a more extensive retroperitonitis and septicaemia. A mild vaginitis has little effect on subsequent fertility unless accompanied by endometritis, pneumovagina or urovagina. However, severe cases of vaginitis may cause extensive scarring leading to infertility or in some instances to dystokia at the subsequent parturition.

Treatment should be based on the severity of the lesions and correction of predisposing factors. The vagina should be gently douched with normal saline or a mild antiseptic solution, following administration of an epidural anaesthetic. The duration of activity of the epidural anaesthesia can be extended by the addition of xylazine to the anaesthetic solution (Caron & Le Blanc, 1989). Douching of the vagina may be repeated on several occasions. In addition, infection of deeper tissues should be treated using systemic antibiotics. Inflammation can be reduced and analgesia provided using NSAIDs.

Acute puerperal metritis

Microbial contamination of the uterine lumen at parturition is a normal event (Elliot *et al.,* 1968) (see p. 509), and in most cows this contamination is eliminated and does not result in severe infection. For this reason acute puerperal metritis is relatively uncommon. However, in those cases where it does occur acute inflammatory changes are seen in the endometrial, myometrial and peritoneal layers of the uterus within ten days of calving. Pathogenic bacteria produce toxins and result in the development of septicaemia, toxaemia and possibly also pyaemia. Cows with acute puerperal metritis have a very serious life-threatening condition that requires intensive treatment.

Diagnosis

A foetid, reddish to brown discharge flows from the vulva and abdominal straining is noted. Affected cows also commonly exhibit pyrexia, tachypnoea, tachycardia, anorexia, rumen stasis and dehydration. Severe cases may have a toxaemia-induced diarrhoea and develop signs of shock including a subnormal rectal temperature. The infection may extend through the uterine wall causing a localized or generalized peritonitis. Therefore internal examination of suspected cases of acute metritis must be undertaken with extreme care. The uterus is often friable and liable to trauma, and therefore uterine exploration should be minimized in the acute stages of the condition. Vaginal or rectal exploration of cases of metritis often results in acute discomfort and may be followed by persistent straining.

It is probable that in the future the diagnosis and monitoring of response to treatment of acute infections such as metritis will be aided by the use of acute phase protein estimations going some way towards removing the need for internal examinations (Eckersall, 2000; Sheldon *et al.*, 2001).

Aetiology

The physiology of the response to normal postpartum infection suggests that there are two main factors that lead to a pathological result.

(1) The uterus is exposed to an unusually high polymicrobial challenge that includes some of the more pathogenic organisms such as *A. pyogenes*, coliforms and anaerobes such as *F. necrophorum* and *Prevotella melaninogenicus*. In rare cases *Clostridium* spp. may cause severe disease and rapid death. The risk of postpartum intrauterine infection may be increased by:
 (a) Dystokia with resultant trauma inside the uterus;
 (b) The use of dirty equipment and dirty calving boxes;
 (c) The delivery of an emphysematous calf, resulting in the uterus being heavily infected with anaerobic organisms;
 (d) Retained fetal membranes;
 (e) Synergistic action between infectious agents, such as *A. pyogenes* and anaerobic organisms (*F. necrophorum* and *Prevotella melaninogenicus*).

(2) The natural defence mechanisms are less effective than normal. Factors that may cause this include the following:
 (a) Dystokia;
 (b) Manipulation within the uterus after calving, such as inappropriate and rough attempts to remove RFMs;
 (c) Uterine inertia;
 (d) Concomitant infection with immunosuppressant agents such as bovine virus diarrhoea virus.

The effect of diet before calving is unresolved; it is possible that dietary energy intakes that result in fatty infiltration of the liver, insufficient protein and micromineral deficiency may also impair uterine defence mechanisms.

Treatment and prognosis

Good nursing is vitally important. The cow should be placed in a well-bedded, comfortable warm box and encouraged to eat and drink. Systemic broad-spectrum antibiotic treatment applied in the correct dose, and maintained for a minimum of 5 days, is essential. Suitable antimicrobials include cephalosporins, potentiated amoxycillin or possibly tetracyclines. However, for good genital tract penetration postpartum oxytetracycline should be prescribed at a dose of 10 to 15 mg/kg b.i.d. This 'off-label' use is above the normal recommended dose and would require additional precautions to be taken to prevent problems with milk or meat residues. See also the section on antimicrobial treatment of endometritis (p. 522) for a fuller explanation of the efficacy of antimicrobials in the treatment of intrauterine infections.

Severely affected cows should also be treated aggressively with intravenous fluid therapy using either high volumes (20–30 litres or more) of isotonic fluid or low volumes of hypertonic fluid (3 litres of 7.2 per cent saline) to combat the effects of the toxaemia and to reduce the development of shock. Non-steroidal anti-inflammatory drugs (NSAIDs) such as flunixin meglumine are also indicated both to provide analgesia and to reduce the effects of endotoxins (see p. 1050). It might be expected that the administration of flunixin meglumine would inhibit normal uterine involution in cows with metritis, due to reduced biosynthesis of $PGF_{2\alpha}$. However, at least one study suggests that the administration of flunixin meglumine to cows with metritis accelerates uterine involution and shortens the calving to first oestrus interval (Amiridis *et al.*, 2001).

If the cow is continually straining, caudal epidural anaesthesia can be used; it may be advantageous to include xylazine in the epidural in order to prolong its duration of action (Ko *et al.*, 1989; Holden, 1998).

Any manipulation of the uterus should be avoided while the cow is systemically ill. However, after the acute phase of the disease a technique of gentle flushing and fluid withdrawal reduces the quantity of infected material in the uterus and may facilitate myometrial contractions and uterine involution. This can be done using a wide diameter smooth ended tube, such as a stomach tube attached to a funnel. The operator (taking extreme care not to traumatize the uterus) passes the tube through the cervix and pours in several litres of a flushing solution made up of warm sterile normal saline. The funnel is then lowered below the level of the uterus and the fluid along with debris from within the uterus is siphoned out. This procedure can be repeated several times to remove as much as possible of the uterine contents (Parkinson, 2001). While removal of the uterine contents in this way seems logical, and has been undertaken many times by these authors, it should be noted that controlled studies to evaluate this form of therapy are lacking. Flushing the uterus in this way also has inherent risks: the uterus may be punctured or damaged and irrigation fluid may flow in a retrograde direction up the oviducts, resulting in salpingitis and adhesions of the ovarian bursae.

Many clinicians introduce antibiotics into the uterus once the cow has responded to parenteral treatment, but the points discussed regarding the use of intrauterine antibiotics for the treatment of endometritis (see p. 522) should be borne in mind.

With acute metritis the prognosis refers to the possibility of death, adverse effect on health, milk yield and future reproductive function. Most cases make a fairly slow recovery as regards body condition, milk yield and return to cyclicity and pregnancy. In the worst affected cases, if the cow survives the acute metritis episode treatment can be considered a reasonable success.

Consequences of metritis

A small proportion of metritis cases develop embolic pneumonia, polyarthritis or endocarditis (see p. 726) as a consequence of a bacteraemia or laminitis following the toxaemia. In those cases that do respond to treatment, after recovery there may be adhesions affecting the uterus, the oviducts and ovarian bursae, resulting in reduced fertility. The majority of cases of acute metritis will also progress to endometritis.

In a meta-analysis of papers published since 1960, metritis was shown to be associated with a seven-day increase in time to first service and a 20 per cent reduction in conception rate to first service, resulting in a delay to conception of 19 days (Fourichon *et al.*, 2000).

Endometritis

Introduction

Endometritis is defined histologically as an inflammation of the endometrium. However, it is normally characterized clinically by the presence of a mucopurulent vaginal discharge, 21 days or more after calving, and associated with delayed uterine involution. The incidence of endometritis is about 10 per cent in dairy cattle, although the incidence in beef herds is less clear. However, there is wide variation in the incidence of endometritis between herds, ranging from a few cases to more than 40 per cent of the herd affected. Endometritis causes considerable subfertility and infertility. The presence of uterine bacterial contamination disrupts the delicate hormonal milieu of the hypothalamic–pituitary–ovarian axis (see p. 489; Chapter 67) and disrupts follicular growth and development. Uterine infection has been reported to be associated with an increased incidence of cystic ovarian disease. Furthermore, the presence and persistence of pathogenic organisms causing endometritis is assumed to preclude the establishment of pregnancy. Thus, endometritis has a detrimental effect on fertility, extending the calving to conception interval, and increasing the number of services per conception and the proportion of culls for failure to conceive.

The economic cost of endometritis depends on the detrimental effect on fertility, increased culling rate and, to a lesser extent, the cost of treatment. The estimated direct cost of a case of vulval discharge was £71 for treatment and a 300 litre reduction in milk yield (Kossaibati & Esslemont, 1997). However, the total cost was £160, including an increased calving interval of 18 days and an increase of 0.3 services per conception.

Aetiology

It is assumed that the uterus and its contents are sterile during a normal pregnancy and prior to parturition. Then at the time of parturition or just afterwards the uterine lumen becomes contaminated by micro-organisms from the animal's environment, skin and faeces, through the relaxed perineum, vulva and dilated cervix.

There are a variety of predisposing factors for endometritis (Box 34.5). Cows with a uterine infection associated with *A. pyogenes* more than 21 days postpartum develop a severe endometritis and are almost invariably subfertile to the first service. In addition, there is synergism between *A. pyogenes*, *F. necrophorum* and *Prevotella melaninogenicus*, causing more severe cases of endometritis. Interference with uterine defence mechanisms such as uterine involution or neutrophil function will delay the elimination of bacterial contamination. Dystokia, the delivery of twins or a

Box 34.5. Predisposing factors for endometritis.

- Retained fetal membranes
- Dystokia and/or assistance at calving
- Caesarian section
- Twins
- Stillbirths
- Induced parturition
- Dirty calving environment
- Postpartum ovarian inactivity
- Diet–possibly vitamin E/selenium deficiency

dead calf and assistance at calving increase the opportunity for faecal contamination of the genital tract. Retained fetal membranes are a predisposing factor for endometritis and are associated with an increase in severity of endometritis (Sheldon & Noakes, 1998).

Uterine infection has a seasonal incidence, being highest during the housed period, presumably because of environmental contamination. A dirty calving environment may increase the risk of endometritis. Noakes *et al.* (1991) described two hygienically contrasting farms: on one with a relatively clean environment the incidence of endometritis was 2–3 per cent, compared with an incidence of 15 per cent for one with a dirty environment. However, there was no difference in the quantitative or qualitative uterine bacterial flora in cows calved on either farm.

A delay in the return of cyclical ovarian activity after calving appears to predispose to endometritis. Conversely, if the interval from calving to first ovulation is too short, it has been suggested that pyometra could occur because *A. pyogenes* and Gram-negative anaerobic bacteria would remain within the uterus after ovulation, allowing bacterial growth to continue following corpus luteum formation (Olson *et al.*, 1984).

Diagnosis and assessment

Clinically, endometritis is characterized by the presence of a mucopurulent discharge in the vagina, associated with delayed uterine involution. The definitive diagnosis of endometritis would be made based on histological examination of endometrial biopsies. However, under field conditions, examination of the vagina and palpation of the genital tract *per rectum* are the most useful techniques for the diagnosis of endometritis. Visual or manual examination of the vagina for an abnormal uterine discharge is essential for the diagnosis of endometritis, although the contents of the vagina do not always reflect the contents of the uterus. Flakes of pus in the vagina could come from the uterus, cervix or vagina and slightly cloudy mucus is often regarded as normal. A number of scoring systems have been used to assess the degree of uterine and cervical involution, and the nature of the vaginal discharge. The majority of systems use a combination of uterine horn and cervical diameter and a score for the contents of the vagina (Fig. 34.4) (Sheldon & Noakes, 1998).

Treatment

The treatment of endometritis has caused considerable debate and has been reviewed extensively in the literature (Bretzlaff, 1987; Sheldon, 1999). The value of treatment of clinical cases has not been accepted by all clinicians, despite evidence that cows administered a placebo, rather than an accepted therapy, had longer intervals from calving to conception and higher culling rates (Steffan *et al.*, 1984). Treatment success rates are higher for mild cases of endometritis compared with severe cases and the success rate is reduced if the vaginal discharge has a foetid odour.

The three treatments most often used are parenteral $PGF_{2\alpha}$ or analogues (see p. 524), oestrogen (see p. 523) and intrauterine antibiotic. There are a limited number of products licensed for endometritis; in addition, a nil milk withholding period is usually demanded in dairy cattle.

Antimicrobial treatment: A number of antimicrobial selection criteria have been suggested for endometritis including efficacy against the causal organism in the uterine environment, but without inhibiting natural uterine defence mechanisms. Fluid and tissue debris reduce the effect of sulphonamides, aminoglycosides and nitrofurazones, and aminoglycosides are ineffective in an anaerobic environment, such as the uterine lumen. The chosen antibiotic must reach appropriate concentrations at the site of infection and persist a sufficient length of time to eliminate the infection. At less than 30 days postpartum, mixed bacterial infections may render intrauterine infusion of penicillin ineffective, due to penicillinase produced by bacteria. In contrast, oxytetracycline and cephalosporins are broad spectrum, and are effective in the uterine lumen in the presence of pus and reduced oxygen tension. In addition, pharmaceutical preparations of oxytetracycline and cephalosporins produce effective antimicrobial concentrations in the endometrium, but with minimal concentrations in milk. Any milk withdrawal period would make a treatment for endometritis unattractive under practice conditions; for example, parenteral tylosin gave effective concentrations in genital tract tissues and the uterine lumen, but has a significant milk withdrawal period (Cester *et al.*, 1993). Metronidazole and chloramphenicol are prohibited in food producing animals in the UK. The use of the intrauterine route of administration has prevailed for many years and the pharma-

Clinical sign				Point score
Vaginal discharge	Smell	Foul		3
		No smell		0
	Character	Bloody		3
		>50 ml pus		3
		<50ml pus		2
		Flecks		1
		Normal		0
External diameter of largest uterine horn	Pregnancy	Primiparous	Multiparous	
	Large	> 5.5cm	> 6.0cm	2
	Medium	3.5 to 5.5cm	4.0 to 6.0cm	1
	Normal	< 3.5cm	< 4.0cm	0
External diameter of cervix	Pregnancy	Primiparous	Multiparous	
	Large	> 7.0cm	> 7.5cm	2
	Medium	4.5 to 7.0cm	5.0 to 7.5cm	1
	Normal	< 4.5cm	< 5.0cm	0
Clinical assessment from total score				
Severe				**8–10**
Moderate				**4–7**
Mild				**1–3**
Normal				**0**

Fig. 34.4 Scoring system for the assessment of the severity of endometritis, suitable for use from 21 days postpartum.

ceutical industry continues to develop antibiotic products administered by this route, despite the widespread use of systemic antibiotics for treatment of other bacterial infections in cattle.

Hormones: The hormonal treatment of endometritis is based upon observations that the genital tract is more susceptible to infection when under progesterone dominance and more resistant under the influence of oestrogens (Rowson *et al.*, 1953).

   Oestrogens: Rowson *et al.* (1953) demonstrated that the bovine uterus was more resistant to infection with

A. pyogenes when either endogenous or exogenous oestrogen was present compared to during dioestrus, and suggested that exogenous oestrogen may be used therapeutically. Despite the potential of oestrogens for the treatment of endometritis, results have been equivocal and vary with the pharmaceutical preparation and dose administered. The treatment-to-conception interval was longer for cases of endometritis treated with a single intramuscular injection of 3mg oestradiol benzoate per 500kg body weight, compared with those treated using prostaglandin or intrauterine oxytetracycline (Sheldon & Noakes, 1998). Furthermore, regulatory authorities have prohibited the use of oestrogens in several countries.

Prostaglandins: The parenteral application of $PGF_{2\alpha}$, or its analogues, has been used widely for the treatment of endometritis. The majority of authors report that the presence of an active corpus luteum is required for optimal results when using prostaglandin to treat endometritis, which supports the hypothesis that the subsequent induced oestrus increases the uterine resistance to bacteria (Jackson, 1977; Sheldon & Noakes, 1998). Conversely, Pepper and Dobson (1987) reported that the efficacy of prostaglandin therapy for endometritis did not depend on the presence of an active CL, as determined by measuring milk progesterone concentrations. An alternative hypothesis for the mechanism of action of prostaglandin as a treatment for endometritis is a direct myometrial effect, with physical expulsion of uterine detritus.

A number of clinical trials have studied the possibility of using the direct myometrial effect of prostaglandin therapy, to reduce the incidence of endometritis and improve subsequent fertility. A routine injection of prostaglandin shortened the calving-to-conception interval in normal cows compared with control animals (Etherington et al., 1988). However, a number of subsequent trials gave conflicting results. Meta-analysis of 24 trials where $PGF_{2\alpha}$ was administered to cattle within 40 days of calving reported no beneficial effect on first-service pregnancy rate, although there was a small reduction in days open for treated cows (Burton & Lean, 1995).

Other treatments: A variety of antiseptics have been administered by intrauterine infusion for the treatment of endometritis including solutions of Lugol's iodine, polyvinyl pyrrolidine iodine, povidone-iodine, chlorhexidine and metakresol sulphonic acid. Many of these solutions cause a necrotic endometritis within 24 hours of infusion that may stimulate release of $PGF_{2\alpha}$ in addition to possible direct effects on pathogenic organisms. However, despite clinical resolution of the endometritis using antiseptic solutions, the effect on fertility may not be beneficial. Nakao et al. (1988) administered a 2 per cent polyvinyl pyrrolidine iodine intrauterine infusion and reported that treated cows, particularly those with a purulent discharge, had an increased calving-to-conception interval compared with controls. In addition, some of these antiseptic products are not licensed for use in food producing animals.

Pyometra

Pyometra is associated with the accumulation of pus in the uterus and by the persistence of functional luteal tissue on one or both ovaries. Affected cows do not appear ill; however, they are anoestrus and may be presented to the veterinarian as 'not-seen-bulling' or for pregnancy diagnosis.

Pyometra may be a sequel to the conditions discussed earlier in this chapter and therefore those factors that predispose a cow to RFM, metritis and endometritis can also be considered to predispose to pyometra. In addition pyometra may also be seen in cows after service (either natural or by AI).

In most cases pyometra is a sequel to chronic endometritis as the uterus ceases to release the endogenous luteolysin $PGF_{2\alpha}$. Research has shown that the persistence of the CL in cows with pyometra is not due to an insufficiency in the synthesis of uterine $PGF_{2\alpha}$ but is associated with inadequate secretion of luteal oxytocin (Vighio et al., 1991). The result is that the dioestrus CL persists and the genital tract remains under the influence of progesterone. The infection is thus not eliminated and the cervix remains closed, resulting in the accumulation of large quantities of purulent exudate in the uterine lumen. Occasionally there will be slight leakage through the cervix, resulting in a small amount of pus accumulating in the anterior vagina and an intermittent purulent vaginal discharge. In a small number of cases the persistent luteal tissue is a progesterone secreting (luteal) cyst rather than a persistent CL. In some instances the introduction of infection during dioestrus, such as occurs when a cow is artificially inseminated at an incorrect time, results in pyometra. Pyometra may also occur secondary to the death of a fetus, either caused by, or followed by, bacterial invasion by *A. pyogenes* and persistence of the CL of pregnancy. Infection with *Tritrichomonas fetus* also causes embryonic death and pyometra formation (Bon-Durant, 1997).

When examined *per rectum*, cases of pyometra have enlarged uterine horns and must be accurately differentiated from a normal pregnancy before treatment can be administered. There are a number of distinguishing points:

- The uterus feels 'doughy' and the uterine wall is thicker than during pregnancy.
- It is not possible to palpate the amniotic vesicle or 'slip' the allantochorion membranes.
- Placentomes are not palpable or visible on ultrasound examination, although the caruncles of the previous pregnancy are occasionally detected.
- Ultrasonography will demonstrate the absence of a fetus and the presence of pus rather than normal fetal fluids.

The best and most appropriate treatment of pyometra is to bring about luteolysis with $PGF_{2\alpha}$ or $PGF_{2\alpha}$ analogues. However, this treatment should never be administered if there is any suspicion that the cow may be pregnant, as it will cause abortion in early pregnancy.

The administration of PGF$_{2\alpha}$ to cases of pyometra usually results in dilation of the cervix and expulsion of the purulent uterine contents, with oestrus occurring three to five days later. There is evidence to suggest that treatment of pyometra is improved by the administration of two doses of PGF$_{2\alpha}$ 8 hours apart (Archbald et al., 1993). This is probably due to the fact that a single dose of exogenous PGF$_{2\alpha}$ has only a very short duration of action, as the inadequate release of ovarian oxytocin from the CL in these cases is insufficient to maintain the normal positive feedback loop that brings about luteolysis by the release of further endogenous PGF$_{2\alpha}$.

Many cases of pyometra go on to become pregnant, despite having a prolonged first luteal phase and a prolonged calving to pregnancy interval of 125 days compared to 74.8 days (Etherington et al., 1991). However, longstanding cases are associated with endometrial degeneration, which may increase the rate of late embryonic and early fetal losses. Comparison between pregnancy rates at first pregnancy diagnosis 33 to 70 days postservice and a subsequent diagnosis 120 to 150 days postservice have shown that attrition rates are 2.6 times higher in cows with previous pyometra than in cows without the condition (López-Gatius et al., 1996).

Postpartum anoestrus

Introduction

Postpartum anoestrus is a greater problem for beef cattle than dairy cows, and it is often evident in specific herds.

Aetiology

The two main predisposing factors are inadequate nutrition, specifically energy deficiency, and suckling or the maternal bond. Other associated factors are that it is more common during late winter, in the absence of a bull and following dystokia. Rarely, anoestrus may be associated with pituitary or ovarian damage.

Negative energy balance (NEB) is common to most postpartum cows and is the difference between the dietary intake of metabolizable energy and the expenditure for maintenance and lactation (see p. 103). Consequentially, the balance between milk yield and feeding (including diet composition, feed supply and appetite) is an important determinant of the severity of NEB. However, in first lactation an animal's metabolizable energy may also have to contribute to continued growth. The effect of NEB is most easily identified by monitoring body condition score (BCS). Cows that lose

>1.0 BCS points during the first 30 days after calving take longer to the first postpartum ovulation than those losing less than one unit (Beam & Butler, 1999). However, monitoring BCS over periods greater than 6 weeks postpartum often has a less clear association with the length of the anoestrus period. The pituitary secretion of FSH appears to be insensitive to NEB. Thus, successive waves of follicular growth start within 10 days of calving. However, in the anoestrus cows, dominant follicles fail to ovulate because of inadequate LH pulse frequency. Insulin-like growth factor-1 (IGF-1) is a likely hormonal mediator between nutrition and fertility. However, the precise mechanisms and how they may be modulated are not yet clear. Shortening the postpartum interval to the NEB nadir is a more tangible management objective to reduce the incidence of anoestrus in a herd.

The suckling calf inhibits the release of GnRH from the dam's hypothalamus, so suppressing LH pulse frequency. However, this inhibitory influence occurs as a consequence of the maternal bond between cow and calf, and it is not dependent upon sensory innervation of the udder (Williams & Griffith, 1995). The frequency and duration of suckling by a single calf are unrelated to the period of anoestrus, although suckling following adoption of an additional calf will delay the return of ovarian cyclicity. If the single calf is removed from its dam there is a corresponding increase in the frequency of LH pulses within two to six days. The inhibition of GnRH release is dependent on the cow being suckled by her 'own' calf, which she identifies by sight and smell. The mechanisms underlying this effect are unclear; in part, they may involve increased opioid tone within the brain.

Diagnosis

At least two examinations, 10–14 days apart, are required to make a clinical diagnosis of anoestrus. Both ovaries are small and there is no CL detectable at either of the examinations; however, follicles up to 18mm diameter may be identified. An alternative or additional method of diagnosis is to use milk progesterone analysis; two low values, at 10–14-day intervals, is indicative of anoestrus.

Treatment

The most important consideration when presented with an anoestrus animal is to correct the underlying causes, in particular dietary deficiencies. The quantity and quality of feed supplied to the animal in relation to its milk yield should be determined. In addition, dry-cow management should be examined, paying particular attention to the transitional period. Monitoring BCS during the dry period and early lactation will help to quantify the severity of dietary energy deficiency. Two groups of pharmaceutical products may be used to treat anoestrus: GnRH and analogues, and progestagens.

GnRH: The pituitary LH content and responsiveness to GnRH are complete by day 10 postpartum and so exogenous GnRH administered to the anoestrus cow will induce a transient LH and FSH release. However, the response to treatment depends on the stage of ovarian follicular wave. If there is a dominant follicle present, ovulation will occur. So, when daily ultrasound monitoring was used to identify a suitable dominant follicle, administration of GnRH consistently induced ovulation (Roche *et al.*, 1992). However, the majority of animals did not express oestrous and had short luteal phases after ovulation. Gonadotrophin releasing hormone administered in the absence of a dominant follicle is ineffective, so overall blind-treatment success rates are variable.

Progesterone: Administration of progesterone, using an intravaginal device or norgestamet by injection and implantation, is an alternative treatment for the anoestrus cow. In the absence of severe NEB, once the progesterone treatment is removed, there is an induced ovulation and such treatment overcomes the absence of behavioural oestrous that often occurs at the first postpartum ovulation. However, if the NEB is severe, progesterone treatment requires supplementation with 400–700iu equine chorionic gonadotrophin (eCG) by intramuscular injection at the time of implant removal. An alternative to eCG is the administration of 1 mg oestradiol benzoate 24 hours after a seven-day progesterone treatment which increased oestrus expression and ovulation (MacMillan *et al.*, 1995).

Cystic ovarian disease

Cystic ovarian disease can be a major problem in the postpartum dairy cow resulting in an increase of 6 to 11 days to first service and an increase in the calving-to-conception interval of 20–30 days (Fourichon *et al.*, 2000). However, this subject is dealt with elsewhere in this book in Chapters 35 and 36.

Prevention of postpartum disease problems

The key to controlling postpartum disease problems is to recognize that they are interlinked (Peeler *et al.*, 1994) and that their control is related to breeding management, nutrition, the management of the transition cow and management at and immediately after calving.

Control of these conditions is not simply a matter of good management at the time of calving.

Breeding decisions and the management of the pregnant and periparturient cow

The most important way of reducing puerperal problems is to avoid dystokia. Where dystokia does occur it is essential that it is dealt with correctly at an early stage and that any developing problems observed after calving are also treated as soon as possible. Attention to all aspects of hygiene is also a basic requirement.

If it were purely a veterinary matter it would be relatively simple to reduce the incidence of dystokia in the majority of herds. However, the measures required may not be acceptable to the farmer. Simple modifications such as improved supervision of calving and better housing may be judged to be too expensive. Selecting an easy calving breed of bull or individual bull within a breed may not produce calves with the desired conformation or genetic potential.

The consequences of several synergistic adverse effects tend to be particularly serious. Therefore, if a client chooses to use a bull that is liable to produce a high rate of dystokia it is particularly important to avoid any other factor that predisposes to dystokia.

Application of the following precautions will reduce the incidence of dystokia in a herd.

(1) Selection of sires that produce calves of suitable size and conformation for the dams concerned. This refers to the breed and to the individual bull within the breed. Special care is needed for heifers (see Chapter 5).

(2) Induction of premature calving, if the fetus is likely to be too large at full term for a normal calving (see p. 687).

(3) Control of energy intake and avoidance of macromineral and trace element imbalances.

   (a) Do not let the dams get too fat, as the perirectal and perivaginal fat will narrow the birth canal, the dam may be less capable of forceful labour and the calf may also be larger. This is also an important way of avoiding necrotic vaginitis and other damage to the vagina. At calving a condition score of 2.5 (see p. 10) is advised.

   (b) Avoid undernutrition as cows in very poor condition also have problems of dystokia.

   (c) Regular body condition scoring and careful attention to the late lactation, dry period and particularly the transition period ration are required. This may be aided by the use of metabolic profiles (see Chapter 47). Specific dietary manipulations such as the use of salts to manipulate the dietary cation–anion balance (DCAB) of the transition cow ration may also be useful in reducing the incidence of periparturient problems (see p. 787).

(4) Provision of a suitable environment, especially for cows that calve inside or in a restricted area. This should be clean, well bedded, with a good water supply, properly lit and with enough space to get at the cow if need be and to allow observation without disturbance. There also need to be facilities to safely restrain the cow.

(5) Avoid stress and disturbance of the calving cow (Hindson, 1976).

(6) Suitable supervision and timely intervention at calving will reduce the severity of those cases of dystokia that do occur (Hodge *et al.*, 1982).

(7) Proper training of the farmer and stockworkers in how to assist at calving should be supplied by the veterinarian.

(8) When veterinary assistance is needed, the farmer and his staff must decide at an early stage to call for help. It is important that the veterinarian and the farmer should agree before the start of the calving season how these problems will be dealt with and at what stage the farmer will call for professional help.

Therapy immediately postpartum

In addition to specific therapies such as those described above for uterine prolapse, cows that have had obstetrical interventions at calving may benefit from a course of systemic antibiotic.

Metabolic diseases, such as milk fever, should be dealt with appropriately and if these cases are common, investigation into their causes is essential. This aspect of bovine medicine is dealt with elsewhere in this book (Chapter 46).

The routine administration of agents such as $PGF_{2\alpha}$ (see p. 524) and oxytocin (see p. 517) to postpartum cows is not justified by improvements in subsequent fertility; reports of the benefits in the published literature are inconsistent. Their use postpartum should therefore be restricted to animals where a specific indication exists, as described earlier in this chapter.

Conclusions

The key to good fertility in multiparous cattle is to maintain a high level of stockmanship at all times, and to manage cattle in such a way as to minimize postpartum problems. The preparation of cattle for breeding begins well before the expected service date. Preparing the cow for parturition and particularly dry cow and transition cow management in the previous gestation period are crucial stages in this preparation. However, parturition is the key event, and it must be managed to minimize the development of abnormalities of the genital tract in the postpartum period, which may lead to problems of subsequent oestrous cyclicity, depression in conception rates, increased embryonic loss and subfertility.

References

Adams, G.P., Matteri, R.L., Kastelic, J.P., Ko, J.C.H. & Ginther, O.J. (1992) Association between surges of follicle-stimulating hormone and the emergence of follicular waves in heifers. *Journal of Reproduction and Fertility*, **94**, 177–88.

Amiridis, G.S., Leontides, L., Tassos, E., Kostoulas, P. & Fthenakis, G.C. (2001) Flunixin meglumine accelerates uterine involution and shortens the calving-to-first-oestrus interval in cows with puerperal metritis. *Journal of Veterinary Pharmacology and Therapeutics*, **24**, 365–7.

Archbald, L.F., Risco, C., Chavatte, P., Constant, S., Tran, T., Klapstein, E. & Elliot, J. (1993) Estrus and pregnancy rate of dairy cows given one or two doses of prostaglandin F2 alpha 8 or 24 hours apart. *Theriogenology*, **40**, 873–84.

Beam, S.W. & Butler, W.R. (1997) Energy balance and ovarian follicle development prior to the first ovulation postpartum in dairy cows receiving three levels of dietary fat. *Biology of Reproduction*, **56**, 133–42.

Beam, S.W. & Butler, W.R. (1999) Effects of energy balance on follicular development and first ovulation in postpartum dairy cows. *Journal of Reproduction and Fertility Supplement*, **54**, 411–24.

Bon-Durant, R. (1997) Pathogenesis, diagnosis and management of trichomoniasis in cattle. *Veterinary Clinics of North America: Food Animal Practice*, **13**, 345–61.

Borsberry, S. & Dobson, H. (1989) Periparturient diseases and their effect on reproductive performance in five dairy herds. *Veterinary Record*, **124**, 217–19.

Bretzlaff, K. (1987) Rationale for treatment of endometritis in the dairy cow. *Veterinary Clinics of North America: Food Animal Practice*, **3**, 593–607.

Brooks, G. (2001) Comparison of two treatments after retained fetal membranes on clinical signs in cattle. *Veterinary Record*, **148**, 243–4.

Bulman, D.C. & Lamming, G.E. (1978) Milk progesterone levels in relation to conception, repeat breeding and factors influencing acyclicity in dairy cows. *Journal of Reproduction and Fertility*, **54**, 447–58.

Burton, N.R. & Lean, I.J. (1995) Investigation by meta-analysis of the effect of prostaglandin F2α administered post partum on the reproductive performance of dairy cattle. *Veterinary Record*, **136**, 90–4.

Caron, J.P. & Le Blanc, P.H. (1989) Caudal epidural analgesia in cattle using xylazine. *Canadian Journal of Veterinary Research*, **53**, 486–9.

Cester, C.C., Ganiere, J.P. & Toutain, P.L. (1993) Effect of stage of oestrous cycle on tylosin disposition in genital tract secretions of cows. *Research in Veterinary Science*, **54**, 32–9.

Cook, N. (1998) Bovine herpes virus 1: clinical manifestations and an outbreak of infectious pustular vulvovaginitis in a UK dairy herd. *Cattle Practice*, **6**, 341–4.

Correa, M.T., Erb, H.N. & Scarlett, J.M. (1992) A nested case-control study of uterine prolapse. *Theriogenology*, **37**, 939–45.

Darwash, A.O., Lamming, G.E. & Woolliams, J.A. (1997) The phenotypic association between the interval to post-partum ovulation and traditional measures of fertility in dairy cattle. *Animal Science*, **65**, 9–16.

Eckersall, P.D. (2000) Acute phase proteins as markers of infection and inflammation: monitoring animal health, animal welfare and food safety. *Irish Veterinary Journal*, **53**, 307–11.

Eiler, H. & Hopkins, F.M. (1993) Successful treatment of retained placenta with umbilical cord injection of collagenase in cows. *Journal of the American Veterinary Medical Association*, **203**, 436–43.

Elliot, L., McMahon, K.J., Gier, H.T. & Marion, G.B. (1968) Uterus of the cow after parturition: bacterial content. *American Journal of Veterinary Research*, **29**, 77–81.

Etherington, W.G., Christie, K.A., Walton, J.S., Leslie, K.E., Wickstrom, S. & Johnson, W.H. (1991) Progesterone profiles in postpartum holstein dairy cows as an aid in the study of retained fetal membranes, pyometra and anestrus. *Theriogenology*, **35**, 731–46.

Etherington, W.G., Martin, S.W., Bonnett, B., Johnson, W.H., Miller, R.B., Savage, N.C., Walton, J.S. & Montgomery, M.E. (1988) Reproductive performance of dairy cows following treatment with cloprostenol 26 and/or 40 days postpartum: a field trial. *Theriogenology*, **29**, 565–75.

Fourichon, C., Seegers, H. & Malher, X. (2000) Effect of disease on reproduction in the dairy cow: a meta-analysis. *Theriogenology*, **53**, 1729–59.

Ginther, O.J., Wiltbank, M.C., Fricke, P.M., Gibbons, J.R. & Kot, K. (1996) Selection of the dominant follicle in cattle. *Biology of Reproduction*, **55**, 1187–94.

Gross, T.S., Williams, W.F. & Moreland, T.W. (1986) Prevention of the retained fetal membrane syndrome (retained placenta) during induced calving in dairy cattle. *Theriogenology*, **26**, 365–70.

Halpern, N.E., Erb, H.N. & Smith, R.D. (1985) Duration of retained fetal membranes and subsequent fertility in dairy cows. *Theriogenology*, **23**, 807–13.

Hernandez, J., Risco, C.A. & Elliott, J.B. (1999) Effect of oral administration of a calcium chloride gel on blood mineral concentrations, parturient disorders, reproductive performance, and milk production of dairy cows with retained fetal membranes. *Journal of the American Veterinary Medical Association*, **215**, 72–6.

Hindson, J.C. (1976) Retention of the fetal membranes in cattle. *Veterinary Record*, **99**, 49–50.

Hodge, P.B., Wood, S.J., Newman, R.D. & Shepherd, R.K. (1982) Effect of calving supervision upon the calving performance of Hereford heifers. *Australian Veterinary Journal*, **58**, 97–100.

Holden, D. (1998) Local analgesia for surgery of the head, distal limbs and mammary gland. *Cattle Practice*, **6**, 233–6.

Hooper, R.N., Crabill, M.R., Taylor, T.S. & Roussel, A.J. (1999) Managing vaginal and cervical prolapses in cows. *Veterinary Medicine*, **94**, 375–89.

Jackson, P.S. (1977) Treatment of chronic post partum endometritis in cattle with cloprostenol. *Veterinary Record*, **101**, 441–3.

Joosten, I., Stelwagen, J. & Dijkhuizen, A.A. (1988) Economic and reproductive consequences of retained placenta in dairy cattle. *Veterinary Record*, **123**, 53–7.

Kaidi, R., Brown, P.J. & David, J.S.E. (1991) Uterine involution in cattle. In *The Veterinary Annual* (ed. by C.S.G. Grunsell & M.E. Raw), Vol. 31, pp. 38–50. Blackwell Scientific Publications, Oxford.

Ko, J.C.H., Althouse, G.C., Hopkins, S.M., Jackson, L.L., Evans, L.E. & Smith, R.P. (1989) Effects of epidural administration of xylazine or lidocaine on bovine uterine motility and perineal analgesia. *Theriogenology*, **32**, 779–86.

Kossaibati, M.A. & Esslemont, R.J. (1995) *Daisy. The DAIRY Information System Report No. 4 – Wastage in Dairy Herds*. University of Reading.

Kossaibati, M.A. & Esslemont, R.J. (1997) The cost of production diseases in dairy herds in England. *The Veterinary Journal*, **154**, 41–51.

Laven, R.A. (1995) The treatment of retained placenta: a survey of practitioners. *Cattle Practice*, **3**, 267–79.

Laven, R.A. & Peters, A.R. (1996) Bovine retained placenta: aetiology, pathogenesis and economic loss. *Veterinary Record*, **139**, 465–71.

Leslie, K.E., Doig, P.A., Bosu, W.T.K., Curtis, R.A. & Martin, S.W. (1984) Effects of gonadotrophin releasing hormone on reproductive performance of dairy cows with retained placenta. *Canadian Journal of Comparative Medicine*, **48**, 354–9.

López-Gatius, F., Labèrnia, J., Santolaria, P., López-Béjar, M. & Rutllant, J. (1996) Effect of reproductive disorders previous to conception on pregnancy attrition in dairy cows. *Theriogenology*, **46**, 643–8.

McDougall, S. (2001) Effects of periparturient diseases and conditions on the reproductive performance of New Zealand dairy cows. *New Zealand Veterinary Journal*, **49**, 60–7.

MacMillan, K.L., Taufa, V.K., Day, A.M. & McDougall, S. (1995) Some effects of using progesterone and oestradiol benzoate to stimulate oestrus and ovulation in dairy cows with anovulatory anoestrus. *Proceedings of the New Zealand Society of Animal Production*, **55**, 239–41.

Markusfeld, O. (1984) Factors responsible for post parturient metritis in dairy cattle. *Veterinary Record*, **114**, 539–42.

Mee, J.F. (1991) The incidence of retained fetal membranes on nine dairy research farms over a ten-year period (1978–1987). *Irish Veterinary Journal*, **44**, 48–52.

Moller, K., Newling, P.E., Robson, H.J., Jansen, G.J., Meursinge, J.A. & Cooper, M.G. (1967) Retained fetal membranes in dairy herds in the Huntly district. *New Zealand Veterinary Journal*, **15**, 111–16.

Nakao, T., Moriyoshi, M. & Kawata, K. (1988) Effect of post-partum intrauterine treatment with 2% polyvinylpyrrolidone–iodine solution on reproductive efficiency in cows. *Theriogenology*, **30**, 1033–43.

Noakes, D.E. (2001a) Injuries and diseases incidental to parturition. In *Arthur's Veterinary Reproduction and Obstetrics* (ed. by D.E. Noakes, T.J. Parkinson, & G.C.W. England), 8th edn, pp. 319–32. W.B. Saunders, London.

Noakes, D.E. (2001b) Postparturient prolapse of the uterus. In *Arthur's Veterinary Reproduction and Obstetrics* (ed. by D.E. Noakes, T.J. Parkinson, & G.C.W. England), 8th edn, pp. 333–8. W.B. Saunders, London.

Noakes, D.E., Wallace, L. & Smith, G.R. (1991) Bacterial flora of the uterus of cows after calving on two hygienically contrasting farms. *Veterinary Record*, **128**, 440–2.

Oakley, G.E. (1992) Survival and fertility of dairy cows following uterine prolapse. *New Zealand Veterinary Journal*, **40**, 120–2.

Olson, J.D., Ball, L., Mortimer, R.G., Farin, P.W., Adney, W.S. & Huffman, E.M. (1984) Aspects of bacteriology and endocrinology of cows with pyometra and retained fetal membranes. *American Journal of Veterinary Research*, **45**, 2251–5.

Parkinson, T.J. (2001) Infertility in the cow: structural and functional abnormalities, management deficiencies and non-specific infections. In *Arthur's Veterinary Reproduction and Obstetrics* (ed. by D.E. Noakes, T.J. Parkinson, & G.C.W. England), 8th edn, pp. 383–472. W.B. Saunders, London.

Peeler, E.J., Otte, M.J. & Esslemont, R.J. (1994) Interrelationships of periparturient disease in dairy cows. *Veterinary Record*, **134**, 129–32.

Pepper, R.T. & Dobson, H. (1987) Preliminary results of treatment and endocrinology of chronic endometritis in the dairy cow. *Veterinary Record*, **120**, 53–6.

Peters, A.R. & Laven, R.A. (1996) Treatment of bovine retained placenta and its effects. *Veterinary Record*, **139**, 535–9.

Peters, A.R. & Riley, G.M. (1982) Milk progesterone profiles and factors affecting post partum ovarian activity in beef cows. *Animal Production*, **34**, 145–53.

Plenderleith, B. (1986) Prolapse of the uterus in the cow. *In Practice*, **8**, 14–15.

Roche, J.F. & Boland, M.P. (1991) Turnover of dominant follicles in cattle of different reproductive states. *Theriogenology*, **35**, 81–90.

Roche, J.F., Crowe, M.A. & Boland, M.P. (1992) Postpartum anoestrus in dairy and beef cows. *Animal Reproduction Science*, **28**, 371–8.

Rowlands, G.A. & Lucey, S. (1986) Changes in milk yield in dairy cows associated with metabolic and reproductive diseases and lameness. *Preventive Veterinary Medicine*, **4**, 205–21.

Rowson, L.E.A., Lamming, G.E. & Fry, R.M. (1953) The relationship between ovarian hormones and uterine infection. *Veterinary Record*, **65**, 335–40.

Sandals, W.C.D., Curtis, R.A., Cote, J.F. & Martin, S.W. (1979) The effect of retained placenta and metritis complex on reproductive performance in dairy cattle – a case control study. *Canadian Veterinary Journal*, **20**, 131–5.

Savio, J.D., Boland, M.P., Hynes, N. & Roche, J.F. (1990) Resumption of follicular activity in the early postpartum period of dairy cows. *Journal of Reproduction & Fertility*, **88**, 569–79.

Savio, J.D., Keenan, L., Boland, M.P. & Roche, J.F. (1988) Pattern of growth of dominant follicles during the oestrous cycle of heifers. *Journal of Reproduction and Fertility*, **83**, 663–71.

Sheldon, I.M. (1999) Bovine endometritis: a review. *Journal of Animal Breeding*, **2**, 2–14.

Sheldon, I.M. & Noakes, D.E. (1998) Comparison of three treatments for bovine endometritis. *Veterinary Record*, **142**, 575–9.

Sheldon, I.M., Noakes, D.E. & Dobson, H. (2000) The influence of ovarian activity and uterine involution determined by ultrasonography on subsequent reproductive performance. *Theriogenology*, **54**, 409–19.

Sheldon, I.M., Noakes, D.E., Rycroft, A. & Dobson, H. (2001) Acute phase protein responses to uterine bacterial contamination in cattle after calving. *Veterinary Record*, **148**, 172–5.

Smith, M.C.A. & Wallace, J.M. (1998) Influence of early post partum ovulation on the re-establishment of pregnancy in multiparous and primiparous dairy cattle. *Reproduction Fertility Development*, **10**, 207–16.

Steffan, J., Adriamanga, S. & Thibier, M. (1984) Treatment of metritis with antibiotics or prostaglandin F2α and influence of ovarian cyclicity in dairy cows. *American Journal of Veterinary Research*, **45**, 1090–94.

Stevens, R.D. & Dinsmore, R.P. (1997) Treatment of dairy cows at parturition with prostaglandin F2α or oxytocin for prevention of retained fetal membranes. *Journal of the American Veterinary Medical Association*, **211**, 1280–84.

Stevens, R.D., Dinsmore, R.P. & Cattell, M.B. (1995) Evaluation of the use of intrauterine infusions of oxytetracycline, subcutaneous injections of fenprostalene, or a combination of both, for the treatment of retained fetal membranes in dairy cows. *Journal of the American Veterinary Medical Association*, **207**, 1612–15.

Stocker, H. & Waelchli, R.O. (1993) A clinical trial on the effect of prostaglandin F2α on placental expulsion in dairy cattle after a caesarean operation. *Veterinary Record*, **132**, 507–508.

Vighio, G.H., Liptrap, R.M. & Etherington, W.G. (1991) Oxytocin–prostaglandin interrelationships in the cow with pyometra. *Theriogenology*, **35**, 1121–9.

Waelchli, R.O., Thun, R. & Stocker, H. (1999) Effect of flunixin meglumine on placental expulsion in dairy cattle after a caesarean. *Veterinary Record*, **144**, 702–703.

Williams, G.L. & Griffith, M.K. (1995) Sensory and behavioural control of gonadotrophin secretion during suckling-mediated anovulation in cows. *Journal of Reproduction and Fertility Supplement*, **49**, 463–75.

Wischral, A., Verreschi, I.T.N., Lima, S.B., Hayashi, L.F. & Barnabe, R.C. (2001) Preparturition profile of steroids and prostaglandin in cows with or without fetal membrane retention. *Animal Reproduction Science*, **67**, 181–8.

Chapter 35

Problems Associated with Oestrous Cyclicity

H. Boyd, D.C. Barrett and M. Mihm

Manifestation   530
Aetiology   532
Diagnosis   535
Treatment   541
Prognosis   542
   Long interservice interval   544
Prevention   544

Manifestation

Normal oestrous cycles, clear oestrous expression and efficient and accurate detection of oestrus with a predictable interval to ovulation are still essential for the successful management of reproduction in cattle. Failure to observe oestrus or lack of oestrus adversely affects the efficiency of production and profitability by interfering with the reproductive markers shown in Box 35.1 (see also Chapter 41 (b) page 678). Inaccurate oestrous detection, i.e. identification of a cow as being in oestrus when she is not, leads to cows being inseminated when fertilization is not possible because there is no ovulation at the expected time after insemination, and to pregnancies being lost when already pregnant cows are inseminated using artificial insemination (AI).

Missed heats that result in longer than planned intervals from calving to first service cause considerable economic loss. A missed oestrus will cause a delay of about 21 days until the next chance for service and this loss in milk production time and delay in producing a calf results in a loss of income. Assessment of the real loss (litres of milk/year; calves/100 cows per year) and the economic loss is complex. Where possible, herd-specific economic estimates should be undertaken to determine the cost–benefit of alterations in the various elements of herd fertility (Dijkhuizen *et al.*, 1997). However, in herds with a conventional breeding strategy it may be useful to consider a rule-of-thumb value to estimate losses occasioned with every day the calving interval is extended beyond the target of 365 days. A figure that has remained remarkably constant over the last decade (to 2002) is £2.50 to £3.00/day for every day over the planned calving interval. In beef suckler cows, delay in achieving pregnancy causing very prolonged calving seasons results in a similar loss; this is partly due to management problems, such as loss of the seasonal calving pattern, but also because at weaning the calf is younger and therefore weighs less. The marketing advantage of being able to sell uniform batches of calves may also be lost if the calving season is extended much beyond nine weeks.

Clients may present individual cases of cows that have not been seen in oestrus when due or overdue for service, but mostly the problem is seen on regular fertility visits when post service anoestrus is also detected in animals diagnosed not pregnant. It is important to differentiate as far as possible those cows that have not been in oestrus from those that have simply not been seen in oestrus either because of poor expression of heat or poor oestrous observation. This may require an assessment to be made of the efficiency of oestrous detection in the herd and careful examination of 'anoestrus' cows on more than one occasion. Regular milk progesterone assays may also be useful when attempting to determine whether an individual cow is undergoing oestrous cyclicity or is truly anoestrus. Suckler cows running with the bull may be presented as failure to conceive towards the end of the breeding season. The problem of abnormal oestrous cyclicity, which is most serious when it occurs on a herd or group basis, is often picked up retrospectively on herd record analysis.

Heifers

Delayed puberty may affect targets for breeding age or date. It occurs mainly as a group problem because heifers are handled and fed in groups and the cause of anoestrus is nearly always related to the environment or to the management, particularly feeding (Webb *et al.*, 1997). Occasionally, anoestrus is manifested in a group of heifers after natural service, which the farmer erroneously thought was successful because of lack of returns to service.

Cows after calving

An extended interval between calving and first service, calculated on a herd basis, is the most important

Box 35.1 Aspects of reproduction affected by failure to observe, or lack of, oestrus.

Heifers
Age at first calving
Season of first calving

Cows
Interval from calving to first service (and thus calving to conception)
Timely observation of returns to service

Table 35.1 Percentage of cows with various calving-to-first-service intervals in days, based on 1595 cows in 15 herds.

	Calving-to-first-service interval (days)			
	0–55	Target 56–77	78–99	>100
Percentage of cows	15.9	32.2	24.7	27.1
Cumulative percentage	15.9	48.1	72.8	99.9

manifestation of dysfunction of cyclicity and oestrus or oestrous detection. A farmer with a serious problem may not be aware of it because of poor records or good ones that are not used properly. In the example given in Table 35.1, in 15 herds that were not in fertility control programmes, the target for calving interval was 12 months and to achieve this target, cows should have had their first services 56–76 days after calving. The distribution of days from calving to first service for the 1595 cows served in these herds shows that about half of the cows were first served after the target date (Boyd & Munro, 1980). Recent data from the National Milk Records (NMR) representing approximately 1 million dairy cows shows that between January 1997 and September 2000 the mean calving to first service interval rose from 84 to 88 days (Barrett, 2001), therefore the majority of cows are probably now served after the target 56–76-day window (assuming a target calving index of 365 days). However, the voluntary waiting period, i.e. the number of days postpartum waited until first service, may be deliberately increased in high-yielding cows, where the decision is taken to extend their lactation for economic and welfare reasons (Knight & Sorensen, 1998). On the best farm illustrated in Table 35.1, 67 per cent of the cows were served within 77 days of calving and on the worst farm only 21 per cent of cows reached that target.

The situation in this group of herds is quite typical of the results obtained in many surveys carried out in different countries and demonstrates the seriousness of the problem. Within herds the incidence of the problem is quite variable at different times and there may be periods of four to six weeks during the year when a high proportion of cows appear to stop cycling or exhibit poor oestrous signs. This may be a direct seasonal effect in certain climates, but in temperate regions is probably largely a nutritional effect (Butler, 1999).

The number of cows treated by veterinarians for anoestrus and suboestrus was reported to be low in the 1980s. Saloniemi et al. (1986) gave the incidence as 5.2 per cent of cows, falling from first calvers (6.3 per cent) to older cows (3.7 per cent). Markusfeld (1987) diagnosed inactive ovaries after two rectal examinations in 8.5 per cent of 7751 lactations. However, more recently 20 per cent of high-yielding cows have been shown to exhibit a delayed interval to first ovulation postpartum based on progesterone profiles (Opsomer et al., 1996).

Another manifestation of absence of oestrus is the cow that starts cycling and then stops, a situation recorded in 5.2 per cent of cases in a survey based on progesterone assays by Bulman and Lamming (1978). In a similar study (Kassa et al., 1986), cyclicity started and then stopped in four (3.2 per cent) of 125 lactations. Once again this situation seems to have worsened over time; in a recent Dutch study, true return to anoestrus was seen in only 3 per cent of high-yielding cows, however, 20 per cent of cows showed a prolonged first luteal phase of more than 20 days based on their progesterone profiles (Opsomer et al., 1996). Royal et al. (2000) have shown an increase in the proportion of animals with one or more atypical ovarian hormone patterns from 32 per cent of cows in the period 1975–82 to 44 per cent in the period 1995–98. During the same period pregnancy rate to first service declined from 55.6 per cent to 39.7 per cent, again suggesting that fertility in dairy cattle has declined over time.

Cows after service

Analysis of data from approximately 35 000 cows in 255 British herds (Warren, 1984) showed that 26 per cent of interservice intervals were greater than 48 days, i.e. more than two cycles (Table 35.2). These results are similar to the results obtained in other surveys. For example, in the 15 herds discussed above (Table 35.1), 25 per cent of the returns to service were after a delay greater than 48 days and in Boyd and Reed's (1961) study in smaller herds at a time when management was less intensive, 23 per cent of returns were greater than 48 days.

In Warren's (1984) report the average interservice interval was 39 days, possibly due to a delay in the return to service of 39 – 21 days = 18 days. In some other surveys there were rather fewer very long intervals,

Table 35.2 Percentage of cows with various intervals between services in days (Warren, 1984)

	Interservice interval (days)					
	1–17	18–24	25–35	36–48	49–90	91+
Percentage of cows	6	37	13	18	18	8

possibly due to different culling patterns or more efficient heat detection. In New Zealand, Moller *et al.* (1986) reported that only 8.6 per cent of return-to-service intervals were greater than 36 days. Nowadays in New Zealand and other locations where dairy farming is highly seasonal, repeats are often resynchronized which increases the submission rates for the first and second repeat cycles of the breeding season.

While survey data do not explain why a cow has not been served, discussion with farmers makes it clear that in the majority of cases the reason is that the cow has not been seen in heat. In conclusion, failure to have cows served because they have not been seen in season is a widespread and important problem.

Aetiology

The aetiology of anoestrus in the cow and heifer is complex because as presented to the veterinarian it includes several different conditions, as shown in Box 35.2. Because there is a wide range of types of anoestrus there is also a wide range of causes, some unknown. Moreover, a variety of management and environmental factors contribute to poor oestrous detection rates.

Physiological anoestrus

It is important to bear in mind that during certain phases of the reproductive cycle, the absence of oestrus is physiological. These phases are prior to puberty, during pregnancy and for at least two weeks after calving. It is not uncommon for a cow that is pregnant to be presented to the veterinarian as a case of anoestrus. This occurs if there is unknown access to a bull, or unrecorded insemination or misidentification of the cow inseminated.

In dairy cows, from which the calves are removed a day or so after birth, ovulation rarely occurs earlier than 15 days after calving; in general first postpartum ovulation occurs 17–21 days after calving in medium-yielding dairy cows calving in appropriate body condition and experiencing no major loss in body condition subsequently (Savio *et al.*, 1990). This postpartum interval to

Box 35.2 Aetiology of anoestrus.

- Physiological anoestrus: prepuberty, pregnancy, puerperium
- True anoestrus: no oestrous cycle and no ovulation or blocked cycle (prolonged luteal phase, such as with pyometra)
- Silent oestrus: better termed silent ovulation, i.e. ovarian cycles occur but no oestrous behaviour is detected
- Weak oestrus: poor oestrous expression (reduced length or intensity)
- Unobserved oestrus: oestrus normal, human error

first ovulation may be prolonged to 60 days in high-yielding cows (Opsomer *et al.*, 1996). In cows that are suckling, usually beef cows, the duration of non-cyclicity may be extended from 25 to beyond 100 days, depending on body condition score at calving and post-partum nutrition (Stagg *et al.*, 1995). The effect of suckling of one or more calves is to inhibit the return to cyclicity via neurohormonal routes, which can be modified by nutritional factors. This is demonstrated by the observation that some well-fed, well-managed beef suckler herds achieve a tight calving pattern at the same time each year, which requires an early return to cyclicity while the cows are still suckling their calves. For a list of factors that affect the onset of puberty, see Chapter 5.

True anoestrus

The major causes of true anoestrus characterized by lack of ovulation are summarized in Box 35.3.

(1) In heifers, bilateral gonadal aplasia, which causes permanent anoestrus and sterility, occurs in the common condition of freemartinism, found in the majority of female calves that are cotwins with males. It is also observed in bilateral ovarian hypoplasia, a rare inherited condition, in which the genes are passed on through fertile individuals with unilateral gonadal hypoplasia. Poor nutrition is important and discussed below.

Box 35.3 Major causes of true anoestrus.

Heifers
  Freemartinism
  Ovarian hypoplasia
  Inactive ovaries (poor nutrition)

Cows
  Dystokia and postpartum problems
  Delayed involution (inactive ovaries)
  Pyometra (persistent corpus luteum)
  Cystic ovarian disease
  Poor nutrition prepartum, severe energy deficit postpartum, especially first calvers
  Age-related factors

(2) In cows a variety of abnormalities at or around calving, such as dystokia, retained fetal membranes, hypocalcaemia, metritis, endometritis and other postpartum abnormalities may result in delayed return to cyclicity (for a full discussion of this see also Chapter 34).

(3) Ovarian cysts, traditionally defined as fluid-filled structures >25 mm in diameter and present for more than 10 days in the absence of a corpus luteum (CL), are quite commonly recorded in cases of anoestrus and in fact the majority of cows with cystic ovarian disease exhibit anoestrus. This traditional definition implied that cysts were static structures; however, this is now known not to be the case, and cysts should be considered dynamic both in structure and function (Cook et al., 1990). The likely hormonal mechanism of cystic ovarian disease is failure of the preovulatory luteinizing hormone (LH) surge. In some cases there may be failure of the ovary to respond to LH at the start of oestrus (Brown et al., 1986). Cystic ovarian disease is a very complex condition and in many cases the cyst produces a mixture of steroids, which are variably absorbed into the general circulation.

In the postpartum period, particularly during the first six weeks, some cows (approximately 20–25 per cent) experience ovulation failure followed by the development of palpable but functionally transient cystic structures that may not interfere with subsequent cyclicity. Towards the end of this period many farmers become concerned about lack of oestrus and so the cow is presented for veterinary examination. Cystic ovaries were associated with 6 to 11 more days to first service and with 20 to 30 more days to conception in a meta-analysis of papers published between January 1987 and January 1999 (Fourichon et al., 2000). By about six weeks after calving an ovarian cystic structure should be regarded as pathological. Cysts are often classified as either follicular (about 70 per cent; single large cyst or multiple smaller cystic structures) or luteal and it is

easy to understand why the cow with the luteal cyst, which is predominantly progesterone producing, does not exhibit oestrus, though it is less clear why she fails to cycle. However, follicular cysts with oestrogen production are also found in cases of anoestrus. This may be due to the low level of the steroid produced in some cases, while in other cases it may result from the negative effect on the behavioural centre of high levels of oestrogen circulating more or less continuously. Another explanation for the lack of oestrus in cows with follicular cysts is that the behavioural centres in the brain, which control the expression of oestrus, respond better to oestrogens if they have been primed by progesterone.

Garverick (1997) in the USA and Dobson et al. (2001a) in the UK have both reviewed cystic ovarian disease. Factors associated with the occurrence of cystic ovarian disease are discussed further in Chapter 36.

(4) The role of nutritional deficiencies in anoestrus is relatively straightforward in heifers but is complex in adult dairy cows.

(a) In heifers it has been shown in many field trials that low energy intake that causes slow growth rate is associated with delayed puberty. Onset of puberty tends to be related to body weight rather than age. The mechanism is discussed in Chapter 5.

(b) In adult lactating dairy cows it is not clear how feeding affects return to cyclicity after calving, even when only energy is considered; however, evidence is growing to suggest that the effect may, at least in part, be mediated by insulin-like growth factor-1 (IGF-1) levels (Taylor et al., 2001). It is clear that dairy cows experience a metabolic crisis early postpartum, as energy loss cannot be compensated for by energy intake and stored energy is utilized. Factors that exacerbate the negative energy balance including the feeding levels before and after calving, particularly the energy density of the ration, excessive energy loss due to high milk yield and increased body condition loss after calving (body condition score loss of more than 0.5) will prolong the interval to first ovulation, as will associated metabolic or other diseases postpartum. A clear relationship has been shown between the timing of the negative energy balance nadir (the lowest point of the negative energy balance postpartum) and the interval to first ovulation, the LH pulse frequency and the LH-dependent fate of the first dominant follicle selected postpartum (Canfield & Butler, 1990; Beam & Butler, 1997). First ovulation occurs 7–14 days after the energy balance nadir; thus, if the lowest point of the negative energy balance is reached between the first to second week postpartum, cows can be expected to ovulate by 21–30 days postpartum. However, in cows in which body condition score loss exceeds 1, the interval to first ovulation may be prolonged to 60 days and beyond. One method to try to take into account these many interacting factors is regularly to measure the body condition score of cows (Anon, 1984); particularly important times include drying off, calving and service times.

(c)   In the beef suckler cow, prepartum nutritional deficits leading to reduced body condition at calving delay the interval to first ovulation by more than 40 days to 90 days and beyond (Stagg *et al.*, 1995, 1998). The delay in resumption of ovulatory activity is associated with continued atresia of recurrently selected dominant follicles; instead of ovulation of the 2nd to 4th dominant follicle postpartum, it is on average the 9th dominant follicle which eventually secretes sufficient oestradiol to induce the gonadotrophin surge and ovulation. As circulatory concentrations of FSH are not affected by pre- or postpartum diet, the detrimental effects of low body condition score at calving on the fate of dominant follicles selected early postpartum are attributed to reduced LH secretion, which reduces dominant follicle oestradiol production.

The relationship between nutrition and fertility is a complex one which is still not fully understood. There is a vast body of literature on this subject which is too extensive to review here. However, the reader may find the following reviews of interest: Britt (1995); Webb *et al.* (1997, 1999); Wathes *et al.* (1998); O'Callaghan and Boland (1999); Garnsworthy and Webb (2000) and O'Callaghan *et al.* (2000).

Several studies have shown that cows in their first lactation exhibit a disproportionately high incidence of true anoestrus, with lack of ovulation. A variety of explanations for this have been put forward, in particular the inhibitory effects of lactation and growth on the recovery of the LH pulse frequency early postpartum, preventing dominant follicle maturation and ovulation. Another suggestion is that this is mainly the result of the high incidence of dystokia that occurs in first calvers.

However, the high incidence of anoestrus in first calvers is often attributed to nutritional and environmental factors. Excessive weight loss and very poor body condition result in cessation of ovulation and cyclicity, presumably through hypothalamic–pituitary dysfunction (see Chapter 67). Cows continue to grow until their second or third lactation and therefore young animals have to carry out the tasks of milk production, growth and reproduction simultaneously, at a time when adult dentition has not been fully developed. In dairy cows it is also the time when the young, smaller cow is introduced to the highly competitive environment of a herd, which, particularly during the housing period, makes it difficult for small animals to compete

for food. It is also presumably a stressful experience being low within the herd hierarchy.

(d)   In many cases first calvers may exhibit a high incidence of lameness. Lameness (see Chapters 31 and 32) is a cause of weight loss that can result in true anoestrus and also, because of the associated pain, can cause poor oestrous expression in animals that are cycling. Various other forms of stress such as surgery, changes in social grouping, transport and heat stress may all affect fertility, thus stress on breeding cattle should be minimized whenever possible (Dobson *et al.*, 2001b).

(5)   Among miscellaneous causes of persistent corpus luteum is the rare condition of uterus unicornis, in which one horn of the uterus is absent. Ovulation on the side without a uterine horn results in a corpus luteum that is not exposed to locally produced prostaglandin and therefore does not regress after 16 or 17 days.

Silent ovulation and unobserved oestrus

First ovulation postpartum is generally silent (80 per cent), but once cycles have been established, silent oestrus is not a common phenomenon, as was clearly demonstrated by Williamson *et al.* (1972), who carried out continuous observation of 107 cows for 21 days and concluded that four demonstrated silent oestrus. This has been confirmed by others in field trials in herds in which silent oestrus was thought to be a problem. Generally, when oestrous detection methods are improved, there is a corresponding reduction in the number of cases regarded as silent oestrus. Many cases previously diagnosed as silent oestrus are in fact unobserved oestrus.

Incidence figures for silent ovulation are most reliable when based on serial progesterone assays, as in the study of 1400 cows by Ball and Jackson (1984) in which 21 per cent of the cows had ovulated but had not been seen in oestrus. This level of non-detected oestrus is in agreement with other studies. McLeod *et al.* (1991) reported 78 per cent of ovulations in their study were correctly identified by conventional oestrous detection, confirming that approximately 20 per cent of those cows ovulating are not seen in oestrus.

To what extent delayed return to service is due to unobserved oestrus is not clear, but Humbolt (1982), using milk progesterone assays, calculated that only 29 per cent of delayed returns were due to embryonic death and that 73 per cent were due to anoestrus (including true, silent and unobserved oestrus).

However, ovulation without the accompanying signs of oestrus (that is, silent oestrus) does occur. The best documented situation relates to the first ovulation after

Box 35.4 Causes of silent and weakly expressed oestrus.

- Social
- Pain and fear
- Weight loss
- Genetic factors
- Presence of calf and suckling

calving, particularly if it occurs within the first 20 days. Otherwise it is almost impossible to distinguish between silent and unobserved oestrus. Some instances of oestrus are so weak or last for such a short time that detection by conventional observation is a matter of chance.

Standing oestrus lasts for about 8–12 hours in cows and 6–8 hours in maiden heifers. However, 20 per cent of heats last less than 6 hours (Esslemont *et al.*, 1985). Increasing herd sizes and decreasing availability of skilled manpower on many farms is probably exacerbating the problem of poor oestrous detection. It may also be the case that high-genetic-merit, high-yielding modern dairy cattle exhibit oestrous behaviour either less intensely or for a shorter duration, making oestrous detection more difficult.

The causes of silent oestrus, weak oestrus and short oestrus are not well understood, but those considered to be the main factors are presented in Box 35.4.

(1) Social factors within the group of cows, the size of the group and the reproductive status of the rest of the group all play a role in oestrous behaviour and in the frequency of mounting (Britt, 1987). Mounting requires that there is both a cow in oestrus and a cow that is willing to mount.

Cows that are usually bullied or are low in the pecking order are less likely to stand to be ridden when they are in oestrus than more dominant cows. A small group of cows, say fewer than four or five, may be less effective at stimulating mounting behaviour than a larger group of sexually active cows. Cows at different stages of the reproductive cycle vary in their likelihood of trying to mount a cow in oestrus. The most likely to jump are those in or near oestrus, followed by non-pregnant cows in the early luteal phase followed by pregnant cows. At the end of an intensive breeding season when most cows are pregnant the remaining cows to be served may be more difficult to detect because of the absence of cows willing to mount. In the main, oestrous detection is therefore easier in tight seasonally calving herds, where a large number of cows are eligible for service within a given time period, than in a herd with a wide calving spread and fewer non-pregnant cows in the herd at any one time.

The presence of a bull inhibits cow-to-cow interaction, but this may be made up for by the bull's own sexual monitoring of the herd. However, a bull may not choose to serve all cows in oestrus if several are in season at the same time.

(2) Pain and fear. As oestrus is a behavioural phenomenon that is subject to psychological influences, it can be inhibited by discomfort, pain or fear. Severe adverse weather conditions such as driving rain and cold reduce cows' interest in sexual behaviour. Slippery flooring produces fear of falling and may inhibit oestrous behaviour. The pain caused by lameness inhibits oestrous expression.

(3) Weight loss. It has been suggested that weight loss is associated with an increase in silent heats.

(4) Genetic factors are almost certainly involved. The subjective nature of the measurement of oestrous expression makes it difficult to gather enough reliable data to evaluate the hereditary influence. Reports from progeny testing stations, where large groups of daughters from bulls under test were kept, showed that different daughter groups exhibited oestrus in characteristic ways. There may also be differences between breeds in expression of oestrus. Currently, there is much anecdotal evidence to suggest that the modern high-genetic-merit Holstein exhibits oestrus less well than the traditional British Friesian, or some other dairy breeds.

(5) Presence of calf and suckling. The presence of a suckling calf may reduce expression of oestrous behaviour in some cows as well as affect oestrous cyclicity.

Epidemiological data

In a study of 70775 lactations in Finnish Ayrshire cows in which only cases treated by veterinarians were analysed (Saloniemi *et al.*, 1986) it was noted that the chance of a cow being presented to the veterinarian as anoestrus was affected by parity (highest risk in first calvers), calving season (highest risk in cows that calved from September to February), herd milk yield (highest incidence in high-yielding herds) and the occurrence of metritis (Chapter 34), mastitis (Chapter 23) and ketosis (Chapter 46).

Diagnosis

A systematic approach to diagnosis is essential and the clinician should follow the steps outlined in Box 35.5.

If the anoestrous cow is in a herd in which the veterinarian is running a fertility control programme involving regular visits, diagnosis will be both easier and more reliable because there will be historical informa-

Box 35.5 The diagnosis of anoestrus.

- History (including records)
- General clinical examination (including condition score)
- Special examination of the reproductive system
- Rectal palpation and transrectal ultrasound examination
- Vaginal specular examination
- Laboratory tests, e.g. progesterone assays

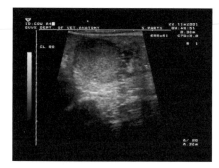

Fig. 35.2 Cyclic solid CL.

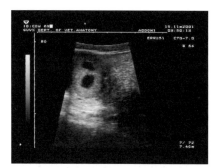

Fig. 35.1 Cyclic CL with lacunae on right ovary.

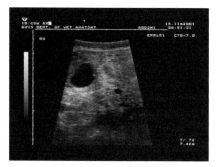

Fig. 35.3 Dominant follicle on right ovary bordering the CL.

tion available and it will be simpler to introduce routine sampling where this is indicated.

There are two separate but overlapping aspects of diagnosis:

- *Stage 1*: assessment of ovarian status to determine whether the case is true anoestrus, in which there is no ovulatory activity, or in which cyclicity is prevented by a persistent corpus luteum or other progesterone producing structure; or silent or unobserved oestrus, in which ovarian cycles are taking place.
- *Stage 2*: assessment of the causes of the condition.

Stage 1: assessment of ovarian status

Since the word 'cycle' implies repetition, theory would dictate that assessment of whether or not a cow is cycling necessitates repeated examinations over an interval that should allow the observation of two oestrous periods. Under practical conditions it is usually assumed that the animal is cycling if it is possible to prove that ovulation has recently taken place. Another common assumption concerns a group of animals. It is usually considered that the group as a whole is cycling if two-thirds of the cows are in the luteal phase, i.e. the same fraction of the oestrous cycle that the luteal phase occupies. Furthermore, the description of the 'luteal phase' given in Chapter 33 presents some difficulties in connection with diagnosis. This is because a corpus luteum is unlikely to be palpable until approximately seven days after oestrus, but

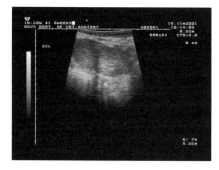

Fig. 35.4 Two corpora lutea in a 6-week pregnancy.

may be functional before that time. However, positive detection of a functional corpus luteum via ultrasound examination (size and echogenicity, Figs 35.1–35.4) is usually closely related to its progesterone secretion. Progesterone assay of milk or plasma will only produce a definite, recognizable rise after a similar delay; to confirm cyclicity a sequence of progesterone assays two or three days apart showing a pattern consistent with a luteal phase followed by a period of low progesterone level and another luteal phase should be seen.

Accordingly, for clinical purposes 'luteal phase' is defined as from day 5 to day 17 and the normal 'period

Box 35.6 History taking for anoestrus cows.

- Date of calving
- Any abnormality at and after calving
- Has the cow been seen in oestrus since calving?
- Could the cow be pregnant?
- Oestrous detection methods in the herd
- Are there other cows in the herd with similar problems?

Table 35.3 The accuracy of corpora lutea detection by rectal palpation based on comparison with milk progesterone assay.

	Corpus luteum	
	Present	**Absent**
Number of cases	244	158
Accuracy (%)	82	70

of low progesterone' is expected to be from day 18 through oestrus (day 0) to day 4. This definition applies to the majority of cows in a normal population and is needed to form a basis for rational diagnosis, but its use should be tempered by the realization that no definition will fit all cases (Bloomfield *et al.*, 1986).

The first step is to take a history of the case. Relevant information, required for both stages of diagnosis, is shown in Box 35.6.

The next step is to find out if there is functional luteal tissue present in the ovaries. The traditional way to do this is to palpate the ovaries per rectum, but there are now several choices. One is to carry out a single or a series of milk progesterone assays, which gives a quick, reliable result. Another is ultrasound scanning, which allows the user to observe functional luteal tissue in the ovary (Figs 35.1–35.4) (Omran *et al.*, 1988; Boyd & Omran 1991).

The choice of method will depend on circumstances as each method has advantages and disadvantages. Rectal palpation is immediate, simple, requires little restraint of the cow and, if part of a regular visit, is relatively cheap. It also allows other observations to be made on other parts of the reproductive tract and on the animal's general condition. There is minimal risk of misidentification of the animal, a danger always present when samples are taken for analysis. On the other hand, it is a less accurate indicator of luteal function than a progesterone assay. Real-time ultrasound scanning is a valuable tool that, in experienced hands, is capable of giving a very accurate picture of ovaries and uterus (Figs 35.1–35.13).

Rectal palpation alone, when undertaken by an experienced clinician, can be relatively accurate. For example, Dawson (1975) compared the findings made by rectal palpation shortly before slaughter with post-mortem observations. He identified accurately 125 (89 per cent) of 141 ovaries with corpora lutea. The errors were mainly in cows with small corpora lutea and also some with cysts or follicles. However, others have suggested that rectal examinations alone are less accurate. On the basis of milk progesterone assays (which were assumed to be correct) Ott *et al.* (1986) summarized their own and other workers' results, as shown in Table 35.3.

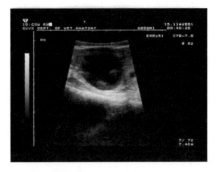

Fig. 35.5 Long-standing follicular cyst.

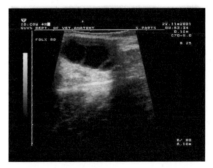

Fig. 35.6 Follicles on right ovary.

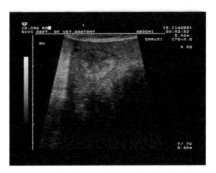

Fig. 35.7 Non-pregnant right uterine horn during the luteal phase.

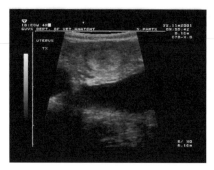

Fig. 35.8 Non-pregnant left uterine horn during the luteal phase with bladder ventrally.

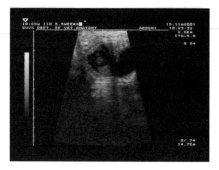

Fig. 35.11 Early PD 5.5 weeks.

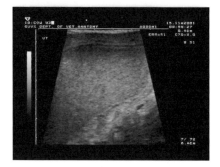

Fig. 35.9 Pyometra.

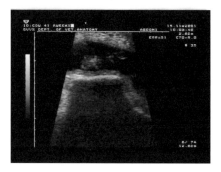

Fig. 35.12 Early PD 6 weeks.

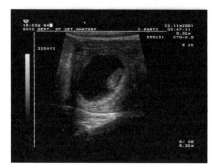

Fig. 35.10 Early PD 4.5 weeks.

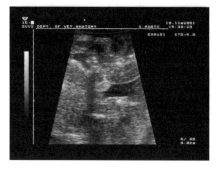

Fig. 35.13 Male fetus (3 months).

The use of progesterone assays has the advantage that they can be incorporated into a fertility control programme and used prior to a visit, so that the clinician has information available before the examination of the animal. They can also be used after the visit to give extra information about the case. There may be slight problems in deciding the level of circulating progesterone that can be taken as indicative of luteal function and caution needs to be exercised in interpretation of absolute values, as these may change depending on time from milking (Waldmann *et al.*, 1999).

The accuracy of ultrasound scanning was investigated by Pieterse *et al.* (1990), who examined the ovaries of 59 cows by rectal palpation, ultrasound scanning (5 MHz linear array transducer) and dissection on the day of slaughter, and concluded that for the detection of a mid-cycle corpus luteum the sensitivity of rectal palpation was 83 per cent and for ultrasonography the sensitivity was 80 per cent. For the detection of follicles, ultrasonography was considered to be significantly better than rectal palpation, with ultrasonography detecting 95 per cent of follicles over 10 mm in diameter whereas rectal palpation only detected 71 per cent. These results obviously reflect in part the quality of the ultrasound equipment used and the skill of the clinician palpating the ovaries and interpreting the ultrasound images. In another study comparing the use of ultrasound and rectal palpation (Fishwick, 1993), the accuracy of palpation and ultrasonography in detection of luteal tissue was compared to contemporaneous plasma progesterone concentrations. In this study the overall accuracy of manual palpation was 62 per cent compared with 83 per cent for ultrasound examination. In cows with high progesterone status, manual palpation (60 per cent) was significantly less accurate than ultrasound imaging (94 per cent), whilst in cows with a low progesterone status manual palpation (65 per cent) and ultrasound imaging (70 per cent) were both equally accurate.

In general it would be expected that imaging of the ovaries using modern ultrasound equipment, for example using a 7.5 MHz transducer, would be more accurate than manual palpation. However, individuals highly skilled in rectal palpation may be able to detect luteal tissue with an accuracy comparable to ultrasound, but will not be able to palpate small follicles that are readily detected by ultrasound scanning. Reduced cost of equipment and improved image quality combined with practice and much increased use within veterinary medicine have made transrectal real-time ultrasound examination of the bovine reproductive organs the examination of choice in regular fertility visits.

If there is evidence of functional luteal tissue, the possibilities shown in Box 35.7 exist.

The simplest way to decide whether the animal is pregnant or has a pathological condition is to carry out rectal palpation or ultrasound examination of the ovaries and genital tract, plus in some cases a vaginal examination. This will, however, fail to reveal very early pregnancy before 25–28 days after service using ultrasound and below 35–40 days using manual palpation. Figures 35.10 to 35.12 show examples of ultrasound images of early pregnancy. Figure 35.13 shows an image of fetal sexing in a three-month-old fetus. The most common finding is that ovaries and uterus appear to be normal and these cases are usually regarded as normal cycling cows that have simply not been seen in oestrus.

Box 35.7. Likely reasons for the presence of functional luteal tissue.

- Cycling (days 5–17 inclusive)
- Pregnancy
- Ovarian pathology (luteal cyst)
- Uterine pathology (pyometra with persisting corpus luteum)

Box 35.8 Likely reasons for no luteal tissue being present.

- True anoestrus
- Cycling (day 18 through oestrus to day 4)
- Ovarian pathology
  Freemartin: heifer
  Cystic ovarian disease

Booth (1988) has investigated the accuracy of diagnosis of luteal cysts using rectal palpation, and the clinical finding of luteal cysts was confirmed by progesterone assay in only 54 per cent of cases. This accuracy can be improved by transrectal ultrasound scanning. For example, Douthwaite and Dobson (2000) reported that diagnostic criteria for follicular cysts using ultrasound examination and plasma progesterone assays agreed in 92 per cent of cases; a similar comparison for luteal cyst diagnosis gave a 74 per cent agreement. The rapid on-farm diagnostic method of choice should thus be transrectal ultrasonography, supported by milk progesterone assay where required.

If initial examination shows there is no functional luteal tissue, there are also the various possibilities shown in Box 35.8.

When the initial examination reveals no luteal function and apparently normal ovaries and tract, and no evidence of mucus or mucohaemorrhagic discharge on the tail to indicate recent oestrus or ovulation, the cow's ovarian status is unresolved. If she is cycling normally and in the low progesterone phase of the cycle, a corpus luteum will become palpable and visible by ultrasound examination in the ovary within approximately 7 days from the first examination. A second examination at 7–10 days after the first will detect this corpus luteum. This second examination must not be delayed too long, as some cows (those at day 5) will go into the low progesterone phase again in about 12 days after the first examination. These calculations can be upset by the considerable variations in cycle lengths and progesterone patterns that occur in a normal population of cows, as detailed by Bloomfield et al. (1986). It is also very useful to carry out a vaginal examination at the time of the first examination, as the presence of copious, clear mucus is strongly indicative of the peri-oestral stage of the cycle. In this way vaginal examination may allow a diagnosis to be made without the need for a second progesterone assay or a second rectal palpation.

If a second examination or sampling is required it is best done 7–10 days after the first. It is even better if serial sampling for progesterone assays can be arranged. It is necessary to work out a satisfactory regimen of sampling. This involves making a compromise between the biological ideal, which might be daily samples, and what is acceptable to the farmer because of the cost, labour and interference with the milking routine. For example, a sampling regimen of two to three samples per week, which will give a useful picture of the oestrous cycle but is not frequent enough to time oestrus exactly, may be unacceptably frequent for a farmer. This situation may change in future if accurate and reliable automated systems to assess the cows' physiological state using biosensors can be developed (Koelsch *et al.*, 1994; Mottram, 1997; Scully *et al.*, 2000). New developments in this area of technology may allow automatic milk progesterone assays, and other assays, to be performed while cows are being milked, allowing the timing of ovulation to be accurately predicted and removing the need for oestrous detection.

Detection of antral follicles in the ovary, the observation of uterine tone and assays for oestrogens are all of limited value because they do not give clear indication of exact timing of oestrus to predict ovulation. There are a number of aids to detection of oestrus that can aid diagnosis (Boyd, 1984).

The veterinarian now knows whether the cow or group of cows is exhibiting true anoestrus or is undergoing ovarian cycles. If a conclusion of anoestrus has been reached an important question is whether (i) the cow is in 'deep' anoestrus, which means that she is not likely to start cycling soon and may revert to an anoestrous state following treatment, or (ii) whether she is in 'shallow' anoestrus and liable to begin cycling soon and be responsive to therapy. Unfortunately, it is almost impossible to predict accurately the 'depth' of anoestrus. However, if the cow is in extremely poor condition and if she has small hard ovaries she is probably in deep anoestrus and may require a combination of treatments to induce first ovulation, with the possibility of subsequently reverting to an anoestrous state.

Detection of the LH pulses that occur in the cow about to start cycling and are absent in those in deep anoestrus requires a series of samples taken at short intervals. At present (2003) LH assays cannot be done in a practice laboratory but are routinely carried out in affiliated research laboratories.

Stage 2: assessment of the cause of anoestrus or silent ovulation

This section deals with the difficult question of how to find out what has caused the abnormal ovarian status or the problem of oestrous expression or detection.

To some extent procedures followed for diagnosis of ovarian status also give the clinician an understanding of the causes of the ovarian dysfunction. Examples of these are listed in Box 35.9. Three of the causes of inactive ovaries: nutritional deficiency causing metabolic stress and severe negative energy balance, delayed

Box 35.9 Causes of dysfunction of the ovarian cycle.

- Freemartinism (congenital)
- Ovarian hypoplasia (inherited)
- Uterus unicornis (congenital)
- Pyometra (periparturient problems)
- Some cases of inactive ovaries
- Nutritional and metabolic stress
- Systemic disease
- Delayed involution

involution and concomitant disease, present some problems in diagnosis.

In cases of delayed involution, the enlarged uterus and particularly the enlarged cervix, which involutes more slowly, usually make the diagnosis of the immediate cause easy. However, on some occasions, by the time the cow is examined the uterus may well have returned to normal size and the veterinarian will have to depend on a history of periparturient problems and possibly of abnormal vaginal discharges noted by the farmer (see Chapter 34 page 523 for details of an involution scoring system).

The clinician should look for any other disease condition in the cow examined for anoestrus. Especially important is any disease that causes loss of body condition or pain.

There is a complicated series of factors, such as actual and potential milk yield, feeding before and after calving and weight change after calving, which are very difficult to assess. Body condition of the cow should be noted at the time of examination for anoestrus, but this deals with only part of the problem (Anon., 1984). If body condition is poor or loss of body condition score has been extreme, or if there are many cases of inactive ovaries, feeding should be investigated. Feeding analysis and metabolic profiles are discussed elsewhere in this book (see Chapters 9 and 47).

On occasion there is no clear reason for the occurrence of inactive ovaries, either in the individual cow or when the condition affects a group of animals.

When investigating silent oestrus and unobserved oestrus, the veterinarian should find out about the following:

- Organization of oestrous detection.
- Ease of cow identification.
- Method of recording.
- Layout of the buildings.
- State of the floors and levels of lighting.
- The way the cows are handled, moved around and assigned to groups.
- Amount of knowledge of oestrus and the oestrous cycle among the people who are detecting oestrus.
- Motivation for oestrous detection.

- Time made available for oestrous detection.
- Personalities of the people involved.

Treatment (see also Chapter 42)

When using proprietary products, the clinician should consult the data sheets, produced by the manufacturers, for details of use, contraindications and other guidance. Successful treatment, leading to oestrus, service and pregnancy, depends not only on veterinary therapy but on husbandry and breeding management, some aspects of which are described in the data sheets and also on page 525. Different manufacturers of apparently similar products often give slightly different advice about their use and users should be aware of the major differences between some of these products. Some of the therapeutics, for example Prostaglandin $F_{2\alpha}$ ($PGF_{2\alpha}$) are dangerous for humans and could cause return to service and abortion in cows, and therefore the veterinarian must handle them responsibly and with care.

Where drugs that result in oestrus are used, efficiency of oestrous detection will be enhanced as the clients are told to concentrate on a specific time for oestrous detection; their attention is focused on the cows treated and aids to oestrous detection such as tail paint are often used.

True anoestrus: no functional luteal tissue

Two points should be remembered when dealing with these cases:

- All healthy, suitably fed cows will start cycling in the first two months after calving.
- There must be an underlying reason for the occurrence of this type of true anoestrus and an attempt should always be made to find the cause and deal with it. Where the cause appears to be nutritional, improved feeding should be part of the treatment of the affected individual and should also be considered for other recently calved cows. Consideration should also be given to the body condition changes and feeding regimen of the dry cows as well as the management and nutrition of the transition cow. Particular care should be taken to ensure that high-genetic-merit dairy cows do not become too fat during the dry period (Rukkwamsuk *et al.*, 1999).

At present there are two main hormonal treatments for inactive ovaries: (i) administration of gonadotrophin-releasing hormone (GnRH) or analogues with GnRH activity and (ii) insertion of a progesterone-releasing device (see p. 681).

Administration of an adequate dose of GnRH results, in the majority of cases, in luteinization or ovulation of healthy dominant follicles present at the time followed by a transient period of progesterone production that can first be identified about five days after treatment. The duration of this progesterone phase is very variable, ranging from one or two days to the lifespan of a normal cyclic corpus luteum, and therefore the interval from treatment to oestrus is very variable, about 8–22 days. It is desirable to follow up these cases to ensure that luteinization or ovulation has taken place; this is best done by ultrasound scanning or by progesterone assay.

If there is luteal tissue present at the follow-up examination 7 days later, it is useful to treat the animal with $PGF_{2\alpha}$ or an analogue, as this will make the resulting oestrus more predictable. Regular fertility control visits at weekly intervals are ideal for this regimen; however, visits are often at fortnightly intervals and this may be a less suitable period between the initial and follow-up treatment when using the GnRH–$PGF_{2\alpha}$ regimen.

If, on the follow-up examination, there is no luteal tissue the cow should be dealt with as a new case.

The use of a progesterone or synthetic progestagen slow release device also mimics the progesterone rise before first ovulation. This device is left in the vagina or implanted subcutaneously at the base of the ear for 8–12 days and the animal should be served at the oestrus that occurs in many cases about two or three days after withdrawal. Fixed-time insemination 48 and 72 hours (or a single insemination at 56 hours) after withdrawal may be carried out (follow data sheet recommendations for whichever product is selected). If oestrus is observed later another insemination should be carried out. Avoid stress and drastic change of diet during and after treatment (see p. 683).

In those animals in which increased negative energy balance, poor body condition or very strong behavioural effects inhibit LH pulse frequency and thus dominant follicle maturation, final differentiation of the preovulatory dominant follicle or the preovulatory oestradiol rise may have to be enhanced. The addition of equine chorionic gonadotrophin (eCG) given at the end of the progesterone or synthetic progestagen treatment will induce oestrus 48 hours later. Similarly, treatment with a very low dose of oestradiol benzoate 24 hours after device withdrawal will induce oestrus 12–20 hours later, but consideration will have to be given to the national legislation relating to the use of these drugs in dairy or beef cattle.

The treatment of follicular cysts involves either using intravaginal progesterone releasing devices (PRID or CIDR) or establishment of endogenous luteal tissue with chorionic gonadotrophin or GnRH (Dobson *et al.*, 2001a). There is evidence to suggest that the success of treatment of follicular cysts depends on whether the cyst is producing oestradiol or not, as reflected by the presence or absence of other follicles >5 mm in diameter. Treated with either an intravaginal progesterone releasing device or GnRH, cystic follicles in the presence of other follicles had a pregnancy rate to all inseminations of 91 per cent compared with 69 per cent if no other follicles were present at the time of treatment (Tebble et al., 2001).

True anoestrus: functional luteal tissue

The therapeutic approach is to cause luteolysis by parenteral administration of $PGF_{2\alpha}$, or an analogue, followed by intensive oestrous detection up to one week after injection and insemination at observed oestrus. In the case of pyometra (Fig. 35.9), the client should be advised to delay service until it appears that the infection has cleared up, as indicated by an oestrus at which the mucus from the vulva is free of pus. It is advisable that the veterinary surgeon should examine these cases at a follow-up visit to ensure the uterus has returned to normal (Figs 35.7 and 35.8).

The treatment of cystic ovarian disease depends largely on whether the structure is progesterone producing or not. If considered a luteal cyst with functional luteal tissue, as judged by ultrasound examination or milk progesterone assay, the logical treatment is to administer $PGF_{2\alpha}$, although alternative therapies such as the use of intravaginal progesterone releasing devices may also be successful (Douthwaite & Dobson, 2000).

Silent oestrus/unobserved oestrus: corpus luteum present

There are two standard approaches in these cases, the choice being between (i) the induction of luteolysis using $PGF_{2\alpha}$ or an analogue and (ii) leaving the animal untreated to be observed when she comes in heat. The method chosen will depend on many variable factors, such as the season, the time since calving, the herd calving pattern and the inclination of the client, and therefore the decision has to be made individually for each case.

Treatment with $PGF_{2\alpha}$ or an analogue should, in the majority of adult cows, result in oestrus in 2 to 7 days, with the peak period being days 3 and 4 after treatment. Service should be at observed oestrus and aids to oestrous detection should be used. Enhanced oestrous expression may be observed when combining a progesterone or synthetic progestagen device with $PGF_{2\alpha}$.

Cows that are not seen in oestrus after treatment should be re-examined after 14 days (Young, 1989)

with a view to treating with $PGF_{2\alpha}$ or an analogue, if appropriate.

Conservative treatment is preferred in the first instance by some clients who would rather leave the animal untreated, are content to know that she is cycling and hope to observe the next oestrus. In these cases aids to heat detection should be used and the animal re-examined if she is not seen in season within the next two weeks.

Silent oestrus/unobserved oestrus: no corpus luteum present

These cases do not benefit from immediate drug therapy as animals are showing ovarian cycles but have either just regressed their CL or are in the early luteal stage following ovulation. Improvements in husbandry, i.e. oestrous detection, and, possibly, feeding may be required to enhance detection and oestrous expression, and it may be useful to enhance oestrous expression hormonally by using eCG or oestradiol benzoate following treatment with a progestagen device (see above).

Because diagnosis is uncertain until the second examination (7 or 14 days later), it is questionable whether these cows should be treated at the first visit. If there is no corpus luteum on the second examination, the condition is to be regarded as true anoestrus and dealt with accordingly.

Prognosis

In considering prognosis, primary attention has to be paid to the return to cyclicity, which can be measured either by observation of oestrus or, more reliably, by one or more progesterone assays at planned times after treatment. The outcome of treatment is influenced by both the veterinarian and the client (and perhaps also by the cow), as presented in Box 35.10.

Factors influenced by the veterinarian, which affect the outcome of treatment for anoestrus, are as follows:

Box 35.10 Contribution of farmer and veterinary surgeon to influencing prognosis.

Prognosis influenced by veterinarian
  Accuracy of diagnosis
  Selection of cases
  Choice of therapeutic intervention
  Follow-up examination

Prognosis influenced by farmer
  Oestrous detection
  Herd pregnancy rate
  Culling rate

- The accuracy of diagnosis is the basis for correct treatment. There is good evidence that identification of a corpus luteum by palpation by experienced veterinarians is over 80 per cent accurate (see p. 537) and that differentiation between follicular and luteal cysts is much less accurate (see p. 539); however, such a diagnosis can now be more specific due to the routine use of ultrasound scanning, and can be enhanced via using milk progesterone assays.
- Selection of cases for treatment has an important influence on the outcome. For example, the corpus luteum early in the cycle is less responsive to PGF$_{2\alpha}$ or an analogue than is the mid-cycle corpus luteum. Accurate assessment of the stage of the cycle will aid in the correct selection of animals for treatment. Similarly, if treatment is confined to cases in which corpora lutea are positively diagnosed, better results may be obtained than if less critical selection of cases is undertaken. However, when PGF$_{2\alpha}$ treatments based on the presence of a corpus luteum were compared with 14-day fixed treatments, the fixed treatments were still superior resulting in better reproductive performance (Heuwieser et al., 1997).

Other factors that influence the success of luteolysis and whether the cow comes in season after successful luteolysis are not well documented. However, it is possible that nutritional factors are involved in the subsequent expression of oestrus.

- None of the luteolytic products commercially available achieve 100 per cent luteolysis (Ball & Jackson, 1984; Martinez & Thibier, 1984).
- Re-examination and retreatment in good time of all cases that do not respond to the initial treatment will affect the time from initial treatment to oestrus, service and conception.

The farmer also affects the outcome of the treatment in important ways.

- The efficiency of detection of oestrus in the herd is crucial to the effectiveness of treatment when measured by the number of cases that come into season within a certain number of days.
- The first-service pregnancy rate in the herd which is to some extent under the control of the farmer, not least because correctly timed insemination is essential for conception, will have a great effect on the success rate as measured in time to conception.
- High culling rate and willingness to cull may result in apparently good results because the failures are culled, but depending on the economic factors pertaining at the time this may be a false economy (Esslemont & Kossaibati, 1997; Whitaker et al., 2000).

Heifers

Freemartins and cases of bilateral ovarian hypoplasia are sterile and will never cycle or become pregnant.

Groups of heifers with delayed puberty due to low energy intake will return to cyclicity after restoration of a suitable energy intake level and other correction of the feeding. How long this will take depends on many things. Under the best possible circumstances, i.e. where the animals are in not excessively poor condition and where there is no complicating disease factor, it will take approximately two months of good feeding before most of the group start cycling (Imakawa et al., 1986). Hormonal treatments to induce and thus advance first ovulation can be used if the management system is seasonally restricted; introduction of a bull may also aid in the induction and synchronization of first ovulation.

True anoestrus after calving in cows

In cases of pyometra with a corpus luteum, the failure to cycle is very effectively dealt with by using PGF$_{2\alpha}$. Ott and Gustafsson (1981) reported that more than 80 per cent of treated cows emptied the uterus and came in season a few days after treatment. If one treatment fails to produce luteolysis, then a second injection almost certainly will be successful. There is evidence to suggest that treatment of pyometra is improved by the administration of two doses of PGF$_{2\alpha}$, 8 hours apart (Archbald et al., 1993) (see p. 524).

Inactive ovaries are treated with either GnRH to cause ovulation and thus a progesterone rise, which then primes the animal to express heat at the next ovulation, or a progesterone or progestagen releasing device. Some indications of the results that can be obtained were shown in a field study involving 62 acyclic cows (Ball & Lamming, 1983). There were two main differences between the two methods. Firstly, ovarian response to the progesterone intravaginal releasing device (PRID) was better, as 89.7 per cent of cows ovulated compared to 73.9 per cent of those treated with GnRH. Secondly, after the PRID, fixed-time insemination resulted in 59 per cent conceptions (measured by milk progesterone) whereas after GnRH, a number of cows that responded successfully were not seen in heat so that only 26 per cent of the cows treated became pregnant at the ovulation after treatment. One problem with GnRH treatment is that the luteal tissue produced has a very variable lifespan with the result that the timing of heat and the next ovulation cannot be predicted and may occur from 8 to about 20 days after treatment. In order to cause more predictable onset of oestrus and next ovulation following GnRH treatment, a luteolytic dose of PGF$_{2\alpha}$ can be given 6–7 days after GnRH. Such a protocol can be further combined with a second injection of GnRH or an injection of human chorionic gonadotrophin (hCG) 48 hours after $PGF_{2\alpha}$ to time the next ovulation in all animals and use fixed-time insemination (De Rensis & Peters, 1999). Occasionally, cows will come into oestrus quickly after GnRH treatment and this may be due to treating an animal that was just about to start cycling spontaneously.

In all reports on treatment of inactive ovaries there are some animals that do not respond to conventional treatment. It is obvious that cows that are still under the influence of the original aetiological factors (such as poor condition) are unlikely to respond well. Similarly, cows in deep anoestrus may not respond satisfactorily to hormonal treatment. It appears that those cows with inactive ovaries, lacking any detectable structures, respond poorly to treatment and may revert to an anoestrous state.

In considering the outcome of treatment of cows with cystic ovarian disease associated with anoestrus there are a number of relevant points to note:

● With the important exception of cases seen within six weeks of calving, spontaneous resolution of these cases is not to be relied upon (Garcia & Larsson, 1982).
● The condition tends to recur unless treatment results in ovulation of a healthy new dominant follicle and conception occurs.
● To the extent that there is a familial predisposition to cystic ovarian disease, the use of offspring from affected dams for breeding purposes is not advisable.
● Results have to be looked at in two stages. The first stage is the resolution of the cystic condition and the induction of normal oestrus and ovulation. The second is getting the affected cow pregnant.

Where diagnosis is correct and appropriate treatment is given the return to ovarian normality is good. The majority of luteal cysts respond to $PGF_{2\alpha}$ or an analogue; in one study (Booth, 1988) 79 per cent of cows had low levels of circulating progesterone within 7 days. In the same field trial, 73 per cent of cases with follicular cysts that were treated with GnRH or hCG plus progesterone had functional luteal tissue by 14 days after treatment.

The pregnancy rate achieved again depends very much on the ability of the farm staff to detect oestrus and have the cow served at the correct time. This, plus the difficulty in accurate diagnosis of the type of cyst present, means that on many farms an unacceptably high percentage of cows with cystic ovarian disease are eventually culled.

Silent and unobserved oestrus after calving in cows

Prognosis for unobserved oestrus is good and pregnancy rate is not greatly different from that for cycling cows in the same herd that have been observed in oestrus. Seguin (1981) compiled results from six trials in which 886 cows were treated; 67 per cent were in oestrus after treatment and pregnancy rate to service at that oestrus was 54 per cent. Seguin (1981) also cited trials in which controls and treated cows had the same pregnancy rate, whereas O'Farrell and Hartigan (1984) obtained a statistically significantly poorer pregnancy rate in the suboestrus cows treated with an analogue of $PGF_{2\alpha}$ than in controls. This latter finding is supported by an analysis of more than 10 000 cases of unobserved oestrus in Israel and 30 000 normal controls (Mayer *et al.*, 1987). First-service pregnancy rate for unobserved oestrus cows was 35.2 per cent compared with 60.3 per cent for the controls.

In an interesting study (Ball & Jackson, 1984) in which non-detected oestrus cows were treated with an analogue of $PGF_{2\alpha}$, and monitored by observation and progesterone assays, 84 per cent of the cows had complete luteolysis after a correctly timed injection. Of all the cows treated 42 per cent were seen in oestrus within 4 days of treatment and 60 per cent within 14 days.

One factor that makes prognosis difficult is the effect of the age of the corpus luteum on the response to $PGF_{2\alpha}$ or an analogue. Luteolysis is unlikely to occur in cows treated before day 5 of the cycle and it may be day 7 before maximum effect results. Even when luteolysis occurs, the time from treatment to ovulation varies greatly depending, in a complex manner, on the stage of dominant follicle development when the cow is treated (MacMillan, 1983; Kastelic *et al.*, 1990). If there is a healthy dominant follicle present, oestrus will usually occur on the third day after treatment; should there be no dominant follicle present at the time of $PGF_{2\alpha}$ injection, 5–7 days will pass until induction of oestrus occurs.

Prognosis is improved if the veterinarian actively follows up all cases, both those treated and those left untreated, within two weeks.

Long interservice interval

Prognosis in these cases is similar to preservice cases, but because of the longer time since calving the urgency to get the cow reserved is greater.

Prevention

The economic importance of prevention of anoestrus in all its forms can hardly be overstated. The cost-effective application of preventive measures, however, calls for careful consideration, and a balance has to be achieved between undue intervention in cows that would resume normal cycles spontaneously and unnecessary loss of time due to leaving intervention too late. For example, the majority of cows that are not cycling by six weeks after calving will be coming in season by eight weeks, i.e. in time for service within the target period. On the other hand, cows that are left without examination and treatment until the end of the target period for first service, say 11 weeks after calving, will lose a great deal of production time. However, with the increase in milk yield and genetic merit of dairy cows, more prolonged voluntary waiting periods may be economically viable and of benefit to the individual animal.

Heifers

Prevention of delay in the onset of puberty depends on good nutrition and the avoidance of diseases that interfere with growth rate (see also Chapter 5).

The first step is establishment of clear targets. The farmer should decide at what age, or at what time of the year, the heifers should have their first calves. It is a simple calculation from that target to decide when the service period should start, so that the majority of the heifers calve within the planned period. The exact timing for the start of the service period will depend on how critical both the beginning and the end of the calving period are held to be. If conditions are good, such as a healthy, fertile young bull running with well-grown, healthy, cycling heifers, more than 80 per cent of heifers should be in calf after six weeks of the service period and practically all by nine weeks.

To ensure that the majority of the heifers are cycling at the beginning of the service period it is necessary to aim for a growth rate that achieves the appropriate body weight, taking account of the breed involved. Puberty occurs around 280 kg in large Holsteins and Holstein/Friesians, around 260 kg for Friesians and around 230 kg for Jersey heifers; these weights equate to approximately 40–45 per cent of the expected adult weight. A rough rule-of-thumb for the rearing of heifers to calve at 2 years of age is to aim for prepubertal growth rates in g/day that equal the adult body weight in kg. For example, if the expected adult weight is 650 kg, rear at a rate of 650 g/day. Target growth rates and the key target weights for dairy heifers in the UK are given in Chapter 5.

The veterinarian has a number of roles to play. Initially, it is necessary to make the farmer aware of the need to plan for a specific calving season or age and what this implies in terms of growth rates. Thereafter, the job is mainly to give advice and to make sure that the client monitors the growth rate of the heifers and onset of puberty. The farmer should consult the veterinarian at an early stage if it looks as though not enough animals are starting to cycle at the expected time, and hormonal treatments to induce first ovulation and synchronize oestrus and ovulation in a group of heifers may be considered.

Avoidance of disease conditions that will interfere with growth is also the veterinarian's responsibility and is described elsewhere in this book. This should not only assist the attainment of the target for age at puberty but should also help to reduce the high mortality rate that occurs between birth and puberty.

Most farmers are aware that female calves born twin to a bull calf are very likely to be sterile freemartins. Few realize that measurement of the vagina in the very young calf and comparison with a normal calf can be used to decide if a suspect calf is a freemartin. Alternatively, in valuable animals blood sampling both twins for karyotyping will usually clarify the issue and allow early culling if desired. However, this procedure is too expensive for use in most commercial cattle.

Prevention of anoestrus in adult cows after calving

The foundations for early return to normal cyclicity and getting cows served are listed in Box 35.11. All these factors are very much under the farmer's control, although the veterinarian has an important part to play in ensuring that the husbandry is up to standard, that intervention, if required, at and after calving is timely and appropriate and that cyclicity is monitored and aberrations are treated.

● *Prevention of dystokia and postpartum abnormalities* is a basic requirement for optimal cyclicity and fertility and has been discussed on p. 526.
● *Routine veterinary postpartum examination and treatment* can effectively limit the adverse effect of abnormalities around calving and delayed involution. It is essential to examine all cows that experienced dystokia or postpartum problems by not later than 28 days after calving. Many veterinary practitioners incorporate routine examination of all cows two to four weeks after calving, as this allows them to deal with problems early (see also Chapter 34).

Box 35.11 Factors likely to prevent postpartum anoestrus.

● Appropriate body condition and nutrition in the dry period
● Normal calving
● Disease-free puerperium, or adequate rapid treatment of diseases in the puerperium
● Suitable transition period feeding and regular checking of body condition score postpartum
● Efficient oestrous detection

Table 35.4 Effect of various treatments on interval from calving to first service.

Calving – service interval (days)				Reference
PGF$_{2\alpha}$	GnRH	Both	None	
–	81	–	77	Langley & O'Farrell (1979)
–	88/89	–	83	Nash *et al.* (1980)
–	72/74	–	73	Nash *et al.* (1980)
–	–	61	63	Richardson *et al.* (1983)
92	108	85	84	Etherington *et al.* (1984)
61	67	64	58	Benmrad & Stevenson (1986)
73	–	–	69	Young & Anderson (1986)
81/51	–	–	91/58	Schofield *et al.* (1999)

There is an attractive concept that by routinely administering PGF$_{2\alpha}$ or an analogue, GnRH or both in the early postpartum period it is possible to improve return to cyclicity and pregnancy rate. It is clear that GnRH given before day 20 after calving will initiate early cycles and PGF$_{2\alpha}$ or an analogue given a little later increases the number of cycles in the first six weeks after calving (Benmrad & Stevenson, 1986). The effect of these treatments on overall fertility is less well defined; Table 35.4 shows results obtained in several field trials.

Meta-analysis of data from 4052 cows in 24 trials published in 10 papers looking at the effect of injecting PGF$_{2\alpha}$ in dairy cattle within 40 days of calving on the rate of pregnancy at first service and the number of days open came to the following conclusions. Treatment with PGF$_{2\alpha}$ during this early postpartum period had no effect on the first service pregnancy rate of cows with a normal or abnormal puerperium. An analysis of those data for the number of days open showed that a significant percentage (54 per cent) of the treated cows had fewer days open than the untreated cows, and that this difference tended to be greater for cows with an abnormal puerperium. The weighted average reduction in days open between treated and control cows was 2.6 days for trials with abnormal cows and 3.3 days for trials including normal and abnormal cows (Burton & Lean, 1995). This effect is probably largely due to improvements in the submission rate; it is questionable whether any improvement in calving-to-first-service and calving-to-conception interval justifies the treatment costs and the cost of the extra semen that would be used if PGF$_{2\alpha}$ were administered routinely to postpartum cows. Thus the routine administration of PGF$_{2\alpha}$ (or other hormone preparations) to cattle without a specific therapeutic indication probably cannot be justified.

In addition to the routine application of these treatments to normal cows not conferring any benefit in terms of reproductive efficiency, there is the danger that induction of a corpus luteum with GnRH in a cow that still has an infected uterus after calving can lead to pyometra. Selected treatment of cows with uterine or ovarian pathology is on the other hand entirely justified.

● *Nutrition.* For normal reproductive function it is vitally important that nutritional levels before and after calving are correct. It has been suggested that condition score at calving should not exceed 3.0 and 2.5–3.0 should be the target at service.

Oestrous detection

Once the foundation for good fertility has been established it is essential to ensure that oestrous detection is as good as humanly possible.

Before discussing how oestrous detection can be improved it is worth asking the question: why is oestrous detection inefficient? After all, many stockworkers who carry out this task have worked with cows for years and know the signs of oestrus well. However, in a recent study of stockworker's attitudes, oestrous detection was recognized as being an important task, but was generally a task that was disliked (Seabrook & Wilkinson, 2000). This may be because it is time consuming and often requires the stockman to spend time watching cows at antisocial hours. The decreasing availability of labour on farms is resulting in reduced labour hours per cow per year and overworked staff often do not have the necessary time to dedicate to oestrous detection.

Good oestrous detection requires regrouping and possibly moving animals as well as accurate observation and recording of behavioural events several times a day over months on end and is therefore a very demanding task. It is made more difficult because of the short duration of oestrus exhibited by many cows, the time of the night or day when oestrus occurs, the weak and indefinite nature of signs shown by some cows when in season and the fact that some animals not in season exhibit some of the signs of oestrus. Veterinarians who wish to educate dairy workers on heat detection would be well advised to attempt to carry out heat detection themselves, so that they may understand the practical difficulties.

If oestrous detection is not a priority for staff and is impossible to organize even with the assistance of oestrous detection aids, then the use of hormonal treatments to synchronize oestrus and ovulation should be contemplated and discussed (see p. 678). This will reduce oestrous detection periods to very specific times, or allow the use of fixed-time artificial insemination with no heat detection. However, pregnancy rates to single fixed-time insemination may be low, and this will also have to be discussed with the client. The details of the various oestrous synchronization regimens for cattle are discussed elsewhere in this book (see p. 684).

The stockworker's dilemma occurs when a cow exhibits signs of oestrus just short of actually standing to be ridden and the decision is taken to have the cow inseminated. If the cow is not in season this decision is criticised. However, if the cow is not inseminated, a cow in season may have been missed. In a large herd these critical decisions have to be made many times a year.

Good heat detection is based on the following facts.

- The definitive sign of oestrus is standing freely to be ridden. It has been proposed that a cow that mounts onto another cow's head is in pro-oestrus. Cows in oestrus, of course, also mount other cows.
- There may be an interval of as much as 30 minutes between bouts of riding.
- Oestrus rarely lasts for more than 18 hours and in many cases lasts for less than 6 hours.
- Oestrus often starts during the night.
- Oestrous expression is greatest during quiet times of the cow's day and night. This means oestrus is seen less often around milking times and when cows are fed.
- As well as a willingness to stand on the part of the cow in oestrus, it is necessary to have a cow that wants to and can mount as discussed above (see aetiology, p. 532). This can cause particular problems when most cows in the herd are pregnant.
- When cows are loose housed there is often a particular area that cows prefer to use for oestrous expression.
- Stalled cows may have reduced physical expression of oestrus (Claus et al., 1983).

A rational system of oestrous detection should be based on these facts and the following points are required for a good heat detection system:

(1) The cows should be observed three times per day for 30 minutes each time. The periods of observation should be when the herd is peaceful after milking and feeding. Often these times are:
 (a) briefly before collecting the cows for morning milking;
 (b) in mid-morning;
 (c) before the evening milking; and
 (d) late in the evening, a very good time for detection of oestrus.
(2) The housing conditions must be suitable for cows and observer. Good non-slippery floors on which the cows feel secure are essential. The observer must be able to see all the cows clearly, should be comfortable and should have a paper and pen to write down details of the cows' behaviour. Good lighting is required.
(3) The cows must be clearly identifiable from a distance.

There are many aids to oestrous detection; however, there is at present no one substitute for close observation of the cows' behaviour (review by Boyd, 1984; Stevenson, 2001). Aids to heat detection either detect unobserved standing to be ridden or depend on the fact that cows in oestrus are likely to behave in ways that, although not unique to oestrus, occur with greater frequency during oestrus. Increased frequency of bellowing, increased restlessness, reduced milk yield, change in routine behaviour such as order of coming into the milking parlour for milking, and increased body temperature are non-specific, oestrus-related events. There are also a number of physical changes in the genitalia related to oestrus that can be measured, such as change in electrical resistance and viscosity of the vaginal mucus.

Marking systems fixed on the cow's pelvic region to detect standing to be ridden when the cows are not being observed can be valuable in suitable circumstances. Examples are tail paint, tail flags and detectors that contain dye that is squeezed out under sustained pressure from another cow. All of these suffer from the defect that rubbing or pressure that is not caused by the cow standing freely to be ridden may trigger them.

Television cameras with video recording have also been used to observe cows continuously and can be viewed later, at increased speed. There are problems of identity (very big numbers on shoulders and rumps are needed) and replaying the recordings is a tedious chore.

Milk progesterone assays, which can be used either as an aid to or as a replacement for oestrous detection, are discussed later (see p. 548).

Pedometers that automatically monitor and record the cow's level of activity can also be used to detect behavioural changes that are consistent with oestrus in some management systems.

It is probable that in future sophisticated decision support software integrated into computerized milking parlour systems will be developed to detect cows likely to be in oestrus and automatically shed them from the main herd for the attention of the stockman. These decision support tools will use various data automatically generated from a number of sources such as pedometers, milk yield, milk temperature, order of milking and milking frequency (fully automated milking systems only), and data detected by integrated biosensors such as in-line milk progesterone assays and assays of other milk constituents. Cows will be identified by implanted microchips. These may also advance beyond the current static data-specific microchip that simply holds the data it was implanted containing, to a new generation of smart chips that record the animal's health and disease history along with other information such as its movement history. It may even be possible in future to develop integrated implanted biosensors that analyse and record the animal's physiological state, including data related to reproduction.

Anoestrus after service

In the majority of cases, delayed return to service is due to unobserved oestrus, as has been shown in the reduction in the number of long return-to-service intervals when oestrous detection is improved. One problem, in a case where the return-to-service heat signs are not clear, is that the result of inseminating by AI a cow that has been served, and could be pregnant, may be loss of the conceptus.

Improved efficiency by the use of aids for heat detection is particularly useful in these cases because the service date can be taken as the start of the oestrous cycle. Clearly, in those cases where insemination takes place in the luteal phase this starting point is erroneous, a fact that will become clear to the stockworker as heat detection aids and substitutes are used.

Use of a three-week calendar and the application of a marker such as tail paint shortly before expected return to service can help efficiency of observation.

Systematic use of milk progesterone assays at about the expected time of return to service can help in overcoming problems of long interservice intervals. High progesterone followed by two successive days of low progesterone is an indication that service should be carried out on the next day. Eddy and Clark (1987) demonstrated, in four large dairy herds, that the efficiency of heat detection after service could be improved greatly by the use of milk progesterone assays. The preferred sampling regimen was every second day from days 18 to 24 after service. The financial benefit to cost ratio was 7.5:1. Some veterinarians report improvements based on a single progesterone assay on day 19 after service. For good results it is necessary for the stock personnel to understand the test and to be willing to carry out the extra work carefully and conscientiously. Very poor pregnancy rates have been reported to result if progesterone assays are used as the only basis for insemination without the active incorporation of oestrus detection (Foulkes & Goodey, 1988). However, the use of milk progesterone assays to confirm that cows are in oestrus before inseminating them can improve pregnancy rates and reduce the number of mis-timed inseminations (McLeod *et al.*, 1991; Watson, 1996). Strategic milk progesterone monitoring as a diagnostic and management tool in dairy cattle is discussed by Darwash and Lamming (1997). Under experimental conditions milk progesterone monitoring has also been used in suckler cow fertility investigation and management (Mann *et al.*, 1998); however, logistical problems will almost certainly prevent widespread use of this technology in the field.

Resynchronization of repeats following an initial synchronizing treatment using a progesterone device is used successfully in New Zealand and other locations where the breeding period needs to be kept short; used progesterone devices are re-inserted on day 16 to days 21 or 22 following first service, and return oestrus detected on days 23 or 24 (Van Cleeff *et al.*, 1996; McDougall, 2001). This increases submission rates in the first three weeks of the breeding season and focuses heat detection periods to a specific time following first service. A similar regimen has been successfully used in the UK in beef suckler herds (Penny *et al.*, 2000).

Acknowledgement

The ultrasound images were produced at the University of Glasgow Veterinary School using digital acquisitions from Toshiba Medical Systems.

References

Anon. (1984) *Dairy Herd Fertility*. Ministry of Agriculture, Fisheries and Food, Reference Book 259, pp. 1–80. HMSO, London.

Archbald, L.F., Risco, C., Chavatte, P., Constant, S., Tran, T., Klapstein, E. & Elliot, J. (1993) Estrus and pregnancy rate of dairy cows given one or two doses of prostaglandin F2 alpha 8 or 24 hours apart. *Theriogenology*, **40**, 873–84.

Ball, P.J.H. & Jackson, P.S. (1984) The use of milk progesterone profiles for assessing the response to cloprostenol treatment of non-detected oestrus in dairy cattle. *British Veterinary Journal*, **140**, 543–9.

Ball, P.J.H. & Lamming, G.E. (1983) Diagnosis of ovarian acyclicity in lactating dairy cows and evaluation of treatment with gonadotrophin-releasing hormone or a progesterone releasing intravaginal device. *British Veterinary Journal*, **139**, 522–7.

Barrett, D.C. (2001) Cattle Fertility Management in the UK. *Cattle Practice,* **9**, 59–68.

Beam, S.W. & Butler, W.R. (1997) Energy balance and ovarian follicle development prior to the first ovulation postpartum in dairy cows receiving three levels of dietary fat. *Biology of Reproduction*, **56**, 133–42.

Benmrad, M. & Stevenson, J.S. (1986) Gonadotrophin-releasing hormone and prostaglandin $F_{2\alpha}$ for postpartum dairy cows: estrous, ovulation and fertility traits. *Journal of Dairy Science*, **69**, 800–11.

Bloomfield, G.A., Morant, S.V. & Ducker, M.I. (1986) A survey of reproductive performance in dairy herds. Characteristics of the patterns of progesterone concentrations in milk. *Animal Production*, **42**, 1–10.

Booth, J.M. (1988) The milk progesterone test as an aid to diagnosis of cystic ovaries in dairy cows. *Veterinary Record*, **123**, 437–9.

Boyd, H. (1984) Aids to oestrus detection – a review. In *Dairy Cow Fertility* (ed. by R.G. Eddy & M.J. Ducker), pp. 60–7. British Veterinary Association, London.

Boyd, H. & Munro, C.D. (1980) Experience and results of a herd health programme – rectal palpation and progesterone assays in fertility control. In *IX International Congress on Animal Reproduction and AI*, Vol. 2, pp. 373–80.

Boyd, H. & Reed, H.C.B. (1961) Investigations into the incidence and causes of infertility in dairy cattle. Fertility variations. *British Veterinary Journal*, **117**, 18–35.

Boyd, J.S. & Omran, S.N. (1991) Diagnostic ultrasonography of the bovine female reproductive tract. *In Practice*, **3**, 109–18.

Britt, J.H. (1987) Detection of oestrus in cattle. *Veterinary Annual*, **27**, 74–80.

Britt, J.H. (1995) Relationship between postpartum nutrition, weight loss and fertility. *Cattle Practice*, **3**, 79–83.

Brown, J.L., Schoenemann, H.M. & Reeves, J.J. (1986) Effect of FSH treatment on LH and FSH receptors in chronic cysticovarian-diseased dairy cows. *Journal of Animal Science*, **62**, 1063–71.

Bulman, D.C. & Lamming, G.E. (1978) Milk progesterone levels in relation to conception, repeat breeding and factors influencing acyclicity in dairy cows. *Journal of Reproduction and Fertility*, **54**, 447–58.

Burton, N.R. & Lean, I.J. (1995) Investigation by meta-analysis of the effect of prostaglandin $F_{2\alpha}$ administered post partum on the reproductive performance of dairy cattle. *Veterinary Record*, **136**, 90–4.

Butler, W.R. (1999) Nutritional effects on resumption of cyclicity and on conception rate. Fertility in the High-Producing Dairy Cow, BSAS Occasional Meeting, Galway, Ireland, September 1999, pp. 13–14.

Canfield, R.W. & Butler, W.R. (1990) Energy balance and pulsatile LH secretion in early postpartum dairy cattle. *Domestic Animal Endocrinology*, **7**, 323–30.

Claus, R., Karg, H., Zwiauer, D., von Butler, L, Pirchner, F. & Rattenberger, E. (1983) Analysis of factors influencing reproductive performance of the dairy cow by progesterone assay in milk fat. *British Veterinary Journal*, **139**, 29–37.

Cook, D.L., Smith, C.A., Parfet, J.R., Youngquist, R.S., Brown, E.M. & Garverick, H.A. (1990) Fate and turnover rate of ovarian follicular cysts in dairy cattle. *Journal of Reproduction and Fertility*, **90**, 37–46.

Darwash, A.O. & Lamming, G.E. (1997) Strategic milk progesterone monitoring. *Cattle Practice*, **5**, 353–5.

Dawson, F.L.M. (1975) Accuracy of rectal palpation in the diagnosis of ovarian function in the cow. *Veterinary Record*, **96**, 218–20.

De Rensis F. & Peters A.R. (1999) The control of follicular dynamics by $PGF_{2\alpha}$, GnRH, hCG and oestrus synchronization in cattle. *Reproduction in Domestic Animals*, **34**, 49–59.

Dijkhuizen, A.A., Huirne, R.B.M., Jalvingh, A.W. & Stelwagen, J. (1997) Economic impact of common health and fertility problems. In *Animal Health Economics – Principles and Applications*. (ed. by A.A Dijkhuizen & R.S. Morris) pp. 41–58. Post Graduate Foundation in Veterinary Science, University of Sydney.

Dobson, H., Douthwaite, R., Nobel, K.M., O'Donnell, M.J., Ribadu, A.Y., Tebble, J.E. & Ward, W.R. (2001a) Cystic ovaries in cattle. *Cattle Practice*, **9**, 185–9.

Dobson, H., Tebble, J.E., Smith, R.F. & Ward, W.R. (2001b) Is stress really all that important? *Theriogenology*, **55**, 65–73.

Douthwaite, R. & Dobson, H. (2000) Comparison of different methods of diagnosis of cystic ovarian disease in cattle and an assessment of its treatment with a progesterone-releasing intravaginal device. *Veterinary Record*, **147**, 355–9.

Eddy, R.G. & Clark, P.L (1987) Oestrus prediction in dairy cows using an ELISA progesterone test. *Veterinary Record*, **120**, 31–4.

Esslemont, R.J., Bailie, J.H. & Cooper, M.J. (1985) *Fertility Management in Dairy Cattle*, pp. 1–143. Collins, London.

Esslemont, R.J. & Kossaibati, M.A. (1997) Culling in 50 dairy herds in England. *Veterinary Record*, **140**, 36–9.

Etherington, W.G., Bosu, W.T.K., Martin, S.W., Cote, J.F., Doig, P.A. & Leslie, K.E. (1984) Reproductive performance in dairy cows following postpartum treatment with gonadotrophin releasing hormone and/or prostaglandin: a field trial. *Canadian Journal of Comparative Medicine*, **48**, 245–50.

Fishwick, J.C. (1993) An assessment of the accuracy of manual rectal palpation as compared with ultrasound imaging of the genital system, milk and plasma progesterone concentrations, and the response to therapy in cows not observed in oestrus. RCVS Diploma in Cattle Health and Production Dissertation, pp. 1–47. Royal College of Veterinary Surgeons Library, London.

Foulkes, L.A. & Goodey, R.G. (1988) Fertility of Friesian cows on the second, third and fourth days of low milk progesterone concentration. *Veterinary Record*, **122**, 135.

Fourichon, C., Seegers, H. & Malher, X. (2000) Effect of disease on reproduction in the dairy cow: a meta-analysis. *Theriogenology*, **53**, 1729–59.

Garcia, M. & Larsson, K. (1982) Clinical findings in post partum dairy cows. *Nordisk Veterinaer Medicin*, **34**, 255–63.

Garnsworthy, P.C. & Webb, R. (2000) Nutritional influences on fertility in dairy cows. *Cattle Practice*, **8**, 401–5.

Garverick, H.A. (1997) Ovarian follicular cysts in dairy cows. *Journal of Dairy Science*, **80**, 995–1004.

Heuwieser W., Oltenacu P.A., Lednor A.J. & Foote R.H. (1997) Evaluation of different protocols for prostaglandin synchronization to improve reproductive performance in dairy herds with low estrus detection efficiency. *Journal of Dairy Science*, **80**, 2766–74.

Humbolt, P. (1982) Respective incidence of late embryonic mortality and post insemination anoestrus in late returns to oestrus in dairy cows. In *Factors Influencing Fertility in the Postpartum Cow* (ed. by H. Karg, & E. Schallenberger), pp. 298–304. Nijhoff, The Hague.

Imakawa, K., Day, M.L., Garcia-Winder, M., Zalesky, D.D., Kittok, R.J., Schanbacher, B.D. & Kinder, J.E. (1986) Endocrine changes during restoration of oestrous cycles following induction of anestrus by restricted nutrient intake in beef heifers. *Journal of Animal Science*, **63**, 565–71.

Kassa, T., Ahlin, K-A. & Larsson, K. (1986) Profiles of progesterone in milk and clinical ovarian findings in postpartum cows with ovarian dysfunctions. *Nordisk Veterinaer Medicin*, **38**, 360–9.

Kastelic, J.P., Knopf, L. & Ginther, O.J. (1990) Effect of day of prostaglandin $F_{2\alpha}$ treatment on selection and development of the ovulatory follicle in heifers. *Animal Reproduction Science*, **23**, 169–80.

Knight, C.H. & Sorensen, A. (1998) Fertility parameters of cows with extended lactations. *Cattle Practice*, **6**, 379–82.

Koelsch, R.K., Aneshansley, D.J. & Butler, W.R. (1994) Milk progesterone sensor for application with dairy cattle. *Journal of Agricultural Engineering Research*, **58**, 115–20.

Langley, O.H. & O'Farrell, K.J. (1979) The use of Gn-RH to stimulate early resumption of oestrous cycles in dairy cows. *Irish Journal of Agricultural Research*, **18**, 157–65.

McDougall S. (2001) Reproductive performance of anovulatory anoestrous postpartum dairy cows following treatment with two progesterone and oestradiol benzoate-based protocols, with or without resynchrony. *New Zealand Veterinary Journal*, **49**, 187–94.

McLeod, B.J., Foulkes, J.A., Williams, M.E. & Weller, R.F. (1991) Predicting the time of ovulation in dairy cows using on-farm progesterone kits. *Animal Production*, **52**, 1–9.

MacMillan, K.L. (1983) Prostaglandin responses in dairy herd breeding programmes. *New Zealand Veterinary Journal*, **31**, 110–13.

Mann, G.E., Keatinge, R., Hunter, M., Hedley, B.A. & Lamming, G.E. (1998) Milk progesterone monitoring of suckler cow fertility. *Cattle Practice*, **6**, 383–4.

Markusfeld, O. (1987) Inactive ovaries in high-yielding dairy cows before service: aetiology and effect on conception. *Veterinary Record*, **121**, 149–53.

Martinez, J. & Thibier, M. (1984) Fertility in anoestrous dairy cows following treatment with prostaglandin $F_{2\alpha}$ or the synthetic analogue fenprostalene. *Veterinary Record*, **115**, 57–9.

Mayer, E., Francos, G. & Neria, A. (1987) Eierstocksbefunde und Fertilitaets-Parameter bei Kuehen mit 'unbeobachteter Brunst'. *Tieraerztliche Umschau*, **42**, 506–9.

Moller, K., Lapwood, K.R. & Marchant, R.M. (1986) Prolonged service intervals in cattle. *New Zealand Veterinary Journal*, **34**, 128–32.

Mottram, T. (1997) Automatic monitoring of the health and metabolic status of dairy cows. *Livestock Production Science*, **48**, 209–17.

Nash, J.G., Ball, L. & Olson, J.D. (1980) Effects on reproductive performance of administration of GnRH to early postpartum dairy cows. *Journal of Animal Science*, **50**, 1017–21.

O'Callaghan, D. & Boland, M.P. (1999) Nutritional effects on ovulation, embryo development and the establishment of pregnancy in ruminants. *Animal Science*, **68**, 299–314.

O'Callaghan, D., Lozanot, J.M., Fahey, J., Gath, V., Snijders, S. & Boland, M.P. (2000) Recent developments in the effect of nutrition on fertility in dairy cows. *Irish Veterinary Journal*, **53**, 417–25.

O'Farrell, K.J. & Hartigan, P.L (1984) The treatment of non-detected oestrus (NDO) in dairy cows with cloprostenol. *Irish Veterinary Journal*, **38**, 23–8.

Omran, S.N., Ayliffe, T.R. & Boyd, J.S. (1988) Preliminary observations of bovine ovarian structures using B-mode real time ultrasound. *Veterinary Record*, **122**, 465–6.

Opsomer G., Mijten P., Coryn M. & de Kruif A. (1996) Postpartum anoestrus in dairy cows: a review. *Veterinary Quarterly*, **18**, 68–75.

Ott, R.S., Breulaff, K.N. & Hixon, J.E. (1986) Comparison of palpable corpora lutea with serum progesterone concentrations in cows. *Journal of the American Veterinary Medical Association*, **188**, 1417–19.

Ott, R.S. & Gustaffson, B.K. (1981) Therapeutic application of prostaglandins for post partum infections. *Acta Veterinaria Scandinavica* (Suppl.), **77**, 363–90.

Penny C.D., Lowman, B.G., Scott, N.A. & Scott, P.R. (2000) Repeated oestrus synchronisation of beef cows with progesterone implants and the effects of a gonadotrophin-releasing hormone agonist at implant insertion. *Veterinary Record*, **146**, 395–8.

Pieterse, M.C., Taverne, M.A.M., Kruip, T.A.M. & Willemse, A.H. (1990) Detection of corpora lutea and follicles in cows: a comparison of transvaginal ultrasonography and rectal palpation. *Veterinary Record*, **126**, 552–4.

Richardson, G.F., Archbald, L.F., Galton, D.M. & Godke, R.A. (1983) Effect of gonadotropin-releasing hormone and prostaglandin $F_{2\alpha}$ on reproduction in postpartum dairy cows. *Theriogenology*, **19**, 763–70.

Royal, M.D., Darwash, A.O., Flint, A.P.F., Webb, R., Woolliams, J.A. & Lamming, G.E. (2000) Declining fertility in dairy cattle: changes in traditional and endocrine parameters of fertility. *Animal Science*, **70**, 487–501.

Rukkwamsuk, T., Kruip, T.A.M. & Wensing, T. (1999) Relationship between overfeeding and overconditioning in the dry period and the problems of high producing dairy cows during the postparturient period. *The Veterinary Quarterly*, **21**, 71–7.

Saloniemi, H., Groelm, Y. & Syvaejaervi, J. (1986) An epidemiological and genetic study on registered diseases in Finnish Ayrshire cattle. II. Reproductive disorders. *Acta Veterinaria Scandinavica*, **27**, 196–208.

Savio, J.D., Boland, M.P., Hynes, N. & Roche J.F. (1990) Resumption of follicular activity in the early post-partum period of dairy cows. *Journal of Reproduction and Fertility*, **88**, 569–79.

Schofield, S.A., Kitwood, S.E. & Phillips, C.J.C. (1999) The effects of a post partum injection of prostaglandin $F_{2\alpha}$ on return to oestrus and pregnancy rate in dairy cows. *Veterinary Journal*, **157**, 172–7.

Scully, A., Hunter, M., Gregson, K., Lamming, G.E. & Darwash, A.O. (2000) The use of on-farm software for automatic interpretation of milk progesterone data: an aid to dairy fertility management. *Cattle Practice*, **8**, 407–10.

Seabrook, M.F. & Wilkinson, J.M. (2000) Stockpersons' attitudes to the husbandry of dairy cows. *Veterinary Record*, **147**, 157–60.

Seguin, B.E. (1981) Use of prostaglandins in cows with unobserved oestrus. *Acta Veterinaria Scandinavica* (Suppl.), **77**, 343–53.

Stagg, K., Diskin, M.G., Sreenan, J.M. & Roche, J.F. (1995) Follicular development in long-term anoestrous suckler beef cows fed 2 levels of energy postpartum. *Animal Reproduction Science*, **38**, 49–61.

Stagg, K., Spicer, L.J., Sreenan, J.M., Roche, J.F. & Diskin, M.G. (1998) Effect of calf isolation on follicular wave dynamics, gonadotropin and metabolic hormone changes, and interval to first ovulation in beef cows fed either of two energy levels postpartum. *Biology of Reproduction*, **59**, 777–83.

Stevenson J.S. (2001) A review of oestrous behaviour and detection in dairy cows. In *Fertility in the High Producing Dairy Cow*. Occasional Publication No. 26, pp. 43–62. British Society of Animal Science London.

Taylor, V.J., Beever, D.E. & Wathes, D.C. (2001) Plasma IGF-1 levels in relation to ovarian function in high producing dairy cows. *Cattle Practice*, **9**, 197–201.

Tebble, J.E., O'Donnell, M.J. & Dobson, H. (2001) Ultrasound diagnosis and treatment outcome of cystic ovaries in cattle. *Veterinary Record*, **148**, 411–13.

Van Cleeff, J., Macmillan, K.L., Drost, M., Lucy, M.C. & Thatcher, W.W. (1996) Effects of administering progesterone at selected intervals after insemination of synchronized heifers on pregnancy rates and resynchronization of returns to service. *Theriogenology*, **46**, 1117–30.

Waldmann, A., Ropstad, E., Landsverk, K., Sørensen, K., Sølverød, L. & Dahl, E. (1999) Level and distribution of progesterone in bovine milk in relation to storage in the mammary gland. *Animal Reproduction Science*, **56**, 79–91.

Warren, M.E. (1984) Biological targets for fertility and their effects on herd economics. In *Dairy Cow Fertility* (ed. by R.G. Eddy & M.J. Ducker), British Veterinary Association, London. pp. 1–14.

Wathes, D.C., Robinson, R.S., Pushpakumara, A., Cheng, Z. & Abayasekara, D.R.E. (1998) Nutritional effects on reproductive performance in dairy cows. *Cattle Practice*, **6**, 371–7.

Watson, C.L. (1996) Milk progesterone analysis – an underused asset in fertility control of the dairy cow. *Cattle Practice*, **4**, 277–80.

Webb, R., Garnsworthy, P.C., Gong, J.G., Gutierrez, C.G., Logue, D., Crawshaw, W.M. & Robinson, J.J. (1997) Nutritional influence on subfertility in cattle. *Cattle Practice*, **5**, 361–7.

Webb, R., Royal, M.D., Gong, J.G. & Garnsworthy, P.C. (1999) The influence of nutrition on fertility. *Cattle Practice*, **7**, 227–34.

Whitaker, D.A., Kelly, J.M. & Smith, S. (2000) Disposal and disease rates in 340 British dairy herds. *Veterinary Record*, **146**, 363–7.

Williamson, N.B., Morris, R.S., Blood, D.C. & Cannon, C.M. (1972) A study of oestrous behaviour and oestrus detection methods in a large commercial dairy herd. 1. The relative efficiency of methods of oestrus detection. *Veterinary Record*, **91**, 50–8.

Young, I.M. (1989) Dinoprost 14-day oestrus synchronisation schedule for dairy cows. *Veterinary Record*, **124**, 587–8.

Young, I.M. & Anderson, D.B. (1986) First service conception rate in dairy cows treated with dinoprost tromethamine early post partum. *Veterinary Record*, **118**, 212–13.

Chapter 36
Failure to Conceive and Embryonic Loss

D.C. Barrett, H. Boyd and M. Mihm

Manifestation	552
Aetiology	554
Stage 1 Failure of ovulation after oestrus	554
Stage 2 Fertilization failure	557
Stage 3 Embryonic death	559
Stage of failure not known	562
Diagnosis	563
Treatment	566
Prognosis	569
Prevention	572

Manifestation

Return to service or detection of non-pregnancy up to six weeks after insemination/natural service are the ways in which poor pregnancy rate due to failure to conceive and embryonic losses are presented. This can have a major economic impact in any herd, but is particularly noticeable where a tight seasonal calving pattern is sought.

Interservice intervals

The interval in days that has elapsed between the unsuccessful service and the next oestrus is part of the manifestation of the condition of return to service. The concept of normal and abnormal interservice intervals has been discussed in connection with postservice anoestrus (see p. 531). While the distribution of interservice intervals varies greatly between herds, reflecting in part the management efficiency in the herd, in many cattle populations fewer than 50 per cent have a normal interservice interval of 18–24 days.

Observable abnormality

Another manifestation of return to service is the normality or otherwise of the cow at the return oestrus. The farmer can observe certain deviations from normality in these cows, in particular the presence of a purulent discharge from the vulva. The farmer may also report aberrant sexual behaviour. In relevant cases, the observant client may notice some of the changes associated with chronic cystic ovarian disease, such as slackening of the pelvic ligaments and voice change. In general, however, the cow that returns to service presents an apparently normal oestrus as regards both behaviour and visible signs.

The way in which the client presents return to service cases affects the clinician's response to the problem. It is presented either as an individual cow problem or as a herd (or group) problem, and it is presented with or without evidence of past or present pathology.

Individual cows

Individual cases are presented in two quite different ways, which influence how they are dealt with.

In the first way, some cows are presented to the veterinarian that have been served two or three times and are still not pregnant. To understand these cases properly they have to be considered within the context of the entire population of cows and heifers in the herd. In any group of apparently normal cows served correctly by a fertile bull or inseminated properly with good semen, either for the first time after calving or at a repeat service, a considerable number will return to service depending on first-, second- and third-service pregnancy rates in each particular herd. Most of these animals are only temporarily infertile and the majority will become pregnant within an acceptable time. Although there is some understanding of the stage at which these losses occur, i.e. whether there is fertilization failure or early embryonic death, the aetiology is known to only a limited extent. For this reason these returns appear to happen at random.

Field studies show that about 12 per cent of cows are still not pregnant after three services as is demonstrated in Table 36.1, which is taken from a population of 5744 cows with a first insemination pregnancy rate of 60.6 per cent (Boyd & Reed, 1961a). 'Actual results' are compared with the 'expected results' that would have occurred if all subsequent inseminations had had a pregnancy rate of 60.6 per cent. However, in recent years a drop in pregnancy rates of approximately one per cent per annum has occurred in high-genetic-merit dairy cattle populations (Royal *et al.*, 2000; Barrett, 2001). This has resulted in expected pregnancy rates of

Table 36.1 The percentage of cows that required various numbers of inseminations for pregnancy with a first insemination pregnancy rate of 60.6 per cent.

Number of inseminations required for pregnancy	Actual results		Expected results	
	Percentage	Cumulative percentage	Percentage	Cumulative percentage
1	60.6	60.6	60.6	60.6
2	20.4	81.0	23.9	84.5
3	7.2	88.2	9.4	93.9
>3 or culled	11.8	100.0	6.1	100.0

50 per cent or less to a single service, thus increasing the proportion of animals within a herd not pregnant after three services.

Farmers often wait until a cow has had three unsuccessful services before presenting her to the veterinarian and Table 36.1 shows that (with certain reservations) about half of these cows, 6.1% versus 11.8%, are not pregnant because of the same (unknown) factors that establish the level of the first insemination pregnancy rate. It is therefore to be expected that half of these cows will not exhibit any diagnosable cause of return to service and that their expectation of pregnancy at the next service is about the same as that for first insemination. However, pregnancy rates to three or more services are usually reduced due to an accumulation of animals with reproductive problems. Warren (1984) cited published data from four different cattle populations in which pregnancy rates to first service ranged from 47–57%. Within these populations, however, the herd pregnancy rates would vary widely.

In the second instance, other cases, for which the term 'chronic repeat breeder' might be used, are presented because they have returned to service repeatedly over a long period of time. These cases have been differentiated into apparently normal repeat breeders and those with abnormalities on the basis of cycle length, sexual behaviour and detectable abnormality, a differentiation of limited clinical value. These chronic repeat breeders require a different approach from the cases discussed above because they are generally cows that the owners regard as particularly valuable and therefore the clinician can devote more time and money to their diagnosis and treatment. The prognosis in chronic repeat breeders is inevitably poor because they have been given so many opportunities to become pregnant without success. It is animals of this type that may be hospitalized in teaching and research institutions where they are given expensive diagnostic and therapeutic treatment, although this is becoming more and more uneconomic within the UK.

There is no realistic incidence figure for chronic repeat breeders because their retention in the breeding herd is dependent on extraneous factors but clearly is unlikely to be more than 6 per cent of the breeding population, although it may be higher in individual herds. The number in any given herd will be determined by various economic factors which dictate at what point it becomes more economic to cull a cow and replace her rather than persist in attempting to get her in calf. Overall culling rates in UK dairy herds are about 20–25 per cent per annum (Esslemont & Kossaibati, 1997; Whitaker *et al.*, 2000). Poor fertility is the single most important reason for involuntary culling. With 30–40 per cent of cull cows being culled for infertility, this represents almost 10 per cent of dairy cows calving each year (Kossaibati & Esslemont, 1995). The exact cost to the farmer of an involuntary cull will vary from farm to farm and from time to time, depending on the cost of a replacement, the value of a cull cow, the milk price and availability (and cost) of milk quota, loss of genetic merit and many other factors. For this reason it is impossible to give an exact cost here, but on a typical commercial dairy farm it is probably between £600 and £800 per cull cow at the present time (2003).

Herd or group problems

Return to service may affect many animals in the herd in which case the client is very worried about the extent of the problem and the serious effect it will have on production and profits. For an assessment of the condition it is necessary to analyse the breeding records to determine pregnancy rates to first, second and further inseminations (or other measure of the success rate of services) and interservice intervals (see also Chapter 41(b)).

The range of incidence of return to service is very wide. In a population of herds with any given mean herd pregnancy rate there is a tendency for the herd averages to be distributed at random round this mean, as demonstrated in Table 36.2. Just over 40 years ago,

Table 36.2 Distribution (%) of herd average first insemination pregnancy rates in 191 dairy herds (Boyd & Reed, 1961a).

Herd first insemination pregnancy rate (herd average)							Total
<31	31–40	41–50	51–60	61–70	71–80	>80	
3.1%	3.7%	16.2%	25.1%	27.2%	19.4%	5.2%	99.9%

the overall herd first insemination pregnancy rate in 191 herds was 59.9 per cent (Boyd & Reed, 1961a). Although not demonstrated here, it is usual for the distribution to be skewed towards the lower end of the scale. The skewed distribution of these data tends to be seen in all studies, however in more recent surveys the first insemination pregnancy rates are lower than those reported by Boyd and Reed (1961a). For example, the mean first service pregnancy rate in 90 herds in the UK was reported as 47.3 per cent in the 1992/1993 calving season (Kossaibati & Esslemont, 1995). National Milk Records (NMR) data from approximately one million dairy cattle in 9000 herds showed that the pregnancy rate to first service (based on available pregnancy diagnosis data and non-return rates at 48 days) was 52.5 per cent in September 2000 (Barrett, 2001). This will be an overestimate of the true pregnancy rate as a proportion of the data are based on non-return rates which will include some cows culled that were not rebred after failing to conceive. Royal *et al.* (2000) reported that 265 first services out of 667 resulted in pregnancy in their study of Holstein Friesian dairy cows between October 1995 and June 1998. This equates to a first service pregnancy rate of 39.7 per cent. Given these recent data it seems reasonable to accept a target first service pregnancy rate of 50 per cent in modern dairy herds, while accepting that in some high yielding herds this may be difficult to achieve.

It is helpful to think of the pregnancy rate for any individual herd as dependent on the combined effects of the following factors:

- The random variation around the mean of the population of herds.
- The background effect, which is dependent on management and environmental factors that are liable to be constant over a long period. Examples, any of which individually would tend to result in low herd pregnancy rates, are inaccurate oestrous detection, unsatisfactory feeding, a high incidence of endometritis (see p. 521) or poor semen handling and insemination techniques (see Chapter 39).
- Specific pathogenic causes, such as a subfertile bull or venereal diseases such as campylobacteriosis, or other infectious conditions known to affect fertility

Box 36.1 Reasons for unsuccessful services.

Stage 1 Ovulation failure
Stage 2 Fertilization failure
Stage 3 Loss of the conceptus, due to early (3 week return intervals) or late embryonic death (3–6 week return intervals) or fetal death (>6 week return intervals)
Stage of failure unknown

such as bovine virus diarrhoea virus infection (see p. 578) or leptospirosis (see pp. 580, 735).
- The incidence of chronic repeat breeders, which to some extent relates to the background effect.

Aetiology

There are three main stages at which failure to achieve or maintain a pregnancy can occur. Although it is often not possible to assign an individual case to one of these stages this knowledge is useful in understanding the aetiology of return to service. The stages are shown in Box 36.1.

Stage 1 Failure of ovulation after oestrus

The most important condition in which there is oestrus without ovulation is cystic ovarian disease. It is important to define 'cystic ovarian disease' because not all cases of ovarian cysts are pathological (see Box 36.2). This traditional definition implied that cysts were static structures; however, cysts should be considered dynamic both in structure and function (Cook *et al.*, 1990). When studying the aetiology of ovulation failure the conclusions reached are affected by which animals are included as clinical cases. For example, cows identified as having cystic ovarian disease at routine preservice veterinary examination will form a different population from cystic ovarian disease cases detected in repeat breeder cows.

Histological and biochemical examination of ovarian cysts demonstrates that cysts are complex structures. On clinical examination and gross anatomical inspec-

Box 36.2 Definition of cystic ovarian disease (see also Chapter 35).

- Persisting, steroid-secreting follicles >2.5 cm in diameter
- No functional corpus luteum present for more than 10 days
- Abnormal sexual cycle (anoestrus, nymphomania, virilism)
- More than six weeks after calving

Box 36.3 The possible pathogenesis of cystic ovarian disease.

- Insufficient luteinizing hormone (LH) release: hypothalamic–pituitary dysfunction causing lack of GnRH release (commonest cause)
- Insufficient production of LH by the pituitary (rare)
- Failure of the dominant follicle to respond to LH

Box 36.4 Factors that predispose to or cause cystic ovarian disease.

- Heredity
- High yield
- Age
- Exogenous oestrogens
- Nutrition and season of the year
- Dystokia and periparturient disease

tion, however, there appear to be two main types of cysts: follicular cysts, which are like large follicles, and luteal cysts, in which obvious luteal tissue produces a thicker cyst wall. These may be difficult to differentiate from a corpus luteum with a central lacuna, which frequently occurs during the normal oestrous cycle (Okuda *et al.*, 1988).

It is well known that follicular cysts can occur and spontaneously resolve during the first few weeks after calving in some cows that then return to normal cyclic ovarian function, albeit later than normal counterparts (Savio *et al.*, 1990). It is often suggested that cows with cystic follicles up to six weeks after calving should be regarded as normal and not be interfered with unless they are nymphomaniac or show other signs of abnormality.

Box 36.3 is to some extent hypothetical but should act as a reminder that there are several possible routes that can result in cystic ovarian disease, among them long-term exposure to oestradiol or subnormal concentrations of progesterone (Dobson *et al.*, 2001a) and cortisol release following stress (Dobson *et al.*, 2001b). There have also been suggestions that energy imbalance due to high milk yields may be contributory, although this has not been substantiated by correlation with either β-hydroxybutyrate concentrations or body condition score (Dobson & Nanda, 1992; Tebble *et al.*, 2001).

There have been many studies of the causes of cystic ovarian disease and factors that predispose to the condition are listed in Box 36.4. There is lack of unanimity about causes, which may reflect differences between the populations of cattle selected for investigation as well as variations in the definition of cystic ovarian disease.

Heredity: A familial predisposition to cystic ovarian disease through sire or dam has been recognized for many years (Bane, 1964). Other studies have produced less clearcut results or even failed to detect a hereditary effect at all (Dohoo & Martin, 1984a). It is possible that this difference is partly due to the stage at which diagnosis is carried out. If the incidence is assessed at routine preservice checks most of the detected cysts are likely to be attributed to environmental factors rather than heredity; on the other hand, one might expect considerably more evidence of hereditary predisposition if the assessment is made on a sample of repeat breeders.

While most veterinarians are generally aware that there is a hereditary component in cystic ovarian disease, their clients want to know to what extent breeding a replacement heifer from a cow with cystic ovarian disease will increase the risk of that daughter having the disease. It is not easy to answer this because cystic ovarian disease may not occur in a daughter until she has had several calves and so field studies take many years and involve complex statistical analysis.

Early studies carried out by Henricson (1957) helped to answer the question. He analysed data from two artificial insemination (AI) centres of cases presented at the time of insemination and classified cows as:

- Having cystic ovarian disease on more than one occasion in a service period;
- Having only one observation of cystic ovarian disease; and
- Without cystic ovarian disease.

The effect of age was taken into account and the results expressed as an average frequency of the condition, where 1.00 is equivalent to an incidence of 100 per cent (Table 36.3).

Henricson (1957) also studied the effect of the sire and noted that the average frequency of cystic ovarian disease in individual bulls' daughters ranged from 0.00 to 0.258. Whether the low incidence of cystic ovarian disease in beef breeds is directly due to hereditary factors, to the lower milk production or to some other factor is not known.

High milk yield: Cystic ovarian disease may be related to high milk yield. It occurs most frequently at the peak

Table 36.3 Dam effect on incidence of cystic ovarian disease (COD) in daughters (Henricson, 1957).

Number of times COD diagnosed in dam in one service period	Average frequency of COD in daughters	
	Centre 1	Centre 2
>1	0.255	0.228
1	0.170	0.158
0	0.143	0.116

of lactation approximately six weeks postpartum and at the age when the cow has reached her full milking potential, which is why it is more common in pluriparous cows than in first calvers. There is a secondary peak of cases late in lactation; presumably these are cases that have been picked up on the examination of repeat breeders. Bartlett *et al.* (1986b) discussed, without coming to a conclusion, whether high milk yield causes cystic ovarian disease, cystic ovarian disease causes high yield or there is a common cause of both! Saloniemi *et al.* (1986) thought that the relationship between cystic ovarian disease and ketosis was due primarily to high milk yield, leading to greater energy demands that in turn resulted in both ketosis and interference with LH production or release.

Some workers have been unable to find an adverse effect of high milk yield on the occurrence of cystic ovarian disease (Dohoo & Martin, 1984a).

Age: It is widely accepted that cystic ovarian disease is rare in heifers before their first calving, not common in first-lactation cows and then increasingly observed in mature cows, with possibly some slight fall off in old animals.

Exogenous oestrogens: Administration of oestrogens in the follicular phase will cause a premature LH peak. This will not cause ovulation if no dominant follicle is present at the time. If oestrogens are administered shortly before dominant follicle selection, the cow may not be able to produce a second LH peak due to down regulation of the hypothalamic response to oestradiol and consequently the dominant follicle will continue to grow and not ovulate. This may be one explanation why a single large dose of an oestrogen for therapeutic purposes may be followed later by cystic ovaries. Recent transitions to organic farming may involve grazing periods on pastures with a high component of oestrogenic plant material; however, a much increased incidence of cystic ovarian disease in such herds has not been reported to date. An analogous situation may arise when oestrogenic substances, such as those found in mouldy brewers' grains, are eaten.

Seasonal effect: A very definite seasonal effect has been reported by many authors, with most reports indicating that the incidence is highest in winter (Dohoo *et al.*, 1984a,b; Saloniemi *et al.*, 1986). The effect can be so great that Bane (1964) stated that it is meaningless to talk of an incidence figure for cystic ovarian disease if details of season (and age) are excluded. The range in his data was from 2.23 per cent for cows that calved in May to 9.68 per cent for October calvers. The relative frequency of severe cases was higher in autumn calvers. Some authors (Bartlett *et al.*, 1986b) reported high levels in summer and autumn. The causes of the seasonal effect are not clear but may be linked to nutritional effects, and could also include the hours of daylight, temperature extremes and stressors such as housing.

Dystokia and periparturient disease: Some information suggests that dystokia and periparturient diseases may predispose to cystic ovarian disease. It is possible that preparturient factors that cause the postpartum conditions also affect the incidence of cystic ovarian disease, for example overfeeding leading to fatty liver (Reid *et al.*, 1979). It has been demonstrated experimentally that damage to the endometrium can prolong the existence of cystic follicles and so inhibit spontaneous recovery (Fathalla *et al.*, 1978) (see also Chapter 34).

Other causes: It is possible that gross adhesions can bind the ovary so tightly that ovulation does not take place, but this must be a rare phenomenon. Of much greater importance is the concept that in cows which had other reproductive disorders there were possibly more than the expected cases of cystic ovarian disease (Jasko *et al.*, 1984).

Reviews of the literature show that incidence ranges from about 6 to nearly 20 per cent (Bartlett *et al.*, 1986b; Garverick, 1997). However, diagnostic methods affect the reported incidence figure, for example Coleman *et al.* (1985) found that the single most important factor that influenced the incidence was the veterinarian who made the diagnosis! Selection of cases is also important, as has been discussed already.

It is generally agreed that follicular cysts make up about two-thirds of recognized cases of cystic ovarian disease (Booth, 1988; Garverick, 1997) although again this figure depends a little on the diagnostic method and criterion used.

While the most important reason for failure to ovulate is considered to be cystic ovarian disease, there are also a proportion of cows who have a delayed ovulation after oestrus, resulting in an extended period

Box 36.5 Causes of fertilization failure.

- Rectal palpation just before ovulation (bursting pre-ovulatory follicles, interference with egg flow into the uterine tubes)
- Interference with egg transport
- Interference with sperm transport
- Delayed ovulation
- Insemination at wrong time in relation to ovulation
- Service too soon after calving
- Poor quality spermatozoa
- Poor quality oocyte (e.g. from persistent follicles)
- Failure to serve the cow
- Metritis and salpingitis
- Vaginitis and cervicitis

Box 36.6 Causes of ovarian and bursal adhesions.

- Trauma
- Rectal palpation
- (Enucleation of corpus luteum – no longer indicated as a therapeutic practice in cattle)
- Caesarean section – inducing (localized) peritonitis
- Ascending infection
    Postpartum metritis
    Therapeutic infusion of uterus
- Descending infection
    from peritoneum
- Specific infections, e.g.
    Ureaplasma sp.
    Mycoplasma sp.

from insemination to ovulation. The incidence of delayed ovulation can be as high as 11 to 13 per cent, as shown in one study by Lamming and Darwash (1998).

Stage 2 Fertilization failure

To achieve fertilization a number of events in the cow (oestrus, ovulation, gamete transport) and in the bull (spermatozoa production, insemination) have to take place and must synchronize with each other. Failure of any one of these events to occur correctly or at the right time will almost certainly result in fertilization failure. The causes of fertilization failure will be discussed, mainly based on the headings shown in Box 36.5. The first two causes, interference with gamete transport, are relatively rare occurrences.

Interference with egg transport: After ovulation the egg has to be transported to the site of fertilization in the uterine tube. Adhesions affecting the ovary and bursa and blockage of the uterine tube will prevent this happening. Factors that cause adhesions, which are fairly rare, are listed in Box 36.6. The ease with which fluids and small objects can be transported spontaneously up or down the uterine tube is demonstrated in two techniques used to investigate uterine tube patency. In one of these tests, phenolsulphonphthalein (PSP) dye is introduced into the uterus and ascends spontaneously through the uterine tube into the peritoneal cavity and becomes absorbed and secreted in urine. In the other test, starch granules deposited in the bursa descend through the uterine tube into the uterus and vagina (Kessy & Noakes, 1979).

Transport in the uterine tube is under hormonal control and can be affected by abnormal variations in steroid hormone production and by oxytocin, but the role of these factors in field conditions is not known.

As transport of the egg depends on secretory and ciliary activity in the uterine tube, salpingitis will interfere with transport of both eggs and spermatozoa, even when the lumen remains patent.

Interference with transport of spermatozoa: Adhesions in the female tract that block egg transport, and have been discussed above, will generally interfere with transport of spermatozoa. There are rare anatomical abnormalities such as white heifer disease (segmental aplasia of the paramesonephric ducts), which results in blockage of the tubular genitalia at various levels.

Poor AI technique, such as insemination in the anterior vagina or caudal half of the cervix, will result in the majority of cases in the loss of much of the inseminate by reflux through the vulva. In contrast, in natural service the ejaculate is deposited in the anterior vagina and on the external os of the cervix, but the volume of the ejaculate and the enormous number of spermatozoa allow loss by reflux while sufficient spermatozoa are transported to the uterine tube. Returning to AI, a rough operator could damage the uterus with the insemination pipette. While it is unlikely that bad insemination technique is much of a problem with a technician inseminator service, it is very likely that the range of expertise among stockworkers who inseminate their own cows is so great that some gross technical errors may be made.

Hunter (1999) discusses possible modifications of the technique used for AI involving deep intrauterine insemination and the effects this may have on the transport and storage of spermatozoa within the female reproductive tract.

Delayed ovulation: Delayed ovulation is a condition in which the interval from the onset of oestrus to ovulation is so much longer than normal that service at the recommended time does not result in fertilization because of the ageing of the spermatozoa. While many authors are of the opinion that the condition is rare, there are a number of papers that suggest that it occurs quite commonly (Hancock, 1948; Nakao *et al.*, 1984; Lamming & Darwash, 1998). Watson and MacDonald (1984) studied events around insemination using rectal palpation and assays for progesterone and oestradiol-17β. They concluded that in cows with a follicle in the ovaries on the day after insemination (which may indicate delayed ovulation if onset of heat occurred more than 30 hours before) this was often due to erroneous timing of insemination in relation to the onset of oestrus and not to delayed ovulation.

As the condition is so difficult to study, ideas about its aetiology must be theoretical. It is possible that there is an abnormality of the LH surge or response of the preovulatory dominant follicle to the LH surge. It has been hypothesized that deficiency of energy intake may be involved in the aetiology.

The role of stress is also speculative, but it is interesting that corticosteroids can block LH release (Wagner & Li, 1982); also the fact that the adrenal cortex under the influence of adrenocorticotrophic hormone (ACTH) can produce some progesterone may be significant in suppressing the LH surge (Watson & Munro, 1984). The importance of stress in bovine reproduction is reviewed by Dobson *et al.* (2001b).

A little understood condition called prolonged low or suprabasal progesterone was described by Jackson *et al.* (1979) as affecting 18 per cent of cows treated with an analogue of prostaglandin $F_{2\alpha}$ ($PGF_{2\alpha}$) and also about 18 per cent of control cows. After oestrus there was an excessively long period of low progesterone, followed by a rise which seemed to indicate that ovulation took place eventually. The herd incidence ranged from 7 to 33 per cent and appeared to be low in herds with adequate nutrition. Other surveys have not revealed such a high incidence. Some workers think prolonged low progesterone is most commonly associated with treatment with $PGF_{2\alpha}$ or an analogue causing incomplete luteolysis and subsequent recovery of some luteal function. Independent of its cause, it will lead to persistence of a dominant follicle resulting in lowered fertility following its ovulation. This does not appear to be due to poor fertilization rates, but to more losses during early embryonic development (Mihm *et al.*, 1994).

Insemination at the wrong time in relation to ovulation: Service during the luteal phase is only a minor problem with natural service but a major one with AI (Sturman *et al.*, 2000). However, on farms using hand mated natural service, a cow restrained in a service crate may be mated when she is not in oestrus.

Artificial insemination at the wrong time is an important cause of fertilization failure. Progesterone assays of milk or blood taken on the day of insemination will detect insemination during the luteal phase of the cycle but will fail to pick up inseminations that are one or two days too early or too late. The reported incidence of luteal phase progesterone levels on the day of insemination is variable. The incidence of 5.2 per cent in well-run herds reported by Claus *et al.* (1983), with over 20 per cent in problem herds, is typical of several other trials. Laitinen *et al.* (1985), in a large field study, reported that the lowest incidence of luteal phase inseminations occurred in the summer. Oltner and Edqvist (1981) observed that in herds with a high incidence of wrongly timed inseminations, even inseminations apparently at the correct time resulted in low pregnancy rates, presumably because of other aspects of poor management.

The reasons are misidentification of a cow that actually is in season or misinterpretation of sexual behaviour, such as jumping another cow, which is thought incorrectly to indicate oestrus. The stockworkers are often under considerable pressure to get all cows served by a target date and are criticised by veterinarians and others, that cows in oestrus are missed too frequently. This can result in error through an overenthusiastic determination to increase the oestrous detection rate. The importance of inseminating only cows in oestrus was demonstrated by Sturman *et al.* (2000), who reported that in a herd they studied 19 per cent of inseminations were performed when progesterone levels were high in the oestrous cycle or while cows were pregnant. Insemination of pregnant cows led to an estimated 17 per cent induced embryonic death or abortion!

Incorrect timing of insemination in relation to onset of oestrus also occurs. Watson *et al.* (1987) confirmed that insemination 24 hours or more after the cow is first seen in oestrus results in a marked reduction in pregnancy rate, possibly due to ageing of the oocyte before fertilization. It is likely that insemination very early in oestrus also causes reduced fertility, possibly due to reduced sperm survival rates before fertilization. There is a long-established, successful rule of thumb about the ideal time for insemination (Trimberger, 1948). Cows first seen in the morning should be inseminated late that afternoon. Cows first seen in the afternoon or evening should be inseminated next morning. Cows still in oestrus 24 hours after first being seen should receive a second insemination. This pragmatic recommendation takes account of the relatively short lifespan of both spermatozoa and ova within the female tubular tract (about 24 hours), the need for capacitation of bull spermatozoa (about 6 hours) and the interval from the onset of oestrus to ovulation (about 24–30 hours).

Incorrect timing within oestrus is of little significance with natural service in which the service is usually early in oestrus. The large quantity of the ejaculate and the great numbers of spermatozoa deposited in the anterior vagina ensure that there is a long-lasting supply of fertile spermatozoa in the uterine tube at the site of fertilization.

Service too soon after calving: It has been known for many decades that service within six weeks of calving results in reduced pregnancy rates. The expected conception rate increases from approximately 20 per cent, at 20 days post partum, to reach normal rates (at the time the studies were carried out these were 50 per cent calving rates) from 50 days post partum. The reasons are likely to be both ovarian and uterine in origin so in some cases the cause is most probably fertilization failure and in others embryonic death. Elimination of infection and restoration of endometrial structure and function after a normal calving requires 5–6 weeks in most animals.

Poor-quality semen or poor insemination technique: Poor semen quality may result in either low pregnancy rate or no pregnancies at all, mainly through fertilization failure but also to some extent through embryonic death. Again there are marked differences between natural service and AI. Because of laboratory control of the semen and follow-up of the results of insemination it is very unlikely that semen supplied by a reputable AI organization will give poor pregnancy rates. The exception to this is semen that has been poorly stored or incorrectly handled on farm for use in DIY AI systems. Schermerhorn *et al.* (1986) found that a technician inseminator service gave rather better results than farmer DIY insemination, although this may depend on the level of training received by DIY inseminators before they begin inseminating their own cows. Howells *et al.* (1999) showed that the amount of training received with live cows significantly affected future pregnancy rates; for those who spent up to three days training in an abattoir using live cows there was an increase of 5.9 per cent in the calving rate they achieved in their first year for every day they spent training. If AI technique is satisfactory, poor results with DIY inseminations could possibly be related to mishandling of the semen. By contrast a bull used for natural service may be of reduced or low fertility or even sterile and serve a number of cows before the owner realizes that something is wrong. Farmers are often not aware that a bull that has been fertile may become infertile or lose libido (see Chapter 38).

Where fresh diluted semen is used, semen that is stored too long will give poor results.

Failure to serve the cow: In certain circumstances when a bull is used to serve the cows, a cow in oestrus is not served. Bulls can develop abnormalities of the penis that prevent normal service, and lack of libido is not uncommon (see p. 610). When animals are running freely, such as heifers or beef cattle, it is essential to include an adequate number of bulls in the group. If there are too few bulls for the number of cows, some cows in oestrus may not be served. The required cow to bull ratio depends on the type of terrain, the age and libido of individual bulls (see p. 610).

Metritis, salpingitis, vaginitis and cervicitis: Infection of the tubular genitalia may interfere with the survival of the spermatozoa in transit and so reduce the chance of fertilization. Endometritis and metritis are fairly common (see p. 524) but in addition a number of species of organisms have been recovered from the uterine tubes and may cause salpingitis or directly affect fertilization, as for example reported by Grahn *et al.* (1984), in connection with fertilization failure with BVDV infection (see pp. 578, 853). Infectious agents in the uterine tube include *Leptospira hardjo* (see p. 735), *Ureaplasma* spp. and *Mycoplasma bovigenitalium*.

Stage 3 Embryonic death

The stage of the embryo lasts from fertilization of the egg until about day 42 after conception, by which time the organ systems have been laid down and placentation has been established. Failure of maternal recognition of pregnancy will cause early embryonic loss, and the animal returns to oestrus at normal intervals (<25 days). Late embryonic loss occurs after maternal recognition of pregnancy, and animals may show their next heat 25 to 40 days after the previous heat.

In any group of breeding cattle, however normal they appear, there will occur a considerable amount of embryonic death, most of it within the first three weeks after fertilization (Sreenan & Diskin, 1986). Ayalon (1978) produced data to show that in repeat breeders the majority of the losses occurred approximately 5–7 days after insemination, around the time the early embryo enters the uterus and begins to synthesize its own proteins (Table 36.4). However, the exact timing of early pregnancy losses in the modern high-yielding dairy cow is largely unknown. Knowledge of the aetiology of this important condition is still very limited but it is possible to produce a list of factors that have been shown to cause embryonic death or are at least very likely to be involved (Box 36.7). In the vast majority of cases the actual cause is never established.

Factors that may contribute to embryonic death

Extreme environmental temperatures: Controlled experiments have demonstrated that cattle that are mated

Table 36.4 Timing of embryonic death, determined by slaughter and dissection of the cow (number and percentage containing viable embryos) (from Ayalon, 1978).

Time of slaughter (days)	Normal cows		Repeat breeders	
	Number	Percentage	Number	Percentage
2–3	10/12	83	12/17	71
4–5	22/25	88	20/25	80
6–7	10/12	83	5/12	42
8–10	13/18	72	9/18	50
11–13	16/18	89	9/18	50
14–16	16/20	80	10/20	50
17–19	12/21	57	9/21	43
35–42	9/13	69	8/24	35

Box 36.7 Factors that may contribute to embryonic death.

- Extreme environmental temperatures, particularly heat stress
- Specific and non-specific endometritis or metritis
- Specific infections of follicles, gametes and/or embryo
- Maternal pre- and postovulatory endocrine environment
- Aged gametes
- Local trauma
- Genetic factors, resulting in non-viable genetic defects
- Nutrition
- Possible fetal/maternal incompatibility

in a high environmental temperature and kept there after service exhibit a high rate of embryonic death. The dominance of the large preovulatory follicle is suppressed by heat stress, and the steroidogenic capacity of theca and granulosa cells is compromised. Progesterone secretion by luteal cells is lowered during the summer in hot climates, and in cows subjected to chronic heat stress this is also reflected in a lower plasma progesterone concentration. Heat stress has also been shown to impair oocyte quality and embryo development, and increase embryo mortality. In addition to the immediate effects of heat stress, delayed effects have also been detected. These include altered follicular dynamics, suppressed production of follicular steroids and lower quality of oocytes and developing embryos. This may explain why poor fertility may persist for some time after periods of heat stress (Wolfenson *et al.*, 2000).

Poor pregnancy rate is a problem when European cattle are introduced into hot countries where they are exposed to ambient temperatures above 30°C; it is quite likely that increased embryonic death is part of the reason. There is little doubt that genetic factors are involved in this as in other aspects of heat tolerance.

Crosses between indigenous heat tolerant breeds and European breeds are more heat tolerant than the imported animals and they are more fertile (see Chapter 6). The improved fertility appears to be the result of the dam's enhanced ability to control body temperature rather than an inherited ability of the embryo itself to tolerate high intrauterine temperatures. The position is less clear with extreme cold, but there are indications that a corresponding adverse effect occurs. The problem could arise during unusually cold periods in temperate climates where housing tends to provide cover rather than warmth.

Metritis/endometritis: Metritis or endometritis in varying degrees of intensity is a common condition causing infertility in cattle (see Chapter 34). Where caused by infection it can be divided into non-specific, exemplified by *Arcanobacterium pyogenes* infection, and specific, typified by *Tritrichomonas fetus* (see p. 584) and *Campylobacter fetus* (see p. 582) infection. There are also a number of infections that are difficult to classify such as bovine herpes virus-1 (BHV-1), *Ureaplasma* spp. and *Haemophilus somnus*.

Non-specific metritis is the result of either massive infection or of the infective organisms taking advantage of a deficient uterine defence mechanism, usually caused by damage at and after calving. Non-specific infection can be facilitated by the synergistic action of different organisms, for example *A. pyogenes* and *Fusobacterium necrophorum*.

Specific infections colonize the undamaged uterus. Two important specific infective agents are *C. fetus* and *T. fetus*. Campylobacteriosis is spread venereally and causes a mild endometritis in infected females that have not had previous experience of the condition. It has been shown in slaughter experiments that in infected animals fertilization rate is normal and that the infertility is due in the main to embryonic death within three weeks of conception. Loss of the embryo is likely to be due to interference with the uterine environment. Venereal campylobacter infection and its control in the UK has been reviewed by Taylor (2002). Trichomoniasis, a parasitic venereal disease that still occurs in some countries (Clark *et al.*, 1986), is clinically similar to campylobacteriosis with one major difference, the occurrence of pyometra in a number of cases (BonDurant, 1997).

Another infectious agent that is introduced from the vagina into the uterus at insemination, but not at natural service, is *Ureaplasma* (Doig *et al.*, 1979), which causes a purulent metritis and infertility. *Haemophilus/Histophilus* also causes vaginitis and reduced fertility. For detailed discussion of a wide range of infectious agents see Morrow (1986). For more details on both endometritis and metritis see also Chapter 34.

Infectious conditions can cause infertility in at least four ways:

- The febrile reaction raises the temperature of the uterus. Bluetongue (Chapter 43a) is an example of a disease that causes a high temperature resulting in loss of the embryo at about the time of hatching from the zona pellucida, about day 10–12 after service.
- The organism infects the uterus and causes metritis, which presumably interferes with embryo nutrition and may also infect the embryo. Examples are BHV-1 virus (see p. 289) and *Chlamydiales* infections. It is likely that, in general, mild endometritis causes embryonic death whereas in cases of purulent metritis there may be interference with spermatozoa survival and thus fertilization failure.
- Infection of the conceptus can cause its death. The thought that embryo transfer could transmit infectious diseases from the sire or the dam is worrying. In theory, bacterial and fungal infections are less likely than viral infections to be carried by embryos. From experimental studies with many different viruses it appears that if the zona pellucida is intact and the embryo is washed properly, there is little danger of the transmission of viral infections by embryo transfer (Singh, 1987; Wrathall, 1995). However, the advent of *in vitro* technology may increase the risk of disease transmission due to differences in the zona pellucida of *in vitro* derived embryos, enabling easier adsorption of pathogens, and due to the use of biological products for culture which may be contaminated with pathogens (Stringfellow & Wrathall, 1995; Guerin, *et al.*, 1997).
- Endotoxins produced by Gram-negative infections can increase $PGF_{2\alpha}$ production and cause premature luteolysis (Fredriksson, 1984).

Maternal endocrine environment: Mann and Lamming (1995) showed that low plasma concentrations of progesterone resulted in the development of a stronger luteolytic signal. This was taken as an explanation for the fact that cows with lower plasma concentrations of progesterone postinsemination are more prone to embryo loss than those with higher progesterone levels.

Interferon tau (IFN-τ) is a protein produced by the embryo that acts locally within the uterus to block luteolysis and maintain the corpus luteum; it prevents $PGF_{2\alpha}$ secretion by inhibiting the development of oxytocin receptors in the endometrium (Robinson *et al.*, 1999). More recently, further work has shown that successful maternal recognition of pregnancy in cows depends on the presence of a sufficiently well developed embryo producing sufficient quantities of IFN-τ, which is, in turn, dependent on an appropriate pattern of maternal progesterone secretion (Mann, 1997; Mann & Lamming, 2001). Thus the maternal endocrine environment, and particularly maternal progesterone levels within the first one to two weeks after insemination, is likely to be extremely important in determining whether an embryo signals its presence to the dam and survives or is lost as the cow returns to oestrus.

Aged gametes: Fresh chilled semen ages after several days and the inseminated cows have a lower pregnancy rate almost certainly due to both reduced fertilization rate and increased loss of embryos. There is no evidence of adverse effects from ageing of frozen semen stored in liquid nitrogen. Fertilization of ageing eggs following ovulation of persistent dominant follicles (Mihm *et al.*, 1994; Austin *et al.*, 1999) is also likely to result in an increased amount of early embryonic death.

Local trauma: This cause of loss affects the late embryo and early fetus. One source of local trauma to the pregnant uterus is the hand of a person carrying out manual pregnancy diagnosis, or some other palpation of the uterus. In one study the average loss was 2.82 per cent of cows diagnosed pregnant (Beghelli *et al.*, 1986). Franco *et al.* (1987) reported a fetal loss rate of 9.5 per cent in cows diagnosed pregnant on days 42–46. The technique, which was carried out on two days, involved palpation of fetal fluid, identification of the amniotic vesicle and slipping of the chorioallantoic membranes. However, with good transrectal ultrasound examination technique such losses should now be largely preventable.

In a very large field study in which they used milk progesterone assays, Laitinen *et al.* (1985) estimated that 1.8 per cent of cows that returned to service were pregnant at the time of re-insemination. When a pregnant cow is inseminated, the conceptus must be at risk either through direct trauma or by the introduction of infection into a progesterone-dominated uterus. An experienced inseminator may be able to feel the difference in the cervix and uterine horns and avoid insemination into the body of the uterus, electing instead to deposit the semen in the anterior cervix or not to inseminate the cow at all.

Genetic factors: Mention has been made of the variable breed susceptibility to high environmental temperature that causes embryo death.

In some cattle, in the process of cell division, translocation of parts of certain chromosomes without loss of genetic material has taken place, a condition that is passed on to future generations. These individuals can be identified by cytogenetic examination of leukocytes. When semen from bulls with a translocation is used for insemination there is a slight increase in the incidence of return to service, which is believed to be the result of embryonic death, presumably because of lack or excess of some genetic material due to abnormal division at meiosis.

It is also probable that many genetically abnormal embryos are lost early in development, with the advantage that the dam can return to normal breeding at the earliest opportunity. Early embryo development and non-infectious causes of embryo loss are reviewed by Kastelic (1994) and Sreenan *et al.* (1999).

Stage of failure not known

It should be clear from the limited number of factors listed as known to cause embryonic death, that in the majority of cases the cause is unknown. Some factors that result in return to service can affect different stages, for example late insemination can result in fertilization failure in some cases and embryonic death in others. There is a very large grey area concerning the aetiology of return to service, particularly where groups of affected animals are concerned. The difficulty concerning the relationship between (possible) aetiological factors and return to service is twofold.

Some factors almost certainly cause an increased return to service via an unknown mechanism. An example is the aetiological relationship between loss in body condition from calving to service and associated poor pregnancy rate. The possible sites where inadequate nutrition may have detrimental effects on reproductive function include:

- The hypothalamus/pituitary gland to impair gonadotrophin release.
- The ovaries, possibly resulting in altered follicular growth patterns and reduced quality of oocytes and subsequent reduced embryo survival.
- Inadequate uterine environment resulting in impaired embryo survival (Webb *et al.*, 1997).

To complicate matters further, additive effects of two or more types will produce low pregnancy rates. Two or more independent minor adverse factors that occur at the same time will produce a poor result. For example, Boyd and Reed (1961b) observed that variations in three factors (calving-to-first-service interval, age of cow and age of fresh semen) caused a range of pregnancy rates from 22 to 70 per cent. As mentioned above, synergistic action of two or more adverse aetiological factors, for example *A. pyogenes* and *F. necrophorum*, can result in a more severe pathological condition than either alone.

Many of the putative causes of return to service are far from being proven but they cannot be simply dismissed for that reason. Amongst these possibly adverse factors are the following:

- Short-term change in feeding and environment, particularly at turnout in the spring and at housing in the autumn. This has been postulated to be due to an energy–protein imbalance changing the uterine tube and uterine environment (pH and urea concentrations) and thus affecting normal early embryonic development.
- High milk yield leading to excessive metabolic stress.
- Stressful effect of disputes about dominance among cows that are subject to frequent changes of groups in dairy herds.
- Non-reproductive systemic illness.
- Deficiencies and imbalances in minerals and vitamins (almost impossible to generalize because of very local effect of feeding practices, local soil deficiencies and many other variables).
- Other conditions that stress the animal or affect its dry matter intake such as lameness.

There are various reasons why there is so much uncertainty in a field where numerous workers have gathered observations and data for several decades. Because expected pregnancy rate is about 50 per cent, the random variation in fertility in groups is great and this necessitates large, properly controlled groups in trials in order to give reliable results. The possibility of erroneous conclusions from any single trial is so great that only results that are consistently repeated in different populations can be regarded as reliable.

In recent years there have been a number of epidemiological studies of a highly statistical nature on the relationships between various aspects of management and production, disease and reproduction. Because of the complexity of interrelationships very large numbers of observations are needed and these reports are based on data from populations that range from about 2000 to >70000 lactation records. For the practitioner this means that evaluation of fertility in small herds is difficult due to the large impact of small numbers of observations on overall herd results.

While there are considerable differences between the findings certain concepts have emerged:

- Reproductive diseases at and after calving tend to occur as an interrelated complex (see Chapter 34).
- Some diseases that are not specific infections of the reproductive tract have an adverse effect on reproduction, e.g. *Leptospira hardjo*, BVD virus (McGowan & Kirkland, 1995) and BHV-1.
- There is disagreement on the effect of high yield on fertility.
- There is disagreement on the effect of hereditary factors on fertility.

Although the relative importance of the factors listed above, along with other management factors, is still poorly understood, what does seem to be beyond doubt now is that fertility, at least in high producing dairy cows in the UK, is declining over time (Barrett, 2001).

The relationship between nutrition and fertility is a complex one that is still not fully understood. The reader may find the following reviews of interest: Britt (1995); Webb *et al.* (1997); Wathes *et al.* (1998); Webb *et al.* (1999); O'Callaghan and Boland (1999); Garnsworthy and Webb (2000) and O'Callaghan *et al.* (2000).

As an example of the complex interactions affecting fertility, data from the very large study by Saloniemi *et al.* (1986) showed the consequential effects of specific causes described in Table 36.5.

For details of other complex interactions, the reader is referred to some original texts: Andersson *et al.* (1991) and Gustafsson and Emanuelson (1996): hyperketonaemia and fertility; Bartlett *et al.* (1986b) and Garverick (1997): cystic ovarian disease; Bartlett *et al.* (1986a) and Sheldon (1999): metritis/endometritis; Curtis *et al.* (1985): metabolic disease, mastitis; Dohoo and Martin (1984a): age, season and sire; Dohoo & Martin (1984b): mastitis and ketosis; Britt (1995): nutri-

tion, weight loss and fertility; Loeffler *et al.* (1999): time of disease, milk yield and body condition; Dohoo *et al.* (1984): disease, production and culling; Rowlands *et al.* (1986) and Peeler *et al.* (1994): interrelationship of diseases; Saloniemi *et al.* (1986) and Fourichon *et al.* (2000): reproductive diseases.

Diagnosis

Although a herd consists of many individuals, diagnosis of a return-to-service problem that affects a large part of a herd requires a different approach from that taken to investigate the cause in an individual animal. For this reason the individual will be dealt with first, followed by the herd fertility problem.

Diagnosis of the individual repeat breeder cow

One problem with diagnosis is that by the time the cow is recognized as being a repeat breeder the situation that prevailed at the time of reproductive failure may well have changed.

The clinician should take a history and carry out a systematic clinical examination to find out whether any of the factors that are likely to cause return to service are present. The fullness and, therefore, costs of the investigation will need to be discussed with the farmer in advance and a diagnosis may only be pursued in valuable animals.

A systematic approach to diagnosis is essential and the following procedure is suggested (Box 36.8).

History: The history should cover various points as shown in Box 36.9.

General examination: The clinician should carry out a brief general examination looking at the following points:

Table 36.5 The consequential effects of management and disease on problems of fertility (reproduced from Saloniemi *et al.*, 1986 with permission of the publisher).

Cause	Consequential effect			
	Retained fetal membranes	Metritis	Anoestrus/suboestrus	Ovarian dysfunction
Winter calving	No	Yes	Yes	Yes
Highest herd milk yield	Yes	Yes	Yes	Yes
Parturient paresis	Yes	Yes		
Mastitis		Yes	Yes	
Ketosis		Yes	Yes	Yes
Retained fetal membranes		Yes		
Metritis			Yes	Yes

Box 36.8   The systematic diagnosis of return to service.

- History
- Analysis of records
- General clinical examination and body condition
- Examination of the reproductive tract (rectal, vaginal and suitable aids including ultrasound examination)
- Appropriate laboratory tests

Box 36.9   The main factors to be covered in history taking.

- Date of calving.
- Dystokia and puerperal diseases
- Postpartum reproductive disease
- Other diseases (e.g. lameness, metabolic diseases)
- Service details
    Dates
    Bull used
    Natural or AI
- Inseminator service or DIY AI
- Major management or environmental changes
- Is this considered to be a herd or individual cow problem?

- Body condition and conformation;
- Signs of non-reproductive disease;
- Signs of vaginal discharge or dried pus or mucus on the tail or hindquarters; and
- Other signs, for example a raised tailhead.

Rectal examination: The technique of rectal palpation of the genital tract is fully described in various textbooks, as are the characteristics of the various normal and abnormal structures in the ovaries and tract. The purpose of carrying out a rectal examination is to assess:

- The state of the ovaries;
- The condition of the bursae and uterine tubes;
- Uterine abnormality or status (e.g. metritis, adhesions, pregnancy);
- Internal slackness of the pelvic ligaments;
- Absence of fat inside the pelvis (body condition);
- Vulval discharge (stimulated by palpation);
- Evidence of other conditions detectable on rectal examination (e.g. cystitis, pyelonephritis, fat necrosis).

Nowadays it is general practice to supplement, or even replace, the manual rectal examination with a transrectal ultrasound examination. This has the same aims as listed above, but will on the whole give more accurate results. The use of transrectal ultrasound examination as a diagnostic tool and the comparative levels of accuracy of rectal examination and ultrasound

are discussed more fully in Chapter 35 (see p. 536). The use of milk progesterone assays may also improve diagnostic accuracy (see p. 548).

Accuracy of diagnosis of cystic ovarian disease by rectal examination: When undertaking rectal palpation there are obvious difficulties in trying to assess the nature of a cyst without rupturing it. A large, soft corpus luteum with no palpable ovulation papillum can be mistaken for a cyst. Some authors are very sceptical about the accuracy of diagnosis of cystic structures by rectal palpation alone, for example Stolla *et al.* (1980) and Guenzler and Schallenberger (1981). However, accuracy is immensely improved with transrectal ultrasound examination (Douthwaite & Dobson, 2000), and once again milk progesterone assays have their place in confirming whether functional luteal tissue is or is not present (Chapter 35).

Accuracy of diagnosis of endometritis: Clinical diagnosis of endometritis is discussed in some detail in Chapter 34 (see p. 521).

Vaginal examination: There is a choice of two methods of vaginal examination on the farm: manual or visual using a vaginal speculum. In both cases the perineal region and vulva are thoroughly cleaned and the veterinarian uses fresh plastic gloves. With manual examination mucus in the anterior vagina is gathered and on withdrawal of the hand examined visually and olfactorily. Minimum lubrication is used to avoid confusion between clear mucus and the lubricant. The cervix and vaginal wall are palpated for lesions and abnormalities. The vaginal speculum should be introduced with care and, when fully inserted, will give a clear view of the cervix. With both techniques the clinician may have difficulty in passing the vulvo–vaginal junction, which is the narrowest part of the tract at this level. When using a speculum great care should be taken to ensure that the speculum does not transfer infection between cows. This is best achieved by using disposable, single-use specula or autoclaving equipment between cows. If a single speculum is to be used on a number of cows at a single visit, it must be thoroughly disinfected between cows. Box 36.10 shows the factors that should be checked in a vaginal examination.

Selection of samples for laboratory examination: Selection of the appropriate laboratory examinations and the frequency of sampling depend very much on circumstances, including the value of the cow. The items listed in Box 36.11 may be considered.

To extend the physical examination beyond what is possible by palpation and transrectal ultrasound, the patency of the uterine tubes can be investigated using the phenosulphonphthalein (PSP) dye test and/or starch grain test as described by Kessy and Noakes (1979).

Box 36.10 Factors to be checked by vaginal examination.

- Anatomical abnormalities.
  Heifers
- Damage
  Caused by dystokia:
  Rectovaginal fistula
  Pneumovagina/urovagina (see p. 519)
  Damage to the cervix
  Serving injuries caused by the bull
  Sadistic human interference
  Other acquired conditions
  Vaginitis (see p. 519)
  Type and quantity of mucus
  Purulent
  Bloody
  Smelly
  Clear oestrous mucus

Box 36.11 Types of samples required for various laboratory tests.

- Single milk progesterone assay: an adjunct to rectal palpation and ultrasound examination
- Serial milk progesterone assays: monitor events around service, confirm diagnosis, monitor treatment
- Oestrone sulphate from milk, blood (specifically from the placenta: indicates live calf)
- Heparinized blood for cytogenetic analysis
- Clotted blood for serology (e.g. BHV-1, BVDV, *Leptospira hardjo*, *Neospora caninum*)
- Purulent material from the uterus: aerobic and anaerobic culture, antibiotic sensitivity
- Uterine biopsy for histology
- Samples from the cervix and uterus for serology and cytology
- Vaginal mucus for campylobacter diagnosis using the vaginal mucus agglutination test (VMAT)

New technological aids to diagnosis: In recent years advances in biochemistry, electronics and fibre optics, along with skills and materials developed for embryo transfer, have opened up new diagnostic possibilities. There is every reason to believe that new equipment and concepts will continue to be produced, which presents problems as well as opportunities for the veterinarian. Most of the new techniques do not require specifically veterinary skills and so may be used by a wide range of operators, although for best effect knowledgeable interpretation is needed. Choices have to be made about the lasting value of each new step forward as investing capital and training in inappropriate technology is unproductive.

The relatively new aids to diagnosis can be classified as:

Box 36.12. Steps required to diagnose a herd fertility problem.

- History
- Analysis of records
  Breeding
  Health
  Production
- Selected clinical examinations and sampling
- Conclusion

- Quick, cheap and, in some cases, automated hormone analysis;
- Non-invasive (or acceptably invasive) examination of internal organs: hysteroscopy, endoscopy (transrectal ultrasound is already routinely used during on farm fertility examinations);
- Automatic or semiautomatic recording of physical, behavioural and biochemical changes that are related to the animal's reproductive status, such as body temperature, restlessness, changes in milk composition and hormone content;
- Computer analysis of data: compilation over time of various measurements in the individual and analysis of herd records (see Chapter 41b).

Diagnosis of a herd problem

It is necessary to approach the diagnosis of a herd fertility problem systematically. It is not practical to lay out in any detail a series of steps to be followed because as the investigation develops the information obtained guides the continued course of the investigation.

The four main causes of herd problems are poor fertility management, an infertile 'male', nutritional errors and deficiencies and infectious conditions. In general terms the steps required are shown in Box 36.12.

History: The object of history taking is to acquire information on the factors shown in Box 36.13.

Analysis of the records: It is useful, if possible, to examine the breeding records before visiting the herd. If there are no records then establish a recording system. The objectives of record analysis in connection with a herd fertility problem are the following:

(1) To assess the current level of fertility in the herd and to establish whether a problem exists, and if so to determine the seriousness of the situation.
(2) To look for clues to aetiology, by looking at the fertility of subgroups within the herd:
  - Bull, semen or inseminator;
  - Age (lactation) group;
  - Yield group;

- General aspects of the herd and farm
    - Number of breeding stock (male and female)
    - Stocking density
    - Type of housing
    - Details of grazing
    - Targets for reproduction and production
    - Other enterprises
    - Information about the stockworkers
- Definition of the perceived problem
    - Anoestrus
    - Return to service
    - Vaginal discharges
    - Other manifestations
- Duration of problem
- Proportion of herd affected
- Reproductive management
    - Calving management
    - Service management: cows and heifers (heat detection, timing of AI, technician or DIY AI)
    - Bulls
- Nutrition
    - Ration formulation
    - Feeding system
    - Assessment of adequacy of nutrition e.g. yield, milk composition, condition score, metabolic profiles
- Details of 'herd health plan'
    - Disease monitoring
    - Intervention levels
    - Preventive medicine initiatives
        - Vaccination protocols
        - Biosecurity
- Disease status of herd
    - Details of herd status for infectious diseases known to affect fertility, e.g. BVDV, BHV-1, leptospirosis
    - Incidence of conditions that have a direct effect on fertility, e.g. retained fetal membranes, endometritis
    - Other diseases and conditions in the herd, e.g. lameness

- Seasonal effect;
- Familial effect;
- Relevant infectious disease: e.g. non-specific endometritis after calving, *Campylobacter fetus*, *Leptospira hardjo*, *Neospora caninum*, BHV-1, BVDV, etc.

Analysis and interpretation of herd fertility records are discussed in much more detail in Chapter 41a,b.

Once a cause of the infertility is suspected, a valuable technique is to group the records of all animals that are influenced by the suspect factor and compare these with the records from all other cows. It can be difficult to identify the cause of a problem where farmer insemination is associated with poor pregnancy rate. In these cases there may be no comparative data on the bull's fertility; the problem could be due to poor insemination technique or to improper semen handling.

Examination of the animals: It is very useful to examine as many cows as possible to obtain a current picture of the herd, to observe the condition of the cows and to detect or confirm the incidence of obvious reproductive abnormalities. It also reveals the (in)accuracy of the information supplied by the farmer or farm staff. Advice should be given about culling of individuals that have a very poor prognosis.

By this stage the clinician should have a good idea of the type of problem; how the investigation then develops is a matter of clinical judgement which cannot be detailed further.

Treatment (see Chapter 42)

The veterinarian is faced with some difficulties when having to decide on appropriate and effective treatments for cows that are presented as infertile. This is partly because of the complex aetiology of return to service, but also because of the time that has passed since the factors that initiated the problem were present. When using pharmaceutical products the reader is advised to consult the manufacturers' data sheets for details of treatment, withdrawal periods, dangers and contraindications. Wherever possible the treatment should be followed up to see whether it has been successful or not and, if need be, repeated or changed.

Ovulation failure

The most important cause of ovulation failure is cystic ovarian disease. Treatment is based on whether the cyst has been diagnosed as follicular or luteal. In most cases the condition is probably caused by hypothalamic–pituitary dysfunction and it is, therefore, logical to treat the condition systemically. There is little or no benefit in rupturing the cyst manually, which also involves a risk of causing haemorrhage and ovarian adhesions. Nor does there appear to be any benefit from administration of drugs directly into the cyst.

Many cystic structures found less than 42 days after calving are transient and benign, and in general these do not require to be treated. Only if abnormal behaviour indicates that they are pathological or if there is some pressing management need should they be treated.

For follicular cysts the three therapeutics of choice are human chorionic gonadotrophin (hCG), gonadotrophin-releasing hormone (GnRH) or GnRH analogues, such as buserelin, and progesterone-releasing intravaginal devices (PRIDs) and controlled internal drug release (CIDR) (Dobson *et al.*, 2001a). They all work in different ways to achieve the same end, i.e. to put the animal under the influence of progesterone. One effect of this is to allow a build-up of LH in the pituitary so that enough endogenous LH is available after removal of the progesterone devices or regression of the (induced) corpus luteum. This leads to normal preovulatory follicle development and ovulation, and in all cases the cow should be served at the first heat after treatment. The duration of exposure to exogenous or endogenous progesterone is thought to be important in the non-recurrence of the cystic condition, with 14 days being preferable to seven (Nanda *et al.*, 1989). There is also evidence to suggest that the success of treatment of follicular cysts depends on whether the cyst is producing oestradiol or not, as reflected by the presence or absence of other follicles >5mm in diameter. Following treatment with an intravaginal progesterone releasing device or GnRH, animals had a pregnancy rate to all inseminations of 91 per cent when other large follicles were present in addition to the cyst, compared with 69 per cent if no other follicles were present at the time of treatment (Tebble *et al.*, 2001).

Human chorionic gonadotrophin has an LH-like direct action on the ovary to induce luteinization of the cyst or follicles. GnRH stimulates the release of LH from the pituitary to achieve the same result. In both cases the lifespan of the luteal tissue produced is variable, ranging from about six days to about 18 days, and oestrus can be expected about 8–22 days after treatment. It is desirable to examine the treated cows about seven days after treatment for the presence of luteal tissue. If luteal tissue is found, treatment with $PGF_{2\alpha}$ or an analogue is a suitable way of increasing the predictability of the following oestrus. Service should be at that oestrus and aids to oestrous detection should be used. If there is no satisfactory response to the first treatment, the cow should be re-examined and treated again.

For cysts containing functional luteal tissue as judged by ultrasound examination or milk progesterone assay, injection of $PGF_{2\alpha}$ or an analogue followed by insemination at observed oestrus is the most suitable treatment.

An alternative treatment, suitable for both types of cystic ovarian disease, is the insertion of a PRID/CIDR, which can be left in position for 12 days, and after withdrawal the cow should be served, either at a fixed time or preferably at observed oestrus (Douthwaite & Dobson, 2000). If the type of cyst cannot be diagnosed accurately, then administration of $PGF_{2\alpha}$ or an analogue, either on the day of PRID/CIDR withdrawal or

up to three days before, can improve predictability of the oestrous response. If fixed time insemination is used and oestrus is observed later the animal should be inseminated again.

Fertilization failure

Delayed ovulation: For many years one of the standard ways of treating apparently normal repeat breeders on the farm has been to administer hCG or GnRH on the day of service. The theory behind this was that many of these cases were thought to be due to lack of an adequate gonadotrophin surge delaying ovulation, although controlled trials of this type of treatment are lacking and a better approach may be to inseminate the cow again 24 hours after the first insemination.

Interference with transport of egg or spermatozoa: When this is due to bilateral blockage of the uterine tubes (or other parts of the female tract), there is no simple treatment. In some cases the diagnostic dye test may remove a minor blockage and attempts have been made to achieve this by adding antibiotics and corticosteroids to the dye, which is introduced into the uterine tube end of the uterus under gentle pressure using a cuffed catheter.

In valuable animals the use of ovum pick-up techniques using transvaginal ultrasound-guided oocyte aspiration can be used to harvest oocytes for *in vitro* production of embryos. One or more of these embryos could then be implanted back into the uterus of the donor, although it is probably more advisable to implant valuable embryos derived in this way into other healthy heifers. In those animals that are not considered of high enough genetic merit to be used as oocyte donors, but which the farmer simply wishes to get back in calf so as to induce another lactation, the implanting of a low cost embryo may be used as a treatment. This has now become commercially feasible and technically achievable for repeat breeders with no uterine or endocrine abnormalities; single step (in straw) embryo thawing, using embryos frozen in ethylene glycol, is used, which allows embryo transfer with little more equipment and skill than that required for AI (May, 1996).

Other factors that can cause failure of fertilization are:

- Service at the wrong time;
- Poor-quality semen;
- Infertile bull;
- Problems with artificial insemination.

These are dealt with elsewhere under Prevention, in Chapter 38 on the bull, or by common sense.

Embryonic death

Although the aetiology of early embryonic death is listed under nine headings (Box 36.7) only non-specific endometritis (already dealt with in Chapter 34), specific metritis caused by *C. fetus* (see p. 582) and a variety of other infections and possibly maternal endocrine environment are suitable for conventional treatment. All the other conditions should be corrected by management improvements or are dealt with in different chapters of this book.

A number of different *Campylobacter* spp. are associated with infertility and abortion in cattle, the speciation and subspeciation of which is complex and currently under review using modern molecular techniques. However, it is clear that the most common isolates associated with fertility problems in the UK are *C. fetus* subsp. *venerealis* and *C. fetus* subsp. *fetus* (Newell *et al.*, 2000). Infection with either of these subspecies should be thought of as a herd problem. In the case of *C. fetus* subsp. *venerealis* the natural habitat of the organism is the bovine reproductive tract and it does not multiply in the intestinal tract; it is thus transmitted only as a venereal disease (Taylor, 2002; see also p. 582).

In the bull, in which infection with *C. fetus* subsp. *venerealis* is limited to the surface of the prepuce and penis, spontaneous cure does occur but is erratic and unreliable. Moreover, if the bull continues natural service of infected cows he will be re-infected as the superficial nature of the infection does not stimulate an immune response in the bull. The organism colonizes the crypts of the preputial epithelium which increase in both size and number as the bull ages. This means that the prepuce of the older bull provides favourable conditions for the persistence of the organism, giving a higher incidence of carrier bulls among those over 5 years of age. Diagnosis and treatment are also more difficult in the older bull (Taylor, 2002).

The usual treatment of the bull involves preputial lavage with streptomycin in a viscous oily medium and parenteral treatment with the same antibiotic. Taylor (2002) recommends daily systemic (e.g. intramuscular) treatment with a combination of streptomycin and dihydrostreptomycin, each at 150 mg per ml as sulphates at a dose rate of 10 mg per kg body weight. Taylor (2002) gives a detailed description of the technique of preputial lavage. It is important that both systemic and local treatments are carried out thoroughly and are repeated daily for three consecutive days. This needs to be combined with further sampling for the organism not less that 30 days after treatment has finished to confirm success of treatment. In a confirmed outbreak of campylobacteriosis, the bulls should be sampled twice, not less than three days and not more than seven days apart, and this should be repeated a

further 30 days later. Taylor (2002) describes in some detail the technique for collecting samples by preputial washing.

Although there is no natural immune response in the bull, one successful form of treatment depends on vaccination (Clark & Dufty, 1982). The vaccine is licensed for use in a number of countries but not in the UK, although one can be made under licence in the UK for specific herds.

Treatment of cows with local or systemic antibiotics is unreliable and because cows develop resistance to the infection it is usually best to wait for this to develop. Whatever course is followed an infected cow should be regarded as potentially infective for at least two gestations after initial infection. Even after this time a few cows may remain infected. As it takes only one cow to infect a bull when natural service is practised, it is clear that it is hazardous to allow natural service of any cows that have ever been infected. Vaccination of cows (where permitted) is widely and fairly effectively practised in range conditions.

On a herd basis, when campylobacteriosis is diagnosed the best advice is that natural service should stop and all services should be by AI using semen from non-infected bulls. Recently infected cows will continue to return to service for some time. In suckler herds where the use of AI to observed natural oestrus may be problematic this approach can be facilitated by the use of repeated oestrous synchronization and fixed-time artificial insemination as described by Penny *et al.* (2000).

There is a management alternative, which is extremely difficult to carry out successfully over a long period and should be advocated only under special circumstances. This is to segregate the herd and use the infected bull(s) on infected cows and AI or non-infected bulls on non-infected cows and heifers. However, this depends on the accurate identification of the infection status of all animals.

Manipulation of the maternal endocrine environment post insemination by the exogenous administration of progesterone or progestagens has been tried as a treatment of repeat breeder cows or where herd conception rates are particularly poor. However, the results of such studies are variable and seem to be affected by the time of progesterone administration and the initial fertility levels. A meta-analysis of 17 progesterone supplementation studies showed that treatment during the first week of pregnancy resulted in an increase in pregnancy rate, especially on farms with poor fertility, while treatment during the second and third weeks of pregnancy gave no overall significant increase (Mann & Lamming, 1999). At the present time treatments of this type cannot be recommended as a means of improving conception rates, and more research is needed to identify suitable hormonal treatment strategies.

An alternative post-insemination treatment involving the administration of GnRH (or GnRH analogues such as buserelin) to the cow around 11 days after insemination has become popular in recent years. In some studies this has been shown to give very good results. For example Sheldon and Dobson (1993) achieved an improved pregnancy rate to first service of approximately 10 per cent. A recent meta-analysis of studies of the effect of GnRH 11–14 days after insemination concluded that while results were not consistent across all studies, there was a significant improvement in pregnancy rate amongst 2541 cows across six studies (Peters *et al.*, 2000). However, post insemination hormonal treatments remain an unpredictable means of improving pregnancy rate on any one given farm, and in most instances resources would probably be better targeted at improving the management of the herd rather than instigating such treatment regimens.

Stage of failure unknown: non-specific endometritis

The two most common therapeutic approaches are (i) promotion of the cow's normal resistance to infection by inducing oestrus and (ii) the use of antibiotics. There is a tendency for spontaneous elimination of the infectious agents from the uterus, most likely due to the cow going through successive periods of oestrus. The current practical approach to treatment is discussed in detail in Chapter 34 (see p. 521).

Prognosis

From the client's point of view successful treatment means that the cow becomes pregnant; this is a two-stage process. Firstly, the cow has to return to normal reproductive function and secondly she has to conceive and remain pregnant. While the first stage is mainly the responsibility of the veterinarian, the second stage often depends on the farmer and farm staff. Where poor husbandry (i.e. feeding, housing or breeding management) is thought to be causing return to service, prognosis must be guarded because it is often a difficult and slow task for the veterinarian to effect a marked improvement.

Results of treatment reported by different workers are rarely comparable because different criteria for selection of cases and assessment of success may have been applied. In many cases self-cure is a phenomenon and because controlled studies are rare, interpretation of results is problematic. Accordingly it is suggested that, as well as reading published reports, clinicians should analyse their own practice records of diagnosis, treatment and outcome.

The most common situation is the cow presented after a few unsuccessful inseminations (or services), which on examination appears to be normal. These *apparently normal repeat breeders* have an expected pregnancy rate at the first service after examination that is about the same as the first service pregnancy rate in the herd, as indicated in Table 36.6.

This is not to say that the factors influencing fertility in first service and repeat breeder cows are the same. In the first service cows, fertility may be affected by closeness to calving and the stress of peak yield. The population returning to service will have overcome these problems, but will include a higher proportion of cows that will never become pregnant. Unfortunately before their ultimate disposal, cows in the last group will have had two or three different treatments and several examinations at regular visits. In most cases there is no reliable way of identifying these problem cows.

Where economics allow the hospitalization and intensive investigation and therapy of repeat breeder cows in referral centres (now very uncommon in the UK), the owner should be given a definite prognosis as soon as possible to minimize the cost involved in keeping and treating cows over several weeks. Much of this cost is due to the fact that once an animal has been served there is little positive that can be done except to monitor changes until pregnancy or non-pregnancy is confirmed. With modern diagnostic methods such as ultrasound scanning it is now possible to reduce the waiting time from service to diagnosis of non-pregnancy to a minimum of 25–30 days, and milk progesterone analysis can be used to give an indication of pregnancy status as early as 19–20 days post service. Other methods of early pregnancy diagnosis such as assays for bovine pregnancy-associated glycoprotein

Table 36.6 Response of apparently normal repeat breeders served without treatment.

Number of cows	Treatment	Percentage pregnant at first AI after examination	Reference
191	None	59.7	de Kruif (1975)
141	None	60.0	Refsdal (1979)

(bPAG) may also be used to speed up pregnancy diagnosis (Skinner *et al.*, 1996). If the prognosis is favourable, costs are reduced if the cow is returned to the owner's farm where the local veterinarian can treat her.

Accurate prognosis with long-term repeat breeder cows is also difficult. The prognosis for natural conception must always be regarded as poor, but particularly so in cases with blocked uterine tubes, persisting endometritis and anomalous steroid hormone production from the ovaries. For example, of 33 chronic repeat breeders treated by Boyd *et al.* (1984) only eight became pregnant. However, the use of embryo transfer techniques to maintain animals for subsequent lactations may offer some hope and has been shown in some studies to give reasonable results. May (1996) reports pregnancy rates in the region of 50 per cent using-single step (in straw) embryo thawing, with embryos frozen in ethylene glycol. Furthermore, nowadays it is also possible to harvest oocytes from valuable animals for *in vitro* production of embryos, and thus offspring, using transvaginal ultrasound-guided oocyte aspiration of ovarian follicles.

The two most commonly diagnosed specific pathological causes of return to service are cystic ovarian disease and purulent endometritis.

Cystic ovarian disease (see p. 526)

In data collected from a number of veterinary practices Bartlett *et al.* (1986b) recorded that culling rate for cows that had cystic ovarian disease was 26.6 per cent, compared with 21.6 per cent for other cows. Cows with cystic ovarian disease that conceived had an interval from calving to conception 33.5 days longer than cows without cystic ovarian disease. More recently cystic ovaries were associated with 6 to 11 more days to first service and with 20 to 30 more days to conception in a meta-analysis of papers published between January 1987 and January 1999 (Fourichon *et al.*, 2000).

In general, three factors affect the outcome:

- The time that has elapsed since calving. Cases of cystic ovaries that occur up to six weeks after calving have a good chance of spontaneous recovery. Cases that are first seen six months after calving have a very poor prognosis.
- The accuracy of diagnosis. If the type of cyst is misdiagnosed, selection of inappropriate treatment may give poor results.
- The aetiology of the condition affects the outcome. If the cyst is caused by a temporary environmental influence such as poor nutrition, then the prognosis is good even without treatment, once this environmental influence is corrected. At the other extreme, if it is one of the minority of cases caused by deficiency of LH receptors in preovulatory dominant follicles, the prognosis may be poor in the short term as this may be the consequence of events occurring up to months previously.

The results presented in Table 36.7, in most of which diagnosis and outcome were checked by progesterone assays, are typical of earlier published field trials. However, these data do not illustrate the ultimate benefit of treatment, which should be measured in terms of calving or treatment to conception intervals and culling rates (see Table 36.8).

Guenzler and Schallenberger (1981) treated 66 cows in which luteal cysts had been diagnosed by rectal palpation. After treatment with an analogue of $PGF_{2\alpha}$, complete luteolysis occurred in the 35 cows with mid-cycle levels of progesterone and all but three of these started normal cycles. The first service pregnancy rate for these cows was 40 per cent. The two groups of cows with lower levels of progesterone cycled erratically after treatment and had first service pregnancy rates of 20 and 24 per cent. Nanda *et al.* (1988) treated 77 luteal cyst cases with an analogue of $PGF_{2\alpha}$ and 65 per cent of these exhibited initial recovery, i.e. the cyst regressed and a corpus luteum formed;

Table 36.7 The treatment of follicular cystic ovarian disease with GnRH.

Number of cows	Type of cyst	Confirmed by progesterone assay	Treatment	Successful result: progesterone rose within 14 days	Reference
104	Follicular	Yes	GnRH	73 (70%)	Nakao *et al.* (1983)
30	Follicular	Yes	GnRH	25 (83%)	Ax *et al.* (1986)
12	Follicular	Yes	None	3 (25%)	Ax *et al.* (1986)
116	Follicular	No	GnRH	61 (53%)	Nanda *et al.* (1988)
55	Follicular	Yes	GnRH	40 (73%)	Booth (1988)
44	Follicular	Yes	hCG + progesterone	32 (73%)	Booth (1988)

Table 36.8 Fertility parameters of cows treated for follicular and luteal ovarian cysts (mean ± SE).

	Treatment (*n* cows)	Follicular cysts	Matched controls	Treatment (*n* cows)	Luteal cysts	Matched controls
Calving to conception (days)[a]	PRID (*n* = 22)	93 ± 27	90 ± 37	PRID (*n* = 14)	132 ± 49	93 ± 52
Treatment to conception (days)[a]	PRID (*n* = 22)	24 ± 19		PRID (*n* = 14)	60 ± 67	
Culling rate (%)[a]	PRID (*n* = 22)	41	4	PRID (*n* = 14)	11	7
Calving to conception (days)[b]	GnRH (*n* = 16)	82 ± 7	70 ± 6	$PGF_{2\alpha}$ (*n* = 22)	141 ± 15	68 ± 9
Treatment to conception (days)[b]	GnRH (*n* = 16)	48 ± 9		$PGF_{2\alpha}$ (*n* = 22)	20 ± 5	
Culling rate (%)[b]	GnRH (*n* = 16)	44		$PGF_{2\alpha}$ (*n* = 22)	9	
Calving to conception (days)[b]	PRID (*n* = 21)	125 ± 17	70 ± 6			
Treatment to conception (days)[b]	PRID (*n* = 21)	33 ± 8				
Culling rate (%)[b]	PRID (*n* = 21)	29				

[a] From Douthwaite and Dobson (2000).
[b] From Tebble *et al.* (2001).

not all became pregnant and in 18 per cent the cyst recurred.

More recent results from Douthwaite and Dobson (2000) and Tebble *et al.* (2001) are summarized in Table 36.8. In these studies the overall interval from calving to conception was significantly greater than that of matched controls irrespective of cyst type or treatment. Cows treated for luteal cysts took significantly longer to get in calf than those treated for follicular cysts, again irrespective of treatment. Cows treated for follicular cysts had a higher culling rate than those with luteal cysts. It would seem that at least in the herds used in these studies, farmers and veterinarians were prepared to persevere with cows diagnosed with luteal cysts, even at the expense of an extended calving to conception interval, whereas cows with follicular cysts tended to be culled earlier.

Purulent endometritis/metritis (see pp. 519, 521)

Ott and Gustafsson (1981) reviewed reports on over 600 cases and showed that in 85 per cent the uterus was emptied within a few days of treatment with $PGF_{2\alpha}$ or an analogue. In most reports the authors stated that pregnancy rate after successful treatment was lower than in normal cows. Time from treatment to conception was about 75 days.

Factors that affect prognosis have been quantified by Anderson (1985) who modified a system proposed by Studer and Morrow (1978), which was based on a careful analysis of clinical and laboratory observations. Anderson took into account (i) the time since calving, (ii) whether oestrus had occurred since calving, (iii) the amount of pus, (iv) the size of the cervix and (v) the diameter of the larger affected horn. By giving points for these factors a cumulative score was calculated that gave a useful prediction about the eventual outcome of the case. Cows that had been in oestrus had a poor prognosis, presumably because they had not responded to the normal defence mechanism.

Pepper and Dobson (1987) found that the relative amount of pus in the discharge gave a (non-significant) indication of the pregnancy rate after treatment and that time from calving to treatment was significantly related to pregnancy rate after treatment. Cows treated with $PGF_{2\alpha}$ or oestrogen within 40 days of calving had a pregnancy rate of about 55 per cent compared with a significantly poorer result for cows treated later. From Anderson's (1985) data it appeared that in successfully treated cows there was a high incidence of periparturient problems at the resultant calving and a very high culling rate in this group of animals in the year after treatment, observations that warrant further study. The treatment and control of endometritis and metritis are discussed in more detail in Chapter 34.

As regards the outlook for herds with a return-to-service problem prognosis varies and obviously is related to the diagnosis. Some episodes of herd infertility are of short duration and normal fertility returns spontaneously.

In cases where a definite infectious cause is identified, such as campylobacteriosis, the outcome can be completely satisfactory with the elimination of the infection and the return to a normal herd pregnancy rate. This depends on treatment being carried out carefully and the subsequent control of breeding management being optimized.

Where the problem is related to poor husbandry caution should be expressed until clear signs of improved management are noted.

Prevention

Improvement in pregnancy rates is achieved by encouraging good husbandry and avoiding factors that have an adverse effect on fertility. While it is possible to achieve a very high fertilization rate (up to 100 per cent), some embryonic death is inevitable, which is why it is rare for a herd to achieve a pregnancy rate of greater than 70 per cent.

There are a number of items, listed below, which contribute to good fertility, but deficiency in any one of these is likely to produce poor pregnancy rates.

(1) Accurate heat detection.
(2) Proper nutrition and maintenance of suitable body condition before and after calving.
(3) Avoidance of dystokia and post partum abnormalities and timely veterinary intervention where indicated. This should reduce the incidence of delayed involution, non-specific endometritis (Chapter 34), blocked uterine tubes, cystic ovarian disease, etc. (see Chapter 34).
(4) The proper use of records can help to achieve a good pregnancy rate and to avoid long interservice intervals. This is done by:
    (a) not serving cows too soon after calving (not before 42 days);
    (b) being aware of the expected return-to-service date (for example, by using a three-week calendar);
    (c) ensuring early pregnancy diagnosis via transrectal ultrasound and milk progesterone assays;

(d) checking the fertility of the bulls;
(e) checking the efficiency of the inseminators, and the quality of the semen used;
(f) understanding the causes of fertility variations in a specific herd.
(5) Avoidance of service contact outside the herd and ensuring veterinary examination, isolation and testing of bought-in breeding stock, especially bulls will reduce the risk of introducing venereal diseases and other diseases affecting fertility. (See also Chapter 57 for a more in-depth discussion of biosecurity.)
(6) Good housing environment and cattle handling will help to avoid stress, lameness, discomfort and fear in the herd.
(7) Consideration should be given to reproductive dysfunction with a hereditary component, e.g. cystic ovarian disease.
(8) Interventions that may cause embryonic death should be avoided, such as drastic changes in feeding and environment, herd medication and the administration of vaccines in the weeks after service. In the case of vaccines the manufacturer's recommendations should always be followed.
(9) Drug therapy, using either antibiotics or hormones, in the post partum phase has been advocated as a way of improving pregnancy rates. The doubtful value of this is discussed below.

Where specific drug therapy is applied selectively in cows identified as likely to have poor fertility this is obviously a suitable approach. However, it has been proposed that routine treatments should be applied to all cows, normal and abnormal, and this is much more questionable. For example in one study post partum administration of $PGF_{2\alpha}$ 21 days after calving reduced the interval to first oestrus and first service by about 10 days. Pregnancy rates to first service were increased and the number of services to conceptions was reduced from 2.0 to 1.3 (Schofield et al., 1999). However, a number of trials have given conflicting results. Meta-analysis of 24 trials where $PGF_{2\alpha}$ was administered to cattle within 40 days of calving reported no beneficial effect on first service pregnancy rate, although there was a small reduction in days open for treated cows (Burton & Lean, 1995). It is now becoming socially unacceptable to administer hormonal products to cattle as 'routine' treatments, and some sectors of the industry such as organic milk producers and many consumers would rather that hormone preparations were not used at all, or that their use were restricted to individual cows with particular problems that cannot be treated by any other means.

The routine use of antibiotics in both normal and abnormal cows after calving or at the time of insemination should be strongly discouraged; results have shown no benefit to normal cows. Antibiotic usage should be restricted to those animals where there is a specific therapeutic indication, and where failure to treat may compromise the animal's welfare.

In order to overcome problems with oestrous detection, oestrous synchronization and fixed time AI may be employed; Lane et al. (2001) have reviewed methods of synchronization. The technique is best suited for dairy heifers and beef suckler cows. For best results the farmer, the veterinary surgeon and a member of the insemination organization should discuss the whole operation well beforehand. The best results are obtained when only reproductively normal cows at least six weeks after calving (preferably longer) or maiden heifers are included, although it is possible to synchronize cows that have had a shortened post partum period (Penny et al., 2000; Penny & Lowman, 2002). First calvers and animals in poor body condition tend to give poor results and may need additional hormones such as equine chorionic gonadotrophin and nutritional treatments. Results following synchronization of dairy cows can be satisfactory (Biggadike & Mawhinney, 1996; Jobst et al., 2000) and cost-effective (Esslemont & Mawhinney, 1996), but currently still need inseminations at observed oestrus for optimal results. Stress and any change in management and diet should be avoided during preparation and for three to four weeks after insemination. As far as possible other interventions such as vaccination should be avoided during the same period. Some of the oestrous synchronization regimens may be used for the repeat synchronization of cows not in calf to the first service (Penny et al., 2000; McDougall, 2001; Penny & Lowman, 2002); this allows repeated fixed time insemination. However, if repeat synchronization is not to be used it is essential that preparation is made to deal with the cows that return to oestrus, such as an intensive period of heat detection approximately 19–24 days after the initial service. If natural service is to be used on these returns it is essential that the 'sweeper bull' is not presented with an excessive number of cows in oestrus over a very short period of time (see Chapter 38).

References

Anderson, D.B. (1985) A clinical study of chronic endometritis in dairy cows. MVM thesis, Glasgow University.

Andersson, L., Gustafsson, A.H. & Emanuelson, U. (1991) Effect of hyperketonaemia and feeding on fertility in dairy cows. Theriogenology, 36, 521–36.

Austin, E.J., Mihm, M., Ryan, M.P., Williams, D.H. & Roche, J.F. (1999) Effect of duration of dominance of the ovulatory follicle on onset of estrus and fertility in heifers. Journal of Animal Science, 77, 2219–26.

Ax, R.L., Bellin, M.E., Scheinder, D.X. & Haase-Hardie, J.A. (1986) Reproductive performance of dairy cows with cystic ovaries following administration of Procystin TM1. Journal of Dairy Science, 69, 542–5.

Ayalon, N. (1978) A review of embryonic mortality in cattle. Journal of Reproduction and Fertility, 54, 483–93.

Bane, A. (1964) Fertility and reproductive disorders in Swedish cattle. British Veterinary Journal, 120, 430–41.

Barrett, D.C. (2001) Cattle fertility management in the UK. Cattle Practice, 9, 59–68.

Bartlett, P.C., Kirk, J.H., Wilke, M.A., Kaneene, L.B. & Mather, E.C. (1986a) Metritis complex in Michigan Holstein–Friesian cattle: incidence, descriptive epidemiology and estimated economic impact. Preventive Veterinary Medicine, 4, 235–48.

Bartlett, P.C., Ngategize, P.K., Kancene, J.B., Kirk, J.H., Anderson, S.M. & Mather, E.C. (1986b) Cystic follicular disease in Michigan Holstein–Friesian cattle: incidence, descriptive epidemiology and estimated economic impact. Preventive Veterinary Medicine, 4, 15–33.

Beghelli, V., Boiti, C., Parmigiani, E. & Barbacini, S. (1986) Pregnancy diagnosis and embryonic mortality in the cow. In Embryonic Mortality in Farm Animals (ed. by L.M. Sreenan & M.G. Diskin), pp. 159–67. Nijhoff, Dordrecht/Boston/Lancaster.

Biggadike, H. & Mawhinney, I. (1996) Planned breeding routine in dairy cows using a treatment regimen involving GnRH and PGF$_{2\alpha}$. A multi site study (interim report). Cattle Practice, 4, 289–91.

Bon-Durant, R. (1997) Pathogenesis, diagnosis and management of trichomoniasis in cattle. Veterinary Clinics of North America: Food Animal Practice, 13, 345–61.

Booth, J.M. (1988) The milk progesterone test as an aid to the diagnosis of cystic ovaries in dairy cows. Veterinary Record, 123, 437–9.

Boyd, H. & Reed, H.C.B. (1961a) Investigations into the incidence and causes of infertility in dairy cattle – Fertility variations. British Veterinary Journal, 117, 18–35.

Boyd, H. & Reed, H.C.B. (1961b) Investigations into the incidence and causes of infertility in dairy cattle – influence of some management factors affecting the semen and insemination conditions. British Veterinary Journal, 117, 74–86.

Boyd, H., Renton, J., Munro, C., Harvey, M., Isbister, J. & Kelly, E. (1984) Clinical studies of a series of long (term) repeat breeder cows and heifers. Vlaams Diergeneeskundig Tijdschrift, 53, 165–9.

Britt, J.H. (1995) Relationship between postpartum nutrition, weight loss and fertility. Cattle Practice, 3, 79–83.

Burton, N.R. & Lean, I.J. (1995) Investigation by meta-analysis of the effect of prostaglandin F$_{2\alpha}$ administered post partum on the reproductive performance of dairy cattle. Veterinary Record, 136, 90–4.

Clark, B.L. & Dufty, J.H. (1982) The duration of protection against infection with Campylobacter fetus subsp. venerealis in immunised bulls. Australian Veterinary Journal, 58, 220.

Clark, B.L., Dufty, J.H. & Parsonson, I.M. (1986) The frequency of infertility and abortion in cows infected with Trichomonas fetus var. brisbane. Australian Veterinary Journal, 63, 31–2.

Claus, R., Karg, H., Zwiauer, D., von Butler, I., Pirchner, F. & Rattenberger, E. (1983) Analysis of factors influencing reproductive performance of the dairy cow by progesterone assay in milk fat. *British Veterinary Journal*, **139**, 29–37.

Coleman, D.A., Thayne, W.V. & Dailey, R.A. (1985) Factors affecting reproductive performance of dairy cows. *Journal of Dairy Science*, **68**, 1793–803.

Cook, D.L., Smith, C.A., Parfet, J.R., Youngquist, R.S., Brown, E.M. & Garverick, H.A. (1990) Fate and turnover rate of ovarian follicular cysts in dairy cattle. *Journal of Reproduction and Fertility*, **90**, 37–46.

Curtis, C.R., Erb, H.N., Sniffen, C.J., Smith, R.D. & Kronfield, D.S. (1985) Path analysis of dry period nutrition, postpartum metabolic and reproductive disorders, and mastitis in Holstein cows. *Journal of Dairy Science*, **68**, 2347–60.

Dobson, H., Douthwaite, R., Nobel, K.M., O'Donnell, M.J., Ribadu, A.Y., Tebble, J.E. & Ward, W.R. (2001a) Cystic ovaries in cattle. *Cattle Practice*, **9**, 185–9.

Dobson, H. & Nanda, A.S. (1992) Reliability of cyst diagnosis and effect of energy status on LH release by oestradiol or GnRH in cows with ovarian cysts. *Theriogenology*, **37**, 465–72.

Dobson, H., Tebble, J.E., Smith, R.F. & Ward, W.R. (2001b) Is stress really all that important? *Theriogenology*, **55**, 65–73.

Dohoo, I.R. & Martin, S.W. (1984a) Disease, production and culling in Holstein–Friesian cows. III. Disease and production as determinates of disease. *Preventive Veterinary Medicine*, **2**, 671–90.

Dohoo, I.R. & Martin, S.W. (1984b) Disease, production and culling in Holstein–Friesian cows. IV. Effects of disease on production. *Preventive Veterinary Medicine*, **2**, 755–70.

Dohoo, I.R., Martin, S.W., McMillan, I. & Kennedy, B.W. (1984) Disease, production and culling in Holstein–Friesian cows. II. Age, season and sire effects. *Preventive Veterinary Medicine*, **2**, 655–70.

Doig, P.A., Rulinke, H.L., Mackay, A.L. & Palmer, N.C. (1979) Bovine granular vulvitis associated with *Ureaplasma* infection. *Canadian Veterinary Journal*, **20**, 89–94.

Douthwaite, R. & Dobson, H. (2000) Comparison of different methods of diagnosis of cystic ovarian disease in cattle and an assessment of its treatment with a progesterone-releasing intravaginal device. *Veterinary Record*, **147**, 355–9.

Esslemont, R.J. & Kossaibati, M.A. (1997) Culling in 50 dairy herds in England. *Veterinary Record*, **140**, 36–9.

Esslemont, R.J. & Mawhinney, I. (1996) The cost benefit of a planned breeding routine for dairy cows (Ovsync/Intercept). *Cattle Practice*, **4**, 293–300.

Fathalla, M.A., Geissinger, H.D. & Liptrap, R.M. (1978) Effect of endometrial damage and prostaglandin $F_{2\alpha}$ on experimental cystic ovarian follicles in the cow. *Research in Veterinary Science*, **25**, 269–79.

Fourichon, C., Seegers, H. & Malher, X. (2000) Effect of disease on reproduction in the dairy cow: a meta-analysis. *Theriogenology*, **53**, 1729–59.

Franco, O.L., Drost, M., Thatcher, M.J., Shille, V.M. & Thatcher, W.W. (1987) Fetal survival in the cow after pregnancy diagnosis by palpation per rectum. *Theriogenology*, **27**, 631–43.

Fredriksson, G. (1984) Some reproductive and clinical aspects of endotoxins in cows with special emphasis on the role of prostaglandins. *Acta Veterinaria Scandinavica*, **25**, 365–77.

Garnsworthy, P.C. & Webb, R. (2000) Nutritional influences on fertility in dairy cows. *Cattle Practice*, **8**, 401–405.

Garverick, H.A. (1997) Ovarian follicular cysts in dairy cows. *Journal of Dairy Science*, **80**, 995–1004.

Grahn, T.C., Fahning, M.L. & Zeinjanis, R. (1984) Nature of early reproductive failure caused by bovine viral diarrhea virus. *Journal of the American Veterinary Medical Association*, **185**, 429–32.

Guenzler, O. & Schallenberger, E. (1981) The treatment of ovarian cysts in cattle with prostaglandins – possibilities and limitations. *Acta Veterinaria Scandinavica*, **77** (Suppl.), 327–41.

Guerin, B., Nibart, M., Marquant-Le Guienne, B. & Humblot P. (1997) Sanitary risks related to embryo transfer in domestic species. *Theriogenology*, **47**, 33–42.

Gustafsson, A.H. & Emanuelson, U. (1996) Milk acetone concentrations as an indicator of hyperketonaemia in dairy cows: the critical value revised. *Animal Science*, **63**, 183–8.

Hancock, L.L. (1948) The clinical analysis of reproductive failure in cattle. *Veterinary Record*, **60**, 513–17.

Henricson, B. (1957) Genetical and statistical investigations into so-called cystic ovaries in cattle. *Acta Agriculturae Scandinavica*, **7**, 3–93.

Howells, H.M.J., Davies, D.A.R. & Dobson, H. (1999) Influence of the number of days spent training in an abattoir with access to live cows on the efficiency of do-it-yourself artificial insemination. *Veterinary Record*, **144**, 310–14.

Hunter, R.H.F. (1999) Pre-fertilisation events and the fate of bovine spermatozoa in the female genital tract. *Cattle Practice*, **7**, 261–6.

Jackson, P.S., Johnson, C.T., Bulman, D.C. & Holdsworth, R.J. (1979) A study of cloprostenol-induced oestrus and spontaneous oestrus by means of the milk progesterone assay. *British Veterinary Journal*, **135**, 578–90.

Jasko, D.J., Erb, H.N., White, M.E. & Smith, R.D. (1984) Prostaglandin treatment and subsequent cystic ovarian disease in Holstein cows. *Journal of the American Veterinary Medical Association*, **185**, 212–13.

Jobst, S.M., Nebel, R.L., McGilliard, M.L. & Pelzer, K.D. (2000) Evaluation of reproductive performance in lactating dairy cows with prostaglandin $F_{2\alpha}$, gonadotrophin-releasing hormone, and timed artificial insemination. *Journal of Dairy Science*, **83**, 2366–72.

Kastelic, J.P. (1994) Noninfectious embryonic loss in cattle. *Veterinary Medicine*, **89**, 584–9.

Kessy, B.M. & Noakes, D.E. (1979) Determination of patency of fallopian tubes in the cow by means of phenosulphon-phthalein and starch grain tests. *Veterinary Record*, **105**, 414–20.

Kossaibati, M.A. & Esslemont, R.J. (1995) *Wastage in Dairy Herds*. Report No. 4 DAISY – The Dairy Information System. Department of Agriculture, University of Reading.

Kruif A. de (1975) Fertiliteit en subfertiliteit Nj het vrouwelijk rand. Thesis, Utrecht.

Laitinen, E.R., Tenhunen, M., Haenninen, O. & Alanko, M. (1985) Milk progesterone in Finnish dairy cows: a field study on the control of artificial insemination and early pregnancy. *British Veterinary Journal*, **141**, 297–307.

Lamming, G.E. & Darwash, A.O. (1998) The use of milk progesterone profiles to characterise components of subfertility in milked dairy cows. *Animal Reproduction Science*, **52**, 175–90.

Lane, E.A., Austin, E.J. & Crowe, M.A. (2001) Oestrous synchronisation in cattle. *Cattle Practice*, **9**, 211–15.

Loeffler, S.H., Vries, M.J. de & Schukken, Y.H. (1999) The effect of time of disease occurrence, milk yield, and body condition on fertility of dairy cows. *Journal of Dairy Science*, **82**, 2589–604.

McDougall S. (2001) Reproductive performance of anovulatory anoestrus postpartum dairy cows following treatment with two progesterone and oestradiol benzoate-based protocols, with or without resynchrony. *New Zealand Veterinary Journal*, **49**, 187–94.

McGowan, M.R. & Kirkland, P.D. (1995) Early reproductive loss due to bovine pestivirus infection. *British Veterinary Journal*, **151**, 263–70.

Mann, G.E. (1997) Early pregnancy in the cow. *Cattle Practice*, **5**, 349–51.

Mann, G.E. & Lamming, G.E. (1995) Progesterone inhibition of the development of the luteolytic signal in cows. *Journal of Reproduction and Fertility*, **104**, 1–5.

Mann, G.E. & Lamming, G.E. (1999) The influence of progesterone during early pregnancy in cattle. *Reproduction in Domestic Animals*, **34**, 269–74.

Mann, G.E. & Lamming, G.E. (2001) Relationship between maternal endocrine environment, early embryo development and inhibition of the luteolytic mechanism in cows. *Reproduction*, **121**, 175–80.

May, P.J. (1996) In straw thaw bovine embryos: new opportunities. *Cattle Practice*, **4**, 237–40.

Mihm, M., Baguisi, A., Boland, M.P. & Roche, J.F. (1994) Association between the duration of dominance of the ovulatory follicle and pregnancy rate in beef heifers. *Journal of Reproduction and Fertility*, **102**, 123–30.

Morrow, D.A. (1986) *Current Therapy in Theriogenology 2. Diagnosis, Treatment and Prevention of Reproductive Diseases in Small and Large Animals*, pp. 1–143. W.B. Saunders, Philadelphia.

Nakao, T., Shirakawa, J., Tsurubayashi, M., Oboshi, K., Abe, T., Sawarmikai, Y., Sago, N., Tsunoda, N. & Kawata, K. (1984) A preliminary report on the treatment of ovulation failure in cows with gonadotrophin-releasing hormone analog or human chorionic gonadotrophin combined with insemination. *Animal Reproduction Science*, **7**, 489–95.

Nakao, T., Sugiliashi, A., Saga, N., Tsunoda, N. & Kawata, K. (1983) Use of milk progesterone enzyme immuno-assay for differential diagnosis of follicular cyst, luteal cyst and corpus luteum in cows. *American Journal of Veterinary Research*, **44**, 888–90.

Nanda, A.S., Ward, W.R. & Dobson, H. (1989) Treatment of cystic ovarian disease in cattle – an update. *Veterinary Bulletin*, **59**, 537–56.

Nanda, A.S., Ward, W.R., Williams, P.C.W. & Dobson, H. (1988) Retrospective analysis of the efficacy of different hormone treatments of cystic ovarian disease in cattle. *Veterinary Record*, **122**, 155–8.

Newell, D.G., Duim, B., van Bergen, M.A.P., Grogono-Thomas, R. & Wagenaar, J.A. (2000) Speciation, subspeciation and subtyping of *Campylobacter* spp. associated with bovine infection and abortion. *Cattle Practice*, **8**, 421–5.

O'Callaghan, D. & Boland, M.P. (1999) Nutritional effects on ovulation, embryo development and the establishment of pregnancy in ruminants. *Animal Science*, **68**, 299–314.

O'Callaghan, D., Lozanot, J.M., Fahey, J., Gath, V., Snijders, S. & Boland, M.P. (2000) Recent developments in the effect of nutrition on fertility in dairy cows. *Irish Veterinary Journal*, **53**, 417–25.

Okuda, K., Kito, S., Sumi, N. & Sato, K. (1988) A study of the central cavity in the bovine corpus luteum. *Veterinary Record*, **123**, 180–3.

Oltner, R. & Edqvist, L.E. (1981) Progesterone in defatted milk: its relation to insemination and pregnancy in normal cows as compared with cows on problem farms and individual problem animals. *British Veterinary Journal*, **137**, 78–87.

Ott, R.S. & Gustafsson, B.K. (1981) Therapeutic application of prostaglandins for post partum infections. *Acta Veterinaria Scandinavica*, **77** (Suppl), 363–9.

Peeler, E.J., Otte, M.J. & Esslemont, R.J. (1994) Interrelationships of periparturient diseases in dairy cows. *Veterinary Record*, **134**, 129–32.

Penny, C.D. & Lowman, B.G. (2002) Mating beef cows without natural service – a triple synchronisation system. *Cattle Practice*, **10**, 23–6.

Penny, C.D., Lowman, B.G., Scott, N.A. & Scott, P.R. (2000) Repeated oestrus synchronisation of beef cows with progesterone implants and the effects of a gonadotrophin-releasing hormone agonist at implant insertion. *Veterinary Record*, **146**, 395–8.

Pepper, R.T. & Dobson, H. (1987) Preliminary results of treatment and endocrinology of chronic endometritis in the dairy cow. *Veterinary Record*, **120**, 53–6.

Peters, A.R., Martinez, T.A. & Cook, A.J.C. (2000) A meta-analysis of studies of the effect of GnRH 11–14 days after insemination on pregnancy rates in cattle. *Theriogenology*, **54**, 1317–26.

Refsdal, A.O. (1979) Undersoekelse av kviger og kyr utsjaltet paa grunn av ufruktbarhet. Thesis, Oslo.

Reid, I.M., Roberts, C.J. & Manston, R. (1979) Fatty liver and infertility in high-yielding dairy cows. *Veterinary Record*, **104**, 75–6.

Robinson, R.S., Mann, G.E., Lamming, G.E. & Wathes, D.C. (1999) The effect of pregnancy on the expression of uterine oxytocin, oestrogen and progesterone receptors during early pregnancy in the cow. *Journal of Endocrinology*, **160**, 21–33.

Rowlands, G.J., Lucey, S. & Russell, A.M. (1986) Susceptibility to disease in the dairy cow and its relationship with occurrences of other diseases in the current or preceding lactation. *Preventive Veterinary Medicine*, **4**, 223–34.

Royal, M.D., Darwash, A.O., Flint, A.P.F., Webb, R., Woolliams, J.A. & Lamming, G.E. (2000) Declining fertility in dairy cattle: changes in traditional and endocrine parameters of fertility. *Animal Science*, **70**, 487–501.

Saloniemi, H., Groehn, Y. & Syvaejaervi, J. (1986) An epidemiological and genetic study on registered diseases in

Finnish Ayrshire cattle. II. Reproductive disorders. *Acta Veterinaria Scandinavica*, **27**, 196–208.

Savio, J.D., Boland, M.P., Hynes, N. & Roche J.F. (1990) Resumption of follicular activity in the early post-partum period of dairy cows. *Journal of Reproduction and Fertility*, **88**, 569–79.

Schermerhorn, E.C., Foote, R.H., Newman, S.K. & Smith R.D. (1986) Reproductive practices and results in dairies using owners or professional inseminators. *Journal of Dairy Science*, **69**, 1673–85.

Schofield, S.A., Kitwood, S.E. & Phillips, C.J.C. (1999) The effects of a *post partum* injection of prostaglandin F$_{2\alpha}$ on return to oestrus and pregnancy rates in dairy cows. *The Veterinary Journal*, **157**, 172–7.

Sheldon, I.M. (1999) Bovine endometritis: a review. *Journal of Animal Breeding*, **2**, 2–14.

Sheldon, I.M. & Dobson, H. (1993) Effects of gonadotrophin releasing hormone administered 11 days after insemination on the pregnancy rate of cattle to the first and later services. *Veterinary Record*, **133**, 160–3.

Singh, E.L. (1987) The disease control potential of embryos. *Theriogenology*, **27**, 9–20.

Skinner, J.G., Gray, D., Gebbie, F.E., Beckers, J-F. & Sulon, J. (1996) Field evaluation of pregnancy diagnosis using bovine pregnancy-associated glycoprotein (bPAG). *Cattle Practice*, **4**, 281–4.

Sreenan, J.M. & Diskin, M.G. (1986) The extent and timing of embryonic mortality in cattle. In *Embryonic Mortality in Farm Animals* (ed. by J.M. Sreenan & M.G. Diskin). Nijhoff, Dordrecht/Boston/Lancaster.

Sreenan, J.M., Leese, H.J., Morris, D.G. & Dunne, L. (1999) Early embryo development and survival in cattle. *Cattle Practice*, **7**, 267–70.

Stolla, R., Bostedt, H., Wendt, V. & Leidl, W. (1980) Zur Ovarialzyste des Rindes. III. Vergleichende Wertung von Therapieverfahren. *Berliner und Muenchner Tieraerztliche Wochenschrift*, **93**, 4–10.

Stringfellow, D.A. & Wrathall, A.E. (1995) Epidemiological implications of the production and transfer of IVF embryos. *Theriogenology*, **43**, 89–96.

Studer, E. & Morrow, D.A. (1978) Postpartum evaluation of bovine reproductive potential: comparison of findings from genital tract examination per rectum, uterine culture and endometrial biopsy. *Journal of the American Veterinary Medical Association*, **172**, 489–94.

Sturman, H., Oltenacu, E.A.B. & Foote, R.H. (2000) Importance of inseminating only cows in estrus. *Theriogenology*, **53**, 1657–67.

Taylor, A.J. (2002) Venereal Campylobacter infection in cattle. *Cattle Practice*, **10**, 35–42.

Tebble, J.E., O'Donnell, M.J. & Dobson, H. (2001) Ultrasound diagnosis and treatment outcome of cystic ovaries in cattle. *Veterinary Record*, **148**, 411–13.

Trimberger, G.W. (1948) Breeding efficiency in dairy cattle from artificial insemination at various intervals before and after ovulation. University of Nebraska College of Agriculture, Agricultural Experimental Station, Research Bulletin 153.

Wagner, W.C. & Li, P.S. (1982) Influence of adrenal corticosteroids on postpartum pituitary and ovarian function. In *Factors Influencing Fertility in the Postpartum Cow* (ed. by H. Karg & E. Schallenberger), pp. 197–219. Nijhoff, The Hague.

Warren, M.E. (1984) Biological targets for fertility and their effects on herd economics. In *Dairy Cow Fertility* (ed. by R.G. Eddy & M.A. Ducker), pp. 1–14. British Veterinary Association, London.

Wathes, D.C., Robinson, R.S., Pushpakumara, A., Cheng, Z. & Abayasekara, D.R.E. (1998) Nutritional effects on reproductive performance in dairy cows. *Cattle Practice*, **6**, 371–7.

Watson, E.D., Jones, P.C. & Saunders, R.W. (1987) Effect of factors associated with insemination on calving rate in dairy cows. *Veterinary Record*, **121**, 256–8.

Watson, E.D. & MacDonald, B.J. (1984) Failure of conception in dairy cattle: progesterone and oestradiol-17β concentrations and the presence of ovarian follicles in relation to the timing of artificial insemination. *British Veterinary Journal*, **140**, 398–406.

Watson, E.D. & Munro, C.D. (1984) Adrenal progesterone production in the cow. *British Veterinary Journal*, **140**, 300–306.

Webb, R., Garnsworthy, P.C., Gong, J.G., Gutierrez, C.G., Logue, D., Crawshaw, W.M. & Robinson, J.J. (1997) Nutritional influence on subfertility in cattle. *Cattle Practice*, **5**, 361–7.

Webb, R., Royal, M.D., Gong, J.G. & Garnsworthy, P.C. (1999) The influence of nutrition on fertility. *Cattle Practice*, **7**, 227–34.

Whitaker, D.A., Kelly, J.M. & Smith, S. (2000) Disposal and disease rates in 340 British dairy herds. *Veterinary Record*, **146**, 363–7.

Wolfenson, D., Roth, Z. & Meidan, R. (2000) Impaired reproduction in heat-stressed cattle: basic and applied aspects. *Animal Reproduction Science*, **60/61**, 535–47.

Wrathall, A.E. (1995) Embryo transfer and disease transmission in livestock: a review of recent research. *Theriogenology*, **43**, 81–8.

Chapter 37
Fetal Loss

G. Caldow and D. Gray

Introduction	577
Pathophysiology	577
Placentitis	578
Causes of abortion	578
Viral causes of abortion	578
Bovine viral diarrhoea (BVDV)	578
Bovine herpes virus 1 (BHV1)	579
Other viruses	579
Bacterial causes of abortion	580
Brucellosis	580
Leptospirosis	580
Bacillus licheniformis	581
Listeria monocytogenes	581
Salmonellosis	582
Campylobacter	582
Miscellaneous bacteria	584
Protozoal causes of abortion	584
Trichomoniasis	584
Neosporosis	584
Other infectious agents causing abortion	586
Chlamydia and rickettsia	586
Mycotic abortion	586
Non-infectious causes of abortion	586
Investigation	587
Conclusion	589

Introduction

The failure of the cow to carry a calf to full term or to produce a live calf causes financial loss through disruption of the normal pattern of milk production, the loss of genetic material or an absolute loss in output for the beef cow. These losses can have a profound effect at the herd level. For example, neosporosis has been reported to cause abortion rates of 26 per cent (Wouda *et al.*, 1999). Losses on this scale may be relatively unusual, but annual losses of 10 per cent are not uncommon. Assessing the scale of these losses is made difficult by the definitions used and the differing clinical manifestations. In Britain abortion is described as the birth of a live or dead calf before 271 days' gestation and stillbirth as the production of a dead calf after 272 days of gestation (Noakes, 1986). However, agents that infect the conceptus, such as bovine viral diarrhoea virus (McGowan & Kirkland, 1995) or leptospira organisms (Bolin & Alt, 1998) can cause embryonic death or death that occurs shortly after birth. Such embryonic loss or early abortion is difficult to detect and increased neonatal mortality may not be immediately associated with disease processes that affect the fetus.

It is also important to define what is normal or unavoidable loss. Spontaneous chromosomal abnormalities are commonly held to account for the bulk of unavoidable wastage and a loss of 20 per cent of embryos by day 45 of gestation has been estimated (Roche *et al.*, 1981). After this period losses are far lower: an abortion rate of 6.5 per cent was calculated by Forar *et al.* (1995) who reviewed 26 published studies. Stillbirth losses of 4 to 6 per cent have been quoted (Miller, 1988) and a study of more than 2000 beef cow calvings found a mortality rate of 4.5 per cent within 24 hours of birth (Nix *et al.*, 1998). In contrast, the target used in beef production in Britain for live calves born is 94 per cent (MLC, 1998) and the estimate of 1.9 to 2.0 per cent losses after day 42 of gestation (Sreenan & Diskin, 1986) may be a more realistic target for unavoidable fetal loss. This is further supported by a survey of Irish dairy cows that found an abortion rate of 1.7 per cent (Mee, 1992). From this it would seem justifiable to use an interference level of 3 per cent for abortions or losses after confirmation of pregnancy at around 6 weeks and one of 2 per cent for deaths at parturition and in the neonatal period.

Pathophysiology

The clinical manifestation of disease of the conceptus is largely the consequence of the stage of development when exposure to the agent occurs (McGowan & Kirkland, 1995), the difference in virulence between strains of recognized fetal pathogens (Dubovi, 1992) and the degree and duration of exposure in the case of non-infectious causes. The corpus luteum is necessary for maintenance in the first half of gestation (Wendorf *et al.*, 1983) and destruction of the corpus luteum during that time will usually result in the termination of pregnancy and the expulsion of a fresh fetus and membranes. However, fetal death may either cause lysis of the corpus luteum and the expulsion of an autolysed fetus some days later or the corpus luteum may persist and the fetus and membranes then undergo mummification. If bacterial infection is present maceration of the fetus is the result. As a consequence, early abortions are rarely observed and when they are the advanced autolysis limits the examinations that can be carried out.

The fetus and placenta maintain the pregnancy in the later stages. Fetal death removes this support and abortion follows after a period of a few days. Autolytic change is a feature in these cases too, characterized by the presence of bloody fluid in the body cavities (Dillman & Dennis, 1976) and a loss of microscopic cell detail. However, fetal death is not the only consequence of disease processes affecting the fetus and placenta. Fetal stress primarily due to anoxia will trigger the steroid response necessary for normal parturition (Knickerbocker et al., 1986) and a relatively fresh fetus can be expelled in these circumstances; indeed, calves may be born alive and survive from day 260. Signs of prolonged fetal stress include staining of the perineum by meconium and inhalation or ingestion of meconium.

Placentitis

Placentitis is the principal lesion in several infectious disease processes associated with fetal loss, and in cattle the placenta is often retained after abortion in the second half of gestation. The precise reasons for placental retention are not known, but this is a further factor limiting the investigation of many cases.

Causes of abortion

A wide range of infectious and non-infectious causes of abortion have been reported, many of which are associated with only occasional or sporadic fetal loss. The following discussion concentrates on the more prevalent conditions in British herds, with only occasional reference to exotic causes.

Viral causes of abortion

Bovine viral diarrhoea (BVDV) (see p. 853)

Laboratory diagnostic rates of 5.4 per cent (Kirkbride, 1992a) and 6.5 per cent (Caldow et al., 1996) have been reported, but the widespread evidence of infection in English dairy herds (Paton et al., 1998) and the ability

of the virus to cause abortion in the early stages of gestation, at a time when both finding the fetus and achieving a diagnosis are more difficult, suggest that the true rate of fetal loss due to BVDV may be higher.

Infection is most often introduced into the herd by the purchase of a persistently infected (PI) breeding replacement and can be maintained in the herd by the birth and survival to breeding age of further PI animals. In the beef herd infection can be maintained within successive calf crops as the calves are kept with the cows during the breeding period and beyond the first trimester of pregnancy. Persistently infected animals produce the largest amount of virus, particularly in their nasal secretions, while acutely infected animals are also infectious to others for at least 15 days (Duffell & Harkness, 1985). Both persistently infected bulls (Meyling & Mikel-Jensen, 1988) and bulls undergoing acute infection (Paton et al., 1989) can pass the virus in semen.

Acute infection during the breeding season and in the first trimester of pregnancy can result in a range of outcomes from reduced conception rates or fetal death to the persistence of infection in the fetus (Kirkland et al., 1997). Infection in both the first and the second trimester can cause abortion or developmental abnormalities, particularly of the nervous system (Baker, 1987). The virus appears to be less pathogenic to the fetus in the third trimester and from 100 to 120 days of gestation the fetus can mount an immune response to the virus, a response that becomes more effective as the pregnancy progresses.

Following acute infection, the virus multiplies in the placentome, but does not cause placentitis, before moving into the fetus. In the first trimester lesions in the fetus include meningitis with cerebellar cortical destruction and necrotizing bronchiolitis (Casaro et al., 1971), but these are rarely observed due to autolysis. Sublethal damage in the first trimester and beyond can result in the birth of calves with lesions such as retinal dysplasia and cerebellar hypoplasia. The difference in virulence between strains described for both type 1 and type 2 viruses (Dubovi, 1992), along with stage of gestation at which individual cows are exposed to infection and the variation in the level of herd immunity, explain the wide differences seen in the outcome of BVDV infection in breeding herds.

The virus can be isolated from an aborted fetus although the success of this is limited by autolysis. It can also be demonstrated in fixed tissues using immunohistochemistry. This allows the agent to be associated with lesions observed on histological examination (Ellis et al., 1995). Nested reverse chain transcriptase polymerase chain reaction (PCR) techniques have been used to detect viral RNA in tissues and may, in future, become the diagnostic technique of choice (Nettleton & Entrican, 1995). As maternal antibody cannot cross the bovine placenta, antibody detected in fetal fluids indicates fetal infection. However, when antibody is detected in late abortions without the presence of specific pathology BVDV may not have been responsible for fetal death (Brown *et al.*, 1979).

Maternal immunity to infection is not life-long. Infection with heterologous strains of the virus can also overcome natural immunity. Control should therefore be based on a programme that includes best practice biosecurity, identifying and removing persistently infected breeding animals from the herd and screening purchased replacements for the presence of PI animals. Vaccines (p. 1011) now available in Britain have been shown to prevent fetal infection (Brownlie *et al.*, 1995), but vaccination should not be relied upon as the sole preventive strategy. The success of eradication and biosecurity as a means to control BVD can be measured by the progress made by the countries that have embarked on national or regional control programmes (Hult & Lindberg, 1998)

Bovine herpes virus 1 (BHV1) (see also p. 289)

In Western Europe there is little to suggest that BHV1 is a significant cause of abortion. In contrast, in North America BHV1 has been shown to be the most frequently diagnosed viral cause of abortion (Kirkbride, 1992a; Anderson *et al.*, 1997) and experimental challenge models to test vaccine efficacy have resulted in a high rate of fetal loss (Miller *et al.*, 1995). This difference may be the consequence of a variation in virulence between the strains of the virus found on the two continents.

BHV1 exists as two distinct subgroups and causes two clinical syndromes: infectious bovine rhinotracheitis (IBR) and infectious pustular vaginitis (IPV). Neither clinical syndrome is exclusively associated with a particular genotype of the virus and abortions have been observed with both subgroups (Barr & BonDurant, 1997). As with all herpes viruses the agent is maintained in a latent form in infected animals, but can be re-activated at times of stress (Kaashoek *et al.*, 1996). In young animals epidemic IBR often follows the introduction of market purchased animals to the herd. Similar outbreaks of clinical disease may be seen in adults, but subclinical disease is more common in this age group. Infection in breeding herds tends to become endemic, with young cows infected as they enter the breeding herd (Pritchard, 1992).

Experimental infection with the virus at 25 to 28 weeks of pregnancy resulted in abortions between 17 and 85 days later (Miller *et al.*, 1991). In abortions attributed to natural infection with BHV1, fetuses show no typical gross lesion, but histological examination consistently reveals multifocal coagulative necrosis in the liver and less frequently in the lung, lymph nodes, kidney and placenta (Kirkbride, 1992b). These changes and the absence of fetal antibody suggest an acute infection and appear to conflict with the prolonged period between experimental infection and abortion.

Virus can be isolated from up to 50 per cent of fetuses that show histological lesions typical of BHV1 infection with the placenta being the most useful tissue for culture (Kirkbride, 1992b). Other diagnostic techniques that have been described include fluorescent antibody staining on cryostat sections of fetal tissues, immunostaining of lesions observed in fixed tissues and PCR techniques (Rocha *et al.*, 1999).

It seems likely that active immunity ensures that reinfection does not result in significant clinical disease and the use of a live modified vaccine has been shown to prevent abortion following experimental challenge (Cravens *et al.*, 1996). However, it remains unclear how long after infection cows are protected from the abortifacient effects of the virus.

As BHV1 is an insignificant cause of fetal loss in Britain there is little financial incentive to control the disease in breeding herds for this reason alone. However, the virus may be found in the semen of infected bulls and it is illegal to sell semen from antibody-positive bulls to third countries within the European Union (EU). Several continental European countries have successfully eradicated the disease or have national control programmes in place and individual herds within these countries are unable to import seropositive animals. There is therefore a sound argument for pedigree and high genetic merit herds to eradicate the disease by a test and cull programme supplemented by biosecurity measures. Gene deleted vaccines offer an alternative to a test and cull programme and have been used in the Netherlands (Kaashoek *et al.*, 1995). Even where breeding herds do not sell semen or pedigree animals, the apparent difference in virulence between European and North American strains of the virus makes it prudent to exclude exotic strains of BHV1 by implementing biosecurity measures.

Other viruses

While a range of other viruses have been isolated from aborted fetuses there is little to support their role as important causes of fetal death. The exceptions are bovine herpes virus 4 (BHV4) and Akabane virus. There is epidemiological evidence of an association between BHV4 seropositivity and abortion in cows in

Belgium (Czaplicki & Thiry, 1998) and in the USA the virus was the third most frequently isolated from fetal submissions to a diagnostic laboratory over a 10-year period (Kirkbride, 1992b). There is no published record of the agent's involvement in British cattle and relevant diagnostic tests are rarely used. It may be of value to consider BHV4 when the usual investigative procedures in problem herds have been unsuccessful. Akabane virus is an arthropod borne virus that has been shown to cause a range of congenital abnormalities that include arthrogryposis and hydranencephaly as well as abortion. The virus occurs in Australia, Japan, South East Asia, Africa, Israel and Turkey and it would appear to be maintained in a range of mosquito and culicoides species (Charles, 1994). The significance of Akabane virus to British herds is limited, but the trade in live animals that would follow inclusion of countries such as Turkey to the European Union could render this virus something other than an exotic curiosity.

Bacterial causes of abortion

Brucellosis (see also p. 461)

According to EU criteria Britain is officially free of *Brucella abortus* infection, but animals from areas with a lower status for this disease are imported and as a consequence the government continues to carry out post import checks and routine serological monitoring of the herds in Britain.

The organism is an intracellular pathogen that is spread in infected uterine discharges. After infection has occurred, usually by ingestion, an animal remains infected for life and the principal sign of this infection is abortion due to placentitis. This is characterized as a purulent intercotyledonary placentitis with necrosis of the cotyledons. Live calves are produced from subsequent pregnancies although the uterine discharges remain a source of infection. Apart from the severe effects on cattle production the disease is also an important zoonosis.

In Britain there is a legal obligation for farmers to notify the government's animal health service of any bovine abortion and it is then at their discretion to require the collection of diagnostic material by the farmer's veterinary surgeon. Microscopic examination of smears made from vaginal swabs, bacteriological culture of milk and vaginal swab and a range of serological techniques can then be employed to screen for evidence of the disease. It is important for both farmers and their veterinary surgeons to recognize that these procedures are not used to test for other abortion agents.

Control of the disease is the preserve of the State Veterinary Service in Britain and test and cull policies are pursued. Vaccination has been used in many national or regional eradication programmes, often in the early stages of control (see p. 1013).

Leptospirosis (see also p. 735)

The disease in cattle is caused by the organisms collectively referred to as *Leptospira hardjo* (*L. borgpetersenii* serovar *hardjo* and *L. interrogans* serovar *hardjo*, previously named *Leptospira interrogans* serovars *hardjobovis* and *hardjoprajitno*, respectively). These are host-adapted serovars responsible for disease in cattle. In New Zealand there is little evidence that these are significant pathogens of cattle and their importance lies in their zoonotic impact (Bolin & Alt, 1998). Conversely, disease surveillance figures from New Zealand have found *Leptospira pomona*, a serovar that is not adapted to cattle, in 1.3 per cent of abortion cases examined (Thornton, 1991). In Victoria, Australia, experimental infection of pregnant heifers with a locally isolated strain of *L. interrogans* serovar *hardjo* failed to cause abortion or to establish fetal infection (Chappel *et al.*, 1989). In Britain and Ireland leptospirosis is associated with infertility, abortion and milk drop. As it is difficult to detect evidence of infection in the fetus it is also difficult to determine the true significance of leptospirosis as cause of fetal death, however diagnostic rates of 1.7 per cent have been observed in Scotland (Caldow *et al.*, 1996) while in Northern Ireland 42 per cent of aborted fetuses showed evidence of infection (Ellis *et al.*, 1982). The disease is widespread in the national herd and bulk milk antibody testing showed 75 per cent of samples from dairy herds in England and Wales to have antibody present (Pritchard, 1999).

Infection is through exposure to contaminated urine and leptospires penetrate intact mucosal surfaces to establish a bacteraemia. The agent localizes in the urinary and reproductive tracts and is passed in large numbers in the urine in the early stages of the disease and may be passed intermittently for prolonged periods thereafter. Spread of infection within a herd is most rapid during the grazing season, an observation that has been explained by the longer survival times for the organism that occur in the moist neutral pH conditions found at pasture in contrast to the more acid environment that prevails when animals are housed, particularly where ensiled forage is fed.

Infection is generally considered to be introduced to a herd through the addition of infected cattle, but both sheep and horses can maintain the infection and one study has suggested that sheep, the use of natural service and the presence of water courses that have run through other farms may all be risk factors for leptospirosis infection (Pritchard *et al.*, 1989).

As with several other infections, abortion occurs as a chronic sequel, following up to 12 weeks after what is often a subclinical acute infection of the dam. Aborted fetuses and placentas do not show any characteristic pathology that is of diagnostic value, but the time course of infection is such that the fetus may have been able to mount an immune response and produce antibody. This antibody can be detected in fetal fluid by the microscopic agglutination test (MAT). Isolation of leptospires from fetal tissues is a preserve of the specialist laboratory and is not routinely used as a diagnostic test. The fluorescent antibody test performed on cryostat sections or impression smears of fetal tissues found favour for some time but inherent difficulties of such techniques in autolytic tissues mean that these tests too are now less frequently used. Once again the detection of specific DNA may well become the technique of choice and several PCR methods have been described (Smith et al., 1994).

The literature on maternal serological response is extensive and serves to underline the diagnostic limitations of serological techniques. The MAT has long been the standard test and principally detects antibody of the IgM class. These antibodies are produced as an early response to infection and may have fallen to undetectable levels by the time the animal aborts. The enzyme linked immunosorbant assay (ELISA) can be designed to detect a specific subclass of antibody or a mixture, but the commercially available ELISAs usually detect predominantly IgG. After infection an animal produces detectable levels of IgG by 21 to 28 days and these persist for prolonged periods. Serology does not allow the differentiation between vaccinal titres and those that follow natural infection. For these reasons maternal serology is of little value in the individual animal that aborts and is best used as a herd diagnostic technique on the understanding that it may have limited applications in vaccinated herds.

In dairy herds a principal reason for controlling the infection by vaccination is to reduce the risk of zoonotic disease in those milking the cows, but one study has claimed an improvement in fertility indices after vaccination (Dhaliwal et al., 1996). In beef herds the risk of zoonotic infection is low and there is no published study to demonstrate the value of vaccination, although this is a commonly used control strategy. Similarly the use of quarantine, serological screening and antibiotic treatment of animals that are seropositive are measures that have been recommended (BCVA, 1992). A successful national herd control programme based on the application of biosecurity and test and cull exists in the Netherlands. In Britain a programme of accreditation of freedom of disease has operated since 1989 (MAFF, 1989). Both approaches offer the benefit of allowing the sale of breeding replacements accredited free of infection.

Bacillus licheniformis

Bacillus species are saprophytes that are widely distributed in the environment and with the exception of Bacillus anthracis are generally considered to have little pathogenic potential. Species differentiation is not easy, but the principal isolate from bovine abortions is Bacillus licheniformis. Bacillus organisms have been isolated from 9.8% of fetal specimens (Caldow et al., 1996) and outbreaks of abortion associated with this agent are commonly observed (David, 1993). Just how an organism that is considered to have little pathogenic potential can appear to be such an important fetal pathogen is not clear. It has been suggested that the risk of abortion may be related to the weight of infection in the environment, either in silage or in other forage or in contaminated water. However, other factors may be important and in 45 per cent of fetuses where a diagnosis of Bacillus licheniformis abortion was made evidence of fetal infection with Neospora caninum was also found (Caldow et al., 1996). Despite this the experimental infection by the intravenous route alone has resulted in placentitis and abortion with lesions similar to those observed in naturally occurring incidents (Agerholm et al., 1999).

Usually abortion occurs relatively late in pregnancy and lesions of a necrotizing placentitis are observed with thickening of the intercotyledonary areas and adventitious placentation. Suppurative bronchopneumonia and occasionally pericarditis can be found in the fetus. The organism is readily isolated from the placenta, fetal lung and fetal stomach contents, but on occasion the organisms can no longer be cultured from the fetus despite isolation from the placenta and the presence of typical pathology.

There is no indication that the bacteraemia that precedes the abortion is associated with any clinical disease in the dam and no serological test has been developed.

In herds experiencing outbreaks group treatment with antibiotic is sometimes advocated, but there is no evidence of efficacy. It is prudent to screen cows for the presence of other agents that may be acting as cofactors as well as to carry out bacterial counts on silage. A threshold of 10^4 colony forming units/g has been suggested above which forage should not be fed to pregnant cows (David, 1993). Other potential sources of the organism should also be investigated, including drinking water.

Listeria monocytogenes (see also p. 904)

There are similarities between listeria and bacillus as causes of abortion, although Listeria monocytogenes is generally considered to be a more significant pathogen. It may be associated with clinical disease in the dam, but is usually only a sporadic cause of cattle abortion. *Listeria monocytogenes* is a small Gram-positive rod that grows rapidly in aerobic or microaerophilic conditions at temperatures of between 3 and 45°C. It can tolerate pH values as high as 9.6, but is inhibited by pH values lower than 5.6 and exists as a plant saprophyte or as an animal pathogen (Low & Donachie, 1997). It is these characteristics that are crucial to the epidemiology of the disease in ruminants, allowing growth of the organism in poorly fermented silage and infection by ingestion.

The clinical syndromes most commonly observed in cattle are iritis and meningoencephalitis, with abortion an uncommon sequel of either of these. Silage feeding is associated with a risk of listeriosis, however disease can occur when animals are grazing pasture. In addition to *L. monocytogenes*, the closely related *Listeria ivanovii* is also isolated occasionally from cattle fetuses (Alexander *et al.*, 1992).

In listeric abortion the aborted fetus is often autolytic, but non-specific lesions of placentitis and fetal septicaemia may be seen (Barr & Anderson, 1993) and the organism can be readily isolated from fetal viscera, stomach contents and the placenta. Serological tests for exposure to listeria exist, but are not used in the diagnosis of bovine abortion.

The same restraints on treatment and control of bacillus apply to listeria. High-risk forages, which in this case are poorly preserved silages with a pH greater than 5, should not be fed to pregnant cattle. In addition to ensuring conditions that promote good anaerobic fermentation during the ensilage process, measures should be taken to reduce soil and faecal contamination of the grass prior to and during harvesting.

Salmonellosis (see also Chapter 15; p. 850)

According to British diagnostic data, salmonella organisms were isolated from 159 to 300 cases of bovine abortion in each of the years of 1994 to 1998 (MAFF, 1998a). During this period *Salmonella dublin* made up 82 per cent of these diagnoses. In contrast, *S. dublin* accounted for 31 per cent of the non-abortion salmonella cases in adult cattle whereas the figure for *Salmonella typhimurium* was 54 per cent (MAFF, 1998b). These data suggest that *S. dublin* is more likely to manifest as a primary abortion problem than is *S. typhimurium*. There is a variation in the number of *S. dublin* cases diagnosed on a regional basis, indicating an endemic problem in some areas.

Salmonella organisms are members of the Enterobacteriaceae and as such can be found as part of the intestinal flora in many species of domestic animals and wildlife. The carrier state is particularly important in the spread of the disease and *S. dublin* shows a greater tendency towards the carrier state than *S. typhimurium* in cattle. Studies on the epidemiology of *S. typhimurium* determinant type 104 have also demonstrated the important role of newly introduced animals in the spread of this disease (Evans & Davies, 1996). While it remains unclear how important wildlife are in initiating new outbreaks, infection was found to be maintained in rodent and wild bird populations after an outbreak.

Infection of the placenta follows bacteraemia and extension to the fetus can follow from this. However, neither infection of the fetus nor indeed placentitis is required to cause fetal death or abortion. Where fetal infection has occurred gross lesions are non-specific; histological lesions of fetal septicaemia may be found and the organism may be isolated from fetal tissues and the placenta. If the cow is showing signs of septicaemia at the time of abortion it is advisable to attempt to isolate the organism from faeces. Serological tests for salmonellosis are available, but are not used routinely for diagnostic purposes in the investigation of bovine abortion.

Once a diagnosis of salmonellosis has been made control rests on efforts to minimize further spread of infection within the herd through improved hygiene and thorough cleaning and disinfection. There are conflicting reports of the effectiveness of vaccination against *S. typhimurium* in the face of an outbreak (Davies & Renton, 1992; Mee & Malone, 1995), but a *S. dublin* vaccine is available and has been used successfully in endemically infected herds (Wray *et al.*, 1989). The removal of *S. dublin* carriers after an outbreak appears to be an attractive course of action, but this approach is impractical as excretion is periodic. Faeces must be cultured with negative results on three occasions at 14-day intervals before an animal is considered to be free of infection. In addition, animals must be individually housed or stall-tied with this method as there is the possibility of passive excretion if animals are loose housed or at pasture (Radostits *et al.*, 1994).

Farmers should be aware of the risks that purchased breeding replacements pose and added animals should be placed in quarantine and screened by culture as above.

Campylobacter (see also p. 568)

Venereal campylobacteriosis is considered to be an important cause of bovine infertility wherever natural service is used and abortions are a feature of this disease. Recent observations have suggested that the condition may be more prevalent in beef herds in Britain than has been widely presumed (Caldow & Taylor, 1997).

Campylobacter fetus is a microaerophilic, motile bacterium that has two recognized subspecies: *C. fetus* subsp. *venerealis* and *C. fetus* subsp. *fetus*. Differentiation has been based on the variation of antigenic and biochemical characteristics of the subspecies, notably that *C. fetus* subsp. *venerealis* will not grow in 1 per cent glycine whereas *C. fetus* subsp. *fetus* will. This differentiation is important, as *C. fetus* subsp. *venerealis* is considered to be adapted to the bovine reproductive tract and to be the cause of venereal campylobacteriosis, whereas *C. fetus* subsp. *fetus* is a gut commensal causing sporadic abortion in cattle. However, strains of the latter vary in their biochemical characteristics and strains identified as *C. fetus* subsp. *venerealis* have developed tolerance to glycine (Chang & Ogg, 1971). In addition, strains identified as *C. fetus* subsp. *fetus*, when used in experimental studies, have resulted in disease indistinguishable from that caused by *C. fetus* subsp. *venerealis* (Schurig et al., 1973) and field outbreaks of venereal campylobacter infertility associated with *C. fetus* subsp. *fetus* have been identified (MacLaren & Agumbah, 1988). It would therefore appear that strains of both subspecies are capable of causing venereal infertility and whenever *C. fetus* is isolated from abortion material the possibility of herd venereal infertility should be investigated.

In the case of sporadic abortion not associated with venereal infertility, invasion from the intestinal tract is the probable route of infection.

The venereal form of the disease is usually introduced to the herd via an infected mature bull and while younger bulls or breeding females are less likely sources, any animal that has previously been mated constitutes a potential source of infection. The use of hired bulls is considered to be a particularly high-risk practice. Infection in the bull follows natural mating with an infected cow, but is not associated with clinical signs or pathological changes. In mature bulls infection becomes established in the lumen of the epithelial crypts of the prepuce, while bulls younger than 6 years of age are more resistant to infection (Clark, 1971). In natural service the spread of infection is from the penis to the anterior vagina, where the organism becomes established before entering the uterus to cause a mild endometritis and salpingitis. Pathological changes are most pronounced at 8 to 13 weeks after infection and have resolved by four to five months (Dekeyser, 1986). Where conception has occurred embryonic death and a delayed return to oestrus, abortion or the birth of a live full term calf can follow. Of the abortions that are detected the gestational length is usually around four to five months. A marked placentitis and pericarditis may be seen on gross examination of the tissues and histological findings are of fetal septicaemia and pneumonia.

Diagnosis of *C. fetus* as a cause of abortion rests on the isolation of the organism from the fetus. As faecal contamination of the placenta may occur after the abortion, isolation from the placenta should not be considered diagnostic unless reinforced by histopathology.

After venereal infection in the cow, antibody is secreted in the uterine and vaginal fluid. Of this IgG is the most important component and can be detected eight weeks post infection, but is largely undetectable by six months. IgA is produced by three to five weeks and is still detectable for up to a year after infection (Corbeil et al., 1974). Despite recovery, the development of immunity and the establishment of normal pregnancies, *C. fetus* has been isolated from the vaginal mucus more than a year after infection (MacLaren & Agumbah, 1988), creating the potential for cows as well as bulls to maintain the infection in the herd from one year to the next.

The sampling technique most frequently used in bulls in Britain is the collection of sheath washings (BCVA, 1995) and phosphate buffered saline (PBS) is adequate for the lavage fluid provided samples are relatively free from gross contamination and transported to the laboratory within four to six hours. However, where immediate delivery to the laboratory cannot be achieved the use of transport enrichment medium (TEM) has proved to be effective in maintaining the viability of the organism (Hum et al., 1994). A fluorescent antibody test is available, but does not allow differentiation between the two subspecies and it is of limited value in the diagnosis of the disease. Vaginal mucus should also be collected without gross faecal contamination and this can best be achieved by using pipettes with the end closed off and perforations made in the last few centimetres. Twenty ml of PBS are injected through a 60 ml syringe and then aspirated back, bringing with it vaginal mucus (Lander, 1983). As with sheath washings, TEM can be used if there is to be a delay of more than six hours between sample collection and the inoculation of media.

In the vaginal mucus agglutination test (VMAT) antigens prepared from *C. fetus* are used to detect agglutinins in the vaginal mucus. Immunoglobulin A is the antibody present in the mucus, but where serum or blood contaminates vaginal secretions false positives can arise as serum antibody to *C. fetus* is common in cattle (Wilkie & Winter, 1971). In addition, where cattle are in oestrus, large amounts of mucus is produced, IgA is diluted and false negatives can occur. Problems have been reported with the test and it has been suggested that only 50 per cent of infected animals will be positive by VMAT and of those 50 per cent will be negative six months after infection. An enzyme-linked immunoassay has been developed to overcome some of the problems experienced in using the VMAT (Hewson *et al.*, 1985; Hum *et al.*, 1991), but the test is not currently used in Britain.

As a consequence of the delay between infection and investigation in most herds and the cows' ability to clear the infection as well as the limitations of the vaginal mucus agglutination test it is necessary to sample a minimum of 12 cows. Where endemic infection is suspected animals in their first year in the breeding herd should be sampled to offer the best chance of achieving a diagnosis. Bulls should be sheath washed in the course of a herd investigation, but a negative result is of little value as the screening is a relatively insensitive test.

Artificial insemination using semen from campylobacter-free studs offers a simple and successful method of control, but for some herds, particularly where mating occurs at grass, this may not be practical. Vaccination is used in many countries where the disease occurs in range cattle and a vaccination programme to eradicate infection from within a herd has been described (Hum & MacInnes, 1987). Antibiotic treatment of the bulls is suggested as an additional measure (Hum *et al.*, 1993). However, there is no licensed vaccine in Britain and an emergency vaccine must be produced under the authority of the Veterinary Medicines Directorate (see Chapter 59).

Prevention can be achieved by maintaining a strict closed herd policy, but in practical terms the purchase of virgin heifers and virgin bulls does not constitute a risk. Difficulties arise where bulls have to be replaced at short notice. In these situations a synchronization and insemination programme would offer the safest course of action with a young unproven bull used to sweep up. If mature bulls are used these should be screened and treated with antibiotics (BCVA, 1995).

Miscellaneous bacteria

Species of bacteria associated only with sporadic abortions can be split into those that can be readily isolated from the posterior reproductive tract of the normal animal and those that cannot.

The former category includes organisms such as *Haemophilus somnus*, *Arcanobacterium pyogenes*, *Streptococcus dysgalactiae*, *Mycoplasma bovis* and *Ureaplasma diversum*. These may gain entry to the uterus through the cervix as a sequel to some other disease process affecting the fetus. It is possible that strain differences in virulence exist, but at the present time these agents should be considered to be of minor importance. Ureaplasmas have been suggested as important, but isolation methods for these organisms are rarely employed in diagnostic laboratories (Sanderson & Chenoweth, 1999).

The second category includes *Yersinia pseudotuberculosis*, *Mannheimia haemolytica*, *Erysipelothrix rhusiopathiae* and *Staphylocccus aureus* where infection of the fetus follows bacteraemia in the dam. *Arcanobacterium pyogenes* may also gain entry to the conceptus in this way and experimental infection via the intravenous route with this organism has resulted in abortion (Semambo *et al.*, 1991).

These infections are unlikely to represent a herd problem and as such do not merit further discussion.

Protozoal causes of abortion

Trichomoniasis

Bovine trichomoniasis is caused by the protozoan parasite *Tritrichomonas fetus* and is a venereal disease responsible for early embryonic death, infertility, pyometra and abortion. It is a particular problem in range cattle, where as many as 50 per cent of the herds may be infected (Dennet *et al.*, 1974). There is no recent report of the disease from within Britain, but there is no biological barrier that would prevent the disease from occurring here and diagnostic laboratories in Britain do not routinely use techniques that would identify the presence of this agent. Therefore trichomoniasis should be considered in the differential diagnosis in herds using natural service where infertility, abortions and pyometra are observed.

Although most pregnancies are lost at around 17 days after conception, one review reported that death can occur at any time up to the fifth month of gestation (Yule *et al.*, 1989), and fetal infection has also been demonstrated in late abortions and in full term calves (Rhyan *et al.*, 1988).

No specific gross changes are seen in the abortion material. Histological examination reveals lesions of placentitis and pyogranulomatous bronchopneumonia with evidence of tissue invasion with the parasite (Rhyan *et al.*, 1995). The organism can be cultured from vaginal discharges, preputial smegma and fetal tissues by using a specific medium in a pouch system (Kvasnicka *et al.*, 1996).

Trichomoniasis can be controlled through the use of artificial insemination and commercial vaccines are available in the countries where the disease is endemic.

Neosporosis (see also p. 283)

Protozoal abortion has been recognized as a problem in the dairy herds of California since the mid 1980s (Anderson *et al.*, 1991) and around the same time a protozoan parasite of dogs was identified in Norway

(Bjerkås *et al.*, 1984). This was subsequently named *Neospora caninum* (Dubey *et al.*, 1988) and the link was made to the infection of cattle (Thilsted & Dubey, 1989). Since then *N. caninum* has been identified as a cause of abortion in many parts of the world and a major volume of research publications has been generated (Dubey, 1999). Serological studies have found evidence of exposure to the organism in 16 per cent of aborted fetuses in Scotland (Buxton *et al.*, 1997) and in 13 per cent of cows that aborted in Northern Ireland (McNamee *et al.*, 1996). Outbreaks described range from 11 per cent of cows that aborted in one herd in England (Dannatt *et al.*, 1995), to as many as 57 per cent of a herd in The Netherlands (Wouda *et al.*, 1999). While neosporosis is a recently recognized disease there is nothing to suggest that the parasite or the disease is new.

Neospora caninum is an apicomplexan protozoan closely related to *Toxoplasma gondii* and although the complete life cycle of the parasite is still to be determined dogs have been shown to be a definitive host and to pass small numbers of oocysts in faeces from 8 to 23 days after experimental infection (McAllister *et al.*, 1998). Tissue cysts and tachyzoites have been found in cattle, sheep, goats and horses and it is possible that the intestinal stage of the life cycle is not limited to the dog. Vertical transmission occurs in addition to the point source outbreaks, where cows are presumed to be infected for the first time and abort. As post natal infection rates are probably as low as 1 per cent (Hietala & Thurmond, 1999) most cases are due to vertical transmission where an infection rate of 95 per cent has been found (Davison *et al.*, 1999). Infection of the fetus may often be a relatively benign event and care should be taken in attributing significance to evidence of infection in an aborted fetus (Thurmond *et al.*, 1997). Co-infection with other agents is often found and potentiation or the presence of factors that cause immune suppression in endemically infected herds may explain some of the cases that appear as epidemics (Bartels *et al.*, 1999).

Experimental infection of pregnant cattle has resulted in fetal death and lesions indistinguishable from those seen in naturally occurring outbreaks (Barr *et al.*, 1994). Abortion most frequently occurs in the second half of pregnancy and the commonly observed lesions are limited to placentitis, focal non-suppurative encephalitis, non-suppurative myocarditis and myositis and widespread non-suppurative infiltrates in other organs (Anderson *et al.*, 1991). The tissue cysts are well tolerated and the host response is limited to the tachyzoites. Histological examination of the fetus is important in order to determine the severity and therefore the significance of the lesions in terms of fetal death (Thurmond *et al.*, 1999). The histological appearance of the lesions is considered significantly characteristic to warrant a diagnosis and immunohistochemistry gives further specificity to this. Autolysis often hampers examination although tissue cysts do survive and may be recognized. The fetus is capable of mounting an immunological response to neospora infection and detection of specific antibody in fetal or precolostral sera is a reliable indicator of fetal infection, but not of infection causing fetal death (Otter *et al.*, 1997). At present, despite the availability of molecular biological techniques for the detection of neospora DNA they are not routinely used for diagnostic purposes.

Maternal infection is followed by the production of antibodies within 14 days that peak by 46 days and in most cases the time lag between maternal infection and abortion is such that antibody production will have peaked before the abortion and may occasionally have fallen to undetectable levels by two months after the abortion (Wouda *et al.*, 1999). In the congenitally infected individual there is fluctuation in antibody level and at times antibody is undetected. The observations that congenitally infected animals have been found to have a higher risk of abortion at their first gestation compared to the second gestation and that abortions occurred at an earlier stage in the first gestation than subsequently suggest the possibility of a protective immunity developing in infected animals (Thurmond & Hietala, 1997). Given the close relationships between neospora, toxoplasma and sarcocystis species there were concerns that serological cross-reaction could occur, however it has been shown that such cross-reactivity is negligible and of no importance diagnostically (Dubey *et al.*, 1996).

The lack of a complete understanding of the life cycle and knowledge of the range of definitive hosts has led to a cautious approach to control, but there seems a clear argument emerging in favour of culling seropositive animals from the herd. These have been shown to have lower levels of production and suffer a higher risk of abortion than seronegative cows within the herd. By using information from the literature in a mathematical model it has been shown that annual culling of seropositive animals was the most effective and rapid method of control. Effective control at a slower rate could be achieved if the action was limited to excluding the offspring from seropositive cows from the breeding herd (French *et al.*, 1999). At the present time the question of the cost-benefits of these strategies has not been addressed, but given the large outbreaks that can occur, action to prevent a sudden catastrophic, albeit low-risk, occurrence might be justifiable. Irrespective of culling practices, all fetuses, placentas and cattle carcases should be disposed of in a way that prevents recycling of *N. caninum* infection through definitive hosts.

Other infectious agents causing abortion

Chlamydia and rickettsia

Q fever, *Chlamydophila abortus* and *Cytocoetes phagocytophilia* have all been identified as occasional causes of bovine abortion. There is serological evidence of exposure to the agent of Q fever in Britain (Paiba *et al.*, 1999), but no recent report of abortion in cattle due to this agent. Occasionally a purulent placentitis and the presence of elementary bodies in modified Ziehl Neelsen stained smears of placenta and stomach contents are observed. Establishing the precise aetiology in these cases can be difficult, but *Chlamydophila abortus* has been isolated from such material and in one report the strain was found to be identical to that responsible for chlamydial abortion in sheep (Griffiths *et al.*, 1995). The outbreak may have been the result of close contact between cattle and an infected sheep flock on the same premises.

Cytocoetes phagocytophilia, the cause of tick borne fever (TBF), will cause abortion in cattle when first exposure to ticks occurs during pregnancy. Diagnosis can be difficult to confirm, as there is no longer parasitaemia by the time the abortion occurs. A presumptive diagnosis may be based on the herd history and the presence of ticks and antibody to the TBF agent.

Mycotic abortion

Mycotic abortion with placentitis and fetal infection is reported throughout the world. In one detailed study 7 per cent were mycotic abortions and *Aspergillus fumigatus* infection accounted for 62 per cent of these (Knudtson & Kirkbride, 1992). Other species of fungi have been reported and it would appear that most are opportunist pathogens. The source of these infections is often poorly preserved hay or ensiled feed that has undergone aerobic fermentation.

Placentitis follows a septicaemia that has resulted from either ingestion or inhalation of spores from the environment. The placenta is frequently thickened and may be of a leathery appearance. White plaques on the skin of the fetus are an occasional feature of this disease, but apart from this gross lesions are seldom observed. At the microscopic level hepatitis, pneumonia and placentitis are evident and Grocott's stain can be used to reveal fungal hyphae in fixed sections. Fungal elements can be seen on direct microscopy of the placenta and the stomach contents, the latter being diagnostic. These organisms are readily cultured from the fetus and the placenta, but environmental contamination after the abortion has occurred may explain isolation from the placenta alone.

There is little information on the development of immunity after infection or whether the cow is likely to return to normal fertility.

Prevention of mycotic placentitis is by reducing the degree of fungal contamination pregnant cows are exposed to, particularly in preserved forage. Fungal growth occurs in other feedstuffs and bedding materials and after a diagnosis of mycotic abortion the management system should be reviewed in order to identify possible sources of these organisms. A visual examination of suspect materials may be sufficient, but where doubt over the source remains it is also possible to use quantitative culture methods to assess the degree of fungal contamination and to identify the organisms present.

Non-infectious causes of abortion

The failure to identify an infectious cause in many cases has led to the suggestion that non-infectious causes are of importance (Norton & Campbell, 1990). Nutritional factors that may be involved include excess dietary protein or non-protein nitrogen and selenium or iodine deficiency. Twin pregnancies are associated with shorter gestation lengths and an increased rate of abortion (Echternkamp & Gregory, 1999). Various poisonous plants have been implicated, but none is indigenous to Britain. Ponderosa pine (*Pinus ponderosa*) and locoweeds (*Astralagus* sp.) cause significant problems in some areas of North America. Deaths due to aflatoxicosis and to nitrate toxicity may be preceded by abortion, suggesting that either the fetus is marginally more sensitive to any toxic effect than the dam or that fetal death is the consequence of the clinical disease in the dam.

However, the literature fails to support non-infectious causes as a numerically significant cause of abortion in cattle (Norton & Campbell, 1990) and in the UK only iodine deficiency, manifest as hyperplastic goitre in full-term stillborn calves, is of importance. The condition is mainly reported in beef herds or in dairy heifers and is thought unlikely to affect dairy cows due to adequate dietary iodine intake. A threshold of 15 g for the weight of the intact gland, above which goitre is suspected, has been in common use. A better indicator is the ratio of thyroid weight to fetal body weight where the threshold value is 1:3000. However, oedema of the head and neck in stillborn calves can render this unreliable (Gee *et al.*, 1989) and histological examination of the gland to confirm the presence of a colloid goitre is recommended (Capen, 1993). There does not appear to be any suggestion that goitrogenic factors should be considered and the inclusion of iodine in an oral mineral supplement should prevent the condition (see pp. 257, 301).

Investigation

In abortion outbreaks in cattle herds abortions are frequently irregular and the single abortion may mark the start of an outbreak that does not become apparent for several weeks. An observed abortion may also represent a more extensive underlying herd problem and therefore there is justification for investigating every abortion. However, there are concerns over unnecessary costs and the diagnostic rate has been found to be higher in cases where there has been more than one abortion in the herd previously (Caldow *et al.*, 1996). Since there is a statutory requirement to report all abortions in Britain there is the opportunity to discuss the problem with the client and to carry out the investigations considered necessary in each individual case.

Investigations should follow a standard pattern:

(1) History
(2) Clinical examination of the cow
(3) Necropsy of fetus
(4) Collection of samples for the laboratory
(5) Interpretation of results

History

The use of a standard form allows the systematic collection of the important details of the individual cow as well as production system, cow numbers, age structure, biosecurity measures, replacement policy and source of replacements (Fig. 37.1). Details on the feeding system and how feeds are stored are also of relevance. This can usefully be expanded to include details on herd fertility, retained membranes and any background clinical problem that may be of relevance. Careful evaluation of the information is essential to guide the investigation and to indicate the diagnostic tests to be employed.

Clinical examination

In most cases examination does not yield useful information, but it is important to exclude conditions such as acute salmonellosis, summer mastitis or tick borne fever and to allow treatment if the cow is ill. At this time a blood sample for serology should be collected and if salmonellosis is suspected a faeces sample as well. Where stillbirth is the problem the body condition of the cow should be assessed and other cows in late gestation can also be examined in this way. Where the majority of animals in the group have scores of 3.5 and above there is cause for concern over excessive body condition.

Even when it has been decided to limit diagnostic tests to those required for brucellosis, a serum sample can be stored frozen for possible retrospective examination.

Examination of the fetus and placenta

In the ideal situation, the entire aborted calf and fetal membranes with the appropriate samples from the dam should be delivered directly to a veterinary diagnostic laboratory. Where transport difficulties or other delays preclude this, the field veterinarian should collect appropriate samples while carrying out a necropsy of the fetus.

A standard approach to the examination should be adopted and the appropriate information recorded. The measurement of the crown–rump length can give an approximation of gestational age. A formula to estimate the fetal developmental age from the crown–rump measurement is $x = 2.5(y + 21)$, where y is the crown–rump length in centimetres and x is the gestational age in days. Measurement of the weight of the carcase is particularly important in stillbirths to explore the possibility of dystokia due to fetal maternal disproportion and for comparison with thyroid weight, for the diagnosis of hyperthyroidism.

Other important features to be aware of include the presence of white plaques of fungal hyphae on the skin of fetuses where there is fungal involvement. Meconium staining of the perineum or the presence of meconium in the airways or fetal stomach indicate fetal anoxia consistent with placentitis or the prolonged parturition of dystokia. Haemarthrosis of the shoulder or hip joints may be seen in dystokia cases. Traumatic lesions in fetuses where dystokia has not been the problem are occasionally observed and while trauma may be the cause of the abortion other causes should not be excluded too early in the investigation. Lesions of pericarditis, pleurisy, pneumonia or hepatitis can all be found on the gross examination, but none of these changes is specific. In calves that have lived for a short time after birth it is important to record whether the calf has fed as this prevents useful bacteriological examination of the stomach contents, but also means that maternal antibody may have been absorbed, interfering with fetal serological tests.

When the placenta is available as much of the surface area of the allantochorion as possible should be examined. Lesions can be focal and may be overlooked if insufficient care is taken. Commonly observed lesions are intercotyledonary thickening, necrosis of cotyledons and adventitious placentation. The last lesion is considered to be a chronic response to insufficient placental area and is seen following placentitis.

Collection of samples for laboratory investigation

If samples are collected in the course of a necropsy on the farm, the collection and transport of samples to the laboratory should have been discussed with the laboratory personnel. The samples required and the means of

CASE HISTORY

Reference Number: C2.....................................
Date of Abortion/Stillbirth..................................

Ear no. of dam...

Age of dam.................................   Due on.......................

Source of dam..............Home bred ☐   Purchased ☐

Breed...   Dam...   Sire...

Vaccination: BVD ☐   *L. hardjo* ☐   IBR ☐   Other.....................................

No. of abortions.......................   No. of stillbirths.......................   No. of weak calves.......................

Calving starts.........................   Group size...........................   Total cows.................................

Replacements: Home bred   Bought in   Mixture

Method of service   AI only   Natural only   Both

Have hired bulls been used? Yes ☐   No ☐

Production: Beef ☐   Dairy ☐

Body condition score of cows/heifers: ....

HOUSING/MANAGEMENT

Roughage

Concentrate

Mineral/trace element supplements

HERD FERTILITY (Dairy)

Average days to conception

All serves pregnancy rate

% barren after p.d. positive

HERD FERTILITY (Beef)

No. of barren cows

Length of breeding/calving season

DETAILS OF PARTURITION

Degree of assistance required/use of calving aid: ....

Calf alive at onset of assistance: YES ☐   NO ☐

Placenta expelled with calf: YES ☐   NO ☐

Vet involved with calving: YES ☐   NO ☐

Other information: ....
....

Fig. 37.1 A standard form to collect systematically important information when investigating fetal losses.

preservation are determined by the causes of abortion that occur in an area and on the diagnostic facilities available to the laboratory. Nevertheless, basic rules do apply.

The minimum sample required for bacteriology is fetal stomach contents. These can be collected using a sterile vacutainer and needle through the unopened abomasal wall. Where the placenta is available a cotyledon representative of the lesions observed should also be submitted fresh. Samples may also include fetal liver and lung, allowing slightly higher diagnostic success for some bacterial causes of abortion. It has been suggested that in cases where the fetal membranes have been retained a placentome is removed manually *per vaginum* (Johnson *et al.*, 1994) for bacteriological and histological examination. However, this is not required when the fetus is available for examination.

Fetal blood or fluid can be collected from any body cavity, again by using a vacutainer. This sample is used for serological tests for BVD, neospora and leptospira. Fetal thyroid, spleen, kidney and brain are all tissues that can be used for virus isolation for BVD, while the placenta is the sample of choice for BHV1.

Histopathological examination is particularly useful to determine the significance of fetal infection with *N. caninum* or BVD, to confirm the significance of apparent thyroid enlargement and for further investigations where the standard screen for infectious disease is negative. The tissues of most value to collect are brain, lung, liver, thyroid (in stillbirths) and a cotyledon. It is important to be guided by the pathologist as to how these samples should be fixed. Tissues for histology must never be frozen.

The minimum samples are fetal stomach contents for bacteriology and fetal blood or serum for serological tests. These may be the samples of choice when investigating what appears to be a single abortion. If subsequent abortions occur then the range of tests can be extended.

Interpretation of results

When evaluating results it is important to consider them in relation to the diagnostic criteria for each disease. Hence, while the presence of antibody to BVD or to *N. caninum* is considered to indicate fetal infection, it must be remembered that infection of the fetus need not necessarily be lethal, especially as gestational age increases. Similarly, the isolation of foetopathic bacteria or fungal organisms from the placenta in the absence of histopathology is of no value as they may arise from environmental contamination after the placenta has been passed.

In the majority of infections maternal infection precedes abortion so that paired serology is valueless. As many of the infections of importance tend to be endemic and circulating antibody may persist for long periods the presence of maternal antibody at the time of the abortion can only be taken to show that the cow has been exposed to the agent. The converse applies when the MAT is used for leptospirosis as the IgM antibody response can be so transient that the dam may be seronegative at the time of abortion.

In essence, serology tests in the dam are of more value when used to exclude infection with negative results than to attempt to confirm a diagnosis with positive results. This should not discourage the use of these techniques to establish whether or not there is evidence of these diseases in the herd, as control strategies may still be required.

Evidence of the involvement of several infectious agents is often found in the course of an outbreak, underlining the importance of proper evaluation of the results, but also raising the question of a potentiation effect amongst agents.

Prognosis

For the individual cow the prognosis is usually favourable as long as any systemic disease or uterine infection is detected and treated. After abortion, oestrous cycles start quickly and, in general, subsequent pregnancy rates are satisfactory. Prognosis for the rest of the pregnant animals in the herd is a more serious consideration and varies with the diagnosed cause of abortion.

Conclusion

Abortions are often the most obvious manifestation of an underlying herd problem that may be of significant financial importance to the owner of the cattle herd. Failure on the part of the veterinary surgeon to pursue or advise correctly could have a severe penalty for the producer.

References

Agerholm, J.S., Jensen, N.E., Jensen, H.E. & Aarestrup, F.M. (1999) Experimental infection of pregnant cows with *Bacillus licheniformis* bacteria. *Veterinary Pathology*, **36**, 191–201.

Alexander, A.V., Walker, R.L., Johnson, B.J., Charlton, B.R. & Woods, L.W. (1992) Bovine abortions attributable to *Listeria ivanovii* – 4 cases. *Journal of the American Veterinary Medical Association*, **200**, 711–14.

Anderson, M.L., Blanchard, P.C., Barr, B.C., Dubey, J.P., Hoffman, R.L. & Conrad, P.A. (1991) *Neospora*-like protozoan infection as a major cause of abortion in California dairy cattle. *Journal of the American Veterinary Association*, **198**, 241–4.

Anderson, M.L., Reynolds, J.P., Rowe, J.D., Sverlow K.W., Packham, A.E., Barr, B.C. & Conrad, P.A. (1997) Evidence of vertical transmission of *Neospora* sp. infection in dairy cattle. *Journal of the American Veterinary Association*, **210**, 1169–72.

Baker, J.C. (1987) Bovine viral diarrhoea virus: a review. *Journal of the American Veterinary Association*, **190**, 1449–58.

Barr, B.C. & Anderson, M.L. (1993) Infectious diseases causing bovine abortion and fetal loss. *Veterinary Clinics of North America: Food Animal Practice*, **9**, 343–68.

Barr, B.C. & BonDurant, R.H. (1997) *Current Therapy in Large Animal Theriogenology*, pp. 373–82. W.B. Saunders, London.

Barr, B.C., Rowe, J.D., Sverlow, K.W., BonDurant, R.H., Ardans A.A., Oliver, M.N. & Conrad, P.A. (1994) Experimental reproduction of bovine fetal *Neospora* infection and death with a bovine *Neospora* isolate. *Journal of Veterinary Diagnostic Investigation*, **6**, 207–15.

Bartels, C.J.M., Wouda, W. & Schukken, Y.H. (1999) Risk factors for *Neospora caninum*-associated abortion storms in dairy herds in the Netherlands (1995–1997). *Theriogenology*, **52**, 247–57.

BCVA (1992) Guidelines for the diagnosis and control of *Leptospira hardjo* infection in cattle. British Cattle Veterinary Association, Gloucester.

BCVA (1995) *Bull Hiring*. British Cattle Veterinary Association, Gloucester.

Bjerkås, I., Mohn, S.F. & Presthus, J. (1984) Unidentified cyst-forming sporozoon causing encephalomyelitis and myositis in dogs. *Zeitschrift für Parasitenkunde*, **70**, 271–4.

Bolin, C.A. & Alt, D.P. (1998) Clinical signs, diagnosis and prevention of bovine leptospirosis. In *Proceedings of the 20th World Buiatrics Congress*, Sydney, Australia, Vol. 2, pp. 899–904.

Brown, T.T., Schultz, A.D., Duncan, J.R. & Bistner, S.I. (1979) Serological response of the bovine fetus to bovine viral diarrhoea virus. *Infection and Immunity*, **25**, 93–7.

Brownlie, J., Clarke, M.C., Hooper, L.B. & Bell, G.D. (1995) Protection of the bovine fetus from bovine viral diarrhoea virus by means of a new inactivated vaccine. *Veterinary Record*, **137**, 58–62.

Buxton, D., Caldow, G.L., Maley, S.W., Marks, J. & Innes, E.A. (1997) Neosporosis and bovine abortion in Scotland. *Veterinary Record*, **141**, 649–51.

Caldow, G.L., Buxton, D., Spence, J.A. & Holisz, J. (1996) Diagnoses of bovine abortion in Scotland. In *Proceedings of the British Cattle Veterinary Association, XIX World Buiatrics Congress*, Vol 1, pp. 191–4.

Caldow, G.L. & Taylor, D.W. (1997) Experiences with venereal campylobacter infection in suckler herds. *Cattle Practice*, **5**, 327–34.

Capen, C.C. (1993) Hyperplasia of the thyroid gland. In *Pathology of Domestic Animals* (ed. by K.V.F. Jubb, P.C. Kennedy & N. Palmer), pp. 315–18. Academic Press, London.

Casaro, A.P.E., Kendrick, J.W. & Kennedy, P.C. (1971) Response of the bovine fetus to bovine viral diarrhea-mucosal disease virus. *American Journal of Veterinary Research*, **32**, 1543–62.

Chang, W. & Ogg, J.E. (1971) Transduction and mutation to glycine tolerance in *Vibrio fetus*. *American Journal of Veterinary Research*, **32**, 649–53.

Chappel, R.J., Millar, B.D., Adler, B., Hill, J., Jeffers, M.J., Jones, R.T., McCaughan, C.J., Mead, L.J. & Skilbeck, N.W. (1989) *Leptospira interrogans* serovar *hardjo* is not a major cause of abortion in Victoria. *Australian Veterinary Journal*, **66**, 330–3.

Charles, J.A. (1994) Akabane virus. *Veterinary Clinics of North America Food Animal Practice*, **10**, 525–46.

Clark, B.L. (1971) Review of bovine vibriosis. *Australian Veterinary Journal*, **47**, 103–7.

Corbeil, L.B., Duncan, J.R., Schurig, G.G.D., Hall, C.E. & Winter, A.J. (1974) Bovine venereal vibriosis: variations in immunoglobin class of antibodies in genital secretions and serum. *Infection and Immunity*, **10**, 1084–90.

Cravens, R.L., Ellsworth, M.A., Sorenson, C.D. & White, A.K. (1996) Efficacy of a temperature-sensitive modified-live bovine herpes virus type-1 vaccine against abortion and stillbirth in pregnant heifers. *Journal of the American Veterinary Medicine Association*, **208**, 2031–4.

Czaplicki, G. & Thiry, E. (1998) An association exists between bovine herpes virus-4 seropositivity and abortion in cows. *Preventive Veterinary Medicine*, **33**, 235–40.

Dannatt, L., Guy, F. & Trees, A.J. (1995) Abortion due to *Neospora* species in a dairy herd. *Veterinary Record*, **137**, 566–7.

David, G.P. (1993) Abortion in cattle associated with *Bacillus licheniformis* infection – an update. *Cattle Practice*, **1**, 33–7.

Davies, T.G. & Renton, C.P. (1992) Some aspects of the epidemiology and control of *Salmonella typhimurium* infection in outwintered suckler cows. *Veterinary Record*, **131**, 528–31.

Davison, H.C., Otter, A. & Trees, A.J. (1999) Estimation of vertical and horizontal transmission parameters of *Neospora caninum* infections in dairy cattle. *International Journal for Parasitology*, **29**, 1683–9.

Dekeyser, P.J. (1986) Bovine genital campylobacteriosis. In *Current Therapy in Theriogenology*, Vol. 2 (ed. by D.A. Morrow), pp. 263–6. W.B. Saunders, Philadelphia.

Dennet, D.P., Reece, R.L., Barasa, J.O. & Johnson, R.H. (1974) Observations on the incidence and distribution of serotypes of *Tritrichomonas fetus* in beef cattle in North-Eastern Australia. *Australian Veterinary Journal*, **50**, 427–31.

Dhaliwal, G.S., Dobson, H., Montgomery, J. & Ellis, W.A. (1996) Reduced conception rates in dairy cattle associated with serological evidence of *Leptospira interrogans* serovar *hardjo* infection. *Veterinary Record*, **139**, 110–14.

Dillman, R.C. & Dennis, S.M. (1976) Sequential sterile autolysis in the ovine fetus: macroscopic changes. *American Journal of Veterinary Research*, **37**, 403–7.

Dubey, J.P. (1999) Neosporosis – the first decade of research. *International Journal for Parasitology*, **29**, 1485–8.

Dubey, J.P., Carpenter, J.L., Speer, C.A., Topper, M.J. & Uggla, A. (1988) Newly recognized fatal protozoan disease of dogs. *Journal of the American Veterinary Medicine Association*, **192**, 1269–85.

Dubey, J.P., Lindsay, D.S., Adams, D.V.M., Gay, J.M., Baszler, T.V., Blagburn, B.L. & Thullies, P. (1996) Serological responses of cattle and other animals infected with *Neospora caninum*. *American Journal of Veterinary Research*, **57**, 329–36.

Dubovi, E.J. (1992) Genetic diversity and BVD virus. *Comparative Immunology and Microbiology of Infectious Diseases*, **15**, 155–62.

Duffell, S.J. & Harkness, J.W. (1985) Bovine virus diarrhoea-mucosal disease infection in cattle. *Veterinary Record*, **117**, 240–5.

Echternkamp, S.E. & Gregory, K.E. (1999) Effects of twinning on postpartum reproductive performance in cattle selected for twin births. *Journal of Animal Science*, **77**, 48–60.

Ellis, J.A., Martin, K., Norman, G.R. & Haines, D.H. (1995) Comparison of detection methods for bovine virus diarrhoea. *Journal of Veterinary Diagnostic Investigation*, **7**, 433–6.

Ellis, W.A., O'Brien J.J., Neill, S.D., Ferguson, H.W. & Hanna, J. (1982) Bovine leptospirosis: microbiological and serological findings in aborted fetuses. *Veterinary Record*, **110**, 147–50.

Evans, S. & Davies, R.H. (1996) Case control study of multiple-resistant *Salmonella typhimurium* DT104 infection of cattle in Great Britain. *Veterinary Record*, **139**, 557–8.

Forar, A.L., Gay, J.M. & Hancock, D.D. (1995) The frequency of endemic fetal loss in dairy cattle: a review. *Theriogenology*, **43**, 989–1000.

French, N.P., Clancy, D., Davidson, H.C. & Trees, A.J. (1999) Mathematical models of *Neospora caninum* infection in dairy cattle: transmission and options for control. *International Journal for Parasitology*, **29**, 1691–704.

Gee, C.D., Gaden, E.R. & Harper, P.A.W. (1989) An investigation of the causes of parturient calf mortality in Shorthorn heifers. *Australian Veterinary Journal*, **66**, 293–8.

Griffiths, P.C., Plater, J.M., Martin, T.C., Hughes, S.L., Hughes, K.J., Hewinson, R.G. & Dawson, M. (1995) Epizootic bovine abortion in a dairy herd: characterization of a *Chlamydia psittaci* isolate and antibody response. *British Veterinary Journal*, **6**, 683–93.

Hewson, P.I., Lander, K.P. & Gill, K.P.W. (1985) Enzyme-linked immunoabsorbent assay for antibodies to *C. fetus* in vaginal mucus. *Research in Veterinary Science*, **38**, 41–5.

Hietala, S.K. & Thurmond, M.C. (1999) Postnatal *Neospora caninum* transmission and transient serologic responses in two dairies. *International Journal for Parasitology*, **29**, 1669–76.

Hult, L. & Lindberg, A. (1998) The Swedish National Control scheme on BVD – tips, tricks and traps. In *Proceedings of the Australian Association of Cattle Veterinarians, XX World Buiatrics Congress*, Sydney, Vol. 2, pp. 995–1001.

Hum, S., Brunner, J. & Gardiner, B. (1993) Failure of therapeutic vaccination of a bull infected with *C. fetus*. *Australian Veterinary Journal*, **70**, 386–7.

Hum, S., Brunner, J., McInnes, A., Mendoza, G. & Stephens J. (1994) Evaluation of cultural methods and selective media for the isolation of *C. fetus* subsp. *venerealis* from cattle. *Australian Veterinary Journal*, **71**, 184–6.

Hum, S. & MacInnes, A. (1987) *Australian Standard Diagnostic Techniques for Animal Diseases* (ed. by L.A. Corner & T.J. Bagust), CSIRO for the Standing Committee on Agri-culture and Resource Management, East Melbourne, No. 22.

Hum, S., Stephens, L.R. & Quinn, C. (1991) Diagnosis by ELISA of bovine abortion due to *C. fetus*. *Australian Veterinary Journal*, **68**, 272–5.

Johnson, C.T., Lupson, G.R. & Lawrence, K.E. (1994) The bovine placentome in bacterial and mycotic abortions. *Veterinary Record*, **134**, 263–6.

Kaashoek, M.J., Moerman, A., Madic, J. Weerdmeester, K., Maris-Veldhuis, M.A., Rijsewijk, F.A.M. & Van Oirschot, J.T. (1995) An inactivated vaccine based on a glycoprotein E-negative strain of bovine herpes virus 1 induces protective immunity and allows serological differentiation. *Vaccine*, **13**, 342–6.

Kaashoek, M.J., Straver, P.H., Van Rooij, E.M.A., Quak, J. & Van Oirschot, J.T. (1996) Virulence, immunogenicity and reactivation of seven bovine herpes virus 1.1 Strains: clinical and virological aspects. *Veterinary Record*, **139**, 416–21.

Kirkbride, C.A. (1992a) Viral agents and associated lesions detected in a 10-year study of bovine abortions and stillbirths. *Journal of Veterinary Diagnostic Investigation*, **4**, 374–9.

Kirkbride, C.A. (1992b) Etiologic agents detected in a 10-year study of bovine abortions and stillbirths. *Journal of Veterinary Diagnostic Investigation*, **4**, 175–80.

Kirkland, P.D., McGowan, M.R., Mackintosh, S.G. & Moyle, A. (1997) Insemination of cattle with semen from a bull transiently infected with pestivirus. *Veterinary Record*, **140**, 124–7.

Knickerbocker, J.J., Drost, M. & Thatcher, W.W. (1986) Endocrine patterns during the initiation of puberty, the estrous cycle, pregnancy and parturition in cattle. In *Current Therapy in Theriogenology* (ed. by D.A. Morrow), pp. 117–25. W.B. Saunders Philadelphia.

Knudtson, W.U. & Kirkbride, C.A. (1992) Fungi associated with bovine abortion in the northern plains states (USA). *Journal of Veterinary Diagnostic Investigation*, **4**, 181–5.

Kvasnicka, W.G., Hall, M., Hanks, D., Ebel, E. & Kearley, B. (1996) Current concepts in the control of bovine trichomoniasis. *Compendium on Continuing Education, Food Animal Medicine and Management* (Supplement) **18**, S105–112.

Lander, K.P. (1983) New technique for collection of vaginal mucus from cattle. *Veterinary Record*, **112**, 570.

Low, J.C. & Donachie, W. (1997) A review of *Listeria monocytogenes* and listeriosis. *The Veterinary Journal*, **153**, 9–29.

McAllister, M.M., Dubey, J.P., Lindsay, D.S., Jolley, W.R., Wills, R.A. & McGuire, A.M. (1998) Dogs are definitive hosts of *Neospora caninum*. *International Journal for Parasitology*, **28**, 1473–8.

McGowan, M.R. & Kirkland, P.D. (1995) Early reproductive loss due to bovine pestivirus infection. *British Veterinary Journal*, **151**, 263–70.

MacLaren, A.P.C. & Agumbah, G.J.O. (1988) Infertility in cattle in South West Scotland caused by an intermediate strain of *C. fetus* subsp. *fetus*. *British Veterinary Journal*, **144**, 27–44.

McNamee, P.T., Trees, A.J., Guy, F., Moffett, D. & Kilpatrick, D. (1996) Diagnosis and prevalence of neosporosis in cattle in Northern Ireland. *Veterinary Record*, **138**, 419–20.

MAFF (1989) Cattle Health Scheme. ADAS.

MAFF (1998a) *Veterinary Investigation Surveillance Report 1998 and 1991–1998*. Veterinary Laboratories Agency, Weybridge.

MAFF (1998b) *Salmonella in Livestock Production 1998*. Veterinary Laboratories Agency, Weybridge.

Mee, J.F. (1992) Epidemiology of abortion in Irish dairy cattle on six research farms. *Irish Journal of Agriculture and Food Research*, **31**, 13–21.

Mee, J.F. & Malone, A. (1995) An outbreak of *Salmonella dublin* abortion in outwintered dairy cows. *Irish Veterinary Journal*, **48**, 314–15.

Meyling, A. & Mikel-Jensen, A. (1988) Transmission of bovine virus diarrhoea virus (BVDV) by artificial insemination with semen from a persistently infected bull. *Veterinary Microbiology*, **17**, 97–105.

Miller, J.M., Whetstone, C.A., Bello, L., Lawrence, W.C. & Whitbeck, J.C. (1995) Abortion in heifers inoculated with a thymidine kinase-negative recombinant of bovine herpes virus 1. *American Journal of Veterinary Research*, **56**, 870–4.

Miller, J.M., Whetstone, C.A. & Van Der Maaten, M.J. (1991) Abortifacient property of bovine herpes virus type 1 isolates that represent three subtypes determined by restriction endonuclease analysis of viral DNA. *Americal Journal of Veterinary Research*, **52**, 458–61.

Miller, R.B. (1988) Reproductive failure in domestic animals: a discussion on the pathogenesis. In *11th International Congress on Animal Reproduction and Artificial Insemination*, Dublin, pp. 284–92.

MLC (1998) *Making Money Out Of Beef: A Way Forward For Beef Producers*. Meat and Livestock Commission, Winter Hill, Milton Keynes.

Nettleton, P.F. & Entrican, G. (1995) Ruminant pestiviruses. *British Veterinary Journal*, **151**, 615–42.

Nix, J.M., Spitzer, J.C., Grimes, L.W., Burns, G.L. & Plyler, B.B. (1998) A retrospective analysis of factors contributing to calf mortality and dystokia in beef cattle. *Theriogenology*, **49**, 1515–23.

Noakes, D.E. (1986) *Fertility and Obstetrics in Cattle* (ed. by E.A. Chandler, P.G.C. Bedford & J.B. Sutton), pp. 65–9. Blackwell Scientific Publications, Oxford.

Norton, J.H. & Campbell, R.S.F. (1990) Non-infectious causes of bovine abortion. *Veterinary Bulletin*, **60**, 1137–47.

Otter, A., Jeffrey, M., Scholes, S.F.E., Helmick, B., Wilesmith, J.W. & Trees, A.J. (1997) Comparison of histology with maternal and fetal serology for the diagnosis of abortion due to bovine neosporosis. *Veterinary Record*, **141**, 487–9.

Paiba, G.A., Green, L.E., Lloyd, G., Patel, D. & Morgan, K.L. (1999) Prevalence of antibodies to *Coxiella burnetii* (Q fever) in bulk tank milk in England and Wales. *Veterinary Record*, **144**, 519–22.

Paton, D.J., Christiansen, K.H., Alenius, S., Cranwell, M.P., Pritchard, G.C. & Drew, T.J. (1998) Prevalence of antibodies to bovine virus diarrhoea virus and other viruses in bulk tank milk in England and Wales. *Veterinary Record*, **142**, 385–91.

Paton, D.J., Goodey, R., Brockman, S. & Wood, L. (1989) Evaluation of the quality and virological status of semen from bulls actively infected with BVD. *Veterinary Record*, **124**, 63–4.

Pritchard, D.G., Allsup, T.N., Pennycott, T.W., Palmer, N.M.A., Woolley, J.C. & Richards, M.S. (1989) Analysis of risk factors for infection of cattle herds with *Leptospira interrogans* serovar *hardjo*. In *Proceedings of the Society for Veterinary Epidemiology and Preventive Medicine* (ed. by G.J. Rowlands), pp. 130–8.

Pritchard, G.C. (1992) Epidemiology of BHV1 infection in cattle breeding herds in Norfolk. In *Denary Proceedings, Society for Veterinary Epidemiology and Preventive Medicine*, pp. 168–85. Edinburgh.

Pritchard, G.C. (1999) Bulk milk antibody testing for *Leptospira hardjo* infection. *Cattle Practice*, **7**, 59–61.

Radostits, O.M., Blood, D.C. & Gay, C.C. (1994) *Veterinary Medicine*, 8th edn, pp. 730–46. Baillière Tindall, London.

Rhyan, J.C., Blanchard, P.C., Kvasnicka, W.G., Hall, M.R. & Hanks, D. (1995) Tissue-invasive *Tritrichomonas fetus* in four aborted bovine fetuses. *Journal of Veterinary Diagnostic Investigation*, **7**, 409–12.

Rhyan, J.C., Stackhouse, L.L. & Quinn, W.J. (1988) Fetal and placental lesions in bovine abortion due to *Tritrichomonas fetus*. *Veterinary Pathology*, **25**, 350–5.

Rocha, M.A., Barbosa, E.F., Guedes, R.M., Lage, A.P., Leite, R.C. & Gouveia, A.M. (1999) Detection of BHV-1 in a naturally infected bovine fetus by a nested PCR assay. *Veterinary Research Communications*, **23**, 133–41.

Roche, J.F., Boland, M.P. & McGeady, T.A. (1981) Reproductive wastage following artificial insemination in catttle. *Veterinary Record*, **109**, 95–7.

Sanderson, M.W. & Chenoweth, P.J. (1999) The role of *Ureaplasma diversum* in bovine reproduction. *Compendium on Continuing Education for the Practicing Veterinarian*, **21**, S98–102.

Schurig, G.C., Hall, C.E., Burda, K., Corbeil, L.B., Duncan, J.R. & Winter, A.J. (1973) Persistant genital tract infection with *Vibrio fetus fetus* associated with serotype alteration of the infecting strain. *American Journal of Veterinary Research*, **34**, 1399–403.

Semambo, D.K.N., Ayliffe, T.R., Boyd, J.S. & Taylor, D.J. (1991) Early abortion in cattle induced by experimental intrauterine infection with pure cultures of *Actinomyces pyogenes*. *Veterinary Record*, **129**, 12–16.

Smith, C.R., Kettereer, P.J., McGowan, M.R. & Corney, B.G. (1994) A review of laboratory techniques and their use in the diagnosis of *Leptospira interrogans* serovar *hardjo* infection in cattle. *Australian Veterinary Journal*, **71**, 290–4.

Sreenan, J.M. & Diskin, M.G. (1986) The extent and timing of embryonic mortality in cattle. In *Embryonic Mortality in Farm Animals* (ed. by J.M. Sreenan & M.G. Diskin), pp. 142–58. Martinus, Nijhoff, CEC.

Thilsted, J.P. & Dubey, J.P. (1989) Neosporosis-like abortions in a herd of dairy cattle. *Journal of Veterinary Diagnostic Investigation*, **1**, 205–209.

Thornton, R. (1991) Bovine abortions – laboratory diagnoses 1991. *Surveillance*, **19**, 24.

Thurmond, M.C. & Hietala, S.K. (1997) Effect of congenitally acquired *Neospora caninum* infection on risk of abortion and subsequent abortions in dairy cattle. *American Journal of Veterinary Research*, **58**, 1381–5.

Thurmond, M.C., Hietala, S.K. & Blanchard P.C. (1997) Herd-based diagnosis of *Neospora caninum*-induced endemic and epidemic abortion in cows and evidence for congenital and postnatal transmission. *Journal of Veterinary Diagnostic Investigation*, **9**, 44–9.

Thurmond, M.C., Hietala, S.K. & Blanchard, P.C. (1999) Predictive values of fetal histopathology and immunoperoxidase staining in diagnosing bovine abortion caused by *Neospora caninum* in a dairy herd. *Journal of Veterinary Diagnostic Investigation*, **11**, 90–4.

Wendorf, G.L., Lawyer, M.S. & First, N.L. (1983) Role of the adrenals in the maintenance of pregnancy in cows. *Journal of Reproduction and Fertility*, **68**, 281–7.

Wilkie, B.N. & Winter, A.J. (1971) Bovine vibriosis: the distribution and specificity of antibodies induced by vaccination and infection and the immunofluorescent localization of the organism in infected heifers. *Canadian Journal of Comparative Medicine*, **35**, 301–12.

Wouda, W., Bartels, C.J.M. & Moen, A.R. (1999) Characteristics of *Neospora caninum*-associated abortion storms in dairy herds in the Netherlands (1995 to 1997). *Theriogenology*, **52**, 233–45.

Wray, C., Wadsworth, Q.C., Richards, D.W. & Morgan, J.H. (1989) A three-year study of *Salmonella dublin* infection in a closed dairy herd. *Veterinary Record*, **124**, 532–5.

Yule, A., Skirrow, S.Z. & BonDurant, R.H. (1989) Bovine trichomoniasis. *Parasitology Today*, **5**, 373–7.

Chapter 38
Bull Infertility

D.N. Logue and W.M. Crawshaw

Introduction	594
Bull use in the UK	595
The role of the veterinarian in bull use	596
Preventing infectious infertility and other diseases	596
Preputial washing	597
Infectious disease control	598
Investigation of bull infertility	598
History	598
Examination of the bull for breeding soundness	599
Manifestations, aetiology, treatment and prognosis of bull	
infertility	610
Failure to mount	610
Failure to achieve intromission	612
Failure to thrust and ejaculate after intromission	616
Normal service with a poor pregnancy rate	617
Conclusion	624

Introduction

Since the domestication of cattle the bull has been a talisman and the desire to own a special bull a particular urge in all stock rearing countries. The bull is a symbol of power in the East, where Indra the sky deity is represented in myth as a mighty bull, while in the West as an example there is the Celtic legend of the Brown Bull of Quelgny stolen by Queen Mae of Connacht from Dara in Ulster only to be retrieved by the hero Cuchulain. Time has not diverted man a great deal from this interest in bull lineage and the performance of his offspring! The development of methodologies to assess the transmission of superior economic traits from bulls to their progeny over the last 50 years has been one of the success stories of the cattle industry. However, like the Brown Bull the truly outstanding sire is still very rare and the purchase of a young unproven bull is a gamble. Despite this the repeated need for young bulls (no bull is immortal) means that many are bought with this vision in mind, despite the difficulties in achieving it.

When all breeding was by natural service the potential for genetic improvement by a good bull was very limited. Furthermore, selling, sharing and hiring animals resulted in the spread of venereal disease with some disastrous results for those affected farms. Artifi-

cial insemination (AI) has proved to be one of the most successful reproductive technologies and it became a commercial reality in the UK just before the end of the Second World War. AI has fulfilled two objectives: firstly, it set in motion more focused genetic improvement coupled with the widespread use of good bulls and secondly, it has limited the spread of venereal diseases. Unfortunately, the expression of oestrus in the cow varies in time of occurrence, duration and intensity and many farmers find accurate and, more particularly, efficient oestrous detection difficult and time consuming. Furthermore, particularly in large beef suckler herds under essentially range conditions, oestrous detection and the handling of cattle for AI are less practical. These factors ensure that many farmers continue to use natural service entirely or partially even though, due to the genetic improvement from AI, dairy farmers in particular could afford to have a longer calving interval and yet still expect to have the same financial returns (Hillers *et al.*, 1982; Stott *et al.*, 1999).

The problem is illustrated by a study of UK national cattle population statistics where only approximately half the cows are bred by AI (Logue & Isbister, 1992), this figure being considerably higher for the dairy herd. Although confidentiality has stopped many of these statistics being easily available in the UK we have no reason to believe the proportion has changed. However, this figure may increase following the 2001 foot and mouth disease outbreak. In the USA the proportion bred by AI is probably a little higher (70 per cent). In addition, there have been a number of factors that have counteracted the undoubted improvements in the efficiency of AI.

(1) The economics of dairy and beef production have resulted in a general trend to larger herds with fewer staff and so less time available for oestrous detection. Furthermore, the continuing financial pressure to cut costs has also made many dairy farmers economize by changing from paying for a technician AI service to inseminating their own cows (DIY AI). Many of these people keep a bull as a precaution against poor fertility arising from a doubtful insemination technique. Unfortunately, no figures are produced for the number

Table 38.1 Number of cows in DIY AI herds (Anon. 1988).

	England and Wales	Northern Ireland	Scotland	Total
DIY licences	3 300	1 000	700	5 000
Average herd size	69	37	89	–
Number of cows	227 700	37 000	54 300	319 000
Cows inseminated (assuming 75%) by DIY AI	170 775	27 750	40 725	239 250

Table 38.2 UK dairy cattle statistics (Anon. 1979, 1988, 1998).

Year	Cow numbers $\times 10^6$	Herd size
1960	4.01	20
1970	4.55	31
1980	4.69	55
1990	4.43	67
1997	4.41	72

of cows inseminated in the DIY AI sector in the UK. However, census data, the number of DIY AI licences issued by area and the assumption that 75 per cent of the cows in each herd are inseminated does allow an estimate (Table 38.1). It can be seen that DIY AI probably accounts for less than one in five of all dairy cow inseminations in the UK.

(2) The gradual increase in herd size has meant that the added costs of keeping one or even several bulls are relatively lower per unit of production. For example, in the UK, dairy herd size has increased dramatically over the last 30 years (see Table 38.2), and this has been mirrored in Europe and in virtually all countries with an advanced dairy industry.

(3) A further effect of the larger number of cows per herd has led to a more predictable production of heifer replacements because the male:female ratio remains nearer to the expected 50:50 as the numbers increase. This has meant that a definite block of heifers of similar age can be released for natural service.

(4) In many beef and dairy herds, calving, and thus breeding periods, are concentrated into relatively short periods of time for production and management reasons. This leads to a requirement for high oestrous detection rates and high fertility, both of which are best achieved by using a combination of AI and natural service.

(5) Finally, in the past an important reason for using AI was to reduce the introduction of disease. With the increasing improvement in the health status of the national herd in many countries there is less pressure for AI use for this reason alone. However, this confidence is likely to be misplaced unless the farm takes adequate precautions when acquiring bulls.

Bull use in the UK

It is worthwhile defining the various types of herd breeding policy since this will influence the management of the bull and may give a guide to the needs of the unit with regard to disease control.

Four basic types of policy can be recognized:

(1) *Beef suckler herd.* The principal demand is to produce calves for finishing. The cows are mated while suckling. For many years and in most geographical locations it has been axiomatic that this system operates at highest efficiency when there is a short (but efficient) breeding period (Kilkenny, 1978). Ideally this should be less than 10 weeks and demands very high levels of fertility in both bull and cow.

(2) *Dairy heifers.* A considerable proportion of dairy herds use natural service when breeding heifers. This is mainly to avoid oestrous detection and the need to gather the individual heifer for AI when often these are run on a more remote area of the farm.

(3) *Sweeper bull.* This term usually refers to the running of a bull after a fixed period of 'AI-only' breeding. Generally, in dairy cattle, the bull used is a beef breed and thus any calves born are easily distinguished from purebred dairy calves. The use of synchronization and fixed-time AI with batches of maiden heifers using an easy-calving sire has to some degree replaced natural service in both dairy and beef heifers, but in many herds those heifers that return are served by a sweeper bull. The timing of the introduction of the sweeper is paramount since mating pressure will obviously depend on the number of non-pregnant cows or heifers left after the AI breeding period. Clearly a

drop in the pregnancy rates achieved with AI can result in an increase of mating pressure.

(4) *Modified sweeper.* The sweeper bull is utilized for mating selected cows throughout the breeding season, for example cows of low genetic potential, repeat breeders, cows not exhibiting firm signs of oestrus and cows with a history of being difficult to get in calf. Subsequently, the bull is used as a 'true' sweeper.

Finally, a minority of dairy herds still primarily use natural service.

The role of the veterinarian in bull use

The role of the veterinarian in the control and monitoring of bull fertility is three-fold (see Box 38.1). Veterinarians should be authoritative in these roles for their clients or be able and willing to refer matters to another veterinarian with the appropriate resources if the occasion demands.

Preventing infectious infertility and other diseases

Before considering the reproductive performance of the bull on the farm the first priority must be to keep disease out! No veterinarian or farmer should be without some appreciation of the risks that are being taken by the purchase of a bull (or even semen or embryos). In addition to the notifiable diseases (such as foot-and-mouth disease) there are a whole plethora of others that can cause economic loss. Unfortunately in the past, farmers in the UK, and for that matter elsewhere, have been pretty cavalier in their attitude to introducing disease. Veterinarians, by discussing these issues with their clients, can do much to reduce the risks of introducing disease and so protect the viability of their clients' farms. The loss of output arising from the

Box 38.1 Role of the veterinarian in bull fertility.

(1) Preventing the introduction of infectious infertility and other diseases to the farm
(2) Assessing fertility and the level of investigation that is needed:
  (a) before purchase
  (b) after purchase
  (c) before use each breeding season
  (d) after poor fertility results
(3) Monitoring herd fertility (including the bull) by the assessment of breeding records

damaging effects of infectious disease impacts significantly on efficiency.

The most important source of infectious disease for cattle is other livestock, particularly cattle. Uncontrolled movement of a bull into a herd carries a significant risk of introducing disease. This can be minimized by the following measures but presupposes that other biosecurity precautions are in place:

(1) Bulls (and any other cattle) should be purchased only from herds certified free from specific diseases of concern by reputable cattle health schemes such as those registered with the Cattle Health Certification Standards (CheCS) body in the UK. While individual farm programmes can be undertaken or declarations made by the farmer and his veterinarian to the effect that a particular disease has not been seen, clearly these will have less certainty. The latter point is illustrated by Kallis *et al.* (1999) who revealed by faecal culture that 40 per cent of 100 Dutch dairy herds considered to be free of Johne's disease on the basis of owner and veterinary declaration were actually infected.

(2) Quarantine incoming cattle before entry into the main herd to allow testing for diseases that may be carried and development of any incubating diseases. In most cases four weeks should suffice, but this depends on circumstances and the diseases under consideration. Quarantine could also be applied to other species of livestock entering the farm that potentially carry diseases infectious to cattle.

(3) During the quarantine period an adequate testing programme and/or prophylactic treatment against diseases of concern should be employed. The latter may be necessary where testing is unreliable or gives an equivocal answer (e.g. for venereal campylobacteriosis and *Leptospira hardjo*).

The diseases of importance vary with country and area and are determined by the economic or practical importance of the disease, an assessment of the risk of introducing the disease, the availability of low cost and reliable tests and whether or not the disease is already present in the herd. In the UK the following non-statutory diseases are suggested as being worthy of consideration based on their prevalence and the economic impact that they may have on the herd.

Bovine virus diarrhoea virus (BVDV)
Infectious bovine rhinotracheitis virus (IBRV) (bovine herpes virus 1 [BHV-1])
Leptospira hardjo
Johne's disease (paratuberculosis)
Venereal campylobacteriosis
Salmonellosis (especially *S. dublin*)

Whilst neosporosis is a significant cause of bovine reproductive failure any epidemiological role of the bull is undetermined and the reliability of current laboratory tests for detecting carriers remains questionable. However, the precautionary principle suggests it is unwise to acquire bulls bred in herds infected with *Neospora caninum* at least until more is known about this infection. Outside and unfortunately even within the UK, diseases considered notifiable in the UK such as brucellosis and tuberculosis also need to be considered.

The two most important true venereal diseases are trichomoniasis and campylobacteriosis, although there is evidence for the venereal transmission of some *Ureaplasma* sp., *Mycoplasma bovigenetalium*, BHV-1, brucellosis and even *Haemophilus somnus*. Bovine trichomoniasis is a venereal disease characterized by early to mid-gestation pregnancy losses, reduced calving rates and pyometra; it is caused by the flagellated protozoan *Tritrichomonas fetus*. As far as is known, it is transmitted by venereal contact only. Campylobacteriosis, which also presents as a large increase in returns to service with early to mid-gestation pregnancy losses, is classically caused by *C. fetus venerealis*. However, there is evidence that this organism does not always follow the classic laboratory identification procedures and this has led to the proposition of *C. fetus intermediatus*, which also appears to cause the same clinical problems in cattle. This organism has many of the properties of *C. fetus fetus*. In these two venereal infections the bull is the long-term carrier of the organism, apparently without ill effects (i.e. no visible lesions are evident in recently or chronically infected bulls) and a distinct correlation exists between age and infection, with older bulls being far more likely to sustain an infection than younger bulls. Infection of the female occurs at the time of coitus. Diagnosis of campylobacteriosis in the female is by examination of vaginal mucus, collected by the method of Lander (1983), for antibody by the vaginal mucus agglutination test (VMAT) and for the bacterium by culture. Since antibody takes some time to appear after an infected service and false negative VMAT results are common, at least 12 cows should be sampled at least 50 days after a potentially infected service. Cows with blood in the mucus can give false positive results and cows in oestrus are more likely to give false negative results and such animals should not be sampled. In the bull, demonstration of the *Campylobacter fetus* bacterium in preputial washings by fluorescent antibody test and culture is used in the UK for diagnosis. Where samples of vaginal mucus or preputial washings are collected with a view to culture they should reach the laboratory within six hours of collection due to the fragility of the bacterium. Alternatively, samples can be submitted in transport enrichment medium. Negative laboratory results in the face of a strong history of infertility and natural service and no other obvious causes should be viewed with suspicion.

Preputial washing

The method of preputial washing used routinely by the Scottish Agricultural College is summarized below.

Protocol for sampling bulls for Campylobacter fetus *sp. screen*

Materials required:

- Recovery fluid: 60 ml phosphate buffered saline (PBS) (sterile).
- Sampling catheter: 10 cm length of 3.5 × 6.5 mm portex tubing (sterile).
- 60 ml syringe: attached to catheter (sterile).
- 3 × 20 ml sterile sample bottles.
- Individual set of sampling materials for each animal sampled.

Procedure:

- Clip preputial hairs.
- Wash preputial orifice with warm water. Do not disinfect.
- Load syringe with 60 ml warmed PBS.
- Insert catheter as far into prepuce as possible. Clamp one hand over preputial orifice to seal around catheter and hold it in place (use hand nearest bull's head to facilitate massage with the other hand).
- Pass 60 ml warmed PBS through catheter. Leave syringe in place.
- Retain fluid and catheter in prepuce by continuing to clamp one hand over preputial orifice and massage thoroughly along full length of prepuce to scrotum for one minute.
- Collect fluid into the original syringe by withdrawal using the plunger as the catheter is slowly withdrawn.
- Dispense sample into sterile containers and label.
- If the bull urinates during collection the sample should be discarded and the process repeated.
- All samples should be submitted to the laboratory within 6 hours of collection.

With preputial washings false negative results are again to be expected on a single screening, indeed four screenings have been recommended (Dufty, 1967) before a bull can be confidently declared free of infection. A more practical approach to reducing the risk of introducing this infection may therefore be prophylactic treatment of purchased, previously bred bulls by preputial lavage with penicillin and streptomycin antibiotic (Melrose *et al.*, 1957) during the quarantine period. This could be refined by employing prophylactic treatment after a single negative preputial wash screening. Nevertheless, the most reliable way to prevent introduction of this infection is to acquire only unbred males and females. Control in infected herds is by disposal of infected bulls, suspension of natural service and use of AI with uninfected semen for 2 years (Clark, 1971) for all exposed cows, thus allowing the cows to develop immunity and eradicate the organism. Where this is not practicable, use of autogenous vaccine (there is no licensed vaccine in the UK), only using young bulls (<4 years) or operation of 'clean' and 'dirty' herds should be considered. The problems of diagnosis and control of venereal campylobacteriosis should not be underestimated and the reader is referred to Caldow and Taylor (1997) for a more detailed discussion of the subject in suckler herds.

Infectious disease control

Control of infectious disease is very dependent on an assessment of the risk of introducing the disease and on the quality of diagnosis, either of the disease or the carrier state, using laboratory tests. For example, in the UK bulls are not usually tested for trichomoniasis as it has not been diagnosed in home bred animals for many years. However, other diseases such as BVDV are very common and campylobacteriosis is not usual. In the first instance the background of the bull must be considered with regard to whether it could have been exposed and, as a consequence, be a potential carrier of any disease. Furthermore, when subsequent testing is contemplated the limitations of laboratory testing regimes specific for each disease must be appreciated before exclusion is considered. For example, testing individual healthy animals for antibody and/or by faecal culture for the presence of infection with the bacterium of Johne's disease leads to a high proportion of false negative results. Therefore, exclusion of this disease is best achieved by purchase of bulls from herds monitored free of Johne's disease under a reputable cattle health scheme rather than by individual animal testing and quarantine. Knowledge of the effects of disease, methods of control and the laboratory technology to detect disease is continually advancing. Understanding and awareness of BVDV in particular have improved greatly over the last decade. The infection is widespread in the UK and recent estimates of associated losses, which primarily arise from reduced fertility and abortion, suggest that these can be over £45 per cow annually in an infected suckler herd (Gunn *et al.*, 1998). Relatively recently, truly cost-effective control schemes have become a realistic option for certain diseases

(BVDV, IBRV and Johne's disease in the UK). However, as some may remember, lack of appreciation of the organism and its epidemiology meant that a pilot attempt to control *L. hardjo* by MAFF was not successful. Some hard lessons were learnt which have been applied to these new schemes.

Another consideration is whether the bull might itself be at risk of being infected by cattle in the herd it is being introduced to and so having a period of infertility as a result of illness. Completion of a vaccination programme during the quarantine period for the bull might be considered in light of knowledge of the disease status of the herd.

Investigation of bull infertility

Bull infertility is presented as one, or a combination of the four manifestations, namely:

(1) Failure to mount
(2) Failure to achieve intromission
(3) Failure to thrust and ejaculate
(4) Poor pregnancy rate with normal service behaviour

A wide range of conditions can cause each of these. Not only are the aetiological factors varied and numerous but also the management of the bull can contribute to the infertility. Consequently only by obtaining a good history of the bull (including previous fertility) and his present circumstances can one gain an informed appraisal of the most appropriate way in which to conduct the assessment of fertility.

Diagnosis is based upon a combination of bull and herd history, examination of the bull and the results of the various tests that are undertaken including an examination of a representative ejaculate of semen. Even if the diagnosis is tentative and the aetiology uncertain the findings will probably allow a prognosis and may give a rationale for treatment.

History

All investigations of bull fertility are built upon the usual prerequisite of obtaining a good history of the problem. This clearly involves both records of any bull in question but should also entail assessment of the herd as a whole. Usually the client will have given some information about the bull by telephone and, ideally, will have presented some farm records for perusal prior to the examination. At the outset, ask and record the answers to the questions in Box 38.2. One is looking for an estimate of the extent of the infertility by comparison to other bulls, when it was first manifest, if it has been continuous or varied and so on.

Box 38.2 Information required to define the problem.

Type and breed of bull?
Age?
Demeanour?
Ringed?
Type of herd?
Role of bull in herd?
When and where acquired and time with herd?
Calves previously born to the bull?
Extent and duration of problem?
More than one bull with a problem?
Can the problem be related to introduction of a new male or female?
Are AI figures available for the same period?
Is there an insurance/sale agreement status?

In cases where points (1) to (3) above apply it may be possible to give a firm diagnosis and an accurate prognosis based on the history and visual examination of the bull when presented with a cow in season, i.e. without even collecting and examining a semen sample. However, depending on circumstances it may still be advisable at least to attempt to collect a semen sample, even if only to confirm the history.

Examination of the bull for breeding soundness

The objectives of the visit to the farm are:

- To see the conditions under which the bull is expected to work.
- To confirm that the history is reliable and, if possible, to examine records.
- To examine the bull. In order to study semen for abnormal characteristics the operator must use a technique to obtain and prepare semen for examination that will be representative of the ejaculate of the bull in natural service.
- To ascertain the status of the bull as a possible vector of reproductive disease and possibly other diseases of a less specific nature but just as important from an economic point of view.

Where an infertile bull is suspected the following simple preliminary breeding soundness examination steps are worth considering before conducting a full breeding soundness examination which includes semen collection.

(1) Ascertain by personal observation or a reliable report from the farmer whether or not the bull is serving normally.
(2) Physically examine the bull for any obvious genital or other abnormalities. Bulls aged 2 years or more with a scrotal circumference of 30 cm or less are more likely to be infertile or have a lower than 'normal' fertility.
(3) If the cause of the problem is not clear from (1) and (2) above and/or the bull is under a sale agreement or insured for infertility then it is necessary to consider a full breeding soundness examination. However this is not to be undertaken lightly and firstly we recommend consideration of:
(a) Sale agreement: if the time period for a claim has not elapsed ensure the farmer has contacted the market or vendor, informed them of the complaint and checked that a full breeding soundness examination will support the claim.
(b) Insurance case: ensure that the farmer has contacted the insurance company, informed them of the complaint and checked that the policy covers infertility and that a full breeding soundness examination will support the claim.

The goal is to obtain a cost-effective resolution to the problem. It may be very attractive to examine the semen of the bull but is it really necessary? For example, if there is a clear history of infertility and severe testicular abnormalities are found on physical examination of a commercial beef bull, then clearly one is not going to recommend that the bull is used as a reliable sire. Collecting and examining semen will be of little additional value to the client unless demanded by the insurance company. Once it is clear that a full breeding soundness examination is required a decision as to who will carry this out should be made. Referral within the practice or elsewhere may be needed to access the necessary expertise and equipment.

The order of events for the full breeding soundness examination should be:

(1) Define the problem.
(2) Prepare for the visit.
(3) Set up the on-farm laboratory.
(4) Assess the collection area and ability and reliability of the farmer and other animal handlers.
(5) Introductory examination of the bull.
(6) Semen collection and assessment.
(7) Observation of natural service.
(8) Full physical examination of the bull.
(9) Collection of other diagnostic samples.
(10) Preliminary diagnosis, prognosis and advice (e.g. treatment or sexual rest).
(11) Final diagnosis, prognosis and advice after all test results are known.
(12) Further action for the herd and its future breeding management.

Define the problem

This is often less easy than might be assumed and is based on the answers to the questions in Box 38.2 and on the information derived from the preliminary breeding soundness examination steps described above. On occasion the history is vague and the farmer is uneasy about this and the fact that his records may be inadequate. Careful and sensitive questioning may be needed to avoid missing some obvious point. In most cases where a full breeding soundness examination is being carried out the manifestation will be poor pregnancy rate with normal service behaviour. However, some remain undefined beyond infertility seen as 'too many returns' until semen collection is attempted.

Prepare for the visit

A full breeding soundness examination can go smoothly and efficiently and be completed in a couple of hours or alternatively take most of the day and not achieve a collection. Furthermore, it is potentially dangerous. Success, efficiency and safety all depend on good organization and attention to detail. Generally speaking a convenient date will be set for the examination and all parties involved (man and beast) need to be organized accordingly. The following factors, if they can be arranged, should help to make the visit go more smoothly and efficiently:

(1) For a full clinical examination and for semen collection it is desirable that the bull be restrained, that he can be led on a halter and, ideally, that he should be used to serving while being restrained by a halter or ring-rope. The reasons for this are obvious but in our experience with fewer staff on farms, bulls are much less used to being handled and therefore restraint is often counterproductive. This leads to difficulties in reconciling the safety of the collector and handlers with the desire to obtain a good semen sample.

(2) The bull should be sexually rested for at least one but preferably three weeks prior to the visit. This will enhance his libido and avoid depletion of semen reserves, ensuring the best chance of obtaining a representative sample of semen.

(3) A quiet cow in oestrus, preferably halter-trained and that has not been served at that oestrus, should be available as a teaser. Synchronization with a progesterone releasing intravaginal device of at least six females, in our experience, maximizes the chances of one or preferably more being available on the allotted date. While keen young dairy bulls will usually mount a quiet non-oestrus cow, our experience is that collection can still prove difficult, particularly with inadequate restraint and facilities. For experienced beef bulls it is definitely a case of no cow in oestrus, no collection!

(4) There should be suitable facilities for restraint and examination of the bull, e.g. crush with removable sides to allow access to the penis and prepuce.

(5) A suitable roomy fenced area with a non-slip surface and with an escape route for the collector should be available to allow collection of semen. This can be inside or outside.

(6) Instruct the bull handler or those helping in the sequence of events, especially in relation to the bull mounting for collection.

(7) Any cows that have been running solely with this bull should be nearby for pregnancy diagnosis or sampling (vaginal mucus or blood) should the occasion demand it. Unfortunately, often another bull will have remated these. However, even then examination may allow confirmation that the cows have conceived to the second bull.

(8) If possible, another bull should be available nearby. This can be useful to confirm the teaser

Box 38.3 Check list for breeding soundness kit.

- Artificial vaginas, liners, cones, cord and adhesive tape
- Semen collection tubes (preferably graduated)
- Lubricant for artificial vaginas (e.g. KY jelly)
- Kettle and jug to fill artificial vaginas with warm water
- Thermometers to measure artificial vagina temperature
- Electro-ejaculator(s)
- Two funnels and wire funnel holder for collection of electro-ejaculated semen
- Electric plug adapters and circuit breakers
- Electric extension cable
- Microscope and light source
- Warm microscope stage
- Heated cabinet
- Transformer packs
- Stains: nigrosin–eosin, Giemsa and methylene blue
- Small test tubes and holder for use in staining and diluting semen for examination
- 2.9% sodium citrate, 0.9% NaCl and phosphate buffered saline
- Glass pipettes and rubber bulbs
- Slides, coverslips and slide holder box plus slide labels
- Small sterile bottles for fresh semen samples
- Immersion oil
- Paper wipes, cotton wool and swabs
- 50 ml syringe with tubing, phosphate buffered saline and sterile containers for preputial wash
- Tape measure (for scrotal circumference)
- Vacutainers, needle holder, needles and spirit
- Virus and *Mycoplasma* transport media
- Record sheets, slide markers and pens
- Spare light bulb for microscope

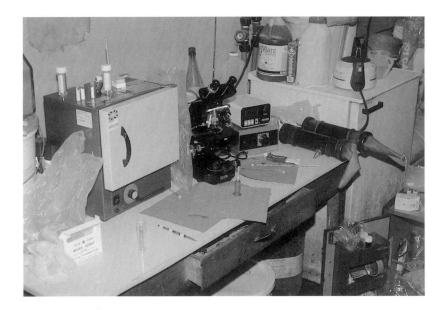

Fig. 38.1 The on-farm laboratory.

cow is in oestrus when the bull under test has failed to mount.

(9) Use a checklist of equipment and materials (see Box 38.3).

Set up the on-farm laboratory

This should be set up on arrival so that there is time for the heated cabinet, solutions, glassware and warm stage to reach the required temperature. Select a small area of bench space, which is covered, has an electricity supply and is not exposed to adverse weather (Fig. 38.1). It should be as near the area of semen collection as possible. Given the standard of some farm electrics a circuit breaker is a wise investment.

The on-farm laboratory should contain the following:

● Microscope with facilities to examine semen by ×50 to ×100 (for initial motility) by ×200 to ×400 (for progressive motility) and ×1000 (for morphology).

● Warm stage (or equivalent). This is a prerequisite for the reliable estimation of motility. Ideally, it should be kept within 1°C of 37°C because either a high or low temperature can have considerable artefactual effects upon sperm motility. Unfortunately, this equipment is quite expensive and therefore many veterinarians use a small prewarmed flat bottle or brass plate as an alternative. If this approach is used then it is best to have two so that they can be alternated and so kept at as steady a temperature as possible.

● Heated cabinet. While it is possible to use the farm kitchen oven to keep slides, coverslips, pipettes and stains, regulation of a reasonable temperature range (35–40°C) is often difficult. For this reason it is preferable to have a small portable cabinet specifically designed for this type of activity.

● Stains. It is well worthwhile using more than one stain routinely. The most commonly used are nigrosin–eosin and Indian ink for sperm morphology, methylene blue for examining the semen for extraneous cells and Giemsa for a combination of the two. Nigrosin–eosin and Indian ink are used directly, i.e. after preheating to 37°C they are mixed with the semen immediately after its collection and a smear is then made. The second stains are used on a direct smear of the semen, which is air-dried and then fixed before staining.

● Solutions to dilute semen for examination of progressive motility. A normal saline solution may suffice, although solutions commonly used for diluting semen are phosphate-buffered saline or 2.9 per cent trisodium citrate. These solutions should also be preheated to as near 37°C as possible.

● Artificial vagina (AV). In general, inexperienced bulls prefer rough liners and younger bulls a shorter artificial vagina, i.e. about 25 cm long. At least two should be assembled (Fig. 38.2) and be filled with warm water (prepared in an electric kettle for example) to a lumen temperature of about 60°C (they will often have cooled to around 45–48°C by the time they will be used). The lumen temperature should be between 42 and 50°C immediately prior to semen collection and this must be checked with a thermometer. In practice it is best to enter the collection area with the AV at 50°C since there will inevitably be some cooling before a collection is made. A sterile lubricant should be applied to the opening of the AV immediately before going to the collection area.

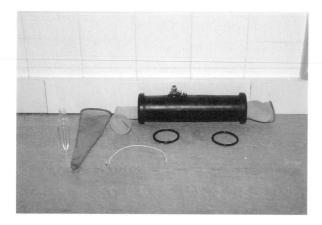

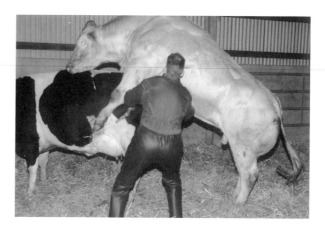

Fig. 38.3 On-farm semen collection in a straw yard using an artificial vagina (AV). The bull is searching for the vulva of the teaser cow. The collector is diverting the penis towards the AV.

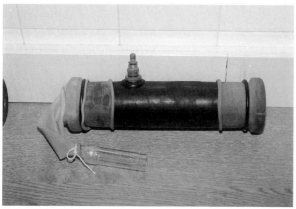

Fig. 38.2 Assembly of the AV. A 30 cm long rubber AV cylinder with latex liner and cone favoured by the authors for collection from adult bulls. A valve on the filling aperture conveniently permits air to be blown in to finely adjust the internal pressure. The graduated collecting tube is anchored to the cone by string and is protected thermally and physically by enclosure in a clear plastic container secured with adhesive tape. A small (1–2 cm) slit can be made in the cone near the AV to act as a safety valve. This reduces the risk of disconnection of the cone or collecting tube that may occur during the thrust if there is too high a pressure in the AV. The AV cylinder is disinfected between bulls and the latex can be sterilized by boiling.

Assess the collection area and ability and reliability of the farmer and other animal handlers

It is worth looking at where the farmer thinks it best for the collection to take place. Remember that while he or she may not understand the needs of collection well they do know the bull much better than you do! Some bulls can be totally inhibited in the wrong surroundings. Ideally, one should work in the place where the bull normally serves the cows. A good surface will encourage a bull to mount, for example a bull with laminitis or an old bull will often work better on a relatively soft

surface such as grass or a firm straw bed rather than on concrete (Fig. 38.3). However, in most circumstances the latter is the preferred surface since it generally gives a sound secure footing. The bull falling causes most injuries to collectors. It is for this reason that most AI centres use service stocks and obviously if these are available they should be used. However, whatever adaptation or compromise is used, the collector must remember that his safety and that of the others involved is paramount. The main prerequisites are common sense, plenty of room and a safe footing. Listen carefully to all remarks about the demeanour of the bull. Be aware that sometimes farmers may be carried away by the novelty of this examination. Try to discourage bystanders!

Introductory examination of the bull

If practical it is worthwhile giving the bull an initial cursory examination prior to collection, gently running one's hands over the bull, touching the prepuce and genitalia. This allows the bull to get used to the personnel involved, particularly the collector of semen, and also allows the collector to judge what size and pressure of artificial vagina might be best and how the bull is likely to react to collection. Remember frightened bulls are dangerous.

Semen collection and assessment of ejaculate

The libido of the bull and the likelihood of a successful semen collection can be enhanced by allowing him to have sight and sound of one or more oestrous cows without physical contact for a short while before collection is attempted. It is important to interfere as little as possible with the normal service behaviour of the bull to obtain a representative ejaculate. The best technique for the collection of semen is therefore the use of an artificial vagina. The teaser cow should be restrained in the collection area. The bull is held separately, but nearby, from where he can be introduced for the collection and returned immediately afterwards to avoid repeated service of the teaser between collections. The teaser cow is an important factor in obtaining a representative semen sample. A teaser cow in oestrus will stand to be mounted. This is very important, particularly with an experienced beef bull, which will generally refuse to mount if the cow does not stand steadily when the bull 'tests' her. Furthermore, since many bulls are not used to being handled and therefore have to be allowed to mount free of control it is wise to have something that they are more interested in than the collector! The cow must be physically capable of bearing the weight of the bull and ideally she should be restrained in the collection area by at least a halter. Unfortunately, many cows have never been haltered so they tend to object to this and thus, by struggling, put the bull off working. Furthermore, in other cases their stubborn lack of initial movement is itself off-putting to the bull and if nothing is happening it is worthwhile trying to lead the cow in front of the bull. In some cases, where it is deemed safe, collection can only be achieved with both the cow and bull running loose and a roomy collection area is essential for this to avoid the collector being knocked over or crushed.

Introduction of the bull to the teaser cow: When the bull is brought into the collection area for service the collector should watch only the bull and make the following mental notes:

● Demeanour – is he interested in the cow?
● Gait – is he lame, if so where?
● Libido – is he keen to work? Watch for the pumping of the ischiocavernosus muscle (this will be apparent by a rippling tail–head movement) and the dripping of clear pre-ejaculatory fluid from the prepuce. The penis may also be seen protruding a little from the prepuce: does this appear normal? Usually before mounting an experienced bull will grunt and make a quick movement at the rear of the cow just to test if she will stand. If the cow is not in season she will move, even if restrained, and this may be quite sufficient to stop the bull mounting.

Penile erection and ejaculation: As soon as the bull mounts the cow the collector should move forward quickly, but without panic, and with one hand on the prepuce guide the erect penis towards the opening of the artificial vagina held in the other hand. Touching the penis directly will generally cause the bull to dismount. The bull will vigorously seek the vulva by rapid backward and forward movement of the penis. The temptation to force the AV over the penis at this point should be avoided as this can reduce the quality of the service. The bull should mount, clasp the cow, erect fully and search for the vulva with the penis, and, on finding the artificial vagina in its place, thrust and ejaculate in one movement. The search should not take more than a few seconds and a good thrust takes both hind legs off the ground in a forward direction. The sound of an explosive exhalation indicates ejaculation. It is important that the bull makes a firm thrust as this reflects stimulation of the full complement of ejaculatory fluids and so ensures that the sample is as representative of the natural ejaculate as possible. A poor quality ejaculate associated with a poor thrust may not be representative, often showing relatively poor motility, and semen collection should be repeated. The ejaculation should take place at the end of the AV, ideally within the cone itself, and thus the semen should be unaffected by the temperature of the AV. However, in some cases this is not what occurs and the sample may have to be allowed to run down from the AV, which is held vertically after collection. In such a case it may not only be affected by the AV temperature but also more contaminated than usual with preputial detritus.

Because of the rapidity of service in experienced bulls and the necessity of examining the semen sample as soon as possible after collection it is often difficult to examine the penis fully and collect semen at the same time. However, an appreciation of its firmness is possible, as is a quick visual assessment of both the penis and the prepuce. Should a more thorough examination be indicated, mounting can be repeated later without a collection being made, the penis (that part within the prepuce) being directed toward the examiner, thereby exposing the protruded portion for a more prolonged examination. This posture can often be held for a few seconds as long as the tip of the penis does not contact the cow. Wherever possible, more than one collection should be made, especially if the first is of poor quality. Moreover, in some cases an even greater number of collections may be required to satisfy the collector that the bull has worked well and that the series of samples obtained is as representative as possible. Only experience allows this judgement.

Experience of collector: There are considerable variations between how bulls cope with the use of an artificial vagina and the experience of the collector can help considerably in obtaining a good ejaculate as opposed to a poor one. It is difficult to rationalize just what the collector does to ensure a good collection. Firstly, there is the judgement as to whether to try and collect when the bull first mounts. Quite often the first mount will be 'premature' with a poor erection of the penis and in most cases it is best just to deflect the penis by using pressure on the prepuce and let the bull dismount. While this carries the risk of putting the bull off mounting again, this is unlikely in bulls with normal libido. Time and effort spent in teasing (even to the point of removing the bull or the cow from the scene temporarily) are usually rewarding and eliminate any doubts that can arise when a poor sample is obtained at the very first mount. Secondly, there is the process of actually allowing the penis to enter the artificial vagina. In some cases, where the bull will not immediately thrust, it may be induced to do so by a short, quick, back and forward movement of the artificial vagina. This should be firm but gentle. Related to this is the decision as to the length of the artificial vagina, the pressure of the water in the liner, the type of liner and temperature. For example, few bulls will thrust well with an artificial vagina temperature less than 42°C, but equally there is no need for it to be more than 55°C. The use of a very warm artificial vagina with a rough liner can leave the penis looking very red! It is vital to remember that the tip of the penis is highly sensitive, and that an ejaculatory thrust is usually induced immediately it enters a properly prepared AV.

Other techniques of semen collection: Occasionally, the collection of an ejaculate by artificial vagina proves impossible and it is deemed necessary to examine a semen sample. In such circumstances, if the bull will mount and serve an oestrous cow then the removal of semen and vaginal mucus from the vagina of the cow and examination of the spermatozoa in the mucus is, in our opinion, more sympathetic to the bull's welfare than electro-ejaculation. It is for this reason that the cow should not be served prior to the visit. Semen can be collected by massage of the ampullae *per rectum* (McGowan *et al.*, 2002) and can be done without a teaser cow in oestrus.

In the last resort, and in our opinion only if it is felt *absolutely* necessary, one should collect semen by electro-ejaculation. This technique depends on electrical stimulation of the sacral segments of the spinal cord, which are mainly parasympathetic nerves emerging from the pelvic plexus. This stimulation will often cause a form of erection (possibly incomplete) and ejaculation. The ejaculate often differs from a 'normal' ejaculate by having a considerably greater volume and a lower sperm concentration (even in the 'sperm-rich' portion). This is due to the excessive contribution of the accessory glands, in particular the seminal vesicles.

Another disadvantage of this technique is that, at least with some machines, the animal shows tetanic con-

tractions with each series of pulses and these increase in strength with voltage. The bull may raise his tail, rock gently to and fro and, if the probe is incorrectly positioned, lift one hind leg and, if excessive stimulation is applied, the bull will go down. It has been suggested that the bull be sedated in some circumstances. However, our experience is that the danger of the bull going down means that the technique is best used without sedation. Sexual rest before electro-ejaculation seems to improve the likelihood of obtaining a representative sample.

In our experience the latter techniques are only of value if one obtains an ejaculate with motile spermatozoa and can study their morphology. Failure to obtain an ejaculate does not mean the bull is infertile! Even then concentration is so variable that at least in our experience it cannot totally be relied upon as representative of naturally ejaculated semen.

Assessment of ejaculate: While there has been, and still is, considerable research into the prediction of fertility on the basis of tests upon semen (Linford *et al.*, 1976; Miller & Hunter, 1987), the general form of on-farm semen examination is still largely based on the pioneering work of the early AI industry. In particular, the reader is referred to the study by Bishop *et al.* (1954).

A full ejaculate examination generally entails observing and recording the following:

● Volume
● Initial motility of semen
● Progressive motility of spermatozoa
● Morphology of spermatozoa
● Presence of other cells
● Concentration of spermatozoa
● Final overall assessment

The first three measurements above are usually carried out on the farm, followed by an initial assessment of the results. Smears of semen are also prepared on farm, but not necessarily examined; this is essential for the nigrosin–eosin stained smears. Samples and smears are then returned to the laboratory for completion of the other tests followed by the final overall assessment. The ejaculate should be returned to the on-farm laboratory as quickly as possible after collection. It must not be allowed to become chilled until after the first three steps and preparation of the nigrosin–eosin smears are completed.

Volume: Use a graduated collecting tube.

Initial motility of semen: A small drop of semen is placed on to a warm slide, which is put on a warm microscope stage (35–37°C) and examined (×100) as soon as possible after collection. It is scored on a scale of 0–5, ranging from 0 being completely static to 5 being vigorously active. In the bull the major criterion of scoring initial motility is wave motion, which is a func-

Table 38.3 Guide to assessment of initial motility.

Score	Motility	Approximate % live, where density and morphology are normal
5	Rapid vigorous waves	90+
4	Good wave motion	80
3	Sluggish wave motion	60
2	Active sample, but no wave	40
1	Some motile sperms	20
0	No movement	0

tion of concentration, proportion of motile sperm and their activity (see Table 38.3). This simple test, if applied correctly, correlates quite well with fertility. Any bull that consistently produces semen with a score of less than 2 should be suspect.

Progressive motility of spermatozoa: Progressive motility, the percentage of motile spermatozoa moving in a forward direction, is best estimated by diluting the semen (roughly 1:50 depending on concentration) in a prewarmed (37°C) physiological solution (see p. 601) and examining this at ×400 magnification under a warm cover slip. A figure in excess of 50 per cent is certainly desirable. High percentage progressive motility generally also means rapid progressive movement. Examination at this power (×400) will also allow some initial observation of the morphology of the spermatozoa and the presence of unusual cells in the semen.

Morphology of spermatozoa: The morphology of the spermatozoa is closely related to testicular function and the appearance of head, midpiece and tail should all be studied. A general morphological examination entails the observation of spermatozoa (and other cells) under high power (×1000), noting any abnormalities and expressing these as the number of abnormal spermatozoa/100 spermatozoa counted. This is best done quietly away from the farm although a cursory on-farm look at ×400 will allow tentative prognosis for the owner and also satisfies the collector that the smear is acceptable. The use of at least two different staining techniques is recommended: one entailing dilution of the semen prior to making the slide and the other using a direct smear, which is stained after fixation. These are described more fully below.

(1) *Nigrosin–eosin stain* (Figs 38.4, 38.5). Freshly collected semen should be mixed with prewarmed stain in a small test tube roughly according to spermatozoa concentration (average 1[semen]:10 [stain]) and allowed to incubate at 35–37°C for one minute. One small drop is then taken and smeared thinly across a prewarmed slide (using the same technique as would be employed

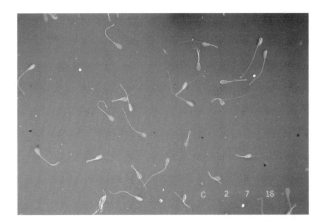

Fig. 38.4 Spermatozoa morphology (nigrosin–eosin × 400). The reflected tails are artefactual, possibly due to chilling during staining and smear preparation. There is no evidence of cytoplasm in the bend of the tail and Giemsa-stained air-dried smears did not show the defect.

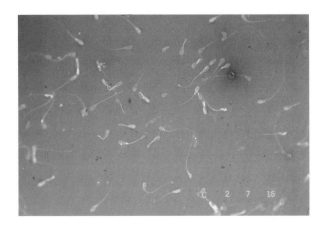

Fig. 38.5 Spermatozoa morphology (nigrosin–eosin × 400). A range of defects including proximal cytoplasmic droplet, dag defect, reflected tail, detached head and microhead.

in the preparation of a blood film) and allowed to dry in the warm cabinet or on the warm stage. Chilling during preparation can lead to artefactual effects on sperm morphology. This stain will also allow the computation of the live:dead ratio since eosin is a vital dye, staining so-called dead (or immotile) spermatozoa pink, but leaving live spermatozoa unstained and pale, almost white. The percentage live figure correlates well with percentage progressively motile and not surprisingly gives similar correlation coefficients with fertility.

(2) *Indian ink smear.* This can be prepared in the same way but does not show 'vital staining'.

(3) *Giemsa (Fig. 38.6) and methylene blue stains.* In this case at least three direct smears of the semen are made on warmed slides and allowed to air dry and this

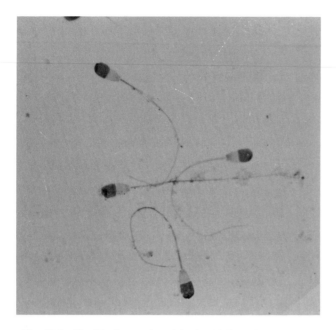

Fig. 38.6 'Knobbed sperm', an inherited defect of the Friesian breed (Giemsa) (×700).

Box 38.4. Spermatozoa abnormalities.

Head abnormalities
  Microhead
  Macrohead
  Pyriform
  Acrosome defect
Neck abnormalities
  Detached head
  Detached tail
  Fractured neck
  Other
Midpiece
  Double
  Swollen
  Abaxial
  Curved
  Distal mid piece reflex
  Other
Tail
  Coiled (dag defect)
  Tail reflected
  Proximal cytoplasmic droplet
  Distal cytoplasmic droplet

would usually be done on the farm. On return to the laboratory one is fixed using 10 per cent formal saline (buffered), one using methanol and the third by gentle heat. After the first two have been washed in water they are stained in a simple buffered 10 per cent Giemsa solution for approximately three hours. Depending on its source, ordinary tap water will do. This stain should highlight the acrosome and allow further identification of any abnormalities of this region in particular. If one brings the slides back to the laboratory before fixation the use of the two different fixes can be of particular value, since often one gives a better resolution of the acrosome than the other, presumably due to differences in the relationship of thickness of the smear, time of air drying and the fix. The heat-fixed slide is stained by methylene blue (see p. 601). Comparison of direct smears with those prepared following mixing of semen and stain (e.g. nigrosin–eosin) allows detection of artefactual morphological effects that can arise from faulty technique in preparing the latter (Fig. 38.4).

Considerable experience is required before reliable counts of morphological abnormalities can be obtained and the reader is referred to Barth and Oko (1989) for authoratative guidance on the procedures required. Overall one is aiming for at least 70 per cent normal spermatozoa. However, this needs to be qualified as the effect upon the fertility of the semen depends upon the type and extent of abnormality (Barth & Oko, 1989); thus head and midpiece abnormalities (including cytoplasmic droplets) are more important than simple reflected tails. Some abnormalities are known to be

Table 38.4 Visual criteria for estimating semen concentration (×10⁶ spermatozoa/ml) (from Logue & Greig, 1987).

Appearance	Estimated number of spermatozoa ($\times 10^6$)
Thick cream	3000
Cream	2000
Milk/cream	1000
Milk	500
Water/milk	250
Cloudy	100

inherited, for example the knobbed sperm. Results of morphological analysis should be presented in tabular form, showing the proportions of the various abnormalities seen (Box 38.4).

Presence of other cells: A variety of cells are normally found in semen and these cells are best observed either in the direct smear stained by Giemsa and/or a direct smear heat fixed and stained by methylene blue. The latter demonstrates leukocytes particularly well. Most of the cells are of preputial or urethral epithelial origin and are of little consequence. However, the presence of large numbers of leukocytes, small darkly staining cells that appear to be degenerating spermatids, multinucleate giant cells and so-called 'round' cells is indicative of spermatogenic disruption.

Concentration: This can be estimated using the criteria in Table 38.4. When a more accurate measurement is needed then resource to a calibrated turbidity meter or a simple haemocytometer is needed.

Final overall assessment: There has been little study of the correlation of these commonly measured semen parameters with the fertility of bulls used under natural service conditions. For semen collected by AV and used for artificial insemination there is evidence for correlation of motility and percentage dead spermatozoa with fertility and that is why we have described these tests (Bishop *et al.*, 1954). In North America, the New Society for Theriogenology Breeding Soundness Evaluation System (Hopkins & Spitzer 1997) is based on examination of semen collected by electro-ejaculation and may not be applicable to AV collected samples. Our experience with an electro-ejaculator is that in some cases perfectly normal bulls fail to give a good sample. However, the Society suggests that to be classified as satisfactory the 'gross motility' must be at least 'fair', the 'individual progressive motility' at least 30 per cent and morphology analysis should show at least 70 per cent normal sperm cells. The Society's 'gross motility' is equivalent to the initial motility assessment described here except that a cover slip is placed on the drop of semen; 'fair' ('generalized oscillation') probably equates with a score of 2 and 'individual progressive motility' is equivalent to progressive motility. Therefore the measurements that correlate best with fertility are generally believed to be initial and progressive motility, percentage dead spermatozoa and percentage morphologically normal spermatozoa. However, volume and density are usually also recorded. Table 38.5 shows minimum reference figures used by the authors when assessing bull semen. They are based on published work and experience and are offered as a guide. However, it must be appreciated that correlation of findings in semen and the fertility of natural service bulls is an inexact science due to the paucity of published information available, which reflects the difficulties of small scale on-farm investigations of fertility. In the final

analysis semen samples tend to fall into one of three categories. Firstly all parameters are well above the minimum reference figures in Table 38.5 (the semen should be of normal fertility). Secondly the important parameters fall well below (the semen is likely to be subfertile or sterile). Thirdly the important parameters are mostly at or just below the minimum reference figures. It is the third category that causes difficulties. If there is a history of infertility and there are no other significant findings, the bull could be re-examined after three months to see if there is improvement in the semen parameters. If the semen picture is normal at this time this suggests the bull was recovering from some form of testicular degeneration at the first examination. If the semen quality has deteriorated further the prognosis is very poor. However, if the quality is similar then test mating to at least ten fertile females followed by pregnancy diagnosis is the only recourse.

Ancillary tests: Research into other attributes of semen, and particularly spermatozoa, that correlate well with fertility has been consistently directed to the development of simple cheap methods to improve the accuracy of our predictions. Unfortunately, to date, such an addition suitable for on-farm use by a practising veterinarian has not been found. The most widespread tests have been the use of sperm motion analysis using a variety of computer based packages, cervical mucus penetration tests and zona pellucida (ZP) penetration tests (the simplest of these being the number of accessory sperm 'trapped' within the ZP). All these measure the ability of the spermatozoa to gain access to the egg for fertilization more objectively. However, only a more accurate evaluation of the acrosome using phase contrast microscopy seems applicable to the practical examinations that we are discussing here and even this seems more relevant to studying the effects of processing damage upon spermatozoa stored for either AI or other reproductive technologies. Finally there are a number of laboratory investigations showing the value of a variety of fluorescent stains which can allow evaluation of the chromosome content (X or Y), DNA variability, membrane integrity, mitochondrial function and vital function (for review see Garner, 1997). In the long term some of these tests may allow an improvement in the accuracy of assessment of semen, but until that time it is still an inexact science!

Observation of natural service

Finally, after semen collection is completed it is very worthwhile standing back and observing the bull serving the cow naturally. Obviously, this is only possible with a cow in season and the consent of the owner, who may not wish to have the cow served. This procedure avoids the risk of declaring a bull fertile on the

Table 38.5 Minimum reference figures (with range) for assessment of ejaculate.

Volume (ml)	4 (2–12)
Appearance	White (some samples have a yellow tinge)
Density (×10⁹/ml)	1.0 (0.3–2.5)
Initial motility (0–5)	≥2
Progressive motility (%)	>50
Total dead spermatozoa (%)	<50
Total morphological abnormalities (%)	<30

basis of normal semen findings when the bull is actually unable to complete natural service.

Full physical examination of the bull

We have already suggested that the first opinion veterinarian may undertake a full examination of the bull as a preliminary to any further investigations. We recommend that even if this was done previously it is always worthwhile going through the examinations again. Hard experience has taught that *no one* is infallible and defects can either be missed or could have become more apparent between examinations! In any event a full examination of the reproductive tract is essential, as is the examination of several other aspects of the clinical appearance of the bull. Obviously, where lameness or some other defect is apparent during collection the relevant area should now be examined more thoroughly.

Mouth: Assess the age of the bull by examining the incisor teeth. This is often very helpful in impressing upon owners how immature their young bulls are. Many bulls of continental breeds have still no adult incisors at two years of age.

Eyes: It is also worthwhile examining the eyes, at the very least to rule out congenital cataracts. Severe cataracts can lead to unpredictable behaviour of the bull and are found in all breeds. A good ophthalmoscope is needed to diagnose less obvious abnormalities such as colobomata of the retina.

Penis and prepuce: Palpate around the orifice of the prepuce, the sheath itself and the penis as it runs back to the scrotum. It is also worthwhile examining the umbilicus for evidence of a hernia.

Scrotum: Palpation of the scrotum allows definition of the following structures:

- Testes
- Epididymes (head, body and tail)
- Spermatic cords
- The scrotal sac itself.

The testes should exhibit freedom of movement within the scrotum and all structures should be of normal size, shape, and free from inconsistency in outline, i.e. bumps and nodules. A simple objective measurement of testicular size is scrotal circumference. This is determined by measuring the circumference of the scrotum at its largest point with a tape measure when the testes are in (or manipulated into) a normal fully descended position. In the normal adult bull this should be between 33 and 45 cm, depending on breed and mature size (see Table 38.6). More recently, the use of real-time ultrasound has been employed as a further diagnostic aid (Figs 38.7, 38.8). It remains to be seen precisely how valuable it will be. However, it is now being used by a number of veterinarians, including the authors, and has highlighted a variety of defects including orchitis and calcinosis.

Pelvis: A rectal examination is needed to examine the accessory sex glands. Some of these are found just under the hand after it has been fully inserted through the anus and the ampullae of vas deferens and seminal vesicles can be identified. The prostate and bulbourethral glands cannot normally be distinguished. The main part of the former is found at the beginning of the root of the penis, while the latter is found just anterior to the ventral bend of the root at the bulbospongiosus muscle. Again ultrasound has an obvious application, in particular for the examination of seminal vesicles.

Confirmation of identity: The breed and physical description of the bull should be recorded along with ear tag numbers and any tattoo numbers where legible.

Collection of other diagnostic samples

The composition of the collection is influenced in part by the health status of the national herd and also by that of the herd the bull is in or has been introduced to. The

Table 38.6 Suggested minimum scrotal circumference measurement (cm) to exert selection pressure for increased testicular size for bulls by breed and age in North America (Reproduced from Coulter *et al.*, 1987 with permission from Elsevier Science).

Age of bull (months)	Simmental	Angus and Charolais	Hereford and Shorthorn	Limousin
12–14	33	32	31	30
15–20	35	34	33	32
21–30	36	35	34	33
Over 30	37	36	35	34

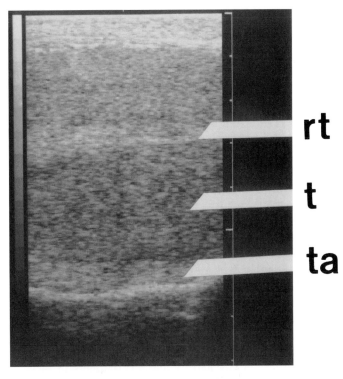

rt

t

ta

Fig. 38.7 Real-time ultrasound of the testis. rt, rete testis; t, parenchyma of testis; ta, tunica albuginea.

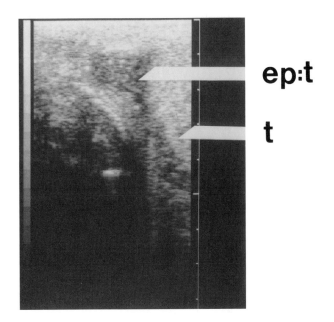

ep:t

t

Fig. 38.8 Real-time ultrasound of the tail of the epididymis. ep:t, tail of epididymis; t, testis.

minimum routine employed by the authors in the UK is as follows (Fig. 38.9):

(1) Preputial washing for culture and fluorescent antibody test for *Campylobacter fetus* sp.

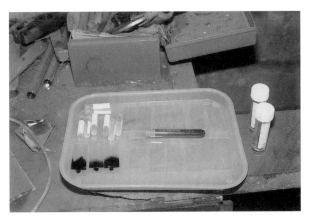

Fig. 38.9 Samples for further laboratory investigation routinely returned from the farm by the authors. From three ejaculates in this case: nigrosin–eosin stained smears, air-dried smears and raw semen; also heparinized blood and preputial wash.

(2) Blood for BVDV antigen and antibody, unless bull previously tested.

If indicated by history, semen findings and/or clinical signs collection of further samples, as detailed below, should be considered:

● Semen for culture of bacteria, virus or *Mycoplasma* sp.
● Blood for serology for IBRV, *Leptospira hardjo* or Johne's disease.
● Blood for biochemistry (e.g. albumin or liver enzymes) or routine haematology.
● Faeces for examination for helminth eggs, culture for *Salmonella* sp. or smear or culture for the bacterium of Johne's disease.

In some cases sampling of the females involved may also be required, e.g. vaginal mucus for VMAT for *C. fetus* sp. antibody.

Preliminary diagnosis and prognosis

Prior to leaving the farm and before all the examinations of semen and further laboratory tests have been concluded the farmer will be keen to hear a verbal preliminary diagnosis and more importantly a prognosis and some advice about what should now be done with the bull. These can usually be given, with the proviso that they are pending the outstanding test results, since any major abnormalities of the semen or physical abnormalities in the bull should be apparent before leaving the farm. Nevertheless, it is wise not to be too dogmatic, particularly with reference to the presence or absence of any form of infectious infertility.

Final diagnosis, prognosis and advice after all test results are known

Having obtained the history of the bull, examined it fully for breeding soundness (and any cows if necessary) and with knowledge of all relevant laboratory test results, a written report should be prepared. This should summarize the history, findings and any laboratory test results. It should then reach a conclusion, which should include a diagnosis, however tentative, and, if available an appropriate treatment and/or management regime to prevent or control the problem should be offered. Finally a prognosis should be given. A discussion of the aetiology of the problem can also be included. In general, the most important aspect of this conclusion is the prognosis. Effectively there are three alternatives:

(1) No abnormality can be detected and the bull should be of normal fertility. If the history is of poor fertility recommend a 'test-mate' with at least 10 fertile females.

(2) An abnormality consistent with a history of poor fertility has been found and the bull is considered long-term infertile or unlikely to return to normal fertility.

(3) The bull is infertile or of questionable fertility, but it may recover. In this case, depending on the diagnosis, the value of the bull and the manner in which the farm use him the bull can be kept, treated if necessary and the situation re-evaluated in two to six months.

Further action for the herd and its future breeding management

Where any findings made in the bull are likely to impinge on the rest of the herd, now or in the future, this should obviously be mentioned in the report. Examples would include the presence of significant infectious agents or evidence of overworking a young bull.

Manifestations, aetiology, treatment and prognosis of bull infertility

The aetiology, treatment and prognosis of infertility in the bull are discussed in more detail below under each of the four manifestations.

Failure to mount

The following factors have an influence on the ability to mount.

● Age
● Genetic factors
● Season
● Social factors
● Overwork
● Nutrition
● Orthopaedic abnormalities and housing conditions.

Age

The age at which a bull is capable of mounting, protruding the penis fully and ejaculating semen (puberty) varies with the bull and breed (see p. 479). However, one would normally expect a bull of a high production dairy breed to be capable of serving a cow at 12 months of age, although usually semen production would have commenced some two months earlier. Indeed mounting behaviour would be normal in the prepubertal state. However, one would not advise use for breeding before 15 months of age. Continental beef breeds tend to mature at a later age than most dairy breeds and so more care is needed with such animals when attempting to use them at a young age, for example less than 18 months. From a behavioural point of view young bulls often display naivety and awkwardness in their approach to an oestrous cow. There is evidence that this can be affected by how young males are reared, so that young bulls raised with female calves are less likely to exhibit sexual naivety than those kept in the presence of their dams until weaning (Kilgour, 1984).

In extreme cases young bulls may go through a pronounced phase of showing no sexual interest even when presented with a cow in oestrus. This 'sexual inhibition' may be heightened by the presence of another bull. While the condition often indicates an inherently poor libido, the problem may correct itself with time. Similarly, despite being clinically normal, bulls can show a considerable lowering of their sexual drive beyond eight to ten years old (Chenoweth, 1983).

Low sexual drive may also be due to overwork or pain, either from an orthopaedic problem or possibly emanating from the reproductive tract (see p. 611).

Genetic factors

There is evidence from work with identical twins that many aspects of mating behaviour, in particular sexual drive and mode of approach to service, are inherited (Bane, 1954). Furthermore, despite the wide variation between individuals there is plenty of evidence that some types and breeds of bulls display better libido than others. For example, dairy breeds tend to show a stronger sexual drive than beef breeds and there is now evidence of a quite high heritability for libido (Chenoweth, 1983).

However, there is little evidence that variation in libido is due to differences in circulating hormone concentrations (Bane, 1954). This was demonstrated dramatically in an endocrinologically abnormal bull with a 60, XXY chromosome complement, in which the mating behaviour was normal (Logue *et al.*, 1979).

There is little firm evidence of any relationship between poor libido in the bull and poor oestrous expression in female offspring, but there is some evidence of a relationship in sheep. Thus libido is a factor that should not be ignored in any selection programme (Chenoweth, 1983).

Season

There is conflicting evidence about the effect of season of the year, largely because of the environmental conditions in which the bulls were kept. A sluggish sexual drive has been related to periods of extreme heat, cold and light reduction (Vincent, 1972; Foote *et al.*, 1976; Gwazdauskas, 1985).

Social factors

Age, genetics and season all interact in the herd situation where the bull is running with a group of cows either as the only male or along with several other bulls as a mating team. Thus generally the oldest and largest bulls are dominant and spend most of their time in the presence of the sexually active oestrous females (Chenoweth, 1983). Subordinate bulls spend considerably less time with that group and in some cases their attempts to serve will be totally disrupted by the dominant bull.

Overwork

Bulls do become satiated. This state varies with the individual and the herd structure and in temperate climates seems more likely to present during the winter than in longer daylight periods. In simple terms, introduction of a young, totally inexperienced, 18-month to two-year-old bull to 20 cycling cows is considered to be risking overwork, while introduction to as many as 40 is foolhardy! Finally, poor female fertility can compound the problem because of returns to service.

Nutrition

High planes of nutrition result in puberty and maturity being reached at an earlier age (Salisbury & Van Demark, 1961). There is also some evidence that high energy intakes in early development are detrimental to subsequent libido. This effect has been described in both dairy and beef bulls, but without looking closely at whether the regime caused the physical defects such as laminitis in the bulls. There does not appear to be a direct relationship between nutrition and fertility in working bulls. Nevertheless, it is widely believed by farmers that performance testing young working bulls is detrimental to their longevity as working sires.

Orthopaedic abnormalities and housing conditions

Often the bull will show intent to mount, moving to the cow and standing behind her, but does not mount because of painful or physically limiting orthopaedic abnormalities. Obviously, the level of libido of the bull mediates the extent of this effect and on some occasions the frustration becomes so great that the bull will strike the cow.

A large number of orthopaedic problems are liable to interfere with the ability to mount and serve a cow. The most common problem areas are in the foot, the hock, the stifle and the back.

The treatment and prognosis of failure to mount depends very much on the diagnosis of the clinician. Many of these problems result from injuries to muscles, tendons and joints caused by the bull slipping when attempting to serve on poor underfoot conditions or foot lameness (see Chapter 31). Thus, adequate housing and service management are prerequisites of good bull fertility. The specific requirements of the bull for service should be borne in mind and thus any prognosis should be guarded. This is because many bulls are prepared to mount before a healing process is complete, thus exacerbating the condition, and also because frequently the bull produces soft, dystrophic bone in and around the site of injury resulting in added healing difficulties with subsequent arthritis (Bartels, 1975; Weaver, 1997). Some injuries appear to be more specific bull problems, such as spinal changes (Bane & Hansen, 1962), stifle injuries (Bartels, 1975) and delayed spastic paresis (Fig. 38.10).

It should also be remembered that other less specific conditions can cause poor libido simply due to the bull feeling unwell or being in pain. This is particularly relevant if the penis and/or prepuce has been damaged (see below). Finally, other diseases such as bovine spongiform, encephalopathy (BSE) (see p. 909) and progressive ataxia (see p. 179) of Charolais cattle (Palmer *et al.*, 1972) should be borne in mind.

As already mentioned, it is most important to introduce the bull gradually to an adult workload and to monitor his progress closely at every stage. In particular, the bull should be introduced initially to quiet adult cows which are clearly in season and virtually hand-mated until the bull and his owner are confident that he can work reliably and fertility is confirmed by early pregnancy diagnosis of those females using real time ultrasound after day 26. Table 38.7 gives some general indications of workload.

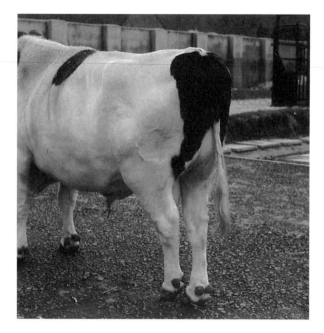

Fig. 38.10 Delayed spastic paresis in the bull.

Table 38.7 Recommended workload of bull with age (running loose with females).

Age	No. of cows
<2 years	10 cows
2–3 years	20 cows
3 years	30 to 50 cows depending on bull

The prognosis for poor libido of indefinable origin must be extremely guarded, since, despite any mitigating circumstances, it is likely that this problem is inherent in the make-up of the bull and will recur. In young bulls of around 18 months to two years of age the prognosis is more hopeful, but a maximum time scale of six months in which to show some evidence of overcoming the condition is appropriate.

Attempts to treat low libido by a variety of hormones, either alone or in combination, have rarely proved of value and there is a dearth of recommendations apart from sexual rest in any of the common texts. In fact, matters remain as described by Lagerlöf in 1951!

Failure to achieve intromission

The majority of bulls that are presented as being able to mount, but then fail to gain intromission, suffer from a variety of conditions, which include penile or preputial defects and orthopaedic problems. It is important not to belittle the problems of diagnosis, for example an early manifestation of either corkscrew penis or a venous drainage defect could conceivably be masked by the overzealous application of an artificial vagina. Observation of the natural service behaviour of the bull should generally avoid this error although some young bulls can display penile abnormalities intermittently. As ever prognosis, treatment and prevention depend upon the exact diagnosis.

In order to understand penile problems fully a brief discussion of the anatomy and physiology of erection in the bull (Fig. 38.11) is necessary.

Intromission can only be achieved if the penis is fully erect. This is a stiffening process brought about by the filling of the corpus cavernosum penis with blood pumped in by the ischiocavernosus penis muscle. Since drainage of the corpus cavernosum penis is very slow in normal bulls, blood pressure in the corpus cavernosum penis builds up well in excess of that in a car tyre (over 200 psi) (Beckett et al., 1974). This is sufficient to harden and straighten the penis and it is consequently forced out of the sheath. The latter, owing to its elastic nature, envelops the erecting penis up to the start of the free end of the penis. As the penis protrudes and reaches the point of ejaculation, it stiffens still further and spirals in an anticlockwise direction. This 'corkscrew' is caused by the fibrous architecture of the glans, in particular the dorsal apical ligament and spiral distribution of collagen fibres along the tip of the penis, allied to the rise in blood pressure in the corpus cavernosum penis at ejaculation. Further distortion may be caused by the very transitory erection of the erectile tissue at the tip of the penis. It is believed that this may be caused by pressure waves in the corpus spongiosum penis (Ashdown, 1973).

Clinically, we suggest that there are two major presentations associated with failure to achieve intromission and each can be further subdivided as follows.

(1) The penis cannot be protruded sufficiently:
    (a) Balanoposthitis
    (b) Short penis
    (c) Rupture of the corpus cavernosum penis
    (d) Persistent frenulum.
(2) Failure to locate vulva or enter vagina:
    (a) Psychogenic problems
    (b) Penile problems: fibropapillomata, drainage defects, corkscrew penis, deviations.

The penis cannot be protruded sufficiently

Balanoposthitis: Some cases of inflammation of the epithelium of the penis and prepuce can result in inabil-

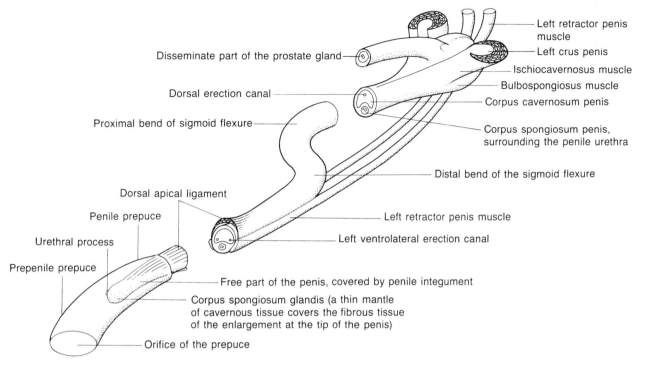

Fig. 38.11 Diagram to show the anatomy of the penis and prepuce of the bull. (Courtesy of Dr R.R. Ashdown.)

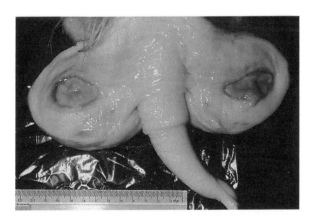

Fig. 38.12 Abcess formation of the preputial epithelium in the bull.

ity to mate because of pain or physical interference. There are three areas of damage:

● The region around the preputial orifice.
● The penile epithelium.
● The reflected prepuce which, by virtue of its extreme elasticity and mobility, stretches and reflects itself along the extended erect penis.

The region around the preputial orifice: Problems in this area may be the result of trauma with subsequent infection (Memon *et al.*, 1980–85). An example is where the bull everts his preputial epithelium, which is then damaged and infected (Long & Dubra, 1972; Fig. 38.12). The breeds most commonly affected are the Aberdeen Angus and polled Hereford, which have no retractor preputiae muscle, and the *Bos indicus* breeds and crosses (Larsen & Bellenger, 1971). Ubiquitous organisms such as *Arcanobacterium (Actinomyces) pyogenes* and *Staphylococcus aureus* can often be isolated from such lesions. The smegma produced by the bull is very tacky and the authors know of at least one case where the problem was caused by the firm matting of the hairs over the preputial orifice due to this substance, with resultant failure to protrude the penis. Others have described hair rings around the free end of the penis, although this usually produces an annular constriction a few centimetres behind the tip of the penis.

The penile epithelium: This can be damaged either traumatically, or by infection, in particular by the virus of infectious pustular balanoposthitis (BHV-1). Damage with subsequent scar tissue can result in a failure to protrude or deviation.

The reflected prepuce: This area is extremely important because it must function properly to allow the penis to protrude (Ashdown & Pearson, 1973a). Any traumatic damage with resulting scar tissue formation

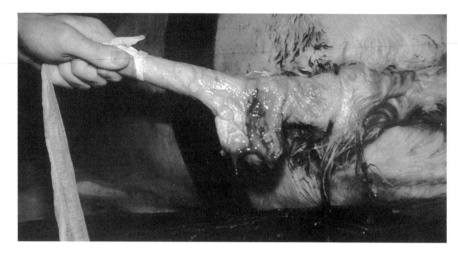

Fig. 38.13 Severe tear of prepuce.

tends to be self-perpetuating since the scar tissue often limits movement, resulting in further tearing. Furthermore, infection at such sites is common with subsequent abscessation. An extreme example of such damage can occasionally be seen after collection with an artificial vagina and in some of these cases the tear is very large indeed (Fig. 38.13). Usually the bull in question is a young inexperienced animal or one returning to work after a prolonged layoff (Monke, 1980). Treatment of this condition is largely symptomatic; however, in cases with severe scar tissue formation, surgery is the only course of action other than salvage (Larsen & Bellenger, 1971; Walker, 1980). Although a guarded prognosis is necessary the chances of recovery will depend on the site, extent and aetiology of the condition. Even in less severe cases sexual rest for at least three months is recommended to ensure adequate healing. Prevention is best effected by good bull management, regular monitoring of the bull when he is serving a cow and recording of his performance. Should the bull be part of an AI stud then the importance of collection technique must be re-emphasized.

Short penis: As the bull grows so the penis should also develop. In some cases it would appear that this does not occur and the bull becomes less and less able to protrude the penis sufficiently to achieve intromission. The exact aetiology of the problem is obscure and this presentation may even be due to several different conditions, but it does not appear to be a defect of erection since the penis appears to firm up quite normally. Fibrous metaplasia of the retractor penis muscle has been described (Arthur, 1960) and this has been successfully treated by myectomy. However, since the condition appears to be heritable surgery is probably not advisable. At its simplest, a grossly enlarged pendulous abdomen may be a cause of the problem, although

usually in such cases some of the penis can be protruded. A severe drainage defect problem could also possibly present in this manner (see later). Diagnosis is based on the increasing difficulty of the bull to protrude the penis after mounting. The penis should be felt to confirm a firm erection because the condition should be differentiated from either a drainage defect of the corpus cavernosum penis or a longstanding balanoposthitis. In our experience the prognosis is hopeless.

Rupture of the corpus cavernosum penis: As mentioned earlier, the pressures erecting and firming the penis are immense and in some unfortunate cases the tunica albuginea ruptures (Fig. 38.14). It is possible that in some cases the tunica albuginea is unable to sustain integrity because of the pressure alone, but it is more likely that it ruptures under additional strains caused by a sudden penile deflection due to an unexpected movement by the cow while service is taking place, or the bull slipping while the penis is in the vagina. Rupture generally occurs in the region of the sigmoid flexure. It is most common on the dorsal aspect of the distal bend of the sigmoid flexure but can also occur on the dorsal surface of the penis between the root and proximal bend of the sigmoid flexure. Such rupture results in a haematoma, which subsequently organizes and prevents the full erection and protrusion of the penis. Diagnosis is based on a sudden onset of an inability to serve coupled with swelling, usually in the inguinal region just above and anterior to the scrotum. Often the bull also presents with a prolapse of the prepuce and because the condition can be painful he may walk stiffly. Where this condition is presented in the acute phase and the surgical approach is adopted, immediate sexual rest followed by surgical removal of the haematoma some five to seven days later, before it can organize (Walker,

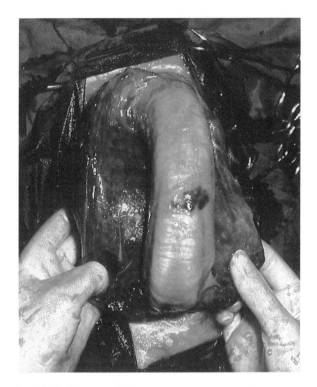

Fig. 38.14 Rupture of the corpus cavernosum penis.

1980), is indicated. In more chronic cases and in those acute cases where surgery is not adopted gradual teasing may eventually result in adhesions being broken down sufficiently to allow mating. Progress may also be assisted by frequent gentle massage in the area of the haematoma. Recurrence is quite common and, if possible, identification of the site of rupture is advisable because the prognosis is more hopeful for a rupture at the distal bend of the sigmoid flexure rather than at the proximal bend. This is because the latter is associated with drainage defects of the corpus cavernosum penis (Ashdown & Glossop, 1983). Prevention is clearly difficult but the introduction of young sexually inexperienced bulls to heifers, especially at grass, should be done with care. Service in slippery surroundings should be avoided if at all possible.

Persistent frenulum: The penile frenulum, which normally attaches the free end of the penis to the prepuce of the prepubertal bull, is normally 'lost' during early puberty, possibly breaking during play and/or masturbation. Occasionally, this does not occur and its persistence prevents the tip of the penis straightening on erection. It is usually bent ventrally and caudally. Although this is not a common condition diagnosis is easy, as is treatment, which involves simple surgery.

Failure to locate vulva or enter vagina

Psychogenic problems: There would appear to be two distinct problems:

● Neck or side mounting;
● Normal mounting, but without success, the bull being incapable of inserting the penis into the vagina despite a good erection and apparently normal seeking movements, even to the extent of touching the vulva.

The aetiology for both these conditions, especially the former, is obscure though neck mounting is not uncommon in young inexperienced bulls. However, they usually quickly move round to the rear of the cow. For the latter one could hypothesise either that this could be an early manifestation of a premature partial drainage defect of the corpus cavernosum penis or that there was an inadequate sensitivity of the penile tip (possibly acquired traumatically or by infection) resulting in a lack of appreciation of the position of the penis relative to the vulva.

A diagnosis of psychogenic depression of libido must be tentative because it is based on a failure to obtain any other. One should always bear in mind that this condition may be the result of penile damage or an early manifestation of a drainage defect of the corpus cavernosum penis, or may be of orthopaedic origin.

There is no known treatment apart from initial sexual rest for at least three to four weeks followed by hand-mating after some considerable teasing. Often collection by a small artificial vagina using a rough liner may obtain an ejaculate and start the bull working. The prognosis is very guarded.

Penile problems:

Fibropapillomata: These are generally found on or near the tip of the penis (Fig. 38.15). They are caused by a virus and are thus transmissible. They can occasionally also cause considerable problems in the female (Meischke, 1979). In the bull they usually only affect the penis of young animals less than four years of age and generally regress after a period of two to six months. In some cases, however, they persist much longer and some become eroded and infected (Walker, 1980). Treatment depends on the extent and severity of the tumour. A small single pedunculated tumour is clearly much easier to deal with than a large, sessile, cauliflower-like lesion. Most authorities advise surgery in severe cases, but it is essential to avoid weakening or rupturing the tunica albuginea (Walker, 1980), since this can result in blood escaping at service and this setback to surgery has been seen by one of the authors. Note that possible leakage from the corpus spongiosum penis (CSP) into the terminal part of the urethral lumen has

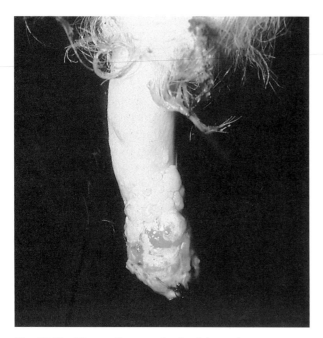

Fig. 38.15 Fibropapilloma on the tip of the penis.

also been described. This could also cause spurting of blood from the penis at service (Ashdown & Majeed, 1978). Since these lesions are transmissible, segregation of affected cattle, especially heifers, from a young bull is advisable. Contaminated bedding may infect young bulls and sexual play between young bulls may result in superficial abrasion of the penis and thus susceptibility to infection. The use of an older bull on infected females reduces the risk of infection of the bull. Prognosis should be guarded as regards both spontaneous recovery and return to service after surgery.

Drainage defects: Careful anatomical studies of the normal and abnormal penis have revealed a number of arteriovenous shunts, which allow the venous cavities of the penis to drain more quickly than usual. This results in an inability to erect fully or to sustain an erection (Ashdown *et al.*, 1979). It is now considered possible to distinguish four different venous drainage defects based on history and clinical findings. However, in the last analysis all are associated with inadequate erection in the bull and a diagnosis of venous drainage defect is probably sufficient in most cases (Logue & Greig, 1985). Diagnosis is dependent on a careful assessment of the history and a thorough clinical examination of the bull while serving. It is advisable not only to attempt to collect semen by artificial vagina but also to palpate the erect penis as much as possible as the bull attempts to mate and finally, if at all possible, the bull should be allowed to attempt to mate naturally and his lack of ability to mate confirmed. Differentiation between the various categories of corpus cavernosum penis

defects is largely academic at present since there is no treatment and the prognosis for all of these is hopeless.

Corkscrew penis: This is one of the most dramatic defects and is often diagnosed by the client. Spiral deviation of the penis within the vagina at ejaculation is physiological but in the clinical condition the spiral deviation precedes intromission and so prevents service. This is most commonly seen in beef bulls of around four years of age (Blockey & Taylor, 1984). In all cases the spiral is anticlockwise and can almost comprise a complete circle. However, it does present with varying degrees of severity from intermittent spiralling (which can present problems with diagnosis) to being so severe that spiral deviation occurs while the penis is still in the prepuce and it may then prevent protrusion. Usually it does not occur until the penis makes contact with the vulva of the cow. It should be remembered that spiral deviation has been described as occurring after entry into the vagina immediately prior to ejaculation in bulls with apparently normal mating behaviour (Ashdown & Pearson, 1973b). The only known treatment is surgical and there are a variety of techniques, all of which depend on either fixing the dorsal apical ligament to the dorsal aspect of the penis or additionally stiffening it by the insertion of fascia lata or carbon fibres. The latter are placed between the ligament and tunica albuginea (Mobini *et al.*, 1982). Postoperative recurrence is quite common after apparent recovery. The problem is said to be heritable but there is little evidence other than anecdotal to confirm this.

Deviations of the penis: These deviations are largely believed to be caused by scar formation such as that following balanoposthitis or surgery (Walker, 1980). As with corkscrew penis, deviations are usually obvious. However, ventral deviations can be confused with a drainage defect of the corpus cavernosum penis and must be differentiated from these. They can usually be distinguished by the flexibility of the erect penis that is apparent in drainage defects. Some bulls can accommodate deviations surprisingly well and if they are not too pronounced, careful hand-mating may allow these bulls to learn to serve again. Surgical treatment is again a possibility (Walker, 1980) for more severe cases. A guarded prognosis is advisable even for relatively discrete deviations.

Failure to thrust and ejaculate after intromission

Occasionally, one encounters a bull that is capable of placing the penis in the anterior vagina but then fails to thrust vigorously and ejaculate. In some cases the cause may be orthopaedic, but in other cases the cause may be neural in origin, whether due to local receptor problems causing a lack of sensitivity of the penis, which may be acquired or congenital, or due to a more general psychosomatic defect. Another possibility is that this problem might be due to either a slight defect in the drainage of the corpus cavernosus penis itself or a defect in the corpus spongosum penis, or even of the erectile tissue in the tip of the glans. The prognosis is poor. Finally, in some cases it may just be due to inexperience where, given time, the problem may resolve but the prognosis should be guarded.

Normal service with a poor pregnancy rate

The vast majority of conditions causing this manifestation are related to problems associated with sperm production and transport. An understanding of the complexity of the mechanisms involved in governing and modifying these processes is essential. There are two basic components in the ejaculate: spermatozoa and seminal fluid. The former are produced in the seminiferous tubules of the testes by spermatogenesis and the latter from the testes, epididymes and accessory sex glands.

The clinician should consider the following items when presented with a bull that is serving normal cows satisfactorily but achieving a low pregnancy rate.

- Age
- Overwork
- Testicular hypoplasia (and testicular atrophy)
- Testicular degeneration and atrophy
- Interference with storage and transport of spermatozoa
- Abnormalities of accessory sex glands

Age

In addition to the influence of age and experience upon libido there is a gradual development towards maximum fertility in the young bull and this is under physiological control. A practical example of these effects can be seen in the increase in scrotal circumference with age (Coulter & Foote, 1978). This parameter is quite valuable as an objective estimate of normal development of the testes and epididymes. Figures from bull examinations suggest that while a scrotal circumference of 35–40 cm is desirable in a young bull (approximately 18 months old), measurements below 30 cm are likely to be linked to infertility or subfertility. However, we have collected perfectly normal semen from young well-grown bulls with scrotal circumferences around this size. We therefore recommend collecting semen from 'borderline cases' if there are likely to be other

parties involved in the future of the bull. One theory for the relatively lower fertility seen in young bulls when compared with adults is related to the development of both testes and epididymis in the young bull, which has roughly half the sperm output of an adult, but less than one-quarter of the storage available in the tail of the epididymis with probably only enough for two to three days' sperm production. Hence it is much easier to deplete the young bull. Furthermore, it will be apparent that relative to the testes the epididymis, particularly the tail, is still enlarging and just how this interacts with sperm maturation in these young bulls is not well understood (Amann & Almquist, 1976; Amann and Schambacher, 1983).

In summary, while the bull may be capable of reproducing quite early in life it is not until after three years of age, or possibly even a little later in the case of late-maturing continental bulls, that one can safely say that the fertility of the bull is unlikely to improve further. While detailed studies are not really available it does appear that fertility also diminishes with advancing age (Amann & Schambacher, 1983). In the older bull poor fertility is associated with degeneration of some of the seminiferous tubules and with the development of testicular calcinosis in the seminiferous tubules resulting in non-productive areas of testes. Testicular calcinosis can be quite marked in some older bulls; however, it can also occur in young animals (Turnbull, 1977). Clearly there is very little that the veterinarian or farmer can do to influence this factor other than limit the mating pressure to both young and old bulls as recommended earlier and this is discussed further below.

Overwork

Much of the information about semen quality and work rates come from AI centres. However, the demands upon bulls running and mating with a herd of cows are obviously very different from those at an AI centre since young active bulls may serve a cow ten times or more during oestrus. This sort of pressure (ten ejaculates in two hours) results in a diminution of total sperm numbers per ejaculate by a factor of around ten (Salisbury & Van Demark, 1961), mainly due to a fall in concentration. Concentration in such circumstances falls to as low as 100×10^6 sperm/ml, a level that, in a semen evaluation as described here, would certainly result in the fertility of the bull being questioned. However, theoretically, a complete rest of around two weeks should allow a return to normal sperm concentrations in the ejaculate. In practice this is generally the case. In other words, the main effect of overuse is to exhaust the epididymal reserves. However, at very high and sustained mating pressures a slower return to normal number of spermatozoa per ejaculate may be found. Furthermore, it has also been noted that as the number of ejaculates increases, sperm motility tends to fall. In addition, the likelihood of an occasional azoospermic ejaculate increases (Salisbury & Van Demark, 1961). Finally, there is some information indicating that young bulls given a diet below maintenance for energy take considerably longer to replenish their sperm reserves. This is particularly relevant to young post sale bulls, which are purchased in very good body condition and then put outside with cows in a hard environment, thereby losing condition rapidly. By inference such bulls take considerably longer to replenish their sperm reserves (Salisbury & Van Demark, 1961). The history, number of cows, frequency of working and the age of the bull will generally indicate this diagnosis. At worst the semen picture will be of low concentration (200×10^6/ml or less), marginal initial motility (2/5), but reasonable progressive motility (60 per cent +) and morphology (<20 per cent abnormal). However, often the bull has been removed from the breeding group and rested before examination so the sample appears normal. As already indicated, treatment is sexual rest since it takes nine weeks for development from the spermatogonia stage to ejaculation as a mature spermatozoon. Hence ideally the bull should not serve for at least nine weeks before being re-examined. There is little point in re-examining a bull after less than three weeks' rest. When this diagnosis is made the prognosis is good. However, one must always be aware that such a diagnosis may be complicated by another underlying cause and so it is advisable to be 'guarded but hopeful'.

Testicular hypoplasia (and testicular atrophy)

Testicular hypoplasia is defined as the congenital presence of either one or two small testes (i.e. bilateral or unilateral). It has been closely studied in the Swedish Highland breed of cattle, where it has been demonstrated to be a heritable defect caused by a recessive gene with incomplete penetrance (Fig. 38.16). In both unilaterally and bilaterally affected cases sexual behaviour and secondary sexual characteristics are normal (Lagerlöf, 1951). It is not known whether a similar inheritance pattern applies to other breeds. It is theoretically possible that toxic or infectious agents affecting the dam at a critical stage of organogenesis of the testes could also cause hypoplasia, either bilateral or unilateral. Mention should also be made of bilateral testicular hypoplasia that is associated with the abnormal sex chromosome constitution XXY, i.e. an 'extra' X chromosome (Figs 38.17 and 38.18). Other cytogenetic abnormalities may be associated with infertility. Thus it

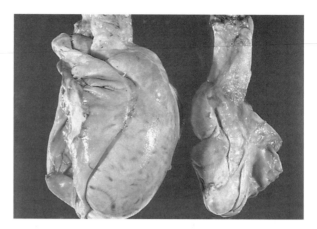

Fig. 38.16 Unilateral testicular hypoplasia in the Ayrshire breed. Note the adhesions on the normal testis caused by needle biopsy.

is believed that chromosomal abnormalities may interrupt the meiotic process to such a degree that infertility or reduced seminiferous tubule output is a result (Chandley, 1979). This does not appear to be as much of a problem in cattle as in man, though there is evidence of reduced fertility in cattle carrying a 1/29 Robertsonian translocation (Gustavsson, 1974; Logue & Harvey, 1978) and bulls with 61 XXY chromosomes are, as might be expected, completely sterile (Logue *et al.*, 1979). However, the nature of the bovine karyotype has meant that identification of reciprocal translocations is not easy and it is likely that, with improved techniques, some will come to light. These abnormalities are more likely to be associated with infertility than the Robertsonian translocations, which are not uncommon in the cattle family.

Although testicular atrophy should be dealt with under degeneration from a clinical point of view it is also being considered here because unless one has a firm history of the previous size of the testes it can be extremely difficult to differentiate between testicular hypoplasia and testicular atrophy, especially in the bilateral state. Both present as the 'small testes syndrome' (Fig. 38.19). Testes that have been affected by atrophy subsequent to a severe local infectious condition or trauma may feel small, firm and nodular on palpation, while those affected by hypoplasia are usually less firm and more uniform. Frequently, one is left in genuine doubt about the diagnosis.

Scrotal circumference measurement can be helpful in giving an objective guide to testis size, as it is a simple, highly repeatable, measurement. In other species it has been related to spermatozoa production and, intriguingly, ovulation rate in the female offspring (Land, 1978). However, from a practical point of view it is sufficient to note that those males with a below normal

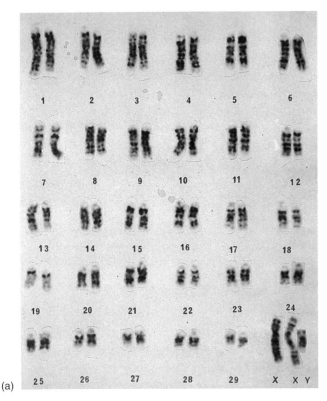

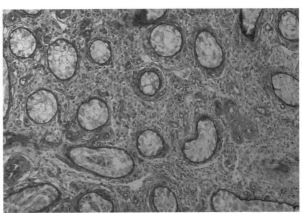

(a)

(b)

Fig. 38.17 (a) G-band karyotype 61XXY. (b) XXY bull. Tubules lined by Sertoli cells only, Leydig cells moderately increased in proportion (Masson ×195). (Courtesy of the *Veterinary Record*.)

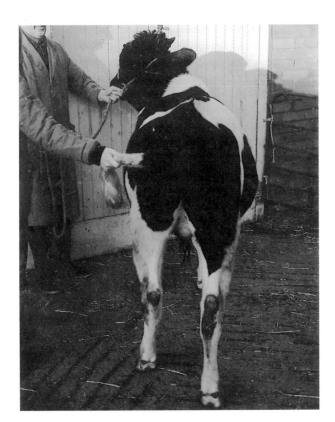

Fig. 38.18 A 61XXY bull with bilateral testicular hypoplasia.

scrotal development have a greater likelihood of being infertile. A further diagnostic aid that may prove of value is the determination of the chromosomal constitution of the animal.

As already mentioned, care must also be taken not to jump to conclusions. Surprisingly good quality semen has been collected from bulls with disappointingly small scrotal circumferences. However, such occasions are rare, so that in general the prognosis for the 'small testes syndrome' is poor. As far as the unilateral condition is concerned this is more problematical since the animal is often fertile. Here every attempt to obtain as reliable a history as possible should be made in order to differentiate between hypoplasia and atrophy because of the strong evidence of the heritable nature of hypoplasia. If the diagnosis is hypoplasia the owner should be advised that such stock are only fit for the production of 'slaughter generation' animals.

Testicular degeneration and atrophy

In many infertile animals the main histological finding is the absence of dividing spermatogenic cells, the Sertoli cells and interstitial cells still being present. This is often the result of testicular degeneration. Evidently,

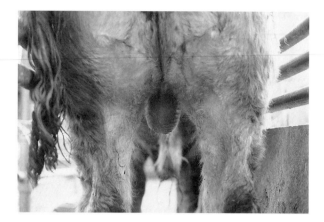

Fig. 38.19 'Small testes syndrome' (scrotal circumference 24 cm) in a Limousin bull aged 2 years with no previous history of fertility. The bull also intermittently displayed spiral deviation of the penis. Semen density was very low (4.0 × 10⁶/ml).

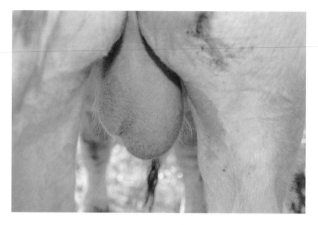

Fig. 38.20 Severe acquired testicular abnormalities in a Charolais bull aged 5 years. Chronic orchitis of the left testis manifested as atrophy, fibrosis and adhesions. The right testis whilst of normal size was very soft in consistency. The bull showed a complete absence of libido.

however, histology does not show the defects of function, in particular the delicate interaction between the cells of the testes and their hormonal influences from, and feedback to, other hormonal control centres. Spermatogenesis is a very sensitive process and can be easily upset. Nevertheless, it can also recover, particularly if the insult has been transient. Studies in the rat have shown firstly that Sertoli cell function was disrupted by a whole variety of noxious stimuli and that one side effect of such damage was an increase in serum follicle stimulating hormone (FSH) concentrations due to a decreased output of inhibin. Secondly, the Leydig cells were also affected since serum luteinizing hormone (LH) concentrations were higher and testosterone concentrations lower. Finally, there was evidence of a reduced response to human chorionic gonadotrophin (hCG) (de Kretser, 1979). The inference is that damage to the spermatogenic epithelium interferes with androgen binding protein (ABP) and inhibin release leading to an increased FSH concentration, which in turn alters the balance of testosterone–oestradiol synthesis towards the latter with a subsequent alteration in LH concentrations. Since there is evidence that LH can directly affect the Leydig cell, testosterone release and so ABP release by the Sertoli cell, it can be hypothesized that if events are prolonged or extreme these effects may accumulate and eventually result in a permanent derangement. However, it is of considerable interest to veterinarians in the field that immunization of bulls to gonadotrophin-releasing hormone (GnRH) is generally reversible (Robertson *et al.*, 1982). This then implies that in many clinical cases where such a regeneration of the seminiferous epithelium does not occur the underlying aetiology is more than just a simple hormonal dysfunction.

Insults to spermatogenesis causing temporary or permanent testicular degeneration can be categorized as either local or systemic.

Local:

Scrotal sac disruption: Obviously, severe trauma to the scrotum can have a direct effect upon the testes and epididymes, but one of the main functions of the scrotum is temperature control and any disruption of this can interfere with spermatogenesis. The first area of spermatogenesis affected is meiosis; the spermatogonia tend not to be affected and, after removal of the insult, regeneration within six weeks is to be expected providing the Sertoli or nurse cells are not damaged also. These are the most resistant to insult (Kumi-Diaka & Dennis, 1978). While weather conditions are capable of insult and cause variations in semen quality (Parkinson, 1987), it really requires trauma, a severe skin infection, an allergic reaction with scrotal oedema, a scrotal hernia or a deformity of the pampiniform plexus (so-called varicocele) to produce serious infertility. Diagnosis should be determined by a clinical examination. The most obvious problems are varicocele and inguinal herniation. Care needs to be taken when making the latter diagnosis as a pad of fat can lie above the pampiniform plexus and feel very like a hernia. The treatment and prognosis both depend on the cause. Thus for a simple skin infection one would be more hopeful of a return to normal fertility than for a variocele or a hernia.

Orchitis/epididymitis: Inflammation of the testes is commonly a purely local problem and frequently it only involves one testicle. However, often the infection so interferes with the temperature gradient of the scrotum that the remaining testicle is indirectly affected (Fig. 38.20). A similar effect is seen with epididymitis, although in this case there is the further problem of obstruction of spermatozoa and testicular fluid on the affected side. Often orchitis and epididymitis are concurrent. The causes of orchitis/epididymitis infection are not well documented. In many cases *Arcanobacterium pyogenes* can be isolated from the affected testes, but whether this is the original pathogen is uncertain. Other bacteria, such as those of the *Haemophilus/Histophilus* group, have been implicated in spermatogenic damage as have a number of viruses.

These conditions should also be relatively easily diagnosed by a clinical examination. Confirmation can be obtained from the semen findings. Generally, there will be low concentration of spermatozoa, poor/marginal motility and poor spermatozoan morphology, especially of the head. There will also be increased numbers of white blood cells and other cells indicative of damage such as large multinucleate cells, so-called 'giant cells'. Culture of semen may allow the identification of a causative micro-organism. However, the findings will to some degree depend on the time scale. Thus a bull with a spermatocele (see later) on the head of the epididymis could have been affected several years previously and the effects of the lesion subsided, allowing the semen quality of the bull to return to normal.

Treatment by antibiotics is usually ineffective and the main aim should be to prevent testicular degeneration of the sound testis and epididymis. The strategy adopted depends on the severity of infection. Thus assuming the remaining testis is not affected the removal of a grossly infected testis is the most straightforward remedy. Unfortunately, even then the local, and possibly systemic, damage to the other testis may be sufficient to cause a permanent derangement of semen production. Thus the prognosis, even in animals that have recovered either after surgery or after conservative treatment, should be guarded. The owner should be reminded that the daily sperm output may be affected in apparently recovered animals and that they should carefully monitor the cows that have been served in the bull's first series of matings to ensure that the proportion of returns to service is acceptable.

Systemic:

Systemic illness: Severe illness can disrupt spermatogenesis by one or all of three routes: firstly, by interfering with the temperature gradient of the testes, secondly as a consequence of toxaemic damage to the spermatogenic epithelium and finally by interfering with the complex hormonal secretions which control spermatogenesis and their interactions. The roles of bacteria and viruses in the aetiology of this condition are not well understood. For example, a few apparently infertile bulls have been found to be persistently infected with BVDV or to have high antibody titres to *Leptospira hardjo*. However, in some cases the animals have subsequently proved fertile; this includes BVDV viraemic animals (Logue, D.N. & Cranshaw, N.M.C., unpublished information). It should again be remembered that the bull might be presented some time after the incident when recovery is taking place. This can take a considerable time – at least some two to three months. Finally one interesting condition, worthy of mention, is idiopathic angioneurotic oedema. This is occasionally seen in young bulls, particularly of continental breeds, and generally occurs soon after introduction to grazing. There is often tremendous oedema of all the dependent areas, especially the scrotum, with consequent azoospermia. The latter is presumably due to a temperature effect. In our limited experience recovery is usually complete, however with other illnesses this is not always the case, especially in older bulls. Treatment and prognosis are dependent on the history, the origin of the insult and the age and type of the bull.

Drugs: Although therapeutic products are subject to very stringent safety screening there are certain drugs that might affect male fertility. Anabolic steroids given to young growing bulls have been shown to have an undoubted effect upon spermatogenesis, resulting in a reduced testicular size and delayed development of the seminiferous tubules and interstitial cells (O'Lamhna & Roche, 1983; Deschamps *et al.*, 1987a,b). Although it was suggested that these effects were temporary, in fact there was a delay in puberty and the effect was more severe in younger animals (these studies have only involved animals of up to 15 months and may not truly reflect the field situation). In addition there was evidence of interference in the hypothalamic–pituitary axis and the size and structure of the testes and epididymis. Finally, the fact that the studies were relatively short term makes one very wary of such a claim. The only problem that might arise is with clandestine and improper administration of a drug, such as an anabolic steroid or β agonist, with the intent of improving the appearance of the bull or even liveweight performance test results. It is possible to test for residues. It is possible that a bull could suffer from an adverse reaction to one of the common treatments, although such cases are rare. The diagnosis is dependent on the history and the treatment. Given the effect of anabolic steroids, by inference treatment with corticosteroids is also likely to affect semen quality (Li & Wagner, 1983), and indeed some slight changes have been described short term. However, administration to adult Holstein bulls did not appear to cause any practical spermatogenic problems (O'Connor *et al.*, 1985). Nevertheless, there is more recent evidence that some non-steroidal anti-inflammatory drugs such as flunixin could have an effect (Archibald *et al.*, 1990). Treatment of such adverse reactions is symptomatic while the prognosis depends on the exact form that the adverse reaction takes. Field experience has also failed to show any fertility effect associated with the administration of the commonly used antibiotics. However, again the periods of administration were relatively short. Abbitt *et al.* (1984) reported that neither dihydrostreptomycin sulphate nor oxytetracycline hydrochloride had any real effect upon reproductive function, even when given in greater than normal therapeutic doses.

The diagnosis of testicular degeneration is dependent upon a history of fertility, followed by infertility with the latter being confirmed by the collection of a semen sample of poor spermatozoa motility, concentration and morphology. In addition there will sometimes also be small, darkly staining, degenerate spermatids, which in some cases 'raft' together in clumps. In the extreme case the sample may be aspermic. In cases of testicular degeneration the testes may be smaller than normal due to atrophy, but often they are within the norm. While collection of semen is the main diagnostic tool many workers have desired to examine the seminiferous tubules. A number of authors have attempted to use a testicular biopsy as a means of obtaining histological evidence of spermatogenic dysfunction (Galina, 1972). This technique is hazardous even when one uses a modern disposable biopsy needle due to haemorrhage (the testis is very vascular), spermatogenic disruption and adhesions. However, with time, good spermatogenic recovery can occur (Galina, 1972; Logue, 1975).

Because testicular degeneration can be either temporary or permanent, it is impossible to be certain of the prognosis on the basis of a single semen examination. However, some guidelines can be obtained by looking at the length of infertility and the semen picture. Should the time scale be relatively short, say three months, and there is evidence of normal motile spermatozoa, albeit at a low concentration, then it is worth waiting another three months for a re-examination. Where the degeneration of the seminiferous epithelium is permanent then this may result in a gradual diminution in size of one or both testes, i.e. testicular atrophy. Unfortunately, unless one had prior knowledge that the affected bull had previously had normal-sized testes in the bilateral condition this small size could quite easily be considered to be testicular hypoplasia. Where there is good evidence of testicular atrophy being present then the prognosis is very poor.

Interference with transport and storage of spermatozoa

It is generally impossible to differentiate clinically which of the local and systemic effects mentioned earlier have an effect solely upon the epididymes, since, as already mentioned, any disruption of testicular function frequently interferes with epididymal function.

The epididymis, unlike the testis, develops from the mesonephric (Wolffian) ducts and is prone to several congenital malformations (Blom & Christensen, 1960). Aplasia of part of the epididymis, ductus deferens and seminal vesicles has been described as a congenital defect in the bull. The aplasia is usually unilateral and can be very specific. It is generally associated with spermatocele formation (so-called sperm granulomas) proximal to the aplasia (Blom & Christensen 1960). These are swellings of the epididymis reflecting a rupture of the tubules and the consequent foreign body reaction to the escaped products of the testes and are most commonly seen on the head of the epididymis. While they have been described as being a result of segmental aplasia (see above), in some cases spermatoceles arise in this position apparently spontaneously. Spermatocele formation has been diagnosed in the field following a sudden failure to mount and thus, by inference, it is painful in the acute phase (Logue & Greig, 1986). Since this was the only behavioural demonstration of pain it could be that any discomfort is only appreciated during sexual arousal. The exact relationship of the spontaneous condition to segmental aplasia is uncertain but one cannot ignore the possibility of an infectious condition causing an epididymitis and subsequent spermatocele. However, epididymitis resulting from infection by *Brucella* sp. and the *Haemophilus/Histophilus* group appears to occur most frequently in the tail of the epididymes. *Mycoplasma* infections have also been implicated in epididymitis (La Faunce & McEntee, 1982).

Unilateral spermatoceles need not necessarily cause sterility since once the inflammatory reaction has settled the remaining testicle can produce an apparently normal ejaculate. However, it is clearly not advisable to use such an animal with a large number of females, as in two cases known to the authors, where the bulls involved were at an AI centre and the concentration of the ejaculate never returned to the level seen before the incident. In one of these bulls the epididymis of the other testis also later suffered the same problem and the bull had to be destroyed. No significant microorganism could be found (Logue, D.N. & Hignett, P.G., unpublished information). Ease of diagnosis depends on the site and the extent of the problem. Should there be a spermatocele then this is generally easily palpated provided one is careful and palpates the entire epididymis. However, some defects can be very small and ultrasound may well prove a very useful diagnostic aid. Treatment is usually symptomatic and certainly in the early stages antibiotic administration is probably worthwhile.

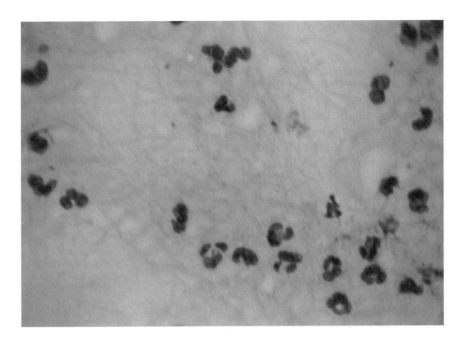

Fig. 38.21 White blood cells in semen (methylene blue) (×700).

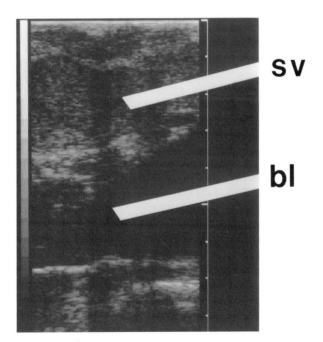

Fig. 38.22 Real-time ultrasound of the seminal vesicle. sv, seminal vesicle; b, bladder.

In some cases small compact masses up to the size of a pea, so-called cysts, can be felt both on the epididymis and on the spermatic cord itself. They are developmental in origin and of no consequence as long as they do not interfere with sperm transport.

Abnormalities of the accessory sex glands

The accessory sex glands consist of the seminal vesicles, ampullae, prostate and bulbourethral glands.

As already mentioned, abnormalities of the seminal vesicles are the most commonly diagnosed condition. Segmental aplasia of the seminal vesicle occurs and often appears to be related to a congenital defect (Blom, 1979a,b). Numerous infectious agents have been isolated and implicated in the aetiology of seminal vesiculitis in the bull, such as members of the *Chlamydia* group, *Mycoplasma bovigenitalium* and *Mycoplasma bovis* (La Faunce & McEntee, 1982). However, in severe clinically recognizable cases the most common organism isolated is *Arcanobacterium pyogenes* (Arthur, 1960; McCauley, 1980). Some authors believe that these infections of the seminal vesicles are secondary to congenital defects. Diagnosis of these abnormalities is firstly dependent upon rectal palpation (where enlargement, firmness, pain and adhesions may be detected in the case of seminal vesiculitis) and ultrasonic scanning; and secondly upon laboratory tests, particularly the examination of semen for white blood cells which indicate the presence of inflammation (Fig. 38.21). Hopefully, ultrasound scanning will prove of value in the reliable diagnosis of severe seminal vesiculitis and also of segmental aplasia of the seminal vesicle (Fig. 38.22). However, as mentioned before, the application of the technique is still in its infancy (Little & Woods, 1987). Treatment of an infectious condition obviously requires antibiotic, preferably one with a broad spectrum, and given that there is no evidence of severe effects upon the structure of the seminal vesicles, prognosis is good.

Conditions affecting the other smaller accessory sex glands of the pelvis in the bull have rarely been recognized clinically, but this may yet be possible using ultrasound.

Conclusion

The investigation of infertility in the bull is one of the most interesting examinations in farm animal practice. The approach is standard and success is dependent upon attention to detail in all the facets mentioned in this chapter. One of the main advantages the general practitioner has compared with the specialist is an intimate knowledge of the farm, the ability of those involved as stockworkers and also a fair idea of the reliability or otherwise of the history and records. On the other hand, the major disadvantages are the small number of cases that the practitioner will see in a year, so limiting the experience that can be built up, and the standard of equipment, particularly microscope, required. Finally the amount of time and flexibility of time that need to be devoted to such work must be balanced against other, possibly more remunerative, demands of a busy practice.

References

Abbitt, B., Berndtson, W.E. & Seidel, G.E. (1984) Effect of dihydrostreptomycin or oxytetracycline on reproductive capacity in bulls. *American Journal of Veterinary Research*, **45**, 2243–6.

Amann, R.P. & Almquist, J.O. (1976) Bull management to maximise sperm output. In *Proceedings of the 6th Technical Conference on Artificial Insemination and Reproduction*, pp. 1–10. National Association of Animal Breeders.

Amann, R.P. & Schambacher, B.D. (1983) Physiology of male reproduction. *Journal of Animal Science*, **57** (Suppl. 2), 380–403.

Anon. (1979) *The Federation of UK Milk Marketing Boards Dairy Facts and Figures 1979*, Thames Ditton.

Anon. (1988) *The Federation of UK Milk Marketing Boards Dairy Facts and Figures 1988*, Thames Ditton.

Anon. (1998) *The National Dairy Council Dairy Facts and Figures 1998*, London.

Archibald, L., Gronwall, R.R., Pritchard, E.L. & Tran, T. (1990) Acrosome reaction and concentration of prostaglandin E$_2$ in semen of rams treated with Flunixin meglumine (BANAMINE). *Theriogenology*, **33**, 373–83.

Arthur, G.H. (1960) Reproductive abnormalities of male animal. In *Wright's Veterinary Obstetrics*, 3rd edn, pp. 507–8. Baillière Tindall and Cox, London.

Ashdown, R.R. (1973) Functional anatomy of the penis in ruminants. In *Veterinary Annual* (ed. by C.S.G. Grunsell & F.W.G. Hill), Vol. 13, pp. 22–5. John Wright & Sons, Bristol.

Ashdown, R.R., Gilanpour, H., David, J.S.E. & Gibbs, C. (1979) Impotence in the bull: (i) Abnormal venous drainage of the corpus cavernosum penis. *Veterinary Record*, **104**, 423–8.

Ashdown, R.R. & Glossop, C.E. (1983) Impotence in the bull: (3) Rupture of the corpus cavernosum penis proximal to the sigmoid flexure. *Veterinary Record*, **113**, 30–7.

Ashdown, R.R. & Majeed, Z.Z. (1978) Haemorrhage from the bovine penis during erection and ejaculation: a possible explanation of some cases. *Veterinary Record*, **103**, 12–13.

Ashdown R.R. & Pearson, H. (1973a) Anatomical and experimental studies on eversion of the sheath and protrusion of the penis in the bull. *Research in Veterinary Science*, **15**, 13–24.

Ashdown, R.R. & Pearson, H. (1973b) Studies on 'corkscrew' penis in the bull. *Veterinary Record*, **93**, 30–5.

Bane, A. (1954) Sexual function of bulls in relation to heredity rearing intensity and somatic conditions. *Acta Agricultura Scandinavica*, **4**, 95–208.

Bane, A. & Hansen, H.-J. (1962) Spinal changes in the bull and their significance in serving ability. *Cornell Veterinarian*, **52**, 363–84.

Bartels, L.E. (1975) Femoral – tibial osteoarthrosis in the bull. Clinical survey and radiologic interpretation. *Journal of the American Veterinary Radiology Society*, **16**, 151–8.

Barth, A.D. & Oko, R.J. (1989) *Abnormal Morphology of Bovine Spermatozoa*. Iowa State University Press, Iowa.

Beckett, S.D., Reynold, T.M., Walker, D.F., Hudson, P.S. & Burphit, R.C. (1974) Experimentally induced rupture of corpus cavernosum penis of bull. *American Journal of Veterinary Research*, **35**, 765–7.

Bishop, M.W.H., Campbell, R.C., Hancock, J.L. & Walton, A. (1954) Semen characteristics and fertility in the bull. *Journal of Agricultural Science*, **44**, 227–48.

Blockey, M.A. de B & Taylor, E.G. (1984) Observations on spiral deviation of the penis in beef bulls. *Australian Veterinary Journal*, **61**, 141–5.

Blom, E. (1979a) Studies on seminal vesiculitis in the bull 1. Semen examination methods and post mortem findings. *Nordisk Veterinaermedicin*, **31**, 241–50.

Blom, E. (1979b) Studies on seminal vesiculitis in the bull 2. Malformation of the genital organs as a possible predisposing factor in the pathogenesis of seminal vesiculitis. *Nordisk Veterinaermedicin*, **31**, 293–305.

Blom, E. & Christensen, N.O. (1960) The etiology of spermiostasis in the bull. *Nordisk Veterinaermedicin*, **12**, 453–70.

Caldow, G.L. & Taylor, D.W. (1997) Experiences with venereal campylobacter infection in suckler herds. *Cattle Practice*, **5**, 327–34.

Chandley, A.C. (1979) Chromosomal basis of human infertility. *British Medical Bulletin*, **35**, 181–6.

Chenoweth, P.J. (1983) Sexual behaviour of the bull: a review. *Journal of Dairy Science*, **66**, 173–9.

Clark, B.L. (1971) Review of bovine vibriosis. *Australian Veterinary Journal*, **47**, 103–107.

Coulter, G.H. & Foote, R.H. (1978) Relationship of body-weight to testicular size and consistency in growing Holstein bulls. *Journal of Animal Science*, **44**, 1076–9.

Coulter, G.H., Mapletoft, R.J., Kozub, G.C. & Cates, W.F. (1987) Scrotal circumference of two-year-old bulls of several beef breeds. *Theriogenology*, **27**, 485–91.

De Kretser, D.M. (1979) Endocrinology of male infertility. *British Medical Bulletin*, **35**, 187–92.

Deschamps, J.C., Ott, R.S., McEntee, K., Heath, E.H., Heinricks, R.R., Shanks, R.D. & Hixon, J.E. (1987a) Effects of zeranol on reproduction in beef bulls. Scrotal circumference, serving ability, semen characteristics and pathologic changes of the reproductive organs. *American Journal of Veterinary Research*, **48**, 137–47.

Deschamps, J.C., Ott, R.S., Weston, P.G., Shanks, R.D., Kesler, D.J., Bolt, D.J. & Hixon, J.E. (1987b) Effects of zeranol on reproduction in beef bulls. Luteinising hormone, follicle-stimulating hormone and testosterone secretion in response to gonadotrophin-releasing hormone and human chorionic gonadotrophin. *American Journal of Veterinary Research*, **48**, 31–6.

Dufty, J.H. (1967) Diagnosis of vibriosis in the bull. *Australian Veterinary Journal*, **43**, 443–7.

Foote, R.L., Munkenbank, N. & Greene, W.A. (1976) Testosterone and libido in Holstein bulls of various ages. *Journal of Dairy Science*, **59**, 2011–13.

Galina, C.S. (1972) An evaluation of testicular biopsy in farm animals. *Veterinary Record*, **88**, 628–31.

Garner D.L. (1997) Ancillary tests of bull semen quality. In *Bull infertility* (ed. by S.D. Van Camp). The Veterinary Clinics of North America, WB Saunder, Philadelphia.

Gunn, G.J., Stott, A.W. & Scanlan, S.A. (1998) Estimating the losses associated with bovine viral diarrhoea (BVD) within the Scottish cow-calf herd. In *Proceedings of the XXth World Buiatrics Conference*, Sydney, Australia, 1998.

Gustavsson, I. (1974) Appearance and persistence of the 1/29 translocation in cattle. In *Colloque les Accidents Chromosemiques de la Reproduction* (ed. by J. Bové & A. Bové), pp. 147–53. Institut National de la Santé et de la Recherche Médicale, Paris.

Gwazdauskas, F.C. (1985) Effects of climate on reproduction in cattle. *Journal of Dairy Science*, **68**, 1568–78.

Hillers, J.K., Thonney, S.C. & Gaskins, C.T. (1982) Economic comparison of breeding dairy cows artificially versus naturally. *Journal of Dairy Science*, **65**, 861–5.

Hopkins, F.M. & Spitzer, J.C. (1997) The New Society for Theriogenology Breeding Soundness Evaluation System. *The Veterinary Clinics of North America, Food Animal Practice*, July, 283–93.

Kallis, C.H.J., Barkema, H.W. & Hesselink, J.W. (1999) Certification of dairy herds as free of paratuberculosis using culture of strategically pooled faecal samples. In *Proceedings of the Sixth International Colloquium on Paratuberculosis* (ed. by E.J.B. Manning & M.T. Collins), pp. 55–8. International Association of Paratuberculosis, Madison.

Kilgour, R. (1984) Sexual behaviour in male farm animals. In *Male in Farm Animal Reproduction* (ed. by M. Courot), pp. 108–32. Martinus Nijhoff, Dordrecht.

Kilkenny, J.B. (1978) Reproductive performance of beef cows. *World Review of Animal Production*, **14**, 65–74.

Kumi-Diaka, J. & Dennis, S.M. (1978) The Sertoli cell index as a measure of testicular degeneration in the bull. *Veterinary Record*, **103**, 112–14.

La Faunce, N.A. & McEntee, K. (1982) Experimental *Mycoplasma bovis* vesiculitis in the bull. *Cornell Veterinarian*, **72**, 150–67.

Lagerlöf, N. (1951) Hereditary forms of sterility in Swedish cattle breeds. *Fertility and Sterility*, **2**, 230–42.

Land, R.B. (1978) Genetic improvement of mammalian fertility: a review of opportunities. *Animal Production Science*, **1**, 109–35.

Lander, K.P. (1983) New technique for collection of vaginal mucus from cattle. *Veterinary Record*, **112**, 570.

Larsen, L.H. & Bellenger, C.R. (1971) surgery of the prolapsed prepuce in the bull: its complications and dangers. *Australian Veterinary Journal*, **47**, 349–57.

Li, P.S. & Wagner, W.C. (1983) *In vivo* and *in vitro* studies on the effect of adrenocorticotrophic hormone or cortisol on the pituitary response to gonadotrophin releasing hormone. *Biology of Reproduction*, **29**, 11–24.

Linford, E., Glover, F.A., Bishop, C. & Stewart, D.L. (1976) The relationship between semen evaluation methods and fertility in the bull. *Journal of Reproduction and Fertility*, **47**, 283–91.

Little, T.V. & Woods, G.L. (1987) Utrasonography of accessory sex glands in the stallion. *Journal of Reproduction and Fertility*, **35**(Suppl.), 87–94.

Logue, D.N. (1975) A study in bovine cytogenetics. PhD thesis, Glasgow.

Logue, D.N. & Greig, A. (1985) Infertility in the bull. 1. Failure to mate. *In Practice*, **7**, 185–91.

Logue, D.N. & Greig, A. (1986) Infertility in the bull. 2. Infertility associated with normal service behaviour. *In Practice*, **8**, 118–22.

Logue, D.N. & Greig, A. (1987) Infertility in the bull. 3. Collection and examination in semen. *In Practice*, **9**, 161–70.

Logue, D.N. & Harvey, M.J.A. (1978) Meiosis and spermatogenesis in bulls' heterozyos for a presumptive V29 Robertsonian translocation. *Journal of Reproduction and Fertility*, **54**, 159–65.

Logue, D.N., Harvey, M.J.A. & Lennox, B. (1979) Hormonal and histological studies in a 61 XXY bull. *Veterinary Record*, **104**, 500–503.

Logue, D. & Isbister, J. (1992) Bull infertility. In *Bovine Medicine* (ed. by A.H. Andrews, R.W. Blocrey, H. Boyd & R.G. Eddy), p. 483. Blackwell Scientific Publications, London.

Long, S.E. & Dubra, C.R. (1972) Incidence and relative clinical significance of preputial eversion in bulls. *Veterinary Record*, **91**, 165–9.

McCauley, A.D. (1980) Seminal vesiculitis in bulls. In *Current Therapy in Theriogenology: Diagnosis, Treatment and Prevention of Reproduction Diseases in Animals* (ed. by D.A. Morrow), pp. 401–405. W.B. Saunders, Philadelphia, London, Toronto.

McGowan, M., Galloway, D., Taylor, E., Entwistle, K. & Johnston, P. (2002) The veterinary examination of bulls. *Cattle Practice*, **10**, 55.

Meischke, H.R.C. (1979) A survey of bovine teat papillomatosis. *Veterinary Record*, **104**, 28–31.

Melrose, D.R., Brinley Morgan, W.J., Stewart, D.L. & Thomson, D.M. (1957) The treatment of *Vibrio fetus* infected bulls. *Veterinary Record*, **69**, 691–3.

Memon, M.A., Dawson, L.J., Vsenik, E.A. & Rice, L.E. (1980–85) Preputial injuries in beef bulls: 172 cases. *Journal of the American Veterinary Medical Association*, **193**, 481–5.

Miller, D.J. & Hunter, A.G. (1987) Individual variation for *in vitro* fertilization success in dairy bulls. *Journal of Dairy Science*, **70**, 2150–3.

Mobini, S., Walker, D.F. & Crawley, R.R. (1982) An experimental evaluation of the response of the bull penis to carbon fibre implants. *Cornell Veterinary Journal*, **72**, 350–60.

Monke, D.R. (1980) Avulsion of the bovine penile epithelium at the fornix. In *Proceedings of the 8th Technical Conference on Artificial Insemination*, pp. 48–65. National Association of Animal Breeders.

O'Connor, M.L., Gwazdauskas, F.C., McGilliard, M.L. & Saake, R.G. (1985) Effect of adrenocorticotrophic hormone and associated hormonal responses on semen quality and sperm output of bulls. *Journal of Dairy Science*, **68**, 151–7.

O'Lamhna, M. & Roche, J.F. (1983) Effect of repeated implantation with anabolic agents on growth rate, carcass weight, testicular size and behaviour of bulls. *Veterinary Record*, **113**, 531–4.

Palmer, A.C., Blakemore, W.F., Barlow, R.M., Frazer, J.A. & Ogden, A.L. (1972) Progressive ataxia of Charolais cattle associated with a myelin disorder. *Veterinary Record*, **91**, 592–4.

Parkinson, T.J. (1987) Seasonal variation in semen quality in bulls: correlation with environmental temperature. *Veterinary Record*, **120**, 479–82.

Robertson, I.S., Fraser, H.M., Innes, G.M. & Jones, A.S. (1982) Effect of immunological castration on sexual and production characteristics in male cattle. *Veterinary Record*, **111**, 529–31.

Salisbury, G.W. & Van Demark, N.L. (1961) *Physiology of Reproduction and Artificial Insemination*. W.H. Freeman, San Francisco, London.

Stott, A.W., Veerkamp, R.F. & Wassell, T.R. (1999) The economics of fertility in the dairy herd. *Animal Science*, **68**, 1148–54.

Turnbull, P.A. (1977) An abattoir survey of bull genitalia. *Australian Veterinary Journal*, **53**, 274–9.

Vincent, C.K. (1972) Effects of season and high environmental temperature on fertility in cattle. *Journal of the American Association of Veterinary Medicine*, **161**, 1333–8.

Walker, D.F. (1980) Genital surgery of the bull. In *Current Therapy in Theriogenology: Diagnosis, Treatment and Prevention of Reproductive Diseases in Animals* (ed. by D.A. Morrow), pp. 370–401. W.B. Saunders, Philadelphia, London, Toronto.

Weaver, A.D. (1997) Joint conditions. In *Lameness in Cattle* (ed. by P.R. Greenough & A.D. Weaver), 3rd edn, pp. 162–80. W.B. Saunders, Philadelphia.

Chapter 39

Artificial Insemination and Diseases Transmitted by Semen

G.H. Wentink

Introduction 627
Semen processing 627
Technique of artificial insemination 627
Disease transmissible by semen (and/or mentioned
    in trade certificates) 628
Semen safety 632

Introduction

Large scale artificial insemination (AI) for cattle was started in Russia at the beginning of the twentieth century (1909) by the stimulating impetus of Professor Ivanovich Ivanov. Verbal history says that it was used for genetic improvement, but mainly to avoid transmission of venereal diseases. These diseases were transmitted from infected cows to cows on different farms by travelling bulls used for natural service. Using extended (diluted) semen the great number of offspring by one bull also produced more information on its breeding value. The main goal of AI is to improve the genetic potential of cattle, and considerable progress has been made since its applications.

Semen is shipped all over the world, and consequently must be free from infectious diseases. Relevant regulations apply in all parts of the world, but may differ slightly between countries. The EU regulations concerning semen production are laid down in Directive 88/407; semen imported into the EU from other countries must also conform to this standard.

Semen is only safe beyond doubt if produced by bulls that were proved to be free of infectious diseases 21 days after its production. International regulations current at the start of the twenty-first century do not fulfil this requirement.

Semen processing

After collection and application of extenders (specific diluents), semen must be cooled to 5°C over a period of 2–5 hours before freezing in liquid nitrogen. During this period metabolism of the spermatozoa continues and metabolic products are excreted into the liquid of the ejaculate. Extenders are applied to improve the buffering action of the media surrounding the spermatozoa for protection against toxic metabolic substances (mainly lactic acid), and secondly to increase the volume in order to serve as many cows as possible with one ejaculate.

Between 300 and at least 1000 straws can be produced from one ejaculate, depending on the concentration needed in one dose. Fertility after insemination is often expressed as the non-return rate (NR): the percentage of cows that are not rebred within a certain period (usually 56 days). This information can be used to optimize the concentration of spermatozoa per dose. Each dose is delivered in a straw (0.25 ml in Europe, 0.5 ml in the USA) containing on average 15×10^6 sperm cells. However, fertility results differ between bulls. The average NR in the Netherlands is 68 per cent; some bulls score above and others below the average. Thus the semen concentration of each bull is altered to produce the average NR and thereby allow an optimal number of cows to be served and become pregnant with each ejaculate. Fertility of bulls can only be judged after insemination based on NR. The criteria in the laboratory do not have predictive value for fertility: very often disappointing results are obtained with semen that was considered of excellent quality in the laboratory, while conversely excellent fertility has been obtained after natural service with bulls that did not fulfil the standards for AI bull approval.

Technique of artificial insemination

The technique in itself is easy to perform, cheap and applied world-wide rather uniformly by technicians and veterinarians. Insemination is routinely performed by the recto-vaginal technique. One arm is introduced into the rectum of the restrained cow in heat, grips the cervix and stretches the vagina. After careful cleaning of the vulval area, the AI gun is inserted into the vagina and through the cervix for the deposition of three quarters of the semen into the corpus uteri (uterine horns are too deep) and, after limited withdrawal of the AI gun, the remaining quarter is deposited in the cervix at the first insemination after parturition. At the second or higher number of inseminations the semen must be deposited in the cervix only, because a limited number of cows show signs of heat in the presence of an embryo. Introduction of the gun into the corpus uteri might interrupt the integrity of the embryo and thus interfere with pregnancy.

The proper time for insemination is in the last period of the standing heat. Cows are selected for insemination by observation of the herd at least twice daily during moments of quiescence: observation during periods of even limited excitation (for example during collecting for milking) can lead to the insemination of cows not in heat and thus to disappointing fertility results. Several aids have been applied to improve heat detection such as electronic pedometers, heat mount detector pads, spotter bulls, etc. However, careful observation of the herd and proper records of heat periods undoubtedly form the backbone of good fertility results (see Chapter 41b). Harmful side effects of improper insemination are infections and/or injuries of the genital tract, which are dealt with in Chapter 36.

Diseases transmissible by semen (and/or mentioned in trade certificates)

Table 39.1 summarizes the diseases in this category.

Foot-and-mouth disease (FMD) (see also p. 700)

This is a highly contagious disease of cloven-hoofed animals characterized by high fever followed by vesicles on the mucosa of mouth and tongue, the feet and the udder. FMD is caused by a picornavirus comprising seven serotypes; infection with one serotype does not induce immunity to other serotypes. In order to prevent spread of the disease in a country immediate recognition of the clinical picture is essential. For a positive diagnosis the demonstration of FMD viral antigen by indirect sandwich ELISA techniques, preferably in the epithelium of unruptured or freshly ruptured vesicles, is sufficient. The agent is very resistant to environmental factors and may be spread over long distances by air and/or vehicles and/or man. FMD virus is easily transmitted by semen.

Infectious bovine rhinotracheitis/infectious pustular vulvovaginitis (IBR/IPV) (see also pp. 289, 579)

This is a disease of the upper respiratory tract or of the genital tract, respectively. IBR is characterized by clinical signs such as high fever, nasal discharge, ocular discharge and abortion in up to 30 per cent of pregnant animals. The disease has a high morbidity but a low mortality. However, the disease might follow a more severe course if complicated by bacterial infections. IPV is characterized by erosion in the vagina or on the penis, leading to adhesions. The disease is caused by bovine herpes virus type 1 (BHV1) which can be subdivided in strains with preference for the respiratory or genital tracts respectively. Diagnosis is made by demonstration of the virus in secreta from respiratory and/or genital tracts up to 14 days after infection, and by serology. However, sensitivity and specificity of serological tests applied in various countries differ considerably. The agent may survive in favourable conditions (high relative humidity, low temperatures) for 30 days in the environment. BHV1 is easily transmitted by semen. AI centres in the EU must be free of IBR: only serologically negative animals are allowed as BHV1 infections lead usually to latency. Latently infected animals are the source for new epidemics. Latently infected animals are serologically positive for BHV1, but some seronegative latently infected cows have also been reported. However, the sensitivities of the tests applied in these animals are doubtful. Straub (see Horzinek, 1990) described seronegative latently infected animals after the application of a one hour incubation serum neutralization test with a limited sensitivity: the animals would probably have been positive with sensitive tests. It is thought that seronegative latently infected animals develop during the period of maternal immunity after an infection with a very low dose of BHV1 and they should exist in very low prevalence in endemic areas. However, Switzerland, Denmark and Austria became free of IBR: these countries eliminated the virus from their cattle populations without unexpected disease outbreaks caused by serologically negative latently infected animals. The straightforward isolation of positive animals was successful. So the problem of serologically negative latently infected animals is very limited or even non-existent.

Bovine virus diarrhoea (BVD) (see also pp. 578, 853)

BVD is observed clinically as transient diarrhoea during three to ten days after infection in at maximum 5 per cent of infected animals; in exceptional cases severe diarrhoea, fever, ulceration of the buccal mucosa, haemorrhages and death occur. The remaining 95 per cent of the infections pass unnoticed. When infected in the first four months of pregnancy, cows may deliver persistently infected (pi) calves that shed the virus during their lifetime. The disease is caused by the pestivirus bovine virus diarrhoea virus (BVDV). Bovine virus diarrhoea is endemic world-wide. Diagnosis is by antigen ELISA or culture of the virus from

Table 39.1 The main characteristics of infectious diseases that could be transmitted by semen or artificial insemination.

Disease	Incubation period	Reservoir	Excretion mainly by	Period of transmission/ viraemia	Transmission by semen/AI[a]
FMD	2–8 days	Animals in the acute phase Chronic carriers (cattle)	Saliva Other secreta	<14 days Carriers for up to 2 years	++
IBR/IVP	2–5 days	Latently infected animals	Nasal discharge	2–20 days	++
Rinderpest	4–15 days	Cattle in the acute phase	All secretions and excretions	21 days or longer	++
BVD	2–15 days	Persistently infected (pi) cattle Cattle up to 56 post infection	Saliva All secretions and excretions of pi animals	Variable, usually 2–15 (but up to 56) days	++
MCF	From a few days to year(s)	Sheep during lambing period	Unknown	Unknown, not cow to cow	0
Akabane virus	??	Biting insects	Viraemia	Viraemia during prolonged periods	0
Bluetongue	3–6 days	Biting insects	Viraemia	Viraemia, mostly <14 days	0
Enzootic bovine leukosis (EBL)	Up to 35 days	Chronically infected cattle	Intact blood Lymphocytes	During lifetime after infection	0
Genital campylobacteriosis	<3 days	Chronically infected cattle: bulls without symptoms	Copulation	During lifetime after infection	++
Bovine brucellosis	14–120 days	Chronically (latently) infected animals	Vaginal discharge Fetal membranes	Prolonged periods	+
Bovine tuberculosis	>3 weeks	Chronically infected cattle	Nasal discharge	During lifetime after open tuberculosis	+
Leptospira hardjo	<7 days	Chronically infected cattle	Urine	Prolonged periods after infection	+
Johne's disease	Occasionally 12; usually 24 months	Chronically infected cattle	Faeces	From 18 months before overt clinical disease onwards	0
Mycoplasma mycoides (contagious bovine pleuropneumonia: CBPP)	2–6 weeks	Chronically infected cattle	Nasal discharge Urine	During lifetime after infection	+
Haemophilus somnus	??	Harboured in genital and respiratory tracts in healthy animals	Nasal discharge Effluents from genital tract	During lifetime after infection	+
Genital tritrichomoniasis	<3 days	Chronically infected cattle: bulls without symptoms	Copulation	During lifetime after infection	++
Query-fever (Q-fever)	??	Ticks Environment (dust) Chronically infected cattle (animals)	Fetal membranes Vaginal discharge	Prolonged periods	0
Bovine spongiform encephalopathy (BSE)	4 years	CNS of contaminated cattle	Contaminated food	No transmission reported	0

[a] 0, unlikely; +, possible; ++, easily.
??, no experience and no information found in the literature.

the peripheral blood or organs after death, and by serology. Persistently infected animals transmit the virus during their lifetime and infect sentinel animals easily. Transiently viraemic animals, however, transmit the disease to a limited extent. These primary infections might lead to prolonged periods of viraemia (up to 40 days), the presence of virus in bronchoalveolar washings (up to 56 days after infection) and in semen even after seroconversion has taken place. Therefore, the risk for transmission of BVDV by semen is substantial. One exceptional bull has been described that shed BVDV in the semen over prolonged periods (11 months), although the animal was serologically positive. This unusual pattern might be explained by a primary infection during puberty or an intrauterine infection around the time of maturation of the immune system. There is information that this phenomenon might occur more frequently. The agent survives for some days in the environment. Transmission by semen is easy. AI centres only accept bulls that are not persistently infected. However, because some infectious routes for the introduction of BVDV are not completely understood, in endemic areas BVDV might infect bulls in an AI station. Where there is unintended infection of AI bulls the infection passes subclinically and, as this disease is easily transmitted by semen, it is very important to test for BVDV. Monthly tests for serologically negative donor bulls and, in the case of seroconversion, ensuring the semen is free from BVDV might be the only solution.

Enzootic bovine leukosis (EBL) (see also p. 693)

EBL is found clinically by enlarged lymph nodes or other lymphosarcomas, or by lymphocytosis in the peripheral blood in the minority (some 30 per cent) of infected animals. Infections for the greater part pass completely unnoticed. The disease is caused by the retrovirus bovine leukemia virus (BLV), which may be demonstrated in the blood by PCR techniques. Routine diagnosis is performed by serology (ELISA, AGID). The agent does not survive in the environment. Only intact lymphocytes are infective: the infection is transmitted by blood. Transmission by semen is very unlikely.

Rinderpest (see also p. 707)

This is a very contagious disease of mainly cattle and buffaloes. The disease is characterized by high fever, erosions on the gums, tongue and palate together with nasal and ocular discharge, and diarrhoea. Rinderpest is caused by a Morbelli virus that can be demonstrated in blood or lymph nodes and spleen, mainly by culture. Transmission is mainly directly by infected animals and can occur via the semen. The virus survives in the environment for limited periods.

Malignant catarrhal fever (MCF) (see also p. 935)

MCF is a sporadically, almost invariably fatal disease of cattle of all ages. The disease is characterized by high fever, bright red coloration of all mucous membranes, enlarged superficial lymph nodes and very often diarrhoea. A herpes virus (BHV3) causes the disease. Diagnosis in live animals is by clinical signs, and by PCR on heparinized blood. Culture of the virus is not possible, therefore information on the resistance of the virus against environmental influences is not available. Cow to cow transmission has never been reported. Transmission by semen is therefore very unlikely.

Bluetongue (BT) (see also p. 691)

BT occurs mainly in small ruminants but may occur in cattle as well. If clinically overt (many infections pass unnoticed in cattle) the disease is characterized by fever, facial oedema, haemorrhages and ulceration of the mucous membranes. An orbivirus consisting of 24 serogroups causes the disease. The virus is identified by culture and by PCR techniques on blood samples of febrile animals. The agent is transmitted by insects of the genus *Culicoides*; transmission from cow to cow has not been reported. Transmission by semen is very unlikely.

Akabane virus (see also p. 580)

Infections of Akabane virus were shown to cause sporadic epizootics of premature births and developmental deformities in the new born (arthrogryposis-hydranencephaly) in cows, sheep and goats. The disease has been reported in Southeast Asia, the Arabian Peninsula and the Middle East and African countries. Diagnosis is done retrospectively by serology in adult animals, and by culture techniques in abnormal fetuses and calves. Biting insects transmit the agent. After experimental infection in bulls, Akabane virus was not demonstrated in the semen; transmission by this route is therefore unlikely.

Bovine genital campylobacteriosis (see pp. 568, 582)

This is a venereal disease characterized by infertility, early embryonic death and abortion. In bulls, infections are inapparent. The disease is caused by *Campylobacter fetus* ssp. *venerealis*, which in bulls can be cultured from preputial washings. Serological methods are unreliable. The organisms survive in the environment for limited periods (hours). Mating and/or semen mainly cause transmission. Virgin bulls are absolutely free of this agent. This agent was the impetus for the world-wide application of AI techniques and for the obligatory addition of antibiotics to the semen. If this procedure is properly executed, semen is free from this bacterial agent. Bull stations should be free of this agent, but the low transmission rate makes testing more often than once a year useless. However, when a positive result is obtained, all semen batches after the last negative result should be checked for the presence of the agent and positive ejaculates destroyed.

A very similar agent, *Campylobacter fetus* ssp. *fetus*, is associated with abortion storms in sheep. In cattle, after oral uptake, this agent infects the gastrointestinal tract and is shed by the faeces. In exceptional cases, oral infections in adult pregnant cattle may lead to bacteraemia and in limited numbers to infection and expulsion of the fetus. This agent is not transmitted by mating or semen. Giacoboni *et al.* (1993) isolated *Campylobacter fetus* ssp. *fetus* from the faeces in 26.5 per cent of young calves, and in 15 per cent of older cattle. Excretion by the faeces leads inevitably to contamination of the environment and thus to the risk of contamination of the prepuce. In The Netherlands, *Campylobacter fetus* ssp. *fetus* was isolated from the prepuce of AI bulls ranging in age from 10 months to 5 years that had never served naturally.

Brucellosis (see also p. 580)

This is manifested by abortions in the last third of pregnancy. The causative organisms are excreted in abundance with uterine discharges and with milk. The disease, which is a zoonosis, is caused by *Brucella (B.) abortus*, occasionally by *B. melitensis* (lower numbers of aborting cows in the herd) and exceptionally by *B. suis*. The disease is diagnosed by culture of the causative organism from uterine discharge and milk, by serology (CFT, BUA, ELISA) or by a specific skin test. The organisms survive in the environment in favourable circumstances for prolonged periods. Transmission by semen is possible.

Bovine tuberculosis (see also p. 862)

This passes unnoticed in the early phases after infection, but in advanced cases emaciation, coughing and enlargement of the lymph nodes develop. It is caused by *Mycobacterium (M.) bovis* and occasionally by *M. tuberculosis* (the human tuberculosis strain) when an infective human source is present. Tuberculosis in live animals is diagnosed by a specific skin test, gamma-interferon assay using peripheral blood lymphocytes, serology (ELISA) and by culture from nasal secretions. The organism is resistant to environmental influences

and may survive for several months and transmission by semen is possible. Tuberculosis is a zoonosis.

Leptospirosis (see also p. 735)

Leptospirosis is a contagious disease of animals and humans. Many *Leptospira* species exist, each with their specific carrier host (reservoir) in which infection leads to diseases of limited severity and prolonged excretion. Infection in other animal species (end hosts) leads to very severe, life threatening disease symptoms. Clinically, infections in susceptible end hosts are characterized by fever, icterus, haemorrhages, uraemia and blood tinged urine. After recovery, the *Leptospira* are completely eliminated from the end host's body and transmission by semen is very unlikely. Infections in the carrier hosts pass with minor clinical problems and may even pass unnoticed.

Cattle are carriers for *Leptospira hardjo*, but end hosts for other *Leptospira* species. Infection with *L. hardjo* in cattle leads to prolonged or intermittent excretion with urine (and semen) and therefore may be transmitted by semen. *Leptospira* may survive in the environment in humid and warm conditions (summer) for longer periods. Attention in AI stations should be concentrated on *Leptospira hardjo* infections. *L. hardjo* is a zoonosis and causes milker's fever in man.

Contagious bovine pleuropneumonia (CBPP) (see also Chapter 49b)

CBPP is characterized by fever, dyspnoea, coughing, nasal discharges and anorexia. It is caused by *Mycoplasma mycoides* ssp. *mycoides*, which can be demonstrated in nasal secreta and bronchoalveolar washings or in pleural fluids collected after puncture by culture in appropriate media. The agent is vulnerable for environmental influences and is transmitted by infective animals over limited distances. Transmission by semen is possible.

Johne's disease (paratuberculosis) (see also p. 857)

This disease is chronic enteritis of ruminants, characterized in cows by severe diarrhoea, emaciation and submandibular oedema. It is caused by *Mycobacterium (M.) avium paratuberculosis*, which only leads to clinical disease and excretion after infection at a very young age. Infection leads to progressive thickening of the gut wall, causing a protein losing enteropathy with diarrhoea in the final stages after 24 months or longer. *M. paratuberculosis* was found in the semen of bulls that suffered from severe clinical disease.

In the clinical stages, the agent can be demonstrated in faeces and exceptionally in milk and the fetus by culture and/or PCR techniques. The use of PCR on the faeces lacks sensitivity. For the detection of subclinically infected animals a skin test, ELISA and CFT are applied. Each method has the disadvantage of limited specificity and sensitivity.

Transmission by contaminated semen or semen from contaminated bulls has never been demonstrated. Johne's disease is endemic in most countries of the world. The prolonged incubation period and test systems with low sensitivity lead inevitably to the introduction of infected calves into the AI centres. However, excretion by semen does occur only after prolonged excretion by the faeces, and shedders can be traced by the application of annual faecal culture tests from the age of two years. Furthermore, there is no evidence that contaminated semen infects cows after insemination. Johne's disease might be a zoonosis (Crohn's disease in man).

Haemorrhagic septicaemia (HS) (see also p. 728)

HS is a highly fatal disease characterized by initial fever, respiratory signs and terminal septicaemia leading to recumbence. It has been reported from Asia and Africa, and is caused by certain strains of *Pasteurella multocida*. The agent can be cultured from blood and from internal organs. *P. multocida* is moderately resistant to environmental influences. Transmission by semen is very unlikely.

Query fever (Q-fever) (see also p. 586)

In cattle, Q-fever is characterized by abortion, retained placenta, metritis and infertility. The disease is caused by *Coxiella (C.) burnetti*. Diagnosis is established by microscopy of fetal membranes or aborted fetuses, or by culture of this agent in embryonated eggs from uterine effluents. Routine diagnostic tests are made by serology (CFT, ELISA). The agent is extremely resistant to environmental influences. Transmission is caused by biting insects or by inhalation of contaminated dust. Transmission by semen is limited or unlikely. Q-fever is a zoonosis.

Bovine genital tritrichomoniasis (see also p. 584)

This is characterized by infertility and abortion. Bulls may be infected without clinical signs. The disease is caused by the protozoan *Tritrichomonas fetus*, which comprises three serotypes of equal pathogenity. The agent can be cultured from uterine discharges and preputial washings. *Tritrichomonas* is rather resistant to environmental influences. Mating and/or semen mainly cause transmission. Virgin bulls are free of this agent. However, if an infection with tritrichomoniasis is diagnosed, no treatment is available and the bull and its semen must be destroyed.

Bovine spongiform encephalopathy (BSE) (see also p. 909)

BSE is a fatal neurological disease of cattle with a long incubation period. Clinically, behavioural changes and locomotion disturbances such as ataxia manifest the disease. Feed is generally regarded as the most likely source of infection. After (oral) uptake of abnormal protein some of the body protein is stereometrically altered, making the protein invulnerable to proteases and thus leading to intracellular accumulation of prions. This stereometrical change leads to death of brain cells, resulting in the aforementioned. No diagnostic tests for live animals are available, although some promising results have been reported. The prions are extremely resistant to environmental factors. BSE prions have never been demonstrated in the genital organs of diseased bulls or in the semen and experimental insemination of susceptible cows with semen from BSE-contaminated bulls has not been shown to induce BSE in the cows or progeny. There is no proof that prions might be present in the semen. At present the risk of BSE transmission by semen is thought to be negligible and so restrictions on semen trade due to BSE should be minimal or none. BSE is considered to be a zoonosis (new variant CJD).

Other infectious agents

Ubiquitous agents that might be or are present in semen, e.g. *E. coli*, *Proteus* spp., *Pseudomonas* spp., *Haemophilus* spp., *Campylobacter* spp. except *C. fetus* ssp. *venerealis*, *Mycoplasma* spp., and *Ureaplasma* spp., should not hinder the semen trade: the addition of appropriate antibiotics after proper procedures is a sufficient guarantee for safety.

Semen safety

For safety testing of semen, two approaches can be applied: examination of the end product or continuous surveillance of the bulls before and after semen production. The tests for the presence of infectious agents in the semen completely depend on one single investigation and therefore rely on the sensitivity of the test methods only. The continuous surveillance of the semen donors for infectious diseases before and after semen collection is based on sequential investigations, increasing the reliability by the application of multiple tests. In terms of semen safety, testing the donor for the absence of infectious diseases 21 days after semen collection is beyond doubt the best method. Therefore the bulls in AI centres must be negative for the diseases mentioned above. The very first step is to accept only virgin bull calves negative for these diseases. Most AI centres in Europe that release semen for the EU market collect their bull calves before the age of six months. There are no concerns about diseases from which the area is officially declared free. An annual check on the health status will suffice if the country in which the AI centre is situated remains negative. However, if diseases are endemic, theoretical risks exist for the introduction of disease agents into AI studs. Preventive measures should concentrate on optimal hygiene for humans entering the premises (showering and changing clothes), on 48-hour storage periods (including forage) or on disinfection of materials before admittance into the station, the use of mains water, and on the eradication of vermin. One risk factor remains, however infectious particles transported by air and/or birds. Only large distances (more than 1 kilometre) between the AI station and other cattle in the area will suffice.

The next step is to minimize the consequences of the unintentional introduction of agents into AI centres. Regular checks must be performed for the presence of disease agents that might be transmitted by semen: animals found positive must be separated or destroyed immediately. The system for checking the disease-free status of the bulls depends on the transmission routes and transmission rate. Highly contagious diseases with a high risk for transmission by semen should be checked regularly (monthly). The rates at which diseases are transmitted to other animals depend on a number of characteristics of the pathogen, the host and of the contact structure between animals. An important parameter related to transmission is the basic reproduction ratio, i.e. the number of animals that are infected by one typical infectious animal during its entire infectious period. This number depends greatly on the number of effective contacts between animals. A contact is effective when the pathogen is transmitted from one infected animal to another (excretion titre above the minimal effective dose). These contacts might be either direct (animal–animal) or indirect (by air, people, equipment, etc.). High transmission rates in AI stations will be achieved when the number of effective contacts is high and the length of the incubation period is short. For diseases with high transmission rates (e.g. IBR) monthly checks of 20 per cent of the donor bulls give a certainty of 99.9 per cent for semen safety. This method is applied in one centre in The Netherlands.

References and further reading

Berchovich, Z. (1998) Maintenance of *Brucella abortus* free herds: a review with emphasis on the epidemiology and the problems in diagnosing Brucellosis in areas of low prevalence. *Veterinary Quarterly*, **20**, 81–8.

Bruschke, C.J.M. (1998) Pathogenesis and vaccinology of bovine virus diarrhoea virus infections. Thesis, Utrecht.

Chen, S.S., Redwood, D.W. & Ellis, B. (1990) Control of *Campylobacter fetus* in artificially contaminated bovine semen by incubation with antibiotics before freezing. *British Veterinary Journal*, **146**, 68–74.

Council Directive (88/407/EEC) (1993).

Den Daas, J.H.G. (1997) Prediction of bovine male fertility. Thesis, Wageningen.

Eaglesome, M.D. & Garcia, M.M. (1997) Disease risks to animal health from artificial insemination with bovine semen. *Revue Scientifique Office International des Epizooties*, **16**, 215–25.

Giacoboni, G.I., Itoh, K., Hirayama, K., Takahashi, E. & Mitsuoka, T. (1993) Comparison of fecal *Campylobacter* in calves and cattle of different ages and areas in Japan. *Journal of Veterinary Medical Science*, **55**, 555–9.

Herman, H.A., Mitchel, J.R. & Doak, G.A. (1994) *The Artificial Insemination and Embryo Transfer of Dairy and Beef Cattle*, 8th edn. Interstate Publishers, Danville.

Horzinek M.C. (1990) *Virus Infections in Vertebrates*. In *Viral Infections in Ruminants*. (ed. by Z. Dinter & B. Morein) Elsevier; Amsterdam, Oxford, New York, Tokyo.

Merkal, R.S., Miller, J.M., Hintz, A.M. & Bryner, J.H. (1982) Intrauterine inoculation of *Mycobacterium paratuberculosis* into guinea pigs and cattle. *American Journal of Veterinary Research*, **43**, 676–8.

OIE (1996) *OIE Manual of Standards for Diagnostic Tests and Vaccines*, 3rd edition. Office International des Epizooties, 1997. ISBN 92-9044-423-1.

Thrusfield, M. (1995) *Veterinary Epidemiology*, (2th edn). Blackwell Science, Oxford.

Wentink, G.H., Frankena, K., Bosch, J.C., Vandehoek, J.E.D. & van den Berg, Th. (2000) Prevention of disease transmission by semen in cattle. *Livestock Production Science*, **62**, 207–20.

Chapter 40
Embryo Transfer

A.K. Smith

Introduction	634
The principles of embryo transfer	634
Results	637
Donors	637
Recipients	637
Embryo collection: practicalities	638
Donor selection criteria	638
Nutrition	638
Superovulation	638
Insemination	639
Embryo collection	641
Embryo processing	642
Embryo freezing	642
Embryo thawing	643
Embryo transfers: practicalities	643
Recipient selection criteria	644
Nutrition and management	644
Disease control	644
Oestrous synchronization	644
Transferring the embryo	644
Hormone supplementation	645
Record keeping	645
Legislation	645
Troubleshooting	646
Advanced technologies	646
Embryo splitting	646
In-vitro fertilization (IVF)	647
Ovum pick-up (OPU)	647
Embryo sexing	648
Cloning	648

Introduction

Although considered a recent technology, Walter Heap performed the first successful embryo transfer (ET) in rabbits over a hundred years ago. A further six decades elapsed before the first embryo transfer calf was produced in 1951, in the USA, by Willet and his colleagues. The first commercially acceptable results were recorded in cattle in 1969 by Rowson and his colleagues. In 1973 Wilmut and Rowson produced the first calf born from a frozen-thawed embryo and five years later Willadsen succeeded in producing commercially acceptable results for cattle embryo freezing.

Now ET technology is widely used in pedigree cattle breeding offering breeders a number of opportunities:

- Increased numbers of progeny from genetically superior dams.
- The possibility of progeny of the other sex from dams that previously may have only produced calves of one sex.
- Increased diversity for marketing herd genetics including international trade.
- Banking of frozen embryos to accommodate seasonal breeding or longer term breeding strategies.
- As a diagnostic technique for infertility cases, especially in diagnosing blocked oviducts.
- As a method of continuing breeding from animals unable to do so naturally.
- Improved disease control applicable to high health status herds and international trade by reducing the number of individual animal movements.

The principles of embryo transfer

As previously described (see Chapter 33), follicular dynamics result in either two or three waves of follicle development during the oestrous cycle. In each wave a dominant follicle suppresses the development of subordinate follicles until at the end of the cycle the corpus luteum (CL) is lysed, allowing the dominant follicle of the last wave to become the ovulatory follicle.

Superovulation utilizes commercially prepared follicle stimulating hormone (FSH) to encourage a group of developing follicles to overcome the dominant follicle suppression and continue developing to ovulation with concomitant maturation of the oocytes. The FSH is commonly administered as a twice-daily injection regime over four days, commencing mid-cycle (days 9–14). Incorporated in this regime is a prostaglandin $F_{2\alpha}$ ($PGF_{2\alpha}$) injection, usually given alongside the fifth FSH injection, to return the donor cow to oestrus. The onset of oestrus and subsequent ovulation are accelerated in superovulated animals and oestrus occurs usually 48–56 hours after the $PGF_{2\alpha}$ treatment, with ovulation occurring as early as the onset of oestrus (cf 12–18 hours post oestrus in non-superovulated cows). Accordingly it is usual to inseminate the donor cow soon after the onset of oestrus (e.g. the afternoon of the day of oestrus, with a second insemination the following morning).

Embryo collection is performed on day 7 of the oestrous cycle (day 0 = day of oestrus). Embryos enter the uterine lumen from the oviduct at approximately day 4 of the oestrous cycle and, although embryos can be collected successfully from the uterus between days 5 and 9, a day 7 collection allows recovery of the most flexible stages of the embryo for both freezing and fresh transfer. Collection (flushing) is a non-surgical procedure requiring catheterization of the uterine horns.

Two types of embryo collection catheter exist:

- Two-way, which has two tubes within it. One allows inflation of a latex cuff near the tip of the catheter, whilst the other enables the flushing media to enter and leave the uterine horn. Greater volumes of media are required as a larger segment of the uterine horn is flushed (Fig. 40.2).
- Three-way, which consists of three tubes. One allows inflation of the cuff situated 10 cm behind the tip. Another tube allows media to enter the uterine lumen from the tip of the catheter and a one-way flow is created by the media returning down the third tube via its entry hole at the level of the cuff (Fig. 40.3).

The flushing media, Dulbecco's phosphate buffered saline (PBS), is infused into the uterine lumen to allow slight distension before drainage by gravity flow along with the embryos and ova into a collection filter. The filter contains a metal or plastic micromesh with a pore diameter approximately half that of an embryo (embryo diameter 140–170 μm), allowing excess media to run through whilst retaining the embryos.

Embryo searching is performed once both uterine horns have been flushed. The contents of the filter are emptied into a petri dish and examined under a stereoscopic microscope at between ×6 and ×10 magnification. Recovered embryos are placed in embryo holding solution (Dulbecco's PBS with bovine serum albumin, glucose and antibiotics), classified (Fig. 40.1; Plate 40.1) and graded (Box 40.1). Embryo holding solution is also known as ovum culture medium (OCM). Embryo evaluation is by subjective visual assessment under ×50 stereoscopic magnification. Embryos can survive on the bench at ambient temperature (20°C) for up to eight hours with little drop in pregnancy rate, but they are best frozen or transferred within three hours of collection (Wright, 1985).

Embryo freezing involves, initially, partial dehydration of the embryo in a cryoprotectant to prevent freezing damage. Two main factors influence the success or failure of freezing cells:

- Solution effects: the solute concentration within a cell increases due to dehydration and causes cell

Box 40.1 Description of embryo grading. Source: *IETS Manual*, 3rd edn (Stringfellow & Seidel, 1998).

Grade 1: Symmetrical and spherical embryo mass with individual blastomeres (cells) that are uniform in size, colour and density. The embryo is consistent with its expected stage of development. Irregularities should be relatively minor and at least 85 per cent of the cellular material should be an intact, viable embryonic mass. This judgement should be based on the percentage of embryonic cells represented by the extruded material in the perivitelline space. The zona pellucida should be smooth and have no concave or flat surfaces that might cause the embryo to adhere to a petri dish or a straw.

Grade 2: Moderate irregularities in overall shape of the embryonic mass or in size, colour and density of individual cells. At least 50 per cent of the cellular material should be an intact, viable embryonic mass.

Grade 3: Major irregularities in shape of the embryonic mass or in size, colour and density of individual cells. At least 25 per cent of the cellular material should be an intact, viable embryonic mass.

injury, particularly when cooling is slower than optimum.

- Intracellular ice: this results in physical damage when cooling is faster than optimal.

Cooling rates of 0.3°C/min to 0.6°C/min are considered rapid whereas 0.1°C/min is considered slow. The cryoprotectants lower the temperature at which intracellular ice forms, reduce the amount of ice present in extracellular fluid, moderate the solute effect and help stabilize the cell membrane. Some cryoprotectants themselves may cause osmotic injury to cells and need to be added or removed gradually. The cryoprotectants most commonly used commercially are 10 per cent glycerol and 1.5 M ethylene glycol. Stepwise addition or removal is required for 10 per cent glycerol in increasing or decreasing gradients of concentration respectively, whereas one-step thawing of embryos frozen in ethylene glycol can be performed as it crosses cell membranes more rapidly. Embryos are frozen in 0.25 ml plastic straws which must be identified with the donor name, sire name, collection team code, breed code and date code. The straws are sealed either by a plastic plug or are heat-crimped.

The cooling curve to be used is preprogrammed into the freezing machine and the straws are subjected to a controlled rate of freezing as this progresses to ensure optimal survival of the embryo. A process called 'seeding' is performed when the freezer chamber temperature is at –6°C (some programmes –7°C). This nucleates the freezing medium with an ice crystal when

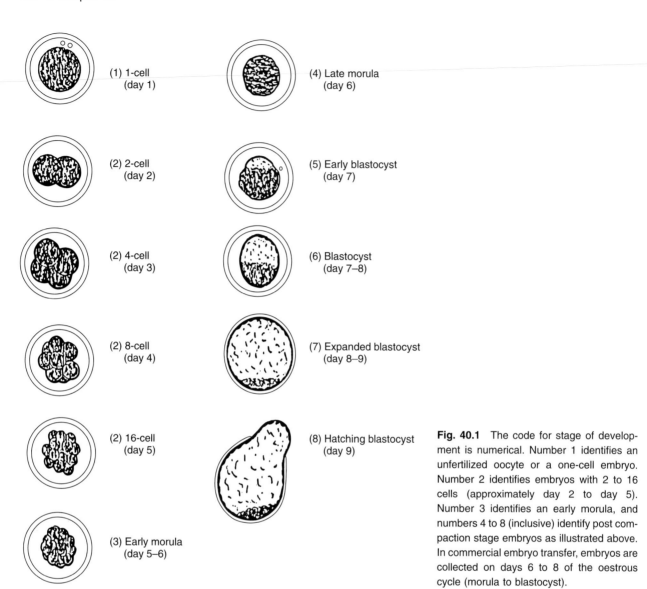

(1) 1-cell
(day 1)

(2) 2-cell
(day 2)

(2) 4-cell
(day 3)

(2) 8-cell
(day 4)

(2) 16-cell
(day 5)

(3) Early morula
(day 5–6)

(4) Late morula
(day 6)

(5) Early blastocyst
(day 7)

(6) Blastocyst
(day 7–8)

(7) Expanded blastocyst
(day 8–9)

(8) Hatching blastocyst
(day 9)

Fig. 40.1 The code for stage of development is numerical. Number 1 identifies an unfertilized oocyte or a one-cell embryo. Number 2 identifies embryos with 2 to 16 cells (approximately day 2 to day 5). Number 3 identifies an early morula, and numbers 4 to 8 (inclusive) identify post compaction stage embryos as illustrated above. In commercial embryo transfer, embryos are collected on days 6 to 8 of the oestrous cycle (morula to blastocyst).

1 or 2°C below its freezing point, preventing supercooling and excessive temperature rise from the release of latent heat in the cooling process. At the end of the freezing programme the straws are plunged directly into liquid nitrogen before being placed in plastic goblets and stored under liquid nitrogen in cryogenic flasks.

Thawing of the straws is a reversal of the previous procedures. The straws are thawed in a flask of warm water and if frozen in 1.5 M ethylene glycol are then ready for immediate transfer. Those frozen in 10 per cent glycerol must first have this extracted from the embryo. The embryos are removed from the straws they are frozen in and passaged through decreasing concentrations of glycerol until finally they are placed in embryo holding solution, re-examined, their grades checked and then they are reloaded into straws for transfer.

The *embryo transfer* procedure for the recipient is the same for fresh or frozen embryos. Recipients need to have been synchronized to display oestrus on the same day as the donor cow or within a 24-hour period either side of that day. For frozen embryos the recipients are synchronized to be in oestrus six, seven or eight days prior to the day of transfer. Before transfer of the embryo the recipient's ovaries are examined by manual rectal palpation or ultrasound scanner for the presence of a CL. Note is also made of which ovary has the CL. Recipients receive an epidural anaesthetic and, after the perineum has been cleaned, the transfer gun is passed through the cervix and guided along the uterine horn ipsilateral to the corpus luteum before depositing

Table 40.1 Analysis of results achieved from 1110 commercial embryo collections. Source: Ovaflo Embryo Transfer.

Overall results per collection	
Total ova (includes unfertilized ova, degenerate embryos and viable embryos)	10.08 (mean)
Total viable embryos	5.03 (mean)
Fertilised ova (includes viable and degenerate embryos)	58.6%
By classification	
Blastocysts	11.3%
Early blastocysts	15.2%
Morulas	73.5%
By grades	
Grade 1 embryos	88.0%
Grade 2 embryos	11.7%
Grade 3 embryos	0.3%

Table 40.2 Analysis of pregnancy results for 3820 embryos transferred commercially. Source: Ovaflo Embryo Transfer.

By classification	
Blastocysts (grade 1)	62.3%
Early blastocysts (grade 1)	62.4%
Morulas (grade 1)	62.4%
By procedure	
Fresh transfers (grade 1)	64.8%
Frozen transfers (grade 1, 10% glycerol)	58.8%
By freezing method (purchased embryos)	
10% Glycerol	53.4%
1.5 M Ethylene glycol	55.4%
By embryo grade	
Grade 1	62.4%
Grade 2	44.5%
By dam breed	
Beef (grade 1)	59.3%
Dairy (grade 1)	64.5%

the embryo. Historically embryos were transferred surgically, involving paravertebral anaesthesia and laparotomy of the sublumbar fossa, but for welfare reasons surgical transfers have been superseded by the non-surgical technique.

Results

Donors

In superovulated animals an estimate can be made of the likely number of ova by counting the corpora lutea on the ovaries. Manual estimation is poor if there are more than ten CLs on an ovary, but if there are fewer then estimates have a higher accuracy. Some discrepancies can be accounted for by luteinized follicles which histologically show an enclosed oocyte with the cumulus cells dispersed and luteinization in the granulosa cells (Monniaux et al., 1983). Heifers can exhibit large responses to superovulation (based on palpated CLs) with high fertilization rates of the recovered ova but lower recovery rates than parous animals (Hasler et al., 1983). Examples of results achieved commercially are given in Table 40.1.

Recipients

Successful pregnancy rates are influenced by a number of factors, both embryonic and maternal.

Embryonic factors

Although some young embryos (days 3–6) have been shown to have abnormal karyotypes (7 per cent) no anomalies were found in day 7, 8 or 9 embryos, suggesting embryos with abnormal karyotypes were non-functional by that stage. Whilst embryos from donors over 15 years old have shown lower pregnancy rates (Hasler et al., 1987), the biggest single embryo factor affecting pregnancy rates is embryo quality. Good quality embryos give better pregnancy rates (Donaldson, 1985). By day 16 well-developed embryos produce significantly more interferon, thus fully inhibiting luteolytic $PGF_{2\alpha}$, than do poorly developed embryos at that stage.

Maternal factors

The best pregnancy rates are achieved when the synchrony is close (±24 hours) between the embryo's stage of development and the recipient's uterine environment (Donaldson, 1985; Newcomb & Rowson, 1975). Transfer of the embryo to the uterine horn ipsilateral to the corpus luteum with deep placement of the embryo, rather than placement at the level of the intercornual ligament, gives the best pregnancy rates (Christie et al., 1979). The CL ensures a source of progesterone but maternal progesterone concentrations can show considerable diurnal fluctuations. Progesterone is required in the first half (approximately 12–14 days) of the oestrous cycle to suppress the oxytocin receptors. Inhibition of the oxytocin receptors is less effective in cows with a low progesterone concentration, meaning that the luteolytic mechanism develops earlier allowing less time for the conceptus to produce sufficient trophoblastic interferon to create an adequate block to luteolysis. Remsen *et al.* (1982) and Northey *et al.* (1985) demonstrated maximal pregnancy rates (PR) when plasma progesterone concentrations were in the ranges 2–5 ng/ml (PR 74 per cent) and 2–6 ng/ml (PR 68 per cent), respectively. However Hasler *et al.* (1980) and Smith *et al.* (1996) found no correlation between pregnancy rates and progesterone concentrations. A review of mean pregnancy rates that can be achieved commercially is given in Table 40.2.

Embryo collection: practicalities

Forward planning is the key. Careful animal preparation and attention to detail will improve success.

Donor selection criteria

Donor heifers:

- Body condition score approximately $2\frac{1}{2}$ (assessed over the range 1–5; Lowman *et al.*, 1976; see also Chapter 2);
- Regular oestrous cycles;
- Age 15–18 months.

Donor cows:

- At least six weeks calved;
- Clean uterus and returned to regular oestrous cycles;
- Preferably two heats since calving;
- Maintaining or increasing liveweight (body condition score 2–3).

Nutrition

It is now recognized that the time required for a primordial follicle to develop to an ovulatory follicle is 60–90 days and the environment that the cow is in during that time can influence not only the vitality of that oocyte but also the subsequent embryo (Webb *et al.*, 1999). In particular there is a correlation between follicular development and plasma levels of insulin and peripheral levels of insulin-like growth factor-1 (IGF-1), with elevated levels of insulin being associated with enhanced ovulation rates. Research continues into identifying the mechanisms and pathways involved in

this relationship, but since diet supplementation can raise insulin levels nutrition has an important role. Donors should be on a rising plane of nutrition for six to eight weeks before flushing. All adjustments must be gradual without any sudden changes. The timing of housing and turn-out needs to be planned carefully as either event occurring in the middle of a superovulation programme can have a disastrous effect on the success rate. Careful attention to mineral supplementation is also important. Apart from ensuring a balanced level of minerals, consideration should be given to molybdenum toxicity. Embryo donors on a high molybdenum diet (15–20 mg Mo/kg dietary DM) produce greater numbers of abnormal embryos, suggesting that elevated dietary molybdenum will retard embryo development. In addition, diets containing 5 mg Mo/kg DM decrease conception rates and cause anovulation and anoestrus in cattle. Protection against molybdenum toxicity is achieved by providing adequate supplies of copper. Although copper can be supplied by injection or orally as powdered mineral, drenches and capsules it seems, from some studies, that the use of intraruminal boluses is more efficacious (p. 298).

Superovulation

Gonadotrophins such as equine chorionic gonadotrophin (eCG) and human menopausal gonadotrophin (hMG) have been used in the past to superovulate cows, but due to the undesirable effects from extended activity of the luteinizing hormone (LH) fraction they have been superseded by purified FSH. This is available as a freeze-dried product with diluent which, when mixed, produces a solution with controlled amounts of LH activity. These commercial FSH products are sourced principally from ovine and porcine pituitaries.

It is best to start superovulation from a known reference heat so that the injections commence at a known point in the oestrous cycle. A superovulated response can be achieved starting anywhere in the cycle, given good control of the follicular wave, but the most repeatedly consistent results are achieved when the FSH injections commence between days 9 and 14 (Hasler *et al.*, 1983). This same review found no differences in the number of ova (11.6 versus 10.2) or viable embryos (6.2 versus 6.4) recovered from donors superovulated following prostaglandin-induced reference heats versus natural reference heats, respectively. The use of intravaginal devices to mimic the hormone levels found mid cycle can supply an exogenous source of progesterone. Although less consistent than starting from a known reference heat, the results from this method are satis-

Table 40.3 Examples of commercial superovulation regime for cattle.

		Maiden heifer	Mature cow
day 12	am	2.25 ml FSH solution	3.0 ml FSH solution
	pm	2.25 ml	3.0 ml
day 13	am	1.75 ml	2.5 ml
	pm	1.75 ml	2.5 ml
day 14	am	1.25 ml + double dose of $PGF_{2\alpha}$	2.0 ml + double dose of $PGF_{2\alpha}$
	pm	1.25 ml	2.0 ml
day 15	am	0.75 ml	1.5 ml
	pm	0.75 ml	1.5 ml
Total dose		**12 ml**	**18 ml**

Note:
At the time of publication there is one licensed FSH product in U.K. This is an ovine FSH (Ovagen, ICP, NZ) containing 0.88 mg/ml NIADDK-oFSH-17 ovine pituitary FSH.
$PGF_{2\alpha}$ = Prostaglandin $F_{2\alpha}$
These protocols are included as examples of regimes used in commercial embryo transfer practice. Alternative protocols do exist with variations in total volume, volume of individual injections and rate of decline of dosage regime.

factory even if few or no behavioural signs are seen at the time of the reference heat.

When a twice-daily injection regime is used the injection interval is ideally 12 hours, but as long as the interval is no less than eight hours satisfactory results will still be achieved. Product manufacturers advocate that the total dose be split into eight equal injections, but the use of a declining regime with higher dose volumes at the start gives superior results. Responses to the same superovulation regime will vary from donor to donor and there are also breed differences in sensitivity to the treatment with the Simmental breed being particularly sensitive. In addition, body condition, nutrition and environmental factors will all influence the response to treatment. A generalization can be made that maiden heifers will respond satisfactorily to a lower total dosage of FSH than that required for a mature cow. Although aged cows can be successfully superovulated the oocyte quality may be compromised in these cows, especially if over 15 years old, so that fertilization rates of these ova or pregnancy rates of subsequent embryos may be poorer. An example of a standard commercial programme used for maiden heifers and mature cows is shown in Table 40.3.

Between animals there can be a substantial variation in their superovulatory response to a given dose of FSH. What can be an effective dose in one animal may result in either too low or too high a response in another. Animals which fail to respond sufficiently (fewer than two ova is a non-response and fewer than five ova is a low response) can usually be improved by increasing the dose on a subsequent occasion. Increasing the total dose in 2 ml increments (0.25 ml per injection) is usually an acceptable approach. The objective is to improve the superovulatory response without creating an over-response, because as the number of follicles stimulated increases there is a negative effect on the viable percentage of the recovered ova. Generally this happens once the total CL count rises above 20. As numbers increase above this level there is a tendency for a rise in numbers of unfertilized and degenerate embryos and a decline in viable embryos, often to zero. However, some donors can still perform successfully with CL counts in the range of 20–30. It is, however, the author's opinion that a preferred target is a superovulatory response yielding a total ova count in the mid teens, which can result in 8 to 12 viable embryos (fertilization rate 50–60 per cent). As Table 40.1 demonstrates real results are lower than this. This can be partly attributed to some donors being consistently successful, but others being consistently poorer performers. Studies of donor populations corroborate this, but such profiles can only be built up over time and on the strength of a single flush a donor cannot be categorized simply as good or bad other than for that single event.

Cleanliness at the time of injection is important as contamination of the stock solution can result in loss of potency of the FSH. New sterile syringes and needles should be used for each injection. In animals that have high body condition scores the superovulatory response is improved if the injections are given into the neck muscle.

Insemination (see also Chapter 39)

The number of straws of semen recommended can vary from operator to operator, but given good quality semen three straws given in two insemination periods

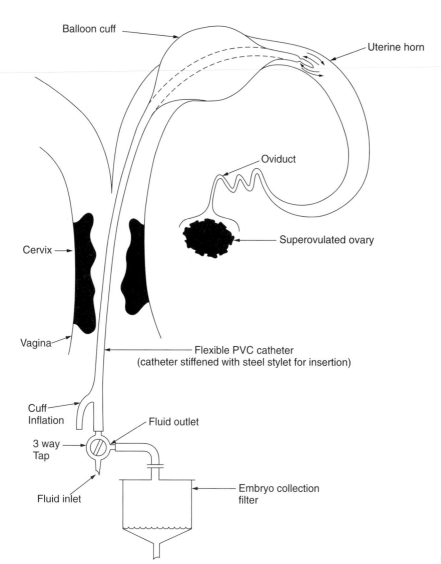

Fig. 40.2 Two-way embryo collection catheter.

are usually adequate, firstly the afternoon of the day the donor is in oestrus and again the following morning. The precise timing of this action can be dependent on the time of onset of oestrus. If the donor is in standing oestrus in the morning then artificial insemination (AI) at mid afternoon that day with two straws and again the following morning with one straw is sufficient. If the donor only comes into standing oestrus later in the day then the first AI can be delayed. This is easily done if DIY AI is used, but may be awkward with a technician service. The time of onset of heat is usually directly proportional to the size of the superovulatory response. If a cow is in standing oestrus the night before she is expected then a large superovulatory response can be assumed and an extra AI session using an additional two straws of semen should be planned for the morning of the first day of AI. If, through

previous experience, the semen is known to be of poor quality then extra straws may be used (e.g. three sessions utilizing two, two and one straws of semen). A mix of semen from two different bulls can also be used when quality is questionable. It should be confirmed that the Breed Society rules permit this practice and all progeny produced will need to be either blood-typed or DNA tested to confirm parentage. Equivocal evidence exists as to whether heterospermic interaction in this scenario will synergistically enhance fertilization rates. Published data suggest enhancement in a range of 2 to 10 per cent, dependent on whether two bulls (same breed) or three bulls (different breeds) were used respectively. Natural service can also be used and the bull should be allowed to serve the donor as soon as she comes into oestrus. Consideration must be given to the health status of bulls used

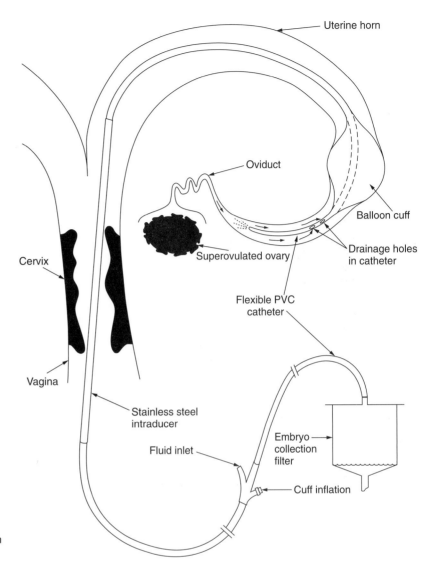

Fig. 40.3 Three-way embryo collection catheter.

for natural service to avoid transmission of venereal and other diseases.

Embryo collection

Cleanliness of the epidural site and the perineum is important and cotton wool swabs dampened with surgical spirit are ideal for this. All instruments, catheters, tubing and filters must be sterile. Metal instruments, silicone tubing and glass tubing can be autoclaved, whereas catheters and filters are usually gas sterilized with ethylene oxide. No disinfectants or harsh cleansing solutions that may persist on surfaces and be harmful to the embryos should be used. All equipment sterilized by ethylene oxide must be aired for a minimum of seven days before use.

A successful recovery rate requires good catheter position and good media flow. These conditions are most easily met if the epidural completely abolishes rectal peristalsis. The ideal position for a two-way catheter is to have the cuff inflated at least 5 cm past the level of the intercornual ligament (ICL) (Fig. 40.2). In the three-way system the stainless steel cannula, down which the catheter passes, is inserted to the level of the ICL. Upon removal of the centre, the catheter is passed down the cannula and along the uterine horn until the tip is about 10–15 cm from the end of the horn (Fig. 40.3). Inflation of the cuff should be enough to anchor it in position without damaging the endometrium; usually 2 ml of air and 4 ml of sterile water will be sufficient in most donors. The two-way system will use more media than the three-way because a larger

(a) 10% Glycerol

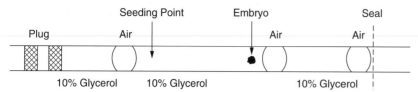

(b) 1.5 M ethylene glycol

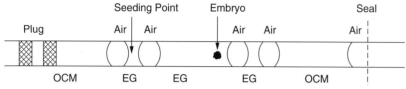

OCM = Ovum culture media
EG = 1.5 M ethylene glycol

Fig. 40.4 Methods of loading straws for freezing.

volume of uterine horn is being flushed. Generally the two-way system will require about 350–500 ml per horn compared to the three-way system using 180–200 ml per horn. Care must be taken not to overdistend the horn and aliquots of approximately 30 ml in a three-way system would be sufficient. To aid successful drainage of the media down the catheter it is important to lift the tip of the uterine horn gently so that it is not curled under the body of the uterus. The bovine uterus is a fragile organ and rough handling or excessively forceful actions can result in damage to the endometrium or perforation of the wall.

Best practice is to return the donor animals to normal cycles after the flush. This ensures termination of skulking embryos and reduces opportunities for development of cystic ovarian disease after superovulation. This can be done by injection of $PGF_{2\alpha}$ or by using a combined progesterone releasing intravaginal device with $PGF_{2\alpha}$. When using $PGF_{2\alpha}$ alone a higher dose than normal is required to lyse the luteal tissue present on superovulated ovaries. Consequently a one-and-a half times or double normal dose of $PGF_{2\alpha}$ is used. If donors are to be repeat flushed they should be allowed two oestrus events between flushes to optimize the repeat results (Hasler *et al.*, 1983). In practice this translates to an eight-week interval between flushes.

Embryo processing

Examination of the embryos requires a good quality stereoscopic dissecting microscope with at least ×10, ×25 and ×50 magnification. Disposable plastic Petri dishes should be used. Once retrieved from the flushing solution, embryos should be kept in embryo holding solution at a constant ambient temperature (approximately 20°C) and out of strong light until the next procedure. Ideally, embryos should be frozen or transferred within three hours of collection. Although the law requires embryos to be washed ten times prior to freezing it is good practice to wash all embryos whether destined for freezing or fresh transfer. An outline of this procedure is given in Box 40.2 and a more detailed account can be found in the *Manual of the International Embryo Transfer Society* (IETS) (Stringfellow & Seidel, 1998). The ten-times washing regime will remove a number of viruses from the zona pellucida whilst other more persistent ones can be removed by including a wash with trypsin in the procedure. Box 40.3 lists viruses and bacteria which can be successfully removed by standard washing procedures and trypsin washing.

Embryo freezing

Prior to freezing the embryos are partially dehydrated in cryoprotectant. Ready-to-use 10 per cent glycerol

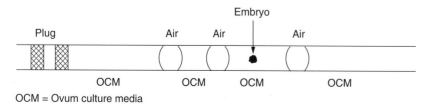

OCM = Ovum culture media

Fig. 40.5 Method of loading straws for transfer.

- Only embryos from a single donor should be washed together
- Ten or fewer embryos should be washed at one time
- Only zona pellucida intact embryos should be washed
- Only embryos free of adherent material should be washed
- A minimum of ten washes is necessary, ensuring gentle agitation in each wash
- Use a new sterile micropipette each time embryos are moved from one wash to the next
- Regulate volumes so that each wash is at least a 100-fold dilution of the previous wash, achieved by using 1 ml droplets of Dulbecco's PBS and a 10 μl micropipette to move embryos

Box 40.3 Pathogens not found after washing of embryos previously exposed to these agents. Source: *IETS Manual*, 3rd edn (Stringfellow & Seidel, 1998).

Normal ten-times washing:	Akabane virus
	Bovine leukaemia virus
	Bluetongue virus
	Bovine viral diarrhoea virus
	Foot-and-mouth disease virus
	Brucella abortus
Trypsin washing:	Bovine herpes virus 4
	Infectious bovine rhinotracheitis virus
	Vesicular stomatitis virus

and 1.5 M ethylene glycol are available commercially, which have the benefit of being quality controlled and screened for viruses. Prior to freezing the embryos need to be allowed time to equilibrate in the cryoprotectant. This state is achieved after 5 to 10 minutes immersion in 1.5 M ethylene glycol, but with the 10 per cent glycerol the embryo needs to be passaged step-wise through increasing concentrations of the solution. A common method is to allow 5 minutes in 5 per cent glycerol (10 per cent glycerol diluted with an equal volume of embryo holding solution) followed by 15 minutes in 10 per cent glycerol. After the required equilibration time in the cryoprotectant the embryos are loaded into straws (Fig. 40.4), sealed and labelled before being put in the freezing machine. It is important not to greatly overextend the equilibration time as the cryoprotectants themselves are embryo-toxic if overexposure is allowed. At the appropriate time in the freezing protocol the cooling process is paused to allow seeding.

Seeding is easily performed using a metal rod, e.g. brass; the rod is supercooled in liquid nitrogen then gently and briefly touched against the straw (Fig. 40.4). The seeded medium immediately becomes opaque as it nucleates. Embryo damage can occur if too long a period of time elapses at seeding (overseeding) or if too large an area is seeded. The use of a brass rod is therefore preferable to tweezers for this reason. Once all straws are seeded the cooling process continues and at the end the straws are swiftly plunged into liquid nitrogen (−196°C). Straws containing embryos (especially the column of medium in the straw in which the embryo lies) should be kept submerged in liquid nitrogen and should not be exposed to air until thawing. The straws should be handled with tweezers, not fingers. The easiest method to check identities on the straw labels is to place the whole goblet containing the straws in a wide-mouthed insulated flask containing liquid nitrogen. Thus the labels/plugs can be read while the

straws are still submerged. If long-term storage is envisaged, separate into two groups and store in different cryogenic flasks.

Embryo thawing

Thawing of the straws is a reversal of the previous procedures. Once the straws have been removed from the liquid nitrogen they are placed in a flask of warm water. Some protocols require a short period of air thawing prior to entering the water. The water temperature (22–37°C), the duration of submersion (7–30 seconds) and the inclusion of air thawing (none–10 seconds) are all dependent on the method and programme protocol used for freezing. Most embryo transfer companies provide recommended thawing protocols along with the embryos. Labels must be checked and the details recorded. Straws with embryos frozen in 1.5 M ethylene glycol can be loaded into the transfer gun for immediate transfer. Embryos frozen in 10 per cent glycerol must be removed from the straws they were frozen in and passaged through decreasing concentrations of glycerol; they are then placed in embryo holding solution, re-examined and their grades checked before they are reloaded into straws for transfer (Fig. 40.5). This step-wise removal of the 10 per cent glycerol is aided by the inclusion of sucrose in the solutions to prevent too rapid an ingress of water to the cells. One brand of ready-to-use solutions passages the embryo from 10 per cent glycerol through 5 per cent glycerol, 0.5 M sucrose (5 minutes) then 2.5 per cent glycerol, 0.5 M sucrose (5 minutes) and finally 0.6 M sucrose (5 minutes) before immersion in embryo holding solution/OCM prior to reloading.

Embryo transfers: practicalities

For successful results forward planning is essential.

Recipient selection criteria

Recipient heifers should be:

● At least 15 months old;
● At least 370 kg (dairy heifers);
● At least 400 kg (beef heifers);
● Of a suitable frame size to carry to term and to calve naturally an embryo calf of the breed to be transferred;
● Body condition score 2–2½; (assessed over the range 1–5; Lowman et al., 1976; see also Chapter 2);
● Displaying regular oestrous cycles.

Recipient cows should be:

● No more than a fourth calver;
● Of a good breeding history;
● At least six weeks calved;
● Clean and returned to regular oestrous cycles post calving;
● Maintaining or increasing liveweight;
● Body condition score 2½–3;
● Of a suitable frame size to carry to term and to calve naturally an embryo calf of the breed to be transferred.

Nutrition and management

It is important that recipients are on a rising plane of nutrition for six to eight weeks before transfer and that this continues for at least another six weeks post transfer. This is of particular relevance around the time of housing and turn-out and ideally these two events should not occur in the middle of a programme but should be completed either two months before the transfer date or delayed until at least six weeks post transfer. The ration should be checked to confirm that it is providing an acceptable balance of energy and protein with sufficient levels of roughage. As with the donors, a suitable supply of minerals is important. If molybdenum toxicity is likely to be a problem then a suitable supply of protective copper should be made available (e.g. intraruminal boluses) (see pp. 254, 298).

Purchasing recipients, mixing groups and routine procedures, such as worming, bolussing, vaccination, freeze-branding and foot-trimming, should all be completed at least six to eight weeks before the transfer date to minimize stress.

Disease control

A number of infective agents can severely affect the success of an ET programme. The principal culprits are bovine viral diarrhoea virus (BVDV), leptospirosis and infectious bovine rhinotracheitis (IBR). Vaccination is possible for all three agents but there is a risk of persist-

ence of virus from the live IBR vaccines which may cause problems for ET progeny destined for export (including Northern Ireland) or for entry to semen collection centres. IBR marker vaccines (p. 1010) may alter the situation but this will depend on recognition by the importing country and importer. If BVDV is known to be a problem on a farm then screening of the recipients prior to vaccination may be desirable to identify and remove any persistently infected animals. When leptospirosis is a known problem on a farm then treatment of the recipients with 25 mg/kg of dihydrostreptomycin (British Cattle Veterinary Association (BCVA), 1992) at the time of first vaccination may be required to reduce the infective load of this bacterium. As the epidemiology of Neospora caninum becomes better understood (see Chapters 19, 37) it may be prudent to screen potential recipients for this agent, especially if vertical transmission of this protozoan from recipient to fetus could affect the reproductive performance of any resulting ET heifers.

Oestrous synchronization

(see also Chapter 42)

For successful pregnancy to be achieved the recipients need to be tightly synchronized to come into oestrus one week before the embryo is transferred. Therefore a tight synchrony period is required. A good method is to use a progesterone releasing intravaginal device or progestage implant in combination with a prostaglandin injection. The device chosen can be inserted for 9, 10 or 11 days and the prostaglandin injection given 24, 48 or 72 hours before removal. This gives a tight synchrony with the peak of activity 28–56 hours after device removal. In the author's opinion a double prostaglandin injection protocol will not provide a tight enough synchrony to maximize recipient usage. The stockperson should observe recipients for oestrus the week before transfer. Observation should be performed at least three times a day for a minimum duration of 20 minutes per observation period. Observations should occur for the three days following the day the synchrony devices are removed.

Transferring the embryo

Having checked for the presence of a CL, and recorded which ovary it is on, the recipient is prepared for the embryo transfer. Cleanliness of the epidural site and the perineum is important and cotton wool swabs dampened with surgical spirit are ideal for this. After traversing the cervix the transfer gun is guided along the uterine horn ipsilateral to the corpus luteum. Pregnancies can be achieved if the embryo is placed at the level of the ICL, but results improve if the site of transfer is further up the horn. Ideally a position of 10 cm or more past the ICL is desirable. It is important to be as gentle as possible and avoid manoeuvres which result in endometrial damage. Sometimes in fatter animals with large dependent tracts it is necessary to accept that the site of placement is not ideal in preference to over-handling the tract, resulting in inflammation or physical injury to the endometrium.

Hormone supplementation

Exogenous hormonal supplementation has taken three main forms in an effort to provide support to the pregnancy. Firstly, exogenous progesterone or progestagen has been used. Progesterone injections have improved pregnancy rates in asynchronous recipients. However, the use of progesterone releasing intravaginal devices produced non-significant negative effects on pregnancy rates when these devices were *in situ* from day 7 to 19 and had direct deleterious effects on embryo development when two devices (double dose) were used from day 7 to day 21. The use of exogenous progestagen treatments (Norgestomet), inserted on day 7, increased pregnancy rates (57.3 per cent control vs 67.8 per cent treated). Norgestomet treatment in acyclic cows did support pregnancies, but by day 38 of pregnancy in cyclic animals there were no significant differences between treated and control groups. It has been observed that too much exogenous progesterone can depress the secretion of LH and result in a reduction in luteal mass. This depresses the luteotrophic support of the endogenous CL, leaving it unable to produce sufficient progesterone for continued support of the pregnancy when the devices are removed. The conclusion is that only discrete (as yet unidentifiable) categories of animal may benefit from this treatment and careful consideration will need to be given to the dosage levels and timing of progesterone supplementation before applying it as a blanket treatment.

The second form of hormonal supplementation has been the administration of human chorionic gonadotrophin (hCG) given at various times and for varying durations. Christie *et al.* (1979) used multiple injections between days 13 and 35 of pregnancy, whereas others used a single injection given on either the day of transfer, day 14 or day 15. All showed a non-significant improvement in pregnancy rates in the treated animals over controls.

The third method of supplementation has been the use of a GnRH analogue (buserelin) given between days 11 and 13. This has been shown to increase pregnancy rates significantly (MacMillan *et al.*, 1986). In cyclic cows treated with buserelin on days 11 and 13 of the cycle the plasma oestradiol concentrations were significantly reduced, suggesting that the mode of action is to reduce the strength of the luteolytic mechanisms, so improving the embryo's chance of inhibiting luteolysis; however, the suppression was transient. Thus if the GnRH analogue is given too soon the luteolytic mechanism may have time to recover, resulting in a temporary benefit, but with some pregnancies being lost at a later date.

These observations indicate that although hormonal supplementation has a tendency to improve pregnancy rates, the concept of a blanket treatment for groups of cattle needs to be considered carefully as inappropriate or mistimed treatments may at best have no benefit but at worst could be detrimental to pregnancy results.

Record keeping

Box 40.4 lists the important records that should be kept for donors, recipients and embryos. Legislation requires that records are maintained for 12 months.

Legislation

Trade in embryos between member states of the European Union (EU) and importation of embryos from approved third countries, including the associated collection, processing, production and storage, is governed

---

Box 40.4 List of necessary records to be maintained by licensed ET teams for 12 months after collection/production of an embryo. Source: Ministry of Agriculture, Fisheries and Food (1995).

Donor
Breed, pedigree name, ID no., herdbook no. and date of birth
Superovulation drug, dosage regime, dose, batch no.
Date of collection, place of collection
Superovulatory response, number and category of embryos recovered, number and grades of viable embryos
Details of processing procedures for embryos (including freezing, transfer, micromanipulation and *in-vitro* fertilization and culture as appropriate)

Recipient
Breed, age and ID no. of recipient
Date and place of transfer
Identification of embryo transferred and its source (if known)

Storage
Identification of every embryo stored
Date of entry/departure of every embryo
Place of origin of embryo prior to arrival
Destination of embryo on departure

IVF storage
In addition to above:
  IVF embryos can be identified on a batch basis
  Must contain details of the date and place of collection of the ovaries/oocytes
  Must identify the herd of origin of donor animals

Box 40.5 Troubleshooting: in the event of poor superovulatory responses or embryo recovery.

Problem	Issues to consider	Solution options
No reference heat	Poor heat detection	Abandon programme and restart
	Poor behavioural signs	Provide artificial CL through exogenous progesterone supplementation
	Poor synchrony	Re-attempt
Poor superovulatory response	Nutrition	Check ration and adjust nutrition
	Mineral status	Check mineral status and adjust supplementation
	Type of FSH	Try alternative type of FSH
	Drug dose/regime	Increase drug dose or alter regime
Unfertilized ova	Semen quality	Check bull history/try different sire
	Insemination technique	Check technique
	Semen handling/thawing	Check technique
	Donor/bull interaction	Try different sire
	Insemination timing	Add additional AI session and extra straws
	Poor ovum quality	Check nutrition/mineral status/body condition loss
	Overstimulation	Reduce FSH dose
	Defective uterine environment	Infection – antibiotic therapy and/or return to oestrus
		Hormonal – difficult to identify/resolve
	Superovulation drug	Try alternative product
Poor recovery (normal breeding history)	Catheter position	Check technique
	Leakage past cuff	Check cuff inflation/integrity of cuff
	Inadequate flow	Raise tip of uterine horn higher than cuff position
		If above fails reposition catheter
		(Note: risk of embryo loss in this procedure)
	Luteinized follicles	
Poor recovery ('problem breeder' history)	As above plus	
	Blocked oviducts	
	Defective gamete transport	
	Ovarian/bursal adhesions	

by EU Council Directive 89/556 of 25 September 1989, amended as appropriate by the relevant Council Directives and Commission Decisions. Within most member states this European legislation is supported by domestic legislation.

In the UK the statutory instrument is the Bovine Embryo (Collection, Production and Transfer) Regulations 1995. This covers the licensing of ET teams and premises, legislation relating to disease control and welfare and also record keeping. The above EU and UK legislation along with the *Manual of the International Embryo Transfer Society* (a procedural guide and general information for the use of embryo transfer technology emphasizing sanitary procedures) are essential reading for anyone planning to become involved in practical embryo transfer.

Troubleshooting

Embryo collection results will vary between donors and pregnancy results can fluctuate between batches of recipients. Boxes 40.5 and 40.6 summarize factors that should be considered in assessing poor results in superovulation of donor cows or pregnancy rates in embryo recipients.

Advanced technologies

Embryo splitting

This technology was promoted in the early 1990s as a commercial application. Its appeal was that it could give proportionately more pregnancies from a collection of embryos than could be achieved by simply transferring the embryos whole. It involved bisecting the embryo with a microblade or a specially designed glass microneedle. These instruments were operated via a micromanipulator which converts gross movements by the operator at the controls to very fine micromovements at the level of the embryo. One disadvantage is that this is a relatively expensive piece of equipment. Inevitably the production of these demi-embryos resulted in some blastomere damage of the embryo so that split embryos tended to have lower pregnancy rates

Box 40.6 Troubleshooting: in the event of poor pregnancy rates.

Recipients	Check:	Nutrition
		Mineral status
		Body condition gain/loss
		Health
		Risk of disease challenge
		Vaccination status
Management	Check:	Correct completion of synchrony programme
		Heat detection
		Recipient handling/stress
Embryos	Check:	Grades used
		Freezing protocol
		Thawing protocol
		Quality control of procedures at each step
Miscellaneous	Consider donor effects:	
		• oocyte quality
		• donor/bull interaction (genetic effect)
		• donor uterine environment
		• a percentage of donors are consistently poor candidates
	Consider operator technique/experience	

than contemporary whole embryos (split embryos 57 per cent versus whole embryos 65 per cent). Even though an increased number of calves could be produced (an increase of the order of 13 per cent) the technique was never really accepted commercially by either the ET operators or the cattle breeders.

In-vitro fertilization (IVF)

This technology involves the creation of embryos in the laboratory. A source of immature oocytes is required. These can be harvested from ovaries removed from a slaughtered animal as long as the ovaries are submitted to the laboratory within four to six hours. Alternatively oocytes can be collected from the live animal by ultrasound-guided ovum pick-up (see later). The immature oocytes must first be matured, which takes approximately 18 hours. After this fertilization takes place by mixing capacitated sperm with the embryo. Following fertilization the embryos are cultured to a stage of development equivalent to day 7 *in-vivo* embryos, when they can then be transferred fresh or frozen. Pregnancy results with IVF embryos tend to be lower than from those originated *in vivo* (IVF 40–50 per cent versus *in vivo* 50–60 per cent). Another potential problem linked to IVF is that of the 'large calf syndrome'. Although it can also be associated with asynchronous timing of embryo transfer and progesterone supplementation early in the oestrous cycle of the dam, it was documented in the early 1990s as being associated with IVF calves. The results of various IVF laboratories worldwide showed that a significant number of ET pregnancies could be affected. There was consider-

able variation between laboratories, but the incidence in some cases was up to 20 per cent. The syndrome manifested itself as giving large calves at birth (up to 75 kg) with increased birthweights greater than could be accounted for by extended gestation length alone. This was associated with an increased incidence of dystocia and a higher mortality rate. Another feature was enlarged placentae in some of these pregnancies, on occasion with a mean weight 25 per cent greater than those of untreated contemporaries. Additionally, in some cases, there were congenital malformations and problems with altered allometric coefficients for the liver, kidney and heart which eventually left these calves unable to survive. Interestingly, despite differences in birthweight, the mean liveweight at one year for these animals can be similar to controls. The effects on the pregnancies did vary depending on the laboratories from which the embryos came. Therefore it was deduced that a factor in the maturation or culture method was significant. The resultant worldwide research effort is helping to elucidate the mechanisms involved. To date, one widely observed finding is that the use of synthetic oviduct fluid (SOF) in the system as opposed to serum reduces, or eliminates, the incidence of large calves.

Ovum pick-up (OPU)

This is the technique that allows the collection of oocytes for IVF from the ovaries of live donor animals. It utilizes an ultrasound-guided transvaginal needle. The operator places one hand in the rectum to allow manual manipulation of the ovaries. The ultrasound probe is placed in the vagina so that the ovary can be visualized with only the vaginal wall between the ovary and the head of the probe. Usually a 7.5 MHz curvilinear probe is used. On visualization of a follicle on the ovary a 60 cm needle (18–21 gauge) is passed down a special channel in the probe. It punctures the vaginal wall and enters the follicle on the ovary. A dotted line on the scanner screen indicates the line down which the needle will transect the ovary, allowing the operator to line up the follicle with the intended path of the needle. At the point of entry the operator uses a foot-pedal to apply a vacuum pressure to the collection line attached to the needle. Too high a pressure results in stripping of the cumulus cells from the oocyte and these denuded oocytes are less developmentally competent. On average, ten oocytes can be collected from both ovaries per session and it is possible to perform a collection session weekly or twice weekly (van der Schans *et al.*, 1991). This usually translates, after developmental losses and fertilization failures, to two transferable embryos per collection session. On average, 70–80 per cent of oocytes recovered are suitable for further processing. Of these, 70 per cent will be successfully fertilized and start to cleave and ultimately 40 per cent of the cleaved embryos will blastulate to become transferable embryos. With an average pregnancy rate of 50 per cent this means that approximately one pregnancy will result from each OPU session.

Embryo sexing

Many methods have been tried over the years to find a simple, easy-to-use way of sexing embryos. The most widely used technique in the UK was developed in Finland (Bredbacka *et al.*, 1995). It involves taking a biopsy of a few cells from the embryo and lysing them to release the DNA content. This DNA material is then mixed with enzymes and multiplied using a polymerase chain reaction (PCR). A stain is included in the solutions which binds to the Y chromosomes, making them fluoresce under UV light. On completion of the PCR cycle the tubes containing the biopsies from male embryos are identified by this fluorescence. Non-fluorescing samples are deemed to be female. This technique is 95 per cent successful in identifying females and 100 per cent in identifying males. The discrepancy is due to errors when biopsies are not placed correctly in the sample tubes.

New technology allows the production of correctly sexed embryos through the use of sexed semen. X chromosomes contain more DNA than Y chromosomes. The semen is mixed with a stain which is taken up by DNA and fluoresces in a laser beam. X chromosomes with higher DNA content will fluoresce more brightly. A flow cytometer/cell sorter utilizing a laser can then sort the sperm on the basis of their DNA content (Cran *et al.*, 1993). At present the technique is 90 per cent accurate, but only small quantities of sperm can be processed at a time and the resulting sexed semen is more successful in fertilizing ova if used for deep uterine AI (Seidel *et al.*, 1998). New freezing protocol advances for sexed semen may obviate the need for deep uterine AI.

Cloning

Cloning results in the production of genetically identical offspring. The simplest form of cloning is twinning (bisecting an embryo). Further advances in the technology resulted in the technique of nuclear transplantation. This involves several procedures including enucleation of ova and the electrofusion of blastomeres from donor embryos. In essence, unfertilized ova are used as recipients for new genetic material. The new genetic material is supplied, in the case of embryos, from a donor embryo which is between the 16 and 64 cell stage (32 blastomere stage at approximately day 5). These blastomeres are disassociated and an individual blastomere (genetically identical to the other 31 blastomeres) is introduced into the enucleated recipient ovum. This new blastomere nucleus is then electrofused to the recipient ovum's cytoplasm and the resultant embryo is cultured to day 7 prior to transfer to a recipient animal. Alternatively, at day 5 the whole procedure can be repeated using blastomeres from the cloned embryo to create another generation. There are reports of this recloning process being used to produce second and third generation embryos. The difference between this procedure and that used to produce the late Dolly the sheep is that, for Dolly, the donated nuclear material was recovered from an adult somatic cell which was then 'reprogrammed' to be capable of differentiation and subsequent organogenesis.

Currently, however, these procedures are too inefficient for commercial production of large numbers of cloned animals and are only justified for biomedical applications. This has resulted in some commercial companies utilizing the technology to produce cloned animals for production of specific proteins for biomedical purposes.

Acknowledgement

The author would like to thank all who assisted with research for this chapter and particularly David McNee for the illustrations, George Seidel Jnr and Richard Bowen of Colorado State University for the pictures and Seonaid Grimmer, Mike Kerby and Arthur Redpath for constructive comments on the manuscript.

References

Bredbacka, P., Kankaanpaa, A. & Peippo, J. (1995) PCR-sexing of bovine embryos: a simplified protocol. *Theriogenology*, **44**, 167–76.

BCVA (1992) Guidelines for the diagnosis and control of *Leptospira hardjo* infection in cattle. British Cattle Veterinary Association, Frampton-on-Severn, pp. 13–14.

Christie, W.B., Newcomb, R. & Rowson, L.E.A. (1979) Embryo survival in heifers after transfer of an egg to the uterine horn contralateral to the corpus luteum and the effect of treatments with progesterone or hCG on pregnancy rates. *Journal of Reproduction and Fertility*, **56**, 701–6.

Cran, D.G., Johnson, L.A., Miller, N.G.A., Cochrane, D. & Polge, C. (1993) Production of bovine calves following separation of X- and Y-chromosome bearing sperm and *in vitro* fertilisation. *Veterinary Record*, **132**, 40–1.

Donaldson, L.E. (1985) Matching of embryo stages and grades with recipient oestrous synchrony in bovine embryo transfer. *Veterinary Record*, **117**, 489–91.

European Community (1989) Council Directive 89/556 EEC of 25 September 1989. In *Official Journal of the European Community* No. L 302/10, 19.10.89.

Hasler, J.F., Bowen, R.A., Nelson, L.D. & Seidel, G.E. Jr (1980) Serum progesterone concentrations in cows receiving embryo transfers. *Journal of Reproduction and Fertility*, **58**, 71–7.

Hasler, J.F., McCauley, A.D., Lathrop, W.F. & Foote, R.H. (1987) Effect of donor–embryo–recipient interactions on pregnancy rate in large-scale bovine embryo transfer program. *Theriogenology*, **27**, 139–68.

Hasler, J.F., McCauley, A.D., Schermerhorn, E.C. & Foote, R.H. (1983) Superovulatory responses of Holstein cows. *Theriogenology*, **19**, 83–99.

Lowman, B.G., Scott, N.A. & Somerville, S.H. (1976) Condition scoring of cattle. East of Scotland College of Agriculture, No. 6.

MacMillan, K.L., Taufa, V.K. & Day, A.M. (1986) Effects of an agonist of gonadotrophin releasing hormone (buserelin) in cattle III, pregnancy rates after a post-insemination injection during metoestrus or dioestrus. *Animal Reproduction Science*, **11**, 1–10.

Ministry of Agriculture, Fisheries and Food (1995) The Bovine Embryo (Collection, Production and Transfer) Regulations 1995: Statutory Instrument 1995 No. 2478 Agriculture, Livestock Industries. Her Majesty's Stationery Office, London.

Monniaux, D., Chupin, D. & Saumande, J. (1983) Superovulatory responses of cattle. *Theriogenology*, **19**, 55–81.

Newcomb, R. & Rowson, L.E.A. (1975) Conception rate after transfer of cow eggs in relation to synchronisation of oestrus and age of egg. *Journal of Reproduction and Fertility*, **43**, 539–41.

Northey, D.L., Barnes, F.L., Eyestone, W.E.H. & First, N.L. (1985) Relationship of serum progesterone, luteinising hormone and the incidence of pregnancy in bovine embryo transfer recipients. *Theriogenology*, **23**, 214 (abstract).

Remsen, L.G., Roussel, J.D. & Karihaloo, A.K. (1982) Pregnancy rates relating to plasma progesterone levels in recipient heifers at day of transfer. *Theriogenology*, **17**, 105 (abstract).

Schans van der, A., van der Westerlaken, L.A.J., de Wit, A.A.C., Eyestone, W.H. & de Boer, H.A. (1991) Ultrasound-guided transvaginal collection of oocytes in the cow. *Theriogenology*, **35**, 288 (abstract).

Seidel Jr, G.E., Herickhoff, L.A., Schenk, J.L., Doyle, S.P. & Green, R.D. (1998) Artificial insemination of heifers with cooled, unfrozen sexed semen. *Theriogenology*, **49**, 365 (abstract).

Smith, A.K., Broadbent, P.J., Dolman, D.F., Grimmer, S.P., Davies, D.A.R. & Dobson, H. (1996) Norgestomet implants, plasma progesterone concentrations and embryo transfer pregnancy rates in cattle. *Veterinary Record*, **139**, 187–91.

Stringfellow, D.A. & Seidel, S.M. (eds) (1998) *Manual of the International Embryo Transfer Society*, 3rd edns. International Embryo Transfer Society, Sary.

Webb, R., Gosden, R G., Telfer, E.E. & Moor, R.M. (1999) Factors affecting folliculogenesis in ruminants. *Animal Science*, **68**, 257–84.

Wright, J.M. (1985) Commercial freezing of bovine embryos in straws. *Theriogenology*, **23**, 17–29.

Further reading

Factors affecting pregnancy rates

Armstrong. D.T. (1993) Recent advances in superovulation of cattle. *Theriogenology*, **39**, 7–24.

Arreseigor, C.J., Sisul, A., Arreseigor, A.E. & Stahringer, R.C. (1998) Effect of cryoprotectant, thawing method, embryo grade and breed on pregnancy rates of cryopreserved bovine embryos. *Theriogenology*, **49**, 160 (abstract).

Beal, W.E., Hinshaw, R.H. & Whitman, S.S. (1998) Evaluating embryo freezing method and the site of embryo deposition on pregnancy rates in bovine embryo transfer. *Theriogenology*, **49**, 241 (abstract).

Gayerie de Abreu, F., Lamming, G.E. & Shaw, R.C. (1984) A cytogenetic investigation of early stage bovine embryos – relation with embryo mortality. In *Proceedings of the 10th International Congress on Animal Reproduction and AI*, Illinois, paper 82.

Lamming, G.E. & Mann, G.E. (1993) Progesterone concentration affects the development of the luteolytic mechanism in the cow. *Journal of Reproduction and Fertility Abstract Series*, No. 11, abstract 8.

Mann, G.E., Mann, S.J. & Lamming, G.E. (1996) The interrelationship between the maternal hormone environment and the embryo during the early stages of pregnancy. *Journal of Reproduction and Fertility Abstract Series*, No. 17, abstract 55.

Nutrition

Black, D.H. & French, N.P. (1999) Copper supplementation and bovine pregnancy rates; three types of supplementation compared in commercial dairy herds. In *Proceedings of the Nottingham Cattle Fertility Conference*, 1999, Nottingham University, pp. 29–36.

O'Gorman, J., Smith, F.H., Pook, D.B.R., Boland, M.P. & Roche, J.F. (1987) The effect of molybdenum-induced copper deficiency on reproduction in beef heifers. *Theriogenology*, **27**, 265 (abstract).

Phillippo, M., Humphries. W.R. & Atkinson, T. (1987) The effect of dietary molybdenum and iron on copper status, puberty, fertility and oestrous cycles in cattle. *Journal of Agricultural Science* (*Cambridge*), **109**, 321–36.

Superovulation

Bo, G.A., Adams, G.P., Pierson, R.A. & Mapletoft, R.J. (1996) Effect of progestagen plus oestradiol-17β treatment on superovulatory response in beef cattle. *Theriogenology*, **45**, 897–910.

Broadbent, P.J., Tresgaskes, L.D., Dolman, D.F. & Smith, A.K. (1996) The effects of varying dose and pattern of administration of ovine FSH on the response to superovulation in performance tested, juvenile Simmental heifers. *Animal Science*, **62**, 181–6.

Garcia, G.J.K., Elsden, R.P. & Seidel Jr, G.E. (1983) Efficacy of $PGF_{2\alpha}$, for reducing the return to estrus interval in superovulated cattle. *Theriogenology*, **19**, 129 (abstract).

Greve, T., Callesen, H., Hyttel, P., Høier, R. & Assey, R. (1995) The effects of exogenous gonadotrophins on oocyte and embryo quality in cattle. *Theriogenology*, **43**, 41–50.

Tonhati, H., Lobo, R.B. & Oliveira, H.N. (1999) Repeatability and heritability of response to superovulation in Holstein cows. *Theriogenology*, **51**, 1151–6.

Warfield, S.J., Seidel Jr, G.E. & Elsden, R.P. (1986) A comparison of two FSH regimens for superovulating cows and heifers. *Theriogenology*, **25**, 213 (abstract).

Hormonal supplementation

Broadbent, P.J., Sinclair, K.D., Dolman, D.F., Mullan, J.S. & McNally, J.R. (1992) The effect of a norgestomet ear implant (Crestar) on pregnancy rate in embryo transfer recipients. In *Proceedings of the 12th International Congress on Animal Reproduction*, The Hague, Vol. 2, pp. 782–4.

Diskin, M.G. & Sreenan, J.M. (1986) Progesterone and embryo survival in the cow. In *Embryo Mortality in Farm Animals* (ed. by J.M. Sreenan & M.G. Diskin) pp. 142–58. Martinus Nijhoff, Dordrecht.

Geisert, R.D., Fox, T.C., Morgan, G.L., Wells, M.E., Wettemann, R.P. & Zavy, M.T. (1991) Survival of bovine embryos transferred to progesterone treated asynchronous recipients. *Journal of Reproduction and Fertility*, **92**, 475–82.

Greve, T. & Lehn-Jensen, H. (1982) The effect of hCG administration on pregnancy rate following non-surgical transfer of viable bovine embryos. *Theriogenology*, **17**, 91 (abstract).

Looney, C.R., Oden, A.J., Massey, J.M., Johnson, C.A. & Godke, R.A. (1984) Pregnancy rates following hCG administration at the time of transfer in embryo-recipient cattle. *Theriogenology*, **21**, 246 (abstract).

Mann, G.E. & Lamming, G.E. (1995) Effects of treatment with buserelin on plasma concentrations of oestradiol and progesterone and cycle length in the cow. *British Veterinary Journal*, **151**, 427–32.

Massey, J.M., Oden, A.J., Voekel, S.A. & Godke, R.A. (1983) Pregnancy rate following hCG treatment of bovine embryo transfer recipients. *Theriogenology*, **19**, 140 (abstract).

Peterson, A.J. & McMillan, W.H. (1996) The effect of progesterone supplementation on actual and potential pregnancy rates and embryo survival following the single or twin transfer of cattle blastocysts. *Theriogenology*, **45**, 228 (abstract).

Rosmarin, M.L., Lock, T.F., Dahlquist, T.G., Nash, T.G., Faulkner, D.B. & Kesler, D.J. (1998) Norgestomet implants enhance embryo survival in *post-partum* cows. *Theriogenology*, **49**, 355 (abstract).

Santos-Valdez de los, S., Seidel Jr, G.E. & Elsden, R.P. (1982) Effect of hCG on pregnancy rates in bovine embryo transfer recipients. *Theriogenology*, **17**, 85 (abstract).

Sheldon, I.M. & Dobson, H. (1993) Effects of gonadotrophin releasing hormone administered 11 days after insemination on the pregnancy rates of cattle to the first and later services. *Veterinary Record*, **133**, 160-3.

Tribulo, R., Nigro, M., Bury, E., Caccia, M., Tribulo, H. & Bo, G.A. (1997) Pregnancy rates in recipients receiving CIDR-B devices immediately following embryo transfer. *Theriogenology*, **47**, 372 (abstract).

Embryo splitting

Gray, K.R., Bondioli, K.R. & Betts, C.L. (1991) The commercial application of embryo splitting in beef cattle. *Theriogenology*, **35**, 37–44.

Kippax, I., Christie, W. & Rowan, T.G. (1991) Effects of method of splitting, stage of development and presence or absence of zona pellucida on fetal survival in commercial bovine embryo transfer of bisected embryos. *Theriogenology*, **35**, 25–35.

In-vitro *fertilization*

Sinclair, K.D., Broadbent, P.J. & Dolman, D.F. (1995) *In-vitro* produced embryos as a means of achieving pregnancy and improving productivity in beef cows. *Animal Science*, **60**, 55–64.

Wagtendonk-de Leeuw van, A.M., Aerts, B.J.G. & Daas den, J.H.G. (1998) Abnormal offspring following *in-vitro* production of bovine preimplantation embryos: a field study. *Theriogenology*, **49**, 883–94.

Walker, S.K., Hartwich, K.M. & Seamark, R.F. (1996) The production of unusually large offspring following embryo manipulation: concepts and challenges. *Theriogenology*, **45**, 111–20.

Ovum pick-up

Pieterse, M.C., Vos, P.L.A.M.; Kruip, Th.A.M., Wurth, Y.A., Beneden van, Th.H., Willemse, A.H. & Taverne, M.A.M. (1991) Transvaginal ultrasound guided follicular aspiration of bovine oocytes. *Theriogenology*, **35**, 19–24.

Scott, C.A., Robertson, L., de Moura, R.T.D., Paterson, C. & Boyd, J.S. (1994) Technical aspects of transvaginal ultrasound-guided follicular aspiration in cows. *Veterinary Record*, **134**, 440–3.

Cloning

Campbell, K.H.S., McWhir, J., Ritchie, W.A. & Wilmut, I. (1996) Sheep cloned by nuclear transfer from a cultured cell line. *Nature*, **380**, 64–6.

Takano, H., Kozai, C., Shimizu, S., Kato, Y. & Tsunoda, Y. (1997) Cloning of bovine embryos by multiple nuclear transfer. *Theriogenology*, **47**, 1365–73.

Wolfe, B.A. & Kraemer, D.C. (1992) Methods in bovine nuclear transfer. *Theriogenology*, **37**, 5–15.

Chapter 41
Herd Fertility Management

(a) Beef herds

S. Borsberry

Introduction	652
Determinants of reproductive performance	652
Factors affecting reproductive performance	654
Infectious disease	654
Nutritional management	655
Controlling the length of the calving season	656
Feeding policy	656
Culling policy	656
Post partum onset of ovarian cycles	656
Factors affecting the post partum acyclic period	656
Suckling	656
Nutrition, body weight and condition and the post partum period	657
Season	657
Induction of ovulation in beef cows	657
Gonadotrophin-releasing hormone	658
Oestrus synchronization and AI in beef cattle	658
Methods	659
Management of heifers	661
Monitoring reproductive performance in the beef herd	661
Analysing herd problems	662

Introduction

Beef cattle fertility must be considered as a separate entity from dairy cattle as they are managed under entirely different circumstances. Usually they are managed as a herd or group and so do not receive the same individual attention as do dairy cows. In general, clinical infertility problems do not appear to occur to the same extent. However, with the dairy herd supplying fewer cross-bred female replacements and the ever increasing importance of biosecurity, many herds are breeding their own replacements. This results in a need for careful planning of breeding in order not to lose fertility and longevity that is achieved with heterosis (Table 41.1).

Veterinary involvement in most commercial suckler herds is often limited, as these herds are run as low input and low output enterprises. In the UK, consumer concerns about food safety and the BSE crisis mean that cull cows are of relatively low value and so the main income derives from the progeny, from either sale as store or finished cattle (see Chapter 3). Calving interval is thus one of the most important measures of reproductive performance. One of the main effects on reproductive performance in beef cows is the adverse effect of marginal nutrition. Inefficient suckler herds are unlikely to survive in the present economic climate and, in Britain, marketing of progeny may become increasingly difficult following the 2001 foot-and-mouth disease (FMD) outbreak. There is likely to be increased legislation concerning the movement of FMD susceptible stock which may well affect public auction at livestock markets, thereby reducing the potential number of outlets for farm animals.

In some beef herds cows and bulls are together all the year round and there is little attempt to control fertility or the season of calving. In better-managed herds a seasonal calving pattern is adopted and the calving pattern itself becomes an important assessment of reproductive performance. An excellent review of suckler cow management in the UK has been published (Lowman, 1988) and this paper is recommended if the reader requires further detail after reading this chapter.

Determinants of reproductive performance

In the UK, beef cows traditionally calve either in spring or autumn. The trend in gross margins has decreased over recent years (1995 to 1999); although there has been a marginal increase in stocking rate, sale price has reduced significantly (see Table 41.2).

Autumn-calving herds tend to produce higher gross margins than spring-calving herds under UK conditions (see Table 41.3). Spring-calving herds tend to be stocked more heavily, but there is greater financial output from autumn-calving herds.

The calf is essentially the sole product of the beef herd, therefore the rate of calf production (calves born

Table 41.1 Traits affected by hybrid vigour (Reproduced with permission from Meat and Livestock Commission, 2000).

Trait	Predicted hybrid vigour effect	
Conformation Skeletal size Mature weight	0–5%	Low
Growth rate Weaning weight Milk production	5–10%	Medium
Fertility Health Longevity	10–30%	High

Table 41.2 Trends in gross margin results for upland suckler herds, 1995–99 (Reproduced with permission from Meat and Livestock Commission, 2000).

	Sale price (p/kg lw)	Stocking rate (cows/ha)	Gross margin	
			(£/head)	(£/ha)
1995	124	1.4	313	438
1996	112	1.5	295	445
1997	107	1.7	308	505
1998	87	1.5	214	316
1999	95	1.5	217	380

lw, liveweight.

Table 41.3 Gross margins and performance for upland sucklers (1999) (Reproduced with permission from Meat and Livestock Commission, 2000).

	Spring calving	Autumn calving
Number of herds	43	43
Gross margin (£)		
Per cow	208	227
Per hectare	355	404
Calf age at sale (days)	212	314
Calf weight at sale (kg)	268	335
Stocking rate (cows/ha)	1.7	1.5

Table 41.4 Performance of upland suckler herds (1999) (Reproduced with permission from Meat and Livestock Commission, 2000).

	Bottom third	Top third
Gross margin (£)		
Per cow	151	278
Per hectare	253	493
Cow performance (per 100 mated)		
Calving period (weeks)[a]	12	10
Number barren	6	6
Calves born alive	91	92
Calf mortality	3	2
Calves purchased	1	2
Calves reared	89	92
Calf performance		
Age at sale/transfer (days)	238	287
Weight at sale/transfer (kg)	276	329
Daily gain (kg)		
Male	1.0	1.1
Female	0.9	1.0
Stocking rate (cows/ha)	1.5	1.6

[a] For 90 per cent of calvings.

alive and reared) is even more critical than it is in the dairy herd. In order to illustrate this a comparison between the worst and best performing (in terms of gross margin/cow) suckler herds recorded by the Meat and Livestock Commission (MLC) (2000) is shown in Table 41.4. The most important factors causing the differences were

(1) The number of calves reared/100 cows and
(2) The calf weight at sale/transfer.

Put more simply, the most successful herds sold more heavier calves than the worst.

Calf weight and age at sale/transfer are reflections of health and growth rate; obviously, calf weight is further dependent, to a major extent, on the breed of the sire and breeding programme used. The heavier breeds such as Charolais and Simmental produce calves with a high weight. However, this has to be balanced against a higher risk of dystokia and possible calf mortality (see Table 41.5), but it must be remembered that there is considerable variation within a breed.

Also, the gestation period and hence the calving interval can be influenced, to a limited extent, by the breed of sire.

When breeding replacements for the suckler herd, two aspects must be considered: mature body size and breed composition. Mature body size must be matched by feed resources. The larger the cow, the more difficult it is to maintain good body condition and this will reduce fertility. In order to maximize hybrid vigour the cross breeding system can be worth up to 23 per cent more weight of weaned calf per cow put to the bull (Meat and Livestock Commission, 2000).

An important index of reproductive performance in the suckler herd is the length of calving season. A 365-

Table 41.5 Pure bred results (Reproduced with permission from Meat and Livestock Commission, 2000).

	Birth weight average (kg)		200 day average (kg)		400 day average (kg)		Easy calvings (%)	
	M	F	M	F	M	F	M	F
Aberdeen Angus	37	35	267	238	516	398	92	95
Blonde Aquitaine	41	39	274	238	548	421	80	88
Belgian Blue	45	41	269	245	494	404	17	32
Charolais	44	41	325	281	652	466	70	80
Hereford	41	39	248	223	447	362	87	92
Limousin	39	36	274	242	545	405	89	94
South Devon	46	42	271	245	499	389	73	86
Simmental	42	38	321	278	628	449	81	89
Sussex	39	36	232	214	411	331	94	94
Welsh Black	38	36	227	215	376	329	81	89

M = male, F = Female.

Table 41.6 Theoretical relationship between conception rate and the calving period in a 100 cow herd (adapted from ICI computer simulation by Allen & Kilkenny, 1980).

Herd conception rate (%)	Service period for 90% of cows to be pregnant (days)	Length of calving period (days)	No. of cows calving in first month
30	245	260	12
40	140	155	28
50	100	110	41
60	70	85	54

day calving interval is optimal, but a compact calving season is also desirable because:

- More cows calve early in the period, therefore the age and weight of calves are higher at the time of weaning and sale.
- The impact of calf disease and mortality may be reduced if there is little variation in calf ages.
- Cows are all at a similar stage in the production cycle, therefore feed can be rationed more precisely and the cows managed more conveniently.
- When cattle are sold they can be batched to produce groups of similar size, weight and condition.

The calving season is almost directly dependent on the pregnancy rate to service and the length of the breeding or service period. Obviously, the higher the pregnancy rate, the shorter the service period required to ensure pregnancy of all or the majority of the cows. A theoretical relationship between the conception rate, the service period and the calving period was calculated by ICI and is shown in Table 41.6.

Factors affecting reproductive performance

Infectious disease

In some cases of low herd reproductive performance there may be an underlying infectious disease. Although the UK is officially brucellosis-free there is always the potential for its re-introduction; indeed, this has happened. Following the use of artificial insemination (AI), campylobacteriosis and *Tritrichomonas fetus* have almost been eliminated, but *Campylobacter* may be a problem in some suckler herds where a bull is used (Caldow & Taylor, 1997). Additionally, some viral dis-

Table 41.7(a) Recommended target body condition scores of beef cows at various stages of the reproductive cycle (Lowman, 1988).

	Calving	Mating	Weaning
Autumn-calving suckler cows	3.0	2.5	2.5
Spring-calving suckler cows	2.5	2.0	3.0

Table 41.7(b) Relationship between body condition and reproductive performance (Kilkenny, 1978).

Herd average mating scores	Calving interval (days)	Calves weaned per 100 cows bulled
1–2	418	78
2	382	85
2–3	364	95
3+	358	93

eases may result in poor reproductive performance, for example bovine herpes I (BHVI) infection (see pp. 289, 579) and bovine viral diarrhoea (BVD) (see pp. 578, 853).

Obviously, it is essential to rectify any infectious problem before attempting to improve herd reproductive performance by other means.

Nutritional management

Nutritional status is of major importance in the maintenance of a high rate of reproductive performance. The nutrition of cattle is covered more comprehensively in specialized texts and only the basic principles are described here.

Whilst specific deficiencies of micronutrients are common under particular circumstances and can affect fertility, under normal conditions dietary energy appears to be the main factor limiting reproductive performance. However, other nutritional deficiencies occur but are usually confined to localities or even individual herds. These include problems with manganese, selenium and cobalt (see Chapter 18) and some vitamins, particularly A and E. For a fuller account of this problem the reader is referred to Chapters 9 and 21.

The technique of body condition scoring has been developed as a simple semi-objective monitor of cows' energy status. The principle depends on the manual palpation of the thickness of subcutaneous fat cover on various parts of the body (see p. 10).

Methods have been developed for both dairy (Mulvaney, 1978) and beef cows (Lowman *et al.*, 1976) and although the finer details vary slightly the overall principle is the same. The thickness of fat cover over the lumbar and tailhead area is estimated and assigned a score, usually from 0 (emaciated) to 5 (very fat), although different scales are sometimes used. Descriptions of the various categories on the 0–5 scale are given on p. 10.

An additional guide to body condition can be obtained by palpating over the hip bones, ribs and either side of the tailhead. With a little experience an

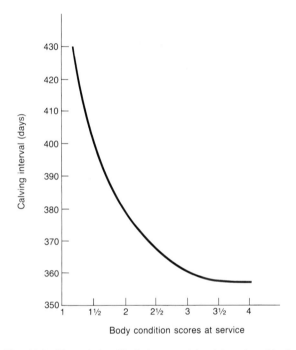

Fig. 41.1 The relationship between calving interval and body condition score at service in beef cows (Kilkenny, 1978).

operator can assess the body condition of cows to within one half-unit. Optimum body condition scores for beef cows have been worked out for the various stages of the reproductive cycle and these are shown in Table 41.7a. The target body condition score at service is the most critical as this is very closely related to overall reproductive performance. The calving interval has been shown to be negatively correlated with body condition at the time of mating in beef cows, although the true relationship is probably curvilinear (see Fig. 41.1) and affects the number of calves weaned (Table 41.7b). This target score is also most difficult to achieve in autumn-calving cows as they are mated during mid-winter when they are lactating and when good quality feed is expensive. In a survey, approximately half of the

Table 41.8 Financial effects of a high culling rate (after Allen & Kilkenny, 1980).

	Normal culling policy	High culling rate		
		Year 1	Year 2	Year 3
No. of cows	90	78	86	88
No. of replacements	13	36	20	16
Calving spread (days)	150	100	100	100
Average calf sale				
Weight (kg)	285	285	305	315
Gross margin/ha (£)	219	174	233	257

autumn-calving beef cows failed to reach the target condition score at mating (Kilkenny, 1978). In contrast, the nutritional drain of lactation is offset in spring calvers by the plentiful supply of grazing.

Cows should be fed to calve at a condition score of 2.5–3 and should lose minimum condition until conception (see Table 41.7a). Cows calving in fatter condition may have calving difficulties, which in turn may lead to delayed involution, reproductive tract damage, susceptibility to infection of the tract or a combination of these problems. Also, cows with a score of 4 or more are likely to mobilize their fat reserves excessively during the early postpartum period.

Beef cows calving in a low condition are also likely to undergo a prolonged period before the re-establishment of ovarian cycles, undernutrition being one of the major causes of failure to ovulate after calving. Consequently, pregnancy is likely to be considerably delayed in such cows.

As pregnancy progresses the lactational demand for a high level of dietary energy decreases. This enables the cow to replace body energy reserves that were lost during early lactation. Thus the cow can be brought back towards the target body condition for the next calving and subsequent mating.

Controlling the length of the calving season

There are a number of ways in which a compact seasonal calving pattern may be established and maintained in a healthy seasonally calving beef herd. These include feeding policy, culling policy and postpartum induction of ovulation.

Feeding policy

It is very difficult to restore compact seasonal calving patterns by nutritional management in herds that have a grossly extended calving season, since this would necessitate the achievement of calving intervals in late-calving cows of well below 365 days. However, it is important to remember that proper nutritional management is vital for the maintenance of a compact seasonal calving pattern.

Culling policy

This is the most extreme but probably the most effective method of modifying a herd's calving pattern. As discussed above, the length of the calving period is highly dependent on the herd pregnancy rate. For example, a five-month calving period is approximately equivalent to a pregnancy rate of 40 per cent. In this situation approximately 70 per cent of cows will calve in the first two months and 30 per cent in the next three months. Therefore, the 30 per cent late calvers should be culled and replaced. Many producers are reluctant to adopt such a high culling rate due to the high cost of purchasing or rearing replacement heifers, particularly during the first year or so. However, such a policy can be of eventual financial advantage due to a decrease in the spread of calving and the consequent management economics as discussed above (see Table 41.8).

Post partum onset of ovarian cycles

A delay in the onset of ovarian cycles can lead to extended calving intervals and possibly increased variation in calving intervals between cows within a herd. This will result in increases in the length of the calving season.

Factors affecting the post partum acyclic period

Suckling

Many studies have shown that the onset of ovulation and/or oestrous behaviour is delayed in either dairy or beef-type cows that suckle calves, relative to milked animals, particularly where more than one calf is suckled per cow. In suckling beef cows kept under UK conditions the average time to resumption of ovarian cycles has been reported as 59.9 ± 2.5 days after calving (Peters & Riley, 1982a), but there was considerable variation both within and between herds. Weaning of calves, either temporary or permanent, or at least the prevention of suckling has been reported to shorten the acyclic period.

Nutrition, body weight and condition and the post partum period

Long post partum acyclic periods in suckling cows may be reduced by the provision of increased dietary energy (e.g. Dunn et al., 1969). Energy intake appears to be more critical than protein intake in the maintenance of reproductive function as positive relationships between energy intake and reproductive performance have been demonstrated in several studies. Low energy intake in prepartum and post partum cows increases the length of the anoestrous period and in heifers it has been shown to result in fewer ovarian follicles, lower progesterone levels and lower conception rates (Hill et al., 1970).

Nutritional status at and before calving appears to be more important than that during the post partum period, since Peters and Riley (1982a), using body weight as an index of nutritional status, found a significant negative correlation between body weight at calving and the length of the acyclic period in beef cows, whilst body weight change after calving had no effect. Also, an increase in energy supply to pregnant beef cows has been shown to accelerate the return of ovarian cycles after calving. Target body condition scores are given in Table 41.7a.

Season

In the temperate latitudes seasonal variations in conception rates and a longer interval between parturition and first oestrus in the winter and early spring have been reported (e.g. Thibault et al., 1966). Furthermore, spring-calving beef and dairy cows have been reported to undergo longer periods between calving and first ovulation than autumn calvers (Bulman & Lamming, 1978; Peters & Riley, 1982a). Most authors have suggested that such seasonal effects are related purely to nutritional management; however, strong effects of season have been demonstrated after adjusting statistically for the effects of body weight at calving (Peters & Riley, 1982b). Evidence for seasonality in cattle has now been accumulated from Europe, North America, Canada and New Zealand. Thibault et al. (1966) have

suggested that photoperiod might play some role in seasonality of reproductive activity in the cow and a negative correlation between daily photoperiod during pregnancy and the onset of ovarian cycles after calving has been demonstrated (Peters & Riley, 1982b). It is possible that a vestigial sensitivity to photoperiod may be present in the domestic cow and that in feral cattle this pattern would predispose towards calving during the late spring to early summer, the optimal time for food supply.

In summary, a variety of factors affect the onset of ovarian cycle in the post partum beef cow. The order of importance is probably nutrition, suckling and season. However, it is normally impossible in the practical situation to quantify these effects so that the time to first ovulation can be predicted.

Induction of ovulation in beef cows

Most evidence to date suggests that delay in ovulation during the postpartum period is mediated by a low rate of gonadotrophin release; most work has been done on luteinizing hormone (LH), but follicle stimulating hormone (FSH) is probably equally important. Such endocrine changes occur as a result of external factors (some discussed above) acting via the hypothalamus to suppress the release of gonadotrophin-releasing hormone (GnRH).

A reliable hormonal method of inducing ovulation in acyclic cows would obviously be advantageous but it is probably true to say that an ideal treatment has not yet been devised.

Gonadotrophins of non-bovine origin in the form of either pregnant mare's serum gonadotrophin (PMSG) and human chorionic gonadotrophin (hCG) have been extensively used for this purpose in the past but results have been variable; hCG has largely LH-like activity whereas PMSG has mainly FSH-like activity and may result in the development of multiple follicles. However, Penny (1998) suggests a dosage of PMSG which in one study did not produce multiple ovulations (see Table 41.9).

The injection of oestrogens in cows results in pre-ovulation surges of gonadotrophin release (depending on dosage) and oestrous behaviour. However, ovulation may or may not follow such treatment. The response is generally too unpredictable for this to be a useful method of inducing ovulation.

Progestagens have been used extensively to synchronize ovulation in cyclic cows, but may also be used to induce ovulation after calving. Roche et al. (1981) reported that 10-day treatment of beef cows with the progesterone-releasing intravaginal device (PRID) resulted in ovulation in about half the cows treated, whereas Bulman and Lamming (1978) reported a 75

Table 41.9 Dose of PMSG at implant removal (Penny, 1998). Reproduced with permission of The British Cattle Veterinary Association.

Type of animal	Conditions	Dose of PMSG at progesterone withdrawal
Beef suckler cow	Calved <55 days	400 iu
	Calved >55 days	Poor body condition score (<2) 400 iu Good body condition score (>2) 250 iu
Beef heifer		None required under normal conditions

PMSG, pregnant mare's serum gonadotrophin.

per cent success rate with a 12-day PRID treatment in dairy cows. However, in the latter study the conception rate in the responding cows was only 50 per cent and treatment did not affect the mean calving-to-conception interval. Other workers (Ball, 1982; Drew *et al.*, 1982) have reported a reduction in the calving-to-conception interval of up to 14 days following the use of PRID; however, the calving-to-conception interval of PRID treated beef cows was reduced only if used before day 30 after calving (Peters, 1982).

Mulvehill and Sreenan (1977) have reported the best success in induction of ovulation in beef cows by injecting 750 iu PMSG at the time of progesterone withdrawal. However, as a small number of twin and triple ovulations did occur, Penny (1998) suggests a lower dose and a maximum of 400 iu (Table 41.9).

Gonadotrophin-releasing hormone

The injection of GnRH in cattle induces release of both LH and FSH. There have been many attempts to induce ovulation in post partum cows by single intramuscular injections of 100–500 µg GnRH and these have given variable results. In order to apply these treatments in practice, more consistent responses would be necessary.

At the above dose levels, LH release of pre-ovulatory surge magnitude usually occurs, depending on the responsiveness of the pituitary. However, ovarian follicles appear to require a two to three day period of rising plasma LH concentrations in order to mature fully prior to ovulation. Therefore, a pre-ovulatory LH surge will induce ovulation only if a follicle at the appropriate stage of development is already present. Alternatively, the induced LH release might cause premature luteinization of an unovulated follicle and transient secretion of progesterone sufficient to initiate ovarian cycles.

Two injections of 500 µg GnRH at an interval of 10 days were advocated by Webb *et al.* (1977). Moreover,

this treatment regime has been particularly successful in large-scale field trials with beef cattle (Mawhinney *et al.*, 1979). A short-lived rise in progesterone concentrations following GnRH injection has been reported by several authors and may be compared to that occurring naturally in some cows prior to the onset of normal ovarian cycles. There has also been interest in longer-acting administration of GnRH, but no product is yet commercially available.

Oestrous synchronization and AI in beef cattle (see also p. 678)

The full exploitation of genetic progress cannot be made in beef cattle without the use of AI. AI is not very widely used in beef cattle, but as oestrus synchronization techniques have improved the number being artificially inseminated has steadily increased. There are several advantages of fixed-time AI (Penny, 1998) in that it:

● Eliminates the practical problems of heat detection in beef cattle;
● Allows the use of superior sires with estimated breeding values (EBVs) (see p. 71) for important traits to improve the quality of the calf crop;
● Allows the use of tested sires to breed replacement heifers;
● Allows the use of sires selected on ease of calving, thus reducing the likelihood of dystokia;
● Helps to create a compact calving pattern;
● Can be used to eliminate venereal disease.

Anecdotal evidence suggests that AI pregnancy rate results on farm have been poorer than expected. Beef cattle tend to be less handled than their dairy counterparts. Mann (2001) suggests poor pregnancy rates in dairy cattle were in part due to impaired ovulation as a

Table 41.10 Pregnancy rates after various treatments and insemination regimens (after Smith *et al.*, 1984, with permission from the American Society of Animal Science).

Treatment	Timing of AI after last treatment	Percentage pregnant
Control	Observed heat	72
6 day PRID plus PG day 6	Observed heat	82
7 day PRID, PG day 6	Observed heat	73
2 × PG	80 hours	52
7 day PRID, PG day 6	84 hours	66

PRID, progesterone-releasing intravaginal device; PG, prostaglandin.

Table 41.11 Summary of oestrous synchronization and breeding protocol (Penny *et al.*, 1997).

Day	Procedure
−12	Insert crestar implants
−4	Inject prostaglandin
−2	Remove Crestar implant ± PMSG
0	First AI
12	Insert crestar implants
21	Remove Crestar implants, take milk samples
23	Second AI if milk progesterone <3–5 ng/ml
35	Insert Crestar implants
44	Remove Crestar implants, take milk samples
48	Third AI if milk progesterone <3–5 ng/ml

PMSG, pregnant mare's serum gonadotrophin; AI, artificial insemination; Crestar, 3 mg norgestomet implant.

Table 41.12 Results of the triple synchrony breeding programme over two years (Penny *et al.*, 1997).

	Year 1	Year 2
Pregnancy rate 1st AI	56% (27/48)	58% (40/69)
Pregnancy rate 2nd AI	69% (11/16)	48% (11/23)
Pregnancy rate 3rd AI	40% (2/5)	33% (4/12)
Pregnancy rate to all services	58% (40/69)	53% (55/104)
Calving rate to all services	58% (40/69)	53% (55/104)
Barren rate	17% (8/48)	20% (14/69)

AI, artificial insemination.

result of 'stress'. In order to maximize the success of synchronized AI, Penny (1998) advises the following:

● Ensure that the animals are handled and that the handling facilities are safe and efficient.
● As nutrition has probably the greatest influence on the success or failure of oestrous synchrony, ensure that target calving condition scores are achieved and minimize body condition score loss between calving and first service. This will result in the majority of cows cycling prior to the synchrony programme. Sudden changes in the plane of nutrition may reduce pregnancy rates due to nutritional 'stress'.
● Avoid major management changes during the programme, e.g. turning out, housing, mixing groups and treatments such as vaccination.
● Ensure that adequate bull power is available for repeats and, to reduce the risk of introducing venereally transmitted diseases, avoid hired or shared bulls.

Methods

Both prostaglandins and progestagens may be used in beef cows (Peters, 1986). Fixed time AI is not generally recommended, however. Programmes which have produced acceptable pregnancy rates utilize a combination of progesterone and prostaglandin (Table 41.10). Prostaglandin administered 24 hours prior to progestagen removal has the effect of synchronizing the decline in progesterone concentrations from endogenous and exogenous sources. Progestagen may either be in the form of a synthetic progestagen implant, e.g. Norgestomet, or a progesterone intravaginal release device.

Penny *et al.* (1997) described a triple synchrony protocol (Table 41.11) in a spring-calving, single-suckled beef herd used over a two year period. Natural service was not used and AI was at fixed times. Repeat insem-

inations 56 hours post progestagen removal were to cows which had a milk progesterone concentration of <3.5 ng/ml. Overall pregnancy rates, for the two years, were 58 per cent and 53 per cent. However, the barren rate was 17 per cent and 20 per cent (Table 41.12).

Stevenson *et al.* (2000) compared combinations of GnRH, Norgestomet and prostaglandin $F_{2\alpha}$. Fig. 41.2 shows the experimental procedure for oestrous synchronization. They found that prior to 60 days post partum, programmes involving GnRH produced a higher percentage of cows in oestrus and higher conception rates compared to the programme involving only two prostaglandin injections (Table 41.13).

Martinez *et al.* (2000) compared oestrous synchronization and pregnancy rates in beef cattle given progesterone in the form of a controlled internal drug release device (CIDR-B), prostaglandin $F_{2\alpha}$ and oestradiol or GnRH. Two experiments were conducted to determine oestrous response and pregnancy rate in beef cattle given a CIDR-B device plus prostaglandin $F_{2\alpha}$

(PGF) at CIDR-B removal, and oestradiol or gonadotrophin releasing hormone (GnRH). In experiment 1, cross-bred beef heifers received a CIDR-B device and 1 mg oestradiol benzoate (EB), plus 100 mg progesterone (E + P group; $n = 41$), 100 µg gonadotrophin releasing hormone (GnRH group; $n = 42$), or no further treatment (control group; $n = 42$), on day 0. On day 7, CIDR-B devices were removed and heifers were treated with PGF. Heifers in the E + P group were given 1 mg EB, 24 hours after PGF, and then inseminated 30 hours later. Heifers in the GnRH group were given

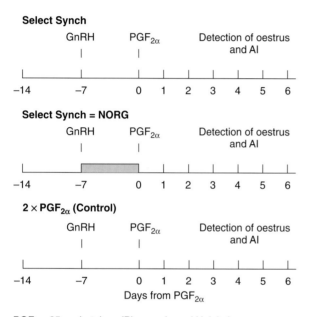

Select Synch

Select Synch = NORG

2 × PGF$_{2\alpha}$ (Control)

Days from PGF$_{2\alpha}$

PGF$_{2\alpha}$: 25 mg Lutalyse (Pharmacia and Upjohn)
GnRH: 100 µg Factrel (Fort Dodge) or Cystorelin (Merial Animal Health)
NORG (indicated by the shaded box): 6 mg Norgestomet – Syncro-Mate-B (Merial Animal Health)

Fig. 41.2 Experimental protocol for oestrous synchronization (Reproduced from Stevenson *et al.*, 2000 with permission from the American Society of Animal Science).

100 µg GnRH, 54 hours after PGF, and concurrently inseminated. Control heifers were inseminated 12 hours after onset of oestrus. The oestrus rate was lower ($p < 0.01$) in the GnRH group (55 per cent) than in either the E + P (100 per cent) or control (83 per cent) groups. The mean interval from CIDR-B removal to oestrus was shorter ($p < 0.01$) and less variable ($p < 0.01$) in the E + P group than in the GnRH or control groups. Pregnancy rate in the E + P group (76 per cent) was higher ($p < 0.01$) than in the GnRH (48 per cent) or control (38 per cent) groups. In experiment 2, 84 cows were treated similarly to the E + P group in experiment I. Cows received 100 mg progesterone and either 1 mg EB or 5 mg oestradiol-17β (E-17) on day 0 and either 1 mg of EB or 1 mg of E-17β on day 8 (24 hours after CIDR-B removal), in a 2×2 factorial design, and were inseminated 30 hours later. There were no differences among groups for oestrus rates or conception rates. The mean interval from CIDR-B removal to oestrus was 44.2 hours, sd = 11.2. Conception rates were 67 per cent, 62 per cent, 52 per cent, and 71 per cent in groups E-17β/E-17β, E-17β/EB, EB/E-17β and EB/EB, respectively. In cattle given a CIDR-B device and estradiol plus progesterone, treatment with either EB or E-17β effectively synchronized oestrus and resulted in acceptable conception rates to fixed-time AI (Table 41.14).

Penny and Lowman (2002) have designed a triple synchrony system for beef cows which relies on fixed-timed AI and not on natural service. The programme allows cows up to three service opportunities over a 46 day period (Table 41.14). Double insemination improves pregnancy rate by 10 per cent compared to a single insemination. GnRH (10 µg Buserelin) at the time of CIDR insertion gave an improvement in pregnancy rate of 12 per cent in treated cows. Cows which were in a body condition score <2 (1–5 scale) or calved <55 days at first AI were injected with 400 iu PMSG. PMSG was administered to maiden heifers and produced a first service pregnancy rate of 74 per cent,

Table 41.13 The effect of oestrous synchronization treatment and number of days post partum on the percentage of cows detected in oestrus and conception rate (Reproduced from Stevenson *et al.*, 2000 with permission from the American Society of Animal Science).

Days post partum	Treatment					
	Select Synch		Select Synch + Norgestomet		2 × PGF$_{2\alpha}$	
	% Oestrus	% CR	% Oestrus	% CR	% Oestrus	% CR
≤60	44.2	50.0	44.1	45.8	25.0	8.3
61–70	62.7	74.4	72.4	60.5	50.6	65.8
71–80	65.1	60.3	84.1	58.9	56.6	61.7
>80	60.0	73.8	72.4	64.0	46.0	72.4

Table 41.14 Triple synchronization programme for beef cows (Penny & Lowman, 2002).

Day	Day	Action
0	Thursday	Insert progesterone + GnRH
7	Thursday	Inject prostaglandin PGF$_{2\alpha}$
9	Saturday	Progesterone out[a] (am) + PMSG[b]
11	Monday	1st AI (am)
12	Tuesday	1st AI (am)
22	Friday	Insert progesterone in late calvers[c] + GnRH
27	Wednesday	Insert progesterone
29	Friday	Inject prostaglandin PGF$_{2\alpha}$ (late calvers)
32	Monday	Progesterone out (am) and tail paint (± PMSG late calvers)
33	Tuesday	Heat detect carefully
34	Wednesday	2nd AI (am) any cows seen bulling + late calvers
35	Thursday	2nd AI (am) any cows seen bulling + late calvers
46	Monday	Scan cows assumed pregnant and insert new progesterone in any non-pregnant + GnRH
50	Friday	Insert progesterone in 2nd AI group
53	Monday	Inject Prostaglandin PGF$_{2\alpha}$ (scanned empty cows)
55	Wednesday	Progesterone out and tail paint
56	Thursday	Heat detect 2nd AI group
57	Friday	3rd AI (am) any cows seen bulling + non-pregnant group
58	Saturday	3rd AI (am) any cows seen bulling + non-pregnant group

[a] Rinse briefly in dilute antiseptic then dry with paper towels and store in cool dark conditions; wear disposable gloves when handling progesterone.
[b] 400 iu PMSG given to thin cows CS < 2 or calved >55 days.
[c] Late calving cows enter the programme for the second AI and therefore only have 2 opportunities for AI. Progesterone CIDR InterAgART. GnRH 10 μg Buserelin Receptal Intervet.

which was better than untreated heifers (pregnancy rate not published). The authors postulate that anoestrus may be a real problem in 15 month-old heifers of later maturing beef breed crosses. They conclude that a target of 90 per cent calving rate is achievable and repeatable in a 46 day breeding period and leads to a sustainable compact calving period.

As beef cattle are less used to being handled they can become fractious when being confined and restrained. At times of hormonal treatments it is essential to provide suitable handling facilities and sufficient experienced labour. If these are not provided there is considerable danger to both animals and humans. Where programmes involve progestogen implants, either as ear implants or intravaginal devices, it must be remembered that these may be lost prior to their planned removal. There are also welfare considerations and consumer concerns when subjecting animals to injections and implants.

Management of heifers (see Chapter 5)

Heifers should be bred to calve three to four weeks before the adult herd. Heavy breeds of bull likely to cause dystokia, e.g. Charolais and Simmental, should be avoided. Oestrous synchronization may be used to

advantage in heifers along with fixed-time insemination if required, although a bull would still be necessary to serve non-pregnant animals subsequently.

Monitoring reproductive performance in the beef herd

This is very much more difficult in beef cattle than in dairy cows because of the nature of the management systems.

Even in the best-managed units, records of reproductive events may be quite rudimentary, possibly including only date of calving. Since bulls are widely used few records of service may be kept. The bull would normally be left with the cows for a length of time that corresponds to the aimed length of the calving season. Whilst it is advantageous to identify barren cows at the end of the bulling period, in many cases it is not desirable to cull those animals because they are still suckling calves. However, methods of early pregnancy diagnosis are highly advantageous in the beef herd so that non-pregnant cows may be identified quickly and appropriate action taken. It is unlikely that the milk progesterone test will become popular in beef herds, even though a 'cow-side' test is available, because of potential difficulties in sample collection. However, the use of real-time ultrasound where embryos/fetuses can be detected by day 30 (White *et al.*, 1985) or earlier offers very exciting possibilities.

It would be desirable for the practitioner to design a 'herd plan' to monitor reproductive performance in beef herds. The following could be used as a guide.

(1) Condition-score cows at least two months before the start of the calving season, e.g. at weaning. Those below target (Table 41.7a) should receive supplementary rations to bring them up to target. Any cows above target should have their condition reduced.
(2) Condition-score cows at calving; those below target should receive supplementary rations.
(3) Special attention should be paid to first and second calvers since these are most likely to be vulnerable to problems, particularly extended periods of anoestrus after calving.
(4) The producer should begin to observe and record oestrus three weeks before the bull is introduced.
(5) Oestrus periods and services should be recorded throughout the breeding season. Particular attention should be paid to the dates when cows are expected to return to oestrus. The use of chinball markers may assist oestrous observation with cows at grass.
(6) Pregnancy diagnosis should be carried out six weeks after the bulls are removed. Barren cows can then be culled when weaned. The findings at pregnancy diagnosis in conjunction with the service records will enable the farmer/veterinarian to estimate the likely calving dates and to plan the nutritional management.

Fertility problems arising in beef herds are likely to result from causes similar to those in the dairy herd. However, investigation is often hampered by the lack of adequate records. Clinical problems such as retained placenta, cystic ovaries and metabolic disease are much less likely to occur, but otherwise the more common problems are similar to those in dairy herds. Similarly, when problems occur they are likely to reflect herd status rather than just involving individual cows.

Analysing herd problems

The following information is likely to be of value in understanding and rectifying problems.

● Cumulative frequency curve of calvings;
● The age distribution of cows;
● The calving dates of first-calving heifers;
● The culling rate and reason for culling;

● An assessment of bull capacity including their ages and clinical histories;
● Evaluation of the other farm enterprises so that the best calving season can be chosen.

Beef cow stockworkers are capable of achieving rates of heat detection equal to those of dairy stockworkers. If reproductive performance is to be optimized then the stockworker must be prepared to observe and record the herd. For those who do so, techniques such as AI, oestrous synchronization/induction and induction of parturition will be much more successful.

The veterinarian should be able to assess the potential of a farmer and to educate and advise accordingly. This should be on a long-term basis, i.e. five years, by which time optimal targets should have been reached and advisory input can be reduced to a surveillance role.

Where herds have an extended calving pattern it may take several years of planning and reproductive manipulation before a herd achieves a two month calving period:

● Calve heifers to an easy-calving bull one month before the adult herd calve.
● Body condition-score cows regularly; if they are too thin increase feed and/or wean calves early.
● For late calving cows, manipulate oestrus and use AI soon after calving.

(b) Dairy Herds

D.C. Barrett and H. Boyd

Introduction	662
Reproductive performance in the UK national dairy herd	663
Components of a fertility control programme	664
Identifying herd-specific goals	664
Planning and setting targets	664
Cow identification, records, data analysis and interpretation	667
Regular veterinary visits	668
Periodic review and regular evaluation of performance	669
Maintaining motivation	672
Advice for veterinarians who wish to start herd fertility control programmes	672
Reproductive record keeping and analysis	672
If the client is aiming for a 12-month calving interval	673
If the client is aiming for a tight calving season	673
Future developments in herd fertility management	675

Introduction

A fertility control programme is a system to monitor and manage reproduction, and is a well-established element of preventive medicine in dairy herd management that is successfully practised in many parts of the world. In a successful programme the farmer gains an improved income more than the cost of implementing the programme (Esslemont *et al.*, 1985). For the veterinarian, a well-managed fertility control programme should represent a profitable outlet for specialist professional skills. In addition, regular farm visits to carry out fertility related work allow the veterinarian the opportunity to promote other aspects of preventive medicine, both within the dairy herd and also to other livestock enterprises on the farm.

Reproduction is particularly suitable for a preventive medicine approach because if intervention is delayed too long there will be an irretrievable loss of production time and thus a financial loss to the producer. Success depends on cooperation between the farmer and the veterinarian, and is based on good husbandry and consistently efficient work by the veterinarian.

Because of the effect of husbandry (feeding, housing and breeding management) and general health on reproduction, a fertility control programme should also incorporate other aspects of preventive medicine and encourage the practice of good husbandry. The development of herd health plans such as the British Cattle Veterinary Association (BCVA) Herd Health Plan over recent years (Anon, 1999) has been a significant step forward in this regard. The instigation of a herd health plan allows the veterinarian to influence all aspects of husbandry and preventive medicine within the herd. Furthermore, as most aspects of husbandry and health care will impact in some way on fertility and reproduction, this holistic approach to preventive medicine will aid and support the fertility control programme. Box 41.1 lists the main components of a fertility control programme.

Reproductive performance in the UK national dairy herd

There has been a general decline in fertility in the UK national dairy herd over recent years, emphasizing the growing need for cost-effective veterinary intervention in the form of well-managed fertility control programmes on dairy farms.

Analysis of approximately 9000 herds (National Milk Records (NMR)) representing data on around 1 million cows, between January 1997 and September 2000, shows that the average herd size has risen from 97 to 112 cows, and that the herd average yield has risen from below 5500 kg to approach 7000 kg per annum. Over the same period the mean calving to first service interval has risen from 84 to 88 days, the mean calving to conception interval from 113 to 121 days (Fig. 41.3) and the mean calving interval from 391 to 399 days (Fig. 41.4). There also seems to be a downward trend in first service pregnancy rate of approximately 3 per cent over the same period (Barrett, 2001). Royal *et al.* (2000) and Esslemont and Kossaibati (2000a) have also reported similar trends of falling fertility performance in the UK and O'Farrell and Crilly (1999) have documented

Box 41.1 The main components of a successful fertility control programme.

Identifying herd specific goals
Planning and setting targets
Cow identification, records, data analysis and interpretation
Regular veterinary visits
Periodic review and regular evaluation of performance
Maintaining motivation

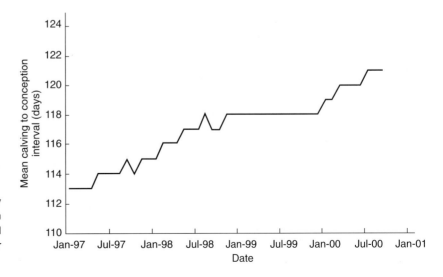

Fig. 41.3 NMR data from approximately 9000 UK dairy herds showing the trend in mean calving to conception interval between January 1997 and September 2000.

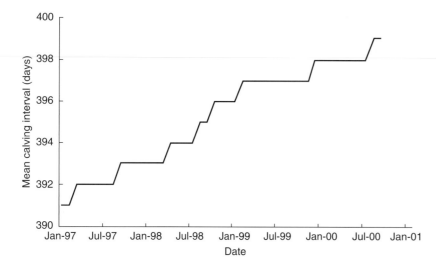

Fig. 41.4 NMR data from appoximately 9000 UK dairy herds showing the trend in mean calving interval between January 1997 and September 2000.

lowered fertility in Irish dairy herds. This declining fertility may be due to a number of factors such as high levels of peri-parturient disease (Peeler *et al.*, 1994a, b), inadequate nutrition (Webb *et al.*, 1997, 1999; Wathes *et al.*, 1998), increasing genetic merit for milk production (Nebel & McGilliard, 1993, Lamming *et al.*, 1997; Lucy & Crooker, 1999), infectious diseases or numerous other independent or inter-related factors. Specific breeding management changes such as the increase in the use of do-it-yourself artificial insemination (AI), with variable amounts of training of personnel, may also be significant (Howells *et al.*, 1999). Increasing milk yields and increasing herd sizes are almost certainly contributing to the problem. It is also highly likely that the decreasing availability of labour on farms is resulting in reduced labour hours per cow per year. The overall effect is greater difficulty in getting cows in calf and increased costs of trying to do so.

Components of a fertility control programme

Identifying herd specific goals

It is no longer possible to assume that every herd owner's reproductive targets are the same. Targets will be determined by various factors fundamental to the production system employed, for example contractual agreement with milk purchaser, seasonal milk price, milk constituent prices, feed costs, availability of labour, other farm enterprises, etc. The ultimate aim of the milk producer will almost always be to maximize financial return within the constraints of milk quota or production economics. Fundamental to achieving this is having a predetermined, and managed, reproductive pro-

gramme for the herd to ensure milk is produced at the most profitable time, maximizing financial margins per litre as well as ensuring an optimal culling rate with minimum involuntary culls and the production of sufficient replacement heifers.

Given that producers will sell their milk to different milk purchasers who have different price structures, it is important to ascertain by discussion with the farmer and his other advisors what reproductive pattern will deliver the best overall profitability. For example, a low input, low to moderate yielding herd of 5000 to 6000 l/cow per year looking to maximize the utilization of grazed grass may be looking for a tight seasonal calving pattern with a calving index (mean calving interval) of 365 days. In contrast, a farmer attempting to produce a uniform supply of milk each month, purchasing a large proportion of the feed used and running an intensive, high yielding herd of 10 000 l/cow per year may desire a year-round calving pattern and a calving index of 420 days. On the other hand a pedigree breeder producing embryos for sale may have general goals for the majority of his herd, but very specific reproductive objectives for his embryo donor cows. Having agreed the overall reproductive strategy that suits a given herd, herd specific reproductive targets can then be set.

Planning and setting targets

A fertility control programme requires reproductive targets. As outlined above, these are usually chosen for economic reasons but are limited by what is physiologically possible. It is the collective responsibility of the farmer, his veterinarian and others in the farm advisory team to choose the targets. However, the veterinarian should ensure as far as possible that the targets are realistic and achievable within an agreed time span.

There is no point producing targets that do not take into account bovine reproductive physiology or that are unduly optimistic concerning pregnancy rate, oestrous detection rate or the standard of husbandry on the farm. It is better to set a realistic target, achieve it and then set a more demanding target than to begin with a target that is unrealistic and totally out of reach, as this reduces stockman motivation. The farmer and his staff have to be in full agreement with the targets set, as only if they really want to achieve the selected targets are they likely to be met. The veterinarian can only help and advise the stockmen on the farm, and cannot achieve the aims of any fertility control programme alone. A team spirit has to be engendered and each member of the team must play his or her part fully.

Heifers

Dairy farmers often aim for seasonal calving for the whole herd. To achieve this, it is essential that the heifers calve early in the chosen season. As *age at first calving* has a major effect on the proportion of a cow's life that is productive, there is an optimal age for first calving and, for modern dairy breeds in Britain and elsewhere, this is usually put at 24 months old (see Chapter 5). However, farmers have to consider conditions in their own herds before they decide at which age the heifers should calve. Seasonal calving herds may have to calve heifers at approximately 24 months of age, as the alternative of 36 months is usually not economically viable (see Chapter 5). However, year-round calving herds or herds with two main calving periods can be more flexible. For example, some may elect to calve their heifers at 27 or 30 months of age.

Having chosen the desired season of first calving and the desired age at first calving, various problems arise that have to be considered. If, for example, the calving season chosen is September, October and the beginning of November and the age at first calving is to be 24 months, what is to be done with heifers that are born late in December, January or February? Will they be left until the next calving season? Will they be sold either as calves or perhaps later as in-calf heifers? Will they be made to calve even younger than 24 months old or will they be allowed to calve in January or February and extend the herd's agreed calving pattern outside the optimum time period? These are important and difficult decisions that have to be considered when the overall goals of the fertility control programme are agreed. Strategic decisions of this type have to be thought through, for example the above scenario can be avoided completely if replacements are only bred from cows and heifers served during the agreed breeding season, and repeat breeders and late calving cows are either culled or bred to a bull of a beef breed.

Once the age of calving has been decided, other consequential targets have to be considered. If a heifer has to calve at 24 months old she must become pregnant at 15 months old. To do this she has to be cycling and well grown (see p. 58). She also has to keep growing to be in a fit condition to calve down and be big enough to thrive in the dairy herd in competition with adult cows, or at least able to lactate, continue growing and get back in calf at the optimum time when managed in a group of first lactation cows. This means the farmer has to plan the growth rate from birth to meet the targets at these critical times (see p. 56). The veterinarian has an important role in reducing calf and growing cattle diseases to allow planned growth rates to be achieved.

Other breeding targets have to be established, for example an acceptable *culling rate* and the choice of sires used. One aim is to avoid dystokia and this should be considered in choosing the breed of bull and perhaps, more importantly, the individual bull to be used for service. Under conventional breeding programmes the generation interval is one of the major constraints to genetic gain. There are advantages in breeding replacement heifers out of heifers as this minimizes the generation interval and thus maximizes genetic gain within the herd (see p. 59). If proven dairy sires are used by artificial insemination (AI) they should be selected for ease of calving and be of higher genetic merit than the heifers being bred. At the present time health traits are gaining in importance in the selection of dairy cattle, and in the future they may be seen as equally, or even more important, than production traits, so in this context genetic merit encompasses both health and production traits.

It may also be a target to use beef sires on heifers, to allow the use of natural service or to avoid replacement dairy animals being produced from dams whose productivity is unknown. This approach may also be used to avoid too many dairy calves being born to the herd, particularly as pure bred dairy bull calves are of little or no value.

Cows

The most important targets are a controlled calving interval and *season of calving*, as these will impact directly on profitability by influencing the mean yield per day of life of the cows and the margin per litre of milk produced. In addition, minimizing the involuntary culling rate and allowing strategic voluntary culling are necessary.

In fertility control work, the *calving interval* is the number of days from the immediately past calving to the next. Farmers are very conscious of the need to have a controlled calving interval, but the ideal target varies from country to country, from farm to farm and indeed

Box 41.2 Factors influencing the choice of calving interval.

Age and breed of the cow
Yield and shape of her lactation curve
Month of the year
Feeding
  Cost
  Availability
Calving and milking facilities
Milk sale contract and differential pricing structures
Milk quota
Calf value

from lactation to lactation. In Britain the normal target for average yielding herds is a 12-month calving interval although, as discussed above, this may on occasions be extended for strategic reasons. Box 41.2 lists factors that influence the choice of calving interval.

There are two reasons why calving interval is important.

(1) Typically, milk yield reaches a peak about five weeks after calving and starts to decline at about eight or nine weeks after calving. This is why the first part of a lactation is more profitable than later parts and the dry period. Short calving intervals result in a greater proportion of a cow's productive life being spent in this early, more profitable part of lactation.

(2) Short intervals produce more calves over a given period of time than long intervals. In a 100-cow herd with a 12-month calving index there will be (approximately) 100 calves born per year; in a similar herd with a 14-month calving index the number of calves per year will be about 86.

However, longer calving intervals should not necessarily be considered a bad thing. If lifetime production could be maintained while reducing the frequency of calving of dairy cows there may be benefits. As many of the disease problems seen in dairy cows occur around the time of calving or in early lactation, having a system of extended lactation that reduces both disease in the cows and the numbers of low value calves produced may bring significant welfare benefits to the dairy industry (Knight & Sorensen, 1998).

It is tempting when marketing fertility control to put a money value on the loss occasioned by every day the calving interval is extended beyond the target. A figure that has remained remarkably constant over the last decade (to 2002) is £2.50 to £3.00/day. It should be realized that this (or any other generalized figure) is not necessarily applicable to any individual herd. Where possible, herd specific costings should be done

to derive the cost-benefit of any alterations in fertility parameters including an extended calving interval; the principles behind this are discussed more fully by Dijkhuizen *et al.* (1997).

Once the target calving pattern and target mean calving interval (calving index) have been chosen a series of consequential targets emerge. If the target calving index is, for example, 365 days, then the target for calving to conception must be 85 days, which is 365 days minus a mean gestation length of 280 days. It should be noted that if the most profitable calving interval for an individual cow is 365 days, then the aim in theory would be to have every cow calve with that interval. In practice what happens is that a herd calving index becomes the target. However, care should be taken to minimize the distribution around this 365-day mean figure, as cows with both longer and shorter calving intervals will be performing below their optimum. As the calving index is the mean interval between two calvings it only relates to those cows that calve again. In a herd with a 25 per cent replacement rate only 50 per cent of the herd will contribute to the calving index, as it takes no account of the fertility of heifers or cull cows, and can be manipulated greatly by culling. It is important therefore always to interpret the calving index alongside the culling rate for failure to conceive. The calving index as a measure of fertility in a herd is also too historical to be of much use in monitoring fertility, as it relates to the fertility of the herd over a year before. A better and more contemporary measure is the calving to conception (more correctly termed calving to establishment of pregnancy) interval as it relates to the current year rather than the previous year.

Account must be taken of the fact that many cows require more than one service per pregnancy when calculating the target interval from calving to first service. In an individual herd this depends on conception rate, oestrous detection rate and culling rate. In many herds a target for calving to first service of 65 days is satisfactory.

It is clear that cows must be cycling by the *target date for first service*. A target that is often taken for the start of cyclicity based on the physiology of the dairy cow is 42 days after calving.

It is quite obvious that a target of first service 65 days after calving has to be modified to become the oestrous cycle that straddles 65 days, often taken as 56–76 days inclusive (eight to eleven weeks) after calving. This modifies the target for calving to conception to the three-week period around 85 days, i.e. up to 96 days after calving. It follows therefore that cows should be served to the first observed oestrus after 56 days post calving. In other words, the voluntary waiting period in this example should be 55 days. Shortening this period will allow cows to be served more quickly, but in general it will result in poorer conception rates.

Many farmers have as their prime target the season of calving, which tends to dictate a 365-day target calving index within a predefined service and calving period. The emphasis tends to be different from farmers aiming for a different calving index, although the method of calculation of target indices is in essence the same. The start and end of the service season is controlled by the targeted calving season. It is essential that as many cows as possible are served in the first three weeks (i.e. one oestrous cycle) of the breeding season. It is particularly important to have all the cows cycling in time and therefore the target for cyclicity is the three weeks before the start of the service period. Submission rates (defined as the proportion of cows eligible for service served in a defined time period, usually 21–23 days) during the breeding season of seasonal calving herds must be optimized, therefore oestrous detection is paramount and every effort has to be made to ensure that cows are served.

Cow identification, records, data analysis and interpretation

A clear, reliable *cow identification system* is needed to run a fertility control scheme. Good identification is needed for accurate records.

Without proper identification there will be no clear system to ensure that cows are served when planned, no way of knowing which animals fail to meet targets and dangerous confusion when animals are presented for veterinary examination. As an example of the latter point, consider a cow that has an unrecorded service, is pregnant and is presented to the veterinarian as 'not yet seen in oestrus'. She will have a corpus luteum, and the usual treatment with prostaglandin or an analogue would cause abortion. Similarly, if a cow that was presented for pregnancy diagnosis on the basis of a known service date had an unrecorded service at a later date, even the most experienced veterinarian could make an erroneous diagnosis of 'not pregnant'.

Although it is now compulsory within Europe that all cattle are tagged in both ears with a unique identification number, this may not allow rapid identification of cattle at pasture or within a large group during routine handling. The veterinarian should encourage the farmer to choose an identification system suitable for the conditions in which the herd is kept. Under most situations this will mean freeze branding, although other methods such as numbered collars may be utilized in some systems. Even with the advent of electronic tagging systems there is still the need for a stockman to be able to identify each animal readily and rapidly in the herd in all housing and pastures used without risk of error or the need to resort to specialist equipment.

Record systems

A great deal has been written about record systems, ranging from simple, individual cow card-based systems, other paper-based systems and wall mounted breeding boards (Anon, 1984) to detailed state of the art computerized systems such as National Milk Records' 'InterHerd' software. Simple systems for beginners are described at the end of this chapter (see p. 673).

Why are records needed?

(1) Records are needed for efficient day-to-day running of the herd, even in herds with no thought-out plans and targets. They tell the stock-worker whether a cow that is in oestrus is due for service or should be left until the next oestrus; they indicate when a cow is expected to come in season from the recorded date of last oestrus or service and they allow the accurate selection of cows for the veterinary visit or for sampling.

(2) Records are needed to monitor progress. It is necessary to keep an eye on herd progress as well as individual cow status. Monitoring will indicate how many cows have started cycling on time after calving, how many cows have been served on time and it will show the success rate of services and the incidence of long and short interservice intervals. Regular monitoring of herd events gives the veterinarian the chance to deal with herd problems at an early stage.

(3) Accurate records analysed and interpreted correctly are an essential aid to the diagnosis of herd fertility problems. Records may be analysed for the whole herd, or if cows are grouped according to factors that may be related to fertility it is sometimes possible to pinpoint aetiological factors which may have temporal or other links. Examples include where one bull has a poor pregnancy rate, or the mean calving-to-first-service interval is very long in first calvers or if a seasonal effect on fertility is noted.

What are records?

Records consist of the following information written down by a farm worker: a cow number, a date and an event. Errors of two sorts occur: items are written down

Box 41.3 The main fertility/reproductive/production events
to record.

> Calving, oestrus, service, result of service, abortion
> Veterinary reproductive findings and treatment
> Other diseases
> Production information
> Milk yield
> Feeding

Box 41.4 Selection of cows for routine visit (the stage for
examination or intervention figures are in brackets).

> Cows with abnormalities at or after calving (21 days after
> calving); some will examine all cows about 21 days after
> calving, although this is probably unnecessary
> Cows not seen in oestrus (≥42 days) after calving
> Cows in target service period but not yet served (56–76 days
> after calving)
> Cows overdue for service (≥77 days after calving)
> Cows due for pregnancy diagnosis (≥42 days after last
> service or earlier if ultrasound examination used)
> Cows seen at the previous visit and not yet served
> Other problem cows, e.g.
>   Purulent vaginal discharge
>   Aberrant sexual behaviour
>   Repeat breeders

incorrectly and events occur and are not recorded. The
main events that are recorded in variable detail are
listed in Box 41.3. Even on farms with the poorest
records, many of the required data should be available.
For example, the number of cows in the herd, culling
records and calving records have to be recorded for
statutory purposes (data required by the British Cattle
Movement Service). If AI is used the AI company can
provide data on service dates. This, along with a veterinary examination of each cow to determine pregnancy
status, will provide enough information to calculate, or
estimate, basic fertility parameters for the herd.

Problems in record analysis: There are two intrinsic,
insurmountable problems in relation to data analysis.

(1) With very few exceptions the amount of data
available, when taking into account the variability
of all fertility measurements, is not enough to give
statistically valid information. This is particularly
the case when the records are subdivided into age
groups, seasonal groups and so on.
(2) Information that is up-to-date is practically always
incomplete (see below) and as a result may
produce incorrect conclusions; complete information is nearly always out-of-date.

Up-to-date, incomplete information will give a more
favourable result than is true in the measurement of the
time from one reproductive event to another. Consider
the calculation of the herd mean and spread of the
interval from calving to first service. If the figure is calculated before all the cows in the calculation have been
served (or marked as 'not to be served') the result will
be biased because it will include only cows served soon
after calving and will exclude those problem cows that
will eventually be served after a long calving to first
service interval. Incomplete pregnancy data based on
non-return rates or on extremely early pregnancy diagnosis using progesterone assays may also distort the
real picture.

These errors matter because decisions can be based
on false assumptions. The actual analysis of records is
further discussed in the section on periodic review and
the regular evaluation of performance.

Regular veterinary visits

At each farm visit, the owner will have selected animals
for examination based on an 'action list' generated
using a system agreed between the client and veterinarian. Where a computerized data management
system is in place the computer software may generate
an action list based on predetermined agreed criteria.
The animals presented for examination will vary from
herd to herd and between practices. The groups of cows
shown in Box 41.4 are examples of cows that may be
presented at the regular visit.

Methods of examination, diagnosis and treatment
have been discussed in Chapter 35. At each visit the
clinician should spend a few minutes looking over
the records with the client to pick up any problems at
an early stage, to modify targets, to give information to
the farm staff and to give them the chance to discuss
any veterinary problem that is worrying them.

Records kept at the visit

Apart from the breeding records the veterinarian
should keep a simple record sheet that records everything done and advised, an example is shown in
Fig. 41.5.

Whatever method is used to transfer the veterinary
findings to the records, care should be taken with cows
that are found to be non-pregnant to make sure that it
is clear to which service 'non-pregnant' applies. Errors
arise when the cow is served later and the result 'non-
pregnant' may be taken to apply to that subsequent
service. Where a bull is present on the farm, a diagnosis
of 'pregnancy not detected' is safer than non-pregnant.

The quality of the work done at the farm visit
together with the informal discussion of progress and

Farm

		Date of visit	30.6.02
		minus 42 days*	19.5.02
		TSP 56 to 77 days**	14.4.02 to 5.5.02

Pregnancy diagnosis

| Date of service | Result | Treatment |

Anoestrus etc.

| Cow | Calving date | Observation | Treatment |

Date of last visit   16.6.02

List of all cows examined at last visit and recommendations (except positive pregnancy diagnosis)

(Check if served or not;
if not served should be in group of cows for the current veterinary examination)

*date for pregnancy diagnosis and oestrus due
**target period for first service

Fig. 41.5   Record of veterinary visit.

problems is very important. It acts not only to detect and treat problem cows and gather fertility and related data such as body condition scores, but also supports the advice given at the periodic review.

Periodic review and regular evaluation of performance

Detailed descriptions of the many different ways of gathering and analysing breeding records are easily obtained in other publications (Anon, 1984; Esslemont *et al.*, 1985; Brand & Varner, 1996a, b; Bailey *et al.*, 1999). Instead of repeating them here, attention is concentrated on what the analysis is trying to achieve and on some of the problems of interpreting records.

While at each visit an eye is kept on the progress of the herd's breeding pattern, periodically it is necessary to look more thoroughly at the fertility of the whole herd. The intervals between periodic reviews will vary with the calving pattern, with the intensity of the client's

interest and with the apparent success rate as noted at each visit. The basis of the periodic review is an analysis of the herd breeding records and an assessment of the effectiveness of all interventions. Cows in the milking herd will be considered separately from heifers.

There are so many ways of recording and analysing herd breeding records that this simple exercise can be unnecessarily confusing. There are two reasons for analysing herd records in these periodic reviews:

● Assessment of current status to establish whether there is a problem that needs attention or whether things are progressing satisfactorily.
● Discovery of any particular areas of weakness.

In the analysis of purely reproductive data (not factors which affect reproduction) there are five analyses that can be carried out, as listed in Box 41.5. The most important of these are marked with an asterisk. Even in herds where overall performance is adequate there may well be subsections of the herd where both

Box 41.5 Analysis of reproductive data.

Intervals in days between calving and subsequent reproductive events
    Calving to first observed oestrus
    Calving to first service*
    Calving to conception*
Pregnancy (conception) rate or services per pregnancy (conception)*
Intervals in days from service to service (interservice intervals)
Involuntary culling rate (reasons for culling)
Submission rate (in herds with short breeding season)*

* Most important reproductive data.

Box 41.6 Measurement of success rate of service.

Percentage (pregnancy rate): 'successful services' of 'all services', e.g. 55%
Ratio (services per pregnancy): 'all services' to 'successful services', e.g. 1.82
Visually: as a cumulative sum (Anon, 1984) – visual and allows a degree of temporal analysis

the farmer and the veterinarian should be concentrating their efforts. Analysis of those data relating to herd subsections may reveal these areas of weakness. However, beware of overinterpreting data from a small number of animals.

The first step is to define clearly which cows are to be included in the analysis. The ideal baseline is all cows that calve in a specified period. This period has to end long enough before the day of analysis to allow every cow to have completed her reproductive cycle to the stage of pregnancy diagnosis or to the decision to cull.

Once the group to be analysed has been selected, it is important that the analysis makes it clear what has happened to every cow in the group.

Calving to subsequent reproductive events
(to first oestrus, to first service, to conception)

It is simple to calculate the number of days from calving to first observed oestrus, to first service and to conception (the date of the service that resulted in a confirmed pregnancy). It is more difficult to express this information in a clear way and to interpret the results correctly.

The first thing to note is how many cows actually had a first observed oestrus, had a first service or became pregnant, in relation to the number of animals that started in the group. Culling rates of about 25–30 per cent are common in dairy herds. If the rate is much greater than this, the veterinarian should establish whether something is going wrong in the herd or whether the records are incomplete.

The next thing to calculate is the mean number of days from *calving to oestrus* (target: cycling by 42 days) to service (target: 65 days) and to conception (target: 85 days). Targets assume that the object is to have a 12-month calving interval. While the means are not completely satisfactory numbers they are worth knowing and comparing with targets.

The mean is of limited value because it may be made up of a wide range of values. For example, a mean calving to first service interval of 65 days may consist of very short and very long intervals (unsatisfactory) or it may be the result of most intervals being close to the target (satisfactory). If the mean is greater than the target, results are certainly not satisfactory and the mean does give some idea of the seriousness of the situation. However, calculation of a mean ± standard deviation for each parameter would be better, with the target standard deviation as small as possible.

Consequently, the concept of a 'target period' has been developed. For example, instead of a 65-day target for a mean interval from calving to first service, the target changes to having as many cows as possible served in the oestrous cycle period around 65 days, i.e. from 56 to 76 days (8–11 weeks) after calving. The target for conception is the period around 85 days, i.e. 76–96 days (11–13 weeks) after calving. For first oestrus it is best to aim for as many cows as possible seen in oestrus by 42 days.

Information about the number of animals that fall into the target period, before the target period and after it can be presented in histogram form. This is very clear, easily understood and puts the extent of the problem into exact numbers. This is particularly easy with modern software spreadsheet programs such as Microsoft (MS) Excel and some of the specialist software available for herd record analysis.

Success rate of services

The success rate of services is again quite simple to work out, but to avoid misinterpretation it is essential to understand the different ways of doing this, as shown in Box 41.6. The difficulty arises because of the different ways of defining 'all services' and 'successful services'. 'All services' can mean literally that; it can also mean all services up to a certain number of services, say five, or it can mean 'all first services' (first service is defined as the first service after calving or in a heifer's life). 'Successful services' can mean services that result in calving, or that result in positive pregnancy diagnosis by rectal palpation or ultrasound examination, or positive pregnancy diagnosis by milk progesterone or by non-return to service at various intervals after calving.

Depending on the definitions used the success rate calculated from the same group of animals can vary enormously.

In most herds that are under veterinary supervision 'success' will be defined as positive pregnancy diagnosis undertaken by the veterinarian using ultrasound examination or rectal palpation. There are several points in favour of basing the success rate on first services rather than on all services, in particular:

- The result can be obtained earlier than if one has to wait for the result of the last repeat breeder in the group.
- Each cow contributes the same weight to the calculation.

Therefore, in herds controlled by a veterinarian, success rate is best defined as the *first service pregnancy rate*, i.e. the percentage of cows that are pregnant to first service. It should he borne in mind that an accurate figure will not be obtained until the result of the last first service is known, which may be about six weeks after that last service.

Once the first service pregnancy rate has been worked out it is compared with the target rate of between 45 and 60 per cent, the target depending on a variety of factors.

In addition to first service pregnancy rate, at the end of a breeding season it is valuable to calculate an *all-service pregnancy rate* as it is this that will dictate the number of straws of semen used and the total insemination charges. The all-service pregnancy rate will give a measure of the overall fertility within the herd, but should be interpreted in light of other information such as the culling policy for failure to conceive.

Interservice intervals

The number of days between services is worked out. These data are presented as one or two normal cycle lengths (18–24 and 36–48 days), or less than one, between one and two or more than two cycles (<18, 25–35 and >48 days). Alternatively, the figures are set out as a histogram with each day represented separately, which is satisfactory for visual presentation but difficult to describe in a report. The object of doing this is to assess the efficacy of heat detection.

- The assumption is made that most cows that do not become pregnant return to service at a normal cycle length of 18–24 days and therefore that returns longer than this represent a missed oestrus. While this is not strictly correct in all cases the proportion

of 18–24-day returns is quite useful for assessing levels of oestrous detection.

- Observation of the incidence of irregular intervals, such as <18 days and between 25 and 36 days, gives an indication of the frequency of inaccurate heat detection. However, it should be recognized that these irregular intervals may be brought about by late embryonic death or may be artefacts due to veterinary intervention to manipulate the oestrous cycle.

The proportion of cows presented for pregnancy diagnosis that are not pregnant also gives an indication of the number of missed oestrous periods because most non-pregnant cows have been in season once or twice before examination and have not been observed in oestrus. Another indicator of oestrous detection efficiency is the submission rate, defined as the proportion of cows eligible for service served in a defined time period, usually 21–23 days. This measure is particularly useful in seasonal calving herds.

Culling rate

The incidence of culling in relation to the total starting population and the stage at which the decision to cull is taken is presented as a percentage and an actual number. It is desirable to record the reason for culling.

Effectiveness of treatment and accuracy of pregnancy diagnosis

Treatment, including conservative treatment, takes place:

- At and after calving
- In the preservice period and
- At and after service.

Lists should be prepared with appropriate dates, diagnosis, treatment and outcome following treatment.

Many veterinarians who have not previously analysed their results will find the effectiveness of fertility treatment disappointing. Better results require more accurate diagnosis, careful selection of cases for treatment and improvement of the client's breeding management, so that practically all cows in oestrus after treatment are inseminated at the right time.

Heifers

Analysis of breeding records for heifers is often restricted because of lack of information, particularly where natural service is employed. Where AI is used analysis is to some extent as for adult cows. The aspects shown in Box 41.7 should be borne in mind.

Box 41.7 Analysis of heifer breeding records.

Starting population
Percentage cycling when put to bull
First service pregnancy rate
Percentage that become pregnant (in defined breeding period)
Length of calving period
Range of ages at first calving (available from milk records)

After the purely reproductive analysis the next stage is to correlate the fertility results with factors that could interfere with reproductive efficiency.

At the periodic review a written report should be presented to and discussed with the client and his other advisors. Targets can then be reviewed and adjusted as considered appropriate.

Maintaining motivation

It is essential if a breeding programme is to be successful for all interested parties to remain focused and motivated at all times. This requires good communication between all involved and regular review of the herd's fertility performance within an economic framework.

There are considerable benefits to be gained from improvements in herd health; for example, a farmer with 77 cows, who adopted a planned approach to herd management, saw his farm profits improve by £13 000 in 2 years. It was estimated that £6000 of this came from improved fertility management alone (Esslemont & Kossaibati, 2000b). This in itself should be enough to motivate farmers to undertake schemes of this type. The economic appraisal of herd health schemes has been extensively reviewed elsewhere and will not be discussed in depth here (Esslemont & Peeler, 1993; Esslemont, 1995). However, it is important to realize that the financial benefits are often hidden and not immediately apparent to the farmer unless the herd records are analysed regularly and benefits quantified in monetary units.

Given the economic pressure on the dairy industry, farmers cannot afford to pay for services that do not bring financial benefits, nor can they afford to tolerate less than optimum fertility within their herds. In the past the uptake of herd fertility programmes has been poor in the UK (Wassell & Esslemont, 1992). If they are to become a regular feature on the majority of dairy farms then it is the responsibility of the veterinarian to ensure that they are cost-effective and to be able to illustrate this fact to his client. The use of spreadsheet programs containing herd specific economic parameters and easily interpreted graphics would make this task much easier.

Advice for veterinarians who wish to start herd fertility control programmes

Problems on the dairy farm that limit herd productivity and profitability such as suboptimal fertility usually have multiple causes and require an integrated, multidisciplinary approach (de Kruif, 1998). The veterinary practitioner will be most effective when he or she is part of a dairy farm consultant team that includes, in addition to the veterinarian, personnel such as the nutritionist, financial consultant and other agricultural professionals who can contribute to a team approach for problem solving. If all the key advisors meet regularly on the farm and collaborate with developing solutions for farm problems, benefits will outweigh those seen if each advisor acts independently. This team approach has been advocated for many years (O'Connor *et al.*, 1985; Kelly & Whitaker, 1999), but has been slow to be recognized by some and barriers are sometime found between the different professionals. The veterinary surgeon should work to break down these barriers for the benefit of his client.

Many veterinarians who are not carrying out fertility control work for any of their clients find it difficult to get started. One problem is lack of confidence as regards skills in rectal palpation or ultrasound examination. If this is the case it has to be overcome by self-education and by undertaking suitable continuing professional development (CPD) training.

Marketing of the service is best done via practice newsletters and a special client meeting to explain to clients all that is involved in control programmes, preferably with the help of a client who is convinced of the benefits talking to others who are more sceptical. Help to arrange a meeting can be obtained from many sources, such as other (specialist) practitioners who run fertility control schemes, commercial firms or colleagues in the veterinary schools.

Beginners often have difficulty in knowing what to do on regular farm visits and particularly how to set up and use a recording system.

Reproductive record keeping and analysis

The first decision to be made on reproductive record keeping and analysis is who is to undertake this. Is it to be the farmer, the veterinarian (or his staff) or a third party? There are distinct advantages if the veterinarian offers a complete package to the farmer including record keeping. This gives the veterinarian control over which cows are presented at the regular farm visits. However, if the farmer already keeps adequate records this may result in duplication of effort and the farmer may be unwilling to pay for something he considers he already has. Whatever system is agreed upon the farmer will be required to collect most of the data and will need some records on farm to make day-to-day management decisions.

It is essential that accurate herd records be maintained and that they are analysed and acted upon regularly (Varner & Brand, 1996; Bailey *et al.*, 1999). A computer-based system of record keeping offers many advantages, including rapid data analysis and the rapid production of action lists and high quality reports. Many dedicated herd fertility record software packages such as DAISY (Agrisoft, NMR), InterHerd (Agrisoft, NMR), Dairy-WIN (Massey University) and DairyCHAMP (University of Minnesota) are now commercially available. These offer distinct functions, which have been produced specifically to handle herd fertility data. In addition, software packages such as Herd Browser (Livestock Services UK Ltd) and Herd Management (Sum-it Computer Systems) offer some fertility recording and analysis functionality within more general software packages that have wider usage to the farmer.

While computers are invaluable in data handling and analysis it is important to realize that specific software is not essential. It is perfectly possible with limited computer skills to maintain and analyse herd reproductive data in a spreadsheet package such as MS Excel, although it will not easily generate action lists and some of the other output available from dedicated herd fertility software. The interpretation and understanding of herd records can be greatly enhanced by the use of computer generated graphs and charts, such as those quickly and easily produced by computer programs like MS Excel (Hendry, 1999).

Computerized recording will allow more in-depth and frequent analysis of data. However, it is vital that the veterinarian (and the farmer) understands fully the output of these systems and recognizes that the output is only as good as the quality of those data being entered into the system.

If for any reason the veterinarian is unwilling or unable to use a computer-based system a written record system is perfectly adequate for small herds, although it lacks the ability to rapidly produce regular record analysis, action lists and reports containing graphical representation of data. The following simple, paper-based system, which can be made up in the practice and photocopied, is suggested as a starting point. One sheet of A4 paper is marked across the top with headings that cover one reproductive cycle for each cow from calving to confirmation of pregnancy or disposal/death. The sheet is lined horizontally and each sheet will take records from about 20 cows (see Fig. 41.6).

This sheet is filled in by the farmer in chronological order of calving. It is usually impossible to obtain accurate records for more than one or two months prior to starting (except those data which are required to be recorded by law) so that recording should be started at the same time as the rest of the programme. The best recording is likely in herds where there is some other recording system used, such as individual cow milk production records. Data kept in this way will require regular analysis which, if done by hand, will be time consuming and thus costly.

Many farmers find that a circular breeding board is useful to supplement this sheet (Anon, 1984; Fig. 4.29). Figure 41.6 could also be used as a template for the construction of a computer spreadsheet for data analysis.

If the client is aiming for a 12-month calving interval

Depending on the calving pattern and herd size, arrange to visit the herd say every 14 days and at each visit examine all cows that:

- Are more than 56 days after calving and have not been served;
- Were served 42 days or more previously and have not returned to service (if unsure of early pregnancy diagnosis, start later);
- Have had any problems.

Keep a record of everything you do on the farm and find out what has happened to all the cows you saw at the last visit (see Fig. 41.5).

It takes a year before the records are complete enough for sensible analysis. Make an initial analysis after six months, bearing in mind the problems discussed above (see p. 672 onwards). After that, analyse the records every six months, or other suitable interval, to show the following as a minimum:

(1) The number of cows that calved.
(2) Calving to service interval:
    (a) The number that have been served since calving;
    (b) The number not served;
    (c) The mean calving-to-service interval;
    (d) A simple, small histogram of distribution of calving-to-service intervals.
(3) The same information for calving-to-conception interval.
(4) First service conception rate (and all service conception rate).
(5) Culling rate (and reason for culling).

If the client is aiming for a tight calving season

Use the same record system. Discuss oestrous detection. Make sure the farmer records all heats in the

Herd breeding record:

Farm:

Sheet no.:

Cow	Calving date	Normal	Lactation no.	Pre-service heat dates		Target	Service dates/bull used					PD	Days from calving to:		
				1st	2nd		1st	2nd	3rd	4th	5th		1st heat	1st serve	Pregnancy
36	6-3-2001	Y	6	8-5-2001		1-5-2001	25-5-2001 GS					P+	63	80	80
20	7-3-2001	Dead calf	3			2-5-2001	12-5-2001 DH	11-7-2001 Char				P+	—	66	126
38	9-3-2001	Y	6	16-4-2001		4-5-2001	3-5-2001 DH					P+	38	55	55
186	10-3-2001	Y	4			5-5-2001	1-7-2001 DH	×		To be sold		P–	—	114	—
148	8-7-2001	CS	1			2-9-2001	13-9-2001 DH						—	67	
148	11-8-2001	Y	I			6-10-2001									
219	12-8-2001	Y	2	15-9-2001		7-10-2001							34		

Fig. 41.6 A simple herd fertility recording system. Y, yes; CS, Caesarean section.

three-week period before the first day of the service period.

Examine, and treat where needed, all animals that have not been in season at the end of the three-week preservice period. Visit at weekly or fortnightly intervals thereafter to examine all cows not yet seen in oestrus and to follow up treatments. Monitor the submission rate.

Carry out pregnancy diagnosis nine weeks after the first day of the service season. Remember this simplified advice covers the first steps to help beginners to get started.

Future developments in herd fertility management

The decreasing availability of staff on farms in the UK is presenting a real challenge to many farmers and veterinarians as they attempt to maintain and improve herd fertility. Over recent years there have been numerous technological developments that can help, particularly aids to oestrous detection such as the KaMaR heat mount detector, pedometers and milk progesterone assays (Peters & Ball, 1995). It is probable that in the future accurate and reliable automated systems to assess the cow's physiological state using biosensors will be developed (Koelsch *et al.*, 1994; Frost *et al.*, 1997; Mottram, 1997; Scully *et al.*, 2000). New developments in this area of technology may allow automatic milk progesterone assays, and other assays, to be performed while cows are being milked, allowing the timing of ovulation to be accurately predicted and removing the need for oestrous detection. In addition, technologies such as automated milking may become more widespread, freeing stockmen from routine mundane tasks and allowing them to concentrate on improving cow care. New methods of data recording, such as the use of palm held computers and mobile phones with internet capability, will allow data collected on the farm to be logged direct to remote computer databases in the farm office or at distant sites.

References

Beef herds

Allen, D. & Kilkenny, B. (1980) *Planned Beef Production*, p. 183, Granada, London.

Ball, P.J.H. (1982) Milk progesterone profiles in relation to dairy herd fertility. *British Veterinary Journal*, **138**, 546–51.

Bulman, D.C. & Lamming, G.E. (1978) Milk progesterone levels in relation to conception, repeat breeding and factors influencing acyclicity in dairy cows. *Journal of Reproduction and Fertility*, **54**, 447–58.

Caldow, G.L. & Taylor, D.W. (1997) Experiences with venereal *Campylobacter* infection in suckler herds. *Cattle Practice*, **5**, 327–34.

Drew, S.B., Gould, C.M., Dawson, P.L.L. & Altman, J.F.B. (1982) Effect of progesterone treatment on the calving-to-conception interval of Friesian dairy cows. *Veterinary Record*, **111**, 103–6.

Dunn, T.D., Ingalls, J.E., Zimmerman, D.R. & Wiltbank, J.N. (1969) Reproductive performance of two year old Hereford and Angus heifers as influenced by pre- and post-calving energy intake. *Journal of Animal Science*, **29**, 719–26.

Hill, J.R., Lammond, D.R., Hendricks, D.M., Dickey, J.F. & Niswender, G.D. (1970) The effects of undernutrition on ovarian function and fertility in beef heifers. *Biology of Reproduction*, **2**, 78–84.

Kilkenny, J.B. (1978) Reproductive performance of beef cows. *World Review of Animal Production*, **14**, 65–74.

Lowman, B.G. (1988) Suckler Cow Management. *In Practice*, **10**, 91–100.

Lowman, B.G., Scott, N.A. & Somerville, S.H. (1976) Condition scoring of cattle. *East of Scotland College of Agriculture, Bulletin No. 6.*

Mann, G.E. (2001) Pregnancy rates during experimentation in dairy cows. *The Veterinary Journal*, **161**, 301–5.

Martinez, M.F., Kastelic, J.P., Adams, G.P., Janzen, E., McCartney, D.H. & Mapletoft, R.J. (2000) Estrus synchronization and pregnancy rates in beef cattle given CIDR-B, prostaglandin and estradiol or GnRH. *Canadian Veterinary Journal*, **41**, 786–90.

Mawhinney, S., Roche, J.F. & Gosling, J.P. (1979) The effects of oestradiol benzoate (OB) and gonadotrophin releasing hormone (GnRH) on reproductive activity in beef cows at different intervals post partum. *Annales de Biologie Animale Biochimic et Biophysique*, **19**, 1575–87.

Meat and Livestock Commission (1986) *Beef Year Book*, p. 55. MLC, Milton Keynes.

Meat and Livestock Commission (2000) *Beef Year Book* pp. 23–4, 31, 44–47. MLC, Milton Keynes.

Mulvaney, P. (1978) Dairy cow condition scoring. Paper No. 4468. National Institute for Research in Dairying, Reading.

Mulvehill, P. & Sreenan, J.M. (1977) Improvement of fertility in post-partum beef cows by treatment with PMSG and progestagen. *Journal of Reproduction and Fertility*, **50**, 323–5.

Penny, C.D. (1998) Practical oestrus synchronisation techniques in beef suckler herds. *Cattle Practice*, **6**, 169–73.

Penny, C.D. & Lowman B.G. (2002) Mating beef cows without natural service – a triple synchronisation system. *Cattle Practice*, **10**, 23–5.

Penny, C.D., Lowman, B.G. & Scott, P.R. (1997) Repeated oestrus synchrony and fixed-time artificial insemination in beef cows. *Veterinary Record*, **140**, 496–8.

Peters, A.R. (1982) Calving intervals of beef cows treated with either gonadotrophin releasing hormone or a progesterone releasing intravaginal device. *Veterinary Record*, **110**, 515–17.

Peters, A.R. (1986) Hormonal control of the bovine oestrous cycle. II. Pharmacological principles. *British Veterinary Journal*, **142**, 20–9.

Peters, A.R. & Riley, G.M. (1982a) Milk progesterone profiles and factors affecting post partum ovarian activities in beef cows. *Animal Production*, **34**, 145–53.

Peters, A.R. & Riley, G.M. (1982b) Is the cow a seasonal breeder? *British Veterinary Journal*, **138**, 533–7.

Roche, J.F., Ireland, J. & Mawhinney, S. (1981) Control and induction of ovulation in cattle. *Journal of Reproduction and Fertility*, Supplement **30**, 211–22.

Smith, R.D., Pomerantz, A.J., Beal, W.E., McCann, J.P., Pilbeam, T.E. & Hansel, W. (1984) Insemination of Holstein heifers at a preset time after oestrous cycle synchronisation using progesterone and prostaglandin. *Journal of Animal Science*, **58**, 792–800.

Stevenson, J.S., Thompson, K.E., Forbes, W.L., Lamb, G.C., Grieger, D.M. & Corah, L.R. (2000) Synchronizing oestrus and (or) ovulation in beef cows after combinations of GnRH, Norgestomet, and prostaglandin $F_{2\alpha}$ with or without timed insemination. *Journal of Animal Science*, **78**, 1747–58.

Thibault, C., Courot, M., Martinet, L., Mauleon, P., De Mesnil du Buisson, F., Ortovant, R., Pelletier, J. & Signoret, J.P. (1966) Regulation of breeding season and oestrous cycles by light and external stimuli in some mammals. *Journal of Animal Science*, **25** (Suppl.), 119–39.

Webb, R., Lamming, G.E., Haynes, N.B., Hafs, H.D. & Manns, J.G. (1977) Response of cyclic and post-partum suckled cows to injections of synthetic LH-RH. *Journal of Reproduction and Fertility*, **50**, 203–10.

White, I.R., Russel, A.J.F., Wright, I.A. & Whyte, T.K. (1985) Real time ultrasonic scanning in the diagnosis of pregnancy and the estimation of gestational age in cattle. *Veterinary Record*, **117**, 5–8.

Dairy herds

Anon (1984) *Dairy Herd Fertility*. Ministry of Agriculture, Fisheries and Food, Reference Book 259, pp. 1–80. Her Majesty's Stationery Office, London.

Anon (1999) *BCVA Herd Health Plan for the Purposes of Farm Assurance*, pp. 1–21. BCVA Office, The Green, Frampton-on-Severn, Gloucester, UK.

Bailey, T.L., Dascanio, J. & Murphy, J. (1999) Analyzing reproductive records to improve dairy herd production. *Veterinary Medicine*, **94**, 269–76.

Barrett, D.C. (2001) Cattle Fertility Management in the UK. *Cattle Practice*, **9**, 59–68.

Brand, A. & Varner, M. (1996a) Monitoring reproductive performance: objectives, reproductive indices and materials and methods. In *Herd Health and Production Management in Dairy Practice* (ed. by A. Brand, J.P.T.M. Noordhuizen & Y.H. Schukken), pp. 283–92. Wageningen Pers, Wageningen.

Brand, A. & Varner, M. (1996b) Monitoring reproductive performance: execution. In *Herd Health and Production Management in Dairy Practice* (ed. by A. Brand, J.P.T.M. Noordhuizen & Y.H. Schukken), pp. 293–311. Wageningen Pers, Wageningen.

Dijkhuizen, A.A., Huirne, R.B.M., Jalvingh, A.W. & Stelwagen, J. (1997) Economic impact of common health and fertility problems. In *Animal Health Economics – Principles and Applications* (ed. by A.A Dijkhuizen &

R.S. Morris), pp. 41–58. Post Graduate Foundation in Veterinary Science, University of Sydney.

Esslemont, R.J. (1995) Economic appraisal of herd health schemes. *The Veterinary Annual*, **35**, 243–80.

Esslemont, R.J., Bailie, J.H. & Cooper, M.J. (1985) *Fertility Management in Dairy Cattle*, pp. 1–143. Collins, London.

Esslemont, R.J. & Kossaibati, M.A. (2000a) Trends in fertility in 52 dairy herds over 11 seasons. In *Proceedings of the XXI World Buiatrics Congress*, Uruguay, December, 2000, pp. 5221–32.

Esslemont, R.J. & Kossaibati, M.A. (2000b) Dairy farming systems: husbandry, economics and recording. In *The Health of Dairy Cattle* (ed. by A.H. Andrews), pp. 299–327. Blackwell Science, Oxford.

Esslemont, R.J. & Peeler, E.J. (1993) The scope for raising margins in dairy herds by improving fertility and health. *British Veterinary Journal*, **149**, 537–47.

Frost, A.R., Schofield, C.P., Beaulah, S.A., Mottram, T.T., Lines, J.A. & Wathes, C.M. (1997) A review of livestock monitoring and the need for integrated systems. *Computers and Electronics in Agriculture*, **17**, 139–59.

Hendry, M.A.W. (1999) Practitioner use and graphical display of dairy cow fertility records to give the farmer/herdsman incentives to improve efficiency of output. *Reproduction in Domestic Animals*, **34**, 203–12.

Howells, H.M.J., Davies, D.A.R. & Dobson, H. (1999) Influence of the number of days spent training in an abattoir with access to live cows on the efficiency of do-it-yourself artificial insemination. *Veterinary Record*, **144**, 310–14.

Kelly, J.M. & Whitaker, D.A. (1999) A multidisciplinary approach to dairy herd health and productivity management. BSAS Occasional Meeting: Fertility in the High-Producing Dairy Cow, Galway, Ireland, September, 1999, pp. 25–6.

Knight, C.H. & Sorensen, A. (1998) Fertility parameters of cows with extended lactations. *Cattle Practice*, **6**, 379–82.

Koelsch, R.K., Aneshansley, D.J. & Butler, W.R. (1994) Milk progesterone sensor for application with dairy cattle. *Journal of Agricultural Engineering Research*, **58**, 115–20.

Kruif de, A. (1998) Modern health care in food producing animals. *Irish Veterinary Journal*, **51**, 588–90.

Lamming, G.E., Darwash, A.O. & Woolliams, J.A. (1997) Subfertility in dairy cattle: potential genetic and environmental influences. *Cattle Practice*, **5**, 357–60.

Lucy, M.C. & Crooker, B.A. (1999) Physiological and genetic differences between low and high index dairy cows. BSAS Occasional Meeting: Fertility in the High-Producing Dairy Cow, Galway, Ireland, September, 1999, pp. 27–8.

Mottram, T. (1997) Automatic monitoring of the health and metabolic status of dairy cows. *Livestock Production Science*, **48**, 209–17.

Nebel, R.L. & McGilliard, M.L. (1993) Interactions of high milk yield and reproductive performance in dairy cows. *Journal of Dairy Science*, **76**, 3257–68.

O'Connor, M.L., Baldwin, R.S., Adams, R.S. & Hutchinson, L.J. (1985) An integrated approach to improving reproductive performance. *Journal of Dairy Science*, **68**, 2806–16.

O'Farrell, K.J. & Crilly, J. (1999) Trends in calving rates in Irish dairy herds 1991–1996. *Cattle Practice*, **7**, 287–90.

Peeler, E.J., Otte, M.J. & Esslemont, R.J. (1994a) Recurrence odds ratios for periparturient disease and reproductive traits of dairy cows. *British Veterinary Journal*, **150**, 481–8.

Peeler, E.J., Otte, M.J. & Esslemont, R.J. (1994b) Interrelationships of periparturient diseases in dairy cows. *Veterinary Record*, **134**, 129–32.

Peters, A.R. & Ball, P.J.H. (1995) *Reproduction in Cattle*, 2nd edn, pp. 47–61. Blackwell Science, Oxford.

Royal, M.D., Darwash, A.O., Flint, A.P.F., Webb, R., Woolliams, J.A. & Lamming, G.E. (2000) Declining fertility in dairy cattle: changes in traditional and endocrine parameters of fertility. *Animal Science*, **70**, 487–501.

Scully, A., Hunter, M., Gregson, K., Lamming, G.E. & Darwash, A.O. (2000) The use of on-farm software for automatic interpretation of milk progesterone data: an aid to dairy fertility management. *Cattle Practice*, **8**, 407–10.

Varner, M. & Brand, A. (1996) Monitoring reproductive performance: decision making and follow-up. In *Herd Health and Production Management in Dairy Practice* (ed. by A. Brand, J.P.T.M. Noordhuizen & Y.H. Schukken), pp. 313–32. Wageningen Pers, Wageningen.

Wassell, T.R. & Esslemont, R.J. (1992) Survey of the operation of dairy herd health schemes by veterinary practices in the United Kingdom. *Veterinary Record*, **130**, 260–3.

Wathes, D.C., Robinson, R.S., Pushpakumara, A., Cheng, Z. & Abayasekara, D.R.E. (1998) Nutritional effects on reproductive performance in dairy cows. *Cattle Practice*, **6**, 371–7.

Webb, R., Garnsworthy, P.C., Gong, J.G., Gutierrez, C.G., Logue, D., Crawshaw, W.M. & Robinson, J.J. (1997) Nutritional influences on subfertility in cattle. *Cattle Practice*, **5**, 361–7.

Webb, R., Royal, M.D., Gong, J.G. & Garnsworthy, P.C. (1999) The influence of nutrition on fertility. *Cattle Practice*, **7**, 227–34.

Chapter 42
Pharmacological Manipulation of Reproduction

J.G. Allcock and A.R. Peters

Introduction	678
Control of the oestrous cycle	678
Induction of luteolysis	678
Trophic hormone and prostaglandin combinations	680
Use of progestagens	680
Factors affecting pregnancy rate after controlled ovulation	682
Synchrony after prostaglandins	682
Synchrony after trophic hormone–prostaglandin combination techniques	683
Synchrony after progestagens	683
Possible methods of overcoming problems of asynchrony	683
Field evaluation of oestrus synchronization techniques	684
Establishment of pregnancy	684
Pharmacological induction of parturition	686
Methods of induction of parturition	687
Delay of parturition	687

Introduction

This chapter aims to cover the manipulation of reproduction in cattle where this is not covered in the chapters on general fertility. The discussion includes control of the oestrous cycle, the establishment and maintenance of pregnancy and induction and postponement of parturition.

Control of the oestrous cycle

The control of the oestrous cycle is dependent on manipulation of the hormonal events occurring during the normal ovarian/oestrous cycle. The over-riding event controlling the development of an ovarian follicle to the point of ovulation in the cyclic cow is believed to be the process of luteolysis or decrease in progesterone secretion occurring between days 17 and 18 of the normal cycle (see Fig. 42.1). This fall in peripheral progesterone concentrations may be manipulated artificially in three ways:

(1) By the artificial induction of premature luteolysis using luteolytic agents, e.g. the prostaglandins.
(2) By attempting to modify the timing of normal ovarian events through a combination of trophic hormones and luteolytic agents.

(3) By the simulation of corpus luteum function, by administration of progesterone (or one of its synthetic derivatives) for a number of days, followed by abrupt withdrawal.

The three methods are discussed in greater detail below.

Induction of luteolysis

The most potent luteolytic agents available are derivatives of prostaglandin $F_{2\alpha}$ ($PGF_{2\alpha}$). Injection of exogenous $PGF_{2\alpha}$ or one of its analogues during the mid luteal phase of the cycle results in premature luteolysis and a consequential fall in peripheral progesterone concentrations. This is followed by a rise in the secretion of pituitary gonadotrophins and eventual ovulation. The fall in progesterone concentration is rapid, often reaching basal levels within 30 hours of injection. There are now several commercial analogues of $PGF_{2\alpha}$. Examples of those currently marketed in the UK and elsewhere are shown in Table 42.1.

Prostaglandins have been used to control the oestrous cycle in several different ways. Some possible methods are given below:

(1) Following rectal examination, only those cows with a corpus luteum are injected. These cows should then show oestrus and ovulate three to five days later. This method has the disadvantage that it is time-consuming and that rectal palpation involves added expense. The results also depend on the accuracy of detection of corpora lutea by rectal palpation.

(2) All cattle are observed for oestrus over a seven-day period, serving any that show oestrus. The rest are injected with prostaglandin on the following day and may be inseminated either once or twice at fixed times or at observed oestrus. The reason for the initial seven-day observation period is that there is a period of about seven days in the cycle (day 18 to day 0 and day 1 to day 4) when the animal is unresponsive to prostaglandin, i.e. when no corpus luteum is present. After seven days, those originally between days 18 and 0 will have shown heat and been served, while those that were between days 1 and 4 will now be between

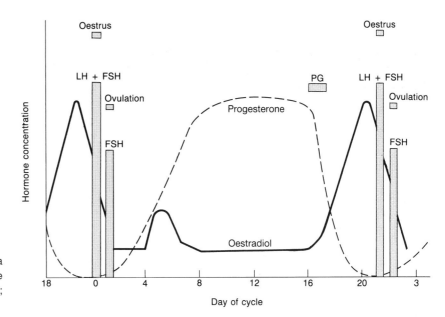

Fig. 42.1 Changes in blood plasma concentrations during the bovine oestrous cycle (schematic): — oestradiol; --- progesterone.

Table 42.1 Examples of prostaglandin analogues available in the UK and elsewhere (2003).

Trade name	Active component	Distributor	Route of injection	Dose rate (mg)	Insemination timing recommendations (hours)	
					Double	**Single**
Estrumate	Cloprostenol	Schering-Plough	im	0.5	72, 96	72–84
Prosolvin	Luprostiol	Intervet	im	15.0	72, 96	72
Lutalyse	Dinoprost	Pharmacia & Upjohn	im	25.0	72, 90	78
Enzaprost	Dinoprost	CEVA	im	25.0	72, 96	No recommendation
Noroprost	Dinoprost	Norbrook	im	25.0	72, 96	No recommendation
Prostavet	Etiproston tromethamine	Bimeda	im	5.0	72, 96	No recommendation

days 8 and 11, i.e. in the mid luteal phase, and therefore responsive to prostaglandin.

(3) The two injections plus two inseminations method. The so-called 'two plus two' technique was designed to synchronize groups of animals cycling at random without prior knowledge of their precise ovarian status. All cattle are injected on day 1 of treatment and the injection is repeated 10 or 11 days later. Artificial insemination (AI) is then carried out usually three and four days later (72 and 96 hours after the second prostaglandin injection).

The principle of this regimen is illustrated in Fig. 42.2. At the time of the first injection some animals will be responsive to the prostaglandin, i.e. between days 5 and 17 of the cycle. These will undergo luteoly-

sis in response to the injection and will ovulate some four days or so later. At the time of the second injection (10 or 11 days later) these cows will be on about days 8 and 15 of the next cycle (Fig. 42.2). The cows that were not responsive to the first injection, i.e. those between days 18 and 4 of the cycle, would now be between days 8 and 15 at the time of the second injection. Therefore all animals are theoretically in the responsive mid luteal phase at the time of the second injection. The technique is popular and quite successful in synchronizing cycles in heifers (Cooper, 1974) and has resulted in pregnancy rates equivalent to control animals. However, pregnancy rates achieved with this technique in adult cows have not always been consistent and some of the reasons for this are discussed later.

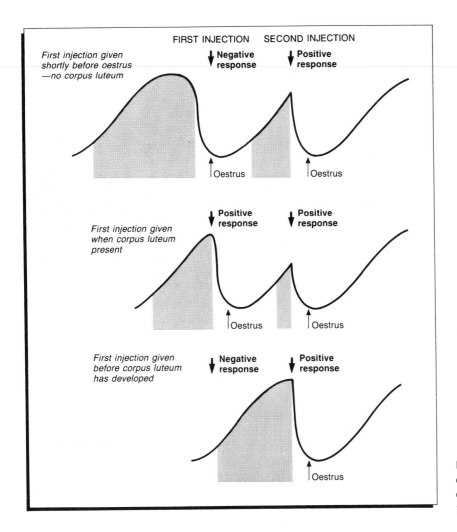

FIRST INJECTION   SECOND INJECTION

First injection given shortly before oestrus —no corpus luteum

↓ **Negative response**   ↓ **Positive response**

↑ Oestrus   ↑ Oestrus

First injection given when corpus luteum present

↓ **Positive response**   ↓ **Positive response**

↑ Oestrus   ↑ Oestrus

First injection given before corpus luteum has developed

↓ **Negative response**   ↓ **Positive response**

↑ Oestrus

Fig. 42.2 The effect on progesterone concentrations of giving two injections of prostaglandin 11 days apart. (MAFF, 1984).

(4) A further method of using prostaglandins that has been quite popular is the so-called '1½ method'. Cows are injected with prostaglandin and those that show oestrus are inseminated. Those that have not been seen in oestrus are injected again 11 days after the first injection and may be inseminated either at a fixed time(s) or at observed oestrus. Although requiring further effort in terms of oestrous detection, this method tends to give better results than the 'two plus two' regimen and is the current method of choice. Its main advantage, however, is the reduction in cost by the reduction of both the number of treatments used and the number of inseminations per cow.

Trophic hormone and prostaglandin combinations

Gonadotrophin releasing hormone (GnRH) or its analogues can be used to reprogram the developing waves of ovarian follicles to maximize the possibility of a dominant follicle being present at the time of induction of luteolysis seven days after the administration of the GnRH. Regimes involving this approach to 'priming' of the oestrous cycle have been tested in the UK (Mawhinney *et al.*, 1996). In most cases a second administration of GnRH has been used in an attempt to further synchronize the timing of ovulation after luteolysis. The second GnRH is administered 48 to 56 hours after prostaglandin administration, with insemination being carried out 18 to 24 hours after the post luteolytic GnRH (Roche, 1999).

Use of progestagens

The third method of controlling the cycle is to simulate the function of the corpus luteum by the administration of progesterone or one of its derivatives. In this method, gonadotrophin release, and hence ovarian follicular maturation, is suppressed until progesterone withdrawal. If progesterone is used to treat a group of cows and then it is withdrawn from all cows simultaneously, this will theoretically synchronize ovulation in the whole group.

In order to synchronize a group of randomly cycling cows effectively, it is necessary to treat them with progesterone for a period at least equivalent to the length of the natural luteal phase, i.e. 16 days. This is because exogenous progesterone has little or no effect on the life span of the natural corpus luteum and therefore, in a small proportion of cases, the natural corpus luteum might outlive a short-term progesterone treatment, resulting in a failure of synchrony. However, it has been shown that longer-term progesterone treatments (18–21 days) result in poor pregnancy rates. It is thought that this is due to adverse changes in the intra-uterine environment that may inhibit sperm transport.

Shorter-term progesterone treatments (7 to 12 days) generally result in more acceptable pregnancy rates, Unfortunately, short-term progesterone treatment does not control the cycle adequately since, if treatment is started early in the cycle, the natural corpus luteum may outlast the progesterone treatment. Therefore, it is often necessary to incorporate a luteolytic agent with short-term progesterone treatments in order to eliminate any existing corpus luteum.

Progestagens (progesterone-like compounds) can be administered in the feed, by injection or by implant. Administration in feed requires that the compound is 'orally active', i.e. it is absorbed into the systemic circulation unchanged. Progesterone itself is relatively inactive orally and thus synthetic analogues, for example medroxyprogesterone acetate (MPA) and melengoestrol acetate (MGA), were developed for this purpose. However, this route of administration presents problems of controlled dosing and the possibility of tissue or milk residues, particularly in dairy cows. Therefore, such techniques are not favoured in the UK for oestrous control in cattle; however, they are used widely in the USA and other countries, particularly in heifers.

Progestagens can be given by injection, but as the half-life of progesterone and its analogues is short, repeated treatments may be necessary. The rate of absorption is often imprecise, so synchronized withdrawal of the compound can be unreliable. Implants appear to be the most suitable method of administration of progestagens since withdrawal can then be precisely controlled by implant removal.

Intravaginal progestagen-containing device (e.g. PRID or CIDR)

The PRID (CEVA Animal Health) or CIDR (InterAg/ART) are specialized forms of implant that are inserted into, and held within, the cow's vagina for a period of 7 to 12 days. The PRID consists of a stainless steel coil

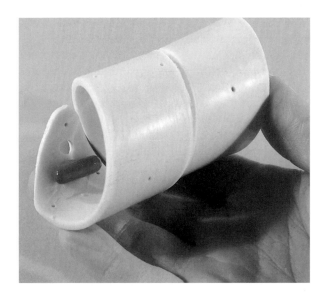

Fig. 42.3 A progesterone-releasing intravaginal device (PRID).

covered by a layer of grey inert silastic (Fig. 42.3) in which 1.55 mg progesterone is impregnated. A gelatin capsule containing 10 mg oestradiol benzoate is attached to the inner surface of the coil. The oestradiol benzoate in the PRID is intended to act us a luteolytic agent. The CIDR is a Y-shaped device consisting of a nylon spine covered by a similar silicone elastomer impregnated with 1.9 g progesterone. These devices are inserted into the vagina by means of specialized applicators and are then left in place for up to 12 days.

The progesterone is continuously released from the elastomer until removal of the device. Removal is effected by pulling on the string (PRID) or plastic 'tail' (CIDR) which is left protruding from the vulva after insertion. Removal after 7 to 12 days causes peripheral plasma progesterone concentrations to fall, thus simulating natural luteolysis. Consequently, the cow should show oestrus 48–72 hours later and fixed-time AI may then be used.

There has been some interest in the use of low doses of oestrogens after the removal of the progesterone delivery device. Doses of 1 mg have been used in an attempt to further synchronize the onset of oestrus subsequent to the fall in plasma progesterone concentrations. Questions remain regarding the fertility consequences of this approach (Roche, 1999).

Norgestomet (Crestar)

Norgestomet, 17α-acetoxy-β-methyl-19-nor-preg-4-ene, 20-dione (Crestar, Intervet), is marketed for planned breeding of beef cows and dairy and beef heifers. It is an example of a synthetic analogue of progesterone and consists of an impregnated silastic subcutaneous implant. The implant is inserted subcutaneously behind the ear for a period of nine or ten days, during which time the progesterone is absorbed into the circulation. The implant is removed by making a small scalpel incision in the skin of the ear over the implant. At the time of the implantation an intramuscular injection of 5 mg oestradiol valerate is given as luteolysin, in combination with an initial injection of 3 mg norgestomet.

Factors affecting pregnancy rate after controlled ovulation

It cannot be overemphasized that in order to maximize results obtained with pharmacological control of the oestrous cycle, nutritional status and general management must be of a high standard. The efficacy of the pharmacological control of ovulation can be considered as two components:

(1) The degree of synchrony obtained following treatment. This may be defined as the proportion of animals beginning to show oestrus or ovulating within a specified time period after the end of hormonal treatment. For the purposes of this discussion the target of synchrony is for the maximum number of animals to show oestrus within approximately 48 hours of progesterone withdrawal or 72 hours after prostaglandin injection (or to ovulate approximately 24 hours later in each case).
(2) Reproductive performance, which may be expressed, for example, as the pregnancy rate achieved after treatment.

Obviously in some circumstances the pregnancy rate may be highly dependent on the degree of synchrony, particularly if fixed-time AI is used. For example, if there is a poor degree of synchrony there will be a wide variation in the timing of ovulation between cows or, more correctly, a proportion of cows will ovulate beyond the specific period anticipated. Therefore insemination would not be accurately timed and the pregnancy rates following fixed-time AI may be poor.

In view of the natural variation in timing of the behavioural and ovarian events around natural oestrus, it is perhaps not surprising that even after hormone treatments there is still considerable variation in the timing of responses between animals. Hence where fixed-time AI is used, two inseminations are usually recommended in order to maximize the probability of conception. In addition, other problems occur that appear to be specific to the particular compounds used and these are described below.

Synchrony after prostaglandins

Three major circumstances in which asynchrony can arise have been reported in the literature (Jackson et al., 1979; Baishya et al., 1980; Peters et al., 1980).

Failure of complete luteolysis

This has occurred in 10 per cent or more of cows treated with prostaglandins. It takes the form either of complete lack of effect on progesterone concentrations or, for example, a fall to half of pre-injection levels, followed by luteal recovery, usually within 24–48 hours. Causes of luteolytic failure are not clear but may be related to several factors including the following:

● Non-responsiveness of some corpora lutea even in the appropriate phase of the cycle.
● Treatment too early in the luteal phase.
● Incorrect injection site or technique: in the case of intramuscular injections, occasionally the material may be injected accidentally into fat or ligamentous tissue.
● Short half-life of the chosen exogenous prostaglandin in the animal.

The extent of these various problems is not known and it must be admitted that all are to some extent speculative.

Long follicular phases after injection

In up to 20 per cent of cows injected with prostaglandin, although luteolysis appears to occur normally, progesterone concentrations remain low for an unusually long period. This may be associated with a delay in the timing of ovulation relative to oestrus. However, extended follicular phases (longer than eight days) also occur in about 17 per cent of untreated dairy cows. Thus it is likely that this phenomenon is related to a natural aberration in the adult cow's ovarian cycle. The problem has not been reported in heifers and certainly the cycles of adult cows would appear to be less uniform than those of heifers.

Acyclic cows

The ovary can only respond to prostaglandin if there is a functional corpus luteum. Therefore, cows with little ovarian activity at the time of injection do not respond. The proportion of cows in this state will vary from herd to herd and the average stage after calving, but it is generally regarded as a more serious problem in suckling beef cows. For this reason some advisors recommend that prostaglandins are not used before day 42 after calving.

Synchrony after trophic hormone–prostaglandin combination techniques

It has been shown that more than 90 per cent of cattle treated with GnRH followed by prostaglandin and a second GnRH (the so-called 'GPG' system) can be induced into a low progesterone phase at the time of planned insemination. The proportion of cattle either failing to respond in this way or failing to show oestrus and ovulation as expected may be influenced by several factors:

- Some cows may fail to be in the luteal phase at the time of prostaglandin administration. This is thought to occur to a greater extent in heifer groups and may be a consequence of a difference in the frequency of follicular waves in immature cattle. The GPG system is usually less effective in heifer groups.
- Failure to respond to prostaglandins as previously discussed.
- Earlier than expected expression of oestrus. The normal recommendation is to serve on observed oestrus should cattle be available for service earlier than the time planned for insemination.
- Failure to exhibit behavioural oestrus due to slow or abnormal follicular development or true anoestrus

Synchrony after progestagens

There are two major circumstances in which synchrony may be incomplete following progestagen treatment.

Ineffectiveness of the luteolytic agent

As discussed above, oestradiol is often used as a luteolytic agent, along with progestagen treatments. If, for example, a nine-day progestagen treatment is started, without a luteolytic agent, at day 9 of one cycle and finishing before day 1 of the next, then these animals should synchronize adequately, since the end of treatment either coincides with, or occurs after, luteolysis (or the progesterone blocks ovulation). However, if treatment is started between days 2 and 8, then the corpus luteum can outlive the progestagen treatment. Hence, it is for cows in the early stages of the cycle that the luteolysin is required. If it is assumed that the group of cows is cycling at random, then one would expect about 30 per cent of them to be in this category and to respond poorly to oestrous synchronization using a progestagen

without a luteolytic agent. Synchronization rates of 70 per cent have been reported in practice (e.g. Drew *et al.*, 1979) Oestradiol is not always an effective luteolytic agent and, like prostaglandins, does not always prevent formation of the corpus luteum when administered early in the cycle (Peters, 1984).

Failure to maintain high blood concentration of progesterone

It has been shown that in some circumstances progesterone concentrations in the cow may fall before withdrawal of the progesterone source (Roche & Ireland, 1981). Obviously this could result in oestrus and ovulation occurring before removal of the device. This premature fall has occurred particularly with the intravaginal method of administration. It has been suggested that this is related to progesterone-induced changes in absorption across the vaginal wall rather than to exhaustion of progesterone in the device.

Possible methods of overcoming problems of asynchrony

Failure to undergo complete luteolysis

An alternative to the use of oestradiol as a luteolytic agent in combination with progestagens is to use a prostaglandin. Whilst problems of prostaglandin usage have been referred to above, they are clearly far more potent luteolytic agents than oestradiol. Prostaglandin is usually injected on the day before progestagen withdrawal. Various studies have shown that such combinations give well-synchronized oestrus and endocrine responses (Beal, 1983; Peters, 1984). However, there have been few reports where fixed-time AI has been used (Smith *et al.*, 1984). Unfortunately, such a treatment combination would obviously add further expense to a controlled breeding programme.

The use of low dose oestradiol

As detailed earlier, low (1 mg) doses of oestrogen have been used in the pro-oestrus period after removal of an intravaginal device. This is said to enhance the positive feedback that promotes the pre-ovulatory surge of the pituitary gonadotrophin, luteinizing hormone, which leads to ovulation. It is also said to enhance the behavioural expression of oestrus.

Prolonged follicular phases

This phenomenon has been associated with a delay in oestrus and ovulation. Therefore a logical approach

Table 42.2 Effect of cloprostenol treatment of cyclic cows that had not been observed in oestrus by day 50 after calving (from Ball, 1982).

Treatment	Time of insemination	No. of cows	Calving-to-conception interval (days)
None until 90 days after calving	Observed oestrus	166	107.4
Cloprostenol[a]	Observed oestrus	61	98.1
Cloprostenol[a]	2 and 3 days after injection	75	104.0

[a] 0.5 mg cloprostenol (Estrumate, ICI) was injected intramuscularly 10–14 days after ovulation had occurred as judged from three times weekly milk progesterone measurements.

might be to attempt artificially to induce ovulation at a standard time after prostaglandin treatment. A single injection of gonadotrophin-releasing hormone (GnRH) administered approximately 60 hours after prostaglandin injection (Coulson *et al.*, 1980) has the effect of inducing a preovulatory-type LH surge normally associated with ovulation. This procedure has been used following synchronization of follicle development with GnRH as described earlier. There are also many reports on using GnRH after observed oestrus to produce a predictable ovulation in order to enhance conception success. This approach is discussed later.

Acyclic cows

This problem may be due to ineffective management in that either the cows are being treated too early after calving or that nutritional management is, and has been, inadequate (see Chapter 9). Assuming these problems are not present, then acyclicity may he overcome in a proportion of cows by the use of progestagens as opposed to prostaglandins.

Effect of the length of progestagen treatment on pregnancy rate

The deleterious effects of long-term progestagen treatment on fertility have already been discussed. However, there is some evidence that even short-term treatments can cause reduced fertility, particularly where the treatment is started during the late luteal phase of the cycle. It is possible that this occurs because the animal has been exposed to an uninterrupted long-term progestagen treatment, albeit a combination of endogenous and exogenous sources.

Field evaluation of oestrous synchronization techniques

Many field trials have been carried out to assess the effect of the various treatments on reproductive per-

formance. These will not be discussed in detail here but they may be summarized as follow:

● In adult cows the calving rate of control groups to single AI at observed oestrus is of the order of 50 per cent. Most studies report equivalent rates in treated cows.
● Fertility results are often up to 20 per cent better in heifers than in cows.
● In general, single fixed-time AI might be expected to result in 10–15 per cent lower pregnancy rates than two fixed-time AIs.
● It is clear that the best reproductive performance is achieved when oestrous cycle control is combined with insemination at observed oestrus. In that situation the reproductive performance of treated cows may often be higher than that of controls. This may happen particularly in a herd where the efficiency of oestrous detection is normally low. Following a synchronization treatment, it is to be expected that the vast majority of cows should show oestrus within 10 days after treatment. Therefore, the effect of treatment in this situation is to concentrate the occurrence of oestrous periods, so that detection efficiency can be increased over a relatively short time. Results of studies on the use of the prostaglandin analogue cloprostenol with either fixed-time AI or observed oestrus are shown in Table 42.2 and help illustrate the advantage of insemination at observed oestrus. Following retrospective analysis of data from 17 published trials McIntosh *et al.* (1984) concluded that prostaglandin treatment combined with insemination at observed oestrus improved conception rates over controls by an average of 7 per cent.

Establishment of pregnancy

The ability to conceive is clearly vital in determining reproductive performance. A low pregnancy rate to first

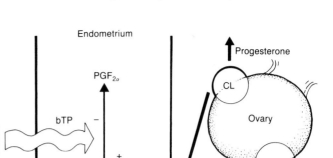

Fig. 42.4 Possible endocrine relationship between the early embryo. endometrium and ovary. BTP, bovine trophoblast protein; AA, arachidonic acid; OT, oxytocin; OTR, oxytocin receptor; CL, corpus luteum; Foll, follicle.

service is a major cause of poor reproductive performance. In the absence of specific infectious disease it has been shown that the major problem here, at least in cattle, is early embryonic death. Total embryonic and fetal mortality is estimated to be around 38 per cent and it is thought that 70 to 80 per cent of that loss occurs between days 8 and 16 after insemination (Sreenan & Diskin, 1986).

Pregnancy establishment involves active and passive communication between the embryo and the uterus. The exact cause(s) of embryonic death is unknown but it is circumstantially related to premature regression of the corpus luteum. In other words, the corpus luteum is normally maintained for the whole of gestation and early embryonic mortality is associated with its early loss. This results in a decrease in progesterone concentrations allowing the animal to return to oestrus, probably at the normal time.

Before examining methods of reducing embryo mortality it might be useful to provide a brief review of findings in relation to the establishment of pregnancy. This is illustrated in Fig. 42.4. In the non-pregnant animal $PGF_{2\alpha}$ secreted by the endometrium causes regression of the corpus luteum. There is evidence that oestradiol-17β from developing ovarian follicles stimulates the synthesis of receptors for oxytocin on endometrial cells. Oxytocin, produced by the corpus luteum (Wathes, 1984; Lamming & Mann, 1995), binds to these receptors, thereby stimulating the synthesis and secretion of $PGF_{2\alpha}$. In early pregnancy a protein of molecular weight of approximately 18 000 is secreted by the embryo. This protein appears to exert an anti-luteolytic effect and has been termed bovine or ovine trophoblast protein 1 (e.g. oTP-1). Stewart *et al.* (1989) showed that the amino acid sequence of oTP-1 has 70.3 per cent similarity, with bovine α2-interferon. Further studies have shown that oPT-1 and bTP-1 bind to receptors on the endometrium and intrauterine infusion of trophoblast proteins or recombinant interferon can extend the

length of the luteal phase in non-pregnant animals (Stewart *et al.*, 1989; Thatcher *et al.*, 1989). This work led to the conclusion that some embryo mortality may be related to a failure of some embryos to produce sufficient trophoblast protein.

A number of methods have been used in the field to improve pregnancy rates in cattle. Diskin and Sreenan (1986) reviewed the studies on comparisons of progesterone concentrations in pregnant and non-conceiving cows before and after insemination and concluded that the data were conflicting and inconclusive in all respects. Progesterone supplementation during early pregnancy has given equivocal results, but does seem to be effective where control pregnancy rates are particularly low, i.e. 40 per cent or below. In summarizing the results of progesterone supplementation during early pregnancy, Mann and Lamming (1999) conclude that while progesterone concentrations during the luteal phase are an important determinant of the outcome of pregnancy, they do not appear to be as important as the timing of the post ovulatory progesterone rise.

More recently attention has been paid to the use of gonadotrophin or GnRH in enhancing early luteal performance in support of the developing embryo. Peters (1996) found that 1500 iu of human chorionic gonadotrophin on day 12 of the cycle resulted in a sustained increase in progesterone concentration and an increased diameter of the corpus luteum.

It has been common veterinary practice for many years to inject cows at the time of service with a 'holding' injection using either human chorionic gonadotrophin (HCG) (luteinizing hormone (LH)-like) or GnRH to stimulate endogenous LH release. The exact physiological rationale for this has not always been clear since such treatment could potentially have at least two effects. Firstly, there is a widely held belief that under some circumstances ovulation may be delayed relative to the timing of oestrus. Administration of GnRH will result in preovulatory gonadotrophin release and subsequent ovulation. Secondly, LH is considered to be the major luteotrophic hormone, at least during the first few days of pregnancy. Therefore, GnRH-induced LH release may facilitate the development and maintenance of the corpus luteum in the post ovulatory period. Numerous trials have been carried out where either HCG (LH) or GnRH has been given on the day of service. In a meta-analysis of many studies Valks (1996) illustrated that a small effect was generally achievable (around 8 per cent) and that the magnitude of any effect was influenced by factors including body condition score. Study results varied, with some showing good responses and others showing no differences from control animals. This could be for one or more of the following reasons:

(1) Poor design of trials, involving a few animals in each study group. This is a common problem where fertility rates are being studied. Due to the fact that pregnancy rate is discrete variable and that rates are very different between farms, very large numbers (several hundred per group) may be required to establish statistically significant differences between groups.

(2) The actual cause of pregnancy failure may differ widely between farms and therefore one may be attempting to rectify many different primary problems by the use of such a treatment. The primary cause is often impossible to diagnose, at least at that time.

(3) Thus it is probably a fair summary to state that the best results for the improvement of pregnancy rates have been achieved where the control or background fertility of the herd is poor, although there are some exceptions to this.

MacMillan *et al.* (1986), attempted to support the corpus luteum when it became susceptible to the luteolytic mechanism, i.e. approaching day 16 after oestrus in the cow. Treated cows (approximately 225) were given a single injection of 10 μg buserelin (a synthetic analogue of GnRH) on day 11, 12 or 13 after AI. Treated and control cows were palpated at six to nine weeks to determine pregnancy status, cows returning to service were re-inseminated. Pregnancy rates at six to nine weeks were 72.5 per cent and 60.9 per cent for the treated and control cows respectively (see Table 42.3). Of those cows returning to service the pregnancy rates to second service were 85.1 per cent and 69.5 per cent for treated and control cows, respectively (see Table 42.4).

In the UK a similar approach was adopted, with 1619 cows studied (Sheldon, 1993). When GnRH was used at 11 days after insemination first service pregnancy rates were enhanced by 9.4 per cent when compared with untreated controls. This benefit rose to 30 per cent in cows treated at third and subsequent services.

Table 42.3 Pregnancy rate (per cent) to first insemination with 10 μg buserelin injected between days 11 and 13 after insemination (from MacMillan *el al.*, 1986).

Trial	Treated	Control
A	75.4	62.2
B	67.5	57.8
Overall	72.4[a]	60.9

[a] $P < 0.01$.

Table 42.4 Pregnancy rates (per cent) to second insemination (from MacMillan *et al.*, 1986).

Trial	Treated	Control
A	78.6	69.0
B	94.7	70.8
Overall	85.1[a]	69.5

[a] $P < 0.05$.

Thatcher *et al.* (1989) suggested that buserelin acts in these situations by disrupting normal waves of ovarian follicular growth and oestradiol secretion, resulting in a failure of the luteolytic mechanism (see Fig. 42.4). Mann and Lamming (1995), however, maintain that GnRH causes a short-lived reduction in oestradiol secretion which reduces the stimulus to the development of the luteolytic mechanism.

Pharmacological induction of parturition

Many attempts have been made to induce parturition artificially in the final days of gestation. These methods have used exogenous hormones to simulate the mechanisms involved in the normal parturition process. These have included the use of corticosteroids, oestrogens and prostaglandins since these are all involved in the endocrine pathway (see Fig. 42.5).

These are several indications for the induction of parturition in cows. Firstly, in countries such as New Zealand, where a tight seasonal calving pattern is often required, this is considered to be an important aid to optimum management and utilization of feed resources. Secondly, cows can be induced to calve at a time when supervision is most readily available. Thirdly, if it is suspected that a high calf birth weight might result in dystokia, early induction may alleviate the problem.

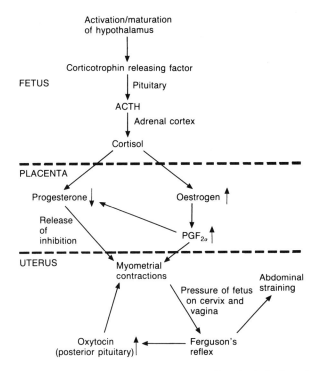

Fig. 42.5 The endocrine pathways controlling the induction of parturition.

Methods of induction of parturition

Corticosteroids

Parturtition can be induced quite reliably from about day 255 of pregnancy onwards by a single injection of a synthetic glucocorticoid, such as dexamethasone, betamethasone or flumethasone. It is assumed that such therapy simulates the effect of the fetal adrenal cortex at term.

Induction of parturition using corticosteroids is an important part of management in many New Zealand dairy herds and considerable experience of the technique has been gained (Welch *et al.*, 1979; Verkerk *et al.* 1997). Both short- and long-acting formulations have been used.

Short-acting formulations, generally in the form of a soluble ester of the steroid, usually result in parturition two to three days later. Although the calves are usually viable, this method has been associated with a high rate of retention of the fetal membranes. Verkerk *et al.* (1997) used 21 mg dexamethasone isonicotinate followed by a short acting formulation of dexamethasone sodium phosphate 10 to 14 days later. Using this regime 35 per cent of cows calved before the second corticosteroid had been administered. This was more common if the cow was in the last 30 days of gestation. A 14 per cent incidence of retained fetal membranes was recorded.

Oestrogens

There is no clear evidence that exogenous oestrogen is effective in inducing parturition in cows, although in one trial cited by First (1979) treatment with oestradiol-17β before corticosteroid treatment shortened the time to delivery and reduced the variation between cows.

Prostaglandins

Prostaglandins, both $PGF_{2\alpha}$ and synthetic analogues, may be used to induce parturition in cows, although treatment before day 270 of gestation is not recommended. Parturition usually occurs between one and eight days after injection, but at an average of three days. A higher incidence of retained placenta compared to non-treated cows may be expected.

A study under UK conditions (Murray *et al.*, 1984) used a treatment regimen whereby cows were injected with 20 mg dexamethasone and those that had not calved 10 days later received an injection of 0.5 mg cloprostenol (an analogue of $PGF_{2\alpha}$). Although there was a high incidence of retained placenta, this did not affect subsequent reproductive performance. It was concluded that, provided management was organized adequately to supervise parturition and to take care of the newborn calves, then this procedure could be carried out to advantage.

A characteristic of early studies on the pharmacological induction of parturition was the high rate of calf mortality and post calving problems, particularly retained placenta. An important determinant of the incidence of retained placenta appears to be the oestrogen status of the cow at the time of induction. As discussed above, oestrogen concentrations rise during late pregnancy, hence the oestrogen status may simply be a reflection of the proximity of term or 'readiness to calve'. From an exhaustive review of the available literature, First (1979) concluded that if induction is carried out when oestrogen levels are elevated, both glucocorticoids and prostaglandins are effective. However, glucocorticoids were the most appropriate treatment if induction was to be attempted earlier. The earlier that interference is attempted, the higher the probability of calf mortality, retained placenta and other related problems.

Delay of parturition

It is also possible to delay parturition for several hours by pharmacological means. This is carried out so that supervision for calving can be more conveniently and readily available. Injection of the potent adrenergic drug clenbuterol inhibits myometrial contractions, thus slowing down the first stage of labour. However, if treatment is started after second stage labour has already commenced, it would have little effect. Clenbuterol is not currently indicated for obstetric use.

References

Baishya, N., Ball, P.J.H Leaver, J.D. & St Pope, O.S. (1980) Fertility of lactating dairy cows inseminated after treatment with cloprostenol. *British Veterinary Journal*, **136**, 227–39.

Ball, P.J.FH. (1982) Milk progesterone profiles in relation to dairy fertility. *British Veterinary Journal*, **138**, 546–51.

Beal, W.E. (1983) A note on synchronisation of oestrus in post-partum cows with prostaglandin PGF$_{2\alpha}$ and a progesterone-releasing device. *Animal Production*, **37**, 305–8.

Cooper, M.J. (1974) Control of oestrous cycles of heifers with a synthetic prostaglandin analogue. *Veterinary Record*, **95**, 200–3.

Coulson, A., Noakes, D.E., Hamer, J. & Cockrill, T. (1980) Effect of gonadotrophin releasing hormone on levels of luteinising hormone in cattle synchronised with dinoprost. *Veterinary Record*, **107**, 108–9.

Diskin, M.G. & Sreenan J.M. (1986) Progesterone arid embryo survival in the cow. In *Embryonic Mortality in Farm Animals* (ed. by J.M. Sreenan & M.G. Diskin), pp. 142–55. Martinus Nijhoff, Dordrecht.

Drew, S.B., Wishart, D.R. & Young, I.M. (1979) Fertility of Norgestomet treated suckler cows. *Veterinary Record*, **104**, 523–5.

First, N.D. (1979) Mechanisms controlling parturition in farm animals. In *Animal Reproduction* (ed. by H.W. Hawk). Beltsville Symposia in Agricultural Research No. 3, pp. 215–57. John Wiley & Sons, New York.

Jackson, P.S., Johnson, C.T., Bulman, D.C. & Holdsworth, R.J. (1979) A study of cloprostenol-induced oestrus and spontaneous oestrus by means of the milk progesterone assay. *British Veterinary Journal*, **135**, 378–90.

Lamming, G.E. & Mann, G.E. (1995) Control of endometrial oxytocin receptors and prostaglandin F$_{2\alpha}$ responses to oxytocin in ovarectomised cows by progesterone and estradiol. *Journal of Reproduction and Fertility*, **103**, 69–73.

McIntosh, D.A.D., Lewis, J.A. & Hammond, D. (1984) Conception rates in dairy cattle treated with cloprostenol. *Veterinary Record*, **115**, 129–30.

MacMillan, K.L., Taufa, V.K. & Day, A.M. (1986) Effects of an agonist of gonadotrophin releasing hormone in cattle: III. Pregnancy rates after a post-insemination injection during metoestrus or dioestrus. *Animal Reproduction Science*, **11**, 1–10.

MAFF (1984) *Dairy Herd Fertility*. Reference Book 259, p. 46. HMSO, London.

Mann, G.E. & Lamming, G.E. (1995) Effects of treatment with buserelin on plasma concentrations of oestradiol and progesterone and cycle length in the cow. *British Veterinary Journal*, **151**, 427–32.

Mann, G.E. & Lamming, G.E. (1999) The influence of progesterone during early pregnancy in cattle. *Reproduction in Domestic Animals*, **34**, 269–74.

Mawhinney, I., Drew, B. & Peters, A.R. (1996) The use of a GnRH and prostaglandin regime for planned breeding of groups of dairy cows. *Cattle Practice*, **4**, 285–8.

Murray. R.D., Nutter, W.T., Wilman, S. & Harker, D.B. (1984) Induction of parturition using dexamethasone and cloprostenol. Economic performance and disease incidence after treatment. *Veterinary Record*, **115**, 296–330.

Peters, A.R., (1984) Plasma progesterone and gonadotrophin concentrations following Norgestomet treatment with and without cloprostenol in beef cows. *Veterinary Record*, **115**, 164–6.

Peters, A.R. (1996) The use of human chorionic gonadotrophin as an antiluteolytic agent in cattle post oestrus on luteal performance. *Cattle Practice*, **4**, 307–11.

Peters, A.R., Riley, G.M., Rahim, S.E.A & Lowman, B.G. (1980) Milk progesterone profiles and the double injection of cloprostenol in post-partum beef cows. *Veterinary Record*, **107**, 74–7.

Roche, J.F. (1999) Reproductive efficiency in post-partum cows. *Cattle Practice*, **7**, 27–43.

Roche, J.F. & Ireland, J.J. (1981) Effect of exogenous progesterone on time of occurrence of the LH surge in heifers. *Journal of Animal Science*, **52**, 580–6.

Sheldon, M. (1983) GnRH on day 11 after insemination to increase pregnancy rates in cattle at first second and subsequent services. *Cattle Practice*, **1**, 93–6.

Smith, R.D., Pomerantz, A.J., Beal, W.E., McCann, J.P., Pilbeam, T.E. & Hansel, W. (1984) Insemination of Holstein heifers at a preset time after oestrous cycle synchronisation using progesterone and prostaglandin. *Journal of Animal Science*, **58**, 792–800.

Sreenan, J.M. & Diskin, M.G. (1986) The extent and timing of embryonic mortality. In *Embryonic Mortality in Farm Animals* (ed. by J.M. Sreenan & M.G. Diskin), pp. 1–11. Martinus Nijhoff, Dordrecht.

Stewart, H.J., Flint, A.P.F., Lamming, G.E., McCann, S.H.E. & Parkinson, T.J. (1989) Antiluteolytic effects of blastocyst secreted interferon investigated in-vitro and in-vivo in the sheep. *Journal of Reproduction and Fertility*, **37**, (Suppl) 127–38.

Thatcher, W.W., MacMillan, K.L., Hansen, P.J. & Drost, M. (1989) Concepts for regulation of corpus luteum function by the conceptus and ovarian follicles to improve fertility. *Theriogenology*, **31**, 149–64.

Valks, M. (1996) Factors influencing the benefit of GnRH on the day of insemination. *Cattle Practice* **4**, 311–17.

Verkerk, G.A., Goble, G., McDougall, S., Woods, M. & Clark, B. (1997) Induction of parturition in dairy cows: a survey from spring 1996 in the Waikato region. *Proceedings of the New Zealand Society of Animal Production*, **57**, 231–3.

Wathes, D.C. (1984) Possible actions of gonadal oxytocin and vasopressin. *Journal of Reproduction and Fertility*, **71**, 315–45.

Welch, R.A.S., Day, A.M., Duganzich, DM. & Featherstone, P. (1979) Induced calving; a comparison of treatment regimes. *New Zealand Veterinary Journal*, **27**, 190–4.

Adult Cattle
Major Infectious Diseases

Chapter 43
Viral Diseases

(a) Bluetongue   691
(b) Enzootic bovine leukosis   693
(c) Foot-and-mouth disease   700
(d) Rinderpest   707
(e) Vesicular stomatitis   710
(f) Bovine immunodeficiency virus (BIV)   713

(a) Bluetongue

R.P. Kitching

Bluetongue (BT) is an infectious, non-contagious disease of ruminants characterized by congestion, oedema and haemorrhage. The disease is caused by strains of orbivirus, within the family Reoviridae.

The genus orbivirus, Reoviridae also contains Ibaraki disease virus of cattle, epizootic haemorrhagic disease virus of deer (EHD), African horse sickness virus and Colorado tick fever virus. The outer shell of bluetongue virus (BTV) has a diameter of 65 nm, within which is an inner shell of 32 ring-shaped capsomers. The genome consists of ten segments of double-stranded RNA which code for the structural and non-structural viral proteins and which can be separated according to their relative sizes by polyacrylamide or agarose gel electrophoresis. Two of these segments (numbers two and five) code for the outer structural proteins (VP2 and VP5) which determine the serotype of the virus. Twenty-four immunologically distinct BTV serotypes have so far been identified by virus neutralization tests; however, it is probable that more types will be identified in the future. BTV is sensitive to low pH and storage at $-20°C$; it is partially resistant to lipid solvents.

Distribution

The distribution of BTV is approximately defined by the latitudes 40°N and 35°S, which includes most of Africa, the Middle and Far East, Northern Australia, United States of America, Central America and South America north from Southern Brazil, Paraguay and Bolivia.

Not all the BTV types are found throughout this enzootic region, and the distribution of the different types can vary between years. BTV types found within a region tend to have greater genome sequence homology, in genome segments other than those which encode the serotype-specific outer capsid proteins, than their designated serotype number would suggest. The type is defined by the outer capsid proteins alone, and while these are found to differ between different serotypes found in a particular region, the remaining genome segments show high levels of sequence homology. The BTV types have therefore been additionally grouped into Australian types and African types, with the North American types being more closely related to the African. The Australian BTV type 1 has more in common with other Australian types than with the African type 1, although sharing with the African type its antigenic determinants. This diversity may explain the marked difference in pathogenicity of the strains of BTV which does not appear to be related to a specific type designation; it also makes epidemiological studies based on serotype determinations of doubtful significance. Recombination can occur between different strains of BTV which adds further to the potential for diversity of BTV isolates.

The closely related EHD group of viruses has been isolated in the USA, Canada, Nigeria and Australia, whereas Ibaraki disease virus is restricted to South Korea, Japan, Philippines and Indonesia.

History

Bluetongue was first diagnosed in South Africa in sheep at the beginning of the twentieth century. It was first seen outside Africa in 1943 in Cyprus, although it had possibly been present in Cyprus as early as 1924. Subsequently BT was diagnosed in Israel in 1951, in Pakistan in 1959 and in India in 1963. A disease at first identified as sore muzzle of sheep in Texas in 1948 and California in 1952 was the following year diagnosed as BT. Between 1956 and 1960, BTV caused a major epizootic in sheep in Portugal and southern Spain, which reportedly resulted in the loss of 180 000 animals, but the virus then disappeared from the region.

Epidemiology and transmission

The distribution of BTV between 40°N and 35°S reflects the distribution of its main biological vectors, certain tropical and subtropical species of *Culicoides* midges, in particular *C. imicola* in Africa and the Middle East, *C. variipennis* in North America and *C. brevitarsis*, *C. fulvus* and *C. wadai* in North Australia.

The adult female *Culicoides* lays her eggs in damp muddy areas containing decaying vegetable material or in cattle dung, two to six days after a blood meal. Depending on the temperature these eggs may hatch in two to three days into larva. The larval stage lasts 12–16 days, followed by pupation and, two to three days later, the emergence of the adult *Culicoides*. In the subsequent 24 hours the adult females take a blood meal and mate, and they will continue to take a blood meal every three to four days until the end of their life, which may last for 70 days, but probably rarely exceeds 10. Optimum conditions are between 13°C and 35°C. Larvae of temperate species can remain dormant over winter and pupate the following spring. Seven to ten days after taking a BTV infected blood meal, vector species of *Culicoides* midge are able to transmit virus.

Culicoides usually feed at dusk, during the night or at dawn, and are subject to being transported, sometimes over considerable distances, by strong wind currents. The passive movement of infected *Culicoides* may be responsible for the introduction of BT into areas usually outside the enzootic region, such as Western Turkey and Cyprus. This introduction of BTV into an area may be associated with abnormal wind currents or may be a regular occurrence. The winds of the Intertropical Convergence Zone annually reintroduce BTV-infected *Culicoides* to South Africa from Central Africa. The movement of BTV into Sudan from Central Africa is also associated with a prevailing wind from the South. However, BTV may also become enzootic in new regions as climatic changes allow the main vectors to extend their breeding sites or, alternatively, virulent strains of new serotypes of BTV may be introduced into an area already infected with mild or avirulent strains.

Within BT enzootic regions the prevalence of sero-positive animals may be very localized around areas particularly suitable for the breeding and survival of *Culicoides*, so called 'hot spots'. The possibility also exists for new species of *Culicoides* to take on the role of BTV vectors; it has recently been shown that some British species of *Culicoides* can biologically transmit BTV under experimental conditions.

Bulls may shed BTV in their semen intermittently during the viraemia following infection. Bowen *et al.* (1985) classified bulls into three categories, those from which virus could not be isolated from the semen (the majority), those from which only low titres of virus were isolated on less than three occasions and those which shed virus over a two to three week period. BTV could only be isolated from the semen when there was a concurrent viraemia. Six out of nine susceptible heifers inseminated with the BTV-contaminated semen became pregnant and three of the nine became viraemic. None of the calves born at term showed any clinical abnormality. Considerable importance has been attached to reports of a bull which was persistently infected but seronegative from birth and intermittently shed virus in semen over an 11-year period (Luedke *et al.*, 1982). Attempts to duplicate the conditions which produce persistently BTV-infected, seronegative calves have been unsuccessful.

Host range

Sheep, goats, cattle, water buffalo, camels and many wild ruminants are susceptible to infection with BTV. BT is predominantly a disease of sheep and has only been reported as a disease of cattle in the USA, South Africa, Israel and Portugal.

Pathogenesis

Infection follows the bite of an infected *Culicoides* midge. The virus is carried to the local lymph node where primary replication occurs before dissemination of virus throughout the body. Viral replication then continues in the spleen, lungs, bone marrow and other lymph glands. In sheep, BTV also replicates in the endothelial cells of the blood vessels and, unlike in cattle, has been clearly shown to cross the placenta and can replicate in the developing fetus causing fetal resorption, abortion or developmental abnormalities. The peak viraemia occurs two to three weeks after infection, its duration and severity depending on the strain of BTV.

Clinical signs

BT in cattle is seen as a transient fever followed by hyperaemia and erosions of the buccal and lingual mucosa and nose and, rarely, the teats. Affected cattle salivate excessively and may walk with a stiff gait. The skin of the nose appears mottled and dark and has been described as 'burnt muzzle', and may completely slough. Fewer than 1 per cent of cattle in the USA infected with BTV show signs, and the lesions may be due to a delayed type hypersensitivity reaction. There is considerable controversy over whether BTV can cross the placenta of the pregnant cow. If the virus is able to cross the placenta it may only do so in association with other placental pathogens, or be restricted to only certain strains of BTV.

Diagnosis

It is not possible to make a diagnosis of BT on solely clinical signs. Cattle infected with BTV develop precipitating antibody detectable on an agar gel precipitation test (AGPT) which is not BTV serotype specific. Type-specific neutralizing antibodies can be titrated in a virus neutralization test using BHK21 cells in a microplate against each of the BTV types present or suspected present in the area. Some cross-reaction is seen on the AGPT with antibodies to EHD virus, however a group-specific competition ELISA using monoclonal antibody which does not cross-react with EHD antibody is now available. The viraemia associated with BTV infection can persist up to 120 days, in the presence of neutralizing antibodies. The virus is attached to the red blood cells and appears to be protected from the developing immune response. Intravenous inoculation of sonicated blood into eight to ten-day old embryonated chicken eggs is a very sensitive laboratory method of isolating virus from blood, whereas the inoculation of suspect material directly into sheep and the examination of sequential serum samples for evidence of seroconversion is the most sensitive test available. Virus can also be grown in the yolk sac of six-day old eggs kept between 33.5°C and 35°C, lamb kidney cells, hamster lung cells, BHK21 cells, some mosquito cell lines and following intracerebral inoculation of day old mice. Chick embryos which die from BTV infection have a characteristic haemorrhagic appearance.

Control

Bluetongue is a non-contagious disease and can only spread by the bite of infected *Culicoides* or the direct transfer of blood or semen from an infected to a susceptible animal. Bluetongue may be controlled by eliminating the vector or vaccinating susceptible animals against the serotypes prevalent in the area. Control of insects has usually been directed towards those insects which carry human disease, and experience gained in these programmes could undoubtedly be of value in BT control. However, there would be little economic justification for attempting to control *Culicoides* solely to prevent BT in cattle

Cattle can be protected against BTV infection by vaccination (p. 1018) with live attenuated vaccine, although it would be extremely unlikely for it to be considered worthwhile. The practice of mixing together vaccines against each of the prevalent serotypes may result in the failure of one or more of the serotypes present in the vaccine to replicate (Jeggo, 1986). However, vaccination against one serotype, followed one month later with a second serotype can provide protection not only against the two serotypes in the vaccines, but can provide an het-erologous protection against a third serotype (Jeggo, 1986). There would still be the difficulty of predicting the probable challenge BTV serotypes. The distribution of the serotypes of BTV tends to be dynamic, with some serotypes being present one year to be replaced the following year by other serotypes.

There is no evidence to indicate that BT can be transmitted during embryo transfer using standard techniques. BTV can be transmitted in the semen collected from viraemic bulls, but reports of a persistently infected, seronegative animal (Luedke *et al.*, 1982) have not been confirmed by further research.

Economic significance

The cost of BTV infection in a 1400 dairy cow herd in California, in terms of reduced fertility was $23 000 over a 52-week study period (Osborn *et al.*, 1986). Of particular interest in this study was that the dairyman responsible for the herd was unaware of the passage of BTV through the herd and the associated increase in return to service of the affected animals. There is, therefore, the possibility that BT has a greater economic significance in cattle than previously thought and should not be considered solely in terms of isolated epizootics.

Animals and semen from BTV enzootic areas are subject to movement and export restriction, the costs of which are of greater significance than the direct effects of disease. Many of these restrictions have been formulated on unconfirmed experiments, but they reflect the cautious attitude of the veterinary authorities of importing countries.

(b) Enzootic bovine leukosis

C. Venables and M.H. Lucas

Two forms of bovine leukosis have been recognized, enzootic bovine leukosis (EBL), which occurs in adult cattle and is associated with bovine leukaemia virus (BLV) infection, and, less commonly worldwide, sporadic bovine leukosis (SBL), which affects calves and young cattle and is of unknown aetiology.

Enzootic bovine leukosis

Enzootic bovine leukosis was first described over 100 years ago in Europe. Clinical disease, in the form of multiple cases of lymphosarcoma, occurs most frequently in animals from three to eight years of age. Tumours may develop in peripheral lymph nodes, and are therefore easily detectable, or they may be confined to internal organs, producing rather ill-defined signs. In some areas of the world appreciable economic losses occur through the tumorous form of the disease. Early workers recognized that the disease could spread slowly from known foci to adjoining regions, and because lymphosarcoma often occurred in familial aggregations it was interpreted as evidence that the disease was heritable. It has since been established that EBL is caused by bovine leukosis virus (BLV). This virus was first isolated from mitogen-stimulated, peripheral blood mononuclear cells by Miller *et al.* (1969) in the USA.

The virus

Bovine leukosis virus is an RNA virus belonging to the Retroviridae family. The family includes tumour and non-tumour inducing viruses of many species including man. The virus particle is spherical, 80–100 nm in diameter and enveloped with surface glycoprotein projections. The virus envelope glycoprotein, gp51, is believed to interact with a cell surface receptor, initiating receptor-mediated endocytosis, leading to entry into the host cell. Within the particle are three non-glycosylated protein structures, the matrix, the nucleocapsid and the core. Three enzymes, reverse transcriptase, integrase and a protease, are also packaged within the virion. The retrovirus genome is composed of two identical copies of positive sense, single-stranded RNA. During replication, viral RNA is converted to DNA by means of the enzyme reverse transcriptase. This enables retroviruses to integrate into the host DNA, establishing infection that persists for the life of the animal. Bovine leukosis virus is present in a subpopulation of circulating B-lymphocytes where its genetic information may be found integrated at multiple sites in the cellular DNA. Lymphocytes of BLV-induced tumours appear to be of the B-cell lineage. Tumour cells are monoclonal or oligoclonal for the site of BLV integration. No evidence has been observed so far for a common integration site for BLV provirus in different tumours.

BLV probably does not remain viable for long outside the host environment. It is readily inactivated by exposure to ultraviolet light, heating at 56°C for 30 minutes and pasteurization. The virus can, however, remain viable in blood stored at 4°C for at least two weeks.

Distribution

BLV is distributed worldwide, but with marked regional differences in prevalence. It is most common in North and South America, Australia and some regions of Africa. In Western Europe BLV has largely been eradicated in recent years, but it continues to be common in many areas of Eastern Europe. In addition to causing significant animal health problems, EBL can also represent a major cause of economic loss.

Transmission

Virus is present in colostrum and milk, in tracheal and bronchial secretions and sometimes in nasal secretions and saliva of infected animals. Virus is also found in the cellular fraction of blood, but not in plasma or serum unless haemolysis has occurred. However, it has not been found in faeces or urine and is probably absent from the semen of most infected bulls. Very small numbers of infected blood cells are capable of transmitting BLV. As little as 0.1 µl of whole blood from an infected cow can be infectious when given intradermally to cattle.

Experimental transmission: Cattle can be infected by the intratracheal route, although not as reliably as by the subcutaneous route. Infection can be transmitted by instillation of infected lymphocytes into the nose and by aerosol exposure to cell-free BLV. A calf can be infected orally when newborn, but is probably resistant to infection by this route by three weeks of age. Adult cattle are not susceptible to infection by the oral route. Adult cows can be infected by the instillation of infected lymphocytes into the reproductive tract. Semen mixed with the inoculum may, however, have an inhibitory effect on transmission, and susceptibility of the genital tract of cows may decrease at the time of oestrus. The virus has been transmitted experimentally to sheep and cattle by rectal inoculation of whole blood from infected cattle.

Sheep can readily be infected experimentally by parenteral routes, but not consistently by the oral route. Between 10^3 and 10^6 lymphocytes from infected cattle, given intravenously, are sufficient to infect sheep. Tumours arise at a higher frequency and after a much shorter time than in cattle and may develop after 10 months to three years. As in cattle, various lymph nodes and visceral organs including heart, abomasum, uterus, kidney and urinary tract are commonly affected. Persistent lymphocytosis is not usual in sheep; once the number of circulating lymphocytes rises it invariably indicates the onset of tumour development. In contrast to cattle, contact transmission does not occur when infected sheep are kept in close contact with uninfected sheep. Goats inoculated with BLV orally and parenterally become infected and develop antibody but do not usually develop persistent lymphocytosis or lymphosarcoma. The incubation period in sheep and goats is variable, ranging from about two to 16 or more weeks. Experimental infection with BLV as indicated by persistent antibody production has been reported for chimpanzees, macaques, pigs, domestic rabbits, cats, dogs, deer and rats. There is no evidence for the production of BLV antibodies following BLV inoculation in the mouse, chipmunk, ground squirrel, Japanese quail and chicken.

Natural transmission: Transmission of virus by contact is one of the most important means of spread of BLV in a herd. The rate of spread of virus is influenced by management and husbandry practices that determine the degree of contact between animals. Because the virus probably does not survive for long in the environment and because infectivity is associated with the cellular fraction of secretions it is therefore assumed that transmission takes place by direct exchange of infected lymphocytes in nasal, saliva and tracheo-bronchial fluids and possibly vaginal discharges. The role of milk in transmission under natural conditions does not appear to be very great. The presence of specific antibody in these secretions inhibits virus transmission, and also the susceptibility of the calf to oral infection decreases with age. Vertical transmission of the virus genome via the gametes does not occur. However, congenital transmission by the transplacental route occurs occasionally. Not all infected cows produce infected fetuses and individual cows may give birth to some infected and some uninfected calves. Fetuses infected *in utero* vary in their serological and virological status, and some may develop neoplastic lesions in the lymphatic tissue. Transmission by biting insects may be important in tropical and subtropical climates, but statistical evidence of seasonal trends is inconclusive.

Iatrogenic transmission is probably one of the main reasons for the high prevalence of infection in some herds. Infected blood transferred from one animal to another on a hypodermic needle can transmit bovine leukosis virus. The use of multidose syringes has been incriminated in virus spread, however there is no published evidence to associate intradermal tuberculin testing with an increased incidence of enzootic bovine leukosis. Dehorning and ear tattooing have been identified as possible methods of transmission. It has been suggested that the technique of rectal palpation to examine the reproductive tracts of cows could be a means of transmission if separate clean gloves were not used for each animal.

Transfer of embryos from BLV-infected cows into uninfected cows is not associated with transmission of virus. Virus has nevertheless been found in uterine flush fluid, but this may be due to contamination with blood cells. Virus has not been found in eggs or embryos from infected cattle. Ova, morulae and blastocysts have been exposed *in vitro* to BLV, but after washing no virus could be detected. Embryos similarly exposed to virus were washed and then transferred to uninfected cows, which did not subsequently develop antibodies to BLV.

It was concluded that it was safe to transfer embryos from infected cows providing that the embryos were washed before transfer. Virus transmission to dam or to progeny is not associated with the use of semen from infected bulls for artificial insemination (AI). Naturally occurring lymphosarcoma in sheep is rare. A retrovirus has been isolated from a diseased sheep and was found to be identical to BLV. Where BLV is found in sheep a bovine origin must be suspected. The virus has also been found in capybaras and water buffaloes. Human beings potentially exposed to BLV do not develop anti-BLV antibodies.

Signs

Following infection of an animal with BLV disease progression depends on genetic, environmental and unknown factors. Over 60 per cent of infected cattle are asymptomatic, however almost all develop detectable antibodies. Between 30 and 70 per cent of infected animals show persistent lymphocytosis, but less than 10 per cent develop lymphosarcoma. Persistent lymphocytosis is seen in 28–85 per cent of tumour cases. In BLV-infected cattle with leukaemia the increase in leukocyte count is due to an increase in B-lymphocytes. The percentage of B-lymphocytes in the blood can rise to 80 per cent, compared with normal values of 15–20 per cent. In clinically normal BLV-infected cattle without lymphocytosis there can still be an increase in B-lymphocytes to 40–50 per cent.

Clinical signs (Figs 43.1, 43.2) in animals that develop tumours depend on the particular organ or organs involved. One or more superficial lymph nodes may be enlarged and these can be felt as lumps beneath the skin, especially in the neck and hind flank areas. However, when the internal lymph nodes are the only ones affected diagnosis may be more difficult. Tumours can occur in the abomasum, right side of the heart, spine, uterus, lymph nodes, central nervous system (Fig. 43.3) and the retrobulbar aspect of the orbit. Clinical signs may include depression, indigestion, chronic bloat, displaced abomasum, lameness or paralysis. Abdominal tumours are sometimes detected by rectal palpation during pregnancy examination. Infection with BLV does not appear to be associated with lower milk production, impaired reproductive capacity in either sex, or with mastitis, lesser longevity or increased susceptibility to other diseases. Bovine leukosis virus does not appear to cause significant immunosuppression in the fetus or adult animal.

Diagnosis

Haematology: Herds with a high incidence of lymphosarcoma often contain many clinically normal cattle with persistent lymphocytosis. The development of

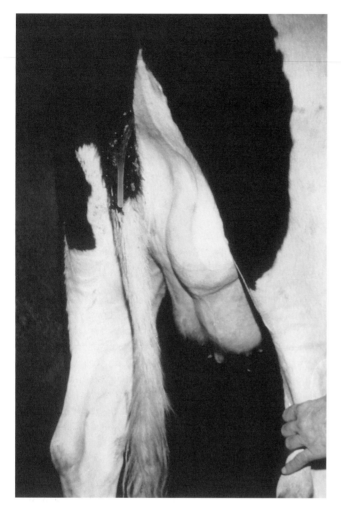

Fig. 43.1   A cow with enzootic bovine leukosis showing enlargement of the mammary lymph nodes. (Courtesy of Dr J. Miller, USDA National Animal Diseases Center, Ames, Iowa, USA and editors and publishers of *Modern Veterinary Production*.)

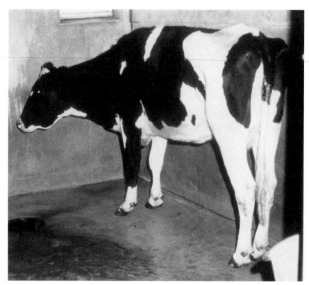

Fig. 43.2   Adult cow with enzootic bovine leukosis showing loss of condition, with wasting of lumbar muscle, brisket and submandibular swelling. (Courtesy of J. Miller, USA.)

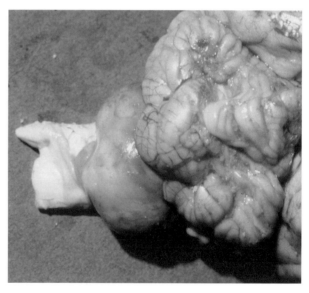

Fig. 43.3   Brain from a cow with neoplasm between cerebellum and medulla. (Courtesy of J. Miller, USA.)

lymphosarcoma is often preceded by persistent lymphocytosis in the absence of any clinical signs. Haematological methods were the main diagnostic tools for a number of years and various 'keys' were developed relating lymphocyte counts and age, presenting maximal values above which an animal was declared to have persistent lymphocytosis. The percentage of B-lymphocytes in normal cattle varies from 18 to 28 per cent. In BLV-infected cattle with persistent lymphocytosis the percentage of B-lymphocytes can increase to as high as 70 per cent. In clinically normal BLV-infected cattle without lymphocytosis the B-lymphocytes are increased to 40–50 per cent.

Serology: The agar gel immunodiffusion test (AGIDT) can be used to detect specific antibody to viral antigens p15, p24 and gp51. The test for gp51 antibody is more sensitive than the p15 and p24 tests or haematology for the detection of infected animals. The test is simple and practical and has been very widely used. The glycoprotein antigen employed in the test is prepared from the supernatant fluid of a cell line persistently infected with BLV.

Using BLV-infected cell monolayers, sera can also be tested for specific antibodies by indirect immunofluorescence or immunoperoxidase techniques. Various neutralization tests have also been described, based on the ability of antibodies to inhibit the effects of BLV in cell cultures. These include a virus neutralization and syncytia inhibition tests. The complement fixation test using viral antigens from a cell line infected with BLV has been used, but seems to be less sensitive than the agar gel immunodiffusion test for antibodies to the gp antigen. A reverse transcriptase inhibition test, based on the fact that serum of some leukaemic cattle inhibits the activity of the reverse transcriptase of BLV, has been described. Radioimmunoassay is very sensitive but has the disadvantage that radiolabelled reagents and special equipment are required.

Enzyme-linked immunosorbent assay (ELISA) is the currently preferred method for the detection of BLV antibodies. The test can be used with milk or tissue fluids as well as serum samples. ELISA is rapid, sensitive and suited to the testing of large numbers of samples. Commercially available ELISA kits, sufficiently sensitive to permit the examination of pooled sera and milk for screening and surveillance, have formed the basis of successful EBL eradication programmes in several European countries.

Isolation and detection of virus: Bovine leukaemia virus particles can be demonstrated by electron microscopy in short-term cultures of lymphocytes from BLV-infected animals. Virus can also be recovered from infected cattle by cocultivation of peripheral blood mononuclear cells with a susceptible indicator cell, e.g. fetal lamb kidney cells. Several passages of the cultures may be required before syncytia can be observed in Giemsa-stained monolayers. Infected cells may be specifically visualized, often in advance of syncytium formation, using immunofluorescence or immunoperoxidase techniques. However, as with other retroviruses, neither electron microscopy nor virus isolation is a particularly sensitive method for demonstrating infection.

Nowadays, techniques including assaying for reverse transcriptase activity or demonstrating the presence of specific BLV nucleic acid sequences are frequently used. Polymerase chain reaction (PCR) assays, generally developed to detect BLV proviral DNA and offering exquisite sensitivity and specificity, are rapidly gaining the advantage over cultural methods in the research, diagnostic and surveillance fields.

Control

Control measures appropriate to any particular situation are largely dictated by local factors. Prevalence of infection is probably the primary consideration, but economics, husbandry practices, cattle movements

and politics may all be significant. Increasingly, driven by trade advantages, EU Member States and other European countries have set in place surveillance and eradication strategies. Many of these have been successful and the countries are now officially EBL-free. The types of actions used, linked with serological monitoring, to produce BLV-free herds are detailed below:

● BLV-positive animals are kept physically separated from BLV-negative animals. Check testing of negative animals is carried out at regular intervals.
● Calves born to negative cows are kept apart from infected animals.
● Calves born from infected cows are reared only on colostrum and milk from negative cows and are kept isolated. If serologically negative at seven months of age these calves join the negative herd.
● Replacement animals should be introduced from sources known to be virus-free, and should be serologically screened. Any originating from herds of unknown status should demonstrate two clear tests at six-month intervals before joining the main herd.
● Embryo transfer and AI are sometimes used as part of a control programme so that new genetic stock can be introduced with minimal risk of introducing BLV.

Where the prevalence of infected cattle has been low, as has been the case in most Western European countries now free of EBL, serological screening followed by slaughter of reactors has been successfully used. However, increased prevalence of infection rapidly makes this approach uneconomic.

Vaccination

Preliminary experiments using inactivated BLV, persistently infected cell lines or purified gp51 indicated that high antibody titres to gp51 could produce some short-term protection to BLV infection. However, no successful vaccine is currently available.

Public health

The structural similarities between BLV and the human T-cell leukaemia viruses, HTLVI and II, have led to speculation about the zoonotic potential of BLV. Serological reactions to BLV p24 in two small studies of people with these diseases and multiple sclerosis have also been reported, but current opinion indicates serological cross-reactions with HTLV proteins to be the cause. This is supported by repeated failure to demonstrate BLV proviral DNA in other studies on human

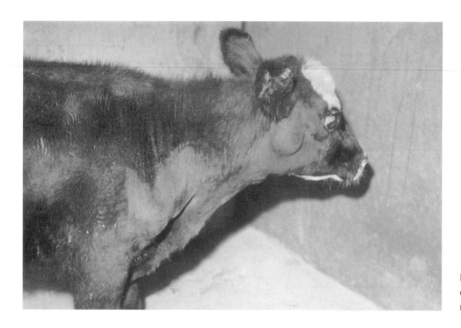

Fig. 43.4 Sporadic bovine leukosis in calf with parotid lymph node enlargement. (Courtesy of J. Miller, USA.)

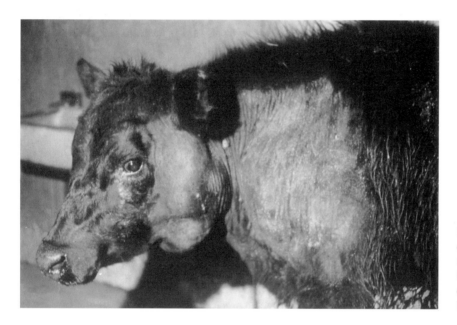

Fig. 43.5 Sporadic bovine leukosis in calf with submandibular, parotid and retropharyngeal lymph nodes on the head and prescapular lymph node enlargement. (Courtesy of J. Miller, USA.)

leukaemia patients and the failure of epidemiological studies to demonstrate a link between BLV and human disease.

Sporadic bovine leukosis

Lymphosarcoma may be found in young animals in the absence of BLV. Three distinct forms are recognized that are collectively classified as sporadic bovine leukosis (SBL):

- The *juvenile* form in calves under six months of age involves lymph nodes, liver, spleen and bone

marrow (Figs 43.4–43.7). During the early stages of disease, marked enlargement of superficial lymph nodes may be the only clinical sign. But as the disease progresses internal organs such as the heart and liver may also become affected, leading to the death of the animal.

- The *thymic* form is seen in animals 6–30-months old. There is massive tumour formation in the thymus and tumorous changes are also seen in the lymph nodes of the neck and thorax (Fig. 43.8). The condition is fatal.

- The *cutaneous* form is a rare condition occurring in animals 18 months to three years of age, in

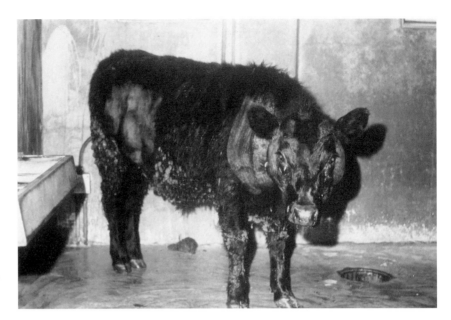

Fig. 43.6 Same calf as in Fig. 43.5 showing gross distension of the head lymph nodes and the prefemoral lymph nodes. (Courtesy of J. Miller, USA.)

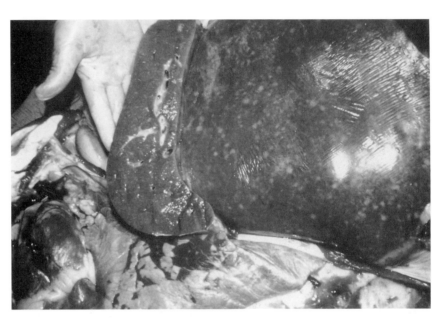

Fig. 43.7 Liver from a calf with sporadic bovine leukosis showing the surface and cut surface with focal neoplastic areas. (Courtesy of J. Miller, USA.)

which nodular lymphocytic neoplasia is seen in the skin. The first signs are urticaria-like nodules (1–2 cm in diameter) in the skin, especially round the neck, back and thighs (Fig. 43.9). These become encrusted with thick scabs, and alopecia and hyperkeratosis follow. Apparent recovery may take place over several weeks (Fig. 43.10). However, the remission is temporary, and lesions reappear together with general lymph node involvement, leading to the death of the animal.

The cause or causes of all forms of sporadic bovine leukosis remains unknown.

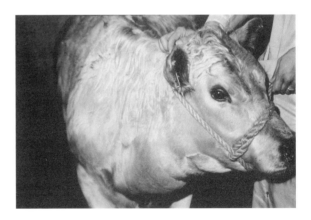

Fig. 43.8 Bullock showing thymic neoplasm. (Courtesy of J. Miller, USA.)

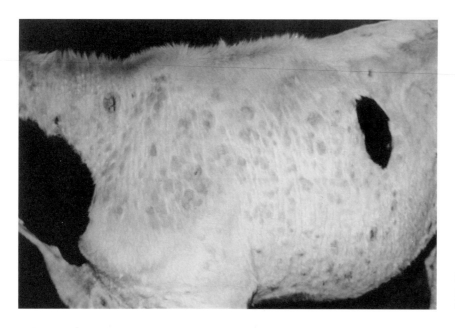

Fig. 43.9 A heifer with acute cutaneous leukosis. (Courtesy of J. Miller, USA.)

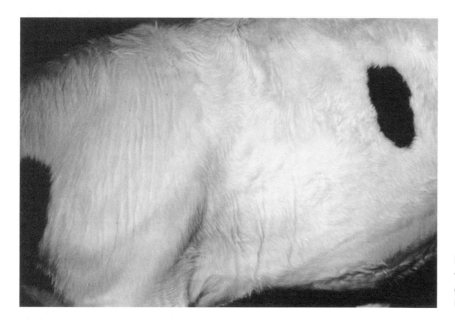

Fig. 43.10 Same heifer as in Fig. 43.9 with cutaneous leukosis lesions subsequently resolving. (Courtesy of J. Miller, USA.)

(c) Foot-and-mouth disease

R.P. Kitching

Foot-and-mouth disease (FMD) is a highly contagious disease of domesticated and wild ungulates characterized by vesicles in the mouth and on the feet. Hedgehogs and very rarely man may also become infected.

Aetiology

Foot-and-mouth disease is caused by infection with a virus of the genus aphthovirus, in the family Picor-

naviridae. There are seven antigenically distinct types of FMD virus, identified as types A, O, C, SAT (South African Territories) 1, SAT 2, SAT 3 and Asia 1. Within each of these seven types there are a large number of strains which form an antigenic spectrum, from closely related strains to strains so antigenically different as to almost justify the establishment of additional types. Attempts to classify the strains into subtypes within the types foundered on the ever increasing number of strains which fulfilled the criteria for creating a new subtype. New isolates of FMD virus are now referred to by the World Reference Laboratory for FMD by their type, country of origin, a sequential number relating to the number of isolates received in that year from the same country and the final two numbers of the year in which they were received, e.g. O India 53/79, Asia 1 India 8/79. The cause of recent infections in Europe, South Africa, Asia, the Far East and the Middle East (Pan Asia strain) was first isolated from an outbreak of FMD in northern India in 1990 (Knowles *et al.*, 2001). Classical subtyping is now only of historical interest.

Aphthovirus has an icosahedral symmetry and a diameter of 24 nm. The outer capsid consists of 32 capsomeres and surrounds a single-stranded molecule of RNA of approximately 8000 bases and molecular weight 2.8×10^6 daltons. This RNA codes for a single large polyprotein which is cleaved into eight non-structural proteins (L, 2A, 2B, 2C, 3A, 3B, 3C and 3D) and the four structural proteins (VP1, VP2, VP3 and VP4), 60 copies of which make up the outer capsid. The RNA base sequence is extremely variable, which is reflected in variations in the amino acid sequence of the proteins for which it codes. The structural characteristics of the outer capsid proteins of the virus stimulate an immune response in the infected host animal. Thus mutations in the genome which change the structure of these proteins can reduce the ability of a vaccinated or previously infected animal to resist challenge with mutated virus.

Distribution

Foot-and-mouth disease is endemic throughout sub-Saharan Africa as far south as Tanzania, and also Equador, Bolivia, Peru, part of Brazil, Columbia and Venezuela in South America and most of the Middle and Far East. Canada, Central and North America, Australia, New Zealand, Japan, Argentina, Chile and South Korea are free of FMD. Most of Europe is also free of FMD, but suffers occasional outbreaks of disease in spite of strict import regulations. When disease occurs, however, it can be severe, as in the European and in particular the British outbreak commencing February 2001. From 1992 routine vaccination against FMD ceased in all countries of the European Union and has since also stopped in Eastern Europe, other than parts of Russia. In Southern Africa FMD virus is usually restricted to wildlife in the game parks, although it rarely escapes into cattle areas bordering the parks.

Types O and A of FMD virus are the most widespread, especially in S. America, the Middle East and Asia; types SAT 1, SAT 2 and SAT 3 are generally restricted to Africa, although they have periodically spread into the Middle East; Asia 1 occurs in the Far East and India, although it also has spread into the Middle East. Type C only rarely causes outbreaks in Asia and has all but disappeared (Kitching, 1998).

Epidemiology

Foot-and-mouth disease is an extremely contagious disease, with as few as ten infectious units being able to initiate disease in a bovine by the respiratory route. The virus can survive in dry faecal material for 14 days in summer, in slurry up to six months in winter, in urine for 39 days and on the soil between three days in summer and 28 days in winter. FMD virus is, however, very susceptible to inactivation by extremes of pH, i.e. below pH 6.0 and above pH 10.0. It is most stable between pH 7.2 and 7.6. Within this range at 4°C the virus can survive in suitable media up to a year but, as the temperature is increased, its survival time is reduced to eight to ten weeks at 22°C, ten days at 37°C and to less than 30 minutes at 56°C. The survival of airborne virus is optimal when the relative humidity is above 60 per cent. Natural ultraviolet light in sunlight has little direct effect on the FMD virus.

Like many diseases, FMD is most commonly spread by the movement of infected animals; of particular significance are sheep, goats and wild ungulates, because disease in them can be mild, and pigs because of the amounts of virus they can excrete. An infected pig excretes up to 400 million infectious units per day, 3000 times more than an infected bovine, sheep or goat. In infected cattle, milk products and semen many contain FMD virus up to four days before the appearance of clinical signs and can also be responsible for the spread of disease. Pigs can carry virus for ten days before disease is manifested. Lorries, fomites and stockmen may also be contaminated with virus from infected carcases, although the reduced pH of the carcase following *rigor mortis* is sufficient to inactivate the virus in the meat.

The possibility of windborne spread of FMD virus has been given considerable significance, particularly in temperate countries where the climate is conducive to the survival of the virus. There is evidence to indicate that FMD virus has been carried up to 250 km over the sea and up to 60 km over land. The spread of disease by the wind is dependent on the amount of virus generated by infected animals, the weather conditions, the topography over which it is carried and the susceptibility of the animals contacting the airborne virus. A plume of virus will be subjected to vertical and horizontal dispersion, which is related to wind speed and turbulence, the vertical air temperature gradient and ground topography; the survival of the airborne virus will depend on relative humidity. Cattle have a large respiratory tidal volume compared with other FMD susceptible stock and can be infected following inhalation of relatively low quantities of virus and thus are most at danger to infection from the airborne virus. Windborne spread of FMD virus is believed to have occurred in 1981 when

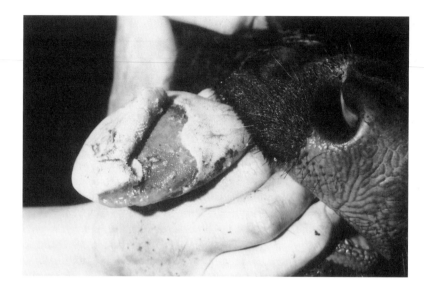

Fig. 43.11 A recently ruptured vesicle in the mouth of a cow with foot-and-mouth disease, showing epithelial separation.

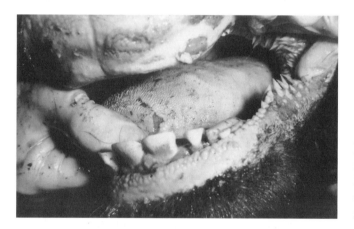

Fig. 43.12 Recently ruptured vesicles on the tongue and dental pad of a cow with foot-and-mouth disease. (Courtesy of A.I. Donaldson.)

infected pigs in Brittany, France, spread disease to cattle in the Isle of Wight, England, over a distance of 250 km, predominantly over sea. Computer models now exist which can predict the likely windborne spread of virus from an infected herd. The maximum daily excretion of virus can be calculated by establishing the number of clinically infected animals and the species infected, and estimating the duration and quantity of airborne virus excreted. The local meteorological office provides information about wind speed and direction, relative humidity and precipitation. When combined with local topographical information and local distribution of livestock holdings, the computer model can give an indication of which herds are most at risk from secondary windborne spread of FMD. Manpower resources for surveillance activity can then be concentrated on the herds adjudged to be at greatest risk.

In tracing the movement of FMD between countries, and identifying specific strains of FMD virus, molecular epidemiology has proved very valuable (Samuel *et al.*, 1997). By precisely characterizing the RNA of an outbreak strain by its nucleotide sequence, it is possible to show its relationship to strains previously isolated in other countries or in use in vaccines. For instance, in Europe between 1970 and 1990 there were a number of FMD outbreaks attributed to the use of improperly inactivated vaccines and escape of virus from establishments producing vaccine. In several instances biochemical analysis of the outbreak strains showed a clear identity with a vaccine strain in contemporary use.

Monoclonal antibodies, which specifically identify some of the individual antigenic determinants on the FMD virus, are becoming important in FMD virus strain characterization. These determinants may change as the virus mutates through the course of an outbreak.

Cattle recovered from FMD and vaccinated cattle in contact with FMD virus may retain virus in their pharyngeal region for many months. This is the carrier state. Vaccinated cattle which have had contact with disease may also develop a pharyngeal infection without showing any clinical signs. The significance of these carrier animals is not clear but, although it has proven difficult to show transmission from a carrier to a susceptible animal under experimental conditions, there is considerable circumstantial evidence supported by sequencing of carrier and outbreak strains suggesting that carriers may have initiated outbreaks.

Transmission and pathogenesis (Figs 43.11–43.13)

Cattle are most susceptible to FMD by inoculation of the virus intradermally into the tongue and this is a

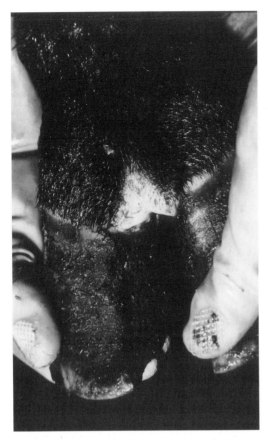

Fig. 43.13 Vesicular lesions of the interdigital skin of the foot in foot-and-mouth disease. (Courtesy of A.I. Donaldson.)

commonly used method of challenging cattle during vaccine trials. However, natural infection is most frequently by inhalation of droplets containing FMD virus or by ingestion of FMD virus contaminated material. One infectious unit of FMD virus is sufficient to infect a bovine by intradermolingual inoculation, while between 10 and 100 infectious units can initiate disease in a bovine following inhalation. Many thousand infectious units may be required to infect an adult bovine by ingestion, although less will be required by a calf following insufflation of infected milk.

The primary site of replication of inhaled virus is in the pharynx and lymphoid tissue of the upper respiratory tract. FMD virus then enters the blood stream, is distributed around the body and following secondary replication in other glandular tissues appears in the body fluids such as milk, urine, respiratory secretions and semen, before the appearance of frank clinical signs of FMD. However, it is during the early vesicular stage of the disease that the majority of virus is excreted into the environment. Milk may contain $\log_{10}6.7$ infectious doses$_{50}$/ml, semen $\log_{10}6.2$ infectious doses$_{50}$/ml, urine $\log_{10}4.9$ infectious doses$_{50}$/ml and faeces $\log_{10}5.0$ infectious doses$_{50}$/g.

An infected bovine can excrete up to $\log_{10}5.1$ infectious doses$_{50}$/day by the respiratory route and can provide a potent source of FMD virus to the remaining uninfected cattle in the herd. This may be sufficient to overcome a waning vaccinal immunity.

The incubation period for FMD can be up to 14 days with low infecting doses and with strains of virus of low virulence. However, as the quantity of virus in the environment of an FMD outbreak increases, the incubation period in cattle decreases. For susceptible cattle in contact with an infected animal it is frequently between two and four days.

Clinical signs

The incubation period is between two and 14 days, depending on the route of infection, the dose, the strain of virus and the susceptibility of the host. Following an initial pyrexia in the region of 40°C (104°F), lasting one or two days, a variable number of vesicles develop on the tongue, hard palate, dental pad, lips, muzzle, coronary band and interdigital space. Vesicles may also be seen on the teats, particularly of lactating cows. Young calves may die before the development of vesicles because of a predilection by the virus to invade and destroy the cells of the developing heart muscle.

The vesicles in the mouth quickly rupture, usually within one to two days of their formation, leaving a shallow ulcer surrounded by shreds of epithelium. The vesicles on the tongue frequently coalesce and a large proportion of the dorsal epithelium of the tongue may be displaced. The vesicles on the feet may remain for two to three days before rupturing, depending on the terrain or floor surface of the cattle accommodation. Healing of the mouth lesions is usually rapid; the ulcers fill with fibrin and by day 10 after vesicle formation they appear as areas of pink fibrous tissue, still, however, without normal tongue papillae. Healing of the lesions on the feet is more protracted and the ulcers are susceptible to secondary bacterial infection. The horn of the heels may become under-run, as a consequence of both the initial vesicle and secondary bacterial infection.

Acutely infected cattle salivate profusely and develop a nasal discharge, at first mucoid and then mucopurulent, which covers the muzzle. They stamp their feet as they try to relieve the pressure on first one foot and then another. They may prefer to lie down and resist attempts to raise them. Lactating cattle with teat lesions are difficult to milk and the lesions frequently become infected, predisposing to secondary mastitis. Affected cattle quickly lose condition; the drop in milk yield can be dramatic and will not be recovered during the remaining lactation. Some animals fail ever to completely regain their previous condition, due to the development of lesions in the thyroid gland – 'hairy panters'.

An outbreak of FMD can be economically devastating in an intensively farmed region. However, in the extensive husbandry systems of South America and Africa, where expectations of cattle productivity are low, FMD may seem insignificant compared with the prevalent clostridial, haemoparasitic and deficiency diseases. This attitude frustrates programmes to completely control FMD and attempts to introduce intensive farming or a dairy industry.

Pathology

The epithelial cells of the stratum spinosum of the skin undergo ballooning degeneration. As the cells disrupt and oedema fluid accumulates, vesicles develop which coalesce to form the aphthae and bullae that characterize FMD. The cells of the squamous epithelium of the rumen, reticulum and omasum may also become involved. In young animals the virus invades the cells of the myocardium and macroscopic grey lesions may be seen particularly in the wall of the left ventricle, giving it a striped appearance (tiger heart). Cells of the skeletal muscles may also undergo hyaline degeneration.

Diagnosis

Initial diagnosis is usually on the basis of clinical signs, with or without a history of contact between the herd and an infected animal or reports of FMD in the vicinity. In a fully susceptible herd the clinical signs are frequently severe and pathognomonic. However, in endemic regions in herds which have a partial natural or vaccinal immunity, clinical signs may be mild and may be missed. All vesicular lesions in cattle should be investigated as potential FMD (OIE, 1996).

The success of the laboratory confirmation of a presumptive diagnosis of vesicular virus infection depends on the submission of adequate material, sent under suitable conditions. A minimum of 2 square cm of epithelium from a ruptured vesicle in a 50/50 mixture of glycerine and 0.04 molar buffered phosphate (pH 7.4–7.6) should be sent to a laboratory designated for handling FMD virus and equipped with the reagents required to type a positive sample.

Diagnosis of FMD is usually controlled by a government department. Where laboratory diagnosis cannot be adequately carried out within a country, samples should be sent by the relevant government department to the regional FMD laboratory or to the World Reference Laboratory (WRL) for Foot-and-Mouth Disease, Institute for Animal Health, Pirbright Laboratory, Ash Road, Pirbright, Woking, Surrey, GU24 ONF, UK. Even

when diagnosis is performed within a country, it is recommended that duplicate samples also be sent to the WRL or regional laboratory for confirmation of diagnosis and strain identification. Details of the method of submission of samples are described by Kitching and Donaldson (1987), although new regulations now also apply to sending pathological specimens by air.

Foot-and-mouth disease virus is very sensitive to pH values away from neutrality and is, for example, quickly inactivated below pH 6. Virus can also be isolated with heparin from vesicular fluid or from whole blood collected from the viraemic animal (up to four days after the initial appearance of vesicles). Although high titres of virus can be recovered from milk and internal body organs such as lymph nodes and muscle, these specimens should only be sent in addition to, and not instead of, epithelium samples. Negative tests on these tissues could be misleading and cause a false sense of security.

On receipt at the WRL, epithelial samples are prepared as 10 per cent suspensions for the enzyme linked immuno-sorbent assay (ELISA). This test identifies virus antigen within the sample and can distinguish between the seven FMD virus types; it has now replaced the classical complement fixation test for FMD diagnosis. Results from this test are available within three hours of arrival. At the same time as the ELISA test is being prepared, samples of the epithelial suspension are inoculated onto primary bovine thyroid cells and pig kidney cells (IB-RS-2 cells). If a clear positive is not obtained from the ELISA test, virus growth on either or both of these two cell systems would provide sufficient antigen after 24 or 48 hours for a second ELISA test. In the absence of virus growth on thyroid or pig kidney cells after 48 hours (first passage) the cells are inoculated onto fresh thyroid and pig kidney cells (second passage). Samples are considered negative following negative ELISA and failure of virus growth after 48 hours on second tissue culture passage, i.e. after a minimum of 96 hours following arrival at the WRL. The polymerase chain reaction (PCR) is also available for detection of FMD virus genome in diagnostic samples.

In countries which use vaccination to control FMD, there is a requirement to relate the outbreak strain to existing vaccine strains. This can be shown using a two-way microneutralization test. Mixtures of field virus and antisera to a vaccine virus, usually prepared in guinea pigs, are incubated at 37°C for one hour and then inoculated with BHK-21 cells into the wells of a microtitre plate. The plates are placed in a 37°C incubator and examined daily for evidence of a virus-induced cytopathic effect in the cells. The titre of serum which neutralizes 100 tissue culture infective dose (TCID)$_{50}$ of virus is calculated and compared with the titre of the same serum which neutralizes 100 TCID$_{50}$ of the vaccine virus. The ratio of titre of serum against field virus to titre of serum against vaccine virus is the r_1 value, and gives an indication of the antigenic relationship between the field and vaccine strains and therefore the probable usefulness of that vaccine in controlling the outbreak of FMD.

A similar r_1 value can be derived using the ELISA (Kitching et al., 1988).

The serum antibody titre against FMD virus of cattle vaccinated against FMD can also be measured using the virus neutralization (VN) or ELISA test. Immunity in cattle to FMD can be correlated with the level of serum antibody at 30 days after primary vaccination, although the relationship is not absolute, being dependent on the challenge dose of virus and the closeness of its antigenic relatedness to the vaccine strain. The VN and ELISA are FMD virus type-specific, so that when used to determine whether an animal has had contact with FMD the tests must be performed separately against each of the FMD serotypes with which the animal may have had contact. In some parts of the world, e.g. Africa, this could be any one of up to six different FMD serotypes. Such testing can be time-consuming, expensive and present results difficult to interpret. A non-type-specific screening test has been developed which estimates the presence of antibody to the non-structural proteins of FMD virus; these are formed in an infected animal as the virus replicates and the non-structural proteins are expressed.

The antigenic characteristics of these proteins are conserved between serotypes. Traditionally the 3D non-structural protein or virus infection associated antigen (VIA antigen or polymerase) was used, but better results, particularly in distinguishing between vaccinated and recovered animals, have been obtained by detecting antibody to the polyprotein 3ABC (Mackay et al., 1998) together with antibody to the 2C protein (Lubroth & Brown, 1995). Both can be produced as pure reagents for an ELISA test by expression in a plasmid vector system. Because animals vaccinated with the dead FMD vaccine produce relatively little antibody to the non-structural proteins (some may be produced against the 3D protein), the tests will also distinguish animals which have been vaccinated – these are positives only for the antibodies to the major structural proteins (see above) – from recovered animals which have antibodies to both structural and non-structural proteins. This would therefore also identify potential virus carrier animals. The problem still remains of how to detect the vaccinated animal which has had contact with live virus and thus become a carrier, but because of its protected status therefore remains negative for antibodies to the non-structural proteins.

Control

The control of FMD depends on prevention of the introduction of virus, prevention of infection of stock and the prevention of spread of virus from infected animals. How this is achieved by individual countries depends on a variety of economic and practical considerations.

Exotic FMD virus may enter an area or country in infected animals and this can include certain zoo animals. Acutely infected animals are usually recognized, but sheep and goats frequently only develop very mild clinical signs. Vaccinated cattle can also develop only local lesions of FMD, particularly in the mouth, and may carry infection if imported to FMD-free areas. The importance of cattle and buffalo that are carrying FMD virus in the pharynx is not proven, although there is ample field evidence of FMD having been introduced with such carrier animals. In order to prevent the introduction of FMD in this manner, FMD-free countries may refuse entry of any ungulate from FMD endemic areas or may insist that any ungulate entering the country has no serum antibody to FMD virus and that oesophageal-pharyngeal scrapings taken by probang are negative for the presence of FMD virus. Any animal vaccinated against FMD is, therefore, prohibited.

FMD virus could also enter in the carcase or products of an animal infected before slaughter. In skeletal muscle the virus is inactivated as the pH of the meat falls as the carcase 'sets', but virus in the bone and lymph glands is not subject to this increased acidity and will escape inactivation. Regulations in FMD-free countries require that meat imported from endemic areas has had the bones and lymph glands removed and may also impose additional requirements such as regular vaccination and certification of the absence of FMD from the farm of origin of the meat, the slaughter house and the surrounding areas. If infected meat should still enter in spite of these restrictions, an additional safeguard is the prohibition of feeding uncooked meat or other swill to pigs. There are many examples of pigs being the first animals to be infected in an FMD outbreak. The Office International des Epizooties (OIE) provides guidelines for trade between countries of different FMD status (OIE, 2001)

The early detection of an FMD outbreak requires the existence of an efficient veterinary service and a rapid diagnostic capability. The World Reference Laboratory, Pirbright, offers a worldwide diagnostic service, although by the time samples are received from abroad an FMD outbreak could be well established. Nevertheless, the service can provide valuable additional support and identify the most suitable vaccine for use to control an outbreak.

Following suspicion of an FMD outbreak the movement of all infected animals must be prevented and local markets and abattoirs closed. The slaughter of all cattle, sheep, goats and pigs on infected premises is practised by countries that do not routinely vaccinate against FMD, and by many countries that do vaccinate, as this will eliminate the source of virus emission and prevent the establishment of a nucleus of potential carrier animals. Cattle, sheep and goats on surrounding farms that have already been vaccinated should be revaccinated with a vaccine antigenically related to the outbreak strain. Pigs are generally also included in emergency vaccination programmes. All previous movement of animals, animal products and other potentially infected material up to 21 days prior to the estimated appearance of the first clinically infected animals must be investigated. This will not only indicate which other farms may develop secondary outbreaks of FMD, but may also identify the source of the infection. Subsequent movement on and off the infected premises must then be kept to a minimum and adequate facilities for cleaning and disinfection provided. Such controllable precautions will identify and considerably reduce the chance of secondary spread. Windborne spread of FMD virus prior to the slaughter of the infected animals is, however, uncontrollable. Numerical models developed to predict this windborne spread can be used to indicate those farms most at risk and have proved their value in helping to control outbreaks of FMD in Europe.

Vaccination against FMD is an effective method for protecting livestock against disease (p. 1016). Only inactivated vaccines are used and they are assessed by their antigen content and the results of potency trials, ideally carried out in fully susceptible cattle (OIE, 2000). An FMD vaccine is most effective against infection with the homologous strain from which the vaccine was prepared. However, a good vaccine must also protect against closely related strains of FMD virus, although its effectiveness will be reduced the more the antigenic characteristics of the outbreak strain differ from the vaccine strain. It is therefore necessary to identify the types and strains of FMD virus that pose the most significant threat. Nowhere has it been necessary to use more than a quadrivalent vaccine, although there are frequent situations when it is necessary to include more than one strain of the same serotype. In addition, the characteristic variability of FMD virus has rendered some vaccine strains no longer effective, and new ones must be introduced.

Maternal antibody can interfere with the development of active immunity in young animals. It is therefore recommended that if calves of immune dams are vaccinated in their first three months of life they should be vaccinated twice more at four and five and possibly again at six months of age. Subsequently cattle should be vaccinated twice yearly, or even three times yearly in areas where FMD is prevalent.

The method used by different countries to control FMD is dependent on a number of factors. Countries free of FMD and protected on their borders by natural barriers such as desert, sea or mountain ranges can maintain their status by strict import controls and can avoid the recurring cost of vaccination or the possibility of initiating an outbreak through the use of improperly inactivated vaccine or escape of FMD virus from a vaccine production plant. In addition, should FMD virus enter a non-vaccinating country it can usually be immediately identified clinically because of the complete susceptibility of the livestock, whereas FMD virus has been known to circulate in countries that do vaccinate without the knowledge of the veterinary authorities. Finally, countries free of FMD which do not vaccinate have a privileged international trading status. However, should FMD virus enter, there is always the possibility of rapid uncontrollable spread, with severe consequences.

Many countries have no choice but to control FMD by mass vaccination. The movement of nomadic people with their animals, and of wild animals across international borders in Africa, the Middle and Far East, makes disease regulations impossible to enforce. The airborne spread of FMD virus cannot be controlled by legislation. Barrier vaccination can reduce the danger of FMD entering a country or area and has been successful in preventing exotic strains of FMD entering Europe through Turkey and Greece, and in allowing South Africa and Zimbabwe to restrict vaccination to their borders and around game reserves. Countries which do not vaccinate or vaccinate against two or three strains may use emergency vaccination to control an outbreak due to a new strain of FMD by slaughtering affected animals and ring vaccinating around the infected area with a monovalent vaccine specifically against the exotic strain.

Economic importance

The economic importance of FMD is hard to quantify accurately. The direct costs of vaccination, slaughter of infected animals, movement restrictions and closure of markets can be measured. The indirect local and national costs, e.g. loss of potential export markets, may be the most significant and yet most uncertain cost.

Assuming that a country wishes to prevent FMD remaining or becoming endemic, two options are available. Either all cattle (and possibly sheep, goats and pigs) are routinely vaccinated or no vaccination is carried out and outbreaks are controlled by slaughter as they occur. Which policy is the most economic can be assessed by critical point analysis or by estimating the critical point at which the cost of one policy equals the cost of the other policy. Costs that must be considered are the cost of vaccine and its administration or its storage as a strategic reserve. If it is also assumed that neither policy will eliminate the possibility of FMD outbreaks, the cost of controlling an outbreak must be assessed and multiplied by the estimated total number of outbreaks.

The cost of an FMD outbreak must include the cost of controlling the outbreak, including ring vaccination, the cost of slaughtered animals, the loss of production and the interruption of domestic and international trade. The international trading status of a country that vaccinates already will be considerably less affected than that of a country that does not vaccinate. Similarly, the status of a country that does not use routine FMD vaccine but vaccinates in order to control an FMD outbreak may be affected by lengthy trade restrictions with other non-vaccinating countries following the cessation of vaccination (OIE, 2001).

The difficulty in assessing these uncertain costs may be illustrated by an analysis of the cost of annual vaccination (policy A) and the cost of a stamping out with ring vaccination (policy B) carried out in the Federal Republic of Germany (Lorenz, 1987). The average annual cost of policy A was estimated to be between 52 and 286 million DM, while the average annual cost of policy B was between 2.5 and 321 or more million DM. The wide range reflected the number of assumed FMD outbreaks that could occur under each regime. The estimates considered most likely, however, were between 183 and 227 million DM for policy A and between 47 and 61 million DM for policy B.

Any scenario for assessing the cost of FMD control must ultimately assume the existence of an efficient veterinary service, capable of diagnosing the disease and with facilities available to control it. Without this infrastructure any, even approximate, estimate of the economic significance of FMD becomes academic.

(d) Rinderpest

by E.C. Anderson

The State Veterinary Service in the UK was brought into being specifically to deal with rinderpest or cattle plague. In the eighteenth and nineteenth century devastating outbreaks of rinderpest were responsible for millions of deaths in cattle in Europe. By 1930, with the exception of parts of Turkey, Europe was free of the disease and since that time only small outbreaks have

occurred. Rinderpest has however continued to persist in Asia and the Indian subcontinent and is still present in Pakistan, India, Bangladesh and Nepal. Occasional outbreaks occur in the Near and Middle East. Rinderpest was introduced into Africa in the early 1800s and was responsible for a massive pandemic between 1889 and 1897. Africa has not been free of rinderpest since, although it has largely been confined to countries north of the Tropic of Capricorn. An international vaccination programme carried out between 1962 and 1975 almost eradicated the disease (Scott, 1985). A second international vaccination programme, commencing in the mid-1980s, has reduced the incidence in West Africa to a level where eradication may be achieved (Rossiter, 1996). Extensive outbreaks have, however, continued in eastern Africa where vaccination coverage has been hampered by civil unrest. The disease is still endemic in the horn of Africa and southern Sudan.

Aetiology

The causal agent of rinderpest is a paramyxovirus of the genus morbillivirus. The other members of the morbillivirus genus are measles, canine distemper, phocine distemper (Osterhaus & Vedder 1988; Mahy et al., 1988; Kennedy et al., 1988) and peste des petit ruminants (PPR) to which rinderpest virus is antigenically related. Recently morbilliviruses have been isolated from diseased marine mammals (Barrett et al., 1993) and a morbillivirus-like agent caused fatal respiratory disease in man and horses in Australia. The morbilliviruses are pleomorphic, enveloped, helical particles of between 150–300 nm diameter and contain a non-segmented negative-strand RNA genome. This codes for six structural proteins and possibly one non-structural protein. The virus structural proteins comprise the nucleocapsid protein (N), which surrounds the genomic RNA, a large polymerase protein (L) and a small polymerase-associated protein (P), a matrix protein (M) associated with the virus envelope and two envelope glycoproteins, the haemagglutinin (H) and fusion protein (F). The P gene shows significant homology between members of the morbillivirus group (Barrett & Underwood, 1985).

There is only one serotype of rinderpest virus and rinderpest virus can be distinguished from PPR virus in reciprocal cross-neutralization tests. Alternatively, the two viruses may be distinguished by comparing their protein patterns in polyacrylamide gels as the N proteins have been shown to have markedly different molecular weights (Diallo et al., 1987). They can also be distinguished by nucleic acid hybridization using cDNA probes to the H gene (Diallo et al., 1989) and by the reverse transcription-polymerase chain reaction (PT-PCR) (Forsyth & Barrett, 1995). It is now also possible to distinguish the two diseases in recovered animals by means of a competitive enzyme-linked immunosorbent assay (ELISA) based on the use of monoclonal antibodies (Mabs) to the haemagglutinin of each virus (Anderson *et al.*, 1991).

The virus is sensitive to lipid solvents, is relatively heat sensitive and is unstable at low pH. It is also labile when exposed to light and survives best at low or high relative humidities but is rapidly destroyed when the relative humidity is between 40–60 per cent. Infectivity is lost when it is suspended in glycerol or water but it is stable in 0.86 per cent sodium chloride at low temperatures with the loss in infectivity rising exponentially with temperature. The use of molar concentrations of magnesium sulphate improves the thermostability of the virus.

Species susceptible

Rinderpest is potentially infective for all members of the order Artiodactyla (Scott, 1964) but in particular infects members of the families Bovidae, Suidae and Cervidae (Plowright, 1968). Of these cattle, water buffalo, Cape buffalo (*Syncerus caffer*) and yak are most susceptible. The disease occurs in sheep and goats and, in India, also in pigs. It also affects camels. It has been recorded in a large number of wildlife species in Africa including eland (*Taurotragus oryx*), lesser kudu (*Tragelaphus imberis*), giraffe (*Giraffa camelopardis*) and warthog (*Phacochoerus aethiopicus*). In 1994 the disease caused significant mortality in buffalo, lesser kudu and eland in the Tsavo National Park in Kenya (Barrett *et al.*, 1998).

Transmission

Rinderpest is spread by direct contact between infected and susceptible animals, by the inhalation of virus-containing aerosols or by ingestion of infected secretions and excretions. On rare occasions it has spread through indirect contact with contaminated fodder and water. Pigs have been infected through eating meat from contaminated carcasses. Different strains of virus vary in their invasiveness and infectivity for different species.

Pathogenesis

Infection is through the upper respiratory tract with primary replication of the virus in the tonsils and local lymph nodes (Plowright, 1968). The virus is disseminated in the blood, where it is closely associated with the mononuclear leucocytes, to all lymphoid tissue and the mucosae of the alimentary and respiratory tracts. The incubation period lasts from two to nine days and viraemia can be detected one to two days before the onset of pyrexia. The prodromal phase usually lasts

from two to five days. The virus is shed in all secretions and excretions, the peak of virus production being during the prodromal fever but continuing after the appearance of erosive lesions. Virus levels fall as antibody begins to be produced with viraemia ceasing before the disappearance of the virus from the tissues, about 14 days after the onset of fever. Viraemia lasts on the average about six days but there is considerable variation between strains of virus. Viraemia can occur following exposure to some strains that lasts four to six days without the development of lesions.

Clinical signs

The clinical signs of rinderpest in cattle and other natural hosts are essentially the same but show wide variations in severity depending on the strain involved, and the resistance of the animal, natural or acquired.

The disease may be hyperacute, acute, subacute or chronic (Plowright, 1968). The typical acute disease can be divided into four phases: incubation, prodromal, mucosal and convalescent.

Incubation phase

Prodromal phase: This is characterized by a sudden onset in fever reaching a peak on the second or third day after onset. It is accompanied by depression or restlessness, loss in appetite and a fall in milk yield in cows. The visible mucous membranes are congested, the muzzle is dry and there may be the beginning of a serous discharge from the eyes and nostrils. There is tachycardia and accelerated respirations, ruminal stasis and constipation. This phase lasts about three days with lesions appearing between two to five days following the onset of pyrexia.

Mucosal phase: The first lesions comprise small foci of necrosis, superficial erosion and capillary haemorrhage in the mucosae of the mouth cavity, which are particularly noticeable on the lower gum and tips of the buccal papillae. They extend to involve the lips, upper gum, hard palate and ventral surface of the tongue. Similar lesions occur in the nasal, vulval and preputial mucosae where they may occur earlier than in the oral cavity. The lesions extend and fuse to produce extensive areas of necrotic erosion with a characteristic fetid smell. There may be excessive salivation and at this stage the lacrimal and nasal secretions become profuse and purulent.

Animals at this stage of the disease are very depressed and respirations are laboured, but pneumonia is rare. Diarrhoea appears usually between four and seven days of pyrexia and one to two days after the appearance of lesions. It is at first watery but later dysentery develops and it may contain pieces of intestinal mucosa. Dehydration is rapid resulting in weakness, prostration and death between six and twelve days after the onset of pyrexia. The mortality rate is over 90 per cent when susceptible animals are infected with virulent strains.

Mild forms of the disease in partially immune animals or following infection with less virulent strains give rise to reduced general signs and less extensive mucosal lesions. However, these may be completely absent with the only sign a transient diarrhoea. Even this may be absent, and some strains of virus result in a complete spectrum of signs from the classical acute febrile disease with extensive lesions and eventual death to a form in which there is fever but no lesions although antigen can be detected in lacrimal secretions (Anderson *et al.*, 1990; Forsyth *et al.*, 2003).

Convalescent phase: Visible mouth lesions may heal within as little as two to three days beginning from the third to the fifth day after their appearance. Diarrhoea may persist for longer. Complete recovery from the acute form takes about four weeks depending on the environment and plane of nutrition.

Pathology

The gross pathology has been described by Maurer *et al.* (1956). The mucosae of the upper alimentary and respiratory tract are eroded and necrotic often being coated with a mucopurulent exudate. Erosions, ulcers and oedema occur in the abomasum, which may also be congested. Peyer's patches in the small intestine are haemorrhagic, oedematous and necrotic. The mucosal surface of the caecum, colon and rectum frequently has characteristic haemorrhagic stripes due to the congestion of the capillaries. Erosion and ulcers also occur in the urogenital tract. The virus has a predilection for lymphoid tissues in which there is extensive necrosis of the lymphocytes of the germinal centres, and the appearance of multinucleated giant cells about eight days after infection. The appearance of cytoplasmic and intranuclear inclusions has been described (Plowright, 1968). The stratified squamous epithelium, particularly of the upper part of the alimentary tract shows syncytium formation and degenerative changes, which are followed by necrosis and detachment to form erosions and ulcers.

Diagnosis

Laboratory confirmation of rinderpest is based on the detection of specific antigens and the isolation of the virus. Retrospective diagnosis is obtained by the detection of specific antibody (Scott *et al.*, 1986).

Antigen detection: Virus is present in the secretions and excretions within two days of the onset of fever. Specific antigen can be detected from this time particularly in the lacrimal secretions but also later in swabs or material from lesions in the mouth, vagina or prepuce. Lymph node biopsies may also be taken.

Early diagnosis is desirable and a rapid chromatographic strip test based on Mab-labelled latex particles is now available for pen-side diagnosis (Buning *et al.*, 1999). The most sensitive method is, however, RT-PCR and this can also be used with lacrimal secretions as well as material from mouth lesions and lymph node biopsies. This method also has the advantage of generating DNA fragments whose sequence may help in defining the origin of the outbreak or differentiating the disease from PPR (Forsyth & Barrett, 1995). Specific antigen can also be detected by the less sensitive immunodiffusion or counterimmunoelectrophoresis (CIEOP) tests in field laboratories. The ELISA is a very sensitive test used in suitably equipped laboratories and is preferable to the complement fixation test (Libeau *et al.*, 1994). Histochemical methods using fluorescein or enzyme-conjugated antiserum may be used on smears, biopsy material or tissue sections (Scott *et al.*, 1986; Saliki *et al.*, 1994).

Virus isolation: Virus may be isolated in tissue cultures of primary or secondary calf or sheep kidney cells or Vero cells. It may be isolated from swabs of lesions or secretions, from the leucocyte fraction of blood collected in EDTA or from lymphoid tissue collected at post mortem. Specimens should be transported on ice but glycerol should not be used as a transport medium, as it inactivates the virus.

Antibody detection: The detection of a rising antibody titre in paired serum samples or in disease surveys may be done using the virus neutralization test. This is suitable for small numbers of diagnostic samples but for disease surveillance requiring the screening of large numbers of samples the ELISA is the test of choice. Other tests that are used include indirect immunodiffusion and CIEOP.

Differential diagnosis

In cattle the one disease that cannot be distinguished from rinderpest without laboratory tests is bovine virus diarrhoea. In sheep and goats peste des petits ruminants is identical to rinderpest. Otherwise there are few conditions that should be confused with the acute form of rinderpest. The mild forms in particular, where diarrhoea is the only clinical sign, are indistinguishable from other enteric conditions.

Control

Rinderpest spreads slowly in endemic countries where it affects mainly immature animals. In these countries control is by vaccination annually of all immatures. In such countries attempting eradication, vaccination of the entire cattle population, as well as sheep and goats in those countries where the disease occurs in these species, for three to five years is practised.

In high risk countries adjacent to endemic regions or those importing livestock from endemic countries quarantine and vaccination are combined (see p. 1013).

All rinderpest vaccines in use are live attenuated vaccines. Most countries use a tissue culture vaccine (Plowright, 1968). New lyophilization techniques have improved the thermostability of these vaccines (House & Mariner, 1995). Goat adapted vaccine and lapinized vaccine are still used in some countries.

(e) Vesicular stomatitis

R.P. Kitching

Vesicular stomatitis (VS) is a vesicular disease of cattle, horses and pigs which can also infect a large range of wild animal species (see p. 366). The virus belongs to the genus vesiculovirus, within the family Rhabdoviridae.

There are two serologically distinct types of VS virus (VSV): New Jersey (NJ) and Indiana (IND). The IND type can be further subdivided into Indiana 1 (Indiana strain), Indiana 2 (Cocal and Argentina strains) and Indiana 3 (Alagoas and Brazil strains). In common with all other rhabdoviruses VSV is a single-stranded RNA virus, the RNA being arranged in an enveloped helical nucleocapsid. The intact virus is bullet shaped, measuring 180 nm by 75 nm, and is covered with 10 nm spikes.

Vesicular stomatitis virus will grow in a wide range of primary cells and continuous cell lines, and laboratory animals such as mice, rats, ferrets, guinea pigs, hamsters and chick embryos. Humans are susceptible to VS, the disease being characterized by fever, myalgia, nausea, vomiting, headaches and occasionally vesicles on the mucosa of the mouth and throat. No deaths have been reported, and the disease rarely lasts more than a week.

Epidemiology

The behaviour of VS in the field has been well documented but in spite of detailed observations there are many aspects of its epidemiology which are still unclear.

Enzootic VS has a limited geographical location, within which the appearance of disease is cyclical, apparently related to season or rainfall. The majority of infections are inapparent and can occur in animals isolated in cages or otherwise separated from other susceptible species. Epizootic spread of VS is associated with simultaneous outbreaks over a wide area, although some herds within this area may remain unaffected. Of the domesticated species, cattle are the most commonly affected, followed by horses and then pigs; sheep and goats never show clinical signs of VS. Few cases are reported in young cattle, most cases appearing in milking cows. Mouth lesions are most frequently reported, although in some outbreaks only teat lesions are seen. Insects have been strongly implicated in the transmission of VS, but this has not yet been conclusively demonstrated. The cyclical appearance of VS suggests the existence of interepizootic reservoir hosts, but these have also resisted identification.

A number of theories have been put forward to explain these observations. It has been suggested that VSV circulates in feral pigs, elk, mule deer and antelope and possibly also in water birds and rodents such as wood rats and deer mice. In support of this theory antibody against VSV has been found in all these species and, in some areas, prior to the onset of a VS epizootic in domesticated animals. It has also been suggested, without much supporting evidence, that VSV could persist in the soil and be circulated by arthropods or even that VSV is primarily a plant virus.

Studies using T_1 oligonucleotide mapping of VSV-NJ (Nicol, 1987) and nucleotide sequencing of VSV-NJ and VSV-IND (Rodriguez, 1999) have helped to identify the origin of VS epizootics in the USA. By precisely characterizing the outbreak strains it has been shown that a VS epizootic is not caused by the simultaneous eruption of many strains of VSV within the United States but the rapid spread of a single strain north from the enzootic region of Mexico. A correlation has been shown between outbreaks of VS in North America and wind direction from VS infected areas, indicating a possible involvement of insect vectors carried by the prevailing wind.

VSV-IND appears to have different epidemiological characteristics from VSV-NJ, and its spread is less associated with clinical disease and has consequently attracted less attention. It is also apparent that the behaviour of VSV need not remain consistent; its mode of transmission, for instance, can vary even during epizootics.

Distribution

VSV is restricted to North, Central and South America and the Caribbean islands. The disease was transported with horses from America to South Africa in 1884 and 1887, and to France in 1915, but did not persist in either country. The first report of VS in N. America was in horses during the American Civil War, and there were further reports in 1889, 1904 and 1907. In South America VS was first diagnosed in Argentina in 1939, in Venezuela in 1941 and in Colombia in 1943.

Indiana 1 and New Jersey strains of VSV are enzootic in southern Mexico and Central America, but a characteristic of both is their periodic movement out of the enzootic areas to cause epizootics in the southern United States and northern South America. VSV-IND has spread as far north as the United States–Canadian border. These seasonal epizootics occur typically at the end of the summer, or in the tropics at the end of the rainy season, and usually finish in the temperate regions at the onset of the frosts. The 1982 VSV-NJ epizootic did not, however, follow this cycle and persisted through the winter. Epizootics which spread into the mid-western and western states of North America tend to occur at intervals of approximately five to ten years, while major epizootics have been occurring every 30 years. The predominant serotype causing vesicular disease in the United States is VSV-NJ, and it is endemic in at least one site in the USA – Ossabaw Island, Georgia. Vesicular stomatitis has not been reported in the New England area, eastern Canada or Alaska.

Transmission

The epidemiological characteristics of VS suggest that the disease is predominantly spread by insects. *Culex* and *Aedes* species of mosquitoes, *Phlabotomine* sandflies, *Culicoides*, *Simulium* blackflies, *Musca* species, *Hippelates* eye gnats and Anthromyidae have all been implicated in the transmission of VS. Transovarial transmission of VSV has been shown in the sandfly *Lutzomyia trapidoi* and biological transmission of VSV-NJ by *Simulium* sp. (Mead & Maré, 1999). However, the very low or possibly absent viraemia associated with VS rules out traditional concepts of vector transmission. The vesicular lesions of clinical VS are rich in virus and could provide a potent source for insect infection, but this fails to explain the transmission of VS between subclinically infected animals. Nevertheless, the climatic conditions which predispose to the spread of VS and the more frequent appearance of VS in animals at pasture strongly implicate the involvement of insects. In addition, the characteristic termination of a VS epizootic with the onset of subzero night time temperatures is typical of many vectorborne diseases. Experimentally inoculated sandflies and *Aedes aegypt* have been shown to transmit VSV to vertebrate hosts (Letchworth *et al.*, 1999). The virus does not appear to be totally dependent on insect transmission, as evidenced by the continuation of the North American 1982/83 epizootic through the winter.

Transmission of VS can also occur by direct contact between infected and susceptible cattle, this being frequently associated with subclinical infections. An association has been made between the feeding of abrasive feeds, which compromise the integrity of the buccal mucous membranes, and the spread of VS.

Clinical signs

Vesicular stomatitis in cattle may be an inapparent, mild or severe disease, animals over nine months of age being most commonly affected. Following an incubation period of two to three days, a usually mild fever develops accompanied by depression, lameness and excessive salivation. The fever reduces as vesicles develop on the coronary bands of the feet, or in the mouth or on the teats; rarely are vesicles seen on more than one of these sites. In severe cases over 50 per cent of the tongue epithelium may be affected and the resultant difficulty in eating can cause dramatic weight loss. Milk yield is depressed. True vesicles may fail to develop, lesions appearing as crusts or ulcers. Recovery is usually rapid, although milk yield frequently fails to recover during the remaining lactation and secondary mastitis may be a problem. Some animals fail to recover fully and remain in poor condition. The lesions produced by vesicular stomatitis virus in cattle are clinically indistinguishable from lesions of foot-and-mouth disease.

Pathogenesis

Vesicular stomatitis virus enters the animal through a skin or mucosal abrasion or it may be inoculated by an infected insect bite. Aerosol infection has been reported in humans and may also occur in cattle. A low titre viraemia has been detected in some experimentally infected animals between 11 and 56 hours after infection, but even this must be considered a rare event. Replication of virus occurs at the site of infection in the prickle cells of the Malpighian layer, but there is no information on subsequent sites of virus replication. As the cells degenerate and transudate from the blood stream accumulates, vesicles develop and the animal becomes febrile. It is not clear why lesions are rarely generalized, but are usually restricted to the teats, mouth or feet. Immunosuppressed or overcrowded animals are more likely to develop lesions. VSV does not cross the placenta and there are no reports of calves from infected dams being viraemic or having pre-colostral antibodies to VSV. However, VSV-NJ has once been recovered from an aborted fetus.

Diagnosis

Diagnosis of VS is by clinical examination of affected animals and the demonstration of the presence of VSV or of a rising antibody titre to VSV. Laboratory confirmation of VS is essential in order to distinguish the disease from foot-and-mouth disease.

VSV has a characteristic appearance under the electron microscope. The virus will also grow on a wide range of primary and continuous cell lines, on the chorioallantoic membrane or in the allantoic cavity of fertile eggs and in many laboratory mammals. The Vero-M (green monkey) cell line is used extensively for the growth of VSV for assay of VS antibodies in the virus neutralization test. The complement fixation test and fluorescent antibody test are also used in the diagnosis of VS, although indirect sandwich ELISA is now considered the most economic and rapid (OIE, 2000). Details given for the submission of samples for FMD diagnosis (see p. 704) apply also to the submission of samples for VS diagnosis, although VSV is much less susceptible to pH outside the range of 7.2 to 8.0. As a differential diagnosis is usually required between FMD and VS, the more stringent requirements of FMD virus should be followed.

Virus neutralization and liquid phase blocking ELISA antibodies may be detected 96 hours after experimental inoculation, and they reach a peak by day 12. These antibodies persist for many years and are valuable in showing evidence of previous infection. Their persistence has led to the suggestion that the virus itself may persist in an animal long after recovery from the disease, although it may remain in a defective, non-infectious form. Complement fixing antibodies recede three to six months after infection. A four-fold or greater increase in VSV neutralizing antibodies between early infection and convalescent serum is diagnostic of infection. The presence of neutralizing antibodies does not appear always to prevent reinfection or the development of clinical signs.

Prior to the establishment of suitable laboratory tests, VS was diagnosed by scarifying infective material into the snout of swine and the tongues of cattle and horses, and by intramuscular inoculation of cattle. VSV produced lesions on pigs, cattle and horses, but not in cattle when given by intramuscular injection. FMD virus produced disease in swine and cattle, but not horses, and vesicular exanthema virus affected only swine, although occasionally lesions were also produced on the tongues of horses.

Control

Measures designed to control VS reflect the poor understanding of its epidemiology, notably the possibility that animals can remain carriers of VSV. It has been observed that recovered cattle have appeared to spread VSV to susceptible animals, and that some of these recovered cattle have again developed vesicles, usually, but not invariably, on a site different from the original area of infection. These recurrent lesions have usually occurred within 48 hours of moving the recovered cattle, and this has led to the suggestion that the recrudescence of clinical disease was brought on by stress. Although it has not been possible to isolate virus from clinically normal animals recovered from VS, the persistence of high levels of neutralizing antibodies in these animals does suggest the presence of a continuous antigentic stimulation.

An additional problem is the high proportion of subclinical cases during epizootics and the possibility that VS could circulate in an area unobserved.

Measures designed to eliminate virus shed in the saliva of infected cattle do reduce transmission; 10 per cent household bleach used on utensils and dairy equipment, and for washing hands, has proved useful. In addition, replacement of hard or abrasive feed with a softer alternative reduces mouth lesions and thereby introduction of the virus.

Within the USA, animals infected with VSV are quarantined for at least 30 days after all signs of VS have disappeared. Countries free of VS are usually considerably more stringent and will not import any animal with virus neutralizing antibodies to VS. This precaution is intended to exclude the possibility of importing a persistently infected animal.

Living and formalin-inactivated vaccines have been prepared against VSV-NJ (see p. 1018). The dead vaccine reduces the incidence of overt disease, while the live vaccine, given by intramuscular inoculation, gives a better protection and does not spread to in-contact susceptible animals. A recombinant vaccine has also been developed by inserting the gene for the VSV glycoprotein into the genome of vaccinia virus. This vector vaccine against VS is reported to be highly effective, but has not been used in the field due to its potential danger to humans (Letchworth *et al.*, 1999).

Economic importance

It is difficult to assess the full economic importance of VS because of the effect the presence of disease has on export markets. Direct losses due to disease can be severe, particularly in high yielding dairy herds, and have been calculated to have been between $97 and $253 per clinical case during the 1982 epizootic in the United States (quoted by Monath *et al.*, 1986). Losses due to reduced growth rates in beef cattle in South America are also reported to be significant. Consequent movement restrictions and the closure of local markets can also cause considerable loss. Nevertheless, it is the exclusion of animals in VS enzootic or previous epizootic areas from countries free of VS that causes the most significant economic losses.

(f) Bovine immunodeficiency virus (BIV)

A.H. Andrews

The virus

The bovine immunodeficiency virus (BIV) is a lentivirus first isolated as strain R29 in the USA from a cow with lymphoproliferative lesions. The organism has also been known as bovine immunodeficiency-like virus, bovine visna virus and bovine lentivirus. The virus is difficult to isolate, thus there have only been two subsequent isolates in the USA and also two in Japan. The virus has a similar morphology to other lentiviruses with a viral envelope of structural gene products and a core of viral nucleic acid, p26 capsid, p16 nucleocapsid, reverse transcriptase and integrase proteins. The RNA genome is 1842 nucleotides in length. While the BIV contains the same non-structural accessory genes as HIV, it lacks the addition gene *nef* found in primate lentiviruses. A genetically related virus to BIV, Jembrana disease virus, has been isolated but is restricted to Indonesia (see p. 766) and causes a severe disease in Banteng cattle (*Bos javanicus*) but a milder problem in *Bos taurus*.

Distribution

Although the virus has been rarely isolated there is serological evidence to suggest that it is distributed worldwide. While it is said to be more prevalent in the southern states of the USA, it is also present in the United Kingdom, Portugal, Switzerland, Croatia, France, The Netherlands, Italy and Germany in Europe. It is also reported to be present serologically in New Zealand, Australia, Canada, China, Korea and Pakistan. It probably is found in other countries but testing is difficult. Serological data suggest the highest prevalence of infection is in the USA and Canada, ranging from 20 to 60 per cent. A recent seroprevalence study in Great Britain suggested a level of 5.9 per cent for dairy cattle and 5.0 per cent in beef cattle (Scobie *et al.*, 2001). While sheep, goats and rabbits have all been infected experimentally, there is no evidence to suggest that this happens naturally. There is nothing to suggest that BIV is of any significant risk to man. It would appear that natural infection is probably confined to cattle. Laboratory workers exposed to infection have not seroconverted. The virus is heat labile and is killed by milk pasteurization.

The disease appears to be expressed in few clinical signs, although in some herds in the USA and possibly in Europe disease can be infrequently expressed. This lack of ability to identify the organism or detect it consistently serologically means that its economic importance cannot be properly assessed. In many instances infection appear to be concomitant with another viral disease, such as enzootic bovine leukosis (EBL) (see p. 693).

In infected animals the infection follows a progression similar to that seen with HIV. Thus the animals have a persistent and chronic lifelong infection. The period of development for natural infection is not known, although following experimental infection cattle become seropositive in two to four weeks. Transmission is thought to be horizontal, although proviral DNA has been detected in the blood and semen of bulls experimentally infected (Gradil *et al.*, 1999). However, transplacental BIV infection has been demonstrated between seropositive dams and their calves (Scholl *et al.*, 2000).

Clinical signs

There is much debate as to the severity of the disease in cattle. It does appear that in many instances the virus causes no detectable signs, although in a few herds it does appear to cause major problems. It has been difficult to define whether the virus caused problems on its own or whether infection predisposes animals to opportunistic infections by other cattle disease pathogens. There is still argument as to whether or not BIV causes true immunodeficiency and this is why it is often referred to as bovine immunodeficiency-like virus.

The main signs in severely affected animals include loss of weight and poor condition, unthriftiness leading to emaciation in some animals. There is a variable degree of lympadenopathy, which may be localized or generalized. Lameness or stiffness may be generalized or result in one or more legs showing lameness. There are nervous signs including changes in behaviour, nervousness, hyperaesthesia and also aggression in some animals, but other cases exhibit depression, dullness and lethargy. Some animals become ataxic and will on occasion fall over. Milk yield is depressed or even absent. A few animals may show prolapse of the third eyelid.

In some infected herds, outbreaks of common disease problems in calves and older animals such as diarrhoea, pneumonia and abortion will result in particularly severe disease in some individuals and not in others.

Pathology

The pathological changes are very variable in extent and severity. In some animals there is lymph node hyperplasia and mild perivascular cuffing in the brain. The most common finding at post mortem examination has involved body lymph nodes which become or contain large spheroidal haemal nodes, black in colour. These haemal nodes vary considerably between infected animals in size, distribution and number (Munro *et al.*, 1998).

Diagnosis

Diagnosis is difficult because the virus is not easily isolated. Thus virus isolation in tissue culture is of limited use as it is of low sensitivity and is also usually complicated by the presence of other viral agents. However, polymerase chain reaction (PCR) techniques have been successfully used to detect the presence of proviral DNA. Very variable results have also been obtained by serological methods. The unreliability of some assay methods has meant that there may have been false positive results during testing in the past. At present, most diagnostic methods involving serology use indirect immunofluorescent antibody (IFA), enzyme linked immunosorbent assay (ELISA) or western blot. The tests most likely to be of use in screening large numbers of cattle would appear to be based on ELISA and one currently in use is based on the TM region of BIV.

Treatment and control

There is no available treatment for BIV infection. The best that can be done at present is to ensure full and adequate treatment of all secondary infections. In some herds where clinical signs have been present it has been the result of management deficiencies such as poor nutrition or poor housing. In some herds where those deficiencies have been improved, the clinical signs have been reduced or become latent.

References and further reading

Bluetongue

Bowen, R.A., Howard, T.H. & Pickett, B.W. (1985) Seminal shedding of bluetongue virus in experimentally infected bulls. In *Bluetongue and Related Orbiviruses* (ed. by T.L. Barber & M.M. Jochim), Progress in Clinical and Biological Research, Vol. 178, pp. 91–6. Alan R. Liss Inc., New York.

Gorman, B.M., Taylor, J. & Walker, P.J. (1983) Orbiviruses. In *The Reoviridae* (ed. by W.K. Joklik), pp. 287–357. Plenum, New York.

Jeggo, M.H. (1986) A review of the immune response to bluetongue virus *Revue Scientifique et Technique d'Office International des Epizooties*, **5**, 357–62.

Luedke, A.J., Jochim, M.M. & Barber, T.L. (1982) Serologic and virologic responses of a Hereford bull persistently infected with bluetongue virus for eleven years. *Proceedings of the American Association of Veterinary Laboratory Diagnostics*, **25**, 115–34.

Mertens, P.P.C., Burroughs, J.N. & Anderson, J. (1987) Purification and properties of virus particles, infectious subviral particles, and cores of bluetongue virus serotypes 1 and 4. *Virology*, **157**, 375–86.

Osborn, B.I., Huffman, E.M., Sawyer, I.N. & Hird, D. (1986) Economics of bluetongue in the United States. In *Arbovirus Reseach in Australia, Proceedings 4th Symposium*, Brisbane, May 1986, pp. 245–7.

Verwoerd, D.W., Els, H.J., DeVilliers, E.M. & Huismans, H. (1972) The structure of the bluetongue virus capsid. *Journal of Virology*, **10**, 783–94.

Enzootic bovine leukosis

Burny, A., Brock, C., Chantrenne, H., Cleuter, Y., Dekegel, D., Ghysdael, J., Kettman, R., Leclercq, M., Leunen, J., Mammerickx, M. & Portetelle, D. (1980) Bovine leukemia virus. In *Molecular Biology and Epidemiology in Viral Oncology* (ed. by G. Klein), pp. 231–89. Raven Press, New York.

Burny, A., Bruck, C., Cleuter, Y., Couez, D., Deschamps, J., Ghysdael, J., Gregoire, D., Kettmann, R., Mammerickx, M., Marbaix, G. & Portetelle, D. (1985) Bovine leukaemia virus: a tantalizing story. In *Viruses and Cancer* (ed. by P.W.J. Rigby & N.M. Wilkie), pp. 197–216. Cambridge University Press, Cambridge.

Burny, A., Bruck, C., Cleuter, Y., Couez, D., Deschamps, J., Gregoire, D., Ghysdael, J., Kettman, R., Mammerickx, M., Marbaix, G. & Portetelle, D. (1985) Bovine leukaemia virus and enzootic bovine leukosis. *Onderstepoort Journal of Veterinary Research*, **52**, 133–44.

Burny, A., Bruck, C., Cleuter, Y., Couez, D., Gregoire, D., Kettmann, R., Mammerickx, M., Marbaix, G., Portetelle, D. & Willems, L. (1986) Bovine leukemia virus as an inducer of bovine leukemia. In *Animal Models of Retrovirus Infection and their Relationship to AIDS* (ed. by L.A. Saizman), pp. 107–19. Academic Press, New York.

Callebaut, I., Burny, A., Krchnak, V., Grasse-Masse, H., Wathetet, B. & Portetelle, D. (1991) Use of synthetic peptides to map sequential epitopes recognised by monoclonal antibodies to bovine leukaemia virus external glycoprotein. *Virology*, **185**, 48–55.

Callebaut, I., Portetelle, D., Burny, A. & Mornon, J.-P. (1994) Identification of functional sites on bovine leukaemia virus glycoproteins using structural and immunological data. *European Journal of Biochemistry*, **222**, 405–14.

Evermann, J.F. (1983) Bovine leukemia virus infection. *Modern Veterinary Practice*, **64**, 103–105.

Ferrer, J.F. (1980) *Bovine Lymphosarcoma*. Advances in Veterinary Science and Comparative Medicine, Vol. 24. Academic Press, New York.

Ghysdael, J., Bruck, C., Kettman, R. & Burny, A. (1984) Bovine leukemia virus. In *Current Topics in Microbiology and Immunology* (ed. by M. Cooper *et al.*), Vol. 112, pp. 1–19, Springer-Verlag, Berlin.

Miller, J.M., Miller, L.D., Olson, C. & Gillette, K.G. (1969) Virus-like particles in phytohaemagglutinin-stimulated lymphocyte cultures with reference to bovine lymphosarcoma. *Journal of the National Cancer Institute*, **43**, 1297–305.

Parodi, A.L. (1986) Enzootic bovine leukosis. Its aetiology, epidemiology and principles of control. *Pro Veterinario*, **i**, 1–4.

Schultz, R.D., Manning, T.O., Rhyan, J.C., Buxton, B.A., Panangala, V.S., Bause, I.M. & Yang, W.C. (1986) Immunologic and virologic studies on bovine leukosis. In *Animal Models of Retrovirus Infection and their Relationship to AIDS* (ed. by L.A. Saizman), pp. 301–23. Academic Press, New York.

Foot-and-mouth disease

Kitching, R.P. (1998) A recent history of foot-and-mouth disease. *Journal of Comparative Pathology*, **118**, 89–108.

Kitching, R.P. & Donaldson, A.I. (1987) Collection and transportation of specimens for vesicular virus investigation. *Revue Scientific et Techniques d'Office International des Epizooties*, **6**, 263–72.

Kitching, R.P., Knowles, N.J., Samuel, A.R. & Donaldson, A.I. (1989) Development of foot-and-mouth disease virus strain characterisation – a review. *Tropical Animal Health and Production*, **21**, 153–66.

Kitching, R.P., Rendel, R. & Ferris, N.P. (1988) Rapid correlation between field isolates and vaccine strains of foot-and-mouth disease virus. *Vaccine*, **6**, 403–408.

Knowles, N.J., Samuel, A.R., Davies, P.R., Kitching, R.P. & Donaldson, A.I. (2001) Outbreak of foot-and-mouth disease virus serotype O in the UK caused by a pandemic strain. *Veterinary Record*, **148**, 258–9.

Lorenz, R.J. (1987) Guide to the economic evaluation of FMD vaccination programmes. Report of the 27th Session of the European Commission for the control of FMD. Appendix 12, pp. 121–36. Rome, 21–24 April 1987.

Lubroth, J. & Brown, F. (1995). Identification of native foot-and-mouth disease virus non-structural protein 2C as a serological indication to differentiate infected from vaccinated livestock. *Research in Veterinary Science*, **59**, 70–8.

Mackay, D.K.J., Forsyth, M.A., Davies, P.R., Berlinzani, A., Belsham, G.J., Flint, M. & Ryan M.D. (1998) Differentiating infection from vaccination in foot-and-mouth disease using a panel of recombinant, non-structural proteins in ELISA. *Vaccine*, **16**, 446–59.

OIE (2000) *OIE Manual of Standards for Diagnostic Tests and Vaccines*, 4th ed., pp. 77–92. Office International des Épizooties, Paris.

OIE (2001) *International Animal Health Code*, pp. 63–75. Office International des Épizooties, Paris.

Samuel, A.R., Knowles, N.J., Kitching, R.P. & Hafez, S.M. (1997) Molecular analysis of foot-and-mouth disease type O viruses isolated in Saudi Arabia between 1983 and 1995. *Epidemiology and Infection*, **119**, 381–9.

Rinderpest

Anderson, E.C., Hassan, A., Burrett, T. & Anderson, J. (1990) Observations on the pathogenicity for sheep and goats and the transmissibility of the strains of virus isolated during the rinderpest outbreak in Sri Lanka in 1987. *Veterinary Microbiology*, **21**, 309–18.

Anderson, J., MaKay, J.A. & Butcher, R.N. (1991) The use of monoclonal antibodies in competitive ELISA for the detection of antibodies to rinderpest and peste des petits ruminants viruses. In *The Sero-monitoring of Rinderpest Throughout Africa, Phase One*. Proceedings of the Final Research Co-ordination Meeting of the IAEA Rinderpest Control Projects, Ivory Coast, November, 1990. IAEA publication TECDOC-623.

Barrett, T. & Underwood, B. (1985) Comparison of messenger RNAs induced in cells infected with each member of the Morbillivirus group. *Virology*, **145**, 195–9.

Barrett, T., Visser, I.K.G., Maemaev, L., Goatley, L., van Bressem, M.-F. & Osterhaus, A.D.M.E. (1993) Dolphin and porpoise morbilliviruses are genetically distinct from phocine distemper virus. *Virology*, **193**, 1010–12.

Barrett, T., Forsyth, M.A., Inui, K., Wamwayi, H.M., Kock, R., Wambua, J., Mwanzia, J. & Rossiter, P. (1998) Rediscovery of the second African lineage of rinderpest virus: its epidemiological significance. *Veterinary Record*, **142**, 669–71.

Buning, A., Bellamy, K., Talbot, D. & Anderson, J. (1999) A rapid chromatographic strip test for pen-side diagnosis of rinderpest virus. *Journal of Virological Methods*, **81**, 143–54.

Diallo, A., Barrett, T., Lefevre, P.C. & Taylor, W.P. (1987) Comparison of proteins induced in cells infected with rinderpest and peste des petits ruminants viruses. *Journal of General Virology*, **68**, 2033–8.

Diallo, A., Barrett, T., Barbron, M., Subbarao, S.M. & Taylor, W.D. (1989) Differentiation of rinderpest and peste de petits ruminants viruses using specific cDNA clones. *Journal of Virological Methods*, **23**, 127–436.

Forsyth, M.A. & Barrett, T. (1995) Evaluation of polymerase chain reaction for the detection and characterisation of rinderpest and peste des petits ruminants viruses for epidemiological studies. *Virus Research*, **39**, 151–63.

Forsyth, M.A., Parida, S., Alexandersen, S., Belsham, G.T. & Barrett, T. (2003) Rinderpest virus lineage differentiation using RT-PCR and SNAP-ELISA. *Journal of Virological Methods*, **107**, 29–36.

House, J.A. & Mariner, J.C. (1995) Stabilisation of rinderpest vaccine by modification of the lyophilisation process. New approaches to stabilisation of vaccine potency, WHO Headquarters, Geneva, 29–31 May 1995 (ed. by F. Brown). Karger, Basel. *Developments in Biological Standardisation* (1996) **87**, 235-44.

Kennedy, S., Smyth, J.A., McCullough, S.J., Allan, G.M., McNeilly, F. & McQuaid, S. (1988) Confirmation of cause of recent seal deaths. *Nature*, **335**, 404.

Libeau, G., Diallo, A., Colas, F. & Guerre, L. (1994) Rapid differential diagnosis of rinderpest and PPR using immunocapture ELISA. *Veterinary Record*, **134**, 300–304.

Mahy, B.W.J., Barrett, T., Evans, S., Anderson, E.C. & Bostock, C.J. (1988) Characterization of a seal morbillivirus. *Nature*, **336**, 115.

Maurer, F.D., Jones, T.C., Easterday, B. & Detray, D.E. (1956) Pathology of rinderpest. *Journal of the American Veterinary Medical Association*, **127**, 512–14.

Osterhaus, A.D.M.E. & Vedder, E.J. (1988) Identification of virus causing recent seal deaths. *Nature*, **335**, 20.

Plowright, W. (1968) *Rinderpest Virus*, Virology Monographs No. 3. Springer-Verlag, Berlin.

Rossiter, P. (1996) Epidemiological and clinical features of rinderpest in the 1990s. *FAO Animal Production and Health Paper*, **129**, 67–9.

Saliki, J.T., Brown, C.C., House, J.A. & Dubovi, E.J. (1994) Differential immunohistochemical staining of peste des petits ruminants and rinderpest antigens in formalin-fixed, paraffin-embedded tissues using monoclonal and polyclonal antibodies. *Journal of Veterinary Diagnostic Investigation*, **6**, 96–8.

Scott, G.R. (1964) Rinderpest. *Advances in Veterinary Science*, **9**, 113–224.

Scott, G.R. (1985) Rinderpest in the 1980s. *Progress in Veterinary Microbiology and Immunology*, **1**, 145–74.

Scott, G.R., Taylor, W.P. & Rossiter, P.B. (1986) *Manual on the Diagnosis of Rinderpest*. Food and Agriculture Organization of the United Nations, Rome.

Vesicular stomatitis

Letchworth, G.J., Rodriguez, L.C. & Barrera, J. del C (1999) Vesicular stomatitis. *Veterinary Journal*, **157**, 239–60.

Mead, D.G. & Maré, C.J. (1999) Vector competence of wild and colonized black flies to the Indiana and New Jersey serotypes of vesicular stomatitis virus. *Annals of the New York Academy of Science* **916**.

Monath, T.P., Webb, P.A., Francy, O.B. & Walton, T.E. (1986) The epidemiology of vesicular stomatitis – new data, old puzzles. In *Proceedings of the 4th Symposium Arbovirus Research in Australia*, CSIRO pp. 193–8. Brisbane, May 1986.

Nicol, S.T. (1987) Molecular epizootiology and evolution of vesicular stomatitis *Journal of Virology*, **61**, 1029–36.

OIE (2000) *OIE Manual of Standards for Diagnostic Tests and Vaccines*, 4th edn. Office International des Epizooties, Paris.

Rodriguez, L.L. (1999) Genetic and epidemiological evidence indicates that vesicular stomatitis virus are not endemic in northern Mexico and south western USA. *Annals of the New York Academy of Science* **916**.

Bovine immunodeficiency virus

Gradil, C.M., Watson, R.E., Renshaw, R.W., Gilbert, R.O. & Dubovi, E.J. (1999) Detection of bovine immunodeficiency-like virus DNA in the blood and semen of experimentally infected bulls. *Veterinary Microbiobogy*, **70**, 21–31.

Munro, R., Lysons, R., Venables, C., Horigan, M., Jeffrey, M. & Dawson, M. (1998) Lymphadenopathy and non-suppurative meningo-encephalitis in calves experimentally infected with bovine immunodeficiency-like virus (FL112). *Journal of Comparative Pathology*, **119**, 121–34.

Scholl, D.T., Truax, R.E., Baptista, J.M., Ingawa, K., Orr, K.A., O'Reilly, K.L. & Jenny, B.F. (2000) Natural transplacental infection of dairy calves with bovine immunodeficiency virus and estimation of effect on neonatal health. *Preventive Veterinary Medicine*, **43**, 239–52.

Scobie, L., Venables, C., Sayers, A.R., Weightman, S. & Jarrett, O. (2001) Prevalence of bovine immunodeficiency virus infection in cattle in Great Britain. *Veterinary Record*, **149**, pp. 459–60.

Chapter 44
Bacterial Conditions

A.H. Andrews and the late B.M. Williams

Anthrax   717
Bacillary haemoglobinuria   719
Botulism   721
Clostridial myositis: blackleg and malignant oedema   723
    Blackleg   723
    Malignant oedema   724
Contagious bovine pyelonephritis   725
Endocarditis   726
Haemorrhagic septicaemia   728
Infectious necrotic hepatitis (black disease)   729
Pericarditis   731
Tetanus   733
Leptospirosis (other than *Leptospira hardjo* infection)   734
Leptospira hardjo infection (flabby bag)   735
Haemophilus somnus infection   737
Pyaemia   737

Anthrax

Bacillus anthracis infection in cattle causes a per-acute or acute disease, which is characterized by a septicaemia and sudden or rapid death. The disease is a zoonosis and is subject to official control measures in a number of countries. Infection in man usually results in the cutaneous form of the disease. Inhalation producing 'woolsorter's disease' is very severe but uncommon.

Aetiology

Bacillus anthracis is a Gram-positive capsulated bacillus and its morphology, together with the staining reaction of the capsula, is of diagnostic importance. When stained by Giemsa's, Wright's or similar stains, the capsule stains a reddish mauve colour, is square ended and its outline is rather ragged or 'shaggy' (Plate 44.1). A similar reaction is produced by methylene blue, but because of the variability in the content of its oxidized products, azur A and B, which have an affinity for the capsule, the staining reaction is less consistent and the staining of the capsule is a less intense mauve colour. The organism produces a lethal toxin that causes death through shock and acute renal failure.

The organism is a spore-forming bacillus, but mature spores are not formed in the animal before death. The vegetative bacilli are not very resistant to environmental conditions or to physical and chemical agents, and are rapidly destroyed by putrefactive processes in unopened carcasses (Sterne, 1959). However, sporulation occurs when carcasses are opened or when discharges containing bacilli are exposed to air. Mature spores are extremely resistant to environmental conditions and certain disinfectants, and in soil they remain viable for many years.

Anthrax has been reported from most if not all cattle rearing countries of the world, but the incidence of disease is dependent on a number of factors, including climate, soil, animal husbandry and disease control methods. Serious outbreaks of disease are more commonly encountered in tropical and subtropical countries. In such areas, infection persists in the soil – spores can survive for decades – and is a major source of infection. The disposal of animal carcasses also presents a serious problem unless whole carcasses are removed. Otherwise cattle and other animals readily come into contact with the tissues, particularly bones, of animals that die from anthrax. This method of infection is very important in phosphorus deficient areas where cattle develop pica and chew bones in an attempt to remedy the deficiency.

In temperate countries sporadic outbreaks occur involving single or a small number of animals, arising from the ingestion of contaminated feedingstuffs. Campbell (1969) reported that the vast majority of anthrax outbreaks in cattle in England and Wales were associated with compound feedingstuffs containing meat and bone meal derived from imported materials from Asia and South America, but he also emphasized that often vegetable protein became contaminated with anthrax organisms in the holds of ships that were being or had been used for the transport of meat and bone meal. Hugh-Jones & Hussaini (1975) confirmed that in Great Britain, contaminated feedingstuffs were the major source of infection, although infection was sometimes derived from tannery effluent and soil at sites where the carcasses of animals had been buried some years previously.

Infection is acquired through the ingestion of soil or effluent-contaminated fodder or contaminated compound feedingstuffs. Schlingham *et al.* (1956) have demonstrated that clinical disease in cattle can be regularly produced by the oral administration of organisms in feed pellets. The spores penetrate the intact mucosa, or through small abrasions in the mucosa of the mouth and pharynx, and are then transported to the local lymph nodes where germination and multiplication occurs, followed by passage via the lymphatics into the bloodstream, leading to a septicaemia with an explosive invasion of all body tissues.

Signs

All ages of cattle are susceptible to infection. The incubation period is thought to be one to two weeks, although in some incidents it would appear to be three to five days.

At the beginning of an outbreak, the peracute form of the disease is more common, animals usually being found dead within a few hours of being seen in normal health. On the rare occasions that animals are seen ailing, fever, muscle tremors, dyspnoea, collapse and terminal convulsions are the predominant signs, with death occurring in 1–4 hours. In the acute form, which runs a course of 24–48 hours, fever, depression, rapid and laboured respirations, diarrhoea or dysentery, haemorrhagic congestion of the visible mucous membranes and in dairy cattle a sudden drop in milk yield are the main signs. Pregnant animals may abort.

Atypical signs have been recorded in calves receiving prophylactic levels of oxytetracycline or chlortetracycline for the control of salmonellosis. In such animals, a mild fever, bleeding from the nose and eyes and melaena were the only signs observed before death, which occurred 48–72 hours after onset (B.M. Williams, unpublished data).

Pathology

Because of the peracute/acute nature of the disease in cattle, there is little opportunity for ante-mortem laboratory examinations. It may be possible to detect organisms in appropriately stained smears of peripheral blood, but sufficient numbers of organisms are only likely to be present during the later stages of the disease. A haematological examination may reveal a leucocytosis and a shift to the left, but because of the relatively short course of the disease, these changes are not marked.

Before a necropsy is carried out on an animal that has died suddenly or after a very short illness, it is essential that anthrax be eliminated, to prevent contamination of the environment and ensure proper disposal of the carcass. Thus a careful evaluation of the circumstances and a thorough preliminary examination of the carcass must be carried out. If anthrax cannot be eliminated, then a blood sample should be taken from a superficial blood vessel and a stained smear examined microscopically. It is more difficult to identify anthrax bacilli if animals have been treated with antibiotics. The procedures for dealing with suspected anthrax cases vary from country to country and those currently in force in Great Britain are discussed below.

Rapid decomposition of the carcass sets in soon after death and in most instances rigor mortis is absent and dark tarry blood exudes from all the body orifices. There is bloodstained fluid in all body cavities and there are widespread haemorrhages throughout the carcass, particularly on the parietal pleura and peritoneum. Unclotted or poorly clotted blood oozes from the cut blood vessels and there is an intense inflammation of the mucosa of the abomasum and both small and large intestine. The spleen is almost invariably greatly enlarged with sometimes a rupture of the capsule, and a dark semifluid pulp. The lesions in animals that have been treated with antibiotics before death are similar but much less spectacular.

Diagnosis

The diagnosis of anthrax is based on the demonstration of capsulated bacilli in peripheral blood and subsequent confirmation by laboratory isolation and identification. In Great Britain and many other countries, anthrax is a notifiable disease and the State Veterinary Service is responsible for confirmation.

There are numerous causes of sudden death in cattle, including clostridial infections, hypomagnesaemia, lead poisoning and lightning strike, all of which can be confirmed by a post-mortem examination and appropriate laboratory examinations. As emphasized earlier, such procedures should not be undertaken until anthrax has been eliminated.

Treatment and prevention

Bacillus anthracis is sensitive to a number of antibiotics and treatment of animals during the early stages of the disease is likely to be successful, although severely ailing animals are unlikely to recover. Greenough (1965) successfully treated animals with 5 megaunits of penicillin alone or with streptomycin. The recommended dosage of penicillin is 10 000 units/kg body weight administered twice daily for at least three to five days. Streptomycin, in 4–5 g doses, should also be administered twice daily for the same period. Lincoln *et al.* (1964) consider that septicaemic anthrax is best treated with a combination of large doses of penicillin and streptomycin twice daily, although oxytetracycline and chlortetracycline are the next antibiotics of choice.

Bailey (1953) also recommends tetracycline for the treatment of anthrax. Anthrax antiserum administered intravenously is effective but the high cost and large volumes required makes its routine use impractical.

When anthrax has been confirmed in a herd, all animals should be carefully observed at frequent intervals and any that are showing signs of ill health isolated, their temperatures taken and, if elevated, immediately treated with antibiotic.

In Great Britain and elsewhere, anthrax is a notifiable disease under the provisions of the Anthrax Order of 1938 for the protection of both animal and human health. An owner or veterinary surgeon must report any suspicion of disease to a police constable, who informs the Local Authority, which then immediately imposes restrictions on the movement of animals onto and off the premises. The carcass(es) of the suspected animal(s) must be detained and the skin must not be incised other than for the removal of a blood sample for diagnostic purposes by the owner's veterinary surgeon or a veterinary officer appointed by the Minister, usually the Divisional Veterinary Manager or a veterinarian acting on his/her behalf.

This State Veterinary Service is responsible for the disease investigation and a stained smear is made from a superficial blood vessel and examined microscopically. If the Veterinary Inspector is satisfied that disease does not exist, the Local Authority is informed and the movement restrictions are withdrawn. If the inspector is not satisfied, an unfixed blood smear and a sample of blood is submitted to the Central Veterinary Laboratory for cultural and biological examination and the Local Authority informed accordingly: On receipt of this information the Local Authority is responsible for disposal of the carcass, usually by burning, and carrying out disinfection of the premises as prescribed in the Order. The disinfectants of choice are 5 per cent lysol, 5 per cent formalin or 5–10 per cent caustic soda. When these procedures have been completed, movement restrictions are withdrawn.

Confirmation of the disease is dependent on the results of the examinations at the Central Veterinary Laboratory, which may take seven or more days. On rare occasions disease is not confirmed; even so the existing procedures are considered effective in view of the serious nature of the disease and the human health implications.

Where enzootic disease exists, then an avirulent spore vaccine is available, and all cattle should be vaccinated on an annual basis. Vaccination is seldom necessary in Great Britain (see p. 1005).

The number of confirmed incidents in Great Britain is now very low. This is largely due to the efforts of feedingstuffs compounders, who no longer use meal and bonemeal (MBM) in their feeds. In other countries, where MBM can be legally used, it is essential to use sterilized meal and minerals in their finished feeds.

Bacillary haemoglobinuria

Bacillary haemoglobinuria or infectious ictero-haemoglobinuria of cattle was described by Roberts (1959) as a rapidly fatal infectious disease, manifested clinically by a high fever and haemoglobinuria, and pathologically by the presence of an infarct in the liver.

Aetiology

The causal organism is *Clostridium novyi* type D, previously designated *Cl. haemolyticum*. Like other clostridia it is a soil-borne anaerobe, the spores of which are resistant to environmental factors and may survive in soil for weeks if not months. The disease is considered to be one essentially of poorly irrigated or wet swampy land, which favours survival of the organism and is likely to harbour *Lymnaea* spp., the host snail of the liver fluke. The principal toxin produced by the organism is beta, which is haemolytic, necrotizing and lethal.

After ingestion the organism is transported from the alimentary tract to various organs. Smith (1957) recovered the organism from the liver, kidneys and bone marrow of normal cattle, where it remains as a latent infection. It is thought that, as in infectious necrotic hepatitis, the latent spore infection is activated by liver damage, especially by migrating immature liver fluke. The disease has been produced experimentally by infecting calves orally with the spores of *Cl. novyi* type D and carrying out a liver biopsy, and by implanting the organism in the liver suspended in calcium chloride solution (Blood *et al.*, 1983). It has also been postulated that telangiectasis may also be a precipitating factor.

When conditions are favourable for the activation of the latent infection, the damaged liver tissue provides a focus for initial multiplication of the bacteria. An organized thrombus develops in a subterminal branch of the portal vein resulting in a large anaemic infarct in which further rapid bacterial multiplication and toxin production occurs. The toxin produces a haemolytic anaemia, and later a bacteraemia develops. The duration of illness may vary from about 18 hours to four days. Bacillary haemoglobinuria has been observed in North and South America, Australia and New Zealand. Few incidents have been reported in Great Britain.

Signs

Cattle at pasture that are inspected at infrequent intervals may be found dead. The onset of disease is usually

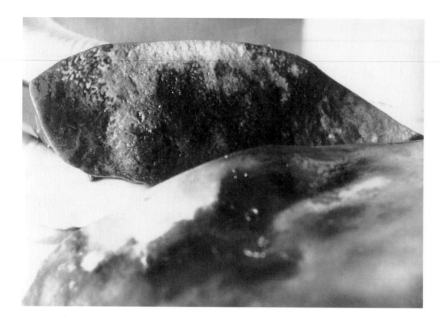

Fig. 44.1 Bacillary haemoglobinuria: a large infarct in the bovine liver caused by *Cl. novyi* type D.

sudden, with cessation of feeding, rumination and defecation. Cows in lactation suffer a sudden and dramatic drop in milk yield. Animals are disinclined to move and the temperature is elevated to 39–41°C (102–106°F). The mucous membranes are jaundiced and there may be oedema of the brisket, submaxillary region and conjunctiva. Small amounts of bloodstained faeces may be passed in the early stages, but later there may be a frank dysentery. Not all these signs may be seen in individual cases and the variation may be due, in part, to different strains of organisms.

Pathology

One of the obvious features of the disease is the profound anaemia that develops before death. Blood samples from ailing animals show a depressed erythrocyte count, which may be as low as 10^6/mm^3 and haemoglobin values are in the range of 40–80g/l. Leucocyte counts are normally elevated to around 20000/mm^3. The organism may be recovered from blood cultures taken during the acute phase. There is a very obvious haemoglobinuria in a proportion of cases, but there are no free red cells in the urine.

In the typical case, the necropsy picture is considered to be pathognomonic, the main features being generalized jaundice often with anaemia; subcutaneous oedema especially over the brisket; accumulation of slightly bloodstained fluid in the pericardial sac, pleural and peritoneal cavities; widespread haemorrhages in the subcutaneous tissues, over the pleural and peritoneal serosa, and endocardium; haemorrhagic abomastitis and enteritis. The liver is usually mahogany coloured with a characteristic yellow infarct, up to 20 cm (8 inches) in diameter, surrounded by a zone of hyperaemia (Fig. 44.1). The kidney cortex is petechiated and deep-red coloured urine may be present in the kidney pelvis and bladder. Evidence of liver fluke damage is not a constant feature.

Diagnosis

Bacillary haemoglobinuria must be differentiated from other conditions in which haemoglobinuria is one of the clinical signs. Acute leptospirosis, due to *Leptospira interrogans* serovar *pomona* (p. 734), is one of these and to confirm a diagnosis in the live animal serological tests and cultural examination of the urine is necessary, although there should be little difficulty in differentiating the two diseases at necropsy. Babesiosis (p. 748) and anaplasmosis (p. 761) can be differentiated by the demonstration of the organisms in blood smears. Post-parturient haemoglobinuria is accompanied by a hypophosphataemia (see p. 792), whilst blood and liver copper levels are elevated in chronic copper poisoning (p. 948). Both these conditions and haemoglobinuria due to the consumption of cruciferous plants (p. 941), such as rape and kale, are afebrile.

Confirmation of diagnosis of bacillary haemoglobinuria is based on the clinical signs, necropsy findings and demonstration of the causal organism in the liver lesion and other sites by fluorescent antibody techniques. It may also be possible to culture the organism from tissue and demonstrate toxins in the liver infarct, but both procedures are time-consuming and laborious.

Treatment and prevention

Bacillary haemoglobinuria can be successfully treated by the administration of wide-spectrum antibiotics in the early stages (Smith & Holdeman, 1968). Early treatment with large doses of penicillin is also effective (Williams, 1964). Supportive treatment by the administration of electrolyte solutions orally and parenterally and the provision of mineral supplements containing iron, copper and cobalt is also necessary, as well as careful nursing.

The disease can be successfully prevented by vaccination with an aluminium hydroxide adsorbed, formalinized whole culture and it is also claimed that infectious necrotic hepatitis vaccines also confer immunity. Annual vaccination is necessary in enzootic areas (see p. 1005).

Botulism

Botulism may be defined as a lethal type of food poisoning in man and several species of animals, caused by the ingestion of *Clostridium botulinum* toxins, which have been produced by the organism in decaying plant or animal tissue.

Aetiology

Smith (1977) defines *Cl. botulinum* 'not as a single species, but as a conglomerate of several distinct culture groups, alike in that they are clostridia and produce toxins with a similar pharmacological action'. There are a number of distinct serological types (A, B, C, D, E, F and G) and although the toxins are similarly designated, the serological specificity of the toxin produced by any strain may not be entirely related to its serological classification.

Like other clostridia, *Cl. botulinum* is a spore-forming organism, which under certain conditions thrives in putrefying animal tissue or decaying plant material. The organism has a world-wide occurrence and is found in the intestinal tracts of herbivores and in soil. It would appear that different soil types favour different types of the organism. Smith (1997) reported that in the USA, type A strains were prevalent in the alkaline soils of the south-west, types B and E in the damp soils of most areas, type C in the acid soils of the Gulf Coast and type D in the alkaline soils of the west.

The toxins of *Cl. botulinum* are neurotoxins, causing motor paralysis without the development of any gross or histological lesions in the nervous system. Although the mode of action is still debated, it appears that the site of action of the toxins is at the synapses of efferent parasympathetic and somatic motor nerves, by interference with the secretion of acetylcholine, which is the chemical mediator of nerve impulse transmission.

Two forms or types of botulism are recognized in cattle. The first is the form that develops after the consumption of, or contact with, carcasses or skeletons of dead animals containing botulinum toxins. The second form of the disease follows the consumption of conserved fodder that is contaminated by the toxins.

The first type of botulism has been widely reported in South Africa (lamsieket), Australia (bulbar paralysis) and in the USA (loin disease). In these countries it has been associated with low phosphorus levels in soil, poor pastures and drought. Under such circumstances animals including the local fauna, which carry *Cl. botulinum* in their intestines, die and the organisms invade the carcass tissues and produce large amounts of toxin. Muller (1961) has demonstrated that the levels of toxin may reach 10^5–10^6 mouse lethal units/g of tissue. Animals that consume tissue from such carcasses, because of a phosphorus deficiency and a subsequent pica, or feed shortage, ingest both toxin and *Cl. botulinum* spores and will subsequently become a source of toxin and spores for other animals. In Europe, similar circumstances may arise after the spreading of litter from poultry houses on to cattle pastures. Investigations into such outbreaks reveal the presence of poultry carcasses in the litter, which are the source of the toxins (Appleyard & Mollison, 1985; Clegg *et al.*, 1985).

The second type of botulism, forage poisoning, occurs in those countries where conserved forage, especially baled hay and silage, is fed to cattle. The source of toxin has usually been identified as the carcasses of small animals (mice, rats, rabbits and birds) accidentally killed and subsequently baled in the hay or ensiled with the grass or cereal crop. Prevot & Sillioc (1955) recorded that more than half of the cattle botulism in France was associated with the presence of cat carcasses in the feed. Fjolstad & Kluna (1969) also reported an outbreak in which the source of toxin was a cat carcass and demonstrated 500000 mouse lethal doses/g of the carcass. A hedgehog, discovered in a hay rack, was the source of toxin in an outbreak in cattle with 20000 mouse lethal doses in its subcutaneous tissue (Ektvedt & Hanssen, 1974). Recently, however, it has been demonstrated that proteolytic strains of *Cl. botulinum* may produce toxin in silage under certain conditions and without the presence of animal tissue (Notermans *et al.*, 1979a, b). It would appear that a low pH prevents toxin formation in silage. The incorporation of poultry manure and poultry waste in cattle feed can also lead to outbreaks of botulism (Egyed *et al.*, 1978) and brewers grains contaminated with *Cl. botulinum* has also been incriminated (Breuknik *et al.*, 1978).

Botulism in any species of animal tends to be associated with certain types of the organism. Ruminants are susceptible to types C and D, although in The Netherlands disease has been associated with type B (Haagsma & Laak, 1977).

Signs

Clinical signs usually appear within two to fourteen days of ingestion of the toxin, although in peracute cases the incubation period may be only a few hours. Illness is afebrile.

In peracute cases the onset of disease is sudden, characterized by a rapid paralysis and death within 12–18 hours. In less acute cases the onset is more gradual, affected animals showing a progressive muscular paralysis of the head, neck and limbs, leading to recumbency, often with the head and neck outstretched or deviated towards the flank.

The majority of cases, however, appear to be of the subacute type. The first signs are periodic periods of restlessness, incoordination especially of the hindlimbs, and an apparent difficulty in chewing and swallowing. These signs progress to ataxia, difficulty or inability to rise, recumbency and in some an obvious paralysis of the tongue, which protrudes from the mouth. There is usually partial or complete anorexia and adypsia. Animals may survive for up to seven days after becoming recumbent, but during the terminal stages respiration becomes laboured and of the abdominal type due to paralysis of the thoracic muscles. An animal often appears to rest its chin on the ground and will lift it when stimulated. A foreleg may be extended. As the condition progresses nominal movements reduce. Later stages often involve lateral recumbency with extended legs which can be flexed. The animal is conscious.

Some animals may recover after showing relatively mild clinical signs over a period of three to four weeks (Clegg & Evans, 1974; Davies *et al.*, 1974). Clegg & Evans reported that surviving animals developed a pronounced respiratory roaring sound, which persisted for three months after recovery.

Pathology

A number of authors have reported on the value of certain biochemical tests on blood and urine from affected animals as aids to diagnosis, but in cattle such tests are of little help in the live animal. However, it is possible in some cases to demonstrate circulating toxins in the serum of clinically affected animals by mouse inoculation tests (Clegg *et al.*, 1985), but such cases are of the peracute or acute type.

As already indicated, the toxins of *Cl. botulinum* do not produce any specific or detectable lesions in the central nervous system, nor do they produce specific changes in the carcass. Those changes that are observed

are non-specific and include haemorrhages on the endocardium and epicardium and congestion of the parenchymatous organs and intestinal mucosa. However, it may be possible to demonstrate toxin in the intestinal contents or liver by mouse inoculation tests. Whilst the presence of the organism in the intestine is of little diagnostic value, its isolation from the liver is of significance. In many cases investigation of outbreaks is unrewarding.

Diagnosis

It must be emphasized that in many instances it is not possible to confirm all suspected cases of botulism by detection of toxin either in the sera of affected animals or in the intestinal contents or liver at necropsy. As *Cl. botulinum* is not normally found in the liver of cattle, isolation from the liver is regarded as significant.

Attempts may be made to demonstrate toxin in suspected feed, but such an approach has its limitations. Suspected feed may be fed to experimental animals of the same species, or an infusion of the feed may be administered to experimental animals. However, toxins in feedingstuffs are not distributed evenly, rather in pockets, and samples of feed for testing must therefore be carefully selected, e.g. from near carcasses or areas of contamination. It is also possible that all the botulinum-contaminated feed will have been consumed before the onset of clinical signs.

Postparturient paresis/hypocalcaemia (p. 781) can be differentiated from the disease by the examination of blood samples and the response to calcium therapy. In some cases of listeriosis (p. 904) there is a paralysis of the tongue, but it is acompanied by fever and other clinical signs such as unilateral facial paralysis and panophthalmia. Bovine spongiform encephalopathy (p. 911) in its later stages might be confused but there is no paralysis and the animal will still eat.

Treatment and prevention

There is little value in the administration of antitoxin, except possibly in the very early stages, and there are conflicting views on the merits of purgatives to remove the toxins from the intestine. However, Breuknik *et al.* (1978) reported that symptomatic treatment for dehydration and acidosis seemed to assist recovery. As a general rule, treatment of subacute cases only should be undertaken, as these are the ones most likely to recover.

Vaccination with toxoid is only necessary in enzootic areas and should be given every two years (p. 1005). Where botulism is associated with the disposal of poultry litter on to pasture, every effort should be made to remove any poultry carcasses in it before application.

All poultry waste should ideally be heat treated before incorporation into compound feeds for direct feeding to livestock.

Clostridial myositis: blackleg and malignant oedema

Two forms of clostridial myositis are recognized in cattle: blackleg, which is caused by *Clostridium chauveoi*, and malignant oedema, which is caused by a number of clostridial species and is nearly always associated with wound infection. It is often difficult or impossible to differentiate between the two conditions at a clinical or post-mortem examination (Williams, 1977).

Blackleg

Blackleg or blackquarter is defined as a gangrenous myositis caused by the activation of a latent *Cl. chauveoi* spore infection (Jubb *et al.*, 1983). These authors also refer to a 'false or pseudo-blackleg' caused by the activation of *Cl. novyi* and *Cl. septicum* spore infection, but this condition is more appropriately designated malignant oedema.

Aetiology

Clostridium chauveoi is a Gram-positive, spore-bearing anaerobic bacillus, the spores of which are highly resistant to environmental conditions and therefore remain viable for many years. It is, like other clostridia, regarded as a soil organism and following ingestion by cattle, sheep and other animals, the spores localize in the spleen, liver and muscles (Kerry, 1964). The vegetative form of the organism produces a number of toxins, which are capable of inducing local muscle necrosis and toxaemia. The trigger mechanisms responsible for the activation of the endogenous latent spore infection are unknown, but it is assumed that a lowered oxygen tension and a degree of muscle damage are necessary. After activation, rapid bacterial multiplication and toxin formation produce the typical muscle gangrenous lesion and systemic toxaemia.

Most cases occur in animals between six months and two years of age at pasture, although incidents may occur in housed animals.

Signs

Often when stock are infrequently inspected animals may be found dead without signs of illness having been observed. The clinical signs that are seen in ailing animals are related to the site of lesion. Limb involvement is manifested as a lameness with a swelling of the upper part which, at first, is hot and painful, but later becomes cold and emphysematous. A lesion of the tongue results in a tongue and throat swelling, with the tongue protruding from the mouth and marked respiratory distress. Stiffness and a reluctance to move is apparent when the sublumbar muscles are involved. In addition to these clinical signs, there is a marked depression, anorexia, rapid pulse rate and high temperature, usually in excess of 40°C (104°F). Later there is dypsnoea, recumbency and coma leading to death within 12–24 hours.

Pathology

The disease usually runs an acute course so that there is little opportunity for collecting specimens for laboratory examination before death. After death the carcass becomes bloated and putrefaction occurs rapidly. Bloodstained froth exudes from the body orifices. It may be possible to palpate the lesion, if it is in a superficial muscle group, but this is usually difficult because of the rapid onset of putrefaction.

Animals dying from blackleg are in good body condition. The body cavities contain bloodstained fluid and the parenchymatous organs show evidence of degeneration and post-mortem decomposition. All the skeletal muscles must be carefully examined by palpation and incision for lesions, which may not be extensive. The lesion produced by *Cl. chauveoi* has a characteristic appearance (Williams, 1977) (Plate 44.2). The muscle is blackened, dry and crepitant with a spongy appearance and a rancid odour. Pale yellow serous fluid surrounds the affected muscle, but this becomes progressively more bloodstained as post-mortem decomposition proceeds.

Diagnosis

A diagnosis can be reached on the basis of clinical signs and necropsy findings, but it is essential that when no clinical signs have been observed, anthrax (p. 717) is eliminated before a necropsy is carried out. *Clostridium chauveoi* can be identfed by the staining of lesion impression smears by the specific fluorescent antiglobulins that are now commercially available. Cultural examination is likely to be unrewarding unless fresh tissue is available and special techniques used.

Blackleg may be confused with other conditions especially when death is sudden. Lead (p. 944) and other chemical poisonings (pp. 941–3) require laboratory examination for confirmation, but the typical lesions of blackleg are absent. Black disease (p. 729) and bacillary haemoglobinuria (p. 719) may also have to be considered in a differential diagnosis, but the characteristic liver infarcts are a diagnostic feature of these two diseases.

Treatment and prevention

Antibiotic treatment of affected animals is likely to be effective only if commenced early. Large doses of penicillin (10 000 units/kg body weight) should be administered intravenously, followed by longer acting preparations, some of which should be given into the affected tissue (Radostits *et al.*, 2000). However, because of the extensive tissue involvement, even if the infection is eliminated, the subsequent muscle loss is so great that recovered animals are of little economic value. Treatment of animals with tongue infection should not be attempted, because even if successful the whole tongue or most of it will be subsequently lost and early slaughter on humane grounds should be considered. Carcasses should be burned or undergo deep burial.

Blackleg can be successfully prevented by the use of commercially available *Cl. chauveoi* vaccines and all animals over six months of age should be vaccinated prior to being turned out in the spring. There are, however, considerable advantages in the use of multivalent vaccines containing the antigens of *Cl. chauveoi*, *Cl. novyi* and *Cl. septicum*, which offer maximum protection to cattle against blackleg, malignant oedema and black disease (p. 1005).

Malignant oedema

Malignant oedema is considered to be an acute wound infection caused by organisms of the genus *Clostridium* (Radostits *et al.*, 2000). However, if blackleg is restricted to cover endogenous *Cl. chauveoi* infection then malignant oedema must also include those incidents, albeit relatively few in number, arising from activation of latent *Cl. novyi* and *Cl. septicum*, which undoubtedly occur.

Aetiology

Clostridium chauveoi, *Cl. novyi*, *Cl. perfringens*, *Cl. septicum*, *Cl. sordelli* and other clostridia have been isolated from, or demonstrated in lesions of clostridial myositis in cattle. Williams (1977) in a survey of 173 cases in Wales demonstrated *Cl. chauveoi* in 75 (43 per cent), *Cl. chauveoi* and *Cl. septicum* in 22 (13 per cent), *Cl. novyi* in 53 (31 per cent), *Cl. novyi* and *Cl. septicum* in nine (5 per cent), *Cl. septicum* in 11 (6 per cent) and *Cl. sordelli* in three (1.7 per cent). In this series *Cl. perfringens* was isolated from about 50 per cent of the lesions, but its presence was not considered to be of sig-

nificance. There is still some uncertainty about the role of *Cl. septicum* in bovine malignant oedema.

Deep puncture wounds, accidentally inflicted, provide ideal conditions for the multiplication of anaerobes and development of malignant oedema. It may also develop after surgical operations, parturition, intramuscular administration of non-antibiotic preparations such as prostaglandlins (Harwood, 1994), anthelmintic and vitamin preparations, and vaccination. The clostridia are soil organisms that persist in the animal environment and therefore readily gain entry to wounds. The tissue damage and low oxygen tension allow rapid multiplication and toxin production so that clinical signs usually develop within 48 hours. Occasionally, malignant oedema may affect a group of animals that had previously been housed or penned for a short period of time and the absence of any form of wound suggests that some factor, perhaps trauma from bruising, may have activated a latent spore infection.

Signs

The disease is usually sporadic involving single or small numbers of animals. All ages of cattle are affected and clinical signs appear within 48 hours of infection. The clinical signs will vary with the site of infection, but in all cases, anorexia, depression and fever are very marked. A local lesion develops at the site of infection consisting of a swelling, which becomes tense and depending on the type of infection may become emphysematous. Lameness, stiffness and muscle tremors may be evident. Animals usually die within 48 hours.

When infection is associated with parturition, the vulva and perineum swell and there is a bloodstained discharge from the vulva. Death is rapid, usually within 24–36 hours after the onset of signs.

Pathology

In malignant oedema there is little opportunity for the laboratory examination of specimens taken from affected animals. As in blackleg, it is necessary for a post-mortem examination to be carried out as soon after death as possible, because of the bacterial invasion of the carcass and rapid onset of putrefactive changes.

The site of infection is surrounded by an extensive oedema of the subcutaneous tissues and intramuscular fascia. It may be possible to identify the initial wound, but tissue damage is usually so extensive that the only trace is a small wound in the skin. The oedema fluid may be clear and gelatinous in *Cl. novyi* infections with very little muscle damage. Infection with *Cl. septicum* produces an extensive bloodstained frothy oedema, with the underlying muscle a dark red colour permeated with gas. *Clostridium sordelli* produces changes similar to those produced by *Cl. novyi* except that the oedema is more bloodstained and has a foul odour. The lesion produced by *Cl. chauveoi* is similar to that described under blackleg.

All body cavities contain bloodstained fluid and the parenchymatous organs show degenerative changes and post-mortem decompostion. If the infection involves the reproductive tract, the uterus will contain a large volume of foul-smelling bloodstained fluid and the uterine and vaginal walls will be greatly thickened, permeated with bloodstained fluid and gas.

Diagnosis

The clinical signs and necropsy findings are so characteristic that diagnosis can be readily reached. It will, however, be necessary to resort to laboratory examination of lesions for the identification of the organisms by fluorescent antibody tests or culture.

Treatment and prevention

Affected animals should be treated with high doses of antibiotics, preferably parenteral penicillin or broad spectrum. In addition, wounds should be drained and irrigated with antiseptic solutions, and packed with a suitable antibiotic preparation.

Trivalent vaccines, containing the antigens of *Cl. chauveoi*, *Cl. novyi* and *Cl. septicum* are available and are effective in preventing malignant oedema (p. 1005).

Harwood (1984) highlights the dangers from intramuscular injections administered to cattle, particularly if infection is introduced and if large volumes are used, and under such circumstances routine vaccination is recommended.

Contagious bovine pyelonephritis

This disease is a specific infection of the urinary tract of cattle, which results in a chronic purulent inflammation of the kidneys, ureters and bladder.

Aetiology

Corynebacterium renale is considered to be the speific causal agent, although other organisms, especially streptococci, staphylococci, *Arcanobacterium* (*Actinomyces, Corynebacterium*) *pyogenes* and *Escherichia coli*, as well as *C. renale* are present in the urine of some animals with pyelonephritis and may also be implicated. *Corynebacterium renale* is an obligate parasite of

cattle and occasionally sheep, and can be readily cultured from the urine of affected and carrier animals.

Goudswaard and Budhai (1975) identified four serotypes, of which type 1 is the most pathogenic.

It has been demonstrated that the pathogenicity of *C. renale* is dependent to a large extent on the presence of pili on the organism, which assist its adhesion to the urinary epithelium. This process is pH dependent and Takai *et al.* (1980) showed that the proportion of piliated organisms adhering to bladder cells is high at a pH above 7.6, but significantly lower at a pH below 6.8, a factor that is important in the pathogenesis of pyelonephritis.

The disease is considered to be the result of an ascending infection, involving successively the bladder, ureters and kidneys. Hiramune *et al.* (1972) established infection in cattle after the introduction of organisms into the bladder and the characteristic lesions developed. Females are far more susceptible than males to infection and the short length of the urethra in the female is thought to be a major factor in the establishment of infection. Stasis of urine is an important predisposing factor in the pathogenesis of pyelonephritis and cystitis and such circumstances may occur when a permanent or temporary obstruction of the urinary tract occurs through the presence of calculi or pressure exerted by a gravid uterus.

The disease is widely recognized in Europe and North America, but the prevalence of infection is largely unknown. Morse (1950) found that *C. renale* could be recovered from the urine of 22.7 per cent of cattle in herds in which pyelonephritis had been confirmed, whereas only 10.7 per cent of cattle in other herds were infected. Clinically infected or carrier cows are the principal source of infection, the disease being mainly transmitted by direct contact, although Morse (1950) reported that infection was transmitted by indirect contact from affected and carrier cows tethered in stalls to those in adjacent stalls. In some herds there is circumstantial evidence to support the existence of venereal spread and the organism has been readily isolated from the prepuce of normal bulls (Hiramune *et al.*, 1975).

Signs

In affected herds, clinical cases appear sporadically with animals under three years of age rarely affected. Most cases occur in dairy herds with the peak incidence usually in winter.

There is considerable variation in the clinical signs observed from case to case, particularly during the early stages. Bloodstained urine may be passed intermittently by an apparently healthy animal over a period of weeks, before other signs appear. In other animals, one, two or more attacks of acute colic lasting up to 6 hours or more may be the first sign. More frequently, however, the onset is insidious. The most common signs are a gradual loss of condition, a slowly declining milk yield, fluctuating or capricious appetite, intermittent fever, and the intermittent passage of bloodstained urine. As the disease progresses, urination becomes more frequent and painful with the passage of small volumes of urine containing blood and tissue debris. During the later stages it may be possible to detect, by rectal examination, enlargement of one or both kidneys, a thickened bladder and enlargement of one or both ureters, particularly the terminal portions where they cross the neck of the bladder. Frequently, palpation of the kidneys induces a pain response. The course of the disease may run from a period of weeks to two or more months, death resulting from a combination of kidney failure and blood loss with an extensive loss of condition.

Pathology

The urine of clinically affected animals is turbid and in the early stages intermittently bloodstained, but in the later stages the urine is almost constantly bloodstained. Microscopic examination of the centrifuged deposit of the urine reveals the presence of erythrocytes, leucocytes and epithelial tissue debris. *Corynebacterium renale* can be readily demonstrated in Gram-stained smears and Ado & Cook (1979) have reported on the value of fluorescent antibody tests for the identification of the organism. It can be readily isolated on blood agar and other media in common use. The clinical signs are so characteristic that haematological examination and blood chemistry estimations are seldom considered necessary. In any case, such examinations are unlikely to reveal any abnormalities until the disease is well developed when anaemia and uraemia are the most prominent findings.

Animals dying from pyelonephritis are usually in poor condition and the carcass pale and anaemic. Specific lesions are confined to the urinary tract. One or both kidneys are enlarged with less well marked lobulation than normal and a markedly thickened capsule. The surface is mottled by greyish white necrotic areas. On section the renal pelvis is greatly dilated and contains varying amounts of blood, pus and mucoid fluid. Greyish white streaks of necrotic tissue radiate from the pelvis towards the cortex and there may be numerous abscesses in the cortex and medulla of each lobule. The ureters are grossly enlarged and distended by blood, pus and mucus. The bladder wall and the urethra are thickened and the mucosa oedematous, haemorrhagic and necrotic.

Diagnosis

The diagnosis of pyelonephritis is based on the clinical signs, the changes in the urine and the presence of *C. renale* in the urine together with the detectable abnormalities in the urinary tract. Enzootic haematuria (p. 947) has some clinical features in common with pyelonephritis, but it is afebrile, lesions are confined to the bladder and the urine from such cases is sterile or negative for *C. renale*. Similarly, non-specific cystitis may also resemble pyelonephritis, but the bladder only is affected and the urine is sterile or negative for *C. renale*.

Treatment and prevention

Corynebacterium renale is sensitive to a range of antibiotics but penicillin remains the antibiotic of choice for the treatment of pyelonephritis in the bovine. A complete recovery can be achieved if treatment is commenced during the early stages, when little tissue damage has occurred. In advanced cases, however, when there is considerable tissue destruction, only a temporary recovery can be achieved through antibiotic therapy, although this may enable an animal to be fattened and subsequently sent for slaughter. Large doses of procaine penicillin G should be administered, e.g. 10000–15000 iu/kg daily for at least 10 days. The acidification of the urine by the administration of monobasic sodium phosphate is still considered by some as useful supportive therapy and 100 g daily for a period of five days during antibiotic treatment is recommened.

There are no specific control measures other than isolation of affected animals and thorough cleansing and disinfection of the contaminated environment. In affected herds where natural breeding is practised, the introduction of artificial insemination may achieve a reduction in the number of clinical cases.

Endocarditis

Endocarditis may be defined as inflammation of the endothelial lining of the heart. The inflammatory processes usually result in valvular insufficiency or stenosis that interfere with the flow of blood into and out of the heart, leading to congestive heart failure.

Aetiology

Most cases of bovine endocarditis appear to be caused by bacterial infection. Several species of bacteria have been incriminated, but streptococci especially enterococci of Lancefield's group D, *A. pyogenes*, staphylococci, *Mannheimia* and *Pasteurella* species are the commonest (Evans, 1957; Larsen, 1963).

It would appear that a persistent bacteraemia is necessary for the development of endocardial lesions and it is significant that in most, if not all, confirmed cases, a primary focus of infection in the form of mastitis, metritis, reticulitis, limb abscesses, etc. can be identified at post-mortem examination (Evans, 1957; Andersen, 1963; Larsen, 1963).

Although it is generally accepted that the causal organisms are transported to the heart via the bloodstream, the method by which they reach the endocardial lesion is still uncertain. It is possible that some bacteria may be able to adhere to the intact endothelium. However, it is more likely that they adhere to damaged endothelium and it is assumed that trauma and debility are the main factors in producing sufficient damage for the bacteria to localize in the endothelium. This hypothesis is based on the fact that the usual sites of the lesions are on the free edges of the valves exposed to the blood flow and that they are in apposition to others. The heart valves of the bovine have their own blood supply and it is thus possible for the bacteria to produce emboli in the capillaries, which form a focus of infection.

The early lesions of endocarditis are seldom seen except in experimental infections. Initially, the leaflet of the valve becomes swollen and an irregular ulcer develops on its surface, in which the bacteria localize. From this ulcerated area the characteristic vegetative structures develop. These have a similar composition to thrombi, except that they contain few platelets. Several layers of thrombus-like material are deposited on the affected valve in response to the bacterial activity, so that vegetations assume a cauliflower or wartlike appearance and the valves become distorted and shrunken and functionally incompetent. Fragments of the vegetation may become detached to form emboli, which lodge in other organs.

Signs

All ages of cattle are affected although Larsen (1963) found that nearly half of the 53 bovine cases he encountered were in animals between two and three years of age. Both Evans (1957) and Biering-Sørensen (1963) found that 3.9 per cent of cattle examined in abbatoir surveys had either died from, or been slaughtered because of, endocarditis.

The published descriptions of the clinical signs of bovine endocarditis are varied and reflect the stage to which the endocarditis had progressed and also the extent to which the clinical signs were attributable to the primary focus of infection (Evans, 1957; Power & Rebhun, 1983). Thus the initial signs may not indicate heart involvement and the onset of the clinical signs of endocarditis may be insidious.

A recurrent or persistent fever of 40–41°C (104–106°F), anorexia, depression and a reluctance to move are the usual early signs. Pinching of the withers and ballottement of the sternum ventral to the heart elicit a pain response. The heart rate is accelerated to 100–120 beats/minute and in due course the jugular vein becomes engorged, which is followed by oedema of the brisket and submandibular areas. The detection of a heart murmur on auscultation is an important clinical feature, but this is not easily detected when the right atrioventricular valves are involved. Lacuta *et al.* (1980) have reported on the value of electrocardiography and echocardiography in the diagnosis of endocarditis. Whilst echocardiography is of value in that it will demonstrate reflected echoes from the vegetative lesions and detect abnormal valve movements, electrocardiography is less so because the abnormalities shown are not diagnostic of endocarditis.

As the disease progresses, secondary involvement of other organs and systems occurs, leading to pneumonia, nephritis, arthritis, etc. Progressive weight loss, anaemia and weakness inevitably is followed by recumbency and death. The course of the disease may extend from one or two weeks to two or three months.

Pathology

Blood samples from affected animals show a leucocytosis and a shift to the left, although in the more chronic cases these changes are less well marked. Plasma fibrinogen levels are elevated (Wuijckhuise-Sjouke, 1984) but this is a feature of inflammation of serous membranes as well as endocarditis. The causal organism can be isolated on blood culture during periods of fever but at least 20 ml of blood are necessary and the cultures may have to be repeated on a number of occasions.

The heart lesions found at necropsy are fairly constant (Plate 44.3). The pericardial sac is distended with varying amounts of oedematous fluid and the heart is enlarged and distorted, due to hypertrophy of the myocardium and dilatation of one or more chambers, because of the incompetence/stenosis of the affected atrioventricular valves. In the majority of cases the right atrioventricular valves are affected. The affected valves are shrunken and thickened, particularly in the later stages, and attached to them there are wart-like or cauliflower vegetations.

The parenchymatous organs may show pathological changes. The lungs are passively congested with frequently a number of embolic infarcts, and the liver is usually enlarged due to passive venous congestion and may show evidence of cirrhosis. Numerous small haemorrhagic foci are scattered over the surface of the kidneys and within the cortex and there may be a number of infarcts or abscesses in the cortex.

Diagnosis

The clinical diagnosis of endocarditis is dependent upon the detection of heart murmurs, which may be extremely difficult when the lesions involve the right atrioventricular valves. Thus it may be difficult or impossible to differentiate between endocarditis and pericarditis (p. 731) (John, 1947) or other causes of congestive heart failure. Cardiac lesions of enzootic bovine leukosis (EBL) (p. 695) may also produce signs of congestive heart failure, but affected animals show a persistent lymphocytosis and are positive to the agar gel immunodiffusion and ELISA tests for EBL.

Treatment

The organisms associated with bovine endocarditis are sensitive to a range of antibiotics. However, the nature of the heart lesions is such that therapeutic concentrations of antibiotic may not penetrate through to the bacteria. Furthermore, the permanent damage inflicted on the heart valves and the embolic lesions in other organs cannot be effectively repaired. Thus treatment of ailing animals is unlikely to lead to complete recovery. Although temporary improvement may occur after intensive antibiotic treatment for seven to ten days, a relapse within seven days is the usual outcome. However, Power and Rebhun (1983) reported that nine cows, in which an early diagnosis had been made, responded to long-term penicillin therapy.

Haemorrhagic septicaemia

Haemorrhagic septicaemia, or more appropriately septicaemic pasteurellosis of cattle, is a peracute disease, which is characterized by a septicaemia and a very high mortality rate.

Aetiology

Carter and Bain (1960) and Carter (1982) highlighted the confusion and conflict in the terminology of diseases attributed to *Pasteurella* infection in bovines. Thus it is difficult to assess the accuracy of many of the early reports on haemorrhagic septicaemia. It is now considered to be a primary pasteurellosis caused by *Pasteurella multocida* capsular serotypes B and E, which appears now to be confined largely to the tropical countries of Asia. Shirlaw (1938) reported on the occurrence of septicaemic pasteurellosis in the Northumbrian area

of Great Britain in 1926. The lesions in the affected animals were those of a bronchopneumonia and although *Pasteurella* was isolated from the lungs it was not fully typed but likely to have been type B. Since then there have been no further reports of haemorrhagic septicaemia in Great Britain. In the USA only four outbreaks, three in bison and one in cattle, have been confirmed and Carter (1982) speculated on its disappearance from that country.

Pasteurella multocida is not a very resistant organism and it is unlikely to survive for long periods outside the animal body. In soil and mud, for example, where competition from other organisms is strong it does not survive for more than 24 hours (Bain, 1963). Toxins have been demonstrated in culture filtrates, but all the evidence suggests that the most significant of these are endotoxins, which are important in producing the clinical disease and rapid death.

The main source of infection is the carrier animal, the organism localizing in the nasopharyngeal mucosa and tonsils. In herds that experienced haemorrhagic septicaemia 44.4 per cent of healthy cattle were carriers, whereas the carrier rates in three herds in which the disease had not been confirmed were 3.89 per cent, 5.5 per cent and nil (Mustafa *et al.*, 1978). Furthermore, the carrier rate was higher in cattle under two years of age than in adult cattle. It is estimated that approximately 10 per cent of carrier animals become immune.

Spread of infection is through the ingestion of feed contaminated by carrier or clinically affected animals. The role of biting and blood-sucking ectoparasites in the spread of infection is still unclear, although Macadam (1962) suggested on the basis of experimental work in rabbits that ticks could transmit the disease.

It is generally accepted that environmental stress is an important factor in precipitating outbreaks of disease. Outbreaks occur when animals are exposed to cold and wet weather, housed under poor conditions or exhausted by prolonged periods of work. Under such circumstances the immunity of carrier animals wanes, allowing a rapid multiplication of the organism and spread within the carrier animal and its subsequent dissemination to susceptible contact animals.

Signs

The disease may be peracute with death frequently occurring so rapidly that few, if any, clinical signs are observed. In the acute form, there is a sudden onset of fever (41–42°C, 106–108°F), severe depression, oedema of the throat, profuse salivation and rapid death, usually in less than 24 hours. The oedematous form of the disease is also acute with the development of hot painful swellings of the head, throat, brisket, perineum and limb(s). Severe oedema of the head and throat may result in dyspnoea and eventually death through asphyxiation rather than death from a septicaemia.

Pathology

Large numbers of *Pasteurella* organisms can be demonstrated in the nasal discharges and saliva of clinically affected animals. The course of the disease is usually less than 14 hours, which limits the opportunities for carrying out laboratory examination on specimens from ailing animals.

On post-mortem examination the most prominent features are widespread petechial haemorrhages on the serous membranes and in various organs, especially the lungs and muscles, and a subcutaneous oedema of the throat region. The lungs are oedematous, may also show an early interstitial pneumonia and often there is a haemorrhagic gastroenteritis. In the oedematous form of the disease, there is widespread oedema of the head, tongue, brisket and/or one or more limbs as well as widespread petechiation. The spleen is not greatly enlarged.

Diagnosis

The regional occurrence of the disease is of some aid in diagnosis, but the clinical signs, rapid course and necropsy findings are similar to those of other diseases, e.g. anthrax (p. 717), clostridial myositis (p. 723), acute leptospirosis (p. 735), so that confirmation can only be achieved by isolation and identification of the causal organism. *Pasteurella multocida* can be readily isolated from heart blood, spleen, liver and other sites, but identification of the specific serotypes may require submission to specialist laboratories.

Treatment and prevention

Pasteurella multocida is sensitive *in vitro* to a range of antimicrobial substances, including oxytetracycline, florfenicol and penicillin/dihydrostreptomycin and, in theory, therefore treatment of clinically affected animals should be feasible. However, the sudden onset and rapid course of the disease are such that treatment during the very early stages only is likely to be successful. Even if all the organisms are eliminated, death from *Pasteurella* endotoxaemia may still occur (Jubb *et al.*, 1985).

The only effective method of control is vaccination of all herds at risk. A dead vaccine in an adjuvant base containing paraffin and lanolin has proved highly effective when used prophylactically and is also of value in reducing losses if used during an outbreak, immunity persisting for at least 12 months. Persistent subcuta-neous swellings may develop in some animals and after the administration of some batches of vaccine, anaphylactic shock has occasionally been recorded. A live streptomycin-dependent mutant of *P. multocida* vaccine has been developed (Wei & Carter, 1978) and successfully tested in field trials (De Alwis & Carter, 1980), but does not appear to be commercially available as yet.

The observations of Sawada *et al.* (1985) on naturally acquired immunity to *P. multocida*, capsular types B and E, are of considerable interest. They found, on the basis of serological and passive immunity tests in mice, that 81 per cent of feeder calves were immune to type B and 91 per cent to type E. The immunity appeared to develop in the absence of either of these serotypes in the microbial flora of the calves.

Infectious necrotic hepatitis (black disease)

Infectious necrotic hepatitis is a highly fatal acute or peracute infectious disease of sheep and cattle, characterized by the presence of one or more necrotic areas in the liver, in which *Cl. novyi* type B has multiplied and produced lethal toxins.

Aetiology

The causal organism is *Cl. novyi*, which like other clostridia is a Gram-positive spore-bearing bacillus, widely distributed in the environment, particularly in soil. The more pathogenic types, however, are more prevalent in those areas where infectious necrotic hepatitis occurs. After ingestion, spores are transported to the liver and other locations, where they remain as a latent infection. On the basis of toxin production a number of types are recognized, but infectious necrotic hepatitis in cattle is caused by type B, which produces large amounts of the lethal alpha toxin.

The disease occurs in cattle and sheep in those areas where liver fluke infection also occurs (p. 276), and it has been demonstrated experimentally in sheep that migrating immature liver fluke produce liver damage and through this an environment suitable for the activation of the latent infection. It is assumed that the same sequence of events occurs in cattle, although Williams (1964) noted the absence of liver fluke damage in some confirmed cases. It has been demonstrated that the survival of *Cl. novyi* and *Fasciola hepatica* is favoured by the same type of soil environment (Bagadi & Sewell, 1973). Other migrating parasites, e.g. the intermediate stages of certain canine cestodes, may also activate latent *Cl. novyi* infection.

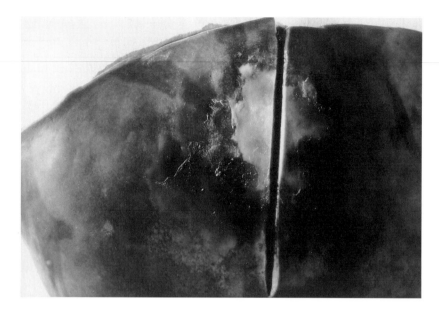

Fig. 44.2 A typical black disease lesion in the vertical lobe of a bovine liver. Note the central necrotic area surrounded by a zone of congestion.

The organism multiplies rapidly in the damaged liver and large amounts of the lethal and necrotizing toxin are formed, which leads to the production of the characteristic lesion. The toxin is rapidly absorbed, leading to a systemic toxaemic and it is only rarely that the organism can be recovered from other organs in the fresh carcass.

The disease has been confirmed in most countries where fascioliosis occurs. Cattle of all ages may be affected; Williams (1964) found that in a series of 46 cases, one was in a six-month-old calf, two were in cows over seven years old and the remainder in bullocks and heifers between one and two years old. There is little information on morbidity rates in cattle, but experience in the UK indicates that in most herds only single animals succumb. It is likely, however, that the disease is becoming more common in some areas.

Signs

Most cattle with infectious necrotic hepatitis are found dead but, in some, illness may last for one to two days (Herbert & Hughes, 1956). Affected animals develop severe depression, are disinclined to move, with a normal or slightly elevated temperature. Signs of discomfort are exhibited on palpation of the liver region.

Pathology

Because of the acute nature of the disease it is not possible to carry out ante-mortem laboratory examinations.

Animals dying from the disease are usually in good condition. The subcutaneous vessels are engorged and clear gelatinous fluid in variable amounts is present in the axillary and inguinal regions, and over the brisket. Fluid, sometimes bloodstained and containing fibrin strands, is present in the pleural and peritoneal cavities and in the pericardial sac. Haemorrhages are scattered over the endocardium and sometimes over the epicardium, parietal pleura and peritoneum. The mucosa of the abomasum is usually congested and often the abomasal wall is distended by a gelatinous oedema. The duodenum and jejunum may show a patchy mucosal congestion.

The pathological changes in the liver are characteristic. The organ is a dark brown colour due to venous congestion and the gall-bladder is usually distended. One, two or more sharply demarcated yellowish necrotic areas up to 8 cm (3 inches) (Fig. 44.2) or more in diameter may be identified, most frequently on the surface but also in the depths of the parenchyma, where they may be missed unless the liver is carefully palpated and sectioned with a knife. The necrotic area is surrounded by an obvious zone of deep congestion. Lesions may be found anywhere in the liver, but the majority tend to be located in the ventral lobe. Evidence of liver fluke migration in the form of subcapsular haemorrhages and greenish yellow scars (accumulations of eosinophils) may be evident near the lesion.

Microscopical examination of sections prepared from the liver lesions show a central core of necrotic tissue demarcated from the congested parenchyma by a leucocytic barrier (Fig. 44.3). Within the barrier and at the periphery of the necrotic tissue, large numbers of vegetative clostridia are evident. The hepatic cells immediately adjacent to the leucocytic barrier show degenerative changes.

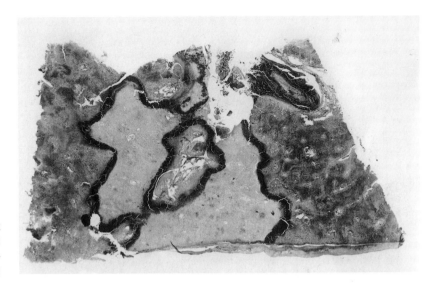

Fig. 44.3 A section through a black disease lesion demonstrating the central necrotic area and the clearly stained leucocyte barrier. (Haematoxylin and eosin, ×5.)

Diagnosis

The post-mortem findings of the characteristic lesions provide a firm basis for arriving at a diagnosis. Fluorescent antibody techniques can be used for the rapid identification of *Cl. novyi* in impression smears made from the periphery of the liver lesion as described by Batty *et al.* (1964). Toxins may also be demonstrated in the liver lesions and peritoneal fluid (Williams, 1964), although the laboratory tests for these are laborious and time-consuming. If the post-mortem findings are inconclusive and the carcass shows evidence of decomposition then the fluorescent antibody and toxin tests cannot be reliably used, since *Cl. novyi* may have multiplied in the liver and other locations after death (Bagadi & Sewell, 1974), and some of the strains found in livers are of low pathogenicity (Williams, 1964) but are detected by fluorescent antibody techniques.

Other cases of sudden or rapid death have to be considered in differential diagnosis and these include anthrax (p. 717), other clostridial infections such as clostridial myositis (p. 723), lead poisoning (pp. 906, 944) and metabolic disorders (Chapter 46). It is vital that blood smears for anthrax diagnosis be examined before post-mortem examination is carried out and thereby prevent environmental contamination with anthrax spores.

Treatment and prevention

There is little opportunity for effective treatment, although in those cattle that are ailing for one to two days, the administration of broad-spectrum antibiotics or penicillin and *Cl. novyi* antiserum may be of value.

Effective vaccines have been developed and in areas where liver fluke occurs their use should be advocated.

Two doses of vaccine at an interval of not less than one month are required to produce a satisfactory immunity (see p. 1005). Because of the association with liver fluke infection, control measures should also be adopted for this parasite. (see p. 278).

Pericarditis

Infection of the pericardial sac by micro-organisms results in a purulent or non-purulent pericarditis with the accumulation of varying amounts of fluid and consequential masking or muffling of heart sounds, and may lead to congestive heart failure.

Aetiology

A wide range of micro-organisms are associated with bovine pericarditis and they include *A. pyogenes*, *Haemophilus somnus*, *Mycobacterium bovis*, *Mannheimia* and *Pasteurella* species, staphylococci, streptococci and *Mycoplasma* species.

Infection with pyogenic bacteria is nearly always primary and frequently associated with traumatic reticulitis. The organisms are introduced during penetration of the pericardial sac by a foreign body originating from the reticulum, or infection may be the result of direct spread from a traumatic mediastinitis. In some instances a purulent infection may be superimposed on an original non-purulent fibrinous pericarditis. Infection of the pericardial sac also occurs through the localization of a blood-borne infection or through the direct extension of a myocarditis or pleurisy.

During the early stages of a purulent pericarditis there is a marked hyperaemia and deposition of a fibrinous exudate on the epicardium. Varying amounts of fluid accumulate within the pericardial sac and, as the volume significantly increases, both atria and the right ventricle are compressed to such an extent that their function is impaired and congestive heart failure results. A severe toxaemia may also develop. In some instances, however, the volume of exudate is small and adhesions develop between the epicardium and pericardium, which become organized, resulting in complete attachment of the epicardium and pericardium, impaired cardiac function and congestive heart failure.

In non-purulent or fibrinous pericarditis, there is seldom a significant exudation of fluid and therefore no marked distension of the pericardial sac. The epicardium is hyperaemic and fibrinous deposits appear at the base of the heart, which subsequently spread over the whole of the epicardium and internal surface of the pericardium. Adhesions develop between the epicardium and pericardium, but these are not sufficiently dense or strong to impair cardiac movement.

Signs

The early clinical signs of pericarditis are often difficult to identify because they are obscured or dominated by those of the primary disease, e.g. pleurisy, traumatic reticulitis, and the onset of pericarditis may therefore be insidious. Arching of the back, reluctance to move, shallow and rapid abdominal respirations and elevation of body temperature to 40–41°C (104–106°F) are the initial signs. The pulse rate is increased, and percussion and palpation over the cardiac area of the thoracic wall elicits a pain response. It may be possible to detect a rough pericardial function sound by auscultation during the early stages, but this is by no means easy and may be missed.

As the condition progresses, fluid accumulates in the pericardial sac and the heart sounds become muffled, although sometimes a splashing sound may be detected. The signs of congestive heart failure, engorged jugular veins, a jugular pulse and subcutaneous oedema of the submandibular space, brisket and inguinal region, develop and most animals die within one or two weeks.

Some animals survive the acute phase with antibiotic treatment, and the signs of congestive heart failure abate slowly. However, complete recovery seldom if ever occurs and recovered animals should be sent for slaughter at the earliest opportunity.

Pathology

Blood samples from animals affected with a purulent pericarditis, especially traumatic pericarditis, show a marked leucocytosis and a shift to the left. However, the overall haematological picture depends to some extent on the causal agent and other lesions that may be present, so that the total white cell count may vary from only marginally above the normal range to more than 30000/μl.

The cardiac lesions found at post-mortem examination depend on the type of infection and the duration of illness. In acute purulent pericarditis the pericardium and epicardium are thickened and covered by a fibrinous deposit, and the pericardial sac distended with fluid, which varies from a dirty grey to a yellowish green colour with a foul odour. The atria and the right ventricle are compressed. When the condition is associated with traumatic injury it may be possible to identify a foreign body, but should this be wire it may have disintegrated. Occasionally, a rupture of one of the coronary vessels, an atrium, or ventricle may occur in traumatic pericarditis and under such circumstances the pericardial sac contains a mixture of blood and purulent fluid. In more chronic cases, the grossly thickened pericardium and epicardium are closely adherent except for loculi containing inspissated or thick creamy pus giving a 'bread and butter' appearance. Signs indicative of congestive heart failure are also identifiable and these include congested liver and lungs, engorged jugular veins and subcutaneous oedema of the submandibular space, brisket and inguinal region. If the pericarditis is associated with other conditions, e.g. traumatic reticulitis, pneumonia or pleurisy, then lesions attributable to them will also be present.

Evidence of a non-purulent or fibrinous pericarditis is sometimes seen in apparently healthy animals dying from other causes. In such animals there is a patchy or diffuse thickening of the pericardium with similarly distributed adhesions to the epicardium, which can be easily broken down. There is no evidence of interference with the cardiac function and the lesions are of no pathological significance.

Diagnosis

The clinical diagnosis of pericarditis is not easy because the signs may be dominated or obscured by those of the primary disease and it may be difficult to recognize the pericardial sounds. The characteristic friction sounds in the early stages may be confused with those of pleurisy, although the latter is synchronized with the respiratory movments. Similarly, the pericardial sounds may resemble the murmurs (p. 727) produced by valvular lesions, but unlike the murmurs, they persist for the whole of the cardiac cycle. The heart sounds may also be muffled by effusion associated with pleurisy but under such circumstances there are signs of respiratory involvement.

Treatment

Although long-term therapy with antimicrobial agents is indicated, it seldom results in complete recovery, especially when the pericarditis is traumatic in origin. Thus Blood and Hutchins (1955) report that only about 50 per cent of cattle with traumatic pericarditis treated with sulphamezathine and/or penicillin responded and were sufficiently recovered for salvage. Surgical drainage of the pericardial sac either by pericardiocentesis or pericardiotomy as described by Horney (1960) may also have to be considered. However, it must be emphasized that pericardiocentesis offers only temporary relief of less than 24 hours duration in most cases. There are a number of reports on the successful treatment of fibrinous and traumatic pericarditis by pericardiotomy (Jennings & McIntyre, 1957; Krishnamurthy *et al.*, 1979; Mason, 1979).

Tetanus

Tetanus has long been recognized as a highly fatal disease of all species of farm livestock. The disease is produced by the toxin of *Clostridium tetani* and is characterized by hyperaesthesia, tetany and convulsions.

Aetiology

Clostridium tetani is a spore-bearing organism and is considered to be one of the least fastidious clostridia as far as growth requirements are concerned. The spores are extremely resistant to environmental conditions. The organism has two main habitats, namely the soil and gastrointestinal tracts of animals and humans. It has been suggested that the main reservoir of infection for animals is soil. The organism produces a number of toxins, but the neurotoxin is the one of principal importance.

The portal of entry is usually through a deep puncture, although in cattle introduction into the genital tract at the time of parturition is also important. The organism may also gain entry into surgical wounds, e.g. after castration, and may be introduced into muscle during vaccination and other injections. There are however outbreaks of disease in cattle in which the organism has not localized in any tissue site but remained within the gastrointestinal tract, and such outbreaks are designated as idiopathic tetanus (Wallis, 1963).

After gaining entry into the tissue, the organism remains localized. Multiplication will only occur if optimal conditions develop at the site of infection. If at the time of initial injury there is sufficient tissue damage

and a lowered oxygen tension, immediate growth and toxin production will occur. However, such conditions may only be attained after healing at the surface has occurred, so that multiplication and toxin production may be delayed. Thus the incubation period may vary from a few days to four weeks or more. In idiopathic tetanus it would appear that the neurotoxin is produced in the rumen (Smith & Holdeman, 1968).

From the site of production the neurotoxin reaches the central nervous system via the peripheral nerve trunks. The exact mechanisms of transport are not known, nor are the means by which the toxin exerts its influence on the nervous system. Smith & Holdeman (1968) state that the neurotoxin can also reach the central nervous system via lymph and blood.

Individual or small numbers of animals are usually affected in a herd, but in outbreaks of idiopathic tetanus many animals may be affected.

Signs

As the incubation period may vary quite considerably it is not always possible to relate the onset of clinical disease to specific incidents of injury or surgical interference. The first signs are those of apparent stiffness and reluctance to move, accompanied by muscle tremors that become more pronounced. Another early sign in some cattle is prolapse of the third eyelid, which becomes more prominent with handling of the head. These signs are progressively followed by the appearance of a slight but persistent ruminal tympany, elevation of the tail, unsteady gait of the hindlimbs, especially when turning, and trismus with saliva drooling from the mouth. Because of inability to adopt the normal urinating posture, urine is retained. Further progression leads to generalized muscular tetany with the adoption of a 'rocking horse'-like posture. Attempts at walking lead to lateral recumbency and an inability to rise. Tetanic convulsions and opisthotonus soon develop. Initially, the convulsions are triggered by external stimuli, but later these occur spontaneously. The duration of fatal disease in young cattle is four to five days, but older cattle may survive for up to 10 days. Non-fatal cases do occur, but generally these do not progress to the convulsive stage and recovery is slow over a period of weeks or sometimes months.

Pathology

There are no tests available for the diagnosis of tetanus in the live animal and any tests undertaken would be for the purpose of eliminating those conditions that produce similar clinical signs. Nor are there any gross or microscopic pathological findings that would confirm tetanus, although attempts should be made to identify the site of infection and culture the organism.

Diagnosis

Because of the distinctive clinical signs, classical tetanus is seldom confused with other diseases. Clinical hypomagnesaemia (p. 255) in calves and cattle (p. 787) is accompanied by tetany and convulsions, but there is no prolapse of the third eyelid or ruminal tympany, and low blood calcium and magnesium levels are diagnostic. Cerebrocortical necrosis (CCN) (polioencephalomalacia) (p. 261, 903) may produce a similar clinical picture, except that again there is no prolapse of the third eyelid and no ruminal tympany. Also, in CCN the erythrocyte transketolase activity is decreased and blood pyruvate and lactate levels are increased, and classical lesions are obvious at necropsy. Some cases of lead poisoning (pp. 906, 944) may also show similar clinical signs, but elevated blood and kidney/liver lead values are diagnostic. Strychnine poisoning is extremely rare in cattle in Great Britain and is usually associated with the ingestion of earthworms treated with strychnine. Strychnine is used for the destruction of moles, and can be identified in the abomasal contents. It is used in other counties, often illegally, to kill wildlife. Bovine spongiform encephalopathy (p. 909) may also need to be differentiated but the signs usually develop over a longer period than tetanus.

Treatment and prevention

Cattle appear to respond better to treatment than horses and sheep, although it is unlikely that fully developed tetanus will respond and therefore under such circumstances euthanasia should be considered.

When treatment is undertaken it should have three objectives: elimination of *Cl. tetani*, neutralization of unfixed neurotoxin and the induction and maintenance of muscle relaxation until all the neurotoxin has been destroyed or eliminated.

Large doses of penicillin administered parenterally is the recommended treatment for *Cl. tetani* infection and this should be supplemented by treatment of the infected site (if located) by irrigation and topical application of antibiotics. Thus treatment should continue for at least seven days.

The administration of antitoxin for the neutralization of unfixed neurotoxin is considered to be of little value unless administered during the very early stages of the disease. If the site of infection has been identified then local injection of the antitoxin may be of value.

A number of drugs have been used to relieve muscle tetany, but because of the need for long-term relaxation some are not suitable because their activity is of short duration. The recommended drugs (Radostits *et al.*, 2000) are chlorpromazine (0.4 mg/kg body weight intravenously, 1.0 mg/kg body weight intramuscularly) three to four times daily and acetyl promazine (0.05 mg/kg body weight), administered twice daily for eight to ten days or until the severe clinical signs have disappeared.

Animals that are treated should be kept in dark quiet surroundings with ample bedding and sufficient space to avoid injuring themselves if convulsions occur.

On farms where tetanus is a problem, vaccinations should be routinely undertaken (see p. 1005).

Leptospirosis (other than *Leptospira hardjo* infection)

Aetiology

There are many different serotypes of *Leptospira interrogans* present in cattle.

Aetiology

Many serotypes do occur but probably the most important are *L. interrogans* serovar *icterohaemorrhagiae* and serovar *canicola*. *Leptospira interrogans* serovar *pomona* has been found in many countries to be the commonest infection of farm animals. It has only recently been found in Britain and the strain appears to be different from the one causing abortion in pigs. In many cases there are carrier animals and often these are rodents. The leptospires survive in the environment if conditions are wet. However, they are inhibited at a pH less than 6 or greater than 8. Temperatures below 7–10°C (44.5–50°F) or above 34–36°C (93–96°F) are detrimental. The organisms can survive over four months under wet conditions but only 30 minutes when the soil is dried. It often survives in the environment in average conditions for about one and a half months.

Most infection is spread via contaminated feed or water. It must be remembered that most serovarieties are able to infect many species including man.

Mortality rate is usually low at about 5 per cent.

Signs

Acute: The cow is often ill with a pyrexia of 40–41°C (104–106°F) with dullness and anorexia. The milk yield drops and often there are haemorrhages under the mucous membranes, and there is often jaundice and haemoglobinuria. In some cases there is synovitis or a necrotic dermatitis. Occasionally, meningitis has been recorded.

Subacute: In this form the signs are milder with a temperature of 39–40°C (102–104°F). The animal has a reduced milk yield and is dull. Jaundice occurs in some cases and there is usually some haemoglobinuria. In some cases abortion occurs about a month later.

Chronic: This is not common and results in abortion.

Necropsy

Acute: There are often submucosal and subserosal haemorrhages, jaundice, anaemia and haemoglobinuria. In some animals there is ulceration of the abomasal mucosa and emphysema. Histological examination often shows an interstitial nephritis as well as centrilobular hepatic necrosis.

Subacute or chronic cases are more likely to show a progressive interstitial nephritis with white foci on the surface of the renal cortex.

Diagnosis

This depends on finding the organism. Otherwise, paired serum samples can be examined for a rise in *Leptospira* titres.

Differential diagnosis

Any form of haemoglobinuria will need to be eliminated, including babesiosis (p. 748), which is usually seen in the summer in tick areas. Kale poisoning (p. 941) and postparturient haemoglobinuria (p. 792) should be partly diagnosed by the history and the low plasma phosphorus levels in the latter. Bacillary haemoglobinuria (p. 719) will be differentiated by the presence of clostridia.

Treatment

The main therapy is usually antibiotics such as dihydrostreptomycin or the tetracyclines. Treatment should be given as soon as signs develop. Blood transfusion often helps. The farmer should be warned of possible human infection.

Control

Separate the infected cow. If it is partly due to rodent build-up, control the rodents. Ensure removal of brackish water and provide good drainage. Vaccination could be used, as with *L. interrogans* serovar *canicola* or *icterohaemorrhagiae*, but as cases are usually sporadic this does not tend to be used.

Leptospira hardjo infection (flabby bag) (see p. 580)

Aetiology

Infection with *Leptospira borgpetersenii* serovar *hardjo* (*Hardjo bovis*) and *Leptospira interrogans* serovar *hardjo* (*Hardjo prajitno*), spiral organisms.

These are a common cause of abortion in Britain, although they have only recently been readily diagnosed. *Leptospira borgpetersenii* sv *hardjo* appears to be better adapted to cattle; it is excreted in large numbers in urine although it is less frequently isolated from aborted fetuses whereas *L. interrogans* sv *hardjo* appears to be less well adapted in cattle (possibly more in sheep), while isolated from Britain, India, Nigeria, Malaysia and the USA, it has not been seen in Australia and New Zealand; urine shedding of organisms is low, but it is more frequently found in aborted fetuses and is relatively more pathogenic.

Up to 50–60 per cent of British farms may be infected. In Northern Ireland 41.6 per cent of randomly selected aborted fetuses were infected (Ellis *et al.*, 1982) and the level rose to 68.9 per cent of fetuses from farms with abortion problems. A very common problem in New Zealand, most cases are in the dairy herd rather than beef cattle. Humans can be infected but they must be exposed to concentrated infection, i.e. contact via urine while milking. Although infection is present in the milk, it quickly dies off once taken from the udder. Meat does not carry infection. Spread occurs more rapidly in wet seasons in low-lying areas. Colostrum-derived protection normally lasts about three months. Serological rises in *L. hardjo* titres following infection tend to be short-lived, i.e. a few months to a year or so. It was originally considered to be a winter disease. However, carriers often stop or reduce excretion on silage. Most infection now occurs in the summer, often with abortion in the summer or early autumn. Serology in individual animals is difficult to interpret because the bacteria are in the lumen of the kidney or uterus.

The spread of infection takes place cow to cow via urine, fetuses and uterine discharge, and from bull to cow by infected semen. The source of infection is via carrier cows or infected calves, which may be chronically infected, but it may possibly be spread by contaminated water or sheep on the farm.

Signs

There are two main syndromes, the udder form and abortion.

Severe udder form: In a cow or heifer the udder signs will not be apparent until the animal has calved. This form occurs soon after the infection enters a herd. There is a sudden drop in milk yield affecting all four quarters, with pyrexia usually between 40 and 41.5°C (104–107°F). The udder secretion becomes thickened and clotted, occasionally it is bloody or it can be yellow and colostrum-like. The udder itself is not swollen or inflamed but tends to be flaccid. In a six to eight-week period, 30–50 per cent of the herd may be infected. The condition usually resolves over seven to ten days (see p. 580).

Mild udder form: Many cows are infected and show only a slight drop in milk yield.

Abortion: This usually occurs six to twelve weeks after the dam is infected. Abortion can occur on its own or be preceded by the milk drop syndrome. Most cases of abortion occur in the second half of pregnancy. If infection occurs late in pregnancy then an infected calf may be born. There may be some apparent infertility in the herd (see p. 580).

Necropsy

Abortion: There are usually no useful macroscopic features in the aborted fetus.

Diagnosis

Udder form: History helps in diagnosis, in particular the sudden onset of the problem. The signs, sudden loss of milk, flaccid udder, are useful. The Californian Milk Test is positive and there is a high milk white cell count. Identification and culture of the organisms from urine (it can occasionally be isolated from milk and blood in the acute stages) is a definitive diagnosis. Paired serum samples can be used for the complement fixation test, microscopic agglutination test and plate agglutination test. High titres over 1/300 indicate recent exposure to infection. Microagglutination titres are found from 10 days after infection; their peak and duration depend on the serotype and route of infection. IgM titres appear first but peak two to three weeks after infection whilst IgG levels appear later and peak 12–30 weeks post infection (G.S. Dhaliwals, pers. com.). Serum and vaginal mucus antibody tests are also available.

Abortion: Identification of the bacterium in the fetus, especially in the lungs, kidneys or adrenal glands, by fluorescent antibody studies, is the main method of diagnosis. It can also be isolated from abortion or post calving discharge. Culture of the bacteria can be undertaken. Fetal serology can also be used. Antibodies may be detected in post calving discharges and cervical mucus. Serology of the dam can help but often antibody titres may be static or falling by the time of abortion. It is very difficult to detect carrier animals, as up to 25 per cent are serologically negative. Bulk herd milk samples can indicate the presence of infection and also give some suggestion of infection levels.

Differential diagnosis

Other leptospiral infections (p. 734), salmonellosis (Chapter 15), foot-and-mouth disease (p. 700), and mastitis (Chapter 23) must all be considered in the udder form. In abortion, (p. 578) salmonellosis, mucosal disease, brucellosis, *Neospora carinum* infection (pp. 283, 584) and infectious bovine rhinotracheitis are some common causes to be differentiated.

Treatment

Large doses of dihydrostreptomycin (25 mg/kg body weight) may help remove the organism and prevent kidney and liver damage. All cattle due to calve should be vaccinated. In countries where dihydrostreptomycin is not available, amoxycillin appears to be equally effective.

Control

Vaccination is possible with a killed strain (p.1015). The vaccines available may contain *Hardjobovis* or *Hardjoprajitno* strains; there is not always cross-protection between the two strains. *Hardjoprajitno* vaccines may produce a longer duration of immunity (G.S. Dhaliwal, pers. comm.). Both vaccines will control abortion and improve fertility in endemic herds. Vaccination of young stock may also produce benefits. Vaccination involves two initial doses at least four weeks apart. If cattle are young when vaccination commences then two doses are required after five months of age. An annual booster is recommended but two vaccinations a year may be required in herds that calve in the autumn. It does not affect animals that already have milk drop syndrome. Vaccination does help prevent abortion but infected cows may still excrete bacteria. It is therefore advisable to treat all adult cattle with dihydrostreptomycin before commencing a vaccination programme.

Any bought-in animals, and especially bulls, should be isolated and treated with antibiotics and vaccine before entering the herd. Reducing exposure to potentially contaminated water supplies and to pasture grazed by sheep is a sensible management control.

Haemophilus somnus infection

(see p. 907)

Aetiology

A Gram-negative small rod-shaped organism. Most strains of the organism are antigenically similar.

Epidemiology

It is seen in North America and Europe. Inapparent infection occurs more frequently than clinical disease. Problems occur more frequently in younger animals. The portal of entry of infections is often via the respiratory tract although it is also found in the reproductive and urinary tracts. Disease is probably a septicaemia with localization. Single or several cases may occur.

Signs

The peracute form often causes sudden death. The acute form is often seen as the sleeper syndrome or thromboembolic meningoencephalitis (TEME) in growing cattle. The animal is depressed, with closed eyes, and recumbent. Usually there is pyrexia (40–42°C, 104–108°F). Nervous signs can be of muscle tremors and hyperaesthesia. The animal may be blind with retinal haemorrhage. Other syndromes include synovitis with initial lameness. Pneumonia is a common finding, particularly in calves, and often associated with pleurisy (see Chapter 17). Abortion can occur and so can chronic bloat.

Pathology

There may be focal or diffuse cerebral meningitis with characteristic haemorrhagic infarcts in the brain. Haemorrhages can occur in other organs. In the joint form the synovial membranes are oedematous with petechial haemorrhages. There is often inflammation of the pericardium, peritoneum and pleura which may be serofibrinous or fibrinous. Histologically there is often a vasculitis and thrombosis, often with infarcts and accumulation of neutrophils.

Prognosis

Recumbent cattle often do not recover and usually, if there is no response after three days' treatment, the condition is irreversible.

Treatment and control

High doses of intravenous tetracyclines for at least three days can be useful. Otherwise ampicillin, amoxycillin, florfenicol, novobiocin, sulphonamides or potentiated sulphonamides can be administered. Once disease is diagnosed, extra observation must be undertaken of in-contact animals. Control is difficult, although in North America an aluminium hydroxide adjuvenated vaccine is now used.

Pyaemia

Pyaemia is defined as a clinical or pathological state characterized by the formation of multiple secondary abscesses in a number of organs and/or tissues.

The primary pyogenic infection may occur in a number of sites and the formation of metastatic lesions in other organs and tissues follows the entry of organisms into the circulation. Small numbers of organisms may intermittently gain entry via the lymphatic drainage of the primary lesion, to produce a bacteraemia, followed by localization and the formation of secondary abscesses. More frequently, however, a septic thrombus is formed within the primary lesion and portions of this become detached to form emboli, which are then arrested in the capillary bed of an organ or tissues to form the metastatic lesions. The most frequent sites for secondary abscess formation are the valvular endocardium, myocardium, lungs and joints, although the liver and kidneys may sometimes be involved.

In cattle, pyaemia is often associated with septic metritis and mastitis, and *A. pyogenes* is the organism most frequently incriminated. Staphylococcal mastitis may also lead, in some cases, to pyaemia. On occasions, hepatic abscesses and foul in the foot caused by *Fusobacterium necrophorum* may also result in pyaemia.

Because pyaemia is a form of generalization of a primary infection, the clinical signs, diagnosis and treatment must be considered in relation to the primary infections referred to above and which are discussed in the appropriate sections of the text.

References

Anthrax

Bailey, W.W. (1953) Anthrax: response by terramycin therapy. *Journal of the American Veterinary Medical Association*, **122**, 305–6.

Campbell, A.D. (1969) Anthrax: A problem of the livestock industry. *Veterinary Record*, **85**, 89–90.

Greenough, P.R. (1965) Anthrax and antibiotics. *Veterinary Record*, **77**, 784–5.

Hugh-Jones, M.E. & Hussaini, S.N. (1975) Anthrax in England and Wales 1963–1972. *Veterinary Record*, **97**, 256–61.

Lincoln, R.E., Walker, J.S., Klein, F. & Haines, B.W. (1964) Anthrax. *Advances in Veterinary Science*, **9**, 327–68.

Schlingham, A.S., Devlin, H.B., Wright, G.G., Maine, R.J. & Manning, M.C. (1956) Immunising activity of alum precipitated antigen of *B. anthracis* in cattle, sheep and swine. *American Journal of Veterinary Research*, **17**, 256–61.

Sterne, M. (1959) In *Infectious Diseases of Animals*, lst edn (ed. by A.W. Stableforth & I.A. Galloway), Vol. 1, pp. 16–52. Butterworth Scientific Publications, London.

Bacillary haemoglobinuria

Blood, D.C., Radostits, O.M. & Henderson, J.A. (1983) *Veterinary Medicine*, 6th end, p. 548. Baillière Tindall, London.

Roberts, R.S. (1959) In *Infectious Diseases of Animals*, 1st edn (ed. by A.W. Stableforth & I.A. Galloway), Vol. 1, p. 200. Butterworth Scientific Publications, London.

Smith, L.D. (1957) Clostridial diseases of animals. *Advances in Veterinary Science*, **3**, 463–524.

Smith, L.D. & Holdeman, (1968) *The Pathogenic Anaerobic Bacteria*, pp. 339–48. Charles C. Thomas, Springfield, Illinois.

Williams, B.M. (1964) *Clostridium* oedematous infections (black disease and bacillary haemoglobinuria) of cattle in mid Wales. *Veterinary Record*, **76**, 591–6.

Botulism

Appleyard, W.T. & Mollison, A. (1985) Suspected bovine botulism associated with broiler litter waste. *Veterinary Record*, **116**, 535.

Breuknik, H.I., Wagenaar, G., Wensing, T., Notermans, S. & Poulos, P.W. (1978) Food poisoning in cattle caused by the ingestion of brewers grains contaminated by *Clostridium botulinum* type B. *Tijdschrift voor Diergeneeskunde*, **103**, 303–11.

Clegg, F.G. & Evans, R.K. (1974) Suspected case of botulism in calves. *Veterinary Record*, **95**, 540.

Clegg, F.G., Jones, T.O., Smart, J.L. & McMurty, M.J. (1985) Bovine botulism associated with broiler litter waste. *Veterinary Record*, **117**, 22.

Davies, A.B., Roberts, T.A. & Bradshaw, P.R. (1974) Probable botulism in calves. *Veterinary Record*, **94**, 412–14.

Egyed, M.N., Shlosberg, A., Klopfer, V., Nobel, T.A. & Mayer, E. (1978) Mass outbreaks of botulism in ruminants associated with ingestion of feed containing poultry waste: Clinical findings. *Refuah. Veterinerath*, **35**, 93–9.

Ektvedt, R. & Hanssen, I. (1974) Outbreak of botulism in cattle. *Norske Veterinaertidsskrift*, **86**, 286–96.

Fjolstad, M. & Kluna, T. (1969) An outbreak of botulism among ruminants in connection with ensilage feeding. *Nordisk Veterinarmedicin*, **21**, 609–13.

Haagsma, J. & Laak, E.A. (1977) Type B botulism in cattle fed grass silage. Report of an outbreak. *Tijdschrift voor Diergeneeskunde*, **102**, 330.

Muller, J. (1961) Type C botulism in man and animals – incidence in cattle and horses. *Medlemsblad for den Danske Dyrlaegeforening*, **44**, 547–57.

Notermans, S., Kozaki, S., Dufrenne, J. & Scothorst, M. van (1979a) Studies on the persistence of *Clostridium botulinum* on a cattle farm. *Tijdschrift voor Diergeneeskunde*, **104**, 707–12.

Notermans, S., Kozaki, S. & Scothorst, M. van (1979b) Toxin production by *Clostridium botulinum* in grass. *Applied and Environmental Microbiology*, **39**, 767–76.

Prevot, A.R. & Sillioc, R. (1955) A biological enigma: resistance of cats to *Clostridium botulinum* toxin. *Annales de l'Institut Pasteur*, **89**, 354–7.

Smith, L.D. (1977) *Botulism, the Organisms, its Toxins, the Disease*, pp. 15, 91–6. Charles C. Thomas, Springfield, Illinois.

Clostridial myositis: blackleg and malignant oedema

Blood, D.C., Radostits, O.M. & Henderson, J.A. (1983) *Veterinary Medicine*, 6th edn, pp. 541–5. Baillière Tindall, London.

Harwood, D.G. (1984) Apparent iatrogenic clostridial myositis in cattle. *Veterinary Record*, **115**, 412.

Harwood, D.G. (1994) Clostridial myositis – an old fashioned disease? *Cattle Practice*, **2**, 323–9.

Jubb, K.V.F., Kennedy P.C. & Palmer, A. (1983) *Pathology of Domestic Animals*, pp. 180–4. Academic Press, London.

Kerry, J.B. (1964) A note on the occurrence of *Clostridium chauveoi* in the spleens and livers of normal cattle. *Veterinary Record*, **76**, 396.

Radostits, O.M., Gay, C.C., Blood, D.C. & Hinchcliff, K.W. (2000) *Veterinary Medicine*, 9th edn, pp. 763–4. W.B. Saunders, London.

Williams, B.M. (1977) Clostridial myositis in cattle: bacteriology and gross pathology. *Veterinary Record*, **100**, 90–1.

Contagious bovine pyelonephritis

Ado, P.B. & Cook J.E. (1979) Specific immunofluorescence of *Corynebacterium renale*. *British Veterinary Journal*, **135**, 50–4.

Goudswaard, J. & Budhai, S. (1975) Some aspects of the immunological response in cattle with *Corynebacterium renale*. Identification of a new serotype, type IV. *Zentralblatt fur Veterinarmedizin*, **22B**, 473–9.

Hiramune, T., Invi, S., Murase, N. & Yanagawa, R. (1972) Antibody response in cows infected with *Corynebacterium renale*. *Research in Veterinary Science*, **13**, 82–6.

Hiramune, T., Narita, M., Tomonari, I., Murase, N. & Yanagawa, R. (1975) Distribution of *Corynebacterium renale* among healthy bulls, with special reference to inhabitation of type III in the prepuce. *National Institute of Animal Health Quarterly, Tokyo*, **15**, 116–21.

Morse, E.V. (1950) An ecological study of *Corynebacterium renale*. *Cornell Veterinarian*, **40**, 178–87.

Takai, S., Yanagawa, R. & Kitamura, Y. (1980) pH dependent adhesion of piliated *Corynebacterium renale* to bovine bladder cells. *Infection and Immunity*, **28**, 669–74.

Endocarditis

Andersen, H.K. (1963) Investigations on pathogenesis, the aetiology and topography of endocarditis in cattle. *Nordisk Veterinarmedicin*, **15**, 668–90.

Biering-Sørensen, V. (1963) Incidence of endocarditis in cattle and its seasonal variation. *Nordisk Veterinarmedicin*, **15**, 691–5.

Evans, E.T.R. (1957) Bacterial endocarditis in cattle. *Veterinary Record*, **69**, 1196–1202.

John, F.V. (1947) Verrucose endocarditis. *Veterinary Record*, **59**, 214.

Lacuta, A.Q., Yamada, H., Nakamura, Y. & Hirose, T. (1980) Electrographic and echocardiographic findings in four cases of bovine endocarditis. *Journal of the American Veterinary Medical Association*, **176**, 1353–65.

Larsen, H.R. (1963) Clinical observations on endocarditis in cattle. *Nordisk Veterinarmedicin*, **15**, 645–67.

Power, H.T. & Rebhun, W.C. (1983) Bacterial endocarditis in cattle. *Journal of the American Veterinary Medical Association*, **182**, 806–8.

Wuijckhuise-Sjouke, L.A. van (1984) Plasma fibrinogen concentration as an indicator of the presence and severity of inflammatory disease in horses and cattle. *Tijdschrift voor Diergeneeskunde*, **109**, 869–72.

Haemorrhagic septicaemia

Bain, R.V.S. (1963) *Haemorrhagic septicaemia*, Agricultural Studies No. 62. Food and Agricultural Organization, Rome.

Carter, G.R. (1982) Whatever happened to haemorrhagic septicaemia. *Journal of the American Veterinary Medical Association*, **180**, 1176–7.

Carter, G.R. & Bain, R.V.S. (1960) Pasteurellosis (*Pasteurella multocida*). A review stressing recent developments. *Veterinary Review Annotations*, **6**, 105–28.

De Alwis, M.C.L. & Carter, G.R. (1980) Preliminary field trials with streptomycin dependent vaccine against haemorrhagic septicaemia. *Veterinary Record*, **68**, 223–4.

Jubb, K.V.F., Kennedy, P.C. & Palmer, N. (1985) *Pathology of Domestic Animals*, 3rd edn, Vol. 2, pp. 488–9. Academic Press, London.

Macadam, I. (1962) Tick transmission of bovine pasteurellosis. *Veterinary Record*, **74**, 689–90.

Mustafa, A.A., Ghalib, H.W. & Shigidi, M.J. (1978) Carrier rate of *Past. multocida* in cattle herds associated with an outbreak of haemorrhagic septicaemia in Sudan. *British Veterinary Journal*, **134**, 375–8.

Sawada, T., Rimler, R.B. & Rhoades, K.R. (1985) Haemorrhagic septicaemia: naturally acquired antibodies against *Past. multocida* types B and E in calves in the United States. *American Journal of Veterinary Research*, **46**, 1247–50.

Shirlaw, J.F. (1938) Haemorrhagic septicaemia: A criticism of the present position with an account of investigations into the problem in the Northumbrian area. *Veterinary Record*, **50**, 1005–9.

Wei, B.D. & Carter, G.R. (1978) Live streptomycin dependent *Past. multocida* vaccine for the prevention of haemorrhagic septicaemia. *American Journal of Veterinary Research*, **39**, 1534–7.

Infectious necrotic hepatitis

Bagadi, H.O. & Sewell, M.M.H. (1973) An epidemiological survey of infectious necrotic hepatitis of sheep (black disease) in Scotland. *Research in Veterinary Science*, **15**, 49–53.

Bagadi, H.O. & Sewell, M.M.H. (1974) Influence of post mortem autolysis on the diagnosis of infectious necrotic hepatitis (black disease). *Research in Veterinary Science*, **17**, 320–7.

Batty, I., Buntain, D. & Walker, P.D. (1964) *Clostridium oedematiens*, a cause of sudden death in sheep, cattle and pigs. *Veterinary Record*, **76**, 115–17.

Herbert, T.G.G. & Hughes, L.E. (1956) Black disease (infectious necrotic hepatitis) in a heifer. *Veterinary Record*, **68**, 223–4.

Williams, B.M. (1964) *Clostridium oedematiens* infections (black disease and bacillary haemoglobinuria) of cattle in mid-Wales. *Veterinary Record*, **76**, 591–6.

Williams, B.M. (1976) Infectious necrotic hepatitis of sheep: An epidemiological survey on Welsh farms. *British Veterinary Journal*, **132**, 221–5.

Pericarditis

Blood, D.C. & Hutchins, D.R. (1995) Traumatic pericarditis of cattle. *Australian Veterinary Journal*, **31**, 229–32.

Horney, F.D. (1960) Surgical drainage of the bovine pericardial sac. *Canadian Veterinary Journal*, **1**, 363–5.

Jennings, S. & McIntyre, W.M. (1957) Pericardiectomy in a cow. *Veterinary Record*, **69**, 928.

Krishnamurthy, D., Nigam, J.M., Peshin, P.K. & Kharole, M.U. (1979) Thorapericardiotomy and pericardiotomy in cattle. *Journal of the American Veterinary Medical Association*, **175**, 714–18.

Mason, T.A. (1979) Suppurative pericarditis treated by pericardiotomy in a cow. *Veterinary Record*, **105**, 305–1.

Tetanus

Radostits, O.M., Gay, C.C., Blood, D.C. & Hinchcliff, K.W. (2000) *Veterinary Medicine*, 9th edn, pp. 754–7. W.B. Saunders, London.

Smith, L.D. & Holdeman, L.V. (1968) *The Pathogenic Anaerobic Bacteria*, pp. 256–81. Charles C. Thomas, Springfield, Illinois.

Wallis, A.S. (1963) Some observations on the epidemiology of tetanus in cattle, *Veterinary Record*, **75**, 188–91.

Leptospira hardjo *infection*

Ellis, W.A., O'Brien, J.J., Neill, S.D., Ferguson, M.W. & Hanna, J. (1982) Bovine leptospirosis: Microbial and serological findings in aborted fetuses. *Veterinary Record*, **110**, 147–50.

Chapter 45

Ectoparasites, Tick and Arthropod-borne Diseases

S.M. Taylor, A.G. Hunter and A.H. Andrews

ECTOPARASITES	740
Insects	740
Hypodermatosis (warbles)	740
Lice (pediculosis)	741
Arachnids	742
Mange	742
Tick infestations	744
Ixodoidea	744
Fly problems	745
Mosquitoes	745
Blackflies	745
Midges	745
Horseflies and deerflies	745
Houseflies	746
Bush flies	746
Face fly	746
Head fly	746
Stable fly	746
Horn flies and buffalo flies	747
Horse louse flies	747
Tsetse flies	747
Tumbu fly	747
Blow flies and screw-worm flies	747
TICK AND ARTHROPOD-BORNE DISEASES	748
Protozoal diseases	748
Babesiosis (redwater)	748
Theileriosis	750
Besnoitiosis	756
Trypanosomosis	756
Rickettsial diseases	761
Anaplasmosis	761
Tick-borne fever	763
Bovine petechial fever (Ondiri disease, ondiritis)	763
Heartwater (cowdriosis or malignant rickettsia, blacklung)	765
Jembrana disease (Tabana disease)	766
Viral diseases	767
Bovine ephemeral fever (BEF)	767
Lumpy skin disease (LSD)	768
Rift Valley fever	769
Tick-borne encephalitides (flavivirus infections)	770
Tick-borne encephalitides (Near East encephalitis)	771
Japanese encephalitis (flavivirus)	771
Other arthropod-borne diseases	771
Parasitic diseases	774
Onchocercosis (worm nodule disease)	774
Stephanofilariosis	774
Thelaziosis	775
Other problems	775
Tick paralysis	775
Sweating sickness	776
Mhlosimge	777
Magudu	777
Stomatitis–nephrosis syndrome	777

ECTOPARASITES

Insects

Hypodermatosis (warbles) (see p. 875)

Hypodermatosis is the term used to describe infection with and the lesions caused by the larvae of two species of the fly genus *Hypoderma*, *H. bovis* and *H. lineatum*. The disease is characterized by damage to dorsal hides, oesophagus, central nervous system and occasionally death due to anaphylaxis (see p. 927).

Aetiology and epidemiology

The adult flies are distributed in the northern hemisphere, excluding the most northerly arctic regions. There are two species, *H. bovis* and *H. lineatum*. *Hypoderma bovis* favours the northern parts of their habitat areas and *H. Lineatum* the southern and warmer areas, but both species can occur simultaneously. The adult flies have a yellow abdomen characterized by a broad stripe of black hairs. They are active in warm weather, generally in Europe between the months of June and August. Their presence upsets cattle, which run to avoid them and in doing so injure themselves on fences or other obstacles. The females of *H. bovis* deposit eggs singly on hairs, frequently above the hocks on the hind legs; the eggs of *H. lineatum* are laid in rows, whence its name was derived, usually on the lower part of the body and in places where both adult and eggs are difficult for cattle to dislodge. The eggs adhere strongly to the hairs. They hatch in four to six days and the first stage larvae crawl down to the skin, which they penetrate, and proceed to migrate through soft tissues towards their overwintering sites. This movement takes several weeks, and by late autumn *H. bovis* has reached the epidural fat within the vertebral column and *H. lineatum* the submucosa of the oesophagus. The larvae remain in these sites during the winter, moulting to their second stage of development. At the end of the winter they resume migration both reaching the subdermal tissue along the back in the spring. They make a hole in the overlying skin through which they respire while developing to the third stage, which reaches a length of 2–3 cm and is characterized by rows of small spines on the posterior margin of most of its segments and posterior spiracles on a terminal tuberosity. The creamy-white larvae emerge from the back of the animal in April and May and fall to the ground to continue development by pupation, eventually emerging as adults five weeks later. They have a short lifespan as adults, mating, laying eggs and dying within two weeks of emergence.

Pathogenesis

The larvae are most pathogenic during two phases of their development. The first is during the late autumn and winter, when they are in epidural fat or oesophageal wall respectively. If present in large numbers, or if treated killed *in situ*, the anaphylactic reactions may cause damage to the spinal cord that can result in either spinal paralysis or difficulty in swallowing and eructation, which can lead to bloat. The second is during their pre-emergence development, where they damage the subdermal tissue and skin of the back and cause subsequent downgrading of hides and trimming of carcasses, and cause irritation and loss of growth in the live animal.

Signs

In the late autumn and winter, occasionally there can be damage to the spinal cord resulting in paralysis, difficulty in standing or bloat. In the spring, there are swellings under the skin 55–75 cm either side of the midline containing pus, a breathing hole and a third stage larva.

Diagnosis

If disease results during their winter development, the symptoms have to be differentiated from other causes of spinal or oesophageal paralysis. There is an ELISA test available that detects antibody to migrating larvae and, although originally designed to aid eradication programmes, it may be helpful in diagnosis. When larvae are in their pre-emergence sites on the back their presence is unmistakeable since no other condition causes similar lesions, especially if a heavy infection is present.

Treatment

The larvae are susceptible during their migration to systemic organophosphorus insecticides and the anthelmintics ivermectin, doramectin, eprinomectin, abamectin and moxidectin. Care should be taken not to treat cattle when larvae are in their overwintering sites, as death *in situ* and subsequent lysis may result in anaphylaxis. For that reason statutory eradication policies have compulsory treatments applied before mid November, coupled where necessary with inspection and further treatments in the following spring.

The organophosphorus treatments are normally applied dermally as pour-on preparations. A large number are available, the most popular currently being phosmet and crufomate. Mass treatment has resulted in eradication from many islands although it has proved more difficult on large land areas. Avermectins, although highly effective, are not normally used in mass eradication campaigns since their primary use is as an anthelmintic, although if a single animal in a herd is found to be infected the entire herd is usually treated with them. Although prophylaxis against adult flies is not actively undertaken, slow-release devices such as ear tags impregnated with organophosphorus compounds or synthetic pyrethroids do reduce the possibility of ovi-position by adults.

Lice (pediculosis)

Lice are ubiquitous parasites of cattle. In large numbers they cause skin irritation and have been associated with anaemia and may act as vectors of pathogenic organisms (see p. 880).

Aetiology and epidemiology

Lice are host-specific parasites and are classified into two types: (i) sucking lice and (ii) biting lice. Five species infest cattle, four sucking and one biting. The former are *Haematopinus eurysternus* and *H. quadripertusus*, 'short-nosed' sucking lice; *Lignognathus vituli*, 'long-nosed' and *Solenopotes capillatus*, 'small blue' sucking lice. The biting species is *Damalinia bovis*. As might be construed the sucking lice have mouthparts adapted for piercing skin and sucking blood; the biting lice ingest skin and hair detritus, blood and scabs. Each species has a preferential area on animals, but if large numbers are present can be found anywhere on the body surface. Normally, *H. eurysternus* and *D. bovis* are found on the poll, neck and head and the latter also along the mid dorsal region of the body. *Lignognathus vituli* and *S. capillatus* also favour the head, neck and frequently the ventral surface of the neck, dewlap and axillae. *Haematopinus quadripertusus* is restricted to subtropical areas and is usually found in the area of the tail and posterior lumbar regions.

The life cycle of lice is direct. Adults live for approximately one month during which time they lay a few hundred eggs, which are tightly attached to hair by a glue-like substance produced by the louse. The eggs hatch within a few days and the first nymph, which resembles a small softer adult, emerges. It undergoes three moults to second and third stage nymphs and finally adults, each nymphal stage taking one week. The entire life cycle from egg to adult occupies approximately three weeks.

There are seasonal variations, especially marked in temperate areas, in the number of lice found on cattle. In these areas numbers on susceptible cattle increase during autumn and early winter, peaking late winter and early spring. There are two reasons for this: (i) cattle are frequently housed in autumn and lice are easily transferred from infested to non-infested animals, and (ii) climatic conditions favour louse activity; strong sunlight and high skin temperatures have been shown to inhibit lice and the converse occurs in winter. Within groups of infested cattle there are always those that carry heavier burdens than others, and it is generally accepted that very large louse populations are indicative of stress or intercurrent illness, poorly fed cattle parasitized by nematodes and trematodes being frequently and characteristically louse infested.

The pathogenic effects of louse infestation have been the subject of much research. It is now considered that light or moderate infections have little effect on cattle. Heavy infestations lead to skin irritation, scratching and rubbing, with resultant damage to hides. Some reports have indicated that large sucking lice burdens may also cause anaemia and weight loss, although it has also been noted that these effects can be prevented by adequate high quality nutrition. Lice may also act as vectors for blood-borne organisms, and have been implicated in the transmission of *Eperythrozon wenyoni*.

Signs and diagnosis

Louse infestations are usually evident by the presence of eggs adhering to hairs, on the edge of bald areas and on parting of hair careful examination of preferential niches with a magnifying lens will reveal adults and nymphs.

Treatment and control (see p. 1030)

Lice are fairly easily killed by the application of organophosphorus, amitraz or synthetic pyrethroid preparations, either as sprays, pour-ons or dusting powders, although resistance to the last of these has been reported. The residual activity of synthetic pyrethroids is generally of longer duration. This aspect is important because for complete removal of all lice the activity must not only kill adults but nymphs emerging from eggs. The anthelmintics ivermectin, doramectin, eprinomectin and abamectin because of their long half-life are also extremely effective, removing all sucking and more than 98 per cent of biting lice. If used as a pour-on preparation they are even more effective, and will remove 100 per cent of both species. For preventative purposes, housed cattle can be treated at housing, sometimes complemented by removal by electric clippers of a 15 cm band of hair from the poll to the root of the tail.

Arachnids

Mange

Mange is the descriptive term used for infection of animals by mites, the smallest arthropods of the order Acarina. They are obligate parasites transmitted from infected non-infected animals by direct contact. There are four species that parasitize cattle and two others which are facultative parasities of them and other animals (See p. 881).

Aetiology and epidemiology

Although of the same order, the mites have different morphologies and habitats, and some are classified as 'burrowing' and others as 'non-burrowing'. For these reasons they are described separately.

Non-burrowing mites: One species, *Chorioptes bovis*, is specific to cattle. *Psoroptes ovis*, although primarily a parasite of sheep, can become permanently adapted to cattle. Non-specific mites are those species of harvest mites present on pasture, the larvae of which can infest many different species of animals: the mite species are *Neotrombicula* and *Eutrombicula*.

(1) *Chorioptes bovis.* The most common mite found on cattle. It reaches a length of 0.75 mm and is recognizable by its cup-shaped suckers on short unjointed pedicels. It is seen most frequently during autumn and winter in housed cattle, frequently on the hind legs but also on the neck, the head and root of the tail. It is a surface feeder and produces mild hair loss, lesions increasing in size only slowly. The lesions are obviously itchy as affected cattle will rub affected areas on walls, doors, etc., incurring damage to the skin and subsequent quality of the hide after death.

(2) *Psoroptes ovis.* The mite is normally found on sheep and is the cause of sheep scab, which is notifiable

and government regulated in many countries. The mite is a similar size to *C. bovis* but is characterized by long jointed pedicels with funnel-shaped suckers on the legs. Although similar to *P. ovis* from sheep, which is transferrable experimentally both to cattle and rabbits, the rarity of cases of mites transferring from sheep to cattle and vice versa in nature has led to the conclusion that some adaptation to specific hosts takes place, and that infection of sheep by cattle strains does not occur.

The mite, although a surface feeder, is much more irritant than *C. bovis* since its mouthparts are adapted for piercing skin, causing the formation of serious vesicles, which can coalesce and eventually become scabs. The life cycle is typical for both *P. ovis* and *C. bovis*. Female mites lay approximately 90 eggs. The hatching of eggs and subsequent development from larva to nymph to adult occupies approximately 10 days. Adult mites can live for a maximum of six weeks.

Affected cattle become restless because of the skin irritation. The areas commonly affected are the abdomen, tail root and perineum, and they can become further damaged by scratching. In extreme cases animals may cease to feed adequately and lose weight.

(3) *Forage mites.* The adults and nymphs of the family Trombiculidae are free-living on pasture. Eggs are laid on soil, and larvae crawl on to vegetation and to animals that lie on or brush through the foliage. The larvae are skin-piercers, causing vesicles. Animals become hypersensitive to their secretions and the subsequent rubbing and scratching increases the damage to skins.

Burrowing mites:

(1) *Sarcoptes scabiei.* Mites of this species are host specific although they are morphologically identical to those infesting other animal species. The adults are slightly larger than half the size of *P. ovis* and *C. bovis*. They are characterized by a rounded shape and the presence of triangular scales on the posterior of the dorsum. Adult females burrow tunnels in the epidermis. They lay eggs in tunnels, hatching taking place within a week. The hatched larvae crawl to the surface and create further epidermal tunnels in which they moult through the stage of nymphs to become adults. Males and females mate either in tunnels or on the skin surface and the cycle resumes, the entire length of which occupies three weeks.

Sarcoptes scabiei infections cause extreme irritation. On cattle the preferred sites are the neck and the lumbar area adjacent to the tail, resulting in the colloquial description of 'neck and tail mange', but it can be found in other areas. Early small lesions exhibit hair thinning and slightly thickened scaly skin, but soon the irritation and resultant rubbing combined with expansion of infected areas result in total loss of hair and thickened, crusted and excoriated skin. Affected animals may become so preoccupied with the irritation that they reduce their food intake, leading to loss of weight or milk production, and secondary bacterial infections may ensue on the most severely rubbed lesion.

(2) *Demodex bovis.* This mite is considered to be a normal commensal found on bovine skin; as for all members of the family Demodicidae it becomes pathogenic only when the efficiency of the immune controls of its host is reduced. The mites are characteristically cigar-shaped, 0.2 mm long, with four pairs of short legs close to the anterior end. Their preferred niches are in hair follicles and sebaceous glands and because of this deep location are not transmitted unless prolonged contact occurs. For this reason it is presumed that the young become infected shortly after birth during feeding from their mother, and as a result lesions are usually seen in cattle on the muzzle, head, neck and back. The lesions take the form of small, 0.75 cm diameter nodules and are follicles or glands filled with mites and caseous pus. In some countries a high proportion of hides may be affected, but in the UK the average prevalence is 17 per cent (Urquhart *et al.*, 1987). The lesions do not normally seriously affect cattle and treatment is not usually necessary.

Diagnosis

All of the mites are too small to be easily seen with the naked eye, and microscopic examination of skin scrapings is necessary, as it is for differentiation of most skin conditions. Mites are normally most easily found in scrapings taken from the edge of lesions. The scrapings are boiled in sodium or potassium hydroxide and centrifuged prior to examination of the sediment by microscope.

Treatment and control (see p. 1030)

Mites are affected by amitraz, some organophosphorus compounds, synthetic pyrethroids and the anthelmintics ivermectin, doramectin, eprinomectin and moxidectin. For topical applications the problem is to ensure that the chemical can come into contact with the parasite and it may be necessary to remove scabs before application. The organophosphorus compounds used frequently are phosmet, propetamphos and diazinon, and the synthetic pyrethroids flumethrin, deltamethrin and cypermethrin. Organophosphorus compounds and ivermectin, doramectin and moxidectin should not be used on dairy cows giving milk for human consumption unless withdrawal periods are observed. Eprinomectin is safe to use in such cattle.

Tick infestations (see p. 1030)

In tropical regions ticks play an important role in causing and spreading disease. Many actively suck blood and can cause death by anaemia. Some ticks cause paralysis, particularly in young animals. The life cycles vary considerably, with some ticks spending all their time on a single host, others are only parasitic at certain stages and some spend each stage of the life cycle on a different host. Those spending all their time on a single host (one-host ticks) are easier to control than those on different hosts for each development stage (three-host ticks)

One-host ticks:	*Boophilus* spp.
Two-host ticks:	*Hyalomma* spp.
	Rhipicephalus bursa
	R. evertsi
Three-host ticks:	*Amblyomma* spp.
	Argaspersicus spp.
	Dermacentor spp.
	Haemaphysalis spp.
	Hyalomma spp.
	Ixodes spp.
	Rhipicephalus spp.

Ixodoidea

Their life cycle involves egg, larva, nymph and adult. Almost all ticks at each development stage require a blood meal. The unfed stage varies in its ability to survive depending on the amount of moisture present.

The engorged stage drops off the host and then does not move from where it is deposited. The group is divided into two main families, the Argasidae ticks and the Ixodidae or hard ticks.

Argasidae family

These have a cuticle without a hardened dorsal scutum and their mouthparts cannot be seen from above. They are mainly found in arid or semi-arid areas. When feeding they rapidly engorge with blood. They are able to survive for long periods, i.e. months or years, without the presence of suitable hosts for feeding. The nymphs and adults can repeatedly feed, which allows greater capacity for transfer of infection.

There are three genera: *Argas*, *Ornithodorus* and *Otobius*.

Ixodidae family

These have a hardened scutum that covers almost all the dorsum in adult males but only one-third of the dorsum in unfed larvae, nymphs and adult females. The mouthparts are visible. There are nymph and larval stages. All stages including the adult females feed only once. Adult males remain on the host and feed often. Up to half the engorged weight can be taken in with one feed.

The family includes one-, two- and three-host ticks and there are ten ixodid genera of which seven have veterinary importance: *Amblyomma*, *Boophilus*, *Dermacentor*, *Haemaphysalis*, *Hyalomma*, *Ixodes* and *Rhipicephalus*.

Control: This can be directed at the ticks on or off the host. The latter is easiest to perform, but is ecologically damaging as other non-dangerous insects are also affected. When off-the-host-control is performed it includes the use of pasture spraying with anti-tick dips, which involves keeping stock off the area for as long as possible to allow death of the ticks. It works best where the ticks are short-lived as in warm arid conditions. It is best performed by treating pastures in rotation. The effectiveness of pasture spraying depends on whether alternative hosts, either domestic or wild, are available. The practice often means underuse of pasture. However, the overuse or intensification in grazing often increases the tick population. Another method of control often under-rated is that of pasture burning.

In most areas the only effective method of tick control is on the host. This is usually done by hand dressing, spraying or dipping, and in some countries by vaccination. Hand dressing is laborious and has to be done efficiently. It can be done by the use of dusting powders, creams, pastes or in a liquid form by hand spraying, paint brushing or application by washes. In large herds sprays or dips are used. In general, dips provide a more effective overall control. Both effective spray races and dips are expensive to install. The compounds used tend to be organophosphates, synthetic pyrethroids and traditional compounds. The last group includes arsenic preparations such as sodium arsenite. It is cheap but has no residual effect and it can be toxic. Resistance to arsenic dips occurs in some areas. Organophosphorus dips are effective but have limited residual activity. They can be toxic, especially when used by unskilled staff. Organochloride compounds are now prohibited in most countries because they are persistent for long periods and affect the human food chain.

Synthetic pyrethroids are good and relatively non-toxic but some resistance to them is developing, and occurs also when ticks are DDT resistant.

The number of dippings depends on several factors and often means the interval between dippings varies according to the season of the year. It depends on the duration of the ixodicide's activity, the toxicity of the dip, the seasonal activity of the ticks, the time the ticks spend on the host and whether it is required to control or try to eradicate the parasite. Thus one-host ticks, which remain on the host for three weeks, are far easier to deal with than three-host ticks, which only feed for a day or two. Generally, at its height, dipping will be once a week for one-host ticks and twice a week for three-host ticks. Such frequent dipping does allow tick selection for resistance. However, often where tick control is not achieved it is more likely due to not dipping frequently enough or the dip being too weak, improperly mixed or the wrong type or concentration for the stage of the tick to be killed. Where resistance does occur it can be overcome by changing the type of agent in the dip. Many farmers alternate the type of dip used on a routine basis.

Vaccination is carried out in Australia and a few other countries to the one host tick *Boophilus microplus*. The vaccine consists of recombinant antigens to the microvilli of the tick intestinal epithelium. As a result ingestion of blood from immunized cattle disrupts the digestion of the tick which leads to death or reduced fertility. After some years of vaccination the local tick population is therefore drastically reduced. Vaccination needs to be repeated at least annually as the immunity is not boosted by antigens from natural infection.

Fly problems (see p. 1030)

Mosquitoes

There are many species of mosquito including *Aedes* spp., *Anopheles* spp., *Culex* spp., *Mansonia* spp. and *Psorophora* spp. They can cause problems when in large numbers due to annoyance of man and animal. Mosquitoes cause some loss of blood by feeding as well as transmitting diseases such as Rift Valley fever and probably other conditions such as lumpy skin disease and bluetongue. The mosquito life cycle is aquatic for the larva and pupa and takes 5–21 days to reach the adult stage.

Control of the insect over large areas involves drainage of still surface water or by treating water with oil, synthetic pyrethroid or other insecticide. Oil is easiest to use and can involve waste engine oil with kerosene or diesel oil. Applying repellents to cattle tends to be too expensive and self-applicators are often used. Otherwise, for small groups of animals the use of mosquito screens will stop contact.

Blackflies

These belong to the family Simuliidae and include blackflies, buffalo flies and sandflies. They are small (<5 mm long) and black or grey in colour. They occur in most countries and when in large numbers they are an annoyance. It is thought that there may be toxic factors in the saliva. The bites result in vesicles and these in turn can result in ulcers and secondary infection. The larvae and pupae are attached to reedy stems and branches in running water. They take about three to four weeks to pass from egg to adult. They are active during the summer months. The flies tend to gather in swarms and annoy animals. They bite the legs, belly and head, causing the animals to stamp and kick their legs. Occasionally they stampede. Cattle may wallow in mud or kick up dust to keep off the flies. Control depends on attacking the larval stages by spraying breeding sites with insecticide. However, rapid reinfection of the areas will occur. Treatment of the adult is difficult but a repellent such as dimethyl phthalate is helpful. Regular dipping of cattle for ticks, etc. also reduces fly levels.

Midges

These are extremely small flies (1–3 mm long) of the family Ceratopogonidae, the important genera being *Culicoides* and *Lasiohelia*. These suck the blood of animals and man. They transmit ephemeral fever, bluetongue and other pathogenic viruses. The larvae are found mainly in swamps, where they live either in wet mud or free-standing water. Some occupy more restricted habitats such as rotting vegetation. Besides acting as vectors of arboviruses they can cause hypersensitivity reactions.

Control is by draining the breeding sites. Otherwise, spraying the areas with oil or DDT gives good results. Repellents, particularly dimethyl phthalate, are effective on a short-term basis. Mosquito screens are of no use. Fires at times of biting activity will assist in herd protection.

Horseflies and deerflies

Horseflies are of the *Tabanus* spp. and are also called March flies or breeze flies. Deerflies are of the *Chrysops* spp., *Haematopota* spp. and *Pangonia* spp. They are large, brown, robust flies that bite and suck blood. They act as vectors of diseases such as anthrax, anaplasmosis and trypanosomiasis. *Haematopota* spp. are thought to help transmit summer mastitis. The eggs are laid on the leaves of plants growing close to or in water. The larval and pupal stages occur in the water or mud and the life cycle takes about four to five months to complete. The flies tend to be active during the day in summer months, particularly when it is hot and sultry, and are mainly found on the ventral abdomen and legs. Control is difficult but depends on drainage of wet areas. Breeding sites can be treated with oil or insecticide. Otherwise, repellents such as dimethyl phthalate and γ-dimethytolumide are useful but last only a few days. Some products are available to apply to the cows' udders.

Houseflies

The common housefly (*Musca domestica*) has a worldwide distribution. They cause worry to animals by settling on them as well as acting as vectors of diseases such as anthrax, erysipelas, brucellosis and possibly summer mastitis. They cause aggravation at wounds or other areas where there is blood, exudate, pus, etc. They cause infections by discharging some of their stomach contents, so-called vomit drop, on to the food to moisten it and often they also defaecate. This means that they are able to transfer many pathogens effectively. Eggs are laid on rotting vegetable material or faeces. The life cycle involves an egg producing a larva (a maggot), which takes about 10 days to mature, thereby completing the cycle in about 12–14 days in warm weather.

Control methods include removing all manure and organic material at least every three days. This can be stacked so as to ferment, ideally in a bunker or pit. Otherwise, it should be turned over every few days or better still treated with insecticide. Faeces can be burnt. Fly traps (Baber's) can be used to collect flies and larvae. Buildings should be kept as clean as possible and can be sprayed with insecticides, or insecticide strips can be placed in areas with little air movement. Electrocutors can be used to which the flies are attracted by an ultraviolet light. Cattle can have insecticide-impregnated ear tags but these are not too effective against the housefly.

Bush flies

These include *Musca sorbens*, *M. fergusoni*, *M. terraeregina* and *M. hilli*. They are found particularly in Australia. They tend to be found all the year round in northern Australia but only in the summer periods in the south. The flies often appear in large numbers and can be found on the lips, eyelids and other mucous membranes and by wounds. They are considered to transmit infectious bovine keratoconjunctivitis. Control is difficult but involves fly spraying cattle and buildings.

A repellant such as dimethyl phthalate can be of use. Synthetic pyrethoids can be successful.

Face fly

This is *Musca autumnalis* a small fly resembling, and slightly bigger than, the housefly, found in Europe, Asia and North America. Numbers tend to be greatest in the summer and particularly cattle outside are worried. Fresh cattle faeces are the only fly breeding grounds. Flies are particularly seen on the face around the nostrils and eyes where they feed on the secretions. They are thought to transmit infectious bovine keratoconjunctivitis. There are no wholly successful control measures although plastic insecticide-impregnated ear tags are useful and powders or cream containing organophosphorus compounds assist.

Head fly

The fly *Hydrotaea irritans* is the same size as the housefly but has an olive abdomen and yellow wing tips. It is found in Great Britain and Europe. It is a nuisance fly and does not bite although it does feed off exudate around wounds. It occurs in large swarms from July to September. The life cycle is annual and it involves periods of development in the soil. Sores on animals are made larger due to self-inflicted aggravation because of irritation. *Hydrotaea irritans* is incriminated in the transmission of summer mastitis (see Chapter 24). It is probably also concerned with infectious bovine keratoconjunctivitis. Control is difficult and involves the use of parasite sprays and dipping. Plastic insecticide-impregnated ear tags are useful.

Stable fly

The stable fly, *Stomoxys calcitrans*, is about the size of the housefly. It is grey in colour, has a sharp proboscis and when it settles it sits with its head upwards. It is a bloodsucker and feeds on the host causing great irritation. Wounds often bleed freely after the flies have fed. The eggs are laid in faeces, rotting hay or straw and the life cycle is complete in two to three weeks. The larval and pupal stages take place in organic matter. Warm damp environments encourage the flies' growth and survival. They cause considerable nuisance and worry with reduced milk and meat production and possibly anaemia. In cattle there can be a hypersensitivity of the forelimb skin, which in turn has blisters that coalesce to form bleeding sores. *Stomoxys calcitrans* can transmit anthrax. Another species, *S. nigra*, occurs in South Africa.

Control of the fly involves the frequent removal and disposal of bedding and faeces from buildings. Destruction of the flies is difficult because they feed for only a short time. It can be helped by the use of insecticide-impregnated plastic ear tags or spraying with suitable sprays, spraying of walls and shaded areas of pens.

Horn flies and buffalo flies

Horn flies include *Liperosia* or *Haematobia irritans, H. minuta* and *L.* or *H. exigua*. This last is also known as the buffalo fly. The flies are greyish, smaller and less active than stable flies. At rest their wings are completely closed but are held away from the body. They thus spend more time on the host except when laying eggs, etc. Many have a limited geographical range. Thus *H. irritans* is found in the USA and Hawaii, *H. minuta* in Africa and *H. exigua* in Australia and south-west Asia. They are most common on cattle and buffalo and occur in large numbers, causing much irritation. Although bloodsuckers they are not known to transmit diseases. Severe infestations lead to weakness and death. They also produce large sores.

The eggs are laid in fresh faeces and can only survive with high humidity and warm temperature. They pupate in the soil and the life cycle takes eight days to three weeks to complete. Control of the flies is difficult but removal of dung is important. The cattle and buildings should be sprayed frequently with insecticide. If tick dipping is undertaken this reduces fly numbers. The anthelmintics doramectin, ivermectin and eprinomectin are effective because of their residual activity, and will protect cattle for periods of up to three weeks. The use of plastic insecticide-impregnated ear tags is helpful. Otherwise, applying insecticide at regular intervals will assist.

Horse louse flies

These include *Hippobasum equina, H. rufipes* and *H. maculata. Hippobasum equina* is the most common, is slightly larger than the housefly and is a reddish-brown, fast, glossy fly that causes problems to cattle and horses. It feeds on blood and is found on the inside of the hind legs and the perineum. The eggs are laid and develop in dry soil. They can act as mechanical vectors of disease. Plastic insecticide-impregnated car tags are of use in control as are spraying or dipping of cattle.

Tsetse flies (see p. 760)

The *Glossina* species are an important African fly that act as the true vector of trypanosomiasis (p. 756). They are 6–13.5 mm long, thin-bodied, yellow or brown flies. The wings are folded over each other and there is a slender proboscis. There are 20 species of *Glossina* and all are found in tropical Africa. They occur in a variety of environments but are usually found in one of three terrains: (i) forest, where they inhabit thickly wooded areas with a high humidity; (ii) riverine, where they live on the edges of forest but by streams, lakes and rivers; and (iii) savannah grasslands, where the tsetse are the most important species for spreading animal disease.

Both the male and female tsetse flies feed on blood and most of the species are attracted to certain host species. In tsetse flies the eggs hatch in the uterus and so they are larviparous. The larvae are deposited on shady dry soil and pupate there. One larva is produced every 10 days and the pupal stage lasts 28–56 days. As the adult female survives three or four months eight to twelve larvae are produced.

Control depends on surveying an area to determine the species of the tsetse fly present and their habitats. Then the possibility of control can be assessed. Methods of eradication or control are direct using insecticides to remove adult flies, removal of pupae and use of repellents on cattle. The indirect approach depends on removal of nesting sites and dry weather refuges, and the use of traps. Insecticides including DDT and dieldrin are of long duration but have been considered by some to cause too much long-term pollution. Shorter term insecticides that are biodegradable such as synthetic pyrethroids. are now favoured (see p. 760).

Tumbu fly

The tumbu or mango fly is *Cordylobia anthropophaga*. It infests man and animals but rarely cattle. It is about the size of a housefly and lays eggs in the soil or sand. The hatched larva attaches to the skin of a host where it produces a painful irritant swelling with a dark central hole. Once mature the larva passes out to the soil where it pupates. The adult lives on food and animal excreta. In light infestations each larva can be manually removed by covering up the airhole with liquid paraffin in Vaseline. The parasite will push its posterior abdomen out of the hole and it can then be pressed out gently. In severe infestations avermectins such as doramectin, eprinomectin and ivermectin will control infection and insecticides, such as organophosphorus compounds, can be applied.

Blow flies and screw-worm flies

These result in blow fly infection or myiasis. The flies involved include several genera: *Calliphora, Callitroga, Chrysomyia, Lucilia* and *Sarcophaga*. Cattle are less affected than sheep. The flies are really scavengers and mainly live on dead meat. However, true screw-worm flies only lay their eggs in fresh wounds. They are, however, attracted to dying flesh on live animals. Even the small wounds of ticks attract the flies. The larvae feed and grow quickly and mature in three to five days.

A local dressing of a larvicide and an antiseptic is useful after clipping away the hair. The most effective treatments are the avermectins doramectin, eprinomectin and ivermectin. They normally promote a complete kill in about 12 hours. All wounds should be treated with an antifly preparation. Dipping or spraying the animals with insecticides can be helpful. Otherwise, the number of flies can be reduced by trapping and quick disposal of carcasses. Chromosomal translocation of males to produce sterile or lethal mutant offspring has been tried with some success. The American screwworm fly *Callitroga americana* has been controlled by the release of irradiated males. They mate with the females, which lay sterile eggs, thereby ultimately reducing or eliminating the fly population.

TICK AND ARTHROPOD-BORNE DISEASES

Protozoal diseases

Babesiosis (redwater)

Babesiosis is caused by a intra-erythrocytic protozoan of the genus *Babesia* transmitted by hard ticks of the family Ixodidae (see p. 744). Unlike many other parasitic diseases, it affects adults more severely than young cattle in which infection is frequently subclinical. It causes fever, haemoglobinaemia, haemoglobinuria, anaemia and death.

Aetiology and epidemiology

The four most important species of *Babesia* that affect cattle are *B. bovis*, *B. bigemina*, *B. divergens* and *B. major*, the first three being much more significant than the last. Two are considered 'small' Babesia and two 'large', and there is one large and one small species for both tropical and temperate climatic areas (Table 45.1).

The parasites are transmitted by hard ticks, which are also affected by their role as intermediate hosts in the babesial life cycle. When an infected tick attaches to the skin of cattle its mouthparts penetrate the skin and it

Table 45.1 *Babesia* spp infecting cattle.

Species	Size	Climatic preference
B. bovis	Small	Tropical or subtropical
B. bigemina	Large	Tropical or subtropical
B. divergens	Small	Temperate
B. major	Large	Temperate

starts to suck blood. Bloodsucking is not continuous but takes place in short periods of activity until the tick becomes fully engorged. Full engorgement for larvae requires three to five days, for nymphs five to six days and for adults seven to ten days. *Babesia* spp. are not transmitted by infected ticks until the end of the engorgement period because the babesial stages in the tick have to develop and move to the salivary gland prior to becoming infective sporozoites. The sporozoites are injected into the host with saliva and then invade erythrocytes. They proceed to divide asexually in red cells, forming two pear-shaped merozoites. Each erythrocyte ruptures when the merozoites leave to infect new cells. The reproduction time in erythrocytes is in the order of 12–15 hours depending on the species. When sufficient multiplication has taken place for parasites to be visible in very low numbers in blood smears the animal will show a febrile reaction. The length of time required is usually approximately one to three weeks after infection, but depends on the number of *Babesia* in the infective inoculum, and in very large syringe-passed infections may be as short as two to three days. Thereafter the parasitaemia may build up and in extreme cases more than 20 per cent of erythrocytes may be infected, although the percentage infected varies with the species involved, e.g. the parasitaemia of *B. bovis* is usually less than 1 per cent in venous blood whereas *B. bigemina* and *B. divergens* on average reach 3–8 per cent. At this point the affected animal has a febrile reaction and may exhibit the characteristic haemoglobinuria that produced the colloquial term of 'redwater' for the disease, and unless treated it may die. After treatment the animal becomes a carrier of the organism and may suffer from occasional recrudescences of parasitaemia. Ticks become infected by feeding on parasitaemic cattle. Infected adult female ticks pass the infection to their eggs, the infection being termed *transovarial*, and the larvae, nymphs and adults up to the F2 generation. Some *Babesia* spp. may remain infected in the absence of feeding on carrier bovines, although for *B. bovis* infection ceases with larvae. Transmission from larva to nymph to adult is termed transtadial infection, and is observed with *B. bigemina* and *B. divergens*.

The epidemiology of the *Babesia* spp. is governed by the local climate and behaviour of its tick vectors. As a result they merit separate consideration as tropical or non-tropical species.

Tropical species: *B. bovis* and *B. bigemina*. These species are found in Australia, Africa, South and Central America, Asia and the very south of Europe. In Australia and the Americas the tick *Boophilus microplus* is the sole vector, in Africa other *Boophilus* and *Rhipicephalus* species. *Boophilus* spp. are one-host ticks, i.e. all stages of the life cycle take place on one animal, only the engorged female dropping to the ground before laying eggs. Some vectors in Africa, e.g. *R. evertsi*, are two-host and *R. appendiculatus* is a three-host tick.

Babesia bovis merozoites in erythrocytes measure $2 \times 1.5\,\mu m$ and those of *B. bigemina* $4.5 \times 2\,\mu m$. Parasitaemia in venous blood is low with *B. bovis* but it may be high in capillaries and cause sludging of blood, which if in the brain causes early death. It also produces enzymes with severe effects on the blood coagulation system, and is generally considered the most pathogenic of the bovine *Babesia* spp.

Babesia bigemina infection results in much higher venous parasitaemia but it has few other effects other than to cause a febrile reaction and straightforward haemolytic anaemia.

Temperate species: *B. divergens* and *B. major*. *Babesia divergens*, the merozoites of which measure 1.5×0.4 μm, is common in areas of permanent pasture in northwestern Europe and is transmitted by the three-host tick *Ixodes ricinus*. *Babesia major* ($3.2 = 1.5\,\mu m$) is found only in south-eastern England and on islands off the coast of The Netherlands and is transmitted by *Haemaphysalis punctata*.

Babesia divergens behaves rather similarly to *B. bigemina*, i.e. it can cause a high parasitaemia, which results in fever and severe haemolytic anaemia. It has little effect on blood coagulation systems in comparison to *B. bovis*. Its epidemiology is closely bound to the ecology of its vector *I. ricinus*. In Europe, *I. ricinus* is generally active only between May and November, and in most areas has spring and autumn population increases, although in the most northerly climates it may only have one in midsummer. The ticks quest more actively in warm conditions and outbreaks of babesiosis are frequently observed two weeks after fine weather. The epidemiology of *B. major* is still only slightly investigated, but such isolations as have been reported have taken place in May and June.

Signs

Early: There is slight dullness with a pyrexia often of 40.5–41°C (105–106°F). The animal shows diarrhoea and because of spasm of the anal sphincter there is a narrow stream of diarrhoea (pipe-stem diarrhoea). There is also haemoglobinuria. Slight dehydration is often seen as a slightly sunken eye.

Mid: After 24–36 hours the mucous membranes tend to become pale and the pulse rate is increased. The animals tend to slow up and there is a reduction in appetite and thirst. The urine tends to become very dark in colour and reduced in quantity. The faeces may return to normal but less tends to be passed although there is still spasm of the anus.

Late: In another 24–36 hours the rectal temperature is often subnormal with the animal having blanched mucous membranes, a poor appetite and drinking little. There is marked constipation and a greatly increased heart rate.

Pregnant cows may abort following infection.

Necropsy

The carcass may be very blanched and there is sometimes jaundice. The liver is often swollen and pulpy, with the kidneys dark and enlarged. The bladder contains red-brown urine. There are ecchymotic haemorrhages under the epicardium and endocardium.

Diagnosis

Cattle suffering from babesiosis frequently have a history of recent movement to tick-infested pastures either through grazing management or after purchase, and in Europe may have suffered from tick-borne fever a week or so before babesiosis is evident. Examination of the cattle, especially the preferential feeding sites of the vector ticks, will reveal evidence of recent tick bites or engorging ticks. Clinical babesiosis is unlikely to be observed in cattle less than nine months old; such cattle can be infected and show febrile reactions but the resultant parasitaemia remains low and haemoglobinuria mild. In areas of large tick populations, most cattle are infected at an early age and become immune thereafter, the situation being described as enzootic stability. In the early stages of the disease, haemoglobinuria may not be present and diagnosis requires careful examination of stained blood smears (see Fig. 45.1). Once haemoglobinuria is present, the parasitaemia may be more obvious. Differential diagnosis requires elimination of other conditions causing haemoglobin uria, e.g. anaplasmosis (p. 761), eperythrozoonosis, leptospirosis (p. 734), postparturient (p. 792) and bacillary haemoglobinuria (p. 719).

Treatment and control (see p. 1029)

There are two aspects to treatment: firstly, treatment with a babesicide and secondly, the need for supportive therapy such as blood transfusion and fluid replacement. There are few babesicides now available. The only treatment now licensed in the UK is imidocarb, which is given at a dose rate of 1 mg/kg body weight. It is used widely in South America and other countries. It is highly effective and relatively non-toxic, but does have tissue residues for several weeks after its use.

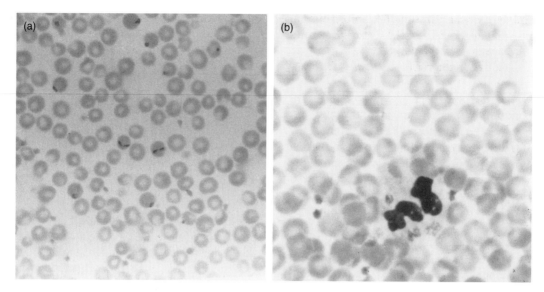

Fig. 45.1 (a) Bovine blood infected with *Babesia divergens* (×630). (b) Bovine blood smear showing *Ehrlichia phagocytophila* in a neutrophil (×630).

It can also be used at twice the therapeutic dose as a chemoprophylactic, giving protection from infection for up to six weeks. It is used in this way to administer to cattle that will be exposed to ticks, or that have been vaccinated with live *Babesia* with the hope that cattle will become mildly affected but protected from clinical illness and immunity to further infection will be stimulated.

Live vaccines for *B. bovis* and *B. bigemina* have been available in many countries for many years, notably Australia and South America. For *B. bovis* the vaccines consist of live organisms made avirulent by repeated rapid syringe-passage through splenectomized calves. In the case of *B. bigemina* rapid passage did not reduce virulence and vaccines available are either developed by 'slow' passage from recrudescences of parasitaemia or are fully virulent organisms, which are used in schemes involving infection and subsequent treatment. There are no vaccines currently available for *B. divergens*, although much research is being carried out to develop inactivated recombinant vaccines for that species and *B. bovis* and *B. bigemina*.

Blood transfusion is frequently required for severely affected adult cattle and is normally achieved by collection of 5 l of blood from an unaffected healthy cow into a 22 per cent solution of the anticoagulant acid citrate dextrose (ACD), the mixture being immediately transfused into the recipient animal. Such single transfusions without cross-matching of blood are usually successful, but repetition can lead to problems of incompatibility of blood antigens.

Table 45.2 Species of the genus *Theileria* in cattle.

Species	Synonym	Disease
T. annulata	*T. dispar*	Mediterranean coast
	T. turkeistomica	infection
T. lawrencei	*T. bovis*	Corridor disease
T. mutans	*T. orientalis*	Benign bovine theileriosis
	T. buffeli	
T. parva		East Coast fever
T. sergenti		Mediterranean coast fever (Russian)

Theileriosis

This comprises a group of infections caused by protozoan parasites of the genus *Theileria* (Table 45.2) and transmitted by ixodial ticks. They occur in a variety of ruminants and wild animals. Both members of the genus *Babesia* and the genus *Theileria* occur within red blood cells. They are collectively called piroplasms and the infections caused by the two are thus sometimes known as 'piroplasmosis'.

East coast fever (ECF) (pp. 73, 753)

The disease is a major constraint for production in countries where it occurs.

Aetiology: The cause is a protozoan parasite, *Theileria parva*. There is some disagreement about its classification. *Theileria lawrencei*, a parasite of buffalo, causes a high mortality in cattle, but if passaged through cattle it reverts to a parasite indistinguishable from *T. parva* and producing a syndrome similar to ECF. Thus it has been suggested that the cattle parasite should be called *T. parva parva* and that of the buffalo *T. parva lawrencei*.

Epidemiology: The disease occurs across a large area of East and Central Africa and is endemic in Burundi, Kenya, Malawi, Sudan, Tanzania, Uganda, Zaire and Zambia. It may also occur in Ethiopia and southern Somalia. It is possible to eradicate the disease and this has been done in Mozambique, South Africa, Swaziland and Zimbabwe, although it can return if preventive measures are not maintained. It is a disease of cattle but can infect Indian buffalo (*Bubalus bubalis*) and African buffalo (*Syncerus caffer*). Infection is restricted to countries with a temperature and rainfall suitable to allow the survival of *Rhipicephalus appendiculatis*, a three-host tick. The tick is found from sea level to 2135 m (7000 feet) provided there is adequate vegetation and a rainfall in excess of 50 cm (20 inches). In many areas where ECF occurs rainfall is seasonal and disease follows the onset of rain and thus tick activity. In some highland areas or close to water or sea, where the rainfall is more or less constant, tick activity and ECF can occur virtually all the year round. Although *R. appendiculatis* is the main arthropod host, eight species of the genus *Rhipicephalus* and three species of the genus *Hyalomma* can be experimentally infected. In areas where there is a constant challenge then the cattle will be continually exposed to infection from the tick. If challenge is heavy then the calves die. However, those that survive are resistant to further challenge and they can thrive in these areas. In marginal areas where challenge is intermittent or seasonal then cattle previously exposed may lose or have reduced immunity. Thus if a heavy challenge occurs at the start of the rainy season the cattle are again susceptible and go down with disease. Immunity is only to challenge by a similar strain. Cattle previously exposed may be partly or totally susceptible to infection by other strains. Recovered cattle have a sterile immunity, which lasts more than three years. Levels of immunity to piroplasm antigens peak often four to six weeks after infection and persist for six months.

Life cycle: The life cycle of *T. parva* is still not completely understood but most of it is now known or extrapolated. Firstly, at the stage of introduction of infection to the cow there is the period of schizogony. Sporozoites from infected ticks are injected with saliva into the cattle while the tick feeds. There is usually a delay of three to five days after attachment before this occurs. If the tick infects a susceptible animal there is a period of five days before the parasite can be detected in the local drainage lymph node closest to the tick bite. What happens during this period is not known but it is likely that sporozoites rapidly enter target lymphocytes. By doing this the sporozoites escape the phagocytic, lytic and immunological defences of the host. Then there is a transformation of the lymphocyte to lymphoblast with larger, less dense nuclei and increased cytoplasm caused by the parasite, which in turn differentiates into a macroschizont in the cell cytoplasm. As the disease progresses the macroschizont grows to an average size of 4.8 μm. The lymphoblasts rapidly proliferate, probably stimulated by the presence of the parasite, which becomes aligned along the spindle and divides by synchrony. As the infected lymphoblast divides both daughter cells are infected. Some macroschizont-infected cells degenerate releasing free macroschizonts, which invade other uninfected lymphoid cells. How this occurs is not known but it may be through membrane fusion of cells in close apposition. From about day 14 after tick attachment macroschizonts differentiate to microschizonts. The mechanism of differentiation is not known. Microschizont-infected cells then rupture and release micromerozoites (1–1.5 μm in diameter). The released micromerozoites enter erythrocytes where they form piroplasms 3–5 μm), which tend to be rod or comma-shaped. The piroplasm-infected erythrocytes are then available to infect ticks feeding on the blood of the cattle host. *Theileria parva* piroplasms rarely divide within erythrocytes, which is different from *T. mutans* and also *Babesia* spp.

Following feeding on the infected bovine the tick, usually *R. appendiculatus*, will inject piroplasm-infected blood that is around the stage of gametogamy. The tick is a three-host tick with all three stages (larva, nymph and adult) feeding on separate hosts. Infection is transitional so an infected larva can transmit infection as a nymph but not as an adult. There appears to be no transovarial transmission as occurs with *Babesia* spp. Once in the tick gut the erythrocytes lyse releasing the piroplasms, many of which are digested but some of the many forms develop into male microgametes or female microgamonts. Fusion of these by processor anisocytosis is then thought to occur to produce zygotes, which invade gut cells and thus differentiate into a motile kinete of about 19 μm. The kinete breaks out from the gut cell and enters the haemolymph. The stage of sporonts is then reached. The kinetes invade the acinar cells (usually type III acinars) of the salivary glands. The kinetes round off and nuclear division occurs to produce a sporont or primary fusion body. The sporont invaginates and forms buds. Further development is delayed until such time as the tick starts to feed in its next instar. When this occurs primary sporoblasts develop from the sporont buds and form cystomeres or the secondary fission stage. There is hypertrophy of the host cell and the cell nucleus. There is then division of the primary sporoblasts to produce secondary sporoblasts or the tertiary fission stage and sporozoites (1–1.5 μm) are produced. This stage is rapidly completed in three days from the onset of the tick feeding. The sporozoites are released into the salivary duct with peak sporozoite production by day 5. The host cell and nucleus degenerate and the parasite residual bodies remain. The sporozoites persist during the whole period of feeding, which may be up to 10 days for female ticks and intermittently over a long period for male ticks.

Mortality in susceptible adult cattle is 80–100 per cent, with an incubation period of 10–15 days.

Signs

Peracute: There is marked pyrexia and death with swollen lymph nodes in a few days.

Acute: Usually the first sign is an enlargement of the lymph nodes for the region draining the area where the infected tick has fed. The preferred feeding sites for *R. appendiculatus* are the ears and so usually the first lymph nodes to swell are the parotids. One to two days after the swelling occurs the animal becomes pyrexic with a temperature rising to 39.5–42°C (103–108°F). The temperature tends to remain high until the animal either recovers or dies. Other lymph nodes begin to swell and this tends to become generalized. Some of the superficial lymph nodes such as the parotids, prescapulars and precrurals become very enlarged. Anorexia gradually develops and there is consequent loss of condition. In many cases lacrimation and nasal discharge occur. The breathing becomes rapid and dyspnoeic, and there is diarrhoea or dysentery. As the animal deteriorates and approaches death, the temperature falls and there is severe dyspnoea and recumbency. Nasal exudate pours out of the nostrils. The animal dies of asphyxiation from lung oedema. Death is usually about 18–24 days after infection, but occasionally this is reduced to 14 days. The mortality tends to be near 100 per cent in susceptible animals.

Occasionally, nervous signs develop and this is known as 'turning sickness'. Foci of Koch's blue bodies are found in the cerebral tissue. The animal appears to turn often rapidly and become giddy with collapse. The less severe form involves slower turning and frequent head pressing. Both nervous forms are fatal and are considered by some to be due to a massive infection in partially immune cattle.

Chronic: This is usually seen in animals that are partially immune or exposed for long periods to low levels of infection. It often occurs in calves in endemic areas. The lymph nodes tend to be enlarged and there is intermittent pyrexia, anorexia and loss of condition. These animals frequently recover. In cases of concurrent helminthosis, malnutrition or other disease and a constant population of *T. parva* some animals become severely retarded and never reach their full production potential.

Pathology: The lesions will depend on the duration of signs. The most consistent finding is one of hypertrophy and hyperplasia of the lymph nodes initially, followed by lymph node oedema and some haemorrhage and necrosis later on. There is destruction of lymphocytes leading to destruction of lymphoid cells. Lymph node biopsy shows hypertrophy of lymphoid cells and often after the 11th day they may show macroschizonts that increase in number and size. Damaged lymphocytes are seen with free schizonts. Microschizonts are then present, either intact or branching out of cells as micromerozoites. Blood examination reveals a progressive panleucopenia. A noticeable rapidly developing anaemia is only seen in the terminal stages.

The examination reveals froth at the nostrils and the most striking feature is massive pulmonary oedema, hyperaemia and emphysema. The alveoli, bronchioles, bronchi and trachea are filled with frothy pulmonary exudate. There can also be pleural and pericardial exudate. There are excessive haemorrhages and these may be present on most serous and mucous membranes. In the abomasum the mucous membrane is red and inflamed and there may be ulceration or erosions, especially in the pyloric region. In chronic cases there are ulcers in Peyer's patches. The cortices of the kidneys show haemorrhage and are often congested, and nodules of lymphoid tissue projecting from the kidney surface may be seen and are a characteristic feature when they occur. The spleen may or may not show changes and it can be enlarged or shrivelled. The liver is often enlarged with mottled grey areas. Degeneration of the organs is rapid after death.

Diagnosis: The signs are relatively specific and infection can be confirmed by the presence of piroplasms in the blood or schizonts in lymph node biopsy smears stained with Giemsa. There is also panleucopenia and then anaemia.

Post-mortem findings are helpful but they are similar to those of malignant catarrhal fever. Differentiation of

T. parva from other *Theileria* spp. depends on the acuteness of the disease, the number of piroplasms present in the blood and the number present in lymph nodes. Complement fixation, capillary titre agglutination and indirect haemagglutination tests have all been used in diagnosis but are less reliable. The indirect fluorescent antibody test (IFAT) is considered more reliable. An enzyme-linked immunosorbent assay (ELISA) test is also being increasingly used.

Treatment (p. 1029): Animals in good condition prior to infection have lower morbidity. Parvaquone and the more recently developed buparvaquone are effective if treatment is not delayed until the animal is too severely affected. Oxytetracycline is effective if given at the same time as infection occurs. It is also able to reduce the severity of clinical disease and appears most effective when given by injection. Chlortetracycline given at any stage of infection at a dose of 10 mg/kg body weight either parenterally or by mouth reduces the severity of parasitaemia and pyrexia.

Control: In endemic areas indigenous calves have a high degree of resistance to disease. However, calves of European breeds are very susceptible to infection and often die. Those that survive often succumb to further attacks. Adult cattle of any breed brought into the areas are highly susceptible to disease and probable death. The immunity is more cellular than humoral.

Thus where disease is endemic there is legislation to control ticks, to slaughter infected animals, quarantine cattle and restrict cattle movement. While it has been shown in South Africa and Zimbabwe that eradication of ECF is possible, it is expensive and in many countries the legislation is not enacted as rigorously as it might be. However, individual farmers can do much to reduce problems on their own premises by sensible cattle management and tick control. Efficient and well-maintained fencing will reduce the access of nomadic cattle or game to the farm. Areas particularly suited to ticks can also be fenced off. Grass burning, rotational grazing, alternate grazing with other species such as goats or sheep, alternate grazing with immune cattle or rotating land between grazing and crop all reduce the problem. Cattle should be quarantined on entry to the farm. Should disease break out its effects can be reduced by slaughtering infected cattle, stopping movement of cattle, other animals, people, hay or feed from infected areas and then creating a buffer area between the infected and clean areas.

It seems that for effective immunization of cattle against ECF it is necessary for the infection to be established in the host. Vaccination is not widely used as it often leads to unpredictable results, with disease breaking out due to poor immunity or deaths due to vaccination. However, animals can be vaccinated with stabilate produced by freezing down emulsions from infected blood. After injection of the stabilate long-acting oxytetracycline or buparvaquone is given; otherwise short-acting oxytetracycline or paravaquone can be used. Cattle so treated become resistant to disease and they show little or no apparent reaction. In some cases more than one strain of *T. parva* is introduced, possibly together with a strain of *T. lawrencei*. A sporozoite vaccine is now being tried.

Mediterranean coast fever

This is in many was similar to East Coast fever but is caused by a different *Theilera* species.

Aetiology: The cause is a protozoan parasite, *Theileria annulata*. Morphologically, the parasite is similar to *T. parva* and the macroschizonts and later microschizonts are found in the lymphoid tissue. *Theileria annulata* piroplasms in the erythrocytes tend to be oval or round in shape. In Russia, there is a similar disease due to *T. sergenti*, which is different from *T. annulata* both morphologically and immunologically.

Epidemiology: The condition is found around the Mediterranean including south-eastern Europe, Russia, the Middle and Far East, India, Sri Lanka, Egypt and Sudan. Both cattle and water buffalo (*Bubalus bubalis*) are susceptible to the infection. The condition involves a development cycle in ticks of the genus *Hyalomma* and seven species are known to be vectors. The ticks involved are one-host, two-host or three-host ticks. It is believed that in most tick species there is no transovarian transmission. Thus infection is acquired in the nymph or larval stages and is transmitted in the adult. When the tick is attached to the host it must feed a considerable amount before infective stages of *T. annulata* are produced and enter the cattle. Piroplasms appear in the erythrocytes shortly after the first detection of schizonts. The intra-erythrocytic form remains in the blood for many years and in natural infections they tend to have a ring or oval shape.

The disease is seasonal, depending on the activity of the ticks, which hide during the winter in crevices between rocks, walls, etc. The result is the infective adult stage being produced in late spring or early summer. Thus infection tends to be seen mainly in the summer and early autumn. Infection can also be transmitted by injecting blood or tissue from ill or recovered animals. Intra-uterine transmission has been recorded on occasion. Infection of calves in endemic areas usually produces a mild disease, although up to one-quarter of calves can die.

In the Russian form involving *T. sergenti*, infection is said to be transmitted by only one species of the genus *Haemaphysalis*.

Signs

Peracute: This occurs in completely susceptible animals entering endemic areas. The animals develop marked pyrexia with anorexia, depression and weakness and they die in three or four days.

Acute: This is most commonly seen in susceptible animals moved into endemic areas and in marginal areas of tick activity. The animals develop pyrexia, which may persist for several days. It is accompanied by inappetence, lethargy, swelling of the superficial lymph nodes, oculo-nasal discharge and ruminal stasis. This is followed in a few days by anaemia with pale mucous membranes, exercise intolerance and a rapid heart rate. Later on jaundice may become apparent. Constipation is common when pyrexia first occurs but later there is diarrhoea and bloodstained faeces. The animals lose condition rapidly and about 90 per cent die over a period of eight to eighteen days after signs occur.

Subacute: There is intermittent fever for two to four weeks with moderate progressive anaemia and jaundice. Many of these animals die but some recover over a long period. Some of these cases change into a more acute phase and die.

Chronic: This is often an even more prolonged form of the subacute disease. Recovery can occur but is very protracted. However, some cases suddenly develop the more acute form and die.

Necropsy: There is a pale, anaemic carcass with the mucous and serosal membranes showing numerous petechial haemorrhages. The lymph nodes are enlarged, cystic and oedematous. The liver tends to be pale brown or yellow, enlarged and friable with an enlarged friable spleen. The kidneys tend to be pale and on occasions show pseudoinfarcts. The abomasum is red, inflamed and may show haemorrhagic ulceration. There are epicardial and endocardial haemorrhages and these may be petechial or ecchymotic. The lungs contain oedema, often red-tinged, and congestion.

A lymph node smear may show schizonts present in lymphocytes but they are more common in the liver and spleen.

Diagnosis: The area, type of animals affected and signs help in diagnosis. Lymph node smears show schizonts. In some cases a liver biopsy is needed to differentiate. Serological tests used for *T. annulata* include the complement fixation test (CFT), indirect fluorescent antibody test (IFAT) and enzyme linked immunosorbent assay (ELISA).

Treatment: Many cases of *T. annulata* infection show spontaneous recovery. There have been few controlled trials of treatment. Both oxytetracycline (by injection) and chlortetracycline (orally) have been claimed to give relief. However, buparvaquone is at present the best therapy.

Control: Following natural infection there exists a premunity that lasts for many years. There is no cross-immunity to other *Theileria* spp. Immunization is practised in several countries by taking blood from recently recovered cattle passaged through susceptible cattle. This is continued until no piroplasmic forms of the parasite occur. Then citrated blood is injected into susceptible stock, usually calves. Most animals show only limited reaction to such vaccination, although a few die. As there are no piroplasms in the blood ticks are not infected. Immunity can then be enhanced by injecting a virulent strain. It has been possible to culture schizonts on various tissue culture cell lines and these have then been used to vaccinate susceptible cattle. They do not produce piroplasms and so the animal cannot infect ticks.

Prevention otherwise involves control of the tick and cattle movements. Cattle can be sprayed or dipped with acaricide. Some walls and buildings can be sprayed to kill off the overwintering stages. Carrier animals still contain infection in their blood and if moved to new farms or countries will take the disease with them to infect local ticks. Thus detection of carriers is of use and can be done by taking blood from the animal and injecting into susceptible cattle.

Corridor disease

This condition is very similar to ECF but it has a different cause.

Aetiology: It is caused by *Theileria lawrencei*, which is primarily a protozoan parasite of buffaloes. However, it is transmissible to cattle and produces a similar type of disease to ECF. The schizonts tend to be smaller and fewer in number and the piroplasms relatively rare in the blood. If *T. lawrencei* is passaged through cattle it quickly reverts to a parasite indistinguishable from ECF. It has therefore been suggested that *T. parva* is a cattle-adapted strain of *T. lawrencei*. It has also been proposed that the nomenclature for the two parasites should be *T. parva parva* and *T. parva lawrencei*.

Epidemiology: The disease has mainly been described in South Africa, Zimbabwe and Kenya. It is transmitted by the three-host tick *R. appendiculatus* and it is possible that distribution of *T. lawrencei* is over the whole area occupied by the tick. The buffalo (*Syncerus caffer*) is considered to be the natural host and cattle brought in to the area tend to be susceptible. Those brought up in the region that survive the first few months are immune but those in marginal areas or where tick levels have only been partially introduced are not. *Theileria lawrencei* is transmissible from carrier buffaloes via ticks to cattle. It can be passed from cattle to cattle via the ticks. The recovered cattle can then act as carriers of infection. Morbidity in susceptible cattle is variable at about 60–80 per cent.

Signs: The signs are similar to those seen with *T. parva*.

Peracute: The animal develops pyrexia, lymph node enlargement and dies in a few days.

Acute: This is the most common form in susceptible cattle. There is pyrexia and swelling of the lymph node closest to the site of the infected tick bite. Other lymph nodes then start to swell and there is general dullness. There is lacrimation, nasal discharge and oedema occurs, particularly of the eyelids, face and throat. The animal becomes weak and develops diarrhoea containing blood and mucus. The respirations become laboured and dyspnoeic.

Mild: In this form there is a mild rise in temperature, swelling of the lymph nodes and some pyrexia.

Pathology: The lymph nodes are swollen and show hypertrophy and hyperplasia followed by oedema and haemorrhage. There are extensive haemorrhages on most of the serosal and mucosal surfaces. The abomasum tends to be red, inflamed and with ulcers, especially in the pyloric region. The spleen may be enlarged. The kidney cortex is congested and may show nodules of lymph and tissue raised above the surface. The liver is enlarged and a mottled grey colour. The lungs are grey and contain blood and fluid with froth in the alveoli, bronchi, bronchioles and trachea. Lymph node biopsy smears show hypertrophy and hyperplasia of the node.

A few lymphocytes contain schizonts and there are one or two piroplasms in the erythrocytes.

Diagnosis: The condition is similar to ECF, anaplasmosis and babesiosis and the peracute form is similar to heartwater. The signs, and area, help in diagnosis, particularly of those cattle associated with buffalo. However, where *T. parva* infection is common then disease caused by *T. lawrencei* may be missed. A lymph node biopsy helps as schizonts in the lymphocytes tend to be few and small in size. Blood samples show only a few erythrocytes to contain piroplasms. There is also no marked anaemia as in anaplasmosis or babesiosis.

Treatment: Use of oxytetracycline by injection reduces the intensity and duration of signs. Similarly, chlortetracycline has an effect and can be given by mouth. The naphthoquinones, parvaquone and buparvaquone are now successfully used.

Control: Infection can be controlled by tick dipping, controlling movement of susceptible cattle, grazing tick areas with less susceptible species such as sheep or goats and ensuring no contact occurs between cattle and buffalo or other game animals. Cattle that are exposed to infection and recover are immune. However, there is not complete cross-immunity with *T. parva* infection, although it does seem that cattle previously infected with *T. parva* have a good immunity to *T. lawrencei*. When cattle are initially infected with *T. lawrencei* there is only limited resistance to *T. parva*. Stabilates of ticks infected with strains of *T. parva* have been injected into cattle followed by treatment with oxytetracycline or parvaquone, which has given some immunity to *T. lawrencei*. Some stabilates have included a *T. lawrencei* strain.

Benign bovine thieleriosis

This disease tends to be less severe than ECF, Mediterranean coast fever or Corridor disease.

Aetiology: The cause is a protozoan, *Theileria mutans*, which is very similar to *T. parva*.

Epidemiology: The condition affects cattle as well as the Indian water buffalo (*Bubalus bubalis*) and the African buffalo (*Syncerus caffer*). It occurs in most parts of the world except countries north of latitude 55°N and South America. It is thought that transmission is by a wide variety of different ticks but it has been proved to be so with *R. appendiculatus*, *R. eventsi* and

Ambylomma variegatum. Injection of parasitized blood can produce infection. The disease is maintained by a premune state of recovered cattle, which allows continued infection of ticks. Infection often occurs with other diseases such as anaplasmosis, salmonellosis, heartwater or babesiosis.

Signs

Acute: This rarely occurs but it has been reported in Australia, India, Japan, Kenya, Korea and South Africa (where it is known as Tzaneen disease). In this case the disease involves fever with swelling of the lymph node closest to the infected tick and then more generalized lymph node swelling. There is a progressive anaemia and some of the cattle die. In Africa there is a cerebral form of the disease known as turning sickness where the animal will tend to walk in circles or head press.

Subacute: There are very few clinical signs other than a mild pyrexia with a swelling of the lymph nodes and a mild anaemia.

Pathology: In acute cases there is hyperplasia and oedema of the lymph nodes. There may be haemorrhages of the serosal and mucosal surfaces. The abomasum may be reddened and ulcerated. The kidney cortex is congested with swollen lymphoid areas. The liver is enlarged and tends to be grey in colour. The lungs contain fluid in the bronchioles, bronchi and trachea. The spleen is swollen.

Usually in the subacute form there is mild hyperplasia of lymph nodes, which contain a few schizonts. Anaemia occurs but is slight. There are only a few piroplasms in the blood and schizonts in lymph node sinuses.

Diagnosis: Diagnosis is helped by the mild nature of the signs but is not helped by the presence of only very few piroplasms in the blood or schizonts in lymph node biopsies. In addition the schizont is morphologically similar to *T. annulata* and *T. parva*. The best method of differentiation is by serology and the most effective test at present is IFAT.

Treatment: Quinoline drugs such as pamaquin are of use in the erythrocytic stage.

Control: As the disease is mild, deliberate control or eradication is not usually undertaken. However, control of ticks will result in control of disease. Cattle maintain immunity by a form of premunity, with piroplasms remaining in small numbers within the blood.

Besnoitiosis

This disease was previously known as globidiosis.

Aetiology

It is due to a protozoan called *Besnoitia besnoiti*.

Epidemiology

It is mainly seen in cattle and horses as intermediate hosts in south-west Europe and in Africa. Transmission has not been elucidated but is probably via the faeces of infected cats which are the final host. Morbidity can be up to 10 per cent and recovery is often protracted.

Signs

In many animals there are no signs. In the cow there may be lesions on the teats. There is pyrexia and warm swellings develop on the ventral parts of the body resulting in reduced movement. The lymph nodes are palpably swollen and there is diarrhoea. Pulse and respiratory rates are elevated. Pregnant cattle may abort. There may be excessive lacrimation and increased nasal discharge, which is at first serous and then purulent. There are small, white, raised nodules on the conjunctiva and nasal mucosa. There then follows severe dermatitis over most of the body associated with infected cutaneous cysts.

Diagnosis

This is based on clinical signs, especially the cysts on the scleral conjunctiva, and on the geographical area and can be confirmed by the detection of cysts containing spindle-shaped spores in scrapings of skin lesions or the conjunctiva.

Treatment

Nothing specific is available.

Control

A vaccine produced by *B. besnoiti* grown on tissue culture is effective.

Trypanosomosis

Trypanosomes are blood-borne protozoa with flagellae. Infections are widespread in wild and domestic animals and cattle are susceptible to infection with several species, the most important of which are those cyclically transmitted by tsetse flies (*Glossina* spp.) throughout much of subSaharan Africa, namely *Trypanosoma congolense*, *T. vivax* and *T. brucei*. *Trypanosoma vivax* infections also occur in cattle in the absence of the tsetse fly in Central and South America and have been recorded in Mauritius. In tropical and subtropical areas other than subSaharan Africa, cattle are commonly infected asymptomatically with *T. evansi*.

Tsetse fly-transmitted trypanosomoses are commonly grouped together under the name 'nagana' (p. 1030). Their distribution lies within the tsetse fly belts of Africa, which extend from 14°N to 20°S in south-west Africa and 29°S in Mozambique, covering an area of 10 million km². Many species of wild animals are symptomless carriers of nagana trypanosomes and provide a sylvatic reservoir of infection in which the trypanosomes are cyclically transmitted naturally from host to host by tsetse flies. The principal carriers of these trypanosomes are wild bovids and suids, e.g. kudu, giraffe, buffalo, warthog and bushpig. Cattle, other domestic animals and man are infected when they come in contact with these wild animal carriers and are bitten by infected tsetse flies as a result.

Tsetse flies can be classified as falling into three groups, namely forest, riverine and savannah. The forest tsetse flies are found in the tropical rainforests of Central and West Africa and in scattered areas of East Africa. Although they are efficient vectors of trypanosomes, they are of least importance as cattle rarely come in contact with them due to the lack of suitable grazing in the forest regions. Riverine tsetse flies, as their name implies, infest riverine vegetation, but virtually only in river systems draining into the Atlantic Ocean. Their distribution is thus confined to Central and West Africa, largely overlapping with that of forest flies. Although they are less efficient vectors of trypanosomes than forest or savannah flies, because they infest vegetation near essential water supplies, riverine flies are important vectors of trypanosomosis of humans (Gambian sleeping sickness) and of domestic livestock including cattle.

Savannah tsetse flies are the most important group of flies because they infest large tracts of land potentially suitable for grazing and browsing by domestic livestock. They are also efficient vectors of trypanosomes and so when cattle and other livestock encroach into tsetse-infested savannah, they are at risk of being bitten by the fly and contracting infection.

Tsetse flies become infected when they take a blood meal from an infected animal. The trypanosomes then undergo cyclical development within the alimentary system, eventually developing to the infective or meta-cyclic forms within the fly mouthparts. These infective forms are then transmitted to another susceptible animal host via the saliva during the next fly feed(s). The development in the tsetse fly is an essential part of

the life cycle and hence nagana is unique to Africa. The one exception of the nagana trypanosomes is *T. vivax*, as mentioned earlier. In Central and South America it is assumed that *T. vivax* is mechanically transmitted by biting flies. This raises the possibility that it may also be transmitted mechanically in Africa, and indeed there is increasing evidence that this is the case.

Infection with *T. evansi* is also transmitted mechanically by biting flies. Infection of domestic livestock is widespread worldwide throughout the tropics and subtropics, but is absent from tsetse-infested areas of Africa. It is an important pathogen of camels, horses, dogs and buffaloes but cattle, although commonly infected, rarely suffer clinical disease. However, they may be important reservoirs of infection for other more susceptible livestock.

Aetiology

Tsetse-transmitted bovine trypanosomoses are caused by *T. vivax*, *T. congolense* and *T. brucei*. All are motile, extracellular, spindle-shaped, flagellated protozoan parasites ranging from about 10 to 30 μm in length. *Trypanosoma vivax* and *T. congolense* are essentially parasites of plasma, although *T. vivax* may leave the circulation in small numbers and invade extravascular tissues particularly of the heart (Losos, 1986). *Trypanosoma congolense* has a predilection for the microvasculature where it attaches to the endothelium of small blood vessels, particularly the heart and brain (Banks, 1978). *Trypanosoma brucei* as well as being a plasma parasite has a predilection for interstitial spaces and tissue fluids.

Trypanosoma evansi is related to *T. brucei* to which it is morphologically similar and has a similar infection pattern in the animal host.

Pathology

The pathogenesis of bovine trypanosomosis is complex and not fully understood but is characterized by a chronic and progressive anaemia. Uncomplicated tsetse-transmitted infection can be considered as following a course comprised of three phases (Murray, 1978).

Phase I (fluctuating parasitaemia and fever): Following an infected tsetse fly bite, trypanosomes multiply locally, causing an inflammatory reaction (chancre) within a few days at the site of the bite. Chancres are a regular feature of experimental infections, but have not been reported in natural infections. About this time, trypanosomes invade the circulation via the lymphatic system, causing reaction and enlargement of locally draining lymph nodes. Trypanosomes then appear in the bloodstream, the prepatent period following initial infective tsetse bite varying with species thus:

T. congolense	12–16 days
T. vivax	8–10 days
T. brucei	5–20 days

A fluctuating but diminishing parasitaemia then develops and parasitaemic peaks at approximately 12-day intervals are associated with febrile responses. Anaemia becomes evident early in infection and is believed to be haemolytic in the first instance, but haemolysis wanes and is superseded by anaemia caused by erythrophagocytosis due to stimulation and expansion of the mononuclear phagocytic system resulting in splenomegaly.

This initial phase of fluctuating parasitaemia and fever may last from a few weeks to a few months during which cattle lose condition and, depending on the severity of infection, some may die. Cattle that survive this phase enter the second phase.

Phase II (low-grade parasitaemia and progressive anaemia): Over the next few months, infected cattle have a low fluctuating parasitaemia during which the parasites may be difficult to detect. Despite the apparent reduction in parasites, the erythrophagocytosis and anaemia continue, although the spleen may return to normal size and cattle continue to lose condition.

Phase III (apparent aparasitaemia but continuing anaemia): Cattle that survive the second phase suffer chronic disease during which the parasites apparently disappear, although anaemia due to erythrophagocytosis continues. Affected animals are cachectic and normally die within six to twelve months of initial infection.

Infection at any stage may lead to congestive heart failure and death due to a combination of anaemia, circulatory failure and myocardial damage. At autopsy, post-mortem findings are not pathognomonic. They include emaciation, visceral pallor and enlargement of the heart. Cattle that die early in disease may have enlarged haemorrhagic lymph nodes and splenomegaly (Stephen, 1986).

Despite the large volume of literature on bovine trypanosomosis, good accounts of the pathology of natural disease are scarce and the above account represents a brief synopsis of the generally accepted picture. Cattle at risk may be infected by several species and strains of trypanosomes and the pathology and clinical signs will be influenced by various factors, e.g. the age, breed and nutritional status of infected cattle, the degree of tsetse challenge and the strains and species of infective trypanosomes. Thus strains of *T. vivax* in West Africa tend to cause a more acute disease in cattle than those of East Africa, whereas strains of *T. congolense* in East

Africa tend to cause a more chronic form of the disease. *Trypanosoma brucei* is the least pathogenic to cattle and normally regarded as of minor importance.

Although infection with more than one species is commonly reported in the field, virtually no studies have been done on mixed infections. Cattle infected experimentally with *T. congolense* and *T. brucei*, either simultaneously or one year apart, developed cerebral trypanosomosis with encephalitis and associated clinical signs and both species of parasites were isolated from the cerebrospinal fluid (Masake *et al.*, 1984). The authors suggested that the higher incidence of cerebral trypanosomosis in mixed infections than in single infections suggests an interdependence between *T. congolense* and *T. brucei* in the pathogenesis of cerebral trypanosomosis, possibly resulting from *T. congolense*'s predilection for the brain microvasculature facilitating the entry of parasites into brain parenchymal extravascular spaces. The possibility of such interaction between different species in natural infections merits further research.

Signs

The clinical picture of cattle suffering from nagana is influenced by several factors, namely breed and health status of cattle infected, pathogenicity of infecting trypanosomes, duration of exposure to infection and level of tsetse fly challenge, which in itself is dictated by several factors. *Trypanosoma vivax* infections in cattle in West Africa are widespread and commonly produce an acute, rapidly fatal disease in which affected cattle die during the initial phase of fluctuating parasitaemia and fever. Stephen (1986) describes acute *T. vivax* infection as resembling septicaemia in which affected animals have body temperatures of 40–41°C (104–106°F), depression, dyspnoea, elevated pulse and respiratory rates and a jugular pulse. Less severe cases show signs of anaemia, loss of condition (Fig. 45.2) and enlargement of superficial lymph nodes. Abortions and stillbirths may occur in pregnant cows.

The situation in East Africa and parts of Central Africa is different in that *T. congolense* tends to be a more serious pathogen than *T. vivax*, although this is by no means absolute as strains of *T. vivax* are known to cause an acute haemorrhagic disease in cattle in the Coast Province of Kenya (Mwongela *et al.*, 1981). *Trypanosoma congolense* in East and Central Africa tends to produce a chronic disease, although the clinical signs are essentially the same as those of *T. vivax* infection and eventual death is the usual outcome in untreated animals. In the early stages of infection appetite may be normal between periods of fever, but as the disease progresses the anaemia becomes more severe, cattle become depressed and lose bodily condition and in the

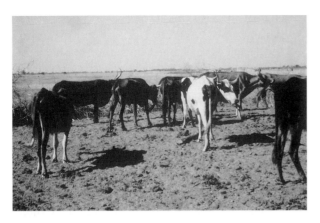

Fig. 45.2 Emaciated cattle suffering from trypanosomosis in northern Botswana (courtesy of A.G. Hunter).

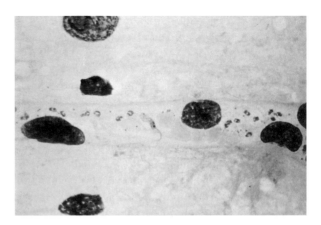

Fig. 45.3 *Trypanosoma congolense* in ox brain capillary (courtesy of CTVM Archives) (×1000).

terminal stages affected cattle are too weak to rise or eat (Stephen, 1986). Superficial lymph node enlargement is not so pronounced as in *T. vivax* infections.

Trypanosoma brucei infections of cattle, though common, are generally regarded as of minor significance and are usually mixed with the more pathogenic *T. congolense* or *T. vivax*. Parasitaemias from *T. brucei* infections are lower than those of *T. congolense* or *T. vivax* and hence infection can be more difficult to detect, raising the possibility that disease caused by *T. brucei* infection may not always be diagnosed. A few reports of meningo-encephalitis have been recorded, and experimental infection produces a severe diffuse meningo-encephalitis resulting in depression, unsteady gait, head pressing and circling (Morrison *et al.*, 1983). There is a greater incidence of cerebral trypanosomosis in mixed *T. congolense* and *T. brucei* infections as mentioned earlier and the involvement of the central nervous system (CNS) in natural bovine trypanosomosis requires investigation.

Trypanosoma vivax infections of cattle are widespread in Central and South America and the West Indies and were probably introduced with imported cattle from Africa. The importance of *T. vivax* in the New World is not clear, but epidemics of serious disease have been recorded in Venezuela and Colombia (Clarkson, 1976). In general, the clinical signs appear to be the same as chronic forms of *T. vivax* infection in Africa and the swaying gait of infected emaciated cattle may be confused with the clinical signs of rabies.

Trypanosoma evansi infections of cattle, though common throughout the tropics and subtropics, rarely cause clinical disease.

Diagnosis

In tsetse-infested areas of Africa, nagana is well recognized and diagnosis is often based on a history of a

chronic wasting condition of cattle in contact with the tsetse fly. Differential diagnoses are babesiosis (p. 748), anaplasmosis (p. 761), helminthosis (Chapter 19) and any condition that causes anaemia and emaciation, notably malnutrition. Nagana can be confirmed parasitologically by demonstrating parasites in the blood of infected animals and various techniques are available (Fig. 45.3). These techniques were reviewed by Paris *et al.* (1982) as follows.

● Microscopic examination of stained thin blood smears. Different species of trypanosomes can be identified by this method.
● Microscopic examination of wet blood films; this must be done at the time of sampling and cannot be used to identify different species of trypanosomes.

These techniques are not particularly sensitive and may not detect animals with low parasitaemias, such as those suffering chronic disease. More sensitive techniques are the following:

● Microscopic examination of the buffy coat–plasma interface of haematocrit-centrifuged blood, either directly through the capillary tube glass or by breaking the capillary tube just below the buffy coat and expressing the contents of the upper part onto a slide for examination by dark-ground or phase-contrast microscopy.
● Microscopic examination of stained dehaemoglobinized thick blood smears.
● Subinoculation of bovine blood into laboratory rodents. This is the most sensitive technique for *T. brucei* and is usually good for *T. congolense*, but most strains of *T. vivax* do not infect laboratory rodents.

In practice, many field programmes of monitoring cattle for infection are based on routine screening of stained thick and thin blood films; thick films are examined to detect infected animals and thin films to determine the species of the infecting trypanosomes.

Trypanosoma vivax infections in the New World may have to be differentiated from conditions causing wasting and anaemia such as anaplasmosis, babesiosis and helminthosis and in addition, as mentioned earlier, rabies (p. 908; Chapter 70). In general the same techniques as described can be used to confirm diagnosis.

Serological tests are not in general use for diagnosis although several are under study. Trypanosomes display the phenomenon of antigenic variation during infection in the mammalian host in which successive parasitaemic populations of trypanosomes have a different antigenic composition. Thus the host mounts successive immune responses to sequences of different antigenic populations and a test developed to detect serum antibodies to one antigenic population may not detect serum antibodies against different antigenic populations of the same strain of trypanosome. These variable antigens are confined to the surface glycoprotein coat of the parasites and, although tests have been developed based on these variable antigens, they are largely confined to research in antigenic variation and have little routine diagnostic use.

Tests based on internal common somatic antigens may have potential diagnostic use as problems of cross-reactions between species become solved by monoclonal technology (Nantulya *et al.*, 1987). Of various tests developed, the IFAT and ELISA appear to have the greatest potential and the ELISA can be used to detect circulating trypanosomal antigens as well as antibodies (Rae & Luckins, 1984).

Treatment and control (see p. 1029)

Because of the phenomenon of antigenic variation, no vaccine has been developed against trypanosomiasis and is unlikely to be in the foreseeable future. In Africa this leaves tsetse control as the main method of prevention. Tsetse control programmes are widespread throughout Africa but will only be considered in summary here. Tsetse control is usually under the direction of the veterinary department and requires specialized expertise. The methods in use are as follows:

● Application of insecticide to tsetse habitat, either on the ground by hand or from the air by helicopters or fixed wing aircraft. This is the main method.
● Use of fly traps. These are used extensively in francophone West Africa and Zimbabwe.
● Removal of the tsetse habitat. Tsetse flies have to rest in certain bushes and trees, which can be cleared by felling and bulldozing, rendering the area unsuitable for the fly. This is expensive, however, and is now largely confined to main-

taining tsetse-free barriers around areas freed of tsetse.
● Settlement of land freed of tsetse. Housing, cropping, etc. may alter the vegetation to a form unsuitable for tsetse flies, so preventing reinfestation.
● Destruction of wild animal hosts. This is now unacceptable except in establishing animal-free corridors, possibly in conjunction with the third method, above.
● Release of sterile male tsetse flies to interfere with breeding of wild tsetse populations. Because of the very low reproductive rate of tsetse flies, only small numbers of flies can be reared in colonies. Therefore this method has limited application, usually in conjunction with other methods.

Thus, the commonest form of prevention is avoidance of the fly by cattle herders who build up local knowledge on when and where pastures are safe to graze. Savannah tsetse flies retreat and disperse during the dry and rainy seasons respectively, so that certain pastures may be tsetse infested for part of the year only. In addition, grazing tends to be safest at midday, when flies are least active, and most dangerous around sunset, when flies are most active (Pilson & Leggate, 1961).

In the absence of a vaccine cattle can be protected prophylactically, although effective prophylactics are now limited to one drug, isometamidium chloride. Isometamidium has certain disadvantages. It causes severe reactions at the site of injection, and there is considerable risk of resistance developing to the drug if cattle are exposed to infection after the active ingredient in blood has fallen to below a trypanocidal level, usually three months after injection. Thus where the risk of infection is constant, injection of the drug must be repeated at regular intervals to maintain effective levels. Despite this, under good management cattle can be efficiently reared in tsetse areas under isometamidium protection, as has been demonstrated on the Mkwaja Ranch in Tanzania over the last 30 years (Trail *et al.*, 1985).

Treatment against trypanosomosis, in order to be effective, should be given early in the disease during the initial phase of fluctuating parasitaemia. As no new drugs have been developed against the disease for nearly 30 years and some have been withdrawn because of resistance, treatment is now essentially limited to two compounds, diminazene aceturate and homidium (either chloride or bromide). Resistance has been recorded against both drugs and undoubtedly will be an increasing problem. As there is little likelihood of pharmaceutical companies developing new trypanocides because of the cost and uncertainty of the market, in many of the countries concerned the management of the existing drugs will require great care in the future.

Trypanosomosis is normally seen as a herd problem and mass chemotherapy is widely used on a herd or area basis, ideally in conjunction with some form of routine monitoring of blood smears of a percentage of cattle to indicate level of infection. Whiteside (1962) pointed out that when drugs are used regularly to treat cattle for trypanosomosis resistance may develop and when this occurs the drug in use must be changed to one against which there is no resistance and that should cure infections resistant to the first, i.e. a 'sanative'.

Resistance was rarely reported against diminazene, which consequently was recognized as the best sanative. The concept of 'sanative pairs' was introduced in which drug usage regimens were devised to alternate diminazene with another trypanocide to minimize the development of resistance. Thus the alternative to diminazene was used for treatment of clinical cases for as long as possible and then changed to diminazene for one year to ensure treatment of any resistant infections in circulation. Thus depending on the level of tsetse challenge, the regimen shown in Table 45.3 for treatment using drugs in current use was advocated.

In practice, it is virtually impossible to rear cattle in areas of very high challenge.

Because treatment is now limited to diminazene and homidium and their use must be managed very carefully, Whiteside's recommendations are possibly more valid today than when first advocated.

Diminazene aceturate is the drug of choice for treatment of *T. vivax* infections in the New World.

Use of trypanotolerant breeds of cattle

It has long been recognized that dwarf humpless breeds of cattle in West Africa have a low susceptibility to trypanosomiasis and can survive in tsetse-infested areas where zebu types or European breeds cannot. Until relatively recently these breeds were regarded as having poor productivity and were of minor significance, however new research indicates this may not be the case; their potential is now under extensive investigation and the situation concerning these so-called 'trypanotolerant' breeds was reviewed by Hoste (1987). Trypanotolerance has also been identified in Orma Boran cattle of East Africa (Njogu et al., 1985) and the future prospects of greater utilization of breeds of cattle with natural resistance to trypanosomosis are very real.

Rickettsial diseases

Anaplasmosis

This is an infectious and transmissible disease of cattle that is seen in most continents of the world. It is non-contagious and is transmitted by ticks.

Aetiology

The cause of the disease is an intra-erythrocytic parasite, usually *Anaplasma marginale*. The red blood cells contain round inclusion bodies called anaplasma and they are peripheral in location, hence the name 'marginale'. There are three *Anaplasma* species and of the other two, *Anaplasma centrale* causes a mild condition in African cattle, as does *Anaplasma caudatim*.

Anaplasma marginale, when mature, is 0.3–1.0 µm in diameter and more than one can be present in the same erythrocyte. The parasite transfers from cell to cell in the form of an inclusion body. This is normally oval in shape and measures 31 µm in diameter and can penetrate the red cell envelope.

A member of the genus *Paranaplasma*, *P. caudatum*, has been found in a mixed infection with *A. marginale* in cattle in the USA state of Oregon. The inclusion bodies of *A. caudatum* can be shown with special staining techniques to have unusual appendages such as rings, loops or beads in the erythrocytes. However, these are not found when deer erythrocytes are infected.

Epidemiology

The disease is particularly seen in tropical and subtropical parts of the world and it exists in some temperate areas. Africa, North, South and Central America, the Far and Middle East, India, Russia and southern Europe all have the disease present. While mainly a bovine disease, buffalo, bison, antelope, deer, gnu and wildebeeste can all be infected. All ages of cattle are susceptible, but calves under six months old show few if any signs. The severity of signs depends on the age and previous exposure to infection. Generally, the older the animal at first exposure, the more severe the signs. Ticks are the natural hosts of the disease and at least 20 species have been shown to transmit infection. Little is known about the developmental life cycle in the tick,

Table 45.3 Regimen for treatment of trypanosomosis to minimize development of resistance.

Tsetse challenge	Drug alternatives	
	Homidium	Diminazene
Very high	6 months	1 year
High	1 year	1 year
Medium	2 years	1 year
Low	As long as possible	1 year

although most infection is transmitted transovarially. The main genera of ticks concerned are *Argas*, *Boophilus*, *Dermacentor*, *Haemaphysalis*, *Hyalomma*, *Ixodes* and *Rhipicephalus*. Horseflies (*Tabanus* spp.) are experimentally and epizootologically the most important insect vector. They directly transmit the disease from an infected to a susceptible animal. Other arthropods that can be involved include stable flies (*Stomoxys*), deer flies (*Chrysops*), housefly (*Musca*) and mosquitoes (*Psorophora*). Cattle can be carriers of the disease as well as deer. The incubation period is usually two to six weeks, but it may be up to 12 weeks.

Signs

Peracute: This usually involves cattle over three years old experiencing infection for the first time. It is most commonly seen in high-producing purebred dairy cattle and is frequently fatal. There is a pyrexia with rapid loss of milk production. Anaemia occurs with very pale mucous membranes. The breathing is rapid with excessive salivation. Some cattle show nervous signs and abnormal behaviour.

Acute: This is seen in cattle up to three years old and is occasionally found in cattle between one and two. Signs often develop unexpectedly. The animal develops a progressive pyrexia over a few days, reaching 41°C (106°F). There is a loss of milk yield with a progressive anaemia and weakness. In addition there is depression, inappetence, dehydration and laboured breathing. The lymph nodes tend to be enlarged. Some cattle will exhibit jaundice, there is frequent micturition of normal-coloured urine and some cows abort. Bulls may show a temporary loss of fertility. Recovery takes a period of weeks. If death occurs it is within one to four days of the onset of signs.

Chronic: The signs may follow an acute infection with gradual emaciation.

Mild: This form is mainly present in cattle infected under one year old. Signs are usually few with a mild pyrexia.

Necropsy

The main signs at post mortem are of an acute anaemia and there is often jaundice. The spleen is enlarged and the gallbladder obstructed. The heart is usually pale and flabby and petechial haemorrhages may be present on the epicardium and pericardium. The lymph nodes are enlarged and oedematous. The blood shows a marked reduction in erythrocytes and haemoglobin. The mor-

phology alters to include anisocytosis and poikilocytosis and leucocytosis is often present.

Diagnosis

In typical cases the signs presented plus the presence of anaplasma inclusion bodies in stained peripheral blood smears are sufficient for diagnosis. Giemsa stain is usually used but toluene blue and acridine can also be helpful. The diagnosis of carrier or chronic cases is more difficult and normally depends on complement fixation, capillary tube agglutination and agglutination tests.

Treatment

The tetracyclines, i.e. tetracycline, chlortetracycline and oxytetracycline, are the only approved drugs that are effective in treatment. Administration can be oral or parenteral. Their use in the acute phase slows down the parasitic life cycle and so reduces the crisis. Latent infections can be eliminated by tetracyclines. They act more effectively and more quickly when given by injection rather than orally. Experimentally, other compounds of the dithiosemicarbazones have been shown to be effective. It is also important to provide good management for the animals and in valuable animals blood transfusions may be necessary.

Control

The main methods of control involve reduction in the vectors of disease, which can be done by ectoparasite dipping, but this does not entirely control the problem. Susceptible cattle can be separated from other carrier cattle and wild animals or carrier cattle can be detected and eliminated, although the tests used are not completely reliable. Otherwise immunization can be undertaken.

It was thought that cattle in indigenous areas do not normally show signs due to an infection immunity or premunity. However, when there is intercurrent infection or the animal is stressed in other ways then signs are evident, although it does seem that in premune animals there is also a cell-mediated immune response. Both cell-mediated and humoral responses are required to provide protective immunity to anaplasmosis. In addition, continuous antigenic response is dependent on a perpetual low-level exposure to infection. Immunity using a live, laboratory-attenuated *A. marginale* ovine-origin vaccine gives good protection. Inactivated *A. marginale* vaccines of bovine and ovine origin require annual boosters. Their protective effect appears to be low. Experimentally, a more effective inactivated vaccine booster has been produced. Recently, a soluble organism-free cell culture derived from *A. marginale* antigen has been developed.

Eradiction is possible where ticks can be removed. Carrier cattle can be detected by a serological test, then the non-infected cattle need to be kept away from potential domestic or wild animal carriers. Movements of the cattle need to be controlled and it is necessary to reduce the level of biting flies. In such circumstances no live vaccination programme must be undertaken.

Tick-borne fever

Tick-borne fever is caused by the rickettsial-like organism *Ehrlichia phagocytophila*. It causes a prolonged febrile reaction, neutropenia and immunodepression in cattle in northern Europe (see Fig. 45.1b).

Aetiology and epidemiology

Ehrlichia phagocytophila is transmitted by the tick *Ixodes ricinus* during engorgement, but unlike babesiosis, infection takes place almost immediately after ticks start to feed. The circumstances and timing of infections are dependent on the ecology of the tick and typically take place most often during spring or autumn tick-activity periods, but can take place at any time between April and November. Infection in ticks persists transtadially, but not to the following generation of larvae.

After infection the organism enters or is phagocytosed by white blood cells, usually neutrophils, but infected eosinophils and monocytes are occasionally observed. The 'elementary body' can be seen in blood smears stained with Giemsa or Leishman stains as a pale blue dot in the cytoplasm of neutrophils. It enlarges to become a morula, after which the neutrophil ruptures and the elementary bodies of which the morula is composed infect further cells (Fig. 45.1b). The disease becomes apparent five to nine days after transmission by infected ticks. The animal develops a high fever, which can persist for up to 10 days. During this period the continuous destruction of neutrophils leads to a severe neutropenia and for as yet unknown reasons to a reduction of packed cell volume (PCV) of 30 per cent. As a result of the neutropenia the animal becomes immunodepressed and susceptible to other infections such as pneumonia, infectious pododermatitis and babesiosis due to *B. divergens*, which is frequently observed in susceptible cattle eight to twelve days after tick-borne fever. The 'parasitaemia' subsides but recrudescences occur periodically thereafter. Immunity develops slowly and persists only for a few months as cattle may be affected, albeit less severely, for some years following their infection.

Signs

Affected dairy cattle suffer an abrupt drop in milk production, which may last despite treatment for four weeks, and beef cattle lose a significant percentage of their body weight.

Diagnosis

The history is usually similar to that of cattle affected with *B. divergens*, i.e. recent purchase or movement to tick-infested pastures. Diagnosis can be confirmed by examination of blood smears for the presence of *E. phagocytophila* (see Fig. 45.1b).

Treatment and control

Tetracyclines are the antibiotic of choice and long-acting preparations have proved most successful.

Treatment of cattle with pour-on synthetic pyrethroids has been used to prevent tick infestation, reducing the tick population for two to three weeks. It has been less successful than when used on sheep, which retain higher concentrations of the pyrethroids on skin and wool for longer than cattle. The fact that transmission of *E. phagocytophila* occurs early in engorgement, in contrast to *B. divergens*, has resulted in the observation that protection of cattle against tick-borne fever using pyrethroids is less successful than against babesiosis, as accumulation of chemicals is more likely to kill the tick before transmission.

Bovine petechial fever (Ondiri disease, ondiritis)

This condition is a rickettsial infection of ruminants, but is restricted in area of occurrence.

Aetiology

The cause is a rickettsia-like organism, *Cytoecetes* (*Ehrlichia*) *ondiri*. The infection initiates in the spleen, and there it parasitizes the circulating granulocytes and, more rarely, monocytes. The organisms are pleomorphic and occur in cytoplasmic vacuoles, particularly in neutrophils. The organisms possess a rippled cell wall and they can be small (0.2–0.4 µm) or large (1–2 µm) bodies. In some cases there are mixed groups of large and small bodies.

Epidemiology

The disease appears to be confined to the highlands of East Africa. It mainly involves cattle exotic to the region. Very well defined areas are often involved. The indigenous cattle and wild ruminants such as the bushbuck (*Tragelaphus*) and duiker (*Silvicapra* spp.) do not show clinical infection. The vegetation common to all sites is the edge of forest or thick bush. Experimentally, infection can occur in cattle, sheep, goats, impala, bushbuck, Thomson's gazelle and wildebeeste. Most of these develop latent infections. Thus carrier animals are produced from which it would seem highly likely infection could be spread by an arthropod vector. However, as yet, despite intensive investigations, the arthropod involved (probably a tick) has not been detected. The incubation period is variable, from four to 14 days, and in natural outbreaks disease has occurred 10 days after entering into an infected area. Mortality is around 20 per cent and occurs within a few days of onset of signs, but some animals will die two or three weeks after disease develops.

Signs

Peracute: These signs are seen in recently imported exotic cattle. They develop marked pyrexia and a drop in milk yield. The signs usually coincide with a parasitaemia. After two or three days petechial haemorrhages occur on mucous membranes, and in some cases that are fatal there is general congestion, with pulmonary oedema, dullness, weakness and a staring coat. Most of the cattle collapse and die within four days.

Acute: These types tend to occur over a longer period. The temperature is high but fluctuates. There is inappetence with reduced milk yield and abortion. Although petechial haemorrhages occur in some animals on the day after the onset of fever, in most animals they have appeared by three days. The haemorrhages disappear to be replaced by fresh ones within seven to ten days. They occur on the vulva, vagina, conjunctiva, labial surface of the gums and ventral surface of the tongue. Any normal discharge and faeces may be bloodstained. In some cases a characteristic 'poached egg eye' occurs with a swollen tense eyeball with the aqueous humour containing blood, the conjunctiva swollen and haemorrhagic and the eyelid everted.

Subacute: Affected animals show a transient, non-fatal condition with pyrexia and petechiation of the mucous membranes.

Inapparent: No signs are present.

Necropsy

The main findings are usually of an animal in good condition with submucosal and subserosal haemorrhages, which may be large and distributed throughout the body. There is oedema and lymphoid hyperplasia. Often there is subcutaneous and intramuscular haemorrhage and melaena. The heart shows large haemorrhages into the epicardium and endocardium. There are also haemorrhages and oedema in the respiratory tract and the mucosa and serosa of the alimentary tract. The lymph nodes show hyperplasia and oedema. Both the liver and spleen may be enlarged and show petechiae. Histologically, there is marked evidence of petechiation. Characteristically, hyperplasia of large areas of the lymphoid sinus are seen. The rickettsiae can be found in impression smears of that surface of the spleen and liver. There is a characteristic absence of eosinophils, followed by markedly reduced numbers of lymphocytes and then neutrophils.

Diagnosis

Diagnosis is often difficult as the condition resembles anthrax (p. 717), bracken poisoning (p. 946), arsenic poisoning (p. 941), haemorrhagic septicaemia (p. 728), heartwater, acute trypanosomosis (p. 756) and acute theileriosis (p. 750). It is usually based on the history plus the area where it has occurred. *Ehrlichia ondiri* can be detected in blood or spleen smears stained with Giemsa, where it is particularly seen in granulocytes and monocytes. Often by the time clinical signs develop the parasitaemia is low or absent. In such cases it may be necessary to collect blood in EDTA or a suspension of spleen or lung and inject this intravenously into susceptible cattle or sheep. The granulocytes and monocytes in blood smears from the recipient, stained with Giemsa, should be examined daily for 10 days after inoculation.

Treatment

The most effective time to treat is during the incubation period when tetracyclines prevent disease. Once overt signs are present, double the usual therapeutic dosage of these antibiotics will reduce clinical signs and limit the parasitaemia. A single intravenous dose of alphaethoxyethylglycoxal dithiosemicarbazone at 5 mg/kg body weight will also reduce signs and the parasitaemia more effectively than tetracyclines.

Prevention and control

Eradication is impossible because wild animals act as a reservoir of infection. Clinically infected cattle are resistant to reinfection for several years, but they probably carry latent infections of *E. ondiri*. Losses due to the disease can be reduced by restricting access to areas of known infection. Clearing the undergrowth and scrub aids this. If susceptible animals are to enter infected areas they should be watched daily and when infection is present a single dose of dithiosemicarbazone may then allow them to recover and become immune to infection.

Heartwater (cowdriosis or malignant rickettsia, blacklung)

This is another rickettsial condition that infects both domestic and wild animals.

Aetiology

The infection is caused by the rickettsia *Cowdria ruminantium* and is transmitted by at least five species of *Amblyomma* ticks. It is first found in reticuloendothelial cells and then parasitizes vascular endothelial cells. It is seen as close packed colonies consisting of less than ten to many hundred cocci. The agent is pleomorphic but the rickettsia in any one group tend to be of similar size. The organism varies between groups from 0.2 μm to greater than 1.5 μm. Division is by binary fission and it produces morula-like colonies in the cytoplasm. The small granules tend to be coccoid, with larger ones looking like rings, horseshoes, rods and irregular masses. It has been suggested that differences in the size and shape of the organisms are the result of a growth cycle.

Epidemiology

The disease has been reported in many African countries south of the Sahara desert. Distribution coincides with that of the *Amblyomma* ticks, which require a warm humid climate and bushy grass. Experimentally, five species of *Amblyomma* are able to transmit infection. These are three-host ticks. Transmission usually appears to be transtadial and so infected larvae are usually free from disease. Transovarian transmission can occur, but is thought to be very infrequent. Infected larvae are found on non-susceptible animals, but if they do become infected it can pass on to both nymph and adult stages. Infected ticks do not transmit infection immediately; they become attached to the animals, but a variable time after they start to feed. In many cases the level of infection is unknown as indigenous domestic and wild animals often show no signs. It is only when susceptible exotic species are introduced that infection becomes apparent. Besides cattle, sheep, goats, Asian buffalo, antelopes and deer are susceptible to infection and disease. Indigenous cattle undergo inapparent infection. Calves under three weeks old, even from susceptible stock, are difficult to infect. Heartwater can occur throughout the year, but incidence declines in the dry season due to reduced tick activity. The incubation period is variable, from 7 to 28 days, with fever starting on average after 18 days. Mortality can be up to 60 per cent in exotic breeds, but less than 5 per cent in local cattle.

Signs

Peracute: This occurs in exotic breeds introduced to the region. The animal appears clinically normal, but if examined will have a marked pyrexia. It may then suddenly collapse, go into convulsions and die. Thoracic auscultation will often reveal oedema in the lungs and bronchi.

Acute: The course of infection is three to six days and consists of pyrexia (often over 41°C, 106°F), with nervous signs that may include ataxia, circling and abnormal posture. In other cases signs develop only to stimuli and there is then an excessive blink reflex, frequent tongue protrusion, a haggard, pained expression and muscular tremors. Pregnant cows may abort. If the condition progresses there are convulsions, paddling movements of the limbs, nystagmus, opisthotonus and chewing movements. Often a fetid, profuse diarrhoea is present or there may be blood in the faeces. A mild cough may be heard. On auscultation hydrothorax, hydropericardium and lung oedema are noted.

Subacute: The signs are like those of the acute form but they are much less severe with a transient fever and sometimes diarrhoea. Disease may last for over a week and the animal usually improves gradually. A few cases progress to collapse and death. 'This is often the most severe form seen in indigenous cattle and those previously infected.

Inapparent: These cattle include almost all the indigenous stock as well as some of those introduced to the region. In addition they often follow cases of reinfection.

Pathology

The lesions present are very variable and not pathognomonic. In the peracute form there are few gross lesions, but in some there is marked lung oedema with tracheal and bronchial froth. In the acute form there is usually ascites, hydrothorax, hydropericardium and lung oedema. The lymph nodes are often swollen. Petechial haemorrhages can occur in the heart, lungs and gastrointestinal tract. The liver is often engorged, with the gallbladder distended. The spleen is occasionally enlarged. There may be congestion of the meningeal blood vessels.

Diagnosis

There is no completely specific method of diagnosis in the living animal. Provisional indication can be from the history and clinical signs. Lymph node material can be aspirated to examine for vacuoles containing organisms in the cytoplasm of the reticular cells. There is a method of taking brain cortex so that the capillaries of the brain can be examined for rickettsia. Blood can be obtained and injected into susceptible animals. Eosinophils also decrease in number during the course of the disease. Serum can be examined using a capillary flocculation test. Diagnosis is easier at post mortem as the organism can be discerned in brain tissue capillaries that have been fixed in methyl alcohol and stained with Giemsa.

Differential diagnosis includes anthrax (p. 717) and acute theileriosis (p. 750) in peracute cases, and in nervous cases rabies (p. 908), tetanus (p. 733), strychnine poisoning, cerebral theileriosis (p. 752), cerebral babesiosis (p. 749) and hypomagnesaemia (p. 787).

Treatment

Therapy is most effective when carried out early in disease. Tetracyclines can be used and do not interfere with development of immunity.

Control

Disease can be prevented by controlling the vector *Amblyomma* by dipping cattle at weekly intervals with reliable acaricides. However, the ticks of this genus are less susceptible than those from other genera. As the tick may transmit infection after a day on the host, better control is obtained by applying acaricide by dipping or spraying every three days. However, *Amblyomma* have in some cases shown resistance to organophosphorus and arsenic. Care should also be taken not to introduce *Amblyomma* on infected animals or in forage to uninfected cows.

In areas where disease is endemic most cattle are immune. A carrier state develops after infection and remains for several weeks. Non-infected resistance persists a variable time, lasting from a few months to several years. After this time reinfection can occur. Ideally, an effective vaccine should be used. However, at present *C. ruminantium* is difficult to culture serially or to adapt to growth in laboratory animals. One method is to inject susceptible stock intravenously with 5–10 ml of blood from an infected animal. As infected animals cannot always be available then infected blood can be stored in a freezer or liquid nitrogen provided it is frozen rapidly after addition of dimethyl sulphonate. The infection can also be retained in deep frozen brain emulsion or, more recently, in a supernatant of homogenized engorged *Amblyomma* ticks. The recipient animal is monitored and then treated with tetracyclines as soon as pyrexia develops. Treatment continues twice a day until the fever subsides. Pregnant cows should not be treated in this way.

Jembrana disease (Tabana disease)

Aetiology

The cause of the condition is not known, but it is thought to be a rickettsial infection. Groups of small coccobacillary organisms have been found in cytoplasmic vacuoles present in circulating monocytes and in impression smears of cut organ surfaces. Some consider the disease may have a viral aetiology.

Epidemiology

The disease was first recognized in the Jembrana District of Bali Island, Indonesia, in 1964. Subsequently, the condition has only been detected in Indonesia. The disease is found in cattle as well as buffalo. Sheep and goats are infected with no apparent signs, but pigs are refractory to infection. In cattle there is apparent age resistance to infection and cattle over two years old rarely die from the disease. Animals that recover are carriers, but the duration of infection is not known. There is no direct infection from animal to animal and so it is not contagious. *Boophilus microplus*, a pantropical cattle tick, appears to be the natural vector and it is believed that infection can pass through the egg phase. The incubation period appears to be about a month to six weeks, although it is considerably shorter after injection of infection. Mortality is about 25 per cent and is usually within a week of onset of signs. Some animals relapse with infection at later dates.

Signs

Invariably there is a pyrexia of about 41°C (106°F) with anorexia, nasal and lacrimal discharge, which can persist for one to nine days. This is soon followed by enlarged lymph nodes. Often there is excessive salivation and erosion of the oral mucosa. Petechial haemorrhages may be found on the visible mucous membranes and haemorrhage is seen within the aqueous humour of the eye. Blood tends to ooze from the skin (so-called 'blood sweating'). Diarrhoea occurs early on and persists; it is often bloodstained.

Pathology

There are widespread haemorrhages and oedema. Usually, generalized lymphadenopathy occurs, with the lymph nodes being hyperplastic and often showing disorganization. Splenomegaly is common and the blood vessels show vasculitis and perivasculitis. Surrounding the blood vessels there is proliferation of lymphoreticular cells in many organs except the liver. Rickettsialike organisms can be detected in impression smears.

Diagnosis

This is based on the area and history. Confirmation depends on the haematological changes, which include a progressive anaemia, thrombocytopenia and transient leucopenia, which particularly involves the lymphocytes. As the disease progresses 'foamy' monocytes appear and large lymphocytes with coarse nuclei are seen. However, confirmation is difficult unless the animal dies. It is then dependent on detection of organisms in impression smears of cut organs and the vascular changes. In some cases blood is taken into EDTA from suspect cases and then injected into susceptible cattle.

Differential diagnosis includes rinderpest (p. 707), haemorrhagic septicaemia (p. 728) and plant poisonings (Chapter 54).

Treatment

Tetracycline injections during the course of the disease appear to have little effect on disease severity or duration, but they do seem to reduce mortality.

Control

Not enough is known about the disease to initiate control measures. Recovered animals are often carriers of infection and so resist further challenge.

Viral diseases

Bovine ephemeral fever (BEF)

This is also known as bovine epizootic fever and three-day sickness. Although signs occur they are quite mild and seem only to affect cattle. It is caused by a rhabdovirus, which can be present in the blood where it appears to be mainly in the leucocyte-platelet fraction and is transmitted by insect vectors. At present there is only a single serological type of the virus, although in Australia several rhabdoviruses with a distinct relationship to BEF have been isolated.

The condition is present in most of Africa except possibly the north. However, the incidence varies widely between regions and countries. It is also present in Asia, Australia and New Guinea. It does not occur in North or South America. The disease is transmitted by vectors from infected host cattle, which explains the seasonality of the condition. If disease enters a new region it can cause epizootic infection with a morbidity of about 100 per cent, but mortality is usually less than 1 per cent. In the enzootic areas the condition is sporadic, with a morbidity of 5–10 per cent.

The cause of transmission is thought to be midges, probably of the *Culicoides* spp. and *Ceratopogonidae* family. Transmission is not direct between animals, indicating the need for maturation in the vector. Spread mainly depends on the number of insects infected and the direction of winds. Viral development in the insect is suspected to be cyclic. More losses occur in adult cattle, although calves from three months old are susceptible. Often the disease seems to disappear only to return again as an epizootic once resistance in the cattle population is reduced.

Signs

The incubation period is two to ten days and is followed by a marked pyrexia of 40.5–41°C (105–106°F). This is often very transient and so is missed. Other animals have intermittent pyrexia. There is a drop in milk yield, which is the main loss caused by the disease, with anaemia, oculo-nasal discharge and increased salivation. Alimentary signs are variable and can include constipation or diarrhoea. Within four days locomotory signs appear, including muscular tremors, which then develop into stiffness and weakness. The animal often becomes lame and the hindlimbs may become stiff. Signs may resemble those of acute laminitis. Occasionally, animals show lateral recumbency.

The animal usually starts to show signs of recovery after two or three days, with appetite and milk yield improving. However, the stiffness and lameness are likely to take several more days to reduce. Recovery is uneventful. Mortality is low and is usually the result of secondary infection, or following aspiration pneumonia after regurgitation of ruminal contents or following lateral recumbency. Abortion does not occur, but semen quality in bulls is often affected for a period.

Necropsy

The lesions are not specific. The main sign is enlargement and oedema of all the lymph nodes. Congestion and petechial haemorrhages of the pleural membranes may occur. Other signs are usually the result of complications such as aspiration pneumonia.

Diagnosis

This depends mainly on the signs of a mild disease with pyrexia and lameness, limb stiffness and muscle tremors. There is a leucocytosis with a neutrophilia. A fluorescent antibody test will detect virus in blood. An agar gel immunodiffusion test has been successfully used on serum. The virus can be isolated by serial passage in Vero or BHK cell cultures or by intracerebral injection of sucking mice.

Treatment

Treatment is symptomatic but can include antibiotics for secondary complications, with the use of non-steroidal anti-inflammatory agents such as phenylbutazone or flunixin meglumine for muscle stiffness. It is best not to drench animals because of the high risk of aspiration pneumonia. Recumbent animals should be provided with adequate shade and water.

Control

Control of the insect vectors has not been successful. Immunity is long lasting after natural infection and has led to the development of vaccines, which are available in Japan and South Africa. Experimentally, live cell culture vaccines in an adjuvant base have been used with success, but give rise to fears of vector transmission between vaccinated and non-vaccinated stock. Control can also be achieved by dipping cows twice weekly during the peak period of infection when conditions are wet, hot and humid.

Lumpy skin disease (LSD) (see also p. 887)

The disease, also called Knopvelsiekte, results in many pox-like skin lesions and has been associated with a virus that is serologically related to sheep pox and on tissue culture produces three different groups of virus. One, an orphan virus (group I), is generally present on the skin of normal cattle but does not appear to cause the disease. The 'Allerton' virus (group II) causes a condition of a mild nature and is isolated from skin nodules, saliva, nasal secretions and semen. This form appears to be identical with the bovine herpes virus 2 of bovine mammillitis. It has often given rise to the name of pseudo-lumpy skin disease (p. 888). The severe disease is caused by a 'Neethling' virus (group III) and is found in blood, mucus, saliva and semen.

The disease is seen in most parts of Africa and is endemic in southern Africa. The virus is present on the skin even when hides are salted, in blood and in saliva and all can transmit infection.

The method of transmission has not been completely established, but it is believed to be by insects, particularly mosquitoes, as spread can occur without direct or indirect contact. Virus has been isolated from *Stomoxys* and *Biomyia* flies. As the saliva is infected, spread can also be by feeding at troughs or sucking milk from infected cows. Indigenous cattle are less susceptible than imported purebreds. Experimentally, giraffe and impala have been infected. All ages of stock are susceptible but calves and lactating cows are most likely to be infected. The duration of immunity is not known and appears variable. Reports suggest it to be from 11 months to five years, or even lifelong.

Morbidity rates are very variable, from 5 to 80 per cent, with less than 2 per cent mortality. There can be a rapid spread of the disease.

Signs

The incubation period lasts from two to five weeks in natural infection but four to fourteen days with experimental infection and is followed by a rise in temperature, which may fluctuate. In severe cases there tends to be anorexia, lacrimation and salivation. There is a clear nasal discharge, which later becomes purulent. There is then the sudden appearance of nodules, varying in number from a few to many hundred. The nodules are firm, raised areas within the skin and vary in diameter from a few millimetres to 4–5 cm. These larger areas often have erect hair over them that exaggerates their appearance. The nodules are usually of a uniform size on individual animals and they occur over the whole body, although they are mainly found on the back, neck, brisket, legs, thighs, scrotum, udder and round the muzzle and eyes. Those on the mucosae of the muzzle, vulva, prepuce, nostrils, eyes and mouth are yellow-grey in colour and soft, and if rubbed off there is an ulcer or erosion. When the eye is affected there is keratitis and conjunctivitis. Respiratory lesions lead to dyspnoea and oral ones to salivation.

The associated lymph nodes tend to be enlarged. In some cases oedema develops. This can be of the lower limbs, brisket, udder, vulva or scrotum. The enlarged skin nodules can later ulcerate. These can then persist for several years or develop a dry surface that is lost. This becomes a deep pit, which heals by second intention. These wounds can become secondarily infected. This secondary infection can then spread to associated lymph nodes, the lungs, liver, kidney, etc. The areas of superficial oedema also remain a long time and can then slough, causing suppurative areas. Involvement of the lung can lead to cicatrization and rupture of the tracheal rings several months after onset of the disease.

The disease results in a chronic loss of condition and milk yield. Secondary infection can lead to mastitis, abortion and sterility in bulls.

The 'Allerton' mild or pseudo-lumpy skin form of the disease is less severe and only lasts a few weeks. There is a mild pyrexia followed by nodule formation mainly on the head, neck and perineum. The nodules are characteristic with a hard, raised, rounded mass with a flat surface and a pit at the centre. Sometimes the skin lesions coalesce. Only the epidermis is affected, unlike the 'Neethling' form. The problem area develops into a hard, dry, necrotic lesion after a week to nine days. This is then lost over the next 10–14 days leaving a hairless area. Hair will grow again.

Necropsy

'Neethling' lesions include the whole depth of the skin, producing a hard white-grey mass. The skeletal muscle may contain grey nodules. Oedema of this is seen as yellow jelly-like liquid. If the oral mucosa is affected it contains soft grey-yellow nodules with necrotic epithelium. Necrotic ulcers with surrounding inflammation can occur in the nasal cavities. In the lungs there are firm grey nodules and the whole tract may show erosions and ulcers. Pulmonary lesions may lead to oedema and a purulent pneumonia. When lymphadenitis is present the nodules are swollen, pale and oedematous. The rumen and abomasal wall can show ulcers and erosions. Microscopically, the stratum papillomis, stratum reticulis and subcutis are involved. Secondarily, the surface epithelium, hair follicles and their associated glands are infected. In the subcutaneous tissues there is oedema, fibroplasia and perivascular inflammation with mononuclear cells, which usually results in thrombosis and overlying necrosis.

Diagnosis

The rapid spread of the disease and the sudden appearance of skin nodules after pyrexia are relatively characteristic signs. However, a biopsy can be taken and inclusion bodies can be found in skin lesions and the virus can be cultured. Other diseases that may be confused are the 'Allerton' form, urticaria (p. 883), dermatophilosis (p. 886), demodicosis (pp. 743, 881), onchocercosis (p. 774), besnoitiosis (p. 756) and severe tick and insect bites.

Treatment

There is no specific treatment but secondary infection may require the use of antibiotics or sulphonamides.

Control

Quarantine has generally not proved to be successful. In some countries a sheep pox virus tissue culture vaccine has been found to be of use. Otherwise, a vaccine produced from attenuated 'Neethling' virus on kidney tissue culture has been used successfully.

Rift Valley fever

This condition, also known as enzootic hepatitis, is a zoonosis but mainly affects sheep and cattle. Camels can be infected and also goats to a limited extent. It is notifiable in many countries. It is caused by an insect-borne RNA virus of one main antigenic strain of the family Bunyaviridae, and genus phlebovirus. The condition is transmitted between animals by insect vectors, usually mosquitoes. The disease was first identified in the East African Rift Valley, which gave rise to its name.

The condition is only found in Africa, particularly the central and southern regions, but the mosquitoes that are responsible for transmission occur on other continents. Thus there is a possibility of spread. Disease is transmitted by various types of mosquito including *Aedes* spp. Other biting arthropods would also cause spread.

Man can be infected by contact with infected animals, such as when undertaking necropsies. Infection may enter skin abrasions. The signs are of an influenza-like disease with pyrexia, severe headache, nausea, joint pains, flushing of the face, sometimes epistaxis and permanently impaired vision due to retinal haemorrhage. Death is rare, but in some instances complications such as sight impairment can occur.

Usually, an epizootic outbreak occurs in cattle followed by long periods, often of five years, between outbreaks. The persistence of infection between epizootics is unknown, but as cattle at the edge of and within forests tend to seroconvert consistently it is considered disease is maintained in wild fauna.

Disease is more common in warm wet seasons. Young animals are more severely afflicted than the adults. Mortality tends to be high in young calves, often reaching 70 per cent. In the adult, a mortality of 10 per cent can occur but the main problem is abortion.

Signs

The signs that develop depend partly on the age of the animals. They tend to be most severe in the calf, where the incubation period varies from 12 hours to three days. Occasionally, death occurs within 24 hours with few characteristic signs other than collapse and colic. Others show high fever, incoordination and collapse. The rare renal form is acute and can occasionally occur in adult cattle. In this type there is pyrexia, a profuse mucopurulent discharge, vomiting and prostration. Up to 70 per cent of affected cattle can die.

In adult cattle abortion is more common than the acute form. However, up to 10 per cent can develop marked pyrexia and die. Other lesions can include erosion of the oral mucosa and dry thickening of the unpigmented areas of the teats, udder and scrotum. Hyperaemia of the coronets also occurs.

Pathology

The main lesion is one of hepatic necrosis with white or grey foci in the subcapsular area. Other lesions are typical of septicaemia with subserous haemorrhages of the pleura, pericardium, endocardium, lymph nodes and gut. There is often also oedema, congestion or haemorrhages of the gallbladder. Microscopically, there is focal or diffuse necrosis of the liver.

Diagnosis

The history of an outbreak is helpful in that it is in a mosquito area, there is an abortion storm plus calves becoming ill with many of them dying. Post-mortem examination of calves may show typical hepatic necrosis. There may also be evidence of human infection and if sheep are present then again in lambs there is disease of high fever, incoordination, collapse and high mortality, with abortion in ewes. There is usually a severe leucopenia. Serological confirmation is by means of a serum neutralization or complement fixation test.

Treatment

There is no known successful treatment, although interferon is effective *in vitro* and may eventually become available.

Control

The passage from country to country is difficult to control without the exclusion of susceptible animal species. Control of the insect vectors would be uneconomic and impracticable. It is possible that humans could act as carriers. A vaccine from neurotrophic virus passage through mouse brain has been used successfully. However, it can cause abortion. In consequence, a killed vaccine produced on BHK cells has been developed (p. 1018). This involves two injections to produce adequate immunity. Good immunity has been produced in sheep and humans by virus grown in rhesus kidney cell cultures and then inactivated by formaldehyde. A human vaccine is now available from virus raised in diploid fetal lung cells and inactivated with formalin.

Tick-borne encephalitides (flavivirus infections)

There are a series of diseases of animals resulting from tick-borne infection and characterized by nervous signs and fever (Chapter 51). The causes are included within a complex of flaviviruses. The infections tend to be contained in various geographical areas. As a result there are a number of diseases that are identified by the area where the disease occurs. Thus, in Europe there is Russian spring-summer encephalitis, Omsk haemorrhagic fever and Central European encephalitis. Tropical problems include Kyasamar Forest fever in India and Lanyot in Malaysia.

In almost all cases the viruses maintain their presence in ticks, small rodents and insectivores. In the endemic cases infection of wild and domestic ruminants is inapparent. However, the introduction of new ruminants can result in disease. As yet the infections of Kyasamar Forest fever, which have been found in man and horses, have not resulted in disease in native domestic cattle. Infection in cattle would be via ixodial ticks. Man can be infected by ticks or, more commonly, via drinking infected goat's or sheep's milk. Infections from material submitted for laboratory diagnosis also occur. Immunity following infection is good and lifelong. Colostrum results in passive immunity being conferred to the young calf.

Signs

Disease is almost always only apparent in animals introduced to the tick area. The incubation period is one or two weeks. Pyrexia suddenly occurs and is usually diphasic. It is not until the second period of temperature rise that nervous signs appear. There is then incoordination, muscle tremors, ataxia, photophobia and hypersensitivity. The nervous signs become progressively worse. There can then be a flaccid paralysis, with death within a week. Those animals that recover are often subsequently debilitated.

Necropsy

There are few gross lesions. On histological examination there is necrosis of the neurones, particularly in the Purkinje layer of the motor nuclei, vestibular nuclei, cerebellum and ventral nerves of the spinal cord. Perivascular inflammation occurs throughout the white matter.

Diagnosis

The diagnosis is based on the area, presence of ticks, signs and lesions. The virus can be isolated from the central nervous system, particularly the brain stem and spinal cord. Differential diagnoses include bovine spongiform encephalopathy (p. 909), rabies (p. 908; Chaptre 70), neuromycotoxins, plant poisoning

(Chapter 54), tetanus, hypocalcaemia (p. 781) and hypomagnesaemia (p. 787).

Treatment

There is no effective form of treatment.

Control

Cattle should not be introduced to endemic areas unless they are vaccinated. The vaccines available provide protection for at least a year. Control of ticks by improving grazing and reducing bracken, etc., is useful.

Tick-borne encephalitides (Near East encephalitis)

This condition is still not fully elucidated. However, there are several diseases that have been recognized for many years. The disease is endemic in some countries including Syria, Lebanon, Israel and Egypt and a similar condition is recorded in India and Russia.

In most cases the accidental infection of ruminants results in few cases of disease. Usually, the virus cycles inapparently within birds and ticks. Most clinical disease is in Equidae, but occasionally problems have been recorded in sheep and cattle. The tick vector of Near East encephalitis is *Hyalomma anatolicum*. Infection passes through all stages of tick life including the egg.

All infection is tick mediated and it cannot be transmitted directly between animals. Immunity follows infection in cattle but its duration is unknown.

Signs

The incubation period for the disease is unknown, but may be four weeks. The severity of signs is variable and in the acute form there is a drowsiness and a pyrexia of about 40°C (104°F). However, in a few horses there are epileptiform fits with a progressive paralysis. Collapse and death can soon occur. In the subacute form pyrexia is usually transient and mild. Nervous signs are slight, but in some cases they can persist. Inapparent infections are common.

Necropsy

The alimentary and urogenital tract of the body show mucosal congestion, but there is meningeal blood vessel congestion. On histological examination there is diffuse lymphocytic infiltration, perivascular infiltration, microglial proliferation and neuronophagia and occasional rarefaction of tissues.

Diagnosis

The signs and post-mortem picture are not specific. However, cerebral injection of infected brain tissue into rabbits will aid virus identification. The major disease to be differentiated is rabies (p. 908).

Treatment

There is no effective form of treatment, only symptomatic.

Control

There are no suitable control measures that can at present be suggested.

Japanese encephalitis (flavivirus)

This is mainly a disease of man and has been given several local names, including Japanese B encephalitis, Russian autumnal encephalitis and summer encephalitis. Infection of animals is often from the human source. Most disease is seen as encephalitis in horses, followed by pigs. Mosquitoes are the natural vectors. Usually, infection in cattle and other ruminants is inapparent and of little overall significance.

Other arthropod-borne diseases

There are well over 300 diseases that are arthropod transmitted. Many are of limited geographical distribution. Frequently areas do not produce overt disease. However, where signs do occur, they can be nonspecific with malaise and pyrexia. Often indigenous animals and wild animals develop inapparent disease that does not cause them any hazards or reduce production. However, the introduction of new animals will frequently result in overt disease, which can reach a high morbidity level.

Akabane virus (Asian virus)

This bunyavirus is mosquito borne and related to Simbu virus. It is recorded in the Far East as well as Kenya and Australia. The condition in cattle is thought to produce arthrogryposis and hydrocephalus as well as abortion.

Bhanja virus (African virus)

This is mainly an infection of goats but it has occasionally been isolated in cattle, particularly in southern Nigeria, and has also been reported in India. Infection has been found in *Haemaphysalis* ticks. Experimentally, calves injected with Bhanja virus have developed a viraemia for several days and leucopenia.

Bunyamwera virus (African virus)

This is mainly a condition of goats, but serological evidence has been found in cattle and sheep. The infection occurs throughout Africa and is considered to be mosquito borne.

Cache Valley virus (American virus)

This is found in mosquitoes in Central and North America. Disease has not been recorded but sera of cattle are often positive.

California encephalitis virus (American virus)

In America there is a high incidence of antibody in the sera of cattle. Evidence of infection can also be found in deer and horses. It is a bunyavirus transmitted by mosquitoes. The virus is the most common cause of human viral encephalitis in the USA.

Calovovirus (European virus)

This is a bunyavirus that is mosquito borne. It results in cattle infection.

Congo virus (African virus)

This is a disease of humans and also affects goats and cattle resulting in anaemia, depression and pyrexia. The virus is transmitted by *Hyalomma* ticks and infection between countries is probably accomplished by migrating birds. It is likely that the condition is related to Hazna virus and others in Europe and Asia. The disease is severe in horses and is often fatal. However, in cattle and goats indigenous to Africa it results in a short period of illness that may be seen as anorexia, fever and depression.

Corriparta virus (Australian virus)

The virus is mosquito borne, particularly by *Culex* spp. The disease level is unknown but antibodies are found in the sera of cattle, horses and man as well as kangaroos and wallabies.

Dughe virus (African virus)

The virus appears to be spread by *Amblyomma variegatum* ticks, *Culicoides* and mosquitoes. It is the most frequently isolated arthropod-borne virus in Nigeria. In most cases there are no signs in cattle, but calves can be infected experimentally and show a short-lasting viraemia.

Germiston virus (African virus)

This is a bunyavirus and is transmitted by mosquitoes. The virus causes infection in humans, usually in laboratories, but in cattle there are usually no signs but seroconversion. The condition is present in cattle, egrets and herons.

Harana virus (Asian virus)

The virus is transmitted by *Hyalomma* ticks and spread to other animals by migrating birds. This virus resembles, and may be identical to, Azo virus. It results in a severe infection of humans, often with haemorrhages and fever. It can be fatal. In cattle the disease is transient and usually results in anorexia, pyrexia and depression.

Ibaraki virus (Asian virus)

It is thought to be arthropod borne and is a double-stranded RNA virus. Antibody surveys show the infection to be widespread in South East Asia and the Far East. The condition is very similar to that of bluetongue. Disease is severe and only recorded in Japan. Signs include pyrexia with oedema and haemorrhaging in the mouth, abomasum and around the horn/skin junction. Degeneration of the muscles follows. There is then dehydration and emaciation due to difficulty in swallowing. Death is commonly due to inhalation pneumonia.

Jos virus (African virus)

This unclassified virus is transmitted by *Amblyomma variegatum* ticks. The disease signs are not really known but the virus has been isolated from indigenous Nigerian cattle.

Kodam virus (African virus)

This flavivirus is found in *Rhipicephalus parvus* ticks. The signs of disease are unknown but antibody is found in cattle.

Kokobera (Australian virus)

The virus has been found in mosquitoes in Queensland. It is a flavivirus. Antibodies have been detected in sera from cattle and horses, although there is no indication that the virus is a pathogen.

Kowanyama virus, Mapputta virus, Trubanaman virus (Australian viruses)

These are all found in tropical Australia and can be isolated from the *Anopheles* mosquito. Their pathogenicity is not known but antibodies are found in the sera of cattle, sheep and pigs as well as kangaroos and wallabies.

Kunjin virus (Australian virus)

This is a flavivirus found in mosquitoes in tropical Australia. There is serological evidence of infection in humans, horses, cattle and poultry. In calves experimentally infected a mild, non-purulent encephalitis develops.

Kotonkan virus (African virus)

This is a rhabdovirus found in *Culicoides*. The disease resembles ephemeral fever virus. The infection is particularly present in Nigeria.

Lokern virus (American virus)

Antibodies to the bunyavirus have been found in cattle, horses and sheep. The infection is found in Californian sandflies and mosquitoes.

Middelburg virus (African virus)

While antibodies can be found in domestic cattle in South Africa, disease has not been recorded. Man is not affected. The virus is spread by *Aedes* mosquitoes.

Murray Valley encephalitis virus (Australian virus)

This is a flavivirus found in mosquitoes and wild birds. It can produce epidemics of human encephalitis in Australia and New Guinea. The infection can be detected serologically in cattle, horses, pigs and dogs. When calves are experimentally infected the disease is symptomless.

Obodhiang virus (African virus)

This is a rhabdovirus found in *Culicoides*. The disease resembles ephemeral fever. It is found in mosquitoes in Sudan and the pathogenicity is not known.

Pongola virus (African virus)

Cattle sera will show antibodies to this virus but disease is not apparent. The name also applies to infection in humans, donkeys, goats and sheep. The condition is spread by mosquitoes. The virus appears to be related to Rwamba virus.

Rwamba virus (African virus)

Cattle sera will show antibodies to this virus but disease is not apparent. The name also applies to infection in humans, donkeys, goats and sheep. The condition is spread by mosquitoes. The virus appears to be related to Pongola virus.

Sabo virus (African virus)

This virus is found in *Culicoides* in Nigeria. It is also frequently isolated from Nigerian cattle and has been isolated from goats. There is a transient fever and listlessness following infection. The virus is a member of the Simbu group of bunyaviruses.

Sango virus (African virus)

This virus is found in *Culicoides* in Nigeria. It is also frequently isolated from Nigerian cattle. There is a transient fever and listlessness following infection. The virus is a member of the Simbu group of bunyaviruses.

Shamondu virus (African virus)

This virus is found in *Culicoides* in Nigeria. It is also frequently isolated from Nigerian cattle. There is a transient fever and listlessness following infection. The virus is a member of the Simbu group of bunyaviruses.

Shuni virus (African virus)

This virus is found in *Culicoides* in Nigeria. It is also frequently isolated from Nigerian cattle and has been isolated from sheep. There is a transient fever and listlessness following infection. The virus is a member of the Simbu group of bunyaviruses.

Sindbis virus (African, Asian and Australian virus)

The life cycle is believed to involve *Culicoides*, mosquitoes and wild birds. In most cases cattle exhibit no signs but they do develop antibody titres. Infection of humans results in illness. It is a species of the alphaviruses.

Thogoto virus (African and European virus)

The virus is found in ticks in Nigeria and in *Boophilus decoloratus* ticks in Kenya. It has also been isolated in the tick *Rhipicephalus bursa* in Sicily. The infection can also involve humans and sheep. Calves, when experimentally infected, show viraemia and leucopenia but usually there are no other signs.

PARASITIC DISEASES

Onchocercosis (worm nodule disease)

Aetiology

This is a filarial infection of the genus *Onchocerca*. In cattle, *Onchocerca gibsoni* affects the subcutaneous tissues, particularly the brisket and lower limbs; *O. liendis* (synonyms *O. gutturosa*, *O. bovis*) is found in the ligamentum nuchae, other ligaments and stifle joints; *O. ochengi* causes a dermatitis and *O. armillata* is found in the aortic wall. The worms are thread-like and often measure 6 cm long with microfilariae 200–400 μm long.

Epidemiology

The condition occurs worldwide, but is more common in the tropics and subtropics. The life cycle is indirect. Transmission is by midges (*Culicoides* spp.), sandflies and blackflies (*Simulium* spp.), which ingest microfilaria in the skin and subcutaneous tissue. They develop to the infective larval stage and then infect the final host when the vector again feeds. The larvae migrate to the predilection site where *O. gibsoni* develops into nodules and the others become enclosed in a fibrous cyst. The females produce microfilariae that remain in the skin or subcutaneous tissue.

Signs

There are few clinical signs except for the presence of nodules up to 3 cm diameter under the skin, particularly in the brisket. In *O. liendis* infections there are few signs in the ligamentum nuchae but the stifle joint may be swollen. Disability can occur due to the supporting ligaments being affected. Infestation with *O. gibsoni* can result in nodules.

Pathology

There are nodules present. *Onchocerca armillata* is present in nodules in the wall of the thrombic aorta; *O. liendis* is found in the ligamentum nuchae, ligaments, stifle, the omentum, splenic ligament and capsule.

Diagnosis

The presence of infection can be detected by examining skin biopsies. Differentiation from skin tuberculosis (p. 743) and demodectic mange (p. 781) is necessary.

Treatment

There is no specific treatment but diethylcarbamazine citrate 4 mg/kg in the food can be helpful, otherwise ivermectin, doramectin and eprinomectin can be used.

Control

The control of insect vectors is not practicable.

Stephanofilariosis

Aetiology

This is caused by parasites of the genus *Stephanofilaria*. These include *S. assamensis*, which occurs in India and Pakistan, *S. kaeli*, found on the legs of cattle in Malaysia, *S. stilesi*, affecting the ventral surface of the body and found in many parts of Asia, and *S. dedosi*, which occurs in Indonesia affecting the head and neck. The parasites are small (2–9 mm long) and filariform in shape.

Epidemiology

The parasite occurs in cattle and buffalo in many parts of South East Asia as well as the tropics. The life cycle is indirect and involves anthomyid flies as intermediate hosts. Open skin lesions develop from which the flies feed and ingest the microfilariae. In the fly they develop to the infective larval stage and are then transmitted to the final host when the fly feeds. There appear to be more flies when conditions are moist either due to rain or presence of rivers, streams or irrigation.

Signs

There are only superficial lesions, seen initially as a papular dermatitis. There is then exudate and haemorrhage lasting many months with the skin becoming thickened and dry.

Diagnosis

This is based on the lesions and recent wet weather. Scrapings or smears from skin lesions reveal adult worms and microfilariae.

Treatment

Topical application of organophosphorus compounds is effective, including trichlorphan 6 per cent and coumaphos 2 per cent.

Control

There is no effective control but in some cases fly repellents are used. However, these are expensive for routine use. In adult animals that have been repeatedly infected with *S. stilesi* there is evidence that further infestation is reduced or stops.

Thelaziosis

Aetiology

Disease is caused by infestation with spirurid nematodes of the genus *Thelazia*, in cattle by *T. rhodesii*. The worms are thin, white and can be up to 20 mm long.

Epidemiology

It occurs in the conjunctival sac of mammals in many parts of the world. In the species that have been studied the worms are viviparous and produce first-stage larvae that are infective for various Diptera, including *Musca* spp. The flies act as the intermediate hosts where the parasite develops to a third-stage infective larva, which is transferred to the final host when the flies feed.

Signs

There are often no signs, otherwise there may be lacrimation that can be unilateral or bilateral and is often purulent. There can be conjunctivitis, keratitis, corneal opacity, ulceration, protrusion of the eyeball and photophobia. Abscesses may develop on the eyelids.

Pathology

There may be conjunctivitis, keratitis and corneal ulceration and scarring.

Diagnosis

This depends on the signs and finding the worms.

Treatment

The most effective treatments are the avermectins ivermectin, doramectin and eprinomectin at 200 μg/kg. Levamisole can be given orally at 5 mg/kg body weight or as a 1 per cent eye lotion. Otherwise, local anaesthetic can be used and the helminths removed manually. Irrigation of the unanaesthetized eye can be undertaken with 1 in 8000 aqueous iodine or 2 per cent boric acid, 3 per cent piperazine adipate or 0.2 per cent diethyl carbamazine.

Control

The condition is not usually severe and so control is not normally undertaken particularly because of the ubiquitous nature of the vector.

Other problems

Tick paralysis

Aetiology

This occurs with a number of different ticks and results in an ascending flaccid paralysis either due to acetylcholine failure at neuromuscular sites or a lack of conduction within the nerve fibres.

Epidemiology

This is seen in ticks in Australia (*Ixodes holocyclus*), North America (*Dermacentor andersoni, D. accidentalis*) and South Africa (*I. pilosus, I. rubicundus, Haemaphysalis punctata*). Most cases coincide with the peak tick populations and particularly at maximum adult activity. At times only one feeding tick may cause the problem.

Signs

The signs involve a change in temperament followed by slight incoordination. Then the animal starts to drag its hindlimbs and as the forelimbs are progressively involved it becomes recumbent. There is respiratory distress and then the animal dies of respiratory failure.

Necropsy

There are no characteristic signs at post mortem.

Diagnosis

If the ticks are removed the animal makes a recovery.

Treatment

Remove as many ticks as possible by hand, then treat with an ixodicide.

Control

Although susceptibility decreases with age, immunity varies from a few weeks to years. Prevention really involves the proper use of dips, sprays, etc.

Sweating sickness (sweetsiekte, notkalersiekte, vuursiekte, schwitzkrankheit, la dyhydrose tropicale, foma, ol macheri)

This appears to be a toxicosis with a dermatotrophic toxin related to tick infestations. Removal of the ticks results in a rapid clinical recovery. The problem is not transferred from animal to animal by the introduction of blood, saliva or tissue from ill animals. Animals appear to be susceptible or non-susceptible. In the former case cattle become ill with each exposure and can die. Only certain strains of the tick *Hyalomma truncatum*, known as the boat-legged tick, are implicated. The disease is seen in Central, East and South Africa. Although cattle are involved, particularly calves, sheep, goats, pigs and dogs are also affected. The signs vary according to individual susceptibility, age of the animal and the number of the correct strain of tick present. The inactive period is about six days, but varies from four to eleven. The morbidity of the condition is very variable and mortality ranges from 30 to 70 per cent. Immediately following recovery from sweating sickness immunity persists for well over a year and in some cases lasts up to four years. There appears to be no passive transfer of immunity to calves in colostrum.

Signs

Peracute: This is fatal in 48–72 hours, with a sudden rise in rectal temperature, hyperaemia, anorexia, dyspnoea, hyperaesthesia of the visible mucous membranes and muscle tremors. There tends to be excessive lacrimation and nasal discharge.

Acute: This only occurs in animals under a year old and presents as a sudden rise in temperature to 40–41°C (104–106°F) for a period of up to eight days. The pyrexia may be continuous or intermittent and lasts longer in the latter case. The mucous membranes become hyperaemic and there is lacrimation, salivation and nasal discharge. The hair is in poor condition and wet eczematous areas develop involving the head, particularly the cheeks under the eyes, nose, ears, then the neck, abdomen and flanks, and especially the groin. In some cases the whole body may be affected and accompanying the eczema there is hyperaesthesia, discharge and loss of the surface epithelium. Many badly affected calves show total hair loss.

Subacute: The signs are a sudden rise in temperature, but to a lesser extent and lasting only two or three days, and the mucous membranes show slight hyperaemia, as can the skin.

Inapparent: These animals show few signs but there is a form of residual immunity to the problem.

Pathology

The lesions depend on the duration of the condition and any concurrent disease. There is a disseminated intravascular coagulopathy with microthrombi (Van Amstel *et al.*, 1987). The oral mucous membranes show ecchymotic dermatitis, inflammation and superficial necrosis. The nasal cavity, pharynx, larynx, oesophagus and omasum show white pseudomembranes. In the thorax there is hydrothorax, hydropericarditis with oedema and emphysema. The liver displays fatty degeneration and the abomasal, small and large intestine mucous membranes show hyperaemia.

Diagnosis

This is dependent on the area and local history of the disease and presence of *H. truncatum* ticks on the animal. Pathological signs are helpful and there is an increased prothrombin clotting time. Peracute cases could be confused with anthrax (p. 717), babesiosis (p. 748), anaplasmosis (p. 761), heartwater (p. 765) and poisonings (Chapter 54).

Treatment

There is no specific drug that will affect sweating sickness, but hyperimmune serum is useful in treatment. The inflammatory nature of the disease suggests the use of anti-inflammatory agents, but corticosteroids are probably contraindicated as there are often high circulating cortisol levels in affected cattle. The use of antibiotics is indicated because of the likely immunosuppression that can occur in the presence of high cortisol levels. As there is severe intravascular coagulation the use of heparin at 10–20 iu/kg body weight may be helpful. The liver is often affected and so multivitamin injections, particularly containing cyanocobalamin, choline and methionine, may be of use.

Control and prevention

Effective control of the ticks responsible with acaricides is helpful. Eradication is usually not feasible and so acaricide regimens should be designed to clear short-term infestation with the ticks, insufficient to produce distress but of long enough duration to allow immunity to develop. As the tick needs to be attached to the animal for at least 7–10 days to produce disease, weekly dipping normally produces reasonable control.

Mhlosimge

This is a less important toxicosis that is transmitted by certain strains of *Hyalomma truncatum*. It affects cattle, sheep and pigs. The signs are usually milder than sweating sickness. Cattle do not die of the disease but show pyrexia and anorexia. There is no cross-immunity between sweating sickness and Mhlosimge.

Magudu

This is also a less important toxicosis transmitted by some strains of *H. truncatum*. Again the disease is non-fatal and can affect cattle, sheep and pigs. The signs are milder than those of sweating sickness, including anorexia and pyrexia. Cattle previously infected with sweating sickness are immune to Magudu.

Stomatitis–nephrosis syndrome

This condition is reported in cattle in Zimbabwe. It is a toxicosis but it is not known whether it is of the sweating sickness type or a different *Hyalomma* toxicosis.

References

Ectoparasites

Urquhart, G.M., Armour, J., Duncan, J.L., Dunn, A.N. & Jennings, F.W. (1987) *Veterinary Parasitology*, pp. 1–286. Longman Scientific, Harlow.

Trypanosomosis

Banks, K.L. (1978) Binding of *Trypanosoma congolense* to the walls of small blood vessels. *Journal of Protozoology*, **25**, 241–5.
Clarkson, M.J. (1976) Trypanosomiasis of domesticated animals of S. America. *Transactions of the Royal Society of Tropical Medicine and Hygiene*, **70**, 125–6.
Hoste, C. (1987) Trypanotolerant livestock and African animal trypanosomiasis. *World Animal Review*, **62**, 41–50.
Losos, G.J. (1986) Trypanosomiasis. In *Infectious Tropical Diseases of Domestic Animals*, pp. 183–318. Longman, Harlow.
Masake, R.A., Nantulya, V.M., Akol, G.W.O. & Musoke, A.J. (1984) Cerebral trypanosomiasis in cattle with mixed *T. congolense* and *T. brucei* infections. *Acta Tropica*, **41**, 237–46.
Morrison, W.I., Murray, M., Whitelaw, D.D. & Sayer, P.D. (1983) Pathology of infection with *T. brucei*: disease syndromes in dogs and cattle resulting from severe tissue damage. *Contributions to Microbiology and Immunology*, **7**, 103–19.
Murray, M. (1978) Anaemia of bovine African trypanosomiasis: an overview. In *Pathogenicity of Trypanosomes*. Proceedings of a workshop held at Nairobi, Kenya, November 1978.
Mwongela, G.N., Kovatch, R.M. & Fazil, M.A. (1981) Acute *T. vivax* infection in dairy cattle in Coast Province, Kenya. *Tropical Animal Health and Production*, **13**, 63–9.
Nantulya, V.M., Musoke, A.J., Rurangirwa, F.R., Saigar, N. & Minja, S.H. (1987) Monoclonal antibodies that distinguish *T. congolense*, *T. vivax* and *T. brucei*. *Parasite Immunology*, **9**, 421–31.
Njogu, A.R., Dolan, R.B., Wilson, A.L. & Sayer, P.D. (1985) Trypanotolerance in E. African Orma Boran cattle. *Veterinary Record*, **117**, 632–6.
Paris, J., Murray, M. & McOdimba, F. (1982) A comparative evaluation of the parasitological techniques currently available for the diagnosis of African trypanosomiasis in cattle. *Acta Tropica*, **39**, 307–16.
Pilson, R.D. & Leggate, B.M. (1961) A diurnal and seasonal study of the feeding activity of *Glossina pallidipes*. *Australian Bulletin of Entomological Research*, **53**, 541–9.
Rae, P.F. & Luckins, A.G. (1984) Detection of circulating trypanosomal antigens by enzyme immunoassay. *Annals of Tropical Medicine and Parasitology*, **78**, 587–96.
Stephen, L.E. (1986) *Trypanosomiasis – A Veterinary Prospective*. Pergamon Press, Oxford.
Trail, J.C.M., Sones, K., Jibbo, J.M.C., Durkin, J., Light, D.E. & Murray, M. (1985) Productivity of Boran cattle maintained by chemoprophylaxis under trypanosomiasis risk. *ILCA Research Report* No. 9, Addis Ababa.
Whiteside, E.F. (1962) The control of cattle trypanosomiasis with drugs in Kenya: methods and costs. *East African Agricultural and Forestry Journal*, **28**, 67–73.

Other problems

Van Amstel, S.R., Reyers, F., Oberem, P.T. & Mathee, O. (1987) Further pathological studies of the clinical pathology of sweating sickness in cattle. *Onderstepoort Journal of Veterinary Research*, **54**, 45–8.

Further reading

Sewell, M.M.H. & Brocklesby, D.W. (1990) *Handbook on Animal Diseases in the Tropics*, 47th edn, pp. 1–385, Baillière Tindall, London.

Adult Cattle
Metabolic Problems

Chapter 46
Major Metabolic Disorders

R.G. Eddy

Milk fever (parturient paresis, hypocalcaemia, eclampsia) 781
Hypomagnesaemia (grass tetany, grass staggers, lactation
    tetany, Hereford disease) 787
Hypophosphataemia 791
    Postparturient haemoglobinuria 792
Acetonaemia (ketosis, slow fever) 793
Pregnancy toxaemia 796
The downer cow 797
Fatty liver syndrome 801

Milk fever (parturient paresis, hypocalcaemia, eclampsia)

Milk fever or hypocalcaemia is probably the most common metabolic disorder affecting cattle. It is normally associated with parturition occurring just before, during or immediately after calving although it has been reported in dry cows and, increasingly, during mid lactation. The incidence of milk fever is higher in dairy cows than beef cows and increases with age and yield. Milk fever undoubtedly increased in incidence during the 1970s and 1980s when levels of around 9 per cent per annum were being reported. More recent studies would suggest that the incidence has fallen to around 5–6 per cent, in spite of increased milk yields, and probably the result of improved nutrition of dry cows. The incidence does vary considerably between seasons as well as between farms. In some years the incidence in September and October in the UK can be as high as 60 per cent on some farms, whereas during the winter months when dry cows are housed 0–6 per cent would be frequently reported. The disease does appear to be more common when dry cows are fed grass rather than conserved fodder. Milk fever is a common cause of death and is probably the most common cause of apparent sudden death in dairy cows. It is also a common cause of dystokia and hence stillborn calves.

Predisposing factors

There are several important predisposing factors that influence the occurrence of milk fever and these account for the wide variation of incidence observed in the UK and other countries worldwide.

Breed: The Jersey and, to a lesser extent, the Guernsey are particularly susceptible to milk fever. This would indicate a genetic predilection for this disease and is probably related to the relatively high production level for a small breed.

Age: It is rare for milk fever to occur at the first calving and relatively uncommon at the second. The incidence does appear to increase with age and incidence levels of 20 per cent or more are common at the sixth calving and beyond. The reason is thought to be that the requirement for calcium at parturition increases as milk yield rises with each lactation and the ability to mobilize calcium quickly from the body reserves, i.e. bone, decreases with age.

Seasonal factors: The incidence in the UK is highest in the months of August to October and at its lowest in the winter months of December, January and February. However, this is more likely to be a result of differing feeding regimens of dry cows than a seasonal effect. In countries where there is little change in dry-cow nutrition during the year, e.g. Israel, there appears to be no seasonal differences in the occurrence of milk fever.

Nutritional factors: The wide range of incidence of milk fever observed between seasons, within a season and between farms in the UK is due to the variation of nutritional input given to dry cows. Dry cows that are fed a diet of hay or silage only, which is now commonplace in the UK, will have a low incidence of milk fever at calving. However, if feeds containing high calcium levels are included in the diet, e.g. sugar beet pulp or high calcium minerals, the incidence will increase.

The incidence of milk fever in cows at grass varies considerably with the season. In dry weather the incidence is low, but during long wet spells the level is high. A diet of grass with a low dry matter (DM), whether in the spring or autumn, can predispose to high incidences of milk fever. There is more than one reason for this. One is that such a diet leads to diarrhoea, which probably reduces the calcium available for absorption. The calcium level of wet grass, particularly in the autumn, can be excessively high, often as high as 1 per cent of

DM. Potassium levels may also be high. It has been shown that low magnesium levels in the diet restrict the cow's ability to absorb calcium (Sansom *et al.*, 1983) and the high levels of milk fever found in the spring and autumn in the UK are often due to low magnesium levels in the grass.

Aetiology

Some degree of hypocalcaemia occurs in all cows at parturition, but only when this becomes severe do clinical signs develop. Frequently, hypophosphataemia and hypermagnesaemia accompany the hypocalcaemia, although when milk fever is due to low magnesium intake the blood levels of magnesium will also be depressed. The normal concentration of calcium in plasma lies within the range 2.2–2.6 mmol/l (8.8–10.4 mg/100 ml), but will fall to 1.5 mmol/l (6.0 mg/100 ml) in most cows at parturition without milk fever signs occurring. Usually, when milk fever is present the plasma level will be in the range 0.75–1.5 mmol/l (3.0–6.0 mg/100 ml).

The predisposing factor in the aetiology of hypocalcaemia at parturition is the sudden increase in the requirement of calcium for the production of colostrum. The daily calcium requirement of a 600 kg cow in late pregnancy is approximately 28–30 g; this comprises 13–15 g required for endogenous loss in faeces and urine and 15 g to maintain the growing fetus. At the onset of lactation, approximately 1–1.5 g of calcium is required for each litre of colostrum produced, so the requirement is increased two- or three-fold in a very short period. In order to meet this enlarged demand and to avoid hypocalcaemia, calcium absorption from the gut is increased and further calcium is available from mobilization of the calcium reserves in bone. This explains why mild hypocalcaemia occurs in all cows at parturition. If the cow does not respond quickly to the sudden increase in calcium requirement the hypocalcaemia deepens and signs of milk fever become apparent.

In the normal cow this adaptation process at parturition is under the hormonal control of the parathyroid hormone (PTH). Hypocalcaemia stimulates the secretion of PTH, which in turn stimulates the production of a hydroxylase enzyme in the kidney that is able to synthesize 1,25-dihydroxycholecalciferol (1,25(OH)$_2$D$_3$), which is produced from vitamin D$_3$. The 1,25(OH)$_2$D$_3$ stimulates increased gut absorption of calcium and probably the mobilization of calcium from bone (Fig. 46.1).

Several factors affect the speed of response to this adaptation process:

- Age of the cow, as already mentioned. Older cows are less able to mobilize calcium from the skeleton.
- Oestrogens also inhibit calcium mobilization and as oestrogen levels rise at parturition this will have a negative effect on the adaptation process to maintain calcium levels. Milk fever does occasionally occur during lactation, usually in association with

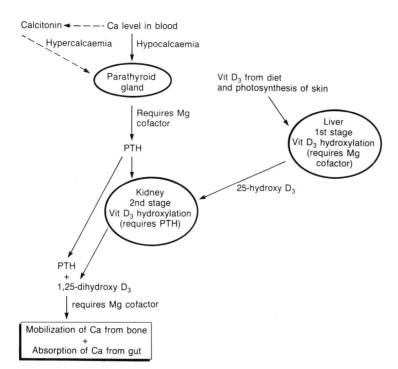

Fig. 46.1 System for mobilizing calcium in cattle. PTH, parathyroid hormone (Kelly, 1988).

oestrus. This again would be due to the inhibitory effect of oestrogens.

● Food intake is often depressed at or around parturition so the total available calcium in the diet will be reduced. This is particularly the case if diets low in calcium, e.g. straw or cereal-based diets, are fed over the parturition period.

● The calcium intake during the dry period. If high levels of calcium are present in the diet the reduced PTH output that occurs reduces the rate of absorption from the gut, so that when the demand for calcium suddenly increases and the cow's appetite is generally reduced absorption does not satisfy the body requirement (Fig. 46.1).

● A low magnesium intake in the diet reduces by various mechanisms the ability of the gut to allow calcium absorption. Therefore, diets that are deficient in magnesium will predispose to hypocalcaemia by reducing calcium absorption. Hypomagnesaemia also inhibits mobilization of calcium from bone (Fig. 46.1).

● Problems associated with digestion, e.g. acidosis and profuse diarrhoea, will reduce the amount of calcium in the gut available for absorption. This could also explain cases of hypocalcaemia that occur at times other than parturition or oestrus.

Signs

The clinical signs of milk fever are progressive. In the first stage there is a loss of appetite, lethargy and the rectal temperature is reduced by 0.5°C (1°F). This progresses to a stage where the cow stands with the hocks straight and sways laterally, particularly when moving. Constipation is normally seen at this stage. Muscle tremors may be present about the head and limbs. Hyperaesthesia is also often evident at this stage and the cow becomes apprehensive. The lateral swaying develops into incoordination and ataxia and the cow will fall over sideways and rise with increasing difficulty until she becomes permanently recumbent.

The recumbent stage is the one most commonly seen by veterinarians in practice. The cow will be sitting in sternal recumbency, often with a noticeable S bend in the neck, progressing to the stage where the head will be resting on her shoulder. The heart rate will be slightly raised but rarely exceeds 90/minute. The pupils will be dilated and the pupillary light reflex will be reduced or even absent. The gut stasis that characterizes this stage of the disease further reduces the availability of calcium for absorption and the disease will progress to the comatose stage. The rumen ceases to function and often becomes tympanic and the cow appears severely depressed. The comatose stage is characterized by lateral recumbency, increased rumen

tympany and total absence of the pupillary light reflex until the cow dies. Death can be due to paralysis of the respiratory muscles, but more often death occurs from bloat. Many cows with milk fever are found in ditches or streams, having fallen in during the incoordination phase of the disease. In these situations death can be due to drowning.

The length of time for the disease to progress from first signs of inappetance to death varies from 10 to 24 hours. Many cows are found dead or near to death by the stockworker at the time of morning milking, having been quite normal the previous evening at 7.00 pm.

If hypocalcaemia occurs at the onset of calving the parturition process will cease due to lack of myometrial contractions. A considerable number of cases of dystokia due to uterine inertia are the result of hypocalcaemia and, if not treated, will result in a stillborn calf or even death of the cow before the calf is born. It is common for the stockworker to find a cow in lateral recumbency in the early morning with the calf presented in the birth canal or even with the head present at the vulva. Frequently, the calf will be dead and occasionally even partially eaten by foxes or other wildlife.

Clinical pathology

The concentration of calcium in plasma is usually below 1.5 mmol/l (6 mg/100 ml) in cows with clinical hypocalcaemia and will fall to as low as 0.25 mmol/l (1.0 mg/100 ml). Phosphorus levels also fall to 1.0 mmol/l from the normal range of 1.4–2.5 mmol/l (4.3–7.8 mg/100 ml). Magnesium levels usually increase to around 1.25 mmol/l (3.0 mg/100 ml), except where the cause of milk fever is related to low magnesium diets when hypomagnesaemia may be present. Hyperglycaemia is also usual during milk fever, but this is frequently seen in normal cows at parturition.

In fatal cases of milk fever there are no gross or histological lesions characteristic of the disease. Bruising of subcutaneous tissue and muscles due to localized trauma may be apparent. The liver is occasionally distended and infiltrated with fat, resulting in a yellow discoloration. Cows with such a fatty liver are thought to be more prone to milk fever, but fatty liver is not pathognomonic of milk fever.

Diagnosis

The diagnosis of milk fever is made on the signs described above and the history of recent or imminent calving. Although blood biochemistry may be considered useful, in practical situations there is not the time available to obtain a result. A cowside test for calcium is now available in some countries but its value is probably limited to differential diagnosis of the downer cow syndrome or cows failing to respond to treatment for milk fever. The most valuable diagnostic aid available is, once the differential diagnoses have been eliminated, the response to treatment. Intravenous treatment with calcium borogluconate will produce a clinical response within minutes. The cow will become more alert, defaecate and eructate, often before the full dose of calcium has been administered.

Differential diagnosis

Although milk fever is an extremely common disease it is essential that a full clinical examination be made for every case. It is common for the new veterinary graduate to diagnose and treat a recumbent cow for milk fever when the cause of the recumbency is toxic mastitis. The clinical examination must therefore include examination of milk from all four teats, the heart rate and the mucous membranes. Misdiagnosis is now more common as farmers treat their own cases of milk fever and frequently confuse the disease with other causes of recumbency.

The differential diagnoses of milk fever are:

- Acute toxic mastitis (Chapter 23);
- Calving paralysis (p. 438);
- Physical injury (p. 446);
- Hypomagnesaemia (p. 787);
- Downer cow syndrome (pp. 439, 789);
- Inanition and other disease (p. 150);
- Pregnancy toxaemia (p. 796);
- Acidosis (p. 829);
- Hypothermia (p. 930);
- Bovine spongiform encephalopathy (BSE) (p. 909).

Acute toxic mastitis: In acute toxic mastitis from whatever cause the temperature may be raised but is sometimes subnormal, the pulse may be in excess of 120/minute, the eyes are often sunken, the mucous membranes injected and, in acute coliform mastitis, they are frequently a purple colour. Abnormal milk secretion will be found in one or more teats, although in acute coliform mastitis this change in milk character may be less than obvious.

Calving paralysis: The history of dystokia due to fetal oversize and recumbency since calving help in the differential diagnosis, but many cases are not clear-cut. Intravenous calcium together with the response noted is probably the best aid to differential diagnosis.

Other physical injury: This can occur at any time of lactation or the dry period and can include fractured limbs, pelvic damage and severe muscle damage. These can be the result of excess riding behaviour during oestrus,

slipping on ice or slippery concrete or even a collision with a vehicle such as a tractor.

Hypomagnesaemia: This can occur at any time of lactation during the spring or autumn but is sometimes present as a complication of milk fever, particularly during the two seasonal risk periods of spring and autumn. Hyperaesthesia is the main differentiating sign of hypomagnesaemia.

Downer cow syndrome: Initially, this may be difficult to differentiate from milk fever but response to therapy and clinical biochemistry will he helpful. This will be discussed in full later in the chapter (see p. 797).

Inanition: Any condition producing severe weight loss will result in recumbency, particularly in pregnant cows, the most common of which is probably starvation. In seasons where insufficient conserved food is available, recumbency due to starvation is common. Body condition is the obvious differentiating feature. However, any disease that causes considerable weight loss will have the same effect, e.g. liver fluke (p. 276). In seasons when liver fluke prevalence is high, this disease can result in extreme weight loss and anaemia and recumbency prior to parturition is common. Weight loss, red cell count and presence of fluke ova in faeces would be the differentiating features.

Pregnancy toxaemia: This can occur, particularly in beef cows, in the last two or three months of pregnancy. The sweet smell of acetone on the breath, poor condition or excessive fat and a history of unavailability of food should distinguish this problem. The rumen will also be functioning in the early stages of this condition.

Acidosis: Acute acidosis as a result of the sudden ingestion of large amounts of carbohydrate material, usually cereal-based concentrates, will result in recumbency, although hypocalcaemia is often a feature of acidosis. Here the history will help and usually acidosis is accompanied by diarrhoea.

Hypothermia: Mild hypothermia (reduction of 0.5°C or 1°F) is a normal feature of milk fever. However, severe hypothermia (reduction of 3–4°C or 5–7°F) occurs in cows that have been recumbent all night in winter out of doors. Although these cows have some other primary disease, e.g. milk fever or mastitis, treatment will be unsuccessful unless steps are taken to raise body temperature as rapidly as possible.

In summary, there are many diseases and conditions that result in recumbency of the cow. However, careful history taking and a thorough clinical examination will eliminate most differential diagnoses and if one is still not sure of the diagnosis, response to intravenous calcium will always be a useful indicator.

Treatment

The treatment for milk fever is the slow intravenous infusion of 8–12 g of calcium as soon as possible after the onset of clinical signs.

A number of licensed preparations are available for the treatment of milk fever and most are based on calcium borogluconate (CBG) at 20 per cent, 30 per cent or 40 per cent strength (see Table 46.1). It has been shown that 400 ml of 30 per cent CBG is adequate to treat milk fever in average size cattle and will provide 9 g of calcium. However, the most commonly used product in the UK is 400 ml of 40 per cent CBG, which will provide 12 g of calcium. During cold weather the CBG solution should be warmed to body temperature. Approximately 85 per cent of cases will respond to one treatment. In many cases cows recumbent from milk fever will rise within 10 minutes of treatment and others will get up 2–4 hours later.

Following the intravenous infusion, which itself should take five minutes, it is essential to sit the cow in a sternal recumbency position and turn her so that she is lying on the side opposite to the one on which she was found. Many cases will eructate and defaecate during the treatment. If the cow does not rise immediately she should be turned to lie on the opposite side every two hours. Following intravenous treatment, milk fever cows should be able to sit comfortably in the sternal recumbent position without the aid of support such as bales of straw. If the cow keeps returning to lateral recumbency following treatment the diagnosis should be reassessed as it is unlikely to be milk fever.

The use of intravenous treatment cannot be overemphasized as it is essential that the blood calcium levels return to normal as quickly as possible to avoid the complications resulting in the downer cow syndrome. Farmers treating their own cases of milk fever commonly use subcutaneous injections of CBG. This is undoubtedly a factor that has increased the incidence

of the downer cow syndrome in recent years. Following intravenous therapy plasma calcium rises rapidly and falls to around 2 mmol/l (8 mg/100 ml) 5–6 hours after treatment. Following subcutaneous therapy, the plasma calcium levels may take 3–4 hours to reach 2 mmol/l (8 mg/100 ml). Furthermore, in severe cases of milk fever the peripheral blood circulation will be impaired, which will inhibit the absorption of any fluid material administered subcutaneously. In practice one is often called to attend cases of milk fever that have not responded to subcutaneous treatment administered by the farmer several hours before and the whole of the treatment solution is still present at the injection site.

As already stated approximately 85 per cent of cows will respond to one treatment. If response is not evident by 5–6 hours, then the cow should be re-examined, the diagnosis reassessed and if necessary a further intravenous infusion of 8–12 g of calcium administered. Some practitioners advocate 400 ml of CBG intravenously plus 400 ml subcutaneously to prevent relapses. Relapse of milk fever occurs in 25 per cent of cases treated and this figure is not affected by additional subcutaneous administration. Blood levels of calcium six hours after intravenous or subcutaneous infusions are similar and by 12 hours after administration all the calcium administered, whether by the iv or sc route, has been eliminated from the body.

Treatment of milk fever should also be accompanied by removal of the calf and advice to the farmer not to milk the cow for 24 hours except to check for the presence of mastitis. As already stated, relapses occur in 25 per cent of cases treated and the likelihood of relapse will be reduced if milk is not drawn from the udder during this 24-hour period. The 8–12 g of calcium given is only a small proportion of the daily calcium requirement, so the treatment is only a holding operation until the normal adaptation process is in full operation. Cases of relapse usually occur at 18–24-hour intervals and should be treated in the same way, i.e. by the intravenous infusion of 8–12 g of calcium. Occasionally cows, particularly Jerseys, have been known to relapse on up to seven occasions.

There is a tendency amongst farmers to give two bottles of 40 per cent CBG, which would amount to 24 g of calcium. Such a procedure is probably counterproductive, as there is some evidence to suggest that too high levels of calcium administration will slow up the adaptation process and actually increase the number of cows that relapse.

Some proprietary CBG preparations also contain magnesium (1.0 g) and phosphorus (2.6 g) in addition to calcium. If hypomagnesaemia is a complicating factor of milk fever then the addition of the magnesium may be helpful. However, in cases of clinical hypomagnesaemia more than 1.0 g of magnesium will be required.

Table 46.1 Licensed products available for the treatment of milk fever in the UK.

Product	Pack size (ml)	Available calcium (g)	Dose required for 600 kg cow (ml)
CBG 20%	400	6	600–800
CBG 30%	400	9	400
CBG 40%	400	12	400
Maxacal[a]	100	4.17	200

[a] C-Vet Veterinary Products.

The presence of the phosphorus has no doubt been added because of the finding that the blood levels of phosphorus in cases of milk fever are also depressed. However, clinical evidence would suggest that the addition of phosphorus has no effect on the percentage of cases that recover or relapse. In fact, it has been shown that plasma phosphorus levels return to normal within a few hours after successful treatment with CBG without the addition of phosphorus.

Historically, the treatment of milk fever was by udder insufflation. This has the effect of slowing down milk production. Plasma calcium levels do rise following udder insufflation and will reach 2.5 mmol/l (10.0 mg/100 ml) by 4–5 hours after treatment. However, the efficacy of CBG intravenously and the danger of mastitis following insufflation have now rendered this mode of treatment almost extinct except that some clinicians have been known to use the technique in cows that persistently relapse.

Prevention

Much milk fever can and should be prevented (see Table 46.2). If an outbreak occurs in any season where more than 10 per cent of cows are needing milk fever treatment the first action the clinician should consider is to blood test a group of six or seven dry cows to measure the concentration of calcium and magnesium. If the magnesium levels are low, i.e. below 0.85 mmol/l (1.8 mg/100 ml), this should be seriously considered as interfering with calcium absorption, in which case supplemental magnesium should be administered to all dry cows within three weeks of calving. Approximately 10–12 g of magnesium administered daily to dry cows will be sufficient to produce normal plasma levels of magnesium and to allow normal calcium absorption. However, this is often difficult to achieve because of the problem of giving supplemental feeds to grazing cows. A supplement of 25 g daily of calcined magnesite mixed with cereal (1 kg/cow) or silage will produce the desired effect, but many farmers are reluctant to give supplemental feeds to dry cows. Recent experience in the UK has shown that the addition of magnesium acetate or magnesium chloride to the drinking water is a practical and effective way to supply magnesium to cows; 40 g daily of magnesium chloride crystals can be added to drinking water if large enough troughs are available. Trough size should be 20 l/cow. If trough size is limited, magnesium acetate can be added to the water supply using a water proportioner plumbed into the water supply pipe.

If the plasma levels of the dry cows are normal then diets restricting calcium intake may be considered, particularly if the plasma calcium levels are at the high end of the normal range. To be certain to prevent milk fever, dry-cow diets should contain less than 30 g/day of calcium. However, in practice, diets producing less than 50 g/day of calcium will prevent most cases of milk fever. Autumn grass in the UK often contains 8–10 g/kg DM calcium. Thus with daily intakes of 12–14 kg DM, 90–140 g/day of calcium will be available in the diet. It is impossible appreciably to reduce this level of intake without removing the cows from grass and substituting a diet based on maize silage, hay or straw. However, some farmers are prepared to do this to reduce the risk of milk fever and incidence levels of 5 per cent or less are possible. It should be appreciated that if low calcium diets are advocated for dry-cow use, just before parturition a diet containing more calcium should be administered to ensure adequate calcium being available over the risk period. This can be achieved by feeding cattle concentrate or feeds that are high in calcium, e.g. sugar beet pulp (see Table 46.3).

Other methods of milk fever prevention involve dealing with individual cows. Maintenance of appetite is essential and, in the past, appetite stimulation by the use of anabolic steroids has been suggested, but the use of these products is now illegal in Europe. Maintaining adequate calcium intake by drenching cows daily with 150 g/day of calcium chloride on the day before calving and for four days thereafter has had some success in

Table 46.2 Approximate requirements of 600 kg cows for dietary calcium, phosphorus and magnesium (g/day). Source: ARC (1980), reproduced with permission of CABI International.

	Ca	P	Mg
Maintenance (non-pregnant)	15	13	9
Maintenance + late pregnancy	28	22	12
Lactation (g/kg milk)	1.65	1.55	0.74

Table 46.3 Approximate calcium, phosphorus and magnesium contents (g/kg DM) of some common feedstuffs.

	Ca	P	Mg
Barley	0.6	3.8	1.4
Wheat	0.5	3.5	0.6
Maize	0.2	2.7	1.0
Sugar beet pulp	10.4	0.9	1.4
Brewers grains	5.0	6.0	1.8
Maize silage	3.7	3.2	3.0
Grass and grass silage (range)	3.0–10.0	1.5–4.5	1.0–3.0
Grass and grass silage (average)	5.9	3.9	1.5

preventing milk fever and might be considered in cows with a known history of milk fever.

The use of vitamin D_3 and its metabolites given by injection has been advocated in preventing milk fever. The administration of 10 million iu of vitamin D_3 given eight to two days before calving will considerably reduce the incidence of milk fever but the practical problem remains of accurately predicting the time of calving, which in practice has proven more difficult than expected. More recently, the analogue of the vitamin D_3 metabolite 1α-hydroxycholecalciferol ($1\alpha(OH)D_3$) has been used in trials to prevent milk fever. Doses of $350\mu g$ given at least 24 hours and not more than five days before calving do reduce the incidence of milk fever, but once again the problem remains of accurately predicting the time of calving. Recently, workers in Israel (Sachs, 1988) have suggested that a single dose of $700\mu g$ of $1\alpha(OH)D_3$ given eight to seven days before expected calving is more effective and that the accuracy of calving date prediction is less important.

Vitamin D_3 or $1\alpha(OH)D_3$ will not be effective if the diet is deficient in magnesium. Before recommending their use the magnesium status of the herd should be assessed by blood testing six or seven dry cows.

It has been found that there is less milk fever when diets are acidic. This is the basis of the dietary cationic–anionic balance (DCAB). It is the balance between cations (Na^+ and K^+) and the anions (Cl^- and S^{2-}) present in the diet. Their levels affect the acid–base balance and thus calcium metabolism. Some diets in the dry period are anionic and the reduction of the balance in favour of a negative balance assists. This is achieved by increasing the feeding of Cl^- and/or S^{2-}, by reducing the amount of Na^+ and/or K^+ present or by feeding maize silage. The target is to achieve in the last two weeks before calving $-200\,mEq/kg$ DM. This can be done by using 200–250 g of anionic salts. Practically this is often achieved by the addition of 100 g NH_4Cl and 100 mg of $MgCl_2$. However, such diets should only be used where there is adequate calcium provision. The system is complex and should only be used on farms with good quality management.

Hypomagnesaemia (grass tetany, grass staggers, lactation tetany, Hereford disease)

Hypomagnesaemia is a common feature of a group of syndromes dominated by hyperaesthesia, incoordination, tetany and convulsions that can occur in all ruminants of all ages. Grass tetany or grass staggers is the name given to the syndrome affecting lactating cattle (beef or dairy cows) when grazing grass in the spring or autumn. Subclinical hypomagnesaemia can occur in lac-

tating or dry cows in the spring or autumn and is usually not accompanied by clinical signs. It usually affects the whole herd. Lactating cows will suffer a slight reduction in milk yield and may have a slight nervous disposition, e.g. reluctance to enter the milking parlour. Dry cows will be more prone to milk fever at parturition. If the herd is affected with subclinical hypomagnesaemia some individuals will develop grass staggers, particularly if stressed. Milk tetany occurs in calves fed predominantly milk, particularly calves suckling cows that are subclinically hypomagnesaemic (see p. 253). The incidence of hypomagnesaemia varies considerably from region to region. Some areas of the UK are particularly high in the incidence of the disease in both beef and dairy cows. Overall, the annual incidence in UK dairy herds is approaching 1 per cent.

The clinical disease is most common around peak lactation, presumably reflecting the secretion of magnesium in the milk. It is also a common cause of sudden death. In 1984 in the UK it was estimated that 0.8 per cent of the dairy cow population died from the disease (Whitaker *et al.*, 1984). This was following the introduction of milk quotas in Europe and a dramatic reduction in the use of concentrate feeds for dairy cows, particularly during the summer months.

Aetiology

As there are no readily available body stores for magnesium, the main factors involved in the aetiology of hypomagnesaemia are the reduction of the amount of magnesium available in the food, and hence available for absorption from the gut, accompanied by a high physiological demand for magnesium. Magnesium is lost from the body in milk, urine and faeces. The endogenous loss in faeces has been calculated to be approximately 1.8 g/day (ARC, 1980). Milk contains 0.12 g/l of magnesium so a cow producing 30 kg of milk would lose 3.6 g daily in the milk. Any excess magnesium absorbed will be excreted via the urine, this being the mechanism for stabilizing plasma magnesium levels. If the plasma magnesium levels rise much above 0.8 mmol/l (2.0 mg/100 ml) the excess will be excreted. If magnesium intake levels are excessive, up to 5.0 g/day may be excreted in the urine. However, if magnesium intake falls to the level to maintain homeostasis or below there will no magnesium identifiable in the urine.

To maintain magnesium homeostasis the absorption of magnesium must be continuous so a constant supply is necessary in the diet. Feeds vary considerably in both the content and the availability of magnesium so the choice of pasture is important. Clovers have higher magnesium content than grasses and grasses themselves vary. Fast-growing Italian ryegrasses have lower levels than perennial grasses. Many broad-leaf plants, such as buttercups (*Ranunculus* spp.), plantains and nettles, have considerably higher magnesium levels than grasses, which probably accounts to some extent for the increasing incidence of hypomagnesaemia seen in recent years in the UK as old permanent pastures have been replaced with ryegrass leys.

Some soils are known to be deficient in magnesium but also the uptake of magnesium by plants may be influenced by cations such as calcium and potassium in the soil. It has been shown that fertilizers containing potassium applied to grazing areas in late winter or early spring will reduce the absorption of magnesium by plants, and soils containing high levels of potassium are particularly prone to producing hypomagnesaemia in grazing ruminants.

Although historically this disease has been one related to spring grass, in recent years it has become increasingly common throughout the whole grazing season from April to October. The occurrence during winter has also increased in the UK; this can be attributed to the increasing use of grass silage made from young leafy grass low in magnesium during May.

Another important factor in the aetiology of the disease is the energy intake of the animals. This is particularly the case in beef suckler cows grazing inadequate pastures, particularly during times of inclement weather. Experiments have shown that reduced energy intake will interfere with the magnesium available for absorption. The availability of magnesium for absorption from the gut is thought to range from 4 to 35 per cent. Calcium, potassium and ammonium (nitrogen) ions are all thought to interfere with body uptake of magnesium.

It is possible to find animals with low plasma magnesium levels but yet clinically normal. It would appear that the critical factor influencing the onset of clinical disease is the level of magnesium in the cerebrospinal fluid (CSF). The speed at which magnesium levels fall also influences the onset of clinical signs. In the spring, magnesium levels fall rapidly and clinical disease may become apparent at blood levels at which in the autumn, when the fall is more gradual, the cows remain clinically normal.

The role of calcium in the onset of clinical hypomagnesaemia is also unclear. Approximately 80 per cent of cows with grass staggers have low plasma calcium levels. It has been shown that cows will develop clinical disease within 24 hours after a fall in plasma calcium levels although they have been hypomagnesaemic for several days.

Milk tetany occurs in calves two to four months old reared on whole milk diets without the addition of magnesium supplementation. In young calves absorption of magnesium is good. However, as the calf grows older the ability to absorb magnesium declines. Thus, if the two to four-month-old calf is denied feed supplementation other than cow's milk, magnesium absorption will decline to less than requirements and clinical signs will appear. This is seen in suckler calves or veal calves reared on milk or milk substitute that has not been supplemented with magnesium (see p. 253).

Signs

The signs of grass staggers may be classified as subacute, acute or peracute. In the subacute form cows will be apprehensive and hyperaesthetic. The head will be held high and tremors may be seen around the head (particularly the eyelids), over the shoulder and on the flank. These tremors will be exaggerated if the animal is touched or the skin pinched. The legs may become stiff and a staggering gait may be evident. Cows can remain in the subacute phase for several hours or progress to the acute or peracute form, particularly in response to noise or some other stimulus such as attempting to herd them. The peracute cases will stagger for a few steps and fall over with tetanic spasms of the head, neck and legs followed by clonic convulsions. The legs will paddle furiously, the eyes roll and there is frothing at the mouth. The heart will pound fast and furious and death can occur at any time. Cows have been known to be grazing one minute and, in response to noise from a vehicle or other stimulus, to stagger, fall over in convulsions and die in two or three minutes.

The signs in the acute case will be similar but may last for up to an hour or more. In these cases a period of convulsions will be followed by a quiescent period in which the cow may attempt to rise, only to walk a few steps and fall over again followed by convulsions. The rectal temperature, if taken, will be elevated by 1 or 2°C (2–4°F). Cows are often found dead with obvious signs that the limbs had been paddling prior to death, thus disturbing the soil around the feet.

In the subclinical form the majority of the herd are usually affected even if acute cases have not been diagnosed. If acute cases are present it can be assumed that the majority of the herd will be affected subclinically. The cows may be slightly nervous, reluctant to enter the milking parlour or be unwilling to be herded. The milk yield will be depressed slightly.

The signs of milk tetany in calves (p. 255) are much the same as for cows with subacute, acute and peracute cases occurring. Often in peracute cases the animals are found dead.

Clinical pathology

Healthy normal cows should possess plasma magnesium levels over 0.85 mmol/l (2.0 mg/100 ml). Any levels below this must be considered a risk and indicative of subclinical hypomagnesaemia, although in acute cases the plasma levels will generally be below 0.4 mmol/l (1.0 mg/100 ml). Magnesium levels in the CSF in acute tetany will generally be below 0.6 mmol/l (1.4 mg/100 ml). Hypocalcaemia is present in at least 80 per cent of acute tetany cases and hyperkalaemia is common. Following tetany or in recovered cases aspartate aminotransferase (AST) and creatine kinase (CK) levels will rise to relatively high levels but return to normal quite soon after recovery.

At post mortem there are no pathognomonic signs. Haemorrhages may be present on the heart muscle and occasionally along the aorta. Regurgitation and aspiration of rumen contents may sometimes be seen. The CSF levels of magnesium will be low and magnesium will be absent from the urine, although the bladder is nearly always empty at post mortem.

Diagnosis

The diagnosis of grass staggers is made on the signs described above. The time of year and type of grazing may help in forming a diagnosis. As there is little or no time in acute cases to conduct blood biochemistry, response to treatment will also confirm a diagnosis. It may be useful for the clinician to take a blood sample before treatment so that analysis can be performed at a later stage should this prove necessary. If animals are found dead then diagnosis must be differentiated from other causes of death. Diagnosis at post mortem is difficult because of the absence of obvious lesions. If quantities of soil have been gouged out of the ground by each of the four feet during the paddling phase this is strongly indicative of acute grass staggers. Absence of magnesium from urine would be a useful indicator, but the bladder is generally empty. Blood and tissues are of no value at post mortem because magnesium levels rise rapidly after death. Levels in CSF may be helpful and recently it has been suggested that magnesium levels in aqueous humour taken after death will be depressed in cows that have died from grass staggers. If a cow is found dead and grass staggers suspected from the history and absence of other lesions at post mortem, the wise clinician will blood sample six to seven cows in the group and test for magnesium levels. It is important to make a diagnosis to be able to offer preventive advice for the remainder of the herd.

Diagnosis of death due to milk tetany in calves is possible by measuring the calcium and magnesium levels in bone. A rib or coccygeal bone is usually used for this purpose. A calcium/magnesium ratio in bone of 70:1 is considered normal and 90:1 considered an indication of severe magnesium depletion.

To diagnose subclinical hypomagnesaemia blood sampling seven cows each from a lactating and a dry-cow group and testing for magnesium is the most useful indicator. Testing urine for magnesium levels has been advocated, absence of magnesium indicating the subclinical state. Urine test strips are available in some countries. However, there are real practical problems in getting a number of cows to micturate on demand.

Differential diagnosis

Acute lead poisoning: In lead poisoning (see pp. 906, 944) there may be excitement and occasional convulsions. Hyperaesthesia, as measured by observing muscle tremors in response to pinching the skin, will be absent and blindness is usually a feature of lead poisoning.

Milk fever (p. 783): Some cows in the early stage of milk fever may exhibit hyperaesthetic signs. The history of being close to parturition is the most helpful aid to this differential diagnosis. Many cows are hypocalcaemic as well as hypomagnesaemic and so treatment involves calcium administration; thus being able accurately to differentially diagnose the two conditions is not important in practice.

Acetonaemia (p. 740): Some cows with acute acetonaemia will have hyperaesthetic signs and appear nervous and apprehensive. However, the depraved actions of these cows, such as licking the walls and floor or biting at gates, will usually distinguish this disease from hypomagnesaemia, as will a Rothera's test on a sample of milk.

Listeriosis (p. 904): Acute listeriosis may be confused with acute grass staggers, but the high rectal temperature and absence of true hyperaesthesia in listeriosis cases should be enough to distinguish this disease.

Bovine spongiform encephalopathy (p. 909): The emergence of BSE in the UK in 1986 has sometimes made the differential diagnosis of the subacute form of hypomagnesaemia more difficult. The ataxia, apprehension and mild hyperaesthesia found in BSE are similar to that found in subacute hypomagnesaemia. Diagnosis is usually confirmed by response to treatment and blood biochemistry, a sample being taken before treatment. If there is any doubt in the clinician's mind it would be wise, in cases of suspected BSE, to take a blood sample to eliminate subacute hypomagnesaemia before notifying the suspicion to the authorities.

Others: Lightning strike (p. 930) as a cause of sudden death, some plant poisonings, and in particular Paspalum staggers (*Claviceps paspali* poisoning), are differential diagnoses but can usually be distinguished on grounds of history alone. Rabies (p. 908; Chapter 70) may cause problems in countries where it occurs, but such animals usually are hyperactive, bellowing and riding other cattle.

Suboptimal production: If production is below expectations, particularly in seasons associated with hypomagnesaemia, then subclinical hypomagnesaemia could be present. Blood biochemistry in the form of a metabolic profile that includes magnesium should be considered (see p. 813).

Treatment

Acute cases of grass staggers must be treated promptly. During the course of treatment the operators should be as quiet and gentle as possible as any sudden stimulus will initiate a bout of convulsions. Hence, actually restraining a staggering acute case will often be difficult and when attempting to place a rope or halter on the animal it will sometimes collapse into a fit of convulsions and may even die before treatment has been administered. The success of treatment is also related to the length of time signs have been present in the recumbent acute case. The longer the cow has been showing convulsions, the less likely it will be to recover.

Intravenous infusions of magnesium salts, e.g. magnesium sulphate, are sometimes recommended for treatment but this procedure is not without its dangers. Intravenous magnesium sulphate may cause cardiac embarrassment or even respiratory failure. If magnesium sulphate is administered intravenously the concentration should be no more than 6 per cent and must be administered very slowly with the heart being auscultated. However, it is also essential to administer calcium in the form of CBG because most cases of grass staggers are also hypocalcaemic.

The treatment protocol favoured by the author is to discard 100 ml of fluid from a 400 ml bottle of 40 per cent CBG, which also contains magnesium 0.2 per cent and phosphorus 0.5 per cent, and replace this with 100 ml of 25 per cent magnesium sulphate solution. The mixture, which then contains 9 g of calcium and approximately 6 g of magnesium, is infused intravenously very slowly, taking 8–10 minutes. The remaining 300 ml of the original 400 ml 25 per cent magnesium sulphate is injected subcutaneously. If during the infusion, or immediately after, the convulsions get worse 10 ml of pentobarbitone sodium 200 mg/ml (euthanasia solution) can be administered intravenously and this will often reduce or even eliminate the convulsions. Following this treatment regimen, if the cow is recumbent, it is important to remain quiet for a further 10 minutes as stimulation even immediately after treatment may initiate convulsions. The recumbent cow should then be raised into sternal recumbency and left for a further 30 minutes before attempting to stimulate the animal to rise.

Treatment is successful, if early, in 80 per cent of acute recumbent cases and nearly 100 per cent in acute standing cases. If the recumbent case is not able to rise within two hours of treatment the likelihood of success is extremely poor and slaughter should be considered. Subacute grass staggers should be treated in the same way and success is usually near to 100 per cent.

Relapses are considered normal unless preventative measures are taken. Blood magnesium falls to pretreatment levels within six hours of intravenous administration, although the subcutaneous injection has a more prolonged effect. Daily subcutaneous injections of 200–400 ml of 25 per cent magnesium sulphate for five days following treatment have been recommended or the oral administration of four magnesium bullets, which are composed of an alloy of 86 per cent magnesium, 12 per cent aluminium and 2 per cent copper weighted with iron shot (Rumbul bullets, Agrimin Ltd), immediately following the intravenous and subcutaneous treatment.

An individual cow suffering from grass staggers is one of a herd and many cows in the herd could be at risk, of or at least suffering from, subclinical hypomagnesaemia. It is important therefore that a group of six to seven cows be blood tested to ascertain the herd magnesium status, and if the blood levels are below 0.8 mmol/l (2.0 mg/100 ml) herd supplementation with magnesium must be instituted.

The treatment of milk tetany in calves is generally academic, as most cases are found dead. However, very slow intravenous infusion of 100 ml of 20 per cent CBG with the addition of 20 ml of 25 per cent magnesium sulphate followed by 60 ml of 25 per cent magnesium sulphate subcutaneously would be the regimen of choice. Oral supplementation of magnesium must also follow if the calf recovers. Suggested daily doses of magnesium oxide would be 1, 2 and 3 g for calves up to five weeks, five to ten weeks and ten to fifteen weeks old, respectively.

Prevention

The simplest method of prevention of hypomagnesaemia is to add calcined magnesite (magnesium oxide) to cattle concentrate that is being fed to the cows. However, the main risk periods in northern Europe for hypomagnesaemia are times when concentrate food is not being fed, e.g. spring grazing and autumn grazing for dry cows. In Australia, New Zealand and Ireland very little concentrates are fed, and in many beef suckler herds other ingenious methods must be devised. The magnesium bullets mentioned above will give protection for four to six weeks. However, although two bullets are recommended, in severe hypomagnesaemic areas experience has shown that four bullets are required to prevent problems.

Dusting the pastures with magnesium oxide has been attempted using 50 g/cow per day of magnesium oxide, or 0.5 kg/week applied in the early morning when the dew is on the grass. This works best when cows are strip grazed and the magnesium oxide is applied every morning. Weekly applications are effective in dry weather, but must be reapplied following rain. However, grass staggers is more common in wet than dry weather.

The increasing practice in recent years in the UK of buffer feeding, where a silage supplement is fed to cows during the grazing season, has meant that magnesium oxide at the rate of 50 g/cow per day can be mixed with or sprinkled on top of the silage and increases feed passage time.

Supplementation of water supplies using magnesium acetate via a water proportioner is effective but expensive. The proportioner has to be adjusted daily to allow for the variation in water intake that occurs under different weather conditions. The expense and management input required have been a disincentive for this method of prevention to become widespread. The addition of magnesium chloride crystals to the drinking water has increased in popularity in the UK in recent years. It is relatively inexpensive but, to be effective, the trough sizes must be large enough for all cows to drink the medicated water. The addition of 40 g/cow per day of magnesium chloride to the drinking water has been shown to give reasonable protection. Addition of magnesium salts to the drinking water will depress water intake if the concentration is too high. Troughs with a volume of 20 l/cow are required for this method of control to work effectively. Mineral licks and powders containing high levels of magnesium are relatively useless in preventing hypomagnesaemia because of the uncertainty of all cows consuming enough material to give them protection when it is required.

When discussing the long-term strategies for controlling hypomagnesaemia, fertilizer policy should be included. All potassium-containing fertilizers should be avoided on soils with high potassium levels and on other soils, if potassium-containing fertilizers are used, they should be applied at low levels in the autumn. If necessary, they can be applied later in the grazing season.

Perhaps plant species should also be considered in long-term control strategies. Clover/grass mixtures should be favoured ahead of grass alone, but perhaps above all the use of selective weedkillers should be discouraged. A few buttercups and other wild plants growing in the pasture may not only be aesthetically acceptable but may reduce the incidence of hypomagnesaemia in grazing animals.

The prevention of milk tetany in calves can be achieved by ensuring magnesium supplementation. Proprietary milk substitute powders are adequately supplied with magnesium. If whole milk is used magnesium oxide at the rates given above should be added to the daily diet (see p. 790).

Hypophosphataemia

Hypophosphataemia is the result of a primary deficiency of phosphorus in the diet (see also p. 792).

Occurrence

Dietary deficiencies of phosphorus are widespread under natural conditions. There is a distinct geographical distribution where large land masses are identified as being deficient in phosphorus and livestock cannot be supported without phosphorus supplementation. These areas will be deficient because of the underlying rock formation. Large areas of southern Africa and Australia are well identified as being deficient in phosphorus. Such areas, however, are unknown or rare in northern Europe and, if they exist at all, will be localized. Although there are areas of Europe where the underlying rock formation contains no phosphorus, continuous application of fertilizers containing phosphorus and cultivation techniques have improved the soil structure and nutritive value. In consequence, primary phosphorus deficiency is probably a rare occurrence in Europe.

Aetiology

Phosphorus deficiency is usually primary, although a severe deficiency of vitamin D (p. 253) may exacerbate the problem. It was once considered that excess calcium would also reduce the availability of phosphorus in the diet and cause deficiencies of phosphorus. Although the calcium:phosphorus ratio in the diet is important in monogastric animals, it is probably of less significance in cattle. The maintenance requirements for adult and growing cattle would be approximately 15 g of phosphorus daily. The lactating cow requires approximately 0.75 g/kg of milk produced, so a cow yielding 30 kg of milk will require 40 g of phosphorus daily. This level of requirement is considerably less than that currently being recommended in the UK by the Agricultural Development and Advisory Service, but nevertheless is supported by experimental evidence from the Agricultural Research Council (ARC, 1980).

Signs

In young cattle phosphorus deficiency results in slow growth and rickets. In adult cattle the principal signs are reduced milk yield, weight loss and depraved appetite. Osteomalacia will result from prolonged dietary deficiency of phosphorus. The depraved appetite or pica results in cows eating earth, licking rocks and, where bones are available, osteophagia. The osteophagia frequently results in a high incidence of botulism (p. 721) and in some areas of southern Africa and Australia death from botulism is the most important consequence of phosphorus deficiency. Reduced fertility has been considered a feature of severe phosphorus deficiency, but experimental work has demonstrated that fertility is independent of either calcium or phosphorus intakes. Reduced fertility is a feature of malnutrition and frequently animals that are deficient in phosphorus are also suffering from malnutrition. Low energy intake in such animals is much more likely to be the cause of reduced fertility than any specific mineral deficiency.

Cows in late pregnancy often become recumbent, particularly in drought seasons. This recumbency is probably a result of general malnutrition rather than a specific phosphorus deficiency.

Hypophosphataemia nearly always accompanies hypocalcaemia in cows with milk fever, but this is not thought to be of any significance. Phosphorus levels rarely fall to the levels of 0.3 mmol/l (1 mg/100 ml) seen in severe clinical cases and in any case calcium therapy will result in the blood phosphorus levels quickly reverting to normal.

Diagnosis

The presence of rickets or osteomalacia and/or pica will indicate a dietary deficiency of phosphorus, which can be confirmed by analysis of serum and the diet for the presence of phosphorus. The normal blood level is 1.3–1.6 mmol/l (4–5 mg/100 ml). Levels of 0.5–1.1 mmol/l (1.5–3.5 mg/100 ml), falling as low as 0.3 mmol/l (1 mg/100 ml) of serum in severe clinical cases, will be found in hypophosphataemic animals.

Most pastures in northern Europe contain 1.5–4.5 g/kg DM of phosphorus and at these levels phosphorus deficiency will not occur. Osteophagia will occur with pasture levels of 0.2 g/kg DM of phosphorus and rickets and osteomalacia at pasture levels of 0.1 g/kg DM.

The only commonly used feedstuffs in the UK that are deficient in phosphorus are sugar beet pulp at 0.9 g/kg DM, kale and other *Brassica* spp. crops. These are rarely used at a proportion of the diet high enough to significantly reduce the phosphorus intake to dangerous levels.

Control

Under range conditions, where phosphorus deficiency is the most common, supplementation of the diet with phosphorus is often impractical. Bone meal, dicalcium phosphate or disodium phosphate may be provided in feed supplements or free access mineral mixtures. The dietary intake of phosphorus should be at least 15 g/day. Top dressing pastures with superphosphate fertilizers will correct any underlying deficiency and have the added advantage of increasing the yield and protein content of the pasture. However, this is often impractical in areas where the problem exists.

In acute cases where phosphorus therapy is urgent, e.g. postparturient haemoglobinuria, the intravenous administration of sodium acid phosphate (30 g in 200 ml distilled water) is advocated (see below).

Postparturient haemoglobinuria

One specific syndrome associated with phosphorus deficiency is postparturient haemoglobinuria. This is a disease of cows one to four weeks after calving. Haemolytic anaemia and hypophosphataemia are consistent features.

Occurrence

Postparturient haemoglobinuria was first described in Scotland in 1853 and has been reported from many countries including Australia, USA and most of Europe. The occurrence is sporadic and when it does arise it usually only affects one or two cows within a herd. In recent years its occurrence in the UK has been extremely rare. In Scotland it has been associated with the feeding of beets and turnips, in Holland with the feeding of lush spring grass and occasionally it has been reported to accompany the feeding of sugar beet byproducts and alfalfa.

Aetiology

Diets low in phosphorus are incriminated in the cause of postparturient haemoglobinuria. However, it is probable that there is some additional factor that precipitates the problem in hypophosphataemic cattle. This is likely to be a haemolytic factor present in sugar beet leaves, alfalfa, kale and other *Brassica* spp. plants.

Signs

The principal clinical signs are those associated with anaemia. The cow may be weak and staggering, with mucous membranes pale and heart rate raised. Haemoglobinuria will be a consistent feature. The faeces are firm and dry. If left untreated the cow will finally become recumbent and may die within two to five days. Less severely affected cases may recover, albeit slowly, in three or four weeks. Pica is frequently observed during the recovery period.

Clinical pathology

Serum phosphorus levels are low, usually 0.15–1.0 mmol/l (0.5–3.0 mg/100 ml). Low phosphorus levels will be encountered in other cows in the herd. Red cell counts, packed cell volume and haemoglobin are all dramatically reduced. Serum bilirubin will increase in the later stages of the disease.

At post mortem the liver will be swollen and infiltrated with fat. The carcass is jaundiced and anaemic and red or red/brown coloured urine will be found in the bladder.

Diagnosis

Postparturient haemoglobinuria must be suspected in any cow that is weak, anaemic and exhibiting haemoglobinuria within four weeks of parturition. The haemoglobinuria must be distinguished from babesiosis (p. 748) and copper poisoning (p. 948). A history of feeding large quantities of kale, beet tops or alfalfa will also be a helpful aid to diagnosis. The diagnosis should be confirmed by demonstrating hypophosphataemia and haemoglobinuria.

Treatment

Intravenous therapy with 30 g of sodium acid phosphate in 200 ml of distilled water followed by the provision of calcium phosphate in the diet is the first line of treatment. In extremely anaemic cases blood transfusion with 5–10 l of blood should be considered. Supportive therapy with large doses of vitamin C intravenously and iron dextran injections will aid the recovery.

Prevention

If brassicas have to be fed to cattle in early lactation their intake should be limited to a maximum of 20 kg wet matter/day. This limitation and an adequate phosphorus intake will prevent the occurrence of postparturient haemoglobinuria.

Acetonaemia (ketosis, slow fever)

Acetonaemia or ketosis is a metabolic disorder of high-yielding lactating cows characterized by reduced milk yield, loss of body weight, inappetance and, occasion-ally, nervous signs. Ketone bodies, e.g. acetoacetate, β-hydroxybutyrate or acetone, are present in all body fluids. Hypoglycaemia together with increased plasma free fatty acids and liver fat and decreased liver glycogen are also a feature of this disease. These changes are associated with an inadequate supply of the energy that is necessary to sustain high levels of milk production in early lactation. Pregnancy toxaemia, a common disease of pregnant sheep and characterized by hypoglycaemia and hyperketonaemia, can also occasionally affect pregnant cows particularly when carrying twins (see p. 796).

Historically clinical acetonaemia was more common in the winter when cows were housed and being fed conserved forage of dubious quality. The annual incidence in dairy herds is around 0.5 per cent and recent reports have indicated an all year round occurrence with a higher incidence in June, July and August than in the winter months. Cows of any age can be affected and Channel Island breeds, particularly the Jersey, appear to be more susceptible than the Friesian or Holstein. Acetonaemia is less common in the UK now than it was 20 to 30 years ago. This is probably due to higher quality feeds being available although the preponderance of the Friesian breed may have some effect on the disease incidence. Outbreaks are usually restricted to one or two cows but varying numbers of cows in the herd may be affected. If the incidence of the disease is high it can become a severe economic problem due to depressed milk production. The disease usually occurs three to six weeks after calving, when the cow is at her peak milk production but her appetite or DM intake has not yet reached its peak. During early lactation the dairy cow is in negative energy balance. The energy intake in feed is insufficient to meet the energy output in milk. This results in the mobilization of fat reserves to meet the energy deficit and a consequent loss in body weight. This should be considered a normal metabolic situation in high-yielding dairy cows. Such cows will have slightly raised blood ketone levels and may even excrete ketones in urine and possibly in milk. The cow in early lactation is therefore in a delicate metabolic balance and any stress that causes a reduction of feed intake can disturb this balance and result in the onset of clinical ketosis. Factors that can influence the occurrence of the disease include excessive feeding of silage that has a high content of butyric acid, a deterioration in forage quality, sudden changes in types of food on offer and excessive fatness at calving. In the UK the butyric acid content of grass silage is of considerable importance in the aetiology of this disease because wet conditions, so frequently encountered during silage making, predispose to butyric fermentation of the silage. The role of such silage in the aetiology of acetonaemia is probably two-fold. Firstly, there is the direct effect of the presence of butyric acid and secondly there is the reduced dietary intake that accompanies such silage. Cows that are too fat at calving have lower DM intakes in early lactation and are therefore more likely to suffer acetonaemia.

Acetonaemia is diagnosed in grazing cattle if the grass has a high moisture content and/or when the energy intake is insufficient. Cobalt is required for rumen microbial synthesis of vitamin B_{12} and is also essential for adequate utilization of propionic acid. In areas of cobalt deficiency acetonaemia will be commonly diagnosed in grazing cows (p. 295).

Secondary ketosis is common, if not more common, than primary ketosis and can result from any disease that causes a reduction in appetite in early lactation. Displaced abomasum (see p. 839) and traumatic reticulitis (p. 837) are two common problems frequently associated with secondary ketosis.

Aetiology

To understand the aetiology of acetonaemia one must realize the precarious metabolic balance that exists in all cows in early lactation. To satisfy the requirements of milk production the cow can draw on two sources of nutrients, food intake and her body reserves. In the first two months of lactation a cow producing up to 45 kg of milk daily will use up to 2 kg of body fat and up to 350 g of body protein per day. As far as the dietary supply of nutrients is concerned 80 per cent of the ingested carbohydrates are fermented by the rumen microflora into the volatile fatty acids, acetic, propionic and butyric acids, which are themselves absorbed. Acetate may be oxidized by various tissues or incorporated into milk fat by the mammary gland.

Glucose is synthesized in the liver and renal cortex by the gluconeogenic pathway. Approximately half of the cow's glucose requirement is derived from dietary propionic acid, which is incorporated into the tricarboxylic acid (TCA) cycle and converted to glucose by gluconeogenesis. Glucogenic amino acids, lactic acid and glycerol can be converted into glucose by this process. Reduced production of propionic acid in the rumen will result in inadequate glucose production and a consequent hypoglycaemia. Hypoglycaemia leads to a mobilization of free fatty acids and glycerol from the fat stores. Hormones such as adrenaline, glucagon, adrenocorticotrophic hormone, glucocorticoids and thyroid hormones all influence this mobilization from the body fat stores. Skeletal muscle and heart can utilize fatty acids for energy production when glucose is short. However, the liver has a limited ability to oxidize fatty acids because acetyl-CoA, which is the end product of fatty acid oxidation, cannot be adequately incorporated into the TCA cycle when levels of oxaloacetate, the result of active gluconeogenesis, are low. The excess acetyl-CoA is converted into the ketone bodies acetoacetate and β-hydroxybutyrate and, to a small extent, acetone. Tissues other than liver can utilize ketone bodies but, if their production exceeds the rate they are used by muscle and other tissues, they accumulate and ketosis is the result. Ketone bodies are excreted in milk and urine.

The reduction of propionic acid production by the rumen is usually a feature of underfeeding or a reduced feed intake caused by inappetance. Cobalt deficiency, as mentioned above, will also have the effect of reducing propionic acid production. Butyrate is a precursor of acetyl-CoA and is therefore ketogenic. An increase in butyrate uptake from the rumen will therefore be ketogenic. This explains why silage high in butyric acid will induce ketosis in apparently normal cows.

Signs

Hypoglycaemia is the major factor involved in the onset and development of the clinical signs of acetonaemia. There will have been a gradual loss of body condition over several days or even weeks. There is also a moderate decline in milk yield over two to four days before the onset of the obvious clinical signs, which are refusal to eat grain and concentrate feeds and a more sudden drop in milk output. At this stage a sweet smell (as in pear drops) of acetone is apparent on the breath and the discerning stockworker will even detect the same acetone smell in the milk. Once appetite is decreased weight loss is accelerated due to utilization of body stores. Rectal temperature, pulse rates and respiratory rates are normal in the early stages of the disease, as are ruminal movements. Faeces will usually be firm with a dark 'waxy' appearance.

A small number of cows with acute acetonaemia exhibit nervous signs, which include excessive salivation, abnormal chewing movements and licking walls, gates or metal bars. Incoordination with apparent blindness will also be a feature. Some cows will even show a degree of aggression and will sometimes charge into walls, occasionally injuring themselves. The other signs observed above are also present. The nervous signs often only last for a few hours with the animals showing more normal behaviour in between.

Clinical pathology

Hypoglycaemia, hyperketonaemia and the presence of ketones in the urine and milk are the features of this disease. Cowside diagnosis is obtained by the detection of ketones in milk and urine using the Rothera's test reaction. A drop of milk or urine is added to a small quantity (which consists of sodium nitroprusside 3 g, sodium carbonate 3 g and ammonium sulphate 100 g) of

Rothera's reagent on a white tile or piece of white card. A pink to purple coloration of the reagent confirms the presence of ketones. Urine normally contains low levels of ketones so a diagnosis is only positive when the milk is also positive.

Blood glucose levels are reduced to below 1.4 mmol/l (25 mg/100 ml). Total blood ketone levels are raised to over 5 mmol/l (30 mg/100 ml). The plasma glycerol and free fatty acid levels (non-esterified fatty acid, NEFA) are also elevated. Subclinical ketosis has become more important in recent years with the introduction of the laboratory test for β-hydroxybutyrate (βHB). The level of βHB is frequently used on a herd basis as a measure of energy balance in both lactating and dry cows. Herds with subclinical ketosis have been identified using this test. Serum levels of βHB in excess of 1.75 mmol/l (10 mg/100 ml) will indicate a severe energy deficit in the diet (see p. 807).

Although mortality is not normally a feature of acetonaemia, affected cows do possess fatty infiltration and degeneration of the liver.

Diagnosis

The diagnosis is made on the history of a cow in early lactation with a sudden fall in milk yield, some weight loss, refusing to eat concentrates, with normal temperature, pulse and respiratory rates and normal rumen movements. Many astute stockworkers will recognize the acetone odour on the breath or in the milk and report this to the attending veterinarian. The diagnosis is confirmed by a positive Rothera's reaction on milk and urine and, if this is not conclusive, a blood sample can be analysed for glucose and ketone levels. It is important to differentiate between primary and secondary ketosis so a complete clinical examination must be performed. Many cases presented by the farmer as acetonaemia are in fact suffering from displaced abomasum (p. 839). Some cows with hypocalcaemia (p. 783) may also show acetonaemia.

The differential diagnosis of the nervous form of acetonaemia can be sometimes confusing. The behavioural changes are similar to listeriosis (p. 904), but usually with listeriosis pyrexia will be present. Hypomagnesaemia (p. 788) should be distinguishable by the presence of hyperaesthesia, particularly the tremors of the eye-lids and muscle tremors over the shoulders and the presence of tetanic convulsions. Bovine spongiform encephalopathy (p. 909) may also be confused with acetonaemia because of weight loss. However, the apprehension, kicking and progressive nature of BSE should be distinguishing features, besides which blood glucose, magnesium and ketone levels will be normal in BSE. Rabies (p. 908; Chapter 70) is characterized by mania, ascending paralysis and is always fatal.

Treatment

There are three main components of successful treatment:

(1) To restore blood glucose levels as quickly as possible.
(2) To replenish oxaloacetate, an essential intermediate in the TCA cycle in the liver, so that fatty acids mobilized from the fat deposits are completely oxidized. This will reduce the rate of production of ketone bodies.
(3) To increase the availability of dietary glucogenic precursors, notably propionic acid.

An intravenous infusion of 500 ml of 40 per cent glucose will cause a transient rise in blood glucose levels that lasts approximately two hours. This should be accompanied by oral administration of glucose precursors such as propylene glycol (150 ml, twice daily). Propylene glycol is preferred to propionate or glycerol because propionate is fermented in the rumen and may cause digestive disturbances and glycerol is converted to ketogenic acids as well as propionic acid in the rumen. Cobalt salts are frequently added to the propylene glycol and in cobalt-deficient areas at least 100 mg/day of cobalt should be administered.

Glucocorticoid drugs are the most commonly used therapy for acetonaemia, either used alone or in combination with glucose therapy or when followed by oral administration of glucose precursors. Glucocorticoid therapy results in a reduction of ketone body formation due to utilization of the acetyl-CoA derived from fatty acid oxidation and raises blood glucose levels due to a greater availability of glucose precursors in the liver. The commonly used glucocorticoids are dexamethasone, betamethasone and flumethasone and all are effective. Frequently, a single dose is administered but this does often result in relapses two to three days after the treatment, when the injection can be repeated. There is one disadvantage of repeated glucocorticoid therapy and that is that appetite and milk yield are reduced.

For successful treatment in most cases of acetonaemia the following regimen is to be recommended:

● 500 ml of 40 per cent glucose intravenously, followed by
● One dose of glucocorticoid, followed by
● Oral treatment twice daily with 150 g of propylene glycol containing cobalt for three to four days.

Anabolic steroids are also a useful treatment for acetonaemia and were used in Europe before their use was prohibited under the EC hormone ban. They are effective by increasing the levels of the intermediates of the TCA cycle in the liver. They also stimulate appetite, which ensures an increased supply of the glucogenic precursors. They do not directly raise blood glucose levels. It is important that the cow's appetite returns to normal as soon as possible after treatment so access to good quality fodder is a prerequisite to successful treatment. If butyric silage is implicated in the cause of the problem this should be removed from the diet and only well-fermented silage or good quality hay offered.

If acetonaemia is affecting a high proportion of the herd it would be wise to obtain a supply of ground maize, as it has been shown that ground maize is readily digested in the small intestine and results in a rapid rise in blood glucose levels.

Prevention

The prevention of acetonaemia starts before calving. Cows should not be too fat at calving, a condition score of 2.5–3.0 would be optimum and anything higher would be considered too fat. Access to a plentiful supply of long coarse fibre to promote good rumen digestion is also important during the dry period. Concentrates used during lactation should be introduced in small quantities (1–2 kg/day) two weeks before calving to allow adjustments in the rumen microflora. Changes to diet in early lactation should be made gradually.

Forage containing ketogenic substances such as butyric acid should be avoided in early lactation. Roughage should comprise at least 40 per cent of the diet. In cobalt-deficient areas measures should be taken to ensure adequate cobalt intake, e.g. by spreading cobalt sulphate on to pastures. The concentrates used need to be of good quality. This statement may seem obvious but unfortunately some concentrate manufacturers, under pressure from farmers, will produce substandard concentrates at a lower than normal price. By and large the quality of a concentrate food is reflected in its price.

The use of metabolic profiles (Chapter 47) measuring blood glucose and BHB levels in groups of dry cows and cows in early lactation can be useful in the hands of the experienced veterinarian. This will often indicate an energy-deficient diet and one that could predispose to subclinical if not clinical acetonaemia.

As already stated, acetonaemia is less common now than in previous years. This is due mainly to improvements in forage conservation techniques and the use of mixed forages, especially maize silage. Thus cows are fed better quality feeds and there is increased awareness that optimum output comes as a result of optimum input.

Pregnancy toxaemia

Pregnancy toxaemia, although primarily considered a disease of sheep, does also affect cattle, particularly beef cattle in late pregnancy. The problem is best described as starvation, but the aetiology and pathogenesis are similar to acetonaemia in that an energy deficit in the diet leads to massive mobilization of fat reserves, resulting in hypoglycaemia and hyperketonaemia. The problem is most common in beef cattle grazing marginal land, but has been seen in dairy cattle in late winter in seasons where there has been a shortage of conserved forage. Cows of all ages are affected, but overfat animals and those carrying twins are the most susceptible. Beef cows often have access to good pastures in the summer months and can get overfat. If the same cows do not have access to good quality forage during the winter months, when they are in late pregnancy they will succumb to ketosis because of the deficit in energy intake. In dairy cows the problem can occur at or around calving and is again the result of insufficient energy intake in excessively fat animals.

Signs

The severity of the clinical signs and their speed of onset are associated with the stage of pregnancy and the degree of nutritional stress. Affected cows are usually seven to nine months pregnant and show the same clinical signs as cows with acetonaemia. They become increasingly dull and depressed and the smell of acetone can be detected on the breath. Many cows become recumbent fairly quickly, within a few days of the onset of hyperketonaemia. Often in poorly supervised herds recumbency is the first sign noticed by the stockworker. Recumbent cows are severely depressed, have an increased respiratory rate and faeces are scanty, hard and covered in mucus. Some cows develop blood-stained or fetid diarrhoea in the terminal stages. Most cows die three to fourteen days after recumbency, having fallen into lateral recumbency. This often occurs two to five days after sternal recumbency. Cows affected close to parturition often die during parturition.

Clinical pathology

Hypoglycaemia, hyperketonaemia and ketonuria are consistent findings. In recumbent cases the blood levels of βHB are much higher than in acetonaemia; levels up to 22 mmol/l (125 mg/100 ml) may be found. Cows affected close to parturition have hypocalcaemia and occasionally hypomagnesaemia. Recumbent cows in the terminal stages have hyperphosphataemia (up to 6.5 mmol/l; 20 mg/100 ml), hyperglycaemia (up to 9.0 mmol/l; 160 mg/100 ml) and raised AST levels. At post mortem the most consistent findings are an enlarged, yellow, fatty liver with fatty changes in the kidney and adrenal cortex.

Diagnosis

Often several cows are affected before veterinary attention is sought. The usual stimulus to seek veterinary help is when one or two cows are dead or close to death. The history, stage of pregnancy and the nutritional status will usually be enough to enable a tentative diagnosis. Raised blood or urine ketone levels and low blood glucose (plus low calcium in cows close to calving) will usually confirm the diagnosis.

Treatment

Treatment as described under acetonaemia (see p. 795) would normally be indicated. However, so severely affected are the majority of these cows that medical treatments almost invariably fail to succeed. Immediate removal of the calf by Caesarean section (p. 1115) may save a valuable cow. This should be followed by the full course of treatment described under acetonaemia.

Prevention

Although the problem is more common in fat cows it is essentially the result of starvation and is predominant in years when insufficient conserved fodder has been made. To prevent further cases developing and becoming recumbent a supply of good quality forage is essential, even if the farmer has to sell a proportion of his herd to obtain fodder for the remainder.

The downer cow

Attending the recumbent cow is one of the more challenging problems encountered by the bovine practitioner (see also p. 439). Often, accurate diagnosis is not possible but prognosis is extremely important and probably more important than accurate diagnosis. It must be remembered that recumbency is the normal course in the terminal stages of any disease so a full clinical examination is essential in every case plus a thorough history, often supported by biochemical examination of blood. Many workers have offered definitions of the downer cow, but the most useful in practice and the one to be used here is: a cow that has been recumbent for 24 hours or more, is in sternal recumbency and is not suffering from hypocalcaemia or hypomagnesaemia, mastitis or any obvious injury to the limbs or spine.

History

It is important that the clinician obtains an accurate history of the case and the following questions must be asked:

(1) How long has the cow been recumbent?
(2) When did she calve and was calving difficult?
(3) Did she rise after calving?
(4) Has she been treated for milk fever, and if so how often and how much CBG has been used?
(5) Has the cow moved recently, either spontaneously or with help from the farmer?
(6) Where did the cow go down, e.g. concrete, ice, in field, in a ditch, and was this likely to affect the pathogenesis?
(7) Is there adequate bedding?

Examination

The first superficial examination will be the position of the animal, position of the legs and degree of alertness. Lateral recumbency, if not due to hypocalcaemia, hypomagnesaemia or bloat, is indicative of a terminal state and slaughter should be advised as soon as possible. This includes cows which, although they will sit in the sternal recumbency position for short periods with the aid of supports such as hay bales, revert to the lateral recumbent position when they struggle free of the supports.

The position of the legs is a useful aid to prognosis. If the hindlimbs are in the normal position and the cow attempts to rise the prognosis is guarded to hopeful. If the hindlimbs are rigidly extended forwards so the feet are touching the elbows of the front legs this indicates severe sciatic nerve damage, upper hindlimb muscle degeneration or hip problems, e.g. fracture or dislocation, and the prognosis is hopeless. If both the hindlimbs are spread laterally, with lateral flexion at the stifle, the cow has probably 'done the splits' and again the prognosis is hopeless. If one hindlimb is in this position then the prognosis is guarded and careful nursing may succeed. If both hindlimbs are extended behind the animal, and when the position is corrected they return to the original position when the cow attempts to move, again the prognosis is hopeless as this indicates severe muscle degeneration.

The full clinical examination will then be conducted (see Fig. 46.2) and may well reveal other diseases present, e.g. mastitis, metritis (vaginal examination is essential), torn vagina, ruptured uterus, pneumonia, septicaemia, hypothermia or abdominal catastrophe. It is essential that a rectal examination be performed.

Assuming there is no abnormality in rectal temperature, respiratory rate, mucous membranes and the heart rate is below 80/minute, then ischaemic necrosis of the hindlimb muscles or, as it is more commonly referred to, pressure syndrome should be considered.

Pressure syndrome (ischaemic necrosis): Experimental work (Cox, 1982) has demonstrated that if a cow is lying in the same position for six hours or more there will be

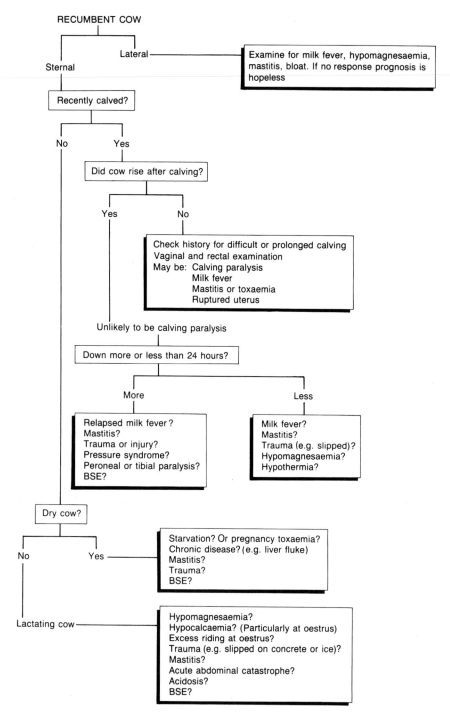

RECUMBENT COW

Lateral —— Examine for milk fever, hypomagnesaemia, mastitis, bloat. If no response prognosis is hopeless

Sternal

Recently calved?

No   Yes

Did cow rise after calving?

Yes   No

Check history for difficult or prolonged calving
Vaginal and rectal examination
May be: Calving paralysis
         Milk fever
         Mastitis or toxaemia
         Ruptured uterus

Unlikely to be calving paralysis

Down more or less than 24 hours?

More   Less

Relapsed milk fever?
Mastitis?
Trauma or injury?
Pressure syndrome?
Peroneal or tibial paralysis?
BSE?

Milk fever?
Mastitis?
Trauma (e.g. slipped)?
Hypomagnesaemia?
Hypothermia?

Dry cow?

No   Yes

Starvation? Or pregnancy toxaemia?
Chronic disease? (e.g. liver fluke)
Mastitis?
Trauma?
BSE?

Lactating cow

Hypomagnesaemia?
Hypocalcaemia? (Particularly at oestrus)
Excess riding at oestrus?
Trauma (e.g. slipped on concrete or ice)?
Mastitis?
Acute abdominal catastrophe?
Acidosis?
BSE?

Fig. 46.2 Aid to diagnosis and prognosis of the downer cow.

damage to the musculature of the leg on which the cow is lying. Cox describes this as ischaemic necrosis as a result of pressure. If the cow is in the same position for 12 hours continuously then the damage to the muscle is irreversible and the prognosis is therefore hopeless. This situation is most common following milk fever, particularly where treatment has been delayed or ineffective subcutaneous treatment has been given. Many

cows first seen with milk fever at morning milking will have been recumbent for six hours, and some for almost 12 hours. Many will be suffering some muscle damage, particularly if they have been lying on unbedded concrete. This is why prompt intravenous treatment for milk fever is essential.

Figure 46.3 shows the pathogenesis of ischaemic necrosis.

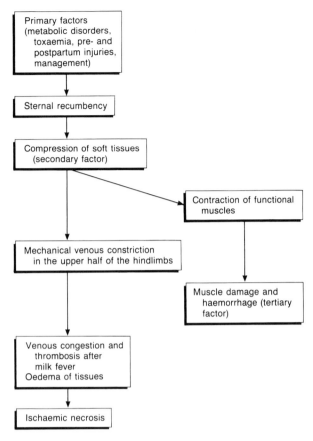

Fig. 46.3 Pathogenesis of ischaemic necrosis (from Andrews, 1986).

Calving paralysis: If the cow has not risen since calving and has not responded to milk fever therapy, and is not suffering from any toxic or septicaemic condition such as mastitis or metritis, then either pressure syndrome or calving paralysis should be suspected. The history should indicate whether calving has been difficult but occasionally a cow will deliver, with difficulty, a large calf but second stage labour may last 3–6 hours. In such cases, calving paralysis may occur. Calving paralysis as a term is preferable to obturator paralysis, sciatic paralysis or other defined nerve paralyses. The damage done to the birth canal during prolonged dystokia will result in a variety of lesions in the pelvic cavity. Generally, the bruising and swelling of the soft tissues of the pelvic cavity will damage the sciatic nerve and occasionally the obturator nerve. Obturator paralysis (p. 438), on its own, whether it is affecting one or both hindlimbs, will not cause recumbency. Such cows can rise, with difficulty, but will show abduction of one or both hindlimbs. Paralysis of the sciatic nerve (p. 439) is more serious and will prevent the cow rising.

Diagnosis and prognosis

Having completed a thorough examination of the recumbent animal that has recently calved and eliminated disease, obvious injury or starvation as a cause of the recumbency, the two most likely problems to be affecting the cow are (i) pressure syndrome (ischaemic necrosis) or (ii) calving paralysis. These cows will be alert, in sternal recumbency, and some will be attempting to rise or crawling along the ground. Appetite for food and water will be good. At this stage it is essential for the clinician to attempt a more exact diagnosis and offer a prognosis. One of the most important inputs that will aid recovery is tender loving care (TLC). The ability and willingness of the stockworker to nurse and attend these cases will be the most important element in successful treatment. So knowledge of the farm and its staff is essential in forming a prognosis, as is the ability to provide soft bedding such as deep litter or a nearby paddock. Diagnosis will be helped if the animal is raised using a Bagshawe hoist and it can be observed if the cow can take weight on one or both hindlimbs and if either or both hindlimbs are abnormal. Abnormalities to observe include the following:

● Flexion of fetlock and extension of the hock, which will indicate paralysis of the tibial, peroneal or sciatic nerve (pp. 438, 439).
● Abduction of one or both hindlimbs will indicate obturator nerve paralysis (p. 438).
● Swelling of the upper hindlimb musculature of one leg would indicate severe pressure syndrome. If the pressure syndrome is so severe that muscle swelling is obvious and one upper hindlimb is larger than the other, prognosis for that limb is hopeless.
● Inability to extend or flex the stifle, hock and fetlock joints.
● The willingness of the cow to take weight on the forelegs. If the cow is so weak she cannot take weight on the forelegs the prognosis is hopeless.

With calving paralysis one can generalize that if both hindlimbs are showing signs of nerve paralysis, e.g. extension of stifle and hocks and flexion of the fetlock, then the prognosis must be hopeless. If only one leg is affected and as long as TLC will be available, the prognosis would be guarded but hopeful. It is surprising how many cows suffering from calving paralysis affecting one hindlimb only will rise seven to ten days after calving.

As an aid to prognosis, several workers have attempted to use blood biochemistry. Serum CK rises to astronomically high levels following muscle damage but its half-life is short and on its own has not proved a reliable indicator of success. Raised serum AST levels will also indicate muscle damage and this parameter is probably more useful than CK levels. As a prognostic indicator in cows that have been recumbent four days or more AST levels can be quite useful. Interest in serum myoglobin levels has been reported from Sweden (Holmgren, 1988), where early work would suggest that in the first three days of recumbency serum myoglobin levels could be a valuable prognostic indicator. Levels below 3 μg/ml would indicate likely recovery.

It is unlikely that any one parameter will be shown to be of value for accurate prognosis. However, a combination of biochemical parameters and clinical signs, particularly attempting to rise, should be useful. Cows recumbent for three days or more must be attempting to rise, as well as bright, alert and eating well, for there to be any likelihood of eventual recovery. The quality of nursing available on the farm must also be considered in making a prognosis. Without good nursing, continual attention to bedding, feed and water, prognosis will be poor. Unfortunately, on many large dairy farms where labour is in short supply, there is often an unwillingness to break from the normal farm routine to provide extra attention to a recumbent cow. This information will be available to the regular attending veterinarian to the farm and will influence the prognosis. On such farms, in the interests of the welfare of affected cows, one will advise immediate slaughter of many cows, while on other farms where TLC is available, they would be likely to recover.

Treatment

Where the prognosis is considered hopeless or where it is known that TLC is absent, all cows should be slaughtered humanely as soon as possible. In some countries, particularly the UK, such animals can be fit for human consumption if they are not suffering from septicaemia, excessive bruising or any other infectious disease. However, in the interests of welfare, slaughter must take place on the farm. This is perfectly legal in the UK as long as the cow is bled on the farm and transported as soon as possible to the nearest slaughterhouse and the carcass is accompanied by a veterinary certificate that complies with the Fresh Meat (Hygiene and Inspection) Regulations 1995. If the slaughterhouse is EC approved, the carcass must reach it within 30 minutes of being bled.

Treatment will of course depend on the diagnosis, but for the cow that has been recumbent for 24 hours or more a soft bed is essential. A box or barn with an earth floor or deep litter bedding would be ideal, but if the weather is reasonable the best place for recumbent cows is in a field. Cows can be transported to the field on a gate, on a buck rake or with a cattle net on a fore-end loader. Wherever the cow is moved it must have continuous access to food and water. It is surprising how many stockworkers will forget to provide water to a cow recumbent for 24 hours or more.

If the hindlimbs are continuously abducted either due to bilateral obturator paralysis or injury from slipping on ice or concrete the application of hobbles (Save A Cow, Arnolds Ltd) or a soft rope to tie the hindlimbs approximately 50 cm apart will prevent further muscle damage. This will sometimes result in the cow rising immediately, the only factor causing the recumbency being the persistent hindlimb abduction.

If there is any doubt as to whether the cow may still be suffering from milk fever, 8–12 g of calcium should be administered intravenously. This situation could occur where farmers, treating their own cows, have administered subcutaneous CBG on two or more occasions within 24 hours, the calcium has not been absorbed completely and a state of hypocalcaemia still exists. Some cows with milk fever that recover will relapse so, if in doubt, intravenous calcium should be administered. A blood sample analysed for calcium levels would provide valuable information, if performed quickly, either as a cowside test or in the practice laboratory.

The most important element of treatment, once the cow is on a soft bed or in the field, is frequent turning so that she does not spend more than three hours in one position or on one side. Cows that are attempting to rise will frequently change their position and will move from side to side. Cows with an injury, whether it is a nerve paralysis or pressure syndrome, can often be turned to lie on the side opposite to which they are found, but at the next attempt to rise they fall back on to the side that is paralysed or injured.

The Bagshaw hoist, which attaches to the pin bones and is lifted using a fore-end loader or pulley blocks, is often advocated for treatment. This equipment will cause muscle damage and its continuous use on the same cow must be questioned on welfare grounds. However, it can be a useful instrument to aid diagnosis. Occasionally, a cow raised by the hoist will take weight on her hindlimbs, remain standing and slowly walk away.

In recent years interest has increased in various inflatable rubber bags (Bovijac, Alfred Cox; Henshaw Airlift, J.M. Henshaw; Downer Cow Cushion, Hamco Products). The reasoning behind the use of these air cushions is to allow improved blood circulation to the affected legs. Unfortunately, with most of the inflatable bags available, once inflated and the cow raised, she frequently struggles and falls off the side of the bag. Cow nets are available and a supportive harness (Downacow Harness, Alfred Murray) can be quite useful.

In Denmark, water flotation is being used. The recumbent cow is hauled into a drop-sided water tank and the tank filled with warm water. The cow will then stand, aided by the water, and is left in the same position for up to seven hours a day. The system is called an Aqua Lift (Rasmussen, 1988).

The use of the Bagshaw hoist (apart from aiding diagnosis) and the various slings and inflatable bags should be questioned. If a cow cannot stand unaided there is little point in raising her to the standing position. Repeated use of the Bagshaw hoist will cause extensive muscle damage and must be discouraged. Until an inflatable bag has been designed that will prevent a raised cow falling off the side, these air bags have only limited use.

The Danish Aqua-lift would appear to be the most practical aid to the recumbent cow, but the capital cost of making the lift and providing transport for it may prevent its widespread adoption.

The only therapeutic agents now licensed for use in cattle which may be of benefit in treating downer cows are the corticosteroids and the NSAIDs with intravenous glucose as supporting therapy. However, there is little or no evidence that would suggest any therapeutic agent may have a beneficial effect and TLC remains the most likely effective treatment.

Prevention

Selecting bulls with known shorter gestation lengths and ease of calving scores can, in part, prevent calving paralysis. Feeding of dry cows should also be monitored and frequently rationed, particularly in seasons where grass is plentiful. Overfat cows (condition score 3.5 or over) more frequently develop dystokia due to relative fetal oversize. If a particular bull has been identified as causing dystokia, then all cows remaining that are pregnant to him should be considered for induced parturition using long-acting corticosteroids (see p. 687).

The pressure syndrome is a preventable problem. The majority of cases are a sequel to milk fever where treatment has been delayed or is inadequate. Intravenous therapy with 8–12 g of calcium as soon as possible after the cow becomes recumbent, accompanied by moving the cow into sternal recumbency and turning her so that she is lying on the side opposite to that in which she was found, will prevent the pressure syndrome occurring. If the cow is down on concrete she should be moved onto a soft bed or into a field. Many pressure syndrome cases are the result of subcutaneous calcium therapy that fails to be absorbed completely.

Fatty liver syndrome

In the 1970s and early 1980s the syndrome of fatty liver (FLS) or fat cow syndrome (FCS) was widely reported in dairy cows at or around calving. Reports of its occurrence came from many countries, including the UK, USA, France, Hungary and the USSR. The syndrome appears to occur in high-producing dairy cattle where overfeeding in the dry period results in overfat cows at calving. Depressed appetite after calving and the consequent energy deficit result in a rapid weight loss and an accumulation of intracellular fat in the liver. The syndrome is associated with an increased incidence of metabolic, infectious and reproductive disorders such as milk fever (p. 781), ketosis (p. 793), mastitis (Chapter 23) and retained placenta (Chapter 34). Fat cow syndrome as described by Morrow (1976) is clinically the most extreme manifestation of the syndrome but is probably only the 'tip of the iceberg' and a much larger number of cows were affected by subclinical FLS, as described by Reid and Roberts (1982).

Occurrence

The FLS was thought to be widespread in UK dairy cows in the late 1970s and was probably related to gross overfeeding of cows during late pregnancy, particularly with the use of high levels of concentrate foods during the late dry period. However, 'steaming up' with concentrates is now out of favour and is rarely practised in the UK, which is probably why the clinical incidence of FLS has apparently declined in recent years. However, in seasons where grass is in abundance there is still a danger of cows becoming excessively fat if their diet is not restricted during the dry period and hence FLS can and still does occur. At worst 50–90 per cent of freshly calved cows can be affected with FLS, although on some farms the incidence was very low or even non-existent. Mortality up to 25 per cent has been reported in herds where severe FCS exists (see also p. 796).

Pathogenesis

As most dairy cows in early lactation are in negative energy balance they mobilize energy reserves of fat and muscle and consequently lose body weight and condition. The mobilization of body weight reserves involves the release into the blood of free fatty acids from fat depots and glucogenic amino acids from protein stores. The fatty acids are transported via the blood to various organs, e.g. the kidney, liver and muscle, where they are deposited as intracellular droplets of triglyceride. Thus at one to four weeks after calving there is an increased level of fat in the liver. There is a rise in liver fat levels occurring two to three weeks before calving. This fat mobilization before calving is probably brought about by the changes in hormonal status as the cow approaches calving. The extent of fat deposition in the liver and other organs after calving is probably determined by a number of factors including high milk yield potential, body fatness or condition at calving and loss of body condition after calving. Excessively fat cows tend to have depressed appetites so the fat mobilization is exacerbated, resulting in even higher liver fat levels and increased weight loss.

Signs

The most common indication of the existence of FLS is a high incidence of peri- or postparturient disease, e.g. retained placenta, milk fever, mastitis and ketosis. Cows with FLS will subsequently prove to be less fertile. However, if FLS is suspected it should be noticed that a high proportion of the dry cows are excessively fat (in excess of body condition score 3.5) and many of the cows four weeks after calving are thin (body condition score less than 2).

Clinical pathology

Cows with FLS one week after calving will have significant alterations in their blood constituents. Free fatty acids, bilirubin and AST will all be increased and glucose, cholesterol, albumin, magnesium, insulin and white blood cell count (WBCC) will all be decreased. In cows with severe FCS the WBCC may fall to as low as 3×10^9/l.

Pathology

At post mortem, cows with FCS will have large deposits of fat around the heart, kidney, pelvis and in the omentum. The liver will be enlarged, with rounded edges and a pale yellow colour. Intracellular droplets of triglycerides will be found in liver cells, kidney, adrenal glands, skeletal muscle fibres and cardiac muscle. In the liver the triglyceride globules are deposited within the hepatocytic cytoplasm. The extent of deposition may be as high as 70 per cent of total hepatocyte volume.

It is important to realize that the findings described above may be seen in animals that have been deprived of food 24–48 hours before death. Therefore, post-mortem findings can only assist in the diagnosis of FCS or FLS when used in conjunction with the herd history and clinical pathology.

Diagnosis

The history of increased disease incidence just after calving followed by examination of body condition of dry cows and cows three to four weeks after calving will often give a strong indication of the presence of FLS. Confirmatory evidence is best obtained by liver biopsy of five or six cows immediately after calving. The liver biopsy samples can then be assessed for fat level percentage. The technique of liver biopsy in cattle is relatively easy to perform and should be used by all cattle practitioners. Levels of fat, as assessed by staining sections of liver with toluidine blue or oil red 0, in excess of 20 per cent would indicate the presence of FLS. Levels in excess of 50 per cent fat would indicate severe FLS.

Blood biochemistry has been widely explored as a measure of fatty liver and various parameters have been explored, e.g. non-esterified fatty acids (NEFA), glucose, AST and glycerol, but these cannot, as yet, be interpreted with great confidence. In the USA another method of estimating liver fat levels is based on the buoyancy of needle biopsy samples in water or copper sulphate solutions.

Treatment

There is no proven treatment for either FCS or FLS. Various empirical treatments have been suggested but there is little evidence that any are of value. The logical approach would be to use the same treatments that are used for acetonaemia. Increasing the glucose supply by the administration of glucose, glycerol or propionate and a glucocorticoid followed by the stimulation of protein synthesis by the administration of an anabolic steroid would appear to be the most logical approach to treatment.

Prevention

Fatty liver is a sign of cows too fat at calving and losing excessive weight in early lactation. The main element of a prevention programme is to restrict the feeding of dry cows so that they calve in a body condition score of 2.5–3.0. The big reduction in the use of concentrates before calving in recent years has almost certainly reduced the number of cows suffering from FLS at calving. Cows in condition score 2.5–3.0 at calving certainly have appetites greater than fat cows and hence lose less weight in early lactation. However, dry cows can become fat on grass diets alone in northern Europe during the spring and early summer, when grass quality is at its best. At such times, therefore, grazing for dry cows should be restricted or supplemented with low quality fibre such as straw or hay. The rules for prevention of FLS are therefore the same as for acetonaemia (p. 796).

References

Andrews, A.H. (1986) The downer cow. *In Practice*, **8**, 187–9.

ARC (1980) *The Nutrient Requirements of Ruminant Livestock*. A technical review by an ARC Working Party. Commonwealth Agricultural Bureau.

Cox, V.S. (1982) Pathogenesis of the downer cow syndrome. *Veterinary Record*, **111**, 67–9.

Holmgren, N. (1988) Immunological determination of myoglobin as a diagnostic and prognostic aid in downers. In *Proceedings of the XV World Conference on Cattle Diseases*, 11–14 October 1988, Palma de Mallorca, Spain, pp. 276–7.

Kelly, J. (1988) Magnesium and milk fever. *In Practice*, **10**, 168–70.

Morrow, D.A. (1976) Fat cow syndrome. *Journal of Dairy Science*, **59**, 1625–9.

Rasmussen, J. (1988) The downer cow. In *Proceedings of the XV World Conference on Cattle Diseases*, 11–14 October 1988, Palma de Mallorca, Spain, pp. 282–5.

Reid, I.M. & Roberts, C.J. (1982) Fatty liver in dairy cows. *In Practice*, **4**, 164–8.

Sachs, M. (1988) The prevention of the periparturient hypocalcaemia syndrome by the use of 1α-hydroxy vitamin D_3. In *Proceedings of the XV World Conference on Cattle Diseases*, 11–14 October 1988, Palma de Mallorca, Spain, pp. 286–91.

Sansom, B.F., Manston, R. & Vagg, M.J. (1983) Magnesium and milk fever. *Veterinary Record*, **112**, 447–9.

Whitaker, D.A., Kelly, J.M. & Smith, E.J. (1984) Hypomagnesaemia increase. *Veterinary Record*, **116**, 451–2.

Further reading

Hibbitt, K.G. (1979) Bovine ketosis and its prevention. *Veterinary Record*, **105**, 13–15.

Spence, A.B. (1978) Pregnancy toxaemia in beef cows in Orkney. *Veterinary Record*, **102**, 459–61.

Chapter 47
Metabolic Profiles

D.A. Whitaker

Introduction	804
Timing of blood tests	805
In relation to feed changes	805
In relation to feeding	805
In relation to calving pattern and seasonal feeding	
changes	805
Selection of cows	805
Early lactation group	806
Mid lactation group	806
Dry cow group	806
Background information	806
Interpretation of results at the farm	806
Written advice	807
Metabolites measured	807
Optimum values	807
Energy balance	807
β-Hydroxybutyrate (BHB)	807
Non-esterified fatty acid (NEFA or free fatty acid)	807
Glucose	808
Bile acids	808
Interpretation of results for energy balance: cows	
in milk	808
Expected forage ME	809
Interpretation of results for energy balance;	
dry cows	810
Protein	811
Urea-nitrogen (ureaN)	811
Digestible undegradable protein (DUP)	813
Albumin	813
Total protein	813
Globulin	813
Minerals and trace elements	813
Magnesium	813
Inorganic phosphate	814
Calcium	814
Sodium and potassium	814
Thyroxine (T_4)	814
Copper	814
Glutathione peroxidase (GSHPx)	814
Manganese	815
Zinc	815
Cobalt	815
Metabolic profiles on milk	815
Metabolic profiles in maiden heifers	815
Metabolic profiles in suckler cows	815

Introduction

The use of metabolic profiles in dairy cattle was pioneered by Payne *et al.* (1970) at the Compton Institute of Animal Health. The approach has been adapted and modified since then (Blowey, 1975; Kelly *et al.*, 1988; Whitaker, 2000) so that it is now widely used in many countries in European-type cows (for example in Italy, Bertoni & Cappa, 1984; in Chile, Wittwer *et al.*, 1987; in Germany, Mansfeld *et al.*, 1996; in Turkey, Sevinc & Aslan, 1998; in Belgium, Opsomer *et al.*, 2000). The approach has also produced useful information in low yielding cows in developing countries (Whitaker *et al.*, 1999) by drawing attention to potential constraints and by confirming that some were not present.

In Britain the system has been developed as a management aid for dairy farmers and their veterinary surgeons (Ward *et al.*, 1995; Kelly & Whitaker, 2000). It contributes information for decision making about nutrition in a more precise and detailed way and more quickly than by other, more conventional approaches. Traditionally forages are analysed, stocks of them measured, targets for productivity set, financial constraints considered – and a ration plan is produced from one of many perfectly satisfactory sets of software. Inevitably such a ration has limitations, starting with those of the reliability of forage analysis and of assessment of intakes. Furthermore, the ration may not be delivered in practice according to the theory of the plan. It may well be that the ration plan is for a cow producing 35 litres of milk at 4.0% butterfat and 3.3% protein, but it may actually be the only one like that in a group of cows, some of which may have just calved and others of which may be 100 days in to their lactations. If the ration is not adequate, a farmer and his advisers can detect this from individual milk yields, from milk constituents, from body weight and condition changes, from weak oestrous signs and from poor conception rates. All of these, with the exception of butterfat percentage, even if measured regularly and carefully, take weeks or months to alter enough for the presence of a problem to be clear. And once it is clear, what actually is it? If the metabolic profile approach is used 'properly', then it can, within two weeks of a ration being started, identify that there is a problem, what it is and what is the best and/or the most economic solution.

The 'proper' use of metabolic profiles depends on care with the timing of blood tests, the selection of cows to be included and the collection and use of background information about the farm, feeding and feeding system and physical state and performance of the cows.

Timing of blood tests

In relation to feed changes

As changes in the diet of ruminants require changes in the character of rumen activity, blood samples for metabolic profiles should not be done until two weeks after a major change and activity has had time to adapt. Minor changes such as an increase in the quantity of an existing component or in access to the same ration do not require a wait of more than 7–10 days. Changes in forage type, such as turnout to grass, housing or the introduction of silage, require the full two weeks, as does the introduction of concentrates or of a new type of concentrates.

In relation to feeding

There can be changes in biochemical values in blood associated with feeding. These are most marked in cows receiving all their concentrate ration at milking time. In such cases two hours should be allowed to elapse after milking before blood sampling. In circumstances where the major part of the concentrate input is mixed with the forages and is available for most of each 24 hours, the timing of tests in relation to feeding is less critical. If lower yielding mid lactation cows are included (see later), their results can be used as a check to see whether there is an effect of feeding on the biochemical values in the blood samples. Cows should not be separated at milking time and confined for hours without access to food when waiting for blood sampling as this can also affect the results.

In relation to calving pattern and seasonal feeding changes

The cow in early lactation is the most important because what happens to her in the first few weeks after calving has the major influence on her subsequent productivity, including her future fertility efficiency. Therefore blood sampling for metabolic profiles should be carried out at the beginning of each new calving season,

with the first cows checked so that the majority can benefit from the information derived.

Of equal importance is the need to test as soon as possible (see previous section) after the introduction of a new ration, so that the judgement of the cows' biochemistry can be made available as quickly as possible, i.e. what the cows, the end users, think of the ration.

Therefore planning of metabolic profile tests needs to be done in advance and should take into account both expected calving pattern and feed changes. Without planning along these lines, time may be lost and productivity with it.

Selection of cows

The selection of appropriate cows for blood sampling is very important. This is because some of the metabolites looked at, particularly those relating to energy balance, can quickly return to the optimum range as cows adapt themselves, including their productivity, to a nutritional constraint. It is possible for cows to experience a significant energy deficit in the first 2–3 weeks of lactation because of intake problems, lose excessive body condition, perhaps modify their milk yield and have their subsequent fertility efficiency suppressed but yet still arrive at four weeks calved with all biochemical measurements within the optimum ranges. This is because the common appetite constraint of the new calved has worked its way out and there is plenty of food available for lower performance than anticipated. If blood were sampled at four weeks calved or longer, a farmer could see thin, underproducing cows with poor fertility but with nothing abnormal about their biochemistry. Thus the farmer would be entitled to feel the metabolic profile test was of no value. However, if those cows had been blood sampled at 14 days calved instead of 27, the blood results would have been quite different and would have identified the nutritional constraint on productivity.

Individual variations in biochemical values are such that single cows should not be tested. Groups of no less than five should be sampled. They should not be picked at random but rather should be typical, average cows of their stage of lactation. Cows with extremes of performance – either very high or very low – should not be selected. Cows with problems should also not be included because the type of analysis carried out is not designed to clarify individual problems. It is important to make all this clear to farmers in advance because they cannot be expected to appreciate the limitations of the analyses made. Experience in the Dairy Herd Health and Productivity Service (DHHPS) (Kelly & Whitaker, 2000) suggests that selecting cows for metabolic profiles may be best done by the veterinary surgeon himself in advance of the test after looking at the calving and production records. If there is a specific concern, such as a poor conception rate, farmers may expect only cows which have failed to conceive to be sampled. This hardly ever delivers helpful information as any nutritional constraints have been compensated for by then and blood biochemical values are usually within optimum ranges. The best approach may be to include such cows as the mid lactation group (see later).

Early lactation group

The definition used for this group is most critical for the reasons given in the previous paragraph. Since the original Compton metabolic profile (Payne *et al.*, 1970), where a high yielding cow was used as the definition, the importance of this group has become increasingly apparent. The definition also has had to be changed to take into account changes in farm practice. The way cows are fed now – total mixed rations, increased out-of-parlour concentrate feeding – has reduced the time after calving by when they can adapt themselves to an unsatisfactory diet. To be sure of detecting the presence of an energy constraint in particular, blood sampling should be carried out between 10 and 20 days calved – less than 10 days and yield is still too far below peak for the test to be a realistic one for early lactation performance; more than 20 days and some cows will be thin, unproductive and subfertile but have compensated for their nutrition and they may have normal blood metabolite values.

Mid lactation group

Some cows which are past the period of peak yield, and so past the greatest period of potential nutritional stress, should always be included. They should be between 80 and 150 days calved so that they are still relatively high yielding. This group provides a within-herd comparison with the early lactation cows. Without this it is very difficult to distinguish between problems caused by constraints on intake of food or protein and energy content, to identify changes in biochemical values caused by mistiming of tests in relation to feeding or by oddities in the diet such as silage with a high butyric acid content and to make judgements on concentrate/forage usage within the herd.

Dry cow group

As the dry period is so important to the success of the following lactation, blood sampling to make sure nutrition is adequate is essential. However, the nature of the measurements which can be made means that primarily cows in the last 7–10 days of pregnancy should be sampled. Cows tested with longer to go than that tend to have normal measurements of energy balance even though they can still get into difficulty. This is because the period of greatest risk is when the volume of the pregnant uterus increases to the point that it can seriously inhibit food intake. It follows that, in a seasonal calving herd, the first dry cows which come in to these last 7–10 days ought to be blood sampled, so that the information can be used for the benefit of the others still to come in to the maximum risk period.

Blood sampling a group of dry cows with a month or longer to go to calving at the same time can sometimes provide a useful within-herd comparison with respect to energy balance. It may also identify the presence of dietary protein inadequacy – specifically rumen degradable – in the early part of the dry period.

Background information

So that full value can be obtained by the farmer from the metabolic profile approach, information about the cows and the farm should accompany the blood samples to the laboratory. This should include cow identification; last calving date for milkers/expected for dry cows; bodyweight – by calculation from heart girth measurement with a weighband pulled to a constant 5 kg tension is the best, because it is not affected by gutfill, and usually most practical, because no mechanical weighing device/crush is required; body condition score by a palpation method; current daily milk yield; expected current daily milk yield; lactation number; daily supplementary feed intakes; daily estimated forage intakes; analytical description of feeds and current herd milk solids percentages. It is useful to have information on herd size, breed, feeding systems and health and fertility. A note of what concerns the farmer has, if any, should also be made.

Interpretation of results at the farm

Circumstances where the diagnosis of a nutritional constraint from blood samples is clearly correct, but the cause is unclear from a distance and there could be many, are common. Therefore it is very important that a final interpretation of what is not working and what are the best and most economic solutions ought to be made at the farm with the information from the laboratory to hand. Farm advisory visits should be made as soon as the results are available and discussions held, including farm staff and any other advisers involved. Experience in the DHHPS suggests that such a team approach produces a more balanced strategy and is more beneficial than each party working in isolation.

Written advice

Any advice given should be recorded concisely in writing and copies given to all participants on the farm. This ensures that the agreed path is followed, keeps a record of it and ensures that the fee is for something tangible.

Metabolites measured

The number of metabolites which could be measured is great. For the sake of cost, not overcomplicating the picture and speed of turn round of results, the number is usually restricted. Metabolites measured should also be confined to those from which reliable, useful and practical information can be derived. Consequent actions will therefore be beneficial. It needs to be borne in mind that aspects of energy and protein nutrition are the most important and constitute, between them, at least 90 per cent of identified constraints (Kelly & Whitaker, 2000).

Chosen metabolites need to be stable in the blood samples after collection for two to three days while in transit to the laboratory. Methods of analysis need to be quick, accurate and automated. Each laboratory must use an outside agency as a continual check on quality control and so reliability of results.

Optimum values

What constitutes a 'normal', or rather optimum, value or range of values for a metabolite in blood is crucial. In the DHHPS (Kelly & Whitaker, 2000) we used originally the values proposed by Payne *et al.* (1970). These were based on population means from 2400 cows plus or minus two standard deviations. The DHHPS laboratory has been operating since 1978, with thousands of blood samples passing through every year, accompanied by information on stage of lactation, feeding, performance and responses to advice based on optimum values used; consequently some of the values have been modified. Account must also be taken of the fact that variation in some metabolites is skewed. For these we have carried out a lognormal transformation (Whitaker et al., 1983) before arriving at an optimum range. For some metabolites, such as urea, the interest primarily is in low values and so in variation only one way from the optimum. Some controlled trials, where detailed measurements of weight and condition change have been made with blood sampling (e.g. Whitaker et al., 1989, 1993), have confirmed the otherwise largely anecdotal evidence for what is optimum. These ranges are the ones quoted in the following pages.

Optimum values should nevertheless not be used too precisely. Small variations from optimum may not be important, depending on the metabolite. Group means should be looked at and compared firstly and then the individual variations and the number of them within each group. Variations which might relate to performance, body weight, condition or stage of lactation need particular attention because they can provide important information on the practical causes of a constraint. Values within the optimum ranges can also be used, in conjunction with the background information, to give advice of economic importance on concentrate/forage usage (see following sections on interpretation).

Energy balance

β-Hydroxybutyrate (BHB)

In cows in milk the optimum level for β-hydroxybutyrate (BHB) in blood is below 1.0 mmol/litre. BHB reflects fat mobilization as an energy source and so higher values are associated with greater degrees of negative energy balance. Values below 0.6 mmol/litre represent a situation where cows are unlikely to be losing body condition. Between 0.6 and 1.0 a low and acceptable rate of fat mobilization may be taking place, depending on the stage of lactation. Above 1.0 mmol/litre health and productivity will be affected. Cows with ketosis will probably have values over 2.0 mmol/litre. In a small proportion of cows BHB results, if very high in early lactation, remain outside the optimum range after energy balance has been restored and body condition is being regained.

Dry cows in the last month of pregnancy should have BHB values below 0.6 mmol/litre because they should be restoring and maintaining energy resources.

BHB is stable in blood after collection for several days. Butyric acid from grass silage, directly absorbed across the rumen wall, has been blamed for increased blood values. In our experience since 1978 this is a rare problem. If it is present, all cows with access to that silage will have high BHB levels in blood. Including lower yielding mid lactation cows receiving the same basic diet, as a within-herd comparison, provides the most reliable means of ruling it out – if those cows have lower results than the early lactation animals which are eating the same silage.

Non-esterified fatty acid (NEFA or free fatty acid)

The optimum level of non-esterified fatty acid (NEFA) in cows in milk is below 0.7 mmol/litre and for dry cows within the last four weeks of pregnancy 0.4 or below. The reasons for the difference are the same as for BHB. NEFA is a more direct measure of fat mobilization than

BHB. It may rise more quickly and it often returns to within the optimum range quite quickly as well, even when negative energy balance is still present. Cows with ketosis have values in their blood above 1.5 mmol/litre.

NEFA is less stable in the blood sample after collection than BHB. It is reputed to start to rise after 48 hours, but we have not seen practical evidence of this in samples analysed four to five days after collection. Severe stress prior to blood sampling is also reputed to cause the level to rise, but this also has not apparently happened in the ten years that we have used this metabolite. Sampling groups of no fewer than five cows and including those in early and mid lactation as within-herd comparisons enable these potential problems to be set aside.

Glucose

Glucose was the first metabolite used in the Compton Metabolic Profile (Payne *et al.*, 1970). Because of the fundamental requirement for glucose in the tissues, homeostatic mechanisms are very strong and variations were not found to be great. Whole blood or serum tended to be used, neither of which are as accurate with respect to energy balance as the plasma content. Added to the difficulties was the fact that glycolytic enzymes start to break down glucose after sampling. So either analysis needed to be carried out very quickly or blood needed to be collected into a tube containing oxalate fluoride as an anticoagulant. This does not mix as easily as other anticoagulants and sample tubes have expiry dates which are easily overlooked. Glucose is also the most likely metabolite to change with delay in transit and it goes down. All this has meant that glucose acquired a reputation as not being very useful in assessing energy balance with certainty.

Our experience suggests that if blood is collected into tubes within their dates, mixing is thorough but gentle and analysis is carried out within four to five days of collection, plasma glucose is a sensitive measure of energy balance – even within the optimum range which is above 3.0 mmol/litre. Sampling groups within a herd, as for BHB and NEFA, allows a check for abnormalities not associated with nutrition.

There are some nutritional circumstances where the predominant finding in a metabolic profile is that plasma glucose levels are low but BHB and NEFA are within their optimum ranges. These appear to be associated often with a dietary shortage of fermentable metabolizable energy (FME), judging by the responses obtained to dietary adjustments.

Plasma glucose does increase sharply to over 5.0 mmol/litre in a cow which is severely stressed immediately prior to sampling.

Bile acids

Some laboratories include bile acid measurement in metabolic profiles as a means of assessing subclinical ill health, with reference in particular to heavy fat infiltration (lipidosis) into the liver in the peri-parturient period as a consequence of severe negative energy balance. There is not firm agreement on the value of this. West (1991) found bile acids to be significantly correlated with the degree of a variety of liver diseases including lipidosis, whereas Garry *et al.* (1994) found no correlation between bile acid level and liver fat content. Schrotter *et al.* (2000) found bile acid levels to be within the normal range in cows with subclinical disorders and chronic hepatopathy. In the DHHPS (Kelly & Whitaker, 2000) we have carried out this analysis on several hundred occasions alongside those for BHB, plasma glucose and NEFA and have found that it did not appear to add sufficiently to the information obtained to justify its regular inclusion.

Interpretation of results for energy balance: cows in milk

Raised BHB and/or NEFA values with or without low plasma glucose results indicate that cows are experiencing a dietary energy problem and not necessarily a dietary energy deficiency. The easy response is to recommend an increase in energy supply through more concentrates. This can be completely the wrong thing to do, which illustrates that identifying that there is a problem is the easy bit and only the start. Identifying the cause(s) and the practical solution(s) is the difficult bit. Using the type of background information described earlier and seeing what is actually happening at the farm are essential parts of the process.

There are a number of possible reasons for dietary energy problems in milking cows, all of which should be considered:

- The forage component of the diet is being expected to contribute more energy than is reasonable, i.e. not enough concentrates are being fed.
- Less concentrate is being fed than supposed because of misunderstanding or feeders are in need of recalibration.
- Too much concentrate is being fed, resulting in a concentrate to forage ratio in the rumen which is in excess of 3:1 on a dry matter basis. This causes underutilization of the energy which is in the diet. For this calculation grazing, silages, hay and straw only count as forages. Often the only way to arrive at a ratio is to add up the amount of dry matter being supplied as non-forages, calculate the theoretical total dry matter intake of the cow and assume the difference is the amount of forage dry

matter being eaten. Another way of looking for this problem is from an expected forage ME calculation (see later). Rationing, which is expecting the forage component to provide less than the equivalent of the energy needs of maintenance (about 65 megajoules), is likely to be threatening this ratio. Loose dung provides supporting evidence.

- The concentrate amount offered each milking is too high – it is either not eaten or, if it is, causes transient rumen acidosis; 4 kg per milking is a reasonable top limit.
- Concentrates supplied contain too much readily soluble carbohydrate, causing rumen acidosis.
- Single feeds of concentrates, unmixed with forages, supplied at times other than milking, may be too great to ensure even intakes between cows – 2 kg per cow per feed is a reasonable limit.
- Not enough conserved forage is being offered – ideally fresh forages should always be readily available to all cows at all times. Empty troughs militate against the cows who are most at risk. Between 5 and 10 per cent more food than the cows are going to eat should be supplied if possible/practical, with the surplus removed at least once daily.
- Silage or silage concentrate mixtures can become stale, because troughs are not cleaned out often enough.
- Loss of nutrients from silage due to secondary fermentation may occur – from exposure to air or water at the clamp face by the way it is handled or because rations are mixed too infrequently. Silages of high dry matter content are more at risk. The ration warm to the hand or with steam rising from it on a still day shows this as a problem.
- Conserved forages may be unpalatable, in UK circumstances grass silages which are very wet or very dry are a risk. Modern forage analytical measures give some indications.
- Access to conserved forages is restricted, e.g. by inadequate trough space and design, troughs not filled evenly, self-feed faces tightly compressed, severe electrified barriers, not enough ring feeders or the feeding facilities or the route to them are exposed to bad weather.
- Different forages fed unmixed – grass silage available as an alternative to maize or whole crop, but not mixed with them, does not deliver the same potential nutritional benefits as a mixture.
- Conserved forage is of low energy content – provided it is palatable this can usually be balanced by other components of the diet, if the problem is recognized. Laboratory analysis of forages can exaggerate the energy content, particularly the fermentable metabolizable energy in maize silage.

- Grass silage can be very low in fibre – uncommon but can occur if of high quality, having been harvested very early in the spring. Mixing 0.5 kg of chopped straw with it may be enough.
- Access to grazing is restricted – strip grazing systems or paddocks not changed often enough; set stocking systems allowing the development of fibrous, less nutritious grass.
- Buffer feeding to grazing may be inappropriate – poor quality forage used; timing of access; substitutes instead of supplements grazing; site of access inappropriate.
- Too much digestible undegradable protein and not enough energy in a ration can occur.
- Salt deficiency is common in some winters.
- Water deprivation is easily overlooked – trough size, site, filling rate and cleanliness can all be constraining.
- Inadequate dry cow nutrition and management can be unnoticed – changes in diet components at calving; failure to allow dry cows to realize their potential appetites in late pregnancy; fat mobilization and body condition loss before calving.
- Lack of reasonable cow comfort and space can contribute considerably to energy problems for new calved cows and especially heifers.

It is important to see the silage clamp, grazing fields and water troughs, to be there when food is put out to see what happens, both with reference to men and cows, and to check troughs and self-feed faces at other times when at the farm. What is said or believed to be happening is not always so!

There are rare circumstances where BHB levels are raised and glucose levels are low which do not reflect an energy problem. Observation of the cows' body condition and their performance can support this, but looking at the results in the different groups should confirm it. If cows in the mid lactation group, producing much less milk, have got the same scale of out-of-range results as cows in early lactation producing a lot more, then some aberration of the timing of sampling in relation to feeding or of a direct effect of a diet constituent, such as butyric acid in silage, is likely to be responsible.

Expected forage ME

More specifically, it is useful to look at the way the rationing is set up for the individual cows and what contribution is being sought from the forage component – the expected forage metabolizable energy (ME) in megajoules. The energy the cow needs, the required ME (AFRC, 1993), is calculated from the cow's body weight, milk yield and milk quality. The energy supplied as concentrates, the fed concentrate ME, i.e. not forages, is calculated from the information obtained from the farm on fed amounts and analysis, actual analysis if available or book values if not. The difference is the energy that the rationing assumes is supplied by the forages. Similar calculations can be made to assess the energy contribution of forages where systems not based on metabolizable energy are used.

$$\text{Expected forage ME} = \text{required ME} - \text{fed concentrate ME}$$

The amounts of concentrates eaten per cow per day are usually the most accurate information available on feeding – certainly more accurate than the amount of forage eaten. Where concentrates are mixed in with silage offered *ad lib*, individual concentrate intakes are less accurate and group means should be considered first, not least because it is these which will have been used to design the ration.

Where metabolite values have been disturbed because cows have been blood sampled too close to a feed, cows will have similar out-of-range levels, even though expected forage ME figures vary widely.

This calculation is of further use when assessing the economic aspects of concentrate/forage usage. Table 47.1 shows an example of a blood test in which all the energy measurements were within the optimum ranges, indicating that all these cows were having their energy needs met. Cows numbered 1–5 are within the second and third weeks of lactation, the period of greatest potential nutritional stress. Because they are in energy balance, they must be achieving from forages the figures shown in the expected forage ME column. If they can, then the rest of the herd can too. This means that cows 6–10, who are being asked to get less from forages, should have their concentrate input reduced so that

their expected forage ME figures are at least the same as those for cows 1–5 or perhaps even greater. So blood tests showing the presence of no nutritional constraint – often looked at by farmers as a waste of money – can be used to guide the important economic management of concentrate usage.

Some further points need to be considered, however. The cost of concentrates and forages may not, in every country, be such that lower use of concentrates is more economic. In addition, a reduction in concentrate input will mean that cows will look to increase forage intakes. So there has to be forage offered/available to them to do this or milk yields will suffer. There may be important implications for forage stocks too because they will be used more quickly. Also it is necessary to consider the protein content of the ration. A reduction in concentrates in this context is of energy supplied, but it may mean that effectively protein input is reduced as well and that could also reduce milk yield. The protein content of the reduced level of concentrate fed may need to be increased to avoid this. Blood urea levels may give some guidance. If they are relatively high, no increase in protein content may be necessary. This is likely to be so where this assessment is being made in cows at grass.

It is worth repeating that optimum levels of BHB, glucose and NEFA can be found in thin, underproducing cows in modern feeding systems after four weeks calved, who have adapted their performance and their metabolic state after experiencing serious energy constraints earlier in lactation.

Interpretation of results for energy balance: dry cows

The dry period needs to be one of maintenance and restoration of resources for cows, especially high yield-

Table 47.1 Examples of individual cow results for assessing concentrate usage/forage contribution to energy needs.

Cow	Days calved	BHB mmol/l	Glucose mmol/l	NEFA mmol/l	Expected forage ME (MJ)
1	10	0.4	3.4	0.5	169
2		0.6	3.2	0.2	175
3	to	0.3	3.5	0.3	135
4		0.4	3.2	0.4	181
5	20	0.4	3.2	0.4	150
6	80	0.6	3.4	0.3	152
7		0.7	3.3	0.4	101
8	to	0.3	3.4	0.2	131
9		0.3	3.2	0.3	95
10	110	0.4	3.3	0.3	121

ing ones, to be able to realize their productivity and longevity potentials. Body condition change during the dry period and body condition score at calving – aspects of energy balance primarily – influence productivity and fertility in the following lactation (e.g. Domecq et al., 1997; Markusfeld et al., 1997). So identifying the presence of undesirable situations during the dry period is important. Body condition scoring, if done once a week, is sensitive enough until the last two weeks of pregnancy. Then blood sampling may be the only way to confirm that there is a problem.

The following is a dry cow management 'best practice' list against which current practice on a farm can be checked where a problem has been found.

From drying off
(1) Look upon the dry period as a unique opportunity for rest and recreation for cows.
(2) Provide a clean, comfortable environment in the first month of the dry period.
(3) Manage cows so that they go dry at body condition score 2.5–3.0 on a scale of 1–5 and maintain it until calving (p. 10). This may mean reducing concentrate inputs in late pregnancy, which is where much overfatness develops. It may mean restricting the quality of forage available in the first month of the dry period to stop excessive increase in condition.
(4) Confine overfat cows at drying off on a diet of straw balanced with adequate effective rumen degradable protein (ERDP) to maintain rumen function. The restriction should be of quality and not quantity of forage so that rumen fill is maintained as far as possible. Only 10–14 days on this regime is advisable and it must be stopped absolutely by the time of one month to go to calving.
(5) Feed overthin cows at drying off generously enough for some condition to be restored.
(6) Provide free access minerals during the first month of the dry period if they cannot be mixed in with the forage on offer, which is preferable.

For the last month of the dry period
(7) Provide the best environment and forages on the farm.
(8) Offer 24 hour access to fresh, quality forages in the last month of pregnancy. All of the forage types which are going to be fed in production should be included. Cows should be challenged to eat between 12 and 15 kg of dry matter each day so that they can eat more and get to maximum intakes more quickly after calving. If more than 0.5 kg of straw is included, total dry matter intakes will be reduced. Expecting cows to 'fill up' even to 12 kg dry matter by providing free access to straw does not work. Failure to provide enough fresh, quality forage, in cows receiving concentrates, is the commonest cause of negative energy balance in late pregnancy.
(9) Feed 2–3 kg of good quality concentrates/cow per day. This increases the energy density of the total food intake, compensating for the dropping appetite. It allows the rumen environment and lining to adapt fully to concentrates by the time cows are in milk. These processes take at least two weeks.
(10) Ensure that these concentrates contain appropriate digestible undegradable protein (DUP) if enhanced milk protein production is desired.
(11) Ensure that the forages contain adequate ERDP and if not compensate through the concentrates. Specialist dry cow concentrates are usually formulated assuming that cows, if getting grass silage, will be getting enough ERDP from that. This is not always the case. A ration with maize or whole crop cereal silage included is more at risk.
(12) Ensure that appropriate minerals are incorporated in the concentrates or silages fed. Production ration minerals are satisfactory for most farms for most of the time and only need changing if cases of hypocalcaemia start. Free access at this stage is not satisfactory.
(13) Include pregnant heifers in this close to calving group, unless to be kept separately in lactation – but even then provide the same ration.
(14) Oversize calves come from overfeeding in the seventh or eighth month of pregnancy, extended gestation length (a function of the genetic make-up of the sire) or an underdeveloped heifer with a genetic potential to be a lot bigger. The rate of growth of the calf in the last month of pregnancy is at its greatest but it cannot be influenced by feeding in that month – either to increase or decrease the eventual size of the calf.
(15) Provide the same fresh concentrates and forages in calving boxes/pens. Also ensure fresh water supplies.

Protein

Urea-nitrogen (ureaN)

If rumen function is satisfactory blood ureaN level is above 1.7 mmol/litre. In some laboratories urea rather than ureaN is measured. This makes no difference except that the values are higher by a multiplication

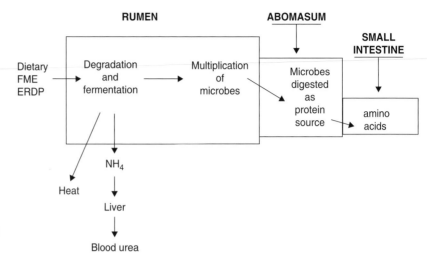

Fig. 47.1 Diagram of degradation and digestion of ERDP and FME by ruminants.

factor of 2.14. So the optimum for urea is above 3.6 mmol/litre.

Blood ureaN reflects the rate of arrival in the rumen of effective rumen degradable protein (ERDP) and the balance there with fermentable metabolizable energy (FME), as illustrated in Fig. 47.1. Low values are the most important from a practical, nutritional point of view but care needs to be exercised in distinguishing between values which are low because of low total food intake or because the diet does not contain adequate ERDP. This is one of the reasons for including mid lactation cows in a metabolic profile test as a within-herd comparison. If the new calved cows, which are the most likely to have appetite constraints, have low ureaN results and so do the mids, who should be able to eat readily, then the diet will be short of ERDP. If the mids have optimum ureaN results though, the diet should be adequate in ERDP but the new calved are not eating as much as they should. If diet intake is the predominant problem, some of the energy metabolites may be out of their ranges too. Obviously the approach to this is different – and importantly so – from a diagnosis of a dietary shortage of ERDP.

On farms where maize and grass silages are not mixed but are offered so that cows can make a choice, or where one silage is fed for 12 hours and the other for the next 12 hours, low blood ureaN may not always relate to an overall diet shortage of ERDP. The best solution then may be to promote mixing of the forages rather than a change in concentrates.

Where an ERDP shortage is diagnosed and more is to be supplied, cows will respond with increased milk yield within 24–48 hours. They will have improved rumen function and so will look for more forage to eat. Therefore for the approach to work, more silage must be made available to them. However, account must be taken of the fact that forage stocks may be depleted more quickly than previously anticipated.

There is a further practical risk arising from the fact that the theoretical ration plan being followed often indicates that ERDP is adequate – the reason is probably a shortcoming in the laboratory analysis of forages. Feed advisers may therefore be reluctant to agree to more ERDP – partly because it is usually cheaper than the existing ration – and often suggest 'higher quality' protein, which is usually digestible rumen-undegradable protein (DUP). That, by definition, passes through the rumen, plays no part in rumen function and does not work where ERDP is short.

Low ureaN results in dry cows are quite common for the reasons indicated in the dry cow/energy section. As a dietary shortage of ERDP inhibits rumen function, reduces potential appetite and enforces a change in rumen function at calving, it is important to identify it.

The same high level of ureaN can reflect (i) an excess of ERDP and adequate FME, (ii) an excess of ERDP and inadequate FME or (iii) adequate ERDP but low FME. Only (ii) and (iii) need action and some other evidence of nutritional imbalance is desirable to make the diagnosis more certain – some energy metabolites outside their reference ranges for example. Where ureaN results are above 3.3 mol/litre and there is evidence of an energy constraint, it is worth increasing the level of FME in the diet. This may mean substituting energy sources not available in the rumen, such as protected fats, with wheat or barley for example, which are high in FME.

It is not advisable to try to correct an excess of ERDP in relation to FME (examples ii and iii) by reducing the amount of ERDP in the diet. This is because it may be impossible not to reduce the DUP supplied as well and so precipitate an unwelcome fall in milk yield. The supposition that high blood urea levels directly affect fertility remains controversial and unproven. Certainly many cows retain good fertility, or even have improvements, when turned onto grass in spring with high blood urea levels. It is possible that observed subfertility in cows with such high levels occurs primarily because of negative energy balance. Therefore care should be taken, if looking at metabolic profile results in herds with fertility problems, before drawing definitive conclusions.

Digestible undegradable protein (DUP)

Higher yielding cows cannot meet their total protein requirements from ERDP and the production in the rumen of microbial protein alone; DUP is required as well. This passes through the rumen unaffected and is digested in the abomasum and small intestine as an additional source to microbial protein. There is no way of directly assessing the dietary adequacy of DUP through metabolic profiles. However, if milk yield is below expectation and cows are maintaining good body condition in early lactation – and if ERDP supplies are adequate – increased dietary DUP should be tried. As with ERDP, the milk yield response should be within 24–48 hours and also as with ERDP cows will be looking for greater forage intakes. More must be made available and account taken of a greater rate of depletion of conserved forage stocks.

Before embarking on this approach a metabolic profile test to confirm satisfactory energy balance and adequate dietary ERDP is strongly advisable. As part of a dietary shortage of DUP is often a complaint that milk protein production is low and as energy constraints are the commonest cause of this, the check metabolic profile test is the first step in such a complaint. Farmers need to be advised as well that feeding more DUP, where there has been a dietary shortage, should result in an increase in milk and milk protein yield but not necessarily an increase in milk protein percentage.

Albumin

Albumin is a protein that is synthesized in the liver. The optimum level is over 30 g/litre. Low levels reflect poor liver health or a poor supply of amino acids from the diet. Any effect from diet is long term. Low levels will only appear after prolonged and severe underfeeding of protein. If the cause is disease, the effect can be more immediate and may involve a raised globulin level as well.

Serum samples as opposed to plasma produce albumin results between 2 and 5 g/litre lower.

Total protein

Measurement of total protein is required to deduce globulin level. This is not directly measured and is the difference between albumin and total protein. As total protein consists of something based on diet and something based on disease and inflammation, it should not be shown on result sheets. If it is, people who are not aware of its content frequently draw exclusively dietary conclusions, which are incorrect.

Globulin

Globulins are produced in response to inflammation of the chronic type. The optimum level is below 50 g/litre. If it is higher, the individual cow concerned has a recent, acute or chronic inflammation problem. The globulin measurement is crude and not specific, consequently a raised value does not indicate with any accuracy the severity of the problem or how recently it took place. In some cases a cow may have some disease process clinically obvious, but the globulin has not risen at the time of blood sampling. The whole value of the measurement is to draw attention to the possibility of individual or herd disease problems and so stimulate discussion and investigation. The commonest individual complaints are mastitis, metritis or lameness. The most likely herd problem in the UK is infection with *Fasciola hepatica*, when albumin levels will be low as well (p. 276).

Minerals and trace elements

Magnesium

Blood magnesium levels should be between 0.8 and 1.3 mmol/litre. This reflects current dietary intake rather than body tissue resources from which magnesium is not readily available. Low blood levels can therefore be a matter requiring urgent action to avoid clinical hypomagnesaemia. A number of slightly low magnesium results may indicate subclinical hypomagnesaemia, which can affect appetite, performance and behaviour.

Because of the complex nature of the dietary factors which interfere with the absorption of magnesium from the diet, a check test 10–14 days after increased supplementation is advisable to make sure that it has worked.

Low dietary magnesium in the dry period may be involved in the incidence of hypocalcaemia, but low blood levels may not be detected until a few days before calving. Clinical hypomagnesaemia is rare in dry cows but it can occur and, if it does, is usually fatal. Underfeeding and exposure to severe adverse weather conditions are the predisposing factors.

Inorganic phosphate

Plasma values also reflect current dietary intake primarily. Optimum levels are between 1.4 and 2.4 mmol/litre. Unlike magnesium and calcium, however, low levels in diet and blood can be tolerated without harm to health and fertility for months (Brodison et al., 1989). A check blood test, a few weeks after some low results occur, is advisable before embarking on potentially expensive and probably useless supplementation. Measurement of this mineral is usually carried out because of the widespread misconception that dietary deficiency is a common cause of poor fertility because of the aggressive marketing of supplements to meet this perceived need.

Hypophosphataemia can be a contributory cause of the downer cow syndrome (pp. 439, 797). However, misdiagnosis can take place because a blood sample taken after a cow has been recumbent and not eating for 24 hours may be low because of that only. Firm diagnosis can only be on response to treatment with phosphate.

Calcium

Homeostatic control of the level of calcium in the blood is so strong that variations are small and do not reflect dietary intake at all. Measurement of calcium should not therefore be carried out as part of a metabolic profile and should only be done as part of clinical diagnosis.

Sodium and potassium

Homeostatic control of sodium and potassium is also too strong to allow measurement in blood to be a reliable indicator of dietary intake.

Thyroxine (T_4)

Thyroxine provides an indication of the iodine status of the cow. The optimum level is above 22 nmol/litre (Whitaker, 1999). Low values have been associated with abortion and stillbirth. Weighing the thyroid gland of stillborn calves does not appear to be sensitive enough to identify an iodine deficiency or the presence of goitrogens, although the iodine content of the gland may be. Histopathology of the thyroid gland should provide confirmation. Iodine deficiency has been associated with poor production as well.

Measurement of inorganic iodine in plasma is also widely practised. Caution is required over interpretation as the level is very sensitive to variation in daily iodine intake. A cow which has not eaten will have a low result primarily because of appetite.

Copper (see also p. 298)

Blood copper levels are not an accurate guide to body and liver status where most of it is found. So, while the optimum level is over 9.3 μmol/litre, clinical copper deficiency can be found with results above or below that. A number of individual results below that in a metabolic profile merit further, clinical enquiry because deficiency, if present, will affect health and productivity.

Recent reports of copper toxicity in cattle, perhaps associated with higher absorption rates from the use of chelates or proteinates in minerals or overzealous supplementation, suggest that blood levels over 20 μmol/litre should be followed up (p. 948).

Much more difficult is assessing the possible primary role of excessive molybdenum on fertility and secondarily on copper status (Phillippo et al., 1987). Suttle (1993) suggested that this problem would not be present unless the forage offered contained more than 5 mg/kg molybdenum on a dry matter basis. Telfer et al. (1996) believe that forage values can be lower than this and the problem may still be present because of molybdenum in concentrates. They have developed a complex system of testing blood involving a ratio between plasma copper and serum caeruloplasmin, trichloracetic acid precipitated copper and superoxide dismutase. This may be too arduous for many laboratories. If this problem is suspected – and forage analysis frequently encourages farmers to think it is – the most practical solution may be to administer for six months an intrareticular copper bolus to alternate cows as they go dry or calve and see what happens.

Glutathione peroxidase (GSHPx) (see p. 302)

The optimum level is over 50 units/g of haemoglobin or over 15 units/ml of red blood cells. As this is an enzyme containing selenium and as it has a half-life of some weeks, GSHPx values reflect historical selenium intake. Low values in early lactation cows, satisfactory ones in mid lactation and lower but still satisfactory ones in dry cows describe a dietary deficiency in the dry period, with production rations taking care of it. GSHPx values can be dropping while selenium intake is rising and *vice versa*. Isolated groups of cattle sampled can therefore produce a deceptive picture. Clinical assessment of possibly related problems is necessary – such as muscular dystrophy, poor fertility in maiden heifers, retained placenta, stillbirth or mastitis in early lactation. Because of the relationship with vitamin E, measurement of this in blood may be advisable as well if a problem is suspected. Blood selenium itself can be measured, but the analysis is too expensive for routine use.

Manganese (see p. 305)

Estimation of blood levels is practised but the relevance of results is questionable. Since Wilson (1966) found no differences in conception rates between supposedly manganese deficient supplemented and unsupplemented herds no published evidence has appeared that this trace element is limiting on fertility. More recently, Gelfert and Staufenbiel (2000) found no evidence of effects on fertility in 70 dairy herds in Germany where, according to published values for the manganese content of hair and serum, deficiency should have existed.

Zinc (see p. 305)

Optimum values for zinc concentrations in blood are equivocal. In UK circumstances the likelihood of primary zinc deficiency is low. Furthermore, specially prepared sample tubes need to be used to avoid contamination from the glass or the cork.

Cobalt (see p. 295)

Levels of vitamin B_{12} in blood below the reference value of 90 ng/litre are commonly found in productive, healthy and fertile cattle. It is probable therefore that what is usually measured is not biologically active or cattle can exist with lower levels than this without coming to harm. It may therefore be preferable to avoid altogether the expense of a laboratory analysis of doubtful practical value.

Metabolic profiles on milk

If the same rigorous 'rules' are applied to the selection of cows, timing of tests and the use of background information as for blood samples, using the more easily collected milk can provide useful information on energy balance and protein intakes. Failure to follow the 'rules' and failure always to check energy and protein together lead to erroneous conclusions. Milk urea can be readily measured and is virtually the same as the level in blood. Methods of assessing energy balance through measurements in milk are available – β-hydroxybutyrate, acetoacetate, ketones. There are technical difficulties, for example because of volatility. The practical value is less clear at the time of writing and measurements may not be as sensitive as for metabolites in blood. Minerals and trace elements can also be measured in milk, but there is no reliable information on reference values. Furthermore, as milk is manufactured for the specific purpose of feeding a young animal, it contains concentrated amounts of many elements, bearing little or no relation to levels in blood, body or dietary intake.

Bulk milk measurements are generally unhelpful. Analysis for urea is widely practised and frequently misunderstood by farmers causing unnecessary concern. A number of milk purchasers have now given this up. The problem is largely because the result is an average for the herd and because of variations in urea in cattle which relate to intake rather than to diet content. Only if bulk milk urea is very low should there be any response and that should be a proper metabolic profile to determine the nature of the constraint.

Metabolic profiles in maiden heifers

In response to complaints of poor conception rates in heifers, blood samplings in housed animals often show diets to be inadequate in ERDP. Sometimes minerals and trace elements do not all fall into optimum ranges either. Anecdotally responses are achieved by correcting the ERDP query. So investigation of this type of complaint should not be confined to minerals and trace elements, which is where feed advisers and farmers often expect the problem to lie.

Metabolic profiles in suckler cows

In the DHHPS metabolic profile samplings are often carried out in suckler herds on cows in late pregnancy and when new calved. While these sometimes suggest the presence of some mineral or trace element shortcomings, it is common to find evidence of considerable negative energy balance at these stages, using the same optimum blood values as in dairy cows, which may inhibit subsequent fertility. As with dairy cows, waiting to blood sample until inseminations are about to start is likely to miss identifying the presence of the most probable nutritional constraint. Equally, if sampling is not done until a problem of low pregnancy rates is apparent, the true cause may not be revealed by it. Then it may be better to wait until pregnant cows are available before the start of the next calving season.

Dietary shortages of ERDP are also common in housed suckler cows fed on low quality conserved forages, resulting in the waning of body reserves when they should be maintained.

A dangerous degree of hypomagnesaemia present in autumn and winter suckling cows is quite commonly revealed. Follow-up tests can assess the success of supplementation.

Summary

The metabolic profile approach in dairy cattle should be used as a way of 'asking the cows what they think of their nutrition'. If the timing of this question is planned for as soon as possible in each new feeding regime, any shortcomings can be quickly identified and corrected before major losses in productivity, including fertility, are inevitable. While the approach may well help in problem solving, continued use as a preplanned exercise in the DHHPS since 1978 in Britain (Kelly & Whitaker, 2000) shows that its most valuable asset is as a means of providing more information to cow managers, more quickly and more precisely, than is possible by any other means.

References

AFRC (1993) In: *Energy and Protein Requirements of Ruminants*, pp. 21–31. An advisory manual prepared by the Agricultural and Food Research Council Technical Committee on Responses to Nutrients. CAB International, Wallingford.

Bertoni, G. & Cappa, V. (1984) Il profilo metabolico nella vacca produzione di latte. *Biochemica Clinica*, **8**, 131–3.

Blowey, R. (1975) A practical application of metabolic profiles. *Veterinary Record*, **97**, 324–7.

Brodison, J.A., Goodall, E.A., Armstrong, J.D., Givens, D.I., Gordon, F.J., McMaughey, W.J. & Todd, J.R. (1989) Influence of dietary phosphorus on the performance of lactating dairy cattle. *Journal of Agricultural Science, Cambridge*, **112**, 303–11.

Domecq, J.J., Skidmore, A.L., Lloyd, J.W. & Kaneene, J.B. (1997) Relationship between body condition scores and conception rates at first artificial insemination in a large dairy herd of high yielding Holstein cows. *Journal of Dairy Science*, **80**, 113–20.

Garry, F.B., Fettman, M.J., Curtis, C.R. & Smith, J.A. (1994) Serum bile-acid concentrations in dairy cattle with hepatic lipidosis. *Journal of Veterinary Internal Medicine*, **8**, 432–8.

Gelfert. C.C. & Staufenbiel, R. (2000) Problems in diagnosis of manganese status in dairy herds by herd supervision. *Tierartzliche Praxis Ausgabe Grosstiere Nutztiere*, **28**, 69–73.

Kelly, J.M. & Whitaker, D.A. (2000) Multidisciplinary approach to dairy herd health and productivity management. *British Society of Animal Science Occasional Publication*, **26: Vol. 1**, 209–22.

Kelly, J.M., Whitaker, D.A. & Smith, E.J. (1988) A dairy herd health and productivity service. *British Veterinary Journal*, **144**, 470–81.

Mansfeld, R., Gruneberg, W., Thiemann, E. & Grunert, E. (1996) Statistical analysis of metabolic profiles of blood and saliva used as a tool for herd diagnostic procedures. *Züchtungskunde*, **68**, 325–45.

Markusfeld, O., Galon, N. & Ezra, E. (1997) Body condition score, health, yield and fertility in dairy cows. *Veterinary Record*, **141**, 67–72.

Opsomer, G., Grohn, Y.T., Hertl, J., Coryn, M. & de Kruif, A. (2000) Protein metabolism and the resumption of ovarian cyclicity post partum in high yielding dairy cows. *Reproduction in Domestic Animals*, Suppl. 6, 54–7.

Payne, J.M., Dew, Sally M. & Manston, R. (1970) The use of a metabolic test in dairy herds. *Veterinary Record*, **87**, 150–8.

Phillippo, M., Humphries, W.R., Atkinson, T., Henderson, G.D. & Garthwaite, P.H. (1987) The effect of dietary molybdenum and iron on copper status, puberty, fertility and oestrous cycles in cattle. *Journal of Agricultural Science, Cambridge*, **109**, 321–36.

Schrotter, G., Mostl, E. & Baumgartner, W. (2000) Determination of bile acid in serum for diagnosis of liver function in dairy cows. *Wiener Tierartzliche Monatsschrift*, **87**, 94–100.

Sevinc, M. & Aslan, V. (1998) The relationship between parturient paresis and fat cow syndrome in dairy cows. *Turkish Journal of Veterinary & Animal Sciences*, **22**, 23–8.

Suttle, N. (1993) Overestimation of copper deficiency. *Veterinary Record*, **133**, 123–4.

Telfer, S.B., Mackenzie, A.M., Illingworth, D.V. & Jackson, D.W. (1996) The use of caerulosplasmin activities and plasma copper concentrations as indicators of copper status in cattle. In: *Proceedings of XIX World Buiatrics Congress*, **2**, 402–4.

Ward, W.R., Murray, R.D., White, R. & Rees, M. (1995) The use of blood biochemistry for determining the nutritional status of dairy cows. In: *Recent Advances in Animal Nutrition*. (ed. by P.C. Garnsworthy & D.J.A. Cole), pp. 29–51. Nottingham University Press.

West, H.J. (1991) Evaluation of total serum bile-acid concentrations for the diagnosis of hepatobiliary disease in cattle. *Research in Veterinary Science*, **51**, 133–40.

Whitaker, D.A. (1999) Trace elements – the real role in dairy cow fertility. *Cattle Practice*, **7**, 239–41.

Whitaker, D.A. (2000) Use and interpretation of metabolic profiles. In: *The Health of Dairy Cattle* (ed. by A.H. Andrews), pp. 89–107. Blackwell Science, Oxford.

Whitaker, D.A., Goodger, W.J., Garcia, M., Perera, B.M.A.O. & Wittwer, F. (1999) Use of metabolic profiles in dairy cattle in tropical and subtropical countries on smallholder dairy farms. *Preventive Veterinary Medicine*, **38**, 119–31.

Whitaker, D.A., Kelly, J.M. & Smith, E.J. (1983) Subclinical ketosis and serum beta-hydoxybutyrate levels in dairy cattle. *British Veterinary Journal*, **139**, 462–3.

Whitaker, D.A., Smith, E.J. & Kelly, J.M. (1989) Milk production, weight changes and blood biochemical measurements in dairy cattle receiving recombinant bovine somatotrophin. *Veterinary Record*, **124**, 83–6.

Whitaker, D.A., Smith, E.J., da Rosa, G.O. & Kelly, J.M. (1993) Some effects of nutrition and management on the fertility of dairy cattle. *Veterinary Record*, **133**, 61–4.

Wilson, J.G. (1966) Bovine functional infertility in Devon and Cornwall: reponse to manganese therapy. *Veterinary Record*, **76**, 562–6.

Wittwer, F., Bohmwald, H., Contreras, P., Phil, M. & Filoza, J. (1987) Análisis de los resultados de perfiles metabólicos obtenidos en rebaños lecheros en Chile. *Archiva Medicina Veterinaria*, **19**, 35–45.

Adult Cattle
System and Miscellaneous Conditions

Chapter 48
Alimentary Conditions

R.G. Eddy

The mouth and associated structures	821
Salivation	822
Simple stomatitis	822
Necrotic stomatitis (calf diphtheria)	822
Papular stomatitis	822
Mucosal disease	822
Mycotic stomatitis	823
Phlegmonous stomatitis	823
Wooden tongue (actinobacillosis)	823
The jaw	824
Fractures	824
Abscesses of the jaw	824
Retropharyngeal abscess	824
Lumpy jaw (actinomycosis)	824
Teeth	825
The oesophagus	825
Emesis or vomiting	825
Disease of the oesophagus	826
Oesophageal trauma	826
Oesophageal stenosis	826
Choke	826
Upper alimentary squamous cell carcinoma	828
Diseases of the rumen	828
Indigestion	829
Rumen acidosis	829
Rumen parakeratosis	832
Bloat (rumen tympany)	832
Vagal indigestion	835
Cold cow syndrome	836
The oesophageal groove	837
Traumatic reticulitis	837
Abomasum	839
Displacement of the abomasum to the left	839
Right-sided abomasal dilatation and torsion	842
Abomasal ulceration	844
Abomasal impaction	844
Abomasal impaction in calves	845
Colic and acute intestinal obstruction	845
Tympanic intestinal colic	846
Torsion of intestines (red gut in calves)	846
Prolapse of intestines through mesentery	846
Caecal dilatation and torsion	847
Intussusception	847
Diaphragmatic hernia	848
Fat necrosis	849
Peritonitis	849
Diarrhoea	850
Salmonellosis	850
Winter dysentery	852
Bovine virus diarrhoea/mucosal disease	853
Johne's disease (paratuberculosis)	857
Tenesmus	858
Diseases of the rectum and anus	859
Rectal prolapse	859
Rectal tears	859
Recto-vaginal fistula	859

The mouth and associated structures

Examination of the mouth, muzzle, mucous membranes, tongue and teeth should form a part of the normal clinical examination. Mouth lesions can be signs of systemic diseases such as foot-and-mouth disease, mucosal disease, bluetongue and various poisonings. Lesions of the muzzle and lips and occasional congestion of the oral mucosa can be a feature of photosensitization. Injuries occasionally occur and there are a number of infections and allergic diseases that produce lesions of the lips, tongue and jaws. Diseases of the gums and teeth are rare in cattle, although chronic fluorosis (see p. 949) where it occurs will cause mottling, discoloration or hypoplasia of the teeth, particularly in growing animals. Even problems associated with excess tooth wear are uncommon, presumably because the majority of cattle are slaughtered well before they reach 'old age'.

The main signs associated with mouth lesions are salivation, excess chewing movements, frequent protrusion of the tongue and licking of the lips and muzzle. Swellings of either jaw will indicate lesions of the jaw, the most common of which are abscesses, infections of the buccal mucosa, e.g. calf diphtheria, or lumpy jaw (actinomycosis). Submandibular swelling may indicate mouth lesions, e.g. wooden tongue (actinobacillosis), or be a sign of cardiac or liver dysfunction, e.g. liver fluke (p. 276) or severe hepatitis (p. 147).

Swelling of the submandibular and retropharyngeal lymph nodes may be the result of infections such as tuberculosis, actinobacillosis or lymphosarcomata. Swollen salivary glands do also occasionally occur due to tuberculosis infection or infections resulting from penetrating wounds.

Salivation

Ruminants normally produce large quantities of saliva, which acts as a buffer in the rumen to maintain the normal ruminal pH. Adult cattle normally produce 5–10 ml/100 kg body weight/minute. A 600 kg cow can therefore produce 60 ml/minute of saliva.

Excess salivation occurs as a result of many diseases:

● Foot-and-mouth disease (p. 700) and infectious bovine rhinotracheitis (p. 289).
● The various causes of stomatitis, e.g. wooden tongue (p. 823), calf diphtheria (p. 250), and teeth-related problems (p. 825).
● Pharyngeal paralysis, although rare in cattle, is a sign of rabies (p. 908), Aujeszky's disease (p. 907), botulism (p. 721) and occasionally tetanus (p. 733).
● Obstruction of the oesophagus, the most common of which is choke (p. 826).
● Eating plants or chemicals that are themselves irritant and cause inflammation in the mouth (Chapter 54).
● Certain chemicals such as copper, lead, mercury and arsenic also stimulate excess saliva production (Chapter 54).

Salivation can be controlled using atropine at a dose of 30 mg for adult cattle and can be used 20 minutes prior to anaesthesia. However, the use of atropine to control excess salivation is not to be recommended or considered necessary. The primary cause of the problem should be diagnosed and corrected.

Simple stomatitis

Inflammation of the oral mucosa is characterized by redness and excess salivation. There are a variety of causes, which include the following:

● Traumatic injuries from the use of balling and drenching guns, mouth gags and stomach tubes may occasionally be encountered.
● Foreign bodies, such as sticks and vegetable roots, may damage the roof of the mouth or be wedged between the teeth and the buccal mucosa.
● Injuries to the tongue may also occur, for example it may be accidentally amputated by sharp metal.

Stomatitis caused by chemicals is more common. Creosote, discarded engine oil, formalin, acids or caustic soda used for forage preservation, chemical dips or sprays are all found on most livestock farms and, if left unprotected from animals, the inquisitive cow may well consume small quantities, resulting in inflammation to the oral mucosa.

Inflammation or infection of the buccal mucosa is occasionally seen. Also, decaying cud may be found wedged between the mucosa and the teeth; this produces a swelling on the side of the face. Removal of the offending material and treatment with a course of parenteral antibiotics (penicillin and streptomycin) results in recovery, although further accumulation of cud material may occur and this has to be removed daily until the lesion heals.

The treatment of these conditions is generally symptomatic. The foreign bodies are removed, antibiotics may be administered and corticosteroids or nonsteroidal anti-inflammatory agents may help to reduce the painful effects of the inflammation. Most conditions recover quickly when removal of the offending material has occurred.

Necrotic stomatitis (calf diphtheria)

Fusobacterium necrophorus will be associated with necrotic lesions of the mouth, tongue and larynx. In calves the condition is extremely common, but it does occasionally occur in growing or adult cattle. A frequent site is the buccal mucosa and this may be a cause of decaying cud accumulating between the teeth and buccal mucosa as described above. The lesions are necrotic and often contain caseous material. Necrotic glossitis has been reported in feedlot cattle with the necrotic lesions present on the tongue. The aetiology is unknown but is probably infectious and may be viral. The signs are of excessive salivation, swollen cheeks when the buccal mucosa is affected and a foul smelling breath. Treatment with parenteral antibiotics or sulphonamides is generally very effective if given over a period of three to five days (see p. 250).

Papular stomatitis

Papular stomatitis is a virus condition producing vesicles that rupture and produce ulcerative lesions. It is a common condition in calves (see p. 252) but is of little economic significance. It is, however, a differential diagnosis of foot-and-mouth disease and lesions caused by mucosal disease, but there are not usually any signs of systemic disease and there is no excess salivation.

Mucosal disease

Erosions or shallow ulcerative lesions of the dental pad, the mucosa below the tongue, the roof of the mouth and occasionally the tongue occur as a sign of mucosal disease, which sporadically affects growing cattle around nine to 18 months of age. The lesions are similar to papular stomatitis, except that vesicles do not precede them. Diarrhoea and wasting are also present. Mucosal disease and bovine viral diarrhoea (BVD) are described in detail on p. 853.

Mycotic stomatitis

Mycotic stomatitis caused by *Monilia* spp. is thought to be a specific disease entity and is characterized by yellow necrotic lesions on the buccal mucosa, which erode, coalesce and become covered in a fibrinous necrotic membrane. It is likely that the fungal infection is secondary and it has been suggested that bluetongue virus (see p. 691) may cause the primary disease. Muzzle lesions similar to mycotic stomatitis also occur occasionally.

Phlegmonous stomatitis

Phlegmonous stomatitis and deep-sited cellulitis occur sporadically in adult cattle. It takes the form of an acute, deep-seated, diffuse, rapidly spreading inflammation of the oral mucosa, pharynx and surrounding structures. It may often follow injury to the mucosa by a foreign body. *Fusobacterium necrophorus*, streptococci and *Escherichia coli* have all been isolated from lesions.

The onset of signs is sudden, commencing with excessive watery salivation and lacrimation. The rectal temperature is raised to 40.5–41.5°C (105–107°F) and the heart rate and respiratory rate are increased. There is marked swelling of the face, mouth, muzzle and the submandibular area. There is a foul or fetid smell to the breath and the oral epithelium frequently peels off. In severe cases death may ensue within 24 hours.

Treatment is successful if commenced early and the condition usually responds to sulphonamides or a course of injections with penicillin and streptomycin.

Wooden tongue (actinobacillosis)

Wooden tongue is a well-defined disease producing stomatitis and glossitis, mainly in adult cattle. The causal agent is *Actinobacillus lignieresi*. The disease is found worldwide but the incidence varies considerably between countries. In the UK the incidence of the disease has declined considerably in recent years; whereas 25 years ago the annual incidence was of the order of 20–30 per 10 000 cattle it has declined to less than 5 per 10 000.

Aetiology and pathogenesis

The aerobic, Gram-negative coccobacillus *A. lignieresi* is the causative organism and it produces small abscesses commonly referred to as 'sulphur granules' in soft tissues. The bacteria do not survive outside the animal host for longer than five days but have frequently been isolated from the faeces of normal healthy animals. It is considered to be a normal inhabitant of the upper respiratory and alimentary tracts.

The organism does not normally invade healthy skin or mucosa but trauma to the mucosal surface from sharp objects such as sticks, dried thistles, straw or barley awns will allow entry of the organism. Although wooden tongue is the most common clinical manifestation of *A. lignieresi*, the organism will produce lesions elsewhere, e.g. the oesophageal groove, the rumen wall, and other soft tissues of the head and neck. It is frequently isolated from cervical and pharyngeal lymph nodes. The organism, once it has gained entry into tissues, produces small multiple swellings that develop into small abscesses 2–5 mm in diameter. The surrounding tissues swell as a result of the inflammation and the tongue may increase in size by 50 per cent.

Signs

Wooden tongue has a sudden onset, with excess salivation, difficult mastication and therefore reduced feed intake. There is considerable submandibular swelling and frequently swollen submandibular and retropharyngeal lymph nodes. The tongue will frequently protrude from the mouth. The tongue (particularly the dorsum) will be swollen, hard to the touch and on the surface will be seen round, discrete, yellow lesions 2–5 mm in diameter. These are abscesses situated just below the tongue epithelium. If left untreated the disease progresses so that eating becomes impossible and weight loss follows. Eventually death will occur due to starvation.

Treatment

If initiated early in the course of the disease, treatment is generally successful. However, if treatment is delayed beyond two weeks it is less likely to be so. Traditionally, treatment consisted of intravenous sodium iodide 7 g/100 kg body weight administered as a 10 per cent solution and repeated in 10–14 days. Oral treatment with sodium or potassium iodide is also effective.

Iodine treatment should continue until signs of iodism occur, such as dry scaly skin rather similar to dandruff. Sodium iodide should not be administered to heavily pregnant animals because of the risk of abortion (see pp. 261, 302).

Antibiotics are effective. Streptomycin at a dose rate of 10–15 mg/kg daily given intramuscularly for 10 days is effective in most cases. However, penicillin is less satisfactory. Some workers advocate the streptomycin should be injected into the lesion. Besides being extremely painful to the animal this does not appear to be necessary.

Animals that have been affected and untreated for two weeks or more and animals that do not recover within two weeks of treatment should be slaughtered.

Prevention

In most situations the disease of wooden tongue is sporadic. However, herd outbreaks have been known to occur, which may be the result of feeding hay or straw containing thistles, gorse or brambles. In any case affected cattle should be isolated to prevent spread of the infection and feeds such as those described above should not be offered. The reduction in UK incidence in recent years may well be related to a sharp decrease in the use of hay and a corresponding increase in silage as a method of grass conservation.

The jaw

A number of conditions affect the jaw of adult cattle, usually the lower jaw or mandible. Fractures of the symphysis (annual incidence 1 per 10000) are a result of falling on ice or slippery concrete and hitting the jaw on a hard surface. Fractures of the mandible usually result from accidental collision with a farm vehicle or occasionally a pathological fracture due to lumpy jaw (actinomycosis) or neoplasia. Jaw abscesses are seen in calves and growing cattle. In calves these are the sequel to untreated calf diphtheria but in growing cattle they may be caused by infections being introduced at the time of tooth eruption. Actinomycosis is a well-defined infection of the mandible, but only occurs rarely.

Fractures

Fractures of the symphysis are presented as an acute onset problem. Some swelling, occasionally blood-stained, of the lower lip will be noticed and some excess salivation. The animal continues to eat, but with obvious difficulty.

Examination of the jaw will reveal bruising of the lower lip and excess mobility of either side of the mandible. The front teeth may or may not be displaced, loose or even lost.

These animals will recover in about three weeks, provided they are isolated from the herd and food is cut and brought to the animal. Grazing or feeding from self-feed silage faces will prove difficult for affected animals. Abnormal positioning of the front teeth may be present after healing has completed.

Trauma-induced fractures of the mandible may be more difficult to manage. If there is no obvious displacement of bone at the fracture site and no dislocation, healing will take place in three weeks providing food is cut and brought to the animal. If there is severe displacement at the fracture site or dislocation is present, casualty slaughter is usually the wisest course of action.

Pathological fractures due to infection will not heal and immediate slaughter should be advised.

Abscesses of the jaw

Jaw abscesses present as round discrete swellings of the cheek and are quite common in calves and growing cattle. Their size varies but frequently they are about the size of a tennis ball (7.5cm or 3 inch diameter). Diagnosis is usually confirmed by paracentesis. Treatment by incising into the abscess, removing the pus and flushing with clean water should only be attempted if a soft area is apparent on the abscess surface. If palpation of the abscess reveals the external surface to be hard all over, treatment should be delayed until a softening and pitting of one area is noticeable. This is called pointing of the abscess. Abscesses that are opened and drained prematurely have a tendency to recur.

Retropharyngeal abscess

Abscesses of the retropharyngeal lymph nodes occur occasionally. These are presented as discrete round swellings the size of a tennis ball (7.5cm or 3 inch diameter) behind the vertical ramus of the mandible. The cause may be actinobacillosis or the result of infection entering a pharyngeal wound. Tuberculosis needs to be considered in countries where it is present. The treatment is the same as for jaw abscesses. There are a few differential diagnoses to consider. However, the author once encountered such a round hard swelling the size of a tennis ball in a Friesian cow. As the swelling was hard with no defined softening the farmer was advised to wait three weeks, by which time lancing the abscess should be possible. Three weeks later, as no softening had occurred and the cow was experiencing some difficulty with swallowing, the animal was anaesthetized and the pharynx explored, where a tennis ball was discovered!

Lumpy jaw (actinomycosis)

Lumpy jaw is a chronic infectious disease characterized by suppurative granulation of the bones of the head, particularly the mandible and maxilla. There is gross swelling, abscesses are present, fistulous tracts and extensive fibrosis all contribute to the granulomatous lesion. Its occurrence is quite rare in the UK (1–2 per 100000 annual incidence) but is said to be more common in the western and mid-western states of the USA. However, it is found at varying incidence levels worldwide where grazing cattle exist.

Aetiology and pathogenesis

The causative organism is *Actinomyces bovis*, a Gram-positive filamentous anaerobe, which is a normal inhabitant of the mucous membranes of the oral cavity, upper respiratory tract and digestive tract of most animals. The organism gains access to the soft tissues as a result of mucosal damage caused by sharp objects or erupting teeth. It generally affects cattle two to five years old.

The organism causes a low-grade inflammatory reaction. There follows a proliferation of connective tissue, invasion with leucocytes and the resulting formation of a walled tumour-like mass. The granuloma then invades the bones of the mandible or occasionally the maxilla. The hard, immovable, circumscribed lesion that results may reach a considerable size (15–25 cm in diameter) and will eventually interfere with mastication. The development of the lesion takes several weeks. Interconnecting abscesses and fistulae breaking to the exterior and discharging small quantities of pus are a frequent sequel. The pus may contain yellow granules that, on compression and staining, will reveal the Gram-positive filaments of *A. bovis*. The granulomatous lesion will continue to invade the soft tissues of the head and neck and the teeth are frequently displaced or become dislodged and the lower jaw may be displaced laterally. Pathological fracture of the mandible may occur (see p. 824).

Pathology

Rarefying osteitis, osteoporosis interspersed with granulomatous tissue and pockets of thin pus-containing, yellow, sand-like granules are the main pathological changes found in this condition. The soft tissues of the head, the oesophagus and oesophageal groove may also be involved. The lymph nodes are not involved.

Diagnosis

Diagnosis is straightforward and based on the clinical signs. Confirmation of diagnosis is made by staining the crushed yellow granules found in the pus and demonstrating the Gram-positive filamentous rods.

Treatment

Treatment with iodides as recommended for actinobacillosis is sometimes advocated (see p. 823). Injecting the swelling with penicillin is also occasionally recommended; however, because of the nature of lesions such treatment is unsatisfactory. Intramuscular injection of penicillin may assist, but once better casualty slaughter should be advised as lesions are likely to recur.

Teeth

Dental problems are rare in cattle. Fractures of the mandibular teeth occur occasionally and traumatic injuries can result in incisor teeth being displaced or lost. Excessive wear of the incisors indicates advancing age. Discoloration of the teeth may result from prolonged treatments with oxytetracyclines during the teeth development phase (see p. 1043). Discoloration and pitted enamel will occur as a sign of fluorosis (see p. 949).

Jaw abscesses may result from infection gaining access during tooth eruption.

Occasionally, heifers will experience problems with feed when teeth are erupting. This will be particularly noticeable if the forage is in the form of self-feed silage and the clamp well compacted.

Foreign bodies do occasionally become lodged between the teeth or between the teeth and the buccal mucosa.

Anatomy

Cattle have both temporary and permanent dentition. The upper front teeth are absent and the premaxilla is attached by a layer of fibrous tissue covered by a thick horny epithelium. There are 20 deciduous teeth with a dental formula of:

$$I\frac{0}{3} \quad C\frac{0}{1} \quad P\frac{3}{3} \quad M\frac{0}{0} \quad \times 2 = 20$$

In the permanent dentition the three pairs of premolars in each jaw are supplemented by three pairs of upper and lower molars:

$$I\frac{0}{3} \quad C\frac{0}{1} \quad P\frac{3}{3} \quad M\frac{3}{3} \quad \times 2 = 32$$

The front teeth, three incisors and one canine are all spatulate and arranged in a broad arch. The fixation of the teeth allows some dorsoventral movement within the alveoli. There is a large gap or diastema separating the front teeth from those of the cheek. The cheek teeth increase in size caudally and the lower premolars and molars are narrower than the upper ones.

The age of tooth eruption varies between *Bos taurus* and *Bos indicus* and also depends on breed, sex and state of nutrition. Examination of the permanent incisors is frequently used to give an indication of age.

The deciduous teeth have little use in age determination. Calves are frequently born with fully erupted incisors and all will be in place by one month of age.

The average age for tooth eruption in European-type cattle is shown in Table 48.1. However, the standard deviation is approximately 10 per cent of the average age. Thus for a given age of development, e.g. 2.5 years, 95 per cent of the population will be 2.5 years ± 0.5 years, i.e. 2–3 years.

The oesophagus

Emesis or vomiting (see p. 139)

Emesis (vomiting) is not a common sign in ruminants. Reverse peristalsis of the oesophagus is a normal physiological process in rumination.

Table 48.1 Average age for tooth eruption in European-type cattle (*Bos taurus*).

Tooth	Deciduous	Permanent
1st incisor	Before birth	22 months
2nd incisor	Before birth	27 months
3rd incisor	Before birth to 2 weeks	37 Months
Canine	Before birth to 2 weeks	44 months
1st premolar	Birth to 3 weeks	27 months
2nd premolar	Birth to 3 weeks	24 months
3rd premolar	Birth to 3 weeks	33 months
1st molar	–	6 months
2nd molar	–	12 months
3rd molar	–	24 months

However, vomiting (when rumen contents are ejected from the mouth) does occasionally occur in actinobacillosis of the oesophageal groove or with painful conditions of the mouth caused by teeth erupting. The ejection of rumen contents is also frequently seen in the terminal stages of milk fever, the result of rumen pressure caused by tympany accompanying oesophageal relaxation that occurs with hypocalcaemia, not by reverse peristalsis. Grain overload (rumen acidosis), traumatic reticulitis, diaphragmatic hernia, vagal indigestion and abomasal impaction have all been reported to produce emesis, but in the author's experience vomiting is not normally associated with these conditions. Emesis as a herd problem has been reported to occur following the consumption of spoiled maize silage. In the UK poisoning with azalea or rhododendron species (see p. 943) is probably the most common cause of vomiting in cattle, although poisoning by lily of the valley (*Convallania majalis*) and sneezeweed (*Helenium loopesii*) has been reported to cause vomiting in cattle in the USA.

Diseases of the oesophagus

Disorders of the oesophagus are relatively rare. Mucosal disease/BVD does produce shallow ulcerative lesions of the oesophagus (see p. 853). Malignant catarrh (see p. 935) also produces characteristic lesions of the oesophagus and occasionally oesophageal lesions may be found in calves suffering from calf diphtheria (see pp. 250, 822). Primary conditions of the oesophagus are:

- Traumatic lacerations
- Stenosis caused by pressure from outside the oesophagus
- Obstruction or choke
- Dilatation (see p. 139)

Oesophageal trauma

The usual cause of lacerations to the oesophagus is the result of careless use of a probang, stomach tube, or bolusing, which can sometimes cause rupture. As the probang is rarely used in cattle practice nowadays this problem is uncommon. If rupture of the oesophagus is suspected, then immediate slaughter should be recommended.

Oesophageal stenosis

Stenosis due to pressure outside the oesophagus can be caused by gross swelling of the mediastinal lymph nodes. This used to be a problem associated with tuberculosis, but more recently it has been reported to be associated with lymphomatosis. Oesophageal stenosis caused by swollen mediastinal lymph nodes resulting in chronic bloat in calves three to six months old is sometimes reported in calves recovering from pneumonia.

Choke

Oesophageal obstruction or choke is a relatively common problem in cattle. As cattle consume food rapidly, incomplete mastication is normal. Regurgitation and remastication of food boluses is relied upon to ensure food is ground into small particles. Apples, potato tubers or portions of root vegetables, such as turnips, fodder beet or mangolds, will all be swallowed in relatively large pieces, often without any mastication. The occurrence of choke therefore mirrors the fashions in feeding cattle. When potatoes are in excess and inexpensive they are used as cattle feed and when mangolds and turnips were widely used choke was common. The presentation of the root crops also affects the occurrence of choke. If large roots such as fodder beet or mangolds are fed whole then choke is uncommon, but if chopped they will attempt to swallow without mastication pieces of root that are too big to pass down the oesophagus. Strip-grazing root crops, such as stubble turnips, also rarely results in choke. Presumably cattle bite relatively small pieces at a time. This is probably why the most common causes of choke are apples and potatoes, which are the right size to obstruct the oesophagus, are difficult to masticate being round and slippery and are rarely chopped before being fed. If potatoes are being fed, ample bunker space is essential for all cows to eat simultaneously. If not, cows trying to barge through to reach the feed bunker may cause the cow eating inadvertently to swallow a whole potato it might otherwise chew.

Signs

Profuse salivation, followed by bloat, are the principal signs of choke because the obstructed oesophagus prevents swallowing of saliva and eructation of rumen gas. Affected cows will look distressed, the head is extended forwards and frequent attempts to swallow are often evident. Excess chewing movements are frequently observed and coughing, due to saliva accumulation in the pharynx, may occur.

The extent of the rumen tympany is related to the length of time choke has been present and the nature of the object. A round object such as an apple or potato will completely obstruct the oesophagus and death from bloat may be a sequel. If the offending object is irregularly shaped, such as a root or a portion of a potato, some gas may escape past the obstruction and death from bloat will be avoided.

Diagnosis

Diagnosis is usually made on the basis of the signs of excess salivation, rumen tympany, forward extensions of the head and the history of the availability of offending feeds. The obstruction is usually at one of three sites:

- Alongside the larynx in the upper oesophagus
- At the entrance to the chest
- In the thoracic portion of the oesophagus.

The cervical sites are more commonly involved than the thoracic oesophagus and occasionally the obstruction will be between the laryngeal area and the entrance to the chest.

Usually the obstruction can be seen and palpated as a discrete swelling, although if it is present alongside the larynx confusion with the thyroid cartilage may occur. If in doubt or an obstruction in the thoracic oesophagus is suspected the passage of a stomach tube will aid the diagnosis. If the stomach tube reaches the rumen and the tympany is relieved, an obstruction, if it existed, will probably have been dislodged. The differential diagnosis should not present problems, although indigestion and tympany may be mistaken for bloat. Bronchitis, because of the cough and protruding tongue, may be, but should not be, confused with choke. Once the obstruction has been located, either by palpation or by stomach tube, diagnosis presents no problems except with rabies (p. 908). Excess salivation is the only sign both rabies and choke have in common so the possibility of rabies must be eliminated by assessing other signs before proceeding along the diagnostic pathway to choke.

Treatment

Before treatment commences, the animal will need to be restrained in a cattle crush or at least tied in a byre stanchion. A bulldog-type nose handler is used by an assistant further to restrain the animal and keep the head from moving. The first element of treatment is to assess the severity of the rumen tympany. If the animal is in distress because of bloat, this is relieved by inserting a cannula into the rumen in the left sublumbar fossa, using a standard bovine trochar and cannula.

If the obstruction is in the cervical oesophagus a spasmolytic such as hyoscine *N*-butylbromide and dipyrone or butylscopolamine bromide and metamizole is administered by intravenous injection and five minutes allowed to elapse before attempting to move the obstruction. The spasmolytic will relax the smooth muscle of the oesophagus, which is in spasm and contracted firmly around the obstruction. Five minutes after the spasmolytic has been administered the operator, using his fingers in the jugular groove with an assistant holding the head forward, gradually pushes the obstruction up the oesophagus until it reaches the laryngeal area. Frequently, when at this position and the spasmolytic has taken effect, upward pressure with the fingers will cause the object to be ejected into the mouth. If this does not happen then a mouth gag has to be applied to keep the mouth open and a second assistant places his forearm into the mouth and pharynx and, simultaneously with the operator pushing the object upwards, will grasp it and be able to remove it. If the object is large and appears reluctant to move, this latter procedure can be carried out under anaesthesia. It is the author's experience that anaesthesia has not been required since spasmolytics have been available.

If the obstruction is in the thoracic oesophagus this will have been detected by the use of a stomach tube. The application of gentle pressure with the stomach tube will dislodge the obstruction and push it into the rumen. Again spasmolytic administration will enable the obstruction to be more readily moved. On occasions the obstruction will move on into the rumen without pressure following the spasmolytic injection. If the efforts described do not remove a thoracic oesophageal obstruction, a probang may be used. However, care must be exercised when using the probang, as the pressure applied must not be too severe for fear of lacerating the oesophagus. If the probang fails to dislodge the obstruction a rumenotomy may be considered and the object removed from the oesophagus manually via the rumen.

In preference to a rumenotomy and if it is certain that the obstruction is caused by vegetable matter, a rumen trochar may be sutured in place in the left sublumbar fossa to prevent bloat and the obstruction allowed to macerate. This may take two to four days but is usually effective.

Prevention

Choke can be prevented by the shredding or chopping of root vegetables into small pieces that will not cause obstruction. If potatoes are fed, ample feeding space is required and if they are offered at pasture they should be placed in the field before the cows enter. Cows will follow a vehicle that is unloading food and will attempt to eat while on the move. If they attempt to eat potatoes or apples while on the move they are more likely to choke. It is rare for apples to be intentionally fed to cattle. However, when cattle graze orchards, windfall apples should be collected before allowing cattle access. This will not only prevent choke but also rumen acidosis (see p. 829) from overeating apples.

Upper alimentary squamous cell carcinoma (see also p. 946)

Occurrence

Squamous cell carcinoma of the upper alimentary tract occurs sporadically in cattle grazing bracken areas. The problem usually affects beef cows and has been reported in Scotland and North Wales. It occurs on farms with a high bracken cover but is less common than another bracken-induced disease, enzootic haematuria (see p. 947). Both conditions have been reported in the same animal. The disease generally occurs in animals over six years old. Almost invariably alimentary papillomata, in which papilloma virus can be demonstrated, occur in animals affected with bracken-induced squamous cell carcinoma. It is thought therefore that the disease is caused by a toxic factor present in bracken that activates papillomata in the alimentary tract to develop into squamous cell carcinomas.

Signs

The clinical signs can be divided into four main syndromes that are related to the site of the carcinoma, which can occur in the pharynx, oesophagus or rumen.

Oropharyngeal syndrome: The presence of the carcinoma in the oropharyngeal region will produce a chronic wasting condition of one to six months' duration. A cough may be present in the last two to four weeks of the disease and excess salivation and drooling will often be evident. Snoring may also be a feature and halitosis is frequent. Examination will reveal a tumour in the mouth or pharynx. Papillomas will also be present. The submandibular lymph nodes may be enlarged.

Oesophageal syndrome: If present in the oesophagus the carcinoma will produce signs similar to choke with partial or complete occlusion of the oesophagus. Halitosis, coughing and drooling may be present and gurgling sounds may be heard coming from the oesophagus. The passage of a stomach tube may prove difficult. The history will include a gradual weight loss over a period of one to three months. Papillomata may be present in the mouth or pharynx. A palpable mass in the oesophageal region will be present.

Ruminal tympany syndrome: Carcinoma of the reticuloruminal cardia or thoracic oesophagus will produce intermittent ruminal tympany following a period of one to six months of gradual weight loss. The passage of a stomach tube will prove difficult. Papillomata of the mouth and pharynx will usually be present and profuse diarrhoea is a common feature.

Wasting and diarrhoea syndrome: If the carcinoma is present in the dorsal pigmented area of the rumen symptoms of rumen indigestion will be present. The tumours in the rumen can reach 30–50 cm (12–20 inches) in diameter. A slow loss of weight over up to nine months is followed by diarrhoea, which contains much fibrous undigested material. Ruminal tympany is usually present and the abdomen is often pendulous. Papillomata are usually found in the mouth or pharynx.

Diagnosis

The diagnosis may at first be difficult, as the signs may resemble choke (p. 826) or rumen indigestion (see p. 829). However, the history of the slow weight loss, the presence of bracken and the occurrence in older beef cows will considerably aid the diagnosis. As papillomata are almost invariably found in the mouth or pharynx of affected animals a thorough examination of the mouth should be made if the other signs are present. Johne's disease (p. 857) may also be confused with this condition but the distinguishing feature is the consistency of the faeces. In Johne's disease the faeces are homogeneous, there being no signs of undigested fibrous material.

Treatment and prevention

There is no treatment and as the condition is invariably fatal affected animals should be slaughtered as soon as possible.

To prevent the condition, cattle should not have access to bracken. Where bracken exists on a farm cows will rarely eat the bracken if adequate food is available.

Diseases of the rumen

There are a number of diseases that affect the rumen, all of which cause inappetence, reduced milk yield and failure to thrive. An essential element in a thorough clinical examination of the bovine is to observe whether the rumen is tympanic by observing distention of the left sublumbar fossa, the animal is chewing its cud, eructating normally and normal rumen contractions are taking place. Rumen contractions can be detected by palpating with slight pressure in the left sublumbar fossa and detecting the rumen movements, which occur approximately every 30 seconds. Eructation will accompany every second rumen contraction.

Indigestion

Simple indigestion is to be suspected if the rumen contractions are weaker than normal, are less frequent and the clinical examination has revealed no other evidence of disease.

Simple indigestion is frequently seen in dairy cows when new feeds are suddenly introduced to the diet. Intakes of large quantities of very wet grass, frosted feeds, sour or spoiled feed, e.g. butyric or soil-contaminated silage, or the sudden introduction of large quantities of concentrate feeds may all predispose to the onset of indigestion. The accidental intake of small quantities of antibiotics, which disturb the rumen flora, will also precipitate indigestion, as is seen in feedlot beef cattle when rations containing monensin sodium are first introduced. Dairy cow concentrate rations containing as little as 0.005 mg/kg dry matter (DM) of lincomycin have been incriminated in causing severe indigestion of whole dairy herds with a consequent 50 per cent reduction in the herd milk production. The lincomycin contamination occurred at the compound mill where the milling equipment was used to produce dairy concentrate immediately following the production of a pig feed containing lincomycin.

Relatively minor changes in rumen pH are likely to cause atony of the rumen. The intake of any indigestible, stale or sour feeds will interrupt the process of rumen fermentation, which changes the pH resulting in rumen atony. The sudden introduction of new feeds to which the rumen is unaccustomed will have a similar effect.

The rumen is a versatile fermentation chamber and will accommodate a wide, variety of feeds, e.g. 100 per cent cereal diets in feedlot beef production, extremely wet grass in some seasons and highly fibrous foods such as hay or straw. However, if changes to the diet are made the rumen flora have to adapt to the new feed and to prevent indigestion occurring, the changes should be gradual. Thus new food should be introduced in small quantities at first, with the intake being gradually increased daily.

Signs

The first clinical sign of simple indigestion will be reduced appetite and in dairy cattle a simultaneous milk yield reduction will be apparent. The reduction in feed intake may be as much as 50 per cent with no other obvious signs. The cow may be slightly depressed. Rectal temperature will be normal and heart rate raised slightly to around 80/minute. There may be mild diarrhoea and a mild rumen tympany may be present. In chronic cases of indigestion undigested fibre may be present in the faeces. Rumen contractions will be reduced in strength and frequency, often to as few as one contraction every 3 or 4 minutes.

Diagnosis

Diagnosis of simple indigestion will be based on the clinical examination and the elimination of any other disease. There is very little in the way of laboratory tests that can be useful. An increase or decrease in rumen pH may be a useful guide but tends not to be used in practice because of its impracticability. The history may be the most useful clinical indicator and may suggest a 'feed problem'. If only one cow in the herd is affected the history may not be helpful and the diagnosis more difficult. However, if the whole herd or a substantial part of the herd were suddenly affected with inappetence it would be quite logical to suspect a 'feed problem'.

Other diseases that may be readily confused with simple indigestion are displaced abomasum, traumatic reticulitis, lesions of the oesphageal groove, early milk fever and acetonaemia. A thorough clinical examination will eliminate these other diseases.

Treatment

Many animals suffering from indigestion will recover spontaneously in two to three days if they are removed from the offending diet and allowed access to good quality hay.

A large number of treatments for indigestion have been employed and were administered as drenches. Historically mixtures containing nux vomica, gentian, sodium bicarbonate, magnesium carbonate, etc. were frequently used and acted by altering the rumen pH and stimulating appetite and even providing vitamins and trace elements essential for rumen microbial synthesis. However regulations on the use of licensed medicines in food animals have resulted in all such preparations being withdrawn by the manufacturers.

If the rumen is atonic for more than 24 hours the administration of rumen inoculum obtained either from an abattoir or a healthy cow will aid recovery. Probiotics may also be helpful.

Prevention

The prevention of indigestion is not always straightforward. The avoidance of abrupt changes in feeds and of indigestible, sour or putrefied feeds is relatively easy. However, cows will break out into pastures where they should not be and will, if given the opportunity, consume foods of dubious quality in large enough quantities to be harmful. The frequency of occurrence of simple indigestion on a farm is likely to be inversely related to the quality of management that exists.

Rumen acidosis (grain overload, overeating syndrome, barley poisoning)

Wherever intensive livestock production is practised acute indigestion as a result of excessive intakes of grain, beans or compound feed is common, either as a result of cattle gaining accidental access to grain stores or by the sudden introduction of unlimited supplies of grain to the diet. There are two distinct syndromes associated with overeating.

The most common is acute acidosis as the result of consuming excess carbohydrate, which rapidly ferments leading to lactic acidosis followed by acute dehydration and depression. Accidental access to compound feed stores by cattle, who will readily consume 15–20 kg of concentrate, is the most common scenario but the problem is also seen in feedlot beef cattle fed *ad libitum* cereal-based diets, particularly when the diet is first introduced. Excess intake of apples by cattle grazing orchards is also a common cause of rumen acidosis.

Alkalosis: A less common syndrome occurs as a result of excessive intake of highly fermentable proteinaceous feeds, e.g. soya bean, which results in excess ammonia production in the rumen leading to alkalosis with excitement and hyperaesthesia.

Pathogenesis

The rumen can be visualized as a continuous culture fermentation vat. The rumen microflora constitute the culture, which grows on the substrate or medium being provided by the feed the animal consumes. The rumen microflora form a balanced colony of bacteria and various protozoa. If the feed content changes the balance of the microflora will need to change, e.g. increase in intakes of highly fermentable carbohydrate will lead to streptococci and lactobacilli organisms predominating. With a normal balanced microflora the fermentation end products are the volatile fatty acids (acetic, propionic and butyric acids), which are absorbed from the rumen. Bacterial cell proteins for digestion and absorption in the lower intestine and water-soluble vitamins are also products of the fermentation process.

The streptococci and lactobacilli organisms that predominate when excess carbohydrate is ingested produce lactic acid as a fermentation end product. Lactic acid production increases the rumen osmotic pressure and fluid is drawn into the rumen from body tissues. The rumen pH also drops and the majority of Gram-negative bacteria and protozoa are destroyed. The pH may drop to 4.5. The lactic acid is converted to sodium lactate, which is absorbed directly from the rumen into the blood or is passed down the intestinal tract and absorbed from the abomasum or small intestine. The presence of sodium lactate in the small intestine produces an osmotic gradient and draws water into the small intestine, thus contributing to the diarrhoea. The sodium lactate in the blood reduces blood pH.

Chemical damage to the rumen mucosal epithelium results in bacterial and fungal organisms penetrating the rumen wall and in chronic acidosis will lead to the occurrence of liver abscesses, which are frequently seen in beef cattle raised on 100 per cent cereal diets.

Urine output will be decreased as a result of the dehydration and will also be acidic, containing high levels of lactate. The damage to the rumen epithelium leads to a chronic rumenitis, which in turn causes an increased incidence of bloat. This is often seen in feedlots as a cause of sudden death. Although the main signs of acidosis are the result of lactate absorption an additional component may be the absorption of endotoxins released from the destruction of large numbers of Gram-negative bacteria in the rumen.

Signs

The speed of onset and the severity of clinical signs will depend on the quantity and nature of the food consumed and whether the rumen is adapted to that particular feed. Newly introduced feeds may well prove fatal to animals that are not accustomed to the particular feed in quantities that other animals consume regularly. Also, feedlot animals that are apparently accustomed to cereal diets will sometimes overeat for no apparent reason. Feedlot cattle being fed cereal diets are probably in a continuous state of mild acidosis and a relatively small increase in intake will produce enough lactic acid to destroy the remaining Gram-negative bacteria and produce clinical signs of acidosis. Problems also arise should cattle on *ad libitum* feed run out of cereal and then are immediately introduced to the old level. Water deprivation can also produce a problem.

Clinical signs usually become apparent 12–36 hours after the engorgement. Incoordination and ataxia are the first signs to be noticed with the stockworker reporting the cattle as 'drunk'. The animals will be anorexic, they may appear to be blind and will rapidly become weak and depressed. The rumen will be distended producing abdominal pain, which causes the animal to grunt or grind its teeth and ruminal movements cease.

Dehydration becomes apparent within 24–48 hours and severe diarrhoea will be evident in animals that do not die immediately. The faeces will be a pale 'pasty' colour. Respiratory rate will be raised because of the acidosis, the rectal temperature depressed by 1–2°C (2–4°F), the heart rate is in excess of 180/minute and the pulse weak. Severe cases will become recumbent with the head resting on the shoulder, as in milk fever. Death will occur within 24–48 hours in acute cases.

In feedlot cattle that recover some animals fail to thrive even after apparent recovery and this can be due to chronic rumenitis, liver abscesses, or chronic laminitis (p. 420).

Alkalosis: The signs are not completely typical but they do involve muscle tremors, convulsions and slow shallow respiration. In the later stages there may be dyspnoea and hyperpnoea.

Clinical pathology

Affected animals are dehydrated and show haemoconcentration. Blood pH may also be depressed. The pH of rumen contents will be 4 or lower and urine pH around 5.

However, in practice, laboratory tests are rarely performed because of the necessity to institute treatment quickly and the diagnosis is rarely a problem. In order to assess blood pH, bicarbonate and total carbon dioxide levels need also to be measured.

At post mortem of acute cases the rumen will be distended, containing excess fluid with evidence of grain particles present. Rumen pH evaluation at post mortem is of no value unless done immediately after death because post-mortem changes will increase the pH. Chronic acidosis as a result of long-term cereal intake may be characterized by rumenitis, although to observe this the examination must be performed soon after death. Multiple liver abscesses may also be present in chronic acidosis.

Alkalosis: If the less common syndrome of alkalosis is present due to the ingestion of excess soya beans or similar high-protein feeds, the rumen pH may be alkaline and the urine and blood pH will also be raised. On occasions there is a paradoxical acidic urine.

Diagnosis

Diagnosis is not usually difficult and is frequently made on the history together with signs of incoordination and ataxia. In feedlot beef animals it is usual for several of the group to be affected, but with dairy cattle any number may be affected, depending on how many cows had accidental access to the grain store, which is the most common scenario. Cows grazing orchards will consume large quantities of apples, particularly after a storm, and again the history should be of considerable help in reaching a diagnosis.

Laboratory tests are not normally necessary and unless a result can be available within an hour or so are of no value in the practice situation because to be effective, treatment must be administered as quickly as possible. The prognosis for peracute recumbent cases is very poor, but for the less acute standing cases the prognosis is relatively good provided treatment is not delayed.

Treatment

In peracute recumbent cases the rumen should be emptied by rumenotomy (pp. 834, 1106) and the dehy-

Table 48.2 McSherry's solution.

Sodium chloride	4.95 g
Sodium acetate	7.50 g
Potassium chloride	0.75 g
Calcium chloride	0.30 g
Magnesium chloride	0.30 g
Water	1 litre

dration and acidosis corrected using a balanced electrolyte, e.g. McSherry's solution (see Table 48.2), and 5 per cent sodium bicarbonate solution intravenously. Up to 60 l of electrolyte solution will be required for an adult cow over a 24-hour period. Up to 300 ml of 5 per cent sodium bicarbonate solution may also be administered, the quantity required depending on the degree of acidosis present and can be assessed by observing a slowing down of the respiratory rate during its administration, if given slowly. Supportive therapy should include intravenous calcium borogluconate (400 ml of 30 per cent solution) and 400 ml of 40 per cent dextrose solution.

For less acute cases that are still standing, the oral administration of magnesium hydroxide, magnesium carbonate or aluminium hydroxide at a dose rate of 1 g/kg body weight mixed in 10 l of warm water and administered by stomach tube will help restore rumen pH. The dehydration and acidosis is corrected using an electrolyte solution and sodium bicarbonate intravenously as for peracute cases. Intravenous administration of a vitamin B/vitamin C mixture is widely used in the UK with apparent success. Doses of 30–50 ml intravenously are frequently used and are thought to aid detoxification of lactate in the liver.

Antihistamines are also considered to be of value by some clinicians. Calcium borogluconate and 40 per cent dextrose are also useful as supportive therapy when administered intravenously.

Alkalosis: Treatment of alkalosis resulting from soya bean or high-protein engorgement should consist of an electrolyte mixture containing excess chloride such as Ringer's solution. Volumes of 30–50 l will be required over a 24-hour period, but no bicarbonate should be used. All concentrate feeds should be withdrawn from the diet and only hay or silage offered.

Prevention

Bulk storage of concentrates in large bins has reduced the incidence of acidosis in many dairy herds where accidental access of feed stores with concentrate stored in bags was once quite common.

In feedlots where concentrated food is fed *ad libitum*, often to the exclusion of long fibre, introduction to the concentrate must be gradual and the feed bunkers should be of adequate size to allow all animals to feed together. The feeders should not be allowed to empty to avoid excessive intake by hungry animals once the feeders are refilled. Continuous access to the food will allow 'little and often' intakes of food. Ideally, some roughage should always be available even if it only represents 10 per cent of the DM intake. Roughage availability has been shown to reduce the incidence of liver abscesses in cereal-produced beef in the UK. It is also advisable that the grains should not be finely ground, which in itself encourages rapid fermentation. The grain should be cracked or rolled and more recently whole grain has been fed without seriously affecting the digestion of the cereal.

Rumen parakeratosis

Parakeratosis of the rumen epithelium is a common sequel to the feeding of 100 per cent concentrate diets to cattle. The disease is characterized by enlargement and hardening of the rumen mucosa papillae and may affect 100 per cent of animals reared on 100 per cent cereal diets. The disease syndrome also includes the associated lesions of liver abscesses and possibly laminitis. Parakeratosis may occur as a secondary stage of acute rumen acidosis.

Pathogenesis

The association between liver abscesses, lesions of the rumen mucosa and the feeding of 100 per cent concentrate diets to ruminants has long been recognized. The lower rumen pH associated with concentrate diets and the consequent increase in lactic acid production produces an inflammatory reaction of the rumen mucosa. This damage to the mucosa allows debris to adhere to the mucosa causing ulceration and infection and resulting in abscess formation in the rumen wall. The rumen papillae become enlarged and thickened and may clump together to form bundles in response to the inflammatory reaction. The papillae may contain excessive layers of keratinized epithelial cells, particles of food and bacteria. A sequel to the damage to the rumen mucosa is the presence of liver abscesses. Some workers also report that laminitis is a later sequel but, as laminitis has been found in the absence of rumen and liver lesions, the role of acidosis in the aetiology of laminitis is far from clear.

Signs

Rumen parakeratosis does not necessarily produce signs of disease, although it has been reported that the addition of 10 per cent hay or silage to the diet of 100 per cent cereal-fed cattle will improve appetite and weight gain. Some individual animals that are seriously affected with abscesses in the rumen wall and liver may show reduced appetite and reduced growth rate, par-

ticularly towards the end of the feeding period. Complications such as peritonitis, septicaemia or even endocarditis may occasionally be evident.

Diagnosis

The diagnosis in the live animal is extremely difficult because the reduced growth rate and inappetance are signs of many diseases. As it is a group problem the detection of the rumen wall lesions and liver abscesses at post mortem will be the best diagnostic indicator.

Treatment and prevention

The treatment of individual cases by the time they show inappetance and poor growth rates is unrewarding because of the severity of the damage to the rumen wall and liver. However, if the problem is suspected (by the post-mortem examination of some animals from the same farm at the abattoir) feeding 10–20 per cent of the diet in the form of long roughage will prevent deterioration and allow the animals to reach slaughter weight. Prevention depends on the inclusion of 10 per cent long fibre in the diet, although recent experience has shown that feeding whole grains will reduce if not eliminate the problem of rumen parakeratosis and liver abscesses.

Bloat (rumen tympany) (see also p. 234)

Bloat or rumen tympany is a disease easily recognized and feared by cattle farmers. Bloat refers to an excessive accumulation of gas in the rumen and, because of a failure to eructate, rumen distension occurs, frequently resulting in death. It is a major cause of death in cattle in all intensive livestock areas of the world.

There are two types of bloat, gaseous bloat or secondary rumen tympany and frothy bloat or primary rumen tympany.

Gaseous bloat (secondary rumen tympany): Any condition that causes an oesophageal obstruction or that interferes with eructation will produce gaseous bloat. The condition is generally sporadic in occurrence and is less common than frothy bloat. The following conditions will lead to gaseous bloat:

- Lesions of the oesophageal groove, e.g. vagus indigestion, abscessation or infection with *A. lignieresii* obstruct the groove and prevent eructation (pp. 826, 837).
- Physical obstruction of the groove with afterbirth has been reported (p. 836).
- Physical obstruction of the oesophagus with potatoes or other root vegetables causing choke will prevent eructation (p. 826).
- Pressure on the oesophagus by enlarged mediastinal or bronchial lymph nodes prevents gas escaping through the oesophagus. This is a common problem in

growing cattle three to six months old, particularly those that have been affected with pneumonia (p. 239).

- Inability to eructate is also a feature of tetanus (p. 733) and milk fever (p. 781) and gaseous bloat is a frequent feature of these diseases.
- Prolonged lateral recumbency as a result of disease or animals that are cast for prolonged surgery will frequently lead to gaseous bloat because of the inability of the rumen gas to escape. Cattle that inadvertently fall in dorsal recumbency into ditches will generally die of bloat if not retrieved in time.
- Severe damage to the rumen epithelium following acute acidosis may lead to rumen atony and accumulation of gas (p. 829).
- Excess cereal ingestion usually results in gaseous bloat (p. 829).

Frothy bloat (primary rumen tympany): Frothy bloat is much more common than gaseous bloat and usually affects several animals in the group at the same time. Although frothy bloat does occur in feedlot cattle it is more generally associated with pasture feeding. Pastures that are most commonly incriminated in the cause of frothy bloat usually contain high levels of leguminous plants, particularly clover or alfalfa.

Frothy bloat is extremely common in some countries, e.g. New Zealand (p. 127), due to the high content of clover in the sward. In these situations the problem is well recognized and anticipated so that prevention regimens are universally applied. In the UK, frothy bloat can appear suddenly without warning on lush spring or autumn pastures and up to 25 per cent of the herd may be suddenly affected. Some of these pastures may not contain a high clover content. The onset may be extremely sudden, often 4–6 hours after milking and return to the grazing areas. The only warning that the farmer experiences is the bellowing of several cows in extreme pain, and on reaching the field there may be several cows recumbent or even dead, with many others exhibiting rumen tympany to varying degrees of severity.

Pathogenesis

Bloat is the result of the inability to eliminate gas from the rumen by eructation. With gaseous bloat this is secondary to some other condition or disease.

With frothy bloat eructation is prevented by the accumulation of froth, which prevents gas escaping into the oesophagus. The production of froth or foam is a result of the raised viscosity of the rumen fluid and the small bubbles of gas, the natural product of rumen fermentation, cannot coalesce. Under certain conditions some naturally occurring plant substances, e.g. saponins, pectins, hemicellulose and certain proteins, will raise the viscosity of rumen fluid. There also appears to be an individual animal susceptibility. Succulent, high-protein plants, particularly the leguminous plants in the pre-

bloom stage, undoubtedly predispose to the occurrence of frothy bloat. Frothy bloat does also occur in feedlot cattle, particularly if fed on finely ground grain. This may be due to the gases being trapped by the fine particles of feed, but the rapid fermentation that follows the feeding of finely ground grain is undoubtedly a contributory factor. Adaptation to a particular feed is also important. As the rumen microflora adapts itself to the particular pasture or ration there is a tendency towards reduced susceptibility.

Signs

Rumen tympany, as evidenced by distension of the left sublumbar fossa, is well recognized by most stockworkers and should present no problems. With severe tympany the animal will be exhibiting signs of pain, e.g. kicking its ventral abdomen and bellowing. The bellowing can frequently be heard up to 500 m ($\frac{1}{3}$ mile) away. In acute frothy bloat the disease progresses rapidly and the animal soon becomes recumbent and can die in 30–60 minutes from the onset of tympany.

Pathology

Post-mortem bloat in ruminants that die from other causes can be confusing to the diagnosis of the condition. If the animal is seen soon after death, death from bloat will be obvious because of the gross abdominal distension and at post-mortem examination oedema in the inguinal and ventral perineal region together with congestion and haemorrhage in the anterior parts of the carcass will be evident. The liver will be extremely pale due to compression and the rumen will be grossly distended and contain froth. The quantity of froth present declines after death. Rupture of the diaphragm and the abdominal musculature, particularly in the inguinal region, may also be apparent. Death from gaseous bloat is less common, but the absence of froth and the finding of a primary lesion should differentiate it from frothy bloat.

Diagnosis

The preliminary diagnosis presents no problems and is based on distension of the left sublumbar fossa. If only one animal is affected in the herd the bloat is probably a gaseous bloat but if several animals are affected to varying degrees and they are at pasture the diagnosis will certainly be frothy bloat. However, if there is any doubt the passage of a stomach tube will provide the answer. If the problem is one of gaseous bloat and the stomach tube reaches the rumen and possibly removes an obstruction on the way, the gas will escape through the stomach tube and the rumen will rapidly revert to its normal size. If gaseous bloat is confirmed and the bloat relieved, a full clinical examination should be performed to ascertain the cause of the failure to eructate.

If the bloat is due to froth little or no gas will escape via the stomach tube, which will itself become blocked with froth.

Treatment

The traditional treatment for bloat was the passing of a 5 mm diameter trochar and cannula into the rumen via the left sublumbar fossa. Many farmers possess such a trochar and cannula. However, this instrument is of little use because gaseous bloat can nearly always be relieved by stomach tube and only when this is not possible should a rumen trochar and cannula be used. For frothy bloat the cannula itself becomes blocked with froth and does little to relieve the tympany.

Treatment for all but the peracute cases necessitates the passing of a stomach tube and, if this reveals the bloat to be frothy, antifoaming agents that reduce the viscosity of the rumen contents and disperse the froth can be passed down the stomach tube. Vegetable oils such as linseed, peanut, corn or soya bean oil are all useful antifoaming agents. Traditionally, 500 ml of linseed oil to which is added 50 ml of turpentine was effectively used as a bloat drench, but this does tend to taint the milk. Oil mixed with detergent will disperse faster in the rumen ingesta.

Proprietary bloat drenches containing silicone or poloxalene are available (Table 48.3) and are equally effective. Within five minutes of administration of the antifoaming agent the animal will start to eructate and in most cases the tympany will be relieved within one hour. If tympany still exists after one hour, a further administration of an antifoaming agent by drench may be given. If tympany still exists one hour after the second drench the diagnosis should be reassessed and a stomach tube passed to ensure there is no oesophageal obstruction. Once the diagnosis of frothy bloat has been established in a group of affected animals the less acute cases can be treated by drenching alone.

In peracute cases where death is imminent and the animal is recumbent, it will be necessary to conduct an emergency rumenotomy (p. 1106). A 10–20 cm vertical incision is made in the mid point of the sublumbar fossa, using a sharp knife. On incising the rumen there will be an explosive release of rumen contents and marked relief for the cow. Following the release of the frothy rumen contents the wound is cleansed and sutured using the standard surgical closure. Antibiotics are administered postoperatively and recovery is usually uneventful.

Chronic gaseous bloat in calves and feedlot animals is often treated by establishing a 10–15-cm length rumen fistula. Under local anaesthesia the skin and musculature of the sublumbar fossa are incised and the rumen exposed. The rumen is then incised and the rumen wall sutured to the skin. Alternatively, a prosthetic device may be sutured into the abdominal wall and the rumen, allowing gas to escape (see p. 827). This device may be removed two to three months later and the wound allowed to granulate, by which time the primary cause of the bloat will have corrected itself.

Prevention

To prevent further cases of frothy bloat occurring when a sudden acute outbreak is encountered at pasture the cattle should he removed immediately, provided with dry food such as hay or straw and all cows showing any degree of rumen tympany drenched with an antifoaming agent. The pasture should not be used for grazing for at least 10 days.

Where risk pastures exist, e.g. those containing high proportions of legumes, gradual access to the pasture should be practised, starting with 10 minutes a day and increasing by 10 minutes each day. Long fibre should be fed before access is allowed to the pasture. Strip-grazing to restrict intake can be practised, but is not favoured by stock farmers who currently prefer paddock grazing or set stocking. However, during high-risk periods in problem areas these methods alone will not be satisfactory. In New Zealand and Australia, where the risk from bloat can be exceedingly high, during the spring, when the pasture is fast growing, the only satisfactory method of control has been the daily administration of antifoaming agents by drench after milking. Oils may be given at doses of up to 240 ml/day in high-risk periods, although 60–120 ml/day would be more common. Poloxalene, a non-ionic surfactant, is frequently used at 10–20 g/head per day and up to 40 g/day in high-risk periods.

If strip grazing is practised, the antifoaming oils can be emulsified with water and sprayed on the grass daily. Addition to the water supply is sometimes used, but effectiveness does depend on adequate individual intake.

Poloxalene can be added to grain mixtures or compound feed or even mineral blocks. However, in grass-rich areas, grain is rarely fed to cattle, particularly in the bloat-risk season of fast grass growth, and mineral blocks suffer from variable individual intake. Daily drenching has therefore become the preferred method of bloat prevention. The rumen implantation of a slow-release device containing an antifoaming agent has been developed in New Zealand and Australia.

Table 48.3 Treatments available for frothy bloat in the UK.

Name	Active ingredient	Manufacturer
Birp	Dimethicone	Arnolds
Bloat Guard	Poloxalene	Agrimin Ltd

The ultimate objective in bloat control is to develop pastures that have a low bloat-producing potential yet still possess the characteristics for high levels of production. The direction of development will be to develop strains of leguminous plants that have a low bloat-producing potential. To date some progress has been made in identifying the strains of red clover with the ability to produce less bloat, although it is recognized that sainfoin produces fewer tympany problems than clover. At the moment, pastures should not contain more than 50 per cent clover until such strains of clover are developed (p. 128).

Vagal indigestion

Vagal indigestion is a chronic condition of adult cattle with a slow insidious onset, but is still a differential diagnosis of rumen atony, simple indigestion or mild bloat. The incidence of vagal indigestion is now quite rare, the annual incidence being less than 1 in 10000, having decreased in recent years, probably mirroring the decline in the incidence of traumatic reticulitis.

Aetiology

Vagal indigestion is caused by interference with the function of the vagus nerve. The condition has been produced experimentally by severing the vagus (Xth cranial) nerve. The clinical syndromes vary slightly depending on the site of the nerve severence. In practice, the most common cause of nerve damage is the adhesions formed around the reticulum in advanced cases of traumatic reticulitis. The vagus nerve passes through the diaphragm in the region of the reticulum and is susceptible to damage in that area from the inflammation and infection that follow traumatic reticulitis. Other lesions that may damage the nerve would include actinobacillosis of the reticulum, infections of the mediastinal lymph nodes, e.g. tuberculosis, ruptured diaphragm or pleurisy. Sometimes cattle that survive surgery for abomasal torsion (p. 842) later develop signs of vagal indigestion. This could be the result of damage to the nerve caused by the torsion.

Because of the loss of function of the vagus nerve, ingesta are not transported from the rumen to the abomasum or from the abomasum through the pylorus, with the consequent result that the rumen and often the abomasum distend with fluid and ingesta producing abdominal distension.

Signs

The clinical signs are variable in that the abomasum is not always directly involved. Depending on the level at which the vagus nerve is damaged various syndromes can develop that are clinically classed as follows:

(1) Pyloric obstruction and abomasal impaction;
(2) Ruminal distension with atony;
(3) Ruminal distension with hypermotility. In some cases combinations will occur.

Pyloric obstruction and abomasal impaction: If the abomasum is involved there is a pyloric stenosis, which prevents ingesta leaving the abomasum. The ingesta accumulates, the abomasum becomes distended and can be palpated in the abdominal flank. Later the rumen becomes atonic and distends with fluid and ingesta.

Ruminal distension with atony: This is due either to a primary effect of the paralysed vagus nerve on rumen function or it can occur following (1) from a backflow from the distended abomasum. The effect of this is to produce a characteristic shape to the abdomen. The left flank is distended and well rounded as in mild bloat and the right flank is distended in the lower regions of the abdomen, giving the right flank a pear-shape appearance. This shape is characteristic of vagal indigestion. In some cases of vagal indigestion where only the rumen is affected the organ will be grossly distended, containing large quantities of fluid. Rumen contractions are infrequent and no rumen sound will be audible. Faecal output is decreased and the faeces are frequently of a pale pasty consistency. Rectal temperature is normal, the heart rate may be normal but in some cases is markedly decreased to around 40/minute. There is also dehydration, decreased milk yield and a gradual but progressive loss of body condition. Rectal examination will reveal a grossly distended rumen, reaching into the pelvic canal, and also the ventral rumen distended well over to the right side of the abdomen. The abomasum is not usually palpated per rectum. The fluid content of the rumen and the abomasum can be assessed by ballottement of the abdominal wall on both flanks.

Ruminal distension with hypermotility: There is slight ruminal tympany, and frequent and forceful rumen contractions. Recent body weight loss will be evident. Faeces are scant and pasty. Rectal palpation will reveal a gross distension of the dorsal sac of the rumen and the ventral sac will possess a U-shaped distension.

Clinical pathology

The experienced clinician will make his diagnosis on the clinical signs described and there are no laboratory tests that can be considered specific for vagal indigestion. The dehydration will increase the packed cell volume. If pyloric stenosis is present a metabolic alkalosis will be present with the effect of reducing scrum chloride to 40–50 mmol/l. An elevation of rumen chloride concentration (above 30 mmol/l) indicates abomasal reflux into the rumen.

Diagnosis

Veterinary advice is usually sought by the stockworker because it is noticed that the cow has slowly developed an abdominal distension and it is considered that the animal may be affected with bloat. A thorough clinical examination must be performed to establish the differential diagnosis.

If the animal is passing small quantities of pale pasty faeces, the left flank is rounded and distended, the right flank distended in the lower half only and the distension is due to fluid accumulation in the rumen and abomasum, and if the rectal temperature is normal and heart rate normal or slightly depressed, then a diagnosis of vagal indigestion can be made. However, many cases are brought to the veterinarian's attention before all the signs have fully developed and perhaps the right flank distension is not obvious. The insidious onset will distinguish the condition from bloat as will the fluid-filled rumen. Abomasal impaction must be distinguished by ballottement, which will indicate firm abomasal contents in impaction and fluid contents in pyloric stenosis.

Accumulation of fluid within the peritoneal cavity from ascites, peritonitis (p. 849) or ruptured urinary bladder can be differentiated by paracentesis. Hydrops allantois or amnii (p. 1119) will also produce severe abdominal distension, but will be differentiated on rectal examination.

Treatment

The prognosis in vagal indigestion is generally poor to hopeless and in most cases immediate slaughter is advised. If treatment is embarked upon because of the value of the animal the dehydration and any chloride deficit should be corrected. As much as 40–50 l of Ringer's solution may be required over 24 hours and given intravenously. It must be remembered that oral fluid therapy must not be contemplated because of the fluid retention in the rumen.

Following rehydration an exploratory laparotomy and rumenotomy may be performed. Adhesions around the reticulum can be palpated. A rumenotomy partially to empty the rumen is then performed and the reticulum and oesophageal groove examined for tumours or other lesions. The author, on one occasion, found a complete afterbirth wedged in the oesophageal groove in a cow that had not eaten since calving 10 days previously and was showing signs of rumen atony and distension. Removal of the afterbirth led to an uneventful recovery.

Even if tumours, adhesions or oesophageal lesions are discovered the prognosis is still likely to be hopeless so surgery should only be contemplated in valuable animals and a poor prognosis given before surgery commences.

Cold cow syndrome

Another rumen indigestion syndrome that has been reported from different areas of the UK has been named the cold cow syndrome. This syndrome usually occurs in early spring in lactating cows when grazing ryegrass pastures. The onset is sudden but not related to change in pasture use. Both poor and lush pastures have been involved and the occurrence is not related to levels of fertilizer use. The morbidity is high and varies from 8 to 100 per cent of the herd, but mortality is nil. Milk yield may be depressed by up to 50 per cent but recovers within two days. The condition was first recognized in Northern Ireland in the late 1970s and in the southwest of England in 1982 and has been reported in several years since.

Aetiology

The aetiology is unknown but several suggestions have been made. These include unusually high levels of soluble carbohydrate found in grass being grazed by affected herds (Jack, 1985). Other suggestions have been the oestrogenic zearalenone or other metabolites of field microfungi or the presence of high levels of soluble proteins or a protein metabolite. Climatic conditions have been investigated and cases have occurred during periods of frost, cold wet weather and during warm dry springs. Large night/day fluctuations in atmospheric temperature of the order of 17–18°C (30–32°F) accompanied one series of outbreaks.

Clinical pathology

Blood samples from affected cows have been examined for a wide range of biochemical parameters but no abnormalities have been detected.

Signs

A sudden onset of ataxia and incoordination, with a few animals being weak and becoming recumbent, followed by a copious non-smelling acute diarrhoea are the principal clinical signs. The cows behave as though they are drunk. The cows are characteristically cold to the touch as though in a state of shock but rectal temperatures are normal. Appetite is much reduced if not absent and the milk yield falls by up to 50 per cent in the herd and in some individuals by up to 100 per cent. The duration of the disease is short as appetite and milk yield return to normal in two to three days. If cows regraze the same pastures later in the season no disease is seen.

Treatment and prevention

Because of the rapid recovery treatment appears unnecessary, except that the herd should be housed on dry food for 24 hours and then moved to new pasture.

Symptomatic treatment of recumbent cows may be required.

Until the aetiology of this condition is understood, preventative measures will not be possible.

The oesophageal groove

Lesions of the oesophageal groove will interfere with the normal rumen digestion process. Tumours or granulomatous lesions will occlude the oesophagus and prevent eructation and lead to a gaseous bloat or secondary rumen tympany. The same lesions may interfere with normal rumen contractions and cause signs of simple indigestion. Although not common (annual incidence 1 per 10000 cattle) actinobacillosis of the oesophageal groove does occasionally occur. Some lesions of the oesophageal groove may be due to upper alimentary squamous cell carcinoma in bracken areas (see pp. 828, 946).

Signs

The presenting signs of actinobacillosis of the oesophageal groove will be inappetence, reduced milk yield and possibly mild tympany evidenced by distension of the left sublumbar fossa. The rumen contraction will be weak, occurring once every 1 or 2 minutes. Rectal temperature and heart rate will be normal. Examination of the faeces will reveal strands of undigested fibre. Although this latter finding is in itself only an indication of indigestion, and several lesions of the rumen or rumen wall or dental problems may lead to undigested fibre appearing in the faeces, the most common cause is likely to be actinobacillosis of the oesophageal groove.

Diagnosis

Only a tentative diagnosis can be made based on the clinical observations described above. Although diagnosis would be confirmed by performing an exploratory laparotomy and a biopsy of any oesophageal groove lesion discovered, this is unlikely to be performed in practice because of economic considerations.

Treatment

Although the prognosis in these cases must be guarded because of the uncertainty of the diagnosis, cows presenting the above described lesions are worthy of treatment. Treatment using antibiotics over a prolonged period of at least 10 days can be successful. The antibiotic of choice is streptomycin and a dose of 5–6g daily for 10 days is effective in a proportion of cows exhibiting the above described signs.

Traumatic reticulitis (traumatic reticuloperitonitis, hardware disease, wire)

Traumatic reticulitis is a well-described disease affecting mainly adult cattle. Because of the rather undis-cerning eating habits of the cow, it is quite common for cattle to ingest metallic objects with their food. Some abattoir surveys have demonstrated over 50 per cent of cattle reticula to contain foreign objects of metal, wood or stone. If pieces of metal wire or nails 5–10cm long are ingested these will accumulate in the reticulum and when rumen contractions occur may penetrate the reticulum wall. The incidence of this disease varies considerably around the world. The incidence in the UK has declined in the last 30 years and the present annual incidence is around 5 cases per 10000 cows. However, in some areas the disease is still extremely common and may reach an annual incidence of 100–200 per 10000 cows.

This disease is probably related to standards of management that exist on the farm, e.g. rusty, poorly maintained, barbed wire fences are a frequent source of the offending wire. It is thought that the incidence has declined since string has replaced wire to secure bales of hay and straw and much barbed wire fencing has been replaced by electric fences. However, cases of this disease will still be encountered on untidy farms where nails, wire and other metallic objects are left lying around in fields and where they can be accidentally picked up by hay or silage making machinery.

Pathogenesis

Metal objects that are ingested invariably lodge in the floor of the reticulum due to their relative mass and the position of the reticulum. It is only short sharp objects that penetrate the reticulum wall and these are usually 5–10cm long. The penetration occurs as a result of the ruminal and reticular contractions. On entering the wall of reticulum the wire will continue to penetrate until it reaches the peritoneum. Infection from the rumen then follows the wire and a localized peritonitis is produced, causing local abscess formation and adhesions. If the direction of the wire is forward the diaphragm and pericardium may be punctured, which produces a localized pleurisy and pericarditis (p. 731). If the direction of the wire is left or right of the forward direction the diaphragm may not be involved but extensive peritonitis (p. 849) could well develop, with adhesions containing a variety of abscesses being produced. If the peritonitis is extensive, adhesions between the reticulum and liver or spleen may be evident. Sequelae to traumatic reticulitis include localized or diffuse peritonitis, liver abscessation, splenitis, pleurisy and pericarditis. These sequelae may take several weeks to develop.

Signs

The condition is generally progressive and the clinical signs change as the disease progresses from the initial acute phase through a subacute to a chronic phase.

In the initial acute phase the cow is anorexic and milk production is reduced. The cow may exhibit an arched back and the abdomen is tucked up. A grunt may be heard when the animal walks, although on occasions there will be reluctance to move and also a reluctance to lie down.

Rectal temperature will be elevated to 39.1–40°C (102.5–104°F) and although the frequency of rumen contractions may be reduced they are often increased to three or four per minute. Respiratory movements will be shallow, increased in rate and mostly thoracic. Frequently, farmers mistakenly diagnose the condition as pneumonia. The heart rate will be raised to around 75–90/minute.

The acute phase may last three to five days and then the rectal temperature will fall to around 39°C (102°F) or sometimes to normal. The subacute phase will last several weeks, showing signs of mild indigestion. Rumen contractions will be weak and infrequent, there may be a mild tympany and undigested fibrous material may be evident in the faeces. Sometimes apparent recovery from the acute phase will occur and the animal will return to near normal production, but a relapse will occur several weeks later. This relapse is usually associated with the onset of pericarditis. The animal will be reluctant to move, may occasionally grunt but signs of cardiac insufficiency will predominate. A firm pronounced jugular pulse will be noticeable, together with oedema of the brisket and auscultation of the lungs may reveal signs of congestion or even pleurisy. Auscultation of the heart will sometimes be difficult, as the heart sounds will be muffled and difficult to hear. However, splashing and tinkling sounds over the heart region will confirm the presence of pericarditis (see p. 731).

Pathology:

During the acute phase there will be a measurable increase in circulating neutrophils with white cell counts rising to 30×10^9/l (30 000/μl). Ketone bodies may be present in urine or milk indicating a secondary acetonaemia. During the subacute phase, when peritonitis is developing, the white cell count may be subnormal.

At post mortem, the degree of peritonitis can be dramatic with adhesions between the reticulum, rumen, diaphragm, liver and spleen. Incising through the adhesions may reveal multiple abscesses. Abscesses may also be present in the liver. The pericarditis, when present, will also be dramatic with gross thickening of the pericardium and large quantities of pus present in the pericardial sac, so-called bread and butter heart. Pleurisy, and localized pneumonia and abscessation may also be present.

Diagnosis

The diagnosis of the acute phase is based on the signs described and discovered during the clinical examination. Cows with traumatic reticulitis can often be made to grunt by pressing down firmly on the withers, thus making the animal lower its back. However, this test is only an indication of peritonitis and not specific for traumatic reticulitis. Grunting can also be induced by applying sharp pressure just to the left of the xiphoid process using a clenched fist. This will specifically indicate pain in the region of the reticulum.

The most successful diagnostic test is known as the 'reticular grunt' or Williams test (Williams, 1975). This test uses knowledge of the cycle of reticulo-rumen contractions:

(1)   Contractions of the reticulum, followed by contraction of the rumen. There is no eructation at this stage.
(2)   Following relaxation of the reticulum and rumen, an independent contraction of the rumen occurs. This contraction is accompanied by eructation.
(3)   Relaxation of the reticulum and rumen completes the cycle. The 'reticular grunt' is based on the correlation of pain with contractions of the reticulum. Since the reticular contractions occur in conjunction with rumen contractions, the clinician should observe for signs of pain during or just before the non-eructating rumen contractions. These signs of pain will be a mild grunt, and shuffling of the forelegs. To help detect the grunt, observation of the left costal arch may reveal the animal holding its breath just before it grunts.

This test is specific for traumatic reticulitis, but is only effective in the acute phase of the disease.

Diagnosis of the subacute phase may prove extremely difficult, as the signs are often vague and only indicative of a non-specific indigestion. If such cases are encountered and a diagnosis of indigestion made, but a return to normal is not rapidly achieved, subacute traumatic reticulitis/peritonitis must be considered as a differential diagnosis.

The use of metal detectors has been advocated by some workers. However, because metal objects are frequently found in the reticulum a positive metal detector test will often be misleading.

Diagnosis of pericarditis is more straightforward. The jugular pulse and brisket oedema will lead the clinician to auscultate the heart in detail. Muffled heart sounds and splashing, fluid or tinkling sounds around the heart will confirm pericarditis.

Treatment

Various treatment regimens have been advocated for traumatic reticulitis and they can be classified into surgical and conservative.

If a diagnosis is made during the acute or subacute phase and there are no signs of pericarditis, the surgical approach has much to commend it. In many cases the diagnosis is only tentative and the rumenotomy is exploratory to confirm diagnosis or establish another diagnosis. Under paravertebral anaesthesia, an 18-cm vertical incision is made in the sublumbar fossa, the rumen wall exteriorized and a 10–15-cm incision made into which a McLintock ring is fitted, thus temporarily fixing the rumen wall to the exterior and preventing peritoneal contamination with rumen contents. A scrubbed arm is inserted into the rumen and the reticulum located. Each crypt of the reticulum should be explored as the offending wire may have penetrated to the extent that very little is left protruding into the reticulum. Adhesions between the reticulum and diaphragm or abdominal floor can be detected by attempting to lift the reticular wall. Once located, the offending wire should be slowly withdrawn back through the reticular wall and removed from the rumen. The rumen incision is closed using Lembert sutures and the abdominal wall incision closed in the usual way (see p. 1106).

Five days of antibiotic treatment should follow the surgery to prevent the spread of the peritonitis initiated by the foreign body. This operation can be very satisfactory to conduct in practice and the majority of cases make an uneventful recovery.

The conservative treatment involves restricting the animal's movement by tying it in a byre stall with the front feet raised 35–40 cm higher than the hind feet for three weeks. Parenteral antibiotics will also be given for five to seven days, and in some countries a magnet will be inserted into the reticulum using a balling gun.

If pericarditis is evident immediate slaughter must be recommended, as there is little likelihood of recovery. On no account should a rumenotomy be considered because even if the wire is located, removing it may well cause the heart to stop and death during surgery will be the result.

Prevention

The main thrust of prevention must be to avoid leaving wire or nails lying around to be picked up by cattle during feeding. The use of metal detectors on forage harvesting equipment to prevent damage to the equipment has undoubtedly reduced the incidence of metal objects being found in cattle feeds. Some workers have advocated the routine use of magnets. These are inserted into all cattle on the farm. There is no real evidence that these have been successful.

Abomasum

Diseases of the bovine abomasum comprise an interesting group of conditions only really appreciated in comparatively recent years (Pinsent, 1978).

There are three important conditions that probably have a similar aetiology and epidemiology, yet produce widely differing clinical syndromes. These are left displacement of the abomasum (LDA), dilatation and torsion in the right flank (RDA) and ulceration. Impaction of the abomasum has also been reported. The three important conditions (LDA, RDA and ulceration) appear to be the result of intensive management of cattle and have not been recorded in wild ruminants. In fact their occurrence, particularly LDA, is almost entirely restricted to dairy cattle and rarely found in suckler beef cows. Diet undoubtedly has an important role in the aetiology of these diseases, with the use of concentrated cereal-based feeds and low-fibre diets generally being incriminated. In some countries the feeding of root crops that are heavily contaminated with soil, sand and gravel has also been incriminated. In the UK and USA, LDA is much more common than RDA or ulceration. However, reports from Scandinavia would indicate that RDA is much more frequently seen there than in the UK or USA and may be the result of much greater use of root feeds such as fodder beet.

Displacement of the abomasum to the left

Left displacement of the abomasum is by far the most common of the abomasal diseases encountered in cattle in the UK or USA. Its occurrence is almost entirely confined to dairy cattle, although it has very occasionally been seen in bulls, where it is probably secondary to some other condition. The author has, on one occasion only, diagnosed the condition in a Friesian bull and in that case the animal was suffering from severe endocarditis. It was likely that this particular LDA was a secondary condition brought about by the inappetence caused by the endocarditis. The overall incidence varies considerably between years and between seasons. In some years the annual incidence can be as high as 25–30 per 10 000 and in others as low as 4–6 per 10 000.

There appears, in the UK, to be a definite seasonal pattern to the incidence with the majority of cases occurring in late winter–early spring, i.e. January to April, the period of winter housing in the UK. However, it is now being seen throughout the year, although at lower numbers during grazing. In the USA, LDA is reported to be more common in the winter housing period. However, the problem is encountered in countries where spring calving predominates and the cows are at pasture during the susceptible period, e.g. Ireland, Australia and New Zealand, although the incidence varies considerably between farms. The author has experienced the condition in eight cows in a 110-cow herd in one year, all occurring from January to April; yet there are many farms that have never, knowingly, experienced the condition. Breed susceptibility has been investigated and there has been no authoritative confirmation that there is a genetic predisposition. However, it is thought that the condition generally affects the higher yielding cows, mainly in early lactation, although occasionally during late pregnancy.

Aetiology and pathogenesis

The precise aetiology of LDA is not readily understood but the occurrence of the problem soon after, or occasionally just before, parturition would suggest that the presence of the gravid uterus or the process of parturition predisposes to the condition. Certainly it has been observed that in normal cows in late pregnancy the presence of the gravid uterus displaces the abomasum forwards and to the left, and after calving the organ returns to its normal position. To remain displaced after calving, the abomasum must have developed atony and the subsequent accumulation of gas. Atony of the abomasum is likely to be caused by one of four factors:

(1) Feeding of rapidly fermentable concentrate feeds, which have a tendency towards the production of acidosis.
(2) The accumulation of sand or gravel in the abomasum, which damages the abomasal mucosa.
(3) Stress conditions or metabolic diseases that frequently occur around the time of parturition. Hypocalcaemia will itself cause atony of the abomasum.
(4) The occurrence of systemic diseases that produce toxaemia, such as acute metritis.
(5) A lack of a suitable quantity of long fibre roughage.

It is likely therefore that atony of the abomasum and the accumulation of gas within the organ is the prime factor in the pathogenesis of the condition. The mechanical effect of displacement by the gravid uterus may well have some involvement in originally displacing the abomasum. Once displaced to the left and the organ is located between the left abdominal wall and the rumen the atonic nature of the abomasum and the presence of gas will prevent the organ returning to its normal position.

Signs

The clinical signs of LDA can vary considerably, although in general the signs are similar to chronic acetonaemia. Mild cases are encountered that show little more than a slightly depressed appetite, rumination and milk yield. At the other extreme, acute cases can be encountered with complete inappetence, absence of rumination, loss of condition, scanty diarrhoea and grunting with some signs of mild colic. The most common clinical picture is one of refusal to eat concentrates, some reduction in milk yield and scanty soft or pasty faeces. Rectal temperature will be normal but the heart rate may be raised to 80–100/minute. Rumen movements will usually be absent or at least infrequent and in some cases palpation of the rumen in the left sublumbar fossa will be impossible because of the presence of the gas-filled abomasum between the left abdominal wall and the rumen. A Rothera's test on urine or milk will usually be positive and thus in many instances the cow will be presented as a suspected case of acetonaemia. In the more acute cases, which are more common in late pregnancy, distension of the left flank will be evident.

Diagnosis

The diagnosis of LDA is relatively easy, providing the clinician always keeps the condition in mind when making a clinical examination of dairy cows. Confirmation is based on auscultation, percussion and auscultation, or ballottement and auscultation of the left flank. The stethoscope is placed on the last intercostal space in line with the lower limit of the left sublumbar fossa and the penultimate rib is percussed by 'flicking' it with the finger. If a 'ping' or high-pitched resonant sound is heard, this is indicative of a gas-filled organ inside the abdominal wall. Should the first attempt fail to elicit the characteristic 'ping' the stethoscope is moved so that an area representing a 20 cm square forward and below the first stethoscope site is auscultated and the second to last and third last ribs percussed in the same way as described above. If a high-pitched resonant sound is heard over this area, confirmation of the diagnosis should depend on auscultation only and a short series of tinkling sounds reminiscent of raindrops falling on a metal roof will be heard.

The frequency of these tinkling sounds is quite variable and the clinician may have to auscultate for up to 10 minutes in some cases. Ballottement of the lower left flank at the same time as auscultation of the target area described above may frequently elicit the same tinkling sounds. The diagnosis, by auscultation of the tinkling sounds without recourse to ballottement, is to be favoured because ballottement may elicit splashing sounds from the rumen that can be difficult to distinguish from the high-pitched tinkling sounds diagnostic of LDA. However, a negative diagnosis can fairly quickly be achieved by using the percussion and auscultation technique over a 20 cm square area forward of and ventral to the lower limit of the left sublumbar fossa. Only when this technique produces a pinging noise should it be necessary to spend time in auscultation alone.

All cows that are presented with inappetence and have a normal rectal temperature, particularly in early lactation or late pregnancy, should be subjected to the percussion and auscultation technique to eliminate LDA as part of a normal clinical examination. If this is performed the clinician is unlikely to fail to diagnose LDA.

However, it must be said that a small number of cases are not diagnosed at the first examination and a diagnosis of acetonaemia or, occasionally, indigestion is made and the corresponding treatment administered. Such cases will show a temporary recovery but the signs will relapse two to five days later. It is essential when treating acetonaemia or indigestion that the farmer is instructed to seek further veterinary advice if the condition regresses. Many cases of LDA are diagnosed in cows that have been treated for acetonaemia two to five days previously, either by the farmer or a veterinarian.

Following a complete clinical examination the differential diagnosis of LDA is related to whether the high-pitched resonant sounds can be confused with anything else. Once heard, these sounds are never forgotten. However, similar sounds do occur in conditions of the rumen that produce rumen atony, a rumen mildly distended with gas accumulation, as is seen in vagal indigestion, actinobacillosis of the oesophageal groove, localized peritonitis or mild rumen tympany. However, if the tinkling sounds are heard spontaneously and not induced by ballottement, the likelihood of misdiagnosing these other conditions as LDA is slim. The author has on one occasion, having made a diagnosis of abomasal dilatation in the right side of the abdomen by recognizing the tinkling sounds, performed a laparotomy to discover the sounds were produced by a large subperitoneal abscess in the upper right abdomen.

Treatment (see also p. 1109)

The treatment for LDA falls into two categories, conservative or surgical.

Conservative measures include drug therapy and rolling. Drug therapy using calcium borogluconate solution, neostigmine and saline cathartics has been attempted with very little success. The usual conservative treatment is to roll the cow. The cow is cast, using the Reuff's method, on to its right side. The cow is then rolled into dorsal recumbency and kept in this position for 5 minutes. During this time the animal may be rocked to the left and right and the abdomen massaged vigorously to encourage the abomasum to rise into the ventral abdomen. The animal is then rolled over to a left side lateral recumbency and maintained in this position for a further 5 minutes, allowing time for the abomasum to return to its normal position. During this process, splashing and gurgling sounds can be heard coming from the abdomen as the abomasum moves. The animal is then allowed to rise. The left flank is then auscultated to ensure the abomasum is still not present in the LDA position.

One variation of this procedure reported to be successful by one UK practitioner (B. Jeffrey, pers. comm.) is to cast the cow into left-sided lateral recumbency and restrain the animal in this position for 30 minutes. The gas present in the abomasum allows the organ to 'float' back to its normal position.

It is essential if the LDA has been corrected by rolling that the animal is re-examined 48 hours later to ensure that a relapse has not occurred. In the experience of the author, and many others, relapse is to be expected in over 75 per cent of cases of LDA that have been corrected by the rolling technique. Quite frequently if relapse does occur, the signs may not be so severe as those present before the correction and the animal may well complete its lactation, albeit with a reduced total milk yield. In such cases, chronic LDA exists and ulceration of the abomasum with adhesions to the abdominal wall may well develop, thus shortening the productive lifetime of the animal.

The surgical approach to treatment consists of laparotomy, returning the abomasum to the right side of the abdomen and suture fixation of the organ to the abdominal wall. Many different surgical techniques have been described for this procedure but the one favoured by the author is the right flank approach with the animal standing. The animal is starved of water and food for 24 hours prior to surgery to reduce the size of the rumen. Using paravertebral anaesthesia, a 20-cm incision is made in the abdominal wall, starting at the lower limit of the right sublumbar fossa and extending vertically downwards. The left arm then enters the abdominal cavity and moves carefully down the right side of the abdomen, along the floor and up the left side with the hand always in contact with the peritoneum. The hand can then locate the distended abomasum situated high in the left flank between the rumen and the abdominal wall. The hand is then placed over the top of the abomasum and downward pressure exerted. Several attempts at downward pressure may be required to disperse the gas present in the organ. The organ is then pushed down and below the rumen. It is important that contact by the hand is maintained with the abomasum during this stage of the operation because if it is lost it may be difficult to find the abomasum without causing trauma to the small intestines.

When the organ has been brought across to the right side, the pylorus is located and brought to the abdominal wall incision. Using non-absorbable suture material, e.g. monofilament nylon, and a round-bodied needle a suture is placed in the greater curvature of the abomasum close to the pylorus and this is then sutured to the peritoneum and abdomen wall at the base of the incision. The abdominal wall incision is closed in the normal way and postoperative antibiotics administered. Appetite is stimulated by the administration of rumen-stimulant drenches and the animal allowed immediate access to good quality fodder and water. The author has used this technique for over 20 years and on one occasion only has correction not been possible. In this case adhesions were present between the abomasum and the left abdominal wall. A second incision was then made in the left sublumbar fossa, and the adhesions were broken down revealing a perforated ulcer. The ulcer was excised, sutured using a purse string suture and the abomasum returned to the right flank where an assistant located and sutured it as described above. This right-sided approach has been used widely in the UK and is suitable for operating on the farm.

The right paramedian approach is also widely used. The animal is cast into dorsal recumbency and local anaesthesia administered for an incision posterior to the sternum and midway between the midline and the right subcutaneous abdominal vein. The abomasum is located, returned to its normal position and fixed using catgut or monofilament nylon sutures 2–3 cm from the margin of the incision. This technique does return the abomasum to its normal position, whereas in the former the fixation of the pylorus to the abdominal flank wound results in the abomasum being slightly out of position. In the author's opinion the abomasopexy should be performed with non-absorbable suture material as the few cases that have relapsed following abomasopexy were mostly sutured with catgut.

A modification of the right paramedian approach, the Sterner–Grymer closed suture technique, has been gaining popularity in recent years and with considerable success (Gordon, 2001). The cow is cast onto her right side and rolled into dorsal recumbency, as above, and the hind legs restrained. The abomasum is auscultated by percussion using a stethoscope and should be on the right of the midline. A DA Trochar and Cannula (Kruuse UK Ltd) is inserted firmly through the skin, muscle and peritoneum 10 cm caudal to the xiphoid process, 10 cm to the right of midline and into the abomasum, avoiding the right subcutaneous abdominal vein. The trochar is removed and a toggle attached to a suture (Kruuse UK Ltd) quickly inserted through the cannula. Minimal gas should be released when placing the first suture. The procedure is repeated with a second toggle inserted 5 cm cranial to the first, allowing as much gas as possible to escape from the abomasum to reduce tension on the sutures. The two toggle sutures are tied together and the cow rolled onto her left side and allowed to stand.

Another technique involves a left flank approach, pushing the abomasum back to the right side and then entering the rumen as in a rumenotomy to transfix the rumen to the floor of the abdomen by using a large needle and a long suture. The suture needle is passed vertically down through the rumen wall and abdominal wall to the exterior. The needle is removed from the suture and the procedure repeated with the other end of the suture material and the suture tied as a mattress suture on the exterior of the ventral abdomen. This produces an adhesion between the ventral rumen and the ventral abdomen that will prevent a recurrence of the LDA.

Prevention

Advice on prevention is difficult because the precise nature of the aetiology is unknown. Furthermore, most cases occur only sporadically and it is rare for farms to experience more than one or two cases in a season. If the incidence is higher on a particular farm, attention to the feeding regimens may prove worthwhile. Dry cows should be fed a diet of long fibre and very little concentrates. Dry-cow diets should always contain less than 30 per cent concentrate on a DM basis. Maize silage, which itself contains up to 50 per cent grain on a DM basis, should be restricted to no more than 15 kg/day during the dry period. The change in diets that occur at calving should be made as gradually as possible. Ideally, 2 kg daily of concentrates for the last two weeks of the dry period will help the rumen microflora adjust to the increased concentrate intake that occurs in early lactation. The approach to prevention of LDA is much the same as the approach to the prevention of acetonaemia.

Right-sided abomasal dilatation and torsion

Occurrence

Right-sided abomasal dilatation and torsion occurs much less frequently than LDA in the UK and USA, although it appears to be more common in Denmark. The annual incidence in the UK is of the order of 2–3 per 10 000. It normally occurs in early lactation and rarely in the dry cow, but although predominantly affecting dairy cows it has been reported in bulls, young animals, beef cows and feedlot cattle.

Pathogenesis

As with LDA, the aetiology of RDA is not fully understood but the pathogenesis is probably similar to that of LDA. Atony of the abomasum followed by the accumulation of feed, fluid and gas produces a grossly distended organ. The presence of gravel and sand in the abomasum has commonly been observed in affected animals, which may account for the higher incidence in Denmark, where large quantities of fodder beet are fed that often is contaminated with soil. Torsion is frequently a sequel to the dilatation and this is purely a mechanical effect of the increased weight and size of the dilated organ. The torsion can be in several directions, e.g. the organ may be rotated dorsally 90–180°, or counterclockwise up to 180° as viewed from the rear or the torsion may incorporate the omasum.

Signs

The onset of dilatation is insidious with inappetence, milk yield reduction and varying degrees of ketosis.

Rumination ceases and rumen contractions are weak and infrequent. Faecal quantity is reduced but its consistency is usually diarrhoeic, foul smelling and often contains occult blood. Rectal temperature is normal and heart rate raised to 80–100 beats/minute. Mild colic signs may also be evident and there is often a noticeable distension of the right flank. Once torsion occurs, the signs become peracute. Then there is a subnormal temperature, with a heart rate up to 160/minute, cold extremities and extreme dullness. These signs indicate severe shock and frequently colic may be observed. At this stage the animal is anorexic and the rectum will be empty except for some tar-like mucus.

Diagnosis

Diagnosis should not present any problems if the techniques of percussion and auscultation, ballottement and auscultation and auscultation alone are applied to the right flank in the same way as described for the diagnosis of LDA on the left flank. The same 'ping' and tinkling sounds if heard on the right flank will indicate an RDA. Determination of whether torsion exists will rely on the severity of the signs exhibited, e.g. the presence of a very fast heart rate, subnormal temperature, the signs of shock and the consistency of the rectal contents. Rectal palpation may also reveal the presence of a grossly dilated viscus in the right sublumbar region. Differential diagnosis of RDA plus torsion will include all causes of acute abdominal obstruction, particularly caecal dilatation and torsion, torsion of small intestines, intussusception and perforated abomasal ulcer. However, being able to palpate the organ on rectal palpation and hearing the characteristic high-pitched sounds should not cause problems in diagnosis.

Treatment

If torsion is not present there is often a temptation to try conservative treatments using antacids by mouth and spasmolytics, vitamins or antibiotics by injection. This is not to be recommended. Although some cases of dilatation do recover spontaneously, many do not. Many cases will remain dilated and a chronic state of abomasal dilatation develops where the animal loses weight and milk production, and eventually is culled as a 'poor doer'. Often the dilatation progresses to torsion and surgery to correct abomasal torsion is much less successful than correcting dilatation without torsion. This is because of the severe shock that is induced in the animal by the torsion. The decision on whether to attempt surgery in cases of RDA plus torsion will depend on the degree of shock that exists. In severe cases casualty slaughter should be advised. Recently, successful treatment of dilatation without torsion has been reported using metoclopramide hydrochloride, although not licensed for this purpose.

However, in valuable animals and less severely affected cows, surgery can be successful (p. 1112). Intravenous drip therapy should be set up immediately using Ringer's solution or isotonic sodium chloride. Cows with RDA plus torsion will be suffering from metabolic alkalosis and will be short of chloride ions. Sodium bicarbonate or sodium lactate should not be used. To restore normal hydration, 40–50 l of electrolyte are likely to be required over a 24-hour period.

Having set up the intravenous drip, surgery should commence immediately. Under paravertebral anaesthesia an incision is made in the right abdominal wall with the animal standing. If the animal cannot stand it is likely her condition is so severe that surgery would not succeed and casualty slaughter should be advised. On entering the abdomen and the abomasum located the first procedure is to deflate the organ using a wide bore (12G) needle and rubber tube. Having deflated the organ the direction of the torsion should be identified and an attempt made to correct the torsion without removing the fluid. If correction of the torsion is not possible then half of the fluid should be siphoned out of the abomasum. This will ease the recognition of the torsion direction and more readily allow repositioning of the abomasum. Abomasopexy is carried out as for LDA correction. The abdomen is closed in the normal way. If RDA exists without torsion the abomasum should be emptied of fluid by siphoning and then the organ opened and all debris, which may include straw or hairballs, stones or gravel, should be removed. The abomasum incision is then closed, the abomasum is returned to its normal position and the abdomen closed in the normal way. Abomasopexy is not normally required in this situation. Fluid therapy is continued until the animal has rehydrated and postoperative antibiotics are administered for five days. Following recovery diarrhoea will be present for two or three days.

Recovery rates of 75–80 per cent are reported by some workers in hospital situations and around 50 per cent when the omasum is involved in the torsion. Recovery rates for on-farm surgery are likely to be lower and this must be appreciated before embarking on surgery in preference to casualty slaughter. The likelihood of recovery will depend on the length of time that elapses from torsion occurring to operation and the level of shock that exists at the time operation commences.

Prevention

Measures to prevent RDA are the same as for LDA (p. 842) but as the condition is relatively rare, specific measures to prevent RDA are academic. If root vegetables are used in large quantities for fodder they should be washed before feeding to remove the soil contamination.

Abomasal ulceration

Ulceration in the form of small multiple ulcers occurs in the abomasal mucosal surface in a number of systemic diseases but these are rarely diagnosed, their presence being masked by the other signs present of the systemic disease.

However, a syndrome of peptic ulceration in adult cattle does occur sporadically and may result in perforation and peritonitis or haemorrhage, which can be mild and recurrent or acute and be a cause of death. The actual incidence of abomasal ulceration is probably much more common than generally realized as many cases are difficult to diagnose and may produce little harmful effect until perforation or haemorrhage occurs. The aetiology is uncertain, but feeding regimens involving a sudden introduction of concentrate feeds are likely to be implicated much the same as in the presumed aetiology of LDA and RDA. The author has experienced three sudden deaths in a herd of 120 dairy cattle that were caused by perforated abomasal ulcers. The abomasum contained large quantities of sand and gravel, which were the result of a depraved appetite. The cows were constantly eating soil, which was later confirmed to be due to hypocuprosis. The aetiology of peptic abomasal ulceration is therefore similar to LDA and RDA and is considered by some workers to be another manifestation of the same syndrome. Certainly, ulcers are found in the abomasum of both LDA and RDA.

The ulcers occur singly or occasionally in twos and threes and vary in size from 2 to 6 cm in diameter. Fungal hyphae are frequently found in the depths of the ulcers, which tend to extend into the submucosal layers until, in some cases, perforation occurs. If the perforation occurs at a point covered by omentum the ulcer may be sealed by omental adhesion. However, if the ulcer perforates at a point lateral to the omental covering, the abomasal contents spill into the peritoneal cavity and death soon follows. Another complication occurs when the ulcer erodes into a blood vessel producing haemorrhage. This may be only temporary and the blood vessel heals, but more often the haemorrhage does not stop and the animal dies from blood loss. This can be a cause of sudden death. The annual incidence for abomasal ulcers with haemorrhage would be in the order of 5–10 per 10 000.

Diagnosis

The only occasion where the syndrome can be diagnosed with certainty is when haemorrhage occurs. A cow presented with inappetence, reduced milk yield and passing black tarry faeces, which contain large quantities of occult blood, will almost certainly be suffering from a haemorrhaging abomasal ulcer. Severe cases will be anaemic, the heart rate fast and loud and death can occur within 24 hours. The prognosis in such cases is extremely guarded for, although animals do appear to make a recovery, relapses are common.

The diagnosis of abomasal ulcers with perforation is difficult. The signs are of mild colic and pain in the right ventral abdomen. Confirmation will only come from an exploratory laparotomy. Abomasal ulcers may well be present in many apparently normal cows and undoubtedly many do heal, but the sudden onset of signs associated with acute haemorrhage or perforation would indicate that until such dramatic consequences occur the ulcers may not be harmful.

Treatment

Treatment is purely academic. Ulcers without perforation or haemorrhage are unlikely to be diagnosed. The prognosis in haemorrhaging ulcers is so uncertain that casualty slaughter should be advised. Perforated ulcers, if not sealed with omentum, are usually only discovered at post-mortem examination. Ulcers that have perforated and become sealed with omentum are unlikely to be diagnosed, except on exploratory laparotomy in a cow showing signs of right-sided anterior abdominal pain and when discovered they are probably best left undisturbed.

Prevention:

With the current state of knowledge on aetiology, the best advice on prevention is to follow that for LDA and RDA (p. 842).

Abomasal impaction

Impaction of the abomasum may occur occasionally but is certainly of no great significance in adult cattle. Its annual incidence would be less than 1 per 100 000 and appears to be more common in beef cows than dairy cows as a result of feeding poor quality fibrous material. Cases can be the result of lymphosarcoma (p. 693). The impaction occurs with the accumulation of large quantities of fibrous food, sand or gravel close to the pyloric outlet. The onset is insidious, with a gradual loss in milk production and inappetence. Progressively, rumen impaction occurs, rumination ceases and constipation sets in. Rectal temperature is normal but heart rate will exceed 100/minute. At first there is little or no abdominal pain but progressively pain becomes evident in the anterior right ventral abdomen (as distinct from the left anterior abdomen in traumatic reticulitis). Pinching of the withers at this stage may elicit a painful grunt. It is unlikely that a positive diagnosis will be made without recourse to an exploratory laparotomy when an enlarged doughy abomasum will be palpated.

Pinsent (1977) was of the opinion that many cases of abomasal impaction reported in the past may well have been vagus indigestion as workers reported enlargement of the fundus of the abomasum, which contained dry rumen contents, and an accumulation of fluid within the rumen.

However, if such a case is encountered at exploratory laparotomy, abomasotomy and removal of the offending contents can be attempted.

Abomasal impaction in calves

Abomasal impaction does appear to be more common in calves than adult cattle. Calves from three weeks to three months can be affected, although six to ten weeks is the most common period. Depraved appetite, causing the calves to eat bedding and lick hair, is thought to be the cause. Finely ground grains made into pellets have also been incriminated in the aetiology, presumably the result of rapid fermentation. Coarse ration where the grain ingredients are rolled or cracked is preferred to pellets by many calf rearers because fewer 'digestive upsets' appear to occur.

Diagnosis

Affected calves usually have a brown, mild diarrhoea and normal rectal temperature. The most striking feature is the result of ballottement of the lower right abdomen, which will reveal loud splashing noises over a large area, usually indicating an enlarged abomasum containing excess fluid.

Treatment

Treatment using antacids such as magnesium hydroxide or magnesium carbonate or mild laxatives such as liquid paraffin or linseed oil may be helpful. In early cases surgical interference to empty the abomasum can be effective. It is interesting to note that the abomasum of veal calves slaughtered at 14–16 weeks old and reared solely on liquid milk substitute diets frequently contains one or several hairballs many up to 20 cm in diameter without abomasal ulceration or any abnormal effects being noticed before slaughter.

Colic and acute intestinal obstruction

Colic signs are frequently reported in adult cattle. They may indicate a tympanic intestinal colic or they may signal some more serious problem. This section will discuss the differential diagnosis of colic signs and will describe in detail: tympanic intestinal colic, intussusception, caecal dilatation and torsion, prolapse of small intestine through a ruptured mesentery and torsion of small intestine around the root of the mesentery.

Occurrence

Colic is a sporadic condition affecting only individual animals, it being extremely rare for more than one animal to be affected at any one time. Signs of colic are reported quite frequently in all ages of cattle and under all types of management, whether extensive or intensive. A thorough clinical examination will be required to differentiate the many problems that produce colic. By far the most common cause of colic is tympanic intestinal colic, which is very similar to the syndrome so frequently seen in the horse. Intussusception, caecal dilatation and prolapse of the small intestine through the mesentery are much less common and in the UK each would have an annual incidence of less than 1 per 10000.

Signs

The clinical signs of colic in cattle are firstly reduced appetite or even anorexia, reduced milk yield and a noticeable change in behaviour – kicking at the ventral abdomen, shifting weight from one hind foot to the other, licking at the flank or chest wall, frequently lying down and then standing and generally restless. The intensity of the signs exhibited will vary with the degree of pain. On some occasions the signs are quite mild, with only occasional kicking at the ventral abdomen, and may be missed by all but the most astute stockworker. The above signs are all indicative of pain, but not necessarily abdominal pain. Conditions that will produce similar signs include photosensitization (p. 884), particularly if the teats are affected, strangulated scrotal hernia, uterine torsion, urolithiasis (p. 263) and ureter obstruction.

Diagnosis

The diagnosis of the cause of the signs of colic will include a thorough clinical examination. The rectal temperature may be raised, the pulse will certainly be increased and the more acute the problem, the faster and weaker will be the pulse. Abdominal sounds may be present or absent. In intestinal obstruction the sounds will be absent. The mucous membranes will be injected in acute problems and the eyes sunken. Ballottement of the ventral abdomen should always be performed and may reveal splashing fluid sounds. A rectal examination should also be performed. In intestinal obstruction the rectum will be empty and sticky. Enlarged viscera or abnormal positioning of the viscera may be palpated on rectal palpation. A detailed description of the use of rectal palpation in the diagnosis of abdominal disorders has been recorded by Stober and Dirkson (1977).

In many cases of intestinal obstruction diagnosis may only be confirmed on exploratory laparotomy. Exploratory laparotomy as a diagnostic procedure as opposed to its use solely as a surgical treatment is to be recommended (Pinsent, 1978) where the attitude of the farmer and conditions conducive to surgery exist. Many farmers, with their increased education and training, will understand the value of an exploratory laparotomy if the problem is fully explained. Furthermore, exploratory laparotomy may well reveal the cause of acute intestinal obstruction and allow surgical correction and recovery to take place, whereas if surgical intervention is unnecessarily delayed the likelihood of recovery is always reduced. The author has, on two occasions, performed an exploratory laporotomy where an unknown intestinal obstruction was thought to exist to find that on both occasions a thin fibrous strand or adhesion was present in the abdomen and a loop of small intestine had become entwined around the strand, thus causing the obstruction. Severing the strand released the bowel and in both cases the animal made an uneventful recovery.

Tympanic intestinal colic

Tympanic intestinal colic is by far the most common condition to produce colic signs. It can occur at any age and calves are presented with colic signs as frequently as adult animals. The signs are of sudden onset, but in lactating cows they are frequently observed at milking time and in calves during or just after feeding.

Diagnosis

As all the usual colic signs are present the clinical examination will reveal normal rectal temperature, raised heart rate (80–90/minute) and normal mucous membranes. Abdominal sounds will be present, sometimes at an increased intensity. Rectal examination will reveal faeces in the rectum and it is unlikely that any abnormality to the viscera will be palpated. It is important to ensure that the differential diagnoses mentioned above are not present. Uterine torsion will only be present in late pregnancy but photosensitization is fairly common (5–10 per 10 000) and must be eliminated from the diagnosis by careful examination and palpation of any white areas of skin.

In the calf, abdominal palpation should be performed, as intussusception (p. 847) is relatively common and can sometimes be palpated. The diagnosis will be confirmed by response to treatment or spontaneous recovery within 24 hours.

Treatment

The most effective treatment is the intravenous administration of a spasmolytic such as hyoscine-N-butylbromide and dipyrone or butylscopolamine bromide and metamizole. Oral treatment with mild purgatives, such as linseed oil or liquid paraffin, has been used in the past but these are unnecessary and not as effective as spasmolytics and may well be contraindicated.

Torsion of intestines (red gut in calves)

Torsion of the intestines around the root of the mesentery is extremely rare in adult cattle (1 per 10 000), but has been reported to occur spontaneously and the cause is unknown. It has also been reported to occur follow-

ing rolling of cows to correct uterine torsion or left displacement of the abomasum. The entire small intestine twists up to 360° around the root of the mesentery.

In calves, the condition is more common and is known as red gut and is associated with the feeding of milk substitutes. It appears to have increased in incidence in recent years and is more commonly seen in loose-housed, machine-fed, calf rearing systems, where the intake of milk is uncontrolled and can be quite excessive. Although the aetiology is uncertain, the pathogenesis is thought to be the rapid fermentation of lactose in the ileum, which leads to gas production and gross dilatation of the intestine, which then twists at the mesentery root. Affected calves are normally three to six weeks old and are presented showing severe colic signs with death following within 12 hours. It can also be a cause of sudden death. Diagnosis is rare in the live animal, mainly because of the rapid progression of the disease and it is not possible to differentiate it from tympanic intestinal colic.

At post mortem the findings are quite dramatic. The small intestines are grossly dilated with gas, are a bright-red colour and the whole of the intestinal mucosa is bright red. To detect the torsion, the post mortem must be performed with care because if the abdomen is fully opened and the intestine allowed to spill out, the torsion will untwist and therefore not be detectable.

In adult cows the presenting signs of intestinal torsion are those of severe colic. Rectal temperature may be raised, the pulse weak and fast, mucous membranes are injected and the eyes sunken. Rectal examination will usually reveal multiple gas-distended loops of small intestine in the right side of the abdomen and these may distend into the pelvic cavity. The site of the mesentery twist will normally be beyond reach, but tense strands of mesentery may be palpable.

Treatment

Immediate surgery is indicated. Laparotomy is performed under paravertebral anaesthesia in the right sublumbar fossa. Loops of distended bowel may protrude through the abdominal incision. The root of the mesentery will be located in the region of the left kidney and the direction of the twist should be determined. The torsion is corrected by manipulation of the intestines, some of which will need to be exteriorized to allow room in the abdomen to correct the twist. This surgery is certainly of a heroic nature, but nevertheless can succeed if the animal is not too severely shocked when the operation commences. Follow-up treatment with intravenous fluids and antibiotics should always be administered.

Prolapse of intestines through mesentery

This condition is usually only seen in adult cattle and is more common than torsion at the mesentery root. Its annual incidence is still only approximately 1 per 10 000. The acute nature of the signs is identical to torsion at the mesentery root and rectal palpation will reveal gas-distended loops of small intestine, which make it clinically indistinguishable. If untreated, death will occur within 12 hours.

Treatment (see p. 1113)

Immediate exploratory laparotomy will reveal the grossly gas-distended intestine, but it may be difficult to distinguish from torsion of the intestines. Palpation of the root of the mesentery must be performed first to distinguish the condition from torsion. One clue to the problem being one of prolapse of intestine through mesentery will be the presence of normal intestine. Palpation of the gas-distended intestine will reveal that it is protruding through a hole in the mesentery. The hole must first be enlarged and the intestines slowly fed back through the aperture, after which the mesenteric rupture is sutured. It must be emphasized that surgery should only be contemplated if the animal is not too severely shocked. As death can occur quickly with this condition, casualty slaughter is commonly advised.

Caecal dilatation and torsion

Caecal dilatation is a distinct clinical entity in adult cattle. Its occurrence is sporadic (approximately 1–2 per 10 000) and usually occurs in early lactation, although the condition has been reported in bulls. The aetiology is thought to be related to high levels of volatile fatty acids in the caecum, which originate from the rumen or from fermentation of undigested starch in the caecum. The fatty acids cause atony of the caecum and the gas accumulates. Mild dilatation probably causes no signs, but severe dilatation will produce typical colic signs. However, many cases of caecal dilatation progress to caecal torsion. Strictly speaking this is not a torsion but due to the gross size of the dilated caecum and the large quantity of fluid it contains, the distal end falls forward producing a kink in the organ. Occasionally, the weight of the distended caecum produces a torsion at the mesentery root and the colon, caecum and small intestine are involved in a torsion rather similar to the torsion of the small intestines at the mesentery root.

Diagnosis

Diagnosis is based on the presence of the signs of colic, although sometimes the colic signs are quite mild. Ballottement of the right flank will elicit copious splashing and fluid sounds and the right flank may be noticeably distended. Rectal examination will reveal an empty rectum and if a reliable history is available the animal will not have passed any faeces for 24 hours or more.

Usually, the dilated caecum will be palpable at the entrance to the pelvic cavity and many even protrude into the pelvic cavity. If the caecum has 'kinked' rectal exploration of the abdominal cavity will be required to detect the dilated organ.

Treatment

Successful treatment using butylscopolamine bromide and metamizole (Buscopan) has been reported in cases of dilatation where torsion is absent. It would be wise to monitor the effect of treatment by rectal examination at 6-hourly intervals so that surgical intervention can be instigated if there is no response or torsion occurs. If medical treatment fails or torsion occurs, surgical intervention should always be considered in an animal that is not too shocked and where the condition has not been present for too long.

A right-flank laparotomy is performed and, on exploration, the grossly enlarged caecum can be detected. Palpation of the root of the mesentery should be carried out to try and determine whether torsion exists.

The first stage of the operation is to siphon off the fluid present in the caecum, thus reducing its volume to a manageable size. It is possible in some cases to siphon off 30–40 l of dark, foul-smelling fluid. When as much fluid and gas as possible have been removed a purse-string suture is used to repair the incision through which the siphon tube was inserted and an attempt is made to relocate the caecum back to its normal position. If the caecum is kinked or twisted, removal of the fluid may well allow the torsion to correct itself. The laparotomy is closed in the normal way. Postoperative treatment is usual with fluid therapy if dehydration is evident and antibiotics to prevent peritonitis developing. This can be a rewarding operation and most animals make an uneventful recovery.

Intussusception (see p. 1114)

Intussusception or telescoping of the bowel occurs in adult cattle and calves. The annual incidence in adult cattle is around 1 or 2 per 10 000, but may be more common in calves. The condition is caused by strong peristaltic movements of the intestine and either the small intestine telescopes into small intestine or occasionally through the ileo-caecal valve into the caecum. In calves the condition is usually a sequel to profuse diarrhoea, but this appears not necessarily to be the case in adult cattle. Some workers have suggested that a tumour or inflammatory growth in the lumen of the affected part may be a causative factor in adult cattle.

Signs

When the intussusception first occurs there will be mild signs of colic. These signs frequently go unnoticed by the stockworker or if they are seen they are discounted because they do not last for long and the animal makes an apparent recovery. Two to three days later the animal's milk production declines, inappetence sets in and the astute stockworker may notice the animal to be constipated. This is the most frequent time veterinary attention is sought.

Examination will reveal a normal rectal temperature, the heart rate raised to 80–120/minute and auscultation will reveal bowel stasis. A rectal examination will reveal an empty rectum or the presence of scanty bloodstained faeces or thickened mucus. On questioning, the stockworker may admit that colic signs were evident two to three days earlier.

Diagnosis

In many cases rectal palpation will reveal a hard, sausage-shaped mass in the right abdomen. The absence of any dilated organ and complete bowel stasis will indicate a strong likelihood that an intussusception is present, even if it cannot be palpated, although simple rumen indigestion may be difficult to differentiate. Palpation of the offending intussusception may be made easier if the floor of the abdomen is raised using a pole under the ventral abdomen and lifted by two persons. The course of this disease is not as acute as other causes of intestinal obstructions; thus if the clinician is not certain of the diagnosis, mild purgatives such as liquid paraffin or linseed oil may be administered orally and the case re-assessed 24 hours later. These will do no harm if an intussusception exists and, if the problem is one of indigestion, faeces will be passed within 24 hours. It is important to instruct the stockworker to isolate the animal in a clean pen for this period so that any faeces voided will be observed. One of many problems with loose-housing systems is that accurate history of whether an animal is eating forage, defecating or urinating is frequently unavailable.

If no faeces have been voided in the 24 hours of isolation an exploratory laparotomy must be contemplated.

Treatment

An exploratory laparotomy in the right sublumbar fossa should be carried out if the farmer is willing. Failing this, casualty slaughter should be performed. Exploration of the abdominal cavity will reveal the hard mass of the intussusception, although when it is exteriorized it may not be recognizable as such. It may appear more like a bloodstained tumour. Normal gut should be identified entering and leaving the mass, which should then be surgically removed and intestinal anastomosis performed. If the mass is recognizable as an intussusception, as may be the case if diagnosis was prompt, on no account should an attempt be made to unravel the intussusception. Although this may well be possible, the offending length of gut must be considered to be diseased because it will certainly re-form as an intussusception within 24 hours of correction. Some workers have suggested that if intussusceptions are not removed surgically, but conservative treatment principles applied, the necrotic tissues of the intussusception will slough out in 10–14 days and the animal will recover. This approach to treatment is not to be recommended because, in the author's experience, animals that are not treated surgically will die.

The intestinal anastomosis does require some surgical skill but should not be beyond the majority of large animal surgeons. The technique has been performed quite satisfactorily on the farm.

Intussusception in calves

In calves intussusception is a sequel to acute diarrhoea. Signs of colic will be present in the initial stages of the disease, but frequently the animal is presented because it is not defecating or is collapsed. Occasionally, the intussusception can be palpated through the abdominal wall and if the calf is not in an advanced state of shock an exploratory laparotomy may be considered and the offending lesion removed surgically and intestinal anastomosis performed. Unfortunately, in calves the condition is most commonly encountered at post mortem.

Diaphragmatic hernia

Diaphragmatic hernia has occasionally been reported in cattle but the condition is rarely diagnosed and the incidence is probably less than 1 per 100 000 per year. Diaphragmatic hernia can be a congenital or acquired defect of the diaphragm with partial or complete entry of abdominal organs (usually the reticulum) into the thoracic cavity. Congenital defects usually manifest before the animal is 12 months old and acquired defects are usually a sequel to traumatic reticulitis or trauma in adult cattle.

The most commonly prolapsed organ seems to be the reticulum and the result is interference with the motility and function of the rumen and reticulum. Colic signs will be noticed at the time of the rupture but they do not persist. Signs similar to vagus indigestion may be apparent, although low-grade pain in the posterior thorax/anterior abdomen region, rather like traumatic reticulitis, has been noticed. Respiratory signs may be apparent due to reduced thoracic space. A definitive diagnosis is unlikely to be made without recourse to an exploratory laparotomy, although radiography may be useful.

Successful response to surgical correction has been reported, particularly in Indian buffalo, although this is only likely to be successful with relatively small ruptures and in cases where the vagus nerve is not damaged. The cow is positioned in dorsal recumbency and the incision made in the xiphoid area. Having retrieved the reticulum from the thoracic cavity the hernia is repaired with monofilament nylon or by the use of a fine nylon mesh.

Fat necrosis (lipomatosis, peritoneal fat necrosis)

Lipomatosis or peritoneal fat necrosis occurs sporadically (annual incidence 1–5 per 100 000) in old cows with a suggested predisposition towards Channel Island and Aberdeen Angus breeds. Affected cows may not present any signs and the condition is detected at routine rectal examination. Advanced cases of the condition will show signs of weight loss, underperformance and inappetence. The diagnosis will be based on rectal palpation findings when large hard masses can be palpated in the abdominal cavity. Occasionally, fat in the pelvic canal will be affected and the canal will be almost completely occluded and it is nearly impossible to carry out rectal palpation because of lack of space.

There is no treatment and slaughter should be advised. On post mortem as much as 20–25 kg of hard necrotic fat may be present in the omentum and mesentery.

Peritonitis (see also p. 141)

Peritonitis is a local or general, acute or chronic, inflammation of the peritoneal cavity. Peritonitis usually occurs as an accompanying condition of other specific diseases, e.g. traumatic reticulo-peritonitis (p. 837) or metritis (pp. 519, 521). The most common cause of peritonitis is traumatic reticulitis followed by peritonitis as a sequel to metritis, dystokia or retained afterbirth. However, peritonitis may be a sequel to abdominal surgery, a ruptured abomasal or intestinal ulcer, penetration of the intestinal tract by foreign bodies, pancreatic necrosis, rupture of biliary or urinary tracts, an infected umbilicus in calves, rupture of the rectum, uterus or large intestine, tuberculosis, liver abscesses and chronic right- or left-sided displacement of the abomasum. Peritonitis can also be associated with septicaemic conditions such as anthrax and calf septicaemia.

Signs

The clinical signs include a raised rectal temperature, which is frequently in the range 39–40°C (102.5–104°F), respiration is frequently shallow and pulse and respiratory rates are increased. The back is moderately arched,

there is a reluctance to move and walking sometimes instigates grunting. Appetite and milk production are invariably depressed and rumination ceases.

Diagnosis

The diagnosis of peritonitis can be difficult and is based on the history and clinical findings. However, the condition should be suspected in all cows that are presented with the above clinical signs and a thorough examination may reveal which organ is responsible. Ballottement of the lower right flank may reveal splashing sounds, indicating the presence of fluid in the peritoneum, and also may cause the animal to grunt. For a more detailed description of the diagnosis of traumatic reticulo-peritonitis see p. 837. The history may also be helpful in arriving at a diagnosis, e.g. recent dystokia or abdominal surgery. If metritis is suspected, a rectal or vaginal examination will aid the diagnosis. Abdominal paracentesis should reveal the presence of peritoneal fluid, which will be foul smelling and contain a large number of white blood cells.

The severity and extent of the peritonitis are usually reflected in the severity of the clinical signs. If the peritonitis is generalized and acute, the animal groans on expiration. When only a limited area of the peritoneum is involved, as in traumatic reticulo-peritonitis, pain will only be evident when the exact location is percussed.

It is important to attempt to determine the cause of the peritonitis in order to give an accurate prognosis and to determine the line of treatment that should be followed.

Prognosis

Localized peritonitis has a favourable prognosis, providing the offending organ can be identified and corrective action taken. However, in acute generalized peritonitis the prognosis can be poor, particularly if the peritonitis is a sequel to abdominal surgery, dystokia or a ruptured abdominal viscus. The prognosis will be related to the severity of the clinical signs, the degree of depression, the weakness of the pulse and the extent of the signs of toxaemia.

Treatment

Treatment may first be directed to correction of the initial problem. However, the peritonitis itself will be treated with large doses of antibiotics administered intraperitoneally, intravenously and intramuscularly. An initial dose of 5 g of benzylpenicillin and 5 g of dihydrostreptomycin is administered into the peritoneum via the right sublumbar fossa, using a 2-inch 16-gauge needle followed immediately by 5 g of procaine penicillin G and 5 g of dihydrostreptomycin by intramuscular injection and every 12 hours for three to five days. Some workers have reported success using heparin by intramuscular injection at a dose of 50 000 iu twice daily for three days in addition to antibiotic therapy (Breukink, 1980). The author can report successful treatment using intraperitoneal injections of metronidazole (10 g daily for 3–5 days). However, metronidazole cannot now be used on animals intended for human consumption.

Diarrhoea

Diarrhoea in adult cattle is a frequent sign and is present in many diseases. It may occur sporadically, affecting only individual animals, or it may be present in a large number if not the whole of the group. If the whole group is affected, one must consider the feed or the possible presence of a virus infection as in winter dysentery. Blood may be present, in which case dysentery is used to describe the sign. The diarrhoea may be very watery or even projectile as in redwater (pipe stem diarrhoea). The colour and odour may be distinctive. Dark, foul-smelling, liquid faeces would indicate the presence of occult blood and haemorrhage in the upper small intestine. Pale, pasty-coloured faeces may indicate rumen acidosis. Diarrhoea with air bubbles is frequently attributed to Johne's disease. Endotoxaemia from a coliform mastitis or metritis will produce dark, watery faeces. Infections with agents such as *Campylobacter* spp. or BVD/mucosal disease virus will also produce diarrhoea and *Salmonella* spp. often produce dysentery. Intestinal parasitism will produce diarrhoea of varying intensity depending on the severity of the problem, although this more commonly affects growing cattle than adults.

Non-inflammatory diseases, e.g. cardiac failure, lymphosarcoma and systemic amyloidosis, also produce diarrhoea by increasing intestinal secretion into the bowel lumen.

The clinician is frequently presented with an adult bovine where the only sign is an afebrile diarrhoea. Clinical examination may reveal sluggish rumen movements but no other signs of indigestion or of abomasal disease. Many of these cases will be the result of ingestion of toxic plants if the cattle are grazing or being fed conserved fodder and frequently the cause may be a small batch of soiled or spoiled silage.

Some cows with such acute diarrhoea die rapidly and post-mortem examination reveals a severe enteritis, frequently haemorrhagic, but the examination for infections or parasite counts proves unrewarding. One usually assumes that the cause of death is poisoning but frequently the toxic agent is not discovered. When presented with individual cows showing diarrhoea and no

systemic disease or other signs present, the cow must be removed from its present food source, isolated and given only dry feed, such as hay, to eat. Treatment with antibiotics such as streptomycin may be instituted, although the efficacy in these situations is not proven. Spasmolytics may help and oral therapy with gut sedatives such as chlorodyne or adsorbents such as kaolin are frequently used but again their efficacy is not proven. The addition of glycine/electrolytes to the drinking water has more recently been suggested, but in cases where severe dehydration is present intravenous administration of 20–40 l of balanced electrolytes is indicated.

If the whole herd or group is affected, one must remember that lush spring grass will produce diarrhoea as will wet autumn grass in the UK. Wet grass silage will also produce fluid faeces. In some areas of the UK and in other countries molybdenum toxicity is common, e.g. on the so-called teart pastures of Somerset, and this will produce severe diarrhoea in the whole grazing herd but can be corrected by the administration of copper in the form of copper sulphate to the diets.

An infectious cause of a whole group of cattle to be affected with diarrhoea is winter dysentery (see p. 852); infection with *Salmonella typhimurium, S. montevideo* or *S. goldcoast* may spread rapidly through a herd but the animals will also be pyrexic.

Thus diarrhoea is a sign of many disease conditions of cattle but frequently enteritis will occur in individual animals and the cause will remain undetermined. There remains a challenge for the bovine practitioner.

Salmonellosis

Infection of adult cattle with a variety of *Salmonella* spp. is frequently encountered in cattle practice (see Chapter 15). In the UK as many as 100–200 herds per 10 000 may suffer the disease each year where it affects a considerable proportion of the herd. The incidence of sporadic salmonellosis, where only one or two animals in the herd are affected, may be as high as 500–1000 per 10 000 herds. These sporadic occurrences are usually abortions due to *S. dublin*. A variety of *Salmonella* spp. have been known to affect cattle but the two most prominent are *S. dublin* and *S. typhimurium*. *Salmonella newport, S. montevideo* and *S. goldcoast* are less frequently reported and sporadic outbreaks with other species occasionally occur. The most serious problems are associated with enteritis and septicaemia, but sporadic outbreaks of abortion with no concurrent septicaemia or enteritis are frequently encountered due to *S. dublin*. Epidemiologically, abortion appears different from the enteritis and septicaemia syndrome and will be dealt with separately (p. 582).

Epidemiology and aetiology

The aetiological agents *S. typhimurium* and *S. dublin* are those most frequently encountered although other species are reported sporadically. The epidemiology of *S. dublin* appears to differ from that of *S. typhimurium*. It has been known for some time that to establish *S. dublin* carrier status in the adult cow there needs to be damage to the liver and/or bile ducts. The most frequent cause of liver damage is liver fluke and in areas where liver fluke is endemic, the incidence of *S. dublin* enteritis is more common. The source of infection for *S. dublin* is therefore carrier cows, most of which are suffering liver damage from liver fluke and if liver fluke is endemic in a herd, *S. dublin* may spread rapidly. In areas where *S. dublin* infection is unusually high, the organism can frequently be isolated from rivers, streams and ditches. It is difficult to postulate the role this contamination has in the spread of the infection as one would expect the watercourses to be infected if carrier cows exist in the area.

The carrier status probably also exists with *S. typhimurium*, but this is much less common than with *S. dublin*. The majority of *S. typhimurium* outbreaks in adult cattle are of sudden onset and indicate a recent introduction of the infection into the herd. The most common source of infection is probably purchased contaminated compound feeds. These feeds often used to contain processed animal protein, which was frequently infected with *Salmonella* spp. Cross-infection to cereals also occurs when common storage bins and mixing equipment are used. Cross-contamination of animal feeds may also be caused by wild birds or rodents that may live in animal feed production premises. A further source of infection for *S. typhimurium* is rivers or streams. In many rural areas public sewerage facilities do not exist and septic tanks or cesspits are used. If these do not function satisfactorily, raw or part-treated sewage finds its way into rivers. Human infection has also been the cause of infection when cattle have grazed fields in which human defecation is known to have occurred or fields that are situated next to lay-bys on busy main roads.

On occasions cows have been shown to be excreting *S. typhimurium* but yet not show signs of disease, i.e. they are carrier cows. The presence of a carrier cow within a herd may go undetected and no problem exists with the rest of the herd. The reason why the infection does not spread in these situations is not clear. It may be that a minimum infective dose is required to establish disease or the immune system of the animals may be depressed with a virus infection spreading within the herd and this allows *Salmonella* infection to develop into disease.

Signs

The principal signs produced by *Salmonella* infections are acute enteritis and septicaemia with a sudden onset of severe diarrhoea or dysentery. Frequently, the mucous membrane lining of the small intestine is passed with the faeces and, occasionally, blood clots are present.

The rectal temperature is 40.5–41.5°C (105–107°F) and the cow is severely depressed. The severity of the signs varies considerably. If the disease occurs at or near parturition, septicaemia sets in and mortality may be as high as 20 per cent of affected animals, particularly with *S. dublin* infections. *Salmonella typhimurium* produces morbidity varying from 10 to 70 per cent of the herd however mortality is generally not high, although it will be higher if infection occurs at or around calving.

If infection with *S. typhimurium* or *S. dublin* occurs during late pregnancy, seriously affected animals will frequently abort. This is probably a result of the fever and septicaemia rather than the infection directly affecting the fetus or placenta. *Salmonella dublin* will cause abortion without enteritis and septicaemia being present but the epidemiology and pathogenesis is different. This will be discussed under *Salmonella dublin* abortion (see p. 582). Animals that abort following septicaemia and enteritis frequently develop acute septic metritis and peritonitis and frequently die.

Diagnosis

The diagnosis is confirmed by the isolation of *Salmonella* spp. from faeces of affected animals. The faeces of all cattle presented with acute enteritis accompanied with fever should be sampled and tested for *Salmonella* spp. by bacteriological isolation. Affected animals should be kept in isolation until the result is known.

Treatment

Antibiotics administered parenterally are used for the treatment of salmonellosis. Due to resistance to some antibiotics an *in vitro* antibiotic sensitivity test should be performed as soon as possible. Resistance to penicillin, streptomycin, the tetracyclines and ampicillin is widespread with *S. typhimurium*. Neomycin and framycetin are frequently effective and resistance to chloramphenicol and gentamicin is rare. The combination of trimethoprim and sulphadiazine is also frequently used. There is always some controversy regarding the use of antibiotics in treating salmonellosis in adult cattle. Septicaemic cases and complications following abortion should always be treated with antibiotics. However, in a herd outbreak, some animals will be less severely affected than others and will recover spontaneously without the use of antibiotics. Antibiotic therapy will need to be administered for three to five days.

Oral rehydration therapy is indicated where dehydration is evident and if the dehydration is severe, intravenous administration of 30 l of balanced electrolyte solution will prove to be a valuable support to antibiotic therapy. Recovery time can be quite variable. Cattle with mild enteritis will recover within two days, whereas severe septicaemic cases may take one to two weeks to recover their previous appetite and will not normally return to previous levels of milk production.

Control

Once the diagnosis has been confirmed, it is important to limit the spread within the herd. Isolation of affected animals will help but by the time cows are identified with enteritis, *Salmonella* organisms will be isolated from any site on the farm frequented by the cattle. Vaccination of non-affected animals should be considered. In the UK the live vaccine prepared from an avirulent strain of *S. dublin* is no longer available. A dead vaccine prepared from formalin-killed cells of *S. dublin* and *S. typhimurium* (Bovivac S, Intervet Ltd) is available and has been used to control outbreaks of *S. dublin* or *S. typhimurium*. The whole herd should be vaccinated with two doses 21 days apart and booster injections administered two to three weeks before calving to boost the passive immunity available to the calves. If exotic *Salmonella* species are identified consideration should be given to the use of autogenous vaccines using the same protocol as stated above. Control measures should also include monitoring the environment, including the wildlife, and husbandry measures put in place to reduce the risk of spreading infection. Cattle slurry should only be applied on land to be ploughed or on grass for conservation at least three to four months before the grass is cut.

If *S. dublin* is identified as the causal organism, a representative number of faeces samples (usually six to twelve) should be examined for the presence of liver fluke ova and if positive the herd should receive appropriate anthelmintic therapy.

It is essential when salmonellosis occurs on a farm that the utmost care should be taken regarding personal hygiene. All the staff should be made aware of the zoonotic implications and should not consume farm milk during the course of an outbreak. In the UK, *Salmonella* isolation must be reported to the relevant departments of agriculture, who monitor the infection nationally. Very little action is taken against the farmer unless there is a perceived human health risk, e.g. fresh milk is being used for yoghurt, cream or cottage cheese production, in which case the public health authorities may insist on pasteurization of the milk prior to processing. The question is frequently asked: should recovered cases be kept and will they become permanent carriers? Practice experience would indicate that in the

majority of outbreaks of *S. typhimurium* the problem rarely recurs. It is only very occasionally that a herd may become chronically infected and sporadic cases will continue to occur. More usually the infection is confined to the calves in endemically infected herds. In the case of *S. dublin* enteritis the main thrust in control following vaccination is to control liver fluke in the herd. If this is successfully achieved, enteritis caused by *S. dublin* will be infrequent.

Attempts to identify carrier cows within endemically infected herds are sometimes recommended. This is achieved by faeces sampling the entire herd and culturing the samples for *Salmonella* spp. Unfortunately, *Salmonella* spp. are excreted intermittently in carrier cows and animals need to be sampled on several occasions, probably as many as six or seven, to be reasonably certain all carrier cows are identified. This procedure has proved to be neither practical nor necessary in most outbreaks.

Prevention

To prevent infection with *S. typhimurium* may be difficult because of the frequency in which it is found in animal feeds. Contamination of feed can also be caused by rodents and birds. However, legislation has been implemented in the UK to supervise all protein processing plants and to ensure the protein material is sterilized. In recent years infections entering the herd via purchased feeds have become less frequent.

Preventing infection spreading from the human population to cattle can be achieved to some extent by the supply of clean wholesome water for cattle to drink. For the effective control of a variety of infections cattle should not be allowed to drink from natural watercourses. Effective fencing of fields may also be required, particularly alongside main roads and lay-bys to prevent humans using grazing fields as a lavatory.

Winter dysentery

As the name implies, winter dysentery occurs during the period of winter housing and affects cattle of all ages. It is obviously an extremely infectious disease because when it enters a herd it rapidly spreads through all animals in the herd. Also, once infected and the animals have recovered, the herd will not usually experience the problem for four or five years, thus indicating development of a herd immunity.

Moreover, once one herd in an area becomes infected, it appears to spread rapidly to other herds nearby. Perhaps this is a disease that can be spread by veterinary surgeons! However, it is interesting that there has been very little mention of its occurrence in the UK during the last 15–20 years, whereas during the late 1950s and early 1960s it was frequently encountered. It has been reported to be present in several countries in Europe and the northern States of the USA and Canada have experienced large outbreaks in past years. Although the morbidity is almost 100 per cent, mortality is normally absent. Milk production, however, may be reduced by up to 50 per cent and take up to two weeks to recover and so it is of economic importance.

Aetiology

Campylobacter fetus var. *jejuni* was once thought to be the causative organism. But the speed of spread, the short incubation period of around three days and the inability to reproduce the disease using cultures of *C. jejuni* lead one to suspect the aetiological agent is a virus, which to date has not been identified. However, coronaviruses have been encountered in several outbreaks and are now often considered to be involved in the causation of some outbreaks.

Signs

The main sign is of a severe, watery, dark brown diarrhoea with a foul-smelling odour. The faeces may be tinged with blood. The diarrhoea is sometimes described as explosive or projectile. At first only one or two cows in the herd are affected, but within three or four days several cows will show signs and within two weeks all the older cattle on the farm will have become affected. The rectal temperature is usually normal and appetite is reduced in only a small number of more severely affected animals. However, milk yield may be reduced by up to 50 per cent and such animals may show signs of abdominal pain, e.g. colic, arched back or a 'hunched up' appearance may be apparent. The course of the disease in most cows is two to three days.

Diagnosis

The severity and speed of spread of the disease present no real problems in diagnosis except with the initial cases, which may be misdiagnosed as a poisoning (Chapter 54) or non-specific enteritis. Once several cows are affected and the disease is occurring during the housed period, diagnosis is based on the clinical signs present.

Bovine virus diarrhoea would involve fewer animals, which would have pyrexia and characteristic oral lesions. Coccidiosis (see p. 282) normally affects younger animals, but this can be differentiated by the presence of tenesmus and the identification of oocysts in the faeces.

Treatment

Most affected cattle recover spontaneously in two to three days and treatments do not speed recovery.

However, a proportion of the cases are more severely affected and some may become weak enough to become recumbent. Severely dehydrated animals will require intravenous administration of 20–30 l of balanced electrolytes and electrolytes added to the drinking water should prove advantageous. Oral astringents, such as 50 ml of 5 per cent copper sulphate administered every 12 hours, may prove effective. Morphine and chloroform (chlorodyne) reduce intestinal motility and absorbents such as kaolin or bismuth salts have also been recommended. Oral sulphonamides have been reported to be useful by some practitioners.

Prevention

This is an extremely infectious disease and when it occurs in an area cattle or unnecessary personnel should not enter the farm. Veterinary surgeons should take the utmost care in thoroughly disinfecting their boots and protective clothing before entering and leaving farms when this infection is present locally.

Bovine virus diarrhoea/mucosal disease

Bovine virus diarrhoea and mucosal disease are both diseases caused by bovine virus diarrhoea virus (BVDV), which is similar to the viruses causing Border disease in sheep and swine fever in pigs. These three viruses are together classified as pestiviruses within the Flaviviridae. It is worth noting that all three pestiviruses can cross the placenta and damage the fetus.

In 1946, veterinary workers at Cornell demonstrated that a virus was the cause of a transmissible bovine diarrhoea and thereby named BVDV. The virus has since been identified worldwide as a most serious cause of cattle disease, particularly reproductive disease.

Aetiology (Figs 48.1 and 48.2)

Infection with BVD virus is generally a mild or even subclinical event, except on two occasions, i.e. infection of the pregnant animal and in mixed infections, e.g. with other respiratory viruses such as respiratory syncytial virus (RSV), infectious bovine rhinotracheitis virus (IBR) or parainfluenza virus (PI$_3$). Recently a more virulent BVDV type 2 has teen reported in North America.

Many isolates of BVDV occur but all appear to cross-react with convalescent BVDV sera. There are two distinct biological forms of the virus called biotypes, distinguishable in tissue culture, cytopathic and non-cytopathic. This distinction is important in the pathogenesis and understanding of mucosal disease. Cytopathic virus in tissue culture causes severe damage to the cells and complete destruction within 48–72 hours. The non-cytopathic virus causes no cell damage

CALF   COW

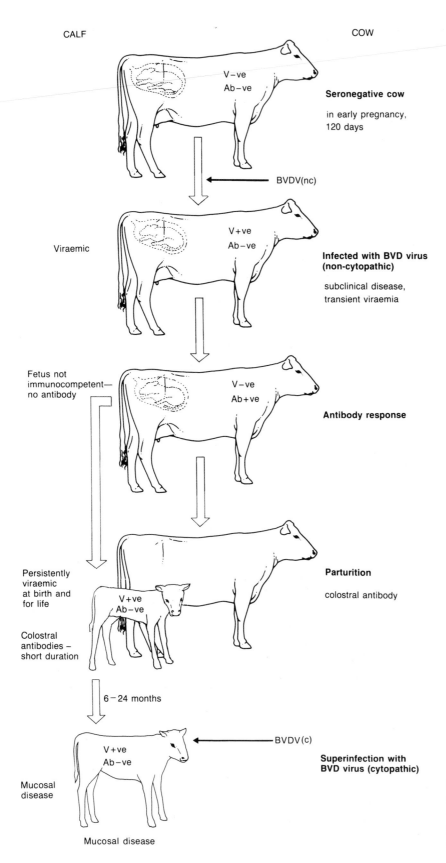

V−ve
Ab−ve

Seronegative cow

in early pregnancy,
120 days

BVDV(nc)

Viraemic

V+ve
Ab−ve

**Infected with BVD virus
(non-cytopathic)**

subclinical disease,
transient viraemia

Fetus not
immunocompetent—
no antibody

V−ve
Ab+ve

Antibody response

Persistently
viraemic
at birth and
for life

V+ve
Ab−ve

Parturition

colostral antibody

Colostral
antibodies –
short duration

6−24 months

V+ve
Ab−ve

BVDV(c)

**Superinfection with
BVD virus (cytopathic)**

Mucosal
disease

Mucosal disease

Fig. 48.1 Hypothesis for the aetiology of mucosal disease. V, BVD
virus; Ab, antibody to BVD virus; nc,
non-cytopathic; c, cytopathic (after
Brownlie, 1985).

Category	Animal	Status	Result of exposure to BVD virus	Final antibody status
1	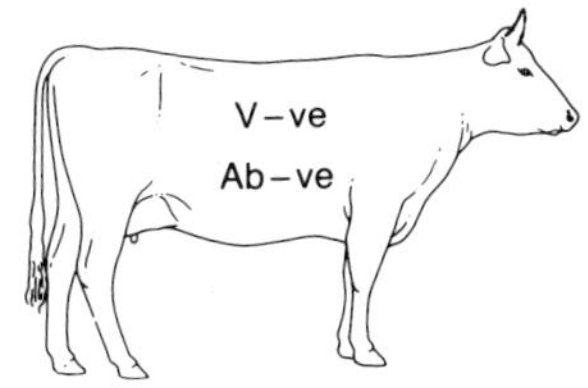 V−ve Ab−ve	No previous exposure to BVD virus	Transient mild infection	+ ve
2	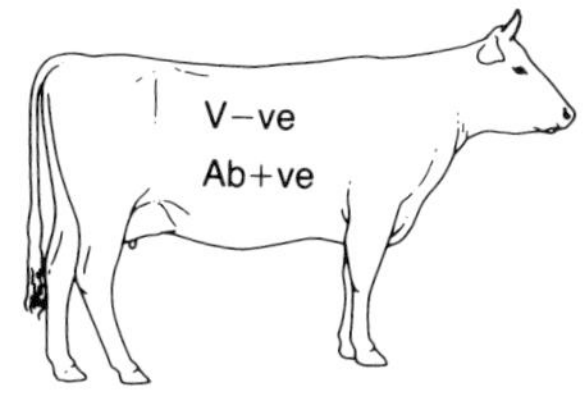 V−ve Ab+ve	Previous exposure to BVD virus from 120 days gestation onwards	Immune	+ ve
3	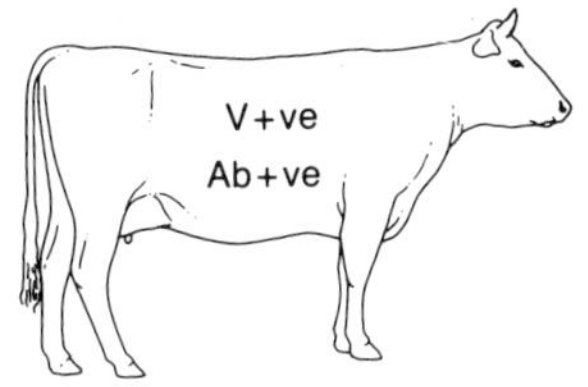 V+ve Ab+ve	(a) Acute viraemia presently sero-converting	Will become immune	+ ve
		(b) Persistently viraemic; occasionally these animals may have low levels of antibody	May later succumb to mucosal disease	± ve
4	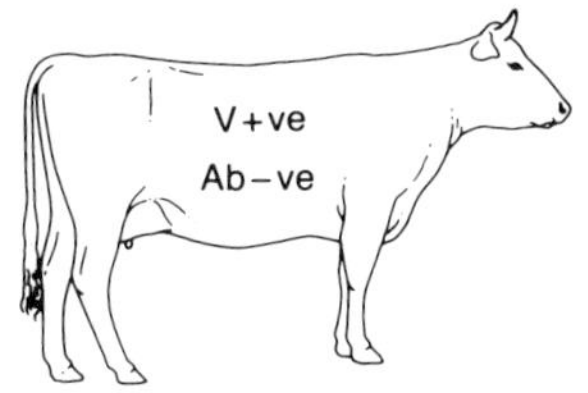 V+ve Ab−ve	(a) Acute viraemia	Will become immune	+ ve
		(b) Persistently infected with BVD virus	May later succumb to mucosal disease	− ve

Fig. 48.2 Combinations of BVD virus and antibody in cattle and their significance (after Brownlie, 1985).

and is identified by staining with fluorescein-labelled BVDV antisera.

Non-cytopathic virus is the major biotype that causes disease, whereas cytopathic virus, isolated from field cases of mucosal disease, is usually only found as a superinfection of a pre-existing non-cytopathic virus infection. Bovine virus diarrhoea virus is shed in nasopharyngeal secretions and urine and perhaps by aerosol droplets. Faeces are a poor source of virus.

Pathogenesis

Postnatal infection of the young or growing animal with non-cytopathic virus is usually a subclinical event. In most herds where the virus is present there is no disease-related problem. However, infection of the seronegative pregnant cow prior to 120 days of gestation, before the immune system of the fetus has become fully developed, can result in disease. When the virus has crossed the placenta, the fetus becomes infected and may result in abortion, mummification or early fetal death. If the fetus survives until neonatal life, it may have developed a state of immune tolerance and then the virus will persist for life. The fetus at birth will be virus positive, but seronegative to the persisting virus. Infection after 120 days will still cause damage to the fetus, but it does not become immunotolerant and viraemic. Such damage would include cerebellar hypoplasia resulting in ataxic calves (see p. 900).

Infertility: Infection of the cow in early pregnancy will cause infertility due to embryo or early fetal death. Evidence of this has been seen in North America, where an infected bull was used on two groups of heifers. One group was seropositive and the other seronegative. The seropositive heifers conceived normally (about 70 per cent pregnancy rate) but the seronegative heifers suffered infertility (in the region of 33 per cent pregnancy rate) that lasted several weeks. These heifers eventually conceived when they had seroconverted some six to eight weeks after the initial infection.

Mixed infections: Bovine virus diarrhoea virus is immunosuppressive. Although infection of calves with BVD virus alone is generally subclinical if RSV, IBR or P13 viruses are also present the pneumonia will be more severe than infection with respiratory viruses alone (see Chapter 17).

Mucosal disease: Mucosal disease occurs as a result of a calf that was born viraemic and seronegative becoming superinfected with cytopathic virus. Mucosal disease is generally sporadic in nature affecting young cattle six to 18 months old. It is usual to find only one, two or three cases occurring on any one farm at the same time; however, larger outbreaks can occur. The disease is characterized by weight loss, severe diarrhoea and inevitably death. Death from mucosal disease usually occurs two to three weeks after infection with cytopathic virus.

Signs

The first signs to appear are anorexia accompanied by reddening and erosions around the dental pad, along the gingival border and under the tongue. These are followed by reddening and erosion around the muzzle. The erosions are shallow, varying sizes and shapes and frequently coalesce. These are to be distinguished from ulcers following vesicular damage, e.g. in foot-and-mouth disease (p. 693) or vesicular stomatitis (p. 710), which are deeper than mucosal disease erosions. Diarrhoea then follows and sometimes lameness may be apparent due to heat and reddening on the coronary band and erosions present in the interdigital space. Because of the sudden onset, diarrhoea is often the first sign that is noticed although salivation is frequently present. The animals are occasionally pyrexic. Weight loss is rapid and death inevitably occurs five to ten days later. Acute infections in adult cows can lead to diarrhoea and agalactia.

Necropsy

The post-mortem findings are usually strongly suggestive of mucosal disease. Oval erosions or shallow ulceration may be seen in the buccal cavity, oesophagus, abomasum, the small intestine beneath the Peyer's patches and in the colon. Oedema and erythema in the intestinal epithelium may also be a feature. The prime sites are the oesophagus, small intestine and abomasum. Care must be exercised in opening the small intestine, which must be opened at the mesenteric attachment in order not to incise through the lesions. Tissue culture can be used to grow virus from all the lesions, as well as from mesenteric lymph nodes, spleen, thymus and tonsil.

Diagnosis

The diagnosis of mucosal disease will be based on the clinical signs and laboratory tests. Pyrexia, diarrhoea, erosions in the mouth and on the muzzle and recent weight loss in an animal six to 18 months old should be highly suggestive of mucosal disease. In the live animal, clotted and EDTA blood samples and a nasopharyngeal swab should be taken and must be submitted to the laboratory within 24 hours for both virus isolation and for BVDV antibodies. It is also helpful to submit fresh spleen, mediastinal lymph node, thymus and small intestinal tissue (particularly with Peyer's patch tissue) for virus isolation. Bulk milk antibody levels can be ascertained.

Differential diagnosis

The main features of mucosal disease are mucosal erosions, diarrhoea and death. Foot-and-mouth disease (p. 693), malignant catarrh (p. 953) and rinderpest (p. 707) are the principal differential diagnoses. With foot-and-mouth disease, morbidity is 100 per cent and vesicles precede the mucosal ulcerations. With malignant catarrh, corneal opacity is a feature; there is also gastroenteritis and enlarged lymph nodes. Lymph node enlargement is not a feature of mucosal disease. Rinderpest has vesicles preceding the erosions, morbidity is high and intestinal oedema and lymph node enlargement are common. *Salmonella* (pp. 225, 850) enteritis should not present a problem with differential diagnosis as it generally affects either young calves or adult animals and there are no mouth lesions. Acorn poisoning can look similar on post mortem, but biochemistry and histology of the kidney should distinguish it from mucosal disease (see p. 951). Other poisoning events may also be considered as a differential diagnosis, but the characteristic oval erosions are generally absent.

Treatment

There is no effective treatment for mucosal disease. If the disease is suspected all efforts should be towards a diagnosis so that effective control measures may be instituted.

Control

When a positive diagnosis has been made, the dam of the affected animal and all the animals in the same group as the affected animal should be blood sampled and the blood cultured for the presence of virus. Persistently viraemic cows invariably give rise to viraemic calves so all dams of viraemic offspring need to be identified. If infection is a recent introduction then several calves in the same age group as the affected one may also be persistently viraemic. Most of these are likely to succumb to mucosal disease at some time in the future.

When testing for BVDV, one should be aware of the possibility of sampling a calf that is only acutely infected and not persistently viraemic. To differentiate this possibility all virus-positive animals should be retested at an interval of six weeks. Persistently viraemic calves should be slaughtered. In the USA and elsewhere vaccines prepared from attenuated cytopathic virus are available, but it is believed that these have occasionally caused disease. Inactivated BVD vaccines are now available in the UK for injection in cows prior to pregnancy (p. 1011) and in calves for respiratory disease control (p. 1007).

It is important to recall that surveys have suggested that 1 per cent of adult animals in the national herd are persistently viraemic. The retention of viraemic animals in the herd is one strategy used to maintain herd immunity. However, there is always a risk that susceptible cows in early pregnancy can become infected. Therefore, once persistently viraemic animals have been identified they should be slaughtered unless they can, with certainty, be kept away from cows in early pregnancy. All newly introduced animals should be isolated and screened for the presence of antibody and virus before mixing with the herd. Persistently viraemic animals should not be kept.

Control of BVD at herd level

Surveys have indicated that upwards of 60 per cent of UK cattle are seropositive to BVD infection and that economic loss can be caused from infertility when seronegative animals are introduced into a seropositive herd. This can be a common scenario with the introduction of replacement heifers, whether home-bred or purchased. Diagnosis of the seropositive status of the herd can be achieved by testing bulk milk for antibody levels. Recently, inactivated BVDV vaccines have become available in the UK. The vaccines have proven excellent efficacy in preventing the fetus becoming infected if cows are vaccinated before they enter the breeding programme. Recent reports would suggest that significant improvements in fertility can follow the use of vaccination. Therefore vaccination of replacement animals before entering an infected herd is to be recommended. Booster vaccination at yearly intervals will probably be required so in time the whole herd will require vaccination annually. The best control policy should be a combination of vaccinating breeding animals and eradicating all persistently infected animals.

Special regard should be given to bulls as they can transmit BVDV in semen. Any veterinary inspection of bulls must include a blood test to ensure freedom from BVDV. Furthermore, any advice about the use of

'sweeper' bulls on breeding animals must include a caution about the possibility of introducing BVDV into the herd.

Johne's disease (paratuberculosis)

Johne's disease is a chronic, infectious enteritis that results in progressive wasting and eventual death. The disease has been reported worldwide wherever ruminants exist and the causal organism is the acid-fast bacterium *Mycobacterium johnei* (*paratuberculosis*). This is now often called *Mycobacterium avium* var. *paratuberculosis* (MAP). The prevalence of Johne's disease varies between countries and within countries.

There appear to be endemically infected farms on which the incidence can be as high as two or three confirmed cases every year, yet in the same district there will be many farms that do not experience the disease, except occasionally in a purchased animal. In some areas of the UK the incidence has declined considerably over the last 30 years, although the incidence in a number of northern European countries appears to be increasing. Recently concern has been expressed at the similarity of Johne's disease and Crohn's disease in humans. The possibility exists that some cases of Crohn's disease may be caused by *M. johnei*.

Pathogenesis

Infection with *M. johnei* occurs in young calves usually from their dams or contact with faeces of carrier cows. There follows a long incubation period of two to six years during which lesions develop in the small intestine and the animals intermittently excrete the organism in the faeces. Not all infected animals progress to the disease state. Where the disease does develop, the organisms multiply and cause extensive lesions in the small intestine that produce overt clinical disease.

Signs

The usual presenting signs are profuse diarrhoea accompanied by gradual weight loss. Frequently, the stress of calving initiates the onset of signs and affected cows are presented two to four weeks after calving. Rectal temperature, appetite and ruminal contractions remain normal. Submandibular oedema is sometimes present. In advanced cases the weight loss leads to emaciation and the diarrhoea remains profuse often with bubbles in the faeces.

Necropsy

The main pathological features are thickening of the lower part of the small intestine, the ileo-caecal valve and sometimes the colon. The mucosal surface has a corrugated appearance. The organism may be present on the mucosal surface or tissue sections of the intestinal wall may reveal both intracellular and extracellular organisms.

Diagnosis

Any debilitating disease that results in emaciation may be confused with Johne's disease. However, the profuse diarrhoea, frequently containing bubbles, will distinguish the condition from weight loss caused by liver fluke (p. 276), liver disease, chronic traumatic reticuloperitonitis (p. 837) or malnutrition. Johne's disease should always be considered as a possible diagnosis when a cow, four years old or more, and recently calved is presented with weight loss and chronic diarrhoea. The history of the prevalence of the disease on the farm will also be helpful. Diagnosis is best confirmed by the demonstration of clumps of acid-fast bacteria in smears of faeces stained with Ziehl–Nielsen stain. As excretion can be intermittent, repeat testing is sometimes necessary. The faeces sample is best taken from the rectum using a gloved hand, scraping faeces from the rectal mucosal surface. Failure to detect the organism in faecal smears does not rule out the possibility of Johne's disease. PCR tests are now also used for the antigen, but with the same provisos mentioned above. However, the organism can usually be detected at post mortem in stained impression smears of the mucosal surface of the terminal ileum or in histological sections of the same area of ileum.

An ELISA test is now available which has a high sensitivity and specificity in animals with clinical disease, although the sensitivity is reduced in animals infected but not showing clinical signs. PCR tests can be used on milk and are a valuable herd screening test.

In some countries, Johnin is used as a diagnostic test and can be administered intradermally or intravenously. Injected intradermally, Johnin produces an oedematous swelling at the site of injection in some cattle that are infected with Johne's disease. When injected intravenously, Johnin will initiate a rectal temperature rise of at least 0.8°C (1.5°F) 4–8 hours after injection. However, as with the complement fixation test, the use of Johnin as an accurate diagnostic indicator is not to be regarded as reliable.

If a definite diagnosis is required, the organism can be cultured from faeces, portions of terminal ileum or mesenteric lymph nodes, but positive results will not be available for six to eight weeks.

Treatment

Treatment of Johne's disease is not to be recommended, as the clinical signs are only evident in the terminal stages of the disease. Antibiotics effective against Gram-negative bacteria, e.g. streptomycin, have been used but without any long-term success. A short remission of the diarrhoea is sometimes possible following a seven-day course of streptomycin and may be considered if for some reason it is not practical to cull the affected animal immediately. If dehydration is evident, rehydration with intravenous fluid therapy may allow the animal to be sent for human consumption.

Control

As infection with the Johne's disease organism occurs in calfhood the main plank in any control programme is to separate the calves from their dams immediately after birth and rear them completely separate from the adult herd. They should not be allowed access to faeces from adult cows at any time during the growing period and all drinking water should be from uncontaminated sources, namely mains water.

In the UK and elsewhere a live vaccine (p. 1012) is available for use in endemically affected herds. The vaccine used is licensed by the Department of the Environment, Food and Rural Affairs (DEFRA) and can only be used on farms where a positive diagnosis has been made from faeces or post-mortem material. Calves are separated from their dams at birth and the vaccine administered subcutaneously in the brisket area in the first seven days of life. A fibro-caseous nodule 2–5 cm in diameter is produced at the injection site and this remains for life.

Vaccinated animals will produce positive reactions to both the avian and bovine tuberculin administered during tuberculosis testing. Usually, the avian reaction is greater than the bovine so differentiation from tuberculosis is possible if the comparative intradermal tuberculosis test is used.

Vaccination in endemic herds has met with considerable success in reducing the incidence of disease in them, but not necessarily infection. However, to be successful separation of the calves from the adults and good hygiene is necessary in addition to vaccination.

Tenesmus

Tenesmus or ineffectual straining to defecate is commonly a sign of disorders of the pelvic cavity, the rectum and some diseases of the alimentary canal.

Tenesmus can be produced by profuse watery diarrhoea or dysentery, constipation, parturition, prolapsed vagina or rectum, vaginitis, urethral calculi, cystitis, lipomatosis of the pelvic cavity and coccidiosis. Tenesmus is also an important sign of ragwort poisoning. Manual examination of the rectum or vagina will produce tenesmus, which will be all the more severe if diarrhoea is present. Rectal or vaginal lacerations as the result of sticks or broom handles being inserted into the vagina or rectum by sadistic individuals will also cause tenesmus. In practice, the most commonly encountered reason for tenesmus is a cow that continues to strain after calving. This can be due to a second calf in the pelvic canal, a retained afterbirth or lacerations to the vaginal wall. The most effective treatment in these situations is to remove the calf if one is present or administer a local epidural anaesthetic.

A thorough examination is essential in cattle exhibiting tenesmus. Vaginal examination should be carried out using a vaginascope to prevent further damage, although frequently signs of vaginal damage may be apparent by separating the vulval lips. A rectal examination will normally be necessary, particularly if constipation is suspected, but a gloved well-lubricated arm should be used because this procedure may exacerbate the condition. Every effort must be made to identify the cause of the tenesmus so that corrective therapy can then be applied.

Diseases of the rectum and anus

Rectal prolapse

Rectal prolapse is less common in cattle than in other species. However, it may occur as a result of prolonged tenesmus associated with vaginal lesions, or coccidiosis, and it has been associated with laurel poisoning. The condition appears to be more common in the Hereford than other cattle breeds.

Treatment

The rectum, if not excessively swollen, can be replaced under epidural anaesthesia and a pursestring suture using umbilical tape inserted around the anal ring.

In recurrent cases a submucosal resection may be required.

Rectal tears

Rectal lacerations are occasionally produced during rectal examinations. They may also be produced by sticks or poles being inserted into the rectum by sadistic individuals. If the tear is completely through the rectal wall repair via a laparotomy may be possible, although it is not easy to reach the pelvic cavity from a laparotomy incision. Also, to succeed the repair must be effected immediately the laceration occurs, otherwise

faecal material will have entered the pelvic and abdominal cavities. The judicious clinician will advise immediate casualty slaughter in such cases.

Recto-vaginal fistula

Recto-vaginal fistulae are invariably the result of severe dystokia, usually in first-calving heifers. Tearing of the vulva can sometimes involve the anus or occasionally a foot of the fetus punctures the roof of the vagina and the floor of the rectum and a fistula results. These normally heal and the animal thereafter defecates via the vagina. Attempts at surgical repair are sometimes recommended because pneumovagina or vaginal contamination with faeces produces infertility. Although conception will not occur in cows so affected if natural service is used, it may be successful using artificial insemination because the semen is deposited in the anterior cervix or the body of the uterus, thus bypassing the vaginal damage.

References

Breukink, H.J. (1980) The effect of heparin in the treatment of general peritonitis in cows. In *Proceedings of the XIth International Congress on Diseases of Cattle*, Tel Aviv, pp. 1442–5.

Brownlie, J. (1985) Clinical aspects of bovine virus diarrhoea/mucosal disease complex in cattle. *In Practice*, **7**, 195–202.

Gordon, P. (2001) A simple technique for correction of left displaced abomasum. *UK Vet*, **5**, 33–5.

Jack, E.J. (1985) The cold cow syndrome – the Cornish experience. In *Proceedings of British Cattle Veterinary Association Meeting*, London, January 1985, p. 203.

Pinsent, P.J.N. (1977) The diagnosis of the surgical disorders of the bovine abomasum. *Bovine Practitioner*, **12**, 40–57.

Pinsent, P.J.N. (1978) The diagnosis of the surgical disorders of the bovine abomasum. *Bovine Practitioner*, **13**, 45–50.

Stober, M. & Dirkson, G. (1977) The differential diagnosis of abdominal findings (adspection, rectal examination and exploratory laparotomy) in cattle. *Bovine Practitioner*, **12**, 35–9.

Williams, E.I. (1975) The 'reticular grunt' test for traumatic reticulo-peritonitis. *Bovine Practitioner*, **10**, 98.

Further reading

Brownlie, J. (1985) Clinical aspects of bovine virus diarrhoea/mucosal disease complex in cattle. *In Practice*, **7**, 195–202.

Chapter 49
Respiratory Conditions

A.H. Andrews and R.S. Windsor

Acute exudative pneumonia	860
Aspiration pneumonia	860
Bovine farmer's lung	861
Bovine tuberculosis	862
Chronic suppurative pneumonia	864
Peracute pleuropneumonia	865
Diffuse fibrosing alveolitis	865
Dusty feed rhinotracheitis	866
Fog fever	866
Thrombosis of the caudal vena cava	867
Contagious bovine pleuropneumonia (CBPP)	868

Acute exudative pneumonia

Aetiology

This is thought in many cases to be a primary bacterial condition and usually *Arcanobacterium* (*Actinomyces*, *Corynebacterium*) *pyogenes* (Gram-positive rods) can be isolated, or in some cases *Mannheimia (Pasteurella) haemolytica* and *P. multocida* (Gram-negative short rods) (Pirie, 1979).

Epidemiology

This condition is not uncommon and is usually seen as respiratory disease in individual animals. It can be present in cattle of any age, particularly when there has been chronic pneumonia in the housing period. In can be seen in dairy-bred cattle as well as in suckler animals, both indoors and at grass. Individual cases usually occur but outbreaks can follow some form of stress. The condition is one of sudden onset and is mainly differentiated from acute viral pneumonia by the fact that it usually affects individual animals.

Signs

The animal shows signs of suddenly going off its feed and is dull. There is an oculo-nasal discharge which may be mucoid or mucopurulent. The temperature is usually 40–41°C (104–107°F), respiratory rate is between 20 and 60/minute, usually with hyperpnoea. There is often some coughing but this is not pronounced. On auscultation there are usually squeaks, humming and wheezing often at inspiration, particularly the latter. Cranioventrally, there may be moist sounds and there may be pleuritic rub (sandpaper-like) sounds in a few cases.

Necropsy

At post mortem there are dark areas of consolidation in the ventral parts of the apical and cardiac, and in some animals, the thoracic lobes. The areas of pneumonia may be small and scattered, but in more severe cases there are large areas of consolidation and, in some animals, abscess formation. Microscopically, there is exudation and vascular congestion with the bronchioles and alveoli showing infiltration with neutrophils and macrophages (Pirie, 1979).

Diagnosis

Diagnosis depends on the history of usually only a single animal being involved with pyrexia and respiratory signs normally being evident.

Differential diagnoses involve chronic pneumonia but normally the animals are less ill and several are affected. Inhalation pneumonia usually results in a very dull animal and also there is often a history of drenching.

Treatment and control

When treating, the affected animal should be isolated. Antibiotic therapy with oxytetracycline, penicillin and streptomycin, ampicillin, amoxycillin, cephalosporins, sulphadimidine, and trimethoprim and sulphadiazine for three to five days is usually successful. Most cases respond well to therapy, but a few cases relapse and some ultimately develop chronic suppurative pneumonia.

Prevention is by trying to ensure adequate ventilation when housed and to avoid chilling.

Aspiration pneumonia

Aetiology

This is also known as inhalation pneumonia and although not a common condition, it still occurs too frequently. Obtaining an adequate history is important and often the stockworker may realize what has happened, but will be reluctant to admit it or even that the animal has been drenched. Obstruction or paralysis of the larynx, pharynx or oesophagus may produce the problem, as with parturient paresis, or the rupture of a pharyngeal abscess or the products of laryngeal diphtheria. The signs will depend on the nature of the fluid introduced, the quantity and the bacteria introduced. If a large quantity is administered into the lungs, then instantaneous death may occur. If the substance given is soluble, then absorption into the body is rapid because of the highly vascular nature of the lungs, and few, if any signs will occur. Less soluble products will result in a varying degree of toxaemia and respiratory signs, which are often fatal, after between one and three days.

Signs

In the peracute form death occurs rapidly after drenching. However, in the acute form only one animal is usually affected and there is a history of drenching. Signs develop rapidly and include a varying degree of dullness and inappetence, a cough and tachypnoea. The temperature is usually elevated to about 40°C (104°F) and on auscultation there are areas of dullness present, normally in the cranio-ventral parts of the lungs, and moist bubbling and crackles may be heard in the area. There is often also a pleuritic rub sound and some degree of thoracic pain. If the condition progresses, the signs of dullness and anorexia become more pronounced, and there may be a fetid odour to the breath.

In the subacute form there are few signs present except for episodes of coughing and tachypnoea following the introduction of the fluid. Some animals will survive the immediate episode and become chronic cases. These will show ill-thrift and intermittent bouts of respiratory problems.

Necropsy

At post mortem there is often an acute exudative or gangrenous pneumonia of the ventral parts of the apical, cardiac and usually also the diaphragmatic lobes. In some animals there is extensive suppurative necrosis.

Diagnosis

Diagnosis is helped if a true history is obtained and is indicative that the condition is present. Usually only a single animal is affected and the signs are of sudden onset. The respiratory signs are severe and there is usually a leucopenia and neutrophilia present.

Differential diagnoses include septicaemia, which has fewer respiratory signs, enteritis but then diarrhoea is present, and acute exudative pneumonia, but in this case there is no history of drenching and usually the animal is less dull.

Treatment and control

If there is to be a hope of effective therapy, it must be administered as soon as possible after the drenching incident. The use of antibiotics or a sulphonamide is indicated and it is best to give the first dose intravenously. Thus oxytetracycline, amoxycillin, ampicillin, sulphadimidine, sulphamethoxypyridazine or sulphapyrazole can be used. In exceptional circumstances where allowed chloramphenicol might be indicated. Therapy should be continued in most cases for about five days. In addition, fluid therapy may be required. The animal should be encouraged to eat and drink. It should be kept on its own in a well-bedded, airy pen.

Control is by ensuring that all drenching and dosing is undertaken slowly, allowing the animal time to swallow.

Bovine farmer's lung

Aetiology

This is a form of chronic atypical interstitial pneumonia. The condition appears to be a chronic reaction to certain fungi found in badly made hay, such as *Micropolyspora faeni*.

Epidemiology

The problem is quite common during the winter in housed cattle fed poor quality mouldy hay or straw. More cases occur in the wetter western parts of Britain and in other countries with high rainfall. Where much rain falls in the summer months, hay may need to be baled at very high moisture contents. This allows overheating to occur and thermophilic microflora then predominate. Disease is often only seen in adult cattle and in some cases the farmer will also have farmer's lung. In Britain this is defined as an industrial injury and is considered to be due to the inhalation of dust from mouldy hay or other mouldy vegetable produce. It results in a defect in gas exchange due to a reaction in the peripheral parts of the bronchopulmonary system. In cattle the condition is usually a herd problem but occasionally a farmer will consider that there is sudden onset in one animal. In such cases the examination of other animals will show varying lesser degrees of the problem.

Signs

The acute signs follow housing and there is often a sudden onset of dullness, a fall in milk yield and a decreased appetite. The animal shows respiratory signs, normally including some respiratory distress, and coughing. On auscultation there are crackles over the cranio-ventral parts of the lung. Although some cases are pyrexic, most animals will have a normal rectal temperature.

In the chronic form there is progressive weight loss and coughing, often with the production of green mucus, which tends to occur with each winter but resolves during the summer months with outside grazing. Occasionally, such animals will develop a sudden crisis following a stress such as calving, a sudden heavy exposure to the antigen, unaccustomed exercise or due to congestive heart failure. Usually there is obvious tachypnoea and hyperpnoea but no pyrexia or thoracic pain or alteration in the resonance of the thorax. Auscultation may produce harsh crackles over the cranio-ventral aspects of the lung and in some cases there are widespread whistles, squeaks and wheezing. It is uncommon for animals to die of the condition unless there are complications.

Necropsy

At necropsy all lung lobes may be affected and there is often overinflation of the peripheral acini. Small grey-green foci tend to be present in the lobules. Histologically, the alveolar walls show interstitial infiltration with plasma cells, lymphocytes and macrophages. Another change is bronchitis obliterans and also epithelial granulomata can occur.

Diagnosis

Diagnosis depends on a history of occurrence in wet areas and feeding poor quality mouldy hay in winter. The problem improves in the summer. Signs include loss of weight with the respiratory disease. An intradermal skin test with *Micropolyspora faeni* produces a reaction 4–6 hours after injection. On serological examination precipitating antibodies to *Micropolyspora faeni* are found but they may also be seen in unaffected cattle within the same herd.

Treatment and control

The use of long-acting corticosteroids may help reduce signs. Where mouldy hay or straw has to be fed or used for bedding then it must be shaken out outside before being offered to the animals. As human problems can arise, a face mask should be worn.

Control involves improving hay-making, which may mean the use of hay additives to upgrade hay quality. Otherwise, the provision of silage might be useful but this does normally mean investment in new machinery for producing the conserved roughage.

Bovine tuberculosis

Aetiology

This is infection with *Mycobacterium bovis* (Gram-positive, acid-fast rods).

Epidemiology

At one time the condition was very common in many countries. However, following tuberculin testing, pasteurization of milk and adequate meat inspection the disease is uncommon in most countries today, but is still seen periodically mainly in dairy herds. In most cases infection breaks out in the growing heifers or younger cows. The condition is still prevalent in south-west England, but is now being increasingly seen in other areas including the south Midlands, north-west England and Wales. In many regions infection has reappeared and is associated with the finding of tuberculosis in the European badger (*Meles meles*). However, in many cases infection can follow the purchase of a carrier without overt signs. Infection of deer with *M. bovis* can also spread disease and in New Zealand a problem occurs with the brush-tailed possum (*Trichosurus vulpecula*). The organism is killed by sunlight, but is resistant to desiccation and can survive in a wide range of acids and alkalis. It is also able to remain viable for long periods in soil that is moist and warm. In cattle faeces, *M. bovis* can survive for as little as a week or as long as eight weeks. Man can occasionally be infected and the disease can occur in goats and pigs, and very occasionally in horses and sheep. Very occasionally cattle can be infected with *Mycobacterium tuberculosis*, usually because people tending or in close contact with the cattle are infected.

When infection is by inhalation, a lesion often occurs at the point of entry and the local lymph node. When ingestion is the route of entry, alimentary lesions are rare but lesions may be present in the tonsils, pharyngeal or mesenteric lymph nodes. Lesions may then disseminate from the primary areas to others.

When the badger is involved, most infection is thought to be by ingestion, but a higher infection level is necessary to establish alimentary than respiratory infection. In most cases the lesions are respiratory and are thought to be due to the inhalation of ruminal gases.

The organism can be present in sputum, milk, faeces, urine, vaginal and uterine discharges and any discharging lesions. Entry is usually by inhalation (especially if housed) or ingestion (when outside or badgers are the source of infection). Drinking infected milk can infect the calf. Signs can occur in very young calves (under a month old). Intercurrent disease in the herd such as BVD may exacerbate the problem (Monies, 2000). Once in a herd, infection probably spreads from cow to cow by inhalation. However, spread from cows to calves may be via the milk. Occasionally, intrauterine infection has resulted from a coital transfer.

Signs

Various body systems can be infected. Often signs are few and usually are confined to the respiratory tract. There is a soft, productive, chronic cough occurring once or twice at a time. It can be elicited by pressure on the pharynx. If the condition continues there is a marked increase in the depth and rate of respirations as well as dyspnoea. In advanced cases, areas of dullness in the chest are heard on auscultation or percussion. In other cases there are squeaks and whistles. A snoring respiration can occur.

The alimentary form is unusual. There are few signs but occasional diarrhoea occurs. Bloat can arise through enlargement of the mediastinal and bronchial lymph nodes. Bone can be infected and meningitis occurs in calves.

Mammary involvement these days tends to be rare but results in udder induration and the supramammary lymph nodes are enlarged. The udder form can be a serious potential source of spread to humans. The uterine form is also uncommon. Swelling of various lymph nodes can occasionally be seen, and abortion may sometimes occur.

A generalized form can occur with signs following calving. There is a progressive loss of condition with a variable appetite. There may be a variable rectal temperature but usually it is only about 39.7°C (103.7°F). The animals are more docile than normal but still bright and alert.

Necropsy

A focus of infection occurs within a week of bacteria entering the cow and, after the third week, calcification can occur. Depending on the route of entry, and where the condition becomes generalized, one or several lymph nodes may contain tuberculous granulomas. In the respiratory system it is the mediastinal or bronchial lymph nodes that are involved, possibly with abscesses in the lungs. The pus is thick, cheese-like and yellow or orange in colour. Sometimes the pleura and peritoneum contain nodules.

In practice, an attempt is made to determine whether infection is active and if cases are 'open' and therefore likely to infect other animals. Active infection is designated by lung infection with limited encapsulation and hyperaemia. This categorization is now thought to be erroneous and it is considered that most lesions are potentially infective. Other organs often show small, transparent, shot-like lesions and these may also be present in the lymph nodes. Tuberculous cystitis and metritis tend to be open cases. Closed infection is seen as discrete lesions enclosed within well-developed capsules. The enclosed pus tends to be caseous and yellow or orange in colour. In tuberculin reactors the apparent absence of gross lesions of tuberculosis – so-called non-visible lesion (NVL) reactors – does not necessarily indicate that the animal is uninfected.

Diagnosis

Diagnosis depends on the history of an area where tuberculosis occurs in cattle, badgers or other wildlife. The signs often result in chronic respiratory lesions with loss of condition and a soft, productive, single cough. The comparative tuberculin test is useful. It uses avian (0.5 mg/ml) and bovine tuberculin purified protein derivative (1.0 mg/ml) injected into the neck skin. There is a greater skin thickness increase in bovine than avian tuberculin. Interpretation depends on whether there is no history of reactions, one or more reactions without confirmation at post-mortem examination or a herd with a recent history of reactions confirmed post mortem.

Johne's disease (p. 857), skin tuberculosis (p. 886) or avian tuberculosis can result in false positive bovine tuberculin reactions but usually the avian reaction increases more than the bovine. False negatives occur following protracted infection, desensitization following tuberculin testing, early cases of infection, old cows and those animals recently calved.

The single intradermal test is used in many countries. Its main disadvantage is that it will give reactions to avian tuberculosis, skin tuberculosis or Johne's disease. A short thermal test can be used by injecting tuberculin subcutaneously and measuring the animal's temperature every 2 hours. A rise in temperature of 1°C (1.8°F) is considered significant. Intravenous tuberculin also results in a temperature rise. The Stormont test has been used to detect disease in infected cattle. Various serological tests have been used and recently the enzyme-linked immunosorbent assay (ELISA) test has shown promise. A gamma interferon test can be used to determine infected cattle.

Differential diagnosis

Differential diagnosis includes enzootic bovine leukosis (Chapter 43b) but this can be detected by serology.

Chronic lung abscesses can cause problems in diagnosis. Traumatic reticulitis (p. 837) may produce similar signs but there is usually a history of an acute attack. Chronic pericarditis (p. 731) can present problems but will result in a jugular pulse and muffled heart sounds and endocarditis (p. 726) cases usually produce a murmur. Contagious bovine pleuropneumonia (p. 868) can cause problems but can be differentiated by a complement fixation test. Lymph node enlargement due to actinobacillosis (p. 823) may be difficult to detect but can be done with a tuberculin test.

Treatment and control

Treatment is not usually undertaken because of the chronic nature of the disease and its potential zoonotic effects. Control in many countries, including North America and Europe, is by tuberculin testing and slaughter of reactors. Hygiene standards need to be upgraded and efficient meat inspection and tracing back to the farm of origin is useful. Research work on vaccine production is being undertaken and may be directed towards vaccination of wildlife such as badgers and possums.

Chronic suppurative pneumonia

Aetiology

Various initial causes may result in one or more pathological conditions such as bronchopneumonia, bronchiectasis and pulmonary abscesses. These are often encompassed by the term chronic suppurative pneumonia.

Epidemiology

Most cases occur in adult cattle rather than those still growing. It is, however, a very common cause of respiratory signs in the individual animal. Often there has been an outbreak of acute pneumonia in the history. Although most cases seem to progress slowly over a period of weeks or months, the odd case will appear to be of sudden onset, due to a rapid exacerbation of a suppurative area in the chest.

Signs

Severe signs of disease include a sudden marked loss of condition with dullness, obvious thoracic pain, pyrexia (40.5°C; 105°F). In some animals there is halitosis due to a necrotizing bronchopneumonia and pleurisy. Death in these animals often occurs within a few days.

More usually the animal becomes progressively duller and thinner, with a fall in milk yield and intermittent pyrexia, up to 40°C (104°F). A cough is usually present with the production of mucus and there is a variable degree of tachypnoea. Thoracic pain may be obvious by an abduction of the elbows and reluctance to move, but in other cases it is only discernible on ballottement. On auscultation there are usually whistles, squeaks and wheezing sounds in the cranio-ventral part of the chest and there are often areas of dullness.

Necropsy

If the main lesion at post mortem is a bronchopneumonia, there is usually marked consolidation of the cranio-ventral parts of the lung, with exudate filling the bronchi and bronchioles. On histological examination, inflammatory cells pass the alveoli and bronchi. When the main problem is a bronchiectasis, often bronchi in the cranial and middle lobes, with dilated air passageways, contain mucus and fibrous tissue. In severe cases the histological sections show complete destruction of the alveolar tissue. When lung abscesses are the main feature, these are usually found in the ventral lung border. Necrotic tissues and pus-containing structures are found within a fibrous capsular wall.

Diagnosis

Diagnosis is based on a history of a chronic loss of condition with respiratory disease in a single animal with signs such as pyrexia, thoracic pain and cough.

Differential diagnosis needs to include acute pneumonia (p. 860), which may be in a single animal or several animals; salmonellosis (p. 850; Chapter 15), but at this age there is usually diarrhoea; infectious bovine rhinotracheitis (IBR) (p. 289) infection, but this usually results in a marked conjunctivitis. Inhalation pneumonia (p. 860) on the other hand has a specific history and tuberculosis (p. 862) will probably have a history of herd infection, whereas malignant catarrhal fever will involve ocular lesions and enlarged lymph nodes, etc.

Treatment and control

Often therapy is of limited use. Any treatment may need to be prolonged for 10 days to two weeks or more. Antibiotic therapy with amoxycillin, ampicillin, oxytetracycline, penicillin and streptomycin, sulphadimidine, or trimethoprim and sulphadiazine may be helpful. Most cases that respond are likely to break down again and so infected animals should be slaughtered when convenient.

Control involves culling animals that have had previous bouts of respiratory disease and ensuring all cases are treated early and thoroughly.

Peracute pleuropneumonia

A respiratory problem was described in the 1990s in Great Britain which appeared to be a relatively well-defined syndrome and which at post-mortem examination showed a pleuropneumonia (Harwood *et al.*, 1995). While it looked like contagious bovine pleuropneumonia, the history and epidemiology were not right and *Mycoplasma mycoides* subspecies *mycoides* was not isolated.

Aetiology

Routine bacteriology of lungs when positive routinely isolated *Mannheimia (Pasteurella) haemolytica*, usually of serotype Al. *Arcanobacterium (Actinomyces) pyogenes* has been isolated from the necrotic areas within the lung. No further consistent bacterial or viral synergism has been recognized.

Occurrence

All problems appear to have involved adult animals and calf respiratory problems on the farms did not appear to be unusual or of high incidence. Usually one or a small number of animals are affected and most of these die. The remainder of the herd do not appear to show any signs of disease. Animals in the immediate post calving period were most commonly infected. There was a history of purchase of cows and/or heifers within the last 12 months on all farms and in several there were imports from Europe as well as from the United Kingdom. There was no history of recent transport or movement of the affected animals.

Signs

Severe respiratory problems are seen with dyspnoea, hyperpnoea and tachypnoea. Most animals will die or are humanely destroyed regardless of any antibiotic regime. There are variable lung signs, including pleural rubs, etc.

Pathology

The thoracic cavity contains severe changes with very obvious fibrinous or fibrous pleurisy. There are strong attachments between the thoracic wall and the lungs; pleural deposits can often be 1 cm thick. There are large amounts of pleural effusion and pulmonary oedema. The lungs show marbling with severe interlobular oedema, with parenchymal congestion and consolidation.

Diagnosis

Small numbers are affected with severe disease, which is often fatal. There is no apparent precipitating factor except for calving. Post-mortem examination allows diagnosis.

Differential diagnosis

Contagious bovine pleuropneumonia (CBPP) is an obvious differential and in many countries, as in Britain, CBPP is notifiable and so it will be necessary to report cases to the authorities (see p. 873).

Treatment

Large doses of antibiotics, often with non-steroidal anti-inflammatory agents, can help in a few cases.

Control

At present there is no real advice to offer in herds which for any reason have to buy in animals.

Diffuse fibrosing alveolitis

Aetiology

The cause is unknown but many cases occur in animals with chronic bovine farmer's lung and have precipitating antibodies to *Micropolyspora faeni*. However, it is probable that there are other precipitating causes as some cattle do not possess antibodies to this organism.

Epidemiology

The condition affects individual animals and is uncommon although more frequently seen in herds with a history of bovine farmer's lung. Both dairy and suckler cows are affected and cases can occur indoors or outside, particularly in animals older than six years. The condition is usually a progressive problem and may actually start following a stress such as calving. The condition has normally been present for weeks or months before advice is sought and the animal will have lost condition with coughing or respiratory signs when subjected to mild exercise. Congestive heart failure occurs in about 12 per cent of cases.

Signs

Affected cattle are bright and do not have a raised temperature or pulse rate. The appetite is good but there is a progressive loss of condition. The respiratory signs tend to be quite severe, with a persistent cough always present as well as tachypnoea and hyperpnoea present even in the resting animal. On auscultation of the chest, rhonchi (whistles, squeaks, wheezing) are heard over both lungs and crackling sounds in the cranio-ventral chest. There is no thoracic pain.

Depression and inappetence only occur in the late stages of the condition with congestive heart failure resulting in subcutaneous oedema and an increased heart and respiratory rate. The liver may be palpably enlarged and there may be diarrhoea.

Necropsy

At necropsy alveolar changes predominate but there may be bronchitis with excessive thick mucus in the bronchi. There is thickening and fibrosis of the alveolar walls. Histologically, large numbers of mononuclear cells are seen in the alveolar air spaces. There may be hyperplasia of type 2 pneumocytes or metaplasia of the alveolar epithelium so that it contains ciliated and mucus-secreting cells. Pulmonary hypertension can occur and this results in right-sided heart failure.

Diagnosis

Diagnosis depends on the history, i.e. a single animal, with gradual loss of condition with respiratory signs present at rest, coughing, no thoracic pain or fever and a bright animal.

Treatment

As the cause is unknown, little can be done to alleviate the problem. However, corticosteroids can reduce the cellular changes in the lung. Casualty slaughter of the animal should be undertaken before the loss of condition is too severe.

Dusty feed rhinotracheitis

Aetiology

Particles of different sizes meet varying fates in the respiratory system following inspiration (see Table 49.1). Most of the particles will be in the nasal passages or the trachea, bronchi and bronchioles. The condition results from the introduction of dry, fine-particled feed, or very dusty bedding.

The introduction of a dusty dry feed to animals indoors causes the problem. The signs occur most frequently in the hour or two following feeding. Removal of the feed causes recovery in a few days. The condition occurs most commonly when the relative humidity is low.

Table 49.1 The fate of various-sized particles entering the respiratory system.

Particle size (μm)	Fate
>10	Removed in nasal passages
2–10	Deposited at varying levels in respiratory tract, but above alveoli. The smaller the particle, the further down the respiratory airways it is deposited. Removed by mucociliary action
1–2	Deposited in alveoli
0.5–1	Exhaled with air
<0.5	Deposited in alveoli due to diffusion forces

Signs

Following feeding or bedding, there is the sudden onset of coughing. The cough tends to be dry and can be single or paroxysmal. Several cattle are normally affected. The animals are otherwise bright and alert; they eat well and there are no abnormal lower respiratory sounds. Respirations are normal in rate and extent, and temperature is normal. There is conjunctivitis and usually a copious ocular and nasal discharge, which is mucoid but sometimes slightly purulent.

Treatment and control

Treatment involves replacing the feed or bedding used. Otherwise dampen down the feed before giving it, or molasses can be added to it. In the case of bedding, new bales should be opened up outside before the cattle are bedded.

Control is by not feeding dusty hay. If the feed is found to be dusty then 5 per cent molasses should be added to it. Dusty bedding should not be used. As the particles affecting the animals can affect humans, it is advisable for workers to wear face masks.

Fog fever

Aetiology

This is a form of atypical interstitial pneumonia. Although not fully authenticated, the condition is considered to be a toxicosis following the ingestion of large quantities of L-tryptophan.

Epidemiology

The condition is seen in cattle over two years old, particularly those in suckler herds, and affects several cattle to a varying degree at the same time. Often the cattle have been receiving little nutrition and are put onto a more lush pasture in the autumn (September to November). The field may have been top-dressed with a nitrogenous fertilizer. The condition is normally seen within two weeks of entry to the new pasture. The Hereford and Hereford-cross breeds seem to be particularly susceptible.

It is thought that L-tryptophan in the grass is ingested and metabolized in the rumen to indole acetic acid (IAA), which is decarboxylated by *Lactobacillus* spp. to produce 3-methyl indole (3MI). This metabolite can enter the blood and is usually acted upon by the mixed function oxidase system to produce indoles and other metabolites in the urine. 3-Methyl indole can cause the destruction of pulmonary cells such as type 1 pneumocytes and monociliated bronchiolar secretory cells, resulting in various pathological changes. Mortality in severely affected animals can be high (up to 75 per cent) but usually only a small number (5 per cent) are so involved.

Signs

Several animals will show signs but the degree will vary widely and often the farmer only notices one to be ill at the start. The cattle tend to be much quieter and more approachable than normal and to have a sleepy or tranquil expression. The respiratory signs are usually of distress but vary in degree. Coughing is normally little heard.

In the severe form there is the sudden onset of dyspnoea with a loud respiratory grunt, mouth breathing, and often the animal froths at the mouth. Auscultation reveals little considering the severity of the illness, but it may produce soft, moist sounds and a few crackles. Death can occur as the result of excitement. Less severely affected animals show tachypnoea (rate 50–80/minute) with hyperpnoea and usually there is no dyspnoea. The rectal temperature tends to be normal and the animal is again quiet and tranquil. Coughing is only heard occasionally and in some recovering animals a subcutaneous emphysema may develop. Auscultation may reveal harsh sounds.

Necropsy

Dead animals have haemorrhages in the larynx, tracheal and bronchial mucosae. The lungs tend to be swollen, heavy and dark red in colour. The cut surface glistens, is smooth and has a red appearance. Emphysema may be present in the interlobular septa and pleura. Histological examination reveals severe congestion and oedema of the pulmonary tissue, hyaline membrane formation, severe interstitial emphysema and moderate epithelial hyperplasia of type 2 pneumocytes.

Cattle slaughtered in the later stages do not usually show haemorrhages of the respiratory mucosa. There is an overall pale pink colour with variable amounts of interstitial emphysema.

Diagnosis

Diagnosis involves the history of a group condition, mainly in suckler animals moved to a lush pasture in autumn. The signs help, particularly the acute respiratory signs with little to hear on auscultation, no cough and the animals being more tranquil than usual. Postmortem findings indicate the condition, with pulmonary oedema and emphysema.

Differential diagnoses include husk (p. 272), but a cough is present and there would be a history of no vaccination. Pneumonic pasteurellosis (p. 286) would produce pyrexia and a mucopurulent discharge. Nitrate poisoning (p. 950) would produce some signs but the blood would tend to be brownish and the urine contain methaemoglobin. Infectious bovine rhinotracheitis (p. 289) would usually involve pyrexia and a loud explosive cough. Thrombosis of the caudal vena cava (see below) would usually involve a single animal and eventually haemoptysis would occur. *Brassica* spp. (p. 941) poisoning would have a different history of feeding and would usually be later in the autumn.

Treatment and control

Treatment is to remove the cattle from the incriminated pasture. Most other treatment tends to be empirical. Interference with a severely distressed animal may result in its death. Atropine at 1 g/450 kg (990 lb) body weight intravenously acts as a bronchodilator and corticosteroids may be useful. Flunixin meglumine has been beneficial in experimentally produced acute bovine pulmonary emphysema and in the field.

Control means that if animals are hungry when they enter a new pasture in the autumn, restrict their feed by only allowing grazing for short periods during the first two weeks. This should be for about 2 hours on the first day, increasing by an hour a day so that the cattle can be left out for the whole day after about 12 days. Otherwise the area can be strip-grazed or initially grazed with a less susceptible species such as sheep. If monensin sodium is given at the rate of 200 mg/head per day before and after entering the pasture, this can stop problems.

Thrombosis of the caudal vena cava

Aetiology

The cause is a septic focus, usually in the liver, resulting in a septic thrombus in the caudal vena cava, from which there is the haematogenous spread of infection to the lungs.

Epidemiology

This is an uncommon condition affecting single animals over one year old, although many cases occur in the growing animal. A few cases of thrombosis of the cranial vena cava have been recorded with similar signs. Most cases result from a liver abscess. This causes a localized phlebitis, usually in the area of the vena cava, adjacent to the liver. Septic emboli pass to the lungs where they can produce chronic suppurative pneumonia and multiple lung abscesses, or they can cause pulmonary arterial lesions. Endarteritis, arteritis and thromboembolism occur, resulting in aneurysms of the pulmonary artery, which then rupture causing haemorrhage in the bronchi and alveoli. Usually, there is a history of sudden onset of respiratory disease, although in some cases there is a history of chronic loss of weight and coughing. A few cases show obstruction of the hepatic venous return with chronic venous congestion of the liver, its enlargement and no access to the collateral venous drainage. Bacteriological examination often reveals little because of previous therapy. However, some cases reveal staphylococci, *A. pyogenes* and *Fusobacterium necrophorum* spp.

Signs

Peracute signs result in an animal dying suddenly with no premonitory signs but usually there is a pool of blood in front of it. In the acute case, cattle with the condition show respiratory disease for a few days or some months, with tachypnoea and shallow breathing. The animal develops haemoptysis and frothy blood can be found in the nasal passages and mouth. There are often blood stains around the animal and in many cases there is melaena. There is a variable amount of thoracic pain with abduction of the elbows. On auscultation there is a widespread whistle, with wheezing sounds.

The chronic form involves animals developing congestive cardiac failure and ascites with an enlarged liver, which may be palpated on the right sublumbar fossa. This often occurs some time before haemoptysis is present.

Once animals start to show haemoptysis then death will ensue, usually within a week or two but occasionally it may take up to 40 days.

Necropsy

Following death, often one or more abscesses are found in the liver, and usually the caudal vena cava thrombosis is in the area of the liver. Multiple septic emboli are normally present within the pulmonary artery. In the lung itself there is usually embolic suppurative pneumonia, intrapulmonary haemorrhage, often concentric and globular in shape, and multiple red areas where blood has been aspirated. When there is obstruction of the hepatic veins then there is marked hepatomegaly and ascites.

Diagnosis

Diagnosis involves the history of loss of condition and respiratory signs in a single animal. The signs help, particularly haemoptysis with thoracic pain, and are almost pathognomonic. Post-mortem findings are relatively diagnostic with thrombosis of the vena cava, emboli in the pulmonary artery and intrapulmonary haemorrhage. Haematological examination shows the packed cell volume is often low (11.0–22.5 per cent).

Differential diagnosis includes an accident, but signs would be highly unlikely unless there is an immediate history of trauma. Tuberculosis (p. 863) could also give rise to some of the signs but is usually much slower and the tuberculin test would reveal this.

Treatment and control

There is no effective therapy. Cattle can be casualty slaughtered if necessary after a course of four or five days' antibiotic therapy using a broad-spectrum compound and then leaving the required withdrawal time.

Control is not possible, but any septic focus should be treated adequately as soon as it occurs. Make sure that all changes in feeding are undertaken slowly so as to avoid the possibility of acidosis (p. 829).

Contagious bovine pleuropneumonia (CBPP)

Mycoplasma mycoides is the cause of contagious bovine pleuropneumonia (CBPP), which now that rinderpest has been controlled, is the cattle disease of greatest economic importance on the continent of Africa. CBPP affects only cattle and the water buffalo (*Bubalis bubalis*). Claude Bourgelat, the great French veterinary surgeon and founder of the Lyons Veterinary School, was the first person to differentiate rinderpest from CBPP (in the eighteenth century). It was thought the disease was introduced into Europe from Asia in the seventeenth century and that the wars of the eighteenth and nineteenth centuries resulted in its spread throughout the continent. From Europe it was taken to the rest of the world; South America is the only continent that has never experienced the disease.

New techniques (PCR, DNA fingerprinting, ELISA, among others) in manipulating mycoplasms have led to new thinking about the phylogeny of the group. Where there were individual species, the organisms now have been grouped into 'clusters'. Economically the *Mycoplasma mycoides* cluster is the most important, containing as it does, *Mycoplasma mycoides* subspecies *mycoides*, small colony type (*M. mycoides*), the large colony type that infects goats and to a lesser extent sheep and *M. mycoides capri*, another of the agents that causes contagious caprine pleuropneumonia.

It has been possible to trace the introduction of the infection into many countries. Indeed, in some cases the identity of the infected animal is known! There is, however, some dispute about the entry of the disease into Africa. French workers believe that the infection was introduced when *Bos indicus* crossed into the continent from Asia; it did not get to southern Africa in this way and there is evidence that it did not exist in East Africa before the invasion of General Napier into Ethiopia in 1868.

The Dutch Ambassador to the Cape Colony, with the intention of improving the local stock, imported a bull from his country in 1853. The infection was rapidly disseminated by trek oxen, particularly to the Transvaal where in the space of two years it killed more than 100 000 animals. From South Africa the infection was taken to Namibia, Zimbabwe and Botswana. From Namibia it was taken to Angola and from there to Zambia and the Congo. By 1940, with the exception of Namibia and Angola, the southern African countries had eradicated the infection. The development of an efficient vaccine at Muguga (the T$_1$ broth vaccine) and Joint Project 16 (a research project to improve knowledge of epidemiology, diagnostic techniques and the vaccine) resulted in CBPP being brought under control throughout west, central and east Africa by 1970.

The failure of African governments to invest in veterinary services over the subsequent years has resulted, as was seen with rinderpest, in a resurgence of the disease throughout the continent; by 1995 most countries of Africa south of the Sahara reported the disease (Fig. 49.1). It is said that the vaccine no longer works.

Aetiology

Two types of *M. mycoides* subspecies *mycoides* are recognized: the small colony type (SC) which causes CBPP in cattle and the large colony type which occurs in goats and rarely in sheep. They cannot be differentiated in culture, biochemical or immunological tests; however, they can be separated by PCR. They have a different pathogenicity in cattle, because only the SC types causes CBPP. *M. mycoides* is a micro-organism that lacks a cell wall and will grow under aerobic or anaer-

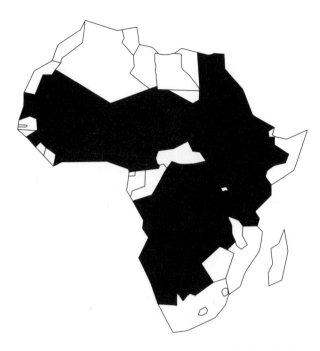

Fig. 49.1 In 1995 most countries in Africa south of the Sahara Desert reported CBPP.

obic conditions. The organism requires a complex medium for growth, containing serum and yeast extract, and growth is slow taking up to 72 hours to reach a maximum. In broth cultures a swirling mucoid mist is produced from the galactan which is attached to the cell membrane.

Epidemiology

Only cattle and water buffalo are susceptible to CBPP; the African buffalo has been infected under experimental conditions, but that same study found that natural transmission did not occur. There is some debate as to whether *Bos taurus* or *Bos indicus* is the more susceptible to infection with *M. mycoides*. An understanding of the epidemiology has been bedevilled by an inability to reproduce the disease in cattle other than by the cumbersome 'in contact' method, in which cattle are artificially infected by having a culture inoculated directly into the bronchi and then these artificially infected animals are mixed with healthy susceptible animals. Normal transmission is by droplet infection from actively infected animals to susceptible animals in close proximity. However, indirect transmission has been demonstrated under experimental conditions.

A second factor that hinders the understanding of this disease is the potentiation of myths and statements of fact that have no basis in experimentation, e.g. 'There is a prolonged incubation period'; 'lungers break down and the animal again becomes infective'. There is no evidence for either of these statements but they are held to be true. In all the vaccine trials carried out at the East African Veterinary Research Institute, Muguga, Kenya, control animals put in contact with diseased animals showed signs of infection (either clinical or serological) at about six weeks (plus or minus 10 days). Under field conditions it may be that the animal has avoided infection for a long period of time. Work at Muguga failed to reactivate disease in recovered animals: stress, corticosteroid treatment and even removal of the spleen were unsuccessful. Until proven otherwise, it is the actively diseased or the animal incubating the disease which must be considered as the main risk to susceptible animals.

CBPP is a disease of the older animal and calves rarely show pneumonic disease. Infection in young animals normally results in lesions in the joints. In consequence, calves play little or no role in the spread of disease.

Although there is no experimental evidence to confirm the observation, it is generally believed that it is the weight of infection in a herd that determines the clinical picture. Under natural conditions, there might be a single animal infected in a herd and this animal will show only mild signs which may well pass unnoticed. Nevertheless, the animal infects several more animals and they in turn yet more. In this way the weight of infection builds within a herd until widespread clinical disease is seen. This picture may explain the long incubation periods referred to in the literature.

When the infection is introduced into a susceptible herd there can be a great variation in response, from a severe, massive, acute outbreak of disease involving up to 60 per cent of the animals in the herd with 40–50 per cent of the affected animals dying, to a much less severe problem, involving less than half of the herd with few animals severely affected and a low mortality. Recovered animals are resistant to further infection. In many of these recovered animals sequestra may be seen: a sequestrum is a piece of diseased lung that has become separated from neighbouring healthy tissue and surrounded by a fibrous capsule. In a closed herd, in which no action is taken, it is not uncommon for the disease to die out. Recently there has been a move towards treating clinically sick animals. The effects of this treatment on sequestrum formation are not known but it is thought that it might prevent the animals from developing a proper sequestrum and so prolong the period in which the animal can pass on the infection.

Pathogenesis

If little is known of the epidemiology of CBPP, even less is known of the pathogenesis of the disease. When infection passes down the respiratory passages there is a bronchiolitis and alveolitis leading to pneumonia and pleurisy. It is thought that the galactan plays a part in attaching the organism to the mucous membrane and so preventing the body defences from eliminating the organism. Some workers believe that hypersensitivity or autoimmune reactions are responsible for the lesions and there is some evidence for this. It is hoped that by use of modern molecular techniques this will be resolved. It has also been suggested that there is a diffusable toxin which stimulates the formation of the fibrous capsule around the necrotic tissue. Some workers believe that the galactan acts as an endotoxin and causes systemic reactions similar to those seen in infection by Gram-negative bacteria; this is not proven. Until recently it was believed that only one lung was affected, which would support the suggestion of an autoimmune phenomenon. However, in recent outbreaks lesions have been seen, in a very few animals, in both lungs. This may be the result of antibiotic treatment. As can be seen from the foregoing, much needs to be done to give a clear understanding of the pathogenesis of CBPP.

Clinical signs

At least these are clearly understood! In the hyperacute form the animal may be found dead, without premonitory signs, but this is not common. The acute disease is characterized by fever, lethargy, loss of appetite and pneumonic signs. The animal stands with elbows abducted and the neck stretched out, the mouth open and the tongue protruding (Fig. 49.2). From time to time it may emit a soft, moist cough. The pleurisy causes severe pain and the animal will grunt if the chest is

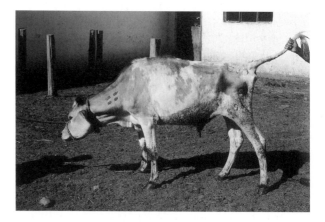

Fig. 49.2 Animal showing signs of acute CBPP – The animal stands with elbows abducted and the neck stretched out, the mouth open and the tongue protruding.

touched. Because the chest is so painful it is uncommon for an animal with the acute disease to lie down and it will remain on its feet until almost the end. Filthy mucus runs from the nostrils and saliva may drool from the mouth. Pregnant cows may abort and the fetal fluids contain vast numbers of mycoplasms. Despite the size and nature of the lung lesions, it is often difficult to identify the site of the lesions by percussion or auscultation. Although there may be massive kidney infarcts present it is rare for an animal to show signs of renal disease. If the animal survives the signs grow progressively less pronounced, the nasal discharge may well become purulent, the animal will lose a considerable amount of flesh and become emaciated. The larger the lesions, the slower the recovery.

There is a great variety of clinical manifestation from this dramatic picture down to almost no clinical signs at all. What determines the size of the lesions and hence the clinical picture is not known. In any outbreak it is possible to see acute, subacute and chronic disease, often all three pictures at the same time. Many workers

state that relapses occur, but there are no published reports of this actually happening.

Although calves can develop the classical lung lesions and show the same signs as the adult, this is uncommon. The more typical picture is one of swollen joints caused by a fibrinous bursitis (Fig. 49.3). For some unknown reason it is more commonly the forelegs that are affected.

Post-mortem findings

In the animal that has died from acute disease, the first thing seen is the vast quantities of straw-coloured pleural fluid in the chest cavity; 10 litres or more have been reported (Fig. 49.4). The fluid may contain pieces of fibrin that have broken off from the pleural adhesions, and up to 10^9 mycoplasmas per ml. A localized or diffuse pleurisy may be present, appearing like an omelette.

Acute lesions vary in size from 1 to 2 cm in diameter to those affecting the whole of the lobe. More than one lesion may be present but they are usually restricted to

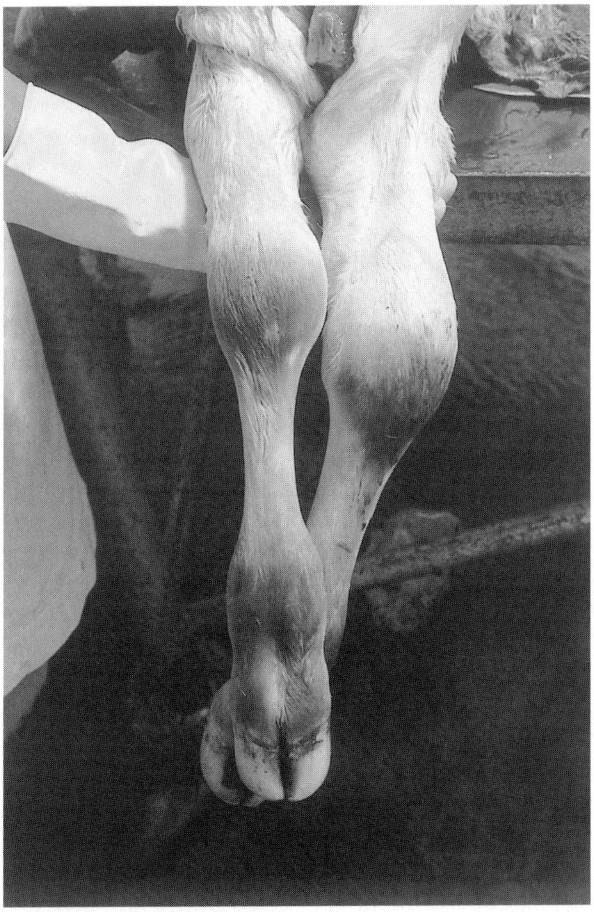

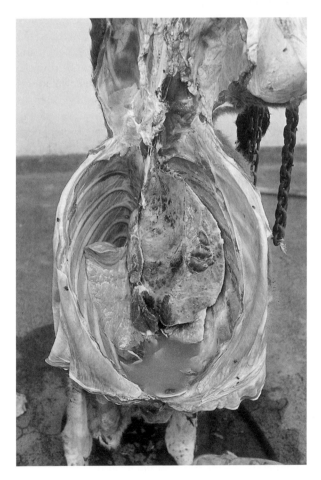

Fig. 49.3 A young calf with CBPP, showing swollen joints caused by a fibrinous bursitis.

Fig. 49.4 Carcass of an animal with acute CBPP, vast quantities of straw-coloured pleural fluid in the chest cavity; 10 litres or more have been reported. Note that one lung is diseased but the other appears normal.

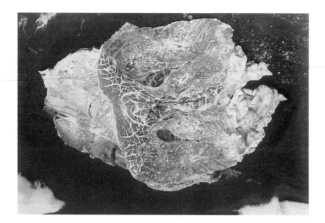

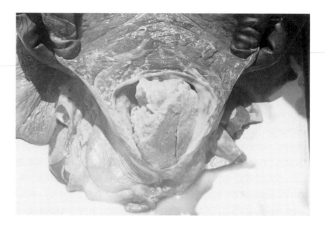

Fig. 49.5 Lungs of an animal with acute CBPP. The characteristic lesion is 'marbling', identical to that seen in acute pasteurellosis.

Fig. 49.6 Lung of animal 27 months after infection, showing a walled-off sequestrum. Thomas Walley, likened the sequestrum to an 'Egyptian mummy in its case'.

one lung. The characteristic lesion is 'marbling', identical to that seen in acute pasteurellosis (Fig. 49.5). Interlobular oedema and fibrin deposits highlight the structure of the lung. The lung tissue itself may be dark red or changing to grey and thrombi may be seen in the vessels. These thrombi result in infarction of the portion of the lung supplied. The tissue dies, separates from the healthy surrounding tissue and becomes walled off into a sequestrum. The nineteenth century Dean of the Edinburgh School, Thomas Walley, likened the sequestrum to an 'Egyptian mummy in its case' (Fig. 49.6). Small sequestra will disappear over time, to be replaced by scar tissue, but the larger ones can remain for life. *M. mycoides* has been isolated from the tissue in a sequestrum up to 27 months after the animal was infected. It was rare for these sequestra to become secondarily infected by other bacteria, but in recent outbreaks such infection has been seen. This may be a result of antibiotic treatment.

Histological examination is not very useful in making a diagnosis as the lesions are not pathognomonic. The lesion commences with a severe hyperaemia of the affected lung and associated pleura with effusion of erythrocytes, neutrophils and macrophages. There is a massive serofibrinous effusion into the alveoli and the interlobular septa. Vasculitis and thrombosis of arteries occur in the affected parts of the lung. This results in the necrosis of that area supplied by the vessel and the onset of sequestration. This commences with a layer of inflammatory cells separating the infarcted area from the surrounding healthy tissue. Granulation and fibrosis separate the infarct from the healthy tissue.

Lesions resembling sequestra may be seen in the mediastinal and bronchial lymph nodes and they are always enlarged and oedematous. Infarcts in the kidney are common in animals with acute disease, and they are thought to be caused by emboli from the lung settling in the kidney. They can be of any size and number and one or both kidneys may be infected; the colour of the infarcts varies from white to red to black. Lesions affecting the joints of calves are normally bilateral, serofibrinous tendosynovitis or occasionally arthritis. Lesions are mostly seen in knees and lower joints of the forelegs. A valvular endocarditis has been reported in calves.

Diagnosis

A presumptive diagnosis should be based on the history, the clinical signs and the post-mortem findings. However, it is essential that the presence of *M. mycoides* be confirmed. The isolation and identification of the mycoplasma gives a certain diagnosis; growth inhibition or immunofluorescent antibody tests can be used to identify the organism once it has been isolated. Under African conditions this may not always be possible, particularly if the outbreak occurs at a great distance from the laboratory. In such cases samples of pleural fluid can be taken onto blotting paper and then dried. These papers can then be examined by an agar gel diffusion test (AGT) or the newer polymerase chain reaction (PCR).

In the live animal serological tests are required to confirm a diagnosis. The simplest crush-side test is the slide agglutination serum or blood test (SAST or SABT) using a stained antigen. It is cheap to produce, easy to carry out and has therefore been discarded! False positive results to this test occur, but they do to all serological tests. The complement fixation (CF) test is the test approved by the Office International des Épizooties (OIE) as the definitive test for the confirmation of CBPP. This workhorse was developed in Australia and has been used successfully throughout Africa for the control of the disease. It does not require expensive equipment or reagents but it is a complicated test to perform, although once mastered, the technique can produce excellent results on a regular basis. The complaint is that CF antibodies do not persist in animals with sequestra. If these animals play no part in spreading the disease, then this is of no importance. The technique has been modified to be carried out in the African bush, but apart from Zambia, this field test is no longer in use in Africa. After vaccination some cattle develop CF antibodies but by 12 weeks these antibodies have gone and at present there is no satisfactory way of determining whether or not an animal has been vaccinated. The new enzyme-linked immunosorbent assay (ELISA) suffers from the same deficiencies. In the absence of post-mortem evidence, it would be a brave veterinarian who diagnosed CBPP on serological findings alone.

Differential diagnosis

Acute pasteurellosis (p. 286) is the condition with which CBPP is most likely to be confused, but the former regularly affects both lungs. A cultural examination of the lesions should identify the cause. Pneumonic lesions of east coast fever (ECF) (p. 750) could be confused with those of CBPP, although pleurisy is not normally a feature of ECF and there are concurrent lesions in the spleen and lymph nodes of animals with ECF. Examination of Giemsa-stained preparations of smears from spleen or lymph node should confirm the diagnosis of EFC.

Sequestra can be mistaken for the cysts of parasitic infestations, particularly echinococcus (p. 281), or aberrant liver flukes (p. 276).

Vaccination (see p. 1011)

There is no treatment for this disease and so vaccination is an important means of protection of the animals. At the turn of the last century, pleural fluid or diseased lung was injected under the skin of the tail to protect the animals. Rider Haggard in his novel 'King Solomon's Mines' refers to this technique for protecting cattle from the 'lungsick'. He points out that this often resulted in the animal losing its tail, which he considered preferable to losing its life. Throughout the twentieth century workers have looked for vaccines. It appears that only live vaccines produce protection. The Australian workers developed the V5 vaccine, which was acceptable in Australia, because there farmers considered that if a few animals did not die after vaccination, then the vaccine had not worked. Such a vaccine could not be used in Africa. In the Sudan the KH3J vaccine was used; although it caused no reactions it also failed to protect cattle. The T_1 vaccine was first used as an 'egg vaccine',

but caused many adverse reactions and some deaths; however, the broth vaccine gave good protection without producing too many adverse reactions. Laboratory and fieldwork showed that it produced a solid immunity for more than a year. The T_1 broth vaccine was then lyophilized, but it was too expensive to test this new vaccine and so it was assumed that since it was a T_1 vaccine it would work! By passage in the presence of streptomycin, a streptocmycin-resistant variety of the T_1 strain was produced. This enabled the vaccine to be mixed with the rinderpest vaccine and so reduce the delivery costs. Again this new vaccine was not tested. Perhaps this is why the new T_1 does not work very well!

Control

CBPP is a disease of cattle movement; stop movement and the spread of disease is halted. Many countries freed themselves from infection by prohibiting movement and slaughtering infected animals or herds. When CBPP was introduced into Botswana in 1995, the disease was eradicated by preventing animals from moving and a stamping-out policy. The price of freedom from CBPP was in excess of $200 million and there are few African countries that can afford such an expense. For Botswana this was an economically sound policy because it protected their markets in Europe.

In almost all African countries CBPP is a notifiable disease and there are official controls on the import of cattle. However, in many countries there are nomadic people who have moved from country to country before the borders existed, e.g. the Fulani in west Africa and the Maasai in east Africa. A recent outbreak of CBPP in Tanzania resulted from the theft of two animals in Kenya by Tanzanian Maasai who moved the animals across the unmarked 'border'. Lack of appropriate action by the Tanzanian authorities has resulted in the disease spreading the length and breadth of the country. Wars, famine and inadequate financing of veterinary departments have resulted in CBPP running riot in east and central Africa. Unless something is done to stop the spread it will not be long before the disease topples over into Malawi and Mozambique, two of the countries in sub Saharan Africa which have never experienced CBPP. From there the whole of southern Africa is at risk. Early warning of the arrival of the disease is imperative for adequate control. To this end, it is essential that all animals that are slaughtered, be it in an abattoir, on a slaughter slab or in the bush, and are examined by a trained member of the veterinary department to ensure that they are not carrying lesions of CBPP.

Rinderpest has almost been eradicated from Africa; it is time that the international community turned its attention to the control of CBPP on the continent. To this end research into vaccines, epidemiology and diagnostic methods are required. Strangely enough these were the topics of investigation for Joint Project 16 over thirty years ago.

References

Blood, D.C., Radostits, O.M. & Henderson, J.A. (1983) *Veterinary Medicine*, 6th edn, pp. 692–6. Baillière Tindall, London.

Harwood, D.G., Otter, A. & Gunning, R. (1995) Peracute pleuropneumonia – adult cattle. *Cattle Practice*, **3**, (Part 2). 149–51.

Monies, R.J. (2000) Tuberculous pneumonia and BVD in housed calves. Cattle Practice, **8**, (Part 2), 119–25.

Pirie, H.M. (ed.) (1979) *Respiratory Diseases of Animals. Notes for a Postgraduate Course*, Glasgow University, Glasgow, pp. 41–2.

Further reading

Bygrave, A.C., Moulton, J.E. & Shifrine, M. (1968) Clinical, serological and pathological findings in an outbreak of contagious bovine pleuropneumonia. *Bulletin of Epizootic Diseases of Africa*, **16**, 21–46.

Currason, G. (1936) Traité de Pathologie exotique vétérinaire et comparée, Vol II, pp. 500–639. Vigot Freres, Paris.

Henning, M.W. (1956) Animal Diseases in South Africa, 3rd edn. Central News Agency, Pretoria.

Hudson, J.R. (1971) Contagious bovine pleuropneumonia. FAO Agricultural Studies No. 86. FAO of the United Nations Organisation, Rome.

Masiga, W.N., Domenech, J. & Windsor, R.S. (1996) Manifestation and epidemiology of contagious bovine pleuropneumonia in Africa. *Scientific and Technical Review*, **15**, 1283–308. Office International des Épizooties, Paris.

Chapter 50
Skin Conditions

L.R. Thomsett

Warble fly   875
Dermatophytosis (ringworm)   878
Parasitic skin disease   880
    Lice (pediculosis)   880
    Mite infestations: mange, scabies   881
Warts (viral papillomatosis)   882
Urticaria   883
Pruritis/pyrexia/haemorrhagic syndrome (PPH)   884
Photosensitization   884
Bovine farcy   885
Atypical mycobacteriosis   886
Dermatophilosis (bovine streptothricosis)   886
Horn cancer   887
Lumpy skin disease and pseudo-lumpy skin disease   887
    Lumpy skin disease   887
    Pseudo-lumpy skin disease   888
Other conditions having skin signs   888

The skin of the ox shows general conformity with the anatomical characteristics of the large domestic animals (Fig. 50.1). Approximately 7 mm in thickness, it consists of epidermis and dermis and their adnexa. The hair follicles are simple and carry a single hair, the colour of which, depending on body site and breed, may be black, white or a wide variety of variants of brown or grey. Single hairs leave the skin surface at an angle, each follicle having an erector pili muscle allowing the hair to be raised to a more upright position.

Hair growth and replacement is a cyclic process of active growth (anagen) when the hair follicle is producing a new hair, and a period of rest (telogen) when the mature hair, which now has a constricted bulb and is referred to as a 'club' hair, is held in the hair follicle before being shed.

Sweat and sebaceous glands are distributed over the body surface and show specialization in certain areas, e.g. the mammary gland, naso-labial glands of the muzzle. At the extremities of the limbs and on the head of horned breeds the skin is specially modified to form the hooves and horns.

Skin diseases of cattle

Primary disease of the skin of cattle is more commonly attributable to parasite infestation or fungal infection.

Bacteria and viruses play a minor role except when skin signs are associated with systemic infection by these organisms. Allergic disorders are also uncommon and genetic diseases rare.

The effect of skin disease on the livestock industry

Where animals are reared to provide food and other byproducts, skin disease, although clinically not in itself serious and rarely life-threatening, may cause significant losses to the agricultural industry through the following effects:

- The debilitating effect of pruritus on the affected animals. Heavy louse infestations or infestation by sarcoptic mites causes irritation, restlessness and weight loss.
- Damage to hides from self-trauma or the migration of parasitic larvae.
- Damage to tissue from bacterial infection or larval migration resulting in condemnation or trimming of meat at slaughter.
- Limitation of sale value or show potential of infected animals and their danger as vectors of disease to other stock.

Warble fly

The insect is also known as warbles, cattle grubs, gad fly or *Hypoderma* infestation and is due to the migrating stages of a parasitic insect (see p. 740). Two species of warble fly are recognized in many countries of the northern Hemisphere, namely *Hypoderma lineatum* and *Hypoderma bovis* and they differ little in their territorial distribution. These parasites are not found in the southern hemisphere as they have not become established, despite importation of infected cattle.

Cattle, particularly young stock at pasture, are the definitive host for the parasitic stages of the life cycle although other species are recorded as occasionally being infested, such as horses, deer, goats and even man. In species other than cattle the life cycle is rarely, if ever, completed.

Life cycle (see Figs 50.2 and 50.3)

Warble flies become active in the spring and on warm days in the summer months adult females (up to 15 mm long) home in on grazing cattle and alight on the hairs of the lower limbs, on which they lay their eggs. *Hypoderma bovis* lays its eggs singly while *H. lineatum* lays a row of six or more on a hair. The egg-laying behaviour of the flies causes irritation and restlessness to cattle and attempts are made to avoid the flies by running away. Characteristically, this is seen as initial apprehension among a group or an individual animal, followed by suddenly taking flight at a gallop, tail in the air, suddenly turning and repeating the movement in an effort to shake off the pursuing flies. This is known as 'gadding'.

Once ova are attached to the hairs they hatch in four days and larvae crawl to the skin surface, through which they penetrate to the connective tissue and wander for four to five months. Migratory patterns within the host differ: *H. lineatum* moves to the submucosal connective tissue of the oesophageal wall while *H. bovis* goes to the region of the spinal canal and epidural fat. At these sites they remain for the autumn and winter. As second-stage larvae they migrate towards the back of the host where further maturation takes place.

Large domed nodules are formed under the skin within 30–45 cm (12–18 inches) on either side of the spine, in which the now third-stage larva produces a ventral breathing pore. Grubs within the nodules progressively increase in size to 25–28 mm in length, depending on species. In the spring the larva emerges from its cyst, falls to the ground and pupates. After a period of four to six weeks the adult fly emerges.

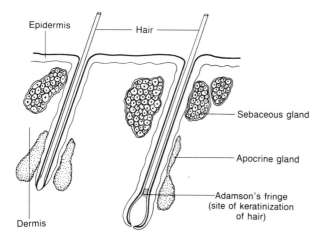

Fig. 50.1 Diagrammatic representation of bovine skin.

Effect of Hypoderma larvae on the host

Fly attacks: Considerable 'worry' is caused to cattle when approached by these flies; this results in restlessness that interferes with grazing and may result in poor weight gain. Milking cattle show a fall in milk yield.

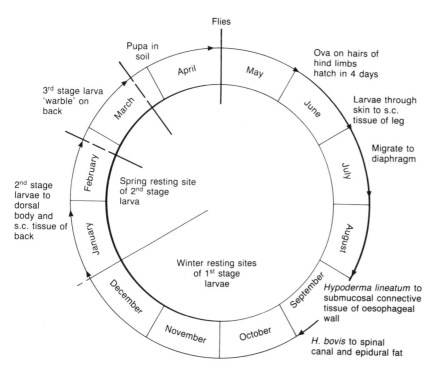

Fig. 50.2 *Hypoderma* spp. life cycle.

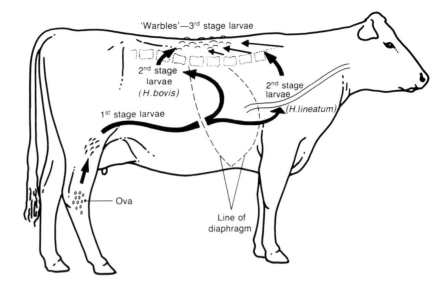

Fig. 50.3 Migration of warble fly larvae within cattle.

Damage by larvae

- Carcasses. The presence of grubs may necessitate trimming of meat at slaughter or, in some cases, condemnation. Trimming makes the carcass less aesthetically acceptable and so it can disproportionately reduce the price when meat is plentiful.
- Hides. Maturation of warble fly grubs to the stage where they make breathing pores causes serious damage to the dermis and results in downgrading of affected hides.
- Rupture of larvae. This occasionally precipitates an immunological reaction.

When migrating in the earlier stage of the life cycle, *H. lineatum* larvae may cause an oesophagitis when they reach the oesophageal wall; *H. bovis* larvae can result in posterior paralysis.

Treatment and control (see p. 1031)

Treatment of lesions associated with the maturation of the migrating larvae has now been superseded by preventive measures.

Since the range of activity of *Hypoderma* flies is limited to 5–14 km (3–9 miles), control of infestation by eradication is feasible provided neighbouring stockkeepers treat their animals.

Organophosphorus preparations. Organophosphate systemic insecticides have been found to be the most effective agents for the eradication of *Hypoderma* larvae, the aim being to destroy them early in the infestation before they reach resting sites near the neural canal or are themselves very large.

Table 50.1 Dose rate for pour-on treatment using Phosmet 13 per cent w/v.

Weight of animal (kg)	Dose (ml)
Up to 130	20
131–200	30
201–260	40
261–330	50
Over 330	60

Preparations used include phosmet, trichlorfon, fenchlorphos, coumaphos and fenthion. All are cholinesterase inhibitors and knowledge of their actions, in particular their toxic effects and antidotes, is essential before using them for warble treatment (see p. 940).

Organophosphorus preparations have been employed by dip, spray and wash. The most satisfactory method of application has been shown to be the 'pour-on' procedure. An example of pour-on treatment, using Phosmet 13.3 per cent w/v solution, is shown in Table 50.1.

Cattle should be treated in autumn (15 September to 30 November) or in the spring (15 March to 31 June). Best results are obtained by autumn treatment and prevent skin nodule formation by the third-stage larvae in the spring. No treatment should be given between 1 December and the following 14 March because of possible reactions at the winter resting sites due to the death of the warbles.

Animals being treated on the above regimen should not be given organophosphorus anthelmintics, levamisole or diethylcarbamazine citrate at the same time.

Special precautions regarding the use and handling of organophosphorus preparations, particularly with regard to wearing protective clothing, are applicable and reference to the manufacturer's data sheet is essential before their use.

In Great Britain warble fly infestation is a notifiable disease. The efficacy of control measures aimed at eliminating warble infestation can now be monitored serologically.

Ivermectin: The systemic parasiticides based on ivermectin are also effective in destroying warble grubs. One per cent ivermectin injection may be used according to the manufacturer's recommendations after the end of the period of fly activity and before the larvae reach their resting sites. The milk of treated cattle may not be used for human consumption, or manufacturing purposes or within 60 days prior to parturition. Meat animals must not be slaughtered within 35 days of their last treatment.

Dermatophytosis (ringworm)

The infection of hair and skin keratin with the dermatophytes *Trichophyton verrucosum*, and less commonly *T. mentagrophytes*, causes lesions commonly referred to as ringworm. This disease has a worldwide distribution, the incidence of which is considered to be high although an accurate figure for its occurrence is not known. It is particularly common in young stock between two and seven months of age and during the autumn and winter months of the year. Adult cattle are also quite frequently affected.

Animals kept in close contact with one another, e.g. under intensive management systems, are particularly at risk. Other species may also be infected, including horses, sheep and also man in whom it may cause serious skin lesions. Although not giving rise to serious systemic debilitating symptoms, the effect of ringworm is on the value of the animal or its hide.

Show animals with the disease may not be shown or sold, infected stock carry a depreciated market value when offered for sale and the hides of animals slaughtered show defects that render them less valuable for top-quality leather manufacture.

Epidemiology

The spores of ringworm fungi survive for many months and in some cases years in the farm environment. They may be transmitted either by fomites or by asymptomatic carrier animals to susceptible hosts.

The *incubation period* of the disease is generally considered to be approximately one week although four weeks has been suggested as the period in some outbreaks. Once in contact with the skin surface of a susceptible animal, the fungus invades the anagen hairs (telogen hairs are not affected) by enzymatic destruction of keratin. Hyphal growth extends only as far as the point at which keratinization of the hair takes place (Adamson's fringe).

The hair, so weakened, breaks off, leading to the partial alopecia seen on clinical lesions of dermatophytosis. A generally mild inflammatory reaction accompanies the infection; only occasionally is this severe in cattle, leading to excess production of skin scale, folliculitis or furunculosis.

Signs

The disease is usually non-pruritic in cattle. Lesions are characteristically greyish-white and have an ash-like surface. Their outline is circular and they are slightly raised due to the accumulation of many layers of scale and the swelling of tissues beneath due to a moderate inflammatory reaction. Some lesions may show areas of mild exudation and yellow crust formation where the skin reaction is more severe. Removal of hair tufts or some of the accumulated crust will often leave a raw bleeding surface. Broken hairs remain as hair stubble encased in scale and crust (Plate 50.1).

The size of lesions varies, 3–5 cm (1–2 inches) diameter being common; in the more severely affected animals lesions become confluent to form extensive areas of infection (Plate 50.2).

The distribution of lesions in calves commonly involves the periorbital skin, ears and back, while in adult cattle the thorax and limbs are the more favoured sites. In show cattle subjected to grooming, multiple small lesions develop over the whole of the body and limbs following the spread of infective spores by contaminated grooming brushes. Very occasionally the udder can be affected (Plate 27.29).

Duration of the disease

Ringworm infection is generally considered to be self-limiting and the course of the disease to be one to four months, although in some cases a period as long as nine months has been necessary for resolution to take place. These periods may be shortened by implementing the appropriate therapeutic measures.

Diagnosis

Diagnosis is made on the clinical signs of classic lesions of dermatophytosis confirmed by the laboratory examination of hair and crust samples.

Collection of samples

(1) By forceps epilation of hair from areas of active infection.
(2) Scrapings of crust, hair and scale using a scalpel blade.

Using either of these procedures the material obtained is collected in a paper envelope (ensuring that the quantity of sample is adequate for the diagnostic procedures to be carried out), sealed and labelled for transmission to the laboratory.

If culture is contemplated, swabbing the area with 70 per cent alcohol prior to collection of material may reduce contaminants in the specimen.

Laboratory diagnosis: Arthrosporic hyphae on hairs can be demonstrated using the microscope.

(1) Wet preparation of suspect material on a microscope slide with coverglass mounted in 20 per cent potassium hydroxide solution and gently warmed.
(2) Wet preparation in lactophenol cotton blue on a microscope slide under a coverglass.
(3) Wet preparation on a microscope slide under a coverglass mounted in potassium hydroxide/Super Quink solution.

In all procedures using the microscope for the examination of wet preparations care is necessary in adjusting the microscope illumination in order to visualize arthrosporic hyphae. This is equally applicable to the examination of portions of cultured material.

Definitive diagnosis of the species of fungus may be obtained by culture techniques using Sabouraud's agar, mycobiotic agar, or dermatophyte test medium (DTM), and observing the characteristics of the organism, i.e. colonial morphology and that of the hyphal growth. In order to arrive at a conclusive answer culture time may need to be extended, i.e. for as long as three weeks.

Using Sabouraud's agar, rapid identification of *T. verrucosum* may be achieved by culture at 30–37°C (34°C), when the colony shows long chains of chlamydospores characteristic of the organism.

The DTM may be used to suggest a positive diagnosis of a pathogen by observation of the indicator colour change.

Definitive diagnosis is only by identification of cultural characteristics.

Treatment

Owing to the difficulty in eliminating the organism from the environment in which many cattle are kept, and the number of animals involved, the reward for treating the disease with such preparations as are suitable (these may only succeed in moderately reducing the duration of the disease) has brought the therapy of ringworm in cattle into question. Scott (1988) refers to 'a sea of antifungals' for the treatment of animal ringworm, many of which are of questionable efficacy. The choice of therapy depends on the availability of appropriate antifungal agents.

Systemic treatment

(1) *Griseofulvin*. An oral feed supplement given at a dose of 10 mg/kg body weight for 7–14 days. In the USA an alternative routine of 15–35 mg per kg body weight for 18–30 days is considered more effective. Pregnant animals should not be treated with this preparation. Milk from treated animals should not be used for human consumption until 48 hours after the last treatment. Cattle should not be slaughtered for human consumption until five days after the last treatment. It is no longer available for cattle in the UK.
(2) *Sodium iodide*. A dose of 1 g/14 kg body weight as a 10–20 per cent aqueous solution is given by intravenous injection, followed by a repeat injection seven days later. Pregnant cattle should not be treated with iodide therapy. Cattle so treated may show signs of iodism (pp. 261, 302, 823).

Topicals

Imidazoles: A wide range of imidazole preparations have been formulated for the treatment of fungal skin infections.

Enilconazole (Imaverol, Janssen Animal Health): Cattle may be treated by spray or wash using a 0.2 per cent w/v emulsion of enilconazole in water. It is recommended that excess scab and crust be removed by scrubbing with a stiff brush soaked in the antifungal emulsion. Subsequent treatments by spraying or wash are made on three to four occasions at three-day intervals.

Other preparations:

Natamycin (Mycophyt, Intervet UK Ltd): A dry powder for the preparation of a 0.01 per cent suspension in water is available for application to cattle by spray or wash. Special care is necessary in reconstituting the powder, for the final suspension reference should be made to the manufacturer's data sheet. Following an initial treatment a repeat application may be made four to five days later. Subsequent treatments can follow at 14 day intervals. Following treatment with natamycin suspension animals should be sheltered from direct sunlight for several hours.

Copper naphthenate (Kopertox): A topical preparation presented as an aerosol containing 2.19 per cent w/v copper naphthenate. Lesions to be treated should be thoroughly soaked with a solution. A repeat treatment may be given after an interval of 10 days if necessary. The product is now not available in some countries.

Iodine: A liquid made up of equal parts of tincture of iodine and glycerin has been used for the treatment of individual lesions of ringworm on cattle.

Note: Special precautions are necessary in the application of topical preparations. Care should be taken to avoid sensitive areas, the eyes in particular and also the transfer of topical applications to other animals in contact with those under treatment.

Prophylaxis

Griseofulvin at a dose of 7.5–60 mg/kg per day for five weeks has been suggested as a prophylactic against dermatophyte infection. Pregnant animals should not be treated. However, animals so treated will not be immune to disease and so may become infected at a later date.

Immunity

The role of immunity in the epidemiology of outbreaks of cattle ringworm remains unclear. Re-infection after natural infection appears to be uncommon.

Vaccination (see p. 1017)

The immunization of cattle against *Trichophyton verrocosum* infection has been practised in Russia and Norway and a vaccine is now available in the United Kingdom (Ringvac Bovis LTF-130, Intervet Ltd). Freeze dried material prepared from an attenuated non-pathogenic stain of *T. verrucosum* is reconstituted for the inoculation of young calves at two weeks of age. Two inoculations are recommended at an interval of 10–14 days by intramuscular injection into the neck.

Disinfection

Viable spores of ringworm fungi may remain in buildings and particularly on porous surfaces, e.g. wood, brick, for months or years, making disinfection difficult.

Cleansing with high pressure water jets, scrubbing down with hot detergent solutions or disinfectants (e.g. benzalkonium chloride) or alternatively, disinfection with 2 per cent formaldehyde solution after prior scrubbing can remove infection. When using disinfection procedures, i.e. spraying and scrubbing walls, doors, etc., special precautions should be taken to prevent contact with the preparation used, e.g. on the skin, in the eyes and by inhalation, particularly when using solutions of formaldehyde. The wearing of appropriate protective clothing in conformation with health and safety regulations is essential.

Parasitic skin disease

Lice (pediculosis) (Plate 50.3)

Lice are somewhat dorso-ventrally flattened insects up to 6 mm in length that are host-specific parasites.

The distribution of lice is world-wide. The species infecting cattle are the biting louse *Bovicola (Damalinia) bovis*, and the sucking lice *Haematopinus eurysternus*, *Linognathus vituli*, and *Solenopotes capillatus*. The biting lice feed on tissue debris while the sucking species suck blood and tissue fluid (see p. 741).

Life cycle

The entire life cycle of approximately three to six weeks' duration is spent on the host. Adult females lay their eggs and attach them singly to hairs. These appear as pearly or opalescent bodies (nits) 1–2 mm long. From the egg immature nymphs emerge, and pass through several moults before becoming adult. Survival off the host is short, usually less than one week. However, under certain conditions lice have been recorded to survive for periods up to three weeks.

On the host, populations of lice vary seasonally, being highest in colder seasons when the coat is long and transmission by contact from animal to animal readily occurs. Lower populations in the warmer seasons are due to the higher environmental temperature of the skin and coat in which lice cannot survive.

In spite of these factors, small populations may survive in protected areas, i.e. the ears, axillae, jowl, tail, ready to multiply when environmental conditions become beneficial.

Distribution of infestation on the host

Biting lice occur mainly on the neck, withers and tail head. Sucking lice are commonly found as a more generalized infestation, occurring on the head, neck, withers, down the brisket, tail, axillae and groin.

Signs

The cardinal sign is pruritus, the resulting restlessness leading to poor feeding and poor weight gain. The coat is poor in condition, often with alopecia and excoriation due to self-trauma, with loss of coat lustre and excess dandruff as well as hide damage. Animals in milk may show lowered production. Infestations with sucking lice may give rise to anaemia and consequent increased susceptibility to concurrent disease.

Diagnosis

This depends on the demonstration of lice and eggs within the coat. Because of pruritis, the only major disease to be differentiated is mange.

Treatment (see p. 1030 onwards)

Louse infestations of cattle may be controlled by the application of antiparasitic sprays, powders, washes, 'pour-ons' and certain injectable preparations. The use of these should be complemented by attention to management and husbandry aimed at eliminating reservoirs of infection and improving nutrition.

Antiparasitics for louse control, of which there are many, are based mainly on organochlorine, organophosphorus and synthetic pyrethroid active principles, e.g. Gamma BHC powder (0.625 per cent), Coumaphos powder (1 per cent), Diazinon wash (2 per cent), Phosmet 'pour-on' (13.3 per cent) and Permethrin 'pour-on' (4 per cent).

Ivermectin 200–300μg/kg subcutaneously is effective against sucking lice but of variable efficacy against the biting species. Before use reference should be made to the manufacturer's data sheet for details of special precautions to be observed, e.g. milk withholding times of dairy cattle, permissible intervals between treatment and slaughter of meat animals.

Mite infestations: mange, scabies

Infestation of the skin of cattle with parasitic mites may be by any of four species: *Sarcoptes scabiei*, *Psoroptes communis*, *Chorioptes bovis* or *Demodex*. The incidence of disease due to these shows variation in different parts of the world in respect of the species of mite and pathogenicity (p. 742).

Sarcoptic mange, sarcoptic scabies

Sarcoptes scabiei (bovis) (Plate 50.4) has a life cycle of 10–17 days and may infest cattle of any age, breed or sex. Infection takes place by direct contact with infected cattle or with environmental fomites, although survival of the mites in the environment is limited to a few days.

Signs: *Sarcoptes scabiei* causes an intensely pruritic papular dermatitis due to the burrowing activities of the female mites within the superficial epidermis and a concurrent hypersensitivity reaction. This results in a non-follicular papular response, exudation and crusting with self-trauma in an attempt to relieve the itching. This produces excoriation, alopecia and thickening of the skin (Plate 50.5).

Lesions commonly commence about the head and spread to become generalized with gross thickening of skin folds. In some animals these lesions may be accompanied by secondary infection with bacteria (Plate 50.6).

The persistent intense pruritus causes debility, loss of condition, poor food conversion, hide and skin damage and in dairy cattle a reduction in milk yield. Workers in close contact with affected animals may show papular skin lesions.

Diagnosis: Physical examination, history, possible human involvement, demonstration of *S. scabiei* in skin scraping material examined microscopically all help the diagnosis. In exceptional cases skin biopsy may be helpful.

The main differential diagnosis is with psoroptic/chorioptic mange.

Treatment and control (see also p. 1030)

(1) Organophosphorus pour-ons, dips, sprays.
(2) Gamma BHC 7.5 per cent (not milking cows) 5–25 ml in 6 l water.
(3) Diazinon 2 per cent wash, 28 ml in 4.5 l water.
(4) Phosmet 20 per cent pour-on.
(5) Permethrin 4 per cent pour on.
(6) Ivermectin 200–300μg/kg by subcutaneous injection.
(7) Amitraz (Taktic, Intervet Ltd). A 0.025 per cent solution in water is applied by spray at 5 to 10 litres per animal to wet the whole body. This should be repeated after an interval of 7 to 10 days in severe cases. Further applications if necessary may be made at two to three month intervals. Special precautions apply to operatives using this preparation in respect of the wearing of protective clothing for which reference should be made to the manufacturer's data sheet. The milk withholding time for milking cattle treated with amitraz solution is 48 hours after the last treatment.
(8) In circumstances where the above preparations are not readily available, lime/sulphur dips can be effective. The disadvantage associated with this treatment is that repeat applications at 7 to 10 day intervals may be required on as many as six occasions.
(9) Synthetic pyrethroids.

These are examples of preparations available. Application routines may vary and response to treatment will determine how many applications may be required. Reference to the appropriate data sheet is essential for information on special precautions and withdrawal times to be observed (see for lice, above).

Psoroptic mange, psoroptic scabies

Psoroptes mites are non-burrowing and have a two-week life cycle. Survival off the host may be as long as three weeks. Transmission of infection is by direct or indirect contact.

Signs: Infection commences over the withers and spreads to the rest of the body. Lesions are papules accompanied by severe pruritus leading to extensive serous exudation and crusting with alopecia and lichenification. Irritability and consequent debility may result in unthriftiness, poor weight gain, hide damage and reduced milk yield in lactating animals.

Diagnosis: The diagnosis is by demonstration of mites by microscopic examination of wet preparations of skin scrapings. Differential diagnosis is with sarcoptic scabies, and chorioptic scabies.

Treatment: Treatment is the same as for sarcoptic scabies, although care is needed to ensure that infection has been eradicated. Resistance to treatment has been recorded.

Chorioptic mange, chorioptic scabies

Chorioptes bovis is a superficial, non-invasive inhabitant of cattle skin. Living on epidermal debris, it has a life cycle on the host of two to three weeks. It survives only a few days off the host under natural environmental conditions although under experimental conditions it may live as long as 10 weeks.

Transmission of infestation is usually by contact. Outbreaks among housed dairy cattle are higher in the winter time when mite populations are greatest.

Signs: Non-follicular pruritic papules result in self-trauma accompanied by erythema, excoriation, exudation, alopecia and the formation of crusts. These mostly involve the limbs, particularly the hindlimbs, the udder, scrotum, perineum and tail. The neck and flanks may also be involved.

Diagnosis: Diagnosis is by the microscopical demonstration of causal mites in wet preparation of skin scrapings. The differential diagnosis is with infestations with lice (p. 880) and other parasitic mites.

Treatment: Treatment is the same as for sarcoptic scabies. Apparent spontaneous regression may occur in the summer months when infestation appears to be confined to the distal limbs.

Demodicosis

Demodectic mites are considered to be normal residents of the skin of many species of wild and domestic animals. They are apparently host specific and live mainly within the hair follicles and sebaceous glands.

Three species of *Demodex* mites have been identified in cattle, the life cycle of which, as in other hosts, is obscure. Transmission of infection occurs from dam to calf by contact during suckling. No age or sex predilection has been established, nor is it clear why an organism living as a commensal should suddenly become a pathogen by its rapid unpredicted multiplication; immunodeficiency has been suggested as one cause.

Signs (Plate 50.7): Multiple nodules, sometimes secondarily infected, result in folliculitis and furunculosis of the face, neck and shoulders, occasionally becoming generalized. The disease is usually non-pruritic but nevertheless results in severe hide damage and consequent economic loss.

Diagnosis: With skin scrapings, wet preparations of expressed nodule contents examined microscopically show caseous sebaceous masses and large numbers of mites.

Histology of skin biopsy shows distended hair follicles packed with mites. Secondarily infected lesions show folliculitis, furunculosis and dermal granuloma formation.

Differential diagnosis is with dermatophytosis (p. 878) and dermatophilosis (p. 886).

Treatment: Demodicosis is often difficult to treat and prognosis is always guarded. Organophosphorus 'pour ons' have in some cases been found to be beneficial.

Warts (viral papillomatosis)

Bovine papillomatosis is commonly thought of as an infectious disease of the skin of mainly young cattle, usually self-limiting, widely distributed about the world, posing little difficulty in diagnosis, prognosis or treatment. The causal agent of the condition is a virus.

This is not, however, the whole story of bovine infection with DNA papovaviruses of which the bovine papilloma virus has certainly five, if not more, strains. Cross-reactivity between strains does not occur.

Papilloma virus appears to be host specific and transmission of bovine warts to humans handling infected cattle and cattle products has not been proven.

Of the strains of virus isolated, it appears that each has an anatomically determined predilection site of infection.

(1) BPV type I causes frond-like lesions on the nose, teats or penis: fibropapillomas in young cattle (Plate 27.31).
(2) BPV type II causes papillomatosis of the skin of the face, head, neck and dewlap, eyelids and occasionally legs of young cattle.

(3) BPV type III causes atypical warts, small smooth white sessile lesions on the udder and teats (p. 367; Plate 27.32).

(4) BPV type IV causes alimentary tract and urinary bladder papillomas and ocular lesions possibly progressing to squamous cell carcinoma.

(5) BPV type V causes non-regressing rice-grain warts on the teats.

Interdigital fibropapillomatosis, although wart-like in character, has no proven viral aetiology.

Epidemiology

Infection may be spread either by direct contact with infected animals or indirectly by fomites, e.g. from fences by trauma through minor abrasions or by direct or indirect effects of ectoparasitism. Following infection lesions appear after a two to six-month incubation period.

Signs

Viral papillomatosis is commonly seen in young cattle and once established lesions will resolve in a period of one to twelve months. Commencing as small, smooth, hairless, firm, button-like elevations projecting slightly above the skin surface, they may be from 1mm to several centimetres in diameter (Plate 50.8). They may develop to become coarse and cauliflower-like (Plate 50.9), sessile or pedunculated and single or multiple in number. Lesions are commonly sited on the head, neck and brisket and extensive generalization may occur.

Diagnosis

On clinical grounds the lesions are characteristic as is their distribution pattern on the skin and also the age group affected.

Histological examination shows epithelial proliferation with or without connective tissue proliferation: BPV I and II produce epithelial and fibrous proliferation; BPV III, IV and V produce epithelial proliferation.

Prognosis

In infection with BPV I and II, spontaneous regression within one to twelve months is the rule, while in the case of BPV III, IV and V and 'interdigital papillomatosis', lesions tend to be persistent.

Treatment and control (see also p. 1030 onwards)

With uncomplicated cases little treatment is required since spontaneous regression in young animals is the rule. Occasional cases of generalization may be encountered and are likely to be due to a failure in cell-mediated immunity.

Autogenous vaccines (p. 1014) for the treatment of bovine papillomatosis are of doubtful value. Where large, persistent growths are present, e.g. on the neck, removal by cryosurgery or cold steel surgery may be attempted.

For the prevention of infection with BPV I and II, commercial and autogenous vaccines are claimed to be effective. The use of lithium antimony thiomalate 6 per cent w/v solution by deep intramuscular injection, 15 ml on each of four to six occasions at 48-hour intervals is claimed to aid enucleation and necrosis of pedunculated warts.

Disinfection

While control of infection by disinfection is not commonly undertaken, where recurrent outbreaks of disease have occurred in housed cattle attempts at disinfection may be justified. Solutions of formaldehyde or caustic soda in appropriate dilution may be used, hosing down all treated surfaces well with water after these solutions have been allowed to act and prior to restocking.

Urticaria

The physical manifestation of urticaria in the form of oedematous skin plaques or of angioneurotic oedema may be caused by a wide variety of factors. These may be immunological, as in Coombs' type I and II reactions, or non-immunological associated with injected irritants or non-immunological histamine release.

Some non-immunologic factors that may precipitate urticarial responses or intensify an already established reaction are pressure, sunlight, heat, exercise, drugs, chemicals, even psychological stress. Certain genetic disorders have also been implicated in the aetiology of urticarial reactions.

Urticaria is usually seen as an acute onset disorder having no age, breed or sex predilection, which runs an acute or chronic course. It mostly affects a single individual or, on occasion, a small group.

Signs

In cattle, urticarial reactions are associated with insect and arthropod bites and stings, infection, the administration of antibiotics, vaccines or other biological products, some feedingstuffs as well as stinging plants.

Lesions of urticaria may vary in size, often being plaque-like wheals, localized or generalized over the neck, body and upper limbs in particular. They are usually cold to touch and may pit on pressure. Pruritus is variable as is the tendency for serum leakage onto the skin surface or for there to be haemorrhage. Urticarial lesions commonly show a well-defined shape or pattern, e.g. being ovular, serpiginous or arciform, or in the case of angioneurotic oedema involve certain structures with extensive oedematous swellings.

Acute onset angio-oedema has been seen in the UK on turning out housed cattle onto spring pasture, manifest as oedematous swelling of the periorbital skin, muzzle, perianal and perivulval tissue and occasionally the udder and teats. The condition is usually transient and apparently causes little distress. More severely affected animals may show evidence of respiratory distress.

In the USA a form of auto-allergic urticaria has been described in Jersey and Guernsey cattle. Affected individuals are believed to have a genetic predisposition to an allergic response when there is unusual engorgement of the udder or undue retention of milk. Clinical signs are of allergic urticarial skin rash and, in some individuals, respiratory distress.

Diagnosis

Diagnosis is mainly on history and lesions of rapid onset. Urticarial-like plaques with superficial exudation and crusting closely resemble the discrete active lesions of dermatophytosis (p. 878).

Treatment

Treatment is with subcutaneous or intramuscular injection of 3–5 ml of 1/100 adrenaline solution. Cattle with milk allergy should be milked out. In urticaria spontaneous resolution is often rapid and may have commenced or taken place by the time a visiting veterinarian arrives to attend the case.

Pruritus/pyrexia/haemorrhagic syndrome (PPH)

A disease of cattle, the pathophysiology of which is unclear, was first reported in cattle in the UK and in The Netherlands in the late 1970s. In The Netherlands the outbreaks were associated with the feeding of concentrates containing a urea compound, diureidoisobutane. In the UK this compound was not implicated and the causal factor has not been identified. Most cases were on self-fed silage, often after the introduction of a different silage additive to the farm. All cases were in cows, with a morbidity of 10.9 per cent and up to 25 per cent mortality, although almost all cases are culled due to loss of condition.

Signs

The systemic response is of a high fever (40–41°C; 104–106°F) with petechiation of the conjunctiva and visible mucous membranes, with general dullness. An extensive papular to exudative dermatitis with pruritus of variable intensity develops over the head, neck, perineum, udder, back and tail-head (Plate 50.10). These signs are accompanied by self-trauma (rubbing, kicking and licking), which leads to excoriation with bleeding and hair loss over a period of days to several weeks. Although the dermatitis may subside, the febrile response may persist for four to seven weeks.

Seriously affected animals may die, while those less so are unthrifty and ultimately have to be destroyed.

Diagnosis

The blood picture shows leucopenia followed by leucocytosis. Skin biopsy shows superficial and deep perivascular dermatitis with eosinophils and mononuclear cells predominating.

The post mortem reveals generalized petechiation particularly subserosal, with some cases showing free blood at external orifices.

The differential diagnosis is with other acutely febrile diseases of dairy cattle, such as anthrax (p. 717), and exudative dermatitis with severe pruritus of parasitic origin.

Treatment

This is non-specific and usually there is little response. A few cases have improved following prolonged use of injectable corticosteroids.

Photosensitization

Aetiology

This biophysical phenomenon occurs when skin becomes sensitized to certain wavelengths of sunlight, particularly within the ultraviolet range of the spectrum, in the presence within skin cells of specific photodynamic agents (see also pp. 370, 943).

Photodynamic agent in circulation → skin → irradiation by sunlight → cell death → necrosis → sloughing

Substances giving rise to these reactions in cattle may be porphyrins originating from defective haemoglobin metabolism, e.g. congenital porphyria, bovine protoporphyria, or they may be substances of plant origin, e.g. hypericin, which is found in the plant St John's wort (*Hypericum perforatum*). This process of photosensitivity is often referred to as *primary* or *direct* light sensitization.

Alternatively, another set of circumstances can lead to photosensitization, referred to as *secondary* or *hepatogenous* light sensitization. Although the final outcome, skin necrosis and sloughing, is the same as in the primary form, the process by which this is brought about differs.

Where liver damage (of diverse aetiology) interferes with the metabolism of the chlorophyll metabolite, phylloerythrin, this latter substance enters the circulation. As with other porphyrins, it initiates a light sensitivity response when present in the skin.

Both of these manifestations of photosensitivity are systemic in origin. A third, localized, form of skin reaction to sunlight may on rare occasions be induced by contact with the sap of certain plants containing psoralens. Localized lesions are more likely to be found on the distal limbs, muzzle or ventrum.

In order for photodynamic cell destruction to take place, the following circumstances are necessary:

(1) The photodynamic agent must be present in the skin at the time of exposure to sunlight.
(2) The exposed skin will be non-pigmented (the greater the density of melanin pigmentation, the greater is the protection against ultraviolet solar radiation).
(3) The density of hair cover should be such that sunlight can penetrate to the skin surface.

Photosensitization leading to photodermatitis is essentially a physical process. The activation of porphyrins within skin cells by ultraviolet irradiation releases energy that causes cell death, the clinical signs of which are erythema, oedema and necrosis of exposed non-pigmented areas of skin. In some animals vesication is present prior to necrosis, sloughing and ulceration of affected areas. Pruritus and pain may also be shown.

Sites most likely to be involved in cattle are those most exposed to direct sunlight, e.g. the head, neck, back and lateral aspects of the body, udder and teats (more extensively when the photosensitive animal is lying down) (Plates 27.23, 50.11 and 50.12).

Diagnosis

The dramatic lesions of skin necrosis and sloughing should not present diagnostic difficulty in the established case. The presence or absence of systemic signs of illness, e.g. jaundice, positive blood screens for hepatic disease, should determine whether the condition is primary or secondary.

Very localized lesions on distal limbs, ventrum or muzzle would suggest a topical plant contact aetiology.

Lesions on the muzzle and udder may suggest a differential diagnosis of bluetongue (see p. 691).

Prognosis

In the primary form of the disease, provided the underlying cause is not genetic, then removal to housed, well-ventilated, shaded and cool conditions should be adequate to allow resolution of the lesions. Where severe liver damage is confirmed, prognosis is poor and may well be terminal.

Treatment

Cool, shaded, fly-free housing to avoid myiasis is necessary. Where necrosis and sloughing has taken place lesion hygiene is essential to prevent fly strike and the application of powder dressing to that end is beneficial. Resolution in severely affected animals is often a long process. Antibiotics to limit secondary infection may be justified, as may the short-term administration of corticosteroids in certain cases. In secondary photodermatitis, the justification of therapy will be determined by the acuteness or chronicity of the underlying disease.

Bovine farcy

A chronic nodular and ulcerative disease of the skin of cattle, the causal organisms of which may be either *Nocardia farcinica* or *Mycobacterium farcinogenes*. The disease is only found in Africa, Asia and South America.

Aetiology

Nocardia farcinica is a soil saprophyte that becomes inoculated into wounds by contamination or enters the skin by inoculation via tick vectors, which themselves carry the organism for long periods of time.

Signs

Once inoculated, slowly developing painless nodules appear more commonly over the head, neck, shoulders, limbs, perineum and groin. Infection may give rise to mastitis and whilst following the lymphatics cause cording of these vessels as well as lymphadenopathy. Ulceration of lesions occurs with the discharge of thick, grey/yellow material.

Infection may be protracted and confined to the skin but generalization, particularly to the lungs and viscera, can occur with a progressive loss of condition leading to death.

Diagnosis

Diagnosis is dependent on the clinical signs. The organism may be demonstrated in smears of exudate (acid-fast filaments, which are beaded). Culture of *Nocardia farcinica* is also possible.

Histopathology shows the presence of pyogranulomatous dermatitis.

The differential diagnosis is with so-called skin tuberculosis due to acid-fast bacilli, particularly nodules found on the lower limbs or cording of lymphatics of forelimbs (see below).

Treatment

Inorganic iodides have been used but the advice given is usually to have the affected animals destroyed.

Atypical mycobacteriosis

Skin infections with environmental mycobacteriaceae are recognized worldwide. Lesions arise from the introduction of organisms through sites of skin trauma. Infection gives rise to nodular lesions on the distal limbs, sometimes discrete, otherwise in chains following the course of the superficial lymphatics. Nodules occasionally rupture to exude creamy pus. The condition is commonly referred to as 'skin tuberculosis'.

Diagnosis is by the demonstration of acid-fast organisms in the smears of pus or by histopathology of biopsied lesions. The importance of this infection is its role in inducing a non-specific reaction to the intradermal tuberculin test (see p. 863). There is no treatment.

Dermatophilosis (bovine streptothricosis)

This is a chronic or acute exudative dermatitis that may affect many species of animals and is of world-wide distribution. It also occurs in humans.

The disease in cattle is of particular importance in Africa, where it is thought to have been known since the nineteenth century, in America, the Middle East and Mediterranean Europe.

In cattle the disease is of importance for its role in causing economic loss through down-grading of hides and skins, reduced milk yield, marked debility in severely affected animals with dehydration and death.

Aetiology

The agent responsible for infection is the actinomycete, *Dermatophilus congolensis*, a Gram-positive filamentous bacterium. Infection with *D. congolensis* is confined to the epidermis where the motile zoospore stage of the organism, activated under suitable conditions of climate and skin damage, grows to form a filamentous mycelium within the epidermis. In dry conditions the spore stage of the bacterium may remain dormant in dry crust, scab and hyperkeratotic skin debris for many months.

A number of factors influence the incidence of the disease, of which high temperature and humidity play an important role. Similarly, breed susceptibility is of importance, indigenous cattle being more resistant to infection than imported exotic breeds.

The initiation of lesions requires skin damage, albeit superficial, by abrasion, e.g. thorn scratches, insect bites (biting flies or ticks may themselves carry the infective organism).

The incubation period may be as short as two weeks.

Signs

Bovine cutaneous streptothricosis commences as a circumscribed moist patch, often with raised or matted hairs, giving a characteristic 'paint brush' appearance. Discrete lesions occur in the initial stages which coalesce to form large areas of hyperkeratotic scab and crust (Plates 50.13 and 50.14). In severe infections as much as half the skin surface may be involved. Scab may be of variable thickness and on removal show a concave underside coated in thick, yellowish exudate, leaving a raw, bleeding epidermis.

Diagnosis

Impression smears of the exudate, fixed and stained by Gram's method or methylene blue, reveal numerous rows of cocci formed into branching filaments. Organisms may not be readily demonstrable in material taken from old lesions or those affected by secondary infection. *Dermatophilus congolensis* may be cultured on blood agar under microaerophilic conditions.

Differential diagnosis is with dermatophytosis (p. 878) and sarcoptic scabies (p. 891).

Treatment

Antibiotic therapy using penicillin and streptomycin as a single dose regimen (70 000 iu penicillin and 70 mg/kg body weight streptomycin intramuscularly) will prevent epidermal invasion by zoospores as well as re-infection. Alternatively, five daily doses of 5000 iu penicillin and 5 mg/kg body weight streptomycin may be given (Lloyd, 1981). Long-acting oxytetracycline by deep intramuscular injection at 20 mg/kg body weight has also been found to be effective (Lloyd *et al.*, 1990). Topical application of solutions of cresols and copper salts in appropriate dilution may have a preventive effect.

Prevention

Since predisposition to the disease is due to skin trauma from vegetation, ectoparasite infestation with poor husbandry resulting in malnutrition and/or the presence of concurrent disease, many of these factors are difficult to control. Efforts directed towards the establishment of herds of breeds resistant to *D. congolensis* may be of long-term benefit.

The quest for an effective vaccine continues but is still in the experimental stage of development (Lloyd, 1984). A combination of improved husbandry with vaccine therapy may eventually be the effective means of control.

Horn cancer

This disease, which results in neoplasia of the horn core, is usually an extension of squamous cell carcinoma that arises from the mucosa of the frontal sinus. Involvement of the horn core causes loosening of the horn, which drops off leaving the tumour exposed. While metastases occur in such conditions as squamous cell carcinoma of the eye, they do not occur in horn core lesions.

Diagnosis

This is by biopsy and clinical examination.

Treatment

Treatment has been found to have variable degrees of success and recurrence is common following surgery. Cryotherapy, surgical excision, radiodiathermy and immunotherapy have all been tried.

Lumpy skin disease and pseudo-lumpy skin disease

(see also p. 768)

Two forms of lumpy skin disease are recognized:

● True 'lumpy skin' disease, the causal agent of which is the Neethling pox virus, infection with which gives rise to acute or subacute disease among cattle in parts of Africa.
● Pseudo-lumpy skin disease due to infection with Allerton virus, bovine herpes virus type 2, which

has a world-wide distribution amongst all types of cattle.

Lumpy skin disease (see p. 768)

A seasonal disease that occurs particularly at times of high insect population and can affect cattle of any age, breed or type.

The mode of transmission of infection has not been fully determined although the association with periods of high insect population and proof that *Stomoxys calcitrans* can carry the virus suggests that the organism is insect-borne. The incubation period is one to four weeks.

Lumpy skin disease causes high economic loss through decreased milk production, abortion, loss of condition and hide damage.

Signs

The initial viraemia is associated with a febrile response, nasal discharge, excess salivation and possibly lameness. After a period of one week the first signs of skin lesions may be seen as papules/nodules with enlargement of the superficial lymph nodes.

Skin lesions can be localized or generalized, circumscribed firm and flattened intradermal nodules up to 5 cm in diameter. While lesions can be confined to the skin of the chest, neck, back, limbs, perineum, udder and scrotum, more severely affected animals may show involvement of the nasal and turbinate bones. Oedema of the ventral chest and abdomen, also the limbs, may occur.

Skin lesions may well ulcerate and be slow to resolve, persisting for months to years in some cases. In most instances the skin lesions necrose, passing through phases of ulceration and scarring before resolution in a period of one to three months.

Morbidity is usually around 50 per cent but may be as high as 90 per cent with mortality in the region of 10 per cent.

Prognosis

This is always guarded. Those animals that progress to respiratory tract involvement may well die.

Diagnosis

History, clinical examination, skin biopsy and virus isolation are all helpful. Apart from other histopathological changes present, eosinophilic intracytoplasmic inclusion bodies may be found in keratinocytes, and glandular and ductal epithelium of the skin glands.

Table 50.2 Other conditions referred to in the text which also show skin signs.

Actinobacillosis	Chronic granulomatous lesions as an extension from infected soft tissues and lymph nodes (see p. 823)
Actinomycosis	Chronic granulomatous lesions eroding skin from underlying bone infections (see p. 824)
Alopecia	Congenital baldness. Baldy calf syndrome (see p. 181)
Albinism	Congenital oculocutaneous absence of pigment (see p. 182)
Bacterial infections	● of the teat – blackspot; *F. necrophorum* (see p. 370)
	● of the udder – folliculitis, impetigo, *Staph. aureus* (see p. 371)
Besnoitiosis	Gross thickening of skin, lichenification, hair loss (see p. 756)
Claw conditions	(See Chapter 31)
Congenital	Epitheliogenesis imperfecta (see p. 181)
	Epitheliokeratogenesis imperfecta (see p. 181)
Copper deficiency	Poor coat, change in black coat colour (see pp. 254, 298)
	Digital disorders see also Claw disorders (p. 427)
Ichthyosis	Congenital hair loss, accumulations of scaly epithelium (see p. 182)
Interdigital dermatitis	See also Claw disorders
Onchocerciasis	Multiple parasitic nodules within the skin (see p. 774)
Selenium poisoning	Hoof cracking, rough coat, hair loss (see p. 305)
Stephanofilariasis	Thickened skin, papules, crusts, ulcers possibly on the udder and teats (see p. 774)
Viral diseases	
Cowpox	Rare, erythema leading to pustule formation on teats (see p. 365)
Foot-and-mouth disease	Vesicles on teats, muzzle, in addition to coronary band and mouth (see p. 700)
Herpes mammillitis	Irregular vesicles on skin of udder and teats, discoloration, ulceration (see p. 363)
Papillomatosis	Warts on teats (see p. 365)
Pseudocowpox	Common, erythema, papules, vesicles and scabs on teats (see p. 364)
Rickettsial disease	Jewbrana disease, petechiation, bleeding through the skin (see p. 766)

Treatment

None is effective. Antibiotics may be given to combat secondary infection. Measures to minimize the possibility of fly strike and subsequent myiasis should also be taken.

Prevention

Some protection is gained by vaccination with modified Neethling virus vaccine. Vaccination with sheep pox virus has also conferred some protection.

Pseudo-lumpy skin disease (see p. 768)

A much milder condition than 'true' Neethling virus lumpy skin disease and due to infection with bovine herpes virus type 2. The organism is also responsible for outbreaks of herpes mammillitis (p. 363).

Signs

There is absence of a systemic response or superficial lymphadenopathy with a clinical course similar to herpes mammillitis, resolution occurring in two to three weeks. In exceptional cases lesions may persist for considerably longer.

Skin lesions have a similar distribution and appearance to those of lumpy skin disease, with limbs, body, neck, back, udder, perineum and scrotum showing superficial raised plaques having a central depression and superficial necrosis.

Diagnosis

History, physical examination, virus isolation and skin biopsy are helpful. Skin biopsy shows, among other changes, eosinophilic intranuclear inclusion bodies in keratinocytes of the stratum spinosum.

Other conditions having skin signs

See Table 50.2.

References and further reading

General

Scott, D.W. (1988) Structure and function of the skin. In *Large Animal Dermatology*, pp. 2–28. W.B. Saunders & Co., Philadelphia.

Warble fly

Fadok, V.A. (1984) Parasitic diseases of large animals. *Veterinary Clinics of North America: Large Animal Practice*, **6**, 3–26.

Scott, D.W. (1988) Parasitic diseases. In *Large Animal Dermatology*, pp. 245–8. W.B. Saunders & Co., Philadelphia.

Soulsby, E.J.L. (1982) *Helminths, Arthropods and Protozoa of Domestic Animals*, 7th edn, pp. 432–7. Baillière Tindall, London.

Dermatophytosis

Scott, D.W. (1988) *Large Animal Dermatology*, pp. 179–82. W.B. Saunders & Co., Philadelphia.

Parasitic skin diseases

Blood, D.C., Radostits, O.M. & Henderson, J.A. (1983) *Veterinary Medicine*, 6th edn, p. 964. Baillière Tindall, London.

Fadok, V.A. (1984) Parasitic skin diseases of large animals. *Veterinary Clinics of North America, Large Animal Practice*, **6**, 3–26.

Linklater, K.A. & Gillespie, I.D. (1984) Outbreak of psoroptic mange in cattle. *Veterinary Record*, **115**, 211-12.

Scott, D.W. (1988) Parasitic diseases. In *Large Animal Dermatology*, pp. 207–30. W.B. Saunders & Co., Philadelphia.

Warts

Gibbs, E.P.J. (1984) Viral diseases of the skin of the bovine teat and udder. *Veterinary Clinics of North America: Large Animal Practice*, **6**, 187–202.

Hunt, E. (1984) Infectious skin diseases of cattle. *Veterinary Clinics of North America: Large Animal Practice*, **6**, 155–74.

Scott, D.W. (1988) Epithelial neoplasms. In *Large Animal Dermatology*, p. 420. W.B. Saunders & Co., Philadelphia.

Pruritis/pyrexia/haemorrhagic syndrome

References to outbreaks are all prior to 1980, since which time there have been no reports in the scientific literature. However, a few outbreaks still occur each year.

Blood, D.C. & Radostits, O.M. (1989) *Veterinary Medicine*, 7th edn, p. 1300. Baillière Tindall, London.

Photosensitization

Manning, T.O. (1984) Non-infectious skin diseases of cattle. *Veterinary Clinics of North America: Large Animal Practice*, **6**, 176–9.

Scott, D.W. (1988) In *Large Animal Dermatology*, pp. 76–83. W.B. Saunders & Co., Philadelphia.

Bovine farcy

Lloyd, D.H. (1981) Bovine farcy. In *Current Veterinary Therapy, Food Animal Practice* (ed. by J.L. Howard), p. 1136. W.B. Saunders & Co., Philadelphia.

Dermatophilosis

Lloyd, D.H. (1981) Streptothricosis. In *Current Veterinary Therapy, Food Animal Practice* (ed. by J.L. Howard), pp. 1134–5. W.B. Saunders & Co., Philadelphia.

Lloyd, D.H. (1984) Immunology of dermatophilosis: recent developments and prospects for control. *Preventive Medicine*, **2**, 93–102.

Lloyd D.H. & Sellers, K.C. (1976) *Dermatophilus* infection in animals and man. Symposium Proceedings, Ibadan. Academic Press.

Lloyd, D.H., Hawkins, J.P. & Pragnell, J. (1990) Efficacy of long-acting oxytetracycline in the treatment and control of bovine dermatophilosis. *Veterinary Dermatology*, **1**, 78–82.

Horn cancer

Bastianello, S.S. (1982) A survey of neoplasia in domestic species over a 40-year period from 1935 to 1974 in the Republic of South Africa. I. Tumours occurring in cattle. *Onderstepoort Journal of Veterinary Research*, **49**, 195–204.

Pachauri, S.P. & Pathak, R.C. (1969) Bovine horn cancer. Therapeutic experiments with autogenous vaccine. *American Journal of Veterinary Research*, **30**, 475–7.

Lumpy skin disease and pseudo-lumpy skin disease

Martin, W.B. (1986) Bovine mamillitis. In *Current Veterinary Therapy: Food Animal Practice II* (ed. by J.L. Howard). pp. 472–3. W.B. Saunders & Co., Philadelphia.

Njoku, C.O. (1986) Lumpy skin disease. In *Current Veterinary Therapy: Food Animal Practice II* (ed. by J.L. Howard). pp. 481–2. W.B. Saunders & Co., Philadelphia.

Scott, D.W. (1988) *Large Animal Dermatology*, p. 108. W.B. Saunders & Co., Philadelphia.

St George, T.D., Uren, M.F. & Melville, L.F. (1980) A generalised infection of cattle with bovine herpes virus 2. *Australian Veterinary Journal*, **56**, 42.

Chapter 51
Neurological Disorders

P.R. Scott

Introduction 890
Development, structure and function of the nervous system 891
  Development 891
  Structure and function 891
The nature and causes of signs of neurological disorder 891
  Endogenous biochemical causes 891
  Exogenous biochemical causes 892
  Genetic causes 892
  Micro-organisms 892
Neurological examination 895
  Cerebral syndrome 895
  Cerebellar syndrome 896
  Vestibular syndrome 896
  Pontomedullary (brainstem) syndrome 896
Collection of CSF 896
General principles of treatment for CNS infections 897
  Summary 900
Specific diseases 900
  Cerebellar hypoplasia/hydranencephaly 900
  Bacterial meningoencephalitis 901
  Brain abscess 902
  Cerebellar abiotrophy (postnatal degeneration) 903
  Unilateral middle ear infections/vestibular syndrome 903
  Polioencephalomalacia (cerebrocortical necrosis, CCN) 903
  Listerial encephalitis 904
  Lead poisoning 906
  Thromboembolic meningoencephalitis (TEME) 907
  Aujeszky's disease 907
  Rabies 908
  Bovine spongiform encephalopathy (BSE) 909
  Idiopathic brainstem neuronal chromatolysis of cattle 911
  Sporadic bovine encephalomyelitis (SBE, Buss disease) 911
  Spinal cord lesions 912

Introduction

Many of the neurological disorders of cattle such as lead poisoning, botulism, hydranencephaly caused by congenital bovine viral diarrhoea/mucosal diarrhoea (BVD/MD) or Akabane virus infections present as outbreaks. It is essential therefore that an accurate diagnosis is reached in order to expedite preventive and control measures. The investigation of possible central nervous system (CNS) involvement in a disease process necessitates a detailed assessment of the animal's history and a complete physical and neurolog-ical examination. A methodical neurological examina-tion allows the lesion to be localized to specific areas of the brain (Braund, 1985). The common diseases and conditions which affect those areas of the brain can then be listed and further investigated. This approach is much more preferable than the undergraduate student or practitioner attempting to memorize long lists of clinical signs for every neurological disease. A logical approach to neurological examination of cattle highlights discrepancies when new diseases arise because it does not limit the differential diagnoses to known diseases.

Such a methodical approach (Scott *et al.*, 1989a, 1995) was not adopted when a vague neurological disease, bovine spongiform encephalopathy (BSE), first appeared in United Kingdom dairy herds during the mid 1980s. The clinical findings were not consistent with any recognized bovine neurological disorder and led to spurious diagnoses such as brain tumours, chronic hypomagnesaemia, listeriosis, hepatic encephalopathy, etc. The lack of a methodical approach to suspected cases of BSE resulted in a correct clinical diagnosis in only 85 per cent of slaughtered cattle. Indeed, many of these cattle were examined twice some weeks apart, which should have excluded many acute neurological diseases. Despite over 15 years' experience of BSE, the clinical diagnosis remains only 85 per cent correct. Despite data collected from over 20000 suspected cases of BSE which were negative on histopathological ex-amination of brain tissue, no summary of these clinical cases has appeared in the veterinary literature. This lack of data indicates the absence of a standard logical approach to neurological disease by many veterinari-ans. Too often the clinical signs are fitted to a limited number of known diseases and it is therefore inevitable that new diseases will not be recognized.

Cerebrospinal fluid (CSF) analysis is the most useful laboratory test in the clinical investigation of neurolog-ical diseases in cattle (Scott & Penny, 1993; Scott 1995a, 1996) but such samples are rarely undertaken in prac-tice. However, lumbar CSF samples can be obtained from affected animals under local anaesthesia on the farm with immediate results available on visual exami-nation, ensuring an accurate diagnosis and specific treatment without further delay (Scott & Penny, 1993). For example, animals may present with neurological signs indicative of cerebellar dysfunction where a neutrophilic pleocytosis and increased CSF protein concentration indicate focal meningitis (Scott et al., 1994a) while normal CSF parameters in another case do not indicate an infectious cause and indirectly support the diagnosis of a developmental abnormality causing dysfunction (Scott et al., 1993a).

In many situations in practice the clinical examination is incomplete and fails to yield sufficient information to make a specific diagnosis. Consequently, in the field situation response to treatment has often been used as an adjunct to diagnosis (Morgan, 1992), despite numerous treatments being administered simultaneously (Power et al., 1985), thereby limiting interpretation of the outcome.

There are specific changes in antibody titre, serum ion, metabolite or enzyme concentration in only a small percentage of bovine neurological diseases and a specific diagnosis is often reached only in fatal cases which are examined in detail at necropsy (Jeffrey, 1992). However, for cost reasons few cattle are subject to a detailed post-mortem examination. Histopathological examination of the CNS is expensive and multiple sections are cost-prohibitive. Accurate lesion localization by the clinician is therefore essential before euthanasia is carried out, otherwise discrete lesions may not be sectioned at necropsy and an incorrect diagnosis reached.

Development, structure and function of the nervous system

Development

Development of the nervous system of mammals takes place as a sequence of intensely active events that occur from early embryogenesis and continue in cattle into postnatal life. During these phases cells undergoing rapid division and differentiation are susceptible to a wide variety of physical, chemical and infectious agents.

The physical factors include extremes of temperature, especially maternal hyperthermia, and direct or indirect trauma. Chemical factors include organic, inorganic and plant poisons, nutritional imbalances and toxic products of microbial activity in the maternal or external environment. The direct invasion of the fetus by microorganisms presents a further hazard and inherited defects or spontaneous errors in nucleic acid templating may produce effects at all stages of development.

Structure and function

Structurally, the nervous system of higher vertebrates comprises neurones and neuroglia. The neurones form the conducting system for neural impulses. The neuroglia are also of two types; the oligodendroglia are responsible for the formation and maintenance of the myelin sheaths of the axons and astrocytes which provide the supporting scaffold of the CNS and also contribute to the blood–brain barrier. In the peripheral nervous system the Schwann cell is the homologue of the oligodendrocyte.

The nervous system is heavily dependent upon glucose and oxygen to sustain functional activity; consequently there is a rich capillary network, especially in regions of high neuronal density. Even brief disruption of blood supply will interfere with membrane function with accumulation of toxic metabolites, such as lipid peroxides, resulting in swelling or cell death. When a nerve cell is lost it cannot be replaced and the circuit containing it is diminished. If substantial numbers of nerve cells are lost, functional deficits will result.

Infectious agents, toxic incidents and traumatic events may damage not only the neurone but also the glial components of the nervous system. Following injury astrocytes can proliferate to produce an astroglial scar, which itself may distort the tissue and further interfere with neural function. Oligodendroglia can also be regenerated from stem cells, but in the mature CNS the ability to replace myelin is to a large extent dependent upon the viability of the neurone.

The nature and causes of signs of neurological disorder

Endogenous biochemical causes
(see also Chapters 21, 46, 54)

This group of conditions includes those metabolic diseases that are associated with the stresses of production and systems of management and includes milk fever, hypomagnesaemic tetany and acetonaemia. These disorders produce no specific pathological changes in the CNS and the clinical condition in most instances can be readily reversed by rapid correction of the specific deficiency.

Inborn errors of metabolism are usually considered to be heritable, mainly with an autosomal recessive mode. A gene may control a specific enzyme or enzyme system and a defect therein will block the normal metabolic pathway. In some cases, however, there may be alternative pathways to modulate or minimize the consequences and these may influence the time of onset and rate of progress of clinical disease.

In inherited congenital myoclonus in the polled Hereford (Harper et al., 1986), affected calves, although bright and alert, are unable to stand from birth and show stimulus-responsive myoclonic spasms. A second genetically mediated disorder, neuraxial oedema, also occurs in Herefords and possibly other breeds. Affected calves appear normal at birth but within a day or two they become dull and recumbent with opisthotonus. The significant pathology is in the CNS and consists of vacuolation at all levels of the neuraxis.

Lysosomal storage diseases comprise an important group of genetically-mediated diseases whereby the products of faulty degradation accumulate in lysosomes and the cell bodies swell. The cells of the heterozygote contain approximately half the normal concentration of enzyme, but the animal itself appears normal, whilst the diseased animal is homozygous for the defect and the enzyme is absent. Heterozygote recognition by appropriate enzymatic assay offers a means of controlling the disease within a population. Examples of lysosomal storage diseases include lipidosis GM_1 gangliosidosis in the Friesian, glycoproteinosis mannosidosis in the Angus, Murray Grey and Galloway and ceroid lipofuscinosis, which has been described in Beefmaster cattle. The clinical signs of GM_1 gangliosidosis are reluctance to feed, dullness, progressive ataxia and ill-thrift, and appear one to three months after birth (see p. 179). Clinically, mannosidosis (pseudolipidosis) presents as wasting, altered behaviour with aggression and progressive ataxia (see p. 179).

Exogenous biochemical causes

There is a wide range of exogenous biochemical causes of neurological disorder. Some compounds, e.g. organophosphorus compounds, organochlorides and carbamates, are specific neurotoxins whose mode of action is known. However, a great many toxicants whose primary targets appear to be gut, liver or the cardiovascular system also cause neurological disturbances. In the early phases these usually take the form of excitement, muscle fasciculations, tachycardia and hyperpnoea, whilst convulsions and coma frequently characterize the terminal phases. The mechanisms of this toxic stimulation and depression of the nervous system are poorly understood (see Chapter 54).

In cattle, intoxication by chemical compounds is not uncommon for reasons that include their innate curiosity, considerable appetite and non-selective habits of grazing and licking. Lead, the organophosphorus compounds, ragwort, copper, urea and sodium chloride are known to cause neuropathological changes. Lead is by far the most important and is considered in detail later. Organophosphorus compounds used as insecticides and herbicides are variably potent inhibitors of cholinesterase (see p. 940). The clinical signs of acute intoxication, miosis, salivation, polyuria, muscle fasciculations, apprehension and ataxia are the consequences of cholinergic overstimulation, but produce no charac-

teristic neuropathology. The clinical signs of hepatic encephalopathy, e.g. ragwort poisoning, may be intermittent and slowly progressive or acutely fatal, depending upon the severity and duration of hepatic overload by nitrogenous compounds. There are behavioural changes, with compulsive walking, circling, twitching of ears and eyelids, blindness and, in severe cases, recumbency with opisthotonus (see p. 945).

Genetic causes

The plurality of genetic neurological disorders in cattle (Table 51.1) is possibly a reflection of intensive selection for particular production traits from within small populations of superior animals and is facilitated by artificial breeding techniques.

Micro-organisms

Neurological disorders in cattle can result from the activities of all types of infective agents. Some invade the nervous system, usually causing inflammation of the brain (encephalitis), spinal cord (myelitis) or the membranous coverings (meningitis). Others that may be present in the alimentary tract or external environment produce neurotoxins or antimetabolites, which cause degenerative encephalopathies and myelopathies.

Viruses

Viruses form an important group of neural pathogens. The oronasal route is the most common portal of entry, but some viruses gain access via the conjunctiva or percutaneously by the bite of an insect vector or infected animal. Initial replication at the site of infection and in local lymphoid tissues is typically followed by viraemia with fever during which the virus penetrates the blood–brain barrier and invades the neural parenchyma. Typical inflammatory responses are focal and diffuse proliferations of microglial cells and perivascular and meningeal infiltrations of lymphocytes. As the CNS is normally impermeable to circulating immunoglobulins, synthesis of antibody by B cells in the perivascular cuffs may play an important role in the recovery of the individual. Other virus infections, e.g. bovine virus diarrhoea/mucosal disease (Trautwein *et al.*, 1987) and Akabane disease (Inaba *et al.*, 1975), generally cause mild or inapparent disease in the adult, but cause severe transplacental infections of the fetus. Fetal meningoencephalitis or gross intracranial malformations from destruction of the granuloprival elements of the developing fetal brain may be the result, depending upon the stage of fetal development at infection.

Table 51.1 Inherited neurological diseases of cattle.

Disease	Mode R/D	Breed(s)	Age at onset	Clinical features	Pathology	Reference
Cerebellar abiotrophy	R	Holstein	3–8 months	Progressive spastic ataxia, dysmetria. Loss of menace response	Degeneration of cerebellar neurones sparing the vermis	White *et al.* (1975) (p. 178)
Hereditary congenital ataxia 'jittery'	R	Jersey	Birth to 3 months	Ataxia and intention tremor	Hypomyelination and oedema of cerebellar white matter	Saunders *et al.* (1952)
Cerebellar ataxia	R?	Shorthorn Hereford	1–3 days	Rapidly progressive ataxia with recumbency	Spongy transformation of cerebellar white matter, shrinkage and loss of neurones	Hulland (1957) (p. 178)
Familial cerebellar hypoplasia and degeneration	R	Hereford	Birth	Recumbent, stuporose, intermittent rigidity	Narrow disorganized cerebellar folia. Paucity of cerebellar cortical neurones	Innes *et al.* (1940)
Familial convulsions and ataxia	D	Aberdeen Angus	Birth to 6 months	Recurrent seizures with gradual development of spastic ataxia and hypermetria	Swelling and vacuolation of Purkinje cells and Purkinje cell axons	Barlow (1980) (p. 178)
Doddler	R	Hereford	Birth	Muscular spasms and convulsions, nystagmus, respiratory difficulties	Calcification of cerebellar and medullary neurones	High *et al.* (1958)
GM₁ gangliosidosis	R	Friesian	1 month	Reluctance to feed, dullness and progressive ataxia	Cerebrospinal lipidosis with ballooning of neurones by accumulations of glycolipid	Donnelly *et al.* (1973) (p. 179)
Mannosidosis	R	Angus, Murray Grey, Galloway	Birth onwards	Wasting, aggression and progressive ataxia, lymphadenopathy	Vacuolation of neurones and fixed macrophages, renal epithelial cells and exocrine pancreas	Hocking *et al.* (1972) (p. 179)
Neuraxial oedema: maple syrup urine disease	R	Hereford and polled Hereford	1–3 days	Dullness, recumbency and opisthotonus: nystagmus. Urine smells of burnt sugar	Raised urine ketones. Vacuolation throughout neuraxis especially white matter	Healy *et al.* (1986) (p. 180)
Inherited congenital myoclonus	R	Polled Hereford	Birth	Stimulus-responsive myoclonic spasms	Contusions of coxofemoral joint with fractures/ deformity of articular cartilage	Harper *et al.* (1986) (p. 180)

contd.

Table 51.1 *Continued*

Disease	Mode R/D	Breed(s)	Age at onset	Clinical features	Pathology	Reference
Bovine generalized glycogenosis	R	Shorthorn	12 months	Muscular weakness, incoordination, deficiency of α-1,4-glucosidase or acid maltase	Accumulation of PAS-positive and Bests carmine plus granules in neurones of midbrain, medullary and cerebellar roof nuclei	Richards *et al.* (1977)
Chediak–Higashi syndrome	R	Hereford, Brown Swiss	Young adults	Partial albinism (ghost pattern colouring). Susceptibility to infection. Premature ageing	Yellow pigmented PAS, LFB and Sudan black B-positive inclusions in nerve cells of brain, cord, myenteric plexuses. Similar to lipofuscin granules	Padgett (1968)
'Weaver syndrome': progressive degenerative myeloencephalopathy	R	Brown Swiss	8–12 months	Motor dysfunction with swinging gait progressing to loss of movement and inability to stand	Axonal degeneration predominantly in spinal white matter, axons in some brain stem nuclei and Purkinje cells of cerebellar cortex. Paramembranous densities and synaptic junctions	Stuart & Leipold (1985) (p. 179)
Neuronal lipodystrophy	R	Beefmaster	12 months	Blindness, circling, recumbency and coma	Neuronal multilamellar and curvilinear inclusions. Similar structures may be found in fixed macrophages in spleen and lymph nodes.	Read & Bridges (1969)
Progressive ataxia of Charolais	R?	Charolais	8–24 months	Progressive weakness and ataxia terminating in recumbency	Segmental demyelination of CNS with retraction of internodes, formation of eosinophilic plaques from oligodendroglial processes	Palmer *et al.* (1972) (p. 179)
Recumbent calf syndrome	R?	Red Danish milk breed	6 weeks	Progressive ataxia, paresis and immobility	Degeneration of neurones in ventral horns of spinal cord	Hansen *et al.* (1988)

R, recessive; D, dominant; PAS, periodic acid shift.

Bacteria

Bacteria, with possibly *Listeria monocytogenes* as the sole exception, do not invade the neuroparenchyma as a primary event. Infection of the neuraxis usually arises from a bacteraemia causing meningitis, which may be purulent or non-purulent depending on the organism involved. Infection of the meninges may also arise directly following local trauma. Subsequent invasion of the neuroparenchyma, however, depends upon damage to the blood–brain barrier, such as may occur following rupture of a meningeal abscess, devitalization of the tissue by toxic products or infarction due to infective emboli as in thromboembolic meningoencephalitis (Ames, 1987).

Other manifestations of bacterial involvement in neurological disease include those caused by the exotoxins of clostridial infections occurring elsewhere in the body, e.g. focal symmetrical encephalomalacia (Buxton *et al.*, 1981) and tetanus, which are discussed elsewhere. Also in this category are the thiaminolytic organisms that proliferate in rumen contents and are implicated in polioencephalomalacia.

Protozoa (see p. 284)

Protozoan infections with *Toxoplasma gondii* and *Sarcocystis* species have been implicated in neonatal necrotizing non-suppurative encephalomyelitis in calves (O'Toole & Jeffrey, 1987). Congenital sarcocystosis infestation has been recorded as a cause of recumbency in newborn calves. Severe coccidiosis in calves is uncommonly associated with neurological disorder in Britain, although more widely reported in North America. Pelvic limb paresis in yearling cattle progressing to tetraparesis over two to three days has been reported, caused by *Sarcocystis zurnii* encephalomyelitis.

Nematodes

The intermediate stage (*Coeneurus cerebralis*) of the dog tapeworm *Taenia multiceps* may occasionally occur in cattle in well-defined regions of Britain, but is much less common than the disease in sheep. The clinical signs are of a slowly progressive, space-occupying lesion in one cerebral hemisphere, circling to the affected side, proprioceptive deficits and contralateral blindness.

Neurological examination

A methodical neurological examination allows central nervous system lesions to be localized to specific area(s) of the brain (Braund, 1985). The common diseases and conditions which affect those areas of the brain can then be listed and further investigated. The most useful and cost effective ancillary test is lumbar cerebrospinal fluid analysis (Scott, 1992, 1995a, 1996). For example, the clinical presentation in a young calf of depression, lethargy, cortical blindness and dorsomedial strabismus is consistent with diffuse cerebral dysfunction; CSF analysis reveals a markedly elevated protein concentration and neutrophilic pleocytosis. These clinical signs are consistent with a diagnosis of bacterial meningoencephalitis which is then confirmed on gross CSF inspection and laboratory findings (Scott & Penny, 1993). There is no need to consider an endless list of obscure differential diagnoses when the neurological findings and lumbar CSF tap yield pathognomic results. The methodical clinical examination explores all aspects of the animal's presentation rather than attempting to fit the clinical signs to a recognized condition/disease. For example, the clinician may believe the calf described above is suffering from bacterial meningoencephalitis because it is four days-old, dull and depressed – this description may equally apply to enterotoxigenic *E. coli*, starvation/hypothermia, polyarthritis, etc. The diagnosis is not confirmed until a lumbar CSF tap is taken and examined, when all potential diagnoses except bacterial meningoencephalitis can be excluded.

Considerable confusion arose with the clinical recognition of bovine spongiform encephalopathy in the United Kingdom during the mid 1980s because practitioners could not assign the clinical findings to any known disease and spurious diagnoses such as tumour, hepatic encephalopathy and chronic hypomagnesaemia were commonplace. The accuracy of clinical diagnosis was approximately 85 per cent with a wide range of diseases incorrectly reported as BSE, including listeriosis. Bovine spongiform encephalopathy presents with clinical signs of cerebral and cerebellar dysfunction with no intrathecal inflammatory response (Scott *et al.*, 1989b); listeriosis shows the classical presentation of the pontomedullary syndrome with an elevated protein concentration in CSF and increased white cell concentration with predominance of large mononuclear cells (Scott, 1996). A methodical clinical examination should readily differentiate these two common neurological disorders of adult cattle in the UK.

While the brain can be conveniently divided into six areas, each with a recognized neurological 'syndrome' (Braund, 1985) only four syndromes concern the veterinary practitioner: cerebral, cerebellar, pontomedullary (brainstem) and vestibular.

Cerebral syndrome

Diffuse cerebral disease is common in ruminants, associated with metabolic disease in adults and bacterial meningoencephalitis in neonates. The cerebrum is concerned with mental state, behaviour and, in conjunction with the eye and optic (II) nerve, vision. Clinical signs which suggest cerebral dysfunction include blindness, but with normal pupillary light reflexes (II, III), compulsive walking, circling, constant chewing movements, severe depression, dementia, yawning, head pressing, hyperaesthesia to auditory and tactile stimuli, and opisthotonus. It is important to note that the clinical signs change as the disease condition progresses; for example, calves with bacterial meningoencephalitis may present with different clinical signs depending upon the duration of CNS infection.

Ipsilateral compulsive circling, sluggish gait, postural deficits, deviation of the head (not a head tilt) and depression with contralateral blindness are variably seen in animals with unilateral cerebral lesions.

Cerebellar syndrome

The cerebellum is primarily concerned with fine coordination of voluntary movement. In cerebellar dysfunction limb movements are spastic (rigid), clumsy and jerky. Initiation of movement is delayed and may be accompanied by intention tremors. Cerebellar disease is characterized by a wide-based stance and ataxia (incoordination), particularly of the pelvic limbs but with preservation of normal muscle strength. In addition to the ataxia, dysmetria may be observed with hypermetria the more common form observed in cerebellar disease. Opisthotonus can occur in animals with severe lesions of the rostral cerebellum.

Vestibular syndrome

In growing cattle unilateral peripheral vestibular lesions are not uncommon. The major clinical signs include ipsilateral (to the same side) head tilt, leaning and drifting sideways when walking. Circling may also be observed. Positional nystagmus may be depressed or absent in animals with a vestibular lesion. There is spontaneous horizontal nystagmus with the fast phase directed away from the side of the lesion. There is frequently ipsilateral ventral strabismus (eye drop) which is exaggerated when the head is raised. Facial nerve paralysis is common in peripheral vestibular disease since both facial and sympathetic nerves fibres pass close to the middle ear. In central vestibular disease the nystagmus may be horizontal, vertical or rotary.

Pontomedullary (brainstem) syndrome

As most of the cranial nerve nuclei are present in the brainstem, dysfunction is characterized by multiple cranial nerve deficits. Depression is also a key sign of brainstem disease which is attributed to a lesion involving the ascending reticular activating system. Circling, ipsilateral hemiparesis and proprioceptive defects are also common. Circling can be observed in diseases affecting the brainstem caused by involvement of the vestibulo-cochlear nucleus. Involvement of the facial nucleus results in ipsilateral facial nerve paralysis. Facial palsy is evident as drooped ear, drooped upper eyelid (ptosis) and flaccid lip. Involvement of trigeminal nerve or the trigeminal motor nucleus results in paralysis of the cheek muscles and decreased facial skin sensation. Listeriosis is the classical brainstem lesion.

Collection of CSF

Collection of CSF forms an integral part of the clinician's detailed neurological examination. Lumbar CSF can readily be collected under local anaesthesia from cattle of all ages (Scott & Penny, 1993; Scott et al., 1995). While it may be preferable to collect cisternal CSF for a more representative sample, this technique is inherently more difficult to perform and is not without risk to the patient. Numerous studies in ruminant species (Scott, 1992, 1995a, 1996) have shown that lumbar CSF samples provide meaningful data which assist the clinician in formulating a more specific diagnosis. Lumbar CSF can be collected under local anaesthesia in the standing animal. Cisternal CSF collection requires appropriate restraint and, in many situations, either deep sedation or general anaesthesia.

Collection of lumbar CSF is greatly facilitated when the animal is positioned in sternal recumbency with the hips flexed and the pelvic limbs extended alongside the abdomen. In adult cattle that are ambulatory the lumbar CSF sample is collected from the standing animal which must be suitably restrained in cattle stocks which prevent lateral movement. The site for lumbar CSF collection is the mid point of the lumbosacral space which can be identified as the mid line depression between the last palpable lumbar dorsal spine (L6) and the first palpable sacral dorsal spine (S2). The site must be clipped, aseptically prepared and 1–2 ml of 2 per cent lignocaine solution injected subcutaneously. Sterile surgical gloves should be worn. A guide to needle length and diameter (Scott, 1996) is included in Table 51.2.

Table 51.2 Guide to needle length and gauge for lumbar CSF sampling in cattle.

Calves <80 kg	1 inch 20 gauge
Calves 100–200 kg	2 inch 19 gauge
Cattle >200 kg	4 inch 18 gauge + internal stylet

When the lumbosacral site has been surgically pre-pared the needle is slowly advanced at a right angle to the plane of the vertebral column or with the hub directed 5–10° caudally. It is essential to appreciate the change in tissue resistance as the needle point passes sequentially through the skin, subcutaneous tissue, interarcuate ligament then the sudden 'pop' due to the loss of resistance as the needle point penetrates through the ligamentum flavum into the epidural space. Once the needle point has penetrated the dorsal subarach-noid space, CSF wells up in the needle hub within 2–3 seconds. There is no justification whatsoever in collect-ing CSF from the ventral subarachnoid space. Between 2–3 ml of CSF is sufficient for analysis and can be col-lected by free flow from the needle hub or by gentle syringe aspiration. Care must be taken not to dislodge the needle point from the dorsal subarachnoid space when the syringe, with the seal already broken, is attached to the needle hub. Sedation of the animal is not usually necessary but intravenous xylazine (0.05–0.1 mg/kg bodyweight) or diazepam (0.04 mg/kg body-weight) can facilitate positioning of the pelvic limbs in recumbent animals. It is not necessary to compress the jugular veins to facilitate CSF collection.

Samples of CSF are collected into EDTA containers. The specific gravity value is determined using a hygrometer. Many cerebrospinal fluid samples have first to be concentrated before CSF protein concentra-tion can be determined using the pyrogallol method. White cell concentration in CSF is determined using a haemocytometer. Cytological examination of CSF is facilitated when the sample is first concentrated by cytospin. The sample is then air-dried and stained with Leishman stain and the differential white cell count based on a minimum of 20 cells. Further laboratory testing, such as protein electrophoresis (Scott, 1993b), adds little additional information and is rarely under-taken for cost reasons.

An assessment of CSF pressure can be made by determining the rate of CSF flow from the needle hub once the needle point has penetrated the dorsal sub-arachnoid space. The normal flow rate is one drop of CSF every 2 to 3 seconds. A steady flow of CSF is obtained immediately following puncture of the arach-noid mater in calves with meningoencephalitis, indicat-ing increased CSF pressure. The use of a manometer has no practical application in farm animal practice.

The analysis of lumbar CSF from a range of neurological disorders, and other conditions which present with abnormal mental state, is presented in Table 51.3.

General principles of treatment for CNS infections

The important factors to consider in the treatment of central nervous system infections include:

- Bacterial pathogen;
- Duration and extent of the disease process;
- Ability of the selected antibiotic to penetrate the blood–brain barrier and achieve concentrations 10 to 30 times the minimum bactericidal concentration in order to sterilize the CSF (Prescott & Baggot, 1988; see also Chapter 61).

Supportive treatments include corticosteroids, diuretics, dimethyl sulphoxide and non-steroidal anti-inflammatory drugs (NSAIDs) e.g. flunixin meglumine, carprofen, meloxicam and ketoprofen. In addition, certain situations necessitate appropriate intravenous and oral fluid replacement therapy to correct second-ary acid–base and fluid disturbances.

For an antibiotic to be effective in bacterial meningi-tis, it must penetrate into the CSF in sufficient concen-tration to be bactericidal to the invading organism (Lambert & Wall, 1991) and achieve CSF concentra-tions 10 to 30 times the minimum bactericidal concen-tration to sterilize the CSF (Sande, 1981; Prescott & Baggot, 1988). Even with successful CSF antibiotic penetration, the intrathecal defence mechanisms are inadequate to control bacterial infection and treat-

Table 51.3 Lumbar CSF results (median, range) for some common bovine CNS diseases.

Disease	Number	Specific gravity	Protein (g/l)	White cells (×10⁹/l)
Control	31	1.007 (1.006–1.011)	0.28 (0.06–0.73)	0.0125 (0.012–0.25)
Meningitis	17	1.010 (1.007–1.017)	2.5 (0.5–7.1)	2.0 (0.012–12.6)
Listeriosis	12	1.009 (1.008–1.017)	1.69 (0.39–10.4)	0.3 (0.012–1.7)
Bovine viral diarrhoea	5	1.007 (1.006–1.010)	0.22 (0.09–0.24)	0.0125 (0.012–0.1)
Septicaemia	11	1.009 (1.007–1.011)	0.77 (0.19–2.04)	0.05 (0.01–0.2)
Acidosis	5	1.009 (1.007–1.011)	0.35 (0.2–1.3)	0.012 (0.012)

ment necessitates the use of bactericidal antibiotics (Landesman *et al.*, 1981; Del Rio *et al.*, 1983).

The blood–brain barrier can be divided into the blood–brain and blood–CSF barriers, although some researchers consider them functionally synonymous because extracellular fluid of the brain is in equilibrium with CSF. Morphologically, the blood–brain barrier comprises the continuous tight junctions (zonulae occludens) of the endothelial cells which form the brain capillaries. The permeability of the blood–brain barrier is dramatically increased by the inflammatory process, whatever the cause (Oldendorf, 1975). The increased permeability of the blood–brain barrier in experimental meningitis models was in part caused by the separation of intercellular tight junctions of the cerebral microvascular endothelium which was augmented by the presence of CSF leucocytes (Quagliarello *et al.*, 1986).

Few broad-spectrum bactericidal antibiotics are capable of penetrating the intact blood–brain barrier, but it has generally been assumed that the disruption of the blood–brain barrier, which occurs in bacterial CNS diseases, increases the degree of antibiotic penetration (Barlow, 1991). Such increased permeability may be sufficient to allow passage of antibiotics which achieve minimum inhibitory concentrations within the CSF (Rings, 1987), but few studies have been undertaken in animals with naturally-occuring CNS infections to support such assumptions.

Antibiotic penetration of the blood–CSF barrier depends upon lipid solubility; the greater the degree of ionization of an antibiotic in plasma, hence reduced lipid solubility, the lower the penetration through the blood–CSF barrier. Antibiotic penetration also depends upon the degree of protein binding. Large molecular weight antibiotics, such as aminoglycosides, achieve very poor CSF concentrations even in the presence of meningeal inflammation (Stone & Wise, 1991).

As well as the selection of antimicrobial agent, there is considerable disagreement regarding the duration of treatment for CNS infections. Prescott and Baggot (1988) quote the experimental findings of Tauber *et al.* (1987), that the single most important factor in achieving a favourable outcome for streptococcal meningitis is the peak concentration of antibiotic in the CSF. Conversely, Rebhun and deLahunta (1982) recommended a six week course of antibiotic treatment for bovine listeriosis. In farm animal practice the cost of antibiotic treatment is an important limiting factor in the animal's treatment and high dose/short duration therapy is perhaps the best compromise in many situations.

Penicillins

In man, penicillin and ampicillin are usually considered the antibiotics of choice for meningitis caused by *L. monocytogenes* (Tuazon *et al.*, 1982). It is strongly recommended that the first penicillin treatment is administered intravenously. The minimum inhibitory concentration (MIC^{90}) of penicillin G for *L. monocytogenes* has been quoted as 0.02 µg/ml (Prescott & Baggot, 1988). While lumbosacral CSF penicillin G concentrations between 0.09 and 1.02 µg/ml were achieved in three cases of bacterial meningitis 48 hours after the commencement of treatment of 44 000 iu/kg procaine penicillin b.i.d. (Scott & Sutton, 1992), the median CSF protein concentration in those animals was higher than values encountered in listeriosis cases (2.5 g/l compared to 1.7 g/l), suggesting greater disruption of the blood–brain barrier. However, it is possible that the CSF penicillin G concentrations achieved in brain tissue were considerably higher than those achieved within CSF. High dose penicillin G or oxytetracycline treatments have been reported to give a good prognosis for listeriosis cases provided the cattle are still ambulatory when treatment commences (Rebhun & deLahunta, 1982). High dose penicillin treatment (44 000 iu/kg procaine penicillin b.i.d.) of cases of ovine listeriosis, where the clinical diagnosis was supported by characteristic lumbar CSF analyses, gave a 24 per cent success rate (Scott, 1993a). It is possible that the optimum daily dose rate of penicillin G to treat acute CNS infections could be as high as 300 000 iu/kg; approximately 15 times the normal dose rate. This dose rate is prohibitively expensive in most cattle except for the first day of treatment. The high cost of appropriate antibiotic therapy for infectious diseases of the CNS further emphasizes the necessity of an accurate diagnosis before commencing therapy. The use of conventional dose antibiotic therapy is unlikely to prove effective in the treatment of bovine listeriosis. Reports of successful treatment of listeriosis with certain antibiotics administered at conventional dose rates raise doubts over the clinical diagnosis and whether the cattle were indeed suffering from a vestibular lesion, which would have responded well to such therapy.

Active removal of penicillins from the CSF can be inhibited by probenicid. In horses the elimination half-life of ampicillin was increased, and total body clearance reduced, following treatment with probenicid (Sarasola & McKellar, 1992). The extent to which probenicid affects the clearance of penicillin from bovine CSF is not known and requires further study before its use can be recommended as an adjunct to penicillin therapy.

Aminoglycosides

Gentamicin is rapidly bactericidal against many potential Gram-negative organisms causing neonatal meningitis but, as a polar antibiotic, is unable to cross the blood–brain barrier, even during meningitis. This lack of penetration into the CSF led to intrathecal and intraventricular administration of aminoglycoside antibiotics for the treatment of meningitis in infants and children, but this technique was associated with an increased mortality rate. Intrathecal injections of gentamicin in the lumbosacral region failed to result in significant concentrations in ventricular CSF (Moellering & Fisher, 1972) and, as a consequence, this technique has not been practised for the treatment of bacterial meningoencephalitis in cattle.

Chloramphenicol

Until withdrawal from the veterinary market in many countries, chloramphenicol was stated to be the antibiotic of choice for the treatment of bacterial meningoencephalitis (Rings, 1987) as it is capable of crossing the intact blood–brain barrier. In field studies 30 per cent of calves responded to chloramphenicol and showed a marked improvement within 24 hours and no relapses occurred after five consecutive days' treatment (Scott & Penny, 1993). There are no published studies of the usefulness of florfenicol, a closely-related molecule, in the treatment of bacterial meningoencephalitis.

Metronidazole

Metronidazole is highly lipid-soluble and capable of penetrating the blood–brain barrier and into brain abscesses. Unfortunately, this antibiotic is not licensed for use in veterinary medicine in Britain and there are no data regarding its use in cattle with CNS infections. In medicine, brain abscesses are frequently mixed aerobic and anaerobic infections and in such situations metronidazole is administered in conjunction with either penicillin or chloramphenicol.

Ceftiofur

Third generation cephalosporins are widely used for the treatment of bacterial meningoencephalitis in medicine but there are no data relating to the field use of ceftiofur in cattle. As chloramphenicol is no longer available to many veterinary practitioners, ceftiofur would present a logical choice for bacterial meningoencephalitis.

Trimethoprim–sulphonamide

Trimethoprim–sulphonamide has been recommended for the treatment of bacterial meningoencephalitis and listeriosis in cattle but there are no published field studies.

Anti-inflammory agents

In certain neurological diseases, particularly polioencephalomalacia and bacterial meningoencephalitis, the control of cerebral oedema is an important factor affecting prognosis (McGuirk, 1987). The increased intracranial pressure in bacterial meningoencephalitis results from cerebral oedema, which may be a factor contributing to death, brain infarction and alterations in CSF hydrodynamics. The development of potentially-serious increased intracranial pressure is indicated by coma, seizures, abducens nerve palsy, persistent bradycardia and respiratory depression. The recommended treatment for the control of cerebral oedema is either 1–2 mg/kg dexamethasone given intravenously, 1–2 g/kg of dimethyl sulphoxide as a 10 per cent solution given intravenously or frusemide 1–2 mg/kg given intravenously (McGuirk, 1987).

There are no comparative field investigations of corticosteroid treatments in bovine CNS disease. While the potential benefits of the concurrent use of dexamethasone with cephalosporin antibiotics have been demonstrated for the treatment of bacterial meningitis in children, it is reported that there may be a number of potential deleterious effects including a reduction in cellular immune function and reduced penetration of antibiotics into CSF (Scheld & Brodeur, 1983).

Non-steroidal anti-inflammatory drugs (NSAIDs)

The potential application of NSAIDs such as flunixin or ketoprofen in the treatment of LPS-induced intrathecal reaction in bovine meningoencephalitis has not been reported. Bacterial meningoencephalitis is commonly associated with septicaemia where intravenous NSAID administration would be of benefit in the treatment of septic shock. The analgesic properties of NSAIDs may also prove of benefit in the treatment of bacterial infections of the CNS. Therefore, there are a number of indications for NSAID administration in calves with bacterial meningoencephalitis, although this statement is not supported by field results. The potential benefits of NSAID therapy in more chronic CNS infections have not been investigated.

Dimethyl sulphoxide (DMSO)

There is no licensed DMSO product for veterinary use in Britain, but analytical quality DMSO has been used in the treatment of cattle with CNS dysfunction. DMSO has many properties, including reduction of cerebral oedema and free radical scavenging (Brayton, 1986), but special handling precautions preclude its use in most situations encountered in general practice. In veterinary practice, DMSO administration would most likely be restricted to the very valuable calf suffering from bacterial meningoencephalitis.

Intravenous/oral fluids

Severe dehydration can be corrected by the intravenous infusion of isotonic saline. Metabolic acidosis, which is commonly encountered in listeriosis cases caused by saliva loss, can be corrected by regular administration of sodium bicarbonate by oro-gastric tube.

Summary

Successful treatment of bovine CNS infections necessitates a rapid and accurate diagnosis. Cerebrospinal fluid collection is a simple procedure and visual inspection can reveal much useful information, particularly in neonatal calves with bacterial meningoencephalitis, permitting a rapid diagnosis and prompt treatment. Encephalitis lesions, such as those caused by listeriosis, result in minor changes in the CSF and laboratory examination is necessary. Ceftiofur, a third generation cephalosporin antibiotic, and trimethoprim–sulphonamide are indicated for the treatment of bacterial meningoencephalitis but field data are limited. The usefulness of florfenicol in the treatment of bacterial meningoencephalitis has not been reported but this molecule is sufficiently similar to chloramphenicol to justify its use and clinical evaluation in the treatment of bacterial meningoencephalitis in calves. Penicillin G (>44 000 iu/kg b.i.d.) is the treatment of choice for listeriosis and peripheral vestibular lesions, with the first treatment administered intravenously. Insufficient data are available to comment upon the efficacy of either corticosteroids or NSAIDs for the treatment of central nervous system bacterial infections.

Specific diseases

Cerebellar hypoplasia/hydranencephaly

The cerebellum is the most common CNS site for in-utero insult. The cerebellum is primarily concerned with fine coordination of voluntary movement. In cerebellar dysfunction, limb movements are spastic (rigid), clumsy and jerky. Initiation of movement is delayed and may be accompanied by intention tremors.

Aetiology

Cerebellar hypoplasia/hydranencephaly can be the result of an autosomal recessive condition or caused by in-utero infection with bovine virus diarrhoea/mucosal disease (BVD/MD; see p. 855) or Akabane virus.

Pathology

In-utero BVD/MD virus infection around 90 to 130 days' gestation causes cerebellar hypoplasia and, less commonly, hydranencephaly. The BVD/MD virus invades the fetus and infects the developing germinal cells of the cerebellum and destroys the Purkinje cells in the granular layer. Microphthalmia is uncommon.

Signs and diagnosis

Cerebellar disease is characterized by a wide-based stance and ataxia (incoordination), particularly of the pelvic limbs, but with preservation of normal muscle strength. In addition to the ataxia, dysmetria may be observed with hypermetria more commonly observed in cerebellar disease. Coarse intention head tremors are frequently observed, particularly during periods of excitement such as feeding times. Opisthotonus can occur in calves with severe lesions of the rostral cerebellum. Such calves present in lateral recumbency with rigid extension of the neck and thoracic limbs and flexion of the pelvic limbs with clinical signs noted soon after birth.

In addition to the cerebellar signs, calves with hydranencephaly exhibit blindness and depression/somnolence (dummies). In extensively-managed beef herds, calves with hydranencephaly may not be detected until the calf is several months old. Often the demeanour of such calves is attributed to another cause and such calves are not presented for veterinary examination. Cerebellar dysfunction in young calves may be the first manifestation of active BVD/MD infection in the herd and it is important that these clinical signs are identified so that control measures can be introduced to prevent further losses.

Treatment and prevention

There is no treatment for cerebellar hypoplasia and affected calves should be culled because they pose a risk to seronegative/unvaccinated breeding cattle in the herd. Biosecurity is an important aspect of herd health which is frequently overlooked on British farms and worldwide. Increasingly, more British dairy and beef herds will become self-contained with high health status, but in the meantime introduction of disease by carrier animals is a major concern. Depending upon the health status of the herd, purchased cattle should either be screened for BVD/MD antibody and antigen status upon arrival or vaccinated during the quarantine period. Establishment of a BVD/MD-free herd is presently included in numerous health schemes packages in Britain but is not without risk from introduction of infection with carrier-status cattle and from adjacent herds via direct contact, water courses, carrion, etc (Chapter 57).

Bacterial meningoencephalitis (see p. 251)

Bacterial meningoencephalitis most commonly affects calves 3 to 8 days old and is associated with poor immunoglobulin status and high bacterial challenge in the environment (Rings, 1987). The early clinical signs of lethargy, depression and failure to suck rapidly progress to hyperaesthesia, opisthotonus and death (Scott & Penny, 1993). Compulsive wandering and head pressing have also been reported (Jamison & Prescott, 1987) but are less common. The prognosis is poor despite intensive antibiotic treatment and supportive care.

Aetiology

Bacteraemia, with subsequent localization within the meninges, results from failure of passive antibody transfer (Jamison & Prescott, 1987) and high levels of bacterial challenge in the calf's environment. The disease is more common in those calves born indoors in unhygienic calving boxes than in those born of cows at pasture. Failure of the calf to ingest colostrum equivalent to 7 per cent of its bodyweight within the first six hours of life may be caused by calf and/or dam factors. Dystokia, weakness, nerve damage, overcrowded calving accommodation, udder shape, dirty teats and an overly-anxious dam may all contribute to poor/delayed sucking behaviour by the calf. Dystokia, nerve damage, hypocalcaemia and weakness may result in prolonged recumbency of the dam. Poor nutrition, short dry period and mastitis cause reduced colostrum accumulation in the udder. Heifers' colostrum contains 25 per cent less colostrum than cows' colostrum. Bacteraemia may result via the oropharyngeal route, respiratory tract, gastrointestinal tract or umbilicus. *Escherichia coli* and *Streptococcus* spp. were the more common isolates from lumbar CSF of calves with meningoencephalitis (Scott & Penny, 1993).

Pathology

Septic foci are prone to localize within meningeal vessels and are either rapidly walled off or may lead to diffuse suppurative meningitis. A combination of synovial, meningeal and intraocular localizations is almost invariably of streptococcal origin; coliform infections rarely cause endophthalmitis (Jubb & Huxtable, 1993). Once bacteria gain access to the leptomeninges there is little resistance to spread and the inflammatory process becomes diffuse.

In the first day or so the meninges are opaque and hyperaemic with pus accumulating in the basal cisterns within two days or so, although this may be difficult to visualize against the surface of the brain. Over the cerebral hemispheres the exudate is largely confined to the fissures. The brain is swollen in the acute stages of disease and may be so severe to cause displacement of the cerebellum into the foramen magnum and coning.

Signs and diagnosis

The early clinical signs include lack of suck reflex, depression, failure to follow the dam (beef calves) and weakness (Green & Smith, 1992; Scott & Penny, 1993). Fever is not a consistent feature. Affected calves stand with the neck extended and the head held lowered. Flexion of the neck is painful and may result in vocalization. In the absence of appropriate treatment the calf becomes increasingly weak over the next 6 to 12 hours with an altered gait, and may be unable to stand. Diligent stockmanship is important when checking young beef calves because the early clinical signs of lethargy and weakness can easily be overlooked, especially when the calves are lying together in a group during adverse weather conditions. Depression and poor appetite are more readily detected in individually-penned dairy calves. As the disease progresses there is lack of menace response and dorsomedial strabismus. Episcleral injection is often present at this stage. Depression progresses to stupor, but the calf is hyperaesthetic to auditory and tactile stimuli which may precipitate seizure activity during handling for intravenous antibiotic injection. Opisthotonus is observed during the agonal stages of disease approximately 24 to 36 hours after clinical signs are first noted. There may be evidence of infection involving other organ systems such as hypopyon, polyarthritis, diarrhoea and omphalophlebitis. Infarcts in the liver and kidney are frequently observed at necropsy. In a study of ten calves with meningoencephalitis, three calves had polyarthritis, three calves showed hypopyon and two calves had omphalophlebitis, but none exhibited diarrhoea (Scott & Penny, 1993).

The important differential diagnosis for bacterial meningoencephalitis is metabolic acidosis resulting from diarrhoea of 2 to 3 days' duration. Septicaemia presents with similar clinical findings to meningoencephalitis as the meninges are a common site for bacterial colonization in neonatal calves.

Lumbar CSF is readily collected under local anesthesia from depressed or stuporous calves. Calves with bacterial meningoencephalitis frequently have a CSF protein concentration above 1.0 g/l (deLahunta, 1983) and greater than 2.0 g/l (Green & Smith, 1992; Scott & Penny, 1993). The normal CSF protein concentration is <0.3 g/l with a white cell concentration less than 0.012×10^9/l. There is also a marked increase in CSF total white cell count in the order of 100-fold and a change in the predominant white cell type from lymphocyte to neutrophil (neutrophilic pleocytosis). These CSF changes cause increased turbidity of the sample which is visible upon gross CSF inspection and affords the veterinary surgeon an immediate diagnosis. One to two days' delay in detailed laboratory examination of the CSF would undoubtedly result in death of the calf if left untreated. However, routine antibiotic therapy of all diarrhoeic calves is not recommended because many antibiotics slow the mitotic rate of enterocytes, which is an important factor in recovery from viral causes of diarrhoea. Bacteriological culture of lumbar CSF is often unrewarding and is unnecessary because of the sporadic nature of the disease and its causation by opportunist organisms.

Treatment and prevention

A successful outcome necessitates early detection of abnormal calf behaviour by the client and prompt clinical diagnosis by the veterinary practitioner supported by visual inspection of lumbar CSF. Any delay in veterinary diagnosis and implementation of treatment has a hopeless prognosis, but prompt treatment with chloramphenicol achieved a 30 per cent recovery rate (Scott & Penny, 1993). Few broad-spectrum bacteriocidal antibiotics are capable of penetrating the intact blood–brain barrier, although it is commonly assumed that the disruption of the blood–brain barrier, which occurs in bacterial CNS diseases, increases the degree of antibiotic penetration. This increased membrane permeability may allow sufficient passage of antibiotics to achieve minimum bactericidal concentrations (MBC) within the CSF. A peak CSF antibiotic concentration 10 to 30 times the effective MBC may be more important than the maintenance of CSF antibiotic MBC (Prescott & Baggot, 1988) and emphasizes that high dose antibiotic therapy is indicated as soon as possible after the onset of clinical signs of bacterial CNS infection.

It is reported that the best treatment for Gram-negative bacillary meningitis in man is the third generation cephalosporins, in particular cefotaxime (Cherubin & Eng, 1986; Feldstein *et al.*, 1987) but no data could be found in the veterinary literature relating to the use of ceftiofur in the treatment of infectious bovine neurological diseases under field conditions.

Chloramphenicol is no longer permitted in food-producing animals in many countries; there are no field studies which report the clinical efficacy of its closely-related successor florfenicol. Other antibiotics which could be administered for bacterial meningoencephalitis include trimethoprim–sulphonamide combination or ceftiofur.

Septicaemia

Calves with septicaemia frequently present with clinical signs similar to bacterial meningoencephalitis because the meninges are simply one site for localization of blood-borne pathogens. The clinical course of septicaemia is generally peracute and affected calves may be found either dead or *in extremis* within 12 hours. Other sites of infection such as eyes (hypopyon), gut (diarrhoea), joints (polyarthritis) and umbilicus (omphalophlebitis) may be identified. Foci in the lung, kidney, liver and spleen are only detected following necropsy.

Enteric infections causing metabolic disturbances

Sequestration of water and electrolytes in the gut lumen, often without overt signs of diarrhoea, caused by the heat stable enterotoxin produced by K99 strains of *E. coli*, can result in recumbency in one to four day-old calves which often rapidly progresses to coma and death. Older calves with severe metabolic acidosis secondary to enteric viral infection, typically 6 to 14 days old, are weak, unable to stand and depressed with deterioration of mental state to stupor. It can prove difficult to undertake a thorough neurological examination, e.g. menace response and spinal reflexes, in such depressed or stuporous calves to differentiate such calves from early cases of bacterial meningoencephalitis. Collection of lumbar CSF on the farm reveals a normal clear sample which allows immediate differentiation from bacterial meningoencephalitis (Scott & Penny, 1993).

Treatment of acidotic calves with intravenous isotonic saline solution, spiked with 400–600 mEq of bicarbonate, is successful with a rapid improvement in demeanour and ability of the calf to stand within 6 to 12 hours.

Brain abscess

Neurological signs of a brain abscess typically appear in 4 to 12 week-old calves following localization of neonatal bacteraemia. Extension of infection through the calvarium following infection of the frontal sinus as a consequence of dehorning, while reported in the literature, is uncommon in Britain.

Aetiology

Arcanobacterium pyogenes is the most common isolate from brain abscesses.

Pathology and pathogenesis

Brain abscesses are usually of haematogenous origin. Most cerebral abscesses are small and track inward to the white matter rather than out to the meninges.

Signs and diagnosis

Affected calves are usually dull and depressed with a sluggish gait. These calves have a poor appetite and as a consequence appear ill thriven. Approximately 90 per cent of efferent nerve fibres cross at the optic chiasma; therefore animals with a left-sided cerebral abscess are blind in the right eye but the pupillary light reflex is normal. As the abscess continues to grow the animal becomes increasingly depressed, sometimes over many months. Ipsilateral compulsive circling may lead to the calf becoming stuck with its head in the corner of the pen or fence. Once in this position, the calf may stand motionless for long periods of time, sometimes hours. The gait is often sluggish and ataxic. There is ipsilateral deviation of the head towards the flank, but this altered head carriage must not be confused with a head tilt. The calf may display ipsilateral postural deficits such as knuckling of the fetlock joints. In most cattle there are no cranial nerve deficits. There is frequently an increased protein concentration and elevated white cell concentration in lumbar CSF, which reflect any accompanying suppurative meningitis.

Treatment and prevention

Treatment with high dose penicillin (minimum 44 000 iu/kg b.i.d.) for 10 days may halt progression of the abscess but the long term prognosis is very poor. Prevention of bacteraemia in neonatal calves necessitates ensuring adequate passive antibody transfer and reducing environmental bacterial challenge by maintaining good hygiene standards in the calving accommodation.

Cerebellar abiotrophy (postnatal degeneration)

Cerebellar abiotrophy is an inherited condition which has been reported in Holstein calves in the UK. The cerebellar abiotrophies are considered to be familial and degenerative but not congenital. Similar clinical signs have been reported in a six month-old Limousin cross heifer caused by selected cerebellar degeneration (Woodman *et al.*, 1993; see also pp. 178, 893).

Signs and diagnosis

Clinical signs of pelvic limb ataxia, especially when turning quickly, wide-base stance and hypermetria appear from around six weeks of age and are slowly progressive over many months, leading eventually to recumbency by one year of age. The preservation of strength and chronicity of the condition differentiates

this condition from cervical spinal lesions which often appear at around 6 to 12 weeks old.

Unilateral middle ear infections/vestibular syndrome (see also p. 252)

The vestibular system helps to orientate the animal in its environment with respect to gravity, and maintains position of the eyes, trunk and limbs during movement. Unilateral middle ear infections (otitis media) are not uncommon in growing calves and yearlings and usually arise from ascending infection of the eustachian tube, often following respiratory disease.

Signs and diagnosis

The major clinical sign in unilateral peripheral vestibular disease is an ipsilateral head tilt of 5° to 10° down to the affected side. There may be loss of balance, leaning and movement/circling toward the affected side. When walking, cattle tend to drift toward the affected side. During the early stages of unilateral peripheral vestibular lesions there is spontaneous horizontal nystagmus with the fast phase away from the side of the lesion. There is often ipsilateral ventral deviation of the eye (eye drop), which is exaggerated when the head is raised. The facial nerve travels close to the middle ear and facial palsy is often seen in conjunction with otitis media.

In central vestibular disease the nystagmus may be horizontal, vertical or rotary, and there may be ipsilateral limb weakness. Depression indicates involvement of the reticular formation.

It is important to differentiate vestibular lesions from listeriosis because of the different treatment regimens and control measures.

Treatment and prevention

The bacterial infection responds well to five to seven consecutive days' treatment with 44 000 iu/kg procaine penicillin s.i.d. The condition occurs sporadically and there are no specific control measures.

Polioencephalomalacia (cerebrocortical necrosis, CCN)
(see also p. 261)

This is a sporadic condition that affects young growing cattle. It is characterized clinically by dullness, bilateral lack of menace response, dorsomedial strabismus and hyperaesthesia to auditory and tactile stimuli, progressing over days to lateral recumbency and opisthotonus.

Aetiology

Healthy ruminants obtain their requirements from thiamine synthesized by the rumen flora. Free thiamine is readily absorbed and is actively phosphorylated to thiamine pyrophosphate (TPP). The brain is critically dependent on carbohydrate for energy and TPP has a coenzyme role in decarboxylation of α-ketoacids for entry into the tricarboxylic acid cycle. Thiamine pyrophosphate is also a coenzyme in the transketolase reaction of the hexose monophosphate shunt and the alternative, glycolytic, pentose phosphate pathway. Outbreaks of PEM have been described in cattle, and sheep (Low *et al.*, 1996), when fed diets high in sulphur.

Pathology

The brain usually appears pale and swollen with flattened gyri, which in the frontal, dorso-medial and parietal regions often show a patchy, bilaterally symmetrical, yellow discoloration. There is swelling of the cingulate and parahippocampal gyri, which may herniate beneath the tentorium cerebelli. The posterior vermis may have herniated through the foramen magnum and appear necrotic. The cut surface of the cerebrum reveals that the necrotic cortical tissues have a laminar configuration and may have separated from the underlying white matter. When viewed in ultraviolet light (wavelength 365 nm) affected regions of cortex have a bright white autofluorescence, which has been attributed to ceroid lipofuscin (Little, 1978).

Histologically, there is increased prominence of capillary endothelium (neovascularization) and dilatation of perivascular spaces with occasional small perivascular haemorrhages. Astrocytes and neurones show hydropic changes and nuclear pyknosis, which proceeds in time to a laminar necrosis. In well established cases there is a massive influx of macrophages into the necrotic areas and adjacent leptomeninges.

Signs and diagnosis

PEM occurs sporadically, affecting weaned calves and young feedlot cattle. It is associated with diets low in fibre, although cases have occurred in animals grazing lush aftermath. Under these circumstances, changes occur in the rumen flora that permit multiplication of micro-organisms such as *Bacillus thiaminolyticus* and *Clostridium sporogenes*, both of which synthesize thiaminase type 1, thereby inducing thiamine deficiency.

During the early stages of PEM there is frequently a brief period of diarrhoea before nervous signs appear. Affected animals are dull and may isolate themselves from others in the group. There is high head carriage and affected cattle may stagger. There is bilateral loss of menace response and dorsomedial strabismus. Affected animals are hyperaesthetic to tactile and auditory stimuli. As the disease progresses animals often head press into corners and there is frequent bruxism (teeth grinding). Twitching, muscular tremors and intermittent opisthotonus are evident, followed by recumbency and clonic convulsions with intermittent periods of spasticity and terminal flaccidity. Untreated cattle die within three to five days.

Diagnosis of PEM is based primarily on the history, clinical signs and response to intravenous thiamine administration. Laboratory tests are of equivocal value and response to treatment of early cases is commonly employed as a diagnostic indicator by practitioners.

Changes in lumbar CSF include a slightly increased protein concentration, but this result is of little diagnostic value.

Treatment and prevention

The response to large doses (10–15 mg/kg) of thiamine hydrochloride given intravenously early in the disease is usually evident within 24 hours. The thiamine should be repeated within 4 to 6 hours, then twice daily for three consecutive days. Full clinical recovery may take one week. Intravenous administration of dexamethasone (1.0 mg/kg) at first presentation may aid recovery.

Prevention of PEM involves the maintenance of normal rumen fermentation with adequate dietary fibre ensuring production of volatile fatty acids which curtail the growth of thiaminase-producing organisms. The efficacy of metaphylactic thiamine injections during an outbreak of dietary sulphur-induced PEM in cattle remains equivocal, although this did appear to halt appearance of new clinical cases in housed lambs (Low *et al.*, 1996).

Listerial encephalitis (see also p. 156)

Listerial encephalitis is the result of infection of the brain substance with *Listeria monocytogenes*.

Aetiology

Listeria monocytogenes is a microaerophilic Gram-positive, flagellated coccobacillus which is present in a wide range of moist environments and may cause disease in man and a variety of domestic species. Listeriosis occurs sporadically in cattle, where most cases are associated with feeding poorly fermented silage during the winter months. Cattle show a similar age incidence to sheep with the majority of cases affecting two to three year-olds, although cattle appear much less susceptible to listeriosis than sheep. Rarely are outbreaks of listeriosis encountered in cattle.

Pathology

The pathogenesis of listerial encephalitis involves centripetal passage of the organism along branches of the trigeminal nerve from minor breaches in the buccal mucosa. Intracranial pathology initially consists of a small focus of necrosis in the lateral part of the pons, which is associated with activation of microglial cells and astrocytes followed by an influx of monocytes and a few neutrophils. The initial focus may be unilateral but thereafter (intraneural) spread results in micro-abscesses forming bilaterally in the mid brain and lower medulla.

Signs and diagnosis

The rectal temperature of affected cattle is within the range 38.5 to 39.2°C. There is reduced appetite with a gaunt appearance, marked fall in milk production in lactating cattle and weight loss. Loss of saliva leads to rumen impaction, causing abdominal pain manifest as an arched-back stance and frequent bruxism.

As most of the cranial nerve nuclei are present within the brainstem, ascending infection of the trigeminal nerve by *L. monocytogenes* is characterized by multiple unilateral cranial nerve deficits, depression and, in some cases, circling to the affected side. Ipsilateral hemiparesis may also be present and should be differentiated from ataxia observed in cattle with BSE.

Involvement of the trigeminal nucleus results in paralysis of the cheek muscles and decreased facial skin sensation. Facial palsy is evident as drooped ear, drooped upper eyelid (ptosis) and flaccid lip. Occasionally, there may be paralysis and protrusion of the tongue. Exposure keratitis may result from paralysis of the *orbicularis oculi* muscle. Loss of cheek and lip muscle tone result in drooling of saliva from the affected side of the mouth. Depression is attributed to a lesion in the ascending reticular activating system. A head tilt toward the affected side is an inconsistent finding. Circling can be observed with involvement of the vestibulocochlear nucleus. Cattle frequently display a 'propulsive tendency' and may be found with the head forced through a gate, under a feed trough or wedged across the front of a cubicle. Indeed, dairy cows have barged through the milking parlour under the cows ahead of them causing chaos and often falling into the milking area; such behaviour in previously quiet cattle led to misdiagnosis of BSE. Caution must be exercised when cattle are found with the head trapped under a feed barrier, etc., because casual examination may attribute the facial palsy to trauma but this would not explain the unilateral loss of jaw tone and facial skin sensation.

Loss of cranial nerves IX, X and XII function results in stertorous breathing and dysphagia, but this presentation is uncommon in cattle with listeriosis. Hypoglossal nerve dysfunction leading to tongue paralysis and protrusion is more commonly observed in ovine listeriosis.

The course in untreated cattle lasts 10–14 days, progressing to coma.

A moderate increase in CSF protein concentration in the range 0.8 to 2.0 g/l is observed in meningo-encephalitis caused by *L. monocytogenes* (Rebhun & deLahunta, 1982).

Listeriosis is frequently associated with the feeding of silage and may be suspected on the basis of the clinical signs and supported by findings of an elevated CSF protein concentration and monocytic pleocytosis. Vestibular lesions (p. 896), lead poisoning (p. 944), brain abscess, BSE (p. 909) and nervous acetonaemia (p. 795) should be considered amongst the differential diagnosis.

Isolation of the causal organism from the brain may require extended periods of 'cold enrichment', but the neurohistopathology is usually sufficiently characteristic to permit firm diagnosis.

Treatment and prevention

Penicillin or trimethoprim-sulpha remain the antibiotics of choice for listeriosis. Oxytetracycline is not considered an appropriate antibiotic for listeriosis because of its large molecular size, although good results have been claimed. A minimum dose rate of 44 000 iu/kg procaine penicillin injected intramuscularly b.i.d. must be considered for at least 10 days in addition to 44 000 iu/kg penicillin G injected intravenously b.i.d. on the first day. Penicillin dose rates as high as 300 000 iu/kg have been recommended for the first day of antibiotic therapy because it is essential to exceed MICs by 10 to 30 times to achieve a successful outcome.

Loss of saliva may lead to dehydration and metabolic acidosis. Care must be taken when replacing fluids by orogastric tube because contraction of the rumen caused by anorexia of some days' duration may result in passive regurgitation of these fluids around the orogastric tube. The amount of fluids administered in this way should be restricted to 15 to 25 litres four to six times daily. Transfaunation with rumen liquor from a healthy cow may promote rumen function and aid recovery.

There are no published studies which have reported the efficacy of prophylactic antibiotic administration in the face of an outbreak of listeriosis, but such epidemiology is unusual in cattle.

Listeriosis occurs sporadically in cattle and is prevented by management practices which ensure the making and storage of high quality silage. Soil contamination is limited by rolling grass fields at the beginning of the growing season. Good fermentation is guaranteed by cutting grass at an early growth stage (digestibility value >72) when it contains a high fermentable sugar content, and the use of various silage additives, whether sugars, organic acids or bacterial cultures. Compaction of the silage clamp is important to expel all air followed by air-tight sealing to prevent aerobic bacterial multiplication. Poor quality or spoiled silage should be discarded. Prevention of listerial encephalitis by vaccination is not an established procedure in ruminant species.

Lead poisoning (see also p. 944)

Cattle, through their innate curiosity, indiscriminate feeding habits and relative susceptibility to lead, are the species most commonly poisoned by lead compounds. Lead poisoning in cattle is characterized by an acute encephalopathy.

Aetiology

The common sources of lead include discarded storage batteries, flaking old lead-based paint, putty, asphalt roofing materials and used motor engine oil. Intoxication may result from a single large dose of lead or from ingestion of smaller amounts over a long period of time. In both forms the neurological signs are acute in onset and similar in type.

Pathology

The severity of neuropathological change in lead poisoning correlates more closely with survival time than with the concentration of lead in the tissues, being most severe in cases that survive longest.

Grossly, the brain appears pale and slightly swollen with flattened gyri, but without herniation of the hippocampal gyrus beneath the tentorium or cerebellar coning (cf. PEM). Some gyri, most commonly those in the occipital region, show a yellow discoloration. The cut surface may show separation of these yellow zones of cortical tissue from the underlying white matter at the tips of the gyri with actual cavitation in the deeper cortical laminae. In cases of longer survival these changes may extend to the tips of almost all gyri and extend down the sides of the convolutions (Christian & Tryphonas, 1971).

Histologically, the earliest changes in affected gyri comprise swelling and prominence of capillary endothelial cells, which is sometimes referred to as neovascularization. Swelling of astrocytes, and fine microvacuolation of the neuropil, also occur at an early stage, advancing to spongy transformation with necrosis of neurones, malacia and infiltration by macrophages. In cattle with long survival periods these cortical lesions may be extensive, and similar lesions may be present also in the thalamus and hypothalamus, medulla and spinal cord.

Signs and diagnosis

Irrespective of the rate of uptake of lead, the clinical signs of intoxication are sudden in onset and characterized by behavioural changes. During the early stages of lead poisoning affected cattle become isolated and depressed. These animals are hyperaesthetic to tactile and auditory stimuli and may show muscle twitching, especially of the palpebral muscles. Affected cattle are blind and may head press forcibly into corners and against walls. The disease progresses and cattle become frenzied, bellow, stagger and crash into obstacles. There may be signs of abdominal pain including kicking at the abdomen and frequent bruxism (teeth grinding). Bloat is often seen and attempts to alleviate this problem often precipitate frenzy. Death may occur suddenly or within days.

The diagnosis of lead poisoning is suspected on the basis of clinical signs and the presence of a source of lead. Confirmation depends upon the histopathological findings and the chemical determination of the concentration of lead in tissues. In kidney and liver concentrations >4 ppm wet weight and blood values in excess of 0.3 ppm are considered diagnostic.

Treatment and prevention

Cattle with severe neurological signs of some days' duration probably have extensive neuropathological changes and are unlikely to respond to treatment. However, if a source can be identified, in-contact animals at risk from a single large dose may be drenched orally with magnesium sulphate (500–1000 g) to precipitate and remove lead from the alimentary tract and injected with calcium disodium edetate at 110 mg/kg by slow intravenous infusion on alternate days for three treatments. The similarity of the pathological changes to those of PEM has encouraged the use of thiamine (10–15 mg/kg intravenously) along with EDTA therapy and is reportedly beneficial. Control of convulsions proves very difficult because drugs such as diazepam have such a short half-life in cattle. Chloral hydrate sedation may be attempted but this drug is not licensed for use in cattle in Britain. Pentobarbitone is frequently used to control seizure activity in cattle with acute hypomagnesaemia and could be used in emergency situations for lead poisoning to control convulsive episodes.

Prevention is a matter of good management, not allowing access by cattle to sources of lead.

Thromboembolic meningoencephalitis (TEME) (see also p. 240)

Under conditions of stress or intercurrent disease a fulminating *Haemophilus somnus* bacteraemia may occur with disseminated intravascular coagulation. Thromboemboli may lodge in meninges, brain, muscles and joints causing depression, blindness and recumbency with muscular weakness. Retinal haemorrhages may be found.

Aetiology

Thromboembolic meningoencephalitis (TEME) is a fulminating *Haemophilus somnus* bacteraemia. TEME is a significant problem in feedlot cattle in North America associated with stresses of weaning, long journeys (often thousands of miles), co-mingling in auction markets and the feedlot, changes in diet, husbandry, altitude and nutrition, and processing on admission to the feedlot. Processing is a collective term used to describe a range of procedures undertaken on admission to the feedlot and may include castration, dehorning, anthelmintic treatment, ectoparasite treatment, vaccination against a wide range of viral and bacterial pathogens including parainfluenza 3 virus, bovine respiratory syncytial virus, infectious bovine rhinotracheitis, *Mannheimia haemolytica* and *Pasteurella multocida*, implantation with hormonal growth promoters and ear tagging. These procedures and stresses render the weaned beef calf susceptible to a wide range of respiratory tract and other infections. Infection with *H. somnus* probably occurs through the respiratory tract from asymptomatic carriers to non-infected cattle. Bacteraemia results in thrombosis in the brainstem, spinal cord, synovial membranes, pleurae and lungs. Outbreaks of TEME are often preceded by respiratory disease, which is all too common in large feedlots where morbidity rates may exceed 40 per cent despite prophylactic antibiotic administration during processing.

Signs and diagnosis

The neurological signs of TEME are sudden in onset and death may occur within 36 hours of onset. Affected cattle are pyrexic (40 to 42°C), anorexic and depressed. The depression may extend to somnolence and has led to the term 'sleeper calves'. Proprioceptive deficits are commonly observed and affected cattle appear ataxic. Cattle may be found recumbent in the pen with the head averted against the chest and are unable to raise themselves. Blindness, nystagmus and strabismus are variably present. Terminally, there is opisthotonus and coma. Lesions are also present in the lungs and auscul-

tation reveals widespread wheezes. Pleural friction rubs are described in some reports but significant pleurisy severely restricts movement of the underlying visceral pleura such that no sounds are generated by this localized pathology. Localization of bacteria within joints causes joint effusion and swelling with associated severe lameness which may result in recumbency. Retinal haemorrhages, hyphaema and hypopyon have also been described in some cattle following localization of the bacteraemia.

Treatment and prevention

Prompt detection of early neurological signs is important to ensure early antibiotic therapy; therefore cattle should be regularly inspected by trained stockmen during the high risk period following introduction of groups of cattle to the feedlot. *H. somnus* is susceptible to a wide range of antibiotics *in vitro* including oxytetracycline, penicillin and ampicillin; however, oxytetracycline does penetrate the blood–brain barrier well. Penicillin offers the most cost effective treatment at dose rates greater than 44 000 iu/kg b.i.d., which should be administered for at least five consecutive days.

Vaccination is not undertaken in Britain due to the sporadic nature of *H. somnus* infections where respiratory disease is the more common clinical presentation. Prophylactic injection with long-acting oxytetracycline and in-feed medication have been described in North American feedlot situations, but these are of doubtful use. Greater attention must be paid to the sourcing of feedlot cattle. Preconditioning including weaning, dehorning, castration, vaccination and introduction of concentrate feedstuffs must be undertaken at least three weeks before sale and transportation. Cattle sourced directly from ranches have a much lower incidence of respiratory disease than those from auction markets or sale barns. Unfortunately, such sensible husbandry practices will not be undertaken until a significant premium is paid for such calves. The use of prophylactic antibiotic administration on admission to feedlots in North America requires urgent review.

Aujeszky's disease

Aujeszky's disease is a herpes virus infection principally of pigs, which can be transmitted to most other mammalian species including cattle.

Aetiology

Infections in cattle are generally sporadic and result from contact with infected pigs, foodstuffs or other materials contaminated with virus. The disease in cattle is extremely severe with self-mutilation necessitating immediate slaughter for welfare reasons.

Pathogenesis and pathology

Infection in cattle is generally by the oronasal route. Centripetal intra-axonal transport of virus causes first a severe ganglioneuritis followed by meningoencephalitis or myelitis. Lesions are most severe in the olfactory lobe, hippocampus and cerebellum, whereas infection of a spinal peripheral nerve results initially in a segmental myelitis. Grey matter is principally affected with degenerative changes in nerve cells and astrocytes in which multiple, small, granular, eosinophilic, intranuclear inclusion bodies may be found. The inflammatory response is essentially non-suppurative and is characterized by lymphocytic perivascular cuffing and focal microgliosis.

Signs and diagnosis

The clinical course is short, rarely extending beyond 48 hours in adult cattle, whilst calves may die without obvious prior signs of illness. Usually, however, there is a brief period of excitement with high fever, bellowing, and aggressive behaviour accompanied by trembling, hyperpnoea, salivation and compulsive licking of the nostrils. Intense pruritus of the neck, trunk or hind legs is accompanied by frantic efforts to relieve the itch to the point of self-mutilation. Affected animals may become bloated and there is incoordination and, terminally, recumbency, convulsions and coma.

Except in calves, the clinical signs are usually distinctive enough for a provisional diagnosis of Aujeszky's disease to be reached. Confirmation is dependent upon demonstration of the characteristic neuropathology or virus isolation from nervous tissue.

Treatment and prevention

There is no effective treatment and affected cattle are killed immediately for welfare reasons. Prevention is dependent upon control of disease in the pig population. Attenuated and inactivated vaccines are available and are effective in preventing disease in pigs. However, they will not protect pigs from infection with field virus, which will replicate and be shed for some time after infection. Thus control in pigs must he through the establishment and maintenance of clean closed herds by serological testing and slaughter. This has been undertaken as a successful national campaign in Britain. The disease in cattle and sheep is notifiable in Britain and in some other countries.

Rabies (see Chapter 70)

Rabies is a neurotropic viral disease that can affect all warm-blooded animals. The virus is excreted in saliva and transmitted by the bite of an infected animal. It is manifested by irritability, mania, hydrophobia and paralysis. It is usually fatal, although recoveries have been documented.

Aetiology

The causal agent is a delicate rhabdovirus readily destroyed by disinfectants and desiccation. It causes pathological changes only in nervous tissue. Rabies occurs worldwide except in certain island territories (Australia and New Zealand) and a few countries from which it has been eradicated, such as the British Isles and Scandinavia. In the western hemisphere the infection is endemic in dogs, foxes, wolves, skunks, raccoons and bats of several species. Infection is transmitted with the bite of a rabid animal.

Pathology and pathogenesis

Cattle are very susceptible to rabies and become infected, usually on the hindquarters or limbs, from the bite of a rabid fox, dog or bat. Following local replication, virus travels centripetally in the axoplasm of a peripheral nerve to reach the spinal cord and thence to the brain. *En route* it replicates in neurones. From the brain, in the later stages of the incubation period, the virus passes centrifugally along nerves to the salivary and lachrimal glands and is present in their secretions. Rabies virus is highly neurotropic and viraemia is minimal or absent.

Signs and diagnosis

The incubation period of rabies in cattle varies from about two to three weeks to several months. Clinical signs classically occur in two distinct forms, the mild paralytic or dumb form and the furious form, depending upon the pathogenicity of the strain of virus. In paralytic rabies there may be partial loss of sensation in the hind legs, knuckling of the fetlocks, locomotor weakness and paralysis of the tail. Flaccid dilatation of the anus may be accompanied by straining and passage of air in and out of the rectum. Drooling of saliva and yawning are common features. The entire clinical course lasts about one week and is terminated by recumbency, generalized paralysis with death probably due to respiratory failure. In the furious form the animal is hyperaesthetic and sexually excited. It bellows hoarsely and becomes violently aggressive towards people, other animals and inanimate objects. Purposeful attacks, however, are frustrated by rapidly progressive incoordination and ataxia. Death occurs quickly following recumbency and paralysis.

Cattle are normally 'end hosts' with respect to rabies, although human infection may follow manual examination of the oral cavity in which virus in saliva is inoculated into scratches caused by teeth.

Clinical diagnosis of rabies is difficult, especially in those countries in which it rarely occurs. The possibility of rabies should be borne in mind in the differential diagnosis of bloat, nervous acetonaemia (p. 795), listerial encephalitis (p. 904) and bovine spongiform encephalopathy (see below). Rabid cattle invariably die and fluorescent antibody staining of impression smears from appropriate parts of the CNS will establish the diagnosis rapidly.

Treatment and prevention

No treatment of clinical cases should be attempted, nor should they be euthanased prematurely as this may prejudice the post-mortem diagnosis. Post-exposure vaccination is a routine procedure in man, but in cattle clinical disease and death would probably occur before an effective immunity had time to develop.

Bovine spongiform encephalopathy (BSE)

Bovine spongiform encephalopathy (BSE) was first reported in the United Kingdom in 1987 as a previously unrecognized spongiform encephalopathy affecting dairy cows (Wells *et al.*, 1987). While the first documented BSE cases were reported in 1987, retrospective case record studies suggest BSE occurred as early as 1985. Some cattle practitioners suggest that clinical cases occurred sporadically over the previous 25 years, but there is no supporting evidence in limited studies of archived pathology material.

Bovine spongiform encephalopathy is a new member of a group of subacute transmissible spongiform encephalopathies characterized by certain physical properties, including long incubation period but relatively short clinical course which is invariably fatal, progressive neurological signs with rapid deterioration terminally, spongiform change visible under light microscopy and presence of scrapie associated fibrils on electron microscopy. All members are transmissible to laboratory animals and many other species by intracerebral injection and other routes. This group includes scrapie of sheep and goats, chronic wasting disease of mule deer, transmissible mink encephalopathy of ranched mink, Kuru and Creutzfeldt–Jakob disease(CJD) of man and new variant Creutzfeldt–Jakob disease (v-CJD) of man.

The postulate that BSE resulted from the ingestion of meat and bone meal contaminated with a scrapie-like agent (Morgan, 1988) has been supported only indirectly by epidemiological data (Wilesmith *et al.*, 1988).

Some change in exposure of cattle to infection in 1981–82 resulted in BSE appearing in the cattle population in 1985–86. A change in rendering practices with an end to hydrocarbon fat extraction of rendered material (NB the scrapie agent is lipotrophic) has been suggested as an important factor in BSE epidemiology. Subsequent studies have demonstrated that operating procedures in many rendering plants during the early 1980s would have been incapable of destroying the BSE agent. To date there are no experimental data which demonstrate that scrapie can be transmitted to cattle by the oral route.

BSE was made a notifiable disease in the United Kingdom on 21 June 1988. Compulsory slaughter with destruction of carcass (incineration since 1991) with compensation was introduced on 8 August 1988. On 18 July 1988 the 'ruminant feed ban' was introduced which prohibited the feeding of ruminant-derived protein to ruminants. Brain, spinal cord, tonsil, thymus, spleen and intestine (specified bovine offals) of cattle over six months old were no longer permitted to be sold for human consumption. In September 1990, specified bovine offals were banned from all other animal feeds.

The introduction of a ban on the inclusion of ruminant-derived protein in cattle rations in July 1988 has resulted in a reduction in the incidence of BSE in younger cattle since 1991 (Wilesmith & Ryan, 1993) which continued throughout the 1990s and into the 2000s.

Aetiology

All the epidemiological evidence presently available strongly suggests that the geographically widespread incidents of BSE are not the result of cow-to-cow transmission but conform to the concept of a single source epidemic, with concentrate feedstuffs containing animal protein as the probable source. Many farms have experienced only one BSE case although many cattle were exposed to the same feed source. In some herds outbreaks have involved the majority of animals in a particular cohort (Winter *et al.*, 1989). It is possible that the transmissible agent was very unevenly distributed in the feed because, unlike sheep, host genotype appears to have little effect upon either susceptibility or the length of the incubation period.

An alternative postulate to the feeding of scrapie-contaminated diets as the origin of BSE is that of spontaneous prion mutation giving rise to histopathological changes and clinical disease of a spongiform encephalopathy of cattle (Scott *et al.*, 1995). The origin of the BSE epidemic could, therefore, have been the inclusion of infected material from 'spontaneous cases' of BSE subsequent to changes in the rendering process, and not contamination of cattle rations with the scrapie agent. The simultaneous widespread appearance of

BSE in the UK could be explained, in part, by the sale and movement of meat and bone meal concentrate derived from cattle. In this respect it is interesting to note that the origins of chronic wasting disease of mule deer and elk have not been determined. It is possible that a scrapie-like disease did occur in cattle from another species (not sheep) and until transmission studies demonstrate classical BSE in cattle after feeding scrapie-contaminated feedstuffs this lack of conclusive evidence remains a serious concern.

Reports of transmissible mink encephalopathy (TME) in ranched mink in Wisconsin, fed from 95 per cent downer or dead dairy cattle and a few horses (Marsh & Hartsough, 1985), raise the question whether an unrecognized spongiform encephalopathy also occurs sporadically in cattle in the USA. However, experimental exposure of mink to BSE produced an encephalopathy with minimal resemblance to TME (Robinson *et al.*, 1994). BSE has recently (2003) been confirmed in Canada. The worldwide sporadic occurrence of CJD, with no obvious reservoir of infection or mode of transmission except for iatrogenic cases, may support the postulate that spontaneous changes of the prion, eventually resulting in clinical disease, do occur. The existence of scrapie in many countries of the world with large sheep populations means that sporadic cases resulting from spontaneous changes in the prion would not be differentiated from those scrapie cases originating from horizontal or vertical transmission of the scrapie agent. In countries that are scrapie-free, such as New Zealand and Australia, 'spontaneous cases' of scrapie, occurring at approximately 0.1 per 100000, could easily be overlooked due to the extensive system of agriculture and unwillingness of sheep producers to employ veterinary services for single sheep. In this respect it is widely regarded that the majority of BSE cases have been overlooked in France and Germany for political as well as animal health reasons.

Experimental transmission of spongiform encephalopathy after intracerebral injection or oral dosing with brain homogenate derived from cattle with BSE has been confirmed in sheep and goats (Foster *et al.*, 1993) and by a combination of intravenous and intracerebral injection to cattle (Dawson *et al.*, 1990). Intracerebral injection of calves with strains of scrapie agent from five flocks in four states in the USA produced neurological signs, brain lesions and distribution of prion protein distinct from BSE (Cutlip *et al.*, 1994), but these differences could be explained, in part, by strain variation in scrapie and route of infection.

Pathology and pathogenesis

The pathological changes consist of bilaterally symmetrical degenerative changes affecting the neuropil and neurones of certain brain stem nuclei (Wells *et al.*, 1987). There is fine vacuolation of the ground substance whilst neurones and neurites develop one or more well-defined intracytoplasmic vacuoles, which may distend the cell body and processes. The nuclei principally involved are the dorsal nucleus of the vagus, the nucleus of the solitary tract, the reticular formation, the vestibular and spinal trigeminal nuclei and in the mid brain the red and oculomotor nuclei.

An additional pathological characteristic of the transmissible spongiform encephalopathies is the presence in extracts of brain prepared for electron microscopy of fibrils 100–500 nm in length that are known as scrapie associated fibrils (SAF).

Signs and diagnosis

Bovine spongiform encephalopathy affects cattle 2 to 13 years of age, with peak prevalence in the four to five year age group. Early epidemiological investigations (Winter *et al.*, 1989) revealed that affected cattle could have had access to feedstuffs containing ruminant-derived protein only during the first four months of life. The disease is less common in beef suckler herds because most replacement heifers are reared naturally with their dam and receive no concentrate feeding. Disease has been commonly reported in beef herds where replacement heifers were sourced from dairy herds, these cattle having received supplementary concentrates containing ruminant-derived protein during calfhood. In dairy cattle the incidence within breeds appears to be a reflection of population size, the majority of cases occurring in Friesian/Holstein cattle.

Early signs include chronic weight loss and decreased milk yield over four to six weeks (Aldridge *et al.*, 1988; Scott *et al.*, 1988a, 1989a). Affected cattle are often isolated from other cattle in the field. Cows stand with an arched (roached) back and a wide-based stance. There is frequent independent ear movement with the ears often directed backwards towards the poll. The abdomen appears drawn up with sunken sublumbar fossae consistent with reduced appetite. During the latter stages, affected cattle spend very little time ruminating. There is a profound change in attitude; affected cattle become anxious, apprehensive and hyperaesthetic to tactile, auditory and visual stimuli. When trotting there is marked pelvic limb hypermetria and ataxia, but normal muscle strength. When in a group, BSE cattle frequently push other cows along with vigorous head butting. Cows have considerable difficulty when encountering obstacles such as steps, ramps and narrow gateways and will frequently attempt to jump over low objects such as slurry scrapers and run through gateways, etc. As the condition progresses cattle frequently slip, especially when turning on wet concrete, have great difficulty raising themselves and excoriation of the carpi results (Scott *et al.*, 1995). When confined for veterinary examination, stimulation often provokes violent kicking (ballism) with the pelvic limbs and bellowing. Repetitive contractions of individual muscle groups (myoclonus) are frequently observed in the shoulder region, ventral neck and proximal regions of the pelvic limbs. There is rapid progression of clinical signs and cattle may become weak and recumbent within two to ten weeks of clinical signs first being detected.

Differential diagnoses include listeriosis, hypomagnesaemia, space occupying lesions, lead poisoning, organophosphorous poisoning, hepatoencephalopathy and rabies. In common with the other transmissible spongiform encephalopathies, there is no immune system response to infection; therefore routine biochemical investigations serve only to exclude other diseases from the differential diagnosis list. There is no intrathecal inflammatory response (Scott *et al.*, 1989b), which assists the clinician to exclude conventional infectious agents from the differential diagnoses (e.g. listeriosis). Confirmation of diagnosis depends upon a neuropathological examination.

Treatment and prevention

There is no effective treatment for BSE. Notification and elimination of affected animals have been in operation in the UK since 1988. The occurrence of approximately 1700 BSE cases per annum 12 years after the implementation of the ban on inclusion of ruminant-derived protein in ruminant rations suggests that vertical/maternal transmission of BSE does occur. A maternal effect resulting in an increased number of BSE cases in the progeny of affected cattle compared to controls was demonstrated (Wilesmith *et al.*, 1997), but the study design was flawed because the progeny were probably exposed to dietary BSE. While the control measures adopted for BSE control, and human safety, were closely modelled on data from scrapie research, regulatory authorities failed to take account of the possibility of vertical/maternal transmission and cull all progeny of confirmed cases. Such short-term monetary expediency has proved extremely costly. Offspring of affected cattle are now culled in the UK.

Idiopathic brainstem neuronal chromatolysis of cattle

Idiopathic brainstem neuronal chromatolysis of cattle has numerous clinical features similar to BSE (Jeffrey & Wilesmith, 1992) and 8 to 27 cattle with this condition have been mistakenly slaughtered annually (Jeffrey & Wilesmith, 1996). The consistent clinical signs include tremor, weight loss and ataxia, but the clinical presentation is claimed to be not dissimilar to BSE (Jeffrey & Wilesmith, 1996). The incidence of disease appears to be more common in beef suckler cows with a mean age of eight years old compared to four to five years old in BSE. The disease is more commonly reported in Scotland than England, despite approximately similar numbers of beef herds.

Brainstem chromatolysis and degeneration of brainstem neurons are found in all cases and are generally associated with a florid and severe lesion (Jeffrey & Wilesmith, 1996). Scrapie-associated fibrils have not been found in the brains of cattle with idiopathic brainstem neuronal chromatolysis nor is there evidence of disease specific PrP (prion protein).

The cause of this disease remains unknown but a toxic or metabolic insult has been suggested (Jeffrey & Wilesmith, 1996).

Sporadic bovine encephalomyelitis (SBE, Buss disease)

Sporadic bovine encephalomyelitis is a generalized inflammatory disorder of serous membranes, synoviae and vascular endothelium. It has no specific neurotropism, the neurological signs being a consequence of inflammation of the mesodermal elements in the CNS.

Aetiology

Sporadic bovine encephalomyelitis is a specific disease of cattle and buffalo caused by a strain of *Chlamydia psittaci*. The disease has been observed in the USA, Eastern Europe, the Middle East, Japan, Australia and South Africa.

Pathology and pathogenesis

The disease is usually fatal within four to five days. The gross post-mortem findings include a serofibrinous peritonitis, pleurisy and pericarditis. A serofibrinous exudate is also found over the surface of the brain, especially the cerebellum and medulla. Histological examination of the brain reveals a predominantly histiocytic and plasma cell infiltration of the meninges.

Signs and diagnosis

Calves less than six months old develop a staggering, stiff gait with circling and stumbling. Affected calves are dull and depressed and may exhibit muscle tremors. About 70 per cent of infected animals recover slowly. Clinical diagnosis of SBE may be confirmed by rising titres of group-specific chlamydial antibody in complement fixation or enzyme-linked immunosorbent assay (ELISA) tests in the live animal or by isolation of the organism from brain and lymph nodes.

Treatment and prevention

Successful therapy depends upon treatment early in the course of the disease using high dosages of tetracycline (50 mg/kg s.i.d.) for five to seven days.

Spinal cord lesions

Spinal cord lesions, whether focal or diffuse, are less common in cattle than sheep but present the veterinarian with a diagnostic challenge as they may result from a wide range of aetiologies including vertebral body abscess, extradural abscess, trauma, protozoan (encephalo-) myelitis and, in those countries where enzootic bovine leucosis virus is prevalent, neoplasia. Bacteraemia occurring during the neonatal period occasionally results in vertebral body abscess and extradural abscess formation causing clinical signs in two to four month-old calves. The neurological signs are frequently sudden in onset despite the chronic nature of the compressive spinal cord lesion.

Accurate localization of a focal spinal cord lesion is important to enable further investigation such as radiography; surgery is rarely, if ever, undertaken in ruminant species. Localization of the lesion(s) relies upon the assessment of simple spinal reflex arcs which indicate the presence of either upper or lower motor neuron signs in the affected limbs.

The simple spinal reflex arc comprises three neurons:

- The sensory neuron (stretch receptor in tendon)
- The internuncial neuron
- The lower motor neuron (contraction of limb muscle)

While the reflex motor response to sensory stimuli can occur without the input of higher centres, the higher motor centres exert control of voluntary movement via the upper motor neurons which synapse on the lower motor neuron. Flexor (withdrawal) reflexes can be determined by pinching the interdigital skin or applying pressure across the coronary band with resultant unconscious flexion and withdrawal of the stimulated limb. Recognition of pain indicates integrity of the spinal cord above the reflex arc. To determine tendon 'jerk' reflexes for the thoracic limb, the triceps tendon is tapped 2–5 cm proximal to its attachment onto the olecranon process. The normal response is extension of the elbow joint. The pelvic limb is gently supported in the mid femoral region and the middle patellar ligament lightly tapped. The normal reflex is extension of the stifle joint.

Lesions affecting the upper motor neurons result in conscious proprioceptive deficits evident as changes in flight of the foot and abnormal placement of the foot on the ground, resulting in stumbling and knuckling of the lower limb joints. Stimulation of the skin over the thoracic wall and flank with a blunt object produces a normal local response of muscle contraction (panniculus reflex). In the case of a spinal lesion the skin caudal to the affected area of the cord has a reduced (hypalgesic) response, with a possible increased (hyperaesthetic) response cranial to the spinal lesion.

The presence of a spinal lesion at the level of the reflex arc results in a lack of muscle contraction in response to stimulation. Denervation of the effector muscle results in flaccid paralysis with atony (lower motor neuron disease). A spinal lesion cranial to the reflex arc removes the normal controlling inputs from higher centres via the upper motor neurons and results in exaggerated responses and spastic paralysis (upper motor neuron disease).

Cervical spinal cord C_1–C_6

The pelvic limbs are more severely affected than the thoracic limbs. There is a range of muscle weakness progressing to complete paralysis. It is important to differentiate weakness from ataxia, which can be achieved by pulling sideways on the tail as the animal is walking. Weak animals can easily be pulled to the side, may stumble and fall over. Spinal reflexes are increased (upper motor neuron signs to all four limbs) but this aspect of the neurological examination may prove difficult in adult cattle which are not recumbent. Cervical pain may be evident as rigidity of the neck with resentment to forced movement of the head. Typically, the neck is extended and the head held lowered. With severe lesions the animal may be unable to maintain sternal recumbency but will make frequent attempts to raise itself from lateral recumbency.

Cervico-thoracic spinal cord C_6–T_2

Spinal cord lesions involving the brachial intumescence may result in equally severe deficits in both the thoracic and pelvic limbs. There is ataxia and weakness of all four limbs. Thoracic limb reflexes are reduced (lower motor neuron signs) with increased pelvic limb reflexes (upper motor neuron signs).

Thoraco-lumbar spinal cord T_2–L_3

Animals with a spinal cord lesion caudal to T_2, but cranial to L_3, have normal thoracic limb function but upper motor neuron signs affecting the pelvic limbs. Affected cattle frequently adopt a dog-sitting posture with normal thoracic limb function (Holmes *et al.*, 1989) but with the pelvic limbs extended alongside the abdomen. The dog-sitting position should immediately alert the clinician because ruminants raise themselves using their pelvic limbs before the thoracic limbs. The withdrawal and patellar reflexes are increased and there are conscious proprioceptive deficits and paresis of the pelvic limbs. The panniculus reflex may be useful when attempting to localize a thoracolumbar spinal lesion.

Lumbo-sacral spinal cord L_4–S_2

A lesion involving the sacral outflow results in lower motor neuron signs of the pelvic limbs with superficial sensation loss, paresis and reduced or absent reflexes.

Sacrococcygeal spinal cord: cauda equina syndrome

The cauda equina syndrome results from lesions involving the sacrococcygeal spinal cord and results in hypotonia, hypalgesia and reduced reflexes of the tail, anus and perineal region, bladder atony and dilation of the rectum.

Once a lesion has been localized to a specific section of the spinal cord a number of ancillary tests can be performed, including radiography and myelography, to define the lesion precisely. Before such examinations are undertaken, which are expensive and may require general anaesthesia to perform, considerable useful information can be obtained relatively easily and inexpensively following the collection and analysis of lumbar CSF.

Lumbar CSF collection and interpretation

A focal inflammatory lesion within the vertebral column involving the leptomeninges results in leakage of protein and some inflammatory cells into the CSF. If the lesion also causes spinal cord compression this will arrest the craniad flow of CSF and prevent equilibration of CSF protein concentration within the lateral ventricles. Such compression results in accumulation of protein within the CSF caudal to the lesion (Scott *et al.*, 1991). In practical terms, where there is a compressive spinal lesion cranial to L_5, collection of lumbar CSF will yield a sample with a marked increase in protein concentration relative to the cisternal sample which is usually normal (Scott & Will, 1991; Scott, 1992).

Typical aetiologies include extradural and vertebral body abscess formation in young calves from which *Salmonella dublin* and *Salmonella typhimurium* are frequently isolated, indicating previous bacteraemia. The isolation of *Arcanobacterium pyogenes* and *Staphylococcus* spp. from ovine vertebral body abscesses (Finley, 1975) has led to the treatment of such lesions with high doses rates of penicillin, but with no success (Scott *et al.*, 1991).

Treatment and prevention

Traumatic lesions in calves following dystokia, indicated by xanthochromic CSF collection, may improve within two weeks with good management and dedicated care with frequent turning of the calf. Treatment of extradural and vertebral body abscesses is hopeless (Scott *et al.*, 1991) and affected calves should be euthanased for welfare reasons.

Prevention of bacteraemia in neonatal calves dictates high hygiene standards in the calving accomodation and ensuring timely ingestion of adequate levels of good quality colostrum by the calf within the first six hours of life. Repeated dipping of the umbilical remnant in strong veterinary iodine BP during the first 12 hours will prevent omphalophlebitis. Control of salmonellosis in calves from endemically-infected herds can be attempted by prior vaccination of the dam and feeding stored colostrum during the first two weeks of life.

References and further reading

Aldridge, B.M., Scott, P.R., Clarke, M., Will, R. & McInnes, A. (1988) Bovine spongiform encephalopathy: clinical signs and extended neurological investigation. In *Proceedings of XV World Buiatrics Congress*, Palma da Majorca, October 1988, pp. 1531–4.

Ames, T.R. (1987) Neurologic disease caused by *Haemophilus somnus*. *Veterinary Clinics of North America*, **3**, 61–73.

Baird, J.D., Johnston, K.G. & Hartley, W.J. (1974) Spastic paresis in Friesian cattle. *Australian Veterinary Journal*, **50**, 239–49.

Barlow, R.M. (1980) Genetic cerebellar disorders in cattle. In *Animal Models of Neurological Disease* (ed. by R. Clifford & P. O'Behan), pp. 294–305. Pitman Medical Series, Tunbridge Wells.

Barlow, R.M. (1991) In *Diseases of Sheep* (ed. by W.B. Martin & I.D. Aitken), 2nd edn. Blackwell Scientific Publications, London.

Berry, P.H., Howell, J. McC., Cook, R.D., Richards, R.B. & Peet, R.L. (1980) Central nervous system changes in sheep and cattle affected with natural or experimental annual ryegrass toxicity. *Australian Veterinary Journal*, **56**, 402–403.

Braund, K.G. (1985) Localizing lesions using neurologic syndromes – 1: brain syndromes. *Veterinary Medicine*, **80**, 40–54.

Brayton, C.F. (1986) Dimethyl sulfoxide (DMSO): a review. *Cornell Veterinarian*, **76**, 61–90.

Buxton, D., Macleod, N.S.M. & Nicolson, T.B. (1981) Focal symmetrical encephalomalacia in young cattle. *Veterinary Record*, **108**, 459.

Cherubin, C.E. & Eng, R.H.K. (1986) Experience with the use of cefotaxime in the treatment of bacterial meningitis. *American of Journal of Medicine*, **80**, 398–404.

Christian, R.G. & Tryphonas, L. (1971) Lead poisoning in cattle; brain lesions and haematologic changes. *American Journal of Veterinary Research*, **32**, 203–16.

Crick, J. & Brown, F. (1976) Rabies vaccines for animals and man. *Veterinary Record*, **99**, 162–7.

Cutlip, R.C., Miller, J.M., Race, R.E., Jenny, A.L. & Katz, J.B. (1994) Experimental inoculation of cattle with US sources of scrapie. *Journal of the American Veterinary Medical Association*, **204**, 72.

Dawson, M., Wells, G.A.H. & Parker, B.N.J. (1990) Preliminary evidence of the experimental transmissibility of bovine spongiform encephalopathy to cattle. *Veterinary Record*, **126**, 112

Del Rio, M.A., Chrane, D. & Shelton, S. (1983) Ceftriaxone versus ampicillin and chloramphenicol for treatment of bacterial meningitis in children. *Lancet*, **1**, 1241–4.

Doherty, P.C. & Reid, H.W. (1971) Louping ill encephalitis in the sheep. 11. Distribution of virus and lesions in nervous tissue. *Journal of Comparative Pathology*, **81**, 531–6.

Donnelly, W.J.C., Sheahan, B.J. & Rogers, T.A. (1973) GM, gangliosidosis in Friesian calves. *Journal of Pathology and Bacteriology*, **111**, 173–9.

Edwin, E.E. (1970) Plasma enzyme and metabolite concentrations in cerebrocortical necrosis. *Veterinary Record*, **87**, 396–8.

Engel, D. (1970) *Populationsgenetische Untersuchungen zur Aetiologie der spastischen Parese beim Schwartzbunten Rind in Kurhessen.* Dissertation, Giessen.

Feldstein, T.J., Uden, D.L. & Larson, T.L. (1987) Cefotaxime for treatment of Gram-negative bacterial meningitis in infants and children. *Pediatrics Infectious Diseases Journal*, **6**, 471–5.

Field, A.C. & Suttle, N.F. (1979) Effect of high potassium and low magnesium intakes on the mineral metabolism of monozygotic twin cows. *Journal of Comparative Pathology*, **89**, 431–9.

Finley, G.G. (1975) A survey of vertebral abscesses in domestic animals in Ontario. *Canadian Veterinary Journal*, **16**, 114–17.

Fletcher, L.R. & Harvey, I.C. (1981) An association of a *Lolium* endophyte with ryegrass staggers. *New Zealand Veterinary Journal*, **29**, 185–6.

Foster, J.D., Hope, J. & Fraser, H. (1993) Transmission of bovine spongiform encephalopathy to sheep and goats. *Veterinary Record*, **133**, 339.

Gallagher, R.T., White, E.P. & Mortimer, P.H. (1981) Ryegrass staggers: isolation of potent neurotoxins lolitrem A and lolitrem B from staggers producing pastures. *New Zealand Veterinary Journal*, **29**, 189–90.

Geerken, C.M. & Figueroa, V. (1971) Cerebrocortical necrosis (molasses toxicity) in beef cattle: some preliminary biochemical parameters. *Revista Cubana de Cienca Agricala* (English edn), **5**, 205.

Green, S.L. & Smith, L.L. (1992) Meningitis in neonatal calves: 32 cases (1983–1990). *Journal of the American Veterinary Medical Association*, **201**, 125–8.

Grundlach, A.L., Dodd, P.R., Grabara, C.S.G., Watson, W.E.J., Johnston, G.A.R., Harper, P.A.W., Dennis, J.A. & Healy, P.J. (1988) Deficit of spinal cord glycine/strychnine receptor in inherited myoclonus of Poll Hereford calves. *Science*, **241**, 1807–10.

Hadlow, W.J., Kennedy, R.C. & Race, R.E. (1982) Natural infection of Suffolk sheep with scrapie virus. *Journal of Infectious Diseases*, **146**, 657–64.

Haig, D.A. (1955) Tick-borne rickettsioses in South Africa. *Advances in Veterinary Science*, **2**, 307–25.

Hansen, K.M., Krogh, H.V., Moller, J.E. & Elleby, F. (1988) The recumbent calf syndrome in the Red Danish milk breed a new hereditary disease. *Dansk Veterinaertidsskrift*, **71**, 128–32.

Harper, P.A.W., Healy, P.J. & Dennis, J.A. (1986) Inherited congenital myoclonus of polled Hereford calves (so-called neuraxial oedema): a clinical, pathological and biochemical study. *Veterinary Record*, **119**, 59–62.

Healy, P.J., Harper, P.A.W. & Dennis, J.A. (1986) Diagnosis of neuraxial oedema. *Australian Veterinary Journal*, **63**, 95.

High, J.W., Kincaid, C.M. & Smith, J.H. (1958) Doddler calves: an inherited disorder of Hereford cattle. *Journal of Heredity*, **49**, 250–2.

Hocking, J.D., Jolly, R.D. & Bait, R.D. (1972) Deficiency of mannosidase in Angus cattle: an inherited lysosomal storage disease. *Biochemical Journal*, **128**, 69–75.

Holmes, L.A., Scott, P.R. & Aldridge, B.M. (1989) Thymic lymphosarcoma with metastases causing spinal cord depression and pelvic limb paresis in a heifer. *British Veterinary Journal*, **146**, 91–2.

Hulland, T.J. (1957) Cerebellar ataxia in calves. *Canadian Journal of Comparative Medicine*, **21**, 72–6.

Humphreys, D.J. (1988) *Veterinary Toxicology*, 3rd edn, p. 8. Baillière Tindall, London.

Inaba, Y., Kurogi, H. & Omori, T. (1975) Akabane disease: epizootic abortion, premature birth, stillbirth, and congenital arthrogryposis-hydranencephaly in cattle, sheep and goats caused by Akabane virus. *Australian Veterinary Journal*, **51**, 584–5.

Innes, J.R.M., Russell, D.S. & Wilsden, A.J. (1940) Familial cerebellar hypoplasia and degeneration in Hereford calves. *Journal of Pathology and Bacteriology*, **50**, 455–61.

Isler, C.M., Bellamy, J.E.C. & Wobeser, G.A. (1987) A neurotoxin in serum of calves with 'nervous' coccidiosis. *Canadian Journal of Veterinary Research*, **51**, 253–60.

Jamison, J.M. & Prescott, J.F. (1987) Bacterial meningitis in large animals. 1. *Compendium of Continuing Education*, **9**, 399–406.

Jeffrey, M. (1992) A neuropathological survey of brains submitted under the Bovine Spongiform Encephalopathy Orders in Scotland. *Veterinary Record*, **131**, 332–6.

Jeffrey, M. & Wilesmith, J.W. (1992) Idiopathic brainstem neuronal chromatolysis and hippocampal sclerosis: a novel encephalopathy in clinically suspect cases of BSE. *Veterinary Record*, **131**, 359–63

Jeffrey, M. & Wilesmith, J.W. (1996) Idiopathic brainstem neuronal chromatolysis of cattle: a disorder with clinical similarity to BSE. *Veterinary Record*, **139**, 398.

Jubb, K.V.F. & Huxtable, C.R. (1993) In *Pathology of Domestic Animals* (ed. by K.V.F. Jubb, P.C. Palmer, & C.R. Huxtable), 4th edn, Vol. 1, p. 385. Academic Press, San Diego.

Kimberlin, R.H. (1982) Scrapie agent: prions or virinos. *Nature*, **297**, 107–108.

deLahunta, A. (1983) *Veterinary Neuroantaomy and Clinical Neurology*, 2nd edn. W.B. Saunders, Philadelphia.

Lambert H.P. & Wall R.A. (1991) Meningococcal meningitis: treatment. In *Infections of the Central Nervous System* (ed. by H.P. Lambert), p. 92. Edward Arnold, London.

Landesman, S.H., Corrado, M.L. & Shah, P.M. (1981) Past and current roles for cephalosporin antibiotics in treatment of meningitis. Emphasis on use in Gram-negative bacillary meningitis. *American Journal of Medicine*, **71**, 693–703.

Little, P.B. (1978) Identity of fluorescence in polioencephalomalacia. *Veterinary Record*, **103**, 76.

Low, J.C., Scott, P.R., Howie, F., Lewis, M., FitzSimons, J. & Spence, J.A. (1996) Sulphur-induced polioencephalomalacia in lambs. *Veterinary Record*, **138**, 327–9.

McCracken, R.M. & Dew, C. (1973) An electron microscopic study of Aujeszky's disease. *Acta Neuropathologica*, **25**, 207–19.

McGuirk, S.M. (1987) Polioencephalomalacia. In *Bovine Neurological Disease* (ed. by J.C. Baker). *The Veterinary Clinics of North America*, **3**, 107–18.

Marsh, R.F. & Hartsough, G.R. (1985) Is there a scrapie-like disease in cattle? In *Proceedings of the 7th Annual Western Conference Food Animal Veterinary Research*, University of Arizona, p. 20.

Menges, R.W., Harshfield, G.S. & Wenner, H.A. (1953a) Sporadic bovine encephalomyelitis. I. The natural history of the disease. *American Journal of Hygiene*, **57**, 1–14.

Menges, R.W., Harshfield, G.S. & Wenner, H.A. (1953b) Sporadic bovine encephalomyelitis. II. Studies on the pathogenesis and etiology of the disease. *Journal of the American Veterinary Medical Association*, **122**, 249–94.

Merz, P.A., Somerville, R.A., Wisniewski, H.M. & Iqbal, K. (1981) Abnormal fibrils from scrapie infected brain. *Acta Neuropathologica*, **54**, 63–74.

Moellering, R.C. & Fisher, E.G. (1972) Relationship of intraventricular gentamicin levels to cure of meningitis. *Journal of Pediatrics*, **81**, 534.

Morgan, K.L. (1988) Bovine spongiform encephalopathy: time to take scrapie seriously. *Veterinary Record*, **122**, 445–6.

Morgan, K.L. (1992) Cerebellar ataxia and head tremor in an Alpaca. *Veterinary Record*, **131**, 216–17.

Morgan, K.T. (1973) An ultrastructural study of ovine polioencephalomalacia. *Journal of Pathology*, **110**, 123–30.

Oldendorf, W.H. (1975) Permeability of the blood–brain barrier. In *The Nervous System* (ed. by D.B. Tower), Vol. 1, pp. 279–89. Raven Press, New York.

O'Toole, D. & Jeffrey, M. (1987) Congenital sporozoan encephalomyelitis in a calf. *Veterinary Record*, **121**, 563–6.

Padgett, G.A. (1968) The Chediak–Higashi syndrome. *Advances in Veterinary Science*, **12**, 239–84.

Palmer, A.C., Blakemore, W.F., Barlow, R.M., Fraser, J.A. & Ogden, A.C. (1972) Progressive ataxia of Charolais cattle associated with a myelin disorder. *Veterinary Record*, **91**, 592–4.

Pienaar, J.G. (1970) Electron microscopy of *Cowdria (Rickettsia) ruminantium* (Cowdry 1926) in the endothelial cells of the vertebrate host. *Onderstepoort Journal of Veterinary Research*, **37**, 67–78.

Power, E.P., Crowley, J.J., Byrne, J.F., O'Keefe, M.P. & Weavers, E.D. (1985) Cerebrocortical necrosis in dairy cows. *Irish Veterinary Journal*, **39**, 81–3.

Prescott J.F. & Baggot, J.D. (1988) *Antimicrobial Therapy in Veterinary Medicine*, p. 71. Blackwell Scientific Publications, Boston, Massachusetts.

Quagliarello, V.J., Long, W.J. & Scheld, W.M. (1986) Morphologic alterations of the blood–brain barrier with experimental meningitis in the rat. Temporal sequence and role of encapsulation. *Journal of Clinical Investigation*, **77**, 1084–95.

Read, W.K. & Bridges, C.H. (1969) Neuronal lipodystrophy occurrence in an inbred strain of cattle. *Veterinary Pathology*, **6**, 235–43.

Rebhun, W.C. & deLaHunta, A. (1982) Diagnosis and treatment of bovine listeriosis. *Journal of the American Veterinary Medical Association*, **180**, 395–8.

Reid, H.W., Buxton, D., Pew, I. & Finlayson, J. (1984) Transmission of louping ill virus in goat milk. *Veterinary Record*, **114**, 163–5.

Richards, R.B., Edwards, J.R., Cook, R.D. & White, R. (1977) Bovine generalised glycogenosis (type II). *Neuropathology and Applied Neurobiology*, **3**, 45–56.

Rings, D.M. (1987) Bacterial meningitis and diseases caused by bacterial toxins. In *Bovine Neurological Disease* (ed. by J.C. Baker), *The Veterinary Clinics of North America*, **3**, 85–98.

Robinson, M.M., Hadlow, W.J., Huff, T.P. *et al.* (1994) Experimental infection of mink with bovine spongiform encephalopathy. *Journal of General Virology*, **75**, 2151–5.

Sande M.A. (1981) Antibiotic therapy of bacterial meningitis: lessons we've learned. *American Journal of Medicine*, **71**, 507–10.

Sarasola, P. & McKellar, Q.A. (1992) Effect of probenecid on disposition kinetics of ampicillin in horses. *Veterinary Record*, **131**, 173–5.

Saunders, L.Z., Sweet, J.D., Martin, S.M., Fox, F.H. & Fincher, M.G. (1952) Hereditary congenital ataxia in Jersey calves. *Cornell Veterinarian*, **42**, 559–91.

Scheld, W.M. & Brodeur, J.P. (1983) Effect of methylprednisolone on entry of ampicillin and gentamicin into cerebrospinal fluid in experimental pneumococcal and *Escherichia coli* meningitis. *Antimicrobial Agents and Chemotherapy*, **23**, 108–12.

Scott, P.R. (1992) Cerebrospinal fluid collection and analysis in some common ovine neurological conditions. *British Veterinary Journal*, **148**, 15–22.

Scott, P.R. (1993a) A field study of ovine listerial meningoencephalitis with particular reference to cerebrospinal fluid analysis as an aid to diagnosis and prognosis. *British Veterinary Journal*, **149**, 165–70.

Scott, P.R. (1993b) Cerebrospinal fluid collection in ruminant neurological disease. *In Practice*, **15**, 298–300.

Scott, P.R. (1993c) Total protein and electrophoretic pattern of cerebrospinal fluid from sheep with some common ovine neurological disorders. *The Cornell Veterinarian*, **83**, 199–204.

Scott, P.R. (1994) Practical application of cerebrospinal fluid analysis in the differential diagnosis of spinal cord lesions in ruminants. *In Practice*, **16**, 301–303.

Scott, P.R. (1995a) The collection and analysis of cerebrospinal fluid as an aid to diagnosis in ruminant neurological disease. *British Veterinary Journal*, **151**, 603–14.

Scott, P.R. (1995b) Differential diagnosis of recumbency in neonatal calves. *In Practice*, **17**, 162–5.

Scott, P.R. (1996) Indications for lumbosacral cerebrospinal fluid sampling in ruminant species in field situations. *Agri-Practice*, **17**, 30–4.

Scott, P.R., Aldridge, B.M., Clarke, M., Will, R. & McInnes, A. (1988b) Bovine spongiform encephalopathy: electroencephalographic studies. In *Proceedings of the XV World Buiatrics Congress*, Palma da Majorca, October 1988, p. 1530.

Scott, P.R., Aldridge, B.M., Clarke, M. & Will, R.G. (1989b) Cerebrospinal fluid studies in normal cows and cases of Bovine Spongiform Encephalopathy. *British Veterinary Journal*, **146**, 88–90.

Scott, P.R., Aldridge, B.M., Clarke, M. & Will, R.G. (1989a) Bovine spongiform encephalopathy in a British Friesian cow. *Journal of the American Veterinary Medical Association*, **195**, 1745–7.

Scott, P.R., Aldridge, B.M., Holmes, L.A., Milne, E.M. & Collins, D.M. (1988a) Bovine spongiform encephalopathy in an adult British Friesian cow. *Veterinary Record*, **123**, 373–4.

Scott, P.R., Henshaw, C.J. & Watt, N.J. (1994b) Cerebellar abiotrophy in a pedigree Charolais ram lamb. *Veterinary Record*, **135**, 42–3.

Scott, P.R., Murray, L.M. & Penny, C.D. (1991) A field study of eight ovine vertebral body abscess cases. *New Zealand Veterinary Journal*, **39**, 105–107.

Scott, P.R. & Penny C.D. (1993) A field study of meningo-encephalitis in calves with particular reference to cerebrospinal fluid analysis. *Veterinary Record*, **133**, 119–21.

Scott, P.R., Penny, C.D. & Sargison, N.D. (1995) Bovine spongiform encephalopathy in a Holstein cow born in the United Kingdom during September 1989. *Canadian Veterinary Journal*, **36**, 310–11.

Scott, P.R., Pyrah, I., Penny, C.D. & Clarke, C.J. (1993b) Post septicaemia focal meningitis causing cerebellar dysfunction in an adult ram. *Veterinary Record*, **133**, 623–4.

Scott, P.R., Sargison, N.D., Penny, C.D. & Pirie, R.S. (1994a) A field study of naturally-occurring ovine bacterial meningo-encephalitis. *Veterinary Record*, **135**, 154–6.

Scott, P.R. & Sutton, D. (1992) A study of some factors which may influence the concentrations of penicillin G in cerebrospinal fluid in some common ovine neurological diseases. In *Proceedings of the XVII World Buiatrics Congress*, St Paul, USA, Vol. 2, pp. 63–8.

Scott, P.R. & Will, R.G. (1991) Froin's syndrome in five cases of ovine epidural abscess. *British Veterinary Journal*, **147**, 582–4.

Scott, P.R., Woodman, M.P., Watt, N.J., McGorum, B.M. & McDiarmid, A. (1993a) Protozoan encephalo-myelitis as a cause of pelvic limb paresis in a Blackface yearling sheep. *New Zealand Veterinary Journal*, **41**, 139–41.

Stolzenberg, V. & Schonmuth, G. (1971) Experimentelle Untersuchungen uber die okonomischen Auswirkungen und die Vererbung der spastischen Parese der Hintergliedmassen. *Wissenschaft zür Humboldt Universität, Berlin*, **20**, 353–70.

Stone, J.W. & Wise, R. (1991) Penetration of antimicrobial agents into the central nervous system. In *Infections of the Central Nervous System* (ed. by H.P. Lambert), p. 40. B.C. Decker, Philadephia.

Stuart, L.D. & Leipold, H.W. (1985) Lesions in bovine progressive degenerative myeloencephalopathy. *Veterinary Pathology*, **22**, 13–23.

Sullivan, N.D. (1985) Cytopathology of the nervous system. In *Pathology of Domestic Animals,* 3rd edn (ed. by K.V.F. Jubb, P.C. Kennedy & N. Paimer), Vol. 1, p. 225. Academic Press, New York.

Tauber, M.G., Shibl, A.M., Hackbarth, C.J., Larrick, J.W. & Sande, M.A. (1987) Antibiotic therapy, endotoxin concentration in cerebrospinal fluid and brain edema in experimental *Escherichia coli* meningitis in rabbits. *Journal of Infectious Diseases*, **156**, 456–62.

Trautwein, G., Hewicker, M., Liess, B., Orban, S. & Peters, W. (1987) Cerebellar hypoplasia and hydranencephaly in cattle associated with transplacental BVD virus infection. In *Pestivirus Infections of Ruminants* (ed. by J.W. Harkness), pp. 169–78. Commission of European Communities, Luxembourg.

Tuazon, C.U., Shamsuddin, D. & Miller, H. (1982) Antibiotic susceptibility and synergy of clinical isolates of *Listeria monocytogenes. Antimicrobial Agents and Chemotherapy*, **21**, 525–7.

Tunkel, A.R., Wispelway, B. & Scheld, W.M. (1990) Bacterial meningitis: recent advances in pathophysiology and treatment. *Annals of Internal Medicine*, **112**, 610–23.

Tyrrell, D.A.J. (1979) Aspects of slow and persistent virus infections. In *New Perspectives in Clinical Microbiology*, Vol. 2, p. 286. Martinus Nijhoff, The Hague.

Wells, G.A.H., Scott, A.C., Johnson, C.T., Gunning, R.F., Hancock, R.D., Jeffrey, M., Dawson, M. & Bradley, R. (1987) A novel progressive spongiform encephalopathy in cattle. *Veterinary Record*, **121**, 419–20.

White, M., Whitlock, R.H. & deLahunta, A. (1975) A cerebellar abiotrophy of calves. *Cornell Veterinarian*, **65**, 476–91.

Wilesmith, J.W. & Ryan, J.B.M (1993) Bovine spongiform encephalopathy: observation on the incidence during 1992. *Veterinary Record*, **132**, 300–301.

Wilesmith, J.W., Wells, G.A.H., Cranwell, M.P. & Ryan, J.B.M. (1988) Bovine spongiform encephalopathy: epidemiological studies. *Veterinary Record*, **123**, 638–44.

Wilesmith, J.W., Wells, G.A.H., Ryan, J.B.M. *et al.* (1997) A cohort study to examine maternally-associated risk factors for bovine spongiform encephalopathy. *Veterinary Record*, **141**, 239–43.

Winter, M.H., Aldridge, B.M., Scott, P.R. & Clarke, M. (1989) Occurrence of 14 cases of bovine spongiform encephalopathy in a closed dairy herd. *British Veterinary Journal*, **145**, 191–4.

Woodman, M.P., Scott, P.R., Watt, N.J., McGorum, B.M & Penny, C.D. (1993) Selective cerebellar degeneration in a Limousin cross heifer. *Veterinary Record*, **132**, 586.

Chapter 52
Ocular Diseases

P.G.C. Bedford

Introduction	917
Anomalies of the orbit and globe	917
Anophthalmia	917
Microphthalmia	918
Multiocular defects	918
Cyclopia	918
Strabismus	918
Nystagmus	918
Orbital neoplasia	918
Anomalies of the eyelids	918
Congenital/paranatal defects	918
Trauma	918
Congenital porphyria	919
Diseases of the conjunctiva and cornea	919
Epibulbar dermoid	919
Infectious bovine keratoconjunctivitis (IBKC)	919
Infectious bovine rhinotracheitis	921
Endothelial dystrophy	922
Neoplasia	922
Diseases of the uveal tract	923
Congenital anomalies	923
Uveitis	923
Neoplasia	923
Disease of the lens	923
Diseases of the retina and optic nerve	924
Congenital defects	924
Inflammation	924
Hypovitaminosis A	925
Male fern optic neuropathy	925
Arthrogryposis	925
Progressive retinal degeneration	925
Glaucoma	925

Introduction

Ophthalmic disorders in cattle are more common than is generally believed, but it is only those that are of considerable economic importance that generally receive much attention. Infectious bovine keratoconjunctivitis (IBKC), variously known throughout the world as New Forest disease, pinkeye, contagious ophthalmia and blight, is undoubtedly the commonest and most important ocular disease that occurs in this species. In the USA alone it is estimated that IBKC is responsible for an annual loss in excess of £25 million (Punch & Slatter, 1984). Approximately three times as many calves are

affected as adults and failure to produce effective vaccines means that this disease will continue to inflict severe economic loss for as long as young cattle are managed intensively. Disease of epidemic proportions occurs all the year round and, while the aetiological controversy may continue, the term IBKC generally embraces all keratoconjunctivitis of infectious nature in this species. Similarly, ocular squamous cell carcinoma of probable heritable nature in breeds with reduced palpebral pigmentation continues to account for a high carcase condemnation rate and runs second only to lymphosarcoma in terms of condemnation for neoplastic reasons. At the other end of the scale there are many congenital, inherited and acquired defects that tend to escape diagnosis on the basis of there being no untoward effect on function, no associated discomfort or pain and no necessity to treat. Were cattle subjected to the same degree of scrutiny as the dog, then it is likely that the literature would indicate a similar incidence of disease. In one study of 500 cattle of all ages, almost 20 per cent overall demonstrated ocular anomalies of one sort or another, the incidence ranging from 3 per cent in young cattle to in excess of 70 per cent in the older individuals (Amman, 1968). Examples of this kind of survey work in cattle are few and far between, but general interest in ophthalmology as a refined discipline in today's veterinary scenario will probably stimulate further ophthalmic studies in animals that are primarily produced for food purposes in our society.

Anomalies of the orbit and globe

Congenital and acquired defects of these structures both occur, some congenital anomalies being inherited while others are probably environmental in origin (see also p. 180). The acquired defects are due to trauma, infection and neoplasia.

Anophthalmia

Absence of the optic vesicle means that an eye cannot develop. Histologically, primordial ectodermal and mesodermal tissues cannot be identified. The condition is rare and is often confused with the type of microph-thalmia in which there has been some early differen-tiation of the optic vesicle but no subsequent maturation.

Microphthalmia

Variable degrees of development can be seen, ranging from minimal differentiation of ocular tissue to the development of a small but otherwise normal eye. Other ocular anomalies may also be present, however, and persistent pupillary membrane (PPM), aniridia, cataract and neuroretinal fold and rosette formation may be seen in association with microphthalmos. Like anophthalmia, the condition is rare in cattle, but inher-itance has been postulated (Gilmore, 1957) and it has been described in calves with vertebral column defor-mation (Leipold & Huston, 1968).

Multiocular defects

Bilateral congenital blindness due to multiocular defects not involving microphthalmos has been recorded in Jersey calves (Saunders & Fincher, 1951). The defects are mainly related to the lens, with microphalmia, ectopia lentis and cataract being seen in association with iridaemia. A recessive mode of inheritance has been suggested, but subsequent literature contains no further references to this condition in this breed.

Cyclopia

The development of one eye in calves is extremely rare (Plate 52.1), but the condition has been induced teratogenically in sheep.

Strabismus (see p. 181)

Bilateral convergent squint (esotropia) has been described as a recessively inherited defect in Jersey cattle, and it is probably inherited in Shorthorn and Friesian cattle too (Willoughby, 1968; Bedford, pers. obs.). A degree of exophthalmos may or may not be additionally present. The condition is usually noticed at four to eight weeks of age (Plate 52.2a) and the degree of convergence increases until the sixth or seventh month when only sclera presents within the palpebral fissure (Plate 52.2b). Impaired vision gives way to total blindness, and attempts at corrective surgery may be ill perceived in the presence of possible optic nerve, central visual pathway and visual cortex anomalies.

Nystagmus

Nystagmoid movement of the globe is most commonly associated with congenital or paranatal blindness. It is

also seen in adult cattle, with various causes including brain tumour and abscess formation. It has been noted as an occasional feature early in the course of BSE.

Orbital neoplasia

Retrobulbar and periorbital lymphosarcoma can result in exophthalmos and possible squint. The lesions may be seen unilaterally or bilaterally. Squamous cell carci-noma of the membrana nictitans may invade the orbital tissues to produce a similar clinical picture.

Anomalies of the eyelids

Congenital/paranatal defects

Unlike other species, inherited and non-inherited con-genital palpebral defects are few and far between in cattle. Eyelid colombomata and agenesis are of rare incidence. Although primary conditions in sheep, both entropion and ectropion occur most commonly as secondary defects in cattle and are associated with microphthalmia, blepharitis, keratoconjunctivitis and trauma. Correction of the cause alleviates the lid dis-tortion except where there is palpebral or orbicularis oculi damage and where cicatrization has occurred.

Congenital supernumerary openings of the proximal part of the nasolacrimal duct and the canaliculi at the medial canthus have been described in calves, heredi-tary predisposition or intra-uterine dacryocystitis being the suggested possible aetiology.

Trauma

Laceration of the eyelid occurs infrequently, but when the palpebral fissure is involved repair is essential. Such wounds left to granulate or inadequately sutured may result in distortion of the margo-intermarginalis, and secondary entropion, secondary ectropion and an incomplete blink can result in conjunctival or corneal disease. Delayed closure is complicated by the problem of wound contraction. Repair is easily effected using manual restraint and the same seventh nerve block as that used in disbudding and dehorning can be employed should blepharospasm be a problem. Such wounds may require debridement, but the removal of tissue should be avoided whenever possible. The sutures are placed at two levels (Fig. 52.1). Tarsal plate and subconjuncti-val tissue are first repaired without penetrating the palpebral conjunctiva, and the knots are buried in the substance of the eyelid such that no suture material can cause corneal irritation. The margo-intermarginalis must be accurately reformed, the first suture ensuring precise apposition at this level. The second row of

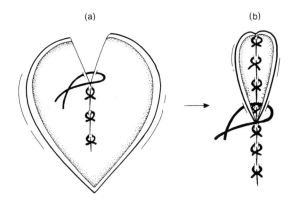

Fig. 52.1 Repair of an eyelid wound by two-layer closure. (a) Tarsal plate and subconjunctival tissue apposed; (b) subcutis and skin apposed.

sutures involves the subcutis and skin, and single interrupted sutures are used to ensure accurate repair and reduce the chance of wound breakdown. Absorbable material is used for the buried sutures and nylon is preferable for the cutaneous repair.

Congenital porphyria

Congenital porphyria is a rare, recessively inherited defect of haemoglobin metabolism which results in the production of abnormal porphyrins. Clinical signs associated with photosensitization are seen in light-skinned cattle upon exposure to sunlight. Adenexal inflammation is characterized by oedema, photophobia, blepharospasm and excessive lacrimation.

Diseases of the conjunctiva and cornea

The occurrence of IBKC and squamous cell carcinoma renders this part of the eye important in economic terms, and as the two disease conditions commonly involve both structures it is convenient to discuss them both under the same section.

Epibulbar dermoid

Dermoid formation (choriostoma) is due to the poor differentiation of the palpebral tissue with the result that plaques of hair-bearing skin and subcutis may be found involving the lateral aspect of the globe (Plate 52.3). Both the cornea and episcleral tissues can be affected, the dermoid replacing the corneal epithelium and bulbar conjunctiva, respectively. Bilateral involvement is unusual, and dermoids are only of clinical significance if they impair sight, cause trigeminal irritation

and conjunctival inflammation or they physically interfere with effective blinking and lid closure. Removal is then advocated, and topical and regional anaesthesia can be complemented by using the auriculopalpebral nerve block. The lesion must be removed in entirety to prevent recurrence. While a suprascleral lesion is easily excised, care is required with the superficial keratectomy needed to remove the corneal dermoid.

Infectious bovine keratoconjunctivitis (IBKC, New Forest eye, pinkeye)

Aetiology

This disease has been recognized for at least 100 years (Billings, 1889) since when it has demonstrated both common incidence and worldwide distribution. It is highly contagious, and outbreaks of epidemic proportions can affect grazing herds during the summer and autumn months, and housed cattle the whole year round. Young animals are more severely affected, dictating the development of possible local immunity to the disease in those previously exposed. Over the years IBKC has been attributed to several organisms (Bedford, 1976), but currently *Moraxella bovis* is still regarded by most authorities to be the cause. The root of the controversy lies in the fact that *Moraxella bovis* can be found in the normal conjunctival sac, and attempts to produce the disease using pure cultures of this bacterium have not always been successful. In addition, infectious bovine rhinotracheitis (IBR) virus, known to cause conjunctivitis in addition to rhinitis, and *Mycoplasma bovirhinitis* and *M. laidlawii* have been isolated with *Moraxella bovis* from IBKC patients. Rather than representing cause, however, these organisms may act synergistically as enhancing factors. Undoubtedly, other enhancing factors can be at work, and the increased incidence of IBKC during the warmer months has indicated that ultraviolet light, flies and dust play potentially important roles in the overall picture. Certainly flies of the *Musca* and *Stomoxys* species have been incriminated as mechanical vectors, but the occurrence of epidemic disease among winter-housed cattle suggest that flies and the other environmental factors are not essential.

Epidemiology

Variation within the clinical picture of the disease may be related to the input of the several possible enhancing factors, but may also be due to the susceptibility of the animal to infection and the type of *Moraxella bovis* present in its conjunctival sac. Older cattle are more resistant to infection, it being calves and cattle of less than two years of age that demonstrate the highest morbidity and the most severe disease. Such resistance may be the result of previous exposure, but local factors as well as antibody formation may be involved (Pugh, 1969). It has been demonstrated that two forms of the bacterium exist: a smooth non-haemolytic form that is avirulent and can usually be isolated from recovering and clinically normal carrier animals, and a rough haemolytic virulent form that causes the acute disease (Pedersen, 1973). The rough form is fimbriated for adherence (Sandhu *et al.*, 1974), and repeated passage has demonstrated its conversion into the smooth form. The presence of fimbriae would appear to be necessary for disease to occur and for immunity to develop. The difficulties experienced in the production of an effective vaccine against *Moraxella bovis* may be overcome as the result of further structural studies to determine the possible immunogenic status of the fimbriae. In the past, alteration of the surface components of bacterial cells in the preparation of vaccines may have been wholly responsible for the ineffectiveness of such vaccines. The economic importance of IBKC demands that an effective vaccine be developed, but it could be many years before the solution is finally produced.

Signs

Epidemics occur as the result of the introduction of incubating, chronically affected or carrier animals into the herd. The presenting clinical features may vary considerably depending on the immunity of the exposed individual and the level of enhancing factors present. This variation is not only seen on a herd-to-herd basis, but between individual animals within the same herd. Both unilateral and bilateral cases will be seen; in the latter a variation in the degree of severity may be noted between the two eyes. Usually, inflammation of the bulbar and possibly the palpebral conjunctivae precedes the keratitis, but occasionally the conjunctival involvement is not seen until after corneal inflammation has made its appearance. Blepharospasm, photophobia and copious ocular discharge herald anterior segment pain, the discharge, primarily clear and thin, becoming purulent quite rapidly to mat the lashes and circumorbital hair. The conjunctiva is chemotic and swelling of the eyelids may occur. Corneal changes usually develop within 48 hours, a 3-mm wide, slightly raised area of cloudiness normally making its appearance centrally. Epithelial loss can be demonstrated using fluorescein stain, and the lesion itself may take on the yellowish blue of pyogenic necrosis. The surrounding cornea becomes oedematous and hazy, and a low-grade anterior uveitis with aqueous flare may be noticeable in some animals. Corneal vascularization from the limbal blood vessels is well established by the sixth day, the new vessels rapidly progressing towards the central lesion in the anterior

stroma (Plate 52.4a). Throughout this stage of the disease the eye is extremely painful, and a bilateral involvement means that the patient is either blind or experiencing impaired vision. Inappetance, suppressed weight gain and reduced milk production are related to the severity of involvement. At this stage, and particularly in young animals, loss of epithelium and anterior stroma in the central lesion may occur, and this ulcer may rapidly enlarge to involve deeper stromal tissue. Less severe forms of the disease resolve within two or three weeks, the cornea gradually clearing from its periphery towards the centre as the vessels cease to transmit blood to the healing ulcer site. Recovery takes longer when extensive ulceration has occurred and deep stromal scarring and keratoconus may result. In some patients descemetocele formation may complicate deep ulcers and actual rupture may lead to panophthalmitis (Plate 52.4b). Blindness may result, and the eye may become glaucomatous but will eventually shrink (phthisis bulbi). The occasional death has been attributed to meningitis following presumed ascending infection of the optic nerve.

Treatment

Moraxella bovis is susceptible to most antimicrobial agents including many antiseptics, and this, combined with uncertainties concerning the aetiology of the condition and a tendency for spontaneous resolution in some patients, renders the accurate assessment of any treatment difficult. It is generally agreed, however, that the earlier the treatment the less severe the disease and the greater the chance of controlling the outbreak. In the absence of isolation facilities, it is suggested that treatment of the entire herd will protect the unaffected cattle. Consideration of potential carrier status dictates the use of antibiotics in newly acquired stock before they are introduced into the herd.

Antimicrobial drugs may be administered topically, by subconjunctival injection and parenterally. The ideal therapy for a herd problem demands effective one-time dosage and, as such, topically applied preparations, which require frequent administration to maintain therapeutically effective levels in the precorneal tear film (PCTF), cannot be very effective. Their short contact time is reduced further by the presence of ocular discharge and lacrimation, and blepharospasm renders their application difficult. Currently, increased contact time as the result of specific formulation is claimed for several antibiotic preparations including cloxacillin, cephalonium and a penicillin and streptomycin combination. The subconjunctival injection of antibiotics can be used as an alternative to the topical route, but the antibiotic must be placed beneath the dorsal bulbar conjunctiva. This is difficult to do for the unpractised hand and a topical analgesic agent (proxmetacaine hydrochloride) must be used. From this site the antibiotic leaks into the PCTF and thus has an effect. Intrapalpebral injections of various antibiotics are used commonly, but there is evidence to demonstrate that a drug deposited in palpebral muscle gets into the lacrimal gland or the PCTF. Long-acting ampicillin, oxytetracycline and penicillin may be used parenterally for repeated good effect. *Moraxella bovis* is usually resistant to lincomycin, tylosin and erythromycin but has variable susceptibility to cloxacillin (George, 1990). In an original study, Pedersen (1973) claimed that intravenous sulphadimidine was the treatment of choice for IBKC. He showed that although *Moraxella bovis* is present on the corneal and conjunctival surfaces, it colonizes the lacrimal and tarsal glands, and that any treatment must effectively penetrate these tissues. A single injection of sulphadimidine at dose rate of 100 mg/kg bodyweight will do this, and the drug will remain in the RCTF at a therapeutically active concentration for 24 hours. It is still surprising that this method of treatment is not utilized to any great extent for it seems to answer both theoretical and practical aspects of therapy. However, some strains of *Moraxella bovis* have proved resistant to sulpha drugs (Pugh & McDonald, 1977). In the future other delivery systems may be evaluated and ocular inserts that allow prolonged drug release would appear to be of potential value in this respect.

Surgery can have a part to play in the treatment of IBKC. The membrana nictitans can be used to support the severely ulcerated cornea or protect a ruptured anterior chamber, and this technique is preferred to a temporary tarsorrhaphy in which the eyelids are sutured together. Using local anaesthesia together with an auriculopalpebral nerve block to overcome any blepharospasm, the membrana nictitans and the loose bulbar conjunctiva can be apposed to cover the cornea (Fig. 52.2). Mattress sutures of non-absorbable material are used, and the cornea is left covered for two to three weeks. The sutures should not penetrate the membrana's full thickness, otherwise corneal erosion will occur. Should a more resilient method of repair be required then under a general anaesthetic a pedicle of bulbar conjunctiva can be sutured directly into the corneal defect (Fig. 52.3). The pedicle is separated from its bulbar conjunctival attachment several weeks later and the residual conjunctival tissue is usually involved in the scar. This technique offers the advantages of directly strengthening the cornea and introducing a blood supply to the ulcer site.

Vaccination (see p. 1018)

There have been considerable difficulties experienced by those attempting to produce an effective vaccine

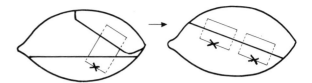

Fig. 52.2 The membrana flap. The membrana is sutured into the loose dorsal bulbar conjunctiva using two or three mattress sutures.

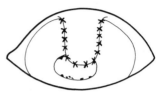

Fig. 52.3 The bulbar conjunctival pedicle flap used in the repair of deep corneal ulceration.

against *Moraxella bovis*, but some recent results are quite optimistic (Lepper, 1993). The research has concentrated on the fimbriae or pili found in the rough form of the organism and recombinant DNA technology has been involved. Certainly pilus-antigen vaccines have demonstrated acceptable levels of protection in several studies (Lepper, 1988; Moore & Rutter, 1989) and workable protocols are now possible. Calves are vaccinated at approximately one month of age, with a second vaccination three weeks later. There is no evidence that colostrum derived antibodies will negate this procedure. Adult cattle should have yearly boosters.

Infectious bovine rhinotracheitis
(see also p. 286)

The role of infectious bovine rhinotracheitis virus in anterior segment disease is not fully understood. The virus is thought to enhance the effects of *Moraxella bovis* in some patients with IBKC, but it is also known to cause conjunctivitis in its own right. Respiratory disease may or may not be present, and abortion rates may be high in IBR-affected herds.

The ocular involvement may be unilateral or bilateral. Varying degrees of chemosis may be present, and a number of white plaques may be found in both the bulbar and palpebral conjunctivae. The discharge may vary from serous in early disease to a mucopurulent type later. Anterior uveitis and corneal opacity are occasional findings, and this latter should not be confused with the corneal abscess or ulcer that routinely occurs in IBKC. Confirmation of diagnosis is not always easy, for it requires virus isolation from swabs taken only in the early part of the disease. Seroconversion from negative to positive or a rising titre for IBR antibody will provide the final proof. There is no specific treatment for the condition, but antibiotics will help control any bacterial secondary infection. Normally, the disease takes three to four weeks to complete its course.

Endothelial dystrophy

Bilateral neonatal corneal oedema has been reported in several breeds including the Friesian (Deas, 1959). The oedema is uniformly present throughout the whole stroma, and its persistent nature ensures permanent impairment of sight. Treatment is not possible, but short-term clearing of the cornea can be obtained using topically applied glycerol or hypertonic saline. Signs of possible precursor or accompanying anterior uveitis and other ocular abnormalities are not present, and defective endothelial function alone is the indicated cause. The defect is considered to be inherited as a recessive trait, and affected animals and their carrier parents should be avoided in any breeding programme.

Neoplasia (see p. 1126)

Ocular squamous cell carcinoma (SCC) or 'cancer eye' is the commonest bovine neoplasm, and its economic importance has already been stressed. Although SCC has worldwide distribution, its incidence increases in countries where cattle experience long-term exposure to intensive sunlight. The Hereford would appear the most commonly affected breed, and tumour formation is rarely seen before five years of age. A presumed inherited predisposition is postulated, and genetic analysis has suggested that it is a recessive trait (Anderson & Chambers, 1957; Vogt & Anderson, 1964). However, several contributory facts seem to be involved, perhaps one of the most important being the role of melanin in palpebral, conjunctival and scleral tissues. Pigmentation is determined genetically, and undoubtedly the presence of melanin protects tissue from SCC development. As such ultraviolet light is considered to be a significant contributory factor in the development of SCC, its absorption by melanin being the significant protective factor. Much SCC finds origin in the bulbar conjunctiva at the lateral and medial limbi, but other areas where pigmentation may be reduced (the palpebral conjunctiva, the membrana nictitans and eyelid skin) can also be affected. Other possible contributory factors are IBR virus, dust, flies and high levels of nutrition.

The indications that ultraviolet light may be an important aetiological factor are the actual tumour sites

and the marked geographic variation in incidence. Squamous cell carcinoma occurs in ocular tissue where there is little or no pigment, and the bulbar conjunctiva at the lateral and medial limbi is more exposed than conjunctiva elsewhere on the globe or lining the eyelids. The incidence of ocular SCC is greater in those parts of the world with high levels of ultraviolet light, and at high altitude. The IBR virus and its inclusion bodies may be found in the neoplastic tissue (Taylor & Hanks, 1969) and it has been postulated that the virus may play a part in initiating tumour growth or be involved in the transformation of precursor lesions into carcinoma. Surprisingly, perhaps, the incidence of SCC is greater in cattle on higher levels of nutrition, but this may be associated with enhanced age changes induced by such diets (Anderson, 1970).

Several stages of development are described in SCC formation. Conjunctival plaques of hyperplastic epithelium (Plate 52.5a) or hyperkeratosis of palpebral skin represent the initial lesion. Regression may occur, but the plaques are generally replaced by papilloma formation, and this in turn is replaced by non-invasive carcinoma. Eventually, most of these carcinomas become invasive, and the whole globe can be involved (Plate 52.5b). Invasion of orbital bone can occur, and with long-standing SCC, metastasis via the lymphatics to involve the lungs, heart, liver and kidney is possible (Cordy, 1978).

Treatment is related to the extent of tumour involvement, and the possibility of metastasis may dictate a policy of early slaughter. Excision of the neoplasm, removal of the membrana nictitans, enucleation or exenteration of the orbit represent possible early treatment. Alternative techniques of cryosurgery, hyperthermia, radiation therapy and immunotherapy have all been tried with some success, again early in the course of tumour development. Small neoplasms can be excised irrespective of site, but recurrence and subsequent extension should be expected. Large lesions of the membrana nictitans may already have invaded the orbit. Premalignant lesions and small carcinomas can be destroyed using liquid nitrogen sprays, but adequate freezing demands the use of thermocouple assessment. Limbal-based lesions can be difficult to treat effectively. Again neoplastic cells can be selectively destroyed by heating tissue to 45°C, and early SCC will respond to hyperthermic therapy. Various forms of ionizing radiation therapy have been used successfully. Beta-irradiation will destroy small lesions, and radioactive caesium, cobalt or gold implants can be similarly effective if the dose rates can be adequately calculated. Immunotherapy offers potentially effective treatment, with the parenteral use of modified or whole-cell tumour cell suspensions having demonstrated considerable promise (van Kampen et al., 1973).

Diseases of the uveal tract

(see also p. 180 onwards)

Both congenital and acquired disease of the uveal tract occur in cattle, with uveitis presenting the clinician with as much difficulty in treatment as it does in the other domestic species.

Congenital anomalies

Several congenital anomalies occur in cattle, including aniridia, colobomata, polycoria, persistence of the pupillary membrane and anterior uveal cyst formation. Aniridia is seen as part of a multiocular defect in Jersey calves, in which bilateral partial absence of the iris is accompanied by microphakia or lens luxation (Saunders & Fincher, 1951). Vision can be affected to the point of blindness, and the defect is inherited as a simple recessive trait. Iris colobomata, polycoria and uveal cysts are of no clinical significance, but persistence of the pupillary membrane may be associated with lens and corneal opacities. The vascular mesoderm in which the pupil develops should be resorbed by the time of parturition, but strands of this tissue may persist to span the pupil or become adherent to the anterior lens capsule or the corneal endothelium. Cataract or corneal endothelial and deep stromal opacities mark the areas of adherence, the size of these opacities varying with the amount of the attaching remnant tissue. Heterochromia iridis, due to a reduction or absence of melanin, is seen in the colour dilute breeds, and it may occasionally be accompanied by photophobia, nystagmus and typical papillary coloboma formation.

Uveitis

Inflammation within the uveal tract occurs in association with systemic disease, corneal ulceration, keratitis, trauma and intraocular neoplasia. Anterior uveitis can accompany IBR infection, toxoplasmosis, tuberculosis and neonatal coliform septicaemia; panophthalmitis in which the whole uveal tract is involved may be seen in malignant catarrhal fever. Infectious bovine rhinotracheitis virus may be involved in IBKC and will cause conjunctivitis; occasionally there is an associated uveitis. In calves with coliform septicaemia, acute anterior uveitis characterized by episcleral congestion, miosis and hypopyon formation may be seen in association with septic meningitis in which paresis, ataxia and convulsions are the obvious clinical features. Occasionally, the choroid is involved, and haemorrhage and exudate will be seen in the vitreous. In peracute malignant catarrhal fever severe photophobia, marked palpebral and corneal oedema, mucopurulent discharge and panuveitis may all be seen. Anterior uveitis, choroiditis and retinitis may all be present as a result of vascular necrosis and vasculitis (Plowright, 1968). A recurrent uveitis, referred to as specific ophthalmia (Marolt et al., 1963) has been described for cattle. It is similar clinically to equine recurrent uveitis (periodic ophthalmia) with corneal oedema, anterior chamber and intravitreal exudates, and retinal haemorrhage being seen in the acute stage. A viral aetiology is suggested, with IBR and other respiratory viruses isolated from affected animals.

Listeria monocytogenes has been previously associated with outbreaks of keratoconjuntivitis and uveitis in housed cattle in the UK (Morgan, 1977), but more recently this organism has been isolated from housed cattle fed on silage, presenting with anterior uveitis as the only clinical feature (Watson, 1989). It has been considered that the organism in the silage gains entry to the eye either directly from conjunctival sac contamination or from the gingival margins by trigeminal migration. The uveitis presents clinically in the same way as any other anterior segment inflammation; it is usually unilateral with marked miosis, thickening and folding of the iris, keratic precipitate (KP) and hypopyon formation and vascularization of the limbal cornea being the presenting signs (Plate 52.6). Treatment includes the use of systemic antibiosis, but subconjunctival corticosteroids and topical atropine are essential for effective resolution.

Neoplasia

Primary uveal tract tumours in cattle are rare, but secondary involvement with squamous cell carcinoma occurs not infrequently.

Disease of the lens

Ectopia lentis (lens luxation) occurs as part of a congenital multi-ocular defect syndrome in Jersey and Friesian cattle, and cataract probably enjoys higher incidence than the literature dictates. Intraocular examinations are not commonly practised in cattle, and cataract is only diagnosed if it is large enough to be noticed initially with the naked eye, has an effect on sight or is present with other noticeable ocular anomalies.

Congenital cataract has been recorded in several breeds (Odorfer, 1995) and in Jersey and Friesian cattle its inheritance is as a simple recessive trait (p. 181). There would appear to be a particularly significant incidence of this lesion in the Friesian and Friesian crosses in the UK, demonstrating marked regional variation. In congenital cataract the nuclear part of the lens is always involved, but cortical extension may severely affect vision (Plate 52.7). There may also be a posterior polar cortical opacity with posterior lenticonus and possible hyaloid attachment. Nystagmoid movements of the globe may accompany the larger opacities. In both these breeds and in the Shorthorn other ocular anomalies including buphthalmia, microphakia, lens luxation and retinal detachment may accompany cataract.

Cataract may be secondary to uveitis, but the aetiology of other capsular and cortical lens opacity remains obscure (Gelatt, 1971).

The treatment of cataract is by surgery, and two techniques are possible. In young calves of several weeks of age lens discission can be successful if the attendant uveitis is minimal (P.G.C. Bedford, pers. obs.). The technique is a simple one in which the anterior capsule of the lens is disrupted using a Bowman's needle inserted into the anterior chamber at the dorsal limbus (Plate 52.8). Normal and cataractous lens material is released into the anterior chamber and is usually almost completely resorbed, leaving the posterior capsule *in situ* to retain the vitreous behind the pupil. Corticosteroids are used to suppress the possible phacoanaphylactic inflammatory reaction, but in young calves this is minimal. After the operation cataract reformation is unusual, despite the retained presence of the anterior capsule and the lens epithelium. In older animals the attendant uveitis renders this technique unacceptable, and extracapsular lens extraction or phacoemulsification offers the best chance of success. In the former the anterior chamber is opened either through a corneal or limbal section, the anterior capsule removed and the cataractous material dislocated from the posterior capsule out through the section. The postoperative therapy must include corticosteroids and, just as in other species, loss of pupil as the result of iris spasm and posterior synechiae formation is the common complication that may render the eye blind. However, the uveitis is usually controllable, and the overall prognosis for sight is good. In phacoemulsification the cataract is removed from within the confines of its capsular bag and then the anterior capsule is removed. This kind of surgery is less intrusive and the degree of associated uveitis is usually minimal.

Diseases of the retina and optic nerve

Both congenital anomaly and acquired disease can involve the bovine fundus but, as with cataract diagnosis, such lesions are not normally detected unless there is an associated effect on sight or other more noticeable ocular defects are present.

Congenital defects

Papillary and peripapillary choroidal colobomata, persistence of the hyaloid artery, retinal dysplasia and maternal hypovitaminosis A induced papilloedema and optic nerve atrophy are seen in the neonate. Choroidal colombomata are reported to be commonplace but may be of no clinical significance. Typical papillary colobomata in Hereford cattle with incomplete albinism are seen bilaterally but have no reported noticeable effect on vision. However, the same bilateral defect in Charolais may blind the affected animal (Plate 52.9). In both breeds the lesion is considered to be inherited, and genetic studies in the Charolais have indicated that it is a polygenic trait (Barnett & Ogden, 1972) (p. 181).

The hyaloid artery is part of the primary vitreous, but with the development of the ciliary vasculature it regresses and becomes non-functional. Large remnants of this vessel can be seen commonly in cattle (Plate 52.10), but they are of no clinical importance. The vessel overlies the optic disc and extends forward from this structure into the posterior vitreous. Blood is often seen within its lumen in young calves up to eight weeks of age, and remnants of the avascular vessel will persist throughout the animal's life.

Retinal dysplasia, in which there is typical rosette formation and usually non-attachment of the neuroretina, is seen in Shorthorn cattle with hydrocephalus and multiple ocular defects, and in Herefords with microphthalmia, cerebellar hypoplasia and hydrocephalus (Blackwell *et al.*, 1959; Green & Leipold, 1974). Congenital retinal degeneration and optic nerve atrophy have been seen in association with microphthalmia, cataract and cerebellar hypoplasia in calves born of dams infected with bovine viral diarrhoea/mucosal disease. Congenital optic nerve degeneration and papilloedema can be produced by maternal hypovitaminosis A.

Inflammation

Retinal and optic nerve lesions will accompany several systemic infections including the neonatal pyosepticaemias, bovine viral diarrhoea/mucosal disease, thromboembolic meningoencephalitis, toxoplasmosis, tuberculosis and rabies.

Septic chorioretinitis characterized by haemorrhages, exudate and bullous retinal detachment can accompany septicaemia in young calves caused by *Escherichia coli*, streptococci, *Mannheimia* spp. and *Arcanobacterium pyogenes* infections. Maternal infection with bovine viral diarrhoea/mucosal disease can cause congenital optic neuritis among other ocular anomalies, and in thromboembolic meningoencephalitis caused by *Haemophilus somnus* conjunctivitis and corneal oedema may be accompanied by retinal vasculitis and detachment. Blindness is usually due to septic thrombosis of the visual cortex. Both anterior and posterior uveitis with possible retinal detachment can accompany tuberculosis (p. 862). Focal retinitis has been reported in bovine rabies (p. 1164).

Hypovitaminosis A (see also p. 256)

Hypovitaminosis A has been described in three situations with variability of the presenting clinical features. It occurs congenitally, and here either papilloedema or optic nerve atrophy is present. In the growing calf there is obvious papilloedema in which the disc becomes very swollen, and the resultant papillary vascular congestion may cause focal superficicial haemorrhage (Plate 52.11). Optic nerve atrophy will occur if the deficiency is maintained. The papilloedema is due to compression of the optic nerve by bony overgrowth within the optic canal, and the accompanying vascular occlusion results in ischaemic necrosis of the nerve (Hayes *et al.*, 1968). Early papilloedema is reversible and optic nerve atrophy preventable if the diet is suitably adjusted. Nyctalopia due to rod degeneration also occurs. Vitamin A is essential in the formation of the visual pigment rhodopsin, and without rhodopsin the photoreceptors degenerate. This process is also reversible should vitamin A be supplemented soon enough. It is likely that the sight problems experienced by the calf are more likely to be caused by the optic nerve lesions rather than the retinal degeneration. In the adult deficient in vitamin A papilloedema is much less noticeable and optic nerve atrophy does not occur. Here the outer segment degeneration is probably more significant in terms of the effect on sight.

Male fern optic neuropathy

Permanent or transient blindness will accompany weakness, malaise and constipation in the early stages of male fern (*Dryopteris filix mas*) poisoning. The toxic effect is on the optic nerve, and varying degrees of papilloedema and associated haemorrhage are seen ophthalmoscopically. In severe cases optic nerve atrophy follows the papilloedema.

Arthrogryposis (see p. 177)

The aetiology of arthrogryposis is open to speculation, and inheritance, fetal lupin toxicosis, manganese deficiency and maternal viral infection have all been considered to be involved. Joint deformities, syringomyelia and cleft palate may be seen, and blindness is due to abnormal photoreceptor development.

Progressive retinal degeneration

A form of retinal degeneration characterized by nyctalopia, progressive pigmentation within the tapetal fundus and attenuation of the superficial retinal vasculature has been described in cattle, and compared with canine progressive retinal atrophy (PRA). It would appear to be a rare condition, and the comparison with PRA may have been somewhat premature.

Glaucoma

Glaucoma is the process of ocular degeneration caused by an elevation of the intraocular fluid pressure (IOP) beyond its physiological upper limit. The incidence is less than 1 per cent in cattle. All bovine glaucomas are due to the impairment of aqueous drainage through a defective or diseased iridocorneal angle, and in the majority of cases the glaucoma is secondary to inflammation or neoplasia. Uveitis may result in pupillary block due to extensive posterior synechiae formation. This results in the forward displacement of the peripheral iris, the so-called pathological iris bombé, and closure of the ciliary cleft. The presence of exudation speeds the transformation of the trabecular meshwork into an impervious physical barrier to aqueous outflow. Alternatively, these peripheral anterior synechiae and ciliary synechiae may form directly to deny bulk aqueous drainage. Tumour cells and the products of any associated inflammation will block the iridocorneal angle to produce secondary glaucoma.

A primary glaucoma has been recorded in the Friesian (Carter, 1960); the condition is inherited as a dominant trait and is seen in association with cataract formation and lens luxation.

Treatment of glaucoma in cattle is determined on the basis of whether the enlarged blind eye is of nuisance value, and enucleation may be necessary in the presence of associated corneal damage or degeneration.

References

Amman, K. (1968) Eye diseases in ruminants. In *Veterinary Encyclopaedia*, Vol. II (ed. by E.A. McPherson), pp. 931–45. Medical Book Co, Copenhagen.

Anderson, D.E. (1970) Cancer eye in cattle. *Modern Veterinary Practice*, **51**, 43–7.

Anderson, D.E. & Chambers, D. (1957) Genetic aspects of cancer eye in cattle. *Miscellaneous Publications of the Oklahoma Agricultural Experimental Station*, **MP48**, 28–33.

Barnett, K.C. & Ogden, A.L. (1972) Ocular colobomata in Charolais cattle. *Veterinary Record*, **91**, 592.

Bedford, P.G.C. (1976) Infectious bovine keratoconjunctivitis. *Veterinary Record*, **98**, 134–5.

Billings, F.S. (1889) Keratitis contagiosa in cattle. *Nebraska Agricultural Station Bulletin*, **10**, 247.

Blackwell, R.L., Knox, J.H. & Cobb, E.H. (1959) A hydrocephalic lethal in Hereford cattle. *Journal of Heredity*, **50**, 143–8.

Carter, A.H. (1960) An inherited blindness (cataract) in cattle. *Proceedings of the New Zealand Society for Animal Production*, **20**, 108.

Cordy, D.R. (1978) Tumours of the nervous system and eye. In *Tumours in Domestic Animals* (ed. by J.E. Moulton), 2nd edn, pp. 443–53. University of California Press, Los Angeles.

Deas, D.W. (1959) A note on hereditary opacity of the diseased cornea in British Friesian cattle. *Veterinary Record*, **71**, 619–20.

Gelatt, K.N. (1971) Cataracts in cattle. *Journal of the American Veterinary Medical Association*, **159**, 195–200.

George, L.W. (1990) Antibiotic treatment of infectious bovine keratoconjunctivitis. *Cornell Veterinarian*, **80**, 999–1002.

Gilmore, L.O. (1957) Inherited defects in cattle. *Journal of Dairy Science*, **40**, 593–5.

Green, H.J. & Leipold, H.W. (1974) Hereditary internal hydrocephalus and retinal dysplasia in Shorthorn calves. *Cornell Veterinarian*, **64**, 367–75.

Hayes, K.C., Nielsen, S.W. & Eaton, H.D. (1968). Pathogenesis of the optic nerve lesion in vitamin A deficient calves. *Archives of Ophthalmology*, **80**, 777–87.

Kampen van, K.R., Crisp, W.E., Martin, J.C.D. & Ellsworth, H.S. (1973) The immunologic therapy of squamous cell carcinoma. *American Journal of Obstetrics and Gynaecology*, **116**, 569–74.

Leipold, H.W. & Huston, K. (1968) Congenital syndrome of anophthalmia–microphthalmia with associated defects in cattle. *Pathologia Veterinaria*, **5**, 407–18.

Lepper, A.W.D. (1988) Vaccination against infectious bovine keratoconjunctivitis: protective efficacy and antibody response induced by pili of homologous and heterologous strains of *Moraxella bovis*. *Australian Veterinary Journal*, **65**, 310–16.

Lepper, A.W.D. (1993) A *Moraxella bovis* pili vaccine produced by recombinant DNA technology for the prevention of infectious bovine keratoconjunctivitis. *Veterinary Microbiology*, **36**, 175–83.

Marolt, J., Burdnjak, Z, Vekelic, E. & Andrasic, N. (1963) Specific ophthalmia of cattle. *Zentralblatt Veterinarmedizin*, **10**, 286–94.

Moore, L.J. & Rutter, J.M. (1989) Attachment of *Moraxella bovis* to calf corneal cells and inhibition by antiserum. *Australian Veterinary Journal*, **66**, 39–42.

Morgan, J.H. (1977) Infectious keratoconjunctivitis in cattle associated with *Listeria monocytogenes*. *Veterinary Record*, **100**, 113–14.

Odorfer, G. (1995) Occurrence and frequency of eye diseases among cattle in Austria. *Wein Tierarztliche Monatsschrift*, **82**, 170–8.

Pedersen, K.B. (1973) *Infectious keratoconjunctivitis in cattle*. PhD thesis, Royal Veterinary College, Copenhagen, Denmark.

Plowright, W. (1968) Malignant catarrhal fever. *Journal of the American Veterinary Medical Association*, **152**, 795–804.

Pugh, G.W. (1969) *Characterization of* Moraxella bovis *and its relationship to bovine infectious keratoconjunctivitis*. PhD thesis, Iowa State University, Ames, Iowa.

Pugh, G.W. & McDonald, T.J. (1977) Infectious bovine keratoconjunctivitis: treatment of *Moraxella bovis* infections with antibiotics. *Proceedings of the Annual Meeting of the United States Animal Health Association*, **81**, 120–30.

Punch, P.I. & Slatter, D.H. (1984) A review of infectious bovine keratoconjunctivitis, *Veterinary Bulletin*, **54**, 193–208.

Sandhu, T.S., White, F.H. & Simpson, C.F. (1974) Association of pili with the rough colony type of *Moraxella bovis*. *American Journal of Veterinary Research*, **35**, 437–9.

Saunders, L.Z. & Fincher, M.S. (1951) Hereditary multiple eye defects in grade Jersey calves. *Cornell Veterinarian*, **41**, 351–66.

Taylor, R.L. & Hanks, M.A. (1969) Viral isolations from bovine eye tumours. *American Journal of Veterinary Research*, **30**, 1885–6.

Vogt, D.W. & Anderson, D.E. (1964) Studies on bovine ocular squamous cell carcinoma ('cancer eye'). XV. Heritability of susceptibility. *Journal of Heredity*, **55**, 133–5.

Watson, C.L. (1989) Bovine iritis? *Veterinary Record*, **124**, 411.

Willoughby, R.A. (1968) Congenital eye defects in cattle. *Modern Veterinary Practice*, **49**, 36–9.

Chapter 53
Other Conditions

A.H. Andrews

Anaphylaxis	927
Amyloidosis	928
Congestive heart failure	928
Diabetes mellitus	930
Hypothermia	930
Lightning strike/electrocution	930
Stray voltage	931
Meloidosis	932
Mycotic diseases	932
Mucormycosis	932
Cryptococcosis	932
Rhinosporidiasis	933
Candidiasis (moniliasis)	933
Aspergillosis	933
Histoplasmosis	934
Teat burns	934
Water availability	934
Heat stress	935
Acute heat stress	935
Chronic heat stress	935
Malignant catarrhal fever	935

Anaphylaxis

Aetiology

Anaphylaxis is the result of antigen–antibody reaction and when severe it can cause anaphylactic shock.

Epidemiology

The condition is usually very uncommon. Most cases follow the parenteral injection of drugs or biological products such as blood. Occasionally, the problem can arise through exposure via the alimentary tract or lungs. Signs may be seen in the system exposed, or they may be generalized. Most cases follow the introduction to the blood of an antigen to which the animal has already been sensitized, but reactions can occur where the animal is not known to have been exposed previously. More anaphylactic reactions occur in some herds and families of cattle than others. Reactions are most prevalent in Channel Island breeds. Initial signs tend to be largely of a respiratory nature, but other areas affected can be the alimentary tract and skin.

Signs

Reaction can occur about 20 minutes after the introduction of the antigen. The animal exhibits pronounced dyspnoea with, on auscultation, bubbling and emphysematous sounds. Muscle tremors can occur, which cause pyrexia to 40°C (104°F). Other reactions include bloat, diarrhoea, increased salivation, urticaria and rhinitis. Occasionally laminitis occurs. Death is due to anoxia. Following i.v. blood transfusion, there are usually hiccoughs and then dyspnoea, muscle tremors, salivation, coughing, lacrimation and fever.

Necropsy

At necropsy usually only the lungs are involved in acute cases, with marked pulmonary oedema and vascular engorgement; some animals develop emphysema. Longer-standing cases show hyperaemia and oedema of the abomasum and small intestines.

Diagnosis

Diagnosis depends on the history of recent introduction of an antigen to which the animal may previously have been exposed. The signs are helpful, being sudden with severe dyspnoea, urticaria, etc. Haematological examination shows increased packed cell volume, leucopenia and thrombocytopenia. Biochemical changes include a hyperkalaemia and blood histamine levels are raised in some cases. Finally, there is a response to therapy.

Differential diagnoses are few because of the rapid onset but acute pneumonia could be confused, although usually there is toxaemia and lesions are more pronounced in the arterio-ventral parts of the lungs.

Treatment and control

The most effective method of treatment is an intramuscular injection of adrenaline (4–5 ml of 1 in 1000 solution) and if necessary a fifth of the dose (0.5–1.0 ml) can be given intravenously, diluted to about a 2 per cent solution. Otherwise, corticosteroids can be administered or they may be given immediately following adrenaline as they potentiate the latter's activity. Antihistamines give variable results, partly because most histamine is released early in the reaction and also there are other mediators of the anaphylactic reactions. Various other compounds have been shown to alter the reaction of mediators and these include sodium meclofenamate, acetylsalicylic acid and diethylcarbamazine.

Once a reaction has occurred in an animal, the antigen causing the problem should not be reintroduced. If a blood transfusion is given, introduce up to 200 ml in a 450 kg (990 lb) animal and wait for about 10 minutes before injecting the remainder.

Amyloidosis

Aetiology

The aetiology of amyloidosis is uncertain but it is the result of a hyperglobulinaemia, probably causing an abnormal antigen–antibody response.

Epidemiology

Is a rare condition that is not fully understood. A few cases occur as the result of repeated antigen usage in the production of hyperimmune sera. However, most animals are affected sporadically and spontaneously following prolonged suppurative infections. The origin of amyloid, which is a glycoprotein, is not certain, but is thought to be due to an abnormality of the antigen–antibody reaction. Renal amyloidosis is the most commonly recognized condition, but amyloid can also be deposited in the liver and spleen. When the main organ affected is the liver, there tends to be proteinuria. This leads to hypoproteinaemia and then oedema of the organ, resulting in marked anasarca. The diarrhoea produced is partly due to amyloid deposition and oedema of the intestinal wall. Many of the animals affected are still growing. Foci of inflammation found can include traumatic reticulo-peritonitis, traumatic pericarditis, salpingitis, mastitis, metritis (Johnson & Jamison, 1984) and nephritis. Cases have occurred following repeated hormonal injections in donor cows which are superovulated several times.

Signs

Usually, the affected animal is thin and emaciated. In most cases there is marked anasarca with an enlarged liver palpated in the right sublumbar fossa and an enlarged kidney with loss of its lobular structure when palpated via the rectum. There is usually polydipsia and a profuse watery diarrhoea. The animals later become uraemic, recumbent and comatosed. Death occurs two to five weeks after the onset of signs. Almost all cases will eventually die unless slaughtered.

Necropsy

At necropsy there are usually one or more chronic suppurative processes present in the organs. The carcass is emaciated, usually with marked oedema. The affected organs are enlarged and pale in colour. The kidney and liver have diffuse amyloid infiltration, while in the spleen it is more localized. The amyloid can be shown by aqueous iodine staining.

Diagnosis

Diagnosis depends on signs, including an enlarged kidney, diarrhoea and oedema. There is hypoproteinaemia, proteinuria and hyperfibrinogenaemia. Blood biochemical examination shows hypomagnesaemia and a serum calcium level at the lower end of the normal range. There are also a high serum urea nitrogen and high serum creatinine. The specific gravity of the urine is low and there is a prolonged bromsulphthalein (BSP) clearance test.

Differential diagnoses are few but include pyelonephritis where there is pus and haematuria, and congestive heart failure in which there is an increased heart rate, respiratory embarrassment and dyspnoea.

Treatment

No successful therapy: cattle should be slaughtered.

Congestive heart failure

Aetiology

The condition can follow diseases of the pericardium, myocardium or endocardium.

Epidemiology

It is relatively uncommon and mainly affects older cattle. Pericarditis or hydropericardium can interfere with the normal filling of the heart during diastole. Pulmonary hyperaemia, which may occur in diffuse fibrosing alveolitis, can result in right-sided congestive heart failure. In cattle, the main cause of myocardial disease is foot-and-mouth disease. Endocardial diseases are the most common and are usually due to infection or inflammation.

When extra demand is placed on the heart, or the myocardial activity is reduced, then compensation can occur by an increased heart rate, increased filling of the ventricles and improved cardiac performance. There are also dilatation and hypertrophy. Venous return increases in speed and blood distribution changes so that there is an increase in blood volume, a decrease in renal blood flow and sodium retention. Cardiac response is reduced and the animal is less able to cope with unusual exercise or other emergencies (Blood *et al.*, 1983). There is a decrease in exercise tolerance and once the compensating mechanisms have been overcome then the heart cannot cope and congestive heart failure develops. Many of the signs of cardiac insufficiency are the result of increased venous pressure. They result in congestion of organs or oedema and the decreased output produces tissue hypoxia.

Failure of the right-sided ventricle causes congestion of the major circulation with reduced blood flow through the kidney, resulting in anoxic damage to the glomeruli and venous congestion of the portal system of the liver, and eventually there is transudation into the intestinal lumen giving rise to diarrhoea. Left-sided ventricular failure results in engorgement and oedema of the lungs. Both left and right-sided failure can occur together.

Signs

Early signs are of reduced exercise tolerance with increased respiratory effort and tachypnoea following light exercise. Pulse and respiratory rates take a long time to return to normal. On percussion the heart area may be enlarged.

In left-sided failure: lungs are mainly affected so that there is a cough, tachypnoea and hyperpnoea. The heart rate is increased and a murmur may be present in the region of the aorta or left atrioventricular valve. On auscultation there are moist noises at the ventral edges of the pulmonary field and on percussion increased dullness on the lower borders of the lung. Later on there is cyanosis and dyspnoea.

In right-sided failure or cor pulmonale: appetite is poor and the animal is dull with a rapid loss of condition. There are marked areas of oedema often affecting the skin of the lower part of the body, the neck and the submandibular space. There is ascites, hydropericardium and hydrothorax. The liver may be enlarged enough to be palpated in the right sublumbar fossa. The heart rate tends to be increased and there is hyperpnoea and often slight tachypnoea. There is a marked jugular pulse. Prognosis usually poor in all cases.

Necropsy

At post-mortem examination there are abnormalities of the pericardium, myocardium or endocardium. Usually, there is pulmonary congestion and oedema. In left-sided failure there is subcutaneous oedema, hydrothorax, ascites and hydropericardium.

Diagnosis

Diagnosis is by the signs, particularly those of oedema. The heart rate is elevated and there is an increased area of cardiac dullness; abnormal heart sounds may be present, depending on the cause. Insertion of a needle into a vein shows a markedly increased venous pressure. Aspiration of fluid from oedematous areas shows it to be a transudate containing large amounts of protein. There is also a proteinuria.

Differential diagnosis

Differential diagnosis includes amyloidosis but diarrhoea tends to be marked and the kidneys are enlarged without heart abnormality. In chronic peritonitis there is often some pain and the aspirated abdominal fluid contains many leucocytes. In bladder rupture there is a normal heart and urine is present in the abdomen. In liver fibrosis the heart is normal and there is usually jaundice or photosensitization. Parasitic gastroenteritis occurs in a younger animal and there is oedema, mainly of the submandibular area, with a high faecal egg count. Fascioliosis could confuse, but again there is usually only submandibular oedema and a faecal egg count. Fog fever (p. 866) could cause problems in diagnosis but usually several animals are affected quite suddenly in the autumm. Anaphylaxis is also a sudden problem with no cardiac signs.

Treatment

The primary cause should be treated as effectively as possible, but with most cases the prognosis is poor. Where oedema is present it is partly due to sodium retention and so the salt intake should be kept as low as possible. Diuretics such as frusemide or hydrochlorothiazide are useful and they can be given by injection or orally. The heart can be treated to improve contractility by use of etamiphylline camsylate, theophylline or digitalis derivatives. The use of digitalis by mouth is probably of limited value because of breakdown in the rumen. Parenteral administration of digitalis extracts is little used for several reasons: intravenous use could result in toxicity whereas intramuscular administration gives variable results. There are no licensed preparations. Little can be done to control the congestive heart failure except to treat all infections quickly and adequately.

Diabetes mellitus

This is a very unusual condition in cattle compared with its relatively frequent occurrence in dogs and cats. However, lesions can occur in the pancreas resulting in this condition. It is usually seen in old cattle and often animals will have had other problems such as fatty liver. The signs are loss of condition with polydipsia and polyuria. There is no rise in temperature and the urine contains both ketones and glucose. Biochemical examination of the blood shows hyperglycaemia. Usually treatment is not contemplated.

Hypothermia

Aetiology

This is also called cold stress and is mainly seen in young calves in severe climatic conditions, particularly where there is wind chilling as well as a cold ambient temperature. The problem is not encountered anything like as commonly as in lambs.

Epidemiology

Exposure to cold conditions mainly occurs in calves of cows calving outside in the winter months with no shelter. It is particularly prevalent in suckler calves and occurs more frequently in countries such as Canada and Australia than say Britain. Mortality is usually higher in calves born in winter and early spring. There is a delay in the onset and rate of immunoglobulin absorption from colostrum in cold-stressed calves. Primary hypothermia with no associated disease can be seen in young calves, and secondary hypothermia with no other disease has been recorded in older calves.

Signs

The rectal temperature may be low and can be defined as a temperature less than 37°C (98.5°F) and there is shivering. Shivering appears to be more intense during the initial period following exposure to cold. Most calves have no problems in the cold but some are depressed and stand or walk about stiffly. A few animals may remain in sternal recumbency. The heart rate tends to be raised but respiratory rate is low.

Necropsy

At post mortem the most common lesions involve the limbs and include subcutaneous oedema and haemorrhage. Experimentally, more haemorrhages occur in the hindlimbs. Some animals show oedema of the ventral sternum. The joints may show mild to severe haemorrhage and acute synovitis. Some cases show haemorrhages of the adrenal glands and oedema of the iliac and jejunal lymph nodes.

Diagnosis

Diagnosis depends on the history and signs. Increased serum glucose and phosphorus levels occur with cooling but fall during recovery.

Treatment

Treatment is by immersion in warm water, which results in quicker rewarming than use of a heat pad or heat lamp. A hot air environment could be constructed with a straw bale shelter and a hot air heater. Control is by ensuring that adequate shelter is provided or by housing cattle during the bad weather.

Lightning strike/electrocution

Aetiology

This is exposure to high voltage electric currents, either natural or generated by man.

Epidemiology

The condition is uncommon but it is often of interest as it is one of the few problems that farmers have usually insured against. Problems arise from lightning, exposure of electrical wires or faulty wiring or earthing in farm buildings. Cases may be single or a group. In many instances, damp ground or floors help to conduct the electricity. Low voltages of 110–220 V are sufficient to kill cattle. Outside, trees such as oak, poplar, elm and conifers are all prone to lightning strike.

Signs

The signs in the severe form are such that animals die without a struggle. Burns or singeing may be seen because of the severity and often they involve the muzzle and feet. Death is usually due to paralysis of the medullary centre, accompanied in some cases by ventricular fibrillation. In the less severe form the animal becomes unconscious for a varying time and there is usually some sign of a struggle. After regaining consciousness there may be dullness, blindness, paralysis of one or more legs, and surface hyperaesthesia. The signs may persist or slowly disappear over a period of up to two weeks. If burns are present, sloughing of the skin in the area is seen. Minor problems may occur such as the animal may jump, be restless, show periodic convulsions or be knocked down.

In lightning strike the animal is usually close to a fence, barn, trees or a pond. Often there are signs of burning affecting these objects. The animal itself may show singeing of the hair or burn marks on the muzzle and feet. Half-chewed food may be present in the mouth. The animal quickly becomes distended with gas and decomposes rapidly. Blood often exudes from the nostrils, rectum and vulva. The pupils are dilated and the anus relaxed. There tend to be petechial haemorrhages throughout the body and the viscera are congested. The superficial lymph nodes are often haemorrhagic.

Diagnosis

Diagnosis depends on the history of a storm, position of the animal near trees, etc. and sudden death of a group of animals. The signs may also be helpful such as singeing of the hair, burns on the muzzle and feet and evidence of sudden death.

Differential diagnosis

Differential diagnosis includes anaphylaxis but there is marked pulmonary involvement. Acute heart failure can cause problems but there is engorgement of visceral veins and macroscopic or microscopic myocardial lesions. Brain trauma can occur but usually there is a haemorrhagic lesion of the brain. Nitrate/nitrite poisoning results in sudden death but methaemoglobin is present. Anthrax can be confused, but stained blood smears assist in determination. Bloat is a possibility but on necropsy the front part of the animal is congested, there is a distended rumen and sometimes froth present. Blackleg results in swelling of the part affected with the causal organism present.

Treatment

No treatment is usually given as often the cattle are either better or dead before any therapy can be administered. Central nervous system stimulants can be given. Artificial respiration may be helpful. Although nothing can be done about lightning strike, all electrical installations should be properly fitted and earthed.

Stray voltage

While not a very common problem, the signs are often difficult to determine and also the origin is hard to find. These stray electrical currents result in mild electric shocks to the animals and cause discomfort, often resulting in apparent behavioural problems.

Occurrence

There are a large number of different origins for this problem. Stray voltage is an electrical current passing between two points. Should an animal come into contact with these points the current will pass through the animal. Cattle are more sensitive to electrical voltages than human beings, who often do not feel any shock due to wearing clothes and boots which can insulate them from the problem. While there is individual variation in the susceptibility to electricity, most cases will only be detected when several animals show similar signs. The most common place for this to occur is in the milking parlour, although feed and water troughs as well as other farm building equipment can be involved. The history may contain the fact that there has been some alteration or modification of the electrical supply or there has been some building. Otherwise most problems result from old and exposed wiring, often with damage to the insulation covering or vermin damage.

Signs

These will vary and are related to the area of the stray voltage. If the source is in the parlour, the cattle are often reluctant to enter, are fidgety during milking and will rush out of the parlour after milking. If the source is a water trough it may be avoided by the cows or they may lap rather than drink normally. Other signs include restlessness, muscular twitching, etc. Milk production may suffer and feed intake as well if the feed area is affected.

Diagnosis

This is often difficult; any behavioural change will usually only be seen in the area of the stray current. If several animals are showing similar discomfort or behavioural changes then diagnosis is made more easy. Confirmation will depend on a qualified electrician and will require a sensitive voltmeter. It may also be necessary to set up the conditions that cause the shock, i.e. have the milking equipment working.

Differential diagnosis

Behavioural changes will usually only affect a single animal and will be less likely to be related to a particular area of the farm. BSE can result in signs such as reluctance to enter the parlour and difficulty in milking, but would always involve the same animal. Other signs would also occur.

Control

Ensure all electrical installations and equipment are properly earthed and maintained. Have wiring checked periodically.

Meloidosis

Aetiology

The cause is *Pseudomonas* (*Malleomyces*) *pseudomallei*. It can survive for long periods in the soil and water.

Epidemiology

The condition is primarily a disease of rodents but occasionally it spreads to man and farm animals such as sheep, goats, horses and pigs. It is very rare in cattle. The disease was first recognized in South East Asia but it is now seen in Australia, Malaysia, Papua New Guinea and Nigeria. Infection is passed in the faeces of rodents and is spread by ingestion of contaminated feed or water, by insect bites, wounds and possibly inhalation. Mortality is high and disease lasts about two to eight weeks.

Signs

The main signs are a marked pyrexia with anorexia and a thick yellow exudate from the eyes and nose. Nervous signs may be exhibited. Some cattle have infection without signs.

Pathology

There are multiple abscesses in many areas of the body as well as in the subcutaneous tissues and associated lymph nodes. The size of the abscesses is variable from a few millimetres to over 2.5 cm in diameter.

Diagnosis

This depends on demonstrating the causal organism by culture from pus, nasal discharges or blood.

Treatment

There is little information available on satisfactory treatment of meloidosis. Chloramphenicol is used in man and *in vitro* tests suggest oxytetracycline may be of use in animals, and perhaps novobiocin, chloramphenicol and sulphadiazine. Treatment is to be discouraged because of the possibility of spread to humans.

Control

Infected animals: slaughtered, disposed of by burning. In-contact animals: slaughtered, the premises disinfected.

Mycotic diseases

Mucormycosis

Aetiology

There are various fungi of the family Mucoracae that can cause infection, including the genera *Absidia, Entomophthora, Mortierella, Mucor, Rhizopus.*

Epidemiology

The fungi occur usually in soil and water and are often plant pathogens and food decomposers. They are opportunistic.

Signs

Infection can cause a necrotic placentitis in cattle resulting in abortion at three to seven months' gestation. There is necrosis of maternal cotyledons and yellow, raised, leathery lesions on the intercotyledonary areas. Granulomatous lesions of the mesenteric and mediastinal lymph nodes can occur. Calves can develop alimentary tract lesions after prolonged antibiotic therapy. Following acidosis the ruminal wall can be invaded with *Rhizopus* spp.

Diagnosis

Hyphae are present on smears of cotyledons, fetal stomach and skin. The lymph nodes need to be examined. There may be a history of antibiotic usage and on post mortem there may be abomasal ulceration. The animal will become black tinted.

Prevention and control

As the fungi are ubiquitous it is impossible to control properly. There are no satisfactory antibiotics.

Cryptococcosis

Aetiology

The cause is *Cryptococcus* (*Saccharomyces*) *neoformans* (synonyms *C. hominis, Torula histolytica*).

Epidemiology

The incidence is worldwide and is high in areas of warmth and moisture.

Signs

Latent: There is a mastitis in many cases with no visible signs in the udder or milk.

Severe: The quarter(s) swells slowly and becomes firm and swollen. The subcutaneous tissue also develops oedema, which persists for several weeks. There is often some discomfort with the legs held apart. Pyrexia occurs up to 40°C (104°F) with anaemia. The supra-mammary lymph nodes are enlarged. Milk production is reduced but the milk itself shows few changes except a few flakes. Later, in persistent cases, there is a watery secretion.

Mild: A swelling of the quarter(s) is seen with little effect on the milk. Occasionally a granulomatous meningoencephalitis may develop or the nasal mucosa may show nodular lesions.

Pathology

Infection is mainly confined to the udder, although there may also be reddening and thickening of the brain tissue and oedema, and naso- or oropharyngeal nodules.

Diagnosis

Diagnosis is by direct examination of the fluids.

Prevention and control

Ensure proper disinfection.

Rhinosporidiasis

Aetiology

The causative organism is *Rhinosporidium seeberi*.

Epidemiology

The disease is distributed worldwide.

Signs

There is the formation of large polyps in the posterior nares and this interferes with respiration. The lesions are small, about 0.5–3cm in diameter. They are soft, friable and bleed. The surface of the polyp shows many small white specks. The nasal discharge results in dyspnoea with mucopurulent and bloody discharge.

Pathology

There is a polyp of papillomatous epithelium, which is hyperplastic and contains numerous sporangia.

Diagnosis

Isolation of the organism provides the diagnosis.

Treatment

Polyps are best removed surgically.

Candidiasis (moniliasis)

Aetiology

The main causal agent is *Candida albicans* but *C. tropicalis*, *C. krusei*, *C. parapsilosis* and *C. guillermondii* can also initiate disease.

Epidemiology

The organisms are worldwide and found in animal faeces.

Signs

A chronic pneumonia can occur with dyspnoea plus only a moderate fever. There is a profuse stringy salivation and brown-streaked nasal discharge. Abortion can occur and there can also be mastitis with mild transient signs that are self-terminating. Where there is severe mastitis it may follow the use of intramammary tubes. The udder is swollen and spongy and the animal's temperature is 40–41.5°C (104–107°F).

Diagnosis

Isolation of the organism provides the diagnosis.

Treatment and control

There is a limit to what can be done but amphotericin B can be successful. An iodine in liquid paraffin intra-mammary infusion can be left in the udder for 10–15 minutes, and then stripped out. This is repeated in seven days, and oral iodides may be given if necessary.

Aspergillosis

Aetiology

There are many *Aspergillus* spp. including *Aspergillus fumigatus*, *A. flavus*, *A. niger* and *A. terreus*.

Epidemiology

The organisms are widespread. Placental infection of cattle is thought to be via abomasal ulcers or from the respiratory tract. It also occurs following inhalation of spores from mouldy straw, hay and sugar beet pulp. Outbreaks of abortions can occur following the feeding of mouldy silage.

Signs

Aspergillosis is a quite common cause of abortion with a placentitis. Abortion is in the sixth to eighth month of pregnancy. Another form is a fatal gastroenteritis with ulceration of forestomachs and oesophagus. Pulmonary aspergillosis also occurs in animals subjected to diarrhoea and poor ventilation. There is fever and dyspnoea.

Diagnosis

Examine placental direct smears for fungi. Culture stomach contents or cotyledon.

Treatment and control

Nystatin can be used in the treatment of diarrhoea. There is no effective preventive but avoid feeding mouldy silage to cows in mid to late pregnancy. Definitely mouldy straw or hay should not be used in enclosed buildings, and preferably not at all.

Histoplasmosis

Aetiology

There are two species causing infection, *Histoplasma capsulatum* and *H. duboisii*.

Epidemiology

Whereas *H. capsulatum* is found worldwide, *H. duboisii* is only found in Africa. It is a rare condition but can occur in man and other species. *Histoplasma capsulatum* is found in the soil. Infection follows inhalation of contaminated dust and entry to the lung.

Signs

Affected cattle may show chronic emaciation, dyspnoea, diarrhoea, swelling of the brisket and grinding of the teeth. At post-mortem examination there is an enlarged liver, ascites, oedematous thickening of the large intestine and interstitial emphysema. Histologically, eosinophilic round bodies can be found in endothelial cells.

Diagnosis

Diagnosis is from the signs, and samples should be taken for culture and histology.

Treatment and control

Amphotericin B given intravenously at 1 mg/kg body weight daily has been effective but a prolonged course may lead to side-effects. The imidazoles may be satisfactory.

Teat burns

Epidemiology

In parts of the world where forest and grass fires are common, burns can result in damage necessitating the slaughter of cattle. However, in other cases the animals will survive but there may be injury to the teats or udder. In such cases it is necessary to provide an accurate prognosis. Often several teats are affected.

Signs

The lesions can be assessed according to the severity of the burn (Morton *et al.*, 1987).

Mild burns: These are reddened with a loss of the outer, white, paper-thin tissue, which sloughs. A teat may have normal tissue interspersed with multiple small black areas over the teat surface or a uniform relatively thick black or red–brown surface layer. There may be areas of sloughing or crusts that develop in the tissue and milk is apparently normal. In all cases the teats are pliable on palpation.

Severe burns: The teats tend to be dull brown or black, dry and often are corrugated. If sloughing has occurred then a thick layer (over 1 mm thick) of tissue is sloughed. Underneath there is red haemorrhagic tissue. On palpation the teat is leather-like and lacks pliability. In some cases the teats tend to be distorted, especially in heifers.

Prognosis

With mild lesions prognosis is good. In severe lesions prognosis is variable but tends to be better in cows than heifers. Some cows only show partial return to function with reduced milk flow.

Treatment

Treatment can increase recovery. Application of 0.5 per cent cetrimide in lanolin daily is helpful. However, healing is slow, taking about 14 weeks. When the surface skin starts to peel antibiotic ointment is helpful. Teat orifice restrictions often respond to surgery.

Water availability

Water debility need not necessarily damage cattle in the dry season in semi-arid regions. Some breeds are obviously less susceptible. They are less affected when they are on pastures containing a very low crude protein level. If fed a high plane of nutrition without water, problems could arise, but in practice this is unlikely to occur. The amount of water required varies but is obviously higher in a dairy cow than a beef animal. Animals are capable of being watered only once every three days if necessary but they should not have to walk more than about 2.5 km to it. If water deprivation occurs there is a reduction in milk or meat deposition. If dehydration persists there is circulatory collapse when the level of sodium reaches 170 mEq/l.

Heat stress (see Chapter 8)

Acute heat stress

If the heat produced by the animal and the heat absorbed from the atmosphere are higher than the heat lost then the animal's temperature will rise. It thus develops hyperthermia and if the rise is great and sudden the animals will pant, salivate excessively, become restless and then prostrate. Problems often occur if cattle are made to walk long distances. Heat stroke can occur at a normal outside temperature if animals are packed tightly in poorly ventilated vehicles travelling during the hottest parts of the day.

If action is not quick death occurs. Affected animals should be sprayed with cold water. They should be kept in the shade and attempts made to increase the air flow. Clipping the hair, particularly along the mane, withers and backbone, will assist but such animals are then susceptible to direct sunlight and so they should be kept in the shade.

Chronic heat stress (see Chapter 8)

The chronic or subacute form occurs more frequently than acute heat stress. When exposed to high temperatures cattle compensate by increasing their loss of heat by panting and sweating. They can also reduce heat production by reducing food intake, drinking more and reducing activity. Cattle are able to accept high midday temperatures if the evenings and nights are cool.

In chronic heat stress there is decreased milk production, reduction in weight gain and sexual maturity. There is also some loss in fertility, particularly involving spermatogenesis in the bull. When animals are affected they should be provided with shelter or otherwise given access to well-ventilated shady areas. Oestrus suppression may also occur. When cattle are grazed in very hot conditions grazing should be restricted to the evenings, nights and mornings. If necessary zero-grazing may need to be adopted. In such circumstances, where the air is hot and humid, then every attempt must be made to ensure good air flow by louvred windows, fans, etc. The cattle should receive an adequate amount of water. Feeding at night will also ensure maximum heat production is during the cool period.

Malignant catarrhal fever

Aetiology

Also known as bovine malignant catarrh and malignant head catarrh. Caused by two different agents but clinically identical. In many countries only one of the agents is present. The African strain, (alcelaphine herpes virus 1 and 2 or bovid herpes virus 3) is wildebeest-associated. The European, North American and Asian strain has not been characterized but is sheep-associated.

Epidemiology

Malignant catarrhal fever (MCF) has a sporadic worldwide distribution. It mainly affects single animals, although outbreaks have occurred. The wildebeest strain is seen in Africa and in zoological gardens. The sheep-associated strain occurs when sheep associate with cattle, which are considered 'dead-end' hosts. The African form is more easily transmitted, transferred via the placenta into the fetus. Soon after birth, the wildebeest calf sheds infection which can be contracted by other species. Transmission of the sheep form is not known, although cattle have usually been in contact with pregnant or lambing sheep. The virus is fragile and does not survive more than a day outside the host. There may be many distinct MCF virus forms.

The incubation period is shorter for the African form. Following infection, there is an eclipse phase of nine to seventeen days, then viraemia continues until death. After a further three to fifteen days, signs develop, followed by death five to ten days after their onset. Transmission is probably by inhalation or possibly blood transfusion.

Signs

Cases are sporadic. Animals are very ill with anorexia, pyrexia (40.5–41.5°C; 105–107°F), depression and loss of condition. An early pathognomonic sign is an intense scleral congestion with bilateral keratitis and corneal opacity starting at the edge of the sclera, causing blindness. Early lesions also involve the buccal mucosa, with reddening of the lips, gingivae and muzzle. Erosions develop, including necrosis of the tips of the labial papillae and the mouth corners.

Other signs vary. They can include nervous signs such as muscle tremors and hyperaesthesia. The superficial lymph nodes are grossly enlarged. There is profuse mucopurulent oculo-nasal discharge which can encrust around the nostrils and eyes. There is often excessive salivation, followed by dyspnoea and stertor due to exudate accumulation. Faeces vary between profuse diarrhoea and soft, scanty faeces. Laminitis and dermatitis can occur in the sheep-associated form.

At later stages, more prominent nervous signs may occur, such as incoordination, leg weakness and nystagmus followed finally in some by head pressing, convulsions or paralysis.

Uncommonly, a mild form occurs with mild, transient fever and some oral and nasal mucosal erosions. These animals can recover.

Necropsy

Lesions occur in many parts of the body including the respiratory, alimentary and urinary tracts. They include varying degrees of haemorrhage, hyperaemia and discrete or extensive erosions. The eyes show scleral congestion and keratitis. The lymph nodes show marked enlargement. The skin around the coronets may show lesions. Histologically, the epidermis shows extensive hydropic degeneration and vesicle formation with rupture. The dermis shows vasculitis with proliferation and necrosis and marked lymphoid cuffing.

Diagnosis

History helps with a record of other species contact and one animal affected. Nervous signs, lymph node enlargement, scleral congestion, corneal opacity and diffuse mucosal erosion are indicators. At necropsy the histological presence of vasculitis confirms diagnosis. There is leukopenia. Serological tests can be used in the African form. Viral isolation or transmission can be attempted.

Differential diagnosis

Differential diagnosis includes mucosal disease, but ocular lesions are not severe and there is no lymph node enlargement. Rinderpest and foot-and-mouth disease are herd problems with no severe ocular lesions. Infectious bovine rhinotracheitis usually affects several animals, with mainly respiratory signs. Calf diphtheria does not produce ocular signs.

Treatment and control

There is no treatment or suitable vaccine. Infected animals should be separated from others. Cattle should not be grazed with sheep, particularly at the time of lambing, nor near wildebeest. Bought-in sheep should come from disease-free farms.

References

Blood, D.C., Radostits, O.M. & Henderson, J.A. (1983) *Veterinary Medicine*, 6th edn, pp. 273–5. Baillière Tindall, London.

Johnson, R. & Jamison, K. (1984) Amyloidosis in six dairy cows. *Journal of the American Veterinary Medical Association*, **185**, 1538–43.

Morton, J.M., Fitzpatrick, D.H., Morris, D.C. & White, M.B. (1987) Teat burns in dairy cattle – the prognosis and effect of treatment. *Australian Veterinary Journal*, **64**, 69–72.

Chapter 54
Major Poisonings

C.J. Giles and A.H. Andrews

Introduction   937
  Diagnosis of poisoning   937
  Relationship between the veterinary clinician and the
    diagnostic laboratory   939
  Principal toxicoses   940
Organophosphate and carbamate poisoning   940
Lead poisoning   944
Ragwort poisoning   945
Bracken poisoning   946
Yew poisoning   947
Copper poisoning   948
Fluoride poisoning (fluorosis)   949
Nitrate/nitrite poisoning   950
Oak poisoning   951

Introduction

The nature of many farming practices such as the widespread and increasing use of agrochemicals and the wide variety of potentially toxic plants, coupled with the innate inquisitiveness of cattle to investigate (often by licking) new or unusual substances, means that many cattle live in a potentially toxic environment. It is perhaps surprising therefore that despite this, incidents of poisoning remain comparatively uncommon in cattle. Most toxic dangers to cattle are well understood and documented. This fact, together with the usually responsible and diligent approach to the handling of toxic chemicals and the correct and proper management of pasture, considerably reduces the risk of cattle gaining access to poisonous substances. Most instances of poisoning arise, therefore, by accident, usually as the result of human error, ignorance, neglect or, rarely, malice. Such errors, of course, may not always be under the direct control of the stockworker, for it may be the actions of a third party, often unconnected with livestock that are to blame for a poisoning incident. As an example, the environment and feed of cattle, like all livestock and indeed humans, may be subjected to the effects of industrial pollution. However, incidents where there is gross contamination of the environment or where an accident results in the release of highly toxic substances are very uncommon and for the maintenance of such a state the livestock farmer, like the population

in general, must rely on the vigilance and safety standards of industry and the monitoring authorities.

Most instances of poisoning in cattle therefore are not the result of large-scale incidents but arise from accidental access by cattle to toxic substances at the local farm level either by cattle moving from a safe to a toxic environment or by the inadvertent introduction by man of a toxicant into the animals' previously safe environment.

Poisoning in cattle can vary greatly in severity, morbidity and mortality. In the most severe cases, where a large number of cattle have consumed toxic quantities of poison very high morbidity and mortality can result. In contrast, mild episodes occur where the clinical effects are transient and few animals suffer harmful effects. Some of such cases are often so insignificant that they are missed or misdiagnosed.

Diagnosis of poisoning

The diagnosis of poisoning in cattle is not easy, as often it is the last thing a clinician will consider when presented with an outbreak of disease and not infrequently it is a subject about which he knows little. In many cases the evidence of intoxication is merely circumstantial, the materials required to establish a definitive diagnosis have long disappeared and in many cases the clinical signs are vague and confusing. However, poisoning incidents are often serious, potentially litigious and hence must always be handled with care and vigilance.

There are essentially three stages in establishing a diagnosis of poisoning:

(1) Recognition that the incident is probably a case of intoxication.
(2) Reaching a presumptive diagnosis of the toxicant or class(es) of toxicant.
(3) Establishing a definitive diagnosis of the intoxication.

It is not possible in many cases for all three stages to be accomplished.

Recognition of apparent intoxication

Rarely is an outbreak of disease in cattle immediately attributable to poisoning on clinical or pathological grounds alone. Before the clinician comes to such an opinion he needs to consider fully the history, epidemiology and clinical signs presented and consider carefully the differential diagnosis in order to exclude the more common non-toxic causes of the condition.

Poisoning incidents should be suspected in the following circumstances:

- The onset of disease is clearly associated with a change in management of the affected animals, for example a change in feed, movement to a new environment or a concurrent agricultural management practice, e.g. spraying or dipping.
- The epidemiology of the disease is not that expected of an infectious disease, for example the condition may quite obviously arise simultaneously in several animals or groups rather than appear to be the result of spread.
- The clinical signs as presented are not typical of the more common infectious, parasitic or metabolic diseases with broadly similar clinical pictures.
- There is circumstantial evidence that animals may have had access to unusual materials.
- The differential diagnosis of the disease as determined by clinical and post-mortem examination includes poisoning as a possible cause.

Presumptive diagnosis of the toxicant

Having established the incident may be a case of intoxication the clinician needs to consider what agent or type of agent might be responsible. In some cases this may be straightforward as the history and circumstantial evidence of poisoning may direct the clinician immediately to the probable cause. More frequently, however, it is far from obvious and requires a detailed consideration of the clinical signs, the post-mortem findings (if appropriate) and the circumstantial evidence. The overall aim should be to answer the question: What possibly could the cattle have had access to that could account for the signs and post-mortem picture as observed? This inquiry needs to be wide-ranging. A full history should always be taken; the clinician should examine the animals in the housing or pasture in which they developed the condition but should not merely concentrate on the animals themselves as it is necessary also to inspect the environment for possible sources of toxicants. It is vital, of course, always to inspect the feed but this should not automatically be viewed as the prime suspect source, although a recent change in feed is strong supportive circumstantial evidence that it may be the source of intoxication. In grazing animals the pasture should be thoroughly inspected for the presence of known toxic plants.

Any recent use of agrochemicals should elicit questioning of farm staff as to their correct usage and the disposal and storage of concentrate. Anything in the environment of the cattle that would not normally be present should be investigated with suspicion; for example, old farm machinery or rubbish left in fields, lead from old batteries and discarded sump oil may be the sources of various toxicants. The water supply must always be critically examined, especially if the supply is provided by means other than a piped mains supply. Could the supply have been contaminated by local dumping of toxic rubbish, or run-off from nitrogenous fertilizers from fields? Only when there is no known indication of local contamination should more distant sources, e.g. industrial sites, be considered.

The clinician's best initial guide to the type of toxicant involved is detailed appraisal of the clinical signs and post-mortem findings, where appropriate, and to correlate these with the known effects of the major types of toxicant (Table 54.1). However, few toxicants produce a clinical picture not shared with other poisons or non-toxic causes and several can produce a wide array of clinical signs.

Establishing a definitive diagnosis

Having attempted to form an opinion as to the type of toxicant involved, the veterinary clinician is now in a position to attempt to reach a definitive diagnosis. To achieve this, in most cases, especially when chemical rather than plant toxicants are involved, he will require the assistance of a diagnostic laboratory. In some cases a routine thorough gross and histological examination by the laboratory may provide strong supportive evidence of the toxicant as may the botanical examination of rumen contents in cases of plant poisoning, but in the majority of instances a definitive diagnosis of poisoning is dependent on the finding, by chemical analysis, of toxicant in the tissues, ruminal or intestinal contents or food of the poisoned animal. The results of such chemical analyses must always be interpreted carefully and in conjunction with the history, clinical picture and post-mortem findings. The question to be answered is: Would the observed level of chemical (as determined by analysis) in the particular tissue at the time of examination account for the signs and disease picture originally observed? Only when this question can be answered in the affirmative can a definitive diagnosis result. This is not always possible, especially with the economic constraints usually imposed on veterinary laboratory examination, and the clinician must view attempts at establishing a definitive diagnosis in this light. The required evidence is often not available; for example, a suspect batch of feed may have long since disappeared and despite a diligent examination the analyst is unable

Table 54.1 Initial linking between clinical abnormality and type of poisoning.

System	Abnormality	Suspected class of poison	
		Chemical	Plant
Alimentary	Diarrhoea	Heavy metals, organophosphates, ionophores	Solanine containing, oak, GI irritants, ragwort
	Colic abdominal pain	Heavy metals, formaldehyde, urea	Oak, GI irritants
	Hypersalivation, vomiting	Organophosphates, urea	GI irritants, rhododendron
Central nervous system	Depression, coma	Ionophores	Oxalate containing, solanine containing
	Hyperexcitability, hyperaesthesia, convulsions	Heavy metals, nitrofurans, organochlorines	Atropine containing
Eye	Mydriasis	Lead	Atropine containing, Hemlock, *Cicuta* sp.
	Miosis	Organophosphates	
	Blindness	Lead	
Respiratory	Dyspnoea	Nitrate/nitrite	Cyanide containing
Skin	Photosensitization		St John's wort, ragwort
	Gangrene		Ergot
Locomotor	Lameness	Fluoride	Ergot
Urinary	Haematuria		Bracken
	Haemoglobinuria	Copper	*Brassica* spp.
			Allium spp.
All	Wasting		Pyrrolizidine containing
	Sudden death		Cyanide containing, yew, water dropwort

GI, gastrointestinal.

to determine a chemical cause of the signs observed. The veterinarian at this stage must conclude the case, after referral if necessary, as merely one of *suspected* intoxication.

Relationship between the veterinary clinician and the diagnostic laboratory

If a significant number of investigations are to be concluded beyond the stage of 'suspected intoxication' by the clinician, a working cooperation must develop between the veterinary clinician and the diagnostic laboratory. Once intoxication is suspected the golden rules are to contact the laboratory earlier rather than later and to take too much material for examination rather than too little. When the clinician suspects intoxication and has concluded the initial clinical and environmental assessments contact should be made with a laboratory experienced in diagnostic toxicology. The clinician should inform the laboratory of the following: history, clinical signs, post-mortem findings (if appropriate) and the results of the environmental assessment, indicating an opinion as to possible toxicants. The clinician must then be guided by the laboratory as to what samples to submit, the size of specimens, how they

Table 54.2 Specimens submitted for toxicological examination.

Tissue	Amount usually required
Serum (separated from clot, not haemolysed)	up to 10 ml
Urine	50 ml
Liver	100 g
Kidney	100 g
Other tissues	100 g
Rumen contents	500 ml
Feed	minimum 100 g

should be packaged or sent and any special instructions. Accompanying all specimens must be the clinical information as above together with details of any treatments given and the time of death. As a general rule, containers should be glass or plastic and tightly sealed, different organs should be packaged separately and no preservative added. As tests for different toxicants require different samples the need for prior discussion between the clinician and the laboratory is paramount. Detailed discussion is not warranted here. Table 54.2 serves as a guide.

Principal toxicoses

There are a vast array of potentially toxic chemical compounds and toxic plants which can, theoretically at least, cause poisoning in cattle due to the fact that they contain known toxic agents and/or have been proven as toxic by experimental observation. In practice, a few principal toxicoses are commonly observed in a given region or country and the majority are rarely, and a few almost never, encountered.

Local, regional and geographic factors greatly influence the importance of the various toxicoses in different regions and countries, so much so, particularly with toxic plants, that attempting to define the principal toxicoses is fraught with difficulty. Nevertheless, certain types of toxicant are encountered much more frequently than others. These common toxicoses, based generally on the position in the UK, are accorded detailed treatment in the text, whereas for those considered of lesser importance a summary of the principal facts is given in Table 54.3.

Organophosphate and carbamate poisoning

The organophosphate compounds are widely-used agrochemicals in agriculture, horticulture and livestock production, and accidental overdosage or overexposure can lead to toxicosis.

Source of toxicant

The principal uses of organophosphates are as insecticides and acaricides, and preparations are made for animal treatment (dusting powders, sprays, washes, dips, pour-on, etc.), sprays for application to plants and granules for application to soil. Carbamates, which have a similar mode of action, are used as molluscicides and herbicides.

Cattle may become poisoned by a variety of methods, principally due to human error, negligence or ignorance. The compounds can be absorbed orally, dermally or by inhalation. Cattle may gain access to stored compounds, they can be mistaken as feed ingredients, and they may also consume treated seed. Containers may be used for feed or water without cleaning. Sprays for pest control in crops may directly contaminate animals or pollute feed or water courses. Inadvertent overdosage can occur with insecticidal sprays, dips or topical pour-on preparations or by a combination of topical and oral therapy or by rapid retreatment.

Signs

The organophosphates and carbamates block the action of cholinesterases (by phosphorylation or carboxyla-tion, respectively) at cholinergic nerve endings and myoneural junctions. The continued presence of acetylcholine at these sites produces continued nerve stimulation and accounts for the clinical signs observed. The time of onset of clinical signs varies with the dose and route of absorption from five minutes to a few hours. Clinical signs are similar for both organophosphate and carbamate toxicoses and are broadly threefold, namely stimulation of the parasympathetic nervous system (muscarinic effects), stimulation of the skeletal muscles (nicotinic effects) and central nervous effects. The muscarinic effects in general precede the nicotinic. The first effects are excessive, followed by profuse salivation. This is accompanied by nasal discharge, cough, dyspnoea, colic, diarrhoea, excessive lacrimation, frequent urination and miosis. These are then joined by the nicotinic signs, muscle fasciculations, stiffness, adoption of a 'saw-horse posture', which then progresses to muscle paralysis. Cattle usually show marked central depression although rarely they may show central nervous excitation. As the condition progresses the muscarinic signs become very pronounced with profuse salivation, severe colic, sweating and dyspnoea progressing to collapse and death. Death is the result of hypoxia due to severe bronchoconstriction with respiratory hypersecretion and irregular slowing of the heart.

Diagnosis

The history and characteristic clinical signs of parasympathetic stimulation are suggestive of poisoning. This will be reinforced if there is circumstantial evidence of exposure to organophosphates or carbamate compounds. Particular attention should be paid to the possibility of inadvertent therapeutic overdosage, for example by combinations of oral and topical exposure. Chemical analysis of blood or tissue for the toxicant is usually of no value due to the fast breakdown of organophosphates; the analysis of contaminated feed or rumen contents is likely to be more successful. However, the preferred method of confirmatory diagnosis is by the determination of the reduction in cholinesterase activity. This test is often performed, for convenience or necessity, on whole blood, but examination of brain tissue is better. The test is a specialized laboratory procedure and the testing laboratory should preferably be consulted before the submission of samples.

Principal differential diagnoses

The respiratory signs may resemble fog fever (p. 866) in which the muscle fasciculations are not, however, usually observed. The syndrome is similar to acute urea

Table 54.3 Summary of the less commonly observed toxicoses of cattle.

Poison	Usual source(s)	Clinical signs	Management guidelines
Aflatoxin	Feeds containing groundnut, cottonseed or maize contaminated with the toxigenic fungi *Aspergillus flavus* and *A. parasiticus*. Growth of toxigenic fungi is only possible when moisture content of stored grain exceeds 15%, feed levels should not exceed 50 ppb.	Reduced feed intake, poor weight gain (or decreased milk yield), inappetence, rough hair coat, reduced resistance to infectious disease. Less commonly acute severe signs may be observed especially in calves less than 6 months, including nervous signs, circling, blindness, convulsions, death.	No specific treatment. Remove all suspect feed, submit samples of feed for analysis (permitted levels of dietary aflatoxin controlled).
Arsenicals	Accidental contamination of feed with inorganic arsenicals or organic (herbicides, pesticides). Formerly in dips and weedkillers, industrial chemicals, horticultural sprays.	Often sudden death. Acute – severe colic, salivation, teeth grinding, weakness, incoordination, rapid collapse and death. Subacute – similar with ruminal stasis, diarrhoea, severe thirst, dehydration, collapse and death.	Rarely successful. Adsorbents orally, sulphur compounds, e.g. dimercaprol (4 mg/kg im) or sodium thiosulphate 15–30 g in 100–200 ml water i.v. and up to 60 g orally (adult).
Atropine-containing plants	Deadly nightshade (*Atropa belladonna*), black or stinking henbane (*Hyoscyamus niger*), thorn apple (*Datura stramonum*).	Those of atropinization, dilation of pupils, dryness of mouth progressing to excitement, incoordination, convulsions and death.	Uncommon, often little can be done; pilocarpine can be given by injection but is not widely available and can itself be dangerous.
Brassica	Conversion of S-methyl cysteine sulphoxide in the plants to dimethyl disulphide. Kale (*Brassica deracea*) fed as fodder crop, rape (*B. napus*) and cultivated cabbages. Usually need to eat kale as sole fodder for about three weeks.	Peracute – collapse and death; acute – haemaglobinuria, pallor, weakness, jaundice, tachycardia, diarrhoea, low haematocrit. Heinz–Ehrlich bodies in RBCs. Can be fatal. Within a group usually a high prevalence of subclinical anaemia.	Stop feeding kale, blood transfusion, vitamin injections, iron. Feed good quality hay before and as well as kale.
Cyanide	Cyanide release by hydrolysis from cyanogenetic glycosides in plants including cherry laurel (*Prunus laurocerasus*), linseed cake, sudan and sorghum grasses, couch grass, white clover.	Dyspnoea, bright red mucosae, recumbency, convulsions, opisthotonus, rapid death. Often less acute; depression, staggering, muscle tremor, dyspnoea, death within 2 h, fresh blood is bright red.	Inject sodium nitrite 16 mg/kg iv followed by sodium thiosulphate (40 mg/kg iv). Repeat only thiosulphate, 30 g doses of sodium thiosulphate orally.
Ergot	Ergots (sclerotia of *Claviceps purpurea*) are found on rye and also on other cereal grains and rye grasses particularly in warm wet seasons.	Acute (convulsive) rare – depression, staggering, blindness, convulsions. Chronic (gangrenous) – lameness, abnormal gait, extremities swollen, reddened, gangrenous, particularly tail, ear tips, distal limbs.	Remove from feed source, avoid heavily ergotized pastures or uninspected stored grain following warm wet summers.
Formaldehyde (formalin)	Formalin used for agricultural purposes, e.g. foot baths. Usually associated with a lack of available drinking water.	Mild – salivation, inflammation of buccal mucosae. Severe – dullness abdominal pain, weak pulse, coma, death.	Do not leave cattle unattended near source of diluted formalin. Symptomatic therapy.
Furazolidone (see p. 260)	Accidental overdosage following therapeutic or prophylactic use, improper mixing in milk substitute.	Acute – hyperaesthesia, convulsions, death. Chronic – haemorrhages, necrotic lesions in mouth, dysentery.	Stop administration of furazolidone, sedatives to control hyperaesthesia.
Hemlock; spotted hemlock, *Conium maculatum*	Umbelliferous plant common in wasteland and neglected pasture, characterized by permanganate-coloured spots on stems and mousey odour when crushed. May be eaten when grazing is sparse; palatability decreases as plant gets woody in late summer.	Dilation of pupils, weakness, staggering, muscle tremor, death from respiratory failure.	Avoid contact with plant and overgrazing, especially in early part of the grazing season.

contd.

Table 54.3 *Continued*

Poison	Usual source(s)	Clinical signs	Management guidelines
Hemlock; water hemlock, cowbane, *Cicuta virosa*	Plant grows in wet ditches and on edges of ponds and swamps. Contains the very toxic cicutotoxin, the roots being the most dangerous.	Dilated pupils, frothing at the mouth, abdominal pain, violent convulsions, rapid death.	None, awareness of the potential danger.
Mercury	Organic mercury compounds from grain dressed with fungicide, no longer common due to control of seed dressings.	May not appear for three to four weeks after feeding dressed grain; inappetence, blindness, staggering, weakness, nervous signs.	Poisoned animals can be treated with sodium thiosulphate (20 mg/kg i.v. and orally) or dimercaprol (BAL) 2.5–5 mg/kg iv 4× daily.
Metaldehyde	Molluscicide for slug/snail control.	Incoordination, hyperaesthesia, salivation, tremor, dyspnoea, fever, ataxia, convulsions, opisthotonus, cyanosis, death.	Sedation or anaesthesia to control hyperaesthesia and convulsions. Consider rumenotomy.
Molybdenum	High soil levels on teart pastures, exacerbated by low copper and high sulphate levels. Induces a relative copper deficiency; high dietary molybdenum and low available copper are interlinked.	Diarrhoea, often green or black with offensive odour, depigmentation, poor condition, stiff gait in young, anaemia, osteoporosis, fractures, poor milk yield.	Test group for low blood copper, careful administration of copper supplements or injections. A perennial problem on known pastures and prophylactic measures should be introduced.
Ionophores (monensin, salinomycin, lasalocid)	Accidental overdosage or incorrect mixing in cattle diets.	Anorexia, depression, diarrhoea, ataxia, recumbency, dyspnoea, can be fatal. Signs develop in up to two days or longer with lower toxic doses.	History of recent access to changed feed useful in presumptive diagnosis. Feed assays, remove ionophore from feed of affected group, ensure correct levels in feed.
Onion, wild garlic, *Allium* sp.	Large quantities of unwanted onions fed to stock, access to wild garlic in woodlands.	Haemolytic anaemia, haemoglobinuria, pallor, possibly jaundice. Can be fatal.	Remove from source, feed well, multivitamin and iron by injection.
Organochlorine compounds	Accidental access or overexposure to insecticides for animal or agricultural use.	Acute and chronic syndromes occur – abdominal problems and typically salivation, incoordination, muscle tremor, clonic spasms, convulsions, possibly aimless or frenzied movements, clonic–tonic convulsions, collapse, death.	Give adsorbents orally and/or wash skin contamination with soap and water. Control excitation with pentobarbitone or sedatives. Exposure of food-producing animals to these chemicals may result in high and persistent tissue residues, particularly in fat.
Oxalate-containing plants	Unwilted leaves of sugar beet, fodder beet, mangels, also fat hen (*Chenopodium album*), docks and sorrells (*Rumex* sp.). Oxalate is detoxified by ruminal microflora and hence previous sublethal exposure will increase tolerance to oxalate. Large quantities of unwilted leaves need to be consumed over a short period.	Rapid ingestion of soluble oxalates induces hypocalcaemia, paresis, muscle tremor, recumbency, coma, death. Ill-thrift due to chronic renal damage.	Treatment of clinical cases with calcium borogluconate as in milk fever. The response is not as certain and is often unsuccessful. Affected forage should be introduced gradually, is best fed wilted, and not as the sole feed source.
Plants causing gastrointestinal signs	In addition to those described elsewhere there are a large number of hedgerow and wild plants which will induce salivation, colic and diarrhoea, these include: cuckoo pint (*Arum maculatum*), black bryony (*Tamus communis*), autumn crocus (*Colchium autumnale*), monkshood (*Aconitum napellus*), hellebores (*Helleborus* sp.), buttercup (*Ranunculus* sp.), spindle tree (*Euonymus europaeus*), white bryony (*Bryonia dioica*), dog's mercury (*Mercurialis perennis*), box	Generally salivation, teeth grinding, abdominal pain, severe diarrhoea, may be accompanied by nervous signs. Fatal in some cases.	Uncommon, symptomatic treatment of colic and diarrhoea, remove from access to suspect plants.

Table 54.3 *Continued*

Poison	Usual source(s)	Clinical signs	Management guidelines
	(*Buxus sempervirens*), greater celandine (*Chelidonium major*), charlock (*Sinapis arvensis*).		
Plants causing photosensitization (see p. 884)	St John's wort (*Hypericum perforatum*) is a common plant in hedgerows and rough grazing and is the most frequently implicated in primary photosensitization. It contains the photodynamic hypericin which is retained when dried. Buckwheat (*Fagopyrum esculentum*) is also photodynamic. Several plants including the ragworts (*Senecio* sp.) and bog asphodel (*Narthecium ossifragium*) cause secondary photosensitization following liver damage.	Photosensitization, erythema, swelling, necrosis of skin in white areas only, pruritus, oedema, later sloughing and self-inflicted injury.	House animals out of direct sunlight, debride raw areas, protect against infection and blowfly strike.
Rhododendron	*Rhododendron ponticum* grows as a cultivated shrub but also extensively in the wild on acid soils where it can form large thickets. Poisoning usually occurs when hungry cattle break out into woodland or gardens or from hedge clippings dumped in fields.	Salivation, staggering gait, abdominal pain, collapse, death in a few days. Projectile vomiting, green froth around mouth.	Symptomatic treatment, purgatives, ensure adequate fencing of stock. Rumenotomy?
Selenium (see p. 305)	Toxic levels of selenium may accumulate in certain plants including certain forage plants and grasses growing on high selenium soils. Increased levels may occur accidentally in feeds; the diet should contain under 5 ppm.	Acute (rare) – blindness, depression, circling, head-pressing, colic, paralysis, death. Chronic – loss of condition, lameness, emaciation, hair loss from base of tail, hoof damage.	Test forage for selenium levels and withdraw suspect feed (>5 ppm is suspect). Levels in blood >2 ppm indicate excessive exposure.
Solanine-containing plants	Plants of the genus *Solanum*. Green tubers and leaves of the potato (*S. tuberosum*). The woody nightshade (*S. dulcamara*) is common in hedgerows; this plant together with the black nightshade (*S. nigrum*) are common in neglected pasture. All parts of the nightshades are toxic, the berries being the most dangerous.	Salivation, dyspnoea, diarrhoea, depression, prostration, coma. Can be fatal.	Symptomatic treatment, green potatoes should not be fed to livestock but boiling and feeding at less than 25% of diet reduces risk.
Tremorgenic mycotoxins	Certain fungi of the genera *Penicillium* and *Aspergillus* which grow at the base of the grass sward produce tremorgens. Toxicity is most likely to occur in hot, dry summers with cattle grazing at the bottom of the grass plant.	'Ryegrass staggers', usually not observed until animals are disturbed, muscular tremors, stumbling, swaying; when forced to run develop a high-stepping gait, staggering, sternal recumbency, will then recover if left undisturbed.	Recovery is usually uneventful when removed from suspect pasture and given alternative feed.
Urea	Inadequate mixing or diluting of dietary urea, accidental access to concentrated amounts, feeding to unadapted animals, or with high-fibre, low-energy rations. Overconsumption of urea-containing blocks or licks.	Begin within 1 hour, excessive salivation, frothing at mouth, bellowing, bloat, muscle fasciculations particularly of the head, colic, dyspnoea, death.	Drenching with vinegar (4–7 l daily) together with cold water (20–40 l). Ensure adequate mixing of urea, continuous access is preferred; tolerance will build up in cattle accustomed to urea feeding, but is short-lived on withdrawal.
Water dropwort (*Oenanthe crocata*)	Root tubers from the plant which grows commonly in ditches and marshes. Usually exposed tubers on pasture following ditching or drainage operations.	Often sudden death, salivation, dilated pupils, convulsions, death.	No treatment, awareness of potential danger to grazing animals when ditches are cleared.

poisoning (p. 943), and it may clinically resemble nitrate toxicosis (p. 950) but without the cyanotic mucosae. The nicotinic effects may resemble hypomagnesaemia (pp. 253, 787).

Treatment and prevention

Atrophine sulphate is the specific antidote to organophosphate or carbamate toxicosis. It acts by blocking the effects of acetylcholine at nerve endings and will thus only counteract the muscarinic effects. The recommended dose is 0.1 mg/kg bodyweight by slow intravenous injection followed by 0.4 mg/kg given subcutaneously. The effects are usually observed within minutes. Treatment may need to be repeated during the first 48 hours depending on clinical response. Cattle should be removed from the suspected source and washed with soap and water if exposed via the skin. Intestinal adsorbents such as activated charcoal given by drench or stomach tube are also useful. Prevention is dependent on recognition of the wide diversity of uses of organophosphates and carbamates in the environment and the possibility of accidental exposure or overdosage.

Lead poisoning (see also p. 906)

Poisoning by lead is one of the most common intoxications of cattle, which are more susceptible to this toxicant than other farm species.

Sources of toxicant

There are many potential sources of lead in the environment and accidental access by cattle to a lead-containing product is the usual predisposing cause which, combined with their natural inquisitiveness and a tendency to lick foreign objects, means that a toxic dose is soon ingested. Common sources of lead include old flaking paint, batteries, discarded engine sump oil, grease, putty, plumber's materials, linoleum and mine washings. Grass from verges of heavily used roads can also contain significant amounts of lead from leaded petrol. Lead poisoning is more frequently observed in calves than adults. Poisoning can result from a single ingestion of a toxic amount or from a continued ingestion of lead from the environment with accumulation in the body tissue.

Signs

The onset of disease and, to some extent, the clinical picture that ensues depends on the dose of lead ingested. Both neurological and gastrointestinal signs

are seen. Ingestion of large quantities, particularly by calves, tends to lead to an acute syndrome with the neurological signs predominating. Ingestion of lesser amounts results in a subacute pattern. In very acute cases sudden death may be the presenting sign. Acute cases are characterized by sudden onset of muscle fasciculations, particularly of the head and neck, frothing at the mouth, teeth grinding, jaw champing and abnormal movements of the head and eyelids. There is a staggering gait and apparent blindness with pupillary dilation. Colic may be observed. This may progress to collapse, tonic/clonic seizures, hyperaesthesia and death. In adults, abnormal patterns of behaviour, including pushing through fences, charging or mania can be seen.

Subacute cases are dull and anorexic and are apparently blind. There may be aimless wandering, there is muscular tremor and a staggering gait, tooth grinding, signs of colic and a ruminal stasis resulting in constipation followed by diarrhoea. The palpebral eye reflex is absent. Rarely, a more chronic form may be observed with poor growth and anaemia.

Necropsy

In very acute cases there may be no gross lesions but the lead-containing material, such as flaked paint, oil or grease, may be found in the reticulum and rumen. In less acute and subacute cases lesions of the gastrointestinal tract are frequently observed including abomasitis and enteritis. The liver and kidneys may be abnormally pale and show some degeneration. There are frequently epicardial and sometimes endocardial haemorrhages. The brain may be oedematous. Histological changes may be observed in the brain depending on the length of exposure. The hepatic and renal cells may also show degeneration.

Diagnosis

Often the history and circumstantial evidence (suspected lead-containing material in the environment) strongly support a tentative diagnosis of lead poisoning particularly when the neurological signs are observed in calves. This being the case treatment should be instituted immediately, a successful outcome of which is highly supportive of the diagnosis. A confirmatory diagnosis in the live animal rests on a measurement of blood lead levels. A heparinized blood sample should be submitted, and levels in excess of 0.4 ppm are considered diagnostic. From the dead animal, kidney, liver and stomach contents should be submitted. Measurement from the kidney is most reliable and levels in excess of 20 ppm are diagnostic.

Principal differential diagnoses

In the absence of compelling circumstantial evidence of poisoning, lead intoxication can closely resemble several other disorders of calves characterized by neurological signs. These include infections, e.g. listeriosis (p. 904), *Haemophilus somnus* infection, brain abscess, rabies, coccidiosis (p. 282), together with hypomagnesaemia, tetanus, cerebrocortical necrosis (pp. 261, 903), vitamin A deficiency, other poisoning (e.g. mercury) (p. 942) and in older animals nervous acetonaemia (p. 794) and bovine spongiform encephalopathy (BSE) (p. 909).

Treatment and prevention

Treatment is threefold: (i) supportive and symptomatic, (ii) oral salts to precipitate soluble lead and (iii) intravenous administration of lead-chelating agents, which can increase by up to 50 times the rate of lead excretion.

Convulsions and nervous signs can be controlled by the use of tranquillizers and sedatives including acepromazine and xylazine. Magnesium sulphate, egg whites and strong tea will precipitate any soluble lead remaining in the gut as insoluble salts of lead. Calcium disodium edetate should be given by slow intravenous injection at a dose of 110–220 mg/kg body weight. This dose should preferably be divided between two or three separate injections per day. Treatment should be given for two to three days, withheld for two days and then repeated, repeating this pattern again if necessary. Good nursing care and oral fluid replacement is required to combat dehydration. Clinical improvement may take two or three days to be apparent and blindness can persist for up to three weeks. Prevention of poisoning by lead is largely a matter of education of those responsible for the care of livestock. A knowledge of the common lead-containing commodities and the need to be vigilant about accidental access should be stressed.

Ragwort poisoning

Poisoning of cattle by the pyrrolizidine alkaloids found in certain genera of plants is a common problem in many parts of the world and can result in severe losses.

Sources of toxicant

The principal genus of plants containing pyrrolizidine alkaloids is *Senecio* of which there are in excess of 1200 species. The quantity and type of alkaloid varies between species, for example the widespread groundsel (*Senecio vulgaris*) is much less harmful than the most important single species the common or tansy ragwort (*S. jacobaea*). In temperate regions the ragwort is widespread in wasteland and neglected pastures and poses a serious potential toxic threat to livestock. Plants of the genera *Crotalaria*, *Heliotropium* and *Amsinckia* also contain the toxic alkaloids.

Circumstances of poisoning

Common ragwort is not attractive to grazing animals and cattle will usually avoid eating the fresh vegetative plant. However, this is not always the case and should never be relied upon. The plant is relatively late in emerging through the sward in the spring and, particularly following widespread seeding from the previous year, small, young plants can become finely distributed within the grasses. This is then non-selectively grazed. In dry conditions and where grass growth is poor, cattle may also be attracted to ragwort. The unattractiveness of the plant is lost, but its toxicity largely retained, when it is dried in hay or ensiled and this represents the single most important cause of intoxication. Cattle will readily consume hay or silage containing ragwort.

Pathogenesis

The pyrrolizidine alkaloids are hepatotoxic, damaging the hepatocytes. The speed at which this cell damage occurs and the consequences thereof are dependent on the dose of alkaloid and the duration of consumption. The liver has a large functional reserve and thus can withstand the functional loss of many hepatocytes before gross dysfunction occurs. An animal would therefore only rarely ever ingest sufficient quantities of alkaloids over a sufficiently short period to result in acute poisoning. Much more commonly cattle will ingest smaller amounts of the toxicant over a period of weeks or even months resulting in a more gradual loss of hepatocyte function, it only being when the functional reserve of the organ has been exceeded that gross hepatic dysfunction and hence clinical disease results.

Signs

The clinical picture can vary: although the principal cause is a subacute to chronic intoxication, acute clinical syndromes may be observed, although more usually a subacute pattern is seen in cattle. Affected cattle will lose weight and usually develop a mild to moderate jaundice, and may show photosensitization. Diarrhoea, colic and straining characteristically occur. Subcutaneous oedema and ascites may be present due to hypoalbuminaemia. Affected cattle are usually dull and depressed. They may show signs of hepatic encephalopathy, resulting from the effects of raised blood ammonia levels on the brain due to the inability of the damaged liver adequately to remove urea arriving via the portal circulation. Signs of encephalopathy include an unawareness of surroundings, staggering gait, aimless wandering, circling and apparent blindness. Head pressing and aggressive syndromes are rare in cattle. Death usually occurs a few days after the commencement of such clinical signs.

Necropsy

The carcass may be jaundiced and in poor condition, and ascites may be present. The liver is characteristically shrunken, fibrosed, slate-grey or mottled. The histological picture of the liver in pyrrolizidine alkaloid toxicosis is characteristic and highly suggestive of the condition but not pathognomonic. The lesions are a fine pericellular cirrhosis, bile duct proliferation and hepatocytomegaly.

Diagnosis

The history and circumstantial evidence are extremely important. It is vital to understand the chronic nature of the intoxication; in most cases animals will often have eaten the plants for several weeks or months prior to the development of clinical signs. Bearing this in mind, examination of hay, silage and pasture for the plants is vital, but their absence does not necessarily eliminate pyrrolizidine alkaloid toxicosis unless a history of an unchanged, uncontaminated diet can be positively established. Histological examination of the liver is the method of choice in establishing a diagnosis and, in the live animal, liver biopsy is the most useful diagnostic aid. Serum biochemistry will usually demonstrate an elevation of γ-glutamyl transferase (GGT), and in some cases an elevation in aspartate amino-transferase (AST). Chemical analysis for the alkaloids is not often of value.

Principal differential diagnoses

Particularly where hepatic encephalopathy is marked, ragwort poisoning can resemble rabies, BSE (p. 909), brain abscess/tumour (p. 902), encephalomyelitis (p. 901) or lead poisoning (pp. 906, 944). Where wasting, jaundice and diarrhoea are the dominant clinical signs, intestinal parasitism (p. 267), fascioliosis (p. 276), hepatitis and biliary obstruction should be considered.

Treatment and prevention

Once the clinical picture has developed there is no worthwhile treatment for pyrrolizidine alkaloid toxicosis, but clinically normal cattle in the same group should be immediately switched to a non-contaminated food supply. Prevention relies upon control of the plant and an understanding of the syndrome. Hand pulling and burning of plants before seeding and the use of herbicide sprays is to be recommended on affected pastures. Sheep are less susceptible than cattle and can often graze affected pasture or eat hay if not too heavily contaminated. Hay or silage should never be prepared from ragwort-infested grassland.

Bracken poisoning

The bracken fern (*Pteridium*) is widely distributed in the UK, the USA and in many other temperate hilly and forested areas. It can relatively quickly become dominant in a grassland pasture. Where cattle have continued access to bracken-contaminated grazing, toxicosis can result.

Source of toxicant

Cattle are often reluctant to eat bracken and will usually only do so when grassland grazing is sparse. Cattle need to graze bracken as a significant constituent of the diet for several weeks or months before clinical disease may become apparent. The rhizomes, exposed after ploughing of bracken-infested pasture, are more attractive and dangerous as are newly sprouted young fronds. Some of the toxicity remains when bracken becomes dried in hay. Bracken contains a thiaminase but, unlike the situation in herbivorous non-ruminants, cattle are largely unaffected by it. Bracken also contains a variety of other toxic chemicals including a cyanogenetic glycoside (which is only usually present in harmless amounts), toxins that depress bone marrow and a carcinogen (ptaquiloside). These last two can cause disease in cattle.

Signs

Acute poisoning: Acute or subacute toxicosis is the result of bone marrow depression producing leucopenia and thrombocytopenia and occurs following consumption of comparatively large amounts of bracken. Clinical signs may develop for up to several weeks after the exposure to bracken has ended. Signs may be sudden in onset and include anorexia, depression and dysentery, and there may be pyrexia; various signs of capillary fragility and haemorrhage become obvious including petechiae on mucosae, bleeding from nose, vagina and conjunctiva. Trauma may produce haematomata. Heart and respiratory rates are increased. Progressive weakness ensues and death may occur in one to five days. In calves there is often pyrexia, dysentery, frank haemorrhage and petechiation of visible mucosae. Death is often the result of heart failure. There may be laryngeal oedema and marked dyspnoea. Due to the leucopenia, a bacteraemia or other secondary infections are often complications.

Enzootic haematuria: Where cattle have consumed comparatively small quantities of bracken over prolonged periods, neoplastic changes can develop in the transitional cell epithelium of the bladder. Various tumour types may occur including haemangiomas, transitional cell carcinomas, adenocarcinomas and haemangiosarcomas. The resulting clinical picture is termed enzootic haematuria. The condition varies from a mild, persistent haematuria as the only clinical sign to severe cases in which there is pallor of the mucosae, dysuria and tenesmus. The urine in severe cases has visible blood clots in it (see p. 154).

Upper alimentary squamous cell carcinoma (see also p. 828): A third less common clinical syndrome resulting from prolonged exposure to bracken is upper alimentary squamous cell carcinoma, which may accompany changes or tumour formation in the bladder wall. The disease has strong regional incidence, e.g. in western Scotland and Wales, often in suckler cows. Four clinical syndromes are recognized depending on the site of tumour formation. Oropharyngeal tumours produce loss of condition, drooling of saliva, coughing or snoring, halitosis. The nasal discharge may contain ingesta, submandibular lymphadenopathy and diarrhoea. Oesophageal tumours produce diarrhoea, halitosis, coughing, drooling and palpable masses in the oesophagus. Ruminal tympany can result from tumours in the lower oesophagus; there is initially intermittent bloat with loss of condition, then diarrhoea and resistance to the passage of a stomach tube. Tumours in the dorsal rumen produce loss of condition, diarrhoea, distended abdomen and bloat. Oropharyngeal papillomas may often accompany tumours at any site.

Diagnosis

This is based on the clinical signs and an association with bracken feeding or of prolonged exposure to bracken. In acute or subacute cases, bone marrow depression results in thrombocytopenia and leucopenia, prolonged bleeding time and clot formation time.

Necropsy

In acute or subacute cases there are multiple internal haemorrhages of varying size and petechiation. The bone marrow is pale. Tumour changes are evident in the bladder wall and/or carcinomas may be found in the upper alimentary tract.

Principal differential diagnoses

Acute disease can resemble leptospirosis, kale anaemia, or babesiosis. Enzootic haematuria should be differentiated from babesiosis (p. 748) and postparturient haemoglobinuria (p. 792). The syndromes caused by upper alimentary squamous cell carcinoma can resemble Johne's disease (p. 857), copper deficiency (p. 298) and mucosal disease (p. 853).

Treatment and prevention

In acute cases the clinical outcome is probably more influenced by the degree of bone marrow damage than by treatment. Broad-spectrum antibiotics should be administered to counteract bacteraemia and secondary infections. Blood transfusions can be considered. The use of bone marrow stimulants including DL-batyl alcohol has been described. There is no successful therapeutic management of urinary bladder or alimentary neoplasia. Despite its widespread abundance in certain areas the bracken fern should always be viewed as a potentially toxic plant to cattle. Access to bracken-infested pasture should be always limited, especially if grass growth is poor. In particular, cattle should never be allowed access to recently ploughed land with bracken present and where the rhizomes are exposed, especially if they have started to reshoot. Limited areas of bracken infestation can be fenced off, and burning, ploughing and reseeding or herbicide control are all measures that can reduce the level of bracken contamination.

Yew poisoning

Cattle that gain access to yew trees (genus *Taxus*) are frequently fatally poisoned.

Sources of toxicant

The various species of yew (*Taxus baccata*, English yew; *T. lineata*, Irish yew; *T. cuspidata*, Japanese yew) are common ornamental trees or hedgeing plants particularly of old established gardens. The leaves and woody twigs of the yew contain various toxic alkaloids collectively termed taxines. The taxines are also present in the seeds but not the fleshy red outer part of the fruit.

Circumstances of poisoning

Yew is well known as a toxic plant among the agricultural and rural community, and poisoning is thus usually the result of neglect, ignorance or (rarely) malice. Cattle will often consume the fresh plant if they are allowed access and will also eat fresh hedge clippings or trimmed branches dumped into their field. The taxines are severe cardiac depressants.

Signs

If moderate amounts of yew have been ingested, sudden death is often the presenting sign. If seen alive, cattle may show dyspnoea, abdominal pain, muscle tremor, weakness and collapse. The pulse later becomes slower before finally disappearing with the heart stopping in diastolic arrest. Recovery is rare and is dependent on ingesting only relatively small amounts of the plant.

Necropsy

Frequently, there are no significant gross findings except the presence of yew leaves and twigs among the ruminal contents or sometimes still in the mouth. The characteristic leaves of the yew when separated by careful washing from the general ruminal contents are thus highly suggestive of poisoning.

Diagnosis

History or circumstantial evidence of access to yew, and presence of leaves and twigs in the rumen contents will usually establish a diagnosis.

Principal differential diagnoses

Yew poisoning should be distinguished from other causes of sudden death, for example lightning strike (p. 930), anthrax (p. 717), blackleg (p. 723), etc.

Treatment and prevention

There is no specific therapy. Symptomatic treatment can be offered to clinically affected animals but the likelihood of recovery or death is principally influenced by the amount of the plant already ingested. Rumenotomy is possible immediately after observing cattle consuming yew. Generally, yew is well known as a toxic plant but the necessity of preventing cattle from gaining access to the plant should be constantly stressed.

Copper poisoning (see p. 300)

Sources of toxicant

The normal problem is an extensive intake of copper, usually from the diet and particularly where there is an absence of uptake inhibitory factors such as molybdenum, iron or sulphur. The acute form follows a single large dose of copper, but more commonly it is the result of mineral ingestion over a long period of time. The copper is retained and accumulates within the liver. It has also been seen with improper use of copper supplements. Some problems have arisen from industrial contamination, and from copper addition to the pasture. There are some areas in the world with copper-rich soil. While the problem of copper poisoning is common in sheep, it is much less seen in cattle. Problems have increased in North America, Britain and other countries in recent years.

Circumstances of poisoning

Cattle are less susceptible to copper toxicity than sheep and are able to ingest higher levels than the latter without any deleterious effect. Animals with intercurrent liver disease may be more susceptible. Chronic intoxication occurs when there is a build-up of the element within the liver until the maximum level which the organ can contain is exceeded. Then the copper is released into the blood and causes an acute intravascular haemolytic crisis. Problems of copper intoxication were reported to be increasing in the first years of the twenty-first century (Bidewell et al., 2000). In their findings grossly increased copper intakes were not always found. However, points to consider include the duration of feeding a copper supplement and the type of supplement (it is claimed that the copper in many amino acid chelated minerals is many more times available than that in inorganic compounds). Jerseys have been said to be more susceptible, possibly because of genetic susceptibility or perhaps related to a lower bodyweight.

Signs

The problem can be either acute, which is rare, or chronic. The latter is more common but often also appears as a sudden presentation.

Acute: The animal shows pronounced depression with colic, rapid collapse and death. In some cases there is a green diarrhoea when the animal has had access to the excess copper within the diet.

Chronic: The average length of illness before death is one to three days, although individual animals may show signs for up to three weeks. There is an acute haemolytic crisis following a prolonged access to excess copper. The signs again often rapidly develop with anorexia, depression, rumen stasis, cold extremities, haemolytic jaundice, anaemia with pale mucous membranes, cyanosis of the teats, haemoglobinuria, methaemoglobinaemia and death. Some animals have shown abortion, ataxia, photosensitization and other signs. Recumbency is common before death.

Necropsy

In acute cases there is a severe gastroenteritis with ulceration and erosion. The abomasum is particularly affected. The chronic signs are those of a haemolytic crisis. Jaundice is present but may be variable in degree; there is hepatomegaly. In sheep there is usually dark discoloration of the kidneys, but this is not so common in cattle. Histologically there is a necrotizing hepatopathy and nephropathy.

Diagnosis

The signs and post-mortem picture are helpful. Usually there will be a known source of copper which has been ingested, although this may not always be the case. The liver will contain more than 8000 μmol/kg dry matter (DM) (although often levels are between 10000 and 20000 μmol/kg DM). Plasma copper levels are usually very high (normally over 50 μmol/l). Blood biochemistry usually shows elevated liver enzymes such as aspartate aminotransferase, glutamate dehydrogenase and gamma glutamyl transferase, and this assists in diagnosis.

Principal differential diagnoses

Nitrate poisoning (see p. 950) may need to be eliminated. There are also many causes of haemolytic anaemia including babesiosis (p. 948), kale poisoning (p. 941) and post-parturient haemoglobinuria (p. 792). In most cases the history should be helpful. However, the use of blood copper examination should provide good evidence of the cause if due to copper toxicity.

Treatment and prevention

First remove the animals from the copper source, if known. While treatment is often of limited value, calcium versanate iv at a dose of 70 mg/kg bodyweight (see p. 945 for details) has been used in calves. Oral sodium thiosulphate at a dose of 1 g daily has resulted in some recoveries. Oral ammonium thiomolybdate at 100 to 400 mg daily can also be of use. In sheep, iv injection of ammonium tetrathiomolybdate at a dose of 2.7 mg/kg bodyweight on three to six occasions at intervals of two to three days has been successfully used. While not licensed, it might also be of benefit to cattle.

If cattle are suspected of having a copper deficiency, blood samples should be taken to estimate the copper levels before any supplementation is given. The normal minimum dietary copper level for adult dairy cattle is 12 mg/kg dietary DM. This level often has to be raised, especially where there are inhibitory factors present such as molybdenum (see p. 298). However, in many countries there are restrictions on the amount of copper supplementation. Thus in Britain the Medicated Feedingstuffs Regulations allow dairy cattle to receive up to 35 mg/kg dietary DM (about 800 mg copper/head per day) without restriction. However, higher supplementation levels can be licensed up to a maximum of 2000 mg/head per day, but with certain restrictions.

Fluoride poisoning (fluorosis)

At normal levels the ingestion of fluorides causes no harm or is even beneficial to cattle. However, at higher levels a chronic (or rarely acute) intoxication results.

Sources of toxicant

Cattle normally gain access to excess fluoride from grazing contaminated pasture. Historically, this commonly arose from industrial effluent, for example from brick manufacture, aluminium smelters, steel works or phosphate production. More recently, other sources of excess fluoride have been recognized including geothermal spring water (when used either as a source of drinking water or for pasture irrigation) and high fluoride-bearing soils. Inorganic rock phosphate is often highly toxic and requires defluorination prior to use as a phosphorus supplement.

Circumstances of poisoning

Rarely will cattle consume sufficient fluoride to result in acute intoxication, but this may result following heavy pasture contamination. More commonly, the grazing of fluoride-contaminated pasture over months or years results in an insidious chronic disease.

Signs

In the acute disease there is anorexia, depression, restlessness, dyspnoea, excessive salivation and muscle tremor leading to convulsions, collapse and death.

Chronic fluorosis: The developing teeth of young cattle are sensitive to excessive fluoride and dental lesions are common in animals exposed before the full adult dentition has developed. The dental abnormalities observed are: increased attrition and liability to fracture, mottling of enamel with white areas, abnormal pigmentation, and yellow or brown discoloration. Teeth may be poorly developed and mineralized.

Bones are also affected by excessive fluoride intake. Although the bones of young cattle are more susceptible, the bones of cattle of any age can be affected by fluoride-induced changes. These are principally periarticular calcification and the formation of exostoses resulting in an intermittent lameness and stiffness of gait, particularly of the hind legs. Palpable exostoses appear on the metacarpals and metatarsals, ribs and mandible and these are painful on pressure. In severe cases fractures of the third phalanx are not uncommon. Affected cattle are unthrifty and have a dull staring coat.

Necropsy

Dental lesions are found, as described above. Bones have a roughened surface and are chalky white, and new bone formation is evident.

Diagnosis

The history, clinical signs and post-mortem findings, together with circumstantial evidence of access to suspect sources of fluoride, are usually suggestive of fluorosis. Radiographic examination of lower limb bones may demonstrate the presence of exostoses. Chemical analysis of urine, blood and bone for fluorine content may be useful. The levels in bone rise with age and elevated levels are indicative of previous exposure to fluoride. Fluorides are chiefly excreted via the urine and do not accumulate in soft tissues.

Attempts should be made to identify the source of fluoride, and feed, water and pasture analysed for fluoride content. As a guide the diet should contain less than 50 ppm fluorine on a dry matter basis, and drinking water less than 8 mg/l.

Principal differential diagnoses

The dental and bone lesions are fairly characteristic of fluorosis but in their absence other causes of ill thrift including mineral deficiencies, parasitism and the common forms of lameness must be differentiated.

Treatment and prevention

There is no specific antidote and dental lesions are permanent. After removal from the source of excess fluoride the bones of affected cattle will gradually be remodelled, with normal bone deposition ensuing, but severely affected cattle will never completely recover. Mildly affected cattle should be removed from the source and given a good quality balanced diet. Where ingestion of high or suspect levels of fluoride is unavoidable, aluminium sulphate or calcium carbonate added to the diet may be beneficial in reducing fluoride deposition in teeth and bone.

Nitrate/nitrite poisoning

Under certain circumstances various types of grazing and forage crops may accumulate toxic levels of nitrate within their foliage. In addition, the widespread use of inorganic nitrate fertilizers poses a potential threat of nitrate poisoning in grazing cattle.

Source of toxicant

The *Brassica* plants, green cereals (wheat, barley, rye and maize) as well as the *Sorghum* and Sudan grasses, docks, nightshades and sweet clover may accumulate excess levels of nitrate in their tissues. Nitrate accumulation may occur after excessive use of inorganic nitrate fertilizers or following heavy rain after a period of drought, which leaches accumulated nitrate into the water table. Water run-off from heavily fertilized fields or excess application of nitrogenous fertilizers are the commonest dangers in intensively managed pastures and can lead to problems on grassland pasture or even hay made shortly after exposure of the sward to high nitrate levels. Cattle thus become poisoned by consuming normal amounts of the fresh pasture containing the abnormal nitrate load.

Nitrate ions in the rumen are reduced by the ruminal microflora to nitrite ions, which are subsequently absorbed. The nitrite ion oxidizes the iron in haemoglobin (to its ferric state) producing methaemoglobin, which is unable to bind oxygen. A single intake of nitrate over a short period is more toxic than accumulating the same amount over several days or weeks. A degree of tolerance may also build up in stock receiving sublethal amounts over a prolonged period. High grain diets tend to be somewhat protective against the effects of excess nitrate.

Signs

The condition is usually acute, less commonly subacute. In the acute condition, signs are seen within a few hours of consuming high levels of nitrate. The clinical picture is due to methaemoglobinaemia and the associated anoxia. The visible mucosae become blue and cyanotic, the pulse is weak and rapid, there is drooling of saliva and tachypnoea, exercise is resented and, if forced, may result in severe dyspnoea with mouth breathing. If untreated the condition deteriorates, and there is weakness, ataxia, prostration, coma and death. The rapidity of onset of the clinical signs is dependent on the dose consumed; death can occur in one hour or up to a day following acute intoxication.

Necropsy

High methaemoglobin levels impart a chocolate-brown discoloration to the blood, which is seen particularly in the fresh cadaver. This brown coloration is evident throughout the mucosae, viscera and possibly in the urine.

Diagnosis

The history may be suggestive if a link of known exposure to nitrates can be established. The clinical picture and particularly the post-mortem findings are also highly suggestive. Methaemoglobin can be detected in blood but is not stable and a fresh sample needs to be analysed within 4 hours. Alternatively, a sample of heparanized blood can be preserved, consulting the diagnostic laboratory for the preferred method. Nitrate levels in all sources of feed and water should be analysed but tolerance to nitrate may be apparent in some circumstances as described above. Levels in feed in excess of 1 per cent nitrate on a dry matter basis are highly suggestive of intoxication.

Principal differential diagnoses

Circulatory collapse or severe respiratory conditions can result in tissue anoxia and acute cyanosis, but in few other circumstances does methaemoglobinaemia with its characteristic chocolate-brown blood result. Intoxication with chlorates will also result in methaemoglobinaemia.

Treatment and prevention

The animal should be immediately removed from the suspected source of nitrate. The specific antidote is methylene blue, which restores the iron in haemoglobin to its ferrous state thus again allowing oxygenation of the blood and so reversing the tissue anoxia. Methylene blue should be given by intravenous injection at up to 4 mg/kg body weight in a 2 per cent solution. It can be repeated if necessary. Defining the nitrate source and reducing exposure are the key elements in control. Ensiling will usually reduce the nitrate content of forage as will allowing the pasture to age and set seed, since nitrate is found mostly in stems rather than in grain.

Oak poisoning

Poisoning by the various oaks of the genus *Quercus* can be a serious seasonal problem in grazing cattle.

Sources of toxicant

Cattle may be poisoned at any time when they gain access to quantities of oak leaves or acorns, which contain the toxic tannins. Cattle can consume small quantities of acorns or oak leaves without ill effects.

Circumstances of poisoning

In temperate countries the autumn fall of acorns is the principal source. The acorn crop varies considerably from year to year and hence there is wide variation in prevalence. Storms and windy conditions that cause a heavy sudden drop of acorns are also predisposing factors. Cattle may also be poisoned from browsing on new leaves and buds or oak seedlings.

Signs

Although sudden death may be observed, poisoning is usually seen as a subacute condition. Affected cattle become depressed and anorexic. Early on in the disease constipation occurs, often with marked straining perhaps accompanied by groaning and abdominal pain; small, dry faecal pellets may be observed at this stage. Later on this gives way to a dark coloured or tarry diarrhoea often with blood; straining may be persistent and severe. As the condition progresses polyuria and subcutaneous oedema may be observed. Cattle then become progressively weaker and collapse with death supervening in four to seven days from the onset of clinical signs.

Pathogenesis

The tannins are nephrotoxic and damage the renal tubules but the precise mechanism of their action is unclear. There is a necrosis of the renal tubular cells and the consequent renal dysfunction leads initially to oliguria or anuria, later progressing in the subacute to chronic stages of intoxication to polyuria with the production of a very dilute urine.

Necropsy

Gross signs include those of oedema, particularly hydrothorax, ascites and ventral subcutaneous oedema, oedema fluid may contain blood, and there is often perirenal oedema together with swollen pale kidneys.

The contents of the rumen are frequently doughy in consistency and often contain large numbers of acorns and/or oak leaves, although this is not invariable in the more chronic cases. There may often be colitis, with tarry, bloodstained faecal contents. Histologically, the acute renal lesions include hyaline cast formation and a coagulative necrosis of the tubular epithelium; later mononuclear cell infiltration and fibrosis are observed.

Diagnosis

The history and circumstantial evidence of poisoning together with the clinical signs usually strongly suggest a diagnosis of oak poisoning. This is usually confirmed by finding large amounts of acorns and/or oak leaves in the rumen at post-mortem examination together with the characteristic gross and histological changes. In live animals there will be an elevation of serum urea and creatinine, and glucose and protein will appear in the urine.

Principal differential diagnoses

The main differential diagnoses include clostridial infections (Chapter 44) and other toxicoses.

Treatment and prevention

There is no specific antidote. Cattle may survive poisoning by oak but are frequently left with chronic renal damage, such that they will often perform poorly. The only treatment that is likely substantially to affect the outcome of clinical cases is expensive and specialized involving full-scale renal supportive therapy including measurements and adjustment of plasma electrolytes, oral and parenteral rehydration and the re-establishment of diuresis. Rumenotomy may be indicated. Anticipation of potential outbreaks by the recognition of the seasonal nature of the disease in inspection of pastures (particularly if the meteorological conditions would produce a sudden heavy acorn drop) followed by removing cattle from sources of contact is the key to successful prevention.

Reference and further reading

Andrews, A.H. & Humphreys, D.J. (1992) *Poisoning in Veterinary Practice*, pp. 1–114. National Office of Animal Health, Enfield.

Bidewell, C.A., David, G.P. & Livesey, C.T. (2000) Copper toxicity in cattle. *Veterinary Record*, **147**, 399–400.

Adult Cattle
Welfare

Chapter 55
Welfare

D.M. Broom

Public perceptions of the dairy and beef industries   955
The concept of animal welfare   955
Welfare problem areas   956
Ill treatment and neglect   956
Housing and management   957
   General points   957
   Calf welfare   958
Beef cattle welfare   960
The welfare of dairy cows   960
Farm operations   962
Handling, transport and slaughter of cattle   963

Public perceptions of the dairy and beef industries

Most members of the public who are asked about the dairy and beef industries think of cattle grazing in fields and cows living for some time whilst a series of calves are born and milk is produced. Milk products and beef are considered by the public in relation to their effects on human nutrition and health, their effects on the environment and their effects on animal welfare. If production is perceived to be bad in relation to any of these aspects, sales of the products could be severely affected. Bovine spongiform encephalopathy (BSE) resulted in a substantial but sometimes brief decline in beef consumption. Some people may limit their intakes of milk products because of a desire to reduce cholesterol intake whilst certain aspects of the dairy industry, such as methane production, may be criticized in relation to pollution; however, it is animal welfare rather than these topics which is the subject of this paper. Until recently, the welfare of the dairy cow was not often perceived to be poor and it has been only in calf rearing that dairy production systems have been regularly criticized. However, the dairy industry has been changing. Evidence of poor welfare in cows is accumulating and has had influence on public opinion in several countries. It is important to the dairy industry that welfare problems should be addressed before there is any widespread public condemnation of breeding and management practices. Similarly, beef cattle production is not often criticized on welfare grounds. However, a few critical newspaper articles or television programmes which appear well founded can be very damaging to producers, processors and retailers.

Public concern about animal welfare manifests itself in actual product purchasing and in pressure applied to retailers and to legislators. Major supermarket and cooked food chains can be influenced rapidly by customer pressure and can cause changes to be brought about in the methods used by suppliers. Retailers may impose codes of practice on suppliers and the execution of these codes is checked because the retailers cannot afford public criticism of what they sell (Broom, 1999a). In several European countries, certain housing systems and farm practices have been changed by many farmers because of the standards required by the purchasing companies. For example, the use of crates for calves, stalls and tethers for sows, and castration of pigs slaughtered at 100 kg or less has ceased on many farms.

The effect of public pressure on legislation is usually slower, but legislation makes for more equal constraints on producers. Legislation is becoming more and more international although it is clearly important that where there is legislation on wholly moral grounds, for example in order to prevent poor welfare in animals, there should be restrictions on imports from countries whose moral standards are lower and that such restrictions should be authorized by the World Trade Organization.

The concept of animal welfare

Animal welfare has to be defined in such a way that it can be scientifically assessed and the term can be used in legislation and in discussion amongst animal users and the public. Welfare is clearly a characteristic of an individual animal and is concerned with the effects of all aspects of its environment on the individual. The welfare of an animal is its state as regards its attempts to cope with its environment (Broom, 1986). This state includes the feelings of the individual, various physiological and behavioural responses and its health. The extent of the difficulty which the individual has in trying to cope with its environment, the extent of any failure to cope and the degree of happiness are all components

955

Box 55.1 Indicators of animal welfare (after Broom, 2000).

Physiological indicators of pleasure
Behavioural indicators of pleasure
Extent to which strongly preferred behaviours can be shown
Variety of normal behaviours shown or suppressed
Extent to which normal physiological processes and anatomical development are possible
Extent of behavioural aversion shown
Physiological attempts to cope
Immunosuppression
Disease prevalence
Behavioural attempts to cope
Behaviour pathology
Self-narcotization
Body damage prevalence
Reduced ability to grow or breed
Reduced life expectancy

Box 55.2 Possible causes of cattle welfare problems.

Ill treatment
Neglect: calculated, accidental or due to lack of knowledge
Inadequacies in design of housing/furniture
Inadequate management system or poor husbandry on the farm
Unnecessary or poorly executed mutilations of the animals
Poor conditions and procedures:
   during transport
   at market
   at slaughterhouse

of welfare. Hence welfare varies from very poor to very good and can be scientifically assessed (Broom & Johnson, 1993; Broom, 1998a, 1999b).

Indicators of animal welfare are listed in Box 55.1. These include disease prevalence and reduced ability to grow and breed. As explained by Broom and Johnson (1993), the welfare of a diseased individual is poorer than that of an individual which is not diseased, and reduced ability to produce offspring given appropriate opportunities also indicates poor welfare. Individuals which are finding it difficult to cope with their environment, or which are failing to cope, may be more likely to become diseased, less likely to produce embryos, less likely to carry young to term and more likely to die early.

Welfare problem areas

Whilst cattle management has been changing, our knowledge of cattle physiology and behaviour has been improving. It is clear that cattle have complex regulatory processes, elaborate social structure and sophisticated learning ability (Kilgour & Dalton, 1984; Stricklin & Kautz-Scanavy, 1984; Fraser & Broom, 1990). These results have made many animal scientists reconsider the effects of conditions and procedures on farms, both in terms of their efficiency as regards production and with respect to the welfare of the animals.

The general range of welfare problem areas is the same for cattle as for other farm animals (Box 55.2). Ill treatment refers principally to physical abuse of animals. Neglect includes failing to give food and water, or to clean out, or to treat disease or to assist as necessary at calving. Accommodation for animals may, for example, give insufficient space, poor flooring or poor

food access and conditions indoors or outdoors may lead to risk of injury (Schlichting & Smidt, 1987).

Management methods and husbandry include all aspects of feeding, moving of animals, grouping, milking, serving, etc. Mutilations for the benefit of farming practice or of the animal require some special mention, both as regards the methods used and the consequences for the animals. Methods of handling and moving animals are of importance before and after transport, at markets and at lairage as well as on the farm. There are also special problems of transport vehicle construction and usage, market accommodation and procedures, and slaughter methods. Welfare problems that should be taken into account in cattle practice have been reviewed by Broom (1988).

Ill treatment and neglect

Human actions that can lead to poor cattle welfare include ill treatment, neglect and inadequate production systems. Ill treatment occurs most frequently when animals are being moved around the farm, when they are being loaded into or out of vehicles, or when they are at market or lairage. Those who do ill treat animals can be advised of likely economic effects of their actions as well as being told about the laws on the subject. Neglect includes failure to provide an adequate diet, failure to treat disease and the lack of normal husbandry procedures. The diet may be inadequate in nutrient composition or in quantity. Cattle are sometimes undernourished for a period, whilst food is scarce or expensive, with the expectation that compensatory growth will occur when more food is provided. If the undernourishment amounts to starvation and this is clear from the condition of the animal, then this is serious neglect. Lack of knowledge on the part of the farmer may result in the provision of a poor diet or in failure to treat disease. This is poor husbandry, a very important cause of welfare problems. Advice on good husbandry methods can be an important veterinary service. If animals are diseased and require treatment there is a moral obligation upon the veterinarian to treat them. In the UK, the veterinary oath, which is sworn on admission to Membership of the Royal College of Veterinary Surgeons, includes the promise that 'my constant endeavour will be to ensure the welfare of animals committed to my care'. In certain circumstances, treatment without any prospect of payment may be necessary. In other circumstances it may be best to call in the State Veterinary Service, the police or the RSPCA, even if to do so might mean losing a client.

Housing and management (see also pp. 40–44, Chapter 56)

General points

Feeding of housed cattle may lead to difficulties for the animals because the acquisition of food in housing conditions is very different from that when grazing. Physical difficulties may occur, as described by Cermak (1987), but social factors are also very important. Cattle synchronize their feeding to a large extent (Benham, 1982; Potter & Broom, 1987), so where group feeding is possible enough feeding places for each animal are required (Metz, 1983; Wierenga, 1983). Those animals that cannot find a feeding place may not get sufficient food and it is likely that there are adverse effects on their welfare. The precise effects of the frustration that occurs when food is inaccessible because of competition

remain to be determined. Competitive feeding situations where there are no individual feeding places pose extra problems for cattle. The subordinate individual has to attempt to obtain food despite the attacks or threats of other individuals. Bouissou (1970) found that the greater the extent of the barrier between feeding places for cows, the fewer the attacks that occurred (Fig. 55.1). A trough that requires subordinate cows to come close to dominant individuals results in those subordinates walking greater distances and taking longer to obtain a meal (Albright, 1969; Fig. 55.2). Calves of low social rank obtain less of the favoured food if trough space is restricted (Broom, 1982). In order to minimize such welfare problems, which are often associated with poor weight gain, farmers should provide feeding spaces for all individuals, preferably with barriers between the individual places. Adaptation to food access from a single source is possible for cattle however, for a transponder-operated feeding stall can be quite successful (Albright, 1981), but some individuals in a herd may have difficulties in learning how to reach the feed in such systems.

Another general problem for housed cattle is having to stand on floors that are wet, slippery, uneven or hazardous because of sharp edges. Slippery slats can lead to difficulties in standing or lying (Andreae & Smidt, 1982; Fig. 55.3). These and other inadequacies of flooring can result in limb injuries, foot lameness, tail-tip necrosis and various diseases. Lameness is the greatest welfare problem of housed dairy cows and factors influencing its occurrence include floor quality

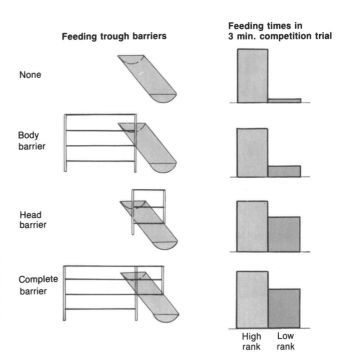

Fig. 55.1 Physical barriers affected feeding times by cows ranking high and low in a competitive order. With no barrier (a) the low ranking cows were scarcely able to feed. A body barrier (b) improved the situation slightly for the low ranking cows but a head barrier (c) and a complete barrier (d) had a much greater effect (redrawn after Craig, 1981; data from Bouissou, 1970).

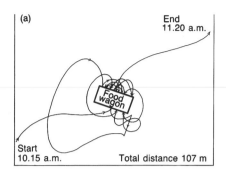

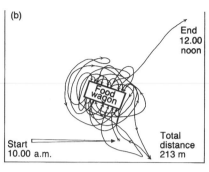

Fig. 55.2 The paths of two cows in a herd after food is provided in a food wagon are shown. Animal (a) was found to be high in a competitive order whereas animal (b), which was low in that order, walked further because of displacement at the food wagon and took longer to feed (after Broom, 1981; modified after Albright, 1969).

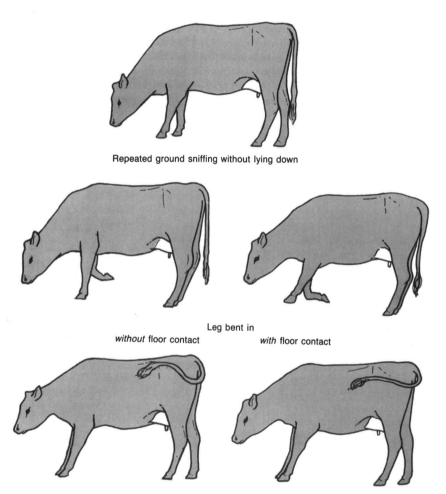

Repeated ground sniffing without lying down

Leg bent in

without floor contact   *with* floor contact

Lying down interruptions

Fig. 55.3 Behavioural alterations in young cattle on a slatted floor (after Andreae & Smidt, 1982).

and poor drainage, which results in cows standing in slurry (Wierenga & Peterse, 1987).

Calf welfare

In the first few days after birth the major calf welfare problems are enteric and respiratory diseases. The calves of dairy cows may fail to obtain sufficient colostrum for a variety of reasons (Edwards, 1982; Edwards & Broom, 1982; Broom, 1983). Management practices that maximize the chance that colostrum will be obtained and minimize contact with pathogens have important beneficial effects on calf welfare. If calves of dairy cows are normally left with their mother for the first 24 or 48 hours, the risk that the calf will not suckle early enough to obtain and absorb the immunoglobulin from colostrum can be minimized by the stockworker placing one of the mother's teats in the mouth of the calf as early as possible after the calf stands. Group-calving situations where several cows calve during a short period can lead to a cow's colostrum being drunk by a calf other than her own or to calves being rejected by their own mothers. Such occurrences can be prevented by providing separate calving boxes, which should ideally allow the cows some visual contact with other cows. The provision of soft bedding for the calf is also desirable and is easier where special calving accommodation is available.

Dairy calves are deprived of their mother from an early age and many are individually housed so that they are confined in a small space and deprived of all or most social contacts.

The needs of calves

A need is a requirement, which is a consequence of the biology of the animal, to obtain a particular resource or respond to a particular environmental or bodily stimulus. The needs of calves are described in detail by Broom (1991, 1996) and examples are given here.

The calf needs to ingest colostrum very soon after birth and milk thereafter. It also needs to show sucking behaviour and if a calf is not obtaining milk from a real or artificial teat, it sucks other objects (Broom, 1982, 1991; Metz, 1984; Hammell et al., 1988).

Calves need to rest and sleep in order to recuperate and avoid danger. They need to use several postures which include one in which they rest the head on the legs and another in which the legs are fully stretched out (de Wilt, 1985; Ketelaar-de Lauwere & Smits, 1989, 1991).

Exploration is important as a means of preparing for the avoidance of danger and is a behaviour shown by all calves (Kiley-Worthington & de la Plain, 1983; Fraser & Broom, 1990). Calves need to explore and it may be that higher levels of stereotypies (Dannemann et al., 1985) and fearfulness (Webster & Saville, 1981) in poorly lit buildings are a consequence of inability to explore.

Exercise is needed for normal bone and muscle development and calves choose to walk at intervals if they can, show considerable activity when released from a small pen and have locomotor problems if confined in a small pen for a long period (Warnick et al., 1977; Dellmeier et al., 1985; Trunkfield et al., 1991).

Normal calf anatomical, physiological and behavioural development occurs only if the calves have some fibre-containing material to eat (van Putten & Elshof, 1978; Webster, 1984; Webster et al., 1985a) so it is clear that they need fibre in their diet after the first few weeks of life.

Grooming behaviour is important as a means of minimizing disease and parasitism and calves make considerable efforts to groom themselves thoroughly (Fraser & Broom, 1990). Calves need to be able to groom their whole bodies effectively.

A variety of nutrients are needed by calves. Sufficient iron is needed to allow normal activity and to minimize disease.

The needs of young calves are met most effectively by the presence and actions of their mothers. In the absence of their mothers, calves associate with other calves if possible and they show much social behaviour. The need to show full social interaction with other calves is evident from calf preferences and from the adverse effects on calves of social isolation (Broom & Leaver, 1978; Dantzer et al., 1983; Friend et al., 1985; Lidfors, 1994).

Comparisons of veal calf housing and management systems

The major housing systems which have been compared in studies of calf welfare are individual crates (Fig. 55.4), group housing on slats and group housing on straw. Where calves are housed individually, the size of the crate and whether or not the sides are solid have been varied. All aspects of diet are important in relation to welfare. For example, if inappropriate proteins or carbohydrates are fed, the calf may be unable to utilize them and if milk is acidified too much, calves may

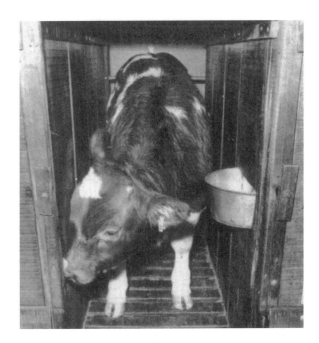

Fig. 55.4 Veal calf in crate with slatted floor. The front of the crate has been removed.

find it very unpalatable. However, the two aspects of diet which have been of greatest concern in relation to calf welfare have been the amount of fibre and the amount of iron.

The incidence of disease in young calves is too high, for example, 25 per cent of veal calves had to be treated for respiratory disease in a study by van der Mei (1987). The use of antibiotics to prevent disease is also a problem. It is important for calf welfare and for farm economics that disease levels be lowered.

One aspect of management which causes problems is the practice of mixing calves from different sources. Webster (1984) found that calves purchased and brought into a unit were five times more likely to require treatment for disease. A second aspect is hygienic practice by farm staff and a third is early detection of disease. These variables seem to be more important than the housing system in exacerbating disease.

As a consequence of the evidence of poor welfare in veal calves, the European Union passed a directive in 1997 which required group housing of calves after 8 weeks of age, individual pens at least as wide as the height of the calf at the withers, no tethering of calves except for <1 h at feeding time, sufficient iron to ensure an average blood haemoglobin of 4.5 mmol/l and fibre in the diet increasing from 50 g/day at 8 weeks to 250 g/day at 20 weeks. Many EU calf producers have found group housing of calves to be more successful economically than the old crate system and white veal can still be produced from systems which comply with the new law.

Beef cattle welfare

The housing conditions for calves destined for beef production are sometimes similar to those kept for veal production so they have similar welfare problems. Older beef animals are kept in small individual pens or are tethered in some countries and they then show much stereotyped behaviour. Riese *et al.* (1977) reported that stereotyped behaviour included tongue rolling, weaving movements and self-licking. Wierenga (1987) reported that one-third of young, individually housed bulls spent several minutes in every hour showing tongue rolling. Physiological responses to confinement also occur. Ladewig (1984) reported that tethered bulls showed more frequent episodes of high blood cortisol levels than did bulls able to interact socially in groups. Such abnormal behaviour and physiology are probably exacerbated by both social deprivation and inability to perform behaviours because of spatial restriction. Tethered animals lack exercise and have different patterns of muscle fibres from those free to walk (Jury *et al.*, 1998) and more osteochondrosis (de

Vries *et al.*, 1986). Individual housing of beef animals is more frequent when they are bulls than when they are steers. In Germany almost all beef animals are bulls, but in the UK most were steers before the ban on growth promoters.

Fighting and mounting can lead to welfare problems when beef animals, especially bulls, are kept in groups. The most important way of minimizing such problems is to keep the animals in stable groups, since social mixing leads to much fighting with consequent injuries, bruising and extreme physiological responses (Kenny & Tarrant, 1982). In stable groups, mounting may lead to more injury than does fighting (Appleby & Wood-Gush, 1986). Animals that are frequently mounted become bruised and may suffer severe leg injuries. Mounting can be greatly reduced by the use of overhead bars, which physically prevent it, or an electrified grid, which deters animals that wish to mount. The brief initial experience of an electric shock has a relatively small adverse effect on welfare as compared with the serious effects on animals that are repeatedly mounted.

The stocking density of beef animals and the flooring provided also have considerable effects on welfare. High stocking densities lead to more aggression, injury and bruising. Beef animals increase rapidly in bodyweight, but they have little exercise if they are housed in small pens and their leg growth may not be able to keep pace with that of the rest of the body. The final weights reached are much higher now than they used to be so the legs are scarcely adequate to support the body. The consequence is cartilage damage, clear indications of limb pain and obvious difficulties in standing and lying (Dämmrich, 1987). Graf (1984) found that these problems were absent if fattening bulls were reared on deep straw and that such conditions also led to fewer behavioural problems. Beef cattle have a strong preference for straw or other bedding.

All of these issues are reviewed in the EU Scientific Committee on Animal Health and Animal Welfare Report on the Welfare of Cattle Kept for Beef Production, 2001.

The welfare of dairy cows

The major welfare problems of dairy cows are lameness, mastitis and any conditions which lead to impaired reproduction, inability to show normal behaviour, emergency physiological responses or injury (Broom, 1999c).

Leg and foot problems (see Chapters 31, 32)

For a review of lameness, including the extent to which it is a welfare problem, see Greenough and Weaver (1996). Almost all animals which walk with a limp, or reduce walking to a low level or avoid walking whenever possible suffer from some leg or foot pain. Their ability to carry out various preferred behaviours is generally impaired and there may be adverse consequences for various other aspects of their normal biological functioning. Lameness always means some degree of poor welfare and sometimes means that welfare is very poor indeed.

Measurements of the extent to which some degree of lameness occurs in dairy cows include 35–56 cases per 100 cows per annum in the USA, 59.5 cases per 100 cows per annum in the UK and more than 83 per cent of examined cows in The Netherlands. The actual figures depend upon the method of assessment and most of these cases were not treated by veterinary surgeons, but there is no doubt that lameness is often a severe welfare problem (Broom, 1999c).

Mastitis (see Chapter 23)

Mastitis in mammals is a very painful condition. The sensitivity to touch of affected tissues is clearly evident and there is obvious damaging of normal function. Mastitis prevalence should have declined greatly with improved methods of prevention and treatment, but it has not declined as much as it should have done. Webster (1993) reports 40 cases of mastitis per 100 cows per year as an average for the UK.

Reproductive problems (see Chapters 34, 35 and 36)

Reproductive problems in dairy cows have become very common in recent years with large numbers of cows being culled because of failure to get in calf. In a study of 50 dairy herds in England, Esslemont and Kossaibati (1997) found that farmers reported failure to conceive as the predominant reason for culling, with 44 per cent of first lactation, 42 per cent of second lactation and 36.5 per cent of cows in total being culled for this reason. However, mastitis, feet and leg problems, ketosis and other disease conditions can lead to reproductive problems and it is difficult to discover their initial cause from farmers' records. A report by Plaizier *et al.* (1998) concerning Canadian herds indicated that reproductive culling risk varied between 0 and 30 per cent, with a mean of 7.5 per cent.

Housing systems and welfare (see pp. 40–44, Chapter 56)

The incidence of lameness is much worse in housed cows than in cows at pasture. Cows at pasture may have stone damage to hooves if they do not have a suitable place to walk, but wet cubicle houses or poorly maintained straw yards can result in very high levels of lameness. Even the best cubicle housing systems seem to have some lameness problems which are exacerbated by social factors (Bickert *et al.*, 1997). Since the best straw yards, with an abrasive area on which normal hoof wear occurs, have little lameness, these may be the best solution for housed cows. Mastitis incidence is affected by hygiene at milking and various other conditions of management. Poorly designed housing systems can result in a variety of welfare problems and these can be exacerbated by high stocking density. Most of these problems, such as those resulting from cubicles being too short for the length of the cows now occupying them or of poor design of cubicles which do not allow adequate movements in the cow, are well known so are mentioned briefly here. In general it seems that many dairy cow housing systems, and cubicles in particular, do not provide an environment to which cows can adapt easily. The best straw yards seem to be the most successful as they give the cows more opportunity to control their interactions with their environment.

Milk yield and welfare in dairy cows

The dairy cow of 1998 could produce 18 000 l or more of milk per annum with a peak milk yield of 75 l per day. This compares with UK figures of 6000 l and 30 l per day 10 years ago (Webster, 1993) and a beef cattle average of 1000–2000 l and 10 l per day. The dairy animal is producing considerably more than its ancestor would have. This raises the questions of whether it is at or beyond its maximum production level and the extent of any welfare problems.

The peak daily energy output of the dairy cow per unit bodyweight is not very high in comparison with some other species such as seals or dogs, but the product of daily energy output and duration of lactation is very high indeed. Hence long term problems are the most likely to occur (Nielsen, 1998). This is what we see because, although some cows seem to be able to produce at high levels without welfare problems, the risk of poor welfare indicated by lameness, mastitis or fertility problems is greater as milk yield increases.

The steady increase in reproductive problems as milk yields have increased is well known. As Studer (1998) states, 'despite programmes developed by veterinarians to improve reproductive herd health, conception rates have in general declined from 55–66% 20 years ago to 45–50% recently (Spalding *et al.*, 1975; Foote, 1978; Ferguson, 1988; Butler & Smith, 1989). During the same periods, milk production has greatly increased.'

Studies showing that milk yield is positively correlated with the extent of fertility problems have come from a range of different countries (van Arendonk *et al.*, 1989; Oltenacu *et al.*, 1991; Nebel & McGilliard, 1993; Hoekstra *et al.*, 1994; Pösö & Mäntysaari, 1996; Pryce *et al.*, 1997, 1998). Studer (1998) explains that high

Table 55.1 Positive correlations between milk production level and indicators of poor welfare (from Pryce *et al.*, 1997 with permission of the American Society of Animal Science).

Milk yield from 33 732 lactation records:	
calving interval	0.50 ± 0.06
days to first service	0.43 ± 0.08
mastitis	0.21 ± 0.06
foot problems	0.29 ± 0.11
milk fever	0.19 ± 0.06

Table 55.2 Positive correlations between milk production level and indicators of poor welfare (from Pryce *et al.*, 1998 with permission of the American Society of Animal Science).

Milk yield from 10 569 lactation records:	
calving interval	0.28 ± 0.06
days to first service	0.41 ± 0.06
mastitis	0.29 ± 0.05
somatic cell count	0.16 ± 0.04
foot problems	0.13 ± 0.06

producing cows which are thin and whose body condition score declines by 0.5–1.0 during lactation often experience anoestrus. A loss of condition score of about 1.0 during lactation was normal in the review presented by Broster and Broster (1998). Data on the relationships between milk yield and reproduction measures from two large scale studies are presented in Tables 55.1 and 55.2.

In some studies, effects of health problems on reproduction are evident, for example, Peeler *et al.* (1994) showed how cows which were lame in the period before service were less likely to be observed as being in oestrus. The lameness could be more likely in high producing cows. Direct links between level of milk production and extent of disease conditions are also evident from a range of studies, positive correlations being reported by Lyons *et al.* (1991), Uribe *et al.* (1995) and Pryce *et al.* (1997, 1998; see Tables 55.1, 55.2). In addition to mastitis and leg and foot problems, which are often measured in such studies, the occurrence of other clinical conditions can also be affected by production level. Modern, high producing cows with good body condition have a high incidence of milk fever, retained placenta, metritis, fatty liver and ketosis (Studer, 1998).

The high yields of modern dairy cows are a consequence of genetic selection and feeding. Cows are adapted to high fibre, low density diets. The ways in which they have been modified genetically do not change these basic characteristics much. Cows do not adapt easily to high grain diets or to manufactured diets with high protein and low fibre. Genetic selection has not taken adequate account of the adaptability and

welfare of cows. Current trends towards ever greater milk production and feed conversion efficiency should not be continued unless it can be ensured that welfare is good (Broom, 1994; Phillips, 1997). Bovine somatotropin (BST) (see p. 1073) results in high milk yields and higher levels of mastitis, lameness, reproductive disorders and other problems such as those at the injection site (Broom, 1993; Willeberg, 1993; Kronfeld, 1997; Willeberg, 1997; Broom, 1998a). Whether or not much of the effect of the genetically engineered hormone is a consequence of the milk yield, the poorer welfare caused by the BST is unacceptable.

The Report of the EU Scientific Committee on Animal Health and Animal Welfare (1999) on animal welfare aspects of the use of bovine somatotrophin concluded as follows:

'BST is used to increase milk yield, often in already high-producing cows. BST administration causes substantially and very significantly poorer welfare because of increased foot disorders, mastitis, reproductive disorders and other production related diseases. These are problems which would not occur if BST were not used and often results in unnecessary pain, suffering and distress. If milk yields were achieved by other means which resulted in the health disorders and other welfare problems described above, these means would not be acceptable. The injection of BST and its repetition every 14 days also causes localized swellings which are likely to result in discomfort and hence some poor welfare.'

The Committee also made the following recommendation:

'BST use causes a substantial increase in levels of foot problems and mastitis and leads to injection site reactions in dairy cows. These conditions, especially the first two, are painful and debilitating, leading to significantly poorer welfare in the treated animals. Therefore from the point of view of animal welfare, including health, the Scientific Committee on Animal Health and Animal Welfare is of the opinion that BST should not be used in dairy cows.'

Farm operations

Certain mutilations of cattle are performed on farms by staff with no veterinary qualification. In most cases, no anaesthetic is used. The most widespread of these operations are disbudding or dehorning, castration and various sorts of individual marking. Some of the procedures used must also cause pain to the animals, but there is little precise information about this. The use of caustic materials that remain in contact with living tissue for any length of time is likely to cause severe pain and should be avoided. Any use of hot irons on living tissue must also cause pain and hot iron branding is a painful and unnecessary form of marking. Castration is often carried out by applying a rubber ring around the testicles until the tissue in them dies and it seems likely that this is also very painful for a long period. Even the ubiquitous ear notching and punching must be painful for a few days and it would be better if alternative marking methods such as freeze branding or tattooing could be used.

More extensive mutilations should only be carried out under anaesthetic by qualified veterinarians and should be permitted only if the animal will benefit. Any practices that necessitate the use of operations should be avoided. An example of a problem area is the breeding of cows such that their calf cannot be born normally. No animal should be made pregnant if there is a likelihood that caesarean section or a difficult birth will occur.

Handling, transport and slaughter of cattle

Every dairy farmer has to be able to move dairy cows in milk to and from the milking parlour. If the races and collecting yards that are used or the methods of moving the animals are inadequate and disturbing to some or all of the cows, there will be welfare problems. Such welfare problems will often be associated with reduced milk yield. Cows may be reluctant to enter a milking parlour because of the behaviour of the stockworker or because of design faults in the parlour that result in uncomfortable milking stalls or stray voltages. Such problems can lead to the use of excessive force by stockworkers in the collecting yard or to forcing animals towards the parlour entrance using gates or an 'electric dog'. The 'electric dog', which is a row of electrically live wires hanging downwards and moved towards the cow in the rear of the yard, has a marked

adverse effect on some cows so that their milk let-down may be prevented and they may become extremely unwilling to move towards the parlour.

The problems associated with the design of races for moving cows to the milking parlour are very similar to those of designing races used for other purposes, such as movement towards vehicles prior to transport. The most extensive study of how to design good races is that of Grandin (1983, 2000). She reported that cattle often balk if they encounter dark areas or areas of extreme lighting contrast. Races with sharp angular turns in them may also pose problems for cattle that are being driven and long straight races may result in animals being either reluctant to move or moving too fast. As a consequence of these observations, Grandin recommends that races should be evenly lit, have solid walls if animals unfamiliar with them have to use them and should be gently curved rather than having sharp corners or long straights (Fig. 55.5). Other studies also suggest that if animals are being loaded into vehicles, the ramp should be long and sloping not more than 1 in 7, should allow a good grip for the feet of the cattle and should have solid sides, and the interior of the vehicle should be well lit.

Vehicles are often not well designed as regards flooring, ventilation and ease of subdivision. Just as important as vehicle design, as regards the welfare of animals during transport, is the behaviour of the transport staff. Problems arise because of rough treatment during loading, over- or understocking of compartments on the vehicle, inconsiderate driving or leaving the animals in conditions that are too hot or too cold and windy for them. The other major transport problems are the effect of very long journeys, especially where there are no stops for food and water, and contact between transported animals or their products which results in disease transmission and poor animal welfare. This area has been reviewed in a Commission of the European Communities (CEC) Report (1984) (also see Broom *et al.*, 2002).

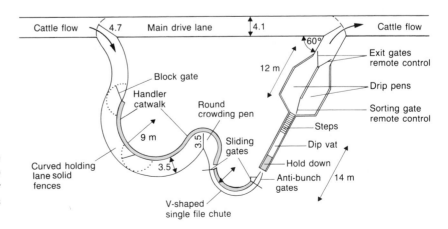

Fig. 55.5 Races for cattle should have no long straights or sharp corners so Grandin (1980) designed this race for movement to vehicles. (Measurements are in metres.)

When cattle arrive at an abattoir they are often injured or bruised during unloading because of too much haste on the part of animal handlers or inadequate ramps. Grandin (1979, 1980) reported that 66 per cent of bruises of the loin area occurred during loading or unloading of trucks. At lairage, animals are often mixed with individuals that are strange to them. This causes much fighting amongst bulls and considerable emotional disturbance in other cattle. Studies of bulls by Kenny and Tarrant (1982) show that mixing at lairage causes much fighting, high levels of bruising and other injury and a great increase in the incidence of dark firm dry (DFD) meat. Both bruising and DFD meat are of economic importance as well as indicating severe welfare problems prior to slaughter.

In an efficient slaughterhouse the period during which animals are moved from pens to the point of slaughter can be very brief and the stunning and slaughter procedure itself can result in no pain for the animal. Welfare is worse if the animals are kept in a confined race for a period of more than one or two minutes before stunning, if stunning is carried out inadequately or if there is inversion before slaughter or no stunning. Poor equipment or lack of care by slaughter staff can result in extreme pain and discomfort for the animals. Extreme pain and discomfort are also inevitable if animals are not stunned, for example in the Jewish schechita or the Muslim halal ritual slaughter procedures. There is a period during which evoked potentials in the brain can still be produced after the throat is cut that may last for from a few seconds to two minutes, during which the animal must be in great pain and distress. As the heart still beats after stunning and blood drains from the animal just as effectively whether or not the animal is stunned there is no logical reason why stunning should not be carried out before the throat is cut.

References

Albright, J.L. (1969) Social environment and growth. In *Animal Growth and Nutrition* (ed. by E.S.E. Hafez & I.A. Dyers). Lea & Febiger, Philadelphia.

Albright, J.L. (1981) Training dairy cattle. In *Dairy Sciences Handbook*, Vol. 14, pp. 303–70. Agriservices Foundation, Clovis, CA.

Andreae, U. & Smidt, D. (1982) Behavioural alterations in young cattle on slatted floors. In *Disturbed Behaviour in Farm Animals* (ed. by W. Bessei), Hohenheimer Arbeiten, Vol. 121, pp. 51–60. Eugen Ulmer, Stuttgart.

Appleby, M.C. & Wood-Gush, D.G.M. (1986) Development of behaviour in beef bulls: sexual behaviour causes more problems than aggression. *Animal Production*, **42**, 464.

Arendonk, J.A.M. van, Hovenier, R. & Boer, W. de (1989) Phenotypic and genetic association between fertility and

production in dairy cows. *Livestock Production Science*, **21**, 1–12.

Benham, P.F.J. (1982) Synchronisation of behaviour in grazing cattle. *Applied Animal Ethology*, **8**, 403–404.

Bickert, W.G., Shaver, R.D., Galindo, F.A., Broom, D.M. & Cermak, J. (1997) Laminitis and factors predisposing to lameness: nutrition, behavior, and housing. In *Lameness in Cattle*, 3rd edn (ed. by P.R. Greenough & A.D. Weaver), pp. 293–307. W.B. Saunders, Philadelphia.

Bouissou, M.F. (1970) Role du contact physique dans la manifestation des relations hierarchiques chez les bovins: consequences pratiques. *Annales de Zootechnie*, **19**, 279–85.

Broom, D.M. (1981) *Biology of Behaviour*. Cambridge University Press, Cambridge.

Broom, D.M. (1982) Husbandry methods leading to inadequate social and maternal behaviour in cattle. In *Disturbed Behaviour in Farm Animals* (ed. by W. Bessei). Hohenheimer Arbeiten, Vol. 12b. Eugen Illmer, Stuttgart.

Broom, D.M. (1983) Cow–calf and sow–piglet behaviour in relation to colostrum ingestion. *Annales de Recherches Vétérinaires*, **14**, 342–8.

Broom, D.M. (1986) Indicators of poor welfare. *British Veterinary Journal*, **142**, 524–6.

Broom, D.M. (1988) Welfare considerations in cattle practice. In *Proceedings of the British Cattle Veterinary Association 1986–87* (ed. by M. Vaughan), pp. 153–64. British Cattle Veterinary Association, London.

Broom, D.M. (1991) Needs and welfare of housed calves. In *New Trends in Veal Calf Production. Proceedings of the International Symposium on Veal Calf Production* (ed. by J.H.M. Metz & C.M. Groenestein), EAAP Publication No. 52. Pudoc, Wageningen.

Broom, D.M. (1993) Assessing the welfare of modified or treated animals. *Livestock Production Science*, **36**, 39–54.

Broom, D.M. (1994) The effects of production efficiency on animal welfare. In *Biological Basis of Sustainable Animal Production. Proceedings of the 4th Zodiac Symposium* (ed. by E.A. Huisman, J.W.M. Osse, D. van der Heide, S. Tamminga, B.L. Tolkamp, W.G.P. Schouten, C.E. Hollingsworth & G.L. van Winkel), EAAP Publication 67, pp. 201–10. Wageningen Pers, Wageningen.

Broom, D.M. (1996) Scientific research on veal calf welfare. In *Veal Perspectives to the Year 2000, Proceedings of the International Symposium, Le Mans*, pp. 147–53. Fédération de la Vitellerie Francaise, Paris.

Broom, D.M. (1998a) The effects of biotechnology on animal welfare. In *Animal Biotechnology and Ethics* (ed. by A. Holland & A. Johnson), pp. 69–82. Chapman & Hall, London.

Broom, D.M. (1998b) Welfare, stress and the evolution of feelings. *Advances in the Study of Behaviour*, **27**, 371–403.

Broom, D.M. (1999a) Welfare and how it is affected by regulation. In *Regulation of Animal Production in Europe* (ed. by M. Kunisch & H. Ekkel), pp. 51–7. KTBL, Darmstadt.

Broom, D.M. (1999b) Animal welfare: the concept and the issues. In *Attitudes to Animals: Views in Animal Welfare* (ed. by F.L. Dolins), pp. 129–42. Cambridge University Press, Cambridge.

Broom, D.M. (1999c) The welfare of dairy cattle. In *Proceedings of the 25th International Dairy Congress, Future Milk*

Farming (ed. K. Aagaard), pp. 32–9. Danish National Committee of the International Dairy Federation, Aarhus.

Broom, D.M. (2000) Welfare assessment and problem areas during handling and transport. In *Livestock Handling and Transport*, 2nd edn (ed. T. Grandin), pp. 43–61. CABI, Wallingford.

Broom, D.M. & Johnson, K.G. (1993) *Stress and Animal Welfare*. Kluwer, Dordrecht.

Broom, D.M. & Leaver, J.D. (1978) The effects of group-rearing or partial isolation on later social behaviour of calves. *Animal Behaviour*, **26**, 1255–63.

Broom, D.M., Barton-Grade, P., Ferlazzo, A., Hartung, J., Mantela, X. & Warriss, P. (2002) *The Welfare of Animals, during Transport*. Report of the Scientific Committee for Animal Health and Welfare, European Commission. D.G. Sanco, Brussels.

Broster, W.H. & Broster, V.J. (1998) Body score of dairy cows. *Journal of Dairy Research*, **65**, 155–73.

Butler, W.R. & Smith, R.D. (1989) Interrelationships between energy balance and post partum reproductive function in dairy cattle. *Journal of Dairy Science*, **72**, 767–83.

Ceppi, A. & Blum, J.W. (1994) Effects of growth hormone on growth performance, haematology, metabolites and hormones in iron-deficient veal calves. *Journal of Veterinary Medicine A*, **41**, 443–55.

Cermak, J. (1987) The design of cubicles for British Friesian dairy cows with reference to body weight and dimensions, spatial behaviour and upper leg lameness. In *Cattle Housing Systems, Lameness and Behaviour* (ed. by H.K. Wierenga & D.J. Peterse), *Current Topics in Veterinary Medicine and Animal Science*, Vol. 40, pp. 119–28. Martinus Nijhoff, Dordrecht.

Commission of the European Communities (1984) International transport of farm animals intended for slaughter. EUR 9556 EN. CEC, Luxembourg.

Craig, J.V. (1981) *Domestic Animal Behaviour*. Prentice Hall, Englewood Cliffs.

Dämmrich, K. (1987) The reactions of the legs (bone; joints) to loading and its consequences for lameness. In *Cattle Housing Systems, Lameness and Behaviour* (ed. by H.K. Wierenga & D.J. Peterse). *Current Topics in Veterinary Medicine and Animal Science*, Vol. 40, pp. 50–5. Martinus Nijhoff, Dordrecht.

Dannemann, K., Buchenauer, D. & Fliegner, H. (1985) The behaviour of calves under four levels of lighting. *Applied Animal Behaviour Science*, **13**, 243–58.

Dantzer, R., Mormede, P., Bluth, R.M. & Soissons, J. (1983) The effect of different housing conditions on behavioural and adrenocortical reactions in veal calves. *Reproduction, Nutrition and Development*, **23**, 61–74.

Dellmeier, G.R., Friend, T.H. & Gbur, E.E. (1985) Comparison of four methods of calf confinement. II. Behaviour. *Journal of Animal Science*, **60**, 1102–109.

Edwards, S.A. (1982) Factors affecting the time to first suckling in dairy calves. *Animal Production*, **34**, 339–46.

Edwards, S.A. & Broom, D.M. (1982) Behavioural interactions of dairy cows with their newborn calves and the effects of parity. *Animal Behaviour*, **30**, 525–35.

Esslemont, R.J. & Kossaibati, M.A. (1997) Culling in 50 dairy herds in England. *Veterinary Record*, **140**, 36–9.

EU (1999) Report of the EU Scientific Committee on Animal Health and Animal Welfare. Aspects of the use of bovine somatotrophin. CEC, D.G. Sanco, Brussels.

EU (2001) Report of the Scientific Committee on Animal Health and Animal Welfare on the welfare of cattle kept for beef production. CEC, D.G. Sanco, Brussels.

Ferguson, J.D. (1988) Feeding for reproduction. In *Proceedings of the Dairy Production Medicine, Continuing Education Group Annual Meeting*, pp. 48–56. Vet. Learning System Co, Trenton, NJ.

Foote, R.H. (1978) Reproductive performance and problems in New York dairy herds. *Search Agriculture (Geneva NY)*, **8**, 1.

Fraser, A.F. & Broom, D.M. (1990) *Farm Animal Behaviour and Welfare*. CABI, Wallingford.

Friend, T.H., Dellmeier, G.R. & Gbur, E.E. (1985) Comparison of four methods of calf confinement. I. Physiology. *Journal of Animal Science*, **60**, 1095–101.

Graf, B.P. (1984) *Der Einfluss unterschiedlicher Laufstall systeme auf Verhaltensmerkmale von Mastochsen*. Doktor Dissertation der Eidgenossischen Technischen Hochschle, Zürich.

Grandin, T. (1979) The effect of stress on livestock and meat quality prior to and during slaughter. *International Journal for the Study of Animal Productions*, **1**, 313–37.

Grandin, T. (1980) Observations of cattle behaviour applied to the design of cattle-handling facilities. *Applied Animal Ethology*, **6**, 19–31.

Grandin, T. (1983) Welfare requirements of handling facilities. In *Farm Animal Housing and Welfare* (ed. by S.H. Baxter. M.R. Baxter & J.A.C. MacCormack), *Current Topics in Veterinary Medicine and Animal Science*, Vol. 21, pp. 137–49. Martinus Nijhoff, The Hague.

Grandin, T. (ed.) (2000) *Livestock Handling and Transport*, 2nd edn. CABI, Wallingford.

Greenough, P.R. & Weaver, A.D. (1996) *Lameness in Cattle*, 3rd edn. Saunders, Philadelphia.

Gygax, M., Hirni, H., Zwahlen, R., Lazary, S. & Blum, J.W. (1993) Immune functions of veal calves fed low amounts of iron. *Journal of Veterinary Medicine A*, **40**, 345–58.

Hammell, K.L., Metz, J.H.M. & Mekking, P. (1988) Sucking behaviour of dairy calves fed milk *ad libitum* by bucket or teat. *Applied Animal Behaviour Science*, **20**, 275–85.

Hoekstra, J., Lugt, A.W. van der, Werf, J.H.J. van der & Oueltjes, W. (1994) Genetic and phenotypic parameters for milk production and fertility traits in up-graded dairy cattle. *Livestock Production Science*, **40**, 225–32.

Jury, C., Picard, B. & Geay, Y. (1998) Influences of the method of housing bulls on their body composition and muscle fiber types. *Meat Science*, **4**, 457–69.

Kenny, F.J. & Tarrant, P.V. (1982) Behaviour of cattle during transport and penning before slaughter. In *Transport of Animals Intended for Breeding, Production and Slaughter* (ed. by R. Moss), *Current Topics in Veterinary Medicine and Animal Science*, Vol. 18, pp. 87–102. Martinus Nijhoff, The Hague.

Ketelaar-de Lauwere, C.C. & Smits, A.C. (1989) *Onderzoek naar de uit ethologisch oogpunt minimaal gewenstle box-maten voor vleeskalveren met een gewicht van 175 tot 300 kg*. IMAG Rapport 110. IMAG, Wageningen.

Ketelaar-de Lauwere, C.C. & Smits, A.C. (1991) Spatial requirements of individually housed veal calves of 175 to 300 kg. In *New Trends in Veal Calf Production. Proceedings of the International Symposium on Veal Calf Production* (ed. by J.H.M. Metz & C.M. Groenestein), EAAP Publications No. 52. Pudoc, Wageningen.

Kiley-Worthington, M. & Plain, S. de la (1983) *The Behaviour of Beef Suckler Cattle*. Birkhäuser Verlag, Basel.

Kilgour, R. & Dalton, C. (1984) *Livestock Behaviour: A Practical Guide*. Granada, London.

Kronfeld, D.S. (1997) Recombinant bovine somatotropin: ethics of communication and animal welfare. *Swedish Veterinary Journal*, **49**, 157–65.

Ladewig, J. (1984) The effect of behavioural stress on the episodic release and circadian variation of cortisol in bulls. In *Proceedings of the International Congress on Applied Ethology of Farm Animals* (ed. by J. Unshelm, G. van Putten & K. Zeeb), pp. 339–42. KJBL, Darmstadt.

Lidfors, L. (1994) *Mother–young behaviour in cattle*. PhD thesis, Swedish University of Agricultural Science, Skara.

Lindt, F. & Blum, J.W. (1993) Physical performance of veal calves during chronic iron deficiency anaemia and after acute iron overload. *Journal of Veterinary Medicine A*, **40**, 444–55.

Lyons, D.T., Freeman, A.E. & Kuck, A.L. (1991) Genetics of health traits. *Journal of Dairy Science*, **74**, 1092–100.

Mainsant, P. (1996) Les consommateurs de veau en France et en Europe. In *Le veau a l'horizon de l'an 2000*. Le Mans.

Mason, G.J. (1991) Stereotypies: a critical review. *Animal Behaviour*, **41**, 1015–37.

Mei, J. van der (1987) Health aspects of welfare research in veal calves. In *Welfare Aspects of Housing Systems for Veal Calves and Fattening Bulls* (ed. by M.C. Schlichting & D. Smidt), p. 99. CEC, Luxembourg.

Metz, J.H.M. (1983) Food competition in cattle. In *Farm Animal Housing and Welfare* (ed. by S.H. Baxter, M.R. Baxter & J.A.C. MacCormack), *Current Topics in Veterinary Medicine and Animal Science*, Vol. 24, pp. 164–70. Martinus Nijhoff, The Hague.

Metz, J.H.M. (1984) Regulation of sucking behaviour of calves. In *Proceedings of the International Congress on Applied Ethology of Farm Animals*, Kiel (ed. by J. Unsholm, G. van Putten & K. Zeeb), pp. 70–3. KTBL, Darmstadt.

Morisse, J.P., Cotte, J.P. & Huonnic, D. (1995) L'anémie chez le veau de boucherie. Evolution maîtrisée on probleme pathologique. Seminaire International sur le Veau de boucherie. A. paraître.

Moser, M., Bruckmaier, R.M. & Blum, J.W. (1994) Iron status, erythropoiesis, meat colour, health status and growth performance of veal calves held on and fed straw. *Journal of Veterinary Medicine A*, **41**, 343–58.

Nebel, R.L. & McGilliard, M.L. (1993) Interactions of high milk yield and reproductive performance in dairy cows. *Journal of Dairy Science*, **76**, 3257–68.

Nielsen, B. (1998) Interspecific comparison of lactational stress: is the welfare of dairy cows compromised? *Proceedings of the 32nd Congress of the International Society of Applied Ethology* (ed. by I. Veissier & A. Boissy), p. 80. INRA, Clermont Ferrand.

Olsson, S.O., Viring, S., Emanuelsson, U. & Jacobsson, S.O. (1993) Calf disease and mortality in Swedish dairy herds. *Acta Veterinaria Scandinavica*, **34**, 263–9.

Oltenacu, P.A., Frick, A. & Lindhe, B. (1991) Relationship of fertility to milk yield in Swedish cattle. *Journal of Dairy Science*, **71**, 264–8.

Peeler, E.J., Otte, M.J. & Esslemont, R.J. (1994) Interrelationships of periparturient diseases in dairy cows. *Veterinary Record*, **134**, 129–32.

Perez, E., Noordhuizen, J.P.T.M., Van Wuijkhuise, L.A. & Stassen, E.N. (1990) Management factors related to calf mortality and mortality rates. *Livestock Production Science*, **25**, 79–93.

Peters, A.R. (1986) Studies of mortality, morbidity and performance in intensive calf rearing. *World Review of Animal Production*, **22**, 83–8.

Phillips, C.J.C. (1997) Review article: animal welfare considerations in future breeding programmes for farm livestock. *Animal Breeding Abstracts*, **65**, 645–54.

Piquet, M., Bruckmaier, R.M. & Blum, J.W. (1993) Treadmill exercise of calves with different iron supply, husbandry and work load. *Journal of Veterinary Medicine A*, **40**, 456–65.

Plaizier, J.C.B., Lissemore, K.D., Kelton, D. & King, G.J. (1998) Evaluation of overall reproductive performance of dairy herds. *Journal of Dairy Science*, **81**, 1848–54.

Pösö, J. & Mäntysaari, E.A. (1996) Genetic relationships between reproductive disorders, operational days open and milk yield. *Livestock Production Science*, **46**, 41–8.

Potter, M.J. & Broom, D.M. (1987) The behaviour and welfare of cows in relation to cubicle house design. In *Cattle Housing Systems, Lameness and Behaviour* (ed. by H.K. Wierenga & D.J. Peterse), *Current Topics in Veterinary Medicine and Animal Science*, Vol. 40, pp. 129–47. Martinus Nijhoff, Dordrecht.

Pryce, J.E., Veerkamp, R.F., Thompson, R., Hill, R.G. & Simm, G. (1997) Genetic aspects of common health disorders and measures of fertility in Holstein Friesian dairy cattle. *Animal Science*, **65**, 353–60.

Pryce, J.E., Esslemont, R.J., Thompson, R., Veerkamp, R.F., Kossaibati, M.A. & Simm, G. (1998) Estimation of genetic parameters using health, fertility and production data from a management recording system for dairy cattle. *Animal Science*, **66**, 577–84.

Putten, G. van & Elshof, W.J. (1978) Zusatzfuttering von Stroh an mastkalber. *Aktuelle Arbeiten zur artgemäßen Tierhaltung*, **233**, 210–19. KTBL, Darmstadt.

Riese, G., Klee, G. & Sambraus, H.H. (1977) Das Verhalten von Kälbern in verschiedenen Haltungsformen. *Deutsche Tierarztliche Wochenschrift*, **84**, 388–94.

Schlichting, M.C. & Smidt, D. (eds) (1987) *Welfare Aspects of Housing Systems for Veal Calves and Fattening Bulls*. EUR 1977 EN. Commission of the European Communities, Luxembourg.

Spalding, R.W., Everett, R.W. & Foote, R.H. (1975) Fertility in New York artificially inseminated Holstein herds in dairy improvement. *Journal of Dairy Science*, **58**, 718–23.

Stricklin, W.R. & Kautz-Scanavy, C.C. (1984) The role of behaviour in cattle production: a review of research. *Applied Animal Ethology*, **11**, 359–90.

Studer, E. (1998) A veterinary perspective of on farm evaluation of nutrition and reproduction. *Journal of Dairy Science*, **81**, 872–6.

Trunkfield, H.R., Broom, D.M., Maatje, K., Wierenga, H.K., Lambooy, E. & Kooijman, J. (1991) Effects of housing on responses of veal calves to handling and transport. In *New Trends in Veal Calf Production. Proceedings of the International Symposium on Veal Calf Production* (ed. by J.H.M. Mnetz & C.M. Groenestein), EAAP Publications No. 52. Pudoc, Wageningen.

Uribe, H.A., Kennedy, B.W., Martin, S.W. & Kelton, D.F. (1995) Genetic parameters for common health disorders of Holsteins. *Journal of Dairy Science*, **78**, 421–30.

Vries, F.W.K. de, Wierenga, H.K. & Goedegebouve, S.A. (1986) *Een orienterend onderzoek naar het voorkomen van afwijkingen aan het carpaalgen wrichtbijvleestieren en naar het vereand met de wijze van opstaan en gaan liggen.* Instituut voor Veeteelkundig Onderzoek 'Schoonoord'. IVO Report B-278.

Waltner-Toews, D., Martin, S.W. & Meck, A.H. (1986) Dairy calf management, morbidity and mortality in Ontario Holstein herds. III. Association of management with morbidity. *Preventive Veterinary Medicine*, **4**, 137–58.

Warnick, V.D., Arave, C.V. & Mickelsen, C.H. (1977) Effects of group, individual and isolated rearing of calves on weight gain and behaviour. *Journal of Dairy Science*, **60**, 947–53.

Webster, A.J.F. (1984) *Calf Husbandry, Health and Welfare.* Collins, London.

Webster, A.J.F. & Saville, C. (1981) Rearing of veal calves. In *Alternatives to Intensive Husbandry Systems*, pp. 86–94. Universities Federation for Animal Welfare (UFAW), London.

Webster, A.J.F., Saville, C., Church, B.M., Gnanasakthy, A. & Moss, R. (1985a) The effect of different rearing systems on the development of calf behaviour. *British Veterinary Journal*, **141**, 249–64.

Webster, A.J.F., Saville, C., Church, B.M., Gnanasakthy, A. & Moss, R. (1985b) Some effects of different rearing systems on health, cleanliness and injury in calves. *British Veterinary Journal*, **141**, 472–83.

Webster, J. (1993) *Understanding the Dairy Cow*, 2nd edn. Blackwell, Oxford.

Wierenga, H.K. (1983) The influence of space for walking and lying in a cubicle system on the behaviour of dairy cattle. In *Farm Animal Housing and Welfare* (ed. by S.H. Baxter, M.R. Baxter & S.H. MacCormack), *Current Topics in Veterinary Medicine and Animal Science*, Vol. 24, pp. 171–80. Martinus Nijhoff, The Hague.

Wierenga, H.K. (1987) Behavioural problems in fattening bulls. In *Welfare Aspects of Housing Systems for Veal Calves and Fattening Bulls* (ed. by M.C. Schlichting & D. Smidt), pp. 105–22. CEC, Luxembourg.

Wierenga, H.K. & Peterse, D.J. (eds) (1987) *Cattle Housing Systems. Lameness and Behaviour. Current Topics in Veterinary Medicine and Animal Science*, Vol. 40. Martinus Nijhoff, Dordrecht.

Willeberg, P. (1993) Bovine somatotrophin and clinical mastitis: epidemiological assessment of the welfare risk. *Livestock Production Science*, **36**, 55–66.

Willeberg, P. (1997) Epidemiology and animal welfare. *Epidemiol. Santé anim.*, **31**, 3–7.

Wilt, J.G. de (1985) *Behaviour and welfare of veal calves in relation to husbandry systems.* Thesis, Agricultural University, Wageningen.

Adult Cattle
Therapy and Disease Prevention

Chapter 56
Health, Housing and Hygiene

D.W.B. Sainsbury

Introduction   971
The essentials for good health   971
  The size of livestock farms   971
  Depopulation   971
  Group size   972
  Isolation facilities   972
Housing types and systems   972
  Climatic housing   973
  Controlled environment house   973
  'Kennel' accommodation   973
The environmental requirements of cattle   974
Environmental factors affecting susceptibility to disease   975
  Intensification and immunity   977
Disinfection   977
  Natural disinfectant agents   977
  Chemical disinfectants   977
  Disinfectants   979
  Recommended procedure in disinfection and
    disinfestation of animal buildings and equipment   980
Ventilation   982
  Underlying principles and calculations   982
  Natural ventilation   983
  Mechanical ventilation   984
  Open-fronted yards and kennels   985
  Dangers from gases in farm buildings   985

Introduction

Good health is the birthright of every animal. Considerable progress has been made towards achieving improved health in cattle but the disease pattern has changed radically in recent years. The most acute, specific, diagnosable and preventable or treatable diseases, using vaccines, sera and medicines for their control, have been largely controlled. In their place have emerged more chronic, insidious and complex diseases not infrequently caused by organisms that are the normal inhabitants of the animal body but which circumstances allow to become pathogenic. These disease conditions may be difficult to diagnose, have a large and confusing number of causal agents, create a massive morbidity and economic loss and require for their control great expertise in the exercise of husbandry, hygiene, housing and management skills rather than recourse to the use of medicines or biological products.

This chapter is concerned with those underlying principles of the management, hygiene and housing of cattle that are essential to assist in the prevention and control of disease.

The essentials of good health

The size of livestock farms

From the point of view of animal health, the smaller the livestock unit the better; nevertheless, the current trend, which appears likely to continue, has been towards increasing the size of units to achieve economies of scale – in manpower, buildings and services. However, in dealing with biological material, in this case cattle, there is clear evidence to show that if the farm becomes too large, efficiency generally decreases and health and productivity are adversely affected. Economic surveys have shown that very small farms as a group are generally less efficient but once the three-man unit has been reached, further improvements in performance are small or nonexistent (Britton & Berkeley Hill, 1975). This knowledge often goes unheeded and overlarge livestock enterprises are a cause of great health and management problems and enormous economic loss. It is, however, pertinent to emphasize that it is the young immature animal which finds itself at greater risk from disease and mismanagement. Therefore, whilst there should be a limit on unit size at a reasonably low level for the young animal, it may be much higher for the adult. The main reason for this, apart from the extra vulnerability of the young animal to stress caused by bad management, is the varying immunity to infectious disease among the stock that is unavoidable on a large unit with a mixture of animals of different ages and possibly of various sources of origin. The adult presents a more stable picture in both respects, being rather more resistant to management changes or errors and very much more uniform in its disease resistance or susceptibility.

Depopulation

So far as possible the principle of periodic depopulation of a building or, if possible, even a site should be followed. The benefits of eliminating the animal hosts to disease-causing agents are well understood and the virtue of being able to clean, disinfect and fumigate a building is also accepted. Nevertheless, in practice the whole concept of the 'all-in, all-out' policy is more complex than the preceding sentences would indicate. For example, it is in the young animal that it is particularly important to consider this and far less so in the older beast, which has achieved an immunity to many of the local diseases. Much also depends on whether the herd or flock is a 'closed' one with few or no incoming animals, or an 'open' one with a constant renewal of the animal population. If the latter is the case, then the depopulation principle is of much greater importance as there is little or no opportunity for natural immunity to develop, and there is a constantly running risk, and usually a near certainty, of introducing animals that are either clinically infected or carriers of disease. Basic design specifications for 'open' herds should be quite different from those of the closed herd.

Group size

One of the principal ways of putting the housing on a firm footing is to keep the animals in groups of *minimal* size. At first sight this sounds an old-fashioned and even reactionary concept that may eliminate all those advantages from automation that large units can give us, but this certainly need not be the case. If groups are small it is easier to match the animals in them for size, weight and age. Under these circumstances it is well established that fighting and bullying are kept to a minimum, if not completely prevented.

There is yet another very important advantage in keeping animals in small groups. It is obviously good practice for a farmer to keep his livestock somewhere near the level that has been shown to be the densest possible for optimal productivity yet still satisfying the welfare essentials. If livestock are kept in a house at a high density it is essential that they spread across the house uniformly, so they do in actual practice occupy and use the whole area. Regrettably, this is very rarely the case in practical experience and especially so when large numbers are housed together without any subdivision at all. If the animals crowd in certain parts of the building there may be grossly overstocked floor areas. This is bad enough in itself but it has further unfortunate side-effects. If they crowd excessively in a part of the house, this part may become polluted with dung and exhalations to an abnormal and harmful degree; the humidity becomes high, proper air movement is impeded and the animals may soon become ill. Sick animals feeling cold tend to huddle together even more, so the vicious circle is perpetuated and there is seem-ingly no end to it unless some measures are taken to ensure a better distribution of the stock.

When animals are kept together in large numbers the effects of a fright caused by an unusual disturbance can be extremely serious. It is almost impossible to guard against all the extraneous sounds and sights that may adversely affect the stock. The best safeguard, therefore, is once again to have the animals in small groups so that the effect of a panic movement will be more limited and will never build up into highly dangerous proportions.

Isolation facilities

There is a critical need for farmers to give better consideration to the isolation of sick and incoming animals. There are numerous reasons why this should be done. First and foremost, isolation removes some of the dangers of contagion to the normal animals; it also makes it much more likely that the sick animal will recover without the unwelcome attentions of the other animals who will always tend to act as bullies. In nature, the sick animal usually separates itself from the rest of the herd, but it is often impossible for the housed animal to do this. Also, under the more intensive systems of management, more animals are likely to suffer from the aggression of their pen-mates and it is essential that such animals are removed to prevent them from suffering or being killed. It is also easier, with an isolated animal, to give it such therapy as it needs and to give it any special environmental conditions, such as extra warmth or adjustments to comfort requirements. For new entrants to the farm it will also enable such tests to be carried out to ensure the animals are free from infection before they can be safely introduced into the herd.

Many modern livestock units completely ignore the provision of facilities to isolate animals and much greater attention should be given to this need. It is also an essential part of helping the attendant to do a satisfying job.

Housing types and systems
(see pp. 40–44)

There are three essentially contrasting types of housing: 'climatic', giving only a cover and protection to the animals; 'controlled environment', which regulates the microclimate as completely as is required for the particular stock being housed; and the 'kennel', which is in a sense a half-way house between the other two forms and gives two environments in the one building allowing some free and appropriate choice for the animals. The methods of use of each of the types and their suitability

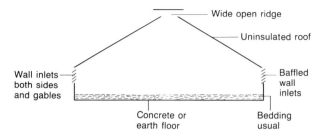

Fig. 56.1 Cross-section of 'climatic' livestock house with open ridge and baffled wall ventilators.

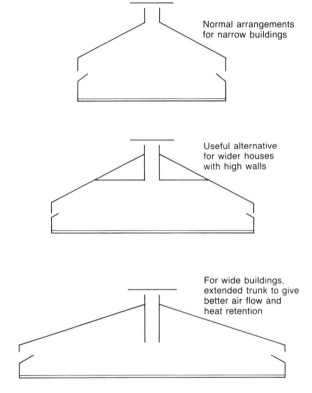

Fig. 56.2 Alternative arrangements suitable for natural ventilation of various widths of buildings and using outlet ('chimney') trunks.

for different countries, climatic regions and forms of livestock vary enormously and must be carefully defined.

Climatic housing (Figs 56.1 and 56.2)

The climatic house is ideal for the adult beast that has developed a large measure of adaptability to climatic stress. The house can be cheap because it is basically a cover alone but because of the lack of control of the climate the space given to the animals must be much greater, especially since there usually is no powered ventilation.

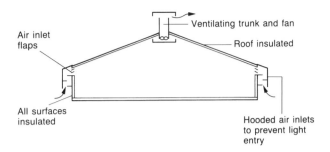

Fig. 56.3 Cross-section of a typical conventionally ventilated controlled environment house with roof fan extraction and hooded wall inlets.

In general, stocking densities tend to be half or less those in the controlled environment house. A major problem is created by agriculturists when they attempt to apply the high stocking rates that are suitable for the controlled environment house to the climatic house, as the building is unable to cope with the demands of the stock and poor productivity and high disease incidence can result. Climatic housing is usually the correct choice for cattle over about six months of age. Such housing usually requires deep bedding for its success, particularly in cooler climatic areas.

Controlled environment house (Fig. 56.3)

The controlled environment house is in great contrast. It has a limited use for cattle, being sometimes used for young calves and to a lesser extent for cattle kept on any bare surfaces, solid or slotted, without bedding. It is most economically viable with livestock that are fed largely concentrate food rather than substantial quantities of roughage, since the former is too expensive to be utilized as a form of energy. The housing is expensive and because of the cost it is usually necessary to stock the buildings as densely as possible to make them viable economically, and this can place a great strain on health control. To cope with the special requirements, management needs to be of the highest standards and unless these criteria can be observed it is the wrong type of housing to have. The rewards can be great but the dangers are greater.

'Kennel' accommodation (Fig. 56.4)

This is an increasingly popular system of accommodation that is in a sense half-way between the climatic and controlled environment housing. It attempts to combine the virtues of both, but at low cost, and often succeeds. The essence of the system is that the animals are kept in pens or groups that are sufficiently small to allow them to be closely confined, at least while resting,

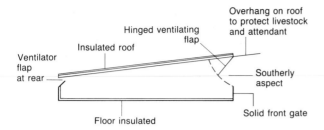

Fig. 56.4 Cross-section of a mono-pitch ('kennel') naturally ventilated stock building.

Table 56.1 A guide to the minimal space allowance for cattle at different stages of growth in strawed yards.

Age	Area/animal (m^2)
Up to 14 days	0.9–1.4
14 days to 3 months	1.4–1.8
3–6 months	1.8–2.4
6–9 months	2.4–2.7
9–18 months	2.7–3.8
Adults	
small	5
large	7

without too great a danger from respiratory or other disease. The close confinement makes it possible to keep the groups warm and draught-free by utilizing their own body heat and by good insulation of the kennel and a limited cubic air space. This part of the accommodation is a simple form of controlled environment house: the rest is the climatic house and can be justified as this is an area where the animals will be moving about freely and will not normally be inactive or lying down. It is likely to contain the dung and often the feeding and watering arrangements and so must be very adequately ventilated, usually by non-mechanical means. In harsh climatic areas it is covered; in milder regions there is no need for this and the 'yard' can, with benefit to health and productivity, be left uncovered.

It is instructive to examine the logic of the 'kennel' system.

- The cost of the housing can be as low as any system, especially with uncovered yarding, and such buildings are also the easiest type of building for the farmer himself to erect.
- Good health is promoted by separation of the animals into small groups. The separation of the kennels one from another should be as absolute as possible as this will limit the build-up and spread of respiratory disease. It will also be a great assistance to the health of the animals if the muck is not allowed to accumulate in the warmth or the closely confined resting area. It is often possible as well, by good design, to keep the dunging areas separate so that the muck from different pens does not come together until after it is out of reach of the animals.
- The cheapness of the housing is largely due to the fact that the environment is controlled only where it is absolutely necessary.

It is certainly a distinct virtue if the dung can be in an area where the air is moving more freely and the temperature and the humidity possibly much lower, at least in temperate climates. Feeding in an outside yard achieves this objective. Controlled environment housing is becoming more and more expensive and there is no possible justification for this control to embrace the effluent from the animals, which is not only a considerable expense but is also likely to intensify the disease risk.

Whatever the system, the principal practical faults in livestock housing systems are as follows:

- Having too close a confinement of the animals.
- Placing too many animals in one common air space.
- Reducing both cubic area and floor space.
- Failing to remove muck from close proximity to the animals.
- Transferring muck through pens, aiding the transfer of disease.
- Failing to separate age groups.
- Neglecting clean feeding and water arrangements.
- Having poor or sometimes no drainage.
- Neglecting the comfort of the stock.
- Inefficient ventilation systems.

Table 56.1 shows the space allowances for cattle in strawed yards.

The environmental requirements of cattle

In most cool, temperate environments, ruminants maintain a stable body temperature by regulating evaporative loss, at little metabolic cost. Ruminants have a very marked ability to alter their zone of thermal neutrality in response to previous thermal history. Thus there are no absolute criteria for the thermal requirements of any class of ruminant livestock, except perhaps the newborn animal; they depend to a large extent on what the animal has grown accustomed to.

Some examples of the lower critical temperatures for cattle under conditions of varying air movements are shown in Table 56.2. This table illustrates a situation where the beasts are standing up, in a dry enclosure, under two variations in air movement (Webster, 1981).

Table 56.2 Lower critical temperature of ruminants housed in a building with very low air movement (0.2 m/s) and in a draught (2 m/s). Source: Webster (1981).

Type of animal	Liveweight (kg)	Lower critical temperature (°C)	
		Low air speed	Draught
Calf			
Newborn	35	+9	+17
1 month old	50	0	+9
Veal	100	−14	−1
Store cattle (maintenance)	250	−32	−20
Beef cow (maintenance)	450	−17	−9
Dairy cow	500	−26	−13

In an unheated building at low air movement the only cattle likely to experience cold sufficient to elevate the heat production are newborn calves or young calves whose metabolic rate is low by virtue of starvation, sickness or emaciation. Such animals can undoubtedly be stressed by cold and may require special attention. Increasing air movement to 2.0 m/s, which is not uncommon in draughty buildings, increases the critical temperature in the newborn calf from +9 to +17°C. This emphasizes the necessity of ensuring that adequate ventilation for calf houses is achieved without allowing excess air movement (or 'draught') to impinge on the calves.

By one month of age the healthy calf with a good appetite and access to an adequate feed source has a critical temperature close to 0°C and is not likely to be stressed by cold while indoors. Well-grown veal calves, by virtue of their very high energy intake and heat production, are particularly tolerant to cold and by the same criteria sensitive to heat. The traditional belief that veal calves should be kept in a warm environment because they are not ruminants and are therefore somehow more sensitive to cold is unscientific and untrue.

No other class of cattle is likely to experience a systemic stress of cold when standing up in a dry enclosure unless air movement is exceptionally high. However, problems do arise in damp conditions. For the dairy cow, however, cold stress should not be considered as a systemic but as a local problem. Heat production in the high-yielding cow is again very high and so the critical temperature is low. Milk synthesis, however, depends on blood flow to the mammary gland, which is reduced by local cooling. The production of dairy cows has been shown to fall at temperatures below about 0°C, although it is obvious that direct chilling of the udder depends as much on the thermal properties of the floor as on the temperature.

It is worth stressing that European cattle tend to be tolerant to cold but intolerant to heat. Their 'comfort zone' is between about 0 and 20°C. The critical temperature leading to a decline in milk yield at the higher level is approximately 21–25°C for most European cattle, including Friesians and Jerseys, but as high as 30–32°C with Brown Swiss (see Chapter 8).

The effect of high temperatures may be ameliorated in practice in a number of ways. The provision of shade makes a great difference, also of wallows and artificial showers. For example, great benefit has been found in tropical climates with cattle kept under a so-called desert-cooler consisting of a three-sided shelter open to the north, with an upper roof of aluminium, which reflects the heat rays, a ceiling underneath of three layers of old hay and an evaporative cooler under the roof at the south end of the shelter. There are a number of highly effective methods of reducing heat stress by the use of water atomizers. In some cases atomizing units are suspended under the roof of the buildings whilst more sophisticated arrangements utilize a series of mist propagators above the stock connected by a pipe-line carrying the water. Provided the humidity of the ambient air is not too high, significant cooling effects can be achieved at a modest running cost (see Chapter 8). True refrigeration plants are very occasionally used but are rarely economic. At high temperatures farm stock also attempt to reduce their heat production by reduced feed intake. This leads to less production and often also to metabolic and fertility problems. Under hot sunny conditions the temperate breeds, particularly, spend less time in grazing and, in fact, under these conditions most of the grazing will be done at night. There are very marked breed differences, as might be expected, the tropical breeds being least affected.

In loose housing systems with open fronted barns, protection from solar radiation and maximum provision of air movement represents the limit of environmental improvement. With closed buildings, such as the cowhouse, mechanical air cooling may be used and, in parts of the world where climatic temperatures warrant it, has been found worthwhile. For a comprehensive consideration of the effects of the environment on cattle the reader is referred to Clark (1981).

Environmental factors affecting susceptibility to disease

Many of the organisms that cause ill-health in intensive livestock units are normally present in the animals and their surroundings and it is environmental stress that acts as a trigger, inducing their multiplication to such an extent that clinically obvious disease breaks out. There are numerous examples, such as respiratory diseases, diarrhoea and mastitis. Whilst these diseases may always become clinically obvious in the long term, there may be a lengthy period beforehand when their effects are limited to poor growth or productivity and an inefficient conversion of feed by the animal. It is an essential feature of a farmer's recording system that records of productivity are kept which should allow the detection of results that are beginning to deteriorate, and this can well be a warning that urgent action is needed to stop a slide in results leading eventually to disease. Most of the conditions of this nature are insidious, chronic and difficult to diagnose by any of the popular methods that are so effective with the well-described diseases. Very limited use can be made of vaccinations or antisera, nor are antibiotics or drugs more than a short-term answer. The only effective way is to attend to the whole environment of the animal by such methods that are known to reduce the risk of disease.

It is extremely difficult to reproduce clinical disease by experimental infections even when huge doses of mixed organisms are used. Whether or not an animal becomes clinically affected depends on non-specific factors of climate, housing and husbandry, which together form the total environment that is considered in this chapter. Above all it should be made clear that the state of health of the animals can transcend all other factors in determining the economic viability of a livestock enterprise. Disease at its worst kills the animal, but even in sublethal infections seriously affects productivity.

The factors influencing the dispersal, survival and deposition of airborne pathogens in farm animals have been reviewed comprehensively by Donaldson (1978). Droplet nuclei are the primary mode of spread of a variety of contagious diseases and many pathogens have been shown to have been spread in this way via the animals' breath and also from secretions and excretions of the infected animals (see p. 242).

Referring specifically to virus particles, the ambient temperature has little effect on their survival in an animal house but a general trend is that high temperatures are more harmful to their survival than low ones (Sanger, 1969). In fact it has been suggested that the inactivation of viruses immediately after exhalation and aerosol formation is dependent on the relative humidity and any temperature effect occurs secondarily (Donaldson & Ferris, 1976). The effect of relative humidity on viruses in general is that viruses with a lipoprotein envelope survive best at a low relative humidity, whereas non-enveloped viruses are unstable in dry conditions but survive best at a high relative humidity. Rhinoviruses appear to survive better at high humidities but infectious bovine rhinotracheitis (IBR) and parainfluenza 3 (PI$_3$) viruses at low humidities. In these last examples the differences in survival time reflect the association between seasonal patterns of relative humidity and disease incidence. There is the further possibility that at high relative humidity there is accelerated sedimentation of airborne pathogens in large aerosols. *Mycoplasma*, on the other hand, tends to be stable at very low and at high relative humidities but sensitive to mid range relative humidity.

So far as bacteria are concerned, a rise in temperature produces an increasing destruction of bacteria but airborne spores are highly resistant. *Escherichia coli* survives and multiplies best at about 15°C, as also does *Mycoplasma*. Bacteria tend to be resistant to low and high relative humidity but sensitive to mid range relative humidity; bacterial spores, however, are resistant almost totally to relative humidity effects.

It is important to be aware that in airborne infections the size of the infecting dose will determine whether or not disease will result. Also, its severity and the likelihood of infection making headway will depend on the animal's overall resistance; for example, chilling can markedly lower an animal's resistance to inhaled pathogens by depressing lung clearance mechanisms (Whittlestone, 1976).

Systems in which the air is recirculated are being favoured as a means of reducing heating costs, but in such systems some form of air cleansing, e.g. filtration, may be necessary to avoid a build-up of pathogens.

It is known from the work of Honey and McQuitty (1976) that animal buildings are often very dusty, but the factors affecting dust production are ill defined. Small changes in relative humidity have been found to have significant effects on settled dust; lower humidities result in more settled dust. There is, however, mounting concern about the deleterious effect of dust on livestock health, and good systems of ventilation should be able to remove it from the building in the same way and as efficiently as other environmental pollutants.

The disposal of large accumulations of animal excrement, bedding and litter is a further problem and can, in some instances, be the limiting factor in determining the size of unit. It is common practice to dilute the effluent from farm buildings into a slurry and then spray it over farmland as a fertilizer. The hazard from the dissemination of slurry-associated pathogens over a wide area in this way can be considerable, particularly in windy weather (Wray, 1975). A dairy herd of 50 cows causes a potential pollution load as large as that of a village of over 500 people, yet frequently the manure is carelessly disposed of without thought of its potential dangers to man or animal.

Intensification and immunity

There are some underlying truths in connection with disease and immunity that need to be explained as they have a close bearing on the incidence of disease and its relationship to the environment.

An animal at birth has a degree of passive immunity to local disease that is passed from the dam to the offspring, partly *in utero* and partly from the colostrum or first milk. Such immunity is, however, only practically effective to local infections to which the dam has been challenged. If the birth takes place in a 'foreign' environment, then the young may have little or no passive immunity to the infective organisms in their new local environment. In many cases the young are housed during the early stages of life in such a 'foreign' environment and it is therefore most important that the challenge of disease-causing organism is reduced to a minimum.

Perhaps the first and foremost methods for reducing this challenge are by the processes of depopulation, cleansing and disinfection. This can obviously be understood to be most important in the case of the younger animal, which has a poor or uncertain resistance to disease. Whilst it can never be said to be other than advantageous, it is most important on sites that have a large population of animals in an area where there are substantial numbers of animals since many diseases, especially viral ones, can pass a great distance by the airborne route. Whilst small infective particles can be carried directly by dust particles moved by the wind, other pathogens are carried indirectly by vectors, especially birds.

Disinfection

The disinfection of a building implies the elimination from the house of all micro-organisms that are capable of causing disease, thus converting the place from a potentially infective state into one that is largely free from infection. A disinfectant is the agent that is capable of achieving this and in livestock farming it is usually a chemical agent.

The processes of disinfection of a building can take place by the action of nature (natural disinfection) and by artificial means (artificial disinfection). Before discussing these processes in some detail, it should be emphasized at the outset that 'cleansing' is an essential preliminary to disinfection. Organic matter has the ability considerably to reduce the effectiveness of disinfectants, so without good cleansing the action of disinfectants is often readily diluted.

Natural disinfectant agents

Most pathogenic micro-organisms do not survive long outside the animal body, but unfortunately sufficient may always remain to cause renewed infection. Some vegetative bacteria and viruses can live several months if protected with organic matter and the spores of bacteria can live almost indefinitely in the soil or protected in cracks and crevices of the building. For example, *Clostridium tetani* and *Bacillus anthracis* can live for many years. Even coccidial oocysts may survive for years in infected quarters.

The factors contributing towards natural destruction of microbes are nevertheless important as they do reduce the numbers and this in itself is a worthwhile aid to the artificial processes. Sunlight, heat, cold, desiccation and agitation all contribute. Sunlight is the most potent and its powers of destruction are enormous; its efficiency is entirely due to the ultraviolet range of wavelengths. Unfortunately, these ultraviolet rays have little penetrating power and cannot pass through glass or translucent roofing sheets or through clouds of industrial haze; the value of sunlight in animal buildings is therefore wholly unreliable. Desiccation, from fresh air and wind, will also contribute to the destruction, particularly when the micro-organisms are exposed to this by prior cleansing of the building.

Another process is antibiosis; many bacteria and fungi produce substances that are antagonistic to other organisms. Penicillin and streptomycin are agents of this nature whose antibacterial action is well known. In the soil, in floors and buildings generally, pathogenic organisms will be acted upon by antibiotics produced by non-pathogenic organisms that are normal inhabitants of the soil. Warm moist conditions will assist the action of such saprophytic agents.

The action of heat

For many years heat has been used for disinfection, dry heat being used with the 'flame-gun' and moist heat in the form of the 'steam-jenny', but both tend to be inexact and uncontrolled methods of applying the agents.

Many bacterial spores can easily survive the transitory attention of the heat source and pathogenic organisms may readily be protected from the heat in cracks and crevices of the building.

Chemical disinfectants

Disinfection on the farm is generally carried out by using chemical agents. The lethal action of disinfectants is due in the main to their ability to react with the protein and, in particular, the essential enzymes of micro-organisms. Therefore, any agents that will coagulate, precipitate or otherwise denature proteins will act as general disinfectants. Among these agents are phenols, alcohols, acids, alkalis, aldehydes, halogens, chloramines and quaternary ammonium compounds, as well as heat and certain radiations.

Selective action

Many disinfectants have a selective action on different types of microbes. For example, Gram-positive and Gram-negative bacteria differ in the structure of their membranes, the latter being of a more complex nature. Micro-organisms also respond to changes in pH and as every protein has its own characteristic isoelectric point, each responds individually and will be influenced by the acidity or alkalinity of the disinfectant; for example, fungi are extremely acid-resistant, whereas viruses tend to be more susceptible to acid disinfectants, such as the iodophors. Another factor affecting the behaviour of a disinfectant is the lipoid content of the cells; in some the content is high, as in acid-fast organisms, and it will thus attract a lipophilic moiety in a disinfectant substance and dissolve it more readily, thereby increasing the germicidal activity. Some disinfectants, which are called broad spectrum, are almost equally active against most species of micro-organisms, while others show specificity and are only active against a restricted number of species.

Disinfection of viruses

For disinfection purposes viruses can be classified into two groups, lipophilic and hydrophilic. Lipophilic viruses have lipid envelopes, which make them sensitive to the majority of disinfectants. Most of the animal pathogenic viruses are in this group. Hydrophilic viruses are enveloped and are less sensitive to disinfectants in general. Some very important viruses are in this group and these have a tendency to become dangerously persistent on farms and in animal buildings; examples are the enteroviruses and reoviruses. Against this latter group quarternary ammonium compounds have a poor effect, but are very good if associated with formaldehyde, gluteraldehyde, chloramines and certain organic acids.

Disinfection of prions

The various infective prions, such as those causing bovine spongiform encephalopathy or scrapie, have a number of common characteristics. They are extremely resistant to heat and, whilst some loss of infectivity occurs at temperatures above 100°C, temperatures greater than 120°C over long periods are needed to inactivate the finely divided material. Resistance to common sterilants and other chemical agents is very high, as is resistance to extremes of pH and to ultraviolet or ionizing irradiation. The only chemical treatment so far found to be effective against all transmissible spongiform encephalopathies is sodium hypochlorite at 20 000 parts per million of available chlorine, for about one hour (see p. 909).

Dynamics of disinfection

Disinfection is not an instantaneous process; it takes place gradually. However, many more microbes are killed at the beginning of disinfection than at the end, although there is an initial lag period before activity commences. The lag phase is normally only a few seconds, but may be seriously prolonged if the environment is unfavourable, for example extreme cold, high humidity or excessive organic matter. An examination of the number of organisms surviving at different stages during disinfection shows that the number of bacteria killed in unit time bears a constant relationship to the number of surviving organisms. Thus, after the lag phase, destruction of the bacteria is very rapid at first but tends to slow up so that eventually destruction of all the organisms takes a considerably longer time. The usual time–survivor curve is of the sigmoid type.

The concentration of disinfectant and temperature of disinfection influence the rate of death and also alter the shape of the time–survivor curves. As the death rate is increased by using higher concentrations of disinfectant, the initial lag phase is eliminated or, in fact, is so quick that it goes undetected. The action of most disinfectants is increased, often quite markedly as the temperature rises.

The effect of organic matter

Almost invariably when disinfection is carried out on the farm, organic matter will be present. It can be said that organic matter always interferes with the action of the disinfectant and may do so in the following ways:

(1) The organic matter may protect the cell by forming a coating on it and preventing the ready access of the disinfectant.
(2) The disinfectant may form an insoluble compound with the organic matter to remove it from potential activity.
(3) The disinfectant may react chemically with the organic matter giving rise to a non-germicidal reaction product.
(4) Particulate and colloidal matter in suspension may absorb the antibacterial agent, so that it is substantially removed from solution.

(5) Fats, etc. in serum and milk may deactivate the disinfectant.

Approval of disinfectants

There is no completely satisfactory method of assessing or standardizing disinfectants and an enormous number of different techniques have been used in the past. There is also no universally effective disinfectant, so that different disinfectants are required for different purposes.

In the UK, approvals for disinfectants are under five headings, as follows:

Group 1A are active against foot-and-mouth disease;
Group 1B are active against swine vesicular disease;
Group II are active against fowl pest;
Group III are active against tuberculosis;
Group IV are for general farm use, the test organism being *Salmonella cholerae suis*.

The official test lays down a rigid procedure for specified reduction of the organisms in the presence of organic matter. The most recent lists of approved disinfectants list over 300 of them for livestock use.

Disinfectants

Phenols, cresols and related compounds

The phenols, cresols and related compounds are an important group of disinfectants that were once the most popular of all such agents.

All phenols can act bactericidally or fungicidally but generally are neither sporicidal nor particularly virucidal. They have high dilution coefficients, i.e. small concentration changes give rise to large differences in their killing rates. They are always more active as acid solutions. Organic matters can severely interfere with their efficiency and even small quantities of faeces can reduce their effectiveness to 10 per cent. There are many proprietary 'coal tar disinfectants', phenolic in nature, and in view of their inevitable low solubility in water they are either solubilized or emulsified. The solubilized types, known as 'black fluids', are those in which the phenol fraction is dissolved in a soap base and the emulsified types, known as 'white fluids', are those in which the phenol is emulsified into a permanent suspension with the aid of gelatin or dextrin.

In more recent years a number of synthetic phenols have been marketed. These may be a chloroxylenol, *o*-phenylphenol or one of the other diphenyl derivatives. Such preparations, in contrast to the cresols or coal tar disinfectants, are non-toxic, non-irritant and have a more pleasant odour, arising chiefly from their purer contents.

Formaldehyde and glutaraldehyde

Formaldehyde is a widely used disinfectant in both the gaseous and the aqueous forms, being bactericidal, virucidal and fungicidal. In aqueous solutions, formalin, which is a solution of formaldehyde gas containing 40 g of formaldehyde in 100 ml of the solution, is widely used at 5 per cent strength as a general disinfectant, but it does need to be in contact with the surface for some time to be effective. Its action is greatly affected by temperature (i.e. it has a high temperature coefficient) and the warmer it is the better, blood heat being most satisfactory. It also acts more efficiently when the surface is wet. In agricultural use formalin is largely used as a gas or an aerosol spray.

A very active complex disinfectant, which is useful against the most persistent viruses, is one containing formaldehyde, glutaraldehyde and a quarternary ammonium compound. This is active at much lower temperatures than formaldehyde.

Quarternary ammonium compounds

These are cationic neutral detergents available as aqueous solutions, powders or pastes. They are effective against a wide range of bacteria and moulds and have a high surface activity. Generally, when dissolved in water, they have a high wetting power and the ions adhere to the surfaces, giving a long-lasting residual effect. They also have low toxicity and lack odour or taste. Combined with other disinfectants they can give a wide spectrum of activity.

Oxidizing disinfectants

Hydrogen peroxide and other oxidizing agents including peracetic acid and propionic acid are emerging as increasingly popular disinfectants. At quite low concentrations they are active against bacteria, their spores, viruses and fungi. Several new proprietary forms are marketed for use in livestock buildings.

The halogens

In agriculture, chlorine is widely used for disinfecting water and in the cleansing of dairy and other farm equipment. Chlorine-releasing compounds containing up to 90 per cent available chlorine are available and have an important use in the formulation of bactericidal detergent powders of the alkaline variety. Products of this type are suitable for use in the washing down of an animal house. The inorganic chloramines, being a concentration of chlorine and ammonia, are used in water and sewage treatment; organic chloramines, such as halazone, are excellent water sanitizers.

The normal use of chlorine in cleaning milking and other utensils is to use a detergent wash with a solution containing 250–300 ppm of available chlorine followed by a rinse with a weaker chlorine solution. Failure of the chlorine disinfectant is more likely due to the presence of organic matter, which does seriously interfere with its action, so that it is not normally used where much dirt is present. In favourable circumstances it is best used warm and will act quickly. Chloramines are much more active in the presence of organic matter and have found a secure place as general disinfectants.

Iodine and iodophors

Iodine is an effective germicide, although like chlorine its action is much depressed by organic matter. It is effective against vegetative organisms and spores. The most widely used iodine preparations are the iodophores in which iodine is mixed with surface-active agents, which act as carriers or solubilizers for the iodine. They lack any real odour and are not irritant.

Iodophors have been used at dilutions of around 25 ppm available iodine for utensils. They have built-in indicators that reveal quickly the approximate concentration of the use dilution; a yellow tinge or pale amber colour is imparted by an iodophor even when only a few parts per million of free iodine are present in the solution. High concentrations give deeper shades of amber or brown to the solution. The use dilution of 25 ppm is equivalent to available chlorine concentrations up to 200 ppm. Iodophors are an ideal germicide to use in water utensils.

Ammonia

A 10 per cent aqueous solution of ammonia is an effective agent for the destruction of coccidial oocysts. This is the only use for ammonia as a disinfectant.

Ectoparasites

It is of great importance to control ectoparasites in and around the farm buildings. They are a nuisance both to the attendants and the animals, may be the cause of direct irritation and disease and may indirectly spread disease; indeed any infectious agent can be carried by ectoparasitic vectors. These ectoparasites include flies (the ordinary housefly, the lesser housefly and the stable fly), mites, ticks, lice, fleas, bugs, beetles and cockroaches.

For the control of external parasites of animals a variety of compounds are available, such as gamma-benzene hexachloride (lindane), piperoxyl-butoxide pyrethrum (pybuthrin) or *O,O*-dimethyldithiophosphate of diethylmercaptosuccinate (malathion) and *O,O*-

dimethyl-*O*-2,3,5-trichlorphenyl phosphorathroate (fenchlorphos 12 per cent) (see Chapter 60).

Health and safety

There are certain dangers to people and mammals in the use and disposal of disinfectants and ectoparasiticides and the residues of their applications. For this reason alone it is advised that only officially approved products should be used and the health and safety regulations attached to them are followed rigidly. An awareness of the possible harm to those using the substances and their effect on polluting the environment has increased immensely lately so that the manufacturers have been forced to update the health and safety data regularly. There are particular dangers with some ectoparasiticides as well as certain disinfectants and it is vital that protective clothing is worn.

Rotation of hygiene products

There are no products that are ideal. All of the disinfectants and ectoparasiticides have their strengths and weaknesses. To minimize the adverse effects of this fact, it is recommended that a rotational programme is instituted so that regular programmed changes are made in the type of product used, thereby reducing the chance of certain pathogens escaping destruction.

Recommended procedure in disinfection and disinfestation of animal buildings and equipment

Basically, two procedures should be adopted. The first is used between batches of livestock within a building in the absence of overt disease, and the second after an outbreak of a contagious and infectious disease.

Procedure of disinfection with no disease present

(1) All equipment and fittings that are removable should be demounted and taken out of the building. It is advisable for them to be soaked in a bath of disinfectant where the materials are able to stand up to this treatment. Alternatively, they may be power-sprayed or steam sterilized. They should be left outside exposed to the elements and away from animals and their products for as long as possible.
(2) All litter should be removed (Fig. 56.5).
(3) The roof and structural elements of the house should be dusted and cleaned, preferably with a vacuum cleaner.
(4) The lower part of the walls and all the floors should be thoroughly cleaned, preferably using a

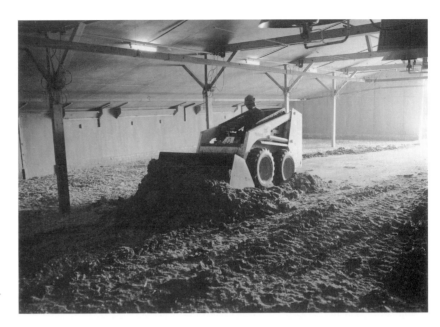

Fig. 56.5 Cleaning out the litter after removal of the animals.

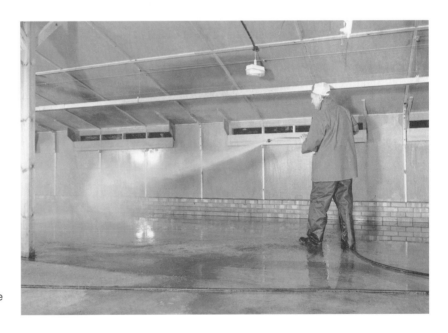

Fig. 56.6 Washing down with a pressure hose using a detergent disinfectant.

pressure washer, with a heavy duty, wide-spectrum detergent/disinfectant mixture (Fig. 56.6).

(5) The surfaces must then have a disinfectant applied (Fig. 56.7) with a wide spectrum of activity, capable of killing all the pathogens that are likely to be present.

(6) In some cases, if there is a heavy insect infestation, it will be necessary to apply a special insecticide spray.

(7) As a final measure a disinfectant is often sprayed over all the surfaces to give a residual effect. Thermal 'fogging' machines are widely used.

Procedure after contagious and infectious disease

(1) The building should be closed and isolated from all visitors.

(2) The bedding, litter and all areas in intimate contact with the stock should be sprayed with a strong disinfectant.

(3) The litter should subsequently be removed from the building and may be burnt or buried so there is no possible contact with livestock.

(4) Portable equipment and fittings should be given the same treatment as previously suggested and

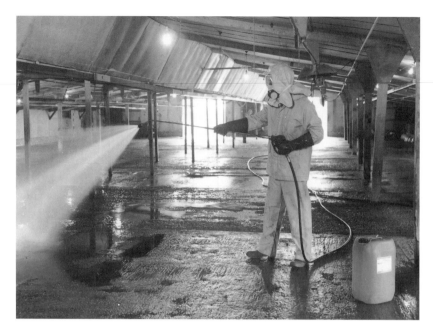

Fig. 56.7 Spraying with a disinfectant.

preferably in the house, later to be taken out and aerated.

(5) The floors and lower part of the walls should be cleaned with detergent disinfectant.
(6) The house should then be treated in the same way as suggested in the previous section.
(7) It may sometimes be advisable to skim off the top few inches of the soil around a heavily infected area.
(8) The approaches to the building should be treated with disinfectant and foot-dips provided (Fig. 56.8).

Ventilation

There are few topics in animal husbandry where there have been more totally erroneous statements made than on the reasons why housed livestock require ventilation or 'air-change'. For example, for many years it was accepted that the main deleterious effect of having too little ventilation was due to the build-up of harmful concentrations of the gaseous products of respiration, and in particular carbon dioxide, combined with a depletion in the oxygen content of the air. It is now known that this is far too simple and usually quite an incorrect hypothesis.

Underlying principles and calculations

In any badly underventilated building the stagnant air gradually becomes both warmer and more humid and there is a rising concentration of dust, other particulate

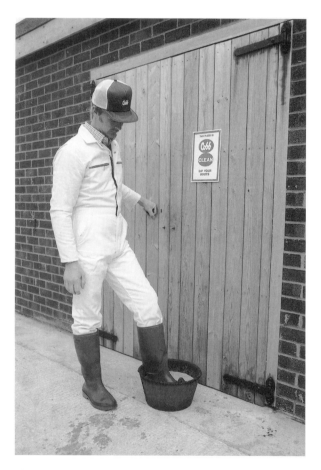

Fig. 56.8 Using protective clothing and dipping boots in disinfectant to reduce the risk of introducing infection.

matter, ammonia and other gases and any pathogenic microorganisms the livestock may be carrying. The end result is that the animals suffer from 'heat stagnation', involving a susceptibility to chilling. Along with this will go poor productivity and a likelihood of disease, particularly respiratory, which modern experience shows to be of the greatest danger in intensive forms of housing.

In addition, in a badly ventilated building, condensation on the surface is often likely and bedding and floors may become wet and the animals uncomfortable. This will tend to exacerbate the effect of disease conditions, respiratory or enteric in nature, or infections such as mastitis.

In recent years a new hazard to livestock and their attendants has been the risk of gaseous intoxication of livestock due to the gases arising from slurry pits or channels under the animals. The risk is very great and has caused the death of many animals and several stockworkers.

The object of ventilation, therefore, is to remove the stale air in a building and replace it with fresh air and remove any danger of toxic gases. But while too little ventilation is obviously serious, so also is too much. In cold weather much valuable animal heat will be wasted. Further, overventilation may be synonymous with draught. Draughts are themselves responsible for causing many deaths by direct chilling and they may also act indirectly by lowering the animals' resistance to disease-producing organisms.

In planning a ventilation system allowance has to be made for all the factors that can influence the ventilation required, i.e. type, age and number of livestock, their management, the construction and locality of the house and finally the weather conditions.

Natural ventilation (see p. 40)

If natural ventilation is to be effective, it must function well in all weathers. To try to avoid too great a dependence on external wind and weather, it is best to make use of the so-called 'stack effect' as its foundation. The warm stale air around the body of the animal, being lighter than cold fresh air, will rise to the top of the building. Outlet ventilation is therefore provided at a suitable point or points in the ceiling or roof. The greater the difference between inside and outside temperatures, and the greater the distance between inlets and outlets, the greater the stack effect. Therefore, if an area of outlet ventilation is provided to cope with difficult conditions (i.e. a small difference between inside and outside temperatures) it can easily be restricted when temperature differences are greater or appreciable winds help in the ventilation. As mentioned, in houses where no great control is necessary, such as climatic housing for cattle, a fixed open ridge with a pro-

tective cap may be sufficient. But in other controlled-climate accommodations far more control is needed and down-draughts, which can be common with the fixed open ridge, must be avoided. Experience has shown that for the latter, good results are obtained by the use of a limited area of controlled outlet ventilation and for this purpose a simple chimney type or insulated 'flue' is satisfactory. It is good practice to have one or a few outlets, but a much larger number of smaller air inlets, as the fresh air should come in slowly all round the building, diffusely and carefully baffled. The basis of a useful inlet system consists of hopper-type windows, fitted with gussets to prevent direct draughts, serving as principal inlets, and small baffled openings between the windows which alone are left open during cold or windy weather. Since cold air coming into the building falls naturally towards the floor, there is no necessity to site inlets at floor level, where the danger of chilling draught is considerable.

The totally covered yard

In practice the following major faults are commonly found in the construction of covered yards:

- Either there is no ridge outlet for stale air or it is inadequate.
- Eaves openings are either absent or, where present, uncontrollable and at the mercy of the weather, causing chilling draughts in cold weather.
- The extreme width of many yards (20 m upwards) prevents natural ventilation functioning properly. This problem is often combined with multispan construction and low eaves and roofs, so that the flow is generally impaired.
- The gable ends are closed and sealed.
- There is no insulation of the roof. While insulation is not usually necessary it may be a desirable 'extra' under a few circumstances, particularly where younger stock are housed or where the roof is low and natural air flow is difficult.
- Poor drainage under or around the yard leads to excessive straw usage and contributes to the humidity of the atmosphere.
- Bad construction of the walls leads to excessive moisture penetration at all points.

Natural ventilation works most satisfactorily on open sites; it is always useful to have it controllable, but this is not usually done. An open ridge 300 mm wide, with a flat continuous top at least 150 mm above, is a simple answer to extraction in narrow yards, and a 600 mm wide ridge in yards above 14 m width.

An even more satisfactory arrangement is to have a series of chimney-type ventilators along the ridge, allowing 0.09 m²/animal. A useful size of chimney is

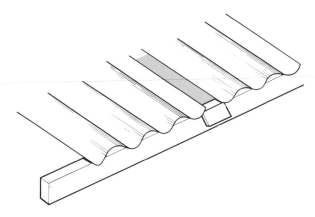

Fig. 56.9 The 'breathing' roof: ventilation achieved by leaving a gap between the roof sheets.

$1 m^2$; this is sufficient for 11 animals. The throat can be controlled by a butterfly valve or hinged flap.

Alternative ways of achieving good 'top' ventilation are as follows:

(1) Raised sheets, consisting of conventional steel sheets fitted with a batten or washers raising the overlapping, allowing air to pass between the sheets. A spacer batten of treated timber measuring $50 mm \times 25 mm$ is suitable.

(2) Upturned corrugated sheeting. Conventional galvanized corrugated steel sheeting is fixed upside down with a gap between each sheet, forming a Venturi flow between each sheet. Typically, a 25 mm gap may be used, which would give 3.75 per cent opening of the roof. (Fig 56.9).

Systems (1) and (2) are often described as 'breathing roofs'.

Mechanical ventilation

This has a place in some cattle yards as it has for other forms of intensively housed stock. With a system of chimney trunks, fans can be added as a complementary arrangement, since an extractor fan may be fitted at the base. If a 600 mm fan running at a maximum of 900 rev/min is fitted, $10\,194 m^3$ hour will be extracted. A maximum allowance of $510 m^3$/hour per beast (or approximately $0.42 m^3$/hour per kg bodyweight) is found satisfactory, so that one fan will serve approximately 30 beef animals to slaughter.

Automatic or semi-automatic control can be achieved if a proportion (one-half to two-thirds) of the fans are put on a thermostatic control, with a thermostat that is easily seen and adjusted. Fans thus operated should have automatic antiback-draught flaps fitted to prevent down-draughts when they are switched off. All fans should be speed controlled. Alternatively, a system

of variable fan speed on a motorized thermostat or electronic control will give full automation on all fans.

Fan ventilation halves the number of roof outlets that need to be installed. The total capital cost of a fan-operated system will hardly be more than £30 per animal-place, an economical cost for automatic environmental control. Running costs may be a rather more daunting charge.

The main use of fan ventilation in cattle yards is in those cases where extremely high stocking rates are used, as with slatted floor units, or where the topography of the site or restriction of wind around the building makes natural flow all but impossible.

The inlet of fresh air is no less important, and it has been found satisfactory to provide inward-opening hopper flaps along both side walls, bottom-hung and 700–900 mm deep, with gussets and variable control through casement stays or remote control from the feeding passage. Alternatively, the hoppers may be controlled from the ends with horticultural glasshouse type fittings. It is preferable if the inlets are not closer than 600 mm to the eaves, to prevent incoming air 'bouncing' off exposed purlins and causing an irritating down-draught on the animals. The flaps should be made so that they can be removed or hinged down flat in the summer; they should extend along at least one-half and preferably two-thirds of the wall length.

With wide-span yards over 21 m, slatted boarding (100 mm boards and 12 mm gaps or 150 mm boards and 25 mm gaps) should be fitted at the gable ends and part of this area made as hinged doors that can be opened in the summer. This is normally not necessary, however, in narrow-span yards. In addition, there are a number of other excellent techniques for achieving good inlet ventilation for cattle and other yards.

'Spaced boarding' is excellent all around a yard – at the gable ends and along the walls above 'animal height' (Fig. 56.10). It gives an opening area of about 20 per cent of the total but is uncontrollable; an alternative is to have an adjustable system with fixed outer slats and inner sliding slats. There are also various other arrangements, such as the Ventair steel sheet with patented louvres (13 per cent open); slatted hardboard with slats $5 mm \times 25 mm$ giving 30 per cent opening; Netlon polypropylene mesh (45 per cent open); Ventrex steel sheet with louvres (0.7 per cent open) and a common device of a space left between the outer sheet and the wall, giving a baffled protected inlet.

It is in no way suggested that the systems outlined are the only satisfactory methods of ventilating intensive cattle yards. For example, other mechanical means have been used, often with equal success. These do, however, often need more careful designing and management to prevent draughts and to give adequate control. The systems suggested are logical and generally understood

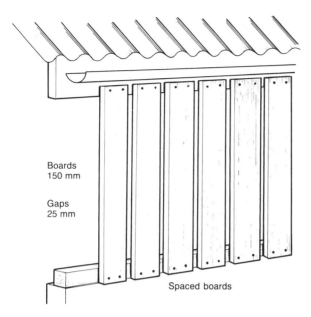

Boards
150 mm

Gaps
25 mm

Spaced boards

Fig. 56.10 Wall ventilation with spaced boarding.

and easily controlled by the stockworker. Mechanical assistance with the designs shown is complementary to natural flow and indeed may be used as an additional stage in the development and improvement of a design. Draughts are least likely where there is the fullest control of the system. Ventilation continues to function at a reduced rate in the event of power failure with the system advocated, since natural stack-effect ventilation takes over from the fans to tide the stock over this period.

If the trend towards high stocking rates continues it is inevitable that the farmer will turn increasingly to thermal insulation of the surfaces, especially the roof. Farmers who have used insulation of the roof have recorded considerable benefits in terms of liveweight gain and feed conversion efficiency, but above all because it helps also to solve environmental problems. A popular way of arranging the insulation is by using two skins of metal or fibre-cement sheeting for the roof separated by a vapour-sealed layer of mineral wool or glass wool. For the latter, a 50 mm thickness is minimal but 100 mm is very much better. A cheap treatment for an existing uninsulated building is to build a false ceiling of wire mesh supporting vapour-sealed insulation. It is an economical way of insulating the building, though somewhat temporary. It must be emphasized that individual attention does need to be given to each yard according to the site and locality. It is one of the advantages of fan ventilation that with mechanical ventilation this statement is much less true. The use of fans partially rules out the dependence on site and weather. It is generally better to have yards in exposed positions because it is easier to restrict the open area if too much

air comes in than to open up the ventilation space in a sheltered site. Sometimes the proximity of other buildings makes it impossible to increase the airflow at all.

Livestock yards are now often made very wide, of the order of 40–50 m. These are invariably the most difficult units to ventilate. From the point of view of ventilation it is desirable to limit the span to some 30 m. Indeed, if the trend towards the use of thermal insulation continues, views on what constitutes an adequate cubic area may change. In an uninsulated yard a large cubic area helps to buffer the outside weather extremes. But in an insulated construction, the roofing area must be reduced to a minimum to cut costs and more economical dimensions would be a height of 3.6 m to eaves with a maximum yard span of 21 m. These recommendations widely used and required for cattle buildings apply, with only minor modifications, to climatic yard accommodation generally, including that for pigs, sheep and turkeys.

Open-fronted yards and kennels

A fundamentally different approach to climatic housing is the 'lean-to' or open-fronted yard, often called the mono-pitch building. This is attractive in several respects and continues to gain in popularity as an alternative to the span roof yard. For a start it is usually cheaper. Also, by its very nature, it is impossible to make it very wide – a depth of 10 m being about the limit – so the enormous problems of ventilation created by wide spans are avoided and stock concentrations in one air space are limited. Best of all, such a system gives a cheap isolation of groups by carrying vertical partitions to the roof and if necessary supporting it every 3–6 m. With an open-fronted design animals have a choice of environment, as they can go towards the lower back part in colder conditions to keep warm, or come to the front for sunlight and more fresh air in warmer weather. Control of airflow can be by simple hinged flaps on the front and kennels can be incorporated if desired. It is most desirable that open-fronted yards in the northern hemisphere face in a southerly direction only; it is preferable not to face two rows together, since there is a risk of the passage-way between becoming a wind tunnel and in this situation one side at least will face north or east and so may get little sun and indeed may suffer from distinctly cooler conditions.

Dangers from gases in farm buildings

Problems associated with gases in and around the livestock farm have been highlighted recently, particularly in association with gas effusion from slurry channels under perforated floors, but it would be wrong to regard these as the only dangers. While there have been numerous fatalities of livestock recorded, and indeed of man, due to gas intoxication, there is also mounting evidence that there may be concentrations of gases in many livestock buildings that may affect production adversely by reducing feed consumption, lowering growth rates and increasing the animals' susceptibility to invasion by pathogenic micro-organisms.

The most serious incidence of gas intoxication arises from areas of manure storage in slurry pits or channels under the stock, usually but not always associated with forms of perforated floors. The greatest risk arises when the manure is agitated for any reason, usually when it is removed. There is also an ever-present danger if a mechanical system of ventilation fails and this is the only method of moving air in the house. Several cases of poisoning have been reported when sluice-gates are opened at the end of slurry channels and the movement of the liquid manure has forced gas up at one end of the building.

High concentrations of gases, chiefly ammonia, may also arise from built-up litter in animal housing. The danger has undoubtedly been exacerbated within more recent years owing to the mistaken insistence of maintaining relatively high house temperatures in order to reduce food costs. The farmer has often attempted to achieve such temperatures by restricting ventilation and in the absence of good thermal insulation of the house surface, so that the result may often be generally harmful if not actually dangerous.

References

Britton, D.K. & Berkeley Hill (1975) *Size and Efficiency in Farming*, pp. 132–47. Saxon House Studies, Farnborough.

Clark, J.A. (ed.) (1981) *Environmental Aspects of Housing for Animal Production*. Butterworth, London.

Donaldson, A.I. (1978) Factors influencing the dispersal, survival and deposition of airborne pathogens of farm animals. *Veterinary Bulletin*, **48**, 83–94.

Donaldson, A.I. & Ferris, N.P. (1976) The survival of some airborne animal viruses in relation to relative humidity. *Veterinary Microbiology*, 413–20.

Honey, H.F. & McQuitty, J.B. (1976) *Dust in the Animal Environment*. Departement of Agricultural Engineering, University of Alberta, Canada.

Sanger, J.R. (1969) Influence of relative humidity on the survival of some airborne viruses. *Applied Microbiology*, **15**, 35–42.

Webster, A.J.F. (1981) Optimal housing criteria for ruminants. In *Environmental Aspects of Housing for Animal Production* (ed. by J.A. Clark), pp. 217–32. Butterworth, London.

Whittlestone, P. (1976) Effect of climatic conditions on enzootic pneumonia in pigs. *International Journal of Biometerology*, **20**, 42–8.

Wray, C. (1975) Survivial and spread of pathogenic bacteria of veterinary importance within the environment. *Veterinary Bulletin*, **45**, 543–57.

Chapter 57
Biosecurity

D.C. Barrett and A.J. Taylor

Introduction   987
Benefits of improved biosecurity   988
Routes of infection   988
Infectious diseases that can be introduced into cattle herds   989
General principles of biosecurity   989
The 'closed' herd   990
Introduction of purchased stock   990
Risk of disease in the herd affecting an incoming animal   991
Principles of biosecurity planning   991
Producing a biosecurity plan   991
Herd biosecurity: where *is* the final frontier?   994
Conclusions   994

Introduction

Biosecurity means a multitude of things to different people. In its broadest interpretation in relation to human health it is defined as 'those cumulative steps taken to prevent transmission of pathogens and other harmful agents to individuals or populations of human beings' (Gillespie, 2000). Gillespie (2000) further states that the harmful effects of these agents may be direct (e.g. smallpox virus causing disease) or indirect, by disrupting the food supply (e.g. animal or plant pathogens), and that any substance that disrupts biological systems necessary for human health and well-being is a threat to biosecurity. In addition to pathogens, it is also suggested that naturally produced poisons, such as aflatoxin, toxic chemicals and pesticides, all have the potential to disrupt beneficial and necessary biological systems and can therefore also be considered to threaten biosecurity.

From the point of view of human health, the ultimate aim of biosecurity is therefore to safeguard the human food chain. While major epidemic diseases of cattle such as foot-and-mouth disease and rinderpest may threaten food supplies, they do not have direct public health implications. However, most foodborne illnesses are the result of inadvertent contamination of foods by pathogens, including viruses, bacteria, protozoa and perhaps also prions. These organisms may be zoonotic, causing disease in cattle and humans e.g. *Salmonella* spp., or foodborne pathogens that are non-pathogenic in cattle, e.g. *Escherichia coli* O157.

While the public health aspect of biosecurity is obviously extremely important, the prime role of the veterinary surgeon is to safeguard the health of food-producing animals, because disease will reduce productivity and/or be detrimental to animal welfare (Barrett, 2001a). It is this animal health aspect of biosecurity which will be dealt with in most detail in this chapter.

From the point of view of cattle health, biosecurity can be defined as 'the efforts put forth to prevent the introduction of pathogens or toxins that have the potential to damage the health of a herd of cattle or the safety and quality of a food product' (Sanderson *et al.*, 2000). An interrelated concept is that of biocontainment, which is the 'effort to contain the spread of disease or intoxication within a herd' (Sanderson *et al.*, 2000). For the purposes of this chapter, we will concentrate on the infectious disease components of both biosecurity and biocontainment, and use the term biosecurity in a generic sense to cover both concepts.

In the past, efforts to use biosecurity principles to control diseases of cattle in the UK have been largely confined to the statutory control and eradication, or attempted eradication, of notifiable diseases such as foot-and-mouth disease (FMD), bovine tuberculosis (TB) and brucellosis, or specific diseases such as bovine herpes virus-1 (BHV-1), the cause of infectious bovine rhinotracheitis (IBR) (p. 286), and leptospirosis (*L. borgpetersenii* serovar *hardjo* and *L. interrogans* serovar *hardjo*) (p. 735) within non-statutory cattle health schemes. This has resulted in an attitude amongst many cattle producers that infectious disease control is either something that government should take charge of, and pay for, on their behalf, or is something that is only relevant to a small number of herds who may benefit from having an 'elite' health status. The majority of commercial herd owners have considered that endemic infectious diseases are always going to be present within their herds. This has resulted in many of them tolerating the infections and acting in a reactive way to treat disease when it occurs while living with the associated depression in productivity, rather than taking a proactive disease control and/or eradication stance.

This is in contrast to the attitude in the UK pig and poultry industries where there are pyramidal structures, designed amongst other things to help control infectious disease. Pig and poultry producers, whether they are breeding companies or commercial units, would not entertain the idea of introducing new stock without taking specific precautions to protect both the newcomers and the indigenous herd or flock from infectious diseases. Although the cattle industry is structured very differently from the pig industry, cattle producers could learn a lot from the biosecurity principles that have been developed for pigs over many years (Moore, 1992). Even so, the outbreak of classical swine fever in Eastern England in 2000 (Sharp *et al.*, 2001) and the spread of new diseases such as post weaning multisystemic wasting syndrome with the movement of pigs between farms (Done *et al.*, 2001) has shown that disease transmission between pig units remains a problem.

Even before the devastating outbreak of FMD in the UK in 2001, the challenge to enhance biosecurity on cattle units was already very real. Biosecurity had become an increasingly topical issue in relation to cattle production, prompted by suggestions that TB control measures would be enhanced if biosecurity were improved (Anon, 1999a,b, 2001a; Collins, 2000; Phillips *et al.*, 2000; Barrett *et al.*, 2001), reducing both cattle-to-cattle (Menzies & Neill, 2000) and badger-to-cattle transmission of *Mycobacterium bovis* (see p. 857). More generally, much needed to be done at a herd level to improve herd health and productivity by implementing well-designed 'biosecurity plans' that were proactive in preventing the spread of numerous infectious diseases endemic within the UK.

The 2001 outbreak of FMD, which affected France, The Netherlands and the Republic of Ireland as well as the UK, emphasized the need to safeguard the national herd from exotic diseases, particularly in these times of a single European Market. The last frontier for disease control must be the farm boundary; cattle farmers have to take responsibility for disease control in their own herds, and, with advice from their veterinary surgeons, decide what precautions they need to take to reduce the risk of disease transmission.

Benefits of improved biosecurity

Improving biosecurity on cattle units, both to control infectious diseases already present and to prevent the introduction of new infections, has a number of potential benefits at the farm level (Box 57.1). If improved biosecurity measures are widely adopted such that increased numbers of cattle herds become free of

Box 57.1 The benefits of improved biosecurity to an individual farmer.

Increases in production, productivity and profit
Improved animal welfare
More efficient utilization of resources
Reduced use of medication, such as antibiotics and anthelmintics, with an associated reduction in the risk of resistant pathogens emerging
Enhanced value of the individual herd, with livestock, and livestock products, of known health status commanding premium prices

Box 57.2 The benefits of improved biosecurity to the wider farming community.

Maximizing export markets by the prevention of disease-orientated barriers being put in place by importing countries
Possible limitation of imports by creating disease-orientated barriers to the importation of livestock, and livestock products, from countries of lower health status

selected infectious diseases, there will be potential benefits related to international trade (Box 57.2).

Farm biosecurity is also an important first step in safeguarding the human food chain with benefits to the community at large. It is an important part of any hazard analysis and critical control point (HACCP) plan to safeguard human health. Food retailers are taking much more interest in this area as a means of combating potential risks to human health (Noordhuizen & Wentink, 2001), for example the possible link between *Mycobacterium avium* subsp. *paratuberculosis* (Johne's disease) (p. 862) in cattle and Crohn's disease in humans (Hermon-Taylor, 2000). The general population is now much more sensitive to disease epidemics and food scares, e.g. salmonella in eggs and bovine spongiform encephalopathy (BSE) (p. 909), and farmers may in future need to show that they have adequate biosecurity measures in place to minimize such risks in order to sell to certain retailers.

Routes of infection

There are many ways in which an infectious agent can enter a herd of cattle. These are summarized in Box 57.3. The greatest risk for most diseases is by contact with infected cattle, either by the introduction of infected cattle into a herd or by contact with neighbouring herds via cograzing or across boundaries. Attendance at shows and the return of unsold cattle from sales also risks the introduction of disease. These infected animals may be either asymptomatic 'carriers' of a specific disease such as bovine herpes virus-1 (BHV-1), bovine virus diar-

Box 57.3 Common routes by which infectious agents can enter a herd of cattle.

> Introduction of infected cattle or direct cattle-to-cattle contacts
> Feed or water, contaminated with pathogens such as *Salmonella* spp. or the prion responsible for BSE
> Visitors, including those regularly working with cattle on other premises, such as relief milkers, foot trimmers, AI technicians and veterinary surgeons
> Mechanical vectors such as vehicles and farm implements
> Wildlife, including badgers, rabbits, rodents, deer and birds
> Other species of livestock such as sheep
> Airborne transmission, notably FMD

rhoea virus (BVDV) (p. 853), *Neospora caninum* (p. 584), *Streptococcus agalactiae* (p. 333) or cattle incubating a particular disease such as *Salmonella typhimurium* DT 104 (p. 850). In the case of cattle incubating disease, it may be possible to prevent the introduction of a pathogen by imposing quarantine measures of a duration that exceeds the expected incubation period. However, some pathogens may not cause infected animals to exhibit overt clinical signs, e.g. *Leptospira hardjo* (*L. borgpetersenii* serovar *hardjo* and *L. interrogans* serovar *hardjo*). Others may have excessively long incubation periods, making simple quarantine impractical without the use of accompanying diagnostic testing, e.g. *Mycobacterium avium* subsp. *paratuberculosis* (Johne's disease). In the case of 'carrier' animals that do not exhibit clinical signs, detection is reliant on diagnostic testing, either of the individual animals or of the herd from which they have been obtained. The reliability of diagnostic tests and the design and implementation of testing regimens have been discussed in detail by Caldow *et al.*, (2001). With or without adequate isolation and quarantine measures, appropriate diagnostic tests will need to be undertaken to ensure, as far as is realistically possible, freedom from disease in introduced animals or at least to define their health status and prior exposure to certain pathogens.

To prevent direct or indirect contact between herds of neighbouring cattle, there should be a 3 m gap between boundary fences and hedges. This should minimize the risk of short-distance airborne disease transmission such as is possible for BHV-1, the cause of IBR. Long-distance airborne transmission, as is classically seen with FMD, is almost impossible for an individual farmer to guard against.

Infectious diseases that can be introduced into cattle herds

The numerous infectious diseases that can be introduced into cattle herds can be divided into three cate-

Box 57.4 Diseases endemic in the UK and elsewhere, which may be controlled in part by enhanced biosecurity measures.

> Bovine virus diarrhoea (BVD)
> Infectious bovine rhinotracheitis (IBR)
> Leptospirosis[a]
> Salmonellosis[a]
> Johne's disease[b]
> Mastitis, e.g. *Streptococcus agalactia*
> Digital dermatitis
> Parasitic diseases[a]
> Ringworm[a]
> Udder skin infections
> Venereal *Campylobacter* spp. infection
> Neospora infection (causing abortion)
>
> [a] Zoonotic diseases transmissible to humans.
> [b] There is some evidence that links this disease with Crohn's disease in humans and its importance may therefore increase further in the future.

Box 57.5 Diseases notifiable in the UK.

> These are the diseases subject to national control policies and/or international trade rules and include:
> Anthrax[a]
> Aujeszky's disease[b,c]
> Bluetongue[a]
> Bovine spongiform encephalopathy (BSE)[b]
> Brucellosis[b,c,d]
> Contagious bovine pleuropneumonia (CBPP)[a]
> Enzootic bovine leukosis (EBI)[a]
> Foot-and-mouth disease (FMD)[a]
> Lumpy skin disease
> Rabies
> Rift Valley fever
> Rinderpest
> Tuberculosis (TB)[b]
> Vesicular stomatitis
> Warble fly[a]
>
> [a] Those diseases considered by the authors to pose the greatest threat of re-emergence or introduction into the UK.
> [b] Diseases known to be present in the UK in early 2002 ([c]Northern Ireland only).
> [d] Occurred in the UK in 2003.

gories: diseases endemic in the UK and elsewhere, examples of which are shown in Box 57.4, notifiable diseases both present in the UK and exotic (Box 57.5) and other diseases not considered present in the UK (Box 57.6).

General principles of biosecurity

Biosecurity is not a new concept; the introduction of 'cattle plague' (rinderpest) (p. 707) into the UK in 1865 resulted in the Cattle Disease Prevention Act of 1866.

Box 57.6 Other important diseases not widely present in the UK that may be introduced.

If cattle are purchased from another country, there are diseases that are currently not present or at minimum levels in the UK but which are also currently not subject to national control measures or importation rules. For example:
Trichomoniasis
Some species of *Leptospira*
Type 2 BVD virus*

*Recently found in Great Britain.

This Act enforced the use of what we would now consider biosecurity measures to eradicate rinderpest from the British Isles after an estimated 400 000 cattle had died of the disease; the last cases were seen in 1877 (Dunlop & Williams, 1996). The basic principles for the prevention and control of many infectious diseases in cattle have therefore been well recognized for over 125 years.

Duncan (1990) set out the principles of infectious disease control in cattle in the early 1990s. At a meeting of the British Cattle Veterinary Association (BCVA) in 1994, three papers related to this subject were presented (Duncan, 1994; Taylor, 1994a,b), followed by a further paper in 1996 (Pritchard, 1996). Duncan (1990) set out a seven-point plan, subsequently modified slightly as follows:

(1) Maintain a closed herd, with no introduction of animals and no contact with outside cattle.
(2) If introduction of cattle is unavoidable, operate an isolation and testing policy for introduced stock, including other species such as sheep.
(3) Ensure feed and water are free from contamination.
(4) Control visitors and vehicles, and operate a policy to reduce the risk of transmission of pathogens from visitors and vehicles.
(5) Control direct and indirect contact between wildlife and cattle, particularly rodents and birds.
(6) Define and monitor the health status of the herd.
(7) Establish and operate an agreed disease control programme or biosecurity plan.

The 'closed' herd

Maintenance of a closed herd is the main plank of a biosecurity programme. No animals must be purchased, borrowed or hired. New genetic material must only be introduced to the herd by artificial insemination (AI) or embryo transfer (ET), but even these introductions can present some risk (see Chapters 39 and 40). When using ET, embryos must be transferred into home-bred recipients; pregnant recipients or animals for use as recipients must not be purchased. No animals must be loaned or hired out. No animals must be returned to the herd from shows or sales. There must be no contact with other cattle when grazing.

Introduction of purchased stock

It will not be appropriate for many herds to be closed, due to management constraints such as cograzing or a production system based on the rearing of purchased stock. It is therefore essential to minimize the risk of introducing infectious diseases into the herd when buying new stock. The introduced animals may bring with them an infectious organism not previously present on the unit, leading to disease in the indigenous population, e.g. Johne's disease. They may also introduce a different strain of a pathogen, e.g. anthelmintic-resistant gastrointestinal nematodes, or virulent BHV-1, or may themselves succumb to a disease endemic in the indigenous population. Even where there is no desire to achieve or maintain a high health status herd, the risk of introducing more virulent strains of a pathogen, or drug-resistant pathogens, is a very real threat whenever cattle move between herds.

The safest source for new stock is a herd certified free of specific diseases, usually by a cattle health scheme. If such stock are not available, the next safest route is to buy from farms of known health status. In order of increasing risk:

(1) A health scheme herd being monitored for specified diseases.
(2) A single source herd of known disease status.
(3) Multiple source herds of known disease status.

The highest risk is to purchase from multiple sources of unknown disease status or herds in which the disease is known to have occurred. Animals from livestock markets or dealers where cattle from multiple sources are mixed together should be considered a very high biosecurity risk.

Unless from certified disease-free herds, incoming animals should be isolated and tested before they enter the herd, preferably on the farm of origin before purchase. Use of the farmer's own transport minimizes the risk of contact with sources of infection in transit, particularly if the haulier cannot guarantee not to mix stock in the lorry. The incoming animals should ideally be isolated on arrival and tested according to a specific pre-agreed protocol before entering the herd.

Some suggested control measures for diseases that may be introduced to a UK herd with the introduction of cattle are outlined in Table 57.1.

Risk of disease in the herd affecting an incoming animal

While many farmers will realize that introduced cattle may transmit disease to their herd, few consider the risk to the incoming animals from pathogens within the indigenous population. This can be a particular problem with breeding bulls, as breeding capacity can be severely depressed by many generalized illnesses as well as by specific infections of the reproductive tract. In addition, pregnant females may abort if infected with many pathogens during gestation. For this reason, the disease status of all incoming animals should be established with regard to pathogens endemic in the herd and, whilst in isolation, they should be treated and/or vaccinated as necessary.

In the specific case of an introduced bull, it is worth remembering that there is a time lag of approximately two months from the start of spermatogenesis to the ejaculation of the sperm. This means that an insult to the testes may not result in deterioration in semen quality for many weeks and, conversely, it can take months for semen quality to recover following a disease episode. Many diseases may also reduce conception rates in cows and heifers if they become infected around the time of conception. Therefore new bulls should be introduced to a herd only after an appropriate isolation and testing regimen has been undertaken. However, this may prove extremely difficult to achieve when bulls are purchased through commercial sales, as the timing of bull sales is often close to the time they are required for breeding, especially in seasonally-calving suckler herds.

Principles of biosecurity planning

An effective biosecurity programme needs to be decision-focused and flexible enough to adapt to the unique situation of the individual enterprise. This requires an understanding of biosecurity principles and the goals of disease prevention, as well as specific information relating to the biology and epidemiology of the particular pathogens of interest.

When considering the construction of a biosecurity plan, it is important to establish which infections are worth concentrating on, to ascertain the current disease status of the herd and then to assess the risks associated with the use of certain management practices in relation to the target infections. The next step is to assess the benefits of risk reduction within the specific biosecurity plan. In an ideal world, this would involve a quantitative risk analysis for each target infection. However, this is usually not practical on an individual herd basis, as many of the required data are often unavailable and gathering these data and undertaking the required modelling would not be cost-effective. This is not the case at a national level and it is now the norm when policy decisions are made on international livestock trade to employ quantitative risk assessment (Wooldridge, 1996; Murray, 2002). Nevertheless, a qualitative risk assessment, using what limited information is available for an individual herd, may be very helpful when beginning to construct a biosecurity plan. The basis for risk assessment is not to eliminate all risk, but to divide risks into various levels to assist informed decision-making (Wells, 2000). Focusing on the major hazards and major areas of risk will allow the cost-benefits of a biosecurity plan to be maximized.

Producing a biosecurity plan

A farmer needs help and advice from his veterinary surgeon if he is to make rational decisions to protect the health of his herd. This advice is best given in the form of a written biosecurity plan for the farm. This could be a stand-alone document or a component of a general Herd Health Plan such as the BCVA Herd Health Plan (Anon, 2001b).

The safest policy will always be to ascertain the disease status of the indigenous herd and then produce a considered biosecurity plan based on a qualitative (or if possible quantitative) risk assessment, looking at all likely hazards for disease transmission. Particular care needs to be taken when animals are to be introduced into a herd or where members of the herd are known to have had contact with outside animals, such as at a show. The action to be taken when new stock are to be introduced to the herd must be decided in advance. This should include details of where animals are to be obtained from, the provision and management of isolation facilities, the testing, treatment and vaccination strategy and what is to happen if an animal fails to meet the predetermined health criterion.

The written plan must have some flexibility built into it and it must be agreed by both the farmer and his veterinary surgeon. It must be reviewed regularly and both parties must work together to maintain interest and motivation.

A possible future aid to biosecurity planning in Great Britain may come from the British Cattle Movement

Table 57.1 Examples of infectious conditions likely to be introduced to UK herds with added animals, with brief suggestions of measures to prevent disease introduction. (Modified and extended from Pritchard, 1996.)

Disease/infection	Preventive measure			Vaccines available in UK	Comments
	Clinical examination	Prophylactic treatment	Laboratory tests		
BVDV	(+)	~	+	Yes	It is essential to test for BVD virus (up to 1.8% of cattle may be virus positive); serology also useful. Calve pregnant females in isolation and test calves at birth for virus if dam seropositive; or isolate calves and test when over 4 months of age for virus and antibody. Bulk milk tests available.
IBR (BHV-1)	(+)	~	+	Yes	Significance of adding seropositive (potentially infectious) animals depends on virus strain, vaccination type if used, existing herd status and possible implications for sale of cattle, semen and embryos. Bulk milk tests available.
Leptospirosis	(+)	+	+	Yes	Test animals using ELISA, 25 mg/kg dihydrostreptomycin given twice within 14 days of entry reduces risk of excretion. Bulk milk tests available. Zoonotic.
Salmonellosis	(+)	(+)	+	Yes	Repeated culture of faecal samples should help to detect carriers. Positive SAT titre for *S. dublin/S. typhimurium* on serum may indicate recent exposure. Zoonotic.
Johne's disease	(+)	~	(+)	Yes	Individual animal screening to detect subclinical infection is hampered by a lack of suitable tests. Tests such as adsorbed ELISA may be useful on a group basis. Request certification of clinical freedom in the herd of origin for a substantial period of time, e.g. 5 years. If diarrhoea develops in isolation examine faeces repeatedly for acid fast organisms and undertake culture. Consider rejecting animals with intermittent/ persistent diarrhoea regardless of test result. (Zoonotic?)
Streptococcus agalactiae	(+)	+	+	No	Should be readily preventable by using CMT, culturing positive quarters and/or treating. Bulk milk screening may be of use.
Digital dermatitis	+	(+)	~	No	Good clinical examination. If in doubt treat with topical antibiotic spray/ footbath.
Ectoparasites	+	+	(+)	No	Use appropriate treatment.

Disease/condition				Comments
Gastrointestinal parasites	~	(+)	No	Use carefully selected, appropriate anthelmintics.
Lungworm	+	(+)	Yes	Use carefully selected, appropriate anthelmintics. Vaccine will not totally prevent infection.
Liver fluke	+	(+)	No	Use carefully selected, appropriate treatment.
Ringworm	(+)	(+)	Yes	Can cause quite serious problems in naïve herds, particularly amongst adult animals. Zoonotic.
Miscellaneous udder/skin conditions	(+)	(+)	No	Troublesome and best avoided. Some are zoonotic.
Venereal campylobacteriosis	+	(+)	No	Treatment probably more cost-effective than laboratory tests, although not 100% effective especially in older bulls.
Trichomoniasis	~	(+)	No	Probably absent from UK, but check imported bulls and remain vigilant.
Tuberculosis	(+)	(+) Skin test	No	Increasing incidence in UK making the introduction of infected cattle into a herd more likely than in the past. Consider isolation and private testing.
Brucellosis	~	+	No	Present in Northern Ireland but absent from Great Britain except for a small outbreak in 2003.
Neospora caninum	?	(+)	No	Problematic, epidemiology complex and not fully understood. Consider not retaining calves from seropositive cows and not introducing seropositive cows or youngstock into a herd. Antibody titres wax and wane, likely to be highest around time of calving. Control dogs on farms.
Other exotic diseases, e.g.				
Foot-and-mouth disease	+	+	No	Major threat if national biosecurity is breached.
Contagious bovine pleuropneumonia (CBPP)	(+)	+	No	Threat if national biosecurity is breached.
Enzootic bovine leukosis (EBL)	(+)	+	No	Threat if national biosecurity is breached.
Warble fly	(+)	+	No	Threat if national biosecurity is breached.

CMT, California mastitis test; ELISA, enzyme linked immunosorbent assay; SAT, serum agglutination test.
+, Indicated; (+), possible benefit; ~ not indicated.
Note: All animals entering a herd should have a period in isolation; this is assumed in the table.

Service (BCMS). Introduced in 1998, it gave British farmers, for the first time, information on the origin and movement of all cattle they may be considering purchasing. This allows some assessment of disease risk to be made based on the animal's movement history. This can be enhanced by declarations of health status by farmers, supported where applicable by veterinary certificates and copies of laboratory test results. In future, there may be an opportunity to include health information on cattle passports, including vaccination history and the health status of all herds in which the animal has previously resided.

Herd biosecurity: where *is* the final frontier?

For many years, efforts to use biosecurity principles to control diseases of cattle in the UK were largely confined to control and eradication of statutory diseases. Cattle imported into the UK were required to be kept in official quarantine premises before being allowed to move to the destination farm. The general attitude therefore was that the frontier was the UK border.

When the single European Market came into force in January 1993 the quarantine requirement was dropped and it become much easier to import cattle, not only from other EU member states but also elsewhere. It was only then that farmers started to realize that 'The farm gate is the frontier' (Taylor, 1994b). That principle still holds today, 'The primary frontier for disease control must be the farm boundary' (Gibson & Andrews, 2000).

Responsibility for biosecurity at farm level is the joint responsibility of the farmer and his veterinary surgeon. However, prior to the outbreak of FMD in the UK in 2001, only a small number of herds were members of voluntary non-statutory cattle health schemes such as the Premium Cattle Health Scheme and Herdcare. Standards for such schemes are set by the Cattle Health Certification Standards (CHeCS), which is a self-regulatory body established in 1999 by the UK cattle industry. The CHeCS technical document (Anon, 2000) includes rules on biosecurity, which are mandatory for members in the accreditation and screening and eradication programmes and are recommended as good practice for all cattle herds. Other high status herds include commercial bull studs, which operate under EU Directives and UK Regulations (Barrett, 2001b).

The 2001 FMD outbreak in the UK brought home to the whole cattle industry the absolute necessity of good biosecurity to control the spread of the disease. In this outbreak, there was very limited airborne spread of the virus. The initial spread was due to movement of animals, but even when animal movements were banned in the early days of the outbreak, the disease continued to spread due to movement of people and vehicles (Gibbens *et al.*, 2001). Increasingly stringent rules were introduced in the worst affected areas and it was only when these rules were rigidly enforced that the spread of the disease was stopped.

Elimination of the FMD virus from the UK and the EU does not, however, reduce the need for good biosecurity. On the contrary, it emphasizes the need for continued vigilance so that the impact of any future outbreaks of disease, whether at farm, local or national level, is kept to a minimum.

Conclusions

In an ideal world all herds would be maintained as closed units of known and preferably high health status, with the introduction of genetic material only by the use of AI and ET following strict quality control standards to minimize the disease risk. However, we do not live in that world. We live in a world of widespread, frequent, long distance transport of animals and animal products, often with little regard for biosecurity. Nevertheless, there is a lot that can be done, even on commercial units, to manage and reduce the risk of infectious disease.

The principles of biosecurity are applicable at some level to all cattle units and each and every one stands to gain by the implementation of a specific tailor-made biosecurity plan. However, it is important for veterinary surgeons to evaluate the risks of various hazards on each cattle enterprise and use this to design and implement an appropriate biosecurity risk management plan specific to the individual farm.

References

Anon (1999a) *Farm biosecurity – protecting herd health*, pp. 1–5. MAFF PB 4517. MAFF, London.

Anon (1999b) TB in cattle – reducing the risk, pp. 1–5. MAFF PB 4516. MAFF, London.

Anon (2000) *Cattle Health Certification Standards (CHeCS)*. Technical document. CHeCS, Dairy House, 60 Kenilworth Road, Leamington Spa, Warwickshire CV32 6JX.

Anon (2001a) TB and cattle husbandry – government response to the report of the independent husbandry panel (TBF 51). Available at http://www.defra.gov.uk/.

Anon (2001b) *BCVA herd health plan for the purposes of farm assurance* (revised), pp. 1–21. BCVA Office, The Green, Frampton-on-Severn, Glos GL2 7EP.

Barrett, D.C. (2001a) Biosecurity and herd health – a challenge for the 21st century. *Cattle Practice*, **9**, 97–103.

Barrett, D.C. (2001b) Biosecurity and its importance in non-regulated venereal diseases of cattle. In *Proceedings of the*

5th Annual Conference of the European Society for Domestic Animal Reproduction (ESDAR), Vienna, Austria, 13–15 September 2001, pp. 28–29.

Barrett, D.C., Sibley, R.J. & Taylor, A.J. (2001) British Cattle Veterinary Association – TB isolation and test protocol. *Cattle Practice*, **9**, 147–50.

Caldow, G., Gunn, G., Humphry, R., Crawshaw, M. & Rusbridge, S. (2001) Herd health security: the role of laboratory tests. *Cattle Practice*, **9**, 105–10.

Collins, J.D. (2000) Tuberculosis in cattle, reducing the risk of herd exposure. *UK Vet*, **5**, 35–9.

Done, S., Gresham, A., Potter, R. & Chennells, D. (2001) PMWS and PDNS – two recently recognised diseases of pigs in the UK. *In Practice*, **23**, 14–21.

Duncan, A.L. (1990) Health security in cattle herds. *In Practice*, **12**, 29–32.

Duncan, A.L. (1994) Health security in cattle herds. *Cattle Practice*, **2**, 415–23.

Dunlop, R.H. & Williams, D.J. (1996) Some animal plagues unmasked. In *Veterinary Medicine – An illustrated History*, pp. 377–93. Mosby, London.

Gibbens, J.C., Sharpe, C.E., Wilesmith, J.W., Mansley, L.M., Michalopoulou, E., Ryan, J.B.M. & Hudson, M. (2001) Descriptive epidemiology of the 2001 foot-and-mouth disease epidemic in Great Britain: the first five months. *Veterinary Record*, **149**, 729–43.

Gibson, L.A.S. & Andrews, A.H. (2000) Disease security. In *The Health of Dairy Cattle* (ed. by A.H. Andrews), pp. 328–50. Blackwell Science, Oxford.

Gillespie, J.R. (2000) The underlying interrelated issues of biosecurity. *Journal of the American Veterinary Medical Association*, **216**, 662–4.

Hermon-Taylor, J. (2000) *Mycobacterium avium* subspecies *paratuberculosis* in animals, food products and in water supplies and its impact on human health. *Cattle Practice*, **8**, 355–60.

Menzies, F.D. & Neill, S.D. (2000) Cattle-to-cattle transmission of bovine tuberculosis. *The Veterinary Journal*, **160**, 92–106.

Moore, C. (1992) Biosecurity and minimal disease herds. *The Veterinary Clinics of North America – Food Animal Practice*, **8**, 461–74. W.B. Saunders, Philadelphia.

Murray, N. (2002) *Import risk analysis; animals and animal products*, pp. 1–188. Ministry of Agriculture and Forestry, Wellington, New Zealand.

Noordhuizen, J.P.T.M. & Wentink, G.H. (2001) Developments in veterinary herd health programmes on dairy farms: a review. *The Veterinary Quarterly*, **23**, 162–9.

Phillips, C.J.C., Foster, C., Morris, P. & Teverson, R. (2000) The role of cattle husbandry in the development of a sustainable policy to control *M. bovis* infection in cattle. Report to MAFF, available at http://www.defra.gov.uk/.

Pritchard, G.C. (1996) Added animals: the challenge to preventive medicine. *Cattle Practice*, **4**, 253–7.

Sanderson, M.W., Dargatz, D.A. & Garry, F.B. (2000) Biosecurity practices of beef cow-calf producers. *Journal of the American Veterinary Medical Association*, **217**, 185–9.

Sharp, K., Gibbens, J., Morris, H. & Drew, T. (2001) Epidemiology of the 2000 CSF outbreak in East Anglia: preliminary findings. *Veterinary Record*, **148**, 91.

Taylor, A.J. (1994a) Bull hiring. *Cattle Practice*, **2**, 425–32.

Taylor, A.J. (1994b) Herd health security at Genus bull studs. *Cattle Practice*, **2**, 537–40.

Wells, S.J. (2000) Biosecurity on dairy operations: hazards and risks. *Journal of Dairy Science*, **83**, 2380–6.

Wooldridge, M. (1996) Risk analysis, risk assessment, animal health and the decision-making process. *State Veterinary Journal*, **6**, 4–6.

Chapter 58
Immunological Fundamentals

W.P.H. Duffus

Introduction   996
Innate immunity   997
  Humoral   997
  Cellular   997
Acquired immunity   998
  Humoral   998
Cell-mediated immunity   1001
  T lymphocytes   1001
  B lymphocytes   1002
Maternal immunity   1002
Homeostasis and stress   1003

Introduction

What does the word 'immune' mean? The derivation of the word stems from 'exempt from burden'. In reality the word was coined to explain what we now term immunological memory. Populations, both human and domestic stock, suffered and continue to suffer from epidemic disease; the old observation was that individuals recovering from a clinical syndrome were 'exempt' at the appearance of the next epidemic.

This ability of the vertebrate immune system to 'remember' a previous exposure to a foreign or non-self material is at the very heart of preventive medicine. The response is normally termed an *adaptive immune response*. This is in contrast to the *innate immune response* which covers the mechanisms pre-existing within an individual. The division between these two main areas of the immune system is not absolute; there is much interaction and interdependence between effector mechanisms in both camps. What do we mean by effector mechanisms? The term usefully describes the sharp end of the immune response: the antibody that actually causes the destruction of a bacteria, the cell that actually destroys another, but potentially malignant, cell.

There are three other broad concepts to consider at an early stage. First, the immune response can itself be harmful. The millions of individuals suffering from allergy will know this fact only too well. The second main concept is one of specificity/recognition. The immune system is exquisitely specific and has the ability to recognize millions of different combinations

of molecules that make up the myriad of different types of 'non-self' material that individuals are exposed to constantly. These are termed *antigens*, each site on the antigen that retains the ability to be recognized by the immune system being termed an *epitope*. Note the use of the word 'non-self'; this is a useful term as 'self' means the immune system has lost the ability to recognize that particular antigen within an individual and therefore the latter remains free of potentially harmful effector mechanisms. Unfortunately this protection can break down leading to an increasing plethora of autoimmune disease. The third main concept is the division of both the acquired and innate immune response into *cellular* (e.g. lymphocyte, etc.) and *humoral* (e.g. antibody, etc.) components.

A study of immunology as it relates to bovine medicine is artificially skewed towards two of the four main areas that cause sickness/death: injury and infection. The other two main areas are degenerative disease and cancer but these are problems of the older individual; subsequently defence mechanisms against these latter two are not as important within a population, such as cattle, with a fast turnover of generations.

The majority of the mechanisms, both cellular and humoral, that make up the ruminant immune system are common to all mammals. The highly developed mammalian immune system is the culmination of evolutionary pressures with effector mechanisms that are traceable in the lower animal kingdom. However, there are aspects of this mammalian immune system that are specifically enhanced and specialized within ruminants (such as the passive transfer of lactogenic antibody). These differences will be discussed within the relevant sections. An important conceptual point to get across early on is one of balance between two conflicting points of view. On one side is the animal trying to preserve its integrity against a variety of potential pathogens by utilizing the effector mechanisms themselves comprising the innate and adaptive immune response. On the other side are the organisms that are trying to survive in the face of these mechanisms, relying on a fast turnover of generations and natural selection. This balance is at the heart of almost all host–pathogen interrelationships. With cattle and intensive husbandry we are tilting this balance in favour of the organism and allowing them to replicate and cause diseases such as mastitis, enzootic pneumonia, etc. Intensive husbandry is here to stay for production reasons and we will have to turn to artificial means to restore the balance. This scenario will involve research to ascertain which 'batch' of effector mechanisms is applicable to a particular pathogen, and then how can we artificially boost this immunity.

Innate immunity

These immune mechanisms pre-exist in an individual and are not improved by repeated infection. Like acquired immunity they can be divided up into humoral and cellular components.

Humoral

Complement

The word 'complement' is a collective term for 15 or so plasma proteins (enzymes) which can be activated sequentially into functional units that then have three major effects:

(1) Production of peptides which are active in inflammatory processes.
(2) Production of C_3b which, by its ability to 'opsonize' micro-organisms or other particulate matter, is a powerful incentive for phagocytosis.
(3) Attachment to cell membranes to create lysis and destruction of the target.

After immunoglobulins, albumin and transferrin, C_3 is the most abundant of bovine serum proteins (in excess of 1 mg/ml).

How is complement activated? The combination of immunoglobulin with antigen will often cause activation, but enzymes such as trypsin and bacterial components such as endotoxin will all activate complement. The normal route of activation by such agents is termed the *classical pathway* and as far as the antibody–antigen reaction is concerned it relies on the availability of the Fc portion of the antibody molecule. In the cow it used to be thought that of the two major subclasses of IgG (IgG_1 and IgG_2) only IgG_1 could fix complement by this route. Recent research using a homologous bovine IgG_2/complement system, has clearly shown that both subclasses can fix complement. Another pathway of complement activation is via the *alternative route*. This is a more primitive pathway and does not require the Fc portion of the antibody and can indeed be activated by antibodies such as IgA which is not effective by the classical route. Certain isolates of *E. coli* and virus-infected cells can all set the alternative

pathway going, an important point in assessing complement as a defence mechanism.

Lysozyme and other serum proteins

Lysozyme, a protein with a molecular weight of approximately 14 000, is highly active against bacteria and is found in many biological fluids and is sometimes called the 'natural antibiotic'. It is not often realized that Fleming discovered both penicillin and lysozyme!

Neutrophils can be stimulated to produce lactoferrin. This protein works by competing with bacteria for the available iron molecules. Milk contains approximately 6 mg/ml.

Acute phase proteins appear within hours of tissue damage or infection. The best known one is C reactive protein which binds to phosphorylcholine on the surface of certain bacteria thus promoting phagocytosis by complement fixation.

Interferon (IFN)

These glycoproteins are a family of cell-regulating proteins produced by many cell types in response to stimuli. Although viruses are well known as interferon (IFN) inducers, others include endotoxin, bacteria and a variety of other antigenic stimuli. Interferons are classified as follows:

(1) IFN-α is produced by leucocytes.
(2) IFN-β is produce by fibroblasts.
(3) IFN-γ is produced by T lymphocytes.

Interferon offers a rapid protection to viral infection. It induces an antiviral state in cells by firstly triggering a receptor (IFN-$\alpha\beta$ share a receptor, IFN-γ remains separate). This stimulates the cell itself to produce proteins to block the transcription of viruses, so protecting them from infection.

Interferon can be produced within hours of stimulation and the antiviral state can last several days. Interferon also has a number of other effects both on the immune system (such as stimulation of cytotoxicity and increased expression of major histocompatability complex (MHC) products), as well as other functions such as cell division.

All three types of bovine IFN have now been genetically engineered and are being investigated for their potential as therapeutic agents. There may well be a role in diseases such as enzootic calf pneumonia.

Cellular

Phagocytic cells

These include neutrophils, macrophages and other cells of the reticuloendothelial system. Free-living bacteria are fairly easy to kill without antibody or complement, but bacterial pathogens such as streptococci with large capsules can alter the surface tension between the phagocyte and the bacteria so preventing phagocytosis. It is for this reason that specific antibody and/or complement is needed to 'coat' or 'opsonize' the bacteria, altering the surface tension and allowing phagocytosis to proceed. Bovine neutrophils and macrophages/monocytes have C_3 and Fc membrane receptors. Cattle have unusually high numbers of monocytes in circulation.

The phagocytic cells have several agents such as acid hydrolases, peroxidase and cationic proteins which can kill micro-organisms after phagocytosis. The cationic proteins come into play first when the pH goes up and in fact these mechanisms are now thought to be at least or even more important than the traditional peroxidase-dependent pathways involving H_2O_2.

Several pathogens such as *Brucella abortus*, *Salmonella* spp., *Listeria* spp. and *Mycobacterium* spp. can live intracellularly and thus pose a problem for the immune system. The solution is by activation of the macrophage, usually by specific protein messengers released especially by T lymphocytes, called cytokines. Activated macrophages are basically a lot 'meaner', more efficient and, for example, contain more lysosomes; they are quite capable of dealing with these more awkward pathogens.

We must also consider another vital, indeed pivotal, role for macrophages. This is one we term *antigen presentation*. These antigen presenting cells (APCs) are found throughout lymphoid tissue, the archetypal one being the Langerhans' cell in the skin. Other specialized APCs are found in the gut, respiratory tract and mammary gland. These cells basically phagocytose the antigen, process it and then deliver it as a neat package to lymphocytes of the immune system. They combine this 'antigen presentation' with MHC products on their membrane and by the release of a soluble mediator such as interleukin-1 (IL-1).

Natural killer (NK) cells

It is only in the last five years or so that natural killer or NK cells have come into their own. They are basically lymphocytes with a separate lineage from T and B lymphocytes. The genealogy of NK cells remains unclear: they share membrane determinants with both monocytes and lymphocytes. They have Fc receptors and are quite large cells, often with noticeable granules. Two fascinating things about NK cells are that: (i) they pre-exist within individuals and do not require antigenic stimulation; (ii) they can kill innumerable targets from virus-infected cells to tumour cells without the need for antibody. Therefore, they could operate a type

of 'policing' role within the body, ready to destroy spontaneous tumour cells when they arise or help clear up virus infections. Cattle have NK cells, although the term almost certainly covers a heterogeneous population. Natural killer cells can easily be recruited (stimulated by cytokines such as IFN and IL-2). Interestingly in cattle, NK activity is quite low in stock reared outside in extensive systems but is often very high in intensive systems. Whether this is caused by the greater prevalence of microbial infection in such individuals is not clear.

Natural killer activity can also be down-regulated by agents such as prostaglandins. Do NK cells have any *in vivo* relevance? They certainly will kill virus-infected cells such as IBR-infected fibroblasts and tumour cells, but the real clinical relevance requires further research.

Acquired immunity

Humoral

Acquired humoral immunity is mediated through immunoglobulin, or antibodies as they are commonly known. These are a group of glycoproteins that have combinations of incredible variety and specificity. The basic units are two identical polypeptide chains, termed light chains, linked to two further identical polypeptide chains, heavy chain, by several disulphide bonds (Fig. 58.1).

The Fc portion of the molecule is responsible for linking to the Fc receptor on leucocytes, while the other end, Fab, carries the actual antigen-combining site itself. This latter site is also called the hypervariable region simply because it is variation in amino acid sequence in this region that produces the incredible diversity of antibodies.

An explanation of the plethora of titles that accompany a description of immunoglobulins is given in Table 58.1.

IgM

IgM has five of the basic units forming a pentamer structure and represents an early stage in the evolution of antibodies. All vertebrates (with the exception of cyclostomes such as the lamprey) have an IgM closely resembling that of mammalian IgM except for the number of units polymerized into the complete molecule. The level of IgM in normal cattle is in the range of 2–3 mg/ml from the age of 4 months. Levels of IgM in calves is complicated by the amount absorbed in colostrum. The actual amount in bovine colostrum is about 6 mg/ml which drops to approximately 0.1 mg/ml in milk. Interestingly the bovine fetus is quite capable

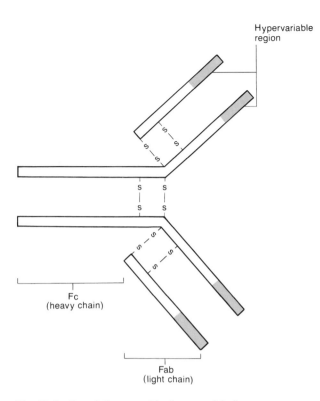

Hypervariable region

Fc
(heavy chain)

Fab
(light chain)

Fig. 58.1 Descriptions used for immunoglobulins.

Table 58.1 Descriptions used for immunoglobulins.

Class	Five major classes are distinguished in mammals: IgM, IgG, IgA, IgE and IgD. These are distinguished in structure and major variations within the heavy chains.
Subclass	Several of the individual classes are further split into subclasses, e.g. IgG$_1$ and IgG$_2$. These are very similar in structure, but vary in the amino acid sequence of the heavy chain.
Allotype	This is a term used to refer to genetic variation within a given animal species involving alleles at a given locus; the variants normally occur within heavy chains. Allotypes in domestic animals could well be linked to disease resistance/production efficiency.
Idiotype	This term describes the product of a single clone of B cells, a unique antibody with a unique antigen combining site. Monoclonal antibodies consist of a single idiotype.

of producing IgM from about the third or fourth month of gestation.

It is, of course, well established that in a primary immune response the major antibody produced early on is IgM. What is not so well recognized is that certain antigens can bypass many of the normal T cell interac-

tions and stimulate B cells directly. Such antigens, including bacterial lipopolysaccharides, normally stimulate only IgM production. The efficacy of specific IgM should not be underestimated. Not only is IgM highly efficient at aggregating antigen, it can bind with the secretory component (see below under IgA) and act as a protective antibody at mucosal surfaces. In diseases, such as *Escherichia coli* enteritis in calves, IgM has been shown to be a major protective mechanism.

In cattle suffering from infection with trypanosomes, IgM levels can rise in serum to over 20 mg/ml, although the majority of this overproduction is not particularly useful against the trypanosomes. On the other hand, in bovine leukaemia IgM levels can fall quite dramatically.

IgG

IgG predominates over other immunoglobulin classes in serum and contributes in excess of 85 per cent of all circulating immunoglobulins. Its structure is based on the usual immunoglobulin model, and it has a molecular weight of approximately 180000.

IgG occurs in two subclasses: IgG$_1$ and IgG$_2$. Adult serum contains approximately 11 mg/ml of IgG$_1$ and 9 mg/ml IgG$_2$. In colostrum the figure is well in excess of 50 mg/ml IgG$_1$ and 3 mg/ml IgG$_2$; this reflects the incredible selective concentration of IgG$_1$ in colostrum (more details are given in the section Maternal immunity, p. 1002). Twenty-four hours after successful suckling the calf has approximately 20 mg/ml IgG$_1$ and 1 mg/ml IgG$_2$, underlining the obvious and often reiterated importance of successful colostral transfer.

As mentioned above, both subclasses can fix bovine complement; IgG$_1$ somewhat more so than IgG$_2$. As for their reaction with leucocytes exhibiting Fc receptors, a somewhat paradoxical situation exists. In experiments involving freshly purified monocytes or neutrophils, IgG$_2$ was always much more efficient at mediating phagocytosis or antibody-dependent cell-mediated cytotoxicity (ADCC). Yet IgG$_1$ is the predominant subclass that the calf receives from the dam.

In the cow and calf IgG$_1$ has a highly significant presence at the mucosal surfaces. While IgA is the predominant immunoglobulin in nasal secretions in the adult, IgG$_1$ is the predominant immunoglobulin in the calf up to at least the 6th week of life. In the lower respiratory tract, for instance the bronchoalveolar secretions, IgG$_1$ becomes the dominant immunoglobulin in all ages. Even infections at mucosal surfaces will produce high levels of circulating and specific IgG$_1$ equal to those achieved by intramuscular injection. When one considers that the main site of the IgG$_1$ synthesis is in the respiratory tract mucosa, it underlines the important potential of this immunoglobulin subclass in local defence mechanisms.

IgA

IgA is recognized as a major immunoglobulin associated with mucosal surfaces. It is basically a dimer (consisting of two of the basic units) joined by another molecule called the J chain (molecular weight of approximately 15 000). This structure is combined with a secretory component (molecular weight of approximately 60 000) to form secretory IgA or SIgA for short.

Individuals with mucosal surfaces have to have a selective system that can decide which antigen to ignore and which to respond to. It is not in the animal's interest to respond to dietary antigens, although of course this can occur, leading to disease. Conversely the mucosal immune system must be able to respond quickly and effectively against a pathogen. One of the most important mechanisms in this decision-making process is distinctive epithelial cells called 'M cells' that overlie Peyers patches and other mucosal lymphoid aggregates. These cells have a tubulovesicular system with pits in the lumen surface and cytoplasmic processes on the opposite surface enfolding lymphocytes and other mononuclear cells. These cells can actively 'sample' the micro-environment within the lumen and pass information on to the proactive cells of the lymphoid system.

The stimulation and subsequent expansion of the plasma cells that are responding to a particular antigen take place within the local lymphoid tissue itself. These IgA-producing cells migrate to the submucosa where they assemble and secrete the complete dimer and J chain. The epithelial cells on the microvilli have a receptor for IgA on their internal side that is probably the secretory component itself. The whole molecule, now the complete SIgA, is transported across the cell in endocytic vesicles and discharged into the mucus itself. This process can also take place in the liver where hepatocytes can make secretory component; therefore bile has high levels of SIgA.

What is the function of the secretory component? It can be found free within normal gut contents or saliva, with large amounts in the newborn calf when very little IgA is being produced. It seems to increase the resistance of the complete SIgA to proteolytic enzymes, although there is little evidence for any direct antipathogenic role. One of its major roles may be to help anchor the SIgA on the mucous layer on top of the epithelium, creating a high concentration of antibody activity at this crucial site.

The IgA part of the SIgA is not particularly effective at 'traditional' roles of antibody such as opsonization, aggregation and complement fixation. Its major, and highly successful role, is simply to block adherence. Micro-organisms *must* attach before penetration of mucosal barriers, e.g. the filamentous K antigen of *E.*

coli. So by a simple steric hindrance such microbes are unable to attach and are excreted.

This local stimulation does underline the necessity to consider vaccination via a local mucosal route when dealing with diseases where a major defence mechanism involves secretory immunoglobulin. Many of the currently successful vaccines are given via the mucosal route and even more are under active research.

Another property of IgA lies in the dimer itself rather than the complete SIgA, or as one famous immunologist put it 'IgA can be more important beyond its laudable but essentially unglamorous role in intestinal sanitation'. Thus, if a dietary or microbial antigen penetrates the mucosal barrier, a high-affinity IgA attaches to it. There is no complement fixation or inflammatory process, so the whole complex is carried off in the blood to the liver where the IgA dimer reacts with the secretory component on hepatocytes with subsequent release into bile.

IgE

This immunoglobulin was first described for humans in the mid 1960s, and is sometimes called the reaginic antibody. It is, of course, associated with immediate hypersensitivity reactions. The structure of IgE is based on the usual immunoglobulin model but has a higher molecular weight than IgG (196 000 as compared with 180 000). This is due to an additional structure in the heavy chain, which is thought to help in the high affinity this immunoglobulin has for Fc receptors on mast cells. IgE normally exists in very low concentrations in serum (e.g. 20–400 ng/ml in dogs). Reliable and specific reagents are not yet available for the cow but by sensitive *in vivo* tests like the passive cutaneous anaphylaxis (PCA) test, potent IgE-like activity can be demonstrated in cattle.

The antigens that can elicit a specific IgE response are called allergens. The allergens are processed in the normal way and plasma cells in lymph nodes local to the area through which the allergen gained access, produce the specific anti-allergen IgE. Mast cell precursors also migrate to the lymph node and they take up the IgE via their Fc receptors. The mast cells now coated with the IgE migrate back to areas underlying the skin and/or mucosal surfaces. When the allergen again gains access it reacts with the IgE and this causes the mast cell to release the contents of its granules, a whole range of pharmacologically active substances. These latter include 5-hydroxytryptamine, histamine, prostaglandins and cytokines such as eosinophil chemotactic factor. The outcome is smooth muscle contraction, increased permeability of capillaries and, through the chemotactic agents, migration of leucocytes. In fact the latter function is a component of the mechanisms that 'dampen down' the reaction: eosinophils contain many factors such as phospholipase D and histaminase that will inactivate the products of the mast cells.

Although such IgE reactions are considered a real clinical nuisance both by humans and their animals, there must have been an evolutionary advantage to develop and then retain this hypersensitivity reaction. One clue for this is a possible mechanism against parasites, especially intestinal nematodes. Although there is a lot of experimental evidence in rodents, using parasites such as *Nippostrongylus brasiliensis*, there is some evidence for nematodes of ruminants such as *Haemonchus* spp. The antiparasite mechanism works by antigens secreted by the nematode (often those associated with their mouth parts) being recognized as allergens by the host. This results in suitably and specifically sensitized mast cells migrating back to the gut. When the worm feeds again the freshly released allergens activate the mast cells. The resultant smooth muscle contractions, and increase in permeability allowing through other factors such as IgG, and the possible direct action of the mast cell mediators themselves, cause a mass expulsion of the worms. Prostaglandin might be one of the important effector mechanisms. A lot of research needs to be done to extend our knowledge of this intriguing immunoglobulin before it could be confidently stated that it is a main mediator of intestinal immunity.

IgD

A brief and quite basic chapter such as this cannot go into details of this immunoglobulin which, although presumed to occur in the cow, has yet to be convincingly demonstrated. IgD is linked to B lymphocytes and appears on the surface of B cells after the initial expression of IgM. The IgD will co-express with IgM and subsequently other immunoglobulin classes. The IgD is lost when the B cells respond to antigen by differentiating into immunoglobulin-producing plasma cells or memory B cells. The exact role of IgD remains unclear.

Cell-mediated immunity

This is an often used 'catch-all' phrase that by strict definition could cover most of the immune system. Early on in fetal development the ubiquitous haemopoietic stem cells produce two distinct progenitors: a common myeloid and a common lymphoid. It is the eventual offspring of the latter cell population that are often considered to constitute cell-mediated immunity.

The lymphoid progenitors produce several different populations of lymphocytes. The rapid development of

monoclonal antibodies has meant a highly specific and accurate assessment of these lymphocyte subpopulations. These are in today's parlance called CD (or cluster determinant) markers, each CD classification describing an identifiable membrane molecule which helps identify subpopulation. The major groups of lymphocytes to consider are:

(1) T lymphocytes, especially the major subsets coded for by the CD4 (T helper) and CD8 (T cytotoxic) markers.
(2) B lymphocytes; lymphocytes involved in delayed-type hypersensitivity.
(3) An increasingly well-researched group of lymphocytes lacking the classical T and B cell markers. The average human adult has about 10^{12} lymphoid cells, representing approximately 20 per cent of all leucocytes.

T lymphocytes

The thymus is central to immunological function. The T-cell precursors migrate there from the bone marrow via the blood. The thymus extends a complicated but highly effective 'education' of these immature T cells, after acting through a cascade of thymic-derived hormones such as thymosin and thymopoietin. The precursor T lymphocytes undergo about eight to ten cell divisions before they leave the thymus. A lot of the cells die within the thymus (maybe up to 90 per cent) and it would be a neat solution to claim that this is how the host rids itself of all potential self-reactive lymphocytes. Unfortunately there is much conflicting evidence as to how exactly the thymus does its job.

What is certain is that when the lymphocytes eventually leave the thymus they can be classified as CD4+ve or CD8+ve cells, two populations that are mutually exclusive in peripheral blood. The lymphocytes have an amazing ability to migrate from blood to secondary lymphoid tissue (within lymph nodes, spleen, gut, skin, respiratory tract, etc.) and often back again to blood. This thorough 'mixing and movement' of lymphocytes is essential for them firstly to respond to antigen when it first appears, and then to be able to contact other cells with a view to initiating and finally curtailing an immune response. T lymphocytes tend to mass into their own areas within secondary lymphoid tissues, quite distinct from B lymphocytes.

CD4 T cells are often called 'helper T cells', which does underlie their important role. The antigen-presenting cells or APCs are responsible for the initial processing and presentation of antigen to the CD4 cells. The latter then further present the antigen to other lymphocytes such as the CD8 population and B lymphocytes. The whole business of presentation is not only dependent on cytokines such as Il-1 and Il-2 but it is also MHC-restricted at the class II level. Crucial to the immune reaction is the T-cell receptor (TCR). The identification of the TCR remained a mystery until a few years ago when the TCR was shown to consist of two chains which clearly belong to the immunoglobulin supergene family. This structure is closely linked to another CD marker: CD3. The human immunodeficiency virus (HIV) preferentially binds to CD4 cells and it is the gradual destruction of this population that is an important factor in the marked immunosuppression that is such a feature of HIV infection.

The CD8 population is also MHC restricted but at the MHC class I level. This is useful as a major function of CD8 cells is cytotoxicity. Like other T cells, CD8 cells are highly specific for antigen, and for cytotoxicity to occur the CD8 cell needs to recognize antigen and MHC. As most body cells express MHC class I then any cell expressing say a virus antigen could be attacked and destroyed by the appropriate CD8 effector cell. In cattle diseases such as *Theileria parva* or IBR infection, these CD8 effector cells, or cytotoxic T lymphocytes (CTL), have been shown to be important.

A single CTL can kill several individual target cells and there is evidence that in virus infection, for example, recognition and then destruction of the target cell can occur before fully infectious virus is assembled inside the cell. The molecular basis behind the actual destruction itself remains poorly understood. Certainly it is vital to have the all-important recognition and close contact. The killing probably involves the release of more than one soluble 'mediators'.

B lymphocytes

B cells develop initially in the fetal liver but production then shifts to the bone marrow. The pre-B cell has IgM heavy chains within the cytoplasm. On a commitment to B cell lineage the B cell acquires surface IgM, the initial antigen receptor. A second phase of development allows the B cells to express immunoglobulins of a different class or subclass (plus IgD). On meeting its pre-ordained antigen the B cell retains only the immunoglobulin it is programmed actually to produce and then enters the terminal stage of immunoglobulin-secreting plasma cells. A proportion of the antigen-specific cells remain as an enlarged population of memory cells.

Although B and plasma cells produce the immunoglobulins, they are under the tight control of the CD4 helper T cells for the majority of antibodies; a proportion of T-independent antigens can avoid this control but at a cost of only IgM production and no immunological memory.

Maternal immunity (see p. 211)

This is an important area for cattle. In the harsh economics of farm animal practice, death in the neonate is a major problem, and the passive protection provided by the mother is vital. Ruminants have five tissue layers between maternal and fetal circulation, so there is little or no transfer of immunoglobulin during pregnancy.

In bovine colostrum the level of IgG is up to a massive 75 mg/ml with 4 mg/ml IgA and 6 mg/ml IgM. Why does the neonate actually need all this antibody? The newly born calf has a somewhat limited capacity to mount a fully effective immune response. It can produce IgM and some IgG_1 at birth; from 36 hours old it will start producing a lot of IgG_1 at a rate of approximately 1 g/day (depending on antigenic challenge). From one to two weeks SIgA starts production and it is several weeks before IgG_2 production starts in earnest.

The neonate is thus basically immunocompetent but has not 'tuned' its immune system to deal with the environment, and it is in this period of tuning and massive primary antibody responses that the neonate needs passive protection. How does this concentration of immunoglobulin in the bovine colostrum occur? The major constituent of the immunoglobulins in colostrum is IgG_1 which is *selectively* transferred from serum. For example, a sheep can produce up to 2500 g of colostrum in the first 48 hours after parturition of which 90 g will be IgG_1. When one considers that the concentration of IgG_1 in her own serum is probably less than 0.015 g/ml, it is a major transfer. This transfer of IgG_1 occurs via receptors on the heavy chain which binds to the acinar epithelial cells. This receptor interaction is under hormonal control and only occurs during late pregnancy. There is no such selective concentration for the much smaller amounts of IgG_2, IgM and IgA.

The specificity of the immunoglobulins is also of obvious importance, not only reflecting the microenvironment of the dam herself, but also as a result of deliberate immunization policy. The neonatal calf has a greatly increased intestinal permeability due to specialized epithelial cells capable of pinocytosis. These cells are activated by the presence of macromolecules and eventually slough off after releasing their contents into the circulation. This spontaneous closure starts in the calf at 12 hours postparturition with a mean complete closure time of approximately 30 hours. Degradation of this colostrum in the neonatal calf is minimal because it contains a trypsin inhibitor, and pancreatic activity itself is low. Abomasal pH is between 6 and 7 due to the delayed development of parietal cells, but by 36 hours postparturition the pH has dropped to between pH 3.0 and 4.0, and pepsin is then active. A final point concerning immunoglobulin in colostrum/milk is that in some diseases in cattle, such as rotavirus in calves, the passive protection is better obtained by the *ingested* immunoglobulin rather than systemic immunoglobulin being re-excreted into the gut. Therefore, it would make more sense to feed diluted colostrum from vaccinated dams during the first week of life rather than relying totally on the protection acquired passively during the first 24 hours of life.

As well as the immunoglobulins in colostrum there is a high concentration of other effector proteins such as lactoferrin. In addition, there are leucocytes, with the macrophage and other mononuclear cells predominant in the resting mammary gland and at parturition. During lactation, however, the predominant leucocyte is the neutrophil, possibly reflecting the constant, although usually non-clinical, bacterial presence. The importance of leucocytes in mammary secretions is as yet unclear for the neonate, but of obvious use for the mammary gland itself; the area of local and effective immunity in the working mammary gland will continue to be a goal for researchers.

Homeostasis and stress (see Chapter 67)

In any book involving diseases of cattle, environmental stress must be a major consideration. Every living organism in an effort to cope with its environment attempts to reach *homeostasis* which can be defined as the steady state achieved by the optimum action of physiological regulation. Stress can be achieved by changes in the animal's environment such as restraint, handling, housing, weather, etc. Although there are many definitions of stress, one of the most useful is 'the cumulative response of an animal resulting from interaction with its environment via receptors'.

This is therefore an adaptive response and is primarily directed at coping with changes in the environment and, perhaps most importantly it is to a large extent an *automatic* response. The response is switched on in three main areas:

(1) A voluntary motor response, which operates via the lower brain centre → spinal cord → peripheral nerves and results in fight/flight, etc.
(2) The adrenal medulla. This works via the autonomic nervous system and adrenal medulla releasing catecholamines, inducing the alarm reaction.
(3) The hypothalamus, which is probably the most important for cattle.

This latter mechanism involves the neuroendocrine system, with the hypothalamic stimulating adenohypophysis, which in turn stimulates (via ACTH) the adrenal cortex, which releases cortisol. The latter hormone has an alarmingly high number of effects such as vasoconstriction in skin and intestine, vasodilatation in muscles, raising blood glucose, raising pain threshold, reducing secretions, etc. The integrity of lysosomal membranes is enhanced by cortisol, so although phagocytosis of bacteria and other particulate matter still occurs, it is more difficult for the enzymes to be released from the lysosomes into the phagosomes. Clinically this can manifest itself as muscle weakness, trembling, impaired immune response, poor wound healing, weight loss, etc. Cortisol normally inhibits the production of adrenocorticotrophic hormone (ACTH) in a feedback mechanism; however, this latter mechanism can be overridden by highly stressful conditions.

Summing up this section: the body attempts to respond to stress by a variety of means to restore homeostasis. These responses evolved to occur in an open environment where the individual can move, seek shelter, etc. But in a crowded calf pen there is no escape, the stress conditions remain with the inevitable consequences.

Chapter 59

Vaccines and Vaccination of Cattle

I.D. Baker

Definitions	1004
Anthrax	1005
Clostridial disease	1005
Salmonellosis	1006
Neonatal calf diarrhoea	1006
Respiratory disease	1007
Bovine respiratory disease complex	1007
PI3 and IBR	1007
Bovine respiratory syncytial virus (BRSV) and	
Mannheimia haemolytica	1009
Infectious bovine rhinotracheitis	1010
Haemophilus somnus infection	1010
Contagious bovine pleuropneumonia	1011
Parasitic bronchitis	1011
Bovine virus diarrhoea	1011
Johne's disease	1012
Rinderpest	1013
Brucellosis	1013
Strain 19 vaccine	1013
Strain 45/20 vaccine	1014
Louping-ill	1014
Papillomatosis (warts)	1014
Erysipelas	1014
Leptospirosis	1015
Mastitis	1016
Coliform mastitis	1016
Foot-and-mouth disease	1016
Ringworm	1017
Rabies	1018
Other vaccines	1018

There are many vaccines available for use in cattle in the UK and worldwide. This chapter is an attempt to summarize some of those available.

Definitions

Vaccination is the introduction of a vaccine into the body to produce immunity to a specific disease. The vaccine may be administered by subcutaneous, intradermal or intramuscular injection, by mouth, by inhalation (intranasal) or by scarification.

Vaccine

A vaccine is a suspension of attenuated or killed microorganisms administered for the prevention or treatment of infectious disease. In cattle practice a vaccine should produce herd resistance to minimize the economic effects of infectious diseases. They are usually administered to healthy animals. There are various types of vaccine.

Modified live vaccines (MLV): There produce high levels of immunity from a single inoculation. Their virulence is reduced by attenuation, which is achieved by either serially passaging the organism through tissue cultures or by genetic manipulation when those genes associated with virulence are removed. These types of vaccine induce immunity by causing a mild infection in animals, often showing mild disease signs and occasionally causing unwanted side-effects.

Inactivated vaccines: These are killed vaccines; the infectious agent is inactivated but retains its antigenic properties, although these are often weaker than live preparations. As a result, two inoculations are needed initially to provide adequate immunity. The antigenicity is often enhanced by using various adjuvants. These adjuvants may cause a local reaction at the site of the injection.

Genetically modified vaccines: These are vaccines where specific genes have been removed or added to the DNA of the infectious agent. Apart from the attenuation of vaccines these techniques have enabled the development of marker vaccines. These are useful in distinguishing between vaccine protected and infected animals.

Autogenous vaccine: This is a vaccine prepared from cultures of material derived from a lesion of the animal to be vaccinated.

Toxoid: This is a toxin that has been treated by heat or chemical agents to destroy its deleterious properties without destroying its abilities to stimulate the formation of antibody.

Serovaccine: This is a combination of an antiserum with a vaccine to produce passive and active immunity.

Anthrax (see p. 717)

Many types of vaccines are available internationally. No commercial vaccine is currently available in the UK. The disease is notifiable and DEFRA should be contacted if emergency supplies of this vaccine are needed. The vaccine that was available was a live vaccine prepared from a suspension of living spores of an encapsulated strain of *Bacillus anthracis*. The vaccine was stable for long periods.

Vaccines have been produced by overcoming virulence using saponins or saturated saline to delay absorption (Carbozo vaccines). In the UK the Stern vaccine contained an avirulent strain.

Dosage and administration

A dose usually of 1 ml is given by subcutaneous injection. This confers an immunity in seven to ten days that lasts for nine months. Annual booster doses are recommended except in areas of increased risk when they should be given at six-monthly intervals.

Contraindications

The use of antibiotics should be avoided from shortly before to 14 days after vaccination to avoid any interference in the production of immunity. Animals in the last stages of pregnancy should not be vaccinated unless there is a serious risk of infection.

There may be a slight reaction at the site of injection and animals may have a mild pyrexia for one to two days and milk yield may be depressed. These side effects will subside.

Empty or part-filled vials must be destroyed by incineration.

Other vaccines

Another vaccine incapable of producing disease is a cell-free filtrate of a culture of a non-encapsulated spore-forming strain of *B. anthracis*. This requires two injections to produce immunity but it is long lasting.

Clostridial disease (see pp. 719, 725, 733)

The clostridial organisms are common and responsible for many serious diseases in cattle (see Table 59.1). Vaccines against these diseases are available individually, for example blackleg and tetanus, but they are often combined as polyvalent vaccines. In general, the vaccines are prepared from formalin-killed cells adsorbed on to aluminium hydroxide producing a

Table 59.1 *Clostridium* spp. and disease syndromes in cattle.

Causative organism	Disease
Cl. chauvoei	Blackleg
	Postparturient gangrene
Cl. septicum	Braxy
Cl. novyi type B	Black disease
Cl. haemolyticum type D	Bacillary haemoglobinuria
Cl. tetani	Tetanus
Cl. botulinum	Botulism
Cl. perfringens (*welchii*)	Enterotoxaemia
Mixed species of *Clostridium*	Gas gangrene

toxoid. Vaccines for *Cl. chauvoei* are often a mixture of formalin-killed cells and a purified toxoid.

Dosage and administration

Usually 2 ml is give by subcutaneous injection. The initial course is two inoculations separated by four to six weeks followed by an annual booster unless there is great risk, when it should be every six months.

Specific vaccines

Blackleg (see p. 723): If this disease is identified at pasture then cattle should be removed from the pasture until the vaccination course is complete. Some veterinarians give a concurrent dose of long-acting procaine penicillin at the same time as the initial vaccination to avoid further disease outbreaks during the period of developing immunity.

Tetanus (see p. 733): Immunity usually lasts for three years following an initial course of vaccination and one annual booster. For especially valuable animals, there is a tetanus vaccine that carries a minimum risk of hypersensitivity; whilst primarily designed for horses it can be used in cattle. It is prepared from purified tetanus toxin converted to toxoid by treatment with formalin and then adsorbed onto aluminium phosphate. A polyvalent vaccine that is commonly available contains the following organisms: *Cl. chauvoei*, *Cl. septicum*, *Cl. novyi*, *Cl. haeamolyticum* and *Cl. tetani*. It seems eminently sensible to use a polyvalent vaccine such as this instead of an individual vaccine since all these diseases occur commonly.

Botulism (see p. 721): Vaccination is practised in enzootic areas with either a combined *Cl. botulinum* types C–O or a type-specific toxoid vaccine.

Salmonellosis (see also Chapter 15)

Many species of *Salmonella* can cause disease in cattle, e.g. *S. dublin*, *S. typhimurium*, *S. newport* and *S. arizona*. The two commonest species in the UK are *S. typhimurium* and *S. dublin* and these can be endemic in a herd. The so-called exotic *Salmonella* species are not usually endemic.

Live vaccine

A live *Salmonella dublin* vaccine prepared from an avirulent strain (HWS 51) used to be available in the UK. It was a freeze-dried vaccine, which was reconstituted immediately before use. This vaccine was very effective both in calves and in adults. It was especially useful in controlling the disease in the face of an outbreak.

Inactivated vaccine

An inactivated vaccine containing *S. dublin* and *S. typhimurium* is licensed in the UK and can be used in the face of a disease outbreak. When the disease has been confirmed, all at-risk stock not showing overt clinical salmonellosis can be vaccinated. Calves are given a 2 ml dose subcutaneously and can be vaccinated from 21 days old. A second dose must be given after 14–21 days. Adult cattle require a 5 ml dose; again this is repeated after 21 days.

Pregnant cows should be vaccinated six and three weeks before calving. All cows that have not calved within eight weeks of the second inoculation should be vaccinated again three to four weeks before calving. This will then confer passive immunity to the calves via the colostrum.

Risks

A small number of animals may not show an adequate response to vaccination. Ideally, healthy animals should be vaccinated. Adequate immune levels will not be reached until two weeks after the second injection. Avoid stress when vaccinating pregnant cows or abortion or metabolic disease may occur.

Serovaccines

Commercial serovaccines have been available containing mixed antisera to *S. dublin* and *S. typhimurium* together with polyvalent strains of *E. coli* and *P. multocida*. These are designed to give passive immunity to calves for prophylaxis and treatment of enteric and pneumonic infections caused by *E. coli*, *S. dublin*, *S. typhimurium* and *Pasteurella multocida*.

Dosage and administration

For prophylaxis in calves, up to 20 ml is given subcutaneously and repeated at 10–14-day intervals during the period of risk. For therapy up to 40 ml is given subcutaneously and repeated at 24 hours if required. In the author's experience these products are not always cost-effective.

Neonatal calf diarrhoea

Neonatal calf diarrhoea is a multifactorial disease complex involving managemental and infective factors. Several bacteria, viruses and protozoa are associated with the disease, for example enterotoxigenic *E. coli* (ETEC) (see p. 201), *Salmonella* spp. (see p. 215), rotavirus (see p. 191), coronavirus (see p. 199) and cryptosporidia (see pp. 204, 282). Pathogenic infections with *E. coli* are most common in the first four days of life, whereas rotaviruses are most pathogenic from 7–14 days and coronavirus causes disease from 7–21 days. Vaccines are available (Table 59.2) and are very successful in practice; they contain inactivated strains of bovine rotavirus with coronavirus and *E. coli* K99 antigens. It is important that the *E. coli* component contains both K99 pilus antigen and K99 capsular antigen. The K99 antigen enables *E. coli* to adhere to the villi of the calf's small intestine where rapid bacterial multiplication causes the production of toxins that are responsible for the diarrhoea.

Dosage and administration

The pregnant cow is vaccinated between 12 and 4 weeks of the expected calving date. Calf protection is dependent upon the calf receiving adequate (3 litres) colostrum within the first six hours of life. They must then continue to receive colostrum or milk from vaccinated cows for the first two to three weeks. This is no problem in the suckler herd. In the dairy herd, milk from the first six to eight milkings should be collected, pooled and stored in a cool place. The calves should then be fed, according to size, 2.5–3.5 litres/day of this milk for the first two weeks of life. In a seasonal calving dairy herd with a close calving pattern it is common practice to vaccinate one cow in four and use her colostrum and milk for the calves. However, the best results are achieved if all the cows in the herd are vaccinated; in this way infection and the level of excretion of infected organism are kept to a minimum.

Oral vaccines have been used and are available in some countries (for example the USA). They are combined MLV of rotavirus and coronavirus and must be given as soon as possible after birth. The suggestion that colostral antibody may interfere with these oral

Table 59.2 Neonatal calf diarrhoea vaccines available in the UK, 2003.

Vaccine	Manufacturer	Type of vaccine	Dosage and administration	Vaccination programme	Duration of immunity
Lactovac	Intervet	Inactivated strains bovine rotavirus (str 1005/78 and Holland), bovine coronavirus (str 800) *E. coli* K99 and F41	5 ml sc	2 doses 4–5 weeks apart to pregnant cows and heifers, 2nd dose 2–3 weeks before calving	Single annual booster given 2–6 weeks before calving
Rotavec K99	Schering-Plough	Inactivated strains bovine rotavirus, *E. coli* K99	1 ml sc in neck	Single injection 12–4 weeks before calving	Single annual booster
Rotavec Corona	Schering-Plough	Inactivated strains bovine rotavirus (str UK – Compton) serotype G6P5 bovine coronavirus (str Mebus) *E. coli* F5 (K99)	2 ml im in neck	Single injection 12–3 weeks before calving	Single annual booster
Trivacton 6	Merial	Inactivated strains bovine rotavirus, bovine coronavirus *E. coli* – enterotoxogenic (ETEC) strains K99, F17 (= Y), F41 – septicaemic strain 31A	5 ml sc	2 doses to pregnant cows and heifers, 1st dose 4–8 weeks precalving, 2nd dose 2–4 weeks later – at least 2 weeks before calving	No data but suggested annual single dose booster given 2 weeks before calving

All these vaccines depend upon the calf receiving passive immunization from the cow via the colostrum – adequate colostrum must be fed for at least 10–14 days.

im, intramuscular; sc, subcutaneous.

vaccines has cast doubt on their effectiveness. The *in utero* vaccination of the fetus has been achieved experimentally with some success, but this is not a practical method at present.

Serovaccines containing mixed antisera to *E. coli*, *Salmonella dublin* and *Salmonella typhimurium* used to be available and details of their use can be found under salmonellosis in the first edition of Bovine Medicine.

Respiratory disease

Bovine respiratory disease complex (see Chapter 17)

Bovine respiratory disease complex (BRD) is a multifactorial disease which can be summarized as follows. The disease complex is triggered by various stresses such as transport, housing, the weather, general cattle handling or by immunosuppression by bovine virus diarrhoea virus (BVDV). These stresses lead to infection by primary pathogens which cause lung damage and disease. These primary pathogens are bovine respiratory syncytial virus (BRSV), parainfluenza-3 virus (PI3), infectious bovine rhinotracheitis virus (IBR) or *Mycoplasma bovis*.

Following these primary pathogens, damaged lungs are invaded by secondary bacterial pathogens of which the principal organism is *Mannheimia haemolytica* (formerly *Pasteurella haemolytica*) which causes severe lung damage, pneumonia and even death. Further bacterial involvement follows, usually *Pasteurella multocida* and *Arcanobacterium* (*Actinomyces*) *pyogenes*, resulting in chronic lung pathology.

BRD can be controlled by the strategic use of vaccines. There are many and those that are available in the UK are summarized in Table 59.3. Often the use of one or two vaccines is sufficient to control the disease.

PI3 and IBR

There are individual live vaccines available against PI3 and IBR. These are freeze-dried preparations which are administered intranasally. The calf is held with its head inclined and the 2 ml reconstituted dose is instilled into one nostril. A short time is allowed for the vaccine to flow into the upper respiratory tract where it stimulates the development of local immunity (IgG) in the upper respiratory mucosa. These vaccines are temperature specific and will not replicate at the high temperatures of the inner tissues. The live PI3 vaccine can be used in the face of an outbreak as a therapeutic agent.

Table 59.3 Vaccines against BRD complex available in the UK, 2002.

Name of vaccine	Company	Type of vaccine	Method of administration	Vaccination programme	Comment	Duration of immunity
Bayovac IBR-Marker Vivum	Bayer	Live IBR marker (gE negative)	in im	Calves from 2 weeks of age 2 doses 3–5 weeks apart (1 × in, 1 × im) Calves from 3 months of age 2 doses 3–5 weeks apart (2 × im)	Intranasal dosage if specific local protection needed in acute infections For use in herds with uncertain infection status and new reactors	Booster every 6 months
Bayovac IBR-Marker Inactivatum	Bayer	Inactivated IBR marker (gE negative)	sc	Cattle from 3 months of age 2 doses 3–5 weeks apart	For use in non-infected herds	Booster every 6 months
Bovilis IBR	Intervet	Live avirulent strain of IBR virus	in (preferred) or im	From 4 weeks of age, 2nd dose at 12 weeks or single dose from 12 weeks	Full protection in 2 days (in), 7 days (im)	Annual booster
Bovilis IBR and PI3	Intervet	Live avirulent strains of IBR and PI3	in	From 4 weeks 2nd dose at 12 weeks or single dose from 12 weeks, special situation for early protection from 1 week		Annual booster
Bovilis IBR-Marker	Intervet	Live IBR marker (gE negative)	in or im	From 2 weeks with second dose at or after 3 months, or single dose given if over 3–4 months old		Booster every 6 months
Bovipast RSP	Intervet	Inactivated strain BRSV PI3 *Mannheimia haemolytica* serotype AI	sc	From 2 weeks of age 2 doses separated by 4 weeks		BRSV – 5 months *M. haemolytica* 6 weeks
Immuresp	Pfizer	Live PI3 virus strain RLB 103	in	From 3 weeks with second dose at 10 weeks or single dose after 12 weeks, special situation from 1 week		
Immuresp RP	Pfizer	Live PI3 virus strain RLB 103 live IBR virus strain RLB 106	in	From 3 weeks with second dose at 10 weeks or single dose after 12 weeks		Animals may remain seropositive to IBR
Pastobov	Merial	Inactivated adjuvanted *Mannheimia haemolytica* type AI	im or sc	From 4 weeks with second dose 3–4 weeks later		Booster dose before each risk period at least annually
Rispoval RS	Pfizer	Modified live bovine respiratory syncytial virus	im	From 7 days of age, repeat doses at intervals of 3 weeks and then at 16 weeks or over 16 weeks with second dose after 3 weeks		

Table 59.3 *Continued*

Name of vaccine	Company	Type of vaccine	Method of administration	Vaccination programme	Comment	Duration of immunity
Rispoval Pasteurella	Pfizer	Inactivated adjuvanted *Mannheimia haemolytica* biotype A serotype 1	im	Single dose from 12 weeks of age	Full protection in 7 days	4 Months
Rispoval 4	Pfizer	Live strains of BRSV and PI3 virus inactivated adjuvanted IBR and BVD virus	im	From 3 weeks of age with 2nd dose 3 weeks later and 3rd dose at 12 weeks or from 12 weeks 2 doses 3–4 weeks apart	Full protection in 2 weeks	
Tecvax Pasteurella 1/6	Vetoquinol	Inactivated *Mannheimia haemolytica* serotypes A1 and A6	im	From 4 weeks, 2 doses separated by 3 weeks, vaccination of pregnant or lactating animals is not recommended		6 Months
Torvac	Vericore	inactivated ajuvanted BRSV	sc	Calves under 9 weeks 3 doses at 3 week intervals Calves over 9 weeks 2 doses 3 weeks apart		
Tracherine	Pfizer	Live IBR virus strain RLB106	in	From 3 weeks with 2nd dose at 10–12 weeks or single dose after 12 weeks		Annual booster
Grovax	Intervet	Polyvalent serovaccine containing serotypes of *E. coli, Salmonella dublin, Salmonella typhimurium Pasteurella multocida* (Roberts) type 1, 2, 3 and 4)	sc	Calves from 1–2 days old or on arrival also weaner calves Pregnant cows, dosages repeated at 10-14 days or 14 days before calving, provides active and passive immunity, increase dose to debilitated or infected calves		

in, intranasal; im, intramuscular; sc, subcutaneous.

Bovine respiratory syncytial virus (BRSV) and Mannheimia haemolytica

There are both live and attenuated vaccines available against BRSV.

Mannheimia haemolytica types A1 and A6 are the principal secondary invaders of damaged lung and also the most frequently isolated organisms from cases of transit or shipping fever. *M. haemolytica* is a common commensal of the pharynx of normal calves. Stress and viral infection lead to the invasion of the lung by this organism. Multiplication of the organism causes the release of leucotoxin which lyses responding leucocytes with the corresponding release of toxic cytoplasmic proteins which cause further lung damage. There are vaccines available against *M. haemolytica*. They are

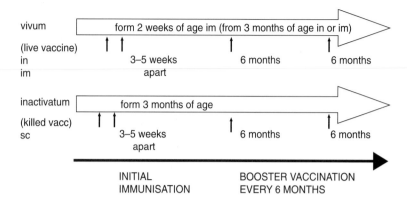

Fig. 59.1 The vaccination schedule with IBR marker vaccines.

inactivated, can be used at various ages and produce immunity of varying duration. They are all effective.

Combined and multifactorial vaccines are also produced. The live vaccines for PI3 and IBR are combined. These are very useful and can be used in conjunction with the live BRSV vaccine to give a more complete cover. From Table 59.3 it can be seen that there are several multifactorial vaccines available. From the author's experience these are all very effective and a vaccination programme can be produced to cover most on-farm situations. It is important to be sure that full protection is in place before the period of stress or risk; for example, before the housing of spring born suckler calves and their dams in the autumn in the UK.

Infectious bovine rhinotracheitis (see p. 289)

Infectious bovine rhinotracheitis (IBR) is caused by bovine herpesvirus 1 (BHV-1) and is responsible for enormous economic loss in worldwide cattle production. BHV-1 is responsible for various clinical syndromes:

- Infectious bovine rhinotracheitis (IBR)
- Infectious pustular vulvovaginitis (IPV)
- Infectious balanoposthitis (IBP)
- Abortion
- Conjunctivitis and keratoconjunctivitis
- Meningo-encephalitis (now classified BHV-5)
- Enteritis
- Dermatitis

Vaccines against IBR have been available for some years and are listed in Table 59.3. Whilst they are useful for the protection of all ages of cattle, they will not protect cattle incubating the disease and animals may remain seropositive after vaccination. The latter point is important when the animal's disease status needs to be considered in the future, for example with the export of animals or in cattle health schemes.

The recent development of IBR-Marker vaccine is a real step forward in the control and eradication IBR.

The vaccine is based on a glycoprotein E (gE) deleted herpesvirus 1 strain. A killed virus as well as a modified live virus marker vaccine have been developed; this enables differentiation between immunized and BHV-1 infected cattle. The vaccine is based on the principle that animals do not form antibodies to the deleted glycoprotein whilst animals infected with the field strain do produce antibodies to gE. By using a gE antibody ELISA test, animals can be distinguished by testing serum or milk. This marker vaccine and the serological diagnostic kit can be used to eradicate IBR both on farms and nationally.

There are four steps to establishing an IBR-free herd:

(1) *Determine the status quo* – all animals are tested using gE-ELISA to ascertain the serological status of the herd.

(2) *Immunization* – all animals are vaccinated with the marker vaccine and so given protection against clinical signs (Fig. 59.1). Where there is an acute risk of infection the live vaccine should be used.

(3) *Stabilization* – natural wastage steadily reduces the number of 'field virus' infected animals in the herd. The natural herd replacements are 'field virus' free.

(4) *IBR freedom* – once the last serological positive animals leave the herd, the herd is IBR negative but protected by the vaccine.

Haemophilus somnus infection
(see pp. 240, 737, 907)

Haemophilus somnus is considered by many to be the aetiological agent of *Haemophilus* septicaemia in cattle. The disease is recognized in the USA and also in the UK and Europe. A vaccine is available in America. It is a killed bacterin containing whole bacteria adhered on to an aluminium hydroxide adjuvant. It is administered by subcutaneous injection and two doses are given at a two to three week interval. Immunity is not long-lasting.

Various vaccination programmes have been tried in feedlot conditions and their efficacy is difficult to evaluate. Some success is claimed for protection in the face of an outbreak. No claims are made on the efficacy of the vaccine in the reproductive form of the disease.

Contagious bovine pleuropneumonia
(see p. 868)

Contagious bovine pleuropneumonia (CBPP) is a highly infectious disease causing septicaemia with localization in the lungs and pleura. It is common in many countries of the world. Control by vaccination is possible and several vaccines are available. They are all live vaccines and are considered by some people to be responsible for some spread of the disease. The vaccines (p. 873) available include the following:

- Pleural exudate from natural cases. This is not a satisfactory vaccine since it can cause severe reaction and spreads natural disease.
- Vaccines produced from culturing the organism *Mycoplasma mycoides* var. *mycoides*.
- Vaccines produced by attenuating the organism in avian egg cultures.

Administration

Vaccination in the tail is the route of administration using a high pressure syringe. Severe reactions can occur in the tail, both generalized and localized. Intranasal vaccination is now being developed with some satisfactory results. Antimycoplasmal drugs should not be used during vaccination as they will possibly reduce the immune response. However, if the side-effects are very severe then treatment may be essential. The immunity to the vaccine varies from six to ten months for some of the cultured broth vaccines to three to four years for the avian egg attenuated vaccines. All vaccines against CBPP are light susceptible and should therefore be stored in the dark.

Parasitic bronchitis (see p. 272)

There is a very successful oral vaccine available. It is a live vaccine consisting of an aqueous suspension of third-stage infective larvae of *Dictyocaulus viviparus* partially inactivated by exposure to ionizing radiation. Each dose contains at least 1000 irradiated larvae (see p. 274).

Administration

Each dose comes in a bottle that should be shaken well and the contents then given orally. Calves should be at least eight weeks old when dosed and a second dose is given four weeks after the first. Calves should not be exposed to any potential source of lungworm infection for at least two weeks after the second dose. During the following grazing season exposure to lungworm infection reinforces this initial immunity. Vaccinated stock should not be grazed with unvaccinated animals or follow behind unvaccinated stock in a grazing system since any increase in pasture lungworm burden may cause a vaccine breakdown. Only healthy calves should be vaccinated. Careful consideration should be given to calves suffering from any respiratory disease before dosing. It is advisable not to use any other live vaccine for a period of two weeks either side of vaccination.

The use of anthelmintics should be avoided for at least two weeks after the second dose, particularly the use of sustained-release boluses. Similarly, the use of any avermectin must be avoided for eight weeks before and ten days after the dosing regimen is complete. The routine use of other anthelmintics and parasiticides must also be avoided for seven days before and at least ten days after treatment. This is due to the residual effects of modern anthelmintics.

Following vaccination it is not uncommon for there to be transient periods of coughing; this occurs after some seven to ten days. Indeed on rare occasions vaccination can initiate an outbreak of calf pneumonia by activating latent infection (see p. 239).

It has been suggested that where ivermectin is used to control lungworm and gastrointestinal worms in a control programme then cattle may enter the second grazing year with no immunity to lungworm. In this case vaccination against lungworm may be carried out before the second grazing season. This is a suggestion only as, at present, no trial work on this has been carried out.

Bovine virus diarrhoea (see pp. 579, 853)

Bovine virus diarrhoea virus (BVDV) is widespread throughout the UK. At the present time there are two vaccines available (see Table 59.4), both containing inactivated strains of BVD virus, and one combined vaccine where inactivated BVDV is combined with IBR, PI3 and BRSV (see Respiratory disease on p. 1007).

BVDV is endemic in the UK and in many if not most countries of the world. The arrival of the inactivated BVDV vaccines has allowed the development of control programmes. The BVDV status can be established by the ELISA testing of bulk milk or blood samples and the results of these tests can direct the control/vaccination strategy. Table 59.5 shows the interpretation of bulk

Table 59.4 Bovine virus diarrhoea vaccines available in the UK, 2003.

Vaccine	Company	Type of vaccine	Route of administration	Vaccination programme	Duration of immunity
Bovidec	Vericore	Inactivated non-cytopathic strain of BVDV	sc	Two doses 3 weeks apart, to protect the fetus the vaccination programme should start in the 3 months prior to service and be completed 1 week before service	14 Months – booster vaccination recommended annually
Bovilis BVD	intervet	Inactivated cytopathogenic BVD virus strain C86	im	From 8 months of age 2 doses 4 weeks apart; fetal protection if primary inoculation is at least 4 weeks before gestation	Annual
Rispoval 4	Pfizer	See Table 59.3			

im, intramuscular; sc, subcutaneous.

Table 59.5 Interpretation of bulk milk BVDV serology and appropriate action. (After Pritchard, 1998.)

Category	OD ratio	Approximate % seropositive	Interpretation	Action
Negative	<0.10	<5	Naive	Maintain high level of herd biosecurity; test all new arrivals in herd; monitor herd every 3 months; vaccinate if biosecurity poor
Low positive	0.10–0.35	<25	Basically naive; few older animals immune	As above; test pooled samples from 1st and 2nd calved cows; if naive, vaccinate them
Mid positive	0.35–0.70	25–65	Some naive animals (probably youngest half of herd); some immune animals (probably older cows)	
Positive	>0.70	>65	Likelihood of PI animals increases with increase in OD ratio	Check for active Infection by checking each age group; bulling heifers using paired serology of 6 animals; 1st, 2nd, 3rd calvers using pooled milk samples; vaccinate whole herd if active infection found

OD, optical density.

milk serology and possible action to be taken. Serology in BVD-positive herds (suckler or dairy) interpretation and action are given in Table 59.6.

In all circumstances if herd biosecurity is poor consider vaccinating the whole herd. After several years of vaccination the older cows, some of which would be persistently infected, will have left the herd and the temptation would be to stop vaccinating. If this happens the herd soon becomes naive and unprotected. Under these conditions there must be complete confidence in the biosecurity of the herd or regular booster vaccination must continue. In Europe and the USA live vaccines, which have originated from strains of cytopathic BVDV, are in use and there is evidence that these vaccines can precipitate mucosal disease.

Johne's disease (see p. 857)

Vaccines are available for the control of the disease. Two vaccines are commonly available: the Vallee vaccine, which contains live *Mycobacterium paratuberculosis* organisms in a paraffin oil/pumice stone vehicle, and the Sigurdsson killed vaccine. In the UK the only vaccine available contains live non-pathogenic strains of *Mycobacterium avium* subsp. *paratuberculosis*. This vaccine is only available from the Veterinary Laboratories Agency in Weybridge. The vaccine causes interference in the interpretation of the tuberculin test. It causes a positive reaction to tuberculin, particularly to the avian component. It obviously also causes a positive reaction to the Johne's intradermal test where it is used.

Table 59.6 Results of cohort serology in BVD positive herds. (After Pritchard, 1998.)

9–18 m Heifers	1st Lactation cows	2nd Lactation cows	Interpretation and action
All negative	All negative	Some or all positive	Active infection unlikely unless 1st lactation cows are recently calved; PI animals probably died or culled from herd; monitor 1st lactation cows – maintain biosecurity
All negative	Some or all positive	Most or all positive	Active infection (acute infection/PI animals in milking herd but no PI heifers): (1) vaccinate heifers (2) test milking herd for PI animals
Some or all positive	Most or all positive	Most positive	Active infection in herd, as above; PI animals present in heifers: (1) screen heifers for PI animals (2) test milking herd for PI animals (3) vaccinate herd

PI, persistently infected.

The vaccine is given to calves under one month of age. It is given by subcutaneous injection, usually in the dewlap. The dewlap is used as an injection site because the vaccine usually produces a localized reaction; indeed such a reaction should be looked for two weeks after inoculation as it indicates that the vaccine has 'taken'. Johne's disease vaccine has a very short shelf life of 14 days.

Rinderpest (see Chapter 43d; pp. 707–10)

Vaccination against this disease is common practice in areas where it is endemic. There are several good vaccines available and in theory complete eradication is possible with a vaccination programme.

Tissue culture vaccine

Attenuated vaccines manufactured from cell culture have largely replaced other attenuated vaccines. They are safe and effective and produce a long-lasting immunity suitable for all cattle.

Goat-adapted vaccine

This is an attenuated vaccine that produces life-long immunity. It is useful for Zebu-type cattle. It is a fairly virulent vaccine, which produces severe generalized reactions in susceptible stock. The signs seen are severe gastroenteritis with high temperatures and loss of milk.

Rabbit-adapted vaccine

This vaccine produces a good immunity that lasts for two years. It can be attenuated to a point where it will not cause severe side reactions, but then is not effective in Zebu-type cattle.

Chicken embryo vaccine

A cheap, stable and safe vaccine that is unfortunately difficult to manufacture and produces variable degrees of immunity.

Measles vaccine

Measles, rinderpest and distemper are antigenically related and human measles vaccine will produce good immunity to rinderpest in all ages of cattle. It is especially useful in very young calves, which can be vaccinated at an earlier age than with normal vaccines. Measles vaccine is not affected by the calf's colostral immunity.

Brucellosis (see p. 580)

Abortion and infertility in cattle caused by *Brucella abortus* can be very successfully controlled by vaccination. There are two vaccines available, strain 19 (S19) and strain 45/20 (45/20). Once eradication is in progress the use of either is limited or prohibited as it interferes with the interpretation of blood and milk antibody tests.

Strain 19 vaccine

S19 is a live vaccine and is presented in freeze-dried form, which is reconstituted with diluent immediately prior to use.

Dosage and administration

The dosage is 5 ml given subcutaneously. It can be given to any age of stock from two months of age onwards. The ideal time is in calves from two to six months of age; at this time it confers a good immunity for approximately seven years.

Inoculation of adult cattle is very successful in controlling severe outbreaks of abortion. In an infected herd the incidence of abortion will begin to subside 40–60 days after vaccination and most herds will be free of infection within two years.

Bulls should not be vaccinated with S19; it does not seem to protect them from infection and has been known to be responsible for the development of an orchitis with *Brucella abortus* S19 present in the semen.

Side-effects

Vaccination reactions: Localized swellings at the site of injection can occur, especially in adult cattle. These reactions are sterile, do not rupture and persist for many months as fibrous nodules. Generalized systemic reactions can also occur with high temperatures and loss of milk in lactating cows. Heavily pregnant cows have been known to abort and should not be vaccinated. Idiopathic gonitis (see p. 458) may be caused by vaccination.

Serological reactions: Following vaccination the serological titres can remain very high for a long period of time and therefore they can interfere with the interpretation of serological testing in an eradication programme. The complement fixation test becomes negative sooner than the serum agglutination test and can be used to identify a post vaccinal reaction from an uninfected cow.

Zoonotic risk: The vaccine is live and accidental injection into cattle handlers and veterinary surgeons can cause severe illness (undulant fever) and so great care must be taken when handling the vaccine.

Strain 45/20 vaccine

Strain 45/20 is a killed vaccine.

Dosage and administration

Two inoculations are given by subcutaneous injection to animals over six months of age. There are often large localized reactions at the site of injection. Although said to be non-agglutinogenic there is usually a rise in serum titres, but these are such that they never reach conclusive levels. Brucellosis has been eradicated from many countries by a programme of initial vaccination followed some years later by serological screening.

Louping-ill (see p. 770)

A vaccine is available for use in cattle in tick-infested areas where louping-ill is a problem. It is an inactivated tissue culture vaccine prepared from the arbovirus and is a thick oily emulsion.

Dosage and administration

A dose of 2 ml is given subcutaneously. Because of the thickness of the vaccine, prewarming can facilitate its use. This prewarming must not exceed 37°C for 30 minutes because the vaccine is heat labile. Initially, two inoculations are given, not less than three weeks and not more than six months apart, with annual boosters. The initial course should be completed at least two weeks before exposure and in pregnant cows before the last month of pregnancy.

Accidental injection of the vaccine into the operator can cause severe localized reactions and immediate medical attention should be sought. The oily vehicle can sometimes cause localized vaccination reactions in animals, which may persist for some time.

Papillomatosis (warts) (see p. 883)

Autogenous vaccines can be prepared for the treatment of warts in individual animals. In the author's opinion their efficacy is doubtful as warts have a tendency to regress spontaneously. Individual vaccines can be prepared by removing 5 g of the lesion from the animal, grinding it up and extracting the virus using glycerine. After sterilization the autogenous vaccine is administered to the affected animal in two doses, one month apart.

Erysipelas (see p. 455)

Erysipelas is a rare disease of cattle but has been associated with clinical arthritis of calves and isolated on post mortem from adults. In an outbreak of disease, vaccination is possible using the available porcine vaccines. The vaccine is killed and produced from cultures of *Erysipelothrix insidiosa* inactivated with formalin and adsorbed on the aluminium hydroxide gel.

Table 59.7 Vaccines against leptospirosis available in the UK.

Vaccine	Company	Type of vaccine	Route of administration	Vaccination programme	Duration of immunity
Leptavoid-H	Schering-Plough	Formol killed *L. interrogans* serovar *hardjo*	sc neck, chest wall	For vaccination against *Leptospira interrogans* serovar *hardjo, prajitno* and *Leptospira borgpetersenii* serovar *hardjo bovis*; two doses 4–6 weeks apart completed before period of risk; calves from 5 months old	Annual; give booster before period of risk, maternal immunity interferes before 5 months so if very young calves are vaccinated the complete course must be repeated at 5 months
Spirovac	Pfizer	Inactivated *L. borgpetersenii* serovar *hardjo*	sc neck	For vaccination against leptospirosis caused by *Leptospira borgpetersenii* serovar *hardjo bovis*; 2 doses 4–6 weeks apart before period of risk, calves from 4 weeks old	Annual; give booster before period of risk

sc, subcutaneous.

Dosage

A dose of 2 ml is given by subcutaneous injection. Two doses are given, separated by two to six weeks. If pregnant cows are vaccinated, with a second dose being given three weeks before the expected calving date, then there is good passive immunity in the calves via the colostrum.

Leptospirosis (see p. 735)

Leptospira serotypes are found in all farm animals; they are distributed worldwide and are an important zoonosis. In cattle the important species are *Leptospira interrogans* serovar *hardjo (hardjo prajitno)* and *Leptospira borgpetersenii* serovar *hardjo (hardjo bovis)* of which *L. borgpetersenii* serovar *hardjo* is the predominant strain. It is only recently, using genetic typing techniques, that the strains previously classified as *hardjo prajitno* and *hardjo bovis* have been identified as separate species. They are both responsible for abortion and they have been identified as one cause of the milk drop syndrome and can also be involved as a cause of infertility. In the UK there are two vaccines available, both are inactivated. These vaccines are summarized in Table 59.7.

When planning a vaccination programme ideally cattle should be vaccinated before the period of greatest risk, which in the UK is when they are out at grass. Cows in the UK should, therefore, be inoculated in the

spring before turn-out. If it is necessary to vaccinate a herd at other times of the year the first booster dose should always be given the following spring and thereafter repeated annually. Calves can be vaccinated, but if they are less than five months old then a further initial course must be given after five months as maternal antibodies may interfere with their immune response. All stock (including bulls) of unknown leptospiral immune status which are brought into a vaccinated herd should be isolated, treated with antibiotics and vaccinated. Antibiotics are used to remove leptospiral infection from the kidneys. The recommended antibiotic is dihydrostreptomycin at a dosage rate of 25 mg/kg (not currently available in the UK) or amoxycillin at a dosage rate of 15 mg/kg of the long acting preparation. Ideally the new stock should be kept isolated until seven days after the second vaccination.

It has been suggested that the two vaccines are not compatible and it is not possible to predict what protection will be afforded when there is a switch from one to another. Cows can be vaccinated during an outbreak to good effect; they are less likely to become infected and shed organisms in their urine. The time for immunity to develop and have its effect on the syndromes associated with leptospirosis varies:

● The response with milk drop is rapid.
● Abortions may continue for some months – as the incubation period associated with leptospiral abortion is 3 months.

● Infertility – once diagnosed as a cause of infertility the herd should be vaccinated as soon as possible but it can be 12 months for the full effect to develop.

Cattle that have been vaccinated may still be carriers of leptospires as a result of prevaccination infection and as such are still a zoonotic risk. They will also show positive to diagnostic serology, which may be important when cattle are to be exported or screened in a health scheme.

Mastitis

Coliform mastitis (see pp. 334, 383)

The development in the USA in the early 1990s of the *E. coli* J5 vaccine and its subsequent release in the UK in 2000 has been a great advance in the control of coliform mastitis. The principle of the J5 vaccine is the mutation of *E. coli* 0111:B4. This strain lacks the O antigen found in the outermost part of the cell wall and so the core polysaccharide antigen is exposed. This core antigen is strongly immunogenic and is common to many Gram-negative bacteria. The bacteria most often associated with coliform mastitis are *Escherichia coli*, *Klebsiella* species and *Enterobacter aerogenes*, but *E. coli* is predominant.

The vaccine is given by subcutaneous injection in the neck and three doses are recommended (see Fig. 59.2). The first dose is given to cows at drying off and heifers two months before calving. This is followed by a second dose four weeks later and a third dose two weeks after calving. The protection afforded by this regime increases with each inoculation and is 10 per cent, 30–40 per cent and 60–80 per cent, respectively. Field studies in the USA have demonstrated the value of this vaccine (see Tables 59.8 and 59.9). In another trial involving 845 cows over one year after vaccination relatively similar results were obtained (see Table 59.9).

The vaccine does not claim to totally prevent intramammary infection in the first 100 days of lactation, but it does significantly reduce the severity of clinical signs. It is best considered as an aid to the control of coliform mastitis, but there will never be a substitute for good dairy cow management. The cost-benefit of its use has been assessed. Herd vaccination has been shown to be profitable when more than 1 per cent of cows in the herd are affected with clinical coliform mastitis.

Foot-and-mouth disease

(see Chapter 43c; pp. 700–707)

This is an acute and very contagious viral disease of cloven footed animals. The aetiological agent of foot-and-mouth disease (FMD) is a picornavirus of which there are seven serotypes and very many subserotypes (>80). The three commonest serotypes are A, O and C, whilst the others are SAT1, SAT2, SAT3 and Asia1. Vaccines are available and many cattle throughout the world are vaccinated. All the vaccines are produced from virus grown in tissue culture, on bovine tongue epithelia or more commonly on baby hamster kidney cells. The virus is inactivated using formalin or other agents and adjuvanted.

A single dose gives immunity in 7 to 21 days; this is followed by a booster after one month and then immunity lasts from four to eight months. Young stock can be vaccinated from a very early age (<3 months). However, if they come from vaccinated cows they

Table 59.8 The response to vaccination with J5. The trial involved 460 cows in the first 90 days of lactation.

	Vaccinated J5	Non-vaccinated
No. of cows	233	227
No. of cows showing clinical coliform mastitis	6	29
Incidence (%)	2.57	12.77

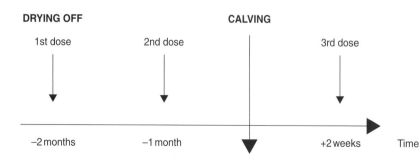

Fig. 59.2 Vaccination schedule for J5 vaccine.

Table 59.9 The number of coliform cases in 845 cows over a one-year period with or without use of the J5 vaccine.

	Vaccinated J5	Non-vaccinated (placebo)
No. of cows	424	421
No. of confirmed cases of *E. coli* mastitis	16	45
Incidence (%)	3.77	10.69

should be revaccinated again at four and five months and possibly again at six months of age. This is due to maternally derived colostral antibody.

The vaccines are usually marketed as monovalent vaccines, for example type A or type O. Ideally, the vaccine used should be homologous with the serotype or strain of the virus found in an outbreak. In many cases, where a new virulent subserotype is isolated the vaccine may be manufactured specifically from this locally isolated virus. In countries where more than one serotype causes disease then bi- and trivalent vaccines are used. Live vaccines are available but are not in common use since there is a narrow safety margin between loss of virulence and loss of immunogenicity.

Vaccination programmes

These need to be planned with specific local knowledge. In some countries adult stock are vaccinated annually and young stock every six months, whereas in others such as South America or Saudi Arabia all cattle are inoculated every four months or less.

Where an outbreak of FMD occurs within a disease-free area a ring vaccination policy can be employed to prevent the spread of infection – for example Holland in 2001. Following a single dose of vaccine, immunity will develop in 7 to 21 days, but if a high potency vaccine is used immunity to aerosol challenge can develop within four days. This immunity would be short lived but may be sufficient to control the disease for long enough to consider the next steps, which may be to give a second dose of vaccine or to slaughter out all the 'ring vaccinates'.

Frontier vaccination can also be employed to prevent transmission from one country or area to another. A buffer zone is created between an infected and a non-infected area.

In Europe, in January 2000, a European vaccine bank was established to hold stocks of FMD virus antigen. Originally in three locations, but now in two, it holds in stock five million doses of type O Manisa vaccine. This is considered to be sufficient for strategic vaccination purposes.

Disadvantages of vaccination

(1) Current vaccines are sometimes not very effective. A high challenge may overcome immunity and there can be partial vaccination breakdown. This has occurred in Saudi Arabia where vaccinated animals were found to have oral lesions.

(2) Symptomless carriers can occur, especially where the disease is very common.

(3) It is difficult to distinguish the immune titre derived from vaccination from that produced by natural infection. It is possible, however, by measuring non-structural protein antibody which is produced in greater amounts following infection, but this is not always reliable.

(4) Vaccination only protects against FMD for a short time (two to six months). The time varies with different vaccines and with individual response.

(5) Repeated vaccination can lead to anaphylactic reactions in some cases, although the reported incidence is low.

(6) On occasions following vaccination lesions similar to FMD may develop.

(7) In an FMD-free country when vaccination is used to control and eradicate the disease then the time taken for international recognition of disease-free status is extended. There are agreed definitions for the designation of FMD disease-free status. These are laid down in Articles of the Office International des Épizooties (OIE). Many countries with endemic FMD have no alternative but to control the disease by mass vaccination.

Ringworm (see pp. 878–80)

A vaccine is available in Europe; it was originally developed in Russia. It is a live attenuated strain (LTF-130) of *Trichophyton verrucosum*, presented in a freeze-dried form. Calves as young as two weeks can be vaccinated. The inoculation is given by intramuscular injection; the neck is the recommended site and two doses are required, 10–14 days apart. Initially the whole herd should be vaccinated and then, in a closed herd, only the young calves need to be injected. All new animals introduced to the herd should be given a full vaccination course. Once vaccinated, booster injections are not required. Heavily pregnant cows (7 months +) should not be vaccinated. Occasionally a small crusty lesion may develop at the site of injection. Cattle infected with or exposed to ringworm should not be vaccinated, as such animals can develop very severe signs of ringworm.

Rabies (see Chapter 70; p. 908)

Rabies is an invariably fatal neurotrophic disease of all warm-blooded animals. A vaccine is available, prepared from inactivated rabies virus adjuvanted with aluminium phosphate. It is used in dogs, cats and horses as well as cattle. Vaccination is advised from six months of age. The primary dose is given by intramuscular injection and boosters are given annually. Calves can be vaccinated from two months of age, but at this age a booster at six months of age is recommended. Immunity develops in 30 days. In cattle, treatment with rabies vaccine after exposure to infection is not successful as death usually intervenes before an effective immunity develops.

Other vaccines

Infectious bovine keratoconjunctivitis (see p. 921)

A vaccine against *Moraxella bovis* is available in some countries. It is made by exposing the pili of *Moraxella bovis* to high frequency sound waves (sonification) and is used to give passive protection. It is not available in the UK.

Bluetongue (see Chapter 43a; pp. 691–3)

Modified live virus vaccines against bluetongue virus are available in some countries. Ideally, the specific serotype vaccine should be used. The practice of using one serotype followed by a different serotype one month later is adopted and is more effective than using mixed vaccines. However, vaccination interferes with diagnostic serology used in health schemes and for export purposes.

Rift Valley fever (see pp. 769–70)

This is a condition found only in Africa, where vaccines are available. One vaccine is prepared from neurotrophic virus passaged through mouse brain. It is known to cause abortions. A killed vaccine is also available and is said to produce good immunity.

Vesicular stomatitis (see Chapter 43e; pp. 710–13)

Vesicular stomatitis (VS) is endemic in Central and South America and also occurs in the southern and western states of the USA. Its importance really lies in its confusion with FMD. Serologically there are two principal strains, New Jersey (NJ) and Indiana (IND). Modified live virus and formalin-killed virus vaccines are available against VS-NJ. The dead vaccine reduces clinical disease whereas the live vaccine conveys better immunity. Inactivated autogenous vaccines prepared from clinical outbreaks have also been used.

References and further reading

Andrews, A.H. (2000) *The Health of Dairy Cattle*, pp. 1–359. Blackwell Science, Oxford.

Andrews, A.H. Blowey, R.W., Boyd, H. & Eddy, R.G. (1992) *Bovine Medicine, Diseases and Husbandry of Cattle*, pp. 1–922. Blackwell Scientific Publications, Oxford.

Bishop, Y.M. (1996) *The Veterinary Formulary*, 3rd edn, pp. 413–25. Royal Pharmaceutical Society of Great Britain and British Veterinary Association, London.

Blood, D.C. & Studdert, V.P. (1988) *Bailliere's Comprehensive Veterinary Dictionary*, pp. 1–1124. Ballière Tindall, London.

Brownlie, J. (1985) Clinical aspects of the bovine diarrhoea–mucosal disease complex in cattle. *In Practice*, **7**, 195–202.

Brownlie, J., Thompson, I. & Curwen, A. (2000) Bovine virus diarrhoea virus – strategic decisions for diagnosis and control. *In Practice*, **22**, 176–87.

Gonzalez, R.N. Cullor, J.S., Jasper, D.E., Farver, T.B., Bushnell, R.B. & Oliver, M.N. (1989) Prevention of clinical coliform mastitis in dairy cows by a mutant *Escherichia coli* vaccine. *Canadian Journal of Veterinary Research*, **53**, 301–305.

Kahrs, R.F. (2001) *Viral Diseases of Cattle*, 2nd edn. Iowa State University Press, Ames.

National Office for Animal Health (2001–2002) *Compendium of Data Sheets for Veterinary Products*, pp. 1–866. NOAH, Enfield.

Pritchard, G.C. (1998) Making the best use of bulk milk antibody tests. *Cattle Practice*, **6**, 133–7.

Radostits, O.M., Gay, C.C., Blood, D.C. & Hinchcliff, K.W. (2000) *Veterinary Medicine*, 9th edn. pp. 1–1877. W.S. Saunders, London.

Rinehart, C.L., Lucas, M.J., Cornell, C.P., Rzepkowski, R.A., Ho, C.H., Peñaredondo, C.C. & Simonson, R.R. (1996) Efficacy against bovine mastitis using a J5 *Escherichia coli* bacterin: Enviracor. In *Proceedings of the XIX World Buiatric Congress*, Edinburgh, 8–12 July 1996, Vol. 1, pp. 285–8.

Chapter 60
Antiparasitics

M.A. Taylor

Introduction	1019
Endoparasiticides	1019
Anthelmintics	1019
Classification of anthelmintics	1019
Others (group 5)	1024
Treatment of parasitic gastroenteritis in cattle	1025
Treatment of parasitic bronchitis	1027
Treatment of trematode infections in cattle	1028
Treatment of cestode infections in cattle	1028
Antiprotozoals	1029
Ectoparasiticides	1030
Introduction	1030
Ectoparasiticide groups	1030

Introduction

The control of parasitic diseases in cattle, as with other domestic animals, relies heavily on the use of antiparasitic drugs. A vast array of drugs has been developed for their antiparasitic activity and these are often classified according to the target parasites they control. For the purposes of this chapter, parasites are classed as either internal parasites (endoparasites) or those on the outer body, the skin, dermal tissues or hair (ectoparasites). Endoparasites include a wide and diverse range of organisms from simple, single-celled protozoa through to large metazoan helminths.

Protozoan parasites are responsible for several major economic diseases globally and are classified into several main groups, the most important of which are the Sarcomastigophora (flagellates and amoebae) and Apicomplexa (coccidia). Protozoa are found in the blood, muscles, internal organs and the gastrointestinal (GI) tract of cattle. Antiprotozoal agents are generally referred to by target parasites and include anticoccidials, trypanocides, theilericides, babesicides, etc.

Helminths are divided into three main groups: roundworms (nematodes), which parasitize the GI tract and lungs, the flukes (trematodes), which parasitize the GI tract and liver, and the tapeworms (cestodes), which parasitize the intestines as adult stages or the muscles and viscera as larval forms. Drugs used in the treatment of helminth infections are generally referred to as anthelmintics, although these can be further subdivided into nematocides, flukicides or taenicides according to the target parasites they control. Some of the more recently introduced anthelmintics have a broad spectrum of activity against a wide range of target helminth parasites.

The external ectoparasites affecting cattle are predominantly arthropods and include insects (flies and lice) and arachnids (ticks and mites). Ectoparasitic treatments (ectoparasiticides) can be classed as pesticides, insecticides or acaricides according to their activity. The more recent introduction of the endectocide antiparasitics, which have activity against both endo- and ectoparasites, has led to new approaches in the treatment and control of parasite infections.

ENDOPARASITICIDES
Anthelmintics

Anthelmintics are widely used in both the treatment and prevention of internal parasite infections of cattle. Their use has been documented from ancient times when it was first recognized that certain disease conditions were associated with parasitic helminth infections. Up to 1938, before the discovery of phenothiazine, few useful drugs existed for the treatment of nematode and trematode infections of domestic animals. Since then, and particularly over the last 30 years, considerable advances have been made in the development of safer and more effective drugs. Modern, highly effective anthelmintics with increased safety margins and ease of application have superseded the potentially toxic chemicals in use less than half a century ago. The introduction in 1961 of thiabendazole, the first of the benzimidazoles, saw the beginning of broad-spectrum anthelmintic therapy that has since led to the development of drugs with activity against GI nematodes, lungworms, tapeworms and liver fluke. The discovery of the avermectins in 1976 has led to the subsequent introduction of a number of endectocidal compounds that has taken parasite therapy one step further.

Classification of anthelmintics

On the basis of chemical structure and mode of action, anthelmintics can be divided into several main groups

(Table 60.1). These include the broad-spectrum groups comprising the benzimidazoles (group 1), imidazothiazoles and tetrahydropyrimidines (group 2) and avermectins and milbemycins (group 3).

Broad-spectrum anthelmintics are highly effective against the majority of nematode species reported in cattle (Table 60.2). Some of the benzimidazoles may also have activity against liver fluke (*Fasciola hepatica*) and cestodes (*Moniezia* spp.). Avermectins and milbemycins (often collectively referred to as endectocides) are active against both endoparasites (nematodes and some larval insects) and certain ectoparasites (species of mites and lice) of cattle.

Narrow-spectrum anthelmintics are more specific in their activity, and are available specifically for liver fluke, although individual compounds may also have activity against some nematode species (Table 60.2). Anthelmintics in this group mainly belong to the salicylanilide and substituted phenol groups of che-

mical compounds, with the exception of clorsulon (available in combination with ivermectin) which is a sulphonamide derivative. Flukicides may be formulated with a broad-spectrum anthelmintic to increase their range of activity to include nematodes and flukes.

Benzimidazoles and probenzimidazoles (group 1-BZ)

Most anthelmintics available for cattle belong to a group of chemicals referred to as the benzimidazoles. Since their appearance in the early 1960s, the benzimidazoles have been subjected to continuous structural modifications to improve their safety and spectrum of activity. Thiabendazole was the first to be introduced in 1961 and was followed by parbendazole (1967), oxibendazole (1973), fenbendazole (1974), oxfendazole (1975), albendazole (1976), triclabendazole (1981) and ricobendazole [albendazole oxide] (1987). Three other chemicals, febantel, netobimin and thiophanate, usually referred to as probenzimidazoles, are also included in this group because they are metabolized in the body by ruminal and hepatic pathways to active benzimidazole metabolites. Netobimin is unusual because, as an ionic salt, it shows good solubility in water, which offers flexibility for its administration. The benzimidazole group is derived from substitution of various side chains and radicals on the parent benzimidazole nucleus, giving rise to individual members of the group. Modification of a particular benzimidazole can affect the pharmacokinetic behaviour of the drug through changes in relative insolubility, slowing the elimination of the parent drug and/or active metabolites (Fig. 60.1). The greater efficacy, and wider spectrum of activity, of the most recently introduced (second-generation) benzimidazoles appears to be due to the relative insolubility of

Table 60.1 Broad-spectrum anthelmintic groups.

Group 1	Benzimidazoles Probenzimidazoles	1-BZ	Affect tubulin polymerization leading to cell starvation
Group 2	Imidazothiazoles Tetrahydropyrimidines	2-LM	Act on acetylcholine receptors causing paralysis
Group 3	Avermectins Milbemycins	3-AV	Affect glutamate-gated Cl⁻ channels and GABA receptors causing paralysis

Table 60.2 Classification and activity of anthelmintics available for cattle.

Chemical group	Gut worms	Lungworms	Liver flukes	Tapeworms	Ectoparasites
Broad-spectrum					
Benzimidazole and probenzimidazole	+	+	±	±	−
Imidazothiazoles	+	+	−	−	−
Tetrahydropyrimidines	+	−	−	−	−
Avermectins/milbemycins	+	+	−	−	+
Narrow-spectrum					
Salicylanilides and substituted phenols	±	−	+	±	±
Diphenoxyalkyl ethers	−	−	+	−	−
Organophosphates	+	−	−	−	+
Chlorinated hydrocarbons	−	−	+	−	−
Piperazines	±	±	−	−	−
Others	−	−	−	+	−

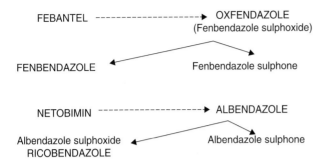

Fig. 60.1 *In vivo* metabolic pathways of the common benzimidazole and probenzimidazole anthelmintics in cattle.

these chemicals, which affects the absorption, transport, passage along the GI tract and metabolism within the host, and ultimately the final excretion of the anthelmintic compound from the host. The longer the persistence in the animal body, the more effective the anthelmintic appears to be.

Pharmacokinetics: Following oral drenching, benzimidazole anthelmintics usually pass to the rumen which acts as a reservoir, allowing gradual release and absorption of the drug into the bloodstream. Thereafter, concentrations of the principal circulatory metabolites can be found in the plasma from where they are extensively recycled between the circulation and the gut wall, along the whole length of the intestinal tract. Nematodes attached to the gut wall may be more exposed to the recycled drug than to a drug present in the digested food passing down the intestinal tract.

Host physiological factors may affect the efficacy of benzimidazoles administered orally. For example, the oral administration of anthelmintic solutions may result in closure of the oesophageal groove in some animals, with subsequent bypass of the rumen and delivery of the anthelmintic to the abomasum. From here absorption, metabolism and excretion of the drug may be rapid, resulting in reduced exposure of the parasite to the drug and lowered efficacy. In some disease and nutritional states, the pH of the abomasum may be altered. This may not only reduce exposure of parasites in the abomasum to some of the anthelmintics, but it may also reduce solubilization of relatively insoluble drugs and thus reduce absorption.

Benzimidazoles are highly effective against most of the GI nematodes of cattle. The range of activity of second-generation benzimidazoles available for cattle, notably albendazole, fenbendazole, netobimin, oxfendazole and ricobendazole (albendazole oxide), also includes arrested (hypobiotic) larvae of nematodes such as *Ostertagia* and also lungworms and tapeworms. Albendazole, netobimin and ricobendazole have activity against adult liver fluke at increased dose rates. Tri-

clabendazole lacks activity against roundworms and tapeworms but is highly effective against immature and adult liver fluke. All benzimidazoles and probenzimidazoles are ovicidal to nematode eggs. This group of chemicals is amongst the least toxic of all the anthelmintics available. However, several members of the group have been found to be teratogenic in cattle (parbendazole, oxfendazole, albendazole and netobimin) and therefore have limitations on their use in pregnant animals.

Benzimidazoles are poorly soluble and are generally given orally as a suspension or as an active ingredient in a bolus. Netobimin can be solubilized and administered via drinking water. Fenbendazole can also be incorporated into drinking water using specialized metering equipment. Benzimidazoles have also been incorporated into a range of controlled release devices, which will be discussed in more detail later (see section on Anthelmintic delivery devices; p. 1026); these include pulse-release devices, containing oxfendazole, and several sustained-release devices available in various countries that contain either fenbendazole or albendazole.

Mode of action: All members of the benzimidazole (BDZ) class have a similar mode of action and act by disrupting energy metabolism in worms by binding to parasite tubulin, a constituent protein present in microtubules (MT) and in plasma and mitochondrial membranes. The formation of MT is a dynamic process involving the polymerization of tubulin rings at one end (Fig. 60.2) and depolymerization at the other end. BDZ anthelmintics bind to β-tubulin causing capping and inhibition of further MT formation. The resultant effect is starvation of the parasite due to inhibition of glucose uptake, protein secretion and MT production. There is also a reduction in enzyme activity such as acetylcholinesterase secretion and in carbohydrate catabolism by the fumarate reductase system.

The mode of action of triclabendazole on *Fasciola hepatica* is at present unknown. It appears to have limited tubulin-binding properties, unlike other members of this group, and it must therefore act along alternative pathways.

Imidazothiazoles (group 2-LM)

The two anthelmintic drugs in this chemical group are tetramisole and levamisole. Tetramisole is a racemic mixture of dextro and levo forms; levamisole is the levo-isomer and it is with this form that anthelmintic potency resides. The dose rate of levamisole is therefore half that of tetramisole, and it has twice the safety index.

Levamisole has good activity against a range of adult and developing larval stages of GI nematodes of cattle, but not against arrested larvae. It is also highly

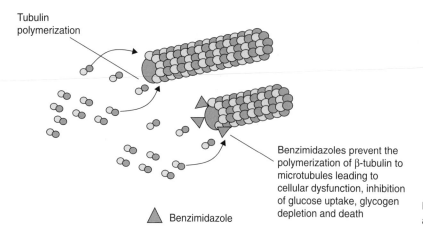

Tubulin
polymerization

Benzimidazoles prevent the
polymerization of β-tubulin to
microtubules leading to
cellular dysfunction, inhibition
of glucose uptake, glycogen
depletion and death

▲ Benzimidazole

Fig. 60.2 Benzimidazoles – mode of action.

effective against lungworms. Unlike the benzimidazoles it is not ovicidal. Levamisole is non-teratogenic and is therefore safe to use in pregnant animals. The therapeutic index in relation to other anthelmintics is, however, low. Animals given levamisole may be hyperactive for a few minutes after receiving the recommended therapeutic dose. Toxic signs, due to a stimulant effect on nerve ganglia, may manifest as salivation, bradycardia, muscular tremors and, in extreme cases, death from respiratory failure. Injectable levamisole may cause inflammation at the site of injection.

Levamisole can be administered orally, by injection or pour-on, according to the formulation, and is active against GI worms and lungworms, but not against tapeworms or liver fluke. A levamisole sustained-release bolus is also available in certain countries. It is combined in a number of products with a specific flukicide (oxyclozanide or triclabendazole) to form a broad-spectrum drench for worms and fluke.

Pharmacokinetics: Levamisole is rapidly absorbed and excreted, most of the dose being lost from the system within 24 hours of administration. Because of the mode of action of these compounds nematode paralysis occurs quickly and removal of the worms is rapid. Unlike the benzimidazoles it is therefore not as essential to maintain high drug levels over a protracted period.

Mode of action: Levamisole appears to act as a selective agonist, mimicking the action of acetylcholine (Ach), and affecting transmission of nerve impulses at synaptic and extrasynaptic nicotinic Ach receptors on nematode muscle cells, causing a rapid, reversible spastic paralysis (Fig. 60.3). Paralysed worms are expelled by normal gut peristalsis. At high concentrations, it has also been shown to affect nematode metabolism by inhibition of the fumarate reductase system. The extent to which this contributes to overall anthelmintic efficacy is unknown. In addition to its

anthelmintic properties, levamisole has been shown to stimulate the mammalian immune system by increasing cellular activity. The relationship between the immunostimulatory and nematocidal properties of levamisole is unknown.

Tetrahydropyrimidines (group 2-LM)

Pyrantel and morantel are the only members of the tetrahydropyrimidine group available for cattle. Morantel, as its tartrate salt, is the more potent and the most widely available in the form of a sustained-release bolus. Morantel has higher activity against adult gut worms and luminal stages, but not against mucosal or arrested stages or against established lungworm infections. Like levamisole, it has no activity against tapeworms and flukes. Neither morantel nor pyrantel are particularly toxic and can be used safely in pregnant and young animals.

Pharmacokinetics and mode of action: The pharmacokinetics and mode of action of this group of chemicals are similar to those of levamisole. They act as nerve ganglion stimulants, causing a spastic reversible paralysis of the worms that results in rapid expulsion from the host.

Macrocyclic lactones: the avermectins and milbemycins (group 3)

Avermectins, and the structurally related milbemycins, are macrocyclic fermentation products of *Streptomyces avermitilis* and *Streptomyces cyanogriseus*, respectively. Avermectins differ from each other chemically in side chain substitutions on the lactone ring, whilst milbemycins differ from the avermectins through the absence of a sugar moiety from the lactone skeleton. The avermectins include abamectin, doramectin, eprinomectin and ivermectin, and are active against a wide range of nematodes and arthropods. Moxidectin is a milbemycin and has a similar wide ranging activity.

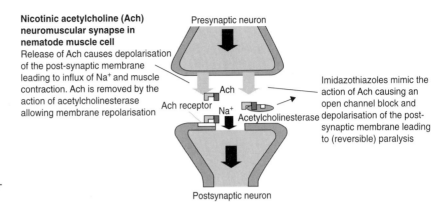

Nicotinic acetylcholine (Ach) neuromuscular synapse in nematode muscle cell
Release of Ach causes depolarisation of the post-synaptic membrane leading to influx of Na⁺ and muscle contraction. Ach is removed by the action of acetylcholinesterase allowing membrane repolarisation

Presynaptic neuron

Ach

Ach receptor

Na⁺

Acetylcholinesterase

Imidazothiazoles mimic the action of Ach causing an open channel block and depolarisation of the post-synaptic membrane leading to (reversible) paralysis

Postsynaptic neuron

Fig. 60.3 Mode of action of imidazothiazoles.

With the exception of eprinomectin, which is only available as a pour-on formulation, these groups of drugs are available as both injectable and pour-on preparations for cattle. Drench formulations of abamectin, and a sustained-release device containing ivermectin, are also available for cattle in some countries. As well as being effective against adult and larval GI roundworms (including arrested *Ostertagia ostertagi*) and lungworms, most have activity against other helminths of cattle such as the eyeworm, *Thelazia rhodesii*, and the filarial parasite, *Parafilaria bovicola*. None of these compounds has activity against tapeworms or liver fluke, although ivermectin is available in combination with the flukicide clorsulon to broaden the spectrum of activity. Ectoparasite activity includes warbles (*Hypoderma* spp.), sucking lice (*Haematopinus, Linognathus, Solenopotes* spp.) and mange mites (*Psoroptes, Sarcoptes, Chorioptes*). More detailed information on the efficacy of the endectocides against ectoparasites is provided in the section on ectoparasiticides (see p. 1030).

Pharmacokinetics: Avermectins and milbemycins are highly lipophilic and, following administration, are stored in fat tissue from where they are slowly released, metabolized and excreted. Ivermectin is absorbed systemically following oral, subcutaneous or dermal administration, but is absorbed to a greater degree, and has a longer half-life, when given subcutaneously or dermally. A temporary depot appears to occur in the fat and liver, from which there is a slow release. Excretion, of the unaltered molecule, is mainly via the faeces, with less than 2 per cent excreted in the urine. The reduced absorption and bioavailability of ivermectin when given orally in cattle may be due to its metabolism in the rumen. The affinity of these compounds to fat explains their persistence in the body and the extended periods of protection afforded against lungworms and stomach worms. Individual variances in these periods of protection reflect differences in drug distribution, metabolism and excretion.

Injectable and pour-on preparations provide protection of 7–42 days for lungworms and 7–35 days for stomach worms, depending on the product and formulation. The ivermectin bolus provides protection against GI worms and lungworms for up to 135 days following administration. The prolonged half-life of these compounds also determines levels of residues in meat and milk, and subsequent compulsory withdrawal periods following treatment. For meat these may vary between 14 and 42 days according to the product and method of administration. With the exception of eprinomectin, which has a zero milk withdrawal period, treatment with this class of compounds cannot be given to lactating cows, or during the last two months of pregnancy.

Mode of action: The mode of action of the avermectins has been studied but has still not been completely elucidated. Ivermectin is known to act on γ-aminobutyric acid (GABA) neurotransmission at two or more sites in nematodes, blocking interneuronal stimulation of excitatory motor neurones and thus leading to a flaccid paralysis (Fig. 60.4). It appears to achieve this by stimulating the release of GABA from nerve endings and

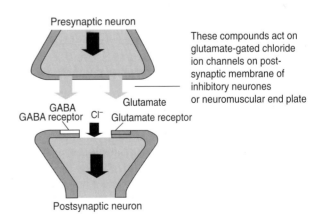

Presynaptic neuron

GABA
GABA receptor

Cl⁻

Glutamate
Glutamate receptor

These compounds act on glutamate-gated chloride ion channels on post-synaptic membrane of inhibitory neurones or neuromuscular end plate

Postsynaptic neuron

Fig. 60.4 Mode of action of avermectins/milbemycins.

enhancing the binding of GABA to its receptor on the postsynaptic membrane of an excitatory motor neurone. The enhanced GABA binding results in an increased flow of Cl⁻ ions into the cell, leading to hyperpolarization. In mammals, GABA neurotransmission is confined to the central nervous system; the lack of effect of avermectin on the mammalian nervous system at therapeutic concentrations is probably because, being a large molecule, it does not readily cross the blood–brain barrier. More recent evidence suggests that ivermectin may exert its effect through action on glutamate-gated Cl⁻ ion conductance at the postsynaptic membrane or neuromuscular end plate.

Salicylanilides and substituted phenols (group 4)

With the exception of niclosamide, the salicylanilides and substituted phenols are usually marketed as flukicides, being highly effective against adult and, to a lesser extent, immature *F. hepatica*. Some also possess activity against blood-sucking nematodes such as *Haemonchus*. Most drugs in this group are given orally to cattle, although nitroxynil is usually given by subcutaneous injection.

The salicylanilides, substituted phenols and bisphenols can be regarded as close analogues and include the bromsalans, clioxanide, oxyclozanide, brotianide, rafoxanide and closantel (salicylanilides), nitroxynil (substituted phenol) and bithionol, hexachlorophene, niclofolan (bisphenols). Niclosamide (salicylanilide) is highly effective against tapeworms and possibly against immature paramphistomes.

Pharmacokinetics: Salicylanilides and substituted phenols appear to be extensively bound to plasma proteins (>99 per cent), which may explain their high efficacy against blood-feeding parasites. Fasciolicidal activity is dependent on the extent to which these drugs persist in the plasma. Rafoxanide and closantel have long plasma half-lives when compared with oxyclozanide. Evidence suggests that the apparent efficacy of these drugs, particularly against immature *F. hepatica*, may be due more to their persistence in the plasma and the effect they have on maturing adult flukes when they reach the bile ducts, rather than the effect they have on the immature stages themselves. Young flukes probably ingest mainly liver cells, which contain little anthelmintic. As they grow and migrate through the liver they cause extensive haemorrhage and come into contact with anthelmintic. Finally, when the flukes reach the bile ducts they are in contact with even greater concentrations of anthelmintic as the bile ducts are important in the excretion of these compounds, as evidenced by the high proportion of these, and their metabolites, excreted in the faeces rather than the urine.

Mode of action: Salicylanilides and substituted phenols uncouple oxidative phosphorylation and therefore decrease the availability of high-energy phosphate compounds such as adenosine triphosphate (ATP) and reduced nicotinamide-adenine-dinucleotide (NADH⁻) in the mitochondria. They have also been shown to inhibit succinate dehydrogenase activity and the fumarate reductase system, which is associated with oxidative phosphorylation. Because of the long half-life of the plasma protein-bound molecules, the parasites experience prolonged exposure to the drugs which reduces the energy available to the parasites. Plasma binding reduces incorporation of the drugs into host tissues and accounts for the selective parasite toxicity. Looseness of faeces and slight loss of appetite may be seen in some animals after treatment at recommended dose rates. High doses may cause blindness and signs of uncoupled oxidative phosphorylation, i.e. hyperventilation, hyperthermia, convulsions, tachycardia and ultimately death.

Others (group 5)

Piperazines

Diethylcarbamazine is still marketed in certain parts of the world, for the treatment of lungworm infections in cattle. It is primarily active against immature lungworms and because it has to be given over a period of three days to achieve its effect, more modern anthelmintics such as the benzimidazoles, levamisole and the avermectins/milbemycins have tended to replace it. It is also active against microfilariae, the mode of action being incompletely understood, but it is thought to enhance phagocytosis of the microfilariae by the host immune system. The action of diethylcarbamazine on immature lungworm larvae is thought to be a flaccid paralysis due to hyperpolarization of neuronal postsynaptic membranes resulting from an increased flow of Cl⁻ ions into the cell. This mode of action, similar to the GABA agonist action of piperazine, is probably unrelated to its antifilarial action.

Organophosphates

Several organophosphorus compounds have been marketed for use in cattle and are still available in a limited number of countries for the treatment of GI nematode infections. Haloxon and metriphonate are usually effective against the adults of some species of GI nematodes, but not against arrested larvae and lungworms. The mode of action of the organophosphates is discussed in greater detail in the section on ectoparasiticides (see p. 1032).

Clorsulon

The sulphonamide clorsulon is available as an injectable solution for cattle and is highly effective against both adult and immature liver flukes over eight weeks of age. It has been shown to inhibit the glycolytic enzyme phosphoglyceromutase in *F. hepatica* by competition with 3-phosphoglycerate and 2,3-diphosphoglycerate, leading to a gradual suppression of motility and paralysis.

Praziquantel

Praziquantel is a quinoline-pyrazine compound and is a highly effective cestodicidal and trematocidal drug for use in both human and veterinary medicine. The drug appears to modulate cell membrane permeability, leading to both spastic muscle contraction and disintegration of the parasite tegument. Praziquantel is active against larval cestodes and schistosomes found in cattle, but the high dosage required is probably uneconomic in these infections.

Treatment of parasitic gastroenteritis in cattle (see pp. 267–72)

The activities of the available anthelmintics have been described under their respective anthelmintic groups and are summarized in Tables 60.2 and 60.3. All are highly effective against adult and developing larval stages of the common GI nematodes. When selecting an anthelmintic for treatment of parasitic gastroenteritis (PGE) in calves during the summer months there is little difference, in terms of efficacy, between any of the currently available anthelmintics. Abamectin, doramectin, eprinomectin, ivermectin and moxidectin injections and respective pour-on formulations have persistent anthelmintic activity against abomasal nematodes and lungworms and can be used at extended treatment intervals in strategic dosing strategies. For treatment of type II ostertagiosis, or for treating animals on housing, it is advisable to use a product with high activity against arrested fourth-stage larvae. An anthelmintic that lacks such efficacy may necessitate repeated treatment as it will only remove adult worms and developing larvae, leaving arrested larvae to resume development and cause damage to the abomasal wall. Here there is some variability in efficacy between products and evidence suggests that at recommended dose rates, albendazole, fenbendazole, netobimin, oxfendazole, ricobendazole, abamectin, doramectin, eprinomectin, ivermectin and moxidectin are more active against arrested fourth-stage larvae than other anthelmintics. The activities of the probenzimidazoles, febantel and thiophanate are increased if they are given in feed over several days.

Strategies for controlling helminth infections of cattle (see p. 271 onwards)

Strategies for the control of parasitic GI nematode infections of cattle are generally targeted at the first year grazing animal, although increasingly control measures are being applied to cattle in their second grazing season. Currently employed control strategies are based on detailed epidemiological studies conducted over several decades. Calves can either be dosed at the onset of disease or used preventatively in the early part of the grazing season, as a means of limiting pasture contamination and subsequent exposure to infective larvae later in the season. This approach is particularly used in temperate climates where there is a fairly predictable cyclical appearance of GI nematode species on the herbage throughout the year. The major disadvantage of strategic single-dose treatments is the labour costs involved in gathering and handling the cattle. As such, the advent of novel methods of presentation of anthelmintics and those with greater persistence in the body has meant that strategic control of PGE in calves can be achieved with the minimal handling of stock. The use of pour-on preparations, for example, is convenient, less traumatic to both animal and handler and is gaining widespread acceptance. The most important development over recent years, and for the foreseeable future, has been the introduction of controlled-release devices which deliver anthelmintic at targeted times throughout the grazing season.

Strategic anthelmintic dosing (see p. 271 onwards)

On farms where 'clean grazing' in the form of new leys or aftermaths is available, GI nematodes can be controlled by integrating systems of grazing management with parasite control strategies. These clean grazing systems can be designed for the effective control of PGE, but offer little protection for the control of lungworm because of the unpredictable nature of the disease. On many conventionally managed enterprises, where cattle are grazed on permanent pasture, control can be achieved through strategic anthelmintic dosing at three and six weeks post turn-out (sometimes referred to as to the 'poor man's clean grazing system'). Further developments of this system include the 3, 8, 13 strategy for ivermectin, the 0, 8 dosing strategy for doramectin, and the use of boluses (see p. 271). Calves dosed with a bolus or treated strategically with anthelmintic should remain set-stocked on the pasture or moved to clean pasture, when available, for maximum benefits. Many of the anthelmintic strategies described claim to protect calves against lungworm disease during their first season at grass. There is much

Table 60.3 Anthelmintics effective against helminth parasites of cattle.

Parasite group	Parasite genus/species	Anthelmintics
Gastrointestinal worms	*Ostertagia, Trichostrongylus, Cooperia, Haemonchus, Nematodirus, Chabertia, Bunostomum, Oesophagostomum, Strongyloides*	Albendazole, ricobendazole, febantel, fenbendazole, netobimin, oxfendazole, thiophanate, levamisole, morantel, abamectin, doramectin, eprinomectin, ivermectin, moxidectin Closantel and nitroxynil (*Haemonchus, Bunostomum, Oesophagostomum* only)
Lungworms	*Dictyocaulus viviparus*	Albendazole, febantel, fenbendazole, netobimin, oxfendazole, levamisole, abamectin, doramectin, eprinomectin, ivermectin, moxidectin Diethylcarbamazine (available in some countries)
Cestodes	*Moniezia expansa, M. benedini*	Albendazole, febantel, fenbendazole, netobimin, oxfendazole Oxyclozanide (some activity against proglottids)
	Taenia saginata (metacestode *Cysticercus bovis*)	Praziquantel
	Echinococcus granulosus (hydatid)	Praziquantel
Trematodes	*Fasciola hepatica* (adults)	Albendazole, ricobendazole, netobimin, triclabendazole, nitroxynil, oxyclozanide, clorsulon, closantel Rafoxanide, bithionol, niclofan
	Fasciola hepatica (immatures)	Triclabendazole, nitroxynil (>6 weeks), closantel
	Fasciola gigantica	Triclabendazole, clorsulon
	Fascioloides magna	Triclabendazole, clorsulon, closantel
	Dicrocoelium dendriticum	Netobimin
	Schistosoma spp.	Praziquantel

debate as to whether these strategies compromise immunity to both GI worms and lungworms and, in part, explain the increasing reports of lungworm in older animals seen over the last few years in parts of western Europe. On farms where lungworm is endemic, or if there is a high risk of introduction of disease, then vaccination is the recommended method of control (see p. 1011).

The two grazing strategies commonly used for the control of PGE in first-year cattle are commonly referred to as 'preventative' and 'evasive'. In a preventative strategy clean grazing is provided at the start of the grazing season, usually in the form of new leys. When weaned, parasite-naïve calves are turned out onto the clean pasture where they should remain set-stocked for the whole grazing season and should not require any anthelmintic dosing. In an evasive strategy, animals are dosed and moved onto clean aftermaths from mid-summer onwards (see p. 271).

Anthelmintic delivery devices

Intraruminal devices represent a new approach to administering anthelmintics for the control of parasitic helminths and are becoming a popular labour-saving means of worming cattle. The reticulo-rumen provides an ideal site for the location of these devices, which can release anthelmintic over an extended period either continuously (sustained-release devices, SRD), or at pulsed intervals (pulse-release devices, PRD). Ruminal retention is achieved either on the basis of density or the variable geometric configuration of the device.

Several devices are available for cattle in certain countries and include:

- A morantel sustained-release device (MSRD);
- A levamisole sustained-release bolus (LSRB);
- A fenbendazole sustained-release bolus (FSRB);
- An ivermectin sustained-release bolus (ISRB); and
- Oxfendazole pulse-release devices (OPRB).

These range in shape and design, each being administered by the use of specially provided dosing guns. Care is required when administering as dosing injuries can easily occur or the bolus may be regurgitated if not swallowed properly.

The MSRD consists of a coiled trilaminate sheet composed of a central core matrix of morantel tartrate. The entire sheet is punched with holes which allow the controlled release of morantel into the rumen from the edges of the perforation as well as the perimeter.

The device is retained in a rolled shape by a special tape. Following administration, the tape releases and the device unrolls and is retained in either the first or second stomach of the animal. The device remains active for about 90 days, after which it gradually disintegrates and is eliminated.

The LSRB bolus consists of a compressed polyvinyl chloride (PVC) matrix containing levamisole encased in an outer impermeable shell. Anthelmintic is released from the internal surface area through a single outer pore over a period of up to 90 days.

The FSRB is a cylindrical bolus consisting of ten flat-faced tablets in two magnesium alloy tubes joined and enclosed by alloy rings. The bolus is designed to release fenbendazole by galvanic erosion over a period of 140 days.

The ISRB consists of an external semipermeable membrane surrounding a semisolid formulation of ivermectin. The bolus is retained in position in the first or second stomach by the presence of an iron densifier at one end. The bolus is designed to release anthelmintic over a period of up to 135 days.

The OPRB consists of either five or seven annular tablets of oxfendazole, mounted on a central metal core with a stainless steel weighted end. The release of each annular tablet is determined by the corrosion rate of the central core. The first dose of oxfendazole is either released within 24 hours (for use in animals already at grass) or at approximately three weeks after administration for either first (seven tablet) or second year animals (five tablet) prior to turnout. Remaining doses are released at regular intervals thereafter (approximately 21 days) giving the boluses active lives of 105, 126, or 147 days depending on the number of tablets and release profile. Devices of this nature are subject to some variation in release intervals dependent on factors such as diet, rumen pH and gut motility, so that release may vary by a few days either side of the optimum.

A novel development from this type of corrosion-based pulse-release system is the electronic bolus based on microchip technology. As well as offering the potential of multiple anthelmintic therapy, the system could be used to pulse release other drugs such as growth promoters and mineral supplements.

Bolus devices are normally administered at the start of the grazing season, although some can be given later in the season. If the animals are turned out early, or moved to pasture grazed by untreated animals during late summer, subsequent protection from infective larvae may be lost, as will any benefits of anthelmintic treatment. The result may be that either the calves experience sufficient challenge to develop clinical disease in the autumn or, alternatively, they acquire large numbers of arrested larvae that may cause clinical disease in the following spring. In this situation calves may require dosing in the autumn while still at grass, or on housing, to remove arrested burdens.

With some delivery system designs the dose/weight ratio reduces as the animals grow, whilst at the same time release rates may decline with time. Both of these factors may result in considerable selection pressure for the development of drug resistance and since these systems are recommended as a form of clean grazing system, the build-up of resistant over susceptible species could rapidly occur.

Anthelmintic resistance

Although widely reported in sheep, anthelmintic resistance appears less of a problem in cattle. This may be a reflection of the relative frequency of treatment and also of differences in parasite population dynamics between the two hosts. It may also reflect the prolonged survivability of free-living larval stages within the bovine faecal pat, thus ensuring a supply of susceptible worms.

The effects of intraruminal devices on the development of resistance, given the selection pressures they exert, are not yet apparent. Until the inheritance of anthelmintic resistance is completely understood, this will remain a matter for speculation. In the meantime, recommendations aimed at limiting the development of resistance in sheep nematodes should be followed wherever possible. The ultimate choice of anthelmintic product may therefore be influenced by a number of factors of which group type or mode of action may become one of the overriding factors, when considered as part of an anthelmintic rotation programme designed to delay the onset of resistance.

Treatment of parasitic bronchitis (see pp. 273–4)

The anthelmintics fenbendazole, oxfendazole, albendazole, ricobendazole, febantel, levamisole, ivermectin, abamectin, doramectin, eprinomectin and moxidectin are all highly effective against developing fourth-stage larvae and adult *Dictyocaulus viviparus*. Diethylcarbamazine (available in some countries) is primarily active against immature larvae if given over a three-day period.

Some degree of control of parasitic bronchitis in calves can be achieved by early season suppression of pasture contamination in much the same way as for the control of GI nematodes. However, the epidemiology of lungworm infection is complex and still not fully understood, and it is the opinion of the author that the vaccination of calves with an irradiated larval vaccine is the most reliable form of control (see p. 1011).

Treatment of trematode infections in cattle (see pp. 276–80)

Fasciolosis

Table 60.4 shows the comparative efficacy of flukicidal drugs against *F. hepatica*. All are effective against adult fluke and are therefore suitable for the treatment of chronic fasciolosis in cattle. Few compounds have activity against immature fluke stages, limiting the choice in suspect cases of acute fasciolosis. As a general recommendation for cattle in temperate countries, housed cattle should be dosed once in mid-winter in average rainfall years. Wherever possible, the most effective drugs with efficacy against mature and immature flukes should be used. Further treatment should then be unnecessary. If a flukicide with activity against mature flukes only is used, a second dose at turnout may be necessary to remove any fluke missed by the first treatment. Where animals were housed for at least eight weeks prior to the first treatment, the second dose should be unnecessary.

In outwintered stock, two doses of anthelmintic may be necessary. The first is given in early winter to remove adult and immature fluke burdens acquired from the autumnal flush of pasture metacercariae. A second dose in early spring may be required to prevent heavy pasture contamination and infection of the intermediate snail host, especially if rainfall has been heavy in previous years. In these situations the treatment interval will depend on the activity of the flukicidal drug against immature stages.

Other Fasciola *spp.* (see p. 277)

The drugs and dose rates given for the treatment of *F. hepatica* are also generally applicable for the treatment of *F. gigantica*. Only triclabendazole and clorsulon are effective against both mature and immature stages of *F. gigantica. Fascioloides magna*, a parasite of deer that can affect cattle, is susceptible to triclabendazole, clorsulon and closantel.

Only limited information is available on the treatment of paramphistomes in cattle (see p. 279). Niclofolan or albendazole has been recommended, but these have only variable activity against intestinal juvenile forms. Oxyclozanide given on two occasions, three days apart, has been shown to be effective against adult flukes in the rumen.

Schistosomes (see p. 280)

In contrast to the chemotherapy of schistosomes in humans, little information is available on the treatment of schistosomosis in cattle. For economic reasons, anthelmintic treatment is not suitable for the control of schistosomosis in cattle, except during clinical outbreaks when praziquantel may be administered orally at 15–20 mg/kg. Repeat doses two to three days apart are usually required or high dose rates (25/mg per kg) at three to five weeks apart.

Treatment of cestode infections in cattle

Adult stages of tapeworms parasitizing cattle are usually of little consequence. Several of the benzimidazoles used in the treatment of GI nematodes are also effective against cestodes (Tables 60.2 and 60.3). Certain flukicidal drugs also have cestocidal activity (Table 60.4). Larval stages of cestodes affecting cattle, notably *Echinococcus* spp. and *Taenia saginata*, are generally refractory to treatment with anthelmintics. However, praziquantel has been shown to have activity

Table 60.4 Activities of anthelmintics against liver fluke in cattle.

Chemical group	Chemical	Recommended dose rate (mg/kg)	Active against			Comments
			A	B	C	
Salicylanilides	Rafoxanide	7.5	+	+	−	No longer available in many countries
	Closantel	NR	+	+	±	Available for cattle in some countries
	Oxyclozanide	10	+	−	−	Some activity against tapeworm segments
Substituted phenols	Nitroxynil	10	+	+	−	Also active against blood nematodes
	Bithionol	30	+	−	−	Also has anticestodal activity
	Niclofolan	3	+			
Benzimidazoles	Albendazole	10	+	−	−	Also active against nematodes and cestodes
	Triclabendazole	12	+	+	+	Do not give to dairy cows within 7 days of calving
Probenzimidazoles	Netobimin	20	+	−	−	Do not administer to cattle in the first 7 weeks of
Sulphonamide	Clorsulon	7	+	+	±	pregnancy

A, adult fluke; B, 6–12 week old fluke; C, 1–6 week old fluke.
NR, no recommended dose rate.

against the intermediate stages of both these parasites, although the cost of treatment may preclude its use.

Antiprotozoals

Ruminants carry large numbers of protozoa in their stomach and intestines, the vast majority of which are entirely harmless. Some species of protozoa, however, are significant as causes of disease in cattle or because of their potential for zoonotic transmission. Antiprotozoal compounds are listed in Table 60.5.

Protozoal diseases of economic importance throughout various regions of the world include trypanosomosis, theileriosis, babesiosis and trichomoniasis. Coccidiosis in cattle is caused by parasites of the genus *Eimeria* spp. and can be a serious cause of disease in young animals (see p. 282). A protozoan disease of increasing importance is cryptosporidiosis. The causative organism, *Cryptosporidum parvum* (see pp. 204, 286), is a significant cause of disease in neonatal calves and is also an important zoonosis.

Haemoparasites

Cattle are infected with a number of haemoprotozoa that include some highly pathogenic species, e.g. the piroplasms (*Babesia* and *Theileria*) (see p. 748) and the haemoflagellates (*Trypanosoma*) (see p. 756). Transmission of these blood parasites normally occurs via a biting tick or insect vector. *Babesia* species occur in most parts of the world where there are ticks. They are of greatest importance in the tropics, but some species occur in temperate climates where they can cause disease in non-immune cattle. The merozoites of *Babesia* occur in the erythrocytes of infected animals where they multiply asexually by binary fission and are described as 'large' and 'small', depending on size.

Table 60.5 Antiprotozoal compounds for cattle.

Compound	Trade name	Manufacturer	Dose rates (mg/kg) Route	Comments
Diminazene aceturate	Berenil	Intervet	3.5–7.0 im or sc	For treatment of typanosomosis (*T. congolense, T. brucei, T. vivax* [nagana]) and babesiosis (*B. bigemina, B. bovis* and *B. divergens*)
Imidocarb	Imizol	Schering-Plough (Mallinckrodt Veterinary)	1–3 sc	For treatment of babesiosis (*B. bigemina, B. bovis* and *B. divergens*). Prophylactic effect for up to 8 weeks depending on dose and species involved. Causes cholinergic effects and is slowly metabolised and excreted
Homidium chloride	Novidium	Merial	1.0 im	Treatment of trypanosomosis (*T. congolense, T. brucei, T. vivax* [nagana])
Isometamidium chloride	Samorin	Merial	0.25–1.0 im or iv	Treatment or prevention of typanosomosis (*T. brucei, T. congolense, T. vivax* [nagana]). Toxic above 2 mg/kg
Suramin	Naganol	Bayer	10 iv	Treatment of typanosomosis (*T. brucei, T. congolense, T. vivax* [nagana])
Amicarbalide	Diampron	Merial	5–10 im	Treatment of babesiosis (*B. bigemina, B. bovis, B. divergens*)
Buparvaquone	Butalex	Schering-Plough (Mallinckrodt Veterinary)	2.5 2 doses at 48h intervals	Treatment of East Coast fever (*Theileria parva*) and Mediterranean Coast fever (*T. annulata*)
Parvaquone	Clexan	Schering-Plough (Mallinckrodt Veterinary)	10–20 2 doses at 48h intervals	Treatment of East Coast fever (*T. parva*) and Mediterranean Coast fever (*T. annulata*)
Halofuginone	Stenoral	Intervet	1.2 po 2 doses at 48h intervals	Treatment of East Cost fever (*T. parva*) and Mediterranean Coast fever (*T. annulata*)

im, intramuscular; sc, subcutaneous; iv, intravenous; po, per os (oral).

Several species are highly pathogenic in cattle and include *Babesia bigemina*, found in Africa, Australia, Europe and Central and South America, and *B. bovis*, found throughout most of the world and being particularly common in southern Europe. Transmission occurs following a bite from an infected tick of the genera *Boophilus*, *Rhipicephalus*, *Haemaphysalis* and *Ixodes*, the species involved varying with geographical location. The species found throughout temperate Europe is *Babesia divergens* (a small piroplasm), transmitted by the tick *Ixodes ricinus*. Clinically affected animals develop a haemolytic anaemia leading to haemoglobinuria, fever and death.

A number of *Theileria* species have been reported in cattle and are significant causes of disease in many tropical countries. The parasites occur within lymphocytic and erythrocytic cells and are transmitted by the bites of various species of ticks. *T. parva* (the cause of East Coast fever) and *T. annulata* (Mediterranean Coast fever) are the main pathogenic species occurring in East and North Africa, southern Europe and parts of the former Soviet States, respectively. Transmission of these parasites occurs following the bite from an infected tick belonging to various species of the genus *Hyalomma*.

Trypanosomosis is one of the most important diseases of domesticated cattle in central parts of Africa. Trypanosomes are broadly divided into two groups depending on the site of development in the insect vector. The salivarian trypanosomes, transmitted in the saliva of biting flies, are responsible for 'nagana' in domestic ruminants (see p. 757), as well as diseases such as 'surra' of horses and other animals, and African Sleeping Sickness in humans. The stercorarian trypanosomes are transmitted by contamination with infected insect faeces and include diseases such as Chagas disease in humans in Central and South America, which is transmitted by reduviid bugs.

Coccidiosis (see p. 282)

At least 18 different species of coccidia are known to infect cattle worldwide. Bovine coccidiosis is primarily a disease of young animals aged between three weeks and nine months, but can occur in older cattle. The disease is usually associated with a previous stressful situation such as shipping, overcrowding, changes of feed, severe weather or concurrent infections. Clinical signs, often presenting as bloody diarrhoea, are associated with the presence of *Eimeria zuernii* or *E. bovis*, which occur in the lower small intestine, caecum and colon. Another species of coccidia, *E. alabamanesis*, has been reported to cause enteritis in yearling calves in some northern European countries.

The incidence of coccidiosis can be reduced by avoidance of overcrowding and stress and increased attention to hygiene. Raising of food and water troughs, for example, can help avoid contamination by reducing the levels of infection. Young animals should be kept off heavily contaminated pastures when they are most susceptible. The anticoccidial decoquinate is licensed in many countries for the prevention of coccidiosis in calves. Other compounds, such as monensin and amprolium, are available is some countries.

Cryptosporidiosis (see pp. 204, 286)

Bovine cryptosporidiosis is often seen as part of the neonatal diarrhoea complex, symptoms of which are profuse watery diarrhoea, dehydration, and death if left untreated. Infections are usually, although not always, associated with the presence of other pathogens such as *Salmonella* spp., *E. coli*, rotavirus and coronavirus. Specific antiparasitic therapy is not available for cryptosporidiosis and treatment relies on the use of supportive antidiarrhoeals and fluid therapy for animals showing dehydration. Recently halofuginone lactate has been licensed for the prevention of diarrhoea caused by *Cryptosporidium parvum* by treating daily for seven consecutive days.

ECTOPARASITICIDES

Introduction (see Chapters 45, 50)

Ectoparasites can cause intense irritation leading to loss of condition and effects on performance such as weight loss, reduced milk yield or hide damage. In addition they may be responsible for transmission of disease. The choice and use of ectoparasiticide chemicals and the method for their control depend to a large extent on husbandry and management practices as well as the type of ectoparasite causing the infestation.

Parasites that live permanently on the host, such as lice and mites, are relatively easily controlled and, once eradicated, reinfestation only occurs from contact with infested stock. Non-permanent parasites (ticks and flies) are less easily controlled because only a small proportion of the population can be treated at any one time and other hosts may maintain them.

Most infestations in cattle are seasonal and predictable and can be countered by prophylactic use of ectoparasiticides. For example, biting and nuisance flies occur predominantly from late spring to early autumn, tick populations increase in the spring and autumn, and lice and mites may increase in winter-housed stock.

Ectoparasiticide groups

Available ectoparasiticides act either systemically or by direct contact with the target parasites and have an effect on the ectoparasite's nervous system. Systemic ectoparasiticides may be given parenterally or applied topically to the skin from where the active ingredient is absorbed percutaneously and taken up into the blood circulation. Topical ectoparasiticides have a direct effect on the target parasite on the surface of the skin. Different formulations of a drug preparation may be indicated for different target parasites (Table 60.6).

Both topical and systemically acting formulations can be applied by various methods including dips, sprays, 'pour-ons', 'spot-ons', dusting powders or ear tags. Typically, a number of formulations are available as liquid concentrates requiring dilution with water to produce an emulsion for application by spray or dip. However, more convenient ready-for-use pour-on and spot-on application methods provide a broad choice of systems depending upon individual circumstances, for example availability of spraying, dipping and animal handing facilities, in addition to labour requirements for such operations.

Organochlorines

Organochlorines (OCs) are no longer in general use but several compounds are still available in some countries. OCs fall into three main groups:

(1) Chlorinated ethane derivatives such as DDT (dichlorodiphenyltrichloroethane), DDE (dichlorodiphenyldichloroethane) and DDD (dicofol, methoxychlor);
(2) The cyclodienes that include chlordane, aldrin, dieldrin, hepatochlor, endrin, tozaphene;
(3) Hexachlorocyclohexane (HCH), also known as benzene hexachloride (BHC), which includes the γ-isomer lindane.

Table 60.6 Chemicals active against cattle ectoparasites.

Ectoparasite group	Parasite species	Ectoparasiticides
Biting flies	Haematobia (Lyperosia) irritans, horn fly Stomoxys calcitrans, stable fly Simulium spp., blackfly	Ivermectin,[a] doramectin,[a] eprinomectin,[a] moxidectin,[a] cypermethrin, deltamethrin, fenvalerate, permethrin
Nuisance flies	Hydrotaea irritans, head fly Musca autumnalis, face fly Musca domestica, house fly Morellia simplex, sweat fly	Cypermethrin, deltamethrin, fenvalerate, permethrin
Warble flies	Hypoderma bovis Hypoderma lineatum	Abamectin, doramectin, eprinomectin, ivermectin, moxidectin, famphur, fenthion, phosmet
Sucking lice	Haematopinus eurysternus Linognathus vituli Solenopotes capillatus	Abamectin, doramectin, eprinomectin, ivermectin, moxidectin, phosmet, cypermethrin, deltamethrin, fenvalerate, permethrin, Amitraz Closantel
Biting lice	Bovicola (Damalinia) bovis[b]	Doramectin,[b] eprinomectin,[b] ivermectin,[b] moxidectin,[b] famphur, fenthion, phosmet, cypermethrin, deltamethrin, fenvalerate, permethrin, amitraz
Mites	Psoroptes bovis Sarcoptes scabiei Chorioptes bovis	Abamectin,[c] doramectin,[c] eprinomectin,[c] ivermectin,[c] moxidectin,[c] phosmet, amitraz
Ticks	Ixodes spp. Boophilus spp. Rhipicephalus spp. Ambylomma spp. Dermacentor spp. Hyalomma spp.	Amitraz Flubenzuron Closantel

[a] Pour-on preparations with activity and protection against horn flies [Haematobia (Lyperosia) irritans]
[b] Efficacy varies depending on method of application. Injectable preparations *aid* in the control of biting lice.
[c] Efficacy varies depending on method of application. Injectable preparations *aid* in the control of chorioptic mange.

Chlorinated ethanes cause inhibition of sodium conductance along sensory and motor nerve fibres by
holding sodium channels open, resulting in delayed
depolarization of the axonal membrane. This state
renders the nerve vulnerable to repetitive discharge
from small stimuli that would normally cause an action
potential in a fully repolarized neuron.

The cyclodienes appear to have at least two component modes of action:

- Inhibition of γ-amino butyric acid (GABA)-
  stimulated Cl⁻ flux and
- Interference with Ca^{2+} flux.

The resultant inhibitory postsynaptic potential leads
to a state of partial depolarization of the postsynaptic
membrane and vulnerability to repeated discharge. A
similar mode of action has been reported for lindane,
which binds to the picrotoxin side of the GABA receptor resulting in an inhibition of GABA-dependent Cl⁻
flux into the neuron.

Organophosphates and carbamates

Organophosphates (OPs) are neutral esters of phosphoric acid or its thio analogue and act by inhibiting the
action of acetylcholinesterase (AchE) at cholinergic
synapses and at muscle end plates. This results in an
accumulation of acetylcholine (Ach) at the postsynaptic membrane, leading to neuromuscular paralysis.
OP compounds include azamethiphos, chlorpyriphos,
coumaphos, dichlorvos, diazinon, fenitrothion, heptenophos, metriphonate, phoxim, propetamphos or
tetrachlorvinphos and there are many preparations
available worldwide for cattle. Carbamate insecticides are closely related to the OPs and are also
anticholinesterases but, unlike OP compounds, are
spontaneously reversible. The two main carbamate
compounds in use in veterinary medicine are carbaryl
and propoxur. OP compounds can be extremely
toxic in animals and humans. Inhibition of AchE, and
other cholinesterases, can occur in higher vertebrates as
well and accounts for host toxicity seen at higher dose
rates. Typical signs of overdosage, or overexposure,
include salivation, miosis, diarrhoea and muscle
tremors. Death may occur through respiratory failure.
Toxic clinical signs can be treated with atropine.
Chronic exposure may lead to damage to the nervous
system and clinical signs including headaches, anxiety
and irritability in operators. OP compounds are generally active against warble fly larvae, flies, lice, ticks and
mites on cattle, although activity will vary between
compounds, formulations and against different target
parasites.

Pyrethrins and synthetic pyrethroids

Natural pyrethrins are derived from pyrethrum, a
mixture of alkaloids from the chrysanthemum plant.
Synthetic pyrethroids (SPs) include bioallethrin, cypermethrin, deltamethrin, fenvalerate, flumethrin, lambdacyhalothrin, phenothrin and permethrin. The content of
some SPs is also expressed in terms of the drug isomers;
for example, cypermethrin preparations may contain
varying proportions of their *cis* and *trans* isomers. Thus,
cypermethrin (*cis* : *trans* 60 : 40) 2.5 per cent is equivalent to cypermethrin (*cis* : *trans* 80 : 20) 1.25 per cent. In
general terms, *cis* isomers are more active than the corresponding *trans* isomers. The mode of action of SPs
appears to be an interference with sodium channels of
the parasite nerve axons, resulting in delayed repolar-
ization and eventual paralysis. The lethal activity of
pyrethroids seems to involve action on both peripheral
and central neurones, while the knockdown effect is
probably produced by peripheral neuronal effects only.

Pour-on, spot-on, spray and dip formulations are
available in many countries with activity against biting
and nuisance flies, lice and ticks. Some compounds are
active against sarcoptic and chorioptic mange mites.
For non-permanent ectoparasites, treatments are generally applied during periods of anticipated peak challenge. Treatments for lice are best administered in
the autumn. Periods of protection against flies vary
between products and methods of application, but generally last for up to one month for most species of flies.
Some SPs are also available as ear tags for use on cattle,
providing protection against biting and nuisance flies
for several months during the fly season. One tag is
usually sufficient but in severe cases of head or face fly
attack, both ears can be tagged.

Amidines

The main member of this group is amitraz, which acts
at octopamine receptor sites in ectoparasites giving rise
to increased nervous activity. When applied as a spray
it is active against mites, lice and ticks in cattle. In severe
cases of mange, lice and tick infestations, treatments
may have to be repeated during the risk period.

Avermectins and milbemycins

Avermectins and the structurally related milbemycins
have been discussed earlier under anthelmintics. As
well as being effective against GI roundworms and
lungworms, all have activity against warbles, sucking
lice and mange mites. Control against the biting louse,
Bovicola (*Damalinia*) *bovis*, the mite, *Chorioptes bovis*,
and the hornfly, *Haematobia* (*Lyperosia*) *irritans* varies
between products and the method of administration.

Insect growth regulators

Insect growth regulators (IGRs) are a group of chemical compounds that do not kill the target parasite directly, but interfere with growth and development. IGRs act mainly on immature stages of the parasite and as such are not usually suitable for the rapid control of established adult populations of parasites. Where parasites show a clear seasonal pattern, IGRs can be applied at the start of the grazing season as a preventative measure. Based on their mode of action they can be divided into chitin inhibitors and juvenile hormone analogues. Chitin inhibitors appear either to interfere with the assembly of chitin chains and microfibrils or to inhibit the deposit of chitin into the cuticle. The juvenile hormone analogues mimic the activity of naturally occurring juvenile hormones and prevent metamorphosis to the adult stage.

IGRs are widely used for flea control in domestic pets and for blowfly control in sheep, but have limited use in cattle. The phenoylbenzyl urea flubenzuron is marketed in Australasia as a tick development inhibitor. When applied as a pour-on it provides long-term protection against the one-host tick *Boophilus microplus*.

Further reading

Anderson, N. (1985) Controlled release technology for the control of helminths in ruminants. *Veterinary Parasitology*, **18**, 59–66.

Armour, J., Bairden, K., Pirie, H.M. & Ryan, W.G. (1987) Control of parasitic bronchitis and gastroenteritis by strategic prophylaxis with ivermectin. *Veterinary Record*, **121**, 5–8.

Barth, D. (1987) Treatment of inhibited *Dictyocaulus viviparus* in cattle with ivermectin. *Veterinary Parasitology*, **25**, 61–6.

Bauer, C., Holtemyer, H. & Schid, K. (1997) Field evaluation of a fenbendazole slow release bolus in the control of nematode infections in first-season cattle. *Veterinary Record*, **140**, 395–9.

Bennett, D.G. (1986) Clinical pharmacology of ivermectin. *Journal of the American Veterinary Medical Association*, **189**, 100–104.

Bishop, Y. (ed.) (1998) Drugs used in the treatment and control of parasitic infections. In *The Veterinary Formulary*, 4th edn, pp. 185–248. Pharmaceutical Press, London.

Boersma, J.H. (1985) Chemotherapy of gastrointestinal nematodiasis in ruminants. In *Chemotherapy of Gastrointestinal Helminths* (ed. by H. vanden Bossche, D. Thienpont & P.G. Jannsens), *Handbook of Experimental Pharmacology*, vol. 77, pp. 407–42. Springer-Verlag, Berlin.

Boray, J.C. (1986) Trematode infections of domestic animals. In *Chemotherapy of Parasitic Diseases* (ed. by W.C. Campbell & R.S. Rew), pp. 401–25. Plenum Press, New York.

Caldow, G.L., Taylor, M.A. & Hunt, K. (1989) Comparison of two early season anthelmintic programmes on a commercial beef farm. *Veterinary Record*, **24**, 111–14.

Campbell, W.C. (1985) Ivermectin: an update. *Parasitology Today*, **1**, 10–16.

Campbell, W.C. (1986) The chemotherapy of parasitic infections. *Journal of Parasitology*, **72**, 45–66.

Craig, T.M. & Hucy, R.L. (1984) Efficacy of triclabendazole against *Fasciola hepatica* and *Fascioloides magna* in naturally infected calves. *American Journal of Veterinary Research*, **46**, 1644–5.

Donald, A.D. (1985) New methods of drug application for control of helminths. *Veterinary Parasitology*, **18**, 121–37.

Eagleson, J.S. & Bowie, J.Y. (1986) Oxfendazole resistance in *Trichostrongylus axei* in cattle in Australia. *Veterinary Record*, **119**, 604.

Egerton, J.R., Suhayda, D. & Eary, C.H. (1986) Prophylaxis of nematode infections in cattle with an indwelling ruminoreticular ivermectin sustained release bolus. *Veterinary Parasitology*, **22**, 67–75.

Eysker, M. (1986) The prophylactic effect of ivermectin treatment of calves three weeks after turnout, on gastrointestinal helminthiasis. *Veterinary Parasitology*, **22**, 95–103.

Fairweather, I. & Boray, J.C. (1998) Mechanisms of fasciolicide action and drug resistance in *Fasciola hepatica*. In *Fasciolosis* (ed. by J.P. Dalton), pp. 225–76. CABI Publishing, Wallingford.

Fairweather, I. & Boray, J.C. (1999) Fasciolicides: efficacy, actions, resistance and its management. *The Veterinary Journal*, **158**, 81–112.

Geerts, S., Brandt, J., Kumar, V. & Biesemans, L. (1987) Suspected resistance of *Ostertagia ostertagi* in cattle to levamisole. *Veterinary Parasitology*, **23**, 77–82.

Grimshaw, W.T.R., Weatherley, A.J. & Jones, R.M. (1989) Evaluation of the morantel sustained release trilaminate in the control of parasitic gastroenteritis in first season grazing cattle. *Veterinary Record*, **124**, 453–6.

Hart, R.J. (1986) Mode of action of agents used against arthropod parasites. In *Chemotherapy of Parasitic Diseases* (ed. by W.C. Campbell & R.S. Rew), pp. 585–602. Plenum Press, New York.

Hashemi-Fesharki, R. (1991) Chemotherapeutic value of parvaquone and buparvaquone against *Theileria annulata* of cattle. *Research in Veterinary Science*, **50**, 204–207.

Jacobs, D.E., Fox, M.T. & Ryan, W.G. (1987) Early season parasitic gastroenteritis in calves and its prevention with ivermectin. *Veterinary Record*, **120**, 29–31.

Jacobs, D.E., Thomas, J.G., Foster, J., Fox, M.T. & Oakley, G.A. (1987) Oxfendazole pulse release intraruminal devices and bovine parasitic bronchitis: comparison of two control strategies in a field experiment. *Veterinary Record*, **121**, 221–4.

Jones, R.M. (1983) Therapeutic and prophylactic efficacy of morantel when administered directly into the rumen of cattle on a continuous basis. *Veterinary Parasitology*, **12**, 223–32.

Kassai, T. (1999) Anthelmintic therapy and control. In *Veterinary Helminthology*, pp. 141–61. Butterworth Heinemann, Oxford.

Martin, R.J. (1997) Modes of action of anthelmintic drugs. *The Veterinary Journal*, **154**, 11–34.

Martin, R.J., Robertson, A.P. & Bjorn, H. (1997) Target sites of anthelmintics. *Parasitology*, **114**, S111–S124.

Peregrine, A.S. (1994) Chemotherapy and delivery systems: haemoparasites. *Veterinary Parasitology*, **54**, 223–48.

Prichard, R.K. (1985) Interaction of host physiology and efficacy of antiparasitic drugs. *Veterinary Parasitology*, **18**, 103–10.

Prichard, R.K. (1986) Anthelmintics for cattle. *Veterinary Clinics of North America: Food Animal Practices*, **2**, 489–501.

Prichard, R.K., Hennessy, D.R. & Steel, J.W. (1978) Prolonged administration: a new concept for increasing the spectrum and effectiveness of anthelmintics. *Veterinary Parasitology*, **4**, 309–15.

Prichard, R.K., Hennessy, D.R., Steel, J.W. & Lacey, E. (1985) Metabolic concentrations in plasma following treatment of cattle with five metabolites. *Research in Veterinary Science*, **39**, 173–8.

Rew, R.S. & Fetterer, R.H. (1986) Mode of action of anti-nematocidal drugs. In *Chemotherapy of Parasitic Diseases* (ed. by W.C. Campbell & R.S. Rew), pp. 321–37. Plenum Press, New York.

Rolfe, P.F. & Boray, J.C. (1987) Chemotherapy of paramphistomosis in cattle. *Australian Veterinary Journal*, **63**, 328–32.

Ryan, W.G., Crawfoes, R.J., Gros, S.J. & Wallace, D.H. (1997) Assessment of parasite control and weight gain after use of an ivermectin sustained-release bolus in calves. *Journal of the American Veterinary Medical Association*, **21**, 754–6.

Schulman, M.D. & Valentino, D. (1982) Purification, characterisation and inhibition by MK-401 of *Fasciola hepatica* phosphoglyceromutase. *Molecular and Biochemical Parasitology*, **5**, 321–32.

Seibert, B.P., Guerrero, J., Newcomb, K.M., Ruth, D.T. & Swites, B.J. (1986) Seasonal comparisons of anthelmintic activity of levamisole pour-on in cattle in the USA. *Veterinary Record*, **118**, 40–2.

Sharma, N.N. & Mishra, A.K. (1990) Treatment of bovine tropical theileriosis with buparvaquone. *Tropical Animal Health Production*, **22**, 63–5.

Taylor, M.A. (1996) Bovine anthelmintics: an overview of current thinking. *Veterinary Practice*, **28**, 7–8.

Taylor, M.A. (1997) Treatment and control of ectoparasites in cattle. *Cattle Practice*, **5**, 279–82.

Taylor, M.A. (1999). Anthelmintics for cattle: a review. *Cattle Practice*, **7**, 157–67.

Taylor, M.A. & Catchpole, J. (1994) Coccidiosis of domestic ruminants. *Applied Pasasitology*, **35**, 83–6.

Taylor, M.A. & Webster, K.A. (1998) Recent advances in the diagnosis of *Cryptosporidium*, *Toxoplasma*, *Giardia* and other protozoa of veterinary importance. *Research in Veterinary Science*, **65**, 183–93.

Taylor, S.M., Malbo, T.R. & Kenny, J. (1985) Comparison of early season suppressive anthelmintic prophylactic methods for parasitic gastroenteritis and bronchitis in calves. *Veterinary Record*, **117**, 521–34.

Wall, R. & Shearer, D. (1997) The control and treatment of ectoparasite infestation, pp. 331–9. Chapman & Hall, London.

Yazwinski, T.A., Featherstone, H., Presson, B.L., Greenway, T.E., Pote, L.M. & Holtzen, H. (1985) Efficacy of injectable clorsulon in the treatment of immature bovine *Fasciola hepatica* infections. *Agripractice*, **6**, 6–8.

Chapter 61
Antimicrobial Agents

A.H. Andrews

Introduction	1035
Identification of the causal agent	1035
Sampling	1035
Sensitivity testing	1036
Penetration	1036
Antibiotic resistance	1038
Dosage	1038
Route of administration	1038
Duration of therapy	1038
Spectrum of drug activity	1040
Bacteriostatic or bactericidal activity	1040
Drug combinations	1041
Cost	1042
Toxicity	1042
Drug withdrawal times	1042
Legal considerations	1042
Frequency of dosing	1042
Possible antibacterial therapy for cattle	1044

Introduction

The choice of a suitable antimicrobial agent is very difficult. It first depends on deciding whether the problem encountered is an infection and even then whether it warrants such therapy. The site of infection needs to be located and the type of microbe established. Then the *in vitro* antimicrobial sensitivity of the organism and the minimal inhibitory concentration need to be determined. The likely ability to penetrate the area, the action of the antibiotic in the local environment and the maintenance of an effective concentration at the area must be considered. The selection also has to include the possibility of any potential toxic side-effects as well as the meat and milk withholding times. Once all these factors have been taken into consideration, the drug to be used, its dosage, route and frequency of administration can be determined. All the above, however, has to be undertaken on an economic basis.

There are various ways of defining antimicrobial preparations. Chemotherapy can be defined as the use in the treatment of a disease of pure chemicals that have a special antagonistic effect(s) on the organism causing the disease.

Antibiotics are complex organic chemicals synthesized by micro-organisms during their growth and which, in minute quantities, have a detrimental effect on other organisms. These chemical compounds are the metabolic products of bacteria and fungi. Most commonly, antibiotics are effective against bacteria but some have activity against viruses, *Rickettsia*, *Mycoplasma*, fungi and helminths (see Table 61.1).

At present all prescribing of antimicrobial agents for therapy, prophylaxis or control of disease is under veterinary control and prescription in the UK. The level of control in some countries is greater than in Britain, e.g. Sweden, although in many parts of the world it is less or almost non-existent.

Identification of the causal agent

Some decisions regarding therapy can only be made once a diagnosis is reached. Clinical examination is used to identify the nature of the infection, its site and possible cause. The signs of some diseases are so clear-cut that diagnosis is easy to establish and the organism is readily identifiable, e.g. wooden tongue, actinomycosis. In such cases the choice of drug is easy to make as well as its dosage, rate and duration of treatment. The likely outcome of therapy can also be predicted with some confidence. However, in many cases the disease signs are not clear-cut, the area of infection is difficult to localize or the sensitivity pattern of the organism is irregular. In such cases the identification of the causal agent is important not only for treatment of the individual animal affected but also for possible future action on a herd basis. However, in many situations, the site of infection and the cause of the condition are not known. In such instances laboratory diagnosis, other than haematological examination to indicate that an infection is present, is of no value. Therapy in these cases usually involves the use of one or more antimicrobial agents to ensure a broad spectrum of activity. Subsequent progress will depend on evaluation of the effect of the chosen treatment.

Sampling

Wherever possible sampling should be undertaken to try to determine the causal organism. This will be

Table 61.1 Non-antibacterial activity of some antibiotics.

Mycoplasma	Chlortetracycline, doxycycline, erythromycin, fluoroquinolones, lincomycin, methacycline, oleandomycin, oxytetracycline, spiramycin, tetracycline, tylosin
Rickettsia	Chloramphenicol, chlortetracycline, doxycycline, fluoroquinolones, methacycline, oxytetracycline, tetracycline
Protozoa	Monensin, sulphonamides, tetracycline
Fungi	
Candida albicans	Amphotericin, nystatin
Dermatophytes	Griseofulvin, natamycin
Ectoparasites and endoparasites	Ivermectin

Table 61.2 Drugs with reasonable penetration of various fluids and tissues.

Bile	Erythromycin
Bone	Chlortetracycline, doxycycline, fucidin, lincomycin, methacycline, oxytetracycline, tetracycline
Cerebrospinal fluid	Chloramphenicol, florfenicol, fluoroquinolones, sulphonamides, trimethoprim and sulphonamides
Eye	Amoxycillin, ampicillin, cephalexin, cephaloridine, cephalothin, chloramphenicol, lincomycin
Milk	Benzylpenicillin, erythromycin, lincomycin (but toxic), oleandomycin, penethamate, spiramycin, tylosin
Prostate	Erythromycin, trimethoprim
Serosal fluids	Chloramphenicol, dihydrostreptomycin, erythromycin, framycetin, gentamicin, kanamycin, lincomycin, neomycin, paromomycin, streptomycin

considered academic by many, but if it is looked at objectively, it has much to commend it. At the first examination and, hopefully, before any therapy has been initiated is the best time to obtain samples to establish the likely cause of the problem. In addition, the cost of micro-organism determination is usually less, or at least no more, than the cost of appropriate therapy. In almost all cases the value of the individual animal will be sufficient to make it worthwhile and this is multiplied many times when problems are encountered on a herd basis. There is virtually no justification for not sampling problems of a herd nature when infections are suspected. In addition, the treatment of chronic conditions or those that have responded poorly is important. Besides positively determining the cause, sampling may help to eliminate other potential agents.

The method of sampling is important in that it should involve fresh clinical cases rather than those of a chronic nature. The sample should be taken from as near the inflamed area as possible. This is difficult with problems such as salmonellosis, as organisms in the faeces may be diluted by those further down the gut, which in themselves may be much faster growing. Sampling of pneumonias is always difficult as the organisms present in the upper respiratory tract may be unrepresentative of those in the lung.

Direct examination of the sample after staining is of use as in some circumstances organisms will not subsequently grow. Rapid staining methods are now available and these allow the shape of the organism and whether it is Gram-positive or Gram-negative to be determined. This in turn can be useful in making a quick decision about the drug most likely to be effective.

Sensitivity testing

Identification of the causal organism allows a decision to be made as to whether or not to test for antimicrobial sensitivity. In many cases there is no need to undertake this. Thus organisms of *Clostridium* spp. are sensitive to high doses of penicillin G. However, in cases involving *Escherichia coli* and *Salmonella typhimurium* there will be considerable variations in the sensitivity pattern, bearing in mind the origin of the organism.

The Kirby–Bauer disc sensitivity test is that most commonly used for *in vitro* testing. The aim is to determine if an organism is likely to be affected by specific antimicrobial agents at the usual therapeutic levels. While the drug concentration reflects levels achieved in the plasma, it does not take into account quantities in various tissues such as the brain or udder. The test organism is usually classified as sensitive, intermediate or resistant to the specific antimicrobial agent. The test was produced for use in human medicine where it provides a quantitative assessment. However, in animals it is a useful guide. Quantitative tests involve determining the minimal inhibitory concentration and usually consist of tube sensitivity tests. In general, an organism sensitive *in vitro* may be sensitive *in vivo*, but one resistant *in vitro* is also likely to be resistant *in vivo*.

Penetration

The ability of a drug to penetrate the infected area needs to be considered (see Table 61.2). Penetration depends on the degree of the pathological process as is seen with abscess or thrombus formation. It also depends on the tissue involved and whether there are natural limits to penetration such as in the brain (see p. 897) or in milk. The location of the organism is also important, i.e. whether it is intracellular or extracellular.

The ability of an antimicrobial drug to cross biological membranes depends on many factors. These include protein binding, lipid solubility, pH of the drug in relation to environmental pH, molecular size and in some cases specific cellular transport mechanisms. Antibiotic is absorbed into the circulation, partly becoming bound to plasma protein. Binding varies, e.g. from less than 50 per cent with amoxycillin, streptomycin or oxytetracycline to more than 80 per cent with cloxacillin or erythromycin. Binding is readily reversible and the bound fraction is in equilibrium with the unbound (active) form. Protein binding can be a disadvantage, as with sulphonamides, which are highly protein bound. As purulent fluids often contain much protein, sulphonamides can be relatively inactive.

Water-soluble drugs are useful for extracellular organisms and where intracellular organisms have a high turnover rate, usually in the lysis of cells and release of the organisms into fluids containing the antimicrobial agent. Lipid solubility does have advantages for organisms that spend most of their time within cells or behind tissue barriers. Inflammation can also alter penetration of drugs. Thus penetration of the central nervous system by many drugs is minimal in the healthy animal although penicillin G and other antibiotics can enter during inflammation. However, the effect of inflammation on the penetration of many drugs is unknown. Thus it can be the local environment in which the organism is present that is important. Most antimicrobial agents do maintain their activity; however, aminoglycosides are more active in aerobic conditions with a slightly alkaline pH. As such conditions do not exist around staphylococcal abscesses this group of drugs is relatively inactive in such circumstances. Activity of antibacterial agent in urine is often influenced by the pH (see Table 61.3.) The problem of sulphonamides and pus has already been mentioned. Some antibiotics do have more effect on anaerobic bacteria than others under such conditions (see Table 61.4).

Table 61.3 Antibacterial drug activity in urine. Urinary infections are relatively uncommon in cattle but can lead to therapeutic problems.

Not affected by urine pH	Most active in alkaline urine	Most active in acid urine
Cephalexin	Colistin	Carbenicillin
Cephaloridine	Dihydrostreptomycin	Chlortetracycline
Cephalothin	Erythromycin	Doxycycline
Chloramphenicol	Framycetin	Methacycline
Nalidixic acid	Gentamicin	Nitrofurantoin
Sulphonamides	Kanamycin	Oxytetracycline
Trimethoprim and sulphonamides	Neomycin	Penicillin G
	Paromomycin	Tetracycline
	Polymyxin B	
	Streptomycin	*Acidifiction*
		D-Methionine (oral)
	Alkalinization	Ascorbic acid (oral)
	Sodium bicarbonate (oral)	

Table 61.4 Antibiotics effective *in vitro* against anaerobic bacteria.

High efficacy	Moderate efficacy	Low efficacy
Amoxycillin	Chlortetracycline	Dihydrostreptomycin
Ampicillin	Erythromycin	Framycetin
Carbenicillin	Oxytetracycline	Gentamicin
Chloramphenicol	Procaine penicillin G	Kanamycin
Clindamycin	Tetracycline	Neomycin
Metronidazole		Paromomycin
		Streptomycin

Antibiotic resistance

The advent of antimicrobial drugs has resulted in the emergence of resistance to these drugs (see Table 61.5). The use of antibiotics in therapeutic concentration results in an alteration of the microflora within the host. There is a tendency for a loss of the sensitive strains with the resistant ones remaining. This selection allows multiplication of resistant strains within the less competitive environment. The resistant organisms can remain in the animal and also contaminate the environment, thereby allowing passage to other animals. The prevalence of the resistant organisms tends to reduce the longer the period since the drug was used.

Spontaneous mutation of organisms can occur but it is probably only of limited importance in practice. However, transferable drug resistance is of significance. This resistance, as determined in the form of plasmids or transposons, is transferred to susceptible strains. Plasmids are extrachromosomal genetic material that can replicate independently of the chromosome. These plasmids can be transferred by conjugation within or between bacterial species and they can also act as vectors for transposons. This allows the transfer of single or multiple antibiotic resistance and has produced many of the resistant bacteria found in enteric calf infections including both *E. coli* and *S. typhimurium* as well as in *Staphylococcus aureus* and some *Pasteurella and Mannheimia* spp. infections. In some countries the use of chloramphenicol in food animals is restricted or banned because of the usage in humans and also due to potential human toxicity from handling it. Increasing concern has been expressed about microbial resistance to antibacterials in human beings caused by contact directly with, or indirectly from food produced from, farm animals. While the risks appear to be minimal in creating human microbial resistance compared with other causes, all veterinarians should bear the problem in mind when treating or prescribing for cattle.

Table 61.5 gives examples of antimicrobials which still have activity in the presence of penicillinase.

Dosage

When an antimicrobial agent is selected it must be in a high enough concentration and used for a long enough period to result in contact with the organism and its consequent demise. Various factors influence this, including the dose, formulation and rate of administration. Doses are usually based on body weight. The recommended dose usually provides good blood and tissue

Table 61.5 Penicillinase (β-lactamase) active antimicrobials.

Penicillins	Cloxacillin, methicillin
Cephalosporins	Cefoperazone, cephalexin, cephalonium, cephaloridine, cephalothin
Aminoglycosides	Amikacin, framycetin, gentamicin, kanamycin, neomycin, paramomycin
Macrolides	Erythromycin, oleandomycin, spiramycin, tylosin
Nitrofurans	Furazolidone, nitrofurantoin, nitrofurazone
Fluoroquinolones	Danofloxacin, enrofloxacin, marbofloxacin
Others	Bacitracin, chloramphenicol, florfenicol, lincomycin, novobiocin, sulphonamide and trimethoprim, vancomycin

levels that are effective against most susceptible organisms, with minimal side-effects. In most cases the recommended dose is the minimal dose. This is particularly so for farm animals where both the interval between therapy and the suggested dose level tend to be lower than for man or small animals due to cost.

Less susceptible organisms require higher levels to ensure success. Increasing the dose needs to be considered carefully, but it is of little danger if the drug has a low toxicity. However, when the antimicrobial agent is of high toxicity any increase in dosage should be undertaken with caution. Different dosages may also influence the drug withdrawal time. It should be remembered that when different companies produce the same antibiotic it may well contain different amounts of the drug and the vehicle in which it is presented may vary.

Route of administration

The choice of administration route depends on the speed with which infection has to be counteracted as well as the volume to be given, ease of administration, etc. The principal routes used are given in Table 61.6.

Duration of therapy

In general terms, most injections are used for three to five days and for at least one day after normality is reached. However, there is a tendency not to treat for long enough in chronic conditions such as some cases of chronic joint or thoracic infections when therapy should be continued for at least 10–14 days. If it was a

Table 61.6 Routes of administration of antimicrobial drugs.

Intravenous (iv): always give slowly

Advantages

  Rapid high blood and tissue levels, therefore useful for
    septicaemias

  Always higher circulating levels than im or oral

  Increased levels at areas where levels usually low, e.g.
  necrotic areas, chronic abscesses

  Useful for large volumes

  Useful for painful injections

  Useful for irritant injections

  Only method of obtaining accurate blood and tissue
  levels

Disadvantages

  Acute toxic reactions more common

  Specific formulations necessary

  Requires good technique

  Perivascular and intravascular thrombosis can occur

Intramuscular (im)

Advantages

  Most common route

  Only 20 ml per injection site

  Peak blood and tissue levels within 2 hours

  Slightly less irritant injections than those given iv can be
    given by deep im injection

  Allows a reasonable level to be maintained over a period
    of time

Disadvantages

  Muscle damage

  Try not to do within 3 weeks of slaughter

  Severe reactions to some drugs

  Some injections painful

  Accurate blood and tissue levels not obtained

Intraperitoneal (ip)

Advantages

  Speed of absorption similar to im injection

  Usually well absorbed

  Useful for peritonitis

  Useful if very toxic

  Useful for irritant drugs

  Useful in severe respiratory distress (especially
    tetracyclines)

  Large volumes can be given

Disadvantages

  Possible sepsis

  Accurate blood and tissue levels not obtained

Subcutaneous (sc)

Advantages

  Little used for antimicrobials except sulphonamides

  Large volumes can be given

  Less irritant than im

Disadvantages

  May provoke marked fluid reaction

  Only slowly absorbed

  Speed of absorption less than im

Intra-articular

  Increased level in joint

  Must be sterile technique

Intrapleural

  Increased level in thorax

  Must be non-irritant

  Must be a sterile technique

Subconjunctival

  Useful for ocular conditions

  Must be non-irritant

  Must be sterile technique

Oral (water or feed)

Advantages

  Easiest method of administration

  Can be undertaken by owner

Disadvantages

  Blood and tissue levels less than for comparable parenteral dose

  Higher doses usually used

  Absorption is variable (depends on gut motility, type of feed,
    volume of feed, drug binding, e.g. calcium, kaolin impair
    absorption of tetracycline, oxytetracycline, chlortetracycline,
    methacycline, doxycycline, ampicillin, lincomycin)

  Blood levels do not peak for 12–18 hours

  Antibiotics may influence normal ruminal flora

  Some antibiotics not absorbed, e.g. streptomycin,
    dihydrostreptomycin, neomycin, framycetin,
    phthalylsulphathiazole

  Some antibiotics destroyed, e.g. benzylpenicillin

Topical

  Ointments, powders, aerosol sprays

Ophthalmic preparations

  Ointments and drops. Limited retention at site except some
    special preparations

Aural preparations

  Drops and ointments

Intramammary (use aseptic technique)

Advantages

  Convenient

  Good efficacy

Disadvantages

  Often diffusion reduced by blocked lactiferous ducts, etc.

  Used for clinical treatment

  Dry-cow therapy used for subclinical mastitis and prophylaxis

  If intramammary tube used in one quarter all milk should be
    withheld

human or small animal there would often be no dispute about such a length of therapy. Many antibacterial preparations are now available that can be injected at extended intervals to provide adequate drug concentrations for several days. However, in some cases the duration of effective therapy can be overestimated.

Spectrum of drug activity

Antibacterial drugs vary in their degree of activity against various classes of organism. They are usually considered narrow spectrum if they are only active against bacteria, but broad spectrum if they also have activity against *Mycoplasma*, *Rickettsia* and *Chlamydia*. The antibacterial activity of drugs can also vary (see Table 61.7): some have a narrow spectrum, only inhibiting either Gram-negative or Gram-positive organisms; others have most activity against Gram-positive organisms but will inhibit some Gram-negative agents. However, some have a broad spectrum inhibiting both Gram-positive and Gram-negative bacteria.

Bacteriostatic or bactericidal activity

At times it is important to know the activity of a drug. Some drugs are bactericidal, e.g. penicillin,

Table 61.7 Antibacterial activity other than for anaerobic bacteria.

Gram-positive bacteria	Gram-negative bacteria	Broad spectrum: Gram-positive and Gram-negative bacteria
Penicillins	*Penicillins*	*Penicillins*
Cloxacillin	Carbenicillin	Amoxycillin
Methicillin		Ampicillin
Penicillin G	*Polymyxins*	Clavulanic acid and amoxycillin
Penicillin V	Colistin	
	Polymyxin B	*Sulphonamides*
Macrolides		Many forms
Erythromycin	*Aminoglycosides*	
Oleandomycin	Amikacin	*Tetracyclines*
Spiramycin	Dihydrostreptomycin	Chlortetracycline
Tylosin	Framycetin	Doxycycline
	Gentamicin	Methacycline
Others	Kanamycin	Oxytetracycline
Bacitracin	Neomycin	Tetracycline
Lincomycin	Paromomycin	
Novobiocin	Streptomycin	*Cephalosporins*
Tiamulin		Cefquinone
Vancomycin	*Others*	Ceftiofur
	Apramycin	Cephalexin
	Spectinomycin	Cephaloridine
		Cephalothin
		Nitrofurans
		Furazolidone
		Nitrofurantoin
		Nitrofurazone
		Fluoroquinolones
		Danofloxacin
		Enrofloxacin
		Marbofloxacin
		Others
		Chloramphenicol
		Florfenicol
		Halquinol
		Sulphonamide and trimethoprim

Table 61.8 Bactericidal and bacteriostatic drugs.

Bactericidal	Bacteriostatic
Penicillins	Halquinol
Amoxycillin	Novobiocin (high concentration)
Ampicillin	Spectinomycin (occasionally)
Carbenicillin	Sulphonamide and trimethoprim
Cloxacillin	Vancomycin
Methicillin	
Penicillin G (benzylpenicillin)	*Macrolides*
Penicillin V (phenoxypenicillin)	Carbomycin
	Erythromycin (low concentration)
Macrolides	Oleandomycin
Erythromycin (high concentration)	Spiramycin
	Tilmicosin
Nitrofurans	Tylosin
Furazolidone (high concentration)	
Nitrofurantoin (high concentration)	*Sulphonamides*
Nitrofurazone (high concentration)	All types
Cephalosporins	*Nitrofurans*
Ceftiofur	Furazolidone (low concentration)
Cephalexin	Nitrofurantoin (low concentration)
Cephaloridine	Nitrofurazone (low concentration)
Cephalothin	
	Tetracyclines
Polymyxins	Chlortetracycline
Colistin	Doxycycline
Polymyxin B	Methacycline
	Oxytetracycline
Aminoglycosides	Tetracycline, etc.
Amikacin	
Dihydrostreptomycin	*Others*
Framycetin	Apramycin
Gentamicin	Chloramphenicol
Kanamycin	Clindamycin
Neomycin	Florfenicol
Paromomycin	Lincomycin
Streptomycin, etc.	Novobiocin (low concentration)
Fluoroquindones	Spectinomycin (usually)
Danofloxacin	Tiamulin
Enrofloxacin	Trimethoprim
Marbofloxacin	
Others	
Bacitracin	
Panfloxacin	

Whether a drug is bactericidal or bacteriostatic needs to be known as problems can occur with combinations.

aminoglycosides, while others are bacteriostatic and require the animal's own defence mechanism to help in the organisms' removal (Table 61.8). These definitions are only relative and some agents are bactericidal in high concentrations but only bacteriostatic at low levels.

Drug combinations

These are frequently used in veterinary practice but are often best avoided. They are of used where infection is due to mixed organisms. They can be helpful where synergism has been shown with the combination, e.g. penicillin and aminoglycosides, or trimethoprim and sulphonamides. Although the bacteriostatic or bactericidal nature of many drugs is dependent on the concentration used, it is still a good ploy to combine antibiotics with a similar activity. This is of particular importance when treating immunocompromised animals. Besides the broader spectrum of activity attained with some combinations, cost may be less and in some cases there may be a reduction in toxicity.

When using combinations it is best to give each drug individually at the correct dose with an interval between administrations. When two drugs are combined in commercial preparations then the dosage of each is fixed regardless of the needs of the particular situation or the interval between doses. Care should be taken in the choice of antimicrobial agent when used in combination with corticosteroids.

Cost

This is a major drawback in that often the best therapy cannot be instituted because of the expense. Repeat doses also cause problems, especially as oral therapy is not often advisable in ruminants. The problem can be overcome by long-acting preparations or providing combination injections for the farmer or stockworker to administer. It must be remembered there is an indirect cost, particularly to the dairy farmer, in the length of time the milk has to be withheld after the end of treatment. The beef farmer encounters a similar problem regarding meat withdrawal time but to a lesser extent.

Toxicity

Except where there is routine usage of antimicrobial drugs in adult animals, few problems of toxicity arise. Some of the more common are give in Table 61.9.

Drug withdrawal times

Following use of an antimicrobial agent there is now usually a period between finishing therapy and the use of the milk or the slaughter of the animal for meat. Milk or meat containing antibiotics can present a public health risk. There is the possibility of allergy to penicillins or other antibacterials following medical prescription. Documented cases are rare and are now almost non-existent in countries with adequate anti-biotic testing. Where they have occurred they involved usage of milk. Another possible hazard is drug resistance in humans but adequate documented evidence for the occurrence of this following consumption of milk or meat is still required. The main effect of antibiotics in milk is a commercial one in that it can affect the starter cultures for cheese or yoghurt.

Various factors influence the withdrawal time and these include the drug dose rate, age, disease, duration and role of therapy. The injection site will obviously contain higher levels than other sites. Depending on how the drug is metabolized, the kidney and liver may have higher levels than other tissues. In all cases it is the duty of the veterinary surgeon to ensure that any withdrawal time is observed and that the owner of the animal is made aware of this. It is always best to write the time down either on the drug vial if doses are to be provided for administration by the farmer, or on an invoice or note to the farmer. Where a withdrawal time is not known then the manufacturer or distributor of the drug should be contacted. However, in general, when no withholding time is stated then milk must be discarded for seven days and cattle may not be slaughtered for human consumption for 28 days. In the USA veterinarians can obtain information on withdrawal times and residues by contacting the Food Animal Residue Avoidance Data book (FARAD).

Legal considerations

The availability of antimicrobial agents in most countries is first dependent on their being licensed for use by a regulatory authority. This can be the Veterinary Medicines Directorate, Food and Drug Administration or another similar body. Some antibiotics are available in certain countries but are banned in others, e.g. chloramphenicol, which is prohibited from use in North America and most of Europe.

Frequency of dosing

The frequency of administering therapeutic preparations varies. Some compounds are placed in slow-release boluses to facilitate this. The rate of absorption also varies between different preparations, dependent on the particle size; thus those with micronized particles are rapidly absorbed. The form of the antibiotic will also influence the level of activity. Thus with penicillin, benzylpenicillin is rapidly absorbed (in minutes) to reach peak levels but only persists for about 6 hours. However, procaine benzylpenicillin

Table 61.9 Toxicity of antimicrobial drugs.

Penicillins	Very low toxicity, hypersensitivity. Occasional severe adverse reactions
Sulphonamides	Toxicity rare, rapid intravenous injection causes collapse and respiratory distress, crystalluria
Macrolides	Pain and reaction following sc or im injections. Crystalluria not a problem in large animals. Erythromycin and tylosin irritant following injection
Lincomycin	Diarrhoea, reduced milk production (oral)
Aminoglycosides	Ototoxicity (unlikely), cardiovascular damage, hypotension (for toxic and shocked animals), renal toxicity
Tetracyclines	Acute collapse syndrome (iv). Alimentary tract dysfunction (if oral). Deposition in bone and teeth
Chloramphenicol	Little toxicity. Superinfection (oral). Anaemia in humans
Polymyxyn B Colistin	Usually only used topically as toxic shock and death can occur following parenteral use
Nitrofurans	Acute – nervous signs
	Chronic – haemorrhagic syndrome

Table 61.10 Some possible antibacterial therapy for infections in cattle.

Calves	
Diarrhoea (acute) bacterial	Amoxycillin, ampicillin, (chloramphenicol), chlortetracycline, clavulanic acid and amoxycillin, danofloxacin, enrofloxacin, framycetin, marbofloxacin, neomycin, oxytetracycline, trimethoprim and sulphonamide
Diarrhoea (subacute) bacterial	Neomycin, nitrofurazone, oxytetracycline, sulphonamides
Joint ill	Lincomycin, oxytetracycline
Meningitis	(Chloramphenicol), danofloxacin, enrofloxacin, marbofloxacin, trimethoprim and sulphonamide
Navel ill	Amoxycillin, ampicillin, clavulanic acid and amoxycillin, oxytetracycline, trimethoprim and sulphonamide
Pneumonia	Amoxycillin, ampicillin, cefquinone, ceftiofur, cephalexin, clavulanic acid and amoxycillin, danofloxacin, enrofloxacin, florfenicol, marbofloxacin, oxytetracycline, penicillin and streptomycin, tilmicosin, tylosin
Ringworm	Griseofulvin, natamycin
Salmonella spp.	Amoxycillin, ampicillin, apramycin, (chloramphenicol), clavulanic acid and amoxycillin, danofloxacin, enrofloxacin, marbofloxacin, neomycin, nitrofurazone, trimethoprim and sulphonamide
Septicaemia	Amoxycillin, ampicillin, (chloramphenicol), clavulanic acid and amoxycillin, danofloxacin, enrofloxacin, marbofloxacin, trimethoprim and sulphonamide
Older cattle – injections	
Actinomycosis	Amoxycillin, cephalexin, oxytetracycline, penicillin, sulphonamides
Anthrax	Amoxycillin, oxytetracycline, penicillin and streptomycin
Blackleg	Benzylpenicillin
Clostridial infections	Oxytetracycline, pencillin
Diarrhoea (acute)	Sulphonamide
Infectious bovine keratoconjunctivitis	(Chloramphenicol), oxytetracycline
Leptospirosis	Amoxycillin, oxytetracycline, streptomycin
Mastitis (peracute) (parenteral)	Amoxycillin, ampicillin, cefquinone, cephalexin, oxytetracycline, trimethoprim and sulphonamide
Metritis	Amoxycillin, ceftiofur, cephalexin, clavulanic acid and amoxycillin, oxytetracycline
Peritonitis	Sulphonamides, trimethoprim and sulphonamides
Pneumonia (acute)	Amoxycillin, ceftiofur, danofloxacin, enrofloxacin, marbofloxacin, oxytetracycline, trimethoprim and sulphonamide
Pneumonia (subacute)	Amoxycillin, ampicillin, ceftiofur, oxytetracycline, penicillin and streptomycin, trimethoprim and sulphonamide
Pyelonephritis	Procaine penicillin
Salmonella spp.	Amoxycillin, ampicillin, (chloramphenicol), danofloxacin, enrofloxacin, marbofloxacin, neomycin, trimethoprim and sulphonamide
Tetanus	Benzyl and procaine penicillin
Wooden tongue	Amoxycillin, oxytetracycline, penicillin and streptomycin, sulphonamide

Note: Not all these drugs are registered for the species or for the use suggested.

Box 61.1 Advantages and disadvantages of slow-release antibiotic preparations.

Advantages
Often used in prophylaxis
Post-operatively
Post calving where there has been intervention
Dry cow therapy: most remain about 3–4 weeks in udder but some persist six weeks or longer
Less stress to animal
Reduced handling
Less pain to animal
Convenience

Disadvantages
Animals may not be examined as regularly as when injected often
Thus animal less monitored
Usually tissue and blood levels lower than routine injections
Increased withholding time for milk or injection-to-slaughter time

reaches a maximum level in 2–4 hours and persists for 24 hours, benethamine benzylpenicillin has a slow absorption (6–24 hours) and may be effective for three to four days, and benzathine benzylpenicillin is slowly absorbed over 6–24 hours and is often effective for four to seven days.

The advantages and disadvantages of slow-release antibiotic preparations are given in Box 61.1.

Possible antibacterial therapy for cattle

A survey of some of the drugs used in the treatment of cattle is given in Table 61.10. It is emphasized that this list is not complete and some preparations are not permitted in all countries.

Chapter 62
Inflammation and Pain

J.L. Fitzpatrick, A.M. Nolan, P. Lees and S.A. May

The nature of inflammation	1045
Mediators and modulators of inflammation	1046
Classification of anti-inflammatory drugs	1048
Non-steroidal anti-inflammatory drugs (NSAIDs)	1050
Classification and mechanism of action	1050
Actions and interactions of NSAIDs and general uses	1051
Pharmacokinetics of NSAIDs	1052
Side-effects and toxicity of NSAIDs	1055
Residues	1056
Steroids	1056
Classification and general properties	1056
Mechanism of action	1057
Administration and pharmacokinetics of steroids	1058
Side-effects of steroids	1059
General uses of steroids	1059
Therapy with anti-inflammatory drugs	1060
Respiratory diseases	1060
Mastitis and endotoxaemia	1061
Metritis	1063
Calf scours	1063
Hypersensitivity reactions	1063
Arthritis and joint diseases	1063
Foot-and-mouth disease	1063
Pain	1063
Conclusions	1064

The nature of inflammation

Inflammation (from the Latin *inflammare*, to burn) is common to many diseases involving injury to living tissues. Inflammation is, in fact, the basis of most pathology. Acute or chronic inflammation occurs as a consequence of chemical, physical or microbiological damage to tissues. Acute inflammation has been described as the response of the living microcirculation and its contents to injury. A range of defence mechanisms including the immune system may be utilized. If the inflammation is caused by micro-organisms, tissue damage may proceed as far as host cell death. An avascular tissue like cartilage, as with dead tissue, cannot respond to injury by mounting an acute inflammatory response, although in some circumstances it may degrade.

The microcirculation therefore plays a crucial role in tissue response to injury. Blood vessels dilate and, ini-

tially, local blood flow increases. Vascular endothelial cells change their shape, with the formation of inter-endothelial cell gaps through which plasma leaks. This leads to the formation of protein-containing exudate (oedema fluid) in the interstitial compartment. At this stage blood flow slows and eventually becomes static.

The contents of the microcirculation include plasma and the cellular elements of blood. The phagocytic leucocytes (neutrophils and monocytes) emigrate from the circulation during the inflammatory process and engulf the tissue irritant, including micro-organisms, in the inflammatory exudate. The initial step is margination and adherence of leucocytes to the vascular endothelial wall, followed by pavementing, the process whereby the cells roll along the wall to the inter-endothelial cell gaps. Passage through the wall and directional movement to the site of injury occurs by the process of diapedesis. Neutrophils are the first cell type to enter the lesion, followed after several hours by mononuclear phagocytes. Other circulating cells (platelets, eosinophils and basophils) may also migrate to the extravascular space.

Inflammation, if associated with infection, may be accompanied by fever, as the result of resetting of the 'thermostat' in the hypothalamus. These changes at the level of the tissue or organ comprise Celsius' four classical signs of inflammation, *rubor et calore cum tumor et dolor* (redness and heat with swelling and pain). To these Virchow added a fifth sign, *functio laesa* (loss of function), many centuries later. The essential features of the acute inflammatory process are outlined in Fig. 62.1.

The suffix '-itis' is appended to the name of the affected tissue to describe organ-based inflammation in the conditions of mastitis, bursitis, colitis, cystitis, metritis, arthritis, tendonitis, laminitis and many others. Severe local inflammation or more widespread inflammation, particularly associated with infection, may be accompanied by fever.

The outcome of acute inflammation may be resolution and hence restoration of normal tissue architecture and function. However, particularly if the stimulus persists, tissue destruction may occur with fibrous tissue formation and repair, potentially compromising normal function. In some cases, there may be delayed healing

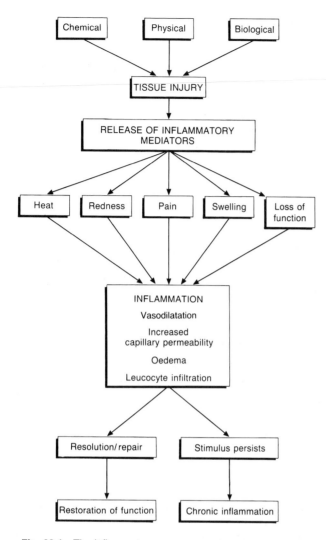

Fig. 62.1 The inflammatory process.

or even persistent chronic inflammation, with local proliferation of connective tissue and mononuclear cell accumulation. The granulation tissue in chronic inflammation comprises highly vascularized connective tissue. In some forms of chronic inflammation lymphocytes are present, suggesting an immune response superimposed on the inflammatory response.

Pain associated with inflammatory disease is probably the major source of pain in ruminant species. The measurement of pain in animals is fraught with difficulties and, to date, pain research in animals has focused primarily on mechanisms of acute pain (e.g. Lascelles *et al.*, 1997; Dolan & Nolan, 2000). Pain is a complex experience, dependent not only on the severity of the insult to pain pathways and the degree of tissue or nerve damage, but also on previous pain experiences and on social position within a herd. The most significant inflammatory diseases likely to be associated with pain in ruminants are mastitis and inflammatory limb

lesions, including sole ulceration, white line disease and acute digital tissue infection, leading to lameness. The pain component of inflammation arises from activation and sensitization of fine unmyelinated and some myelinated sensory fibres to the actions of chemicals released from a variety of sources during inflammation (Ferreira, 1983). Information from the periphery is conducted to the spinal cord and from there to the brain, where pain is perceived. Inflammation induces alterations in nociceptive information processing which may have serious consequences for the animal. Allodynia (perception of innocuous stimuli as noxious) and hyperalgesia (exaggerated responses to noxious stimuli) are common features of inflammatory pain (Coderre & Melzack, 1987; Nolan, 2000).

Mediators and modulators of inflammation

The characteristic pathophysiological changes of acute and chronic inflammation are produced by the action of chemicals, either released from cells such as mast cells, macrophages and fibroblasts or formed by *de novo* synthesis. If there is an immune basis to the inflammatory response, lymphocytes are also involved. Compounds like histamine, that act directly to produce microvascular changes, or like bradykinin, to cause pain are called inflammatory mediators or, if their role has not been firmly established, they are termed putative mediators.

The number of putative mediators identified is considerable. Moreover, there are some species differences in mediators, so that, for example, 5-hydroxytryptamine (5-HT) is probably an acute inflammatory mediator in rodents only. Some mediators, such as complement fragments C5a and C3a, not only act directly on the microcirculation but also cause mast cell degranulation, leading to histamine release and hence reinforcement of the inflammatory response. In addition, there is a sequential release of mediators, such that histamine, 5-HT and bradykinin are involved in the early part of the acute phase, whereas lysosomal and other proteolytic enzymes are involved subsequently. Much is now known about acute inflammatory mediators; information on the mediators responsible for the transition to, and the subsequent persistence of, chronic inflammation is more sparse. Examples of mediators inducing vascular leakage are bradykinin, histamine and platelet activating factor (PAF), which act directly, and leukotriene B_4 (LTB_4) and complement fragment C5a, which exert their effect through neutrophil-dependent mechanisms (Williams, 1983). Mediators of cell migration and accumulation include C5a, PAF, LTB_4, interleukin-1 (IL-1) and many other chemokines and cytokines, whilst mediators responsible for producing tissue damage include the neutral proteases and the highly reactive oxygen (free) radicals, notably the hydroxyl radical.

Mediator interactions are complex, and there are compounds whose principal role is to interact synergistically with inflammatory mediators. For example, the vasodilator prostanoid prostaglandin (PGE_2) enhances markedly both the pain produced by kinins such as bradykinin and the increased vascular permeability produced by simple amines, like histamine (Davies *et al.*, 1984). Those compounds that amplify the actions of others are described as modulators of inflammation. The properties and sources of some important mediators and modulators of inflammation and joint disease are described in Table 62.1. It should be noted that the list is not comprehensive!

Table 62.1 Mediators and modulators of acute and chronic inflammation.

Putative mediator/modulator	Properties and source
Histamine	An amine produced from histidine by decarboxylation. Stored in mast cells, basophils and platelets. Mast cell degranulation leads to release into extracellular environment in immune and non-immune inflammation. Causes vasodilatation and increased permeability of small postcapillary venules. Local administration causes pain and itching
5-Hydroxytryptamine (serotonin)	Another simple amine stored in platelets and mast cells. Increases permeability of small venules in rodents but probably at most a minor mediator in other species
Bradykinin	A peptide containing nine amino acids that act on bradykinin receptors. Synthesized from plasma kinins *de novo*. Produces vasodilatation, increased vascular permeability and pain
Neuropeptides	Main peptides involved are substance P, serokinin A (both tachykinins) and calcitonin gene related peptide. Induce mediator release, contract smooth muscle and induce vasodilation
Complement system	Several complement components including C3a, C5a, C8, C9 exert proinflammatory actions, e.g. vasodilatation, increased vascular permeability, mast cell degranulation, leucocyte chemotaxis and cytolysis
Eicosanoids	
PGE_2	Derived from cell membrane phospholipid, following release of the precursor arachidonic acid. Produces prolonged dilatation of small arterioles and potentiates the increased vascular permeability and pain produced by other mediators like histamine and bradykinin
PGI_2	A potent dilator of small arterioles. Possesses similar properties to PGE_2 but with shorter duration of action
PGJ_2	A derivative of PGD_2. Believed to play a role as anti-inflammatory prostanoid in the resolution of acute inflammation
LTB_4	Potent chemoattractant for polymorphonuclear leucocytes and mononuclear cells. Enhances vascular permeability produced by other mediators such as PGE_2, PGI_2 and bradykinin
Lipoxin A	Produced from cell membrane phospholipid by polymorphonuclear leucoctyes. Stimulates leucocytes to generate superoxide radical and causes release of lysosomal enzymes. Lipoxins also possess anti-inflammatory properties and are probably involved in resolution of acute inflammation
Platelet activating factor (PAF)	An ether-linked analogue of phosphatidylcholine. Derived from cell membrane phospholipid. Produces platelet and neutrophil aggregation, bronchoconstriction, vasodilatation, increased capillary permeability and chemotaxis
Interleukins and other cytokines, e.g. IL-1, TNF-α	Produced by macrophages, chondrocytes and synovial cells. Chemotactic for leucocytes and possess mitogenic and pyretic properties. Stimulate release of PGE_2 and collagenase by chondrocytes, synovial cells and dermal fibroblasts. Possibly involved in cartilage breakdown. Other cytokines possess anti-inflammatory properties
Enzymes	Lysosomal enzymes such as lysozyme and acid phosphatase concerned with lysis of foreign and host cells in acute and chronic inflammation. Non-lysosomal metalloproteinases such as stromelysin, concerned with proteoglycan breakdown in arthritis

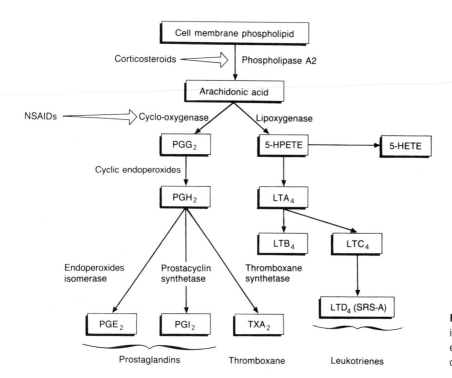

Fig. 62.2 The arachidonic acid cascade illustrating pathways of generation of eicosanoids and proposed sites of action of steroids and NSAIDs.

The eicosanoid group of mediators and modulators is particularly important to a consideration of the two most important anti-inflammatory drug groups in cattle medicine, steroids and non-steroidal anti-inflammatory drugs (NSAIDs). Eicosanoids are formed from the 20-carbon unsaturated fatty acid substrate arachidonic acid (Willoughby, 1968). Arachidonic acid is released from an esterified form in which it is bound as a natural component of the phospholipid of cell membranes. The release is catalysed by phospholipase A_2, an acylhydro-lase enzyme that is activated by tissue injury. Arachidonic acid may act as a substrate for two enzyme groups, the cyclo-oxygenases (COX) and lipoxygenases (LO). Cyclo-oxygenases catalyse the production of prostanoids such as prostaglandin (PG)E_2 and PGI_2 and thromboxane A_2 (TXA_2) from the cyclic endoperoxides PGG_2 and PGH_2 (Fig. 62.2). Lipoxygenases, of which there are three groups, 5-LO, 12-LO and 15-LO, on the other hand, are responsible for the synthesis of hydrox-yeicosatetraenoic acids (HETEs), leukotrienes and lipoxins (Fig. 62.2). The importance of the arachidonic acid pathway in inflammation in general, and in veterinary therapeutics in particular, lies in the fact that the steroids and NSAIDs act, at least partially, by inhibiting enzymes in the arachidonic acid pathway (Fig. 62.2) (Higgs *et al.*, 1981). The NSAIDs act by inhibiting COX and thus they decrease the release of PGE_2 and TXA_2, since COX catalyses the conversion of arachidonic acid released from cell membranes when they are damaged (Vane, 1971).

Classification of anti-inflammatory drugs

In view of the complexity of the inflammatory process and the involvement of many mediators and modulators in determining the time course of inflammatory reactions, it is inevitable that those anti-inflammatory drugs with activity against a single mediator have only limited clinical effectiveness. With currently available drugs, it is easier to inhibit the pain, increased blood flow and oedema associated with acute inflammation than it is to suppress chronic inflammation or the cartilage breakdown that characterizes degenerative joint disease. However, there have been some interesting recent advances in the latter field.

Table 62.2 gives a general classification of drugs that either possess anti-inflammatory properties or that have been used to treat various joint diseases. Drugs that inhibit COX are the classical aspirin-like drugs collectively known as NSAIDs (Higgs *et al.*, 1980, 1981). The first compound of this class in clinical use was salicylate, derived initially from the bark of willow and poplar trees. Aspirin was the first synthetic NSAID; it is the acetyl derivative of salicylate and was introduced into clinical medicine by Hoffman in 1898.

More recently introduced are the drugs that inhibit both 5-LO and COX enzymes, so-called dual inhibitors. By inhibiting the synthesis of leukotrienes such as LTB_4 as well as prostanoids like PGE_2, these novel com-

Table 62.2 Classification of anti-inflammatory drugs and drugs used in the treatment of joint disease.

Drug class	Examples	General properties
Antihistamines	Tripelenamine, mepyramine, diphenhydramine	Classical histamine $(H)_1$-receptor antagonists. Produce some suppression of acute inflammation but limited to early phase of acute inflammation
COX inhibitors	Aspirin, phenylbutazone, flunixin, carprofen, meloxicam, tolfenamic acid, vedaprofen, ketoprofen	Provide analgesia in inflammatory pain and some suppression of vascular changes in inflammation. Little or no effect on leucocyte migration. Gastrointestinal ulceration may occur and blood dyscrasias; hepatotoxicity and renotoxicity may arise occasionally
Dual inhibitors of COX/5-LO	Tepoxalin	Inhibit most changes in acute inflammation, possess fewer side-effects than pure COX inhibitors
Corticosteroids	Hydrocortisone, cortisone, dexamethasone, betamethasone, prednisolone, prednisone, triamcinolone	Suppress all components of acute and chronic inflammation but side-effects associated with medium- to long-term use (adrenal atrophy, immune suppression, decreased bone strength, Cushinoid symptoms, delayed wound healing, muscle wastage, etc.)
Disease modifying agents	Penicillamine, gold salts	Retard the degenerative changes in immune-based arthritides. Very slow onset of effects (several weeks). Potentially severe side-effects, little veterinary use
Cytotoxic agents	Cyclophosphamide, chlorambucil	Used in rheumatoid arthritis in the dog. Immune suppression and other toxic effects to rapidly dividing cells limit clinical value
Free radical scavengers	Orgotein, copper-containing compounds, DMSO, some NSAIDs	Possess superoxide dismutase activity. Scavenge toxic free radicals, e.g. superoxide, hydroxyl
Miscellaneous	Hyaluronic acid, polysulphated glycosaminoglycan, pentosan sulphate	Inhibit prostaglandin synthesis and proteolytic enzymes, e.g. stromelysin. Administration by intra-articular injection may be required for some drugs

pounds may provide the basis for the introduction of agents with a broader spectrum of activity than inhibitors of COX enzymes alone. They may be of use in immune-based diseases such as asthma, chronic obstructive pulmonary disease and insect bite allergies. However, only one compound of this class, tepoxalin, is currently in veterinary use in the dog. An interesting feature of dual inhibitors is their excellent gastrointestinal tolerance.

Corticosteroids are the anti-inflammatory agents that provide a greater control of all elements of both acute and chronic inflammation than any other class of drug. They exert membrane-stabilizing properties on lysosomal and cell membranes. Through this and other actions, they suppress the release of inflammatory mediators and act to preserve cell integrity. Their mode of action is multifactorial. It is attributable partly to their action on the cell nucleus to promote, by protein transcription, the synthesis of a group of endogenous polypeptides with antiphospholipase activity, the lipocortins or annexins (Fig. 62.2). However, they also inhibit induction of one isoform of COX, described as COX-2 (see below).

Of other drug classes listed in Table 62.2 several, including immune stimulants, disease modifying agents and cytotoxic agents, have been used extensively to treat rheumatoid arthritis in man. They slow the progressive degenerative changes in cartilage and soft tissue inflammation in this disease. Some have also been used for similar therapy in veterinary medicine, notably in the dog, but their use has been limited by several factors such as slow onset of action and potentially severe side-effects have prevented extensive veterinary use. They are not used in bovine medicine.

Other drugs which have been used in the therapy of joint disease, especially in the horse, are the free radical scavengers orgotein and dimethyl sulphoxide (DMSO) and drugs with uncertain mechanisms of action, hyaluronic acid and chondroprotective agents. Again, the use of these compounds in bovine medicine has been very restricted to date, mostly due to lack of licensed products for use in food producing species.

Non-steroidal anti-inflammatory drugs (NSAIDs)

Classification and mechanism of action

The organic acid drugs in this important group of compounds can be divided into two subclasses, carboxylic acids (R—COOH) and enolic acids (R—COH). Further subdivisions can be made on the basis of chemical structure. For example, the main enolic acid groups are pyrazolone derivatives, such as phenylbutazone and oxicams, like piroxicam; the carboxylic acid groups include the propionic acid drugs such as ketoprofen. Most non-steroidal anti-inflammatory drugs (NSAIDs) possess three principal types of pharmacological activity: peripheral analgesic and anti-inflammatory actions and central antipyretic, anti-inflammatory and analgesic actions (Table 62.3). Some differences between drugs have been reported for the three types of activity. Paracetamol possesses weak peripheral actions and does not produce significant gastrointestinal irritation. However, it is a relatively weak anti-inflammatory drug and is principally a centrally-acting analgesic (Lees *et al.*, 1991; McKellar *et al.*, 1991).

An important action of NSAIDs, underlying their therapeutic uses, is inhibition of COX and consequent inhibition of production of the eicosanoids, which produce hyperalgesia, inflammation, pyrexia and platelet coagulation (Fig. 62.2). Differences in relative potency between drugs for these activities are probably due to tissue differences in enzyme structure, i.e. the existence of isoenzymes. Two forms of COX have been identified, COX-1, a constitutive enzyme, and COX-2, which is expressed constitutively in some tissues, but is also inducible. The existence of COX isoenzymes may also explain species differences in plasma concentrations required for efficacy. Therapeutic concentrations of phenylbutazone in the horse are of the order of 10–$30\,\mu g/ml$ (Gerring *et al.*, 1981), however, in cattle even higher concentrations produce only limited COX inhibition (Arifah & Lees, 2002).

All NSAIDs can have antithrombotic effects by blocking platelet COX-1, and thus inhibiting production of the proaggregatory eicosanoid, TXA_2. However, at therapeutic doses most NSAIDs do not impair clotting mechanisms or prolong bleeding time. Aspirin is unique in this respect since it irreversibly binds to COX so that production of TXA_2 is inhibited for the life-span of the platelet. Consequently, aspirin is a potent anti-thrombotic drug.

COX-1 may also contribute to the inflammatory process and in particular to the pain component and, consequently, COX-2 selective inhibitors may not be as efficacious as mixed inhibitors in their anti-

Table 62.3 Principal therapeutic and toxic effects of NSAIDs.

Site of action	Pharmacological or toxicological action/therapeutic use
Therapeutic effects	
CNS	Antipyretic. Lowering of body temperature in patients with fever but not in normothermic subjects. Action on temperature regulating centre in hypothalamus Analgesic and anti-inflammatory. Mechanisms poorly understood
Peripheral	Anti-inflammatory in acute inflammation and analgesic against inflammatory, but not against non-inflammatory pain Antithrombotic through inhibition of platelet COX. Aspirin, irreversible inhibitor of COX Anti-endotoxic. Some effects on endotoxin due to release of eicosanoid synthesis being inhibited by NSAIDs
Toxic effects	
Gastrointestinal tract	Ulcerogenic following parenteral as well as oral administration. Blood or plasma loss. Melaena. Emesis in simple-stomached animals only
Kidney	Nephropathies such as renal papillary necrosis
Liver	Both cholestatic and parenchymal cell toxicity
Blood cells and cardiovascular system	Various dyscrasias including aplastic and haemolytic anaemias and agranulocytosis described. Methaemoglobinaemia, hypoprothrombinaemia and prolongation of bleeding time. Small vein phlebopathy. Alteration of acid-base and electrolyte balance
Skin	Urticaria, erythema
Fetus	Teratogenic and embryopathic effects with some drugs. Delayed gestation at term

inflammatory actions. COX-2 is constitutively expressed in kidney, and mice which have the COX-2 gene deleted suffer from renal failure and are poorly viable, while displaying inflammatory responses similar to normal mice. Both COX-1 and COX-2 are constitutively expressed in the central nervous system (CNS) and their relative expression varies depending on species. More work is required to elucidate the role of these enzymes in CNS function. COX-2 generated PGs are also involved in ovulation, parturition and may be involved in the resolution phase of acute inflammation and wound repair.

Until recently, it was considered that the PGs that mediate inflammation, fever and pain were produced by COX-2, while the PGs that are important in gastrointestinal and renal function are produced via COX-1. This led to the belief that the NSAIDs exerted their therapeutically beneficial effects primarily by inhibiting COX-2, while inhibition of COX-1 was considered to be responsible for some of the toxic side-effects associated with these drugs, e.g. gastric ulceration and renal papillary necrosis.

Recent work has indicated that the distinction between the two roles of COX-1 and COX-2 is not as clear as was once considered (for review see Wallace, 1999). Most commercially available NSAIDs at present licensed for use in animals inhibit both enzymes. There is much controversy over the selectivity of these compounds, with conflicting data being obtained depending on the test systems used for assessing COX-1 and COX-2 selectivity and whether these assays were carried out *in vitro*, *ex vivo* or *in vivo*. In addition, drugs may appear selective for one enzyme over the other, while not being highly potent. Currently, there are no truly selective/specific COX-2 inhibitor drugs licensed for use in veterinary medicine. The balance of evidence currently available suggests that phenylbutazone, flunixin and ketoprofen are non-selective, whereas carprofen, meloxicam and tolfenamic acid are COX-2 preferring, depending on the test systems used. There is, however, evidence of specific differences on COX1 : COX2 selectivity in ruminant species.

While most NSAIDs inhibit COX very effectively, other actions, both on the arachidonic acid pathway and on other unrelated enzymes, may contribute to their effects. For example, some fenamate derivatives inhibit some (but not all) actions of PGs by blocking activity at PG receptors in addition to blocking their synthesis. High doses of most NSAIDs also block 5-LO, and thus suppress leukotriene synthesis. However, it is doubtful whether this action contributes significantly to the clinical efficacy of most NSAIDs, although tepoxalin is exceptional in this respect. Finally, some NSAIDs (carprofen is one example), although relatively weak COX inhibitors, are nevertheless effective anti-inflammatory agents and this suggests that the principal mechanism of action, of at least some drugs, is due to some other effect. Carprofen, for example, has been shown to inhibit secretion of interleukin 6 (IL-6) (Armstrong & Lees, 2002).

In general, NSAIDs do not, at clinical dose rates, affect all components of the inflammatory response. They do not affect cellular events or minimize tissue damage, although high doses of some drugs do possess free radical scavenging properties, suggesting tissue healing mechanisms may be impaired, but more research in this field is required.

Other actions of NSAIDs have been described. Recent evidence suggests that some NSAIDs can act by mechanisms other than COX inhibition; for example, aspirin inhibits the transcription factor NF-κB pathway (Kopp & Ghosh, 1994), and recently the R(−)- and S(+)-enantiomers of ibuprofen were reported to inhibit activation of NF-κB (Scheuren *et al.*, 1998), an effect independent of specific COX inhibition. By preventing the translocation of NF-κB into the nucleus, NSAIDs modify the expression of genes such as the COX-2 gene, which is involved in the cellular response to acute inflammation. Furthermore, activation of the glutamate receptor, *N*-methyl D-aspartate (NMDA), a key step in both the induction and maintenance of inflammatory hyperalgesia, activates NF-κB (Guerrini *et al.*, 1995). An action on prostanoid receptors has been described for meclofenamic acid (see above), while some drugs inhibit glucuronidase release from neutrophils. Recent work in humans has indicated a role for COX-2 inhibition in the therapy of colonic cancer. This may represent a new role for NSAID use in the future.

Actions and interactions of NSAIDs and general uses

The analgesic action of most NSAIDs on the CNS is weaker than that provided by narcotic analgesic drugs of the morphine type. To what extent the central analgesic effect accounts for the clinical efficacy of NSAIDs is unclear, but there is increasing recognition of its importance for some drugs. The peripheral analgesic effect is thought to be due to blockade of synthesis of PGs, which exert hyperalgesic actions through synergism with pain-inducing mediators like bradykinin (Ferreira, 1983). Suppression of pain produced by tissue damage is a major use of NSAIDs, together with suppression of the acute inflammation associated with tissue trauma. Post surgical use of NSAIDs to provide analgesia and to reduce oedematous swelling that can lead to wound breakdown is now widespread. These drugs are clearly of value in the former circumstance, but the doses required for anti-oedematous actions may be higher and are less well established in veterinary medicine. NSAIDs have been used increasingly alone to treat acute inflammatory conditions caused by microbial diseases but, more usually, they are combined with antibacterial agents. Endotoxic shock may result from a number of disease states when endotoxin derived from Gram-negative bacterial cell walls is released into the circulatory system. This may occur, for example, in cases of equine colic, acute and peracute mastitis, metritis and in septic peritonitis. Some of the ensuing effects on cardiovascular function and the respiratory system, together with metabolic and gastrointestinal changes, are produced by the release of eicosanoids such as PGI_2 and TXA_2. Hence, the pathophysiological changes associated with endotoxaemia are generally suppressed, though rarely abolished, by NSAIDs such as flunixin. This is particularly so when, in experimental circumstances, the drugs are administered prior to the onset of endotoxaemia. However, the effectiveness of these drugs once shock is established is likely to be less than when pre-treatment is possible. The clinical value of NSAIDs therefore remains to be established; however, anti-endotoxaemic effects have been demonstrated for flunixin meglumine at doses considerably less than those required for anti-inflammatory or analgesic activity (approximately ×0.25).

Prostaglandin E_2 is a pyretic agent released as a result of the action of endogenous pyrogens such as IL-1. The local release of PGE_2 in the anterior hypothalamus leads to resetting of the thermoregulatory centre. NSAID inhibition of PGE_2 synthesis accounts for their antipyretic action when infections are accompanied by fever. The reduction in body temperature gives symptomatic relief in such patients. However, NSAIDs may theoretically influence adversely viral diseases, since the production and release of interferons are increased in pyrexia. In spite of this, NSAIDs have been used in the treatment of respiratory disease produced by parainfluenza type 3 (PI3) virus in calves and in the therapy of acute interstitial pneumonia caused by *Ascaris suum* in pigs (Selman *et al.*, 1984; Selman, 1988). Both the anti-inflammatory action in the lungs and the central antipyretic action may underlie the therapeutic response in these diseases.

Aspirin differs from other NSAIDs in that its inhibitory action on COX is irreversible (Lees *et al.*, 1987). It covalently acetylates the enzyme, which is, in consequence, permanently inhibited. In most body cells new COX enzyme can be synthesized in the cell nucleus. As aspirin concentration falls the cell's ability to form the products of COX metabolism is restored. However, the platelet cannot do this. The platelet is anuclear and the enzyme is thus inactivated permanently, i.e. for the lifespan of the platelet. Partial inhibition may persist for several days since platelet numbers are replaced at the rate of approximately 10 per cent per day. Longer inhibition can occur if significant amounts of aspirin penetrate to the developing megakaryocytes in bone marrow.

This action of aspirin explains its use in preventing clot formation in humans who may be prone to thromboembolic diseases. It is of interest that low doses of aspirin are preferred in these subjects, because inhibition of synthesis of PGI_2, an endogenous anti-aggregatory agent released from endothelial cells, by high aspirin doses could offset blockade of synthesis of TXA_2 by platelets. Low aspirin doses, administered once daily or every second day, very effectively inhibit platelet COX, without seriously impairing COX in endothelial cells. The full potential for the antithrombotic action of aspirin in veterinary medicine has not yet been fully explored, although it is recommended for use in prevention of aortic embolism in cats and may be of value in conditions such as laminitis, navicular disease and disseminated intravascular coagulation.

The use of two, or more, NSAIDs in combination generally has no clear advantages over the administration of a single drug at a higher dose rate. Most NSAIDs probably act by the same mechanisms and they are likely to be additive in their toxic as well as their therapeutic effects. Non-steroidal anti-inflammatory drugs have been licensed for the treatment of inflammation in animal species and, more recently, their potent anti-hyperalgesic activity has been recognized (Welsh & Nolan, 1994; Cheng *et al.*, 1998). Although the measurement of pain in ruminants has not been described frequently, workers have described the occurrence of hyperalgesia in animals suffering from lameness (Ley *et al.*, 1995; Whay *et al.*, 1998; Dolan & Nolan, 2000) and mastitis (Fitzpatrick *et al.*, 1998). While the magnitude of hyperalgesia does not appear to be related to the stimulus intensity, the duration of hyperalgesia does appear to be correlated significantly to the intensity of the inflammatory stimulus (Nolan, pers. obs. supported by Fitzpatrick *et al.*, 1998; Dolan & Nolan, 1999; Dolan & Nolan, 2000). Inflammatory conditions that induce hyperalgesia therefore probably induce spontaneous pain in the first instance, and contribute to adverse welfare over a longer duration (Dolan & Nolan, 2000). Thus, measurement of hyperalgesia is potentially a useful tool in validating disease severity and since it is a consequence of altered pain processing, it provides a pathophysiological link between disease and pain.

Pharmacokinetics of NSAIDs

The pH of fluids within the gastrointestinal tract varies but at all sites it is usually more acidic than plasma. In the stomach of monogastric species, fluid pH can be as low as 1.0. This marked difference from plasma increases, by the mechanism of ionic trapping, the rate at which NSAIDs are absorbed. Being weak organic acids they are relatively less ionized in gastrointestinal tract liquor than in plasma and this facilitates absorption. A similar mechanism, enhancing NSAID absorption, will operate in ruminants in the reticulum and rumen, where liquor pH is also acid relative to plasma. However, the normal pH, approximately 4–5, is less acid than the gastric juice of monogastric species. Moreover, other factors are involved in determining rates of absorption. Low drug solubility in acidic conditions for some NSAIDs, such as aspirin, can lead to precipitation in the stomach and this prolongs and slows absorption and may also increase local irritation. Diet can also be an important factor in horses and ruminants, since some NSAIDs may be adsorbed on to hay. Such binding to feed, with subsequent release of the drug by fermentative digestion within the large intestine of the horse, has been suggested as a cause of the ulcerogenic action of phenylbutazone in the distal parts of the gastrointestinal tract (Lees & Higgins, 1985; Maitho *et al.*, 1986). In spite of these factors, absorption of most NSAIDs is generally good after oral dosing in all species and bioavailability generally exceeds 50 per cent.

Another factor that may potentially markedly influence NSAID absorption following oral dosing in ruminants is operation of the oesophageal groove reflex. Closure of the groove can direct orally administered substances directly to the abomasum and this will generally speed absorption into plasma, since dilution within the vast fluid volume in the rumen inevitably extends the time course of absorption. Double peaks in the plasma concentration–time curve of the NSAID meclofenamate after oral dosing in sheep have been attributed to an initial rapid absorption phase from the abomasum and slower subsequent absorption from the rumen-reticulum of that fraction of the administered dose which enters the rumen (Marriner & Bogan, 1979). A similar mechanism of oesophageal closure does not seem to operate for oral phenylbutazone in adult cattle (Lees *et al.*, 1988). Further studies are required to determine to what extent species, drug substance, drug formulation and age determine operation of the oesophageal groove reflex. NSAIDs are usually administered parenterally. Some NSAIDs are irritant to tissues when injected perivascularly but flunixin, meloxicam and carprofen can be given intramuscularly or subcutaneously when absorption is rapid and tissue irritation is minimal. Species differences in pharmacokinetic parameters, particularly clearance and elimination half-life, have been described for many NSAIDs and within the bovine species elimination half-lives vary between drugs and with different studies. However, it should be noted that plasma half-lives of the NSAIDs do not always relate to the tissue half-lives because of the tissue binding properties of the drugs.

Thus many NSAIDs are retained at the site of inflammation for periods long in excess of those predicted by the plasma half-lives. In consequence, there are significant differences in dosing schedules between species. As well as species differences in pharmacokinetics, the possibility of breed differences should be noted, as has been described for naproxen in dogs. Whether similar differences occur for any NSAIDs in other species, including cattle, is not known, but such information is clearly important to the rational setting of efficacious and safe dosage schedules.

A further factor relevant to the activity of some NSAIDs is the formation *in vivo* of active metabolites. The conversion of aspirin to salicylate is one example. Another is the hydroxylation of phenylbutazone in several positions. One such metabolite, oxyphenbutazone, is of similar potency to phenylbutazone and is formed in the liver in quantities that are sufficient to contribute about one-fifth of the overall activity in the horse. Plasma concentrations achieved in the goat may also be significant, but in both young and adult cattle, concentrations are low or undetectable and no contribution of oxyphenbutazone to efficacy can therefore be assumed in cattle.

Age may also affect NSAID pharmacokinetics. In general, both urinary excretion and hepatic biotransformation of drugs are less efficient in very young animals, aged less than two to six weeks depending on species. Aged animals may also metabolize and excrete NSAIDs less readily than young adults. There is some evidence in support of this for phenylbutazone in the horse (Lees *et al.*, 1985). Reduced capacity to metabolize drugs in the liver is likely to be of greater significance than any decreased renal excretory capacity in the case of NSAIDs, since virtually all are highly bound (usually greater than 98 per cent) to plasma protein. Consequently, less than 2 per cent of the drug in plasma is available for excretion in urine by glomerular filtration. This small fraction is readily excreted in the urine of herbivores, since it is 'trapped' in ionized form in the alkaline urine, i.e. tubular reabsorption is limited or absent. Nevertheless, only a very small proportion of the administered dose will be removed from the body by urinary excretion of parent drug. Reduced dosage or longer intervals between doses is probably required in both young and old animals.

Limited and indirect evidence indicates that at least some NSAIDs are excreted by active secretion in bile in cattle, possibly with subsequent reabsorption to create an entero-hepatic shunt. This is suggested, for example, by the 'kink' in the plasma concentration–time curve that occurs consistently following the administration of flunixin intravenously and intramuscularly to calves (Fig. 62.3). Studies of bile:plasma concentration ratio are required to investigate this possibility further.

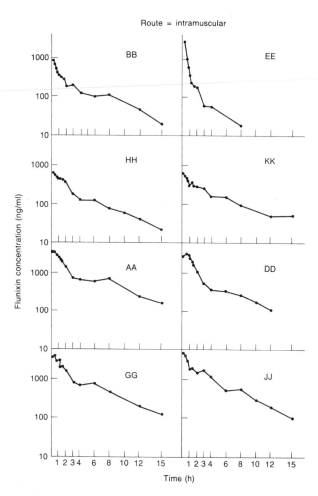

Fig. 62.3 Plasma concentration–time curves for eight calves receiving fluxinin meglumine by intramuscular injection at two dose rates: 2.2 mg/kg body weight (BB, EE, HH, KK) and 8.8 mg/kg body weight (AA, DD, GG, JJ).

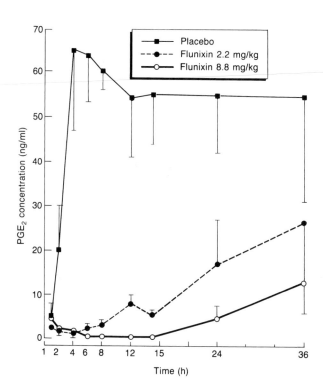

Fig. 62.4 Influence of two dose rates of fluxinin (2.2 and 8.8 mg/kg body weight) administered intramuscularly to calves on the generation of the pro-inflammatory mediator, PGE$_2$, in carageenan-induced inflammatory exudates. Each point is the mean ± SEM for six animals.

Knowledge of the pharmacokinetics of particular NSAIDs cannot be transposed between species since interspecies differences are marked. Pharmacokinetic data in cattle are available for flunixin, tolfenamic acid, ketoprofen, carprofen and meloxicam and these drugs have licensed products in the UK for use in food-producing species (*NOAH Compendium of Data Sheets for Veterinary Products 2000–2001*). Pharmacokinetic data are available for other drugs including aspirin and phenylbutazone, neither of which are licensed currently for use in food producing animals. Phenylbutazone has a long half life (40–60 hours) in both calves and adult cattle (Arifah & Lees, 2002). Even when basic pharmacokinetic data are available, it is not possible to define dosage schedules with such data alone for two reasons. First, different plasma and tissue concentrations of NSAIDs are likely to be required for the various therapeutic effects of analgesic, anti-inflammatory, antipyretic and antithrombotic actions. In calves,

clearance of carprofen was slower in animals aged 8 weeks than in 16 week old animals (Lees *et al.*, 1986; Delatour *et al.*, 1996). Profound differences in ketoprofen pharmacokinetics were demonstrated in young goats compared to adult animals (Eltom *et al.*, 1993). Second, the pharmacological actions may be longer for NSAIDs than might be predicted from plasma clearance data. Studies have shown that relatively prolonged inhibition of production of the inflammatory and hyperalgesic mediator, PGE$_2$, is produced by therapeutic doses of flunixin, tolfenamic acid and ketoprofen, administered to calves (Landoni *et al.*, 1995a, 1996; Lees *et al.*, 1998) (Fig. 62.4) and, moreover, there are likely to be species differences in IC$_{50}$ values for inhibition of COX isoenzymes. This has been shown for example in studies comparing COX isoenzymes from the horse and the dog (Brideau *et al.*, 2001; Armstrong & Lees, 2002). In cattle, tolfenamic acid was shown to significantly inhibit serum TXA$_2$ and inflammatory exudate PGE$_2$, measured as indicators of blockade of the isoforms COX-1 and COX-2, respectively (Lees *et al.*, 1998). Whilst penetration of these drugs into tissue cage fluid was poor, passage into acute inflammatory exudate was good and clearance from the latter fluid was slow, i.e. there was a strong tendency for them to accumulate.

It is likely that three distribution compartments relating to the different sites of action of the NSAIDs exist: a central compartment and shallow and deep peripheral compartments (Landoni *et al.*, 1995b, 1996). The very high degree of binding to plasma protein probably explains both the relatively high concentration in inflammatory exudate, into which plasma protein passes readily, and the low concentration in interstitial fluid into which it does not. Similar considerations apply to most NSAIDs, since almost all are highly bound to plasma protein (Galbraith & McKellar, 1996).

Side-effects and toxicity of NSAIDs

At high dose rates NSAIDs may affect a number of biochemical pathways. However, with clinical doses the toxic effects of most drugs, like the therapeutic effects, are probably caused primarily by inhibition of COX. There are exceptions, however. Carprofen is a relatively weak inhibitor of COX, except in sheep where it produced marked inhibition (Cheng *et al.*, 2002), but it is, nonetheless, an effective anti-inflammatory agent.

The NSAID side-effect reported most commonly is irritation leading potentially to ulceration of the gastrointestinal mucosa. All NSAIDs produce this effect at high dose rates and with most drugs some gastric irritation is associated with oral dosing with therapeutic dose levels. The mechanism of action may involve back-diffusion of acid, although ulceration is not restricted to the stomach; it may occur throughout the gastrointestinal tract and it may accompany intravenous as well as oral dosing. The vasodilator eicosanoid PGI_2, generated in the COX pathway, may be a local hormone controlling blood flow to the gastrointestinal mucosa. By inhibiting the synthesis of PGI_2, NSAIDs may produce ischaemia and hence hypoxia of the mucosal surface. This may be the mechanism that causes erosion and hence ulceration of the gastrointestinal tract mucosa.

The ratio of doses of NSAIDs producing ulcerogenicity relative to anti-inflammatory and analgesic activities seems to be low for some drugs, e.g. aspirin, intermediate for others such as phenylbutazone and high for some selective agents, e.g. COX 2 inhibitors. It is, however, not possible to draw general conclusions concerning particular NSAIDs since many factors have been claimed to influence their ulcerogenicity (Rainsford, 1977); these include species, age, sex and the animal's nutritional status. Moreover, high drug concentrations in bile for some NSAIDs may explain lesions occurring in distal regions of the gut. When severe, the gastrointestinal ulceration induced by NSAIDs can lead to plasma protein-losing enteropathy or to blood losses into the gastrointestinal tract and

melaena. For example, high doses of phenylbutazone administered to the horse can quickly lead to significant plasma loss, haemoconcentration and death from hypovolaemic shock only a few days after the commencement of therapy. The horse may be particularly susceptible to this effect of phenylbutazone (Lees & Higgins, 1985).

Until recently, it was considered that the prostaglandins that mediate inflammation, fever and pain were produced by COX-2, while the prostaglandins that are important in gastrointestinal and renal function are produced via COX-1. This led to the belief that the NSAIDs exerted their therapeutically beneficial effects primarily by inhibiting COX-2, while inhibition of COX-1 was considered to be responsible for most or all of the toxic side-effects associated with these drugs, e.g. gastric ulceration and renal papillary necrosis. Recent work has indicated that the distinction between these two roles is not as clear as was once considered (for review see Wallace, 1999). Thus, highly COX-2 selective drugs (still in development) are gastro-protective and do not induce gastric ulceration. However, COX-2, while expressed in low amounts in a healthy stomach, appears to play an important role in promoting ulcer healing in the stomach. Consequently where gastric ulceration is present, COX-2 inhibitors may delay healing as, indeed, may non-selective COX inhibitors.

Useful data on the ulcerogenic actions of particular NSAIDs in cattle and any relationship to age, dose administered and route of administration are generally lacking. However, there is no reason to suppose that ruminant species are not susceptible to the ulcerogenic action of these drugs. Attempts have been made to reduce the degree of gastrointestinal tract irritation by the use of slow-release formulations, enteric coating and water-soluble salts. The use of such approaches in cattle does not seem to have been described in the literature. In ruminants, in general, NSAIDs are administered parenterally.

Non-steroidal anti-inflammatory drugs may be nephrotoxic. At high dose rates they may produce tubular nephritis. Renal papillary necrosis has also been reported in man. In horses papillary necrosis has been described in animals that received clinical doses of NSAIDs. However, this occurred only when horses on NSAID therapy also had restricted access to water. Retention of fluid leading to oedema is a commonly reported side-effect of NSAIDs in humans. Oedema seems to be uncommon and transient in animals, but has been described in horses receiving phenylbutazone (Lees *et al.*, 1983). Cholestatic and parenchymal hepatotoxicity have also been reported in animals. Since most NSAIDs are metabolized in the liver, any toxicity to parenchymal cells might, potentially, lead to a cycle of drug cumulation and toxicity. Again, evidence for drug-induced hepatotoxicity has been described for horses receiving a high dose rate of phenylbutazone, but whether similar effects occur in cattle has not been reported.

A number of blood dyscrasias have been reported in human subjects treated with NSAIDs, generally over long periods. Similar blood cell effects in dogs, cats and horses have been described. However, the data available are limited and it has not been established whether particular drugs or certain species are especially implicated. With the use of clinical dose rates of NSAIDs, the incidence of blood dyscrasias in animals seems to be low.

At high dose rates some NSAIDs, notably aspirin and particularly when administered for long periods, impair platelet aggregation and thereby affect blood clotting. Potentially, this may lead to internal or external bleeding. Another problem of impaired clotting, through an indirect mechanism, may occur when NSAIDs are used together with anticlotting drugs of the coumarin group. For example, the combination of phenylbutazone and warfarin has been used in the therapy of navicular disease in the horse. Phenylbutazone-induced suppression of warfarin metabolism may lead to warfarin toxicity. Both cardiovascular and respiratory effects result when very high doses of NSAIDs are administered, but acute cardiovascular/respiratory effects do not generally occur with normal dose rates.

Residues

Published data on NSAIDs and their metabolite residues in cattle are sparse. Tissue concentrations of meclofenamate and phenylbutazone are lower than corresponding concentrations in plasma and, for the latter, drug plasma and tissue concentrations decrease in parallel (Toutain *et al.*, 1982). Pharmaceutical manufacturers have submitted residue data to registration authorities to establish meat withholding times for flunixin, carprofen, ketoprofen, tolfenamic acid and meloxicam in cattle. Theoretically, the passage of NSAIDs into milk in healthy cattle will be severely limited by the more acid pH relative to plasma and by the high degree of drug binding to plasma protein. In practice, this has been found to be the case for one drug, phenylbutazone (milk concentration about 1 per cent of plasma concentration), and will almost certainly apply to others. In mastitis, however, the pH of milk is less acid and the 'blood–milk' barrier is much more permeable, so that higher NSAID concentrations in milk may occur and it is necessary therefore that milk withdrawal times following therapy with NSAIDs are adhered to by farmers and veterinary practitioners. Only some of the available NSAIDs are licensed for use in lactating dairy cattle, including flunixin, ketoprofen, tolfenamic acid and meloxicam.

Steroids

Classification and general properties

Three classes of steroid hormone are secreted by the adrenal cortex into the peripheral circulation: sex steroids (generally in small quantities only), mineralocorticoids and glucocorticoids. The latter two groups together comprise the corticosteroid hormones. The mineralocorticoids, secreted by the zona glomerulosa and zona fasciculata, include aldosterone; their principal endocrinological actions are exerted on electrolyte and water balance. They promote sodium and chloride retention and potassium loss by their actions on the renal distal tubule and on parts of the gastrointestinal tract, notably the large intestine. Sodium retention is accompanied by osmotically obliged water. When administered as drugs or secreted in excessive amounts in some disease states, aldosterone and related compounds cause oedema. Glucocorticoids influence lipid, carbohydrate and protein metabolism and some exert weak mineralocorticoid effects also. The principal glucocorticoid hormone secreted by the zona fasciculata and zona reticularis in most species is cortisol (hydrocortisone).

The main veterinary use of glucocorticoids derives from the fact that they are potent anti-inflammatory agents. Cortisol itself is used as an anti-inflammatory agent, being administered systemically or applied locally. In addition, a number of synthetic steroids with much greater glucocorticoid potency than cortisol and with the advantage of reduced mineralocorticoid potency are available for clinical use. For example, prednisone and prednisolone are some four to five times more potent than cortisol as glucocorticoids, but they possess slightly weaker mineralocorticoid activities. Unwanted side-effects on water and electrolyte balance are therefore less likely when prednisone and prednisolone are used at equi-effective dose rates to hydrocortisone. The relative potencies of a number of corticosteroids in producing glucocorticoid and mineralocorticoid effects (in arbitrary units, cortisol = 1) have been reported by Keen (1987) and are presented in Table 62.4. It will be seen that methylprednisolone and triamcinolone are about five times as potent as cortisol as glucocorticoids and both have little or no mineralocorticoid activity. For dexamethasone and betamethasone, effects on electrolyte balance are also slight, but these drugs are 25–30 times as potent as cortisol as glucocorticoids. In contrast, the synthetic corticosteroid deoxycorticosterone acetate (DOCA) is a potent mineralocorticoid with negligible glucocorticoid activity.

Table 62.4 Relative potencies and biological half-lives of some corticosteroids used in veterinary practice (from Keen, 1987).

	Relative potency (hydrocortisone = 1.0)		Biological half-life (h)
	Glucocorticoid[a]	Sodium retaining	
Hydrocortisone (cortisol)	1	1	8–12
Cortisone[b]	0.8	0.8	
Prednisolone	5	0.8	12–36
Prednisone[b]	4	0.8	
Methylprednisolone	5	Minimal	
Triamcinolone	5	None	24–48
Dexamethasone	30	Minimal	36–54
Betamethasone	25	Negligible	
Flumethasone	100	Negligible	

[a] Closely paralleled by anti-inflammatory and HPA-suppressant activity.
[b] Inactive until converted to active drug in the body.

Anti-inflammatory potency of corticosteroids closely parallels glucocorticoid activity. Clinically, this is most important since it means that whilst mineralocorticoid activity has been divorced from anti-inflammatory activity, glucocorticoid effects have not and this dictates the side-effects associated with clinical usage. An appreciation of the general actions of glucocorticoids will therefore assist an understanding of these potential side-effects, which are described in a subsequent section of this chapter. Glucocorticoids are gluconeogenic, promoting the release of amino acids from skin, muscle and connective tissue, and they subsequently increase the conversion of amino acids to glucose. Glucocorticoids produce hyperglycaemia in many species, especially in ruminants, and they promote the storage of glucose as liver glycogen, although both uptake and utilization of glucose by other tissues are reduced. In general, rates of lipolysis are increased, leading to fatty acid and glycerol release from adipose tissue. Subsequently, the glycerol may be converted to glucose. Calcium metabolism is altered by glucocorticoids in several ways. First, calcium absorption from the intestines is decreased and renal excretion is increased. Second, there is increased parathormone secretion and a resulting osteoclast stimulation whilst osteoblast activity is inhibited. These actions together promote calcium mobilization from bone, and bone strength is reduced. Glucocorticoids cause diuresis by dilating glomerular afferent arterioles and thus increasing glomerular filtration rate and also by depressing tubular water reabsorption in the distal nephron.

The main action of glucocorticoids on blood is to promote leucophilia, principally reflecting an increased number of circulating neutrophils. However, circulating lymphocyte and eosinophil numbers are reduced. In addition, glucocorticoids are depressant to lymphoid tissue. For example, in some species (rabbit, mouse) high doses reduce thymus weight and reduction in the size of the spleen and lymph nodes occurs. Immunosuppression by glucocorticoids is reflected in a number of ways, principally by a reduction in cell-mediated immunity and, usually at higher dose rates, by suppression of antibody production. The secretion of mineralocorticoid hormones is regulated in a number of ways, but the principal mechanism involves the renal release of renin from the juxtaglomerular apparatus and subsequent conversion of angiotensin I to angiotensin II, which acts on the adrenal cortex zona glomerulosa cells. Glucocorticoid secretion from the zona fasciculata, on the other hand, is increased in response to stress, but there is also a basal level of secretion that is subject to a diurnal rhythm. In the dog, cortisol secretion peaks during the day, usually late morning, whilst in nocturnal species, like the cat, peak levels occur at night. The regulatory control involves secretion of adrenocorticotrophic hormone (ACTH) from the anterior pituitary, which in turn is regulated by the release of corticotrophin releasing factor from the hypothalamus (Fig. 62.5). There is a negative feedback of cortisol on this system and high levels of glucocorticoid drugs in the circulation similarly suppress ACTH secretion. Long-term suppression induced by steroid drugs leads not only to inhibition of cortisol secretion, but also to reduced cell function to the point of adrenal atrophy.

Mechanism of action

The mode of action of steroids is multifactorial. Unlike NSAIDs, they generally suppress all components of acute and chronic inflammation. Indeed, steroids are the anti-inflammatory drugs 'par excellence'. Steroids inhibit the vascular dilatation in the microcirculation

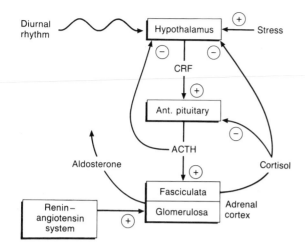

Fig. 62.5 Pathways of mechanisms of control of secretion of adrenal steroids.

and the increased capillary and small vein permeability and they thereby lessen oedema. Steroids also inhibit hyperalgesia and fibrin deposition. The extravascular migration of polymorphonuclear leucocytes initially and subsequent movement of monocytes are reduced. In addition, phagocytic activity of leucocytes is depressed. In the repair stage of the inflammatory response and in chronic inflammation, proliferation and the deposition of collagen are suppressed. In consequence, wound healing and cicatrization are delayed. Glucocorticoids also decrease the production of inflammatory complement components, reduce lymphocyte accumulation and decrease production of interleukin-2 (IL–2) and other lymphokines from lymphocytes.

Glucocorticoids exert a stabilizing action on all biological membranes. Cell, mitochondrial and lysosomal membranes are affected and this suppresses the synthesis or release of acute inflammatory mediators such as PGE_2 and histamine, and subsequently the tissue breakdown arising from the effects of released lysosomal and non-lysosomal enzymes is suppressed. However, these actions, although relevant to the anti-inflammatory effects of steroids, do not explain how they act at the molecular level.

Many studies have shown that one biochemical pathway inhibited by glucocorticoids is the arachidonic acid cascade. Arachidonic acid is released from its esterified form from the phospholipid component of cell membranes by the action of phospholipase A_2 (Fig. 62.2). Anti-inflammatory steroids inhibit this enzyme indirectly by promoting the synthesis of a family of endogenous polypeptides, the lipocortins, which possess antiphospholipase activity. This indirect mechanism of action may account for the lag period of 1–5 hours between steroid administration and the biological

response. Because of this delay, it follows that any relationship between effect achieved and plasma or tissue drug concentration will be complex. Drug effects will generally outlast the period for which they can be detected in biological fluids. This may explain why dexamethasone, which has an elimination half-life of approximately 1 hour in horses and 2.5 hours in cattle (Toutain *et al.*, 1982), possesses a 'biological' half-life of 36–54 hours (Table 62.4).

As discussed earlier, arachidonic acid may act as a substrate for two groups of enzymes, COX and LO. Through the production of lipocortins and consequential blockade of phospholipase A_2 steroids can be expected to block the synthesis of COX-derived inflammatory mediators, including PGE_2 and PGI_2, and LO-derived HETE and leukotriene compounds. One of these, LTB_4, is a potent chemotactic agent for neutrophils and the peptidoleukotrienes LTC_4 and LTD_4 are believed to be important mediators of allergic airway diseases. They may be involved in such conditions as fog fever in cattle and chronic obstructive pulmonary disease in horses. The evidence that anti-inflammatory steroids act through the production of lipocortins and blockade of eicosanoid synthetic pathways is, however, controversial (Lane *et al.*, 1990). High doses certainly do affect eicosanoid synthesis, but whether doses used in veterinary therapy effectively do so is far less certain. Another important action of steroids at the molecular level is inhibition of induction of COX-2 in response to inflammatory stimuli.

Administration and pharmacokinetics of steroids

The application of steroids topically to skin and mucous membranes, e.g. the eye, is commonly used in veterinary practice. It provides high drug concentrations at required sites of action and at the same time minimizes the risks of inducing systemic side-effects, although some systemic absorption is likely. In addition, most steroids are readily absorbed from the gastrointestinal tract, so that licking sites of drug application can lead to significant absorption from the gut. In some topical products local activity is high, but systemic absorption from the site of application is low and systemic side-effects are thus unlikely. Betamethasone-l7-valerate and beclomethasone dipropionate are examples of esters with activity restricted to local sites.

Oral corticosteroid administration is a frequently used route for medium or long-term therapy. There are unavoidable potential risks of significant suppression of the hypothalamic–pituitary–adrenal axis (HPA) (see Chapter 67) when long-term treatment is employed and ways of reducing this to a minimum have been sought.

A short-acting preparation administered at twice the recommended dose rate on alternate days instead of normal dosing once per day has been proposed on the assumption that HPA suppression will decline on the non-treatment days. The therapeutic effects, on the other hand, may persist since steroid biological half-life is generally much longer than the pharmacokinetic half-life (Table 62.4). Another approach has been to recommend drug dosing in the morning in the dog and in the evening in the cat. Then, maximum circulating concentrations of drug can be expected to coincide with peak circulating concentrations of endogenous cortisol. This, in theory, will produce HPA suppression for the minimum time over each period of 24 hours.

Corticosteroids are frequently administered parenterally and generally this will give less variable plasma concentrations than oral dosing for short- or medium-term therapy. Water-soluble formulations include succinates, phosphates and m-sulphobenzoates. They may be administered intravenously or intramuscularly. Pharmacokinetic properties have been reported for commonly used corticosteroids. Thus, with intravenous dosing the half-life of dexamethasone ranges from 290 to 335 minutes in the cow, 53 minutes in the horse to 110 to 130 minutes in the dog (Toutain et al., 1982).

The water-soluble short-acting esters are rapidly absorbed from intramuscular injection sites to give an onset and duration of action almost as quick as and of fairly similar duration to intravenous administration. In addition, water-insoluble esters providing longer duration of action, from 2 to 14 days, are available. These suspensions, providing a depot at the injection site, include acetate, undecanoate, pivalate and phenylpropionate esters. Some very insoluble esters, e.g. acetonide and adamantoate, provide effective concentrations over several weeks, and the use of these esters involves undesirable, but unavoidable, HPA axis suppression.

Intra-articular injection, for the treatment of joint diseases, is another route employed. Intra-articular dosing reduces but does not prevent the risks of systemic side-effects, since some formulations are rapidly absorbed. Long-acting formulations maintaining local concentrations for several days are sometimes used. A careful aseptic technique is required with all intra-articular injections. Steroids are used in this way to suppress soft tissue inflammation, reduce stiffness and pain and allow more joint movement. Disadvantages are that they may suppress natural repair processes and they may induce osteoporosis and osseus metaplasia. Steroids are chondrodepressant and can lead to 'steroid arthropathy'. However, in recent years it has been increasingly recognized that low dose steroids can achieve benefits without the undesirable side-effects of high doses.

Some steroids are prodrugs, requiring metabolic conversion in the body. This is true of cortisone and prednisone which are converted, respectively, to cortisol and prednisolone. Such drugs may be used for systemic therapy, but they are not applied locally.

Side-effects of steroids

The side-effects of those steroids with mineralocorticoid activity, e.g. prednisolone and prednisone, include sodium and water retention and resulting oedema, and hydrogen and potassium loss leading to hypokalaemia and metabolic alkalosis. Effects arising from glucocorticoid action on the kidney include a transient polyuria and a compensatory polydipsia. Hyperglycaemia, possibly leading to glucosuria, also occurs. Protein catabolism with long-term therapy causes muscle wasting and in the short term may delay wound healing. The lipolytic action of glucocorticoids is associated with redistribution of body fat with the characteristic 'moonface' appearance in man and pendulous abdomen in animals. With prolonged treatment, changes in calcium metabolism can lead to osteoporosis and bone fractures. Gastrointestinal side-effects include reduced motility, thinning of the gastric mucosa and reduced mucus production. However, unlike NSAIDs, glucocorticoids are not normally regarded as ulcerogenic. Nevertheless, colonic perforation in corticosteroid treated dogs has been described (Toombs et al., 1986). The immunosuppressant actions involve a reduction in cell-mediated immunity, suppression of lymphoid tissue and lymphocyte movement and activity and, possibly, reduced antibody production.

When long- or medium-term steroid therapy is terminated, the HPA axis suppression present during therapy is restored only over several weeks and animals are susceptible to stress during this period. Stepwise reduction in steroid dose rate and increasing the inter-dose interval may be helpful in assisting restoration of HPA axis function.

General uses of steroids

Anti-inflammatory steroids are widely used for the therapy of immune and non-immune inflammatory conditions. Allergic and non-allergic eczemas respond to steroid therapy and steroids are used in the treatment of inflammatory conditions of the eye and the ear. In dogs and cats, steroids have been used to terminate the itch–scratch cycle in non-specific dermatoses. Steroids have been used extensively in the therapy of anaphylactic, endotoxic and haemorrhagic shock, but there are several disadvantages. The slow onset of action of steroids has been discussed earlier and very large doses are required, making therapy in cattle and other large animal subjects impractical and/or prohibitively expensive. Administration to patients in shock should be by intravenous injection since absorption from intramuscular and subcutaneous sites in shocked patients would be slow.

In inflammatory conditions associated with bacterial infections, steroids are commonly administered with appropriate antibacterial agents. However, the immunosuppressant actions are undesirable and some authorities believe that such combinations are not justified. Where antimicrobial cover cannot be provided, as in some viral infections, corticosteroid therapy is generally totally contraindicated.

Corticosteriods have been used successfully in treatment of bovine iritis, or 'silage eye', a condition that is thought to be associated with infection with *Listeria monocytogenes* (see p. 923) and involves the pathophysiological change iridocyclitis. Corticosteroids are most frequently administered by subconjunctival administration, either alone or in conjunction with antibiotic injections.

There are a number of musculoskeletal conditions for which steroids may be indicated, including traumatic arthritis, osteoarthritis (see p. 453), myositis (see p. 451), eosinophilic myositis, tendonitis (see p. 452) and bursitis (see p. 461). In joint diseases steroids provide relief through their analgesic and anti-inflammatory actions. However, they may suppress natural repair mechanisms and repeated injections or long-acting formulations may produce degenerative changes in cartilage (steroid arthropathy). For this reason, glucocorticoid use in all forms of arthritis is increasingly controversial, and they are definitely contraindicated in septic arthritis. Similarly, in patients with laminitis steroids have fewer and fewer advocates. If they are used, treatment should be limited to the initial 24-hour period after the appearance of signs. Otherwise steroids may exacerbate the condition.

A number of respiratory conditions (see Chapters 17, 20, 49), both allergic and non-allergic, have been treated with systemic steroids. They include acute respiratory distress syndrome in cattle and chronic obstructive pulmonary disease in horses. In these conditions steroids are most useful when disease signs are severe; high doses of water-soluble formulations are administered intravenously. Depot preparations of steroids have been used in severe cases of the equine allergic skin disease 'sweet itch'. Other indications for steroid therapy are ulcerative colitis, cerebral oedema and autoimmune haemolytic anaemia.

In view of the potentially serious side-effects of steroids, guidelines for their use have been recommended and a number of contraindications may be stated.

Guidelines

(1) As animals vary in their response, depending on disease severity, dosing schedules should be established for individual subjects.
(2) Single large doses of steroids or short-term therapy are unlikely to produce serious side-effects.
(3) The incidence and severity of side-effects generally increase with the duration of treatment.
(4) Corticosteroid treatment is usually symptomatic rather than curative.
(5) Cessation of therapy abruptly after a prolonged course of treatment may reveal adrenal insufficiency.

Contraindications

(1) Glucocorticoids are insulin antagonists and may therefore exacerbate or precipitate diabetes mellitus (see p. 930). They should not generally be used in diabetic animals.
(2) Steroids should be used with extreme caution in acute infections because of their immunosuppressant actions and, if used, this should be in combination with bactericidal antibiotics.
(3) Steroids are generally contraindicated in viral infections, in late pregnancy due to the risk that they may induce parturition and in subjects with corneal ulcers.
(4) Administration by intra-articular injection should be avoided when there is sepsis in or close to the joint, in the presence of intra-articular fracture, when the articular cartilage is damaged, when extensive degenerative bony lesions are present, if previous injections were ineffective and when there is any likelihood that the treated joint will be over-exercised.

Therapy with anti-inflammatory drugs

Respiratory diseases (see Chapters 17, 20, 49)

Acute and sometimes overwhelming life-threatening inflammatory conditions occur in cattle and it is possible that the use of anti-inflammatory drugs, especially non-immunosuppressant agents, will reduce morbidity and mortality in such cases. Acute calf pneumonias of viral or bacterial origin and those of mixed aetiology, for example, have been shown to respond to NSAID treatment. Although such treatment is symptomatic it can be effective in life-threatening pneumonias. Selman and coworkers showed that flunixin reduced significantly lung consolidation scores in calves infected experimentally with PI3 virus (Selman *et al.*, 1984). Flunixin also reduced lung lesions, post-mortem lung weights (reflecting an anti-oedematous action) and clinical signs of the disease in an experimental bovine pasteurellosis model based upon challenge with *Mannheimia haemolytica* A1. However, the benefits of flunixin therapy were not apparent when the drug was used alone but when used in combination with oxytetracycline (Selman, 1988). The additional benefits provided by the combination over oxytetracycline by itself comprised a lower body temperature, decreased respiratory rate and improved food intake.

Anderson (1989) confirmed the benefits of a flunixin/oxytetracycline product in comparison with oxytetracycline alone in field cases of pneumonia, with treatment daily for three days. Reduction in coughing, return to normal food intake and weight gain were improved more with the combination product and there were fewer relapses. Since these early studies, other NSAIDs have been used in combination with antibiotics in calf pneumonia; they include ketoprofen, meloxicam, carprofen and tolfenamic acid (Delaforge *et al.*, 1994). The precise way in which NSAIDs act in these subjects is unclear, but it seems likely that the anti-inflammatory action (reduced pulmonary oedema) improves pulmonary function and respiratory gas exchange, while the antipyretic action may improve the clinical status to the point where animals wish to eat and drink. In this way nutritional and fluid requirements will be maintained. Species such as cattle, which rely principally on respiration for temperature regulation, may be under particular stress from infections causing pyrexia, thus the antipyretic actions of NSAIDs may be particularly useful in such species. NSAIDs are also potent analgesics (against inflammatory pain) and when pain is a significant element in cattle pneumonias, this analgesic action of flunixin is likely to contribute to the improved clinical status.

Ingestion of 3-methylindole (3MI) in cattle produces a chemical toxicosis characterized by respiratory signs and pulmonary lesions (congestion, oedema, interstitial emphysema) that are indistinguishable from naturally occurring acute bovine pulmonary emphysema (fog fever). Intoxication with 3MI is accepted as a valid model of the natural disease. Selman and co-workers have shown that parenteral flunixin (2.2 mg/kg) markedly reduces respiratory rate and the extent of lung lesions assessed by lung weights and both pathological and histopathological examinations. Flunixin resulted in a prompt return to normal demeanour and respiratory rate and it reduced the degree and severity of alveolar epithelial hyperplasia.

A study comparing the effectiveness of carprofen to flunixin for respiratory disease showed that a single dose of the former drug had similar beneficial clinical effects to three doses of the latter drug when used as an adjunctive therapy to antimicrobial treatment (Balmer *et al.*, 1997). Meloxicam has been licensed for use in dogs for medium to long term therapy of musculoskeletal pain and inflammation and is available as a suspension and in injectable form. It is available as an anti-inflammatory drug for use in the therapy of calf pneumonia. Further evaluation of NSAIDs in acute life-threatening respiratory infections is needed, since some of the reports have reached conflicting conclusions. Nevertheless, carprofen, flunixin, ketoprofen, tolfenamic acid and meloxicam all possess marketing authorizations for use in pneumonia in calves.

Mastitis and endotoxaemia (see Chapters 22, 23, 24, 30)

Mastitis in cattle also benefits from NSAID treatment. The main indication is in acute and peracute cases in which *Escherichia coli* or other endotoxin-releasing bacteria are involved. Thus, within the udder, the endotoxin-induced increases in PGE_2 and TXA_2 concentrations were significantly reduced by systemic flunixin therapy (1.1 mg/kg at 8-hour intervals for seven doses) (Anderson *et al.*, 1986a) and clinical signs of both udder inflammation and depression as well as pyrexia were suppressed (Anderson *et al.*, 1986b). The enhanced phagocytosis of *Staphylococcus* spp., which occurs in milk neutrophils harvested from endotoxin-inoculated quarters, was not affected by flunixin treatment. However, flunixin did suppress significantly the increased whey IgG_1 and IgM concentrations produced by endotoxin inoculation (Anderson *et al.*, 1986c). The local effects of systemically administered flunixin may seem surprising when the high degree of binding to plasma protein and its acidic nature are considered; these properties should severely limit penetration across the blood–milk barrier. However, in the acutely inflamed udder blood flow is increased and milk pH will be much closer to plasma pH than in non-mastitic milk and the permeability of the blood–milk barrier will be increased. Probably of even greater significance in peracute cases will be antagonism of the acute systemic effects of endotoxin by NSAIDs, since these are mediated in part through activation of the arachidonic acid cascade with release of PGE_2 and TXA_2. Clinically, Anderson *et al.* (1986b) also demonstrated improvement, including reduction in rectal temperature, in mastitic cows with coliform mastitis.

Flunixin in combination with oxytetracycline has also been evaluated in cases of peracute mastitis in comparison with the antibiotic alone and clinical appraisal suggested that the combination product gave better results (Christie, 1988). Similarly, ketoprofen was shown to significantly improve recovery in naturally-occurring clinical mastitis in dairy cows when used in combination with sulphadiazine and trimethoprim (Shpigel *et al.*, 1994). Carprofen has also been evaluated in cows with endotoxin-induced mastitis, at a dose rate of 0.7 mg/kg. Clearance of the drug was slower, elimination half-life longer and penetration into milk greater in endotoxaemic compared with normal cows. In the mastitic animals carprofen reduced heart rate, rectal temperature and quarter swelling significantly (Lohuis *et al.*, 1991), although at the time of writing no licensed product containing carprofen is available for use in lactating cows in the UK. Similarly, flunixin showed antipyretic, anti-inflammatory effects and reduced clinical depression following experimental intramammary infusion with endotoxin.

Mastitis is an inflammatory disease associated with pain (Chapter 23). Indeed bradykinin, a hyperalgesic mediator, has been detected in milk from cases of clinical and subclinical mastitis in cows (Eshraghi *et al.*, 1999). Kinin peptides are released during inflammation and are among the most potent mediators of vasodilation, oedema and pain. Bradykinin was detected in milk from cows with clinical and subclinical disease and the concentrations of bradykinin were shown to correlate with the severity of the disease. Bradykinin concentrations were significantly higher in quarters with high somatic cell counts and from which *Staphylococcus aureus* was isolated compared to high cell count quarters from which no pathogen was isolated. Whether systemically administered NSAIDs are beneficial in clinical cases of mastitis that are not so severe as to be classified as acute or peracute has received little attention to date. However, Pyorala and co-workers (1988) examined the influence of phenylbutazone (10 mg/kg) and flunixin (2.2 mg/kg) administered intravenously in cases of chronic subclinical mastitis. Neither drug influenced bacterial growth, somatic cell count or the levels of inflammatory markers (*N*-acetyl-β-D-glucosaminidase activity and trypsin-inhibitory capacity). Eckersall *et al.* (2001) showed that dairy cows with naturally-occuring clinical mastitis of mild or moderate grades, assessed by farmer observation, had significantly different concentrations of the acute phase proteins serum amyloid A and haptoglobin in serum and in milk compared to normal cows. The cows in this study showed evidence of allodynia for approximately 5 days and 40 days in the case of mild and moderate cases of mastitis, repectively (Fitzpatrick *et al.*, 1998). The allodynia was shown to be abrogated by a single intravenous dose of flunixin (2.2 mg/kg), an effect that lasted for 24 hours, after which the allodynic state resumed. This indicates the potential use of NSAIDs to

provide analgesia in inflammatory conditions in cattle, although further work is required to establish optimal and economical treatment regimens.

There have been few attempts to administer NSAIDs locally by intramammary infusion to establish whether their analgesic and anti-inflammatory effects are of value in providing symptomatic relief in any form of mastitis. No doubt such use has been precluded by the irritant properties of many NSAIDs. One NSAID, ibuprofen, has been administered locally into udders of cows with induced endotoxin mastitis. The drug attenuated reduction in milk yield when compared both with control cows and steroid-treated cows (DeGraves & Anderson 1991), but no licensed product is currently available in the UK. A specially prepared, non-commercial preparation of flunixin was administered via the intramammary route in the study by Fitzpatrick *et al.* (1998), described above. As expected, the somatic cell count increased on infusion of the compound, but there was no evidence of an excessive induced inflammatory response from observation of clinical signs or from milk yield subsequent to the clinical episode. Interestingly, abrogation of the allodynia resulting from the use of intravenous flunixin was not seen when the intramammary route was employed, indicating the possibility that the drug had a central effect on pain processing, probably at the level of the spinal cord.

Steroids with anti-inflammatory actions, such as prednisolone, have been used extensively for the therapy of clinical bovine mastitis. Corticosteroids are incorporated in a number of products containing also one or more antibiotics and used to treat clinical cases during lactation. The popularity of such products is indicated by volume usage; in the UK at the present time the three most widely used lactating-cow intramammary products all contain an anti-inflammatory steroid. The value of steroids in such products is unclear and in view of their potential immunosuppressant actions such usage has been questioned. One suggestion has been that the main value of steroids is not to influence the disease, but merely to suppress the irritancy that inevitably accompanies intramammary infusions and which varies in degree with the product formulation/excipients. However, studies have been undertaken comparing intramammary antibiotic products with and without steroids in bovine models of mastitis induced by *E. coli* endotoxin, *Streptococcus uberis* and *Staphylococcus aureus* (Bywater *et al.*, 1988). Signs of inflammation (swelling, milk consistency) were reduced, but leucocyte infiltration was not impaired. Further studies in this field, for example to establish that the phagocytic capacity of infiltrating neutrophils and immune protective mechanisms are not impaired, would provide confirmation of the value of steroids in some forms of mastitis. In acute and peracute mastitis the slow onset of action of steroids is likely to limit their value, but in the *Streptococcus uberis* model mentioned above, benefit was obtained when treatment was administered 16–18 hours after challenge (Bywater, pers. comm.).

In summary, it seems at least possible that the anti-endotoxaemic effects of systemically administered NSAIDs may be of value (together with other supportive therapy, including fluids and systemic antibiotic administration) in cases of acute and peracute mastitis, whereas reduced swelling and pain provided by intra-mammary infusion of steroid/antibiotic products may assist recovery in less severe clinical mastitis. The latter proposal is compatible with the suggestion of Sandholm and co-workers (1990) that inflammatory changes in the mastitic gland seem to improve bacterial nutrition and growth, with potential adverse effects on the host. However, further studies are needed to examine these proposals concerning both steroids and NSAIDs.

Steroids have also been used, usually systemically, to counteract the life-threatening symptoms of endotoxic shock in cattle, commonly together with large volumes of fluids. In addition to their anti-endotoxaemic effects, steroids promote gluconeogenesis and this may contribute to the therapeutic response. The disadvantages of steroids are the large doses required and consequential high cost of treatment and the latent period prior to onset of action. This can be minimized by the use of water-soluble steroids.

Metritis (pp. 520, 521)

While some studies showed no beneficial effect of NSAIDs in the treatment of reproductive disorders such as retained placenta and post-partal endometritis (Konigsson *et al.*, 2001), flunixin was shown to reduce the incidence of pyrexia in cows with either acute and subacute metritis compared to non-treated controls (Amiridis *et al.*, 2001). Uterine involution and onset of oestrus occurred earlier in cows that received flunixin.

Calf scours (Chapter 14)

Early studies by Jones *et al.* (1977) indicated a possible benefit of flunixin in suppressing inflammation, reducing fluid losses in faeces and suppressing morbidity and mortality in calf scours. Until recently, no drugs were available with licensed indications for such use. However, meloxicam is now licensed for use in calf scours in combination with anti-microbial drugs.

Hypersensitivity reactions (p. 927)

Anaphylaxis can be inhibited both *in vivo* and *in vitro* in cattle by the NSAIDs sodium meclofenamate and aspirin and the actions of these drugs in acute interstitial pneumonia has been described above.

Arthritis and joint diseases (p. 453)

In contrast to the horse and dog, long-term therapy of joint diseases in cattle is not commonly undertaken. This in part relates to economic factors, in part to drug and drug metabolite residue problems in milk and edible tissues and in part to the lack of knowledge of drug pharmacokinetics linked to dosage regimens that are known to be effective and safe. However, some joint diseases of cattle have been treated with phenylbutazone, corticosteroids or NSAIDs but there is, as stated, an urgent need to establish rational dosage schedules. Whether the chondroprotective class of agents, which includes polysulphatedglycosaminoglycans and pentosan sulphate, is likely to be used in the future is not clear. Some increase in therapy in this field can be anticipated, should the economic situation in the farming industry improve, as joint disease is relatively common and can affect individual valuable animals, where treatment may be justified.

Foot-and-mouth disease (Chapter 43(c))

This contagious viral disease is characterized by fever and vesicular eruptions in the mouth and in the interdigital area of the feet. The clinical presentation varies but a proportion of animals suffer severe ulceration with loss of large areas of oral epithelial tissue and under-running of hoof structures. The use of NSAIDs might be of value as adjunctive therapy and one agent, flunixin, has been studied. Artificially infected cattle treated with flunixin showed clinical improvement, indicated by lowered body temperature and increased weight gain, whilst antibody titres were not affected. In light of the recent epidemic of foot-and-mouth disease (FMD) in the UK (2001) and the considerable concerns for the welfare of affected animals prior to slaughter, the role of NSAIDs in palliative therapy could be evaluated and implemented, to allow improved pain management, should future outbreaks of FMD occur.

Pain

Calves that received ketoprofen before and after dehorning following a sedative and a local anaesthetic showed reduced behavioural signs thought to be associated with pain, such as head shaking and ear flicking, compared to untreated controls (Faulkner & Weary, 2000). Different methods of castration such as use of rubber rings, bloodless castrators or surgical methods were shown to result in different levels of pain response, demonstrated by altered behaviour (Robertson *et al.*, 1994). This indicates that there may be the potential to use NSAIDs either pre- or post-procedure to reduce or abrogate pain caused by castration.

Conclusions

It seems likely that both steroids and, in particular, NSAIDs, judiciously used, may be of value in a number of cattle diseases in which inflammation, endotoxaemia and/or pain are major components. Further work is needed if such prospects are to be realized and especially if licensed pharmacological products that will improve animal health and welfare are to result from these studies.

References

Amiridis, G.S., Leontides, L., Tassos, E., Kostoulas, P. & Fthenakis, G.C. (2001) Flunixin meglumine accelerates uterine involution and shortens the calving-to-first-oestrus interval in cows with puerperal metritis. *Journal of Veterinary Pharmacology and Therapeutics*, **24**, 365–7.

Anderson, D.B. (1989) Utilisation de la flunixine dans les maladies respiratoires. *L'Action Veterinaire.* (Suppl.), **1092**, 22–7.

Anderson, K.L., Kindal, H., Smith, A.R., Davis, L.E. & Gustafsson, B.K. (1986a) Endotoxin-induced bovine mastitis: arachidonic acid metabolites in milk and plasma and effect of flunixin meglumine. *American Journal of Veterinary Research*, **47**, 1373–7.

Anderson, K.L., Smith, A.R., Shanks, R.D., Davis, L.E. & Gustafsson, B.K. (1986b) Efficacy of flunixin meglumine for the treatment of endotoxin-induced bovine mastitis. *American Journal of Veterinary Research*, **47**, 1366–72.

Anderson, K.L., Smith, A.R., Shanks, R.D., Whitmore, H.L., Davis, L.E. & Gustafsson, B.K. (1986c) Endotoxin-induced bovine mastitis: immunoglobulins, phagocytosis and effect of flunixin meglumine. *American Journal of Veterinary Research*, **47**, 2405–10.

Arifah, A.K. & Lees, P. (2002) Pharmacodynamics and pharmacokinetics of phenylbutazone in calves. *Journal of Veterinary Pharmacology and Therapeutics*, **25**, 299–309.

Armstrong & Lees (2002) Effects of carprofen (R and S enantiomers and racemate) on the production of IL-1, IL-6 and TNF-alpha by equine chondrocytes and synoviocytes. *Journal of Veterinary Pharmacology and Therapeutics*, **25**, 145–53

Balmer, T.V., Williams, P. & Selman, I.E. (1997) Comparison of carprofen and flunixin meglumine as adjunctive therapy in bovine respiratory disease. *The Veterinary Journal*, **154**, 233–41.

Brideau, C., Van Staden, C. & Chan, C.C. (2001) In vitro effects of cyclooxygenase inhibitors in whole blood of horses, dogs, and cats. *American Journal of Veterinary Research*, **62**, 1755–60.

Bywater, R.J., Godinho, K. & Buswell, J.F. (1988) Effects of prednisolone on experimentally induced mastitis treated with amoxycillin and clavulanic acid. In *Proceedings of the 15th World Buiatric Congress*, Spain (abstract).

Cheng, Z., McKellar, Q.A. & Nolan, A. (1998) Pharmacokinetic studies of flunixin meglumine and phenylbutazone in plasma, exudate and transudate in sheep. *Journal of Veterinary Pharmacology and Therapeutics*, **21**, 315–21.

Cheng, Z., Nolan, A. & McKellar, Q. (2002) Anti-inflammatory effects of carprofen, carprofen enantiomers and Ng-nitro-L-arginine methyl ester in vivo using sheep as a model. *American Journal of Veterinary Research*, **63**, 782–8.

Christie, H. (1988) The veterinary uses of a non-steroidal anti-inflammatory agent: flunixin meglumine. *British Veterinary Journal*, Suppl. No. 1, **8**.

Coderre, T.J. & Melzack, R. (1987). Cutaneous hyperalgesia: contributions of the peripheral and central nervous systems to the increase in pain sensitivity after injury. *Brain Research*, **404**, 95–106.

Davies, P., Bailey, P.J. & Goldenberg, M. (1984) The role of arachidonic acid oxygenation products in pain and inflammation. *Annual Review Immunological*, **2**, 235–57.

DeGraves, F.J. & Anderson, K.L. (1991) Ibuprofen treatment of endotoxin-induced coliform mastitis. In *Proceedings of the International Congress of Mastitis*, Ghent, Belgium.

Delaforge, J., Thomas, E., Davot, J.L. & Boisrame, B. (1994) A field evaluation of the efficacy of tolfenamic acid and oxytetracycline in the treatment of bovine respiratory disease. *Journal of Veterinary Pharmacology and Therapeutics*, **17**, 43–7.

Delatour, P., Foot, R., Foster, A.P., Baggot, D. & Lees, P. (1996) Pharmacodynamics and chiral pharmacokinetics of carprofen in calves. *British Veterinary Journal*, **152**, 183–98.

Dolan, S. & Nolan, A.M. (1999) N-methyl D-aspartate induced mechanical allodynia is blocked by nitric oxide synthase and cyclooxygenase-2 inhibitors. *Neuro Report*, **10**, 449–52.

Dolan, S. & Nolan, A.M. (2000) Behavioural evidence supporting a differential role for group I and II metabotropic glutamate receptors in spinal nociceptive transmission. *Neuropharmacology*, **39**, 1132–8.

Eckersall, P.D., Young, F.J., McComb, C., Hogarth, C., Safi, S., Weber, A., McDonald, T., Nolan, A.M. & Fitzpatrick, J.L. (2001) Acute phase protein in serum and milk from dairy cows with clinical mastitis. *Veterinary Record*, **148**, 35–41.

Eltom, S.E., Guard, C.L. & Schwark, W.S. (1993) The effect of age on phenylbutazone pharmacokinetics, metabolism and plasma protein binding in goats. *Journal of Veterinary Pharmacology and Therapeutics*, **16**, 141–51.

Eshraghi, H.R., Zeitlin, I.J., Fitzpatrick, J.L., Ternent, H. & Logue, D. (1999) The release of bradykinin in bovine mastitis. *Life Science*, **64**, 1675–87.

Faulkner, P.M. & Weary, D.M. (2000) Reducing pain after dehorning in dairy calves. *Journal of Dairy Science*, **83**, 2037–41.

Ferreira, S.H. (1983) Prostaglandins: peripheral and central analgesia. In *Advances in Pain Research and Therapy* (ed. by J.L. Bonica). Raven Press, New York.

Fitzpatrick, J.L., Young, F.J., Eckersall, D., Logue, D.N., Knight, C.J. & Nolan, A.M. (1998) Recognising and controlling pain and inflammation in mastitis. In *Proceedings of the 11th British Mastitis Conference*, pp. 36–44. Stoneleigh.

Galbraith, E.A. & McKellar, Q.A. (1996) Protein binding and

in vitro serum thromboxane B2 inhibition by flunixin meglumine and meclofenamic acid in dog, goat and horse blood. *Research Veterinary Science*, **61**, 78–81.

Gerring, E.L., Lees, P. & Taylor, J.B. (1981) Pharmacokinetics of phenylbutazone and its metabolites in the horse. *Equine Veterinary Journal*, **73**, 152–7.

Guerrini, L., Blasi, F. & Denisdonini, S. (1995) Synaptic activation of NF-kappa B by glutamate in cerebellar granule neurons *in vitro*. *Proceedings of the National Academy of Science USA*, **92**, 9077–81.

Higgs, G.A., Flower, R.J. & Vane, J.R. (1979) A new approach to anti-inflammatory drugs. *Biochemical Pharmacology*, **28**, 1959–61.

Higgs, G.A., Moncada, S. & Vane, J.R. (1980) The mode of action of anti-inflammatory drugs which prevent the peroxidation of arachidonic acid. *Clinics in Rheumatic Diseases*, **6**, 675–93.

Higgs, G.A., Palmer, R.M.J., Eakins, K.E. & Moncada, S. (1981) Arachidonic acid metabolism as a source of inflammatory mediators and its inhibition as a mechanism of action of anti-inflammatory drugs. *Molecular Aspects of Medicine*, **4**, 275–301.

Jones, E.W., Hamm, D., Cooley, L. & Bush, L. (1977) Diarrhoeal diseases of the calf: observations on treatment and prevention. *New Zealand Veterinary Journal*, **25**, 312–16.

Keen, P.M. (1987) Uses and abuses of corticosteroids. In *The Veterinary Annual*, 27th issue (ed. by C.S.G. Grunsell, F.W.G. Hill & M.E. Raw). pp. 45–62. *Scietechnica*, Bristol.

Konigsson, K., Gustafsson, H., Gunnarsson, A. & Kindahl, H. (2001) Clinical and bacteriological aspects on the use of oxytetracycline and flunixin in primiparous cows with induced retained placenta and post-partum endometritis. *Reproduction in Domestic Animals*, **36**, 247–56.

Kopp, E. & Ghosh, S. (1994) Inhibition of NF-kappa B by sodium salicylate and aspirin. *Science*, **265**, 956–59.

Landoni, M.F., Cunningham, F.M. & Lees, P. (1995a) Comparative pharmacodynamics of flunixin, ketoprofen and tolfenamic acid in calves. *Veterinary Record*, **137**, 428–31.

Landoni, M.F., Cunningham, F.M. & Lees, P. (1995b) Determination of pharmacokinetics and pharmacodynamics of flunixin in calves by use of pharmacokinetic/pharmacodynamic modeling. *American Journal of Veterinary Research*, **56**, 786–94.

Landoni, M.F., Cunningham, F.M. & Lees, P. (1996) Pharmacokinetics and pharmacodynamics of tolfenamic acid in calves. *Research in Veterinary Science*, **61**, 26–32.

Lane, P., Lees, P. & Fink, J. (1990) Action of dexamethasone in an equine model of acute non-immune inflammation. *Research in Veterinary Science*, **48**, 87–95.

Lascelles, B.D.X., Cripps, P.J., Jones, A. & Waterman, A.E. (1997) Post-operative central hypersensitivity and pain: the pre-emptive value of pethidine for ovariohysterectomy. *Pain*, **73**, 461–71.

Lees, P. Ayliffe, T., Maitho, T.E. & Taylor J.B.O. (1988) Pharmacokinetics, metabolism and excretion of phenylbutazone in cattle following intravenous, intramuscular and oral administration. *Research in Veterinary Science*, **44**, 57–67.

Lees, P., Creed, R.F.S., Gerring, E.L., Gould, P.W., Humphreys, D.J., Maitho, T.E., Michell, A.R. & Taylor, J.B. (1983)

Biochemical and haematological effects of recommended dosage with phenylbutazone in horses. *Equine Veterinary Journal*, **15**, 158–67.

Lees, P., Delatour, P., Foster, A.P., Foot, R. & Baggot, D. (1986) Evaluation of carprofen in calves using a tissue cage model of inflammation. *British Veterinary Journal*, **152**, 199–211.

Lees, P., Ewins, C.P., Taylor, J.B.O. & Sedgwick, A.D. (1987) Serum thromboxane in the horse and its inhibition by aspirin, phenylbutazone and flunixin. *British Veterinary Journal*, **143**, 462–76.

Lees, P. & Higgins, A.J. (1985) Clinical pharmacology and therapeutic uses of non-steroidal anti-inflammatory drugs in the horse. *Equine Veterinary Journal*, **17**, 83–96.

Lees, P., McKellar, Q.A., Foot, R. & Gettinby, G. (1998) Pharmacodynamics and pharmacokinetics of tolfenamic acid in ruminating calves: evaluation in models of acute inflammation. *The Veterinary Journal*, **155**, 275–88.

Lees, P., Maitho, T.E. & Taylor, J.B. (1985) Pharmacokinetics of phenylbutazone in young and old ponies. *Veterinary Record*, **116**, 229–32.

Lees, P., May, S.A. & McKellar, Q.A. (1991) Pharmacology and therapeutics of non-steroidal anti-inflammatory drugs in the dog and cat: 1 General pharmacology. *Journal of Small Animal Practice*, **32**, 183–93.

Ley, S.J., Livingston, A. & Waterman, A.E. (1995) A field study of the effects of lameness on mechanical nocicepetive thresholds in sheep. *Veterinary Record*, **137**, 85–7.

Lohuis, J.A., van Werven, T., Brand, A., van Miert, A.S., Rohde, E., Ludwig, B., Heizmann, P. & Rehm, W.F. (1991) Pharmacodynamics and pharmacokinetics of carprofen, a non-steroidal anti-inflammatory drug, in healthy cows and cows with *Escherichia coli* endotoxin-induced mastitis. *Journal of Veterinary Pharmacology and Therapeutics*, **14**, 219–29.

McKellar, Q.A., May, S.A. & Lees, P. (1991) Pharmacology and therapeutics of non-steroidal anti-inflammatory drugs in the dog and cat: 2 Individual agents. *Journal of Small Animal Practice*, **32**, 225–35.

Maitho, T.E., Lees, P. & Taylor, J.B. (1986) Absorption and pharmacokinetics of phenylbutazone in Welsh Mountain ponies. *Journal of Veterinary Pharmacology and Therapeutics*, **9**, 26–39.

Marriner, S. & Bogan, J.A. (1979) The influence of the rumen on the absorption of drugs; study using meclofenamic acid administered by various routes to sheep and cattle. *Journal of Veterinary of Pharmacology and Therapeutics*, **2**, 109–15.

Nolan, A.M. (2000) Patterns and its management of pain in animals. In *Pain: Its Nature and Management in Man and Animals. International Congress and Symposium Series*, (ed. by Lord Soulsby & D. Morton), vol. 246, pp. 93–100. Royal Society of Medicine Press.

Pyorala, S., Patila, J. & Sandholm, M. (1988) Phenylbutazone and flunixin meglumine fail to show beneficial effects on bovine subclinical mastitis. *Acta Veterinaria Scandinavica*, **29**, 501–503.

Rainsford, K.D. (1977) The comparative gastric ulcerogenic activities of non-steroid anti-inflammatory drugs. *Agents and Actions*, **7**, 573–7.

Robertson, I.S., Kent, J.E. & Molony, V. (1994) Effects of different methods of castration on behaviour and plasma cortisol in calves of three ages. *Research in Veterinary Science*, **56**, 8–17.

Sandholm, M., Kaartinen, L. & Pyorala, S. (1990) Bovine mastitis – why does antibiotic therapy not always work? An overview. *Journal of Veterinary Pharmacology and Therapeutics*, **13**, 248–60.

Scheuren, N., Bang, H., Munster, T., Brune, K. & Pahl, A. (1998) Modulation of transcription factor NF-kappa B by enantiomers of the nonsteroidal anti-inflammatory drug ibuprofen. *British Journal of Pharmacology*, **123**, 645–52.

Selman, I.E. (1988) The veterinary uses of a non-steroidal anti-inflammatory agent: flunixin meglumine. *The British Veterinary Journal*, Suppl. No. 1, 4–6.

Selman, I.E., Allan, E.M., Gibbs, M.A., Wiseman, A. & Young, W.B. (1984) Effect of anti-prostaglandin therapy in experimental parainfluenza type 3 pneumonia in weaned conventional calves. *Veterinary Record*, **115**, 101–105.

Shpigel, N.Y., Chen, R., Winkler, M., Saran, A., Ziv, G. & Longo, F. (1994) Anti-inflammatory ketoprofen in the treatment of field cases of bovine mastitis. *Research in Veterinary Science*, **56**, 62–8.

Toombs, J.P., Collins, L.G., Graves, G.M., Crowe, D.T. & Caywood, D.D. (1986) Colonic perforation in corticosteroid treated dogs. *Journal American Veterinary Medical Association*, **188**, 145–50.

Toutain, P.L., Brandon, R.A., Alvinerie, M., Garcia-Villar, R. & Ruckebusch, Y. (1982) Dexamethasone in cattle: pharmacokinetics and action on the adrenal gland. *Journal of Veterinary Pharmacology and Therapeutics*, **5**, 33–43.

Vane, J.R. (1971) Inhibition of prostaglandin synthesis as a mechanism of action for aspirin-like drugs. *Nature*, **231**, 271–3.

Wallace, J.L. (1999) Clinical significance and potential of selective COX-2 inhibitors. *Trends in Pharmacological Sciences*, **20**, 389–90.

Welsh, E.M. & Nolan, A.M. (1994) Repeated intradermal injection of low dose carrageenan induces tachyphylaxis to evoked hyperalgesia. *Pain*, **59**, 415–21.

Whay, H.R., Waterman, A.E., Webster, A.J.F. & O'Brien, J.K. (1998) The influence of lesion type on the duration of hyperalgesia associated with hindlimb lameness in dairy cattle. *The Veterinary Journal*, **156**, 23–9.

Williams, T.J. (1983) Prostaglandin E_2, prostaglandin I and the vascular changes of inflammation. *British Journal Pharmacology*, **65**, 577–24.

Willoughby, D.A. (1968) Effects of prostaglandins $F_{2\alpha}$ and PGE_1 on vascular permeability. *Journal of Pathological Bacteriology*, **96**, 387–87.

Chapter 63
Growth Promoters in Cattle

K. Lawrence

Introduction   1067
In-feed additives   1067
    Rumen   1067
    Intestine   1069
Hormonal implants   1071
Growth hormone (BST)   1073
Repartitioning agents   1073

Introduction

Bovine growth promoters are divided into four groups:

- In-feed additives
- Hormonal implants
- Growth hormone (somatotropins)
- Repartitioning agents (β-agonists)

In the European Union (EU) the use of hormonal implants and β-agonists has been banned since 1988, followed in 1990 with a moratorium on bovine somatotropin (BST) that became a ban in 2000. Meanwhile the use of in-feed additives is under close scrutiny with a proposed 'phase out' by 2006. The EU position on growth promoters has been taken in spite of the increased production costs to farmers and the enormous knock-on costs of increased feed usage and slurry production leading to environmental pollution (Verbeke & Viaene, 1996). The other major cattle-producing countries of the world continue to use a variety of growth promoters, as they have done for over 30 years.

In-feed additives

In-feed additives are divided into two types by the site of primary activity: rumen and intestine.

Rumen

The most widely researched of the rumen active growth promoters is monensin sodium (Romensin, Elanco Animal Health). Monensin is an 'ionophore', a group of antibiotics that are used only in agriculture – there are no equivalent products used or in development for use in human medicine, nor do they share a mode of action with any compound in human medicine. Interestingly, in addition, the ionophores do not have antibiotic resistance encoded by transferable genes. Monensin acts on bacteria by facilitating the carriage of sodium ions in to the cell. This causes the cell to speed up the sodium/potassium pump in the cell membrane to redress the ion balance. As the transport mechanism requires energy in the form of ATP, continuous exposure to monensin could lead the cell to exhaust energy supplies, resulting in death by osmotic disruption of the cell, but more usually it prevents the bacteria from competing in a mixed population and numbers decline (Pinkerton & Steinrauf, 1970; Pressman, 1976).

The mode of action of monensin in the rumen has been elucidated and it can act as model for other products in this class, such as lasalocid (Bovatec, Alpharma Animal Health Division) and laidlomycin (Cattlyst, Alpharma Animal Health Division).

The rumen is a fermentation vat that converts carbohydrates into volatile fatty acids (VFAs) such as acetic, butyric and propionic acids that drive the animal's metabolism (see Fig. 63.1). While all three VFAs can be used in the nutrition of the bovine, the production of propionic acid is the most efficient leading to an improved efficiency of usage of both compounded feed and roughage. The key to the efficiency of production of the VFAs is the preservation of the six carbons from the final fermentation substrate, usually a hexose sugar such as glucose. With acetic acid only four of the carbon atoms are retained in the rumen, with two being lost as the gases carbon dioxide and methane; butyric acid is similar although only carbon dioxide is produced. Only with propionic acid is there a complete retention of all six carbon molecules in the fermentation products.

Richardson *et al.* (1976) provided the first evidence of the effects of monensin on VFA production using anaerobic batch fermentation. In this study the propionic acid levels rose from $7.4\,\mu M/ml$ to $12.5\,\mu M/ml$ as the concentration of monensin was increased (Table 63.1).

Similar results were found *in vivo* by Van Maanen *et al.* (1978) in steers being fed both roughage and grain based rations – there was a significant increase in the

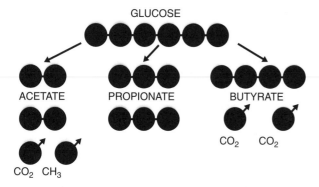

Fig. 63.1 Rumen fermentation pattern for a simple carbohydrate, showing the preservation of carbon molecules.

Table 63.1 The shift of VFA production ratios with increasing levels of monensin, during anaerobic batch fermentation.

Monensin (mcg/ml)	Acetic (μM/ml)	Propionic (μM/ml)	Butyric (μM/ml)
0.0	19.6	7.4	7.1
0.10	20.8	8.6	7.2
0.25	20.2	9.4	6.9
0.50	19.6	10.6	6.5
1.00	19.1	11.1	6.3
5.00	17.5	11.2	5.8
25.00	16.7	12.5	5.6

Table 63.2 The effect of monensin on rumen propionate pool size and production rate in steers consuming roughage or grain based diets.

Treatment	Propionate pool size (g)	Propionate production rate (g/day)
Roughage	32.0 ± 1.3	441 ± 24
Roughage + monensin	56.5 ± 2.1	659 ± 22
Grain	36.5 ± 2.0	510 ± 10
Grain + monensin	66.3 ± 4.1	899 ± 45

Table 63.3 The sensitivity of rumen bacteria to monensin and their related products of fermentation. (After Chen & Russell (1989); Chow & Russell (1990); Dawson & Boling (1983); Dennis *et al.* (1981).)

	Products of fermentation
Monensin-sensitive organisms	
Ruminococcus	Acetic acid
Methanobacterium	Acetic acid, methane
Lactobacillus	Lactic acid
Butyrivibrio	Acetic acid, butyric acid
Streptococcus	Lactic acid
Methanosarcina	Methane
Monensin-insensitive organisms	
Selenomonas	Propionic acid
Bacteroides	Acetic acid, propionic acid
Veillonella	Propionic acid

Table 63.4 The effect of monensin on rumen protozoa and propionic acid production in fistulated sheep.

Monensin feed inclusion (mg/kg)	Total protozoa ($\times 10^5$/ml)	Molar % propionic acid concentration
0	10.1	20.2
11	9.0	23.6
22	6.2	24.4
33	7.1	25.8
44	5.4	28.7

size of the propionate pool and the production rate. The results are summarized in Table 63.2.

The effect of monensin seems to be mediated by changes in the balance of the bacterial population in the rumen. The sensitivity of a range of rumen bacteria to monensin is reviewed in Table 63.3, along with their fermentation output. Monensin clearly inhibits the major acetate- and butyrate-producing bacteria, allowing a proliferation of the primary propionate producers.

Monensin has also been observed to reduce the concentration of rumen protozoa in many experiments. This has also been associated with an increase in the proportion of propionic acid production, as is shown in the sheep study presented in Table 63.4.

Goodrich *et al.* (1984) and Potter *et al.* (1986) have reviewed the expected performance benefits from the use of monensin and highlighted the different nature of the response in grain-based and roughage-based systems. In all performance trials two measurements are made to derive a third. The feed intake (ADF, average daily feed in kg) and the growth rate (ADG, average daily gain in kg) are measured and the feed conversion ratio (FCR) is calculated by dividing ADF/ADG. While the FCR is improved in all the trials, in grain-based diets the ADG often remains unchanged

but the ADF is markedly reduced. This contrasts with the roughage diets where the ADG is increased while the ADF is unchanged. In balanced rations composing both grain and forage the effects on ADF and ADG are less clear, but there is still an 8 to 10 per cent improvement in FCR.

There are additional benefits from the rumen active growth promoters in the control of acidosis (Nagaraja *et al.* 1985, 1987), bloat control (Sakauchi & Hoshino,

1981; Bartley *et al.*, 1983; Lowe *et al.*, 1991) and the prevention of coccidiosis (Watkins *et al.*, 1986).

Intestine

The growth promoters with a more pronounced effect in the intestine are the bambermycins (Flavomycin, Intervet) and virginiamycin (Stafac, Phibro Animal Health). This does not imply that these products have no effect in the rumen and indeed with virginiamycin there have been reports of significant effects on VFA production and the control of acidosis (Hedde *et al.*, 1980).

Likewise monensin is described as a rumen active growth promoter, but this does not imply it has no effect in the intestine. Indeed, as monensin has been shown to be an effective growth promoter in pigs it must also have a more conventional mode of action in this species (Mackinnon, 1987).

The mode of action of in-feed growth promoters in monogastric animals and in the intestine of a ruminant is complex and still open to debate. The comparison of healthy animals with a normal digestive tract bacterial flora to germ-free animals has produced an insight into the role of the gut flora in inhibiting nutrient absorption. This has been built upon by comparing the response of each group to antibiotic incorporated into their diet (Visek, 1979). Conventional animals grow more slowly and use their feed less efficiently than gnotobiotic or 'germ-free' animals because of the presence of the intestinal flora. When antibiotic was administered, the growth response of the conventionally grown

animals matched that of the germ-free group; there was no effect of the antibiotic on the germ-free group. Antibiotics within the digestive tract of animals inhibit the growth and modify the metabolism of susceptible populations of bacterial flora. Since most of the antibiotics used for growth promotion have a Gram-positive spectrum of activity, such bacteria as *Clostridia*, *Enterococci* and *Bacilli* seem likely candidates. The inclusion of growth promoters in cattle feeds serves to allow a conventionally raised animal to grow at the same rate as a germ-free animal.

Studies on the physiological, nutritional, metabolic and immunological effects associated with the use of antibiotic feed additives demonstrate the complexity of their mode of action (Visek, 1979; Hays, 1979; Coates, 1980; Anderson *et al.*, 2000). The reported effects include:

● Inhibition of the growth or modifying the metabolism of harmful gut bacteria;
● Decreased elaboration of toxic substances, including bacterial toxins;
● Reduced bacterial destruction of essential nutrients;
● Increased synthesis of vitamins and other growth factors;
● Improved efficiency of nutrient absorption by modification of the gut wall;
● Reduced intestinal mucosal epithelial cell turnover;
● Reduced intestinal motility.

The net effect of the changes in the intestine listed in Table 63.5 is an increased availability and absorption of nutrients and a reduced cost/kg gain.

Table 63.5 Some physiological, nutritional and metabolic effects ascribed to in-feed growth promoters (after Ewing & Cole, 1994).

Physiological effects[a]		Nutritional effects		Metabolic effects	
Gut food transit time	↘	Energy retention	↗	Ammonia production	↘
Gut wall diameter	↘	Gut energy loss	↘	Toxic amine production	↘
Gut wall length	↘	Nitrogen retention	↗	Alpha-toxin production	↘
Gut wall weight	↘	Limiting amino acid supply	↗	Fatty acid oxidation	↘
Gut absorptive capacity	↗	Vitamin absorption	↗	Faecal fat excretion	↘
Faecal moisture	↘	Vitamin synthesis	↘	Liver protein synthesis	↗
Mucosal cell turnover	↘	Trace element absorption	↗	Gut alkaline phosphatase	↗
Stress	↘	Fatty acid absorption	↗	Gut urease	↘
Feed intake	↗, ↘, →	Glucose absorption	↗		
		Calcium absorption	↗		
		Plasma nutrients	↗		

[a] ↘ denotes a reduction; ↗ denotes an increase; → denotes no change.

In spite of the different emphasis of the mode of action of the rumen and gut-active in-feed growth promoters, their effects on the efficiency of performance is very similar with a 6 to 8 percent improvement in FCR.

Consumer concerns have been raised about the use of in-feed growth promoters in all species. The spectrum of data on this aspect of these products submitted for registration was summarized by Lawrence (1998).

As with therapeutic veterinary medicines, stringent safety studies are necessary for growth promoters. The safety data requirements for registration in the EU are listed below (source: *Official Journal of European Communites* L208-21 T025):

1. Studies on target species
   1.1 Safety studies – Biological
       – Toxicological
       – Macroscopic
       – Histological effects
   1.2 Microbiological studies of the additive
       1.2.1 Antibacterial spectrum of activity
       1.2.2 Cross-resistance to therapeutic antibiotics
       1.2.3 Tests to find out whether the additive is capable of selecting resistance factors
       1.2.4 Tests to determine the effect of the additive:
           – on the microflora of the digestive tract
           – on the colonisation of the digestive tract
           – on the shedding or excretion of pathogenic micro-organisms
       1.2.5 Field studies to monitor bacterial resistance
   1.3 Studies of the metabolism and residues
2. Studies on excreted residues – 'ecotoxicity'
3. Studies on laboratory animals
   3.1 Acute toxicity
   3.2 Chronic toxicity
   3.3 Mutagenicity
   3.4 Carcinogenicity
   3.5 Reproductive toxicity
   3.6 Toxicity of metabolites

Microbiological safety of the use of growth promoters has been included in the registration dossiers from the earliest legislation. All the potential hazards of their use have been well recognized from the very beginning. The microbiological safety is assessed in three areas:

(1) Selection of antibiotic resistance in the gut flora.
(2) Effect on the excretion of enteric pathogens by animals.
(3) Residues in the meat and the effect on human gut flora.

(1) *Selection of antibiotic resistance in the gut flora.* In any population of bacteria, there is a range of antibiotic susceptibility from fully sensitive to solidly resistant – even in the absence of antibiotics (Linton, 1982). Usually, the bulk of the bacteria remain sensitive to an antibiotic, unless a therapeutic dose is administered which kills the sensitive and allows the few resistant bacteria to proliferate; thus a resistant population develops (Evangelisti *et al.*, 1975).

It is a truism that the use of a therapeutic dose of an antibiotic selects for the survival of the few resistant organisms in the population; it does not cause individual sensitive bacteria to become resistant. As the growth promoters are included at levels approximately 10 to 100 times lower than therapeutic doses (Corpet, 1996), there is little, if any, selection pressure on the gut flora. A selection of studies on growth promoters that have demonstrated their low resistance selection capacity at authorised use levels are listed below:

- Flavomycin (Dealy & Moeller, 1977; Devriese, 1980; Mee, 1982; Corpet, 1984; Dutta & Devriese, 1984)
- Monensin (Dutta & Devriese, 1984; Newbold *et al.*, 1993)
- Virginiamycin (Gaines *et al.*, 1980; Devriese, 1980; Mee, 1982; Dutta & Devriese, 1984)

It is usual for the antibiotic growth promoters to have a Gram-positive spectrum of activity; therefore they cannot have a selection pressure on the Enterobacteriaceae and do not contribute to antibiotic resistance in *Salmonella* spp. or *E. coli*.

(2) *Effect on the excretion of enteric pathogens by animals.* An increased number of organisms or an extended shedding time in the faeces could lead to an increased risk of contamination of human food. All current growth promoters have been examined for their effect on *Salmonella* and, in many cases, other bacteria including *E. coli*. All modern studies, undertaken with authorized inclusion levels, have given satisfactory results (Nurmi & Rantala, 1974; Hinton, 1988). Ungemach (1996) considered that the use of growth promoters in animal feeds posed no risk to the indigenous gut flora of human consumers.

(3) *Residues in the meat and the effect on human gut flora.* Growth promoters administered in animal feed do not leave detectable residues in the meat. Indeed, they can be used from birth to slaughter, i.e. they have a zero withdrawal. As there is no detectable residue in the meat, there is unlikely to be a selection pressure on human gut flora (Ungemach, 1996).

The public health implications of the use of antibiotics in animal feeds have been examined on many occasions:

Netherthorpe Committee	1962
Swann Committee	1969
FDA Task Force	1972
Kennedy Report	1977
Office of Technology Assessment (OTA) Report	1979
AVI Conference – "Ten Years after Swann"	1979
National Academy of Sciences Review (NAS)	1980
Council for Agricultural Science & Technology Report	1981
American Society of Animal Science	1986
Office of Technology Assessment (OTA) Report	1995
Scientific Conference on Growth Promotion in Meat Production	1995
Antimicrobial Feed Additives	1997
Office International des Epizooties. The Use of Antibiotics in Animals. Ensuring the Protection of Public Health	1999
Advisory Committee on the Microbiological Safety of Food Report on Antimicrobial Antibiotic Resistance in Relation to Food Safety	1999

All have discussed the hazards but none have proved any risk to human health.

Hormonal implants

Hormonal implants are not currently licensed for use in the European Union. Those listed in Table 63.6 are in use in the rest of the world.

The mode of action of the hormone implants has not been fully elucidated although some work has indicated that changes in serum concentrations of IGF-1 occur in implanted steers, while serum IGF-1 concentration in the control steers remains or changed or, indeed, decreases across time. This suggests that IGF-1, the essential growth hormone, is related to the additional gain of the implanted steers. However, the reason for this linear decrease in serum IGF-1 concentration sometimes reported in control cattle is unclear. For example, it does not appear that the effect can be attributed to the control animals approaching their physiological maturity, because the control and implant animals usually exhibited similar degrees of fatness. The net effect could be an increase in protein synthesis and protein gain, which translates into greater, more efficient liveweight gain and profit for the cattle producer (Simpkins et al., 2000).

The usual explanation is more mundane as bulls grow faster and produce a leaner carcass than steers; steers grow faster and produce less fatty meat than heifers and cows. The differences in growth rate are usually ascribed to hormonal status and the levels of androgen in particular. The hormone implants are used to replace or adjust the circulating hormone levels to achieve optimal growth.

The efficacy of hormonal implants is well accepted, both alone and in combination with in-feed growth promoters (see Table 63.7 for a typical trial). There is some

Table 63.6 Hormonal implants licensed for use as growth promoters in non-EU countries (modified from table in the report of the fifty-second meeting of Joint FAO/WHO Expert Committee on Food Additives (JECFA, 1999)

Product names[a]	Comparison of the composition (mg/implant) of hormonal implants used for growth promotion					
	Oestradiol	Testosterone	Testosterone propionate	Progesterone	Trenbolone acetate	Target cattle
Compudose 200	24					Cattle
Compudose 400	45					Cattle
Synovex S	20			200		Steers
Synovex H	20		200			Heifers
Synovex C	10		100			Calves
Steeroid	20			200		Steers
Heiferoid	20		200			Heifers
Implix BM	20			200		Steers
Implix BF	20	200				Heifers
Torelor	40				200	Steers
Revalor	20				140	Calves
Revalor G	8				40	Steers
Revalor S	24				120	Steers
Revalor H	14				140	Heifers
Finaplix-S					140	Steers
Ralgro	Active ingredient is Zeranol 3 × 12 mg pellets/dose					Cattle

[a] Product names are registered trade marks®.

Table 63.7 The efficacy of an implant in grazing steers used either alone or in combination with supplementary feed and the in-feed growth promoter monensin. (Source: Elanco Animal Health in-house data.)

Treatment	ADG (kg)		Increased ADG (kg)	Total gain in 150 days (kg)
	Control	Compudose®		
No supplement	0.554	0.631	0.077	11.55
Compound feed (1 kg)	0.613	0.709	0.096	14.4
Compound feed (1 kg) + monensin	0.659	0.782	0.123	18.45

®, registered trade mark (oestradiol 17β).

evidence that the response to an implant varies with the start weight, with the greatest response in finishing cattle being reported from the heaviest cattle (see Fig. 63.2).

Some carcass traits can be changed by the use of implants, with lower dressing percentages (Kuhl *et al.*, 1989), reduced marbling (Eversole *et al.*, 1989) and a reduction in top grade carcasses (Foutz *et al.*, 1989) being reported. These changes vary between implants, but have not been associated with any significant changes in the eating quality of the meat.

While the efficacy of hormonal implants is accepted, the consumer safety of implanted meat has been a focus of conflict between the USA and the EU, leading to a complaint to the World Trade Organization (WTO). The USA consider the hormone ban in the EU to be an unjustified barrier to trade and have effectively won this case at arbitration through the WTO Appellate Body. The findings of the case centred round the lack of a proper risk assessment prior to the imposition of the ban on imports of meat from animals treated with hormones.

This whole debate is best followed by reading the full Joint FAO/WHO Expert Committee on Food Additives (JECFA) assessments:

Natural hormones (WHO Feed Additive Series 43–52nd Meeting JECFA)
(http://www.inchem.org/documents/jecfa/jecmono/v43jec05.htm)

Zeranol (WHO Feed Additive Series 44–53rd Meeting JECFA)
(http://www.inchem.org/documents/jecfa/jecmono/v44jec14.htm)

Trenbolone (26th meeting JECFA)
(http://www.inchem.org/documents/jecfa/jecmono/v23je03.htm)
and the Opinion of the Standing Committee on Veterinary Measures related to Public Health (SCVPH) dated 30 April 1999
(http://europa.eu.int/comm/food/fs/sc/scv/out21_en.html)

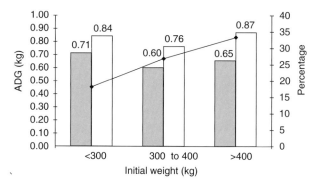

Fig. 63.2 The effect of the initial weight on the percentage response from an implant in finishing cattle.

as well as the recent assessment of the SCVPH report by a subgroup of the Veterinary Products Committee (VPC) of the Veterinary Medicines Directorate (VMD) in the UK on the potential risks to human health from hormone residues in bovine meat and meat products
(http://www.vmd.gov.uk/) see under Publications.

The main areas of concern have been best summarized in the VPC subgroup report and they are reviewed below:

(1) Direct consumer exposure to hormone residues in meat. The residues are all very low compared with the acceptable daily intakes (ADIs) identified by JECFA. Therefore consumer exposure to oestradiol, progesterone and testosterone will be very low compared with those naturally produced in the body (see Fig. 63.3). The ADI is an amount of medicine/hormone that can be eaten every day over a lifetime in the practical certainty that, based on current knowledge, no harm will result.

(2) Hormonal residues can adversely affect the immune system. References used to support this argument in the SCVPH report did not reflect modern physiological understanding of the

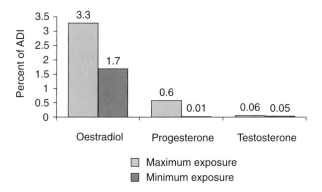

Fig. 63.3 The maximum and minimum consumer exposure to natural hormone residues from implanted meat as a percentage of the JECFA ADI. (JECFA Joint FAO/WHO Expert Committee on Food Additives. ADI (acceptable daily intake) in the amount of a medicine or hormore that can be taken every day during a lifetime in the practical certainty no harm will result.)

immune system. With reference back to the first area of concern, the residues are such a small fraction of daily endogenous hormone production as to be without effect.

(3) Hormonal residues can lead to an increase in certain common cancers. However, epidemiological evidence only shows a direct link between meat and fat consumption; to relate that to hormone residues is a leap in logic. The leap is difficult to support as these tumours are found equally widely in both men and women in countries where hormonal growth promoters are not permitted.

(4) Hormone residues in meat could affect many aspects of human development and reproduction. The only evidence of such an effect comes from high levels of hormones injected into experimental animals. No current data show any ground for these suspicions in respect of residues, even with the intensive research in this area.

The 'hormone' debate is about politics and the role of science to support obviously conflicting views. Even if the science supporting the safety of hormones wins the politicians can still ensure that there will be no consumer acceptance for this technology in the EU. It is not anticipated that there will be a return of the implant in beef production in the EU, but this should not jeopardize its use in other countries with less political interference in product registration.

Growth hormone (BST)

The use of bovine somatotropin (BST) in cattle has primarily been concentrated on increasing milk pro-

duction. This does not mean that the effects of BST on the growth performance and carcass characteristics in beef animals have been neglected. The earliest trial in 1959 (Brumby, 1959) and those in the late 1980s produced consistent effects leading to increased growth rates, improved feed conversion and carcass lean, while decreasing carcass fat. The effects on eating quality of the meat associated with reduced carcass fat were a reduced acceptability because of lower scores on tenderness. The available data in cattle on growth performance were summarized by Enright (1989) and on meat quality by Allen and Enright (1989). As nearly all the data summarized were from trials involving the daily injection of BST, and even sustained-release injectable formulations only last 14 days, there does not currently seem to be a place for its use in the beef industry as a growth promoter.

A direct comparison has been made between anabolic steroids and BST. Untreated controls (UC) were compared with steroid implants (STI) and 160 mg BST injected weekly (Preston *et al.*, 1995). Daily gain was increased by both treatments (UC 1.30 kg/day; STI 1.66 kg/day; BST 1.51 kg/day) and feed conversion was improved (UC 5.92; STI 4.88; BST 5.13). The anabolic effects of STI and BST were considered to be potentially additive.

Repartitioning agents

β-Adrenergic receptor agonists (β-agonists) increase muscle mass and decrease fat mass when fed to cattle. A wide range of compounds has been investigated including cimaterol, clenbuterol, fenoterol, isoprenaline, mabuterol, ractopamine, salbutamol, terbutaline and zilpaterol (see Fig. 63.4). The most extensive review of the use of β-agonists in meat animals was published by Anderson *et al.* (1991), in which nearly 400 papers were reviewed. There are currently no β-agonists registered in the EU for use in cattle as growth promoters, indeed in the EU this class of compound is specifically prohibited under EU Directive 96/22/EU. There is one product registered as a growth promoter in cattle in South Africa and Mexico – zilpaterol (Zilmax, Hoechst Roussel Vet) – and one in pigs in the USA, Mexico, Brazil, Philippines and Korea – ractopamine (Paylean, Elanco Animal Health).

The mode of action is complex, with direct effects on skeletal muscle cells, leading to hypertrophy, and on adipocytes, causing lipolysis, as well as secondary mechanisms mediated by other hormones and changes in blood flow (Mersmann, 1998). Studies attempting to relate the relative density of β$_2$-adrenoreceptors on muscle and the local response to β-agonists have failed to find a useful tool to predict efficacy of compounds

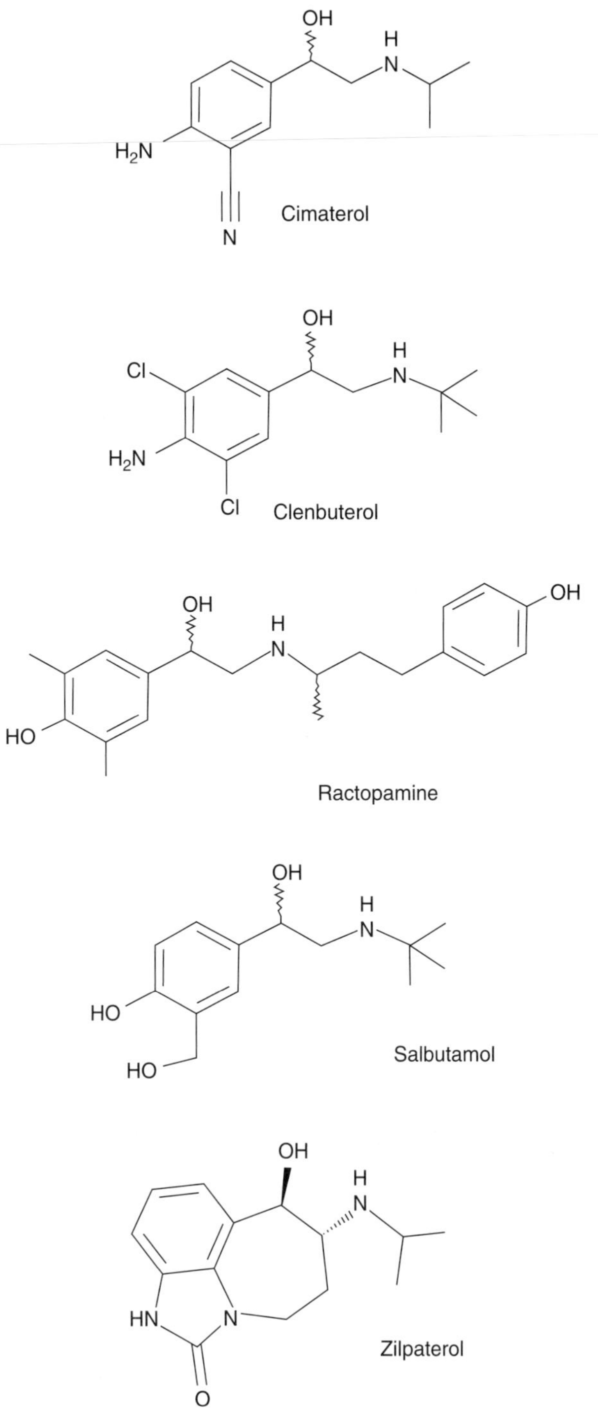

Fig. 63.4 Structural details of a range of β-agonists that have been proposed as growth promoters in cattle

Table 63.8 The effect of ractopamine on growth performance in finishing cattle. A summary of six trials.

Dose (ppm)	ADG (kg)	ADF (kg)	FCR
0	1.26[a]	9.40[a]	7.46[a]
10	1.34[b]	9.31[a]	6.95[b]
20	1.39[b]	9.40[a]	6.76[b]
30	1.48[c]	9.31[a]	6.29[c]

ppm, parts per million; ADG, average daily gain; ADF, average daily feed; FCR, feed conversion ratio; kg, kilogram. Means with different superscripts are significantly different.

Table 63.9 The effect of ractopamine on carcass yield in finishing cattle. A summary of six trials.

Dose (ppm)	Dressing (%)	Protein (%)	Fat (%)
0	60.71[a]	15.16[a]	30.31
10	60.76[a]	15.16[a]	30.24
20	61.02[b]	15.36[a]	29.70
30	61.03[b]	15.54[b]	28.81

ppm, parts per million. Means with different superscripts are significantly different.

and a 'rebound' when the product is removed, leading to an increase in fat deposition and a reduction in muscle mass (Elliot *et al.*, 1993). The most effective use of a repartitioning agent is therefore in the finishing period in the one to two months prior to slaughter. The results from the use of β-agonists in cattle are very consistent and are summarized in Table 63.8, which shows significant increases in growth rates and feed utilization, and Table 63.9, which shows significant increases in dressing percentage, increased carcass lean.

β-agonists are usually divided into two classes (Smith, 1998):

(1) *Halogenated aromatic ring.* This class tends to have a long serum half-life and when coupled with high oral absorption and potency of action in humans there can be a real safety concern from residues in meat. An example of such a compound is clenbuterol (pharmacodynamic dose in man 10 μg/day – Meyer & Rinker, 1991); levels found in contaminated meat in the EU affected humans who consumed as little as 100 g of the product (Kuiper *et al.*, 1998). See Table 63.10 for a summary of some poisoning incidents.

(2) *Hydroxylated aromatic ring.* The metabolism is much simpler with the hydroxylated β-agonists and they tend to have relatively short plasma half-lives and when coupled with a low potency in humans they may pose little risk from residues. An example of this type of compound would be ractopamine, where the phar-

(Hoey *et al.*, 1995). Moody *et al.* (2000) have undertaken a detailed review of the mode of action of the β-agonists in all species. When β-agonists are used as growth promoters, two major problems arise during chronic exposure. Firstly, receptor downregulation leads to a fall off in effect over time (Peters, 1989; Re *et al.*, 1994)

Table 63.10 A summary of some documented cases of β-agonist poisoning in Europe (after Witkamp, 1995).

Year	Source	Compound	No. of people	Symptoms	Country
1990	Bovine liver	Clenbuterol (0.16–0.30 mg/kg)	135	Tremor, palpitations, tachycardia, nervousness	Spain
1990	Calf liver	Clenbuterol (0.38–0.50 mg/kg	22	Tremor, headaches, dizziness, palpitations, malaise	France
1994	Calf liver	Clenbuterol (?)	127	Not specified	Spain
1995	Fillet, rump steak	Clenbuterol (>0.5 mg/kg)	16	Tachycardia, tremors, nervousness	Italy

Class 1 – Halogenated aromatic ring

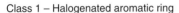

Slow metabolic inactivation

Clenbuterol

Half life in man $T_{1/2}$ = 30 hr

Pharmacodynamic dose in man 10 μg/day

Class 2 – Hydroxylated aromatic ring

Rapid metabolic inactivation

Ractopamine

Half life in man $T_{1/2}$ = 4 hr

Pharmacodynamic dose in man 25 000 μg/day

Fig. 63.5 A comparison with the metabolic deactivation rate and plasma half-life of halogenated and hydroxylated aromatic ring β-agonists.

macodynamic dose in man exceeds 25000 μg/day (Paylean Freedom of Information Summary).

Effective doses of ractopamine and zilpaterol are reported to have negligible to undetectable residue levels in the target species (Anderson *et al.*, 1993; *Zilmax Technical Manual*, 1998). These products have only been cleared for use in food animals after extensive reviews of the safety of residues and it is perhaps unreasonable for a class ban to have been introduced in the EU based on the misuse of clenbuterol when safe alternatives were in development.

The classes of β-agonist are contrasted in Fig. 63.5.

The use of highly active β-agonists as growth promoters should not be pursued because of the potential hazards for human and animal health (Anon, 1996), however this should not preclude the development of safe effective products (Smith, 1998).

References and further reading

Advisory Committee on the Microbiological Safety of Food (1999) *Report on Antimicrobial Antibiotic Resistance in Relation to Food Safety*. The Stationery Office, London.

Allen, P. & Enright, W.J. (1989) Effects of administration of somatotropin on meat quality in ruminants: a review. In *Use of Somatotropin in Livestock Production* (ed. by K. Sejrsen, M. Vestergaard & A. Neimann-Sorensen), pp. 201–9. Elsevier Applied Science, London and New York.

American Society of Animal Science (1986) Public health implications of the use of antibiotics in agriculture. 77th Annual Meeting, Suppl. 3. *Journal of Animal Science*, **62**, 1–106.

Anderson, D.B., McCracken, V.J., Aminov, R.I., Simpson, J.M., Mackie, R.I., Verstegen, M.W.A. & Gaskins, H.R. (2000) Gut microbiology and growth-promoting antibiotics in swine. *Nutrition Abstracts and Reviews. Series B, Livestock Feeds and Feeding*, **70**, 101–8.

Anderson, D.B., Veehuisen, E.L., Schroeder, A.L., Jones, D.J. & Hancock, D.L. (1991) The use of phenethanolamines to reduce fat and increase leanness in meat animals. In *Proceedings of Symposium on Fat and Cholesterol Reduced Foods – Advances in Applied Biotechnology Series* (ed. by C. Haberstroh & C.E. Morris), pp. 43–73. Portfolio Publishing, New Orleans.

Anderson, D.B., Veehuisen, E.L., Smith, C.K., Dalidowicz, J.E., Donoho, A.L., Williams, G.D., Jones, D., Schroeder, A.L., Turbert, M.P. & Guneratne, R.J. (1993) Ractopamine hydrochloride: a unique PLE (phenethanolamine lean enhancer) for swine. In *Proceedings of the 11th World Association of Veterinary Food Hygienists (WAVFH) Symposium* (ed. by P. Ingkaninum & P. Poomvises). pp. 96–102. The Thai Veterinary Medical Association, Bangkok.

Anon (1996) Working Group II – Assessment of health risk. Scientific Conference on Growth Promotion in Meat Production, pp. 19–25. EU Commission DG VI Agriculture.

Association of Veterinarians in Industry (1979) In *Proceedings of the Conference 'Ten Years after Swann'*. AVI, London.

Bartley, E.E., Nagaraja, T.G., Pressman, E.S., Dayton, A.D., Katz, M.P. & Fina, L.R. (1983) Effects of lasalocid or monensin on legume or grain (feedlot) bloat. *Journal of Animal Science*, **56**, 1400–406.

Brumby, P.J. (1959) The influence of growth hormone on growth in young cattle. *New Zealand Journal of Agricultural Research*, **2**, 683–9.

Chen, G. & Russell, J.B. (1989) More monensin-sensitive, ammonia producing bacteria from the rumen. *Applied Environmental Microbiology*, **55**, 1052–5.

Chow, J.M. & Russell, J.B. (1990) Effect of ionophores and pH on growth of *Streptococcus bovis* in batch and continuous culture. *Applied Environmental Microbiology*, **56**, 1588–1561.

Coates, M.E. (1980) The gut micro-flora and growth. In *Growth in Animals* (ed. by T.L.J. Lawrence), pp. 175–88. Butterworths, London.

Commission on Antimicrobial Feed Additives (1997) Report. Stockholm, Sweden.

Corpet, D.E. (1984) The effect of bambermycin, carbadox, chlortetracycline and olaquindox on antibiotic resistance in intestinal coliforms: a new animal model. *Annals of Microbiology (Pasteur Institute)* **135A**, 329–39.

Corpet, D.E. (1996) Microbiological risks for the consumer of antimicrobial growth promoters used in meat production. In *Proceedings of the Scientific Conference on Growth Promotion in Meat Production*, pp. 401–29. European Commission DGVI, Brussels.

Council for Agricultural Science and Technology (1981) *Antibiotics in animal feeds*. Report No. 88. Ames, Iowa.

Craene, A. de & Viaene, J. (1992) *Economic effects of technology in agriculture. Do performance enhancers for animals benefit consumers?* Department of Agro-marketing, Faculty of Agricultural Science, University of Ghent, Belgium.

Dawson, K.L. & Boling, J.A. (1983). Monensin-resistant bacteria in the rumen of calves on monensin-containing and unmedicated diets. *Applied Environmental Microbiology*, **46**, 160–2.

Dealy, J. & Moeller, M.W. (1977). Influence of bambermycins on *E. coli* and antibiotic resistance in calves. *Journal of Animal Science*, **45**, 1239–42.

Dennis, S.M., Naharaja, T.G. & Bartley, F.E. (1981). Effects of lasalocid or monensin on lactate-producing or -using rumen bacteria. *Journal of Animal Science*, **52**: 418–22.

Devriese, L.A. (1980) Sensitivity of *Staphylococci* from farm animals to antimicrobials used for growth promotion and therapy, a ten year study. *Annals of Veterinary Research*, **11**, 399–408.

Dutta, G.N. & Devriese, L.A. (1984) Observations on the in vitro sensitivity and resistance of Gram positive intestinal bacteria of farm animals to growth promoting antimicrobial agents. *Journal of Applied Bacteriology*, **56**, 117–23.

Elliot, C.T., Crooks, S.R.H., McEvoy, J.G.D., McGaughey, W.J., Hewitt, S.A., Patterson, D. & Kilpatrick, D. (1993) Observations on the effects of long-term withdrawal on carcass composition and residue concentrations in clenbuterol-medicated cattle. *Veterinary Research*, **132**, 459–68.

Enright, W.J. (1989) Effects of administration of somatotropin on growth, feed efficacy and carcass composition of ruminants: a review. In *Use of Somatotropin in Livestock Production* (ed. by K. Sejrsen, M. Vestergaard & A. Neimann-Sorensen), pp. 201–9. Elsevier Applied Science, London and New York.

Evangelisti, D.G., English, A.R., Girard, A.E., Lynch, J.E. & Solomons, I.A. (1975) Influence of subtherapeutic levels of oxytetracycline on *Salmonella typhimurium* in swine, calves and chickens. *Antimicrobial Agents and Chemotherapy*, **8**, 664–72.

Eversole, D.E., Fontenot, J.P. & Kirk, D.J. (1989) Implanting trembalone acetate and estrodiol in finishing beef steers. *Nutritional Reports International*, **39**, 995–8.

Ewing, W.N. & Cole, D.J.A. (1994) *The Living Gut*, pp. 67–74. Context, Dungannon.

Food and Drug Administration (FDA) (1972), *Report of the FDA task force on the use of antibiotics in animal foods*. US Department of Health, Education and Welfare.

Foutz, C.D., Dolezal, H.G., Gill, D.R., Strasia, C.A., Gardner, T. & Ray, F.K. (1989) Trembalone acetate effects on carcass traits of yearling feedlot steers. *Journal of Animal Science*, **67**, (Suppl. 1), 434.

Gaines, S.A., Rollins, L.D., Williams, R.D. & Selwyn, M. (1980) Effect of penicillin and virginiamycin on drug resistance in lactose-fermenting enteric flora. *Antimicrobial Agents and Chemotherapy*, **17**, 428–33.

Goodrich, R.D., Garrett, J.E., Gast, D.R., Kirick, M.A., Larson, D.A. & Meiske, J.C. (1984) Influence of monensin on the performance of cattle. *Journal of Animal Science*, **58**, 1484–98.

Hays, V.W. (1979) Benefits: antibacterials. In *Drugs in Livestock Feeds. Vol. 1. Technical Report*, pp. 29–36. Office of Technology Assessment, Congress of the United States, Washington, DC.

Hedde, R.D., Armstrong, D.G., Parish, R.C. & Quach, R. (1980) Virginiamycin effect on rumen fermentation in cattle. *Journal of Animal Science*, **51**, (Suppl. 1), 366.

Hinton, M. (1988) Salmonella colonization in young chickens given feed supplemented with the growth promoting antibiotic avilamycin. *Journal of Veterinary Pharmacology and Therapeutics*, **11**, 269–75.

Hoey, A.J., Reich, M.M., Davis, G., Shorthose, R. & Sillence, M.N. (1995) Beta 2-adrenoceptor densities do not correlate with growth, carcass quality, or meat quality in cattle. *Journal of Animal Science*, **73**, 3281–6.

Kennedy, D.F. (1977) Antibiotics used in animal feeds. *HEW News*. US Department of Health, Education and Welfare, Rockville.

Kuhl, G., Simms, D.D. & Hartman, P.D. (1989) Sequential implanting with Synovex-S or Synovex-S + Finaplix-S on steer performance and carcass characteristics. *Journal of Animal Science*, **67**, (Suppl. 1), 434.

Kuiper, H.A., Noordam, M.Y., van Dooren-Flipsen, M.M.H., Schilt, R. & Roos, A.H. (1998) Illegal use of β-adrenergic agonists: European Community. *Journal of Animal Science*, **76**, 195–207.

Lawrence, K. (1998) Growth promoters in swine. In *Proceedings of the 15th IPVS Congress*, Birmingham, England, pp 337–43.

Linton, A.H. (1982) Host–parasite interactions in health. In *Microbes, Man and Animals* (ed. by A.H. Linton), p. 42. John Wiley & Sons, Chichester.

Lowe, L.B., Ball, G.J., Carruthers, V.R., Dobos, R.C., Lynch, G.A., Moate, P.J., Poole, P.R. & Valemtine, S.C. (1991) Monensin controlled-release intraruminal capsule for control of bloat in pastured dairy cows. *Australian Veterinary Journal*, **68**, 17–20.

Mackinnon, J.D. (1987) The role of growth promoters in pig production. *The Pig Veterinary Society Proceedings*, **17**, 69–100.

Mee, B.J. (1982) The selective capacity of pig feed additives and growth promotants for coliform resistance. In *Proceedings of the 4th International Symposium. Antibiotics in Agriculture: Benefits and Malefits*, pp. 349–58.

Mersmann, H.J. (1998) Overview of the effects of β-adrenergic agonists on animal growth including mechanisms of action. *Journal of Animal Science*, **76**, 160–72.

Meyer, H.H. & Rinke, L.M. (1991) The pharmacokinetics and residues of clenbuterol in veal calves. *Journal of Animal Science*, **69**, 4538–44.

Moody, D.E., Hancock, D.L. & Anderson, D.B. (2000) Phenethanolamine repartitioning agents. In *Farm Animal Metabolism and Nutrition*, (ed. by J.P.F. D'Mello), pp. 65–96. CABI Publishing, Wallingford.

Nagaraja, T.G., Avery, T.B., Galitzer, S.J. & Harmon, D.L. (1985) Effect of ionophore antibiotics on experimentally induced lactic acidosis in cattle. *American Journal of Veterinary Research*, **46**, 2444–52.

Nagaraja, T.G., Taylor, M.B., Harmon, D.L. & Boyer, J.E. (1987) In vitro lactic acid production and alterations in volatile fatty acid production by antimicrobial feed additives. *Journal of Animal Science*, **65**, 1064–76.

National Academy of Sciences, National Research Council (1980) *The effects on human health of subtherapeutic use of antimicrobials in animal feeds*. National Academy Press, Washington.

Netherthorpe (1962) *Report of the joint committee on antibiotics in animal feeding*. Agricultural Research Council/Medical Research Council, London.

Newbold, C.J., Wallace, R.J. & Walker, N.D. (1993) The effects of tetronasin and monensin on fermentation, microbial numbers and the development of ionophore-resistant bacteria in the rumen. *Journal of Applied Bacteriology*, **75**, 129–34.

Nurmi, E. & Rantala, M. (1974) The influence of zinc bacitracin on the colonization of *Salmonella infantis* in the intestine of broiler chickens. *Research in Veterinary Science*, **17**, 24–7.

Office International des Epizooties (1999) The use of antibiotics in animals. Ensuring the protection of public health, In *Proceedings of the Conference*, 24–26 March 1999, Paris, France.

Office of Technology Assessment (1979) *Drugs in livestock feed. Vol. I. Technical Report*. Congress of the United States, Washington, DC.

Office of Technology Assessment (1995) *Impact of antibiotic-resistant bacteria*. Congress of the United States, Washington, DC.

Peters, A.R. (1989) Beta-agonists as repartitioning agents: a review. *Veterinary Record*, **124**, 417–20.

Pinkerton, M. & Steinrauf, K.L. (1970) Molecular structure of monovalent metal cation complexes of monensin. *Journal of Molecular Biology*, **49**, 533–46.

Potter, E.L., Muller, R.D., Wray, M.I., Carroll, L.H. & Meyer, R.M. (1986) Effects of monensin on the performance of cattle on pasture or fed harvested forages in confinement. *Journal of Animal Science*, **62**, 583–92.

Pressman, B.C. (1976) Biological applications of ionophores. *Annual Revue of Biochemistry*, **45**, 501–30.

Preston, R.L., Bartle, S.J., Kasser, T.R., Day, J.W., Veenhuizen, J.J. & Baile, C.A. (1995) Comparative effectiveness of somatotropin and anabolic steroids in feedlot steers. *Journal of Animal Science*, **73**, 1038–47.

Re, G., Badino, P., Novelli, A. & Girardi, G. (1994) Homologous β-adrenoreceptor downregulation and heterologous estrogen and progesterone upregulation induced by repeated β2-adrenergic stimulation in the female reproductive tract of veal calves. In *Proceedings of the 6th Congress of the European Association of Veterinary Pharmacology and Toxicology*, Edinburgh, pp. 7–11.

Richardson, L.F., Raun, A.P., Potter, E.L., Cooley, C.L. & Rathmacher, R.P. (1976) Effect of monensin on rumen fermentation *in vitro* and *in vivo*. *Journal of Animal Science*, **43**, 657–62.

Sakauchi, R. & Hoshino, S. (1981). Effects of monensin on ruminal fluid viscosity, pH, volatile fatty acids and ammonia levels, and microbial activity and population in healthy and bloated steers. *Zeitschrift fur Tierphysiologie, Ticrernahrung und Futtermittelkunde*, **46**, 21–33.

Scientific Conference on Growth Promotion in Meat Production (1995) Proceedings European Commission DGVI, Brussels.

Simpkins, S., McElhenny, W., Rahe, H., Wolfe, D., Mulvaney, D. & Lino, S. (2000) Weighing the advantages. Do growth-promoting implants impact quality beef? *Highlights of Agricultural Research, Auburn Veterinary College*, **47**, 1–4.

Smith, D.J. (1998) The pharmacokinetics, metabolism, and tissue residues of β-adrenergic agonists in livestock. *Journal of Animal Science*, **76**, 173–94.

Swann, M. (1969) *Report: Joint Committee on the Use of Antibiotics in animal Husbandry and Veterinary Medicine*, HMSO, London.

Ungemach, F.R. (1996) Safety aspects of growth promoters used as feed additives. In *Proceedings of the Scientific Conference on growth promotion in meat production*, pp. 333–45. European Commission DGVI, Brussels.

Van Maanen, R.W., Herbein, J.H., McGillard, A.D. & Young, J.W. (1978) Effects of monensin on *in vitro* rumen production and blood glucose kinetics in cattle. *Journal of Nutrition*, **108**, 1002–1008.

Verbeke, R. & Viaene, J. (1996) *Environmental impact of using feed additives. Economic implications and legal environment in Benelux*, Department of Agro-marketing, Faculty of Agricultural Science, University of Ghent.

Visek, W.J. (1979) The mode of action of growth promotion by antibiotics. *Journal of Animal Science*, **46**, 1447–69.

Watkins, L.E., Wray, M.I., Basson, R.P., Feller, D.L., Olson, R.D., Fitzgerald, P.R., Stromberg, B.E. & David, G.W. (1986) The prophylactic effects of monensin fed to cattle inoculated with coccidia oocysts. *Agri-Practice*, **7**, 18–20.

Witkamp, R.F. (1995) The use of β2-agonists as growth promoters in food species. Toxicological aspects and possible health risks to consumers. In *Proceedings of the Scientific Conference on Growth Promotion in Meat Production*, pp. 297–332. EU Commission DG VI Agriculture.

Zilmax© Technical Manual (1998) Hoechst Roussel Vet, GmbH, Rheingaustrasse 190, D-65203 Wiesbaden.

Chapter 64
Injection Damage

J.H. Pratt

Introduction	1078
Damage produced by injection	1078
Intramuscular injection sites	1079
Methods of introducing contamination	1079

Introduction

The faulty administration of veterinary medicines by injection can give rise to complaints from meat wholesalers and retailers and on occasions from consumers. The lesion resulting from the injection of a drug may be aesthetically repugnant to the consumer and commercially unacceptable in the case of abscessation or fibrosis in muscle tissue to the wholesaler, the retailing butcher and the supermarket outlet.

Damage produced by injection

Abscesses deep in the gluteal region of cattle are reported since the site is frequently used for intramuscular injection of drugs. Damage in this area reduces the value of a relatively expensive part of the carcass. Abscessation may render the entire limb unsuitable for human consumption. Intravenous injections can result in haematoma formation and abscess production. In some cases this is due to irritant substances invading the perivascular tissue rather than being delivered properly into the bloodstream. In addition, the deep injection of an irritant substance causing a localized reaction within muscle tissue may elude detection at meat inspection and even later in the cutting premises. The damage may not be revealed until further butchering procedures are performed on the beef in the processing plant or retail shop by which time it may prove difficult to trace the animal back to the farm of origin. Indeed, in countries where complex marketing arrangements exist, the tracing of animals back through marketing chains may prove impossible until unique individual identification of the live animal and the resultant carcass and cuts becomes feasible in all stock. Such an achievement

would constitute a major contribution to future meat quality standards and may now prove possible throughout Western Europe where individual cattle identification is obligatory under European Community law.

Where the farm of origin can be determined, advice on proper injection techniques can be given thereby improving the welfare interests of the animal and enhancing the future profitability of the producer. Losses incurred by the abattoir through the downgrading of affected cuts of beef from incorrect injection procedures would also be reduced.

It is to be regretted that in Britain the use of data collected in the abattoir has not been exploited to its full potential. Such information can play a significant role in future preventive veterinary medicine strategies and in the depiction of regional and national animal disease patterns.

The losses incurred by the meat industry through poor injection technique are spasmodic but nevertheless can be substantial. There are, unfortunately, no reliable figures in UK meat inspection records for condemnation of meat for abscessation due to faulty injection procedures alone. However, on occasions a number of animals within one consignment of cattle exhibit deep muscle fibrosis consistent with damage from injected material, necessitating the rejection of 1.5–2 kg of a high-priced cut of meat. These lesions are formed in the same anatomical area in a number of animals within a group from the same unit. The similarity in age, character and distribution of these lesions suggests a common cause, the introduction of foreign material by injection. Both injectable nemicides and substances used in the regulation of bovine reproduction, e.g. some prostaglandins, may have been responsible for such damage encountered in recent years in this country.

The leather industry also suffers financial loss, as injection damage due to scarring and abscessation can reduce the value of the hide, particularly if the lesion is in a position that prevents the optimal use of the complete hide for large leather or suede items of clothing and upholstery.

Intramuscular injection sites

Alternative siting of injections to that of the gluteal region is therefore desirable. The middle third of the neck, about one-third of the way down from the top, is recommended (see Figs 64.1 and 64.2); this in itself does not reduce the incidence of abscessation or muscle scarring following the injection of drugs but trimming of this less expensive area reduces blemishing of the carcass. This area also tends to be cleaner than the hindquarters and so it is less likely that infection will be introduced with injection.

The factors contributing to muscle damage and abscess formation must therefore be identified to allow the formulation of advice for veterinarians and animal owners to reduce such damage.

The efficiency of the host animal's inflammatory response in removing the foreign protein and devitalized tissue together with the persistence of the stimulus determine the size and progression of the abscess formation. In mild cases no abscess may form, but scar tissue will mark the tissue damage. When an abscess has been formed and the inflammatory stimulus removed the abscess may persist for a prolonged period before resolving to scar tissue.

Methods of introducing contamination

The introduction of foreign protein may occur in a variety of ways.

Contamination of injected drugs: This is most likely to occur prior to administration as a result of poor hygienic procedures employed. To obviate contamination of the contents of a bottle or vial a separate sterile needle to that used for injection must remain attached to the container and used only to refill the syringe. In multiple dosing an automatic injection mechanism avoids this requirement and results in a smoother and more efficient operation. The manufacturer's storage instructions should be followed; unused vaccine should be discarded. When therapeutic agents such as antibiotics are used they should be used up as quickly as possible after opening.

Contamination of needle or syringe: Ideally, a sterile needle should be used for every injection but in practical situations this is often not feasible; however, in special circumstances this approach may be applicable on veterinary advice in certain herds to avoid transfer of specific viral and other infections such as enzootic bovine leukosis (EBL). It is good practice, however, to change needles and syringes regularly, i.e. after every

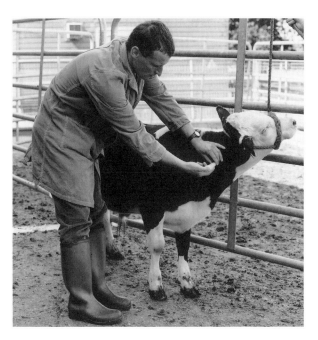

Fig. 64.1 A growing calf being injected into the neck muscle.

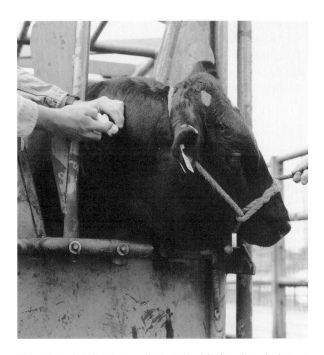

Fig. 64.2 A bull adequately restrained before introducing an injection into the neck muscles.

10–15 cattle, when groups of animals are injected and in any event when contamination of the equipment occurs or is suspected or the needle is in any way damaged.

Punching a fragment of host skin: The introduction of host tissue along with the injection material is most likely to occur when damaged needles are used. The regular changing of needles will reduce the chances of this occurring. When needle damage has obviously occurred a replacement is necessary in order to avoid possible injury to the animal and to maintain good meat hygiene and quality standards.

Irritant injections: The introduction of an irritant substance that devitalizes tissue locally can be responsible for direct or indirect damage to muscle tissue. Examples used in veterinary medicine are: basic and acidic compounds, such as the sulphonamide drugs and spectinomycin; hypertoxic preparations, e.g. long-acting oxytetracycline; and adjuvants, e.g. aluminium hydroxide, saponin.

Vasoactive substances, e.g. local anaesthetic preparations containing adrenaline and some synthetic prostaglandins, lead to ischaemic necrosis.

Contaminated skin: Pathogenic bacteria may be introduced not only when injecting cattle with a contaminated drug or when the needle or syringe is dirty but when the skin surface is not clean; the introduction of pathogens from the site of injection will occur in a proportion of cattle treated. It is therefore incumbent upon the veterinarian and the stock owner to employ hygienic injection procedures at all times using sterile equipment and uncontaminated injectable materials. Preparation of the injection site is an integral part of this hygienic approach; the avoidance of contaminated sites of injection is essential. A clean site should be chosen. If not available an area should be cleaned, or if necessary clipped and cleaned.

There are now available multidose syringes with special sterilization caps to reduce the possibility of infections. Caps can also be placed on the tops of therapeutic agents.

The recommended route of administration and the injection technique outlined in the manufacturer's instructions must be followed. The incorrect route can lead to tissue damage, e.g. drugs recommended for subcutaneous administration must not be given by the intramuscular route or intraperitoneally unless specifically indicated.

Proper restraint of the animal will lessen the likelihood of tissue damage and allow hygienic procedures to be followed. The injection of a fractious or nervous animal can lead to unnecessary suffering and damage to the animal, not to say injury to the operator also. Furthermore, struggling while injecting an animal may preclude the proper administration of the medicine with less than the prescribed dose deposited at the recommended site, the remainder forming a depot with ensuing damage. Thus all animals should be adequately restrained (see Figs 64.1 and 64.2).

Chapter 65
Alternative Medicine

C.E.I. Day

Introduction	1081
Homoeopathy	1082
Principles	1082
How to cure	1082
Conversion to veterinary application	1084
Application	1085
The challenge of herd treatment	1088
Materia medica	1088
Prescribing guide	1090
Acupuncture	1091
Theory	1092
Diagnosis	1096
Treatment	1098
Technique of needling and treatment	1101
Homoeopathy and acupuncture combined	1102
Herbal medicine	1102
Essential oils	1102
Other therapies	1103
Conclusion	1103

Introduction

Alternative medicine, in all its many modalities, was the object of a great resurgence of interest in the latter part of the twentieth century. This phenomenon is consistent with the trend towards environmental consciousness (the so-called 'green' movement), which embraces an awareness of the importance and of the mechanisms of health. A large body of consumers now recognizes the vital role played by diet in the maintenance of health. They have an awareness of the effect of additives and of residues upon the value of food items and an understanding of the potential impact of livestock medication upon the health of food animals and upon the wholesomeness of the products of animal husbandry.

As is suggested by the epithet, alternative medicine is relevant to this trend, in that it provides an 'alternative' to what has become the accepted system of medicine, modern conventional drug medicine. There are many so-called systems of alternative medicine (sometimes now described as 'complementary medicine' in an attempt to attenuate the overtones of conflict embodied in the word alternative). The wide range of such systems can present a baffling array to the casual observer, but they are united in several respects, in that they are:

- Natural, relying on no man-made chemicals for their effect;
- Able to work with and through the body's own mechanisms, stimulating the 'vital force' or 'life energy' in order to achieve health;
- Holistic, embracing the concept of mind and body as a whole in harmony with the environment, and recognizing the interaction of the whole body with each part, and the interaction of the parts with the whole body and with each other; and
- Environmentally and dietarily appropriate, since they give rise to no tissue residues in animals so treated.

Exceptions to this last point are *herbal medicine* and *aromatherapy*, in that they can give rise to residues and taints, thus making the selection and use of herbs and oils, as medicines for food-producing animals, a matter for great caution (see below).

Owing to practical considerations, there are two main systems of alternative medicine that have been developed and refined in the field of bovine medicine and that have become partially accepted by the conventional 'scientific' community. These are *homoeopathy* and *acupuncture*. Of these, the one used to the greater extent is homoeopathy, since it lends itself more easily to rapid, less specialized treatments and is applicable to herd medicine. Acupuncture is more demanding of professional time and is not appropriate to herd applications. Both are very well suited to use on organic farm units, since neither gives rise to any medicinal residues in tissues or in milk.

The title 'alternative' is more appropriate for these therapies than 'complementary', in that each is a complete system of medicine in its own right, demanding a full understanding of its principles and practice for its true value to be manifested. This should embody no contentious sentiments. The following is a brief introduction to the concepts of each of these two, followed by more medical detail. Other therapies, being less appropriate in the context of cattle medicine, are described in very brief format, in order to act as an introduction only.

Homoeopathy

Founded by a German physician, Hahnemann, in the latter part of the eighteenth century (1790), homoeopathy is a system of medicine embodying the principle '*similia similibus curentur*' meaning 'let like be cured by like'. This classical slogan is often enough in itself to deter the casual student, since it constitutes an entirely opposite stratagem to that of conventional 'school medicine'. It is hoped that the reader will keep an open mind, forming opinions only after searching and objective study into the relative merits of each strategy and the part each system may play in the overall fight against disease. The provision of an objective study requires some comparisons with the 'known' to be made, so as to shed light on the 'unknown' which homoeopathy represents.

The principle of like curing like is elevated from the status of an amusing idea or the product of a fertile imagination by the fact that it exploits a *natural law* (*The Law of Similars*). It was not an invention, therefore, that occurred in 1790 but a discovery. Hahnemann hit on his discovery as a result of objective testing of the effects of Cinchona bark (the parent material of quinine and an accepted cure for malaria even today). He dosed a healthy person (namely himself) in order to try to discover the mode of action of Cinchona bark, as he could not accept the current eighteenth-century explanation for its activity. What happened must have been a great shock to him, for he developed symptoms quite indistinguishable from malaria. Cause and effect he objectively established, by alternately withholding and restarting the administration of the substance. This led him to formulate his hypothesis: '*To cure mildly, rapidly, certainly and permanently, choose in every case of disease, a medicine which can itself produce an affection similar to that sought to be cured*' (quotation from *Organon der Heilkunst* by Hahnemann 1790, translation by Boericke & Dudgeon).

Having carried out tests (Prüfungen in German, which became translated as 'provings') on healthy volunteers, with many substances, he started to use this system of medicine on his patients. He soon found that his crude substances evoked quite serious 'aggravations' in his patients, so he proceeded to dilute the remedies. This led to the second great stumbling block for the modern, conventionally-trained observer in that his commonly used dilutions exceeded those that could reasonably be expected to contain even a single molecule of the original substance. His dilutions, called 'potencies', were often to the extent of 30c and beyond

(i.e. diluted 1/100, 30 times over) giving rise to a dilution of 10^{-60} (at 10^{-23} Avogadro's hypothesis suggests that it is unlikely that a molecule could be carried over to the next stage). What Hahnemann found, with his serial dilution and succussion method (succussion is the violent shaking of the solution at each stage of dilution), were two phenomena. Not only was the toxic power of the substance reduced at each stage (easily understandable) but also the curative power was increased (not so readily acceptable). It is a fact of life that this latter phenomenon exists and that science has not yet found the way to explain it. It therefore remains, unexplained, to puzzle the reader and sadly, in so many cases, to act as a complete blockade to further enquiry.

The big advantage of Hahnemann's discovery of the effects of extreme dilutions, made prior to any understanding of molecules and atoms, is that there can be no drug residues in meat or milk. This makes homoeopathy a front-runner in the choice of medicine for organic cattle units. Whereas herbal medicine, using the primary effects of material doses of pharmacologically active plant material, relies on achieving significant tissue concentrations of medicine, homoeopathy exploits the secondary effects (the body's reaction) for the mediation of its medicinal benefit. It depends not upon material doses but upon energy interactions. The result of this is that, as there has been a rapid growth in conversions of farms to organic status, so there has been an increasing demand for skills in farm homoeopathy, stimulating a burgeoning interest among cattle veterinarians for proper training. With the holistic discipline this study brings, cattle welfare can only be a beneficiary.

In more modern times, and in a veterinary context, clinical trials have revealed good results in many fields. Examples are *Caulophyllum* and its use in controlling porcine stillbirths (Day, 1984a), bovine mastitis prevention studies (Day, 1986), bovine dystokia prevention (Day, 1985), reduction of calf rearing losses (Mahé, 1987) and control of canine kennel cough (Day, 1987a).

Principles

A more detailed approach to veterinary homoeopathy is provided by Day (1984b, 1987b).

How to cure

Hahnemann's four steps to cure (a word he used very objectively, to indicate a removal of symptoms/signs with no further need for therapy to maintain that healthy state) were: (i) know the remedies, (ii) know the disease, (iii) match the remedy to the disease and (iv) remove the obstacles to recovery. Our objective in veterinary medicine is to *cure* disease wherever possible, and it is difficult to argue with the logic of Hahnemann's four steps. The fourth is, in particular, a little surprising in a positive way, in view of our modern culture's opinion of the soundness of eighteenth century medical beliefs and practices.

Know the remedies

A working knowledge of the 'provings' and actions of each individual 'remedy' or medicine is the basis of this stage. Obtaining this knowledge requires dedication. The remedies are written up in books of Materia Medica (e.g. Boericke, 1972; Clarke, 1982; Macleod, 1983; Vermeulen, 1997), which may run into several volumes. These books give an account of the properties of the remedies, in terms of source, general properties, 'provings' and clinical findings with applications. This represents a huge body of knowledge on each remedy's known ('proven' by Hahnemannian tests) capabilities. The information is recorded in very fine detail and for each part of the body and mind, with its assumed capabilities (from clinical data).

It is fair to say that, despite our pharmacological knowledge of modern manufactured drugs, there is not the equivalent amount of knowledge of their actions in the body and, for the most part, very little is known of a drug's possible actions apart from the major primary and local effects. It may also be fair to say that not enough pharmacodynamic studies have been made of homoeopathic remedy actions but, if research is never directed this way, that information will never accrue.

Not even the most learned veterinary homoeopath has a *full* knowledge of even the major remedies (let alone of the full range of several thousand available), since there is so much detail to be learnt. A basic knowledge of major remedies is nonetheless essential to good practice, as well as a superficial knowledge of minor remedies. The hard work and dedication required, to obtain the necessary working knowledge, discourages many would-be practitioners.

Know the disease

Since each set of symptoms and signs, displayed by each individual patient suffering disease, is a product of the individual's own reaction to a disease influence, then each disease occurrence encountered is a unique incident (Fig. 65.1).

Knowledge of each disease incident must depend, therefore, upon one's ability to discern as much as possible of its aetiology in broad terms and upon one's ability to read the symptoms/signs shown by the organism, i.e. its reaction to the disease influence. A detailed effort must therefore be made in history-taking and in clinical examination. The findings can be grouped as follows:

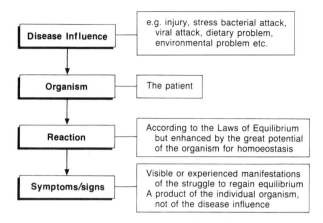

Fig. 65.1 A disease event in an animal.

(1) *Aetiological* or *historical* influences.
(2) *Generals*: symptoms/signs/properties of the whole body, e.g. build, disposition, response to environment, response to food, response to climate, etc.
(3) *Mentals*: symptoms/signs relating to the mind, e.g. demeanour, behaviour, character, responses to various mental stimuli.
(4) *Particulars*: the symptoms/signs displayed in each part of the body, in fine detail (the gleanings of a very thorough clinical examination and enquiry). Also any 'modalities' shown by these signs, e.g. 'worse when cold and wet', 'worse after food', 'better after exercise', etc.

Match the remedy to the disease

The findings of a detailed history-taking plus clinical examination and the body of knowledge contained in Materia Medica each constitute a picture that can be cross-matched, but this is often a daunting task. As each disease incident is considered to be a unique event and several thousand possible remedies exist, the task may appear impossible. Once a basic knowledge of a good number of remedies is obtained, however, then the ability of the human brain to 'compute' at high speed makes the task achievable, in an acceptable number of cases, for the conscientious student, after several years of practice and study. There are also books to aid the process, which are basically computers in print. These are called Repertories (Boericke, 1972; Kent, 1986; Schroyens, 1993) and are basically dictionaries of symptoms (in human terms) listed under 'generals', 'mentals' and 'particulars' (for each part of the body). A dedicated veterinary version of the latter is in preparation. Several remedies are then suggested (with scoring or weighting) that are able to cause the precise symptoms sought and which may therefore be applicable in the particular patient. If one lists enough symptoms and looks up each in a Repertory, the highest scoring remedy (in theoretical terms at least) is the ideal choice. Resort to the Materia Medica will then help to confirm or negate this choice. Obviously, this is a fairly long-winded process and, although helpful in difficult cases, it is not applicable to rapid, on-farm selection of remedies. Thus, for practical clinical application, a basic knowledge of the remedies is required, together with a practised ability to think rapidly in 'picture' format. No equivalent veterinary Repertory yet exists although, in slightly differing form, help can be found in books by MacLeod (1981, 1983), Brock and Nielsen (1986) and Day (1984b, 1987b). Each of these works gives an easily assimilated guide to remedy choices under given conditions, but (therefore?) is less accurate. Computer programs are being developed for this type of work but, again, are not applicable to practical, on-farm use, with the presently available technology.

Remove the obstacles to recovery

Even in the early stages of the twenty-first century, the insight of Hahnemann in the eighteenth century is remarkable. The single most exceptional example of futuristic perspicacity is in the concept of 'removal of obstacles to recovery'. In trying to observe this fourth provision for cure, very modern ideas must be embraced. Not only must there be obvious remedial efforts, such as splinting or fixation of fractures, dietary investigation and correction, removal of an obstructive foreign body from the bowel, etc. but also, in the herd context, the myriad parameters (environmental, management, dietary, etc.) affecting herd health must be considered. The idea that herd factors are important has been practised by forward-thinking veterinarians for *only the last 40 or so years*. However, Hahnemann made clear provision for it 200 years ago. Sadly, however, the most stringent efforts to improve the husbandry of modern cattle farms will never provide truly *ideal* environmental and nutritional conditions for the animals, although meticulous attention to detail can approach the ideal. Thus, however much effort is applied, one is presented, in modern dairy cattle practice, with an imperfectly fulfilled provision for real cure (Hahnemann's definition). This explains the need, sometimes experienced on intensive farms, for repeated medication (or possibly even continuous, in some of the worst examples), but this must not be an excuse for lack of effort. The unattainability of perfection must not be an excuse for failure to achieve the best conditions possible for the cattle nor for failure of removal, to a maximum possible extent, of the obstacles to recovery.

Conversion to veterinary application

Homoeopathic medicine was developed in humans for humans and therefore presents some difficulties in conversion to veterinary practice. The difficulties can be summarized as:

- Lack of speech in animal patients;
- Interspecies differences in reaction to remedies;
- Lack of family history; and
- Intensivism in farm management.

Hahnemann (1814) did, however, advocate its use in animals and so veterinary homoeopathy has a long tradition.

Lack of speech

The lack of speech in animal patients leads to the loss of a large range of symptoms which would be of value to the prescriber in human medicine. The ability to detail *mental symptoms and feelings* is lost, but much of what is needed in that respect can be discerned by extrapolation from the demeanour and behaviour of the patient. However, the finer details of how the mind is affected by the disease influence, or why it responds in the way it does, cannot be determined. Only the end result of behaviour is seen rather than the mental processes behind that behaviour. Since the mental symptoms of disease are a sure guide to the unique individual response to disease, by each patient, a large proportion of diagnostic (remedy-selecting) parameters is therefore lost to the veterinary prescriber. However, deductions about mental symptoms, extrapolated from the external behavioural signs, can provide an invaluable guide to the sensitive observer. Lack of speech also deprives us of the enormous field of *subjective* symptoms. The adjectives used by human patients to describe pain symptoms are legion. They are again an expression of the individuality of each disease incident and are therefore invaluable. Descriptions of pain such as 'tearing', 'cutting', 'burning ', 'aching', etc. are all lost in veterinary medicine. Also hidden, among these symptoms, is the headache in its many forms. We can rarely even diagnose headache in animals, let alone describe it. Approximately 100 pages of Kent's Repertory (1986) are devoted to headache, showing its importance to the prescribing physician.

Interspecies difference

It is not unreasonable to suppose that different species of animals will react differently to the medicines, when compared with *human* reactions. There will also be differences between the individual domestic species. To reconstruct the painstaking 'provings' of Hahnemann and his followers, for each remedy for each species, would involve several laboratories for many generations, then only with an enormous usage of laboratory animals. This exercise would ethically be unjustifiable. Despite the obvious existence of such a problem, as shown by the varying toxicology and pharmacology, known in different species, for many poisons (Garner, 1967), drugs (Daykin, 1960) and foods, homoeopathy is largely transferable *en bloc*. This is a fortunate fact but one that should never be taken for granted. Thus the astute practitioner of the art will need to be aware of the possibility of failure due to species difference and will use pharmacological and toxicological knowledge to advantage.

Lack of family history

Although not strictly applicable to units where pedigree breeding and recording has gone on down the years, the lack of family history of bovine patients, particularly in terms of disease, will lead to loss of some accuracy in prescribing. Known line susceptibilities are an important factor in choosing remedies in such conditions as cancer, mastitis, lameness, etc., but the loss of some of this material is not likely to be as deleterious, to effective veterinary prescribing, as the lack of speech and the potential interspecies differences.

Intensive farming

This factor has been discussed previously (see. p. 955).

Application

Disease can affect an animal to a greater or lesser depth and, therefore, so can the so-called remedies of homoeopathy, since they are also 'disease-producing agents' when administered to a healthy body. These different levels of prescribing can be classified as:

(1) Pathological
(2) Local
(3) Organ-specific
(4) Constitutional
(5) Facilitative /regulatory
(6) Detoxifying
(7) Historical
(8) Specific and
(9) Preventive

These terms require explanation, since their usage in this context is peculiar to homoeopathy alone.

Pathological

To prescribe at the pathological level, one needs to be satisfied that the disease influence has evoked an acute and easily identifiable disease process, that could be easily matched to the actions of a particular remedy. The effects of *traumatic injury*, for instance, are very well covered by the properties of arnica. The administration of arnica, as rapidly as possible after the traumatic insult, will swiftly and effectively initiate a healing process that will reduce the pain, shock, haemorrhage, tissue fluid accumulation and resultant tissue damage that normally follows trauma. The net result is a happier patient, less distortion at the site of injury and, more importantly, less disturbance to the circulation in the area. Therefore there is more effective and rapid restoration of normal tissue integrity and structure. There is also a powerful and often underestimated antiseptic effect of this remedy.

The fact that one remedy covers this process is very convenient for the prescriber and very helpful to the patient. It removes the need to apply the full rigours of the homoeopathic method, in times of emergency. Furthermore, this pathological level of prescribing provides a simple proving ground for homoeopathy to the sceptic and a useful starting point for learning the first steps of the homoeopathic method. Other commonly used remedy/pathological indication pairings are:

Hypericum:	injury to areas rich in nerve endings (e.g. in digit, tail, etc.), injury to nerves, painful grazes, photosensitization
Ledum:	puncture wounds
Aconitum:	sudden shock to the mind or body, sudden disturbances of the body's equilibrium (e.g. sudden-onset fever, sudden haemorrhage)
Calendula:	open wounds – antiseptic and promotes healing

Local

One would apply this level of prescribing when the nature of the disease is acute and fairly superficial, to an otherwise healthy animal with a robust constitution. Examples of this application are: acute-onset mastitis (see p. 326) resulting from a chill, where aconitum is useful, New Forest eye infection (see p. 919), where mercurius corrosivus may be effective, and foul-in-the-foot infection (see p. 426), where hepar sulphuris could be the correct remedy. To prescribe effectively for these conditions, one only needs to take note of the local presenting signs and match these to a remedy. One does not need, again, to delve into the deeper homoeopathic method, discussed in previous pages, in order to achieve a good result. However, it is vital to ensure that the disease is not chronic in nature or an acute exacerbation of an underlying chronic disorder. If this should prove to be the case, satisfactory results will not follow from employment of this simplified technique and one would need to apply the constitutional approach (see below).

Organ-specific

Organ-specific remedies may be used when one organ is particularly embarrassed in an illness, when it is considered important to support that organ. Some remedies have a particular affinity for specific organs or tissues and the most important are:

Rhus toxicodendron:	muscles
Ruta graveolens:	tendons, ligaments, joint capsules, aponeuroses, periosteum
Hypericum:	nerve fibres
Symphytum:	bone
Nux vomica:	liver
Flor de piedra:	liver
Lycopodium:	liver
Berberis:	liver, kidney
Kali chloratum:	kidney
Digitalis:	heart

Constitutional

The concept of a 'constitution' embodies everything that is unique to an individual organism. It embraces the idea of the 'programmed' nature of each body's response to a disease influence. Another way to consider this is to think of predetermined tendencies in each individual. Response to disease is determined by a number of factors: genetic make-up inherited from the parents, *in utero* influences during pregnancy, the birth process, postnatal influences, influences during the growing period and influences during adulthood. In the farm context, one can see how breeding, pregnancy, calving, rearing and general management or dietary regimens can affect the make-up of an adult cow. By reading the response pattern of the animal (signs and symptoms) in the face of disease or situations, and by studying her conformation and behaviour, one can formulate an idea of her 'constitutional type'. This whole picture can be matched to a whole remedy picture, as previously discussed. Not many remedies have a combination of wide enough or deep enough effects on the body to rank as constitutional remedies and, in the world of cattle, the major nine examples can be listed, conveniently classified into three groups:

Aurum Pulsatilla Sepia	Corresponding to a great many cows that suffer typically female or hormonal problems as a rule
Antimonium crudum Nux vomica Lycopodium	Fitting those cattle that suffer digestive or liver problems
Calcarea carbonica Calcarea phosphorica Phosphorus	Matching those cows suffering from lactation-induced disorders

These generalizations are too sweeping to be strictly followed but the pictures of the remedies listed above are suitable to be grouped in the way shown. These are 'big' remedies (Hahnemann's so-called polycrests) and have wide-ranging effects on all parts of the body. They cannot, therefore, be type-cast purely in the roles shown above, but the groupings are useful nonetheless. The groupings represent trends in the relevant animal's disease response patterns and are very useful for short-listing of remedies. These and other useful remedies will be discussed later (see pp. 1088–1090), in fuller detail.

In the case of a patient affected by chronic disease, no real cure can follow treatment unless this method of prescribing is followed. The organism has learnt, in the case of chronic disease, to live in a state of uneasy harmony with the disease. The animal is therefore unable to regain health, often lost a long time previously, unless the deep, powerful and most appropriate stimulus of true holistic constitutional homoeopathy is prescribed.

Facilitative/regulatory

The facilitative level of prescribing exploits the ability of certain 'potentized' substances to facilitate metabolism with respect to those substances. Examples are the use of 'potencies' of calcium phosphoricum to facilitate metabolism with respect to calcium and phosphorus, magnesium phosphoricum to help magnesium metabolism, and cuprum metallicum to assist copper metabolism. It is well known that so-called mineral deficiencies are rarely absolute deficiencies but can be more often a malfunction of the relevant absorptive, metabolic and eliminative processes for that mineral. Cases of 'relative' excesses and deficiencies can both be helped by such methods. In the case of a hormone disturbance, a 'potency' of the hormone may help regulate and balance the body with respect to that hormone.

Detoxifying

The detoxifying method of prescribing echoes very closely the preceding remarks. Should a specific substance be causing a toxic effect, e.g. alkaloid, metal, chemical, etc., then the body's natural ability to break down and/or eliminate such toxins will be enhanced by the administration of the specific substance, or a close relative, in 'potency' (homoeopathic dilution). Examples are the use of plumbum in cases of lead toxicity, coumarin or melilotus in cases of warfarin toxicity, opium or nux vomica in cases of anaesthetic toxicity or even of carbohydrate overdose in the ruminant. Such methods have often been shown to produce unexpected results, even in extreme cases of toxicity.

Historical

The historical method of prescribing utilizes the body's ability to respond to an appropriate curative homoeopathic stimulus, long after the initial disease-producing influence has subsided, should the body still be suffering from the effects of that influence. Examples are: using arnica long after an initial traumatic insult, should the body still be suffering disease from that injury; using aconitum long after a mental or physical shock, if the body is still suffering effects or fears produced by that shock; using a 'specific' remedy (see below) long after a specific infectious disease has passed its acute phase, should the body still be suffering effects from that disease.

All that is necessary, in order to utilize this method, is to detect, in a chronic disease situation, a facet of the history that leads one to believe that the current disease has its origins in a specific historic incident. One can then treat for that incident, as if it were in the here and now, even though it may have occurred years previously.

Specific

The specific method of prescribing would usually be used in an acute infectious disease context, where a known specific infectious disease agent is involved. Generally speaking, this method of treatment would imply use of *nosodes* (remedies made from disease material). Examples are: mastitis nosode in cases of mastitis (see Chapter 23), infectious bovine rhinotracheitis (IBR) nosode in cases of IBR (see p. 286), bovine virus diarrhoea (BVD) nosode in cases of BVD (see p. 853) or salmonella nosode in cases of salmonellosis. In the acute phase of an infectious disease, it may be dangerous to use the nosode in an attempt to produce a cure. For this reason, this form of therapy is usually reserved for use during the recovery phase of the disease, in order to prevent any tendency for the disease to become chronic. During the acute phase it is always better to select an appropriate homoeopathic remedy for cure, according to the Law of Similars in the usual way. This implies that, in each case of acute spe-

cific disease, there will be no remedy specific to the disease but a whole host of possible remedies, the most suitable of which must be selected for each patient. Having said this, it is possible that baptisia could be specific to salmonellosis (Chapter 15), mercurius cyanatus to calf diphtheria (see p. 250), mercurius corrosivus to New Forest eye or even borax to foot-and-mouth disease (see Chapter 43(c)) (in those countries in which it is permitted to treat this disease).

Preventive

In herd medicine it is very important to apply preventive principles, in order to minimize or to obviate the risk of spread of a known or predicted infectious disease within the herd. This is the basis of effective veterinary involvement on the modern bovine farm unit. In an individual animal context, it is important to prevent disease occurring in the face of a predictable challenge or disease-producing event.

The greatest demands on the veterinarian using homoeopathy are on a herd basis. Where infectious disease has either entered the herd, in which case the healthy individuals must be protected, or is threatening the herd, in which case the whole herd must be protected, one would select for prevention a specific remedy. This would generally be a *nosode* (see Specific prescribing, above) although it could be any remedy from the homoeopathic Materia Medica that the prescriber feels specific enough to a certain disease (see Prescribing guide, p. 1091). In conventional medicine one would be reaching for a vaccine in this context, but in the case of some infectious diseases, no effective vaccine is available or no vaccine exists at all. Nosodes may be considered as if they were vaccines, if it helps the reader to understand the principle of their application in this context. However, they do not produce any antibody response in the treated animal, due to the extreme dilutions in which they are usually used (30c). Neither do nosodes carry the potential hazards that vaccination sometimes can, e.g. strain 19 *Brucella abortus* vaccine (Day, 1986, 1987b).

These preventive remedies, in order to be swiftly, effectively and easily applied to the whole group at risk, may be administered via the drinking water. Water troughs should be as clean as possible and should be large enough or well enough supplied with water, so as not to run dry on the day of dosing. The quantity of remedy used does not appear to be very critical but an easy guide is to use 5 ml per drinking trough, unless the trough is unusually large or small. Frequency of dosing would depend upon the estimated properties of the challenge. In an enzootic disease situation within the herd, the frequency would be selected corresponding to the estimated violence and virulence of the disease and according to the animals' estimated ability to withstand it. At times of high risk, when the disease agent is perhaps given the upper hand by management factors or by climate or the animal is compromised by similar factors, then one would dose more frequently. In the case of assumed risk from an epizootic disease, i.e. a disease not yet met by the herd, dosing could be more sporadic.

The second sphere of use of the preventive technique is in the case of the individual animal, which may be threatened by a predictable disease challenge. Thus with impending parturition, caulophyllum could be used to help prevent problems (Day, 1985, 1987b), or for an anticipated stressful journey, aconitum could be used in advance of the challenge. Incidentally, aconitum can be used on a group or herd basis, in order to prevent the production losses consequent on herd stress, such as the periodic tuberculin test.

Thus it can be seen that the application of the homoeopathic method has come a long way, since it was first devised in humans some 200 years ago. Although the rigorous and in-depth diagnostic and prescribing processes may daunt the novice, the classification into different levels at which the method can be applied in bovine medicine makes it easier to start out. They provide scope, for even the newly initiated and hesitant prescriber, to test the principles of homoeopathy and its efficacy at an easier level, without immediately being committed to long-term study or to large and therefore expensive stocks of medicines.

The challenge of herd treatment

Much has been made, in the foregoing pages, of the need to individualize therapy for best results. This high ideal is frankly not practical in a herd or group situation. If we consider, for instance, a group of calves suffering from pneumonia, treating each on an individual basis is not possible. What is needed is a modification of principles, while maintaining the essence of homoeopathic philosophy and methodology. This short section can only be a summary of the techniques involved, in order to show the options. Clearly, homoeopathy will not be a practical therapy on the farm if it is not adaptable to herd applications.

A detailed account of how this can be done is to be found in the Further reading section (Day, 1999). In essence, there are six main possibilities:

(1) To choose a single similimum (a homoeopathic medicine which is similar to the signs and symptoms displayed) for the entire group. This will only be properly effective in an epizootic situation, in which all individuals are likely to be similarly affected.

(2) To select a combination of remedies for the group. This will allow the incorporation of the spectrum of signs shown by the different individuals. A maximum of three different remedies should be incorporated.

(3) To select a number of different remedies (maximum of three) to stimulate the individuals at different levels, as in the foregoing section. A 'constitutional' remedy, say, could work alongside a 'specific' remedy and a 'local' prescription.

(4) A single constitutional prescription may be possible, especially if the group all come from one family or from one breeding line.

(5) A specific or nosode prescription could be selected, as in the above section. This can be very successful in the case of a known infective disease and lessens the need for more detailed homoeopathic knowledge or skill.

(6) The group could be 'repertorized', as if it were a single animal. The technique would be as outlined in the section describing how to match the remedy to the disease. This is an advanced technique and should not be tackled without experience.

The reference given describes how these techniques are compatible with proper homoeopathic philosophy and principles.

Materia medica

There follows a brief summary of the properties of some of the homoeopathic remedies most commonly used in a farm context and some of their possible clinical applications. This is not intended to be an exhaustive source on the subject but an introduction to these 30 useful remedies. Fuller works on this material can be found in the Further reading section. Remedies are presented in alphabetical order for simplicity, not in order of importance nor grouped according to possible application. The way in which these remedies are presented shows the emphasis placed upon the 'picture' presented by the disease rather than upon its usual *name*. Remedies are taken from the plant kingdom, animal kingdom and minerals and are available in tablet, pillule, crystal, powder, tincture, injection, cream, ointment or lotion forms. The thirtieth centesimal (30c) potency is a useful potency of most remedies, for the purposes of beginners.

Aconitum napellus: this is a remedy suitable for use in cases of sudden shock (physical or mental in nature), sudden-onset fevers, disorders from chilling and cold winds, and in cases of profuse bright red haemorrhage.

Affected animals tend to shudder in response to fear or shock, display a rapid pulse, run a fever and suffer conjunctivitis with fluid lacrimation and nasal discharge. Symptoms tend to centre on the chest, so use in 'shipping fever' is an obvious application (see p. 286).

Antimonium tartaricum: this remedy is particularly suited to respiratory signs. Indications are mucoid, rattly breathing or coughing, frothy saliva and a tendency to cyanosis. Animals display minimal thirst and a rapid, weak pulse. Cold, damp weather aggravates the condition and affected animals are unwilling to lie on their sides. This remedy is one of several useful pneumonia remedies and should be considered in cases of fog fever (see p. 866).

Apis mellifica: it is useful in cases characterized by oedema. Urine retention, pulmonary oedema, oedematous swellings of vulva/perineum or udder, ascites, cystic ovaries, etc. may all respond if concomitant signs agree. The patient is usually thirstless and prefers cool open air. Cold bathing of affected areas produces comfort.

Arnica montana: this is a remedy of use in *all* conditions arising from trauma. Bruising, haematoma formation, pain, swelling, shock and even resultant local infection will respond to treatment. Patients often display a fear of being touched.

Arsenicum album: this remedy is a polycrest and therefore of constitutional importance. Restlessness, chilliness and thirst characterize the patient. The remedy can be useful, on a more local basis, in cases of diarrhoea, dehydration and collapse, if concomitant signs agree. Diarrhoea is usually profuse, watery and offensive-smelling.

Belladonna (genus: *Atropa*): a 'fever' remedy, this is useful in cases where there is an acute febrile or inflammatory state characterized by heat, redness, swelling, fullness and pain. The pulse may be full and bounding. There are often delirious or convulsive signs too. The animal is usually thirsty and displays a dilated pupil. Symptoms tend to centre on the chest, making a useful distinction from the usual pattern of *aconitum*.

Bryonia alba: this remedy has an affinity for serous membranes. All suitable conditions are worsened by movement, so a major sign in the affected animal is unwillingness to move. Affected animals are thirsty for long cold drinks. Guided by these three points one may prescribe confidently in cases of pneumonia, mastitis, arthritis, peritonitis, etc. The pneumonic calf will stand still, despite its fear, and will tend to lie on its affected side to prevent movement. The mastitic cow would allow herself and her hot swollen painful udder to be examined, rather than move away.

Calcarea carbonica: another polycrest, this remedy has constitutional applications. Disorders of production are an indication, e.g. fertility, lameness, mastitis. The animal has a heavy skeletal structure, large limbs, large joints and large feet. It usually has a good condition score and is generally peaceful but dominant. Movements tend to be unhurried. The appetite is very good and, if a milking cow, the milk yield is high. The animal is susceptible to chilling and usually shows catarrhal-type responses from the mucous membranes.

Calcarea phosphorica: a polycrest, this remedy is suited to similar conditions to *calcarea carbonica* and the typical animal is similar, although lighter in skeletal structure, quicker

in movement and responses, difficult to handle and more fearful.

Carbo vegetabilis: abdominal distension by gas, flatus, flatulent colic, weakness of circulation and musculature, poor resistance to infection and even collapse characterize this remedy. Its main application is in the treatment of the cold, collapsed individual, in whom its results can be spectacular. It has been dubbed the 'homoeopathic corpse reviver', on account of its prowess in such cases.

Caulophyllum thalyctroides: one of the Native North Americans' so-called 'squaw-root' remedies, it has great application in all disorders of labour, at any stage (Day, 1984a, 1985). It also has an effect on shifting lamenesses, particularly if the origin is in the small joints.

Colocynthis (genus: *Cucumis* or *Citrullus*): this remedy is of particular use in colic. The abdomen is distended and the back arched. Animals will roll and kick at the belly in cramp-like paroxysms.

Hepar sulphuris: if any homoeopathic remedy could be said to fill the role of antibiotics in septic conditions, then this is the one. Suppurative processes in their early stages respond well. In suitable cases, there is always great sensitivity to pain, with relief from warm applications. Pain is aggravated by the least touch. Joint-ill and navel-ill usually respond (see pp. 249, 255).

Hypericum perforatum: injury to nerves or to areas rich in nerve endings is an indication for this remedy. It has a very rapid healing effect, both on the pain and on the physical damage. Not surprisingly (on account of modern knowledge of the physiology involved and of the symptoms) the lesions and pain of photosensitization also respond well (see p. 884).

Lycopodium clavatum: a polycrest, this remedy has an application constitutionally. With an affinity for the liver, the remedy is often used in this context. Possible digestive disturbance, dry, withered appearance to the skin, tendency to flatus, abdominal distension, liver dysfunction, dyspnoea, tachypnoea, movement of the nostrils with every breath and an overall anxiety distinguish this animal type in disease. Problems are often right-sided and the animal prefers warmer water to drink (if offered).

Mercurius cyanatus: a thirsty patient with a paradoxically wet mouth and possibly even drooling saliva may require a mercury-type remedy. *Mercurius cyanatus* patients display offensive breath, offensive-smelling ulceration of mouth and throat and swollen glands. The picture fits that of calf diphtheria.

Mercurius solubilis: as with all mercury remedies, there is a tendency to thirst, to profuse salivation, to offensive breath, to swollen glands in the throat and to ulceration of mouth, bowel or teats. Ulcers will discharge pus. If there is diarrhoea, there will also be a degree of tenesmus. Since the remedy is a polycrest, it has constitutional applications. The preceding disease tendencies in a dominant, usually heavy, animal are an indication for its use.

Nux vomica: as a polycrest, it has wide application in a constitutional context in the bovine. Patients tend to be dull and sluggish in movements, with paradoxically rapid or violent reactions when disturbed, bad tempered and thin. They suffer digestive complaints, characterized by cessation of rumen function and a tendency to constipation, having hard knotty stools. Some cases of 'acid' or fermentative diarrhoea may respond and complaints following from overeating of concentrate will respond well. Conditions tend to be worse in the morning and worse for disturbance or chilling (Mahé, 1987).

Phosphoric acid: in common with all the 'acids', phosphoric acid is indicated in cases of general weakness. More specifically there is debility, dehydration, pale flatulent painless diarrhoea with a dry mouth, thirst and possibly a degree of jaundice.

Phosphorus: because of its extent of action, it is a polycrest and therefore of great value in a constitutional context. Phosphorus conditions are characterized by sudden onset and by their serious nature, e.g. sudden-onset pneumonia, sudden haemorrhages, hepatitis, haematogenous jaundice, etc. The phosphorus animal is also 'sudden' in temperament, being averse to separation from the rest of the herd and apt to panic. The type is of lean build and averse to handling. Conditions are worse for touch and change of weather.

Phytolacca americana: this is the remedy above all others with a reputation in mastitis. This reputation can lead to overuse in this context, as it will only produce results when used in the correct homoeopathic manner. Lymph glands and mammary glands become indurated swollen and painful. There is usually heat too. Milk becomes thickened, stringy and yellowish. Cold wet weather aggravates the symptoms.

Pulsatilla nigricans: this is a common constitutional type in the bovine, particularly in the case of heifers. The type is shy, feminine in appearance, suffers catarrhal complaints and has little thirst. Breeding problems respond well, if it is used in the correct constitutional context. Catarrhal syndromes of respiratory tract, udder, reproductive tract, etc. are typical. The animal prefers fresh, open air and symptoms are aggravated by warm, stuffy atmospheres and in the evening.

Pyrogenium: fevers, particularly those of a septic nature, respond well to this remedy, especially if pulse and temperature are not in agreement. In suitable cases, there is a tendency to toxaemia, offensive secretions, dark blood and offensive, dark-coloured, septic lesions.

Rhus toxicodendron: American poison ivy (the source of this remedy) produces, and is therefore able to help, severe pruritic conditions or conditions characterized by rheumatic or arthritic stiffness and pains with great thirst and an aggravation from cold, wet or damp conditions. Skin lesions are often vesicular in nature, resembling cowpox lesions. Musculoskeletal problems are further characterized by an aggravation when moving from rest, with a subsequent 'loosening' and easing of the stiffness and pain. Suitable diarrhoea cases display dysentery and tenesmus.

Ruta graveolens: with an affinity for fibrous structural tissues such as ligaments, tendons, joint capsules and perios-teum, this remedy is a powerful aid in the treatment of sprains and other damage to such tissues and regions of the body.

Sabina (juniperus): sabina's main sphere of activity is the uterus, where bloody discharges and lack of tone may respond. It is not indicated where sepsis exists. Retained fetal membranes may also be expelled under its influence.

Sepia: a polycrest, sepia has great value as a bovine constitutional remedy. It is predominantly of use in a female context. Lack of tone and lack of tautness typify the conditions and the constitutional type suited by this remedy. The animal takes on a worn-out, tired, sagging appearance and so, also, do individual body regions, e.g. uterus/perineum, limbs, udder, etc. Venous congestion and tendency to prolapse are also characteristic. Fertility problems may respond, if constitutional aspects agree.

Silica: Better known for its ability to stimulate expulsion of foreign bodies from the tissues or to awaken chronic low-grade inflammatory lesions, silica is also a great constitutional remedy. Structural weakness and distortion, whether of skeleton or feet, with a poor immune response, typify the animal able to respond to the remedy.

Thuja occidentalis: The reputation of this remedy rests mostly on its action on papillomatous lesions (p. 882), especially when they occur on neck or abdomen. Ill-effects of vaccination also may respond. The constitutional and other effects of the remedy are not so important in cattle work.

Urtica urens: The lesions of nettle rash are well known to everyone, as is the pain that follows. The remedy is of value in such conditions. Apart from these properties, the remedy has the ability, in high potency, to promote milk flow and, in low potency, to induce suppression of milk. This dual regulatory power gives the remedy great value in bovine medicine. Lesions respond favourably to warm applications and negatively to cold applications, so too does the mastitis helped by urtica.

It is hoped that the foregoing brief account of 30 remedies will allow a start to be made in homoeopathic prescribing. It cannot be expected that, in so few pages, it will provide a comprehensive knowledge of the remedies. The reader must also realize that these few remedies, although forming a good nucleus of prescribing material, actually represent only a fraction of what is available. For each condition or syndrome mentioned, a great many other remedies have a potential value, should they prove to have properties 'similar' to the problem.

Prescribing guide

There follows a small vade-mecum, showing some indicated remedies that may prove effective in the named syndrome. Please be reminded that true homoeopathy does not rely upon the name of a condition for remedy selection but upon the similarity between disease picture and remedy picture, on as many counts as possible. The following list only serves as a pointer to some commonly indicated remedies. Final selection between those remedies mentioned (and many not mentioned) rests with the prescriber. All the remedies mentioned below appear in the preceding section, so that section can act as a brief guide to help selection of the most relevant remedy. (Remedies may be given orally, by injection, topically or orally via the drinking water.)

Acetonaemia (p. 793)	*Lycopodium, nux vomica*
Arthritis (pp. 454–458)	*Bryonia, caulophyllum, phytolacca, rhus tox., ruta graveolens*
Bloat (p. 832)	*Carbo veg., lycopodium, nux vomica*
Calf diphtheria (pp. 250, 822)	*Mercurius cyanatus*
Constipation	*Nux vomica, sepia*
Convulsions	*Belladonna, nux vomica*
Dystokia (Day, 1984a, 1985)	*Caulophyllum, pulsatilla*
Fever	*Aconitum, belladonna, pyrogenium*
Foul-in-the-foot (p. 426)	*Hepar sulphuris*
Haemorrhage	*Aconitum, arnica, phosphorus*
Infertility (Chapter 36)	*Apis mell., aurum, pulsatilla, sepia*
Injury (Chapter 32)	*Aconitum, arnica, calendula, hypericum, ledum, rhus tox., ruta grav., symphytum*
Joint ill (pp. 249, 255)	*Hepar sulphuris*
Ketosis (p. 793)	See Acetonaemia
Mastitis (Day, 1986) (Chapter 23)	*Aconitum, belladonna, bryonia, carbo veg., hepar sulphuris, mercurius sol., phytolacca, silica, urtica*
Metritis (Chapter 34)	*Caulophyllum, pulsatilla, pyrogenium, sabina, sepia*
Navel ill (p. 249)	*Hepar sulphuris, silica*
Papillomatosis (p. 882)	*Thuja*
Placenta (retained) (Chapter 34)	*Caulophyllum, sabina, sepia*
Pneumonia (Chapters 17, 49)	*Aconitum, antimonium tart., bryonia, lycopodium, phosphorus, pyrogenium*

This list is far from complete and is aimed at providing an insight and a starting platform, for deeper homoeopathic prescribing and learning.

Having read this guide to the principles of homoeopathy and having tried out some of the methods and suggestions contained in this chapter, it is hoped that the reader will go on to further study and will venture into more ambitious prescribing, from a position of confidence. Books giving a greater depth of homoeopathic knowledge are listed in the Further reading section and accredited courses in Britain, on veterinary homoeopathy, are conducted under the auspices of the Faculty of Homoeopathy, 15 Clerkenwell Close, London EC1R 0AA. The Faculty has an examination structure, for postgraduate qualifications. On an international basis, the Faculty does help courses in other countries, and the International Association for Veterinary Homoeopathy both runs courses and sets examinations for veterinary homoeopathy.

Acupuncture

Acupuncture is a science of energy medicine, having its origins in ancient China anything up to 4000 years ago. The oldest medical textbook known, the *Huang Ti Nei Jing Su Wen* (Veith, 1972), may have originally been written as long ago as 1000 BC. Its origins are confused, since it has undergone many alterations and commentaries since it was first written. (In fact the *Su Wen* was possibly a later addition to a scaled down *Nei Jing*.) This book has formed the basis of traditional Chinese medicine theory down the centuries, but there have been myriad adaptations and variations applied since its inception, giving rise to traditional Chinese medicine as we know it today. Acupuncture is but a component of this, Chinese herbalism also forming an integral part, along with moxibustion (the application of heat). The practice of traditional Chinese medicine is truly holistic, in that it embraces an understanding of the part played by diet and lifestyle in the health of the individual and it makes a positive effort to optimize these, as an integral part of therapy.

The Chinese have long treated animals with acupuncture, so our veterinary use of this in the West is no new thing. Dogs, cats, horses, cattle and other farm animals can be treated. In countries other than Britain, working animals such as elephants, llamas, donkeys, camels and buffalo are patients. In the UK, acupuncture is much more widely used on dogs and cats than in horses, and more in horses than in cattle. This is more a function of the pattern of specialization in the veterinary profession and that more interest has been shown by those veterinarians who are in small animal practice, than a reflection of the efficacy and value of acupuncture in cattle. Cattle respond very well to the methods but chronic disease is less a feature of bovine medicine than in the other species. This means that there is less call for a specialist second opinion than in equine or pet medicine. The call for acupuncture help in cattle is reduced, compared with the other species, since the species is kept more on a financial (productivity) basis than for emotional, competitive or recreational reasons. The reality is that there is less perceived value in the individual as a result.

Acupuncture is a system of *internal* medicine devised, in ancient times, purely from the outside of the body. In ancient China, the human body was not to be violated, either in life or in death, so post-mortem examinations and anatomical or physiological studies were not performed. The basis of the system is the relationship of points on the surface of the body to the internal organs and their integrated functions. The mechanism of the relationship is not clear to Western science and is unquestioned in the East, where such a different philosophy of life and living pertains as to be incomparable. Clearly, as far as some of the acupuncture points are concerned, there is a cutaneous–visceral reflex at work but this does not satisfactorily explain the mechanism of acupuncture, any more than does the discovery of the release of endorphins or opioids in response to treatments. Our Western way of looking at life leads to a linear thought process, trying to establish 'cause and effect', and an attempt to rationalize, classify and compartmentalize in a way that does not sit well with the oriental philosophy and method.

The Chinese discovered, empirically, a collection of points (some 700 forming the basis of the system) that related to bodily function and to disease patterns or pictures. In order to explain the indisputable facts and verifiable correlations so discovered, they wove a web of philosophical concepts, in harmony, of course, with their philosophy of life (so turning an empirical art into a science). In ancient China, and still today, medical lore, religion and their way of life are inextricably entangled and form a unity not found in any comparable form in Western culture, where it seems that all three tend to be considered as separate entities. This chapter does not argue which view may be the more correct, valid or healthy, but merely presents comparisons.

The philosophical lattice work, developed so long ago, is not there to confuse the would-be student but to explain and elucidate the empirical findings. This is not apparent to the sceptical Western observer, who will undoubtedly find the concepts not only confusing but amphigoric. Atavism and Taoism are indigenous to the oriental way of thinking and are totally foreign to us. However, acupuncture was devised in the East and developed in the light of oriental concepts. It must be taken or left at face value, at present, until some more readily assimilable theory may be formulated that can explain the observable phenomena as well as the original. This development is not in the offing. It is hoped that by presenting a rapid overview of the theory and philosophy, it will not confuse the reader but will serve to give an introduction to the principles and methods of traditional acupuncture and encourage the diligent student to look further into the subject.

Theory

The theory of the science of acupuncture is based upon concepts of energy and forces which are rooted in Taoist philosophy. In this there exists no linear thinking, no cause and effect. The order and pattern of life (and therefore disease, which is a part of life) and of the universe are governed by principles of inevitability. Concepts are not placed one under the other in a deductive sequence or subsumption, but side by side in a picture. Events follow each other, not by cause and effect but by a kind of inductance. Light does not cause darkness and vice versa, one becomes or leads to the other inevitably. Similarly, the concept of light cannot exist without a concept of darkness, nor the concept of good without that of evil.

It has been said of Taoism that it does not deny reason, but that it remains just beyond its grasp. It is a concept of balance, of rhythm, of sustainability, of harmony. It describes a complex web of interrelationships, in which the whole is dependent upon and affected by its parts and in which each part is dependent upon and affected by the whole and each of the other parts. There is an essential understanding of flux, of dynamism and of interconnectedness.

The two forces that maintain the universe, and the life within in it, are called *Yin* and *Yang* and represent philosophical polarities. They are the eternal opposites. They are aligned to other pairings of polarities, ranging over the whole of our existence. Examples are, respectively, dark and light, cold and hot, female and male, low and high, sluggish and fast, lower and upper, night and day, soft and hard, earth and heaven, light and heavy, passive and active, inside and outside, empty and full, water and fire, weak and strong, under- and overactivity, humble and exalted, front and back (more logical in quadruped terms than in the human biped, i.e. ventral and dorsal, in that dorsal is higher, therefore representing Yang) and so forth. It should be becoming clear that these two polarities act both simultaneously and antagonistically within the universe (and within its microcosm, the body). There is, however, no absolute in life and so with Yin and Yang. There is no Yin without Yang. They are forever transforming into one another, on an almost imperceptible basis. Nothing is all Yin, nothing is all Yang. All systems are composed of Yin and Yang. Within Yin there is Yang and within Yang there is Yin. Within any given Yin/Yang system under discussion, there is a further yin/yang system and, within that, another. This applies over and over, *ad infinitum*. Zou Yen, the philosopher of the third century BC, observed: '*Heaven is high, the earth is low, and thus they*

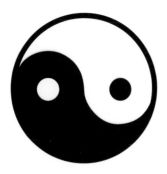

Fig. 65.2 The Taoist *T'ai Chi T'u* symbol.

Table 65.1 The paired (tsang/fu) organs, relating to Yin and Yang.

Yin (*tsang* organ, ventrally/medially-routed meridian)	Yang (*fu* organ, dorsally/laterally-routed meridian)
Heart	Small intestine
Kidney	Bladder
Pericardium	Triple heater
Liver	Gall bladder
Lung	Large intestine
Spleen/pancreas	Stomach

are fixed. As the high and low are thus made clear, the honourable and humble have their place accordingly. As activity and tranquility have their constancy, the strong and weak are thus differentiated.... Cold and hot season take their turn... and Heaven knows the great beginning, and Earth acts to bring things to completion. Heaven is Yang and Earth is Yin' (Kaptchuk, 1983). Thus are embodied the consistencies and (apparent) inconsistencies of the oriental approach and there is no way to determine the beginning or the end. The classic 'chicken and egg' situation holds, and one can only observe the continuum/perpetuum. The Taoist *T'ai Chi T'u* symbol (Fig. 65.2), more correctly a sphere rather than a two-dimensional object, is the traditional and elegant attempt to represent this concept diagrammatically. In this yin-yang model, the dark area represents Yin and the light area, Yang. The dots represent yin-within-yang and yang-within-yin. As the sphere turns, so the interplay of yin and yang are illustrated.

Yin and Yang act together and antagonistically within the body and are components of the life energy – *Qi* (pronounced 'chee'). This energy is said to circulate continuously and rhythmically (to a circadian rhythm) through twelve paired (left and right) channels. These channels are often also called meridians. The correct balance and harmony of Yin and Yang within the body and the even and regular circulation of energy (*Qi*) within the channels maintain perfect health. The converse applies: an imbalance of Yin and Yang and an interrupted flow of energy will imply disease. Thus disease is considered to be more Yin or more Yang, relative to the state of health. This can occur as a relative deficiency of one or the other, or as a relative excess of one or the other. Each would produce an apparent excess of one over the other. There is unlikely to be an absolute deficiency or excess, since life could not then be supported.

Qi itself has many facets. To the Chinese, who did not distinguish between matter and energy, *Qi* could be described as *matter on the verge of becoming energy* or

energy on the point of materializing. They did not trouble to define, merely to observe its function. It pervades the entire universe, so is not simply *life energy*. The *Qi* of the body is called *normal Qi* or *upright Qi*. This is derived in equal parts from each parent, as the *original Qi* or *conceptual Qi*. It is nourished and replenished throughout life by *grain Qi* and *air Qi*, which are combined with each other and with *normal Qi*, to permeate the entire body.

Chinese theory also gives the ultimate power of life to the kidneys, in that the kidneys store the *Jing*. This is an undifferentiated 'substance', which is most closely associated with life itself. It contains the potential for birth, maturation, decay and death. It supplies the potential for differentiation into Yin and Yang, in other words, the capability of life. Since all organs require Jing, the kidney bestows the gift of life on each organ. Since Jing also controls conception, future life is gifted by the kidneys. The anatomical relationship of the gonads to the kidney would have escaped the ancient Chinese. Jing gradually diminishes in quality and quantity with time, so ageing is controlled in this way. Death is inevitable when there is not enough Jing to maintain life. It is said '*The kidneys are the root of life, the residence of Yin and Yang, the channel of life and death*'. This makes a lot of sense in Western terms, since the kidneys, once damaged, cannot regenerate.

The channels are related to organ function, thus the twelve meridians, or channels, have names indicating these relationships. The organs, to which they relate, are each said to be either Yin or Yang in nature and, needless to say, there are six Yin and six Yang organs/channels (Table 65.1) in order to maintain balance. The Yin organs are the solid '*Tsang*' organs, the Yang organs are the hollow or '*Fu*' organs. Each Tsang organ is related to a Fu organ, e.g. (respectively) kidney is related to bladder.

The energy (*Qi*) dwells in any single channel for two hours and the flow pattern follows a '-Yin-Yang-Yang-Yin-' cycle, repeated three times. We are then able to draw a flow chart, built from the preceding lists

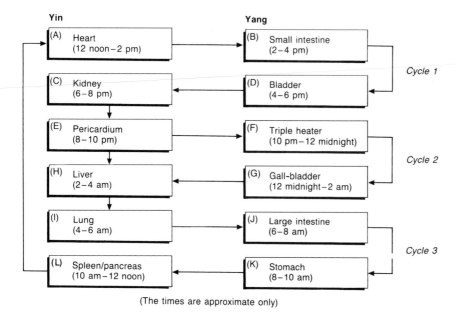

Fig. 65.3 An energy flow chart for the '-Yin-Yang-Yang-Yin-' cycle.

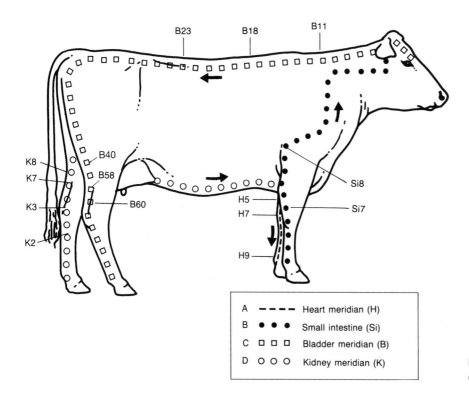

Fig. 65.4 Cycle 1 of the energy flow chart for -Yin-Yang-Yang-Yin-.

(Fig. 65.3). On the body, these are represented in diagrammatic and simplified form in Figs 65.4–65.7. Routes of meridians, and point locations thereupon, are approximate guides only. Accurate point location requires reference to more substantial works; the titles of important reference works can be found in the Further reading section. Owing to the loss of digits on the bovine limb (compared with the human five per limb) the distal sections of some meridians are open to interpretation (Fig. 65.8) and different authors disagree in detail. Experienced practitioners, nonetheless, are able to develop their own working models and to achieve the desired results.

Having read that the channels are each related to an organ, the reader is probably wondering about the triple heater. This 'organ' represents thorax, abdomen and lower abdomen (pelvic), and therefore takes in the functions of respiration, digestion and the urogenital

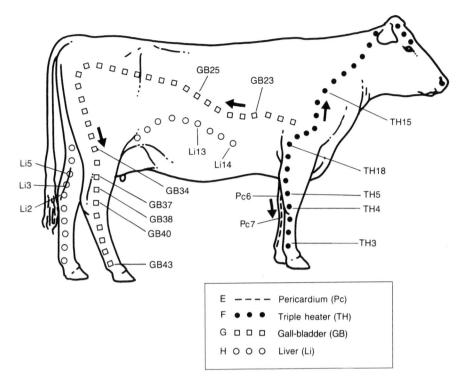

Fig. 65.5 Cycle 2 of the energy flow chart for -Yin-Yang-Yang-Yin-.

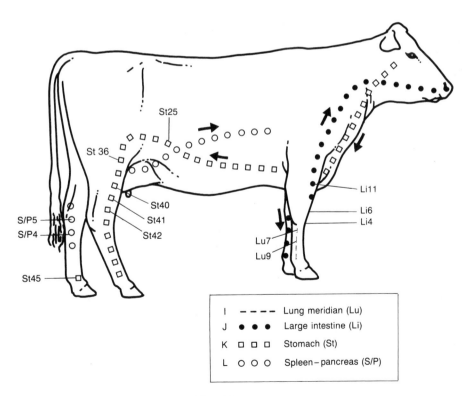

Fig. 65.6 Cycle 3 of the energy flow chart for -Yin-Yang-Yang-Yin-.

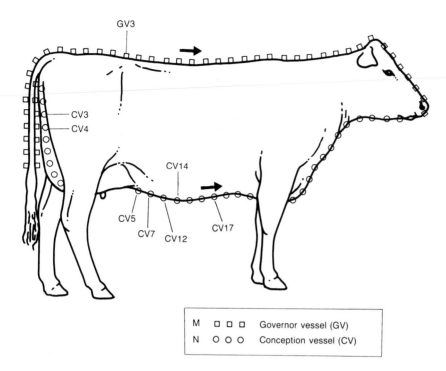

Fig. 65.7 The two extraordinary (unpaired) meridians (Governor vessel [yang] and Conception vessel [yin]).

| M | □ □ □ | Governor vessel (GV) |
| N | ○ ○ ○ | Conception vessel (CV) |

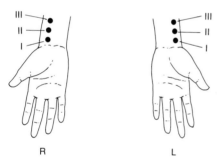

Fig. 65.8 Pulse positions on the human wrists. Each position has a deep and superficial pulse.

system. It can be considered also as the seat of humoral control and interconnections.

There are two other (extraordinary) vessels or meridians, which are of similar importance to the six pairs and these are the conception vessel and the governor vessel. These follow, respectively, the ventral and dorsal midlines. The energy flows from anus to mouth in both and therefore the vessels are not 'paired'. They differ from the other meridians in that they also lack special tonification and sedation points, etc. as described later for the other meridians, and are not an integral part of the circadian energy circulation system. The governor vessel is dorsal and therefore Yang, the conception vessel is ventral and therefore Yin (see Fig. 65.7).

The circulation of the energy (Qi) is allowed to occur through the 12, seemingly-disconnected channels, with apparent open circuits at each end, by means of the deep internal connections, creating continuity proximally and of the exterior 'secondary vessels', creating continuity at the extremities.

The opposing forces of Yin and Yang are constantly at work in the body and are supposed to be in total balance, flowing evenly through the 'channels' that the meridians represent. In fact it is better to picture a constant strife between Yin and Yang with alternating conquest and defeat but, in a state of health, with a balanced result throughout the 'championship'. It is important to note that the 'correct' balance for each individual is unique, and that a female will tend more towards Yin and a male more towards Yang.

Any stimulus that leads to an uneven 'contest', with one or other side in the ascendancy on balance, will lead to disease. The Chinese called such adverse forces the 'pernicious influences'. These are wind, cold, heat/fire, dampness, dryness and summer heat. They also believed disease could originate under the influence of emotions (joy, anger, sadness, grief, pensiveness, fear and fright), way of life (departure from Tao – 'the way'), diet, sexual activity and physical activity. Further factors were recognized, that did not fit into these categories, e.g. burns, bites, stings, trauma, etc.

Diagnosis

Diagnosis of the nature of disorders in the body in terms of the information given in the preceding pages was by pulse diagnosis in the human wrist (Fig. 65.8 and Table 65.4). Kothbauer and Meng (1983) give a method using the midline caudal artery in the bovine (Fig. 65.9), but this is sadly a long way from the complex and refined method developed for the human (through no fault of the authors, more of anatomy and practicality). General quality of pulse can still be determined and can be very helpful. Overall impressions only can be gained by this method.

Inference can be made from the signs of disease, displayed by the body, as to the nature of pernicious influence and which meridians or organs are disturbed by this influence (Kaptchuk, 1983). This requires a great deal of further study, if the reader is to develop these skills and it is too large a subject for this small treatise. Help can, nonetheless, be derived from the following charts of relationships, which provide information on the possible route of pathology, once the disease process has gained entrance (Table 65.2).

An important and functional model for the ancient Chinese was the concept of the 'five elements'. In this abstraction there are cycles of creation and destruction/control, which can be of great help in establishing patterns of pathology and in diagnosis. The five element theory is not respected by all practitioners of acupuncture, but holds the key to many important deductions about health and disease for those who uphold its tenets.

Water destroys *Fire* but creates *Wood*
Wood destroys *Earth* but creates *Fire*
Fire destroys *Metal* but creates *Earth*
Earth destroys *Water* but creates *Metal*
Metal destroys *Wood* but creates *Water*

The (*tsang/fu*) organs and the emotions are related to these elements. Thus, for example:

Liver/gall bladder	–	Anger	–	Wood
Heart/small intestine, pericardium/triple heater	–	Joy	–	Fire
Spleen (+pancreas)/ stomach	–	Pensiveness	–	Earth
Lungs/large intestine	–	Sadness/grief	–	Metal
Kidneys/bladder	–	Fear/fright	–	Water

In addition, the organs and functions of the body are related to each other, for example:

The kidneys are connected with (control) the bones and rule over the spleen
The heart is connected with (controls) the pulse and rules over the kidneys
The lungs are connected with (control) the skin and rule over the heart
The liver is connected with (controls) the muscles and rules over the lungs
The liver nourishes the muscles and the muscles strengthen the heart
The heart nourishes the blood and the blood strengthens the spleen, etc.

These connections are not so far-fetched, even in modern Western terms.

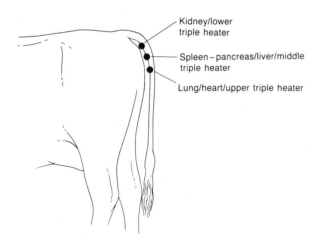

Fig. 65.9 Pulse diagnosis in the bovine (according to Kothbauer & Meng, 1983).

Table 65.2 Pernicious influences on disease.

	Yang	Yang		Yin	Yin
Season	Spring	Summer	Late summer	Autumn	Winter
Climate	Wind	Heat	Dampness	Dryness	Cold
Direction	East	South	Centre	West	North
Organs (Tsang)	Liver	Heart/triple heater	Spleen	Lungs	Kidneys
Organs (Fu)	Gall-bladder	Small intestines/pericardium	Stomach	Large intestines	Bladder
Orifices	Eyes	Ears	Nose	Mouth	Urogenital orifices
Tissues	Ligaments	Arteries	Muscles	Skin and hair	Bones
Elements	Wood	Fire	Earth	Metal	Water
Odour	Rancid	Scorched	Fragrant	Rotten	Putrid
Emotions	Anger	Joy	Sympathy	Grief	Fear
Fluids	Tears	Perspiration	Saliva/mucus	(Mucus)	Spittle

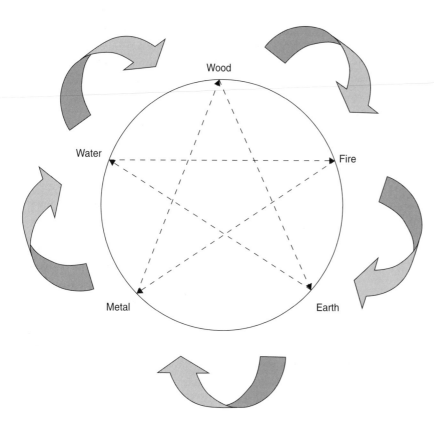

Fig 65.10 The creation (*sheng*) and destruction or control (*ko*) cycles of five element theory. The large arrows denote creation, dashed lines denote destruction/control.

What has been described, although briefly and therefore not to do it full justice, is an attempt on the part of the ancients to explain the rhythm and dynamics of life and disease, albeit often by metaphor, which can be off-putting to the Western mind. The explanation does seem to embrace the reality of the integrity of the whole body and its interconnectedness, both in anatomy and function, and its relationship to the outside world. Disease does not come in tidy parcels, affecting only one part of the body in a single way, but in complex patterns of whole body dysfunction. The philosophy behind traditional Chinese medicine embraces this essential concept very satisfactorily and provides a means of arriving at a 'diagnosis'.

From the platform of the diagnosis, in the traditional Chinese sense, a treatment rationale or treatment principle can then be devised. This will be based on the need to balance Yin and Yang, to restore harmonious flow of *Qi*, to counteract the *pernicious influences* and to support the stressed *organs*. What may be surprising, to the uninitiated, is that this allegorical methodology can provide the clinician with a valid working model for effective diagnosis and successful therapy.

Treatment (Plates 65.1 and 65.2)

The acupuncture prescription for the patient should be devised from the treatment principle, at which the pre-

scriber has arrived by following the foregoing paragraphs. Treatment of the body in traditional Chinese medicine, whether by diet, herbs, moxibustion or needles, attempts to restore the balance in the constant conflict between Yin and Yang. This treatise really only deals with treatment by insertion of needles.

Moxibustion is the application of heat to specific points of the body to supply heat energy (yang) to the system. Usually, *artemisia vulgaris* herb is used for this purpose, as a 'wool'. Heat is applied directly to the area or a few millimetres above it. Needles can also be inserted at the point and heated by burning moxa. It is not a practical method for the beginner, for general farm use. It is mentioned briefly here, merely to put it in context and to introduce the reader to the concept, which may otherwise confuse when it is encountered in other texts.

There are many different categories of points that can be utilized in acupuncture prescriptions, in an attempt to restore the desired balance. The major ones are listed below.

The points

Acupuncture points are not anatomically represented, although there are histological and physiological properties which are peculiar to them. A good account of this phenomenon is given by Kothbauer and Meng

(1983). Their exact positions are described in relation to anatomical landmarks, measurements being expressed in terms of units which relate to the dimensions of specific parts of the body. The measurement units are:

> *Tsun* or *cun*: this is the *acupuncture inch*. In human acupuncture it is traditionally equal to the length of the second phalanx of digit 3 of the human hand.
> *Fen*: One tenth of the above.
> *Finger breadth, thumb width, forearm length, pubis-nates, shin length*, etc. are all as they state, and apply to human measurement, but sources vary as to their relationship to the *cun*. It is usually accepted that a thumb width is 1 *cun*, two finger breadths are 1.5 *cun*, four finger breadths are 3 *cun*, cubital crease to carpal crease is 12 *cun*, etc.

It may be thought strange to have this unique form of measurement, but it allows for measurement proportional to the size of each individual patient. In horses, some texts refer to the 'inch' as the width of the 16th rib, at the level of the tuber coxae. The provision for measurement in animals is not good, so sources can refer to precise anatomical descriptions, rather than measurement units.

The point types

Locus-Dolendi needling, using Trigger (ah-shi) points is the use of points of local pain, which are directly related to the site of injury or illness. The effect is not very long-lasting but provides relief from pain in local conditions. It requires little knowledge on the part of the prescriber, but should probably be reserved for localised locomotor pain or injury.

Master points relate to individual organs or tissues and can be used regardless of the nature of the pathology or dysfunction which that target suffers. These master points may be sensitive to stimulus when there is a dysfunction or injury in the influenced organ/tissue but are unreliable diagnostically, unless taken as part of the wider picture. Effects of using these points alone, as a method of prescribing, will lead to disappointment. There is no deep and lasting influence on disease if the prescriber sticks to this elementary process. The master point of the musculature, for instance, is gall bladder 34.

Symptomatic or influential points have an influence over certain specific functions. For instance, bladder 31 influences female hormonal function very strongly and gall bladder 39 influences the function of marrow. They can be used in a prescription when such problems predominate (Plate 65.1). The action of these points is usually fairly narrow so, again, prescriptions based on these

alone are unlikely to be far-reaching. Like master points, the symptomatic points may also be used in reverse as diagnostic tools, the reliability being questionable unless they are used as part of the whole picture.

Pilot points are used properly to redistribute or balance the Yin–Yang conflict. Main points are the *tonification points*, which increase energy in an energy deficient meridian (gold needles are often used) and *sedation points* decrease energy in overactive meridians (silver needles are often used). Each meridian has one of each of these.

The source (yuan) point on each meridian acts as an adjuvant to one or other of the two above-mentioned points. The metal used for needling is selected according to which function it is wished to augment.

The passage or connecting (luo) points, situated on each meridian, will help to 'shunt' energy from the meridian in question to its partner. Energy usually flows 'downhill' (i.e. from 'mother' to 'son' or from the meridian earlier in the cycle to its paired neighbour).

The alarm (mu) points may or may not lie on the meridian to which they relate but may be used for diagnosis or treatment if sensitive. A sensitive point indicates stress in its related organ.

The association (shu) points, lying on the bladder meridian, are also of value diagnostically or therapeutically and relate to specific organs and meridians. For example, the association point for the spleen/pancreas is bladder 20, for the heart it is bladder 15 and for the stomach it is bladder 21.

It is helpful to list some useful points for earlier selection by the beginner; see Table 65.3 and refer to Figs 65.3–65.7.

Table 65.3 is clearly by no means comprehensive (as can be seen from the numeration), but represents a useful reference list for the main functional points. For more comprehensive point descriptions the reader is referred to much fuller works on acupuncture therapy. Their location, as shown on Figs 65.4–65.7, is a synthesis of information from personal experience and the work of Klide and Kung (1977), Lewith (1982), Kothbauer and Meng (1983), Bishchko (1983), Gilchrist (1984) and Janssens (1984). The nomenclature of the points is in accordance with the IVAS standard, in order to prevent confusion and to enable the reader to compare with all IVAS-derived texts. When reading other texts, many different conventions of nomenclature and classification will be encountered. The reader should not be confused by this, but should develop the

Table 65.3 Useful points.

Heart (HT) meridian
- 5. Passage point
- 7. Sedation point and Source point
- (9.) Tonification point

Small intestine (SI) meridian } (site open to interpretation)
- (3.) Tonification point
- (4.) Source point
- 7. Passage point
- 8. Sedation point

Bladder (BL) meridian
- 11. Bone disorders
- 13. Association point, lung
- 14. Association point, pericardium
- 15. Association point, heart
- 18. Association point, liver
- 19. Association point, gall-bladder
- 20. Association point, spleen/pancreas
- 21. Association point, stomach and master point, stomach
- 22. Association point, triple heater
- 23. Association point, kidney
- 25. Association point, large intestine
- 27. Association point, small intestine
- 28. Association point, bladder
- 31. Master point, female hormones
- 58. Passage point
- 60. Master point for pain
- (64) Source point
- (65) Sedation point } (site open to interpretation)
- (67) Tonification point

Kidney (KI) meridian
- 1/2. Sedation point
- 3. Source point
- 4. Passage point
- 7. Tonification point
- 8. Master point blood
- (II.) Alarm point pericardium (not clearly identifiable in bovine) (in groin)

Pericardium (PC) meridian
- 1. Alarm point pericardium (lateral thorax in posterior axilla)
- 6. Passage point
- 7. Sedation point and source point
- (9.) Tonification point (anterolateral of second digit)

Triple heater (TH) meridian
- 3. Tonification point
- 4. Source point
- 5. Passage point
- 10. Sedation point
- 15. Master point for forelimbs

Gall bladder (GB) meridian
- 24. Alarm point for gall bladder
- 25. Alarm point for kidney (caudal to last rib)

- 34. Master point of muscles
- 37. Passage point
- 38. Sedation point
- 40. Source point
- 43. Tonification point

Liver (LIV) meridian
- 2. Sedation point } (medial hock)
- 3. Source point
- 5. Passage point (postero-medial tibia)
- 8. Tonification point (postero-medial stifle joint)
- 13. Alarm point for spleen/pancreas (caudal to last rib)
- 14. Alarm point of the liver

Lung (LU) meridian
- 1. Alarm point for lung (between shoulder joint and third rib on chest wall)
- 5. Sedation point (medial elbow)
- 7. Passage point
- 9. Tonification point and source point
- (II.) Master point for the throat (not clearly identifiable in the bovine)

Large intestine (LI) meridian
- (1.) Master point for teeth } (site open to interpretation)
- (2/3.) Sedation points
- 4. Source point } (medial carpus)
- 6. Passage point
- II. Tonification point

Stomach (ST) meridian
- 25. Alarm point for large intestine
- 40. Passage point
- 41. Tonification point
- 42. Source point
- 45. Sedation point

Spleen/pancreas (SP) meridian
- (2.) Tonification point } (site open to interpretation)
- (1) Source point
- 4. Passage point
- 5. Master point for connective tissue and sedation point } (anteromedial tarsus)

Conception vessel (CV) (Fig. 65.7)
- 3. Alarm point for the bladder
- 4. Alarm point for small intestine
- 5. Alarm point for triple heater
- 7. Alarm point for lower triple heater
- 12. Alarm point for stomach and alarm point for middle triple heater (caudal to xiphoid, cranial to navel)
- 14. Alarm point for the heart (caudal to xiphoid)
- 17. Alarm point for upper triple heater and pericardium (on sternum, rib 7)

Governor Vessel (GV) (Fig. 65.7)
No main or special points.
20 and 26 are very important points for advanced manipulation of *Qi*.

Table 65.4 The relationships based on the human pulse system.

Position	Right		Left	
	Superficial	Deep	Deep	Superficial
III	Large intestine	Lung	Heart	Small intestine
II	Stomach	Spleen/pancreas	Liver	Gall bladder
I	Triple heater	Pericardium	Kidney	Bladder
	(Yang)	(Yin)	(Yin)	(Yang)

ability to 'translate' these into the 'standard'. In texts on TCM, another potential confusion arises from the use of the various conventions of westernization or romanization of the Chinese language (e.g. *Pinyin* or *Wade-Giles*). Again, it is important not to be daunted by this, but to compare texts in order to find the correlations.

Use of these points

The meridians are interconnected energetically in various 'rules' of therapy. Treatment strategies may be based on these relationships. Again the Chinese show their proclivity towards metaphorical description. The first relationship is based upon the human system of pulse diagnosis and relates to the position of pulse-taking in the human wrist (Table 65.4; see also Fig. 65.8).

(1) The 'husband–wife' rule relates meridians sharing the same positions on either wrist. Tonifying one will sedate its partner and vice versa. They oppose each other.

(2) The 'mother–son' rule relates to the sequence of the meridians in the circadian rhythm. A meridian preceding that in question is its mother and that succeeding it is its son. It is logical to assume that the mother is ready to give energy, the son to receive it. Tonifying the meridian in question *and* its mother will produce extra effects. Similarly, sedating both the meridian in question and its son will increase the effects of sedation. Passage points may be used instead when the meridians in question are partners.

(3) The 'midday–midnight' rule relates meridians most active in a similar time period, am and pm. One will be Yin and one Yang, e.g. lung (Yin), 4 am to 6 am., bladder (Yang), 4 pm to 6 pm. Tonifying a meridian in its active time will sedate its opposite number.

These three rules should always be borne in mind because, even if it is not the intention of the prescriber, the rule will operate upon stimulation of the relevant points with appropriate needles. Using the three rules together can achieve a rapid restoration of harmony within the body. The system of acupuncture thus used is not only complete but also quite simple to apply, providing infinite combinations of therapy. It is sad that pulse diagnosis is not so refined in animals, but the general quality of pulse can still be ascertained. The relationships of the meridians are still valid and so too is the correspondence of disease patterns with the effects from the pernicious influences and other origins of disharmony. Conclusions about meridian malfunction are inferred from the disease patterns displayed by the patient and by the demonstrable point sensitivities.

Technique of needling and treatment

Steel, gold or silver needles are selected according to the effect required. Alternatively, the different effects can be achieved by varying the needling technique or by varying the duration of insertion. The needles should be inserted confidently into the skin, as near to the centre of the point as possible. Depth of insertion is generally up to 1 cm, but varies from point to point. During a treatment the body 'reacts' with the needles in a way that has not been defined physiologically or anatomically. During this time, the needles are firmly held by the tissues. When a treatment is over, perhaps between 5 and 20 minutes later, the needles may be removed with ease.

After treatment there may be a 'slump' in the patient's apparent energy for the next 24 hours. The author has observed this less in cattle than in other species. Treatments may be repeated at intervals of several days to several weeks, but a useful guide for an initial course of therapy is a 3 to 14-day interval for three or four treatments. If no improvement is noted in this period, it is possibly a sign of a poor prognosis. Most of the author's successful cases have shown definite improvement within the initial three treatments. After a good initial result, in chronic conditions, treatment may need repeating at longer intervals (say six monthly, but the patient's condition should determine this).

Up until recently, it has been very difficult to obtain meaningful training in veterinary acupuncture. At the time of writing, however, courses are available run by the combined efforts of the International Veterinary Acupuncture Society (IVAS), the Association of British Veterinary Acupuncturists (ABVA) and Exeter University.

Homoeopathy and acupuncture combined

Since both homoeopathy and acupuncture are addressing the same entity or challenge, the living and interconnected body, in disease, it stands to reason that they must overlap if they are truly effective. The different rationales and strategies merely express the fact that they represent two different windows on the same room. It is possible to combine the two therapies, only if the rationale for selection of treatments is harmonized. Failure to do this will produce disharmony and will inevitably be counterproductive. If in doubt, the best advice is not to attempt it.

It is beyond the scope of this text to go into detail on this facet of therapy, but there is a reference to further study in the Further reading section below (Day, 1993).

Herbal medicine

The use of plants and plant material in medicine is as old as human existence. Those plants which form the basis of herbal medicine are called medicinal herbs, but probably represent only a fraction of the plants which could prove to be of benefit, if researched. They are classified according to origin (whether ayurvedic, traditional Chinese, Western, Australasian, etc.), or according to effect. This latter would be a different classification system, depending upon the culture which devises it. Broadly speaking, in the West, we classify according to the perceived pharmacological effect.

A large proportion of modern conventional drugs owe their existence or their origins to herbal medicine. The rationale of the use of herbs is to exploit their primary effect, rather similarly to the rationale of modern drug medicine and unlike homeopathy, which exploits the secondary effect (the body's reaction), although it uses many of the same plants that are used in herbal medicine. Although there are similarities between drug medicine and herbal medicine, the tradition of herbal medicine is very holistic in the truest sense. The more modern fashion for establishing a supposed active ingredient of a medicinal herb, purifying it

and using it in isolation is not at all in accordance with the holistic principles of herbal medicine. The obvious danger of this practice, leading to potential side-effects, is that the synergistic effect of the other constituents of the plant is lost.

Western herbs are classified according to their perceived actions, as per the following examples.

Alterative, anodyne, anthelmintic, antibacterial, antica-tarrhal, antiemetic, anti-inflammatory, antifungal, antilithic, antispasmodic, aperient/laxative, aromatic, astringent, bitter, cardiac, carminative, cathartic/purgative, cholagogue and anticholagogue, demulcent, diaphoretic, diuretic, ecbolic, emetic, emollient, expectorant, febrifuge, galactagogue, hepatic, hypnotic, nervine, rubefacient, sedative, sialogogue, soporific, stimulant, styptic, tonic, vesicant and vulnerary.

Chinese herbs are classified according to their ability to modify the course of action of the pernicious influences. The usual oriental pictorial language prevails. Examples, with an approximate Western equivalent where appropriate, are:

Release externally (diaphoretic?), *purge down* (purgative?), *clear heat, transform moisture (damp), facilitate urine* (diuretic?), *expel wind-damp, dispel cold*, etc.

Because material doses of herbs are utilized, there is the inevitability of tissue or milk residues. Some of these will be totally harmless or even beneficial to the consumer. Some may be harmful. Because the residue side of the use of herbs is so poorly researched and so beyond our control, it is wiser not to use herbs in food-producing animals unless absolutely sure of the consequences. A fuller account of veterinary herbal medicine is to be found in the Further reading section (Day, 1998).

Essential oils

The use of essential oils in medicine (aromatherapy) is also a very ancient tradition around the world. Further reading is recommended (Grosjean, 1994). The application and rationale are not dissimilar to those for herbal medicine. The active principles are distilled aromatic compounds derived from plants and represent very powerful and effective medicines. The classification of the oils is as for Western herbs.

Since the same caveats apply to aromatherapy for food-producing cattle, as have been detailed for herbs, with the additional worry of powerful taints of meat or milk, the use of aromatherapy in production cattle is not advised.

Other therapies

Two other therapies lend themselves to specialized use in cattle and bring with them no risk of meat or milk residues, they are *Schüssler's Tissue Salts* and *Bach's Flower Remedies*.

Tissue Salts: In the latter part of the nineteenth century, Schüssler, who was a homoeopath, devised a system of medicine based upon the mineral nutrition of cells. His 12 mineral remedies were prepared to the sixth centesimal potency, according to homoeopathic methodology. The 12 remedies are:

> *Calcarea fluorata, calcarea phosphorica, calcarea sulphurica, ferrum phosphoricum, kali muriaticum, kali phosphoricum, kali sulphuricum, magnesia phosphorica, natrum muriaticum, natrum phosphoricum, natrum sulphuricum, silica.*

These remedies, according to the founder, are able to correct cellular chemistry in order to achieve health (Goodwin, 1980). The rationale appears to work in part, and the practice persists in modern times. The author believes that these remedies act as facilitators, regulators or modulators of those cellular processes which involve those minerals. A more detailed description of this action of potentized substances is found in the section on homoeopathy, presented earlier in the chapter. Knowing what we now know about enzymes and their cofactors, this is easily comprehensible in modern terms.

In view of modern knowledge and understanding, and recognizing the adverse effect of artificial nitrogenous fertilizers on the soil mineral content in modern times, it is logical to extend the range of 'tissue salts' to include *chromium, cobalt, copper, iodine, manganese, selenium, zinc,* etc. The potential for helping cattle back to balance, in terms of mineral metabolism, particularly in those situations of relative or marginal insufficiency as can be encountered on farms, is an interesting development. No one could pretend that such dilutions amount to material supplementation, but the aid to absorption and metabolism, which they can offer, can amount to a significant benefit. The use of these potentized salts, in place of some of the mineral supplementation now required by most farm livestock, should be particularly attractive in the case of organic farm units, where outside inputs need to be minimized (Day, pers. comm.).

Bach Flowers: In the 1930s, another homoeopath, Edward Bach, devised a system of medicine which would treat disease more via the psychology and personality of the patient than via the obvious physical signs. This system can be applied well to animals, but it is best used on those animals with which we develop close emotional ties. This is because we are then better able to discern the necessary prescribing clues. There is not much application in farmed cattle, for this reason. Further reading is recommended, for a deeper understanding (Chancellor, 1971; Ball & Howard, 1999)

Bach's 39 remedies include *agrimony, beech, centaury, clematis, elm, holly, oak, olive, rock rose, scleranthus, vine and willow*. The system is included in this chapter, esoteric though it may seem, for two reasons. It introduces the reader to the medical modality and it presents the opportunity to use of one of Bach's medicines, which can be of great value in cattle medicine: *Rescue Remedy*.

Rescue Remedy is composed of Bach's *cherry plum, clematis, impatiens, rock rose* and *star of bethlehem*. It is of great virtue in the treatment of stress, fear and shock situations, and can be used just as well in cattle as in other species. Situations demanding its use are post surgical trauma, disbudding, herding of unhandled cattle, injuries, entrapments or 'casting', bereavement or distress on handling for procedures such as foot trimming. It can be given by mouth or to a group via the drinking water and can represent a very positive welfare input.

Conclusion

It is to be hoped that the reader, having studied this chapter or one or other part of it, will have experienced adequate stimulation to take a deeper look into alternative medicine (see Further reading section). It is also hoped that he or she will have gleaned sufficient information to take the first steps in applying one or both of the main therapies described therein. What should be clear is that either of those systems of medicine is a very large and complex subject. Should the reader wish to go further, it must be said that a great deal of motivation and dedication will be required. If this chapter has provided the motivation, that is good. If not, then it should at least serve to dispel some of the mists of ignorance and suspicion that enshroud the art and science of both homoeopathy and acupuncture. This should allow for more productive cooperation between conventional veterinarians and those who have diverged into 'alternative medicine'. Those who choose to apply themselves to diligent study and to professional application of these methods will be able to enjoy a life full of surprises and rewards commensurate with effort, but will not have chosen an easy option.

References and further reading

Ball, S. & Howard, J. (1999) *Bach Flower Remedies for Animals.* C.W. Daniel, Saffron Walden.

Bischko, J. (1983) *Einführung in die Akupunktur*, 13th edn. Karl F. Haug, Heidelberg.

Boericke, W. (1972) *Materia Medica with Repertory*. Boericke & Runyon, Philadelphia.

Brock, K. & Nielsen, J. (1986) *Veterinær Homøopati*. DSR Forlag, København.

Chancellor, P.M. (1971) *Handbook of the Bach Flower Remedies*. C.W. Daniel, Saffron Walden.

Clarke, J.H. (1982) *Dictionary of Materia Medica*, 3rd edn, Vols 1, 2 and 3. Health Science Press, Saffron Walden.

Day, C.E.I. (1984a) Control of stillbirths using homoeopathy. *Veterinary Record*, **114**, 216.

Day, C.E.I. (1984b) *The Homoeopathic Treatment of Small Animals, Principles and Practice*. Wigmores, London (now republished as an expanded 3rd edition by C.W. Daniel, Saffron Walden, 1998).

Day, C.E.I. (1985) Dystokia prevention. In *Proceedings of LMHI Congress*, Lyon.

Day, C.E.I. (1986) Clinical trials in bovine mastitis using nosodes for prevention. *International Journal for Veterinary Homoeopathy*, **1/1**, 15.

Day, C.E.I. (1987a) Isopathic prevention of kennel cough. *International Journal for Veterinary Homoeopathy*, **2/2**, 57.

Day, C.E.I. (1987b) *A Guide to the Homoeopathic Treatment of Beef and Dairy Cattle*. Beaconsfield Publications, Beaconsfield.

Day, C.E.I. (1993) *Acupuncture and homoeopathy combined*. Lecture delivered to IVAS Conference in Minneapolis, USA.

Day, C.E.I. (1998) Herbal medicines. In *The Veterinary Formulary* (ed. Y. Bishop). Pharmaceutical Press, London.

Day, C.E.I. (1999) Herdenbetreuung (herd treatments). In *Proceedings of the 2nd Workshop: Veterinary Homoeopathy in Organic Herds*. IAVH, Frick, Switzerland.

Daykin, P.W. (1960) *Veterinary Applied Pharmacology and Therapeutics*. Baillière, Tindall & Cassell, London.

Garner, R.L. (1967) *Veterinary Toxicology* (rev. by E.S.C. Clarke & M.L. Clarke). Baillière, Tindall & Cassell, London.

Gilchrist, D. (1984) *Greyhound Acupuncture*. Pro-Prom Pty, Mareeba.

Goodwin, J.S. (1980) *Biochemic Handbook*. Thorson's, Wellingborough.

Grosjean, N. (1994) *Veterinary Aromatherapy*. C.W. Daniel, Saffron Walden.

Hahnemann, C.F.S. (c1814) *Homöopatische Heilkunde der Hausthiere*, Leipziger Universitätsbibliothek.

Hahnemann, C.F.S. (1833/42) *The Organon of Medicine*, 5th/6th edn (transl. by Boericke & Dudgeon). B. Jain, New Delhi.

Hansard (1855) 14th May, pp. 557–8.

Janssens, L.A.A. (1984) *Acupuncture Points and Meridians in the Dog*. Blondiau Print, Beersel.

Kaptchuk, T.L (1983) *Chinese Medicine*. Rider, Melbourne.

Kent, J.T. (1986) *Repertory of the Homoeopathic Materia Medica*. Homoeopathic Book Service, London.

Klide, A.M. & Kung, S.H. (1977) *Veterinary Acupuncture*. University of Pennsylvania Press.

Kothbauer, O. & Meng, A. (1983) *Grundlagen der Veterinär Akupunktur*. Verlag Welsermühl, Wels.

Lewith, G.T. (1982) *Acupuncture, its Place in Western Medical Science*. Thorsons, Wellingborough.

MacLeod, G. (1981) *The Treatment of Cattle by Homoeopathy*. Health Science Press, Saffron Walden.

MacLeod, G. (1983) *A Veterinary Materia Medica and Clinical Repertory*. C.W. Daniel, Saffron Walden.

Mahé, F. (1987) Evaluation of the effect of a collective homoeopathic cure on morbidity and the butchering qualities in fattening calves. *International Journal for Veterinary Homoeopathy*, **2/1**, 13.

Schoen, A.M. (1994) *Veterinary Acupuncture – Ancient Art to Modern Medicine*. Mosby, USA.

Schroyens, F. (1993) *Synthesis, Repertorium Homeopathicum Syntheticum*. Homeopathic Book Publishers, London.

Veith, I. (1972) *The Yellow Emperor's Classic of Internal Medicine*. University of California Press, Los Angeles.

Vermeulen, F. (1997) *Concordant Materia Medica*. Emryss bv Publishers, Haarlem.

Chapter 66
Aspects of Bovine Surgery

G. Wyn-Jones

Introduction	1105
Anaesthesia	1105
Preparation of the surgical site	1105
Surgery	1106
Rumenotomy	1106
Dilatation and displacement of the abomasum	1109
Intestinal obstruction	1113
Caesarean section	1115
Amputation of a digit or claw	1119
Surgical correction of an umbilical hernia	1122
Dehorning of an adult	1124
Eye enucleation	1126
Teat surgery	1127

Introduction

The following chapter deals with those surgical situations which most commonly arise in dairy practice. There are always several ways to achieve the same end and there are probably as many variations in the techniques described here as there are surgeons. The methods detailed in this account are only one variation. However, they are based on many years of experience in practice and in the more rarified environment of the university teaching hospital and every attempt has been made to keep the contents practicable and pragmatic. Although each individual technique is dealt with comprehensively, there are some general points which relate to them all and are most sensibly made at the outset.

Anaesthesia

Most procedures described here will be done under local anaesthesia or regional 'blocks'. The author's guide to success with these is based on several points. Firstly, for most 'blocks' in cattle use 3 per cent lignocaine with adrenaline. The rate of development of the block is faster and it persists for much longer than when a 2 per cent solution is used. However, use the latter alone without adrenaline for subcutaneous infiltration as occasionally the vasoconstrictive effects of adrenaline can lead to local skin ischaemia, necrosis and death.

Secondly, use plenty of anaesthetic solution. It is cheap and the added expense of using 50 per cent more is easily outweighed by better results. For example, most descriptions of paravertebral anaesthesia advocate 15–20 ml spread between the upper and lower branches of each nerve. Increasing the amount to 25 or 30 ml greatly increases the percentage of successful blocks, especially in relatively inexperienced hands. Thirdly, despite the refinement of the techniques nerve blocks are still relatively imprecise methods of inducing analgesia. To offset this, spread the anaesthetic solution more widely to create a larger block of saturated tissue and to increase the chances of affecting the target nerve. Finally, do not 'line-block' at the site of the incision if at all possible as this creates a sodden, jelly-like tissue which is difficult to dissect and which has reduced initial healing properties. Use either a regional block or a field block.

Preparation of the surgical site

Whenever we operate on large or small animals we have to accept that we cannot create a sterile field. At best we can hope to make it 'surgically clean' and reduce bacterial contamination to a level where it can effectively be controlled by antibiotics and body defences. The weakest link in sterility is always the patient itself and this is where most attention should be directed. Physical removal of hair and dirt is important; use proper clippers whenever possible and clip a big enough area to give a good margin around the incision site. Initially wash the area with copious amounts of water and antibacterial soap, although elbow grease is probably more important than antisepsis at this stage. Finish with an antibacterial agent which will persist on the skin; although pure surgical or methylated spirits poured onto the skin is comforting it does not, in fact, achieve very much.

Drape as extensively as possible. For abdominal surgery prepare several large drapes that will hang over the animal's back, each with holes appropriate for a certain technique. Only two variations are really needed, one with two holes for abomasal and rumen approaches and one for caesarean sections. The synthetic material used for tent making is now widely available and is ideal, being impervious to fluids, mouldable and capable of being sterilized. The use of drapes makes the maintenance of a clean site so much easier and imparts a professional air to the operation.

The choice of suitable dress for the surgeon is difficult. Abdominal surgery requires extensive intra-abdominal palpation or manipulation. A long-sleeved gown is inconvenient in that the material abrades the wound edges and rapidly becomes sodden and uncomfortable; in a rumenotomy it also becomes severely contaminated. For the same reasons the use of gloves for these procedures is often impractical too. A good compromise which should be encouraged is a short-sleeved gown worn over a disposable plastic apron. Even if only freshly laundered and not sterilized they are still infinitely preferable to the calving gowns which many practitioners use. If these are the same garments which are used for routine obstetrics they will inevitably be grossly contaminated and will impregnate the wound edges with a good variety of pathogenic organisms.

Having eschewed gloves for abdominal surgery, there are some occasions when they should be used. The hands of a dairy veterinary surgeon are, of necessity, frequently in contact with faecal or septic material and even with a full surgical scrub they are unlikely ever to be surgically clean. For those surgeries where maximum cleanliness is essential, e.g. in an umbical hernia repair where non-absorbable sutures are to be buried, the practitioner should overcome his prejudices, accept the limitations and wear gloves!

Surgery

The old adage 'time is trauma' still holds true; for large animal clinicians it could be supplemented by 'time is infection', 'time is tiredness' and practically 'time is money'. An inexperienced surgeon cannot be expected to be rapid but there are some things which help. Most novices spend more time nerving themselves for the next action than actually doing it and then more time contemplating what they have done. If these delays are omitted then the duration of a procedure can be sharply reduced without spending less time on the actual surgery. In addition, if gratuitous and uneccesary tissue handling is abolished, tissue trauma will be greatly reduced to the benefit of healing.

Another area where a great deal of time can be wasted is that of haemostasis. The concept of a blood-free field is dear to the heart of many surgical teachers and newcomers often devote a great deal of time and effort to stopping every bleeder.

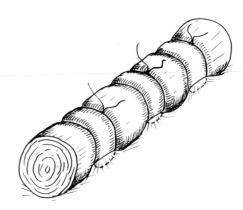

Fig. 66.1 A Stent bandage. The cylinder is made of rolled up gauze swabs; it should be sutured firmly, tenting the surrounding skin at the suture attachment points. It can be left in place for about 48 hours, although it must be removed earlier if it becomes sodden. It protects the wound and exerts inward pressure which prevents fluid accumulation.

Cows can afford to lose a great deal of blood before showing any ill-effects, but even if no haemostasis is done they will never lose more than a few hundred millilitres during a routine procedure. Consequently only those vessels which are a persistent nuisance should have time spent on them. The others will dry up very rapidly. The most efficient method of dealing with them is to clamp them in the tip of a pair of artery forceps then to twist them about eight to ten revolutions. Although this advice may sound heretical to some, it is sound, and surgery which is done rapidly but deftly without unnecessary frills will result in less tissue trauma, less contamination from the environment and substantially better healing.

For suturing, plain catgut is entirely adequate and cheap. Despite purist objections the variety obtainable in long lengths in plastic cassettes is perfectly acceptable. In its thickest size it is suitable for closing even the largest abdominal wounds and should there be infection, its rapid lysis is beneficial in that the sutures do not form a persistent nidus of sepsis. The suture wound can be protected effectively by means of a stent bandage (Fig. 66.1). This will help absorb wound seepage following umbilical hernia repair or eye enucleation, and will effectively reduce post-operative swelling.

Rumenotomy (see p. 837)

The indications for rumenotomy are: confirmation and treatment of traumatic reticulitis ('wire', 'hardware disease') and examination of the cardia, oesophageal groove, reticulo-omasal orifice, reticulum and rumen. The abdominal wall incision is also suitably placed for exploration of the left and caudal abdominal cavity.

Anaesthesia

This procedure must be done with the animal standing. Fractious patients must not be given too much sedation otherwise there is a risk of them going down during surgery with disastrous results. In most cases, local anaesthesia of T13, L1 and L2 spinal nerves using the paravertebral technique is satisfactory without need for sedatives.

Technique

No specialized instrumentation is needed for the technique described here. However, the surgeon should wear a short sleeved gown to avoid gross contamination of the sleeves and, for exploration of the rumen, gloves should not be worn as they promptly fill up with rumen liquor! Surgeons with short arms must recognize that they may not be able to reach the reticulum in a large cow. Under these circumstances there is a definite need for a long-armed assistant.

The site for the incision is high up on the left flank just caudal to the last rib (Fig. 66.2). This is so that the rumen can be entered above the likely level of ingesta and to minimize the distance from the incision to the reticulum. Following routine preparation of the area, start the incision some 6–7 cm ventral to the transverse process and some 5–6 cm behind the last rib and continue ventrally for some 15 cm parallel to it. Remember that the aperture must be large enough to accommodate easily the upper part of the surgeon's arm without traumatizing the tissue. Once through the skin there is no great muscle thickness, though it is important that the three mainly aponeurotic abdominal muscle layers be identified so that the peritoneum can be recognized and dealt with carefully. During this stage, haemorrhage is not usually a problem and only the occasional spurting vessel needs attention.

The peritoneum must be cut carefully to avoid possible damage to the rumen wall, which is often tightly applied to its underside because of the concurrent rumen tympany. The safest method is to pick up a fold of peritoneum in tissue forceps and to incise with a scissor tip. Once a hole is created, air will rush *into* the abdomen with a characteristic sound and the rumen should fall away. Insert two fingers into the hole and, with one each side of the scissor blade acting as tissue guards, lengthen the incision to its full extent.

Prior to entering the rumen it is worthwhile exploring the left cranial abdomen. Pass the right or left arm coated with some sterile lubricant e.g. KY jelly, into the incision and then forward between the rumen and inner left abdominal wall. The ribs can be felt laterally and on the dorsal cranial rumen the free 'tongue' of the spleen can be palpated. In the case of a recent wire penetration the cow will begin to show signs of resentment at this point and the first adhesions may be encountered. In early cases, this feels as if the hand is separating two freshly buttered pieces of bread and their extent is surprising! With time, they become organized and more difficult to disrupt.

If no adhesions are present then the reticulum can be reached and palpated. If this engenders no obvious pain response then it is unlikely that the animal is suffering from traumatic reticulitis and another cause for the symptoms must be sought.

The problem of contamination of the peritoneal cavity during rumenotomy has long worried surgeons and many methods, some extremely complex, have been devised to avoid this. However the bovine peritoneum is remarkably tolerant to the presence of the rumen contents in small amounts and, while excessive contamination is obviously to be avoided, these laborious methods are time-consuming and unnecessary.

In preparation for entering the rumen, place a small folded cloth in the ventral commissure of the abdomi-

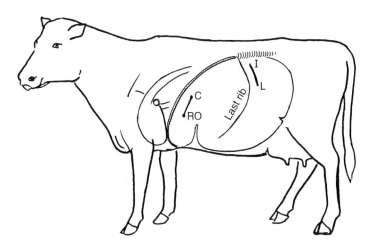

Fig. 66.2 This shows the position of the incision line (IL) for a rumenotomy. Note that the reticulum and heart apex are separated only by the thickness of the diaphragm. C, cardia; RO, reticular-omasal orifice.

nal incision so that half lies between the rumen and peritoneum and half outside on the skin. This will mop up most of the inevitable spillage of rumen contents. Pick up a fold of rumen wall from approximately 5–6 cm caudal to the abdomenal incision and exteriorize it. Retain this vertical fold of rumen by clamping it firmly with two pairs of strong Vulcellum or other tissue forceps, some 15 cm apart. The upper pair is held by an assistant who stands on the right side of the cow and who is instructed to maintain a gentle upwards and outwards traction.

Incise the rumen fold between the two forceps and expose the lumen. There is some haemorrhage from the cut wall but haemostasis is rarely needed. Apply a third tissue forceps to the mid point of the caudal cut edge and ask the assistant to maintain a mild degree of caudal traction to open up the rumen incision. Hold the lower pair of forceps in the left hand and insert the right hand and arm into the rumen. Follow the dorsal wall of the rumen downwards and forwards *over* the mass of contents. The reticulum is identifiable by being at arms length, being full of fluid and having a distinct honeycomb pattern to its mucosa.

Sometimes the wire is immediately palpable, protruding from the reticular wall; if so, grasp it firmly and withdraw it. Note the angle and depth of penetration as these factors can influence the prognosis; e.g. a cranial penetration of even 1 or 2 cm could have impinged on the pericardium; a medial penetration could well result in the localized peritonitis affecting the vagus nerve and inducing 'vagus indigestion'. Bring out the offending wire, holding it firmly all the way, rinse the arm and explore the reticulum again. Further foreign bodies may be found within the silt that invariably lies on the reticulum floor as may all kinds of other, harmless items such as bolts, pebbles etc. Take the opportunity to examine all aspects of the reticulum, cardia, oesophageal groove, etc., for abnormalities and try to assess where the bulk of the adhesions lie. This is best done by attempting to pick up folds of reticular wall. In the normal state this can be done fairly easily, but where induration of the wall and peritonitis exist it is impossible and attempts will be met by evidence of severe discomfort from the patient. The disposition of the inflammatory process also has implication for the prognosis; major involvement of the medial reticulo-rumen wall could well lead to damage to the stretch receptors located there.

If no foreign body or penetrating wire is discovered at the first examination, the reticulum wall must be searched carefully, honeycomb by honeycomb. If no trace of a wire is then found (and fresh adhesions are present) it must be assumed that either the wire has dropped back into the lumen and has been swept into the rumen food mass or, more commonly, the wire has completely penetrated and has begun a migration through the abdominal or thoracic structures. While this is likely to have further grave repercussions, with chronic peritonitis, liver abscesses, pleurisy or pericarditis all being possible, the occasional wire can migrate out through tbe body wall or become encapsulated in omental tissue and be rendered harmless.

At this point, terminate the search, withdraw the arm carefully from the rumen and scrub up again while the assistant maintains traction on the rumen incision, holding it clear of the abdominal wall.

Clean the surface of the rumen by gentle wiping with a moistened swab. Close the incision in the rumen with a continuous inverting pattern of absorbable suture material (Fig. 66.3). Catgut is ideal. Start the inversion several centimetres dorsal to the dorsal commissure and be sure to include the areas traumatized by the forceps in the inversion. Invert at least 2 cm of each margin and continue the inversion pattern for several centimetres ventral to the ventral commissure. Pull the suture material tight as each suture is laid to ensure a watertight seal. One layer is usually sufficient but there is always enough slack rumen for a second inverting layer to be inserted for maximum security of closure.

The rumen is now allowed to fall back within the abdominal cavity. Because the initial fold was taken from caudal to the abdominal incision the rumen suture line now lies several centimeters caudal to its abdomi-

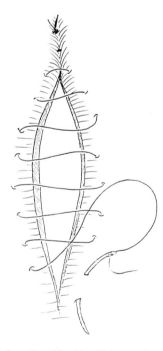

Fig. 66.3 An inverting ('Cushings') type suture pattern which may be used for closing an incision in the rumen, abomasum or uterus.

nal wall counterpart and the risks of adhesions and fistula formation are diminished.

It is the author's practice to close the abdominal incision in three layers: an everting continuous pattern of absorbable material in the peritoneum and transversus, a series of large simple interrupted sutures, again of absorbable material, to close the remaining subcutaneous layers and, finally, horizontal mattress sutures of non-absorbable material for the skin. If the margins of the abdominal wound appear somewhat traumatized, discoloured or contaminated, debridement by slicing a thin sliver of tissue off each incision edge will create fresh bleeding surfaces for apposition and virtually eliminate the potential for major infection and dehiscence.

In the normal course of events, removal of a penetrating foreign body should result in a dramatic clinical improvement over two to three days, recovery being hastened by the use of broad-spectrum, systemic antibiotics. Occasionally the penetrating portion of the wire will have instilled infected material into important sites such as the pericardium and despite foreign body removal the symptoms of pericarditis will progress. Similarly induration of the medial reticulum/rumen can result in the development of 'vagus indigestion' even if surgery was successful (see p. 835).

Locally, the most likely complication is the development of an abscess or abscesses at the incision line. This will show 10–15 days post surgery as a small lump or lumps which can eventually rupture and discharge pus. These abscesses are almost invariably located around the nidus of a buried suture and, for rapid treatment, the abscess is incised, the suture located and removed. This is facilitated by having used interrupted sutures for closure of the bulk of the abdominal wall. Sometimes the sutures are difficult to locate and in this eventuality, if absorbable material such as catgut was used, the suture will lyse and disappear of its own accord, following which the abscess will dry up. If non-absorbable material was used the suture will have to be removed otherwise the infection will persist indefinitely. After two to three weeks there is no risk involved in either searching for or removing these sutures. There will be enough thickening and induration at the site to prevent accidental penetration into the abdomen, and enough healing to prevent dehiscence.

Dilatation and displacement of the abomasum (see also pp. 839–842)

This is a 'production' disease. It is seen primarily in dairy cattle within the first three to four months after calving. The aetiology of condition is still not completely elucidated but is certain to be multifactorial. Any set of circumstances which creates a complete or partial atony of the abomasum will lead to gas accumulation and instability of the organ. Normally the abomasum lies within the right, ventral aspect of the cranial abdomen; when it fills with gas it acts much as a hollow ball pushed down into a swimming pool: it wants to rise and it can do so with some force! Whether the abomasum rises to the right or the left of the rumen probably depends on factors not yet fully understood, but an important one is likely to be the physical size of the rumen relative to the abdominal cavity. In diets deficient in roughage, as are many fed to the modern dairy cow, the bulk of the rumen diminishes; its mesenteric attachments force it to contract dorsally thus creating a potential space ventral to it. Nature and a closed cavity such as the abdomen abhors a vacuum and the nearest mobile organ, the abomasum, becomes drawn down and across to occupy a more ventral mid line position. If distension occurs now, the greater curvature of the abomasum is able to rise on the left hand side. In countries such as the UK, left side displacement seems to predominate while in some European studies, right side dilatation, displacement and associated torsion are much more common.

Factors which have been implicated in the aetiology of atony include a high concentrate, high fat diet, chronic hypocalcaemia, stress of parturition, abomasal ulcers, accumulation of silt within the abomasum and vagus nerve damage. Of these the most important are likely to be the high concentrate, high fat diets commonly fed to parturient dairy cows. Others, such as abomasal ulcers and silt impaction, are probably due to the same aetiological factors or they are a mechanical consequence of the atony.

Left displacement of the abomasum (LDA)

Diagnosis is based on the presence of a non-pyrexic, sudden onset 50–75 per cent drop in milk yield within the first few months after calving, coupled with a very characteristic selective appetite where the cow is reluctant or refuses to eat concentrate food. The heart rate is normal, except when there is severe distension of the displaced abomasum. The faeces are characteristically firm and may be mucus covered, although occasionally and confusingly there may be diarrhoea. A ketonaemia may be present but the condition is distinguished from simple ketosis by the local symptoms related to a distended, abnormally positioned abomasum.

Auscultation over the last two or three ribs on the left side will, when the abomasum is distended, often reveal the characteristic splashing and pinging noises associated with a gas/fluid interface. However, if the cow is immobile these may have to be instigated by firm ballotment. This is best done by placing the right ear over the mid point of the last-but-one rib and using one's knee or fist to rhythmically indent or ballot the left lower abdomen. A second method is to tap the upper last two ribs sharply while listening at the same point as before. If there is a gas distended viscus, i.e. abomasum deep to the ribs, the tapping noise will have a clear resonant quality not heard in the normal cow.

Both tests are easy to perform, take only a few seconds and should be part of a routine examination of any anorexic cow. If positive, they are virtually pathognomic for a displaced abomasum. Although both 'vagus indigestion' and the much rarer pararumenal abscess can under some circumstances produce similar noises, these will extend much further caudally in the flank and be associated with other symptoms.

The absence of these characteristic sounds does not mean that an LDA is not the cause of the problem, only that the abomasum is not distended with gas at the time of the examination. Any previous vigorous movement, e.g. being brought in from the collecting yard, can result in the escape of gas and fluid from the abomasum, either back to the reticulum or forward to the duodenum. If possible, re-examine the animal in about half-an-hour or come back the next day. Sometimes several examinations are necessary.

Treatment: All the techniques described, and there are many, are directed towards returning the abomasum to the right and anchoring it there. The most commonly used techniques will be described here, although the author does recognize that others or variations may be used successfully. The 'toggle' method is described on page 842.

The bilateral flank technique: Of those techniques done in the standing animal, this is probably the most consistently successful. Its great advantage is the ease with which in most cases the abomasum can be returned to the right. This is especially important when the organ is tightly distended and apparently immobile. Its only real disadvantage is that it does need two people, though one can be a lay assistant.

Anaesthesia: Bilateral paravertebral anaesthesia of T13, L1 and L2 spinal nerves. Sedation is usually not required, but if needed it should be used sparingly to avoid the possibility of the animal going down.

Technique: No special instrumentation is needed. Make the left side incision as for a rumenotomy. Incise the peritoneum carefully as the distended abomasum may be lying up against its deep face and an accidental incision in the organ would result in its collapse with serious contamination of the abdomen with acidic and irritant abomasal contents. Through the incision the abomasum is seen lying between the abdominal wall

and the rumen and pushing the latter medially. (This accounts for the hollow looking sublumbar fossa of many LDA patients.) If one surgeon is operating on both sides, open the left flank first, protect the wound with a towel laid across it and then open the right side.

The position of the right incision is critical to the success of the operation. Make a vertical incision about 15 cm long with its centre point about half-way up the flank and some 6–7 cm caudal to the last rib. Higher, and there could be difficulty reaching the abomasum. Lower, and the small intestine will persist in prolapsing through the incision. The internal abdominal oblique muscle is the thickest at this point and its fibres, cut obliquely, hide some large vessels. Only the largest of these need to be dealt with and they can be stopped quickly by clamping with artery forceps. Do not leave these hanging on the wound as they will inevitably fall off or be carried accidentally into the abdomen. Cut the peritoneum carefully with guarded scissors. Visible through the incision will be a curtain of fat-filled mesentery and omentum, with the descending duodenum running horizontally across the middle of the incision and separating them.

Lubricate the right arm and pass it into the incision downwards and slightly forwards between the abdominal wall and the omental sheet. Advance across the mid line and as far over to the left as possible. Simultaneously the assistant on the left starts to deflate the abomasum by rhythmic downwards ballotment using the flat of the hand or a fist. Even if at first the abomasum seems reluctant to empty, persistent intermittent pressure will usually cause release of gas and fluid through the pylorus or cardia with a characteristic burbling sound. As the body of the abomasum becomes slacker it is pushed further and further down the left flank to meet the surgeon's awaiting hand. Grasp a large handful of the tissue which is being pushed ventrally and attempt to draw it across the mid line. Establish a push–pull sequence and continue until the abomasum has completely disappeared from the left flank. Sometimes the tissue being pulled can be felt to tear; this is almost certain to be omental tissue and not abomasal wall. If this happens grasp a fresh handful and try again.

If the abomasum does not collapse with ballotment, relieve the initial tension by puncturing the gas cap with a 14 g needle. Further rhythmic bouncing should then cause it to deflate. If the organ still remains fixed in position it is worthwhile checking for adhesions between it and the peritoneum or rumen. They can form as a consequence of the abomasal ulceration that is present in many cases.

In the majority of cases the abomasum and its abomasal attachments come over easily. Pull a handful of the displaced tissue up into the right incision. First to appear will be folds of fat-filled omentum. Search then for an area where the fat deposits are thickest and firmest. In this region lies the pylorus which is instantly recognizable as an obvious, shiny, serosa-covered blind-ending sac. Occasionally some degree of upwards traction on the omentum is needed before the pylorus comes into view. Palpate the pylorus, the pyloric antrum and the body of the abomasum to determine whether there is any abnormality such as gravel impaction. If all is well proceed with the omentopexy.

The earliest techniques sutured the pylorus to the inner face of the abdominal wound. However, this put too great a tension on the abomasum and animals would take many days to accommodate. Current practice is to allow the pylorus to sink back to a more anatomically correct position and anchor it via its omental attachments.

Grasp a fold of thick omentum some 12–15 cm from the pylorus and fix it with Vulcellum or similar forceps. Start the abdominal incision closure with a continuous simple suture pattern picking up peritoneum and transversus, but with every deep needle pass pick up a deep bite of the omental fold. Do this for the *whole* length of the incision in order to ensure a strong adhesion. Then close both wounds in the routine manner as described for the rumenotomy.

With this technique there is usually a good strong adhesion formed and the recurrence rate is low. However, some do tear away and the owner should be instructed to lessen these chances by feeding a high roughage, low concentrate diet for 7–10 days and keeping the animal quiet, in a loose box if possible.

An alternative technique is performed through a paramedian incision. It has the advantage of needing only one surgeon, though the animal must be heavily sedated or under general anaesthesia. This in itself carries some risk in the cow and the animal *must* be starved of food and water for 24 hours prior to surgery to minimize the risk of regurgitation. Also heavy faecal matting of the ventral abdomen in some cows can make asepsis of the surgical site impossible to achieve.

Position the animal on its back (wedge-shaped supports can be made if this operation is done frequently) and support her firmly. Prepare the area that lies in the triangle between the costal arches, then if necessary carry out a 'field block' to anaesthetize the incision site. This lies some 5 cm from the mid line with its cranial margin some 20–25 cm behind the xiphisternum. Be sure to identify the course of the mammary vein before cutting as this runs within 10 cm of the mid line in places. The 'milk-well' or foramen through which the vein enters the abdomen can usually be easily papated and this gives a guide to the course of the vein which, as the animal lies in dorsal recumbency, is completely collapsed.

Incise the skin parallel to the mid line; below, the abdominal wall at this point is almost entirely fibrous, being composed of rectus sheath and aponeurotic rectus abdominis muscle. On entering the abdomen, identify the abomasum which is likely to have risen to lie at, or near the incision line. Push the organ, probably in a collapsed state, over onto the right side, identifying the attachment of the greater omentum to the greater curvature. Grasp a fold of the greater omentum some 7–10 cm from, and parallel to the insertion of the omentum to the abomasum and incorporate it in the closure of the peritoneal incision. This is done with a continuous simple suture of catgut or similar. This has the effect of interposing a barrier between the abomasum and the left side, preventing displacement in that direction or upwards on the right.

Close the fibrous aponeurosis with strong non-absorbable sutures laid in simple interrupted fashion (absorbable material is unlikely to remain strong enough for long enough in this high stress, poor healing site). Coapt the skin with horizontal mattress sutures and protect the wound with a Stent bandage (Fig. 66.1) sewn firmly in place.

Other techniques: A non-surgical method for correction of LDA is the 'rolling technique'. Although quite effective at correcting the displacement, its major drawback is the very high rate of recurrence. It was popular in the early days following the discovery of the condition, but it does have a place in modern therapy as a means of returning the abomasum to its correct position prior to surgical omentopexy by a surgeon working through a single, right sided incision.

Cast the cow onto her right side and hobble her. Pull her gently onto her back (dorsal recumbency). Rock her gently over this 90° arc for two to three minutes to allow time for the gas-filled abomasum to move from the right to a higher position, i.e. into the ventral abdomen. Finally, allow her to roll into left side recumbency when the buoyant abomasum should slide around to her, now uppermost right side. If this is done as a prelude to sugery, the operation should commence immediately as redisplacement can occur within a very short time.

Another technique used by single-handed surgeons is to deflate the distended abomasum using a 14 g needle attached to a length of giving-set tubing. The needle is taken into the abdomen guarded by the left hand, passed between the abdominal wall and the omentum, lateral to the rumen and up to the abomasal gas-cap. The wall is punctured, as much gas as possible released and the partially deflated organ manhandled into its correct position. The drawback of this method is that the needle often becomes blocked and it is sometimes impossible to deflate the abomasum sufficiently to reposition it. A larger needle gauge would help avoid this, but would increase the risk of subsequent leakage.

Some techniques have been developed which involve operating through the left flank alone. One such method attempts to create a barrier to redisplacement by suturing either the omentum or the actual rumen wall to the peritoneum and musculature of the left mid flank. The abomasum is first repositioned and a series of sutures is laid to create the adhesions. This is a rather imprecise method and the results are distinctly variable. The rumen can occasionally be penetrated resulting in abscess formation. Another method involves placing long, 100 cm (3–4 feet), heavy synthetic sutures through the cranio-ventral fundic area of the abomasum. After deflation, the organ is repositioned whilst keeping the free ends of the sutures outside the incision. These are threaded, one at a time, on to a large straight needle which is then taken into the abdomen and used to penetrate the ventral abdominal wall immediately caudal to the xiphoid process. The sutures are tensioned to bring the abomasal wall into firm contact with the peritoneum and then tied outside. Again, the aim is to create adhesions which, this time, it is hoped will bind the abomasum into its correct position. The sutures are left in place for three to four days before being removed. It is suggested that because of the risk of leakage of abomasal contents, both intraperitoneal and systemic antibiotics are used. Although the author has no personal experience of these techniques, both have their advocates, with the latter method especially being popular in some countries.

A final technique, which is occasionally described is known as the 'ventral abdominal blind approach'. It has few adherents because of its imprecision and the very high risks of serious complications. The cow is cast in dorsal recumbency and an area behind the xiphoid is surgically prepared. The animal is rocked from right to left until the abomasum is auscultated in its normal position. A large, full-curved needle threaded with 6 mm (¼ inch) cotton or synthetic tape is passed blindly through the abdominal wall, hopefully through the abomasal wall and out again. The sutures are pulled tight and tied off. They are left in place for several days to allow adhesions to form before being removed.

Abomasal dilatation and right sided displacement (RDA) (see p. 842)

In the UK this variation is seen much less frequently than left side dilation and displacement. As with LDA the symptoms are usually manifest within the first few weeks after parturition. Insidious in onset, with inappetance, reduction in milk yield and a variable ketosis, the animal's condition soon deteriorates with signs of abdominal pain shown by lifting of the hind legs towards the belly and looking around at the flank. There is elevation of the heart rate to about 100 bpm

and, frequently, diarrhoea and melaena. A marked difference between this condition and LDA is that right side dilatation and displacement frequently progresses to a complete torsion of the organ around either a caudo-cranial, vertical or transverse axis. This leads to compromised blood supply to the organ, sequestration of fluid and gas within the lumen, further distension and a marked increase in the severity of the symptoms. The animal becomes profoundly depressed, totally anorexic and the heart rate increases to between 120–140 bpm.

The aetiology of the condition is probably similar to LDA. However, in many cases of RDA large amounts of sand or silt are found, often impacted into the pyloric antrum. There is still dispute as to whether this is cause or effect, although it does suggest either a high intake of mineral matter, e.g. through the feeding of root crops, or possibly a chronic, low-grade atony which leads to the reduced passage and hence accumulation of this solid material. Other suggested aetiologies are mechanical strictures, or pyloric dysfunction consequent to abomasal ulceration or maybe pyloric nerve damage.

Diagnosis is by detection of a distended viscus on the right side. Auscultation and ballotment of both flanks take little time and should be a routine part of any clinical examination. The sounds are identical to those heard in a case of LDA and they occur in a mirror-image position, i.e. over the last two ribs. If dilatation is severe or torsion has occurred, the distended viscus can often be seen distending the cranial, right sublumbar fossa just behind the last rib. The organ can also be felt per rectum as a spherical, taut structure at arm's reach on the right side of the abdomen. The animal's general demeanour, and especially the heart rate, will indicate whether torsion has occurred.

Anaesthesia: A right side paravertebral block of T13, L1, and L2 spinal nerves or a field block.

Technique: The only special item of equipment needed is a stiff plastic tube, about 1.5 m long and with a bore of some 1 cm. This will be used to syphon off the fluid sequestered within the abomasum prior to correction of the displacement or torsion. If available, a stirrup type pump is also useful to speed up the evacuation.

Make an incision in the right flank as if for an LDA correction. Palpate the swollen abomasum and try to assess visually the condition of its wall. In general terms, the larger the organ and the darker its colouration, the less favourable is the prognosis; where torsion has been present for some hours it can be enormous, contain many gallons of fluid and, when its blood supply has been compromised, it will be a dull, dark reddish-blue in colour.

The first step in the management of this formidable looking organ is to reduce the tension in its gas-cap.

Pierce the most dorsal accessible point with a 14g needle attached to a length of plastic giving-set tube. When the wall is reasonably slack, insert a purse-string suture in the serosa and muscularis layers in a position above the fluid line. Make a small incision within the purse-string and thrust the plastic tube through into the lumen, drawing the suture tightly around it. Foul-smelling, coffee-coloured and often blood-stained fluid will run out of the tube and can be collected for diposal. The stirrup pump will speed up the process and can be reversed to blow out the tube if it becomes blocked.

The next step is to reposition the abomasum, a relatively simple procedure if only dilatation is present. However, in a case of torsion the direction of the twist must first be established.

After removing the evacuation tube and tightening the purse-string suture, try and feel at the extremities of the organ, i.e. the omaso-abomasal junction and the pyloric end, to see if the twisted tissue there gives some indication of the torsion axis. If not, a process of trial and error repositionings often proves successful. In the author's experience most torsions occur along a caudo-cranial axis with the direction of twist being anticlockwise when viewed from behind, so it seems logical to try correcting that version first. Using the flat of the left hand on the most dorsal part of the partly distended abomasum, push downwards and obliquely forwards; if this is the correct direction, the twist unravels itself and the area reverts to a relatively normal anatomical state. If not, the organ will resume its previous abnormal position, begin to distend and another direction must be tried. Fortunately, gentle perseverance usually pays. Once repositioned, the abomasum can be anchored by the standard omentopexy technique.

Unfortunately, there is a high rate of recurrence of this condition. Many authors, believing that pyloric dysfunction contributes greatly to the development and persistence of the syndrome, advocate either a pyloroplasty or a pyloromyotomy with or without evacuation of silt.

Although there is not enough information available to decide which combination is the correct one, it seems illogical not to carry out the relatively simple pyloric surgery and to remove any silt which seems to be forming an obstructive mass. This author has had encouraging results with the simpler pyloromyotomy coupled with silt removal.

To evacuate the sand, exteriorize a portion of the flaccid abomasum, make a 10 cm incision in the wall and, having protected the abdominal wound margins with a sterile towel, manually remove the contents. Close the wound in two layers; firstly the mucosa with a simple continuous pattern and then the muscularis and serosa with a continuous inverting suture, both of catgut. To perform the myotomy, identify the thick muscular spincter (see the section on LDA), grasp it firmly between the thumb and forefinger and incise parallel to the lumen axis through the serosa, circular muscle and submucosal layers until the mucosa bulges from the inside. (If the mucosa is accidentally punctured it can be repaired with a catgut suture.) An alternative method is to carry out the procedure while the abomasal evacuation incision is still open, inserting an index finger into the sphincter lumen and cutting down *very carefully* on to the site indicated. When these procedures are complete the abomasum is anchored in the usual manner.

Some idea of prognosis can be gained by studying the abomasum after its deflation and repositioning. If the discoloured wall assumes a more normal healthy colour and acquires a degree of tone, the outlook is reasonable. If it stays discoloured and flaccid the prognosis is not good. Pre- and postoperative fluid replacement therapy will be of course very beneficial and the choice of fluid should take into account the massive sequestration of sodium and chloride ions that has occurred. Intravenous normal saline or Ringer's (not bicarbonate-containing Hartmann's) solution at 5 l/h to a 450 kg cow has been recommended. This can be 'spiked' with potassium (up to 40 mmol/l).

In the first days after surgery the patient should receive routine antibiosis and be fed small quantities of hay only, though with unlimited access to water. During this period, foul smelling diarrhoea is inevitable but temporary.

Intestinal obstruction (see p. 847)

The theoretical causes of intestinal obstruction include volvulus, gut tie, strangulation in scrotal or umbilical hernias, caecal torsion and others. However, intussusception would seem to be the one most commonly encountered in practice situations. It may be seen in any age of animal, but most often is encountered in young stock.

Acute intestinal obstruction differs from most of the other abdominal conditions in that it causes abdominal pain which manifests as a colic-like syndrome. The bovine reaction to this is much more subdued than the more excitable horse, but it does show in restlessness, with frequent getting up and down, looking around at the flanks and lifting of the hind legs to kick forward at the belly. Some people describe a 'trestle'-like stance which affected animals adopt with a dipped back and spread legs. Rectal temperature can vary and is no guide but as the condition progresses the heart rate will cross the 100 bpm barrier and reach a high of 120–130 bpm. Faeces are passed at first but on the second day only scant, tarry material is seen. The colic phase may only last 12 hours or so and the animal often looks brighter for a time before becoming dull and depressed as the obstruction leads to gut necrosis, peritonitis, toxaemia and shock.

This set of signs presented to the clinician fairly obviously indicates an abdominal problem and in theory there are a number of conditions to consider. However, the absence of a distended single viscus rules out LDA, RDA or torsion. Hernias can be examined externally for signs of strangulation and traumatic reticulitis can be virtually eliminated by, amongst other differences, a failure to elicit pain by ballotment of the xiphoid region and by the fact that it rarely causes such an elevated heart rate or signs of colic.

A rectal examination is important both for elimination and possible positive findings. Where an obstruction is present, some distended small intestinal loops may be palpable in the right abdomen and occasionally, in small cows, an intussusception can be felt as a sausage-shaped mass about 6 cm in diameter and of variable length. However, distended gut loops alone or the presence of taut bands of mesentery are a strong indication of an abdominal catastrophe and the need for an exploratory laparotomy.

Bearing in mind the simplicity and straightforward nature of the procedure, a laparotomy should be regarded as a diagnostic tool; there is an immense amount of diagnostic and prognostic information to be gained and there is the opportunity for immediate corrective surgery; it is therefore surprising how often it is shunned by both veterinary surgeon and owner.

Surgical correction of intussusception: Make the laparotomy incision in the mid point of the right flank, preferably under paravertebral anaesthesia of T13, L1 and L2 spinal nerves. Avoid making the incision too low in the flank otherwise small intestinal loops will persist in prolapsing out of the wound. The small intestinal mass is reached by first going caudally between duodenum and the flank, then medially and finally cranially into the omental sling, or recess in which the bowel loops lie (Fig. 66.4). The intussusception is usually easy to feel and once located it should be exteriorized. Sometimes the mass will not come to the incision. In these cases surgery cannot be performed and the procedure must be abandoned. Most, however, can be exposed although the mesentery is short and access to the affected area and to the surrounding normal bowel is always limited. This fact makes the help of an assisant essential since a constant traction has to be maintained to keep the mass in view of the surgeon.

Several additional problems now have to be overcome. In other species it is usual to remove the intussusception along with a reasonable length of normal bowel each side so as to ensure viability of the anastomosis. In the cow, however, the mesenteric frill is so short that only the intussusception itself and a minimal margin of normal gut can be removed otherwise the two cut ends might not come together.

Before attempting resection, it is worthwhile seeing if the invaginated length (the intussusceptum) can be pulled clear of the enveloping bowel (intussuscipiens). If this can be done easily and the wall looks pink and healthy then there is no need for resection. Usually though, adhesions have fixed the two parts together or

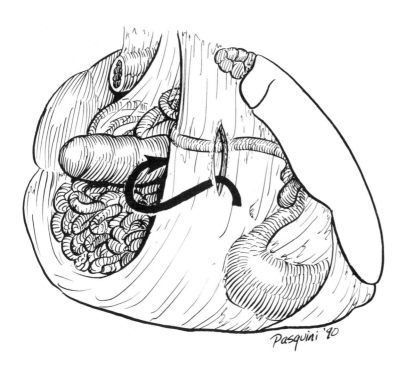

Pasquini '90

Fig. 66.4 This illustrates the route taken to gain access to the small intestine from a right flank laparotomy incision. (Courtesy of Chris Pasquini.)

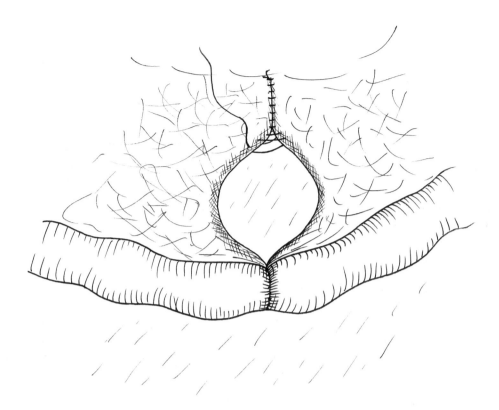

Fig. 66.5 This illustrates the problem in closing the defect in the mesentery following a small bowel resection.

if they are separable the intussusceptum is discoloured and friable and must be removed.

Use bowel clamps to isolate the intussusception. (Use the minimum compression needed to avoid trauma to the remaining gut.) Place each pair about 5 cm apart and try to ensure that the bowel between them has a good blood supply. Again, unlike other species the cow provides unique problems, as the blood vessels to the small intestine, although large, are completely obscured under a thick layer of mesenteric fat; ligating individual vessels supplying the intussusception is therefore difficult. To ensure that all are sealed start the ligation procedure at the level of one of the inner clamps. Take bites of the mesentery and fat with strong absorbable suture material and lay down an arc of overlapping blind ligatures from one end of the intussusception to the other. Occasionally large lymph nodes will get in the way and the ligature line must deviate around these. When all the ligatures have been laid, resect the affected length, cutting the bowel close to the inner set of clamps. This leaves a good length of free bowel protruding from the remaining forceps and makes the subsequent surgery easier.

Either an everting or inverting suture pattern can be used to join the two ends, although the latter gives a more secure union with better healing. Whichever is chosen, insert the first four sutures at the poles of the lumen, the first being inserted at the mesenteric border. There is likely to be a disparity in size of the lumen of the proximal and distal segments and if this disparity is large then apposition may be difficult. If there is enough slack, the distal stump can be cut at an angle to try and equate the circumferences (see Fig. 66.5). An alternative is to take longer bites of the proximal end to try and pull it down to the size of its opposing partner.

When completed, test the seal by removing the clamps and massaging gut contents at pressure through the anastomosis. If it holds, the next step is to close the hole in the mesentery. Use an absorbable material (catgut) and a continuous simple pattern, starting from the inner aspect of the defect and working outwards. Because of its short length that part of the mesentery adjacent to the bowel may not come together (Fig. 66.5) and the hole so formed will have to remain.

Clean the anastomosis, return the bowel to its correct position and close the abdominal incision routinely as described elsewhere in this chapter.

Caesarean section

This is probably the commonest major surgical procedure in cattle practice. It is carried out in all sorts of circumstances; from the ordered serenity of a teaching school clinic to the murky depths of small hill-farm barns at 3 am by torch or car headlight. It is therefore a procedure performed in sometimes difficult and adverse conditions, often by a surgeon tired by the attempt to calve the animal, and frequently under pressure of other calls to attend. It therefore, more than most, requires the establishment of a routine which can be carried out in all forseeable circumstances. The technique described here is a routine which the author has developed over the years and which has worked successfully and consistently.

Indications: These are dealt with exhaustively elsewhere. However, one point needs to be stressed: the decision to carry out a caesarean section is one that should be made at the earliest stage possible. Far too many of these procedures are carried out after heroic attempts at normal delivery and avoiding surgery have failed, with a bone weary clinician operating reluctantly on an exhausted and traumatized patient.

Anaesthesia: A decision must be made early whether to operate on a standing or recumbent animal. The standing position is infinitely preferable so if the cow is tractable, use little or no sedation, merely manual restraint. If the animal is wild enough to require heavy sedation then the author recommends that the animal be cast at the outset and hobbled to keep her down. Nothing is more chaotic than operating on an ataxic cow struggling to keep her feet and collapsing, inevitably on the wrong side during surgery.

Anaesthesia of the flank is best achieved by paravertebral block of T13, L1, L2 and L3 spinal nerves, the latter included because the top 2 cm or so of the incision often intrudes into this dermatome. In addition the author strongly recommends epidural anaesthesia for all caesareans other than early elective cases. If not done, any cervical stimulation, for example by the calf moving aginst it, will trigger abdominal contractions even in exhausted cows. At best these are disconcerting, at worst they can cause massive prolapse of the rumen through the abdominal incision. However, the epidural injection must be done with care since too much volume will cause the cow to start knuckling on her hind legs (usually the right one first) and to become unsteady on her feet. Only the barest minimum, sufficient to stop straining should be given and this is usually the same as that required to produce vulval anaesthesia. A small cow should require no more than 1.5–2 ml of 3 per cent lignocaine (2–3 ml of 2 per cent). Also be sure to carry out the injection with the cow standing or, if already down, with the animal's hindquarters in a horizontal position. If the animal's pelvis is tipped to one side or other to any degree, the block will probably

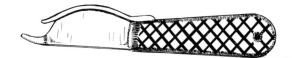

Fig. 66.6 A Charles Roberts embryotomy knife.

not work. This is presumably because gravity causes the anaesthetic solution to affect only the dependent side and the straining reflex is an 'all-or-nothing' phenomenon!

Technique: This technique requires the use of a Charles Roberts embryotomy knife (Fig. 66.6), but no other special instruments.

If the surgery is to be carried out in the standing position, put the patient's right side up against a barrier of some sort to prevent her swinging away. Mild restraint can be achieved with a nose twitch or 'bull-dog' but, if at all possible, always have someone standing at her head to exert control if necessary. If the cow is down, or cast, position her in sternal recumbency with her hind-quarters tipped towards the right. Hobble both fore and the right hind legs together but pull the left hind gently backwards to stretch the left flank. Take care not to put too much traction on the leg as this can cause peripheral nerve injury. Again it is sensible to have someone at the cow's head to restrain her if she attempts to get up. Some surgeons operate with the animal in full lateral recumbency. This provides for good restraint, but lifting a calf out of the abdomen at arms' length with bent back is extremely difficult and uncomfortable, not to say dangerous and the author does not recommend it for this reason alone. In addition there is the distinct impression that abdominal wound closure is more difficult with more tension being required, probably because of the increased upward intra-abdominal pressure and the convexity of the upper flank.

The only technique to be described here will be the sloping, left flank incision principally because the author has had no indication to do any other. Right side 'caesareans' should be avoided because of the propensity of the small intestine to prolapse profusely out of the abdominal incision for the duration of the surgery. Occasionally though, old left side lesions may make this necessary and the surgeon should be aware of this complication of operating on the right side.

Begin the abdominal incision about 12–15 cm ventral to the tuber coxae ('pin-bone') and, at an angle of about 30–35° to the vertical, extend it downwards and forwards. Make the incision long enough to remove the anticipated size of calf at the outset. Extending it later, when the calf is stuck half way out, is difficult; an adequate size makes for easier delivery and much less trauma to the wound edges. Cut through the fatty sub-cutaneous fascia and the external abdominal oblique muscle whose fibres cross the incision at right angles and which, at about this level, merge with the relatively avascular aponeurosis. Deep to this lies the principal muscle layer, the thick internal abdominal oblique with its fibres running approximately parallel to the incision. Reverse the scalpel and with its blunt handle separate a small gap in these fibres at mid incision level. Insert the index finger of each hand into this gap and pull apart. The muscle then splits easily and bloodlessly along the incision line to the required length.

Below lies the transversus muscle whose fibres run, like the external oblique, across the incision. At the mid point there is usually a fairly large segmental nerve and accompanying blood vessels and it pays to ligate this bundle before cutting. For some reason this nerve branch often seems to retain sensation, so it is wise to stand away from the hind leg whilst it is quickly cut. Take care cutting through the peritoneum as the rumen is usually tightly applied to its deep face.

Pass the right hand and arm behind the rumen and then medially to feel the uterus lying in the mid and right caudal abdomen. Palpate it thoroughly to feel the lie of the calf within. If the calf is in anterior presentation relative to the cervix, feel for the distinctive outine of the hocks and, if in posterior presentation, locate the head and nose. Once these are found the uterine incision can be made without delay.

The principles are: begin the incision over the extremity of the calf which is furthest away from the cervix (i.e. over the hocks or nose of the calf) but not too close to the fallopian tubes or ovaries; continue the incision over the dorsum or back of the calf, along the greater curvature of the uterine horn, making the aperture big enough to extract the calf without tearing the uterus in the process. However, the incision must not be so large that it extends too far towards the cervix and therefore to a position which will be difficult or even impossible to reach and suture. As a general rule this means an incision length of between 30–50 cm depending on the size of the calf. Also the more friable the uterus (e.g. after a torsion), the longer it should be to help prevent tearing. If these lengths sound excessive, remember that following removal of the calf, uterine contraction will substantially reduce them within minutes.

Many texts refer to exteriorizing the uterus or visualizing it before making the incision. However, few people are strong enough to manipulate, let alone lift this huge and heavy organ (often 75 kg or more) at arm's length, and in trying to do so, accidental damage is often done. It is far better to learn to use a Robert's knife which has a protected blade and is used to incise the uterus in situ. The prospect of using a knife blindly in a site surrounded by small intestinal loops is daunt-ing at first; however, the novice should take heart from the fact that the author has never experienced or heard of any damage being done with this instrument. Hold the knife in the palm of the left hand with the blunt, probe-headed blade away from the palm and pointing forwards. Push this blunt point vigorously through the uterus wall over the extremity of the calf, then push the knife along the greater curvature of the uterus for the required distance, preventing loops of bowel from possibly straying into the cutting area by using the first two fingers of the same hand extended alongside the knife guard. If the knife is sharp it cuts effortlessly, pushing cotyledons aside with its blunt probe tip and thus minimizing haemorrhage.

To remove the calf grasp a leg, through the fetal membranes if they are not cut, and bring it to the abdominal incision. This may necessitate careful manipulation and flexion of the joints, especially in the case of the hind limbs. Deal with each leg separately, and the head too if the calf is in posterior presentation. Break through the fetal membranes and extract the calf by lifting it as gently as possible from the incision. Remember that some part of the calf may be within the pelvis and traction downwards and cranially may be needed. If the calf is alive, try not to let it fall and snap the umbilical cord precipitously; rather move the calf away from the cow slowly, breaking the cord in a controlled movement. If possible, let someone else deal with resuscitation of the calf and return to the cow.

Even in this short time, the uterus will have contracted considerably, but in the majority of cases it is perfectly feasible now to exteriorize the incised horn to make closure easier. This has to be done carefully to avoid damage to the uterine wall and is best done with flattened cupped palms and a scooping motion. Where the placenta has separated, the membranes can be peeled away easily, but when the calf is delivered alive this is not feasible and attempts to separate the fetal and maternal parts of the cotyledonary attachments will result in severe damage and bleeding. However, if the placenta remains in its entirety, it will make closure very difficult. A simple remedy is to grasp the mass of membranes close to the uterine incision and to cut the bulk away with a scalpel keeping about 10–15 cm away from the cotyledons. Some of the large placental vessels bleed transiently but this is not a problem. By this method, suturing the uterus is simplified and expulsion of the remaining membranes is not affected.

Begin the uterine closure at the cervical end of the incision some 3 cm away from the wound commissure and invert 2–3 cm of the wound edges to bring serosa in contact with serosa. Any continuous inverting suture pattern will suffice but a Cushing's pattern (Fig. 66.3) provides for the most rapid closure. Use an absorbable material such as catgut and penetrate only the serosa and muscular layer. Pull each suture bite snugly as it is laid and be careful not to trap strands of placenta in the closure. If a 'T' or 'Y' tear has occurred suture the branch tear(s) first then treat the remainder as a single incision. If there is any doubt as to the seal achieved, oversew the whole incision with a second inverting layer. Clean the uterus of blood and fibrin tags and replace it in the abdomen.

Close the peritoneum and transversus together with a continuous everting suture to appose peritoneum to peritoneum. This is not a weight-bearing layer so the closure can be rapidly attained with large tissue bites. Oppose the remaining layers of muscle and fascia with a row of large, simple interrupted sutures. As there is tension on this part of the closure the knots can be difficult to tie, with the first throw slackening before the second throw is laid to lock it. If the first throw is made a triple or even quadruple slippage does not usually occur and tissue opposition can be maintained. The skin is closed with horizontal mattress sutures of non-absorbable material.

The choice of suture materials for the deep layers of the abdominal wound is the subject of controversy. However, the author has no doubt that an absorbable material such as catgut is indicated. The thickest gauge is easily strong enough and, in the event of infection, these sutures will not act as persistent, individual foreign bodies, will lyse rapidly and will not have to be painstakingly removed before healing can take place.

As soon as the surgery is over, release the cow and, if it is alive, allow her access to the calf. In an uncomplicated caesarean section there is no indication to use any drugs other than the routine pre and post operative antibiotics. However, if the uterus seemed slow to contract down, as often happens when a dead calf is removed, oxytocin can be given and, of course, if there is any suspicion of hypocalcaemia, appropriate therapy is indicated.

Special cases

Caesarean section in cases of torsion of the uterus: The operation proceeds routinely until the stage of incising the uterus. If this is done without first correcting the twist, suturing will be extremely difficult because in the, by then, untwisted uterus, the incision will lie on the deep face of the horn. It is therefore the author's practice to try and correct the torsion at this stage if at all possible. Use the flat of each hand to start the heavy uterine body swinging in the copious peritoneal fluid that invariably is present in these cases. Be very careful not to allow stray fingers to penetrate the oedematous, friable uterine wall and if this seems likely, or the twist is resistant to correction, abandon the attempt and proceed to incise the twisted horn. Uterine wall tears

are far more likely in torsion cases so make sure that the uterine incision is made long enough to extract the calf easily. Also sutures tend to pull through the soft wall and it is invaluable to have an assistant scrub up to help oppose the edges of the incision. Always oversew in these cases and check that the torsion is completely relieved before closing the abdomen.

Removal of a dead, contaminated calf: The bovine abdominal cavity is, by and large, a tolerant organ, but the gross contamination by infected fluids, membranes, hair, etc. that occurs in a caesarean delivery of long dead fetuses leads to a high incidence of maternal endotoxaemia, peritonitis and abdominal wound dehiscence. However, with suitable modification to the basic technique the level of post operative morbidity and mortality drops to such a low level that surgery becomes a viable alternative to sending the animal for slaughter. These modifications were adopted successfully by the author and others at the Liverpool University Veterinary Field Station.

In anticipation of the massive abdominal contamination give the animal 10 million units of crystalline penicillin G intravenously just prior to surgery. Open the abdomen in the conventional way but then attempt, if at all possible, to bring the gravid horn up to the incision. (Take care not to damage the friable uterine wall in the process.) Incise the horn over an extremity and try to extract the calf and membranes with the minimum of spillage into the abdomen. To make this easier, make sure that both the abdominal and uterine incisions are of adequate length to prevent sticking or tearing. Close the uterus carefully as described for uterine torsion and oversew the first closure. Clean the uterus, reposition it and then begin the task of cleaning out the abdominal cavity. This is achieved by repeated lavage. Use 2 litres of saline each time, warmed and poured through the incision. Use the saline to literally wash the viscera before scooping as much as possible with cupped hands. Repeat this process twice. Instill 10 million units of crystalline penicillin G into the peritoneal cavity and begin the closure.

The margins of the abdominal wound will be severely contaminated so remove a 4–5 mm strip of the incision margin of each muscle layer by sharp dissection. The bleeding edges are then sutured in the usual way using plain catgut. Strip the contaminated fascia from below the skin margins and close the skin with horizontal mattress sutures of a non-absorbable material. Use high levels of penicillin and streptomycin to supplement the initial intravenous therapy for about 5 days and to ensure the maintenance of high concentrations in the peritoneal cavity inject 10 million units of penicillin G directly through the abdominal wall in the right sublumbar fossa on the first and second post operative day.

Despite these precautions, wound infection can occur and can be recognized by a swelling of increasing size at the ventral aspect of the wound which is painful on palpation. Needle puncture will confirm the presence of pus. In these cases remove the sutures from the lower third of the incision and open the wound to allow drainage. Penetration of infection into the abdomen is not likely at this stage and the only treatment needed is daily wound irrigation. It is in these circumstances that the use of catgut sutures is vindicated. The material lyses rapidly in the infected tissue and does not form a series of permanent niduses of infection which would have to be removed before healing could take place. Whilst these open wounds look extremely serious, provided drainage and irrigation are maintained they heal well with minimal long term scarring.

Caesarean section for treatment of Hydrops allantois: Hydrollantois in the cow develops within the last three months of pregnancy. It results in a massive fluid accumulation within the allantoic cavity and caesarean section is the treatment of choice. Initially a two stage operation was devised in an attempt to avoid the splanchic pooling and vascular embarrassment which might occur if the fluid was allowed to escape too quickly. On the first day, a drainage tube was inserted into the uterus and fluid was evacuated slowly overnight; on day two a routine caesarean section was carried out. A development of this technique was to drain fluid through a larger bore tube over an hour or so before completing the caesarean procedure.

The author has modified this technique further so that delay is minimized.

Begin the abdominal incision in the usual way but open only the top or dorsal 50 per cent of the wound. The fluid-filled uterus invariably bulges out of the aperture. Make a small 2 cm stab incision into this bulging portion and slowly release some of the fluid. As the intra-uterine pressure drops, slowly at first, then faster and faster, the abdominal and uterine incisions can be progressively enlarged. If the evacuation of fluid is controlled to take place over 15–20 minutes the animals show no sign of discomfort or vascular embarrassment and the caesarean section can proceed as normal. Bear in mind, however, that the calf is likely to be small, so the incision does not need to be as large as normal, and that the vastness of the uterus and prolificacy of the membranes can occasionally make locating that calf rather difficult!

Amputation of a digit or claw (see p. 430)

The main indications for this procedure are severe trauma to the hoof and associated internal structures and intractable infection of the foot. It is a procedure whose success rate and ease of execution improves considerably, the earlier it is done. Too often the clinician and owner delay the decision to amputate, just in case the animal improves, and are only persuaded that it is necessary when the infection has extended above the hoof and the distal limb is swollen and excruciatingly painful. By this time, the unfortunate patient has lost a great deal of condition and most of her milk, has taken up a great deal of time and money and is a prime candidate for humane slaughter, not surgery.

Probably the commonest instigating condition for this type of deep infection is solar ulceration. Typically the lesion remains unnoticed because of its bilateral nature and only when infection penetrates through the keratogenic layer into the deeper structures does the lameness worsen sufficiently for the farmer to notice and bring the case to the attention of his veterinary surgeon. By this time involvement of the deep flexor tendon (DFT) at its insertion into the pedal bone has usually occurred. This extension of infection to the level of the DFT is easily established by probing down through the granuloma which is always present by this stage at the ulceration site. If the probe tip strikes bone or penetrates to a depth of 2.5–3 cm, then DFT involvement is certain. In these cases it is the author's practice to excise the granuloma and the infected deep tissue once only. If, on a repeat examination some 5–7 days later, the granuloma and sinus have reappeared, then, as the chances of success a second time are minimal, amputation is recommended. At this stage, infection is usually localized within the hoof and has not spread to the soft tissue of the pastern region or, worse, to the flexor tendon sheath.

Done at this relatively early stage, the operation is easy to perform and is usually successful in its aims. The animal heals rapidly and begins to improve in condition almost immediately after surgery. However, a warning note must be sounded: the remaining digit will now be carrying all of the animal's weight. It will therefore be subjected to a great deal of extra wear and tear and is likely to support the cow for only one or two more lactations; in small cows, with a good clean management system it can be much longer.

Anaesthesia: For the technique to be described here, the animal must be sedated and cast to lie in lateral recumbency. For sedation use xylazine or chloral hydrate. The latter drug, now sadly out of fashion, is in many ways superior to modern sedatives for this type of work and is also unlicensed in the UK. Onset of sedation is quiet and unmarred by bellowing or salivation and the depth of sedation can be profound if so desired. Its analgesic effect is good and its duration of action, after oral dosing and a 10–15 minute induction period, is 45 minutes or longer; this allows plenty of time for surgery by even the most inexperienced. The recovery phase is calm and uneventful and it is cheap!

The oral dose is between 60 and 90g, depending on the size of the animal, and it can be given through a stomach tube, dissolved in about 1 litre of warm water, or as a drench. If using the latter method allow the animal plenty of time to swallow and to avoid inhalation of the liquid. Make sure that the solution does not contact the eyes as it is extremely irritant.

Chloral hydrate can also be given intravenously, virtually to effect, although again its irritant nature means that care must be taken to avoid perivascular injection.

Whatever sedative is used, local analgesia of the foot is essential. The method of choice is, without doubt, intravenous regional anaesthesia (IVRA).

The secret of successful IVRA is the application of an effective tourniquet. Use thick (2cm diameter) rubber tubing of the type used in milking machine pipelines, applying it just proximal to the carpus or the hock. To improve compression in the latter case, place 15cm (6 inch) bandage rolls into the lateral and medial depressions which lie just anterior to the Achilles tendon. Wind the tubing around the leg at least 4 times applying *maximum* effort to ensure a high degree of tension and compression; if necessary, use two people. Whilst doing this do not lift the leg above the horizontal or the limb veins will collapse and be difficult to inject. Clip a strip over one of the superficial veins and clean it thoroughly. Using a wide bore (16g) needle inject about 30ml of 2 per cent lignocaine or 20ml of 3 per cent, rapidly into the vein; withdraw the needle and syringe and apply pressure to the injection site immediately. (If the injection is done slowly the animal often kicks after about 50 per cent of the solution is injected and frequently the needle pulls out of the vein.)

Once injection is completed, full analgesia will usually develop in about 10 minutes or so. However, before starting the incision, this must be checked. Within a volume of tissue subjected to IVRA the initial effects are random, with blocks of anaesthetized tissue lying adjacent or deep to other tissue blocks which are fully sensitive. It is therefore essential to check, not just by skin pricking, but by driving a needle down to the bone all the way around the claw. (It needs little imagination to picture the consequences of completing half the operation only to find the deep layers of tissue are entirely sensitive!) The interdigital cleft and especially its caudal aspects seem to be the last tissue to be affected and these areas should be carefully checked. If anaesthesia has only been partially achieved after 10–15 minutes, repeat the intravenous injection using the same amount of local anaesthetic solution. If it is still not fully effective then it is likely to be the tourniquet which is at fault.

Technique: No special instruments are necessary, although a proper curette is a great help.

With the cow in lateral recumbency, and the affected claw uppermost, prepare the foot for surgery. The claws can be difficult to clean and a combination of paring and scrubbing with a stiff brush is often needed. To clean the interdigital area use three or four lengths of cotton bandage soaked in surgical scrub and see-sawed briskly backwards and forwards in the cleft.

Make the incision about 5mm proximal and parallel to the coronary band–skin junction. Extend the incision through the thick skin all the way around the outer hemicircumference of the pastern and into the interdigital cleft. Here, cut the skin 2–3mm axially to the horn–skin junction, carrying the incision through the cleft to rejoin the skin wound. Always take care to cut towards (or into) the affected claw. Some force is needed to penetrate the thick skin of this region and one inadvertent slip of the scalpel blade into the sound claw can ruin the animal. Once through the skin, angle the incision proximally to aim for the proximal interphalangeal joint. This lies in the dorsal (anterior) half of the pastern thickness and some 20mm proximal to the coronary band (Fig. 66.7). Careful dissection is not necessary and the fascia, ligaments, tendons and sheaths can be cut rapidly with fairly bold strokes.

Finding the proximal interphalangal (pastern) joint can be difficult at times, especially if chronic infection has resulted in extensive fibrous reaction or the deposition of periarticular new bone. The easiest way is to put an axial (inwards) force on the claw and then to make a series of cuts parallel to where the joint is believed to be. When one of these cuts is made in the

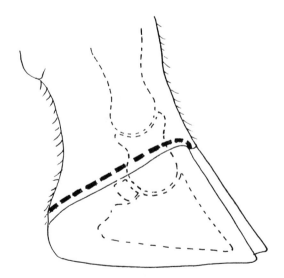

Fig. 66.7 The heavy dotted line shows the course of the initial skin incision when amputating a digit. Note the position of the proximal interphalageal joint relative to this incision.

correct place the tautly stretched collateral ligaments and joint capsule part easily with the release of some synovial fluid and an increase in joint laxity. Carry this incision on and around the articulation, bearing in mind its deeply curved profile. Take care when cutting its deep attachments not to penetrate too far towards the sound digit. During this phase twisting and turning the partially amputated claw can help to expose and tense the tissues for cutting. At this point, scalpel blades are often broken and it is a good idea to have a few spares available. Complete the removal of the claw by severing any remaining attachments.

During surgery, haemorrhage is not a problem because of the tourniquet; however, if some pre-emptive action is not taken it can be quite considerable once the latter is removed. The only vessel of real significance is the dorsal digital artery and its cut end is usually fairly easily found in the dorso-medial quadrant of the wound axial to the stump of the first phalanx (Fig. 66.8). Ligatures should not be used as the wound is to heal by second intention. Instead, grasp the severed end of the artery in forceps and twist it some 8 to 10 times to seal its lumen. Debride the wound if necessary, cutting off any obviously infected or necrotic tissue. Do not remove any of the large interdigital fat pad which prolapses into the wound unless this too is infected. Check the flexor tendon sheath: if the fluid that can be milked out of it is turbid or flocculant it should be repeatedly irrigated with saline and antibiotic solution. Although not disastrous, this finding is a poor prognos-

tic sign as the sheath usually remains infected; it also occasionally communicates with the sheath of the sound claw at the level of the fetlock. The final step is to curette the articular cartilage. This must be done thoroughly to expose the subchondral bone over the entire surface of the articulation. If it is not done carefully, granulation tissue will not grow from the bone end, or adhere to it, and a persistent sinus will develop in the healing tissue. The use of a proper curette greatly simplifies this part of the surgery, but if one is not available a scalpel can be used as a substitute.

Careful bandaging of the wound is vital, not only for its protection but as the only means of post operative haemostasis. Place a layer of non-adhesive dressing on the exposed tissues then overfill the wound cavity with gauze, swabs or cotton wool. Wrap the stump and the entire pastern region with a layer of cotton wool and use a cotton elastic bandage to keep it in place. Finally, apply a 10 cm (4 inch) elastic adhesive bandage. Starting from the tip of the remaining claw, progress upwards, increasing the tension over the stump and continuing up to and above the fetlock. The latter is necessary to anchor the bandage securely; if it were to come off the consequences would be disastrous! Take care not to crush the accessory digits; the bandage can be laid over them, but its tension should be slackened and they should be packed around with liberal wedges of cotton wool prior to wrapping. This will prevent the skin necrosis that can occur deep to them if they are subjected to too great an inward pressure.

Once the bandage is secure, the tourniquet can be removed. By this stage it will probably have been on for at least a half to three-quarters of an hour. This does not seem to be harmful in any way and the author has often seen tourniquets *in situ* for an hour or more without deleterious effect. Remove the hobbles and assist the patient onto her sternum. Do not force her to her feet, rather let her get up in her own time. As soon as she puts weight on the foot blood is frequently forced through the weave of the bandage – if this is minor it can be ignored, but if it persists for 10–15 minutes or is excessive in amount, apply a second elastic adhesive bandage over the first and, if necessary a third. *Do not*, under any circumstances, remove the existing bandage.

Leave the bandage in place for four to five days. If it is taken off before that time the fragile clot is easily disturbed and haemorrhage can be severe. Thereafter, change it every five to seven days depending on the amount of exudate produced by the healing wound.

The wound cavity will begin to contract about seven to ten days after surgery rather like a flower closing and the wound area diminishes rapidly. Concurrently, granulation tissue grows from the cut surfaces and at five to six weeks is usually flush with the skin edge. Skin contraction continues and when the wound is about 30 mm

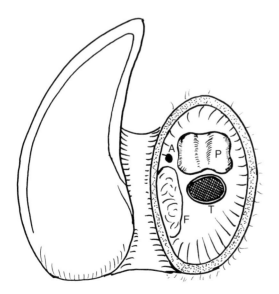

Fig. 66.8 This shows the anatomic relationships of the structures remaining after amputation. A is the arterial stump; F is the fat pad; T is the transected flexor tendon bundle and P is the distal end of the first phalanx.

across the bandage can be left off. Exuberant granulation tissue is not a problem at this site.

Occasionally a cleft persists in the granulation tissue bed and wound closure stops. This usually shows three to four weeks after surgery and the likely cause is incomplete stripping of the articular cartilage. If there is no progress over one week, reanaesthetize the site, cut out the granulation tissue and recurette the bone end.

If surgery has been delayed, infection may have established itself proximal to the amputation site. In these circumstances, and especially where tendon sheath is involved, the lameness and swelling will persist despite some wound closure. No hard and fast rules can be given as to when to give up hope of healing but, if there is no improvement in the condition of the distal limb or the lameness within two weeks of surgery, then resolution is very unlikely and the animal should be slaughtered on humane grounds.

Other techniques: The disarticulation technique described here is somewhat more complicated than those which use an embryotomy wire, either to cut through the phalanges or to carry out the entire amputation. Its use is justified because transection of either the second or first phalanx opens up their medullary cavity to an infected environment, resulting in a fairly high incidence of osteomyelitis following such procedures. In addition the nutrient foramen of the bone may also be destroyed leading to necrosis of the remaining fragment. A second distinct advantage of the disarticulation method is that it produces a cup-shaped wound cavity which maximizes the potential for healing by skin contraction. In contrast, the use of an embryotomy wire for the entire amputation produces a flat wound surface. This does not favour skin contraction and wound closure is often considerably delayed.

However, there is no doubt that this technique takes much less time than disarticulation and it can be performed without casting the cow; for these reasons alone many busy practitioners prefer it. With the foot anaesthetized, locate the wire loop in the interdigital space, checking that it begins to bite above the coronary band. The aim is to amputate through the distal third of P1 (i.e. distal to the nutrient foramen) so initially angle the direction of cut proximally. When the wire is at the correct level, change the plane of incision to lie at right angles to the long axis of the phalanx and complete the amputation. It is worth checking carefully to ensure that it is indeed P1 that has been cut and not P2, otherwise ischaemic necrosis of the remaining fragment of the second phalanx is very likely. Otherwise postoperative management is the same as for disarticulation.

Avoid techniques which call for sutured flaps of skin over the stump. This operation at best can only be regarded as clean and never sterile. Sutured wounds in this environment always succumb to infection and to post operative haemorrhage and swelling and always dehisce.

Surgical correction of an umbilical hernia

The reasons why umbilical hernias develop in some animals are not fully understood. It is presumed that in some there is a failure of the normal closure mechanism (see p. 182), although there is no doubt that many previously normal calves are found to have hernias following a bout of 'navel-ill' or umbilical infection. This also accounts for the incidence of navel abscesses which can mimic hernias and for the fact that hernias and abscesses can co-exist.

Hernias are broadly classified into those where the contents are easily returned to the abdomen, i.e. 'reducible', and those where the contents are not, the 'non-reducible'. The former, which are in the majority, are easily diagnosable and cannot be confused with an abscess. The latter, however, present as a firm swelling which could be either an abscess or a combination of both abscess and hernia. In these suspect cases, use needle puncture and aspiration to determine which is what. Puncture the swelling from both its caudal and cranial aspects, using a separate needle for each puncture to prevent possible transmission of infection. Use a large gauge needle and much suction as the pus in these abscesses is often quite thick.

Small hernias, i.e. those with rings which are two fingers' width or less, do not usually need repair. The animal grows around the hernia and it is insignificant. Some surgeons recommend closure because of the risk of strangulation of herniated viscera; this risk is very small and the author has seen only one case in over 20 years. In addition, the hernial content is almost always omentum rather than the vulnerable small intestine. However, hernias which are 3 fingers' width or more are often quite pendulous and can become traumatized. They can also become significant cosmetic blemishes in later life. Occasionally, the abomasum can become lodged in large hernial sacs although this does not seem to create any clinical problems for the animal.

Technique: No special instruments are needed.

The calf should be prepared by being starved of all food for 24 hours. As well as being a routine preparation for anaesthesia this creates a slack abdomen during surgery which helps with ring closure. The surgery should be performed under general anaesthesia, or under heavy sedation, with the surgical site anaesthetized by a field block. With the patient in dorsal recumbency, excise a fusiform (Fig. 66.9) shaped area of skin centred on the cicatrix at the hernial apex. Try and

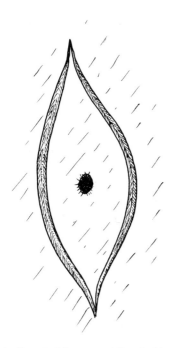

Fig. 66.9 A fusiform incision around the cicatrix.

estimate how much surplus skin is to be removed and adjust the width of the excised portion accordingly; err on the cautious side as more can be removed later. Separate the skin of this area from the underlying fascia by blunt dissection, though at the cicatrix it is firmly attached and may need to be cut. Next, using blunt dissection with a scissors tip, and beginning at the cicatrix, dissect back the multiple layers of fascia in a radial fashion to expose the discrete, thick, peritoneal hernial sac which lies deep to them. This is facilitated by grasping the cicatrix with an Allis or similar forceps and applying upwards traction to tense the tissues. As the fascial layers peel back, the sac becomes more obvious and eventually becomes completely exposed, along with the now easily discernible edge of the hernial ring. Clear the fascia back from the edges of the ring for at least 1.5 cm all the way round so that there is a clear shelf of aponeurosis into which the closure sutures can be laid.

Invert the sac and contents into the abdomen; if they go easily, as most do, there is no need to open the sac. If the contents are irreducible, the ring will need to be enlarged. Carefully, so as not damage the hernial contents, make a small opening in the sac at the caudal or cranial ring margin. Using a grooved blade director if available, or any blunt instrument which can be inserted between the contents and the ring as a shield, enlarge the ring by cutting caudally or cranially as appropriate. In most cases the ring only needs to be enlarged to a small extent before the contents and subsequently the sac can be inverted into the abdomen. There is no need to suture the sac, only to close the now enlarged ring in the usual way.

For closure, use strong, non absorbable suture material which forms a secure knot. Monofilaments are not ideal and the author prefers a sheathed multifilament type of suture. There is no need to use any complicated suture patterns to overlap the ring margins, e.g. the so-called 'vest-over-pants' technique, as a simple apposition with simple interrupted sutures is entirely sufficient. The former creates a bulky mass of tissue which in turn creates a poor cosmetic effect. Also there is no need to 'freshen' the ring edges.

Insert the first suture some 1 cm beyond the caudal or cranial ring edge, then progress along the ring laying sutures every centimetre or so to finish one centimetre beyond the ring edge at the opposite pole (Fig. 66.10). Use the finger of the 'spare' hand to protect the abdominal viscera from the point of the needle. Lay all the sutures before tying and clamp each pair of free ends with artery forceps to prevent them from pulling out or becoming tangled. Tie the sutures one by one, starting with the outer ones and progressing towards the middle. Pull each suture tightly enough to appose the ring margins and then a little more to create a mild compression effect. If tied in the conventional way the first throw often slips as tension comes on it; to prevent this either use a stitch holder while the second throw is being applied or, alternatively, make the first throw a triple rather than a double. This will usually resist the applied tension sufficiently for the locking throws to be completed.

Close the fascial layers over the ring sutures with a simple continuous pattern using absorbable suture, having first trimmed off any excess tissue that may prevent a flat closure. If the skin edges are still apart, put in a subcuticular layer to bring them together. More likely there will be some surplus skin and this too can be trimmed away, being careful to maintain the fusiform shape of the final deficit. Close the skin with either a simple interrupted or interrupted horizontal mattress suture pattern. Finally, to apply pressure to this ventral and dependent wound, and to protect it, sew on a Stent bandage (Fig. 66.1).

The repair of large hernias: To repair hernias which have large rings over four to five fingers in width, most surgery texts advocate the use of stainless steel or synthetic mesh to fill the defect. The author has had little success with these as, no matter how tightly they are sutured in place, they invariably sag under the weight of the viscera so that the final result is little better than the original hernia!

An alternative and effective method is to create a slack abdomen by depriving the animal of roughage for

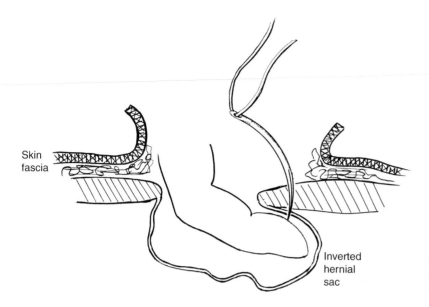

Skin
fascia

Inverted
hernial
sac

Fig. 66.10 Illustration of how the index finger is used to guard the advancing needle tip when laying sutures to close a hernial ring.

some 48 hours prior to surgery and then to carry out the repair as described above. Be sure to use strong suture material and to take good solid bites of the fibrous aponeurotic tissue surrounding the ring. One modification which helps a great deal is to have an assistant apply upwards traction equally and simultaneously on all the laid suture ends to bring the ring edges together before the row is tied off, one suture at a time. Using this technique and preoperative fasting, even the largest hernias can be repaired satisfactorily.

Dehorning of an adult

In the past this procedure was commonplace; nowadays it is done less and less since most cattle are debudded as calves. As a consequence, many students may not see the procedure performed at all.

Dehorning should be done in the winter months when the risk of fly-strike is at its lowest.

Anaesthesia: This is a technique which relies heavily on good restraint of the animal and the use of a 'crush' and the help of a strong and competent assistant are essential if a rodeo is to be avoided.

For most routine cases the standard cornual nerve block is sufficient. A common mistake is to use too little anaesthetic solution: at least 10 ml should be infiltrated across the path of the cornual nerve. Redirect the needle several times during the injection to saturate a large volume of tissue and increase the chances of a successful block. Bleeding from the injection site is normal and a good indication that the needle was in the correct place. Another error which can lead to problems is to attempt surgery too soon after the injection was made. Wait for at least 10 minutes before beginning to cut and,

if several animals are to be done, anaesthetize and operate on them a batch at a time. Be sure to use an anaesthetic solution containing adrenaline which has a long duration of effect, and be sure that there is enough help available to persuade the animals to enter the crush a second time!

Animals with very large horns and therefore a broad diameter at the skin–horn junction often require an additional ring block for full analgesia. If in doubt carry out this procedure at the outset to avoid undue pain and the consequent non cooperation of the patient. The skin at the base of the horn is tightly applied to the skull and infiltration can be difficult. Slide a long, relatively narrow gauge needle (e.g. 19G) under the skin and inject the solution as the needle is withdrawn. Concentrate on the caudal aspect of the horn base as the 1st and 2nd cervical nerves can innervate this area of skin–horn junction and they will not have been affected by the cornual block.

Surgical technique: There are many methods for removing the horns; the commonest are shears, embryotomy wire and the butcher's saw. Shears can be used for young stock where the horn and cornual process is soft, but they are well nigh impossible to use if the horn is mature or the horn base is very wide, as in the Welsh Black breed. They allow very rapid removal of horns, though if used carelessly they may not cut the horn low enough and therefore not amputate a complete circle of the keratogenic tissue which lies at the skin–horn junction. In addition to the long term complication of horn regrowth which may result, there is the more immediate problem that a cut made too high amputates the cornual vessels after they have entered the bone of the cornual process, making haemostasis extremely difficult.

Embryotomy wire is silent in operation, resulting in better patient cooperation; it allows for the direction of cut to be changed and provides good instrinsic haemostasis. However, the push/pull action needed is very tiring, the wire often jams in the cut, especially if it is used too fiercely, and it is very prone to break.

The author's preference is for a heavy butcher's saw which cuts with its own weight and whose use involves a more congenial action than the embryotomy wire.

With the animal in the crush, the assistant should, using a 'nose lead' ('nose grip', 'bulldog'), bend the animal's neck sharply to one side to move one horn away from the crush door. This often causes the head to tilt to one side and it should be straightened as much as possible before cutting begins. At this stage check that the anaesthetic has worked and that the whole of the horn base is desensitized. If it has not been done already, clip the hair from around the base of the horn then position the saw blade some 2.5 cm from the medial horn base. Angle the blade towards the point where the ear meets the head and begin sawing. Occasional animals object violently even when the horn is apparently completely desensitized and the blocks have been repeated or supplemented with a ring block. In these cases it is likely that they are reacting to the noise of the saw in their heads and a change to an embryotomy wire will solve the problem.

Saw swiftly through skin and bone to emerge just above the ear. Take care not to lift the skin from the ear and, if this seems likely, cut the remaining skin tag with scissors.

Haemostasis: When the horn is finally detached from the head, haemorrhage can be impressive. However, it is not life-threatening and can easily be temporarily stopped by finger pressure. Many techniques of haemostasis have been described and advocated but the simplest and most effective is torsion or twisting of the bleeding vessels.

With a robust pair of artery forceps, grasp the vessel ends firmly, apply gentle traction and spin them about six or so revolutions or until they break off. This will, in most cases, completely stop the bleeding or at worst reduce it to a small point of seepage. The largest vessels are always to be found at the ventral, rostral edge of the skin wound and, if the cut is made low enough, will be exposed for several centimetres of their length. If they are not, grasp the bleeding, severed end of the artery and, using gentle leverage over a finger, expose a sufficient length to be twisted. Do not attempt occlusion by snapping off the vessel end, as is occasionally recommended; a high proportion break way below skin level and continue to bleed from inaccessible depths. If these large vessels are occluded in the manner described most

of the remaining bleeding points stop or slow to a level where they can be ignored.

In those cases where the horn and cornual process have been sectioned too high the vessels will continue to bleed from the vascular canals within the bone. They cannot be picked up in artery forceps and are a nuisance. The time-honoured way of dealing with these is to insert a sharpened matchstick point into the hole to plug it. Although seemingly crude in these days of modern technology, it works, and the presence of the wood fragment does not appear materially to affect healing in any way.

Post operative course: Treatment of the resultant wounds with antibacterial powders and aerosols is widely practised. However, its effects are likely to be cosmetic only and the author uses no wound dressing without apparently affecting the speed or course of healing.

Post operative care must involve examining the animals every few hours for the first day or so in case there is secondary haemorrhage; thereafter daily monitoring will be sufficient. Advise the farmer to feed hay off the ground and not from overhead racks as this diminishes the amount of seed and dust contamination of the exposed frontal sinus. In the normal course of events the hole will scab over within one or two weeks, with complete healing by skin contraction and epithelialization taking several months.

Complications: Secondary haemorrhage is not common provided the largest vessels have been dealt with properly. However, fighting or rubbing of the wounds can occur as the analgesia wears off and bleeding can be severe. Identification of the source of the haemorrhage is almost always impossible as the side of the head and the surgical site are covered with a mass of blood clot which effectively hides the bleeding point. The area is now completely sensitive again and the animal usually vigorously resents its handling. The quickest and least painful remedy is to apply pressure. Place a large pad of cotton wool directly over the horn stump and bind it down tightly with several rolls of 10 cm (3 inch) adhesive elastic tape wound around the head. Leave the ears protruding, as they help to prevent the bandage slipping, and take care not to constrict the larynx or trachea. Although apparently crude, it is a very effective method and avoids the need to re-anaesthetize and explore the site in an often fractious animal. Some individuals may be extremely anaemic after such haemorrhage and a small number may require blood transfusion. As a rough guide, if the animal is able to stand and move around without being too ataxic it is not likely to require such measures. However, if in doubt, transfuse.

Long term complications are sinus empyema and fly-strike. Farmers must be instructed to call for veterinary attention if a recently dehorned animal becomes dull or anorexic. In these cases the sinus should be examined, if necessary by lifting the scab. If infected, or affected by fly strike, give systemic antibiotics and treat locally by irrigation with copious amounts of water to remove the pus or larvae. Repeat the irrigation daily until the sinus is clean and healing is progressing well.

Eye enucleation (see p. 922)

(see p. 922)

The common indications for eye enucleation in cattle are panopthalmitis and conjunctival or scleral squamous cell carcinoma. The presence of infected or tumour material within the conjunctival sacs in these cases precludes a subconjunctival approach through the palpebral fissure and so most large animal enucleations are done by a transpalpebral technique. With this method, the eyelids are sewn tightly together to trap infection or neoplastic material with the conjunctival sacs and the globe is removed intact to maintain a sterile wound.

Anaesthesia: In tropical countries where occular squamous cell carcinoma is rife, enucleation is a common procedure and is usually done under retrobulbar block. This is a relatively simple technique which is described in many textbooks but, if only the occasional enucleation is done, and facilities are available, then the lack of movement and relaxation of general anaesthesia makes for much easier surgery!

Technique: Prepare the eye by fine clipping of the eyelashes, lids and periorbital region, followed by removal of debris and discharge from the conjunctival sac. Sew the shorn eyelids together *tightly* with an O or I non-absorbable suture, laying the sutures close to the eyelid margins. The lids and surrounding area can now be prepared for surgery.

Incise the skin of the upper lid in a line parallel to the lid margins and some 4 mm outside the suture line. Deepen the incision carefully to expose the subcutaneous fascia. Using Metzenbaum or other similar scissors blunt dissect under the skin of the eyelid, through the circular muscle of the eye (orbicularis oculi), until a probing finger shows that the dissection plane has reached the boney rim of the orbit. Extend the skin incision the length of the upper lid and the dissection plane to the remainder of the dorsal orbital rim. Repeat the process on the lower eyelid so that the incisions above and below the suture line meet beyond the medial and lateral canthi in a fusiform shape. Make sure that the dissection planes within the lids remain superficial until the orbital rim is reached; this will help prevent acci-

dental rupture of the conjunctival sac and contamination of the wound.

To penetrate into the orbital cavity, retract the upper eyelid skin and use a finger tip to locate the boney edge of the mid upper orbit. With a scalpel cut just below the bone edge and parallel to it. Once an access hole has been created, use a curved-on-flat scissors to extend the aperture laterally and medially, keeping close to the orbit rim all the way round. Leave the medial canthus until last as the largest vessels lie here and their bleeding can be difficult to control. Up to this point haemorrhage is not usually a problem and it can be controlled by conventional means. When the medial attachments are severed the globe becomes free and relatively mobile. If bleeding from the medial vessels is severe then hard finger pressure for a minute or so should reduce it to manageable proportions. These vessels are often difficult to identify and even more difficult to grasp with artery forceps so if first attempts fail, apply pressure to the area for a little longer and then proceed with freeing the globe from its deep attachments. This is done by putting outward traction on the globe, inserting a heavy pair of curved-on-flat scissors into the gap between globe and orbit and cutting the taut tissue. As the globe becomes progressively looser it can be pulled further from the cavity and access improves. Ideally the muscles should be detached close to their insertion on the capsule so that as much tissue as possible is left within the orbit to minimize dead space. Practically, poor access, retrobulbar fat and the inevitable haemorrhage mean that cutting is usually done blind and the muscles, fat and optic nerve are sectioned randomly. As soon as the globe is free lift it away and attend to any haemorrhage. Unlike the dog and cat, bleeding from the optic artery is not dramatic, there is no need for ligation, and at worst blood wells up slowly within the cavity and can be contained by firm finger pressure maintained for four to five minutes. It is not necessary to stop haemorrhage completely so as soon as it has slowed to manageable proportions suture the remaining skin of the eyelids together with horizontal mattress sutures of non-absorbable material. With the suturing completed, squeeze out excess blood from the socket through the incision line and sew a stent bandage (Fig. 66.1) firmly in place over the wound so as to exert a firm inward pressure. This controls residual haemorrhage and protects the wound.

If the conjunctival sacs and globe were removed intact, healing is likely to be uncomplicated. Remove the 'Stent' at two to three days and the sutures at about 10 days. Some authorities recommend instilling antibiotics into the orbital cavity before wound closure, but this is probably not indicated unless there is some contamination and routine prophylactic and post operative antibiotics normally suffice.

Where there is known contamination of the wound, first intention healing may still occur with vigorous antibiotic therapy, but an alternative method is to pack the cavity with sterile cotton bandage coated with antibacterial cream and layered concertina fashion. The free end is laid in the medial commisure of the wound which is sutured in the usual way apart from its medial 1–2 cm. The bandage is removed through this gap after two to three days and the socket eventually fills with granulation tissue. There is a persistent discharge from the drainage hole and routine management involves maintaining the patency of the aperture and clearing up the discharge. Irrigation of the cavity does not seem to materially affect the healing process. When the socket is full the discharge dries up and the medial sinus closes. This process can take several weeks.

Teat surgery (see Chapter 27)

Milk production is the *raison d'être* of the modern dairy cow. Inefficiency in any of the factors involved leads to her becoming unprofitable. The care of teats and the surgery that is frequently involved therefore deserve more attention than they often receive.

There are three enemies of successful teat surgery: the 3 Ms! Milk, milking machines and mastitis must always be taken into account by the surgeon.

A simple way to avoid these problems in the small proportion of surgery which is elective is to delay until the cow's next dry period. Often this option is not open as the majority of surgical procedures are emergencies. In these cases the surgeon must take steps to ensure that milk pressure does not build up within the teat, that the teat and surgical site do not have to bear the trauma of being milked, either by machine or by hand, and that adequate antibiotic cover is given.

In practice the former two requirements are met by using plastic indwelling cannulae, of which there are many designs. Use them liberally; they are relatively cheap and work well. However, bear in mind that as well as being a boon, they can also act as very efficient introducers of infection if used incorrectly. If they drop out, they must never be reintroduced, but must be replaced by a new one from the packet. Supply them in quantity with careful instructions as to their handling and the cleansing of the teat before insertion.

To protect against infection be scrupulously clean when introducing anything into a teat and use intramammary antibiotic preparations routinely after any form of teat surgery or while a cannula is in place. Systemic antibiotics too, although not often used, are indicated in cases of trauma and surgery to aid successful healing.

Restraint: It is impossible to be clean and deft when the patient's hind legs are flying around the surgeon's head! Use restraint and lots of it! For simple examinations, tail restraint, i.e. forcing the root of the tail vertically, is often adequate; it discourages kicking, although it will not stop a reaction if there is a sufficiently painful stimulus. A second level of restraint is a 'nose lead' or 'bulldog' clamp; again its effect is of discouragement rather than prevention of reaction. A more effective method is the 'udder cinch'. This is a length of rope with a loop in one end which is passed around the cow's abdomen just in front of her udder. The free end is threaded through the loop and pulled against it to tighten the cinch around the belly. Pull it tight enough to cause the cow to sway slightly then secure the free end by tucking it partially under the taut portion to form a quick release (Fig. 66.11); do not pull too tightly or the animal may go down! Used in combination these

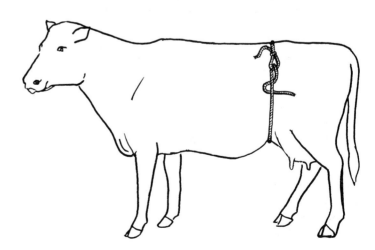

Fig. 66.11 An udder cinch.

three techniques of restraint will dissuade the cow from kicking even in the face of a considerable pain stimulus. Use them routinely as a cow's kick is quite capable of causing major injury!

When there is a need to perform fine surgery, e.g. the closure of a lacerated wound, the success rate will be much better if the cow is first cast, restrained and positioned to allow good access to the wound, better lighting and a more comfortable position for the surgeon.

Local anaesthesia: The usual method is a ring block at the base of the teat or an inverted V block (Fig. 66.12). In the former technique, the cow need only feel one needle prick, as the subsequent injections are made through the area of skin already desensitized. For streak canal and teat sinus surgery, more localized analgesia can be obtained by putting a tourniquet around the base of the teat and infusing local anaesthetic solution up through the streak canal.

Crush injuries: In days gone by when cows were shippen-housed, crush injuries were commonly caused by one cow swinging round to tread on her lying stall-partner's teat. Nowadays most cases are in older cows who tread on the hind teats of their own pendulous udders whilst getting up. These self-inflicted injuries usually consist of gross contusion to the teat walls with much haemorrhage into the substance of the teat, swelling, pain and acute stenosis of the streak canal.

If no major laceration has occurred, the treatment is one of systemic antibiotics for several days and insertion of an indwelling cannula to ensure that milk can be released from the quarter and that milking is avoided. Leave the cannula in place until the swelling and pain have subsided and the streak canal is functioning again; this can take up to 14 days.

Inserting the cannula into the painful and swollen teat can be difficult. After gentle cleansing of the teat and the canal area, locate the latter with a blunt ended probe. Insert the atraumatic end of a tube of intra-mammary antibiotic and lubricate the canal with the

cerate. Also use the cerate to lubricate the cannula before inserting it gently into the canal and spiralling it up into the teat. Once in place remove the cap and, after a pause whilst the lubricant with which the cannula is filled dissolves, the milk and some of the antibiotic will run out.

Streak canal stenosis: This long-term sequel to teat trauma is caused by fibrosis of the sphincter region. It results in an increase in time needed to milk the quarter and is a nuisance in a parlour system which does not tolerate delays.

In the first instance, dilatation of the canal can be tried, using a plastic teat cannula; this is inserted and left in place for 7 to 10 days. If this is ineffective use a teat dilater. This device has two arms which, when the instrument is in a closed position, form a probe-like shape. After insertion into the canal a knurled knob is turned at the end of the instrument and the two arms separate, stretching the lumen of the canal. These two methods are relatively atraumatic and should be used if possible; however, their effects are usually temporary.

A more permanent result is obtained by incising the canal walls with a McLean's knife or similar. This is flat, double-edged (Fig. 66.13) and is used with a push/pull action. The teat is grasped firmly as if for hand milking, tensed and the probe end of the knife inserted into the canal. A sharp push causes the leading edges to cut as the blades pass through the canal. Once inside the blades are rotated through 90° and pulled sharply out, creating a cruciate incision. Use the narrowest blade size first and if after its single use the milk flow is good, insert a plastic cannula and allow the healing phase to take place around it. If the milk still does not run out easily, repeat the procedure with a larger diameter knife.

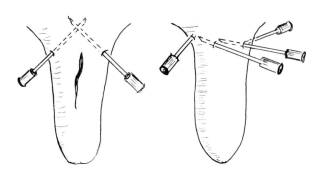

Fig. 66.12 Ring block and field block techniques.

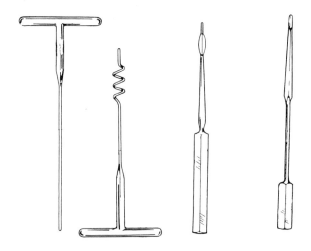

Fig. 66.13 Some common teat instruments; from left to right: a probe, a Hudson's spiral, a McLean's knife and a Hall's knife.

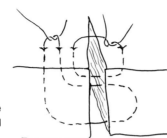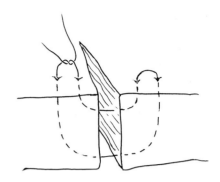

Fig. 66.14 Two suture patterns which provide apposition of both the deep and superficial layers of the teat wall.

Although effective in the short term this is also traumatic to the canal and sphincter, and post operative fibrosis will usually result in a sphincter of varying competence, with contraction of the scar tissue almost always causing a recurrence of the problem at some later date.

Lacerations: For the purpose of deciding on the appropriate treatment, teat lacerations should be divided into 'penetrating', i.e. those where the wound penetrates into the lumen of the teat or canal, and 'non-penetrating', where the deep layer(s) are intact.

Non-penetrating wounds: Teats heal extremely well if given the opportunity. If it is certain that there is no penetration and no leakage of milk through the wound, then allowing the wound to heal by second intention or granulation is less risky than attempting to suture and possibly entrapping ischaemic tissue and infection. There is then the distinct possibility that enclosed sepsis will erode through the deep layers of the wound and create a fistula into the lumen. Only if a non-penetrating wound is very fresh and exceptionally clean should suturing be considered. If there is doubt, treat by physical cleansing of the wound and by inserting a cannula to remove the trauma of milking. Systemic and intramammary antibiotics are indicated and usually healing is rapid with minimal scarring.

Penetrating wounds: Where the lacerations penetrate into the lumen there is not the luxury of deciding whether to suture or not. The wound must be closed to prevent the development of a fistula and inevitable mastitis and, because the surgery involved is delicate and must be done carefully, there is every reason to cast the patient and conduct the operation in a controlled and comfortable manner.

In cases where the cut is recent and is minimally contaminated, simple cleansing and suturing may be all that is needed. However, most wounds are much older when seen and are often badly contaminated. In these circumstances a much better rate of healing is achieved if the cleansing of the wound is supplemented by surgical debridement of the wound margin. To achieve this, trim a thin (0.5 mm) sliver of tissue off each wound edge along the whole of its length, extending the wound commissures slightly at each end. This results in fresh bleeding tissue being apposed and a consequent rise in the chances of primary union.

Use the suture patterns shown (Fig. 66.14) if possible as these compress both the superficial and deep layers, yet can be removed later. Sometimes the teat wall is exceptionally thin and these more complicated patterns are difficult to use; in these cases use simple interrupted sutures. Using fine, non-absorbable material, lay sutures fairly close to each other and do not penetrate the teat lumen.

On completion, allow the cow to rise then apply a bandage to the teat. Degrease its surface carefully with alcohol and allow it to dry. Place a small patch of non-adhesive wound dressing over the incision line and, using a 2.5 cm wide adhesive bandage, start at the sphincter end and layer it directly on to the teat skin. Overlap each winding by about 30 per cent and secure the upper, free end of the bandage to the skin with a single superficially placed suture. Insert a cannula into the streak canal and remove the cap; this will prevent any build-up of milk pressure within the teat. Give systemic, broad-spectrum antibiotics. The use of intramammary cerates within the first few hours is questionable as their base is very pervasive and may penetrate the suture line if they contact it before there is some adhesion between the wound edges. After the first 12–24 hours they are definitely indicated as a barrier to any infection entering the teat.

Special cases: Sometimes the teat is lacerated horizontally near its end so that the cut lies close to or enters the streak canal. To discover whether there has been penetration, hand milk the teat and look for milk emerging from the cut.

Where the streak canal has been spared, the decision to suture or not will be based on the criteria already laid out. In these cases the laceration rarely extends even 180° around the teat circumference and so it usually does not gape too much. With a teat cannula in place to minimize milking trauma, but otherwise left to their own devices, teat lacerations usually heal extremely well, being barely visible in a few months. This makes the possible repercussions of suturing and the trapping of infection much less acceptable.

On the other hand, when the streak canal has been cut its early closure is essential. However, before suturing begins, try to make some estimate of whether the distal tissue flap has an adequate blood supply for survival and healing; there is no point in trying to repair the defect if it has not! Sometimes it is obvious that the attachment of the flap is too small for a good supply to be present and in these it is best to cut it off immediately in the sure knowledge that it is not viable. With a cannula inserted in the remaining streak canal while healing takes place, the resulting slightly truncated teat is likely to be completely functional, although more liable to bacterial ingress and mastitis.

In other instances it is obvious that a good blood supply exists and repair can proceed; in yet others it is not so obvious and in these cases it is wise to give the tissues the benefit of the doubt.

Before beginning to suture, debride the cut surfaces carefully, if necessary cutting a thin sliver off both surfaces of the entire wound. Also, and most importantly, insert a teat cannula through both parts of the streak canal so that they will be aligned during suturing and in subsequent healing. In the post operative period, examine the wound often and remove the sutures from any part that looks as if it may dehisce. In this way pus pressure is not allowed to build up and disrupt healing further.

Transection of the teat: Milking machines need very little length of teat to hold on to, so if after the acci-dental amputation an inch or so remains it is worthwhile attempting some reconstruction. Trim the end of the stump so that it lies roughly at right angles to the long axis of the teat, then insert a purse-string suture around its circumferance close to the cut end. Draw the purse-string tight to compress the sinus opening snugly around a plastic cannula. Fashion two or three stay sutures to anchor the cannula in place and remove its cap or plug. With heavy antibiotic cover the teat end will heal around the cannula into a semblance of a streak canal. There will, of course, be no sphincter and milk leakage and bacterial ingress are major hazards. However, as a salvage operation it will often allow completion of the lactation and even a subsequent one.

Repair of congenital and acquired teat fistulae: Congenital fistulae are usually first noticed when a heifer calves and comes into milk. The most likely explanation for their presence is that they are the streak canals of otherwise vestigial, supernumary teats. Acquired fistulae are the result of wounds to the teat and failed repair of penetrating lacerations. They are a nuisance in that they leak milk, which causes bacterial multiplication on the teat surface and hence milking machine contamination. They also allow ingress of infection into the quarter and attract flies. To avoid the complications associated with open teat surgery, delay if possible until the next dry period. Then with a cast, restrained cow and the maximum cleanliness available, excise the fistula through all the wall layers by means of a fusiform incision. This shape causes the minimum of distortion on closure of the wound. Use the suturing techniques described above, apply a bandage post operatively and give systemic antibiotic cover for several days.

Adult Cattle
The Interaction of the Animal, Environment and Management

Chapter 67
Stress and the Pathogenesis of Disease

P.J. Hartigan

Introduction   1133
The stress system   1134
The stress response   1134
Coping with stressors   1137
The biological costs of stress   1138
The transition to pathology   1138
Concepts of allostasis and allostatic load   1139
Allostatic load and the veterinary practitioner   1140
Clinical implications   1142
Concluding comments   1146
Glossary   1147

Introduction

It is generally believed – and frequently repeated in the literature – that 'stress' is the major challenge to the welfare, health and productivity of animals in intensive commercial cattle enterprises. However, when it comes to drawing practical conclusions from the literature it becomes clear that scientists have been working with paradigms of animal stress that have done little to help the industry to cope with the biological imperatives that it must address as it seeks to manage intensive units with the minimum of animal distress. There is a lack of unanimity and clarity about which stimuli are so stressful that, on occasion, they can undermine the dynamic equilibrium established and maintained by a battery of homeostatic responses. Any stimulus that challenges homeostasis can be described as a stressor. It is a condition of life that homeostasis is under constant challenge by a multitude of stressors. Most of those encountered by cattle in a well-managed enterprise are amenable to the routine coping strategies of the animals; however, there are occasions when particular stressors seem to overwhelm the homeostatic responses, to the detriment of welfare, health and production. Apparently, the amount of stress an animal perceives depends on the intensity and duration of challenging stimuli and on the animal's physiological and psychological state when challenged; as a consequence, the effects of a particular stressor may differ between one animal and another or, indeed, the same stressor may have different effects on an individual animal on different occasions. Hence, when stress has adverse effects on health, different patterns of disease may emerge amongst animals exposed to the same stressors.

Historically, biologists have formulated paradigms of stress based on the concept of an integrated stress response jointly regulated by the sympathetic–adrenal medulla axis (Cannon's fight/flight response to threat) and by the hypothalamic–pituitary–adrenal cortex axis (the general adaptation syndrome described by Selye). The two neuroendocrine axes have the capacity to alter metabolism and to redistribute metabolites to help the animal maintain homeostasis as it responds to stressors. While these feedback systems are capable of coping with the many uncomplicated and discrete stressors that animals encounter every day, it has been realized that the operating characteristics of typical feedback-controlled homeostatic systems are too narrow to account fully for the complexity of the interactive responses that culminate in stress-related pathology. By definition, homeostatic responses serve to maintain the constancy of the internal environment; each strives to return a regulated parameter to a set point that represents the central tendency of that activity. For instance, a fall in serum calcium concentration elicits an immediate increase in the secretion of parathyroid hormone, which should promptly bring the calcium concentration back to set point, its 'normal value'.

Many stress disorders may not be amenable to such a straightforward resolution. Stressors may create perturbations within several interacting organ systems and they may require compensatory responses that elicit changes in the activities of other body systems that are governed by other regulatory actions. In those circumstances, the regulatory systems must have sufficient flexibility to enable them to recalibrate operating set points and to adjust the dynamic ranges of compensatory processes so that the interactions between the brain, the autonomic nervous system and the endocrine system are geared to defend welfare, health and productivity in the face of ongoing and evolving challenges. That type of construct is exemplified by the physiological adaptations of a mother during pregnancy: as gestation progresses the set points and operating ranges of a plethora of homeostatic systems continually readjust in such a manner that the organ systems remain a harmonious team.

In this chapter we provide a synoptic overview of the homeostatic components of the 'integrated stress response' before proceeding to introduce a relatively new paradigm of stress that recognizes that stressors may activate multiple interactive mechanisms, that functional set points are subject to change, that disturbances in one body system may elicit compensatory changes in another and that compensatory changes come at a biological cost which may make the animal vulnerable to other unrelated stressors – which cost is a determinant of the clinical consequences of environmental stressors. We shall then examine the paradigm in relation to aspects of the more common problems encountered in intensive cattle enterprises: lameness, mastitis, infertility, metabolic disorders, welfare, behavioural problems and levels of production.

The stress system

For didactic purposes, it is convenient to refer to the neuroendocrine responses evoked by stressors as the work of the 'stress system' (Fig. 67.1). As mentioned,

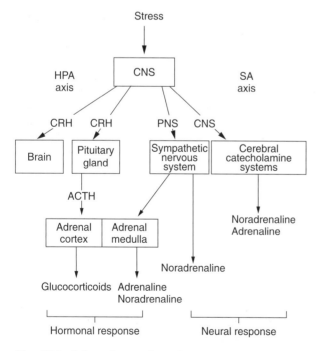

Fig. 67.1 Schematic overview of the stress system. CRH, corticotrophin-releasing hormone; HPA axis, hypothalamic-pituitary-adrenal axis; PNS, peripheral nervous system; SA axis, sympathoadrenal axis; ACTH, adrenocorticotrophic hormone.

the core of the stress system consists of two axes that serve to integrate neural and neuroendocrine activities: in one, a neural pathway links the sympathetic division of the autonomic nervous system with the adrenal medulla (the SA or sympathoadrenal axis); in the other, hormones link the hypothalamus with the adrenal cortex (the HPA or hypothalamic–pituitary–adrenal axis). The stress system is on continuous service: in the absence of significant challenge it has a baseline, circadian pattern of activity that delivers homeostasis at rest; when challenged by perceived stressors it makes the appropriate adaptive changes to maintain physiological equilibrium, delivering what might be described as stress-related homeostasis.

Anatomically, three elements of the nervous system interact to provide the regulatory core of the stress system (Fig. 67.2):

- Groups of noradrenergic neurones in the brainstem (the locus coeruleus–noradrenaline system; LC/NA);
- Peptidergic neurones in the hypothalamus, mainly in the paraventricular nuclei (PVN), that release corticotrophin-releasing hormone (CRH) and arginine vasopressin (AVP);
- Central neural projections that enable the LC/NA neurones and the PVN neurones to innervate and activate each other.

Mutual interactions between the two axes are not restricted to local neurocircuits. They are regulated in parallel by an extensive battery of humoral messengers: hormones, opioid peptides, cytokines, growth factors, metabolites – some stimulatory, some inhibitory and almost all counter-regulated by glucocorticoids (Chrousos, 2000). For instance, the secretion of ACTH (which can be stimulated by hypoglycaemia, social stress, fear, physical stress, exercise, acute illness or inflammatory cytokines) is inhibited by oxytocin, somatostatin and opiates, and is modulated by negative feedback by glucocorticoids. We shall have occasion to return to the importance of counter-regulation again, and again.

The stress response

The principal function of the stress system is to release appropriate amounts of glucocorticoids and catecholamines from the adrenal glands and of noradrenaline at peripheral nerve terminals, specifically to assist the animal to cope with the demands of metabolic, physical, social or psychological stressors. The SA axis elicits responses much more rapidly than does the HPA axis; that is largely because it releases catecholamines

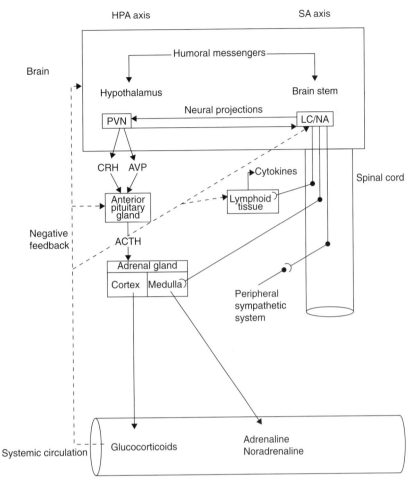

Fig. 67.2 A schematic representation of cross-talk between the neural, endocrine, and immune systems when challenged by stressors. The cell bodies of the peptidergic neurones that govern the hypothalamic-pituitary-adrenal (HPA) axis are located principally in the paired paraventricular nuclei (PVN) within the hypothalamus. They secrete corticotrophin-releasing hormone (CRH) and arginine vasopressin (AVP; also known as ADH), both of which stimulate the release of adrenocorticotrophic hormone (ACTH) from the anterior pituitary gland. ACTH stimulates the adrenal cortex to release glucocorticoids (principally cortisol). The glucocorticoids exert negative feedback at hypothalamic and pituitary levels of the HPA axis and they counter-regulate the activities of both the sympathoadrenal (SA) neurones in the brain stem (locus coeruleus-noradrenaline: LC/NA) and (but not shown) the central humoral messengers that modulate the stress response. Neurones in the PVN and in LC/NA mutually innervate and activate each other. The SA axis releases noradrenaline within the brain (not shown), adrenaline and noradrenaline from the adrenal medulla and noradrenaline from peripheral sympathetic nerves. The cells of the lymphoid tissues release various cytokines that interact extensively with the neural and endocrine systems (see Fig. 67.6). Solid lines represent activation; dashed lines represent inhibition.

that can achieve their objectives by modifying pre-existing substrates within their target cells, whereas the HPA axis releases steroids – hormones that direct the synthesis of new proteins that the target cells must manufacture before they can proceed to do the business. When the stress system is being aroused, the peptidergic neurones at the PVN and the noradrenergic neurones of the LC/NA activate each other and both contribute to the adaptive behavioural and physiological changes that ensue.

Response of the SA axis

When activated by stressors, the SA axis releases noradrenaline from neurones within the brain and from peripheral sympathetic nerve endings; in addition, it releases both adrenaline and noradrenaline from the adrenal medulla. The noradrenaline released centrally results in greater mental acuity ('arousal'), whilst the catecholamines released peripherally promote changes in metabolism and in the activities of

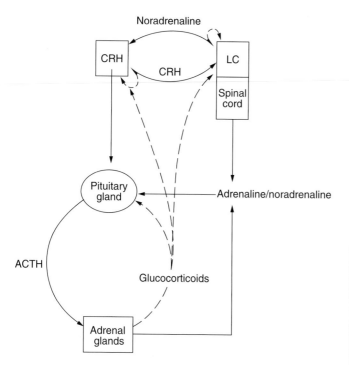

Fig. 67.3 Schematic diagram of the functional inter-relations between corticotrophin-releasing hormone (CRH) and the locus coeruleus–noradrenaline (LC/NA) system. ACTH, adrenocorticotrophic hormone. Adapted from E.O. Johnson *et al.* (1992). Solid lines represent stimulatory effects; dashed lines represent inhibitory effects.

Box 67.1 Metabolic responses to stress.

- Initially, insulin secretion is suppressed
    decreased uptake of glucose by cells: hyperglycaemia
    breakdown of stored triglycerides: increased fatty acids in blood
- Raised concentration of plasma catecholamines
    breakdown of stored glycogen:
      in liver → increased blood glucose
      in skeletal muscle → increased blood lactate
    breakdown of stored triglycerides → increased fatty acids in blood
    increased secretion of glucagon
    decreased secretion of insulin
    increased gluconeogenesis (from glycerol, lactate, amino acids)
- Increased secretion of glucagon
    breakdown of stored glycogen
    breakdown of stored triglycerides
    increased gluconeogenesis
- Rapid rise in secretion of glucocorticoids
    breakdown of skeletal muscle
    breakdown of stored triglycerides
    inhibition of uptake of glucose by tissues (other than brain)
    increased gluconeogenesis
- Increased release of arginine vasopressin (AVP, ADH)
    retention of water
- Increased release of renin
    activation of angiotensin–aldosterone system
    retention of water and sodium ions,
    loss of potassium ions

the cardiovascular and respiratory systems to increase cardiac output, to facilitate oxygenation of blood, to raise blood glucose concentration and to deliver the enriched blood selectively to the tissues upon which the stressors are making the greatest demands.

Response of the HPA axis

The paraventricular nuclei secrete CRH and AVP in response to stressors. In cattle, the two peptides appear to be equipotent in stimulating the pituitary gland to secrete adrenocorticotrophic hormone (ACTH) which, in turn, stimulates the adrenal cortex to secrete glucocorticoids. As the final effectors of the HPA axis, glucocorticoids (chiefly, cortisol) participate in a multitude of activities that maintain whole-body homeostasis, including feedback regulation of both axes of the stress system (Fig. 67.3) and the metabolic readjustments (Box 67.1) required to sustain the physiological adaptations invoked to cope with stressors.

Counter-regulation

The stress response can increase the concentrations of adrenaline and/or glucocorticoids in the circulation.

The secretion of adrenaline is the more rapid response that underpins the flight/fight reaction, whereas the glucocorticoids give a slower response that helps to reallocate resources to meet the challenges to homeostasis and, equally important, to curtail the potentially harmful effects on health and welfare that could be exercised by exaggerated or unregulated autonomic responses. The importance of counter-regulation of the autonomic component of the stress response is brought into sharp focus by the conviction of our medical colleagues that the risk of myocardial infarction is significantly increased in individuals in whom sustained high catecholamine levels cause hypertension by sustained contraction of arterial smooth muscle and at the same time induce metabolic changes (insulin resistance, hypercholesterolaemia, hyperlipidaemia) that predispose to arterial damage and the formation of atheromatous plaques in the coronary arteries.

Counter-regulation of the SA response is a key element in an animal's ability to cope with environmental stressors without incurring a residual physiological toll of inordinate proportions.

Coping with stressors

Animals may employ active coping strategies to reduce the aversive effects of stressors or they may use passive coping strategies to minimize the biological cost of the stress response evoked by the stressors. Moberg (2000) identified four general types of biological responses available to an animal to cope with stress: behavioural, autonomic, neuroendocrine and immunological (Fig. 67.4). Although all four biological defence systems are available to respond to a stressor, an animal does not always call on each of them to deal with each stressor: different stressors elicit very different types of biological responses. Nevertheless, in the vast majority of instances the response will contain some element of all four.

Behavioural responses

Behaviour offers the animal choices: to confront the stressor aggressively, to remove itself from the stressor or to engage in displacement activity that ameliorates the impact of the stressor. In many instances a behavioural response is the simplest and most biologically economic reaction to a stressor; for instance, simply walking away. However, some displacement activities (e.g. stereotypies such as compulsive walking) may expend an enormous amount of energy to no productive purpose.

Autonomic (LC/NA) responses

When the situation is not immediately resolved by a behavioural response, the reaction is directed by a generalized activation of the sympathetic nervous system including the release of adrenaline from the adrenal medulla. The preparation for 'fight or flight' is manifest by a heightened state of arousal, by increases in blood pressure, heart rate, respiratory rate, blood flow to skeletal muscles and consumption of energy and by decreased blood flow to skin, kidneys and digestive tract. Another consequence of general activation of the sympathetic system is the release of renin, leading to activation of the angiotensin–aldosterone system, and consequent conservation of sodium and water, accompanied by excretion of potassium ions.

Neuroendocrine responses

Within minutes of the LC/NA response, the HPA axis is called to arms but, because steroids take longer than amines to elicit responses, there is a time lag before the glucocorticoids begin to exercise dominant control – with adrenaline, growth hormone and thyroid hormones in supporting roles. The combined activities of these hormones result in metabolic adjustments (Box 1) while the animal continues to resist the stressor(s) or until its reserves of energy have been exhausted. The first priority is to maintain blood glucose concentration and to conserve the glucose for utilization by the neural system. The liver can liberate glucose from stored glycogen. Skeletal muscles do not possess the full complement of enzymes necessary to do this; there glycogenolysis yields lactate, which the liver can use to produce new glucose (gluconeogenesis). Metabolic processes are altered so that peripheral tissues use lipids rather than glucose as the prime source of energy; glucocorticoids and growth hormone (GH) act in consort to facilitate that switch by inducing the breakdown of triglycerides stored in adipose tissues to yield the required fatty acids plus glycerol. These glucose-sparing actions are augmented by the synthesis of new glucose from endogenous substrates: the glycerol released from adipose tissues is made available for the synthesis of glucose in the liver (gluconeogenesis), as is the lactate released from muscle glycogen. Concurrently, the same hormones induce proteolysis in skeletal muscle, releasing amino acids that the liver also uses to manufacture glucose. The process of gluconeogenesis is regulated by glucocorticoids (HPA axis), by glucagon and by adrenaline from the adrenal medulla (SA axis).

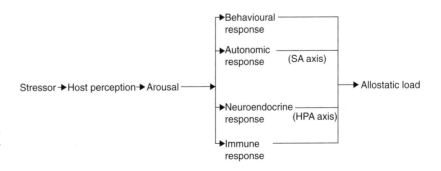

Fig. 67.4 Coping with stressors. SA axis, sympathoadrenal axis; HPA axis, hypothalamic–pituitary–adrenal axis.

Immunological responses

The two axes of the stress system are at all times engaged in bidirectional communication between the central nervous system and the immune system. The cross-talk is intensified during the stress response. The brain issues messages through the SA and HPA axes that affect the activities of the cells of the immune system, while products elaborated by various immunocytes affect the functions of the neurones at the centre of both axes. In brief, the corticosteroids and the catecholamines down-regulate the activities of the immune system: they inhibit many of the functions of leucocytes, macrophages and lymphocytes, and they decrease the production of many cytokines and mediators of inflammation. Also, it is believed that the endogenous opiates released in response to stress are, in general, immunosuppressive. Early in the response to stress there is increased release of growth hormone and prolactin, both of which enhance the immune response; however, the circulating levels of both hormones are decreased later in the stress response and, also, when there is recurrent or chronic stress. Thus, the net effect of stress is immunosuppression and increased susceptibility to some infectious diseases, particularly those that target the respiratory system or the digestive system. There is convincing circumstantial evidence that some bacterial, viral and parasitic pathogens themselves act as stressors that attenuate the immune response.

Physiological toll

If stress is intense and prolonged, the coping strategies may become part of the problem. Rapid production of glucocorticoids in response to a stressor is beneficial, provided an efficient shut-off can occur; chronic elevation of glucocorticoids persisting after the stressor has gone indicates poor adjustment and is detrimental to health. Prolonged elevation of glucocorticoids in the circulation can cause excessive breakdown of muscle protein, depletion of energy reserves, hyperglycaemia, immune suppression, attenuation of the inflammatory reaction, increased susceptibility to infection and delayed healing of wounds. The principal mechanism by which the body is protected from these deleterious effects is feedback inhibition of the HPA axis by the corticosteroids themselves.

The biological costs of stress

All stressors, no matter how innocuous, have some biological costs. There is a price to pay, even when the homeostatic balance is restored promptly. The real questions are: to what extent does the challenge diminish the body's metabolic reserves and how does this impact on health and welfare?

In the first instance, the biological cost of stress is met from the body's reserves of energy. For many short-lived stressors that cost is negligible: it is met from reserves without any impact on other biological functions. As an example, catecholamines secreted during stress stimulate the conversion of stored glycogen into glucose; once the stress has been alleviated, the glycogen stores are quickly replenished by gluconeogenesis; there is no lasting deficit. On the other hand, when there are insufficient biological reserves to meet the costs, resources must be diverted from other biological functions: for example, if a young heifer reared under very stressful conditions has to divert a significant fraction of the energy normally expended on growth and reproduction it is likely that her growth will be retarded and puberty will be delayed. In other words, for some persistent or intense stressors the cost is high, a significant burden on the body that places the animal 'at risk of developing pathologies' (Moberg, 2000). The gap between those two extremes is filled by examples in which the hidden costs of coping strategies so deplete biological reserves that the animals develop 'pathologies' when challenged by what might otherwise be considered to be rather minor, inconsequential factors. Such are the cases that raise the questions that need to be addressed by the clinician in the field: how does stress influence the pathogenesis of disease and what accounts for the variation in susceptibility to stress-related diseases amongst animals in the same, or similar, environmental circumstances?

The transition to pathology

There are several routes by which coping strategies can progress into pathology.

- If stress is intense and long-lived, the coping strategies may become part of the problem. The potential pathological consequences of prolonged elevation of glucocorticoid concentrations have been mentioned above. Persistent activation of the SA axis, which stimulates the renin–angiotensin–aldosterone system, may also translate into pathology: initially, by progressively increasing blood volume and raising blood pressure; later, as a consequence of the alterations in neuromuscular excitability due to hypokalaemia.
- Obviously, whenever coping strategies have exhausted the biological reserves of the animal it is to be expected that further challenge(s), even by inconsequential stressors, may translate into pathology.

- A coping strategy may increase the animal's exposure to environmental factors that damage its health (e.g. the housed subordinate cow that copes with dominant cows by standing and lying at a distance in damp, dirty, unsheltered locations) or it may deny the animal the opportunity to participate in activities that promote its health and welfare (e.g. limit its access to feed or, in the extreme, an animal exposed to chronic, unavoidable stress may develop 'learned helplessness', become recumbent and stop eating).
- A coping strategy may involve a physiological response that directly contributes to a pathological process (e.g. a very thirsty, salt-deprived animal consumes excess water and develops haemolysis and cerebral oedema: water intoxication).
- A coping response may attenuate or suppress an important component of the animal's normal defence system and leave it vulnerable to a disease unrelated to the original stressor (e.g. attenuation of the immune response by transportation stress renders an animal susceptible to respiratory disease).

In each scenario the transition to pathology is predicated on a changed (or changing) internal milieu that cannot be explained in terms of strict homeostatic dogma. The principle of homeostasis is that the body must hold all its regulated parameters within very narrow operating ranges centred on the relevant 'normal' set points. Students of stress are well aware that that is not how things are in the real world. It is recognized that an animal exposed to intense or persistent stressors may have to vary many parameters of its internal milieu and match them appropriately to environmental demands. Sterling and Eyer (1988) referred to this principle as allostasis, meaning 'stability through change'.

Concepts of allostasis and allostatic load

When an animal perceives a situation as stressful it makes the behavioural and physiological responses that it considers most appropriate. Experience will help the animal assess how much of a threat is posed and what it requires to do to ward off that threat. If a particular stressor has been encountered previously and been found to be easily controlled, the response will be measured accordingly; habituation will ameliorate the physiological perturbation and the biological cost will be reduced. The responses are mediated by the SA and HPA axes and, if the stressor is mild and short-lived, homeostatic regulation will modulate the perturbations within tolerable operating ranges until the regulated parameter(s) can be returned to the fixed set point(s). A simple example: if, for whatever reason, blood glucose concentration falls, the neuroendocrine axes will set about correcting the deficit by typical homeostatic responses that implement glucose-sparing measures augmented by gluconeogenesis.

It is entirely appropriate that those components of the internal milieu that are absolutely essential for life (for instance, oxygen tension, pH, body temperature) should be governed according to strict homeostatic principles that operate within narrow ranges about fixed set points. However, life expects the body to be capable of adapting to marked variations in its natural environment and that is possible only if the animal can continuously readjust a number of parameters toward new set points and wider operating ranges that are appropriate to the challenging circumstances in which it finds itself. Put very simply, different circumstances demand that the several interacting systems vary their homeostatic set points to ensure that their activities remain in synchromesh. Allostasis enables the SA axis, the HPA axis and the cardiovascular, metabolic and immune systems to effect the changes in the internal milieu that make the most beneficial use of the animal's biological resources; in brief, they induce a new steady state based on a panel of readjusted set points in counter-balancing systems.

Allostasis is a useful concept but, as McEwen and Stellar (1993) pointed out, it does not take into consideration the strain on the body produced by the activities of physiological systems adjusting to repeated challenges, the consequent changes in metabolism or the impact of wear and tear on a number of organs and tissues that can predispose an individual to disease. They introduced the term allostatic load to describe the aggregate biological costs that result from chronic overactivity or underactivity of allostatic systems.

As McEwen (1998) perceived it, there are three phases in the body's response to challenge: it must mount an adequate allostatic response, it must maintain that response until the stress ceases and it must shut off the response when the threat has passed. Thus, allostatic load can accrue when:

- There is an inadequate response that leads to compensatory hyperactivity of other regulatory systems;
- The body is subjected to repeated challenges from multiple stressors;
- There is failure of habituation to repeated challenges of the same type;
- Delayed shut-down prolongs the response after the threat has passed.

When circumstances improve, with environmental stress consistently at a low level, the animal may discharge much of the allostatic load, to the benefit of its health and production.

On the other hand, if life remains stressful the load will accumulate and the animal will find it progressively more difficult to make effective readjustments in response to further challenges: in a figure of speech, a point may be reached at which all the slack in biological reserves has been taken up and the next coping strategy will propel the animal into overt dysfunction. In many instances, the final challenge that breaches the boundary between the compensated state and 'pathology' may be relatively minor and, if it is identified, it may be assigned an exaggerated degree of causal importance that is an impediment to the exploration of the real sources of allostatic load within the herd, which must be the ultimate target for the dedicated clinician. More immediately, failure to see the 'big picture' may militate against the efficacy of treatment of the diagnosed ailment – it is unlikely that targeting what, in essence, may be just the tip of a dyshomeostatic iceberg will successfully restore the animal to full health and production. Recognition of the bases from which the allostatic load has accrued should enable the clinician to implement a more holistic, more successful, approach to the problem.

In summary, the concept of allostatic load provides a rational hypothesis to account for the contribution of environmental stress to the pathogenesis of dyshomeostasis, a sometimes precarious state of readjusted parameters that, when propelled into decompensation, can be manifest as any of a range of different ailments in individual animals within a herd.

Allostatic load and the veterinary practitioner

How should the concept of allostatic load inform the veterinary practitioner in the field? How does it relate to the major problems encountered in intensive cattle enterprises: lameness, mastitis, infertility, metabolic disorders, welfare, behavioural problems and levels of production?

'Life is stress, stress is life'

Life is a minefield of potential stressors that each creature has to negotiate by recourse to its repertoire of cognitive, behavioural, neural, endocrine and immunological modalities. The ability to adapt successfully to the multifarious challenges of life – or, in the words of Sterling and Eyer (1988), the ability of the 'organism to vary parameters of its internal milieu and match them appropriately to environmental demands' – is called allostasis. When the adaptive responses put those parameters persistently outside their normal operating ranges – whether because of many significant challenges or because the allostatic responses remain turned on when no longer required – the body incurs a cumulative biological burden that constitutes its allostatic load.

The biological costs of each challenge to homeostasis are influenced by the genetic background of the animal, its previous history, the magnitude of the allostatic load it has accumulated already and the functional priorities of the current phase of its life cycle, as well by the nature of the stressor, its novelty, its intensity, its frequency, its duration and the types of responses it elicits.

Thus, when clinical disease is manifest the cascade of environmental factors that have contributed to the current state of the sick animal will have operated at two levels: the proximate and the ultimate. The proximate factors (infectious, metabolic, toxic or whatever) have made the immediate challenges that caused the presenting signs. The ultimate factors have been responsible for the allostatic load, for the depletion of energy reserves and the cumulative wear and tear of vital organs and their regulatory controls that have predisposed the animal to the ravages of the proximate stressors. In brief, allostatic load is the burden of costs that have been paid at several toll-bridges on the road to clinical disease. Increasingly, trends in intensive systems of animal production will force us to bring that toll into sharper focus in our deliberations on the pathogenesis and treatment of ailments and on the husbandry and welfare of farm animals.

The stress response can be mobilized in response to physical or physiological stimuli, and also in expectation of them. As is evident from the early part of this chapter, the brain is the coordinator of the body's responses to the stimuli: it decides whether or not a potential stressor poses a threat, and how the animal should cope with it. The cognitive appraisal of the environmental stimulus determines the response: if it is not perceived as a threat, it does not elicit a stress response. On the other hand, novel stimuli will be perceived as threats *ipso facto*, even though they may not be particularly aversive in character; the intensity of the responses will decline as the novelty wears off. It is neither possible nor desirable to isolate livestock from the aversive stimuli that are a feature of the complex, dynamic environment of the modern intensive cattle enterprise. Some types of mild stimuli are beneficial; for instance, they induce a state of arousal in which metabolic processes are adjusted for rapid expenditure of energy and they 'tune' the cognitive and motor mechanisms that the animal will call upon whenever it is challenged by a significant stressor. Furthermore, there is convincing experimental evidence that when the stress system is activated in that manner, productivity is improved and some immune functions are enhanced, at least in the short term.

Practical considerations

The scientific literature, particularly the medical literature, has concentrated unduly on the negative aspects of stress, on its role in the pathogenesis of disease; in reality, the stress system has evolved as an essential defence mechanism that plays a very positive role in the survival of organisms beset by stressors. The task is to manage the sources of environmental stimuli to the mutual benefit of the animal and of the commercial imperative; that requires attention to the structure and hygiene of the physical facilities, and to the social contexts, metabolism, physiology, vulnerabilities and coping strategies of the animals. Several of those topics are dealt with in some detail elsewhere in this book; here, under several subheadings, we cherry pick some clinical conditions that illuminate the central thesis: that allostatic load is a significant factor in the pathogenesis of many ailments, that sick animals should be seen as sentinels of stress within the herd and that the therapeutic, prophylactic and managerial measures are unlikely to be entirely satisfactory unless that fact is taken into consideration. Although the vast literature on the stress response has yet to generate a unitary paradigm that would inform the clinical judgement of a veterinary surgeon in relation to those decisions, there are two less ambitious constructs, mentioned above, that are relevant to the message of this essay: the partitioning of metabolic fuels and the counter-regulatory activity of the corticosteroids.

Partitioning of metabolic fuel

Each organism has a limited energy budget from which it must allocate resources prudently if it is to maintain the body and perpetuate the species. When the supply of energy falls below total requirement, the available metabolic fuels are partitioned according to priorities set to ensure the survival of the organism (Fig. 67.5). The energy equation can go into negative balance either because the intake has been reduced below normal expenditure, or because the expenditure has been increased to meet special needs, as happens in early lactation or when the animal has to cope with major stressors. In the trade-off between competing energetic requirements, environmental stressors can exercise a defining role. Top priority is given to maintenance of basic cellular functions, thermoregulation and locomotion for foraging (not a problem in a modern cattle enterprise). When the short-fall is severe, less and less of the intake goes to growth, fat storage or reproduction; in extreme circumstances these activities will be suspended until they can be resumed when the energy balance has been restored.

Counter-regulation by glucocorticoids

As mentioned, negative feedback by glucocorticoids plays a significant role in protecting the organism against 'overshoot' by either limb of the stress system (Fig. 67.3). In addition, they contribute to the effort to conserve energy whenever stressors threaten homeostasis: they exert inhibitory effects at more than one point in each of the endocrine axes that regulate growth, thyroid function, reproduction and immune function (Fig. 67.6).

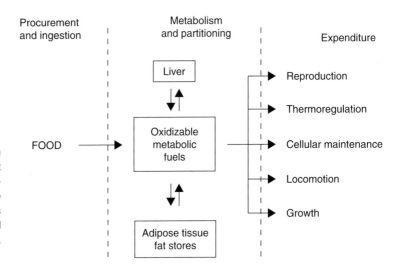

Fig. 67.5 Partitioning of metabolic fuels. When the supply of energy is insufficient to meet demands, non-essential processes such as reproduction and growth are deferred, and fat stores are mobilized to ensure that the essential processes of basic cellular metabolism, thermoregulation and locomotion are maintained. (After G.N. Wade & J.E. Schneider, 1992).

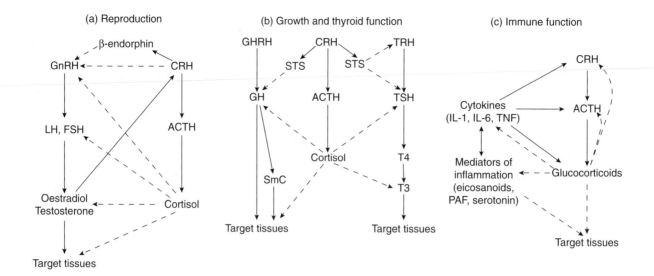

ACTH: Adrenocorticotrophic hormone
CRH: Corticotrophin-releasing hormone
FSH: Follicle-stimulating hormone
GH: Growth hormone
GHRH: Growth hormone-releasing hormone
IL-1: Interleukin-1
IL-6: Interleukin-6

SmC: Somatomedin C
STS: somatostatin
T3 and T4: thyroid hormones
TNF: Tumour necrosis factor
TRH: Thyrotrophin-releasing hormone
TSH: Thyroid-stimulating hormone

Fig. 67.6 Interactions of the HPA axis with the systems that subserve (a) reproduction, (b) growth and metabolism, and (c) immune function. Solid lines represent direct or indirect activation; dashed lines represent direct or indirect inhibition. (After Stratakis & Chrousos, 1997.)

Clinical implications

Social context (see Chapter 55)

Each herd of cattle develops its own social structure, a hierarchy in which social rank is held at a price. Social interactions within the group can be stressful: determined subdominant animals challenge the dominant animals; in turn, dominant animals bully subordinate animals. Several lines of evidence suggest that the magnitude of the allostatic responses to social stressors is influenced greatly by the social rank of the animal: the biological costs are greatest at the two extremes of the hierarchy. The allostatic load – and the loss in productivity – depends on the animal's perception of the threat to its well-being and on its coping strategy. The active coping strategy of the dominant animal can be as costly as the passive coping style of the subordinate animal. When an animal is exposed repeatedly to the same predictable stressors, the intensity of the stress reaction tends to decline progressively. This process of habituation appears to be stressor-specific; the animal retains the capacity to make an acute response to a novel stressor. Therefore, within a settled herd the toll of social stress can be attenuated by good stockmanship that seeks to shield the animals from all that they will perceive as novel, frightening, painful, unpredictable, frustrating or uncontrollable.

Social stress may be a source of significant allostatic load.

Foot lameness (see Chapter 31)

It is accepted that poor quality horn is a significant factor in the pathogenesis of foot lameness in lactating dairy cows. The defect in the horn is associated with impaired keratinization in the epidermis of the horn, a process that is known to be influenced by the dominant hormones in late pregnancy and early lactation. Particularly relevant to the present discussion is the evidence from hoof explants in organ culture that glucocorticoids inhibit the synthesis of hoof protein. It has been suggested that the elevated systemic concentrations of glucocorticoids during lactation could contribute to the deterioration in horn quality in the lactating cow. It is conceivable that other stressors that induce the release of more glucocorticoids would exacerbate that deterioration. For instance, poor quality horn that predisposes to foot lameness is not uncommon in recently-calved heifers joining the milking herd for the first time; in those circumstances, horn is being produced by an immature animal whose endocrine organs are secreting unprecedented quantities of lactogenic hormones augmented by the hormones released in response to the social stress – and whose metabolic stability is being challenged by the unaccustomed demands of her first lactation. Thus, the presenting ailment may be a manifestation of a 'big picture' that incorporates a number of elements of systemic dyshomeostasis – abrupt exposure to a novel hormonal milieu, unrelenting demand for an unprecedented quantity of energy, and social stress.

Allostatic load may find expression in a presenting ailment that has no obvious anatomical link to the systemic dyshomeostasis that has made the host animal vulnerable to 'pathologies'.

Infertility (see Chapters 33–37)

Reproductive functions in the female are more susceptible to the effects of stress than are those of the male, for two reasons: firstly, because she has to budget for a vastly greater investment of metabolic resources over a much longer time; secondly, because stressors are prone to disrupt the precision with which a number of hormones must be secreted in appropriate quantities and in a delicately ordered and exquisitely timed sequence in order to establish a pregnancy. It is known that short-term stressors (such as fear engendered during herding, handling or transport, electric prods or stray voltage) can interfere with fertility if they challenge the cow at a critical juncture. To a considerable degree, the response of the female to stressors is predicated by a desire to conserve energy until the threat is past; clearly, that is the case when she falls into a negative energy balance and suspends her reproductive activities *pro tem.* Fortunately, the suspension leaves the regulatory neuroendocrine apparatus intact and normal business should be resumed when the energy balance has been restored. In reality, spontaneous resumption often takes longer than is ideal for the commercial enterprise; this is particularly significant in relation to the low calving rates achieved in the early post partum period – which can be a cause of considerable economic loss, especially in a herd where a seasonal breeding programme is in operation.

Over the past 20 years, the dairy industry in the UK has switched from a predominantly British Friesian cow population to predominantly North American Holstein cows and, further, it has engaged in intense selection for milk yield. The records show that over that period the pregnancy rate to first service has declined at an average rate of approximately 1 per cent per annum, and that atypical ovarian hormone patterns have been contributing factors to that reduction (Royal *et al.*, 2000). The response to hormonal therapy has not been consistently good; it has fallen considerably short of that which current knowledge of reproductive biology would lead us to expect.

A plausible hypothesis advanced to account for the decline in fertility in high-producing cows was that reproduction is suppressed while the animals are in negative energy balance: that the hypothalamic–pituitary–gonadal (HPG) axis is inhibited while the cow 'milks off her back'. Most high-producing dairy cows enter the breeding season in a negative energy balance; some will not have achieved a positive balance before the end of the third month after calving, at which time they are expected to be in-calf again. From an energetic perspective, this means that the biological costs of reactivating cyclic activity of the HPG axis and its associated organs have to be abstracted from a budget that is in negative balance because it has to support, either in sequence or in parallel, the extensive hormonal changes (qualitative, quantitative and temporal) that accompany the transition from pregnancy to lactation; the biological costs of uterine involution; the extraordinary nutrient demands of lactation and the regulation of the associated metabolic adaptations; the extensive adaptations in cardiovascular and digestive physiology; the biological costs of immune defence of organs newly opened to ascending infection (uterus, mammary gland); the transition from housing to pasture and the associated meteorological and nutritional changes; together with any number of contingency costs. Despite all that massive drain on body reserves, approximately half of the mated cows conceive to first service. It is clear that although the energetic perspective provides a rational account of the drain on body resources, it does not provide a comprehensive explanation for either the infertility of a sizeable number of clinically normal cows or for the relatively poor response to hormone therapy in those animals.

It is likely that much of the infertility reported in clinically normal cows is due to unrecognized allostatic load; in other words, it is not a disease in the traditional sense, rather a suspension of service due to a fault in the signalling system. Therefore, the protocol for clinical assessment of cows being prepared for the breeding season should include a check-list of potential stressors to which the animals due for examination are most likely to have been exposed; the prophylactic management of the breeding herd should take account of the findings.

The effects of stress on reproductive functions are complex; however, it is reasonably close to the truth to say that most of the adverse effects are mediated by interactions between the HPA axis and the HPG axis (Fig. 67.6(a)). Corticotrophin-releasing hormore (CRH) can suppress the secretion of gonadotrophin-releasing hormone (GnRH) via an opioid-mediated mechanism, supranormal levels of androgens from the adrenal glands can distort the negative feedback regulation at the hypothalamus and pituitary gland and glucocorticoids can exercise inhibitory effects at all critical points in the HPG axis (and even as far as the target tissues for gonadal steroids). It is probable that the most important factor in the suspension of reproductive activity is interference with the pulsatile release of GnRH by the hypothalamus, which alters the pulsatile release of LH by the pituitary gland that, in turn, regulates ovarian activity. However, in practice, inhibition at other points in the HPG axis may be just as significant if it reduces the prospects of success when exogenous hormones are used to 'kick start' the inactive axis. For instance, exogenous GnRH may be an adequate stimulus to provide a functional pulsatile release of LH, but its ability to improve calving rates may be constrained if it does not lead to the removal of inhibition or to the acquisition of essential receptors at other points around the HPG axis or in the peripheral target organs.

A plausible alternative hypothesis is that the counterregulatory components of stress responses to various challenges experienced during early lactation exert a residual inhibition on the biochemical activities of the HPG axis and that this inhibition can be of varying duration depending on the magnitude of the allostatic load and the ability of individual animals to cope with it.

Allostatic load may find expression as a biochemical lesion.

Metabolic diseases (see Chapters 46, 47)

The peripartum period is a stressful time in the life of a cow. During the 'transition period' (the last four weeks of gestation and the first four weeks of lactation) cows experience enormous changes in the hormonal milieu, a negative energy balance and a plethora of stressors that arise from changes in feeding and management regimes. Not surprisingly, a considerable proportion of the metabolic and infectious diseases to which cows are subject occurs during the transition phase, many of them having metabolic perturbation as the ultimate source of allostatic load. Metabolic perturbations can both induce and be induced by allostatic load.

It is recognized that absorption of glucose by the intestine contributes little to the energy homeostasis of lactating cows. The large and immediate requirement of the lactating mammary gland for glucose is met by a reduction in utilization by several other tissues and by an increase in synthesis from fats and proteins by the liver (gluconeogenesis). The key role is played by lipid metabolism that provides a rich supply of substrate for gluconeogenesis. The amount of energy reserves upon which the postparturient cow can draw is a product of the feeding regime during the recent dry period. At the onset of lactation there is extensive mobilization of body fat and in many cows this gives rise to a state of subclinical ketosis, a condition that impairs immuno-

logical defences. When the stored fat is mobilized, some is deposited in liver, kidneys, adrenal glands and muscle. The fatty infiltration of the liver can be severe in cows that are overfat at calving and in cows that mobilize fat faster than it can be utilized. Subclinical fatty liver has been linked to increased susceptibility to ketosis, milk fever, mastitis, lameness and infertility.

The important features here are that metabolic perturbation can be a significant primary cause of allostatic load borne by a cow as she enters the transition period and that the magnitude of that load can be a significant factor in determining how she copes with the subclinical metabolic problems that invariably arise in the early weeks after calving. Failure to cope renders her vulnerable to a plethora of stressors that are rife at that time and act as proximal factors in the pathogenesis of several clinical diseases, metabolic or infectious.

Inappropriate nutrition can be a significant factor in the pathogenesis of a variety of metabolic and infectious diseases.

Coping with pathogens

By definition, pathogens are stressors. The magnitude of the biological costs they impose on their hosts is determined by the virulence, infective dose and novelty of the pathogen and by the nature, location, intensity and duration of the host response, together with the pre-existing allostatic load of the host. In turn, stress is a risk factor for a variety of infectious diseases, particularly in the periparturient period and especially in individual cows who enter the transition period with appreciable allostatic loads, and in cows that are genetically predisposed to exaggerated responses of the HPA and SA systems to stressors.

Risk of infection can be increased when the stress response leads to behavioural changes that increase exposure to pathogens, when it impairs the immune response (whether to an invading pathogen or to a latent resident), when it contributes to the progression of an existing pathological process or when it is prolonged unnecessarily.

It is accepted that stress has a negative effect on the immune response and it is often said that the effect is largely due to the corticosteroids released during the stress response. The reality is a very much more complex scenario that involves the nervous, the endocrine and the immune systems. The different types of immune cells possess receptors for the signals issued by the HPA and SA axes; in turn, immunocytes release cytokines that modulate the activities of the stress system.

Recent research indicates that stress may boost humoral immunity as it suppresses cellular immunity – a response that is due to the effects of glucocorticoids and catecholamines on the differentiation of T helper cells. The stress hormones modulate the secretion of different types of cytokines by antigen-presenting cells (macrophages and other phagocytic cells); those cytokines influence the differentiation of antigen-naïve T helper cells (Th0) into two subsets (Th1 and Th2) that, in turn, secrete cytokines that are involved in the acute phase response, in sickness behaviour and in the differential regulation of cellular and humoral immunity. The cytokines secreted by Th1 cells promote cellular immunity, those secreted by Th2 cells promote humoral immunity. The Th1 and Th2 responses are mutually inhibitory; it is thought that the Th2 shift that accompanies a vigorous stress response might have important implications for the course and outcome of infectious, allergic, autoimmune and neoplastic diseases. Some immunocytes secrete hormones: for instance, lymphocytes can synthesize ACTH, growth hormone and prolactin – messengers that probably act locally in a paracrine fashion. In addition, there are functional contacts between nerve fibres and immunocytes: for instance, lymphoid organs are innervated by nerve fibres that release noradrenaline or neuropeptides which interact with the immunocytes to cause changes in cellular trafficking, lymphocyte proliferation, antibody production and cell lysis. The physiological and pathophysiological consequences of all this cross-talk are most evident to the veterinarian in the periparturient cow.

The transition period is recognized as a time of relative immunosuppression and increased susceptibility to infectious diseases – whether viral, bacterial or parasitic. The periparturient cow is at serious risk of infection because, at parturition, the uterus and the udder lose the physical barriers that have protected them from ascending infections; thus, bacterial pathogens may enter while the defences are at their weakest. Leukocytes play key roles in the defence of both organs: prompt migration of neutrophils (PMNL) is essential to overcome the bacteria; however, the activities of the leucocytes are depressed as a consequence of the negative energy balance, the subclinical ketosis, the fatty liver and the raised circulating concentrations of glucocorticoids. Some recently-calved cows develop a severe systemic illness when the influx of PMNL does not materialize in response to invasion of the udder by *Escherichia coli*. However, in most instances the cellular and humoral responses control the proliferation of the invading bacteria without achieving total elimination; for instance, *Staphylococcus aureus* frequently is relegated to subclinical residence in the udder. This is an important adaptive strategy: its immediate effect is to protect the organ from serious tissue damage, while it sets up a mechanism by which the organ can maintain a satisfactory level of local immunity to cope with

future challenges. This strategy is used in dealing with a range of microbes and parasites and, in addition to enhancing the host's immune repertoire, it represents prudent use of energy reserves since the likelihood is that the biological cost of total elimination would be far greater than the net cost of maintaining a resident population to which the host becomes habituated – and which brings such benefits as on-going priming of local immunity to the pathogen and competitive inhibition of other pathogens that might attempt to invade the location.

Given that infectious agents impose an increased metabolic and nutritional load on their hosts, it is astonishing that voluntary reduction in food intake appears to be a beneficial coping strategy in some viral, bacterial and parasitic diseases. For instance, there is experimental evidence that when mice infected with *Listeria monocytogenes* were force fed to the same energy intake as their uninfected controls, they had a higher mortality rate and a shorter survival time than did the infected mice that were anorexic. Clearly, in this instance, force feeding nullified the benefits of a natural coping strategy and became an iatrogenic instrument of death. It is legitimate to question the wisdom of force feeding sick animals.

The two coping strategies just discussed – subclinical infection and anorexia – are somewhat at variance with the thrust of conventional wisdom; nevertheless, their adoption by diverse species indicates that they bring significant benefit to the host. Therapeutic interventions should not run counter to the way of nature.

Therapeutic interventions in infectious diseases should be consonant with coping strategies, including those that appear to be contrary to conventional wisdom and expectation.

Altered behaviour

Changes in behaviour may be evoked as coping strategies (confrontational, submissive or socially neutral) or they may emerge in the course of stress-induced illness – in the form of listlessness, exaggerated sleepiness, weakness, depressed locomotor activity, shivering, diminished social interaction, anorexia, decreased foraging and absence of body-care activities. Current opinion amongst those who study infectious diseases is that those behavioural changes are an integral part of an adaptive response to antigenic challenge and that they are elicited by the pro-inflammatory cytokines that are released from immunocytes to mediate both the local (inflammatory) and the systemic (febrile and behavioural) components of the reaction to foreign antigens. In that interpretation, sickness behaviour and fever share two significant attributes that are of fundamental concern to the therapist: each is an important component of the natural defence system; in excess, each can be detrimental to the host.

Cytokine-induced anorexia can be interpreted as a way to reduce the availability of some nutrients (e.g. iron, zinc) necessary for multiplication of the pathogens. Sleepiness and reduced activity can be interpreted as ways in which to conserve energy that the sick animal will re-allocate to new priorities geared toward victory over the pathogens (e.g. inflammatory and immunological responses). Therefore, as far as is possible, our treatment modalities should not nullify the natural benefits of sickness behaviour – as force feeding did to the *Listeria*-infected mice.

The behavioural changes evoked by the stressors may be transient (e.g. failure to groom during illness), persistent (e.g. stereotypies) or life-threatening (e.g. learned helplessness). Learned helplessness is an unmotivated state in which an animal gives up trying to cope with the exigencies of life, is indifferent to its own well-being and is unresponsive to therapeutic or punitive interventions. Originally, the term was used by scientists who assessed the coping abilities of dogs exposed to repeated electric shocks. They found that dogs that had been subjected to unavoidable shock treatments in a preliminary experiment just sat and took the shocks when the experiment was repeated in a situation from which there was a fairly obvious means of escape. Subsequently, it has been recognized that chronic stress can lead to learned helplessness in other species (including humans), notably when they have endured repeated failed attempts to achieve an objective.

The author believes that he has encountered this cognitive aberration in cattle originally thought to be suffering from metritis, mastitis, acetonaemia or hypocalcaemia, but most convincingly in a subset of downer cows that did not have the physical or biochemical defects to account for their predicament (pp. 439, 797). From clinical experience, he suspected that some of the underlying allostatic load in the helpless downer cow had been brought forward from the dry period and, perhaps, from previous lactation(s). If the conjecture is correct, it follows that a comprehensive record of health and production parameters should reveal more about the bases from which the load accrued than would the most recent metabolic profile. Learned helplessness may be associated with either infectious or non-infectious conditions; it is regarded as a putative animal model of depression. The pathophysiological mechanisms have not been elucidated but some evidence from animal experiments hints at an imbalance between the activities of the two limbs of the stress system, with the HPA axis in the ascendant. It would not be prudent to treat such animals with corticosteroids, as is often advocated for the downer cow syndrome.

Quite often the downer cow syndrome is seen as an incomplete response to treatment for milk fever: it is said that the longer the interval between the time the cow becomes recumbent and treatment for milk fever, the greater the incidence of the downer cow syndrome. One has to entertain another possibility: that some recently-calved cows, already burdened with substantial allostatic loads and with the added stress of acute hypocalcaemia, may find *rapid* intravenous injection of essential ions to be a stressor too many – sufficiently stressful to necessitate a period of recumbency in which to recover the will and the confidence to resume normal activities. When management fails to recognize the cow's immediate need for a period of relative inactivity she will be subjected to repeated premature attempts to force her to stand; this will increase the risk of physical damage and, by the same token, it is likely to reinforce the state of helplessness that now is at the core of her problem.

It is tempting to speculate that the dispirited state may have a morphological basis somewhat analogous to the neuronal damage seen in the hippocampus of chronically stressed humans, shrews and rodents. If that were the case, the evidence from the other species would be reassuring: the neuronal damage is neither terminal nor irreversible. Most of the affected cattle should respond to standard treatment, always provided the clinical problem is not compounded by musculoskeletal damage incurred during ineffectual attempts to get the cow on her feet before she is ready to do so of her own volition or by complications arising from prolonged recumbency.

These observations on altered behaviour highlight two significant aspects of animal health: firstly, sickness behaviour is an adaptive response to infectious or non-infectious stressors; it provides the allostatic base from which the recuperative process develops and it is instrumental in setting the endogenous rhythm for that process; secondly, any therapeutic intervention that jolts the periodicity of the process becomes an additional stressor that is likely to delay or distort resolution.

Sickness behaviour is a strategy that may be invoked to cope with either infectious and non-infectious stressors; interventions that target the behaviour rather than the stressors are liable to delay, distort or prevent the recuperative process.

Concluding comments

The primary aim of this chapter is to draw attention to the concept of allostatic load and to encourage practitioners to appreciate how important a role it plays in the pathogenesis of most of the ailments they encounter. More often than not, clinical disease is the product of a cascade of environmental stressors: some can be designated as ultimate factors that have been responsible for the allostatic load that has made the animal vulnerable to the proximate stressors (infectious, metabolic, toxic) that are the immediate causes of the ailment. If we wish to keep pace with current trends in intensive systems of animal production we will have to take greater stock of ultimate stressors than has been our wont. Increasingly, our task will be to devise and monitor herd health programmes that manage the sources of environmental stimuli to the mutual benefit of the livestock and the profit-and-loss account. In that context, it does not require great insight to realize that curtailment of allostatic load is the key to improvement in the overall health and productivity of the herd.

When the accumulated allostatic load attenuates the animal's ability to cope with further challenges, the host becomes vulnerable to all sorts of stressors, even those that are only mildly aversive. In that situation, a relatively minor proximate stressor may propel the host into clinical disease, particularly one that reflects the functional priorities of the current phase of the animal's annual life cycle. For that reason, the differences in presenting signs shown by herd mates should not obscure the fact that each sick animal has had a significant allostatic load and, in that sense, each clinical case should be seen as a sentinel of stress within the herd.

Allostatic load is not something that can be measured by standard biochemical or physiological techniques. Research scientists use hormone assays and heart rates to monitor responses to acute stressors, but those parameters are not indicative of allostatic load. The best sources of the required information are comprehensive life-time records of health and production parameters. The onus is on the herd veterinarian to ensure that the appropriate records are compiled, that they are used to identify both ultimate and proximate stressors and that the information so gained is taken into account whenever therapeutic or prophylactic interventions are contemplated.

Glossary

AROUSAL: the state of general alertness. It is reflected in conscious state, in cognitive activity, and in behaviour.

AUTOCRINE: hormone (or cytokine) acts on the cells that produce it.

BRAINSTEM: the stem-like region that links the cerebrum with the spinal cord; consists of the midbrain, pons and medulla oblongata.

CYTOKINE: protein or glycoprotein (produced by one or more cell types) that regulates the activity of other cells.

ENDOCRINE: hormone is secreted directly into blood stream and acts on target cells elsewhere in the body.

HABITUATION: extinction of a conditioned response by repetition of the conditioned stimulus; perceived threat diminishes as novelty wears off.

HYPOTHALAMIC–PITUITARY–ADRENAL (HPA) AXIS: the hormonal interplay between those three organs; the principal hormones involved are corticotrophin-releasing hormone (CRH) and arginine vasopressin (AVP; formerly ADH) from the hypothalamus, adrenocorticotrophic hormone (ACTH) from the pituitary gland and cortisol from the adrenal cortex.

HYPOTHALAMIC–PITUITARY–GONADAL (HPG) AXIS: the hormonal linkage between the hypothalamus (releases GnRH), the pituitary gland (releases the gonadotrophins, FSH and LH) and the gonads (secrete testosterone, oestrogens, progesterone).

LOCUS COERULEUS: a small pigmented cluster of noradrenergic neurones in the dorsal brain stem on the floor of the fourth ventricle. It contains more than half of the noradrenergic neurones in the brain; they project widely throughout the CNS and they are highly responsive to alerting/stressful stimuli, including those that activate the HPA axis.

PARACRINE: hormone (or cytokine) acts on a different cell type which lies in close proximity to the producer cells.

PROXIMATE CAUSE: an environmental factor that acts as an immediate stimulus for a biological event (e.g. a disease).

SYMPATHOADRENAL (SA) AXIS: consists of two components: the sympathetic nervous system and the adrenal medulla. The major biologically active products, the catecholamines (adrenaline and noradrenaline), serve both as neurotransmitters and as hormones. Within the CNS they act as neurotransmitters; outside the CNS, adrenaline acts principally as a hormone, while noradrenaline acts principally as a neurotransmitter at sympathetic post ganglionic terminals.

ULTIMATE CAUSE: an environmental factor that increases the probability that a particular biological event will be elicited by another factor that is seen as the immediate stimulus.

References

Chrousos, G.P. (2000) The stress response and immune function: clinical implications. *Annals of the New York Academy of Science*, **917**, 38–67.

Johnson, E.O., Kamilaris, T.C., Chrousos, G.P. & Gold, P.W. (1992) Mechanisms of stress: overview of hormonal and behavioural homeostasis. *Neuroscience and Biobehavioral Reviews*, **16**, 115–30.

McEwen, B.S. (1998) Protective and damaging effects of stress mediators. *New England Journal of Medicine*, **338**, 171–9.

McEwen, B.S. & Stellar, E. (1993) Stress and the individual: mechanisms leading to disease. *Archives of Internal Medicine*, **153**, 2093–101.

Moberg, G.P. (2000) Biological response to stress: implications for animal welfare. In *The Biology of Animal Stress*, pp. 1–21. CABI Publishing, Wallingford.

Royal, M.D., Darwash, A.O., Flint, A.P.F., Webb, R., Woolliams, J.A. & Lamming, G.E. (2000) Declining fertility in dairy cattle: changes in traditional and endocrine parameters of fertility. *Animal Science*, **70**, 487–501.

Sterling, P. & Eyer, J. (1988) Allostasis: a new paradigm to explain arousal pathology. In *Handbook of Life Stress, Cognition, and Health* (ed. by S. Fisher & H.S. Reason), pp. 629–49. Wiley, New York.

Stratakis, C.A. & Chrousos, G.P. (1997) In *Endocrinology: Basic and Clinical Principles* (ed. by P.M. Conn & S. Melmed), p. 205. Humana Press, Totowa, NJ.

Wade, G.N. & Schneider, J.E. (1992) Metabolic fuels and reproduction in female mammals. *Neuroscience and Biobehavioral Reviews*, **16**, 235–72.

Adult Cattle
Global Variation in Cattle Practice

Chapter 68

Diseases Related to Management in Europe

G.H. Wentink and A. de Kruif

European dairy farming trends   1151
Infectious diseases   1152
Metabolic diseases   1153

European dairy farming trends

Europe stretches from the 70th degree of latitude (north of the polar circle) to the 40th degree of latitude into subtropical regions. Many different climatic conditions and huge differences in landscape exist. These differences work out in very variable disease problems and different husbandry systems. In Denmark, northern Germany, The Netherlands, northern Belgium, north west France and in Italy at the borders of the river Po, flat land with fertile pastures is located. These areas are suited for dairy farming. Annual milk production is high and may reach 8000 kg with 4 per cent fat corrected milk (The Netherlands). However, in Sweden, southern Germany, southern Belgium, eastern France and Austria a hilly or mountainous landscape exists. These areas are less suited for dairy cows, but more suited for suckler cows and beef production. Traditionally, in these areas dairy herds with limited numbers of cows occur. Italy, Spain, Portugal and Greece have a rather hot climate during summer time; dairy farming is difficult and of reduced extension. The average annual milk production is 3000 kg (Greece), although exceptionally dairy farms with a high production level occur (Portugal). In this chapter attention will be focused mainly on dairy cattle management in north west Europe.

In 1998 just over 82 million cattle, including 21 million dairy cows over 2 years old, were present in Europe. In Table 68.1 the number of cows and the agricultural area per country are given. In The Netherlands and northern Belgium the ratio of cattle to agricultural area is more than two animals per hectare, in Ireland 1.5, while the other countries have less than one cow per hectare agricultural surface. This quotient applies to the agricultural area and gives an indication of animal density in a country. In countries with a low quotient cows may be kept on a limited part of the agricultural area and in some areas the actual number of animals per hectare may be as high as or even higher than in The Netherlands and Belgium.

Total milk production in Europe is fixed by the quota system introduced in 1983. Placing a ceiling on milk production per country puts a limit on the number of dairy cows. As a result of fruitful breeding programmes and efficient feeding regimes the annual milk yield per cow increased during the last decades. The number of dairy farms and dairy cows will be reduced even more during the next decade, with an increase in the number of cows per farm.

The diets of dairy cows in The Netherlands and Belgium contain substantial levels of concentrates. The constituents of these concentrates are partly grown in Europe, but for the larger part, in particular protein, they are imported into Europe. Nitrogen, phosphate and other minerals are actually imported into these countries, but a limited amount of minerals is exported as milk and meat. Therefore, an imbalance exists between the amount of minerals imported into these areas and the amount exported to other areas of Europe or to other parts of the world. The mineral surplus is applied into the ground as manure. This causes an accumulation of elements (nitrogen) and puts a further stress on the reduction of the number of cows on environmental grounds, especially in The Netherlands and Belgium.

During the last decades, the average education level of the farmers increased sharply and as a consequence veterinarians must take another role. The veterinarian will be called in to take their part in prevention of diseases and to sustain the milk production level on dairy farms rather than to cure sick animals. Therefore a shift in the veterinary skills is inevitable: the veterinarian has to support the management system of the client, mainly by doing the thinking for prevention of diseases and to optimize production levels.

In the past, much attention was paid to certain aspects of food quality, e.g. the cell count in milk, but nowadays the consumer's attention is even more focused on food safety. Although the quality of products for human consumption increased during the last decade, the confidence of the consumer in these prod-

Table 68.1 Cattle population and agricultural area in Europe 15 (source FAO).

Country	Agricultural area × 1 000 000 ha (1999 data)	Number of cattle × 1000 (2000 data)	Cattle/agricultural ha
EU 15	143.018	82.332	0.58
Austria	3.419	2.150	0.63
Belgium-Luxembourg	1.521	3.085	2.03
Denmark	2.644	1.850	0.70
Finland	2.272	1.086	0.48
France	29.900	20.572	0.69
Germany	17.031	14.658	0.86
Greece	9.020	590	0.07
Ireland	4.418	6.708	1.52
Italy	16.268	7.184	0.44
Netherlands	1.967	4.200	2.14
Portugal	4.142	1.245	0.31
Spain	29.980	6.203	0.21
Sweden	3.235	1.713	0.53
UK	17.219	11.133	0.65

ucts continuously declined. The latter aspect is emphasized by BSE. The supposition that BSE prions might have caused the vCJD in man (see p. 909) and the possibility that prions entered the human food chain without appropriate check on the source of the animals for food production caused a shift in public opinion. The threat of disease caused by products of animal origin and the threat of antibiotic resistance in human bacteria due to the application of antibiotics in food animals increase the attention paid by the consumer to the chain in which human food is produced. The chain must be completely transparent and the methods to control the processes must be supervised by independent people.

Furthermore, increasing attention is paid by the public to animal welfare. The consumer demands food from animals that are kept under conditions that allow them to function more or less naturally. Reducing the frequency of microtraumata by comfortable barns beyond doubt increases the durability of dairy cows. In the future veterinarians may participate in the supervision of the production of food from cows by paying attention to their comfort.

Knowledge of diseases, and especially knowledge of their cause and aetiology, the consequent knowledge to prevent problems and the skills to prevent a decline of milk production and disasters on dairy farms must be an essential characteristic of veterinarians in the next decade. Veterinarians may also contribute to the achievements of dairy farmers by increasing the quotient milk production versus manure per surface unit.

Two aspects for veterinary prevention programmes must be considered: prevention of the introduction of infectious diseases and of diseases that are indigenous in all cattle populations, such as mastitis and lameness.

Infectious diseases

In north west Europe a number of major infectious diseases have been eradicated, e.g. rinderpest, BCPP, tuberculosis, brucellosis and EBL. In 2001, FMD re-emerged in north west Europe and caused severe (UK), moderate (Netherlands) or mild (France) epizootics, focusing attention on this disease again. Until this outbreak attention was mainly focused on the eradication of BSE, IBR, BVD and on a limited scale of paratuberculosis (Johne's disease) (see p. 857).

Veterinarians must be fully aware of the agents and their epizootiology. The Achilles heel in the infection chain must be found for each individual pathogen to develop effective eradication strategies.

FMD (see Chapter 43c)

As long as FMD exists somewhere in the world, the risk of introduction of the virus into Western Europe by food products from infected animals remains real. Intensive traffic movements of people over the world increase the risk of accidental introduction of contaminated food products. When the FMD virus is introduced into a West European country, the risk of an epizootic depends on the time lapse between introduction of the virus and the diagnosis, and of the number of animal movements over the country or to other countries during that period (see p. 705).

IBR (see p. 289)

In the 1980s, voluntary eradication programmes for IBR were started in the Scandinavian countries. However, there was no thorough economic basis for the eradication of IBR. IBR is also not a threat for human health, the economic damage is limited and clinical disease can be prevented by an appropriate vaccination programme. However, as Scandinavian countries became officially free of IBR several other European countries were forced to achieve IBR negativity as well. It was mainly a political decision to eradicate IBR.

Eradication programmes were successful in Switzerland, Denmark, Sweden, Finland and Austria. The basis for the success of these programmes was that all serologically positive cows, which might be latently infected, were eliminated. The percentages of animals found serologically positive for IBR in these countries did not exceed 20 per cent of the dairy cows.

However, percentages of serologically positive animals turned out to be as high as 50–60 per cent in The Netherlands and Belgium, and therefore the above mentioned method was not applicable. Vaccination programmes using gene deleted vaccine virus, but with a serological response distinguishable from field virus infections, are applied to all cattle herds that are not proven negative for BHV1. These programmes started recently (1998), so there is no evidence that these schedules will turn out to be completely successful.

BVD (see p. 853)

Bovine virus diarrhoea virus (BVDV) has a real economic impact on infected farms and the disease deserves full attention for eradication. Although some Scandinavian countries have voluntary eradication programmes, the efforts to eradicate this virus are far less intensive than the efforts to eradicate IBR. In Sweden and in Denmark voluntary programmes for the eradication of BVDV have been in progress since 1993. The backbone for the eradication programme is the detection and destruction of all persistently infected animals. A herd has to start with a virological search for the presence of persistently infected animals. After the elimination of these animals a regular serological survey of the animals between 6 and 12 months is performed, and later on by testing for the absence of antibodies against BVDV in bulk milk samples.

Paratuberculosis (Johne's disease) (see p. 857)

Johne's disease is caused by *Mycobacterium avium paratuberculosis*. After infection by the oral route during the first months of life, clinical disease characterized by diarrhoea and emaciation may develop later in life. In the last phases of the disease bacteraemia develops and as a consequence milk and meat might be infected with the bacterium.

In man, Crohn's disease has a pathology that is very similar to paratuberculosis in the bovine. *M. avium* ssp. *paratuberculosis* was isolated from the intestines of patients with Crohn's disease, but not from the intestines of humans suffering from other intestinal disorders. The PCR for *M. avium* sp. *paratuberculosis* is significantly more often positive in patients suffering from Crohn's disease than in those suffering from other gastrointestinal disorders. This does not prove, however, that *M. avium* ssp. *paratuberculosis* is the causative organism for Crohn's disease. The agent might take advantage of the pathological changes in the intestines of human patients with Crohn's disease to colonize the bowel. It demonstrates, however, that the agent must be present in the human environment and probably in human food. Actually, about 6 per cent of milk for human consumption in the UK was contaminated with *M. avium* ssp. *paratuberculosis*, although it is unclear whether the bacteria in milk are viable.

It is, however, important to ensure that the human food chain is free from this bacterium and veterinarians are obliged to pay attention to the eradication of the agent from the cattle population. On the other hand, efforts to eradicate paratuberculosis (Johne's disease) in all countries are limited.

BSE (see p. 909)

Bovine spongiform encephalitis prions are suspected to be the cause of the [new] variant Creutzfeldt Jacob Disease ([n]vCJD). These prions are present in tissues from the central nervous system and jejunum of cattle with overt clinical signs of the disease. Cows are believed to contract the disease by consuming ruminant proteins produced from infected ruminants. The major breakthrough was the total elimination of animal proteins (except fish and poultry proteins) from the ruminant food chain. The consumer requires a guarantee that animals for human consumption have never consumed animal protein and puts emphasis on the source of the meat and its control chain.

Metabolic diseases (see Chapter 46)

The increased capacity for milk production necessitated improved feeding regimes. The quality of grass silage and corn silage increased and facilitated higher production levels. Next to roughage a substantial amount of concentrates are fed. Concentrates are added in the milking parlour or in concentrate stations, where each

Table 68.2 Prevalence of disease problems in 8272 cow years in nine dairy farms in The Netherlands during a 10-year period.

Fertility problems	34.9%
	including 19.0% irregular heat periods
Udder problems	24.6%
	including 22.5% mastitis cases
Locomotory problems	36.7%
	including 6.8% laminitis
	including 17.7% solar ulcers
Metabolic problems	19.7%
	including 5.5% acetonaemia
	including 14.4% milk fever

individual cow can obtain an amount relative to milk production, or a total mixed ration is provided.

Indications for a causal relationship between food, feeding and diseases are increasing and substantiated by experimental work. Metabolic disturbances also significantly influence the health of claws and may exacerbate the consequences of external forces (minitrauma) on claws, causing lameness (see Table 68.2).

Veterinarians should be fully aware of the relationships between food, metabolism and disease, and must be able to translate food changes into possible deviations of the health of the animals in a herd. Thus the veterinarian involved in cattle herd health management must be familiar with food constituents and components and their digestion and metabolism.

Large quantities of rapidly fermentable starches in the diet may cause disturbances of rumen fermentation, resulting in low milk fat percentages, off feed syndrome, laminitis and ruminal acidosis consecutively, depending on the grade and the period of acidosis. These phenomena are mainly observed in herds with high milk production levels being fed high amounts of concentrates in the diet. Although there are no exact data on the incidence of these diseases in Europe, in The Netherlands and Belgium these disturbances have occurred rather frequently in the past, but are now decreasing due to the lower percentage of easily fermentable starches in the concentrates.

If the energy in food is maintained in accordance with the milk production level, cows lose body weight moderately during the first few weeks of lactation. The negative energy balance during the first weeks after parturition is physiological (energy intake by food and energy from reserve fat equals energy demand). If this equilibrium is disturbed by low energy content of the food acetonaemia some three weeks after parturition develops, characterized by high levels of β-hydroxybutyrate and low glucose levels in the peripheral blood. This problem is still known but occurs less frequently than previously due to increased quality of the diet

(roughage). In experimental farms in The Netherlands with a management above average the incidence of this disease was limited to 1 per cent of the cows.

A disease biochemically very similar to acetonaemia may develop within two weeks after parturition. In the peripheral blood high levels of non-esterified fatty acids (NEFAs), high levels of β-hydroxybutyrate and low levels of glucose are found, indicating severe energy deficit, but with very high levels of triacylglycerol in the liver. This phenomenon is known as fatty liver, a very peculiar phenomenon in that the peripheral body is deficient in energy supply, while in the liver high levels of energy (up to 25 per cent of triacylglycerol of wet liver tissue) are available (see p. 801). The cow is ill and may die from energy depletion while abundant energy is present but is not made available for the metabolism. The origin of the disease is considered to be a sequel of excess of energy supplementation in the last part of the lactation period and during the dry period. About 10 to 12 weeks after parturition, the initial decrease in body weight due to the physiological negative energy balance turns and becomes positive. The body weight increases until drying off.

During the dry period the body weight must be kept constant. However, the increasing energy value of the roughage produces an energy surplus during the dry period and as a result many cows increase their body weight and are fat at calving. Although exact mechanisms are poorly understood, many cows in a fat body condition at calving (BCS 4 or higher on a 5 point scale) suffer from a decreased appetite after calving. This reduced appetite may be related to or caused by leptins, by high levels of NEFAs, by a combination of these factors or by other not yet described causes. In these fat animals with often high milk production the energy intake is short in comparison to the energy demand. Increased lipolysis, in order to compensate for energy demand, results in the accumulation of triacylglycerol in the liver, i.e. fatty liver. In the short term this metabolic disease may result in emaciation and death; in the long term it may cause reduced reactivity of the immune system, making the cow more vulnerable to common bacterial infections. There may be a high prevalence of mastitis in the post partum period in animals suffering from fatty liver. Ova mature during an eight-week period and the first ovulation after parturition in these cows produces an ovum matured during the period with high levels of NEFAs in the blood. These ova are less fertile and may result in lowered conception rates. This metabolic disturbance causes decreased ovarian activity with prolonged intervals from calving to heat, resulting in prolonged intervals from calving to conception. The incidence of fatty liver is not known, but it is suspected to occur more frequently than anticipated.

Dietary deficiencies are rarely diagnosed in dairy herds in areas with a high milk production. The diet receives adequate levels of minerals and vitamins from the addition of concentrates, the composition of which is monitored by the manufacturer. However, as many farms start to feed home-produced diets composed from basic substances there is a risk of miscalculation and thus excesses or deficiencies may occur. The veterinarian will be asked to support management decisions taken by the owner and to diagnose failures in management which result in reduced fertility, reduced immunoreactivity or in lameness.

Further reading

FAOSTAT Database Collections; http://apps.fao.org/
Smolders, G. In *Annual Reports of the Research Station for Cattle-, Sheep-, and Horsehusbandry 1990-1999,* Institute edn. Research Institute for Animal Husbandry, Lelystad, The Netherlands.

Chapter 69
Cattle Disease in Africa

R.S. Windsor

Introduction	1156
Epizootic diseases	1156
Rinderpest	1156
Foot-and-mouth disease	1157
Tuberculosis and brucellosis	1157
Parasitic diseases	1157
Trypanosomosis	1159
East Coast fever	1160
Plant poisonings	1161

Introduction

The purpose of this chapter is to indicate some of the differences between cattle problems in Africa and the rest of the world and to highlight some of the conditions that are of major importance to livestock production. North Africa is part of the Mediterranean area and it is separated from the rest of Africa by the Sahara Desert, where there are few cattle. SubSaharan Africa has a variety of climatic conditions, from almost no rainfall to heavy, regular and seasonal rainfall areas, and in consequence there is a variety of environmental types and eco-systems. This in turn has led to many different lifestyles from the sedentary agriculturist to the nomadic pastoralist who moves his herds as conditions dictate, e.g. the Fulani in west Africa would prefer to graze their animals in the south where there is more rain and the grass is better for the cattle. However, during the rainy season the tsetse flies are active, so the cattle are moved north to escape their bites. When the dry weather returns and the pastures in the north become depleted of grass they return their animals south. In large measure the distribution of the human population has been governed by this fly (*Glossinia* spp.). To many African people, the well-being of their animals governs their lifestyle. The differences in the ecology of the continent govern the behaviour of disease agents, parasites and vectors: therefore, cattle diseases to be considered here fall into three main categories:

- *Epizootic diseases* that have mostly been introduced into the continent from Europe – rinderpest (p. 707), contagious bovine pleuropneumonia (p.

868), foot-and-mouth disease (p. 700), rabies (pp. 908, 1164), tuberculosis (p. 862) and brucellosis (p. 280).
- *Parasitic diseases* caused by either by helminths, e.g. *Haemonchus contortus* (p. 275), or *Fasciola gigantica* (p. 276), or by tick-borne protozoa, e.g. *Theileria parva* (p. 750) or *Anaplasma marginale* (p. 761), or by the biting flies (p. 747) (*Glossinia* spp.), or the various species of *Trypanosoma* (p. 756).
- *Plant poisonings* caused by the varied and extensive flora of Africa. Among such a profusion only a few examples can be given.

Epizootic diseases

Rinderpest (see p. 707)

First among cattle diseases is rinderpest, the greatest scourge of cattle, and indeed their owners, that the world has ever seen. When rinderpest was imported into Britain in the mid nineteenth century it ruined farmers, bankrupted insurance companies and was directly responsible for the foundation of what is today the State Veterinary Service. The Royal Agricultural Society considered that rinderpest was responsible for the death of more than 400 000 head of cattle in Britain in six months of 1866 at a cost in 1866 figures of £8 million. It was introduced into Egypt in 1890 and in five years it had travelled to South Africa, killing not just cattle but also huge numbers of game animals as it passed.

Following Macmillan's famous 'winds of change' speech to the South African parliament in 1960, African countries raced towards independence. The cold war was beginning to push America and Russia: both wished to develop spheres of influence in Africa and so they poured money into the continent. Joint Project 15 was set up, with almost limitless funding, to eradicate rinderpest from Africa. A vaccination campaign, using the Muguga tissue culture vaccine, almost succeeded in eradicating the infection. Unfortunately pockets of virus persisted in Chad and Ethiopia and from these the disease 'recolonized' Africa. The Pan African Rinderpest Campaign (PARC) was set up with the aim of eradicating rinderpest within a period of 10 years. PARC has the advantage of superior immunological tests and it would seem that the goal may be achieved. Similar projects in the Middle East and southern Asia also seem to be achieving success: it is possible that early in the new millennium global eradication of rinderpest may become a reality.

Foot-and-mouth disease (see p. 700)

In Africa, foot-and-mouth disease (FMD) is more important for its political impact than for the disease that it actually causes. It is endemic throughout much of the continent and the African buffalo (*Syncerus caffer*) has been shown to be a carrier of the SAT strains. This makes the eradication of the virus from the continent problematical. Control measures follow the normal international pattern, with the exception of Botswana, which has developed its own technique of control. The country is divided by cordon fences (some hundreds of kilometres in length) into different areas of 'infected', 'clean but vaccinated' (buffer) and 'unvaccinated' areas. Movement of cattle from one area to another is strictly controlled, including physical examination of every animal by the Veterinary Department. At each biannual vaccination the animal is branded and only branded animals are allowed into the abattoirs. As a result of this control, Botswana is permitted to export meat into the European Union from the 'unvaccinated' areas.

For many years Kenya was allowed to export meat into the European Economic Community. Movement controls broke down, the disease spread and Kenya is no longer able to export its meat to Europe. Other countries with no export trade outside the continent make little or no official attempts to control the infection.

Tuberculosis and brucellosis (see pp. 280, 862)

Bovine tuberculosis in Africa is complicated by the presence of a large number of 'cold blooded' or atypical strains of *Mycobacterium*. These make the interpretation of the tuberculin test more difficult and today outside South Africa there is little done to control the disease at the official level. In most countries with a commercial dairying industry (e.g. Kenya, Ivory Coast) the industry itself tries to ensure freedom from both tuberculosis and brucellosis, thus enabling producers to market 'attested' milk.

Parasitic diseases

The African continent has the climate, soils and hence ecology to support a great diversity of animals and their parasites. Unlike the Amazon Jungle the tropical forests of Africa are not so large as to make huge tracts of land uninhabitable. Africa has probably more species of tick than any other continent and because of the extensive savannah areas these creatures have had plenty of hosts and time, so that a reasonable equilibrium has built up between animals (including indigenous domestic cattle), ticks and the parasites that they carry. This equilibrium was destroyed when the Europeans imported exotic cattle in an attempt to increase productivity of the native cattle. For some unknown reason cattle, and indeed humans, have failed to build up resistance to the parasites carried by the tsetse flies (*Glossinia* species) (see p. 747) – the trypanosome (*Trypanosoma* species) (see p. 756). In large measure it has been the trypanosome that has determined the distribution of cattle in Africa and consequently it has played a part in the distribution of the human population. Tsetse fly are recorded in 37 African countries and more than 10 million square kilometres of land are infested. There are few breeds of cattle that have developed a trypanotolerance and these are mostly confined to west Africa.

The reason for the difference in resistance may well be associated with the feeding habits of the parasites. Hard ticks (and these are the only ones of importance to cattle) are sedentary and remain on the host, or at least each stage of the parasite remains on the hosts and feeds by sucking blood. There are three types of hard tick: one-, two- and three-host ticks, depending upon whether or not at the completion of each stage of life the tick remains on the host to moult or whether it drops off. A one-host tick spends its life on one animal: the larvae moult to nymphs, the nymphs to adults on the same animal. The gravid female drops off to lay her eggs on the ground. The two-host tick usually moults from larva to nymph on one animal but the nymph drops and moults to an adult on the pasture. The three-host tick drops off at each moult. It is obvious that three-host ticks are more efficient at spreading infections than the one-host variety. By contrast, the tsetse fly takes each meal where it finds it and moves from animal to animal: there is no time for a host–parasite interaction and the parasite moving from host to host has accustomed itself to varying host immune mechanisms.

Each species and genus of tick has a different distribution, a different life cycle and differing host preferences and site predilections. Specific ticks transmit specific infections: e.g. *Rhipicephalus appendiculatus* (the brown ear tick) transmits East Coast fever (ECF) (theileriosis) (p. 750) and other theilerial parasites, whereas *Boophilus decoloratus* (the African blue tick) transmits *Babesia bigemina* (the cause of bovine babesiosis) (p. 748) and *Anaplasma marginale* (the cause of anaplasmosis) (p. 761). By the same token, there are different species of *Glossinia* that inhabit different ecological niches and that transmit different species of *Trypanosoma*. The demonstration by Bruce, at the end of the 19th century, that it was the tsetse fly that transmitted pathogenic trypanosomes to livestock led the way to understanding the role of arthropod vectors in animal disease. The tsetse fly has been a major impediment to the development of a large part of the continent and environmentalists would say that this has been a good thing! With the rapidly increasing population in Africa and the need for more food it is essential that tsetse flies and ticks be controlled.

It has been known for many years that some animals in a herd are more resistant to a specific disease than others, and some more susceptible. Breeders have used these characteristics and, as mentioned above, trypanotolerant breeds of cattle are found in west Africa. It has been demonstrated recently that some cattle have an increased resistance to tick infestation. This increased resistance is associated with immune mechanisms. It has been said that the trypanotolerant Ndama breed is more resistant because the animals are better able to control the parasitaemia, although the mechanism by which this occurs has not yet been demonstrated. Resistance to *Babesia bigemina* (p. 748) has been shown to have more to do with resistance to the tick, than to the parasite itself. Resistance to tick infestation was first demonstrated in Australia. It was also noted in Africa that indigenous breeds kept with exotic animals often showed much lower (down to 1/6) tick burdens. It has been possible to breed cattle with increased resistance to the one-host tick, but so far not to the multi-host ticks.

It is unlikely that tick resistance can be developed to the point where there is no transmission of the protozoal diseases. Consequently a combination of resistance with acaricide treatment will probably always be required. Before deciding upon a programme of tick control by acaricides it is essential to know which ticks are to be controlled, and when. For many years Malawi had a policy of strategic dipping of cattle: in the north of the country it was confined to the wet season when the number of ticks increased dramatically. In the dry winter the tick burden was at a minimum and so the gain was less than the cost. In areas of Africa where ECF is not a problem it is often not necessary to attempt acaricide dipping or spraying of cattle. In areas of Africa where ECF has been introduced, there may be a mortality rate approaching 100 per cent, and then it may be necessary to use chemicals to keep the tick burden to a minimum. In the absence of ECF, there are two options: the first is to control the remaining tick-borne diseases by chemotherapy and vaccination and to ensure that the young animals are exposed to the infec-tions in order to reduce the dipping and work towards endemic stability; the second is to try and control the ticks by intensive dipping.

Over the years there has been a different approach to the control of tsetse flies. Perhaps the greatest natural control of the fly was the epidemic of rinderpest that started in Egypt and moved south at the end of the nineteenth century. Not only were cattle killed, but there was a massive destruction of game animals and hence a lack of food for the tsetse flies: e.g. rinderpest eliminated the tsetse fly from the Limpopo valley between Botswana and South Africa and in almost 100 years the valley has not been recolonized. Human activity has an effect:

- Clearing forests for timber or settlement destroys the habitat of the *fusca* group of flies (*G. brevipalpis* in particular).
- Clearing the savanna has made the greatest impact on the *morsitans* group (*G. morsitans* and *G. pallidipes*). These primarily feed on game animals and clearing the bush results in destruction of the wildlife. At levels of human habitation in excess of 40 per square kilometre, the *morsitans* group dies out completely.
- The *palpalis* group may be beneficially affected by human activity, as these are the flies of the riverbank, and it is rare for human activity to clear the bush by the side of rivers. Cattle graze on the cleared land but pass through the riverine bush to get to the river. The establishment of game parks has provided breeding grounds for tsetse flies and food for them to eat!

Pesticides have been used to control the flies, by knapsack spraying the area of the flies' resting sites. Organochlorine compounds such as DDT and dieldrin were widely used and effective, with synthetic pyrethroids taking over when the organochlorines were banned. A more efficient form of spraying was from the air. Today with the rotary atomizers and night flying equipment, the spraying is much more efficient and in the Okavango Swamp in Botswana, the use of endosulphan has reduced the environmental contamination – only 8 g per square kilometre are used and the drug targets the tsetse fly rather than other insects; so far as is known, the only detrimental environmental effect that it has is to inhibit fish reproduction for a season.

Tsetse flies can be caught in traps and although this was not successful at eliminating flies from an area, work with traps led to the discovery that the flies are attracted by the colour blue. The use of odour to attract the flies only had limited success, but the development of targets impregnated with insecticides has had a striking success. As the fly lands on the blue cloth it receives a dose of insecticide.

Trypanosomosis

This disease occurs in humans, cattle (where it is known as nagana), camels, horses and pigs, but the infection occurs in most wild mammals. Trypanosomes are protozoa that possess a kinetoplast and a flagellum and require two hosts to complete their life cycle: a mammal and an insect (in South America, chaggas the human disease is transmitted by blood sucking bugs). The trypanosomes multiply in the mammalian host and, with the exception of *T. equiperdum* which is venereally transmitted, they are ingested by blood sucking insects: in Africa normally by tsetse flies. Multiplication within the fly varies with the *Trypanosoma* species, but the infective stage ends up either in the salivary gland or in the faeces. Other biting flies are able mechanically to transmit the parasite to a new host.

There are three major species that infect cattle: *T. brucei* (p. 759), *T. congolense* (p. 758) and *T. vivax* (p. 758). The last has become established in South America where there are no tsetse flies and so transmission is by means of other haematogenous flies, and it is assumed that no development of the parasite occurs in these flies. Trypanosomes multiply by longitudinal binary fission in the fly and the mammalian host, although sexual processes occur only in the fly. Mature trypanosomes are ingested by feeding flies and they undergo development in the salivary gland or gut. Development and maturation occur in the vector, after which the parasite is transferred to another mammalian host. Transmission is either by the presence of the trypanosome in the saliva or by contamination of the host's skin by trypanosomes in the faeces of the fly.

A critical factor in the epidemiology of trypanosomosis is that, once infected, a tsetse fly remains infected for life. The development of the parasite in the fly varies from a few days in the case of *T. vivax* up to 45 days in the case of *T. brucei*. The role of game animals cannot be overemphasized; the present policy of game ranching in conjunction with rearing cattle and the increasing numbers of game parks has increased the risk of disease in cattle. Another significant factor in the epidemiology of the disease is the use of trypanocidal drugs, which may in turn lead to the development of resistant trypanosomes.

The pathogenesis is not completely understood: the trypanosome multiplies at the site of infection and local lymph nodes become enlarged, before the parasite is found in the blood. Then the classic intermittent parasitaemia ensues. As the parasites increase in number, so does the febrile response: as they decrease, so does the fever. The body mounts an immunological defence against the parasite and the trypanosome changes its external antigens to defeat the host. The outcome of this battle often depends upon extraneous factors such as the nutritional state of the host. Tissue lesions vary with the species: *T. vivax* and *T. congolense* are mainly intravascular parasites inducing changes in the endothelium of the capillaries, wheareas *T. brucei* has an affinity for tissues. The anaemia seen in trypanosomosis is caused by a multiplicity of factors including haemolysins and enzymes such as proteinases or phospholipases. The trypanosome attaching to the erythrocyte makes it a target for the body defence mechanisms. If the animal does not die in the acute stages it becomes progressively emaciated. Mixed infections tend to cause more severe disease.

In endemic areas the disease causes huge economic losses. Clinical disease is more commonly caused by *T. vivax* and *T. congolense*; *T. brucei* causes much less serious disease. However, there are no specific signs for trypanosomosis and they are dependent upon the degree of damage to specific organs and the severity of the anaemia. Acute disease with death within two to six weeks is seen in animals introduced into an endemic area, but chronic disease with the animal surviving months or even years is more common. Acutely affected animals rapidly lose weight and all the classic signs of fever may be seen. In the chronic form the animals show periods of weakness and lethargy followed by a recovery; the animal becomes pale with raised pulse and respiratory rates. Good nutrition may help an animal to throw off this chronic infection, but the more normal outcome is for the animal to become thinner and thinner. The infection induces immunosuppression, which can allow other infections such as anaplasmosis to take over.

It can be very difficult to diagnose this disease because the parasites are not always present in the blood and there are no specific clinical signs. Moreover there is no relationship between the number of parasites and the severity of the disease. Trypanosomosis must be considered to be a herd problem and so the presence of parasites in the blood of a 'normal' animal should be taken as significant. In many endemic areas there are inadequate laboratory services to assist in making the diagnosis and so many veterinarians consider that response to treatment is a good way to confirm the diagnosis. Serological tests have until recently suffered from an inability to produce specific antigens. However, the indirect fluorescent antibody test and the enzyme-linked immunosorbent assay have recently been introduced into the arsenal of tests used for making a herd diagnosis, and monoclonal antibodies have been produced to identify the three bovine species of trypanosome. The main problems in the differential diagnosis are with the other protozoan infections, i.e. anaplasmosis (p. 761), babesiosis (p. 748) and East Coast fever (p. 750), however, in these diseases it is usually a simple procedure to demonstrate the parasite.

The control of the infection by the use of drugs presents a continuing problem and the Veterinary Departments in many African countries control the use of them to prevent the development of resistant strains of trypanosomes. There is more to treatment than drugs and a good plan of nutrition is essential; all animals, and particularly work oxen, must be rested during convalescence. One of the major problems facing trypanosomosis control is that today there are only four drugs effective in treating the condition, the most recent of which (isometamidium) was introduced in 1961; moreover, no pharmaceutical company is working on this problem. Care must be exercised in using a combination of drugs because some of the drugs have a combined toxicity greater than that of the individual drugs.

Because of the problems of drug resistance it is essential that optimum use must be made of them, that is to say they should be used in a strategic way whenever possible to coincide with the local rainfall and hence fly patterns. However, the most important factor is to reduce the fly population and hence the parasite challenge. The Zimbabwe Veterinary Department has made great strides in vector control going back over a period of more than 50 years. This is well described by Connor (1994). Many countries in Africa have units within their Veterinary Departments (e.g. Botswana, Kenya, Ghana and Zimbabwe) devoted to testse fly control. However, Basil Parsons, the Kenyan parasitologist, was of the opinion that 'when the last man leaves the African continent, he will be bitten on the backside by a tsetse fly'.

East Coast fever (see p. 750)

In 1965, the owner of a 'high grade' (mostly Jersey cross indigenous Kenyan cattle) herd of cattle went on holiday leaving his manager in charge. Because they were 'high grade' they had to be dipped in acaricide every five days to prevent ticks introducing *Theileria parva parva (T. parva)*. Unfortunately the manager allowed the fences to be cut and the neighbour's indigenous cattle were able to mix. The farmer returned to find 75 of his best heifers dead from East Coast fever (ECF). The infection is transmitted by the three-host tick *Rhipicephalus appendiculatus* and the disease is characterized by the multiplication of the lymphoblasts infected with theilerial schizonts throughout the body.

The disease was first recognized in 1897 by Robert Koch, who called it African Coast fever. Following the ravages of rinderpest and the introduction of European stock in an effort to replace the dead animals, ECF spread south from East Africa down to Cape Province in South Africa, killing more than one and a quarter million cattle. The disease was eradicated by a process of dipping in acaricide, movement controls and destocking of infected pastures.

As with trypanosomes, so *T. parva* alternates between its mammalian and invertebrate hosts. The piroplasms in the erythrocytes of an infected bovine are ingested by the tick in its blood meal and these develop via a sexual stage to a stage that invades the gut cells of the tick. Further development results in a motile stage that invades the body cavity and migrates from there to the salivary gland, where large numbers of sporozoites are produced; these are the infective stage for the bovine, being injected when the tick feeds. Because the vector is a three-host tick and because there is no transovarial transmission the infection is transmitted by nymphs infected as larvae, or adults infected as nymphs. Should an infected larva feed on a non-susceptible host there will be no transmission from the larva to the adult.

The disease affects only cattle, the African buffalo (*Syncerus caffer*) and the Asian water buffalo (*Bubalis bubalis*). No other ungulates are infected and the parasite depends upon *Rhipicephalus appendiculatus* for transmission. This tick is widespread in the warm humid areas of Africa, and were the parasite to be introduced to these areas the infection would be rapidly disseminated. The peak incidence of the disease is just after the rainy season. Zebu cattle which carry low burdens of ticks rarely show clinical disease: they are infected as calves and may show a febrile reaction with complete recovery; mortality is low. However, if susceptible animals are introduced into this endemic area and become infested with ticks, acute disease will follow. The disease can be introduced into a clean area if an infected animal is brought in or if conditions are such that an area can be colonized by the tick. In the absence of control measures, the mortality can reach 90 per cent.

The disease is primarily one of the lymphatic tissue. The sporozoite enters lymph cells at the place of entry and within a few days schizonts can be seen in the cytoplasm of the cells. Lymphocyte proliferation occurs at the site and within five days infected cells can be found in the drainage lymph node. Massive proliferation of lymphoblasts ensues and more distant lymph nodes, spleen and thymus become affected. Finally all the parenchymatous organs become involved. Within a few days lymphocyte proliferation is replaced by lymphocyte destruction, resulting in immunosuppression. The outcome of the disease depends upon the survival of sufficient lymphocytes to effect an adequate immune response. Release of piroplasms which then invade the erythrocytes appears to have no specific pathogenic effects.

East Coast fever is characterized by fever with all its complications – lethargy, constipation or diarrhoea, respiratory signs and abortion, together with enlargement of the superficial lymph nodes. Auscultation of the lungs indicates severe pulmonary oedema. Because the ticks live in the ears it is often the parotid lymph nodes that first show enlargement. Death occurs from five days to three weeks after the onset. Exotic animals that recover often become emaciated and can remain unproductive for months.

On post-mortem examination the three classic findings are severe lymph node enlargement, a massive pulmonary oedema and splenomegaly. Congestion and oedema can be found in any of the internal organs. Numerous small white foci may be present in the kidneys, indicating lymphoid hyperplasia in the cortex. There may be emaciation and subcutaneous oedema. Diagnosis is confirmed by the examination of smears stained with Giemsa stain, of lymph node, spleen, blood or almost any organ. The presence of large lymphoblasts is strongly suspicious: the presence of schizonts is conclusive.

In some cases it is possible to observe lymphocytes containing schizonts in blood smears. It may not be possible to demonstrate schizonts in zebu cattle and so demonstration of rising titres of antibodies should be made, using the immunofluorescence techniques. Among the conditions to be considered in the differential diagnosis are rinderpest (p. 707), bovine virus diarrhoea (p. 853), contagious bovine pleuropneumonia (Chapter 49(b)) and trypanosomosis (p. 750); the presence of the schizonts is conclusive. At the Veterinary Research Laboratory, Kabete, Kenya, in the mid 1960s, each morning the staff were confronted by a line of men with bicycles, in the baskets of which were a selection of viscera from a dead animal. The farmers were only interested to know whether or not the animal had died from anthrax (if not, then they could eat the meat!); most animals had died from ECF.

Although tetracyclines have some effect against *T. parva* they are only consistently effective during the incubation period. The development of parvaquone, napthoquinone and febrifugene has resulted in success rates for treatment of over 90 per cent. However, some animals may remain carriers following treatment. Because immunity to the natural disease persists for more than five years, there has been a massive search for a vaccine and millions of pounds have been invested in this work at the Veterinary Research Laboratory, Kabete, the Kenya Agricultural Research Institute (formerly East African Veterinary Research Organisation), Muguga, and latterly at the International Laboratory for Research on Animal Diseases (now ILRE), all in Kenya. The vaccine consists of injecting a controlled number of sporozoites obtained from schizonts, originally from infected ticks but now from tissue culture, and then following this with treatment; initially a tetracycline was used but today the newer drugs have taken its place. Because the vaccine is only effective against homologous strains different preparations must be used

in different places and so the famous 'Muguga cocktail' was developed. This in turn has its problems, in that Directors of Veterinary Services are not happy to use live, virulent strains of *Theileria parva* from foreign countries and this means that it is not possible to produce the vaccine on a large, regional scale. The vaccine is expensive and not without its problems and so it is only used by commercial farmers. Work to improve the vaccine using molecular techniques is in progress.

Because of the behaviour of the tick and the parasite it is possible to control the infection by isolation of susceptible cattle, but they must not be fed purchased hay which might contain ticks. Tick control can keep ECF at bay providing that mistakes are not made in dip strength or dipping interval. Leaving the pasture free from cattle for 18 months or more will 'sterilize' the pasture because the parasite cannot survive that long: the ticks will feed on other animals, but there will be no transmission of the parasite and so it will die out. The control of cattle movement is also a good way to halt the spread of the parasite. Because ECF control requires a comprehensive infrastructure many countries have employed communal dipping as a means of bringing the cost within the grasp of the smallholder. To be effective, control measures for ECF need to be long term, take into account the whole management of the herd and the farmer must be eternally vigilant.

This account has concentrated on the disease caused by *Theileria parva parva*; however, this is not the only theilerial disease. Corridor disease caused by *Theileria parva lawrencei* was first seen in Zimbabwe and is an infection transmitted by ticks from the African buffalo. It is indistinguishable from ECF. Zimbabe theileriosis, caused by *Theileria parva bovis*, is also clinically indistinguishable from ECF, but is treatable with tetracyclines and shows differences in its epidemiology. The cause of 'turning sickness' (p. 752) is a theilerial parasite but its identity is in doubt. The disease is manifested by nervous signs and infected lymphocytes can be found in the brain. None of these conditions has the economic importance of ECF.

Plant poisonings

The foreword to *Plant Poisonings and Mycotoxicoses of Livestock of Southern Africa* (Kellerman *et al.*, 1990) says it all!

'Southern Africa is well known for the diversity and beauty of its flora. It is perhaps ironical, but not entirely unexpected that the sub-continent should be "blessed" with a possibly unequalled variety of poisonous plants and toxic fungi.'

'About 600 indigenous poisonous plants are known to occur.'

'In this part of the world, where livestock are traditionally kept under extensive conditions on veld that is frequently denuded by droughts, overstocking and uncontrolled fires, the animals are often forced to eat poisonous plants which they would normally avoid. Devastating outbreaks have been reported under such conditions, for instance, during 1926–27 about 600,000 sheep died of plant-induced photo-sensitization in the north western Cape Province and during 1929–30 over one million were killed by *Geigeria* spp., in Griqualand West.'

It is only possible to give a few examples with a view to stimulating the reader to carry out his own researches. Among many strange poisonings, perhaps the most odd is that caused by *Pavetta harbori* (Rubiaceae) (gousiekte). The original report concerned a mob of fat cattle waiting in the holding pens at the railside of Mahalapye Station, Botswana. The train came into the station, sounded its horn and 18 beasts dropped dead. The author found it hard to believe until he had a similar experience (on a much smaller scale): when he was investigating an outbreak of this disease, he drove into a kraal, shut the door of his truck and a fat bullock in excellent condition dropped dead. A post-mortem examination revealed no gross abnormalities. There had been a severe drought and the only green plant on the range was *Pavetta harborii* and the animals had been eating it for several months. The lesions produced by this plant are caused by one or more cardiac glycosides and produce a diffuse hyaline degeneration and necrosis of heart muscle, with the muscles being replaced by fibrotic tissue. There is no treatment for this condition and the only control is by preventing access to the plant. Since there are few farm fences in Botswana the only remedy is to dig up the plants – a forlorn hope.

A second plant which kills by means of a cardiac poison is *Dichapetulum cymosum* (Dichapetalaceae) (Mogau [Tswana] or gibflaar [Afrikaans]), the toxic principle of which is monofluoroacetate. In the rumen this is converted into fluorocitrate which interferes with the Krebs cycle. The plant has been likened to an underground tree: the tips of the branches protrude above the soil while the vast majority of the plant is underground, making it very difficult to eliminate. Unlike *Pavetta*, mogau is an acute poison which acts within four to 24 hours of ingestion, but as with *Pavetta* the animal drops dead without any premonitory signs. There are no post-mortem lesions and there are often no histological lesions. The only way to confirm the diagnosis is to demonstrate the leaves in the rumen.

Massive losses occur from this plant; in the Maun District of Botswana in 1984 one farmer lost 34 animals (10 per cent of his herd) and more than 700 cattle deaths were reported in the District. At the same time in the Chobe Game Park more than 70 buffalo were found dead by the side of the Chobe River. If the farmer sees his animals eating mogau he can save them by restricting their access to water for 24 hours. Because of its nature *Dichapetulum cymosum* is even more difficult to eliminate from the pasture than *Pavetta*.

A plant that is found throughout Africa and beyond is the castor oil shrub *Ricinus communis* (Euphorbiaceae). It has been grown as both a crop plant and as an ornamental plant in gardens because of the striking leaves and its red stems. The toxic principle is ricin, a toxalbumen, that is immunogenic and so repeated ingestion of small doses produces immunity. Ricin is found in all parts of the plant, but particularly in the seeds. Pure ricin is one of the deadliest substances known to man (Georgi Markov, the Bulgarian refugee, was murdered by this poison being injected from an umbrella on London Bridge!). The toxin is not so potent when ingested and the author remembers seeing an outbreak in Kenya in which 25 yearling dairy heifers were involved. All recovered, but the moment they were turned back into the field they went straight back to the plant and started eating it: they were removed from the field. The classic signs of the disease are a profuse watery, haemorrhagic diarrhoea, accompanied by inappetence, pain and bellowing. The normal post-mortem picture is of a severe haemorrhagic gastroenteritis. Since there is no way to demonstrate ricin, it is essential that a careful examination of the rumen contents be made for the seed or leaves. The best means of control is to keep the animal away from the plant.

This is just a small sample of the 'unequalled variety of poisonous plants' that are found in Africa. For those whose interest has been stimulated, the books by Kellermann *et al.* (1990) and Watt and Breyer-Brandwijk (1968) make excellent and entertaining reading.

Conclusion

In conclusion it must be said that only a small number of diseases have been discussed from a continent of infinite varieties. There are virus diseases such as lumpy skin disease (p. 887) or bovine malignant catarrh (p. 935); there are protozoal diseases such as elephant skin disease or Ondiri disease (p. 763), rickettsial diseases such as heartwater (p. 765). There are many, many problems and the governments have no money to control the major diseases, how much less these minor infections. Africa is in need of our help.

Further reading

Parasitic diseases

An excellent text covering all aspects of disease vectors with good diagrams and maps is:

Coetzer, J.A.W., Thomson, G.R. & Tustin, R.C. (ed.) (1994) *Infectious Diseases of Livestock with Special Reference to Southern Africa.* Vol. 1, Section 1, 3–163, Oxford University Press, Cape Town. various authors and topics on this theme.

Trypanosomiasis

Connor R.J. (1994) African animal trypanosomiasis. In *Infectious Diseases of Livestock with Special Reference to Southern Africa* (ed. by J.A.W. Coetzer, G.R. Thomson & R.C. Tustin), Vol. 1, pp. 493–552. Oxford University Press, Cape Town.

Murray, M., Morrison, W.L., Murray, P.K., Clifford, D.J. & Trail, J.C.M. (1979) Trypanotolerance – a review. *World Animal Review*, **31**, 2–12.

Murray, M. and Dexter, T.M. (1988) Anaemia in bovine African trypanosomiasis. *Acta Tropica*, **45**, 389–432.

Nantylya, V.M. (1990) Trypanosomiasis in domestic animals. The problems of diagnosis. *Revue Scientifique et Technique de l'Office International des Epizooties*, **9**, 357–67.

East Coast fever

For an early description of the disease see the reports of Koch or Theiler:

Koch, R. (1903) Interim report on Rhodesian redwater or 'African coast fever'. *Journal of Comparative Pathology and Therapeutics*, **16**, 273–80.

Theiler, A. (1904) East Coast fever. *Transvaal Agricultural Journal*, **2**, 421–38.

Modern papers on various topics are given below:

Brown, C.G.D., Malmquist, W.A., Cunningham, M.P., Radley, D.E. & Burridge, M.J. (1971) Immunization against East Coast fever. Inoculation of cattle with *Theileria parva* schizonts grown in cell culture. *Journal of Parasitology*, **57**, 59–60.

Chema, S., Chuomo, R.S., Dolan, T.T., Gathuma, J.M., Irvin, A.D., James, A.D. & Young, A.S. (1987) Clinical trial of halofuginone lactate for treatment of East Coast fever in Kenya. *Veterinary Record*, **120**, 575–7.

Irvin, A.D. (ed.) (1985) Immunization against theileriosis in Africa. International Laboratory for Research on Animal Diseases, Nairobi, Kenya.

Plant poisonings

The classic modern text, which is brilliantly written and superbly illustrated, is:

Kellerman, T.S., Coetzer, J.A.W. & Naudé, T.W. (1990) *Plant Poisonings and Mycotoxicoses of Livestock of Southern Africa.* Oxford University Press, Cape Town.

Apart from this the only book required is a good flora and the finest, although old, is:

Watt, J.M. & Breyer-Brandwijk, M.G. (1968) *The Medicinal and Poisonous Plants of Southern and Eastern Africa*, 2nd edn., E. & E. Livingstone, Edinburgh.

Chapter 70
Rabies

R.S. Windsor

Introduction	1164
Aetiology	1164
Epidemiology	1165
Europe	1165
Africa	1165
North America	1165
The Caribbean, Central and South America	1166
Asia	1166
Transmission	1166
Pathogenesis	1167
Clinical signs	1167
Necropsy and pathological findings	1168
Diagnosis	1168
Differential diagnosis	1169
Vaccination	1169
Control	1170

Introduction

Rabies is the most feared of all diseases. Once humans show signs of disease, they die. This virus disease affects all warm-blooded vertebrates and is usually transmitted by the bite of a carnivore. The virus enters the peripheral nerves and spreads to the spinal cord and brain, a process that might take several months. The nervous disease that ensues may last from a few days to several weeks before the animal dies. In humans one of the characteristic signs is a fear of water – hence its alternative name of hydrophobia.

The disease appears to have had a wide distribution since time immemorial, but it was Louis Pasteur who demonstrated the association between the causal agent and nervous tissue. By serial passage in laboratory animals he transformed the field ('street') agent into a 'fixed' agent with a shortened reproducible incubation period. Not until the twentieth century was it shown that the agent of rabies was a virus which could pass filters that retained bacteria. And in the same year, 1903, Negri demonstrated the intracytoplasmic inclusions in the nerve cells of infected animals. These Negri bodies form the basis of diagnosis even today.

Aetiology (see p. 908)

Rabies virus belongs to the family Rhabdoviridae and is classified as a lyssavirus, from the Greek word for rage. In recent years the rabies-related viruses have been added to this genus. Today the rabies virus is referred to as lyssavirus serogroup 1: the Lagos bat, Mokola and Duvenhage viruses are serogroups 2, 3 and 4, respectively. What previously was thought to be a single, simple agent has been shown to belong to a complex grouping. Studies using monoclonal antibodies have shown that within a given geographical area the virus adapts to its environment, resulting in distinct biotypes. Despite this, the antigenic structure of rabies virus has remained stable, which is a boon for diagnostic workers.

This is not the place to discuss the structure of the virus: suffice it to say that it is bullet shaped, and contains a single-stranded genome of RNA and five structural proteins. Following attachment to a cell the ribonucleoproteins are released and act as a template for replication in the cytoplasm. These accumulations of viral proteins in the cytoplasm give rise to the bodies described by Negri.

The rabies virus is delicate and is destroyed by sun and ultraviolet light, heat and many of the common disinfectants, e.g. 0.2 per cent quaternary ammonium compounds. However, it remains viable in nerve tissue, the length of viability depending upon temperature and storage conditions.

Because of the work of Pasteur, rabbits were used as laboratory hosts for experimental work up to the Second World War, since which time the mouse has been the principal experimental animal. At the same time the virus was adapted to grow in embryonated eggs; these were later used to produce very successful vaccines for use in animals. In 1958 the virus was first grown in tissue culture and there is a multiplicity of cells in which the virus will grow. The rabies-related viruses will also grow in tissue culture. Recently the human diploid cell line has been used for the production of a very successful human and animal vaccine.

Epidemiology

It is mostly island countries that are reported to be free from rabies infection – Great Britain, Ireland, Malta, Cyprus, New Zealand, Australia, Japan, Fiji and certain Caribbean islands. Some mainland countries are also free from the infection – Denmark Portugal, Spain, Sweden, United Arab Emirates and South Korea. These are not exhaustive lists but the majority of the countries in the world have endemic rabies.

Europe

Rabies has been known and feared here since time immemorial. Dogs, foxes and wolves have all played their part in the spread of the disease. From the end of the second world war rabies in foxes has become a serious problem with the disease moving westwards and eastwards from Poland, reaching France in 1968. Vaccination and rigorous control of urban dogs has reduced the disease dramatically in the past 30 years. The upsurge of rabies in foxes has resulted in an increase in the disease in cattle; until today cattle rabies is more common than dog rabies. However, human rabies has been on the decline for many years and today it is a rarity in Western Europe. The move to reintroduce the wolf into Scotland has been halted for the time being by the fear of rabies.

Africa

It is likely that far more rabies occurs in Africa than is reported. In the 1960s rabies was mostly controlled throughout the continent. War, strife and the breakdown of veterinary services have resulted in an upsurge of the disease, but less disease is being reported from many countries. There is some debate about whether rabies existed in subSaharan Africa or whether it was introduced by the European colonists. The answer is probably both: as will be seen below there is some evidence of virus modification in west Africa.

The first outbreak of rabies confirmed on the African continent was in the Cape Province of South Africa in 1892 in a dog imported from England that spread the infection to dogs, cats and cattle. The outbreak was controlled and the disease was not confirmed again for more than 30 years. A rabies-like disease affecting mongeese and humans on the western side of the country was known and, in 1928, rabies was confirmed in two children bitten by a yellow mongoose (*Cynictis penicillata*). Since then rabies has been regularly diagnosed throughout South Africa.

Although suspected for many years, rabies was not confirmed in Botswana until 1938. Workers in Botswana believe that there are four manifestations of rabies:

(1) *The urban dog cycle*: in the towns dogs spread the disease which can spill over into other species, most commonly man. Cattle are not involved in this cycle.
(2) *The jackal cycle*: this is the rural cycle with the disease spreading between the black backed jackal (*Canis mesomelas*) and being transmitted to cattle, small ruminants, wild ungulates and man. It is jackals that infect most cattle.
(3) *The mongoose cycle*: this is seen in the yellow mongoose in south eastern Botswana. The disease mostly cycles within the burrows of these animals but can affect wild and domestic cat populations. The domestic cat is responsible for most human infections in this part of Botswana. Cattle are not involved in this cycle.
(4) *The kudu cycle*: this is really a Namibian problem but may involve Botswana. The kudu (*Tragelaphus strepsisteros*) outbreak was responsible for the death of more than 30 000 kudu between 1975 and 1985, but still continues. The disease spreads from kudu to kudu: herbivores are normally thought to be 'dead end' hosts because they do not spread the disease. Kudu groom each other, which may account for this atypical spread.

In East Africa the disease was first confirmed in 1912, with intermittent outbreaks until the 1960s. The war with Somali insurgents after Kenya's independence resulted in wholesale destruction of the herbivores in the northern districts of Kenya. The jackals and hyenas, being deprived of their prey, moved into the villages and there was an upsurge in human and dog cases. Jackal and urban dog cycles remain a problem to this day throughout east Africa. However, disease in cattle is not a major problem. In central southern Africa, rabies is a problem in cattle when the jackal population is allowed to increase.

Non-fatal rabies-like disease is seen in west Africa and classical rabies does occur. The author will never forget walking into a house in northern Nigeria to find a mother protecting her children from a rabid dog that had entered the house. After dogs, cattle are the animals most commonly seen with rabies in West Africa.

In the countries bordering the Mediterranean, rabies has been known since time immemorial: it is primarily a disease of urban dogs, but it spills over into herbivores, including cattle, and humans. The Saharan countries are sparsely populated by animals and man and in consequence rabies is not a major problem in countries such as Mali, Niger or Somalia.

North America

Was rabies endemic in America or was it brought by the Europeans? The latter may hold good because the disease was not seen until the middle of the eighteenth century. It is also possible that the disease came across the Arctic at the time of the human and animal migration when the Baring land bridge existed. The disease is well reported in Eskimo folklore. It was not common in the USA until the civil war, after which it increased in dogs on a regular basis until the end of the second world war. With increasing vaccination of dogs and consequent decrease in the number of cases there has been a concomitant increase in the amount of sylvatic rabies. Today there are approximately 4000 cases of rabies a year in the USA, of which almost 90 per cent is in wild animals (bats, foxes, raccoons and skunks being the animals principally affected); domestic cats and herbivores (including cattle) make up the remaining 10 per cent of cases. The number of cases of rabies in cattle has remained static over the past 30 years, during which time the disease in dogs and cats has been decreasing, thus demonstrating that it is not the urban dog cycle that involves cattle. Cattle rabies occurs most frequently in those states that have the highest levels of skunk rabies (Iowa, Texas and Minnesota), indicating that it is this sylvatic cycle that involves cattle. The decrease in urban dog rabies with an increase in the sylvatic cycle has also been seen in Canada.

It has been said that some wild species of mammal are natural or 'reservoir' hosts for the virus and that the rabies virus persists in these animals without inflicting harm until the virus is transferred to a different mammalian host. The extension of this theory is that the infection will not be controlled in domestic animals until it is controlled or eliminated from these hosts.

Bats present another problem. In addition to the role of vampire bats in the spread of rabies (an important cause of the disease in cattle), 30 of the insectivorous species of bats have been shown in the Americas to be infected with the true rabies virus (lyssavirus 1). It was originally thought that all true rabies viruses belonged to a single strain. However, recent work has suggested that there are species-specific biotypes of the virus.

The Caribbean, Central and South America

The introduction, from India, of the grey mongoose (*Herpestes auropunctatus*) in an attempt to control rats and snakes in the sugar plantations has not been an unequivocal blessing. It soon became the principal carnivore on the islands. Today almost 50 per cent of the mongoose population has antibody to rabies virus in its blood. Rabies has been eradicated from many of the islands but the mongoose population presents a serious threat should the virus be reintroduced. In Mexico the major problems are urban dog rabies and vampire bat rabies. The vampire bats are of several different genera but the most important is *Desmodus rotondus*. These animals occur from Mexico to Perú and are responsible for huge losses in the cattle population: some authorities quote annual losses of half a million for South America alone. It has been thought for many years that vampire bats are 'true carriers' of the disease, in that they can be infected without being affected and yet still be capable of transmitting the infection. Recent work suggests that this is not so and that the bats have a variable length of incubation period before they succumb. The urban dog cycle is seen in the large South American cities, but it is not important to cattle rabies.

Asia

There are many Asian countries with huge cities as in South America, and again urban dog rabies is a serious problem. As a result, India has an enormous human death toll: some authorities put it as high as 25 000 a year, although this figure is disputed. There is little hard evidence of the level of infection in the dog population in any of these poor Asian countries; there is even less information on the incidence of the disease in the cattle populations. More is known about the disease in India than in other Asian countries and jackal and mongoose cycles are known to occur.

Transmission

Rabies is normally transmitted by a bite, but not all animals bitten contract the infection. Although the virus is present in the salivary glands of infected carnivores for several days before the animal shows signs of disease, it is not normally secreted in the saliva until clinical signs are apparent. There is no convincing evidence of a species' susceptibility to rabies other than epidemiological data. Despite this animals have had their susceptibilities rated, as in Table 70.1.

The site and severity of the bite is also important: the nearer the brain, the more rapid the onset. Non-bite transmission is not common. Transplacental transmission has been demonstrated in cattle, dogs and humans. There are reports of oral transmission from dam to offspring in humans and sheep via the milk. The only

Table 70.1 Susceptibility to rabies.

Very high	High	Moderate	Poor
Foxes	Cattle	Humans	Opossum
Jackal	Cats	Primates	
Coyotes	Skunks	Dogs	
	Rodents	Sheep/goats	
	Mongoose	Horses	

species in which this is a significant route of transmission is the kudu, which transmits the infection by licking. There has been a report of aerosol transmission of rabies virus to two humans in a bat-infested cave in Texas, which was confirmed by placing animals in insect-proof cages in the cave. Transplantation of corneas from cadavers to patients has resulted in the transmission of the disease.

The study of the outbreak in foxes in Western Europe over the past 30 years has shown that normally the infection spreads from one family group to its neighbour, with the occasional jumping of a group. Because fox ranges are much larger in Canada than in Europe, the disease spreads more rapidly there – up to 100 km a year compared with 20–60 km here. Within a wild animal species it is thought that the disease spreads at a rate related to the number of animals available. As the disease kills them so there is less opportunity for spread and the disease becomes quiescent. The number of cases in cattle can indicate the weight of infection in the predator.

The level of urban rabies in a population is controlled by the size of the city and the numbers of dog, the socio-economic status of the people and the efforts of government to control the disease. Rabies was a serious problem in Lima until the Veterinary Department supported by the World Health Organization instituted effective vaccination campaigns.

The understanding of the pathogenicity and spread of rabies-related viruses is as yet incomplete and anything that muddies the waters of rabies control needs investigation. One of the problems is that rabies-related viruses have been isolated from domestic animals vaccinated against rabies. There have also been cases of rabies-related viruses in humans that have no history of a bite by a wild animal. Rabies-related viruses have been demonstrated in bats in Australia, where rabies has never occurred. Recently, bats infected with these viruses have been found in Britain; they are thought to have come from Europe.

Pathogenesis

A skin wound following a bite from an infected animal is the common route of entry of the infection, hence the common route of entry of the virus is the sensory nerve endings in the affected area. With deep bites the virus enters the stretch proprioceptors of the muscle or the motor nerve endings in the muscle. The virus is thought not to enter through the cut surface of damaged nerves. Both sensory and motor nerves may be infected. Experimental work has shown that the virus multiplies at the site of infection and that it remains there for some time (more than two weeks in some cases). Once viral repli-

cation has commenced there is transport of particles of the genome along the axon to the central nervous system. Viraemia can occur but it is thought to be of importance only in animals with damaged immune systems or pregnant animals. The mechanism of spread from neuron to neuron is not properly understood, but the genomic material may complete its maturation or there could be direct transmission of the genomic material at the synaptic junctions. Once it reaches the brain the spread there is rapid, although adjacent structures are thought to be the first affected. The accumulation of virus in particular parts of the brain is thought to be responsible for the clinical signs. Once the virus reaches a particular site in the cord the virus can travel in a centrifugal direction out to the tissues. Thus the virus can be found in a range of tissues and organs. However, it is thought that the spread to the salivary glands occurs once the virus spreads within the brain.

Emaciation or failure to thrive is often seen and this is caused by damage to the hypothalamus and interference with the production of growth hormone. Cell mediated immunity is suppressed. Post exposure vaccination is known to be effective, but the mechanism is still not definitely understood. However, the production of virus neutralizing antibody correlates with resistance. Passive antibody has been shown to be effective in animals that have been infected, if given in large enough doses. While it is in the nervous system it seems that the virus does not stimulate the immune mechanisms but once it has passed into the non-nervous tissues, antibody production is stimulated. It is then too late to help the animal.

Recent workers have suggested that the pathogenicity of rabies is eminently suitable for the persistence of the virus and the spread of the disease. The virus is hidden from the immune system until it is too late. The distribution in the brain spares the neocortex and results in behavioural changes that promote confrontation between rabid and healthy animals and these changes coincide with the arrival of the virus in the salivary glands. The high mortality ensures that there is a minimal accumulation of immune individuals in the population and the occasional long incubation period ensures that the virus survives until there are sufficient susceptible individuals present in the population!

Clinical signs

Man

The incubation period in humans varies from a week to a reported 19 years. However, only 15 per cent of cases have incubation periods in excess of 90 days. Non-specific signs are the first to develop: malaise, headache, anorexia, nausea or diarrhoea. Some patients experience pain or itching at the site of the wound. This is followed after a few days by the acute, agitated form of the disease: the patients are excitable, rush about and undergo convulsive seizures which occur at random or following stimulation. They become unable to swallow and this is followed by hydrophobia. Death may supervene in about 10 days or the patient may slowly develop paralysis and pass into a coma before death. A small percentage of patients develop signs similar to the dumb form of dog rabies. There is a gradual onset of paralysis; once the respiratory muscles are affected the patient dies. There are only three recorded cases of humans recovering from clinical rabies, all from the New World.

Dog

In the dog the incubation period is commonly two to eight weeks, although there is a record of a dog imported into Britain that developed rabies eight months after it arrived. It is likely that the prodromal period seen in humans occurs in dogs but is recognized by few owners, after which the dog passes into the classic 'furious' phase, showing nervousness, restlessness and exaggerated response to stimuli. Self-infliction of injury at the site of bite is not uncommon. They may attack anything – human, animal or inanimate objects – and some will eat anything, including stones and lumps of wood. There is no forgetting the look in the dog's eyes: a fixed stare or a far-away look which is difficult to describe. They may howl between the convulsive seizures and they often die during a seizure, or paralysis ensues, the animal passes into a coma and dies.

Dogs that develop the dumb form of the disease may show periods of furious activity. The muscles of the jaw are often the first to be affected and so the dog lies with its mouth open. The dog is unable to eat and many owners suspect that the dog has a bone in its throat. Argentine veterinarians believe that the disease is caused by two different strains of the virus: the furious form by the strain involved in the urban dog cycle and the dumb form by animals involved in the fox cycle.

Cattle

Much less is known about rabies in cattle than in either humans or dogs. The incubation period is said to be between two and 12 weeks (three to 21 weeks in the USA). Where the disease is transmitted by jackals it is not uncommon to find several animals affected at one time (although this was not the experience when the infection was introduced into Ghanzi District in Botswana, where the single animal was the norm). The affected animal separates itself from the herd, shows anorexia and docility. Usually there is a drop in milk production and bulls become more sexually active. After a few days the aggressive phase may begin with the animal attacking anything. A fixed stare may be seen and the animal grinds its teeth. Inability to swallow in many African animals results in saliva running from the mouth and you put your arm down the throat to relieve the choke at your own risk! Salivation occurs in less than half the bovine cases in the USA. As the disease continues, paralysis of the tail is seen, posterior paresis and a swaying gait are noted and the animal bellows. Loss of condition ensues and the animals go off their legs, develop paralysis and between bouts of convulsions go into a coma and die. In north west Argentina a completely dumb form of the disease is seen in cattle, with the animal showing progressive paralysis. Other domestic animals show variations on the pictures described above.

The classic sign of rabies in wild animals is the loss of fear of humans. This was very dramatically seen in the kudu outbreak in Namibia in which the animals would walk into houses. Jackals become very friendly but have sudden mood swings. Wild cats become more aggressive with rabies, although even some of these animals become docile. Most humans bitten by rabid mongeese are bitten while handling these animals, thinking that they are tame.

Necropsy and pathological findings

No consistent macroscopic lesions are seen. There may be emaciation and self-mutilation. The histological findings are, however, consistent in the central nervous system. There is perivascular cuffing, focal and diffuse gliosis, neuronal degeneration and intracytoplasmis inclusion bodies from 2 to 8 μm in diameter: these are the acidophilic Negri bodies. There is a marked species difference in the presence and distribution of these bodies. In the Ammon's horn (the usual place to look for such bodies) the number of bodies in humans and dogs is variable. In herbivores, particularly goats and donkeys and to a lesser extent cattle, large numbers of Negri bodies of variable size are found. In cats, Ammon's horn is a poor source of Negri bodies and so it is more common to make the smears from the cerebellum.

Diagnosis

The history and origin of the animal will suggest the possibility of rabies and abnormal behaviour of any sort should lead the clinician to suspect rabies. In most countries rabies has to be reported to the state or national veterinary authorities. If they suspect rabies as the cause of the problem the normal action is to keep the animal under observation for up to 10 days and to kill it for laboratory diagnosis if the disease is suspected. With the advent of the fluorescent antibody test it is no longer necessary to wait for clinical disease to progress before the animal is killed for examination. This is particularly so with wild animals or animals of unknown ownership.

The animal should be killed in such a manner that the brain is not damaged; it should be divided sagittally into two halves, one half should be immersed in a large quantity of 10 per cent formol saline (histological examination) and the other half should be put into a large jar of glycerol-saline (viral examination). Both jars are placed in a special container with sufficient absorbent material to soak up the liquids should the bottle break; the parcel should be sealed and all should be sent to the laboratory. In Botswana, where there were daily temperatures of up to 40°C, samples that were delayed for a week *en route* could still be examined with a good chance of success.

The tissue in formalin is used for making histological sections and, in negative cases, may often help to confirm a differential diagnosis, e.g. babesiosis in cattle and distemper in dogs. Smears are made from the Ammon's horn and can be stained by Seller's stain (a Romanovsky stain) in which the eosinophilic bodies stain pink. This technique is rarely used today because it has been replaced by the use of the fluorescent stained antibody test in which the smears along with control positive and negative smears are stained and examined under the ultraviolet light microscope. A definitive test is to make a suspension of the brain and inject this into the cranium of sucking mice. If rabies virus is present, the mice will die within 30 days and Negri bodies can be demonstrated in their brains. Unpublished results from Botswana show the relative value of these tests (Table 70.2).

Complete comparability between the fluorescent antibody test (FAT) and the biological tests was demonstrated. Following this work, biological tests were only carried out on samples that were negative to the FAT. Histological examination was abandoned. Recently an ELISA test has been developed which apparently gives similar results to the FAT. The results can be read with the naked eye and thus an accurate diagnosis can be achieved without the need for expensive equipment. Viral tissue culture, the detection of viral nucleic acid and serological tests are not used in diagnostic laboratories but are restricted to research and investigation laboratories. Monoclonal antibodies have been used in the identification of the rabies-related viruses.

Differential diagnosis

There are many diseases that can be confused with rabies in different animals. Distemper and canine hepatitis are the most common infections in dogs, heartwater (p. 765), cerebral babesiosis (p. 748), cerebral theileriosis (p. 750), meningoencephalitis caused by *Haemophilus somnus* (p. 907) and BSE in cattle and parasites and toxic plants and chemicals in all species. One should first eliminate rabies and BSE and then proceed to the differential diagnosis.

Vaccination (see p. 1018)

Pasteur produced the first vaccine by suspending spinal cords from infected rabbits in an atmosphere of sodium hydroxide for various periods of time. The drawback to this vaccine (used for many years) was that the patient had to receive 14 injections on a daily basis. There was also the possibility of the patient developing a neuropathy (paralytic neuritis) following vaccination. The next vaccine was produced in sucking mice because these immature creatures have less myelin, so reducing the risks of auto-antigenicity. Hen (for animals) and duck (for human) eggs were the next vaccines produced and both were used extensively for upwards of 20 years. In some African countries the Flury strains are used to this day and they work well – high passage for cats and cattle and low passage for dogs. Today the vaccine most

Table 70.2 Results of all brains examined over a period of three years.

Positive			Negative		
FAT	Biological	Histological	FAT	Biological	Histological
207	207	156	235	235	286

FAT, fluorescent antibody test.

commonly used in man and animals is the human diploid vaccine. Post exposure treatment of humans in Botswana is given on days 0, 4, 7, 11, 17 and 84.

Oral vaccines have been developed for use in the control of the disease in wildlife, particularly for foxes in western Europe. It has been shown that foxes will take chicken head bait laced with the vaccine in a capsule. This has proved very successful in controlling the disease in foxes. So far it has not been extended to other species of wild animal. Future research will undoubtedly be into the production of recombinant vaccines using harmless viruses: in this way it might be possible to vaccinate all species of wild animals that carry the rabies virus.

Control

In Britain, as in many other islands free from infection, the perfect control measure was in place, namely the prohibition of importation of carnivorous animals unless they underwent six months' quarantine. This was changed in 2000 to a system of movement controls and vaccination. It is interesting to speculate when the first case of rabies will be diagnosed in Britain. Most countries in the world have laws in place to control this disease. These vary from the strictest in Australia, where carnivores may only be imported from countries free from infection and they are still required to be kept in quarantine for six months, to poor countries such as Tanzania where almost nothing is done (there were 400 human deaths in the Mwanza region a few years ago because there was no money to buy vaccine!).

What is needed to control the disease is an efficient laboratory to diagnose the infection and an efficient veterinary service to undertake field studies to determine the areas of the country in which the infection is most prevalent, the various species of animal that are involved and the populations of these animals. It is necessary to determine whether there are wild-life reservoirs of infection or whether it is purely a problem of urban dogs.

With this information it is possible to plan the campaign of control and budget for its costs. In most Third World countries rabies vaccination is supplied free to dog owners during the campaign, either at predetermined vaccination sites or on house to house visits. Owners who require their animal to be vaccinated outside this time usually have to go to a private veterinary surgeon. In Botswana, at the time of vaccination, the dog is painted on the head. Once the vaccinations are completed then control teams go into the area and capture or shoot all dogs without the paintmark. Other countries do not have such draconian measures. In countries where there is little control of the dog population such slaughter may be counterproductive: rapid reproduction will soon increase the numbers and all the increase will be susceptible. Cats are not usually vaccinated because they play less part in the disease cycle. In countries where there is movement of animals then some form of permanent marking or certification is required. Although the modern vaccines produce immunity that lasts for three years it is normal practice to mount a vaccine campaign on a yearly basis. Movement control from the affected areas is practised and only vaccinated dogs are permitted to leave the area. It is considered that an area can be considered rabies-free if there has been no case of the disease in the last two years.

In Botswana, cattle owners are not permitted to vaccinate their cattle against rabies. A susceptible cattle population acted as a marker for the infection of jackals. The economics of vaccinating cattle in Africa are such that the farmer would not recoup the cost of the vaccine as it is cheaper to let the odd bovine die. This is not the case in South America where the vampire bat can wreak havoc in a herd. The author knows of no country in South America that has a policy of cattle vaccination: it is left to the individual owner.

The presence of rabies-related viruses in a country complicates the control of rabies. It is known that with some viruses the rabies vaccine provides some protection and so this has been used in human patients bitten by bats. In the National Veterinary Laboratory, Botswana, it was the policy that staff were not routinely vaccinated against rabies. It was thought that confidence would breed carelessness. It was known that pre-exposure vaccination even with the tissue culture vaccine would not give adequate protection, if it were not followed up with post exposure vaccination. Over the years several staff members received the treatment course of rabies vaccination.

With rabies eternal vigilance is required.

Further reading

A modern text with a bent towards southern Africa is:
Swanepoel, R. (1994) Rabies. In *Infectious Diseases of Livestock with Special Reference to Southern Africa* (ed. by J.A.W. Coetzer, G.R. Thomson & R.C. Tustin), Vol. 1, pp. 493–552. Oxford University Press, Cape Town.

An older text on rabies in the tropics including vaccination:
Kuwert, E., Mérieux, C., Koprowski, H. & Bogel, K. (eds) (1985). *Rabies in the Tropics*. Springer-Verlag, Berlin.

An older text concerning South America:
Anon (1984) *Septimo Informe*. Comité de expertos de la OMS sobre Rabia. World Health Organization, Geneva. (Control in cities, pp. 39–41; vampire bats, pp. 71–5.)

Rabies in cattle in the USA:

Baer, G.M. (1986) Rabies in cattle. In *Current Veterinary Therapy 2: Food Animal Practice* (ed. by J.L. Howard), pp. 501–504. W.B. Saunders, Philadelphia.

Oral vaccination of wildlife against rabies:

Steck, F., Wandeler, A., Biochel, P., Capt, S., Hafliger, U. & Schneider, L. (1982) Oral immunisation of foxes against rabies: laboratory and field studies. *Comparative Immunology, Microbiology and Infectious Diseases*, **5**, 165–71.

Chapter 71
Dairy Farming in Saudi Arabia

J.C. Fishwick

Introduction	1172
Cattle industry	1172
Dairy farming	1172
Role of the veterinary surgeon	1174
Function of the health team	1176
Summary	1176

Introduction

With an area of approximately 2.1 million square kilometres and an estimated population of over 19 million people, the Kingdom of Saudi Arabia dominates the Arabian Peninsula. Within its boundaries, the country holds the two most sacred sites of the Islamic faith, the Holy Mosques of Mecca and Madinah, and Islam is the all-embracing force which is seen in every aspect of Saudi society. The nation was united into its present form by King Abdul Aziz in 1932 and is still ruled as an absolute monarchy by his descendants.

Saudi Arabia consists almost entirely of desert or semi-desert areas and is one of the driest countries on earth, with an annual rainfall in most areas of around 100 mm. The rainfall that is seen is irregular and unreliable. There are two distinct seasons with summer lasting from March to early October, when daytime temperatures are consistently above 40°C and commonly reach as high as 50°C, while at night the temperature will remain above 30°C. The daytime temperatures during the winter months are usually in the range 20–30°C. Coastal regions suffer with extremely high humidity, especially in the summer, whilst the central regions are characterized by a very dry atmosphere.

Saudi Arabia has the largest known oil reserves in the world, together with vast amounts of natural gas and mineral wealth. The discovery of these natural resources had a dramatic effect on the nation during the latter half of the twentieth century and the health of the economy is now closely linked to the price of oil on the world market.

Cattle industry

The dairy industry is sophisticated and is concentrated in the hands of relatively few large, integrated compa-

nies, both privately and state owned. In addition to farming activities most dairy companies have their own processing plants and distribution systems.

The full range of pasteurized fresh dairy products that would be found in any Western country is readily available. The largest selling product is a traditional Middle Eastern fresh natural drinking yoghurt called *laban*. About 60 per cent of fresh milk production is fermented into *laban* while approximately 25 per cent is processed as fresh milk. The retail price of a litre of milk has fallen rapidly due to competition pressures from the equivalent of 75 pence (US$1.05) in 2000 to about 53 pence (US$0.80) in 2002.

In contrast to Europe, a higher value is placed on fat than protein in milk and this is reflected in the nutrition of dairy cows and in sire selection. This is primarily because of the demand for traditional breakfast cream called *ghiste*. However the demand for skimmed and semi-skimmed milk is increasing and both products are readily available. Milk quality is generally excellent and most companies produce milk with a bacterial count and somatic cell count that would qualify for the highest payment bands offered by UK milk purchasers.

The beef industry is quite small. The majority of locally produced red meat consumed is sheep, goat and camel and the best quality beef is imported. Most local beef is slaughtered at up to 18 months of age and is referred to as veal. Veal cattle are usually castrated Holstein bulls sourced from the dairy sector. There is also a small amount of beef produced by nomadic farmers who keep suckler cows.

There are effectively no private veterinary surgeons working in the cattle industry; veterinary surgeons are exclusively employed directly by individual farming companies.

Dairy farming

Milking cattle are Holsteins which are zero grazed with a diet based on home-grown alfalfa hay and maize silage. Saudi Arabia is fortunate in having enormous underground reservoirs of water and it is this water which is used for both dairy farming and arable production. Certain areas of the desert are extremely fertile if water is provided and the basis of crop and forage production is an irrigation system known as the *centre pivot* (Fig. 71.1). A pivot consists of a bore hole producing water which then passes into a horizontal overhead pipe mounted on wheels which makes a slow circuit and irrigates a circular area of land around the bore hole. Nutrients may be added to the water as required and pivots may have a diameter of up to 800 m. From the air pivots may be seen as 'green circles in the desert'.

Forage is supplemented with imported products such as soya, flaked maize, cottonseed, cottonseed hulls, sugar beet pulp and fishmeal. Feed is usually fed as a total mixed ration off the floor with the cattle in lockable head stanchions. Feeding time provides an opportunity for breeding and other management procedures.

The best dairy units have around 4500 to 5000 dairy cows together with a large youngstock rearing operation. Cows are milked four times a day in a two hundred stall parallel parlour which operates 24 hours a day, with breaks between shifts for cleaning and routine maintenance. A farm of this size has a total staff of about 145 men, including everyone from the farm manager to cooks and administration staff. Rolling herd average milk yield in the best units is over 12 000 litres per head. Lactating cows are housed in groups of 300 and considerable effort is spent to ensure that this number of animals calves in as short a period as possible to fill the house quickly. The spread of calving dates in the house must be minimal so that they can be managed and fed as a single group. First lactation cows are housed separately from older cows.

The extremely high temperatures experienced both day and night throughout the summer months make careful control of the cows' environment essential. Efficient milk production is difficult without effective cooling during the summer months and even during the winter cooling still plays an important role. A good illustration of the high temperatures experienced is the fact that mercury clinical thermometers are of little use in the summer. The air temperature is considerably higher than the normal body temperature of a cow and so it is almost impossible to make an accurate measurement of a cow's rectal temperature.

The technology for cow cooling was originally developed in the arid regions of Arizona, USA. One commonly used cooling system involves a large electrical fan mounted in the roof which blasts air downwards onto cattle. The air may be cooled by evaporating controlled amounts of atomized water into it. A cow house will need a whole series of fans to provide effective cooling and for much of the year these will be operating 24 hours a day (see Chapter 8). Cooling is also essential in parlour collecting yards (Fig. 71.2).

Cows are housed on sand and, over time, the original sand bedding accumulates increasing amounts of dung. This provides a peaty type of bedding which is com-

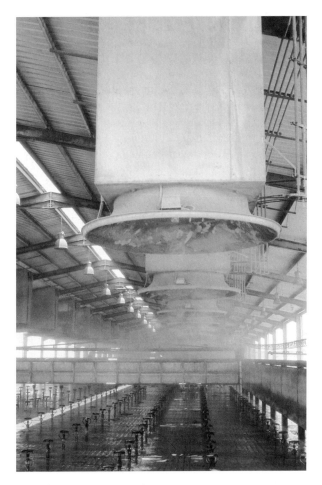

Fig. 71.2 Coolers over a collecting yard. Note the udder washers on the floor.

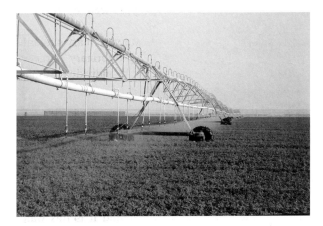

Fig. 71.1 A centre pivot irrigation system.

fortable and works extremely well, provided it remains dry. To maintain the beds in good condition houses are groomed four times a day by scraping the top layer of bedding outside and leaving it in the sun to dry, whilst previously dried material is scraped back inside. It is possible to maintain a house for several years before completely cleaning out and starting with fresh sand. Rain is uncommon, but when it does fall it can cause serious problems with the bedding which is associated with an increased incidence of mastitis and lameness.

Mastitis is maintained on well-run units at a level of less than 20 cases per 100 cows per year, and levels would be considerably lower in some cases. Meticulous attention to the Five Point Plan for many years has been very successful in reducing contagious mastitis to very low levels and most of the cases are environmental mastitis. There is still a lot to be learned in the management of cows and housing in this type of system to reduce environmental mastitis further.

Staff are divided into several teams with responsibility for areas such as milking, feeding, health, breeding, calving and youngstock rearing. Because of the large number of cows being dealt with, members of these teams gain a great deal of experience.

Role of the veterinary surgeon

The veterinary surgeon has an essential, proactive role to play in the productivity and health of the herd.

First and foremost he must establish performance targets, monitor them continuously and intervene immediately when performance starts to deviate from that target. As well as collecting, handling and interpreting data this involves working closely with farm staff at all levels to investigate problems as they arise. Examples include the calving live birth rate, incidence of mastitis, conception rates, incidence of ketosis and cow and calf mortality. If any of these parameters fall below the set target investigations must start immediately.

Secondly, he must establish the optimal working practices for each team and produce written manuals to set these out in a clear and methodical manner. It is important to utilize the very best current knowledge available in an area and produce firm guidelines that can be applied simply on a very large scale.

Thirdly, he has the responsibility for the maintenance of herd disease security. There is probably no other situation in the world where herd disease security takes on such an important role. Foot-and-mouth disease (FMD) and rinderpest are a real risk and if either of these were to enter a large unit the results could be catastrophic.

FMD is endemic in the region and attempts to control it on a national scale are thwarted by the move-

ment of livestock into the region from the Horn of Africa and from more northerly states such as Turkey, Iraq and Iran. The greatest threat to dairy units comes from the large, mobile population of sheep and goats in the region and these may commonly be infected whilst showing only minor clinical signs.

Prevention of FMD is maintained in two ways: physical security of the unit and a stringent vaccination policy. The principle of physical security is that livestock, people and vehicles do not enter the unit unless absolutely necessary. When they do, sensible precautions are taken in terms of disinfection of vehicles and provision of farm overalls and footwear. However, these precautions are no substitute for preventing entry to the unit and this must always be the main thrust of physical security.

Farms are fenced with a single point of entry (Fig. 71.3) which is manned 24 hours a day. Cattle sales and disposals are done through a separate gate at the perimeter so that cattle trucks do not enter the farm (Fig. 71.4). There is a large separation between the perimeter fence (Fig. 71.5) and the cow houses, typically 200 m or more. Essential deliveries are kept to a minimum and lorries are disinfected before entry. Visitors are not allowed and all company staff entering the site must leave their vehicles outside the perimeter fence.

There are special risks when companies with multiple sites have to move livestock between their own farms. The risk is reduced by using lorries exclusively for their own animals, efficient disinfection and ensuring a member of farm staff always accompanies the driver to ensure that cattle are not exposed to any unnecessary risk during transit. Forage is only sourced from suppliers known to have effective fencing to keep their pivots free from livestock.

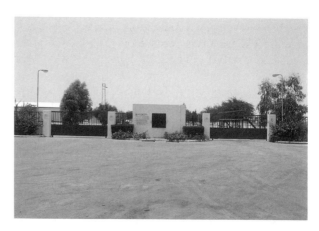

Fig. 71.3 A farm gatehouse, which is controlled to reduce the risk of foot-and-mouth entering the farm.

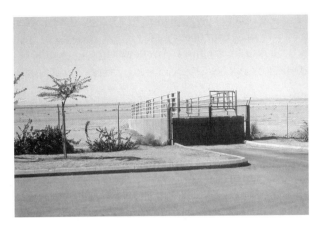

Fig. 71.4 Loading ramp at the perimeter fence for livestock movement. Cattle are moved through a separate gate from the main entrance to ensure that cattle trucks do not enter the farm.

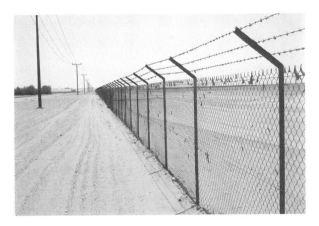

Fig. 71.5 Farm perimeter fence. Security is important in a region where foot-and-mouth is endemic. The perimeter fence is separated from the cattle housing by several hundred metres.

One feature of farming in this region is that a large proportion of farm staff are expatriates from countries such as the Philippines, Kenya, Sri Lanka, Nepal, Pakistan, India, UK and Ireland. Most staff are resident on site and this reduces the chance of staff coming into contact with other local livestock.

Preventing the movement of cattle and personnel does nothing to prevent the chance of airborne spread between units. This is a particular risk if another dairy unit in the region is suffering a clinical FMD outbreak. The chance of infection by airborne spread appears to be greatest when humidity is above 60 per cent.

The second component of FMD prevention is vaccination. The antigenic components included in the vaccine available in Saudi Arabia are authorized by the Saudi Ministry of Agriculture and Water, based on the best scientific advice available from authorities such as the Institute of Animal Health at Pirbright, UK. FMD vaccination is carried out every 75 days in all stock over 6 months old. This routine is carried on a predetermined day and all cattle are included regardless of any other considerations. Calves less than 6 months old are given a course of three vaccinations at 4, 5 and 6 months old before joining the whole herd schedule.

Vaccination against FMD is a tremendous cost to any dairy organization. Apart from the direct costs of vaccination and time involved, milking cows often suffer a significant but short lived reduction in milk yield. Typically total daily milk production may fall by an amount equivalent to between 0.5 kg and 2.0 kg per cow for a 24- or 48-hour period immediately following whole herd vaccination. This cost is, at present, an unavoidable loss associated with the keeping of dairy cattle in the region. Dairy companies do vary in the vaccination schedule employed depending on their own circum-

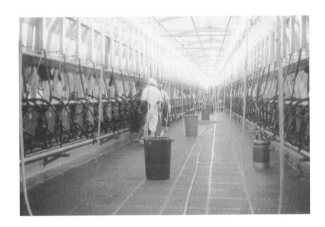

Fig. 71.6 A 100-stall parallel milking parlour.

stances and the schedule described above would be amongst the most vigorous seen in the region.

Despite the great attention given to FMD prevention, outbreaks of the disease do occur sporadically and they will probably remain a feature of dairy farming while the disease remains endemic in the region.

A fourth role is the development of effective control and contingency programmes for a number of diseases which may occur. FMD provides the most obvious example but other diseases such as mycoplasmal mastitis, brucellosis and tuberculosis, all of which may occur, need definite policies in place to deal with them. In the case of mycoplasmal mastitis a control programme must ensure that sensible precautions are in place to prevent it, that sampling and laboratory procedures are effective in continuously monitoring for the disease and that should an outbreak occur a well-organized response can be implemented immediately.

Other roles include the coordination of parlour testing and maintenance, which assumes great importance when cows are being milked around the clock in one or two hundred stall parlours (Fig. 71.6); maintenance and monitoring of raw milk quality, co-ordination with consultant nutritionists and selection of bulls.

Function of the health team

Staff on a large dairy unit are commonly divided into a number of specialist teams, one of which is the health team. The principle of a health team's activity is that problems must be detected early and rapid intervention must ensure that affected cows are returned to full productivity as soon as possible. Any cows that do require treatment are moved to a separate hospital area which has its own dedicated milking parlour. All the milk produced in this parlour is disposed of as waste to prevent any mastitic or drug-contaminated milk from entering the main milk output of the farm.

Health teams concentrate most of their efforts on the observation of cattle in their houses. All cows are locked in their stanchions for feeding four times each day and it is during this 'lock up' period that health teams walk the cows and observe carefully for any signs of abnormality. Particular attention is given to cows within the first three weeks after calving. These fresh cows are checked four times a day whilst others are checked twice a day. Although this type of dairy farming is carried out on a large scale, great attention is paid to the health of individual cows as judged by careful observation and basic clinical skills. Health men have to be satisfied that each and every cow is eating properly and looks healthy at the time of each lock up.

Any cows that show problems are removed and given a full clinical examination in a crush. Cows are then returned to their houses or retained in the hospital for treatment as necessary.

The most common disease identified in fresh cows is ketosis and the diagnosis of this condition is assisted with the use of a urine dipstick. Any fresh cow that is submitted for clinical examination will have a urine test done as a routine. The incidence of diseases such as ketosis and left displaced abomasum is recorded daily and this information is used by nutritionists, the farm manager and the feeding team to assess the effectiveness of their feeding management.

Careful observation of cattle at frequent intervals during the day is a very time consuming activity, but it is considered essential to the effective management of a dairy unit. A successful health team is judged by an empty hospital area and not by the amount of sophisticated treatments being given to cows in it.

Summary

The dairy industry in Saudi Arabia has developed rapidly over a period of about 25 years and has been greatly influenced by the experience gained from dairy farming in arid regions of the USA. It is now probably as efficient and advanced as anywhere in the world. Prevention and control of foot-and-mouth disease is a major challenge and is very expensive.

Regardless of the size and scale of any operation, a herd is comprised of individual cows. A herd can only operate efficiently if full attention is given to the individual members of that herd. This applies as much in a unit of five thousand cows as it does in one of fifty.

Chapter 72

Bovine Medicine in New Zealand and Australia

N.D. Sargison and J.J. Vermunt

New Zealand   1177
   Dairy farming   1177
   Beef production   1177
   Animal health   1178
   Reproductive management   1178
   Major problems   1179
The Australian scene   1182

New Zealand

Dairy farming

New Zealand's dairy herd of slightly over 3.3 million cows is small by comparison with Europe and America. However, about 90 per cent of the milk production is processed for export as butter, cheese and milk powders, making New Zealand a major contributor to the world dairy trade. New Zealand's unique climate favours extremely efficient livestock production from clover and perennial ryegrass pastures, top dressed with phosphatic fertilizers, which enables the unsubsidized dairy industry to compete on the world market.

Dairy farming is concentrated in areas of reliable high rainfall (Northland, Waikato, Taranaki and Southland) and where irrigation is possible and cost-effective (Canterbury). Most production is from New Zealand–Friesian and Holstein–Friesian cows (57 per cent), although there are still a significant number of Jersey (16 per cent) and crossbred herds (19 per cent). The average herd size is about 230 cows and managed by one person, but herds of 800 cows or more are not uncommon. About 30 per cent of the dairy farms are operated on a share milking basis where, for example, the owner is responsible for the farm maintenance and the fertilizer costs, whilst the share milker owns and milks the cows. This system traditionally provided a route of entry to the industry for young farmers, who could eventually accumulate enough capital to buy their own property.

The majority of dairy farms are seasonal producers, traditionally spring calving over a two month period timed with the lush spring growth, and supplying milk processing factories for nine to ten months of the year.

Recently, there has been an increased interest in autumn calving, thereby spreading the workload for both the farmer and the dairy factory. Inputs to factory supply herds are low, with little supplementary feeding, no winter housing, efficient milking plant and a low labour requirement. Farms are subdivided into small paddocks and most lactating cows are mob stocked and shifted daily. The annual production of 3000–3500 l/cow is low by comparison with grain-based systems. Cows are stocked at an average of 2.7/ha and produce 600–1200 kg milk solids (fat and protein)/ha. Only small amounts of hay or silage are conserved for winter feeding and the use of temporary electric fencing enables a variety of winter grazing systems to ration winter pasture and ensure adequate spring growth. A small number of town supply herds have a greater reliance on winter feed and produce milk to quota all year round.

Beef production

The majority of the beef produced in New Zealand is exported to the USA as processing beef, some is exported to North and South East Asia and about a fifth is consumed locally. About 50 per cent of the total beef production is from suckler cows and 50 per cent is derived from the dairy industry, comprising cull cows and Friesian bulls which are reared to between one and two years-old on lowland pasture. The original role of suckler cattle in New Zealand was to improve pasture quality for more profitable sheep grazing and to prevent reversion to bush. Whilst recently the price of beef has improved relative to wool and lamb, most of the country's 1.4 million suckler cows are still kept on steep and rolling hill country farms in a complementary role to sheep. Angus cattle with mature weights of about 475 kg are the predominant breed, although there are many herds of Hereford and crossbred cows. The numbers of Charolais, Simmental and Limousin cattle are low by comparison with Europe, partly because of their high grazing requirements for maintenance relative to production.

Typical herds of 150–200 suckler cows achieve calving percentages of 80–85 per cent depending on the topography of the country. Beef production is wholly dependent on pasture nutrition so virtually all suckler cows are spring calving. The various classes of cattle are kept separate and regularly moved around the farm along with the sheep. Pasture is prioritized depending on the nutritional requirements of the different classes of livestock at different times of year and care is taken to avoid competition with sheep, especially during the late winter–early spring period. Winter grazing is managed by the rotation of mobs around paddocks. Store cattle are mostly finished on intensive lowland farms, where weight gains from about 1 kg/day in spring to 0.5 kg/day in autumn are achieved on a pasture-only diet.

Animal health

The unsubsidized New Zealand beef and dairy industries are very sensitive to world production and market trends. The important economic constraints on production and requirements for veterinary input are, therefore, different when compared to the current situation in Europe. Reproductive performance is the most important determinant of herd profitability and forms the basis of veterinary input to most herds. The treatment of individual sick animals is often uneconomic, especially in extensively grazed beef cattle where early signs of disease may not be seen. However, there is an important role for veterinary advice on the control and prevention of production limiting diseases. Whilst respiratory disease and calf scour are relatively unimportant diseases in animals which are not housed, dependence on a solely pasture diet can predispose to specific animal health problems. New Zealand's volcanic soils are generally deficient in trace minerals and in the absence of supplementary feeding, trace element deficiencies (copper and selenium) are commonplace. Mycotoxicoses such as facial eczema and ryegrass staggers, which are seldom seen in Europe, can also be important production limiting diseases. Most lameness in dairy cattle is associated with the unavoidable need to walk long distances from pasture to the milking shed, and consequently the lameness-causing lesions differ from those seen in winter-housed animals. Problems of winter pasture feeding and management, the metabolic demands of late pregnancy and early lactation and stress associated with prolonged wet spring weather often result in a high incidence of metabolic diseases in dairy cows.

Reproductive management

The pattern of pasture growth in New Zealand means that suckler cows must be spring calving and a mean calving interval of 12 months is therefore essential. Most suckler cows are mated in large groups with two to three bulls per 100 cows, depending on the topography of the farm. Most reproductive problems are associated with an extended calving period and veterinary input is, therefore, based on the achievement and maintenance of a compact calving period.

- Heifers or cows which calve late during one season inevitably calve late during the following season or do not become pregnant before the end of a compact mating period.
- Calves which are born late in the calving period are younger and lighter at weaning than those born earlier and, therefore, of lower sale value.
- The labour requirement for supervision is lower when the calving period is compact.
- Feed budgeting is more accurate for heifers and cows calving over a known short period.

The annual performance of most of the country's beef cows and the published results of field studies of more than 150 000 suckler cows (Hanly & Mossman, 1977) indicate that the average pregnancy rate is 60 per cent for each oestrous cycle, provided that heifers or cows are cycling and the bulls are sound. After calving, there is a post-partum anoestrus period of at least 40 days, which is related to body condition at calving and to the plane of nutrition and is about 20 days longer in calved heifers than in mature cows with the same body condition. Thus, provided that all heifers or cows are cycling at the beginning of the mating period, a 5-oestrus-cycle (105-day) mating period is required for 99 per cent of cows to be pregnant. However, in subsequent years if the bulls are introduced on the same date, not all cows will be cycling at the time of bull introduction and a 99 per cent pregnancy rate will not be achieved by 105 days. Therefore, a mean calving interval significantly greater than 365 days is required to sustain a 99 per cent pregnancy rate. Alternatively, a sustainable 365-day calving interval can be achieved when bulls are removed after three oestrus cycles, although annually about 6 per cent of the cows will not be in calf (Mossman & Hanly, 1977). In the absence of annual cow subsidy support and provided that the difference between cull and replacement cows is low, this not-in-calf rate is more than compensated for by increased weaning weights due to the greater mean age of calves at weaning.

Good heifer management is the key to achieving satisfactory reproductive performance in the whole herd. Provided that heifer management is correct, nutrition is adequate and sound bulls, matched for size, with high libido and low estimated breeding values for calf birthweight are used, the achievement of good reproductive performance in subsequent years is relatively straightforward. Traditional heifer calving at three years of age presents few problems. However, about 30 per cent of

New Zealand beef heifers are first calved as two-year-olds, which necessitates careful management to avoid dystokia and subsequent reproductive problems. Heifers weighing 65 per cent of their mature weight at 14–15 months of age should be cycling and achieve target pregnancy rates when mated. For 15-month-old Angus, Hereford and Simmental heifers, this critical minimum weight is in the order of 270 kg, 290 kg and 310 kg, respectively. Heifers intended for calving as two-year-olds are preferentially managed and regularly monitored to ensure that target weights are achieved through good nutrition and control of growth-limiting diseases, such as parasitism and trace element deficiencies. Heifers which do not reach the critical minimum weight at 15 months of age are usually culled from the breeding herd or mated the following year to avoid the problems of poor pregnancy rates and failure to rebreed as second calvers. On many hill farms, or on lowland farms with heavy breeds of cattle, the achievement of critical minimum weights by the age of 15 months is not possible and calving as two-year-olds is uneconomic.

Bulls are removed from the herd of replacement heifers one cycle ahead of the cow herd to overcome the problem of a longer post-partum anoestrous period in calved heifers. When cows are mated over a period of 63 days, this is achieved by mating replacement heifers for only 42 days or by mating heifers for 63 days, but introducing the bulls 21 days before the start of mating in the cow herd. Forty-two-day heifer mating is suited to calving at two years of age, because animals are three weeks older at the time of bull introduction, which can make a significant difference to achieving critical minimum weights and subsequent herd reproductive performance, while 63-day heifer mating is best suited to traditional three-year-old heifer calving.

Poor body condition at calving results in long calving to conception intervals and a high not-in-calf rate when a short mating period is employed. Furthermore, thin calved heifers that do become pregnant usually conceive late in the breeding season, calve later, wean lighter calves and fail to become pregnant as second calvers. Under intensive grazing conditions, replacement heifers cannot compete with adult cows for nutrients unless managed as a separate group through to their second calving. Having achieved good heifer management, day-to-day management is based on assessing the body condition of cows in accordance with their reproductive status. If feed inputs are below requirements, cows will lose weight and fail to reach target condition score for mating and eventually fail to rebreed.

The same requirement for a compact spring calving period applies to the dairy herd, where 60 to 70 per cent of the cows conceive to proven sires by artificial insemination. About 30 per cent of inseminations are per-formed by the farmer and 70 per cent by trained technicians. Heat detection is assisted by the use of tail paint. Poor reproductive performance in dairy cows is often associated with extended post-partum anoestrous periods due to failure of winter/spring pasture to meet the nutritional requirements of advanced pregnancy and early lactation. Intravaginal progesterone releasing devices (e.g. CIDR, InterAg, NZ; Cue-Mate, Duirs, NZ; PRID, Stockguard, NZ) are routinely used in an attempt to overcome this problem and to induce oestrus in later calving animals.

Major problems

Copper deficiency (see p. 298)

Copper deficiency is an important cause of ill-thrift in cattle over the age of six months. Severe scours and copper-responsive post-parturient haemoglobinuria in dairy cows used to be common in some areas, associated with high spring levels of molybdenum in peat soils or the application of molybdenum to pasture as a fertilizer. There are also reports of poor reproductive performance associated with copper deficiency, although it is unclear whether this is due to copper deficiency, the toxic effects of molybdenum or just secondary to ill-thrift.

Whilst the copper levels of New Zealand pastures vary little throughout the year, the levels of interfering factors, molybdenum and iron, increase significantly throughout the winter and spring. Copper availability is therefore lowest in spring, at the time of year when animal requirements for late pregnancy, lactation and early growth are highest.

Both serum and liver copper concentrations are used in the diagnosis of poor animal performance, but liver is the only useful sample when the reasons for sampling are to determine whether reserves are adequate to last throughout the winter or to monitor a supplementation programme (Ellison, 1992). The correct number of samples is essential (minimum of eight sera or four liver samples), because the laboratory reference values are based on mean values from these numbers. Liver samples are obtained by biopsy or from slaughterhouse or necropsy material.

There are no recipes for trace element supplementation, which depends on many factors including the severity of the deficiency, production system, stocking density and availability of labour (Wakelin, 1992). Short-term supplementation of dairy cattle can be provided by daily drenching with copper sulphate in the milking shed or administration of copper salts through the drinking water, but requires careful monitoring. Intermediate-term supplementation is achieved in both dairy and beef cows by the parenteral injection of copper glycinate or copper edetate, whilst long-term supplementation can be provided by the oral administration of copper oxide particles (capsules or bullets) or pasture top dressing with copper sulphate.

Selenium deficiency (see p. 302)

About 30 per cent of farmed land in New Zealand is considered to be selenium deficient. The most important selenium responsive condition in New Zealand cattle is ill-thrift in growing calves and growth responses of 5–10 per cent can be achieved by supplementation on most deficient pastures. Selenium responsive infertility and poor milk production have been reported on severely deficient pastures (Grace, 1994). The selenium responsive condition of nutritional muscular dystrophy is now quite rare due to the awareness of selenium deficiency and widespread supplementation.

The selenium status of cattle is usually confirmed by the laboratory analysis of blood glutathione peroxidase (GSH-Px) or selenium concentrations in serum, whole blood or liver, all of which provide useful diagnostic information (Wichtel, 1998). Liver samples collected from finished calves at slaughter are commonly used to determine the need to supplement. Within any herd, there is little between-animal variation in the concentrations of selenium in blood, serum or liver, or blood GSHPx concentrations, therefore samples from three or four animals usually provide adequate information. The New Zealand reference ranges for selenium are based on numerous calf growth response trials (Ellison, 1992). Overseas reference ranges are of no value to New Zealand conditions and vice versa, because the vitamin E status of New Zealand cattle is generally more than adequate due to their year-round pasture nutrition. Economically significant growth rate responses to supplementary selenium are unlikely at liver selenium concentrations above 600 nmol/kg (wet weight).

Sodium selenate or selenite administered orally, as a pour-on or by subcutaneous injection can provide a useful method of short-term supplementation. Long-term supplementation is achieved by controlled release subcutaneous injections of barium selenate paste, intraruminal selenium pellets or pasture top dressing with sodium selenate or sodium-barium selenate prills. Pasture top dressing is an efficient supplementation method where stocking rates are high and is the preferred supplementation method on about 30 per cent of selenium deficient properties.

Facial eczema

Facial eczema is an important cause of ill-thrift and hepatogenous photosensitization during late summer and autumn, in many areas of the North Island of New Zealand. Facial eczema is caused by ingestion of the mycotoxin sporidesmin, which is present in the spores of the saprophytic fungus *Pithomyces chartarum*. Under the ideal conditions of high humidity (close to 100 per cent) following a prolonged warm period (>20°C with a minimum night temperature of 12°C), spore numbers can increase rapidly in the mat of leaf litter beneath shaded pasture. Sporidesmin is rapidly absorbed and becomes concentrated in the liver where it causes epithelial necrosis of the bile ducts with periductal oedema and inflammation, leading to cirrhosis. Most affected animals show no outward clinical signs. However, the resulting liver damage causes ill-thrift and a significant reduction in milk production. Photosensitization occurs in about 10 per cent of affected animals and is due to derangement of the biliary excretion of phylloerythrin (Bruère *et al.*, 1990).

Outbreaks of facial eczema are both distressing and expensive, therefore intensive monitoring is performed to assess the risk of disease and expedite preventive measures. Monitoring consists of recording weather conditions and carrying out pasture spore counts using spore trapping or pasture washing methods. When counts rise rapidly, or reach threshold value, the options are to move stock to safer pasture, to instigate protective treatment with zinc salts, to apply fungicides to the pasture or a combination of these practices. Fungicide spraying can provide safe pasture for six weeks, but can be expensive, especially when it has to be repeated due to heavy rainfall or a prolonged risk period. Oral administration of large doses of zinc oxide, before exposure to toxic levels of sporidesmin, effectively reduces the severity of liver damage, although the mechanism is unclear. Milking cows can be dosed daily in the milking shed, but other classes of cattle are usually drenched weekly at a higher dose rate to overcome the impracticalities of yarding and handling. Alternatively, zinc sulphate can be administered to dairy herds through the water supply. Wax-coated, slow-release zinc oxide intraruminal boluses (Time Capsule, AgResearch, NZ) are available for use in calves. The boluses slowly dissolve in the rumen to provide four weeks' protection and are useful when animal handling is difficult. Zinc salts have no therapeutic value when administered after exposure to sporidesmin.

Outbreaks of facial eczema can be avoided by judicious farm management practices such as feeding of hay or other supplements during high risk periods, avoidance of close grazing and removal of stock from high risk areas. Affected animals should be provided with shade or if possible housed in darkness during day light hours. Milking cows should be dried off and skin lesions treated topically.

Ryegrass staggers

Ryegrass staggers occurs under close grazing conditions during summer and autumn in perennial ryegrass (*Lolium perenne*) dominant pasture-fed livestock throughout most areas of New Zealand. The disease is caused by tremorgenic mycotoxins (lolitrem A and B) which are produced by the perennial ryegrass endophytic fungus *Acremonium loliae* and is characterized by tremors, incoordination and depressed growth rates. The prevalence of the endophyte in perennial ryegrass is greatest during summer and autumn, in particular in the plants' lower sheaths, old leaves and seedheads. Many modern ryegrass cultivars have been selected for high levels of the *A. Loliae* endophyte, because it is associated with resistance to attack by the Argentine stem weevil (*Listronotus bonariensis*), an important agronomic pest. Such selection has inadvertently resulted in an increased incidence of ryegrass staggers (Bruère *et al.*, 1990).

Clinical signs develop within one to two weeks after introduction to toxic pasture. At rest, the only visible signs may be fine tremors of the head and neck, but when animals are disturbed, clinical signs immediately become apparent with development of head nodding and jerky movements of the neck and limbs. Moderately affected animals have a wide-based, swaying stance and a high-stepping gait. Severely affected animals show a stiff-legged gait and usually collapse when moved. Whilst the disease is distressing to observe, most losses are associated with misadventure. However, affected animals are difficult to handle, interfering with normal management practices. There is no specific treatment for the disease, but animals recover within days of removal from the toxic pasture. However, the avoidance of close grazing of high endophyte ryegrass dominant pastures can be problematic, especially during dry summer conditions.

Lameness (see Chapter 31)

Lameness is a significant problem in New Zealand dairy herds. Unlike the situation in winter housed cattle, the main problems are excessive wear and bruising of the sole, perforation of the sole (septic pododermatitis) and white line disease. Most herd problems are associated with poor design, construction or maintenance of farm tracks and impatient animal handling.

Observational case-control studies of New Zealand dairy herds have shown that when cows walk at their own pace, each limb is accurately placed to avoid injury. The incidence of claw injury is low in herds which are allowed to drift to and from the milking shed, even on rough or poorly maintained tracks. Significant problems occur when cows are hurried by pushing the animals at the back of the group. The problem is compounded by poorly maintained tracks which cause direct trauma to the sole and slow the herd down, causing further impatient handling. Impatient forcing of cows results in cows skidding as animals from the back of the group are forced against those in the middle; tussling to avoid body contact, resulting in unplanned placement of limbs; abnormal forces being taken on the abaxial wall of the lateral claw as cows attempt to resist being forced off the track; shortening of the stride so that the hind limbs are no longer placed in the same safe spot as the fore limbs and cows being unable to see their lower limbs as their heads are forced up and above the animals in front (Chesterton, 1989).

Most lameness problems can be managed by patient movement of cows along the farm track to the milking shed, proper maintenance of tracks and careful handling in the shed. Congestion points and distractions should be removed and the track surface should be nonabrasive, correctly crowned and well drained, especially the parts closest to the milking shed (Vermunt & Greenough, 1997).

Bloat (see p. 832)

Pasture bloat is a common cause of sudden death in cattle in New Zealand. It is caused by the production of a stable foam which traps the normal gases of fermentation in the rumen (frothy bloat) and inhibits eructation. Pasture bloat occurs most commonly when cattle graze pastures dominated by lush, immature, rapidly growing legumes (clovers, lucerne), but there are also reports of the disease when cattle are grazed on other materials such as turnips, brassica and cereal crops, and young grass with a high soluble protein content. While death is the most obvious loss associated with bloat, subclinical and mild bloat are associated with considerable production losses.

Although bloat susceptibility is heritable, progress in the genetic selection for low bloat susceptibility has been slow (Morris *et al.*, 1991). Outbreaks of bloat with several cows dead and/or stabbed are devastating, and nowadays most farmers take precautions by using antifoaming agents, which are still the only reliable way of controlling or preventing bloat. Historically, farmers have used detergent based products for controlling bloat. These have included oils, marlophens, pluronics or turps, and currently the most favoured are the alcohol ethoxylate derivatives due to their extended persistency of action. Most commercially available products are suitable for daily drenching, trough treatment or pasture spraying. The rumen modifier monensin (Rumensin Liquid and Rumensin Anti-Bloat capsule, Elanco, NZ), is marketed as an effective product in the prevention of milk bloat. Monensin is not a detergent, but acts to reduce the bacterial/protozoal activity that releases foam producing compounds in the normal rumen.

The Australian scene

Dairy farming in Australia is largely confined to those climatic regions which are favoured by higher rainfall and better quality soils, especially in the eastern seaboard states and Tasmania. Flood irrigation is used extensively in areas where rainfall is very seasonal. Although each of the states in Australia maintains its own highly regulated dairy industry, the entire industry is influenced by the dominance of the southern dairy industry, particularly that of Victoria, which produces well over half of the total Australian production. Like New Zealand, the Victorian and Tasmanian dairy industries depend heavily on world markets for their manufactured and export products. The ability of farmers freely to sell market milk contracts (quota) is limited in most states, as is the ability to establish new dairy enterprises. This is in contrast to New Zealand, where dairy conversions are occurring on a large scale. The average milk price to the farmer is slightly higher than in New Zealand, but is still low when compared to Europe or the USA.

Similar to New Zealand, dairy farming in Australia is highly efficient in labour and land usage and is predominantly seasonal with the majority of the herds being spring calving. The average Australian dairy herd is smaller than in New Zealand, but the degree of 'Holsteinization' of the national dairy herd is further advanced. Dairy cows graze pasture all year round and this forms the major portion of the diet. In addition to this, supplementary feed sources such as grain are widely used. Consequently, the average milk production is higher and the average days in milk longer. Grain is fed at a much lower cost, because of the proximity to the main grain producing areas. Certain animal health problems associated with this grain feeding (e.g. abomasal displacement, ruminal acidosis, salmonellosis and laminitis/lameness) are therefore relatively common.

Specific diseases common to Australia but exotic to New Zealand are the insect-borne diseases such as anaplasmosis, babesiosis (ticks), ephemeral fever or 'three-day-sickness' and Akabane disease (midges).

References

Bruère, A.N., Cooper, B.S. & Dillon, E.A. (1990) Mycotoxicoses. In *Veterinary Clinical Toxicology*, pp. 167–84. Foundation for Continuing Education of the New Zealand Veterinary Association, Palmerston North.

Chesterton, R.N. (1989) Examination and control of lameness in dairy herds. *New Zealand Veterinary Journal*, **37**, 133–4.

Ellison, R.S. (1992) A review of copper and selenium reference ranges in cattle and sheep. *Proceedings of the New Zealand Veterinary Association Sheep and Beef Cattle Society*, **22**, 3–27.

Grace, N. (1994) Selenium. In *Managing Trace Element Deficiencies*, pp. 9–23. AgResearch, Palmerston North.

Hanly, G.J. & Mossman, D.H. (1977) Commercial beef production on hill country. *New Zealand Veterinary Journal*, **25**, 3–7.

Morris, C.A., Cockrem, F.R.M., Carruthers, V.R., McIntosh, O.T. & Cullen, N.G. (1991) Response to divergent selection for bloat susceptibility in dairy cows. *New Zealand Journal of Agricultural Research*, **34**, 75–83.

Mossman, D.H. & Hanly, G.J. (1977) A theory of beef production. *New Zealand Veterinary Journal*, **25**, 96–100.

Vermunt, J.J. & Greenough, P.R. (1997) Management and control of claw lameness – an overview. In *Lameness in Cattle* (ed. by P.R. Greenough & A.D. Weaver), 3rd edn, pp. 308–15. W.B. Saunders, Philadelphia.

Wakelin, R.L. (1992) Copper supplementation for ruminants. *Proceedings of the New Zealand Veterinary Association Sheep and Beef Cattle Society*, **22**, 43–51.

Wichtel, J.J. (1998) A review of selenium deficiency in grazing ruminants. *New Zealand Veterinary Journal*, **46**, 47–52.

Chapter 73
North American Dairy Production and Veterinary Involvement

T.W. Graham

Milk production trends 1183
Veterinary involvement 1183
Approaching a herd problem – an example 1184
Veterinary monitoring on the dairy farm 1185
   Disease monitors 1185
   Mastitis monitoring 1185
   Fertility monitoring 1185
   Production monitoring 1186

Milk production trends

Production of high quality nutrient-dense milk and meat is a primary goal of dairy operators throughout North America. As our populations become more aware of human health concerns regarding food safety, they have required that we provide them with products without pathogens or chemical contaminants. As they should, consumers expect their food to be safe, wholesome and highly nutritious. With urbanization, consumers have become less aware of how their food is produced, both as a raw and manufactured product. Animal welfare issues have increasingly become a concern for consumers. Now, more than ever, veterinarians are expected to provide leadership in animal husbandry and care, ensuring that all animals are treated humanely throughout their lives. Veterinarians are in a key position to provide leadership in animal welfare, health and food safety.

As an industry North American dairies are increasing in cow numbers, but the number of facilities continues to decline. Because of increasing animal density it is likely that future dairy owners will face more environmental constraints. Environmental constraints are increasing the operating costs for existing and newly built dairies. Environmental laws are likely to restrict building and expansion of existing and new dairy facilities. Cost of production for meat and milk continues to rise, while the value of raw products sold has increased at a slower pace. The narrowing margin of profit per unit of product sold requires that animals produce meat and milk with high efficiency and that animals remain healthy. Veterinarians are now expected to maintain animal health, give expert advice in milk production, reproduction and growth, help design and modify facilities, design and monitor food safety protocols (pathogen- and chemical-free meat and milk) and provide information to producers on-cost-effective production of meat and milk products sold.

Veterinary involvement

The focus of this discussion is to outline those aspects of dairy production (meat and milk) about which veterinarians can provide information to dairy owners to enhance performance of their enterprise. Clearly our training as veterinarians is focused on animal health aspects of dairy cattle production. Ironically, it is often poorly planned and maintained housing, milking parlour/equipment design and inadequate or unbalanced rations that will curtail production and lead to disease. Understanding the requirements for clean comfortable housing and bedding and then helping producers implement those changes greatly increases animal welfare and performance. The use of inorganic bedding (i.e. sand) in properly designed freestall barns has a positive effect on feet and legs, mastitis and milk production. Reducing the time that cows spend standing on concrete reduces the incidence of laminitis and sole abcess formation. Increasing the time cows spend laying down chewing their cud increases mammary blood flow, with the subsequent effect of increasing milk production. Laying down a manure-free environment greatly reduces exposure to environmental streptococci, staphylococci and coliform bacteria, which helps reduce the incidence of environmental mastitis.

Knowledge of nutrient needs from birth to slaughter greatly increases our ability to reduce health problems and manipulate growth, reproduction and milk production. From our classical veterinary training, knowledge of the pathophysiology of disease allows the attending veterinarian to recognize the conditions being diagnosed and guide therapeutic intervention. Taking diagnostic methods to the population level requires an understanding of the epidemiology and dynamics of diseases in groups of animals. Understanding the aetiopathogenesis of disease allows for intervention on a herd basis after identifying the affected groups and underlying causes of diseases within a herd. Knowing what factors predispose cows to disease and what control methods can be used to remove or attenuate risk for disease in exposed cattle will greatly help dairy owners to produce milk and meat profitably, often with less labour.

Approaching a herd problem – an example

As a case example, an 1100 cow herd had several hundred cows with diarrhoea throughout the lactating herd (900 lactating cows). The incidence of mastitis varied from zero to ten new cases per day. The expected incidence was 0–1/day. In the first 10 days after calving, 30–40 percent of newly calved cows had retained placenta and/or metritis. The expected incidence of retained placenta was 5–8% and was principally associated with dystokia and twin birth. The expected incidence of metritis in newly calved cows was 3–5 per cent and mostly associated with retained placenta. The number of cows with displaced abomasum varied from three to ten per week across all lactating strings, but mostly in the first month post partum. The expected incidence of displaced abomasum was 1–3 per cent of cows calving, with none of the cases coming from cows later than 30 days post calving. Cows dying or being sold as unproductive approached 50 per cent of the milking herd over a 5-month period and the expected rate was 30–35 per cent. The milk production was 30 litres (68 lb) per cow per day and the expected production was 35–36 litres (78–80 lb).

As an approach to the herd problem, cows identified by the herd manager as poorly producing or sick were held for diagnosis of underlying disease. Visual examination of all cows in the herd was done during biweekly fertility examinations. All calving and mastitic cows had composite milk samples collected aseptically for identification of *Mycoplasma* and aerobic bacteria. Approximately 10 per cent of cows in three groups had blood samples collected: cows before calving, in the first 10 days after calving and approximately 100 days after calving. Metabolic profiles (haemograms and serum chemistries) were run to help determine the underlying causes of disease. Faecal cultures for *Salmonella* sp. were collected, as well as blood for determining exposure to or active infection with bovine virus diarrhoea (BVD). Antepartum blood samples were collected to determine serum non-esterified fatty acid (NEFA) levels. Urine pH was determined to evaluate the effectiveness of the anionic dry cow diet. Diets by produc-

tion string were collected directly from the feed wagon as it delivered feed to cows. Rations, as formulated, were evaluated to determine any deviations from governmental recommendations (Subcommittee on Dairy Cattle Nutrition, National Research Council, 2001).

Antepartum cows had elevated NEFA levels, indicating weight loss in the last weeks before calving. Cows had low calcium levels before and after calving with only rare milk fever, suggesting that the antepartum diet was not well balanced for prevention of hypocalcemia. Urine pH was 8.0 in antepartum cows, indicating that the anionic diet was not effective. Non-lactating and lactating cows had high serum magnesium levels, suggesting higher than normal intake of magnesium (Mg). Diet analysis suggested that antepartum cows did not have adequate protein intake and their daily diet intake was low. This suggested that cows should be losing weight before calving, predisposing them to periparturient immunosuppression, retained placenta, mastitis, metritis and displaced abomasum. The lactating cows also had high Mg levels and diet analysis indicated that they were fed a ration containing 0.6% Mg on a dry matter (DM) basis (upper levels recommend 0.4% DM). Lactating cow diets also contained 22 per cent protein in the DM. *Mycoplasma bovis* was discovered in a few cows with mastitis in the early lactating period and several cows were culture positive for environmental streptococci, staphylococci and coliform bacteria.

Ration and feed analysis suggested the milk cows were oversupplemented with Mg and protein, and effective fibre may have been limiting. *Salmonella* cultures were negative and results of BVD serology and PCR probes for BVD suggested that neither *Salmonella* nor BVD were the cause of diarrhea. As formulated, dry cows should have been fed a ration adequate in energy and protein, but intake was low, probably causing weight loss and contributing to periparturient metabolic disease (retained placenta, mastitis, milk fever, displaced abomasum, ketosis, low milk production). The prevalence of diarrhoea was 80–90 per cent of lactating cows. There was no apparent diarrhoea in non-lactating cows.

New rations were formulated to reduce Mg throughout the herd, reduce protein in the lactating cow rations and to increase the effective fibre in the lactating herd. Close-up and far-off dry cow rations were reformulated to reduce feed sorting and to increase intake for all cows. String cultures (emphasizing newly calved and hospital cows) and retrospective reculture of all cows having had mastitis within the past two months were initiated to identify mycoplasma-positive cows. From interviews with the dairy manager it was noted that most cows were administered 40–120 mg of dexamethasone for udder oedema in the first one to four days after calving. Routine use of dexamethasone was greatly curtailed to alleviate the immunosuppression associated with its use.

After reducing the protein and Mg levels to governmental recommendations for level of milk production, diarrhoea in the milking cow herd was reduced to one to two cases/900 cows per week. These were mostly attributed to indigestion. Replacement of long-stem oat hay with corn silage from the dry cow diets and reformulation of the close-up mineral package reduced the urine pH to 6–6.5 and increased diet intake and uniformity of consumption of these two rations. Of cows calving, retained placenta and metritis incidence was reduced to 6–8 per cent and 3–5 per cent, respectively. The incidence of displaced abomasum declined to 0–3 cases/month. Cows at three to five days post calving or identified with mastitis had milk aseptically collected from all four quarters and all cows positive for mycoplasma were removed from the herd. All purchased cows were routinely monitored for contagious mastitis and treated, segregated, culled or returned to the supplier as needed. It was thought that periparturient immunosupression, both from poor feed intake and from use of dexamethasone, facilitated the mycoplasma outbreak. After initial identification of the index mycoplasma-positive cows it took approximately one month to bring the incidence down to zero. Evaluation of the freestall environment and cows in the milking parlour indicated that the freestalls were not well maintained (wet and manure/urine contaminated), but the cows were clean and dry when milked. It was recommended that the freestalls be dug out and refilled with sand to encourage stall acceptance and reduce exposure to organic bedding.

Veterinary monitoring on the dairy farm

In addition to traditional veterinary tasks of routine health care (including biosecurity protocols), surgical and reproductive intervention, and disease monitoring, veterinarians should be involved in facility design, selecting equipment and monitoring its performance (feed trucks, milking equipment), personnel training and management, ration formulation, monitoring milk production and heifer growth, forage production and monitoring of stored feed quality.

Disease monitors

Routine monitoring of disease prevalence and incidence allows the veterinarian to interpret changes in expected levels of disease and whether intervention

may be needed to reduce disease to expected levels. Identifying factors that may contribute to lower than expected levels of disease can advance the science of veterinary medicine. Communicating new ways to reduce disease incidence can allow those of us in practice to contribute to our personal growth, advance our clients' needs and advance the way veterinary practice is carried out.

A traditional and still important area for veterinary intervention is development of cost-effective vaccination protocols and evaluation of their success. This should be done for all stages of life and production. Evaluating calving and calf facilities and performance is a way to begin routine herd health monitoring and intervention. Evaluation of the calving facility cleanliness, calving protocols for ensuring healthy cows and calves after calving (e.g. hygiene in assisting with dystokia or the force applied when pulling calves), colostrum monitoring (bacteria counts, amount, density) and calfhood disease control (cleanliness of the calving and newborn facilities, cleanliness of the feeding utensils, milk and feed and protocols for routine disease treatment) are good starting points. Focusing veterinary care in these areas has a high return on investment for producers as they are areas that are often neglected, yet have a great effect on profitability when well maintained.

Mastitis monitoring (see Chapters 23, 25)

Mastitis control and evaluation of pathogens in milk is still a very important service provided by veterinarians. Evaluation of types of bacteria in individual and bulk tank samples, individual and herd somatic cell counts and total bulk tank bacteria counts can direct where and when intervention is needed to correct a herd/equipment problem. Routine milking equipment evaluation, quality control for teat dips and milker training schools are valuable services to producers to help ensure the sale of quality milk.

Fertility monitoring (see Chapter 41b)

With several strategies of intervention for improving pregnancy rates within a herd (e.g. timed insemination and prostaglandin synchronization programmes), assessing the success and cost-effectiveness of these programs is important. Evaluation of personnel skills on a facility will help determine the likelihood of success and whether these types of programmes should be used in an enterprise. Use of bull breeding may be most appropriate for some herds, while in others highly successful artificial breeding programmes can greatly aid in creating a high quality and uniform genetic base for a herd. Goals for reproductive performance have been well described over the past 40 years, but with the advent of products such as recombinant bovine somatotropin (rBST) some of these goals have changed. Some have suggested that increasing the calving interval in these rBST herds can be economically advantageous. However, maintaining a high proportion of the herd pregnant (50 per cent or more) with good conception rates (2.0–3.0 services/conception) still remains a primary goal to ensure profitability of a dairy enterprise.

Evaluation of body condition at calving, one to two months after calving, at conception and at cessation of lactation can help maintain reproductive performance. Increasing rates of anoestrous cows in early lactation (60–120 days in milk) suggest weight loss in the dry period or early post-parturient period (0–90 days), heat stress or inadequate nutrition in the current ration. High levels of endometritis at 30–45 days' lactation suggest problems in the periparturient period and require that all factors contributing to the endometritis be identified (e.g. nutrition, hygiene practices, dystokia, twinning). Correcting these deficits will help keep the herd reproductively sound, reduce treatment costs, lower culling rates and help maintain profitability.

The use of progesterone assays to verify heat detection accuracy (at the time of insemination) is another tool the veterinarian can use to help monitor herd health, although anoestrous cows can also lack detectable levels of progesterone. Holding breeder training schools to teach or review heat detection techniques, semen handing and proper insemination techniques can maintain high fertility in a herd.

As part of any herd monitoring programme, evaluation of the incidence of periparturient disease allows for a retrospective evaluation of the health of non-lactating cows and cows in the first month of lactation. Recording and evaluating the incidence of ketosis, displaced abomasum, milk fever, diarrhoea, pneumonia, mastitis, etc., are critical so that action or target levels for intervention may be set. Certainly diseases should be monitored at all stages of life (birth to sale) and goals of performance evaluated for each stage of production. Routine monitoring of urine pH and fresh cow metabolic profiling (Ca, Mg, P, K, Na, Cl, liver function, serum protein) will help evaluate the success of non-lactating and early lactating feeding and housing programmes. This will help ensure that cows perform well throughout lactation. Monthly or bimonthly evaluation is appropriate and can be more or less inclusive depending on the frequency of farm visits.

Production monitoring

Routine evaluation of production parameters, such as feed intake, calf growth and milk production (milk flow, butter fat, solids not fat, protein, lactose, somatic cell

count) will help guide decision-making for feeding changes, forage selection, production, harvest, storage and removal for feeding. Examination of foodstuffs can help identify those practices that alter cow health and milk production. Poor quality forage production, harvest, storage and removal for feeding can directly affect both both feed intake and cow health. Overly mature feed that is too dry when ensiled can become mouldy or compost, leading to both an unhealthy feed and one that is unpalatable and poorly available. Too wet a forage or contamination of feed with animal carcasses can lead to high levels of clostridial growth, predisposing animals to diseases such as botulism. Improperly stored corn, barley, canola, cottonseed, soybeans and other protein meals can lead to mould production and subsequent mycotoxicosis. Contamination of feed from bird droppings and wild and domestic animal faeces allows for spread of *Salmonella*, *Leptospira* and other shared pathogens. Cross-contamination of feeds with cattle manure increases the spread of Johne's disease, BVD, *Salmonella* spp., etc. Recommendations for facility design to limit feed transmission of infectious diseases facilitate disease control at the population level. This type of activity is analogous to the design of vaccine and treatment protocols that veterinarians have engaged in for years. Taking steps to reduce exposure of the animals on farms to these agents is also becoming a goal for limiting contamination of food at the consumer level.

Feed sorting, or the selection of high concentrate feedstuffs over forages by cattle, increases the likelihood of lameness, subacute ruminal acidosis, reduction in the production of fat in milk and ultimately lower milk yield. Directing forage production (selecting seed, fertilization, planting density), timing (immature or mature) and method of harvest (e.g. kernel processing or rolling of corn silage as it is harvested, chop length), size and dimensions of storage facilities for forages, management of forage removal (face management of silage) will help producers keep cattle healthier and more productive. Veterinarians, by the very nature of our relationship with producers, often are in the best position to evaluate feeding practices. If we are evaluating those practices it makes sense that we are the ones directing how to feed the cows for health and production. An evolving role of veterinarians is routine ration evaluation and formulation. Because cow health is directly affected by improper nutrition, it is increasingly important that veterinarians become directly involved in ration formulation.

As part of the routine evaluation of cattle health, veterinarians should monitor why cattle are sold from the herd and the number sold in a given time. Culling rates directly affect profitability. While production may appear very good for cows in a herd, this can be deceiving if the number of cows entering and leaving the herd is high. If replacement costs are low and the value of milk high that strategy could be very profitable. Today in North America, cattle prices are high and the average price for milk sold has remained relatively steady. If a producer has a high cull rate (45–55 per cent of the herd/year), milk production per cow can be quite high (13000 litres (£3000) per 305-day lactation). However, because of the high removal rate and high cost of replacements, this strategy can reduce net profitability or prevent a dairy from growing if cows are removed for disease. If the high cull rate is because cows are being sold for dairy production (highly valued cattle) to other herds and the producer has an excellent calf raising programme, this strategy could prove to be very profitable. Helping producers evaluate their return on investment of a given strategy is an appropriate task for veterinarians to engage in.

In summary, the role of veterinarians is rapidly changing in North America. Today more of the focus of veterinarians will be in operations management, including herd health, personnel training, udder health and milking equipment evaluation, facility design, nutritional and financial advice including commodity contracts, crop selection and forage production. The opportunities for veterinarians are ever expanding, allowing several avenues of input into animal agricultural production.

Further reading

Martin, S.W., Meek, A.H. & Willeburg, P. (1987) *Veterinary Epidemiology, Principles and Methods*. Iowa State University Press, Ames.

Radostits, O.M., Leslie, K.E. & Fetrow, J. (1994) *Herd Health, Food Animal Production Medicine*, 2nd edn. W.B. Saunders, Philadelphia.

Sniffen, C.J. & Herdt, T.H. (1991) *Dairy Nutrition Management, Veterinary Clinics of North America, Food Animal Practice*. W.B. Saunders, Philadelphia.

Subcommittee on Dairy Cattle Nutrition, Committee on Animal Nutrition, National Research Council (2001) *Nutrient Requirements of Dairy Cattle*, 7th edn (*revised*). National Academy Press, Washington, DC.

Van Soest, P.J. (1982) *Nutritional Ecology of the Ruminant*. Cornell University Press, Ithaca, NY.

Chapter 74
The North American Beef Industry

D. Sjeklocha and S. Sweiger

Introduction   1188
Cow-calf sector   1188
  Cattle distribution   1188
Cattle feeding sector   1189
Meat packing sector   1190
The practice of beef cattle veterinary medicine in North
America   1190

Introduction

The North American beef industry is very diverse and complex. It is distinctly separate from the dairy industry, with the exception of cull dairy cows and castrated male dairy stock (steers), which are eventually added to the beef supply. 'Dual purpose' breeds are very seldom used for true dual purposes. There are three sectors to the North American beef industry: the cow-calf, cattle feeding and meat packing sectors. A very short synopsis would say that the cow-calf sector provides cattle for the cattle-feeding sector, which provides cattle for the meat packing industry. One may wonder why the meat-packing sector would be included in this discussion. It has become evident in recent years that all three sectors must work together and share information in order to deliver a beef product that provides a good eating experience for the end consumer. So, in this light, each of these sectors will be discussed.

Cow-calf sector

Cattle distribution

This sector is undoubtedly the most diverse. This is due to the fact that it uses grazed forage (primarily grass) as its primary raw material. Grazable forage is available in every geographic region. The landscape and climate throughout North America differ greatly between geographic regions. As the landscape and climate changes, so do the types of forages available in that region as well as the type of herd management. Cattle herds are developed in such a way to best deal with the environment in which they live. For example, in the southern United States, *Bos indicus* breeds are very popular

because of their ability to deal with the extreme heat. In the northern United States *Bos taurus* breeds are used because of their ability to withstand the cold temperatures.

Sixty per cent of the United States' cattle herd is located in the south east. Amongst others, states in this area would include Florida, Georgia, Alabama, Mississippi, Louisiana, Tennessee, Kentucky, North Carolina and South Carolina. In this area, only 1 to 5 acres (0.4–2 ha) are required to sustain a cow and her calf for one year. There are a few very large herds in this region, the vast majority are very small herds. Many of these small herds are either a hobby or a secondary source of income for the producer. Often, these producers simply have a small parcel of grass that would not be utilized at all unless the producer owned a few cows to graze it. These producers are not necessarily in the cattle business to produce beef, but rather use cattle to harvest a forage that would otherwise go to waste. Because of this, genetic control of production is not taken very seriously in many cases. In recent years, producers and veterinarians in this area have taken steps to improve genetic selection and to market cattle in uniform groups.

The remaining 40 per cent of the nation's cattle herd is spread throughout the rest of the United States' grazable landmass. In some regions of this land mass, only one acre (0.4 ha) is required to support a cow and her calf, while in other areas, as much as 100 acres (25 ha) is required to support a cow and her calf. Generally, as the carrying capacity of the land decreases, the size of the herd increases. The regions that have a high carrying capacity are also regions that produce a great deal of cereal grains. Cow-calf producers in these areas take advantage of the crop residues by allowing their cattle herds to graze the fields after they have been harvested, gleaning the grains that were missed by the harvesting machines (combines). In regions where there is very little cereal grain production, there is more reliance on harvested forage (grass hay, alfalfa hay, etc.) for winter feed. Herds in these regions can be as small as one up to as many as 15 000 head or more.

It is generally considered to be good management for cow-calf producers to adhere to a fairly rigid 'calving season'. Producers will turn bulls out with the cattle for 45 to 90 days for breeding. At the end of this time period, the bulls are removed from the herd. This allows for better use of the producer's time and a more uniformly sized calf crop. Some producers do not adhere to this type of calving season, some of whom allow their cows to have calves all through the year. The majority of calves are born in the late winter or spring and are weaned in late summer or in the fall.

Weaning of calves is yet another area of great diversity within the cow-calf sector. Some producers will go through a strict 'preconditioning' programme, in which the calves are vaccinated once while still on the cow (typically against IBR, BVD, PI3, BRSV and clostridial disease). Then, approximately three weeks later, they are revaccinated against the viruses, implanted with a growth-promoting hormone and weaned. The calves are then fed a grain and roughage ration for anywhere from a couple of weeks to several months, depending on the marketing plans of the producer. Other producers will vaccinate their calves once, pull them off the cow and sell them. Still others will simply pull their calves off the cow without vaccinating them and sell the calves. Most bull calves are castrated at some point prior to marketing, becoming known as 'steers'.

Some cow-calf producers will retain ownership of their calves through the feeding period up to harvest. These producers most commonly send their calves to a 'custom' or 'commercial' feedyard and pay the feedyard to feed the calves for them. This will be discussed in more depth in the cattle feeding section. Most cow-calf producers sell their calves at some point prior to the feeding period. The most common form of marketing calves is done through a livestock auction (also commonly known as a 'sale barn'). Calves are taken to the livestock auction, sorted for size or other common characteristic and sold to the highest bidder. Disadvantages of this type of marketing are that cattle are commingled, thus allowing disease transfer. Cattle can also be sold via 'satellite auctions' in which video images of calves are transmitted by satellite all over the country for bidders to view and bid on. Still more cattle are now being sold over the internet/world wide web. These latter two marketing options offer the advantage of not commingling different groups of cattle, as the cattle are marketed directly from the ranch of origin.

Within the cow-calf sector is a group of producers collectively known as 'seedstock producers'. These are producers who specialize in producing breeding stock to be used by the commercial cow-calf producer. Careful attention is paid to fertility, carcass traits, muscling and performance characteristics (average daily gain, weaning weight, yearling weight, feed conversion, etc.). There is a wide range of criteria that cow-calf producers use to select breeding stock and many of these are predicted by the use of expected progeny differences (EPDs). EPDs give the bull buyer an idea of how a particular bull's calves may perform in various traits.

Cattle feeding sector

The cattle feeding sector has become very specialized. In the 1960s, many cow-calf producers fed their own cattle to harvest weight. As more science and technology have been put to use, it has become more efficient and cost-effective for cattle feeding operations to get increasingly larger, and less efficient and cost-effective for the cow-calf producer to feed his own cattle. Many of the modern cattle feeding operations (known as 'feedlots' or 'feedyards') can hold 100 000 head of cattle or more at one time.

A feedyard is a collection of pens that are used to confine cattle while they are being fed a high-energy ration. One side of the pen is lined with a concrete feed trough (feed bunks). Trucks, fitted with a special box that is capable of mixing feed, auger feed into the feed bunks as they drive alongside them. Feed management is considered to be one of the most important and detailed jobs around the feedyard. Calling for the wrong amount of feed can hurt the performance of the cattle in that pen for the rest of the feeding period. Feedyard cowboys ride through each pen of cattle every day looking for sick cattle. Sick cattle are removed from the pen and placed in a hospital pen, where treatment is administered and the animal is given time to recover before being returned to the original pen.

Cattle are usually hauled into feedyards by semi tractor-trailers. These large trucks can carry 50 000 to 56 000 lb (22.5–25.4 tonnes). It is not uncommon for cattle to be hauled for 8 to 24 hours before arriving at the feedyard. This puts the cattle under a great deal of stress and increases the chances that they will become sick. Over the years, feedyards have become very adept at dealing with this stress. Many feedyards have pens that are used especially for receiving cattle. These pens are usually smaller than other pens on the feedyard and have excellent drainage so the newly arrived cattle have a dry place to rest. Fresh feed and clean water are provided at all times. After the cattle have eaten, drunk and rested, they are put through a series of procedures known collectively as 'processing'. Processing may include any or all of the following: vaccination (against pathogens such as IBR, BVD, PI3, BRSV, *Pasteurella/Mannheimia*, spp. clostridial pathogens, *Haemophilus somnus*, etc.), implantation with a growth hormone, eartagging, administration of a parasiticide, administration of a vitamin/mineral supplement, castration of bulls or pregnancy examination of heifers. If a heifer is found to be pregnant, the pregnancy may be aborted.

Upon completion of processing, the cattle are moved to a regular pen on the feedyard. Over the next two to three weeks, the cattle are fed a series of rations designed to acclimate the rumen to starch digestion. The 'finishing' ration will contain approximately 90 per cent concentrate. Feeding concentrates at this level may result in lactic acidosis, thus proper feed management is of the utmost importance.

Historically, finished cattle were sold to meat packing companies simply as a commodity. There were no premiums paid for exceptional quality, so there was no reason for feedyards to feed for quality – just performance. Beginning in the 1970s, consumption of beef declined steadily, year after year. It became apparent that more attention needed to be paid to the quality of the beef produced. Meat packing companies and feedyards started to enter into arrangements that would pay premiums for superior beef quality and yield and would penalize for inferior beef quality and yield. These pricing arrangements are commonly known as 'grids' or 'formula pricing'. Most grids are developed to reward for both beef quality and yield, but there are some that primarily reward for yield or primarily reward for quality. Feedyards enter into grid agreements that best fit their feeding abilities. Even with grid agreements, there are still a large number of cattle sold on a cash basis as a commodity.

This discussion would be incomplete if 'stockers' and 'backgrounders' were not included. Stockers are cattlemen who purchase calves at approximately weaning age and turn these calves out to pasture. These calves gain anywhere from 200 to 400 lb (90–180 kg) while on pasture. The calves are then sold to a cattle feeder or the stocker retains ownership of the cattle through the feeding period. Backgrounders (or preconditioners), on the other hand, are cattlemen who specialize in feeding and taking care of high risk calves (calves that have a high risk of sickness). Many feedyards will send their high risk calves to backgrounders or growyards because the feedyard does not have enough employees to give these calves the level of attention they need. Often, calves in a backgrounding operation are checked two or more times per day for sickness. After a few weeks, the health problems subside. The calves will adjust to a concentrate-based ration and learn to eat out of a feedbunk. After several more weeks, the calves are removed from the backgrounding operation and sent to their respective feedyard, where they are fed out to harvest.

Meat packing sector

Once the cattle have reached the appropriate harvest weight and condition, they are sent to the meat packing plant. While there are several meat-packing companies in the United States, there are three very large ones that control the bulk of the industry. As many as 5000 head per day can be harvested through these meat packing plants. Cattle are humanely harvested and the carcasses are hung on an overhead rail to cool. The United States Department of Agriculture provides quality inspectors and veterinary inspectors to ensure a safe, wholesome food supply.

Possibly one of the most positive changes that the meat packing industry has made in recent years is the implementation of information sharing. It is currently possible for a cow-calf producer to receive information about how well his cattle performed, in terms of quality grade and yield grade. This type of feedback is very important for genetic advancement in the cattle herd.

The practice of beef cattle veterinary medicine in North America

Beef cattle veterinary practice has evolved a great deal in the last 20 years. This evolution has developed from a primarily ambulatory practice in which individual animals were treated to a much more production-oriented approach of veterinary medicine. As American food production has become more and more efficient, American society has become less and less aware of how their food is produced. This has led to many misconceptions among the American people about how food animals are handled and treated for disease. Society is very concerned about animal welfare, antibiotic resistance and food safety. Beef producers are very concerned about these things as well, but are also concerned about production performance, cost-effectiveness and the ever-tightening profit margin.

Individual treatment of animals is still a substantial part of beef cattle practice. Veterinarians are still called upon to treat respiratory disease, lameness, reproductive disorders, digestive and nutritional problems, among other things. However, veterinarians are also taking a more active role in preventing these situations. Beef cattle producers are being economically forced to provide cattle with added value. This means that the cattle must have the genetics and the immune integrity to perform well and stay healthy through each stage of production.

Many new opportunities in veterinary medicine have arisen because of this change from individual treatment to preventive medicine. In the cow-calf sector, many new computer software programs have been developed that can help with production parameters, record keeping and genetic selection. Because of the labour intensity involved in beef production, many producers simply do not have the time to get comfortable with the software and its capabilities, although they still want the information that the software provides. Many veterinarians have taken this opportunity to help their clients by serving as a data analyst. Veterinarians gather the information needed and record the information in the software program. Because the veterinarian has the opportunity to work with several herds, he/she also has the opportunity to understand the software and its capabilities at a deeper level. The veterinarian can then analyse a client's data, work up reports in various areas of production and consult with the client on topics that may include replacement heifer selection, herd sire selection, culling, preventive health programmes, nutrition, effective treatment schedules and the cost-effectiveness of various production practices. There is still plenty of opportunity for some of the traditional services of veterinary practice, such as pregnancy examination, vaccination of calves and cows and treatment of diseased stock, but veterinary consultation has the potential of a wide scope of development in the cow-calf sector.

In the cattle-feeding sector, veterinary consultation already has a tremendous foothold. With the very large numbers of cattle in these feedyards, it is very cost-effective for the feedyard to hire a consulting veterinarian to design health programmes, evaluate treatment protocols, help in the training of new employees and advise on the construction of new facilities and the repair of current facilities. This type of practice can be very satisfying professionally, but there is a great deal of travel involved.

Whether a veterinarian specializes in the cow-calf sector, the cattle feeding sector or both, the issues that the beef industry faces will affect his/her practice. One of those issues is food safety. Food safety has captured the attention of the consumer, the producer and the veterinarian. Veterinarians play a key role in control and/or elimination of pathogens in the food chain. Educating the beef producer and the consumer in areas such as how these pathogens develop and how they can be controlled is important for human health and for the survivability of the industry. Another food safety concern is the use of growth-promoting implants. The European Union has stopped the importation of beef from the United States that has been exposed to growth promoting hormones. The use of growth promoting hormones has been proven to be a safe practice. However, the EU's ban has caused some Americans to question its safety (see Chapter 63). Veterinarians are playing a key role in quelling rumours and misinformation about the safety of American beef and the use of growth-promoting hormones by applying good, sound science.

Beef cattle veterinary practice will continue to move away from individual animal medicine and move toward population medicine. Veterinarians must be cost-effective and must be able to demonstrate their cost-effectiveness. Applying good science to decision-making is a major key to being cost-effective. Skills in critical evaluation of the scientific literature need to be honed to a high level of precision so science-based decisions can be made. This is very important in an increasingly litigious society, as good science is much easier to defend in court than anecdotal decisions.

There are and will be many, many opportunities available in beef cattle veterinary practice in the future. The beef industry is changing at a rapid pace and the same is true of beef cattle practice. Veterinarians must be willing and able to adapt to a changing industry and be able to recognize an opportunity when it arises.

Index

abamectin 742, 1022, 1025, 1026, 1027, 1031
abbatoirs, 1190
abdomen distension, acute 140–42
abdominal pain 139–40, 142–6
Aberdeen Angus breed 8, 9, 10, 30, 1177
  hereditary ataxia 162
  joint hypermobility 178
  osteopetrosis 176
  spastic paresis 458–9
abomasum
  dilatation 141, 237, 1109–13
    right-sided with torsion 141, 842–3, 1112–13
  diseases 839–45
  displacement 141, 1109–13
    to left 839–42, 1109–12
  impaction 144, 835, 844–5
  milk clot failure 212, 231–3
  torsion 140, 141
  ulceration 146–7, 149, 236–7, 844
abortion 577, 578, 587, 588, 589
  aspergillosis 934
  bacterial 580–84, 735, 736
  candidiasis 933
  mycotic 586
  non-infectious 586
  protozoal 584–5
  viral 291, 578–80
  see also Brucella abortus (brucellosis)
abscess
  brain 902–3
  Brodie's 464
  injection damage 1078
  jaw 824, 825
  lameness 465
  liver 148, 150, 832, 868
  muscle, 1078
  myocardial 154
  pulmonary 864
  retropharyngeal 824
acantholysis, familial 182
acaricides 83–4, 1158
acceptable daily intake (ADI) 1072
accidents 152
  see also trauma
acetic acid 117, 1067
acetoacetate 815
acetonaemia 150, 151, 156, 168, 789, 793–6, 1091, 1154
  hypomagnesaemia differential diagnosis 789
  nervous 139, 156
acetyl salicylic acid 246
achondroplastic calves 175

achronchia 177
acid detergent fibre (ADF) 374, 375
acid detergent insoluble protein (ADIP) 109
acidosis 96, 145, 147, 151, 784
  calves 902
  control 1068
  diarrhoea 190–91
  rumen 119, 195–8, 203, 829–32
Aconitum napellus 1085, 1087, 1088, 1091
acrosome reaction 485, 486, 499
ACTH see adrenocorticotrophic hormone
actinobacillosis 139, 150, 261, 821, 823–4, 837, 888
Actinobacillus lignieresi 823
Actinomyces bovis 824
Actinomyces pyogenes see Arcanobacterium pyogenes
actinomycosis 821, 824–5, 888
acupuncture 1081, 1091–4, 1095, 1096
  diagnosis 1096–8
  treatment 1098–9, 1100, 1101–2
acute exudative pneumonia 860
ADI see acceptable daily intake
ADIP 109
adrenaline 246, 884
adrenocorticotrophic hormone (ACTH) 1003, 1057, 1058, 1134, 1135, 1136
Aedes spp 745
aesculin-hydrolysing streptococci see streptococci, aesculin-hydrolysing
Africa
  dairying 76–7
  diseases 1156–61
  plant poisonings 1161–2
  rabies 1165, 1170
air cushions 800, 801
Akabane virus 452, 579, 580, 771, 1182
  cerebellar hypoplasia 900
  transmission by semen 629, 630
alarm points (acupuncture) 1099
albendazole 1020, 1021, 1025, 1026, 1027, 1028
albinism 182, 888
albumin, metabolic profile 813
aldosterone 191
alfalfa see lucerne
alimentary tract
  congenital defects 177–8
  obstruction 140
  upper tract squamous cell carcinoma 828
  see also named regions

alkali disease 305
alkalosis 830, 1059
alleles, multiple 163
allergic eczema 1059
allergens 1000
Allerton virus 768, 887
allostasis/allostatic load 1139–41, 1142
alopecia 181, 888
alternative medicine 52, 84, 1081–103
aluminium hydroxide 831
alveolis, diffuse fibrosing 865–6
Amblyomma spp 744, 756, 765, 1031
amicarbalide 1029
amidines 1032
amikacin 1038, 1040
amino acids 107, 108–9
aminoglycosides 394, 395, 1038, 1040, 1041, 1043
amitraz 742, 743, 881, 1031
ammonia 98, 99, 106–7, 108, 115, 116, 117, 118, 125
ammonium chloride 264
amoxycillin 245, 250, 288, 392, 393, 395, 396, 398, 736, 737, 860, 861, 864, 1036, 1037, 1040, 1041, 1043
amphistomiosis, intestinal 279
amphotericin 1036
ampicillin 245, 250, 288, 291, 392, 393, 394, 395, 456, 458, 737, 851, 860, 864, 1036, 1037, 1040, 1041, 1043
amprolium 1030
amputation of digit/claw 1119–22
amyloidosis 928
anaemia 149, 168, 720, 792, 935
anaemia, haemolytic 735, 792
anaesthesia 1105
  abomasal dilatation/displacement 1110, 1112
  amputation of digit/claw 1119–20
  caesarean section 1116
  dehorning 1124
  eye enucleation 1126
  rumenotomy 1107
  teat surgery 1128
anal diseases 859
Anand pattern of dairying 76
anaphylaxis 139, 153, 927–8, 1059, 1063
Anaplasma caudatum 701
Anaplasma centrale 761
Anaplasma maryinale 761, 762, 763
anaplasmosis 745, 761–3, 1063, 1182
  vaccination 762
androgens 481, 485–7
Angus Breed see Aberdeen Angus

animal production level (APL) 104–5, 106, 108, 110
ankylosing spondylitis 462
anoestrus 531, 532–5, 541–4
  after service 548
  cows after calving 545–6
  diagnosis 535–41, 543
  heifers 530
  ovarian status assessment 536–40
  physiological 532
  postpartum 525–6
  prevention 544–8
  true 532–4, 541–4
Anopheles spp 745
anophthalmia 917–18
anthelmintics 84, 270–76, 1019–29
  cestode infection treatment 1028–9
  dairy heifers 57–8
  delivery systems 1026
  parasitic bronchitis treatment 1027
  parasitic gastroenteritis treatment 1025–7
  plant materials 83
  resistance 1027
  trematode infection treatment 1028
  use in tropics 83–4, 85, 86
anthrax 152, 717–19, 745, 746
anthrax antiserum 719
  vaccination 719, 1005
anti-inflammatory drugs 1060–64
  see also corticosteroids; non-steroidal anti-inflammatory drugs (NSAIDs); steroids
antibiotics 198, 396, 397, 885, 886, 888, 1043, 1044
  deep pedal infections 430
  diarrhoea management 210
  dosage 1038
  endometritis 522–3
  growth promoters 1069–71
  intramammary preparations 393–5
  intrauterine treatments 518
  mastitis 335, 339, 391–403
  metritis 521
  neurological disorders 897–9, 900
  open fractures 443–4
  parenteral 395–6
  pneumonia 244
  postpartum 527
  resistance 217–18, 391–2, 396–7, 1038
  salmonellosis 217–18, 227, 229–30
  sensitivity testing 1036
  slow-release 1044
antibodies 380
anticholinesterase 1032
antihistamines 246, 831, 1049
anti-foaming agents 834
antigens 996
antimicrobial agents 1035–44
  activity 1037, 1040
  administration route 1038, 1039
  antibacterial therapy 1043, 1044
  bacteriostatic/bactericidal activity 1040–41
  causal agent identification 1035–6
  cost 1042

dosage 1038
dosing frequency 1042, 1044
drug combinations 1041–2
duration of therapy 1038, 1040
penetration of infected area 1036–7
sensitivity testing 1036
toxicity 1042, 1043
withdrawal times 1042
see also antibiotics
antimodium crudum 1086
antimodium tartaricum 1089, 1091
antimony thiomalate, lithium 883
antiparasite mechanism 1001
antiparasitic drugs 1019–33
  see also anthelminthics
antiprotozoals 1029–30
antiseptics 524
aortic stenosis 174
Apis mellifora 1089, 1091
APL *see* animal production level
apple pomace 113, 114, 131
apples 131
apramycin 1040, 1041
arachidonic acid 1048, 1058, 1061
Arcanobacterium (Actinomyces) pyogenes 141, 146, 148, 240, 249, 327, 328, 334, 337, 382, 385, 391, 399, 455, 457, 463, 464, 725, 865
  mastitis 327, 328, 334, 337–40, 382, 385
  osteomyelitis 463
  pneumonia 240, 241, 860, 865
  pyaemia 737
  uterine infection 521, 523
Argas 762
Argasidae family 744
Argaspersicus spp 744
Arnica montana 1089, 1091
aromatase 494
arsenicum album 1089
arthritis 1063, 1091
  degenerative 454–5
  infectious (septic) 455–8
  treatment 1063
arthrogryposis 163, 164, 177, 451–2, 925
  congenital 462
arthropod-borne diseases 748–61, 771–4
  see also flies; mosquitoes; tick-borne diseases; tsetse flies
artificial insemination (AI) 29–30, 39, 61, 62, 76, 77, 627–8
  beef cattle 9, 658–61
  closed herds 990
  dairy heifers 59, 61–2
  DIY 559, 594–5
  embryo transfer donor 640
  erroneous timing 558–9
  fixed time 573
  genetic defects 166
  genetic improvement by 48, 49
  level of use 594
  pre-sexed semen 30, 48
  sweeper bulls 595–6
  technique 627–8
    poor 557, 559
  tropical cattle 77

artificial shade 90–91
artificial vagina (AV) 601–2
ascorbic acid 1037
ash 117
aspirin 246, 399, 1048, 1050, 1053
Aspergillus (aspergillosis) 933–4
association points (acupuncture) 1099
assisted calvings 8
astrovirus 200–201
ataxia
  familial 178–9
  hereditary 162
  progressive 179
atlanto-occipital fusion 176
atresia ilei/coli/ani 177, 203
atropine 867
atypical mycobacteriosis 886
Aujesky's disease 907–8
aurum 1086, 1091
Australia 1182
automatic cluster removers (ACRs) 40
automatic parlours 39
avermectins 741, 748, 1019, 1020, 1022–4, 1032
Ayrshire cattle 28, 30, 76
azemethiphos 1032

BHB *see* beta hydroxybutyrate
β-agonists 1073–5
B cells 323, 381, 1001, 1002
Babesia (babesiosis) 748–50, 763, 1029–30, 1182
  Babesia bigemina 748, 749
  Babesia bovis 748, 749
  Babesia divergens 748, 749, 763
  Babesia major 748, 749
  vaccines 750
Bach Flower Remedies 1103
bacillary haemoglobinuria 719–21
  vaccination 721, 1005
Bacillus anthracis 717–19
Bacillus cercus 327
Bacillus licheniformis 581
Bacillus spp 261, 347
bacitracin 393, 1040
backgrounders 1190
bacteria
  disinfection 978
  fermentation in rumen 96, 97, 98
  milk
    counts 345–8
    differential screen 347–8
    total counts 345–7
  uterine cultures 512
  see also infections/infectious disease, bacterial
bacterial endocarditis 144, 726–8
bactericidal antimicrobials 1040
Bacteroides melaninogenicus 385, 425, 426, 457
bactoscan 346–7
Bagshawe hoist 800, 801
balanoposthitis 612–13
baptisia 1087
baquiloprim 245, 280, 395
barley 14, 19, 78, 113, 124

barley beef 14, 19
barley poisoning 141, 147, 829–32
    see also acidosis
barium selenate 304
basophil 1045
BCMS (British Cattle Movement
    Service) 6
bedding disposal 976
beef cattle
    anoestrus 534
    calving 652–4, 656
    heifer management 19–20, 661
    herd fertility management 652–62
    infections 654–5
    nutrition 655–6
    oestrous synchronization 658–61
    ovulation induction 657–8
    parasitic gastroenteritis 269
    post partum acyclic period 656–8
    reproductive performance 652–62
        determinants 652–4
        factors affecting 654–6
        monitoring 661–2
    seasonal effect 657
    welfare 960
    see also suckler cows
beef finishing systems 14–21, 1189
    barley (cereal) 14, 19
    budgeting 14–15, 16
    dairy beef 18–21
    eighteen-month beef 20, 21
    grass 17–18, 20–21
    overwintering 18
    planning 14–15
    sale returns 15, 16
    winter finishing 15–17
beef production 28–9, 68, 69
    feed budgets 121, 122
    housing 960
    New Zealand 1177–9
    North America 1188–91
    public perceptions 955
    ranching in South America 77
    tropical cattle 77
    see also bull beef production; suckler
        herds
beef, sources of 29
beef special premiums (BSP) 15, 18, 20,
    21
BEF *see* bovine ephemeral fever
behaviour changes 1145–6
Belgian Blue breed 8, 30
Belgian Blue cross 19, 20, 21
belladonna 1089, 1091
benchmarking 50
benign bovine theileriosis 755
benzalkonium chloride 880, 1039
benzathene penicillin 288, 395, 400
benzene hexachloride 880, 1031
benzyl penicillin 394, 396, 849, 1036,
    1039, 1040, 1041, 1043
benzimidazoles 1020–21, 1022, 1024
berberis 1086
Besnoitia besnoiti 756
besnoitiosis 756, 888
beta-lactam antibiotics 394

beta-lactamase 391–2, 396, 397, 1038
betamethasone 795, 1049, 1056, 1057,
    1058
beta hydroxybutyrate 794, 807, 810
bezathene penicillin 288, 395, 400
Bhanja virus 771–2
BHB *see* beta hydroxybutyrate
BHU-1 289–90, 519, 561, 579, 613, 628,
    887–8
BHV-4 578–9
bicarbonate sodium 202, 829, 831, 843,
    1037
bile acid metabolic profiles 808
bilharziosis 279–80
bioallethrin 1032
biosecurity 198, 987–94
biothional 1024, 1026, 1028
biotin 422–3
bisphenols 1024
biting flies 1031
biting lice 1031, 1032
BIV 713–14
black disease 729–31
blackflies 745, 774, 1031
blackleg 152, 723–4, 1005
    vaccination 728, 1005
blacklung 765–6
blackspot 370, 371
BLAD 175
Bladder meridian (acupuncture) 1100
blastocyst 499–500
blind staggers 305
bloat 127, 128, 129, 141, 832–5, 1091
    abomasal 237
    chronic 146–7
    clover grazing 128
    control 1068
    feedlot 119
    frothy 832–5, 1181–2
    lucerne grazing 127
    New Zealand 1181–2
    ruminal 141, 234–6, 832
    sudden death 152
blood disorders, congenital 175
bloodletting 83
blood transfusion 261, 749, 794
blowflies 747–8
Blue Grey 9
bluetongue 561, 629, 630, 691–3
    transmission 745
    vaccination 1018
BLUP (best linear unbiased predictor)
    8
BLV 694, 696–8
B-lymphocyte 1002
BMCC *see* bulk milk cell count
body condition/condition scoring 10, 11,
    121–2
    anoestrus 540
    beef cattle 10, 11, 655–6
    conception failure 562, 563
    dairy heifers 56, 58–9, 63
    postpartum 512–13, 525
    suckler cows 10, 11, 121
    tropical cattle 72
body heat *see* heat

BOHB *see* beta hydroxybutyrate
bone cysts, subchondral 454, 455
bones
    fluorosis 950
    foot 413, 429–30
Boophilus spp 744, 748, 762, 766, 1030,
    1031, 1032
    vaccination 745
Borrelia burgdorferi 427
Bos indicus see Zebu cattle
Bos taurus 72, 75–6, 89
botanical trend monitoring in tropics 73
botulism 147, 151, 721–3, 1005
    vaccination 722, 1005
botulin antitoxin 722
Bovicola bovis 880, 1031, 1032
bovine coronavirus 189, 195, 199–206,
    207, 208, 218
bovine ephemeral fever (BEF) 767–8
bovine farcy 885–6
bovine farmer's lung 860, 861–2
bovine genital campylobacteriosis *see*
    Campylobacter fetus
    (campylobacteriosis)
bovine genital trichomoniasis *see*
    Tritrichomonas fetus
    (trichomoniasis)
bovine herpes mammillitis 363–4, 888
bovine herpes virus 1 (BHV-1) 289–90,
    519, 561
    abortion 579
    balanoposthitis 613
    pseudo-lumpy skin disease 887, 888
    transmission by semen 628
bovine herpes virus 4 (BHV-4) 579–80
bovine immunodeficiency virus (BIV)
    713–14
bovine leucocyte adhesion deficiency
    (BLAD) 175
bovine leukosis, sporadic 698–9, 700
bovine leukosis virus (BLV) 694, 696–8
bovine papilloma virus (BPV) 365, 367,
    882–3
bovine papular stomatitis (BPS) 252–3
bovine petechial fever 763–5
bovine respiratory disease (BRD)
    239–48, 287, 1007–9
    vaccination 1007, 1008–9
bovine respiratory syncytial virus
    (BRSV) 239, 240, 241, 247, 287,
    1007, 1009–10
bovine somatotrophin (BST) 56, 100,
    962, 1073, 1186
bovine spongiform encephalopathy
    (BSE) 9, 14, 156, 168, 789, 890,
    909–11
    crisis 6, 9, 14, 29
    Europe 1152, 1153
    Over Thirty Month Scheme (OTMS)
        9, 14, 28, 29
    transmission in semen 629, 632
bovine streptothricosos 886
bovine virus diarrhoea (BVD) 138, 213,
    240, 241, 247, 287, 452, 559, 853,
    854, 855–7, 987, 1184
    abortion 578–9, 589

bovine virus diarrhoea (BVD) (cont'd)
  bovine respiratory disease complex 1007
  bulls 598, 857
  cerebellar hypoplasia 900
  embryo transfer 644
  Europe 1153
  Hereford disease 178
  oesophageal lesions 826
  serology 1013
  transmission by semen 628, 629, 630, 857
  vaccination 644, 857, 1011–12
BPS (bovine popular stomatitis) 252–3
BPV (bovine papilloma virus) 365, 367, 882–3
brachial plexus avulsion 436
bracken poisoning 154, 828, 946–7
bradykinin 1046, 1047, 1051
brain lesions 156
  abscess 902–3
brainstem neuronal chromatolysis, idiopathic 911
brainstem syndrome 896
bran 80, 112, 114
Brassica spp 792
BRD (bovine respiratory disease) 239–48, 287, 1007–9
breathing symptoms 154
Breda virus 191, 201, 206, 208
breeding
  crossbreeding 9, 169
  dairy farming 25, 47–9
  dairy heifers 59
  decisions 526–7
  policy 47
  records 45, 46
  synchronized 59, 61–2, 497–8, 543, 547
    asynchrony 682–4
    pharmacological methods 678–84
  see also repeat breeder cows
brewer's grains 80, 112, 113, 114, 131
Brodie's abscess 464
bromhexine hydrochloride 246
bromsalans 1024
bronchiectasis 864
bronchitis, parasitic 272–4, 1011, 1027
bronchopneumonia 864
Brown Swiss 76
browse material 80
Brucella abortus (brucellosis) 580, 746, 987, 989, 992, 1013–14, 1087
  Africa 1157
  carpal bursitis 461
  transmission by semen 629, 631
brussel sprouts packhouse waste 113, 114
Bryonia alba 1088, 1091
BSE 9, 156, 168, 784, 890, 909–11
BST 57, 962, 1073, 1186
bucket feeding 3, 4–5, 71
budget feed 121, 122
buffalo flies 745, 747
buffer feeding 119, 130, 377, 791

buildings
  dairy farm 38–44
  see also housing; yards, covered
bulk milk cell count (BMCC) 343–5, 399, 401, 402
bull beef production 16–17, 19, 124
bull mothers 169
bulldog calves 175
bulls
  breeding soundness 599–610
  campylobacteriosis 568, 597, 598, 629, 630–31
  dairy 48–9, 59, 60, 595
  failure to serve cow 559
  genetic defects 166, 610–11
  genetic worth 48–9
  herd replacement breeding 9
  high genetic merit 48
  hip dysplasia 453–4
  Improved Contemporary Comparisons 47, 48
  infectious disease control 598
  infertility 594–624
  intromission failure 612–16
  libido 611–12, 615
  nutrition 611, 618
  on-farm laboratory 601–2
  overwork 611, 617–18
  physical examination 608
  poor pregnancy rate 617–24
  preputial washing 597–8
  puberty onset 481
  quarantine 596
  scrotal temperature 481–2
  selection 48–49, 60
  suckler herds 7–8, 594, 595
  sweeper 595–6
  terminal sires 7–8
  UK use 595–6
  see also semen
Bungaviridae 769
Bunostomum phlebotomum (bunostomosis) 275
Bunostomom spp 1026
Bunyamwera virus 772
buparvaquone 1029
burns 934
bursitis
  carpal 461–2
  tarsal 460–61
bush flies 746
butterfat *see* milk fat
butter production 26
butyl bromide 846
butylscopolamine bromide 827, 846–7
butyric acid 117, 794, 1067
BVD 213, 287, 452, 559, 578–9, 589, 628–30, 644, 822, 853, 855–57, 909, 1007, 1013, 1153, 1187

cabbage 131
Cache Valley virus 772
caecum dilatation and torsion 140, 141, 797, 847
caesarean section 1115–19
calcarea carbonica 1086, 1089

calcarea phosphorica 1086, 1089
calcined magnesite 256
calcium copper edetate 255
calcium chloride 831
calcium 264, 462
  deficiency 253–4, 781–7
  metabolic profile 814
  requirements 33
  in feeds 123–9, 131
  see also hypocalcaemia; milk fever
calcium borogluconate infusion 785–6, 790, 800, 831
calcoferal 782
calendula 1085
calf diptheria 139, 250, 822, 1049, 1091
calf pneumonia 239–40
Calf Processing Aid Scheme (CPAS) 28–9
calici-like virus 200, 218
California encephalitis virus 772
California Mastitis Test (CMT) 329
Calliphora spp 747
Callitroga spp 747
Callitroga americana 748
calovovirus 772
calves
  abomasal impaction 845
  achondroplastic 175
  acidosis 902
  cold stress 930
  convulsive syndromes 156–7
  digestive disorders 231–8
  diphtheria 139, 822
  femoral nerve paralysis 437
  housing 3, 959–60
  identification 6
  intussusception 848
  machine feeding 5
  management 69–71
  milk consumption 11
  milk tetany 791
  mortality 3, 4, 8, 63, 64, 66, 71, 1082
  neonatal diarrhoea 1006–7
  performance targets 5, 6
  pneumonia 4, 70, 239–48, 274, 871
  postweaning management 71–2
  pot-bellied 236
  preweaning management 70–71
  rearing 3–6, 11, 69–72
  red gut 846
  respiratory disease 4, 239–48, 274, 871
  restricted suckling 71
  scouring 4, 70, 1006–7, 1063
  septicaemia 204, 902
  sleeper 907
  suckler management 11–12
  twin 545
  veal 959–60
  weaning 3, 5, 70
  weaning weight 8
  welfare 958–60
  see also diarrhoea, calf; suckled calves
calving
  age at 48, 54, 55, 64, 665
  beef cattle 653–4, 656
  culling policy 656

difficulties 9–10, 167
'downer' cow 151
feeding before 373
heat stress 90
management of dairy heifers 64, 65
month 55
nutritional status 657
pattern in tropical cattle 71, 77
planning 545
season 656, 665, 667, 673, 675
seasonality 52, 55
service after 559
subsequent reproductive events 670
suckler herds 7
see also parturition
calving boxes 42, 65
calving interval 50, 55
of dairy cows 49, 665–6, 673, 1177
economic losses 530
to first service 530–31, 559, 670
of suckler cow 8
calving paralysis 438, 784, 799, 801
calving rates 58
calving value index 9
Campylobacter 204
Campylobacter coli 204
Campylobacter faecalis 427
Campylobacter fetus
(campylobacteriosis) 204,
560–61, 568
abortion 582–4
bovine genital 629, 630–31
bulls 568, 597, 598
Campylobacter hyointestinalis 204
Campylobacter jejuni 204
cancer horn 887
Candida (candidiasis) 933
carbamates 1032
poisoning 940, 944
carbaryl 1032
carbomycin 1032
carbo vegetabilis 1089, 1091
carboxylic acids 1050
carbenicillia 1037, 1040, 1041
carbohydrates *see* water-soluble
carbohydrate (WSC)
carcase conformation 15
cardiomyopathy 174
cardiovascular system, congenital
conditions 173–6
carpal bursitis 461–2
carprofen 246, 1051, 1053, 1056, 1061,
1062
carrots 113, 114, 131
castor oil plant 83, 1162
castration 4, 12, 72, 1063
casts 442–3, 456
cataract 181, 923–4
catarrh *see* malignant catarrhal fever
(MCF)
cattle fly 370
Cattle Health Certificate Standards
(CHeCS) 994
cattle passport 6, 45
cattle plague *see* rinderpest
cattle population 23, 25, 69

cauda equina syndrome 913
caudal vena cava thrombosis 868
Caulophyllum thalyctraides 1082, 1089,
1091
caustic soda 883
caustic treated straw 124
CBG *see* calcium borogluconate
infusion
CBPP *see* contagious bovine
pleuropneumonia
CCN *see* cerebro cortico necrum
CD4 and CD8 T cells 1001–2
cefquinone 288, 393, 394, 427, 1040,
1043
ceftiofur 288, 245, 427, 458, 1041, 1043
cell-mediated immunity 1001–7
cellulitis, tarsal 460–61
cellulolytic bacteria 96
cellulose 96, 112
digestible 80
rumen fermentation 96, 98
cellulosic feeds 112
cell wall digestion 96, 101
central European encephalitis 770
cephacetrinine 393
cephalexin 395, 1036, 1037, 1038, 1041,
1043
cephalonium 393, 402, 1038
cephaloridine 1031, 1037, 1038, 1040,
1041, 1043
cephapirin 393
cephalothin 392, 1036–8, 1040–41
Ceratapogonidae 745, 767
cereal beef 14, 19
cereal crimping 118
cereal processing 118
cereal rolling 118
cereals 112, 114
cerebellar abiotrophy 178, 903
cerebellar ataxia, inherited 178
cerebellar hypoplasia/hydranencephaly
178, 900–901
cerebellar syndrome 896
cerebral syndrome 895–6
cerebrocortical necrosis (CCN) 157,
261–3, 903–4
cerebrospinal fluid (CSF) 890–91,
896–7
cervical vertebrae, injury 145
cervicitis 559
cervix
contraction 508
rupture 151
stretch receptors 475
cestodes 280–82, 1028–9
cetaperoxase 394, 1038
CGI *see* cow genetic index
Chabertia spp 1026
Charolais breed 6, 7, 8, 9, 30, 1172
arthrogryposis 6, 9, 14, 15, 19, 20, 21,
163, 177
Charolais x Friesians beef 21
CHeCS 994
cheese production 26
Chlamydia 561
Chlamydophila abortus 586

chloramphenicol 217, 245, 250, 252, 288,
851, 861, 1036, 1037, 1038,
1040–43
chlorinated hydrocarbons 1020
chlorine 33
chlorpyriphos 1032
chlortetracycline 753, 762, 1036, 1037,
1040, 1041, 1043
choke 139, 826–8
cholecystitis 148
Chorioptes spp 742, 881, 882, 1023,
1031, 1032
chromosomal abnormalities 163–4, 577
chromosomal translocations 184
chopping feeds 117
chronic pneumonia 239–48
Chrysanthemum 1032
Chrysomyia 747
Chrysops spp 762
CIDR 1179
cimaterol 1073, 1074
Cinchona bark 1082
ciprofoxacin 393
cirrhosis 148
Citrobacter spp 327, 334
citrus pulp 112, 113, 114
clamp silo 41–2
clauvlanic acid 245, 393, 396, 398, 1040,
1043
claw
amputation 1119–22
conditions 409–32, 888
size disparity 415
cleansing 977
cleft palate 177
clenbuterol 1073, 1074, 1075
clindamycin 427, 1037, 1041
clinical case approach/examination
136–8
clioxinide 1024
cloning 170, 648
clorsulon 1020, 1025, 1026, 1028
closantanel 1024, 1026, 1028, 1031
closed herds 990
clostridial infections 152, 719–25
bacillary haemoglobinuria 719–21
black disease 729–31
infectious necrotic hepatitis 729–31
myositis 723–5
vaccination 722, 724, 734, 1005
see also blackleg; botulism; tetanus
Clostridium botulinum 721–3
Clostridium chauveoi 723–5
Clostridium haemolyticum 719–21
Clostridium novyi type B 723–5, 729–31
Clostridium novyi type D 719–21
Clostridium perfringens 724
Clostridium septicum 723–4
Clostridium sordelli 725
Clostridium sporogenes 261
Clostridium tetani 723–4, 729–31
clover 12, 33, 34, 102, 116, 123, 127–8
cloxacillin 392–4, 1040–41
CMT *see* California Milk Test
coagulase-negative staphylococci *see*
staphylococci, coagulase-negative

cobalt 815
  deficiency 296–8, 794
  disorders 295–8, 810, 1029
  supplementation 72
coccidiosis 282–3, 1030, 1069
coffee grounds 112
cold cow syndrome 836–7
cold stress 930, 975
cold water ingestion 147
colic 139–40, 238, 845–9
  tympanic intestinal 141, 846
coliform bacteria 334, 347
colistin 1037, 1040, 1041, 1043
collagenase 518
colobomata 181, 924
colon torsion 141
colocynthis 1084
colostrum 3, 193, 203, 211–12, 247,
    958–9
  calcium requirement 782
  immune components 999, 1002–3
  rotavirus protection 193
  vitamin A 256
Common Agricultural Policy (CAP)
    23–4
compartment syndrome 439
compensatory growth 17, 71, 79
complement 323, 381, 997, 1046–7
complementary medicine see alternative
    medicine
complete diets see total mixed rations
composite breeds 9
computer records 44
concentrates 103, 119, 124, 130
  dairy cows 30, 31, 32–3, 37, 51, 121, 124
  dairy heifers 56, 58
  early weaning 4, 5
  eighteen-month beef 20
  energy fraction 374
  feeding systems 14, 18, 20, 33, 38, 119,
    120, 376–7
  fermentation in rumen 98
  intake 100–101
  metabolizable energy 810
  suckler calves 11, 12, 17
  suckler cows 12
  tropical cattle 70, 78
  winter finishing beef 17
conception failure 552–73, 1091
  aetiology 554–63
  diagnosis 563–6
  manifestation 552–4
  prevention 572–3
  prognosis 569–72
  treatment 566–9
  see also infertility
conception vessel 1096
conceptus 499–500
  disease 561, 577–8
condensed milk production 26
condition scoring see body
    condition/condition scoring
conformation, lameness 425
congenital conditions 173–84
  alimentary tract 177
  arthrogryposis 462

blood disorders 175
body cavity 182
cardiovascular system 173–6
lymphatic system 177
muscular system 177–8
nervous system 178–80
ocular 180–81
reproductive system 182–4
skeletal defects 175–7
skin defects 181–2, 888
urinary system 184
Congo virus 772
conjunctival diseases 919–22
connecting points (acupuncture) 1095
constipation 142, 148–9, 1091
contagious bovine pleuropneumonia
    (CBPP) 629, 631, 868–74
  vaccination 873, 1011
contagious bovine pyelonephritis
    725–6
contamination by injection 1079
contracted flexor tendons 451–2
contracted tendons 462
controlled breeding see oestrous
    synchronization
controlled internal drug release (CIDR)
    567, 659–60, 681
convulsions 1091
convulsions, familial 178–9
convulsive syndromes 155–7
cooling 1173
  ambient air temperature reduction
    91–2
  evaporative/non-evaporative 89
cooling pads 92
cooling ponds 93
cooling systems 90–93, 1173
cooperative societies 76
Cooperia (cooperiosis) 269, 1026
copper
  biochemical indices 296
  calcium edetate 255
  disorders 150, 298–300, 462
  metabolic profile 814
  methlonine complex 255, 300
  oxyquinoline sulphate 255, 300
  naphthenate 880
  sulphate 255, 462
  supplementation 63, 300, 721
  toxicity 147, 155, 255, 300, 814, 948–9
copper deficiency 150, 254–5, 260,
    298–300, 888, 949
  abomasal ulceration 844
  New Zealand 1179–80
  physeal dysplasia 465
copper ethylene diamine 300
copper glycine 300
copper tetra-acetic acid 300
copra expellar 113
cording see jugular stasis
coriosis 63, 145, 150, 417–19, 420–21
  control 421–5
corium 413
corn see maize
corn oil 834
corn steep liquor 113, 114

corneal diseases 919–22
coronavirus, bovine (BVC) 189, 195,
    199–200, 207, 208, 218
corpus cavernosum penis rupture
    614–15
corpus luteum 492, 493–8, 539
  conceptus role 500
  cyst diagnosis 539
  persistence 524, 534
  uterine involution 504
Corridor disease 754–5
Corriparta virus 772
corticosteroids 245, 288, 290, 292, 398,
    461, 795, 802, 862, 866, 884, 885,
    1049, 1056–60
  neurological disorders 899
  parturition induction 687
  pneumonia 244–5
cortisol 1048, 1049, 1057
cortisone 245, 1049, 1057
Corynebacterium bovis 327, 335, 347
Corynebacterium renale 725–6
cotton cake 113
cotton seed 78, 80, 112, 113
coumaphos 774, 880, 1032
coumarin 1087
cow genetic index (CGI) 48
cow tracks 423–4
Cowdria (cowdriosis) 765–6
Cowdria rumination 765
cowpox 365–6, 371, 888
COX (cyclo-oxygenases) 1048, 1051,
    1054, 1055, 1058
COX inhibitors 1048, 1049, 1051,
    1055
CP see crude protein
cranial nerve paralysis 139, 150
cream production 26
creep feeding of suckler calves 11
Creutzfeldt–Jakob disease, new variant
    1152, 1153
Crohn's disease 1153
crop residues 75
cross-breeding 9, 169
crude protein (CP) 31, 32, 73, 78, 80,
    106–7, 117
  recommended dietary concentration
    111, 112
  tropical cattle feeding 73, 78
crufomate 741
cryptococcosis 932–3
cryptorchidism 163, 164, 182–3
Cryptosporidium parvum
    (cryptosporidiosis) 189, 191, 194,
    195, 204–6, 207, 208, 218, 1029,
    1030
Crysops spp 745
cubicles 40–41, 42, 63, 66
  design 41, 331, 421–2
  training heifers 63
cuffing pneumonia 239, 248
Culex spp 745
Culicoides spp 745, 769
culling
  calving season control 656
  dairy cattle 47–8, 665, 671

mastitis control 335, 336
rate 543, 553, 665, 671
selective 481
cutaneous leukosis 698–9, 700
cyclic AMP 185, 187, 203
cyclo-oxygenase (COX) 1048, 1051,
1054, 1055, 1058
isoenzymes 1054
cyclo-oxygenase (COX) inhibitors
1048–9, 1051, 1055
cyclopia 918
cypermethrin 744, 1032, 1081
cystic ovarian disease 521, 526, 542,
554–7
diagnosis 564
prognosis 570–71
treatment 567
cysts *see* follicle, cysts
Cytocoetes ondiri 763–5
Cytocoetes phagocytophilia 586, 763
cytokines 382, 479, 1047
cytotoxic agents 1049

D valve *see* digestibility valve
daily live weight gain *see* live weight
gain
dairy beef systems 18–21
dairy cattle
beefing characteristics 28–9
bulls 48–9
culling 47–8, 665, 671
heat stress 88–93
herd fertility management 662–75
lameness 41
records 44–7, 50, 667–8, 672–3, 674
service success rate 670–71
veterinary visits 668–9
dairy cows
age at first calving 48
anoestrus 533–4
appetite 32, 33
breed of sire 48
bull use 595
calving interval 49, 665–6
calving season 665, 667
calving seasonality 52
feed budgets 121, 122
feeding 25, 30–33, 37, 41, 1151
fertility 49, 662–75
control programme 665–7
first service 666–7
fodder beet 124
forage crops 35–6
genetic worth of sire 48–9
health 49–50
housing 38, 40–41
identification 44, 667
intensive production 76
interservice intervals 671
kale 126
longevity 169
magnesium supplementation 64
maize silage 124
metabolic disease 168
parity effect on performance 59
pregnancy diagnosis 671

rations 123, 124, 131
root crops 125
rye 129
selection 169
semi-intensive production 76
stocking density 34, 35
tropical management 77–8
water requirement 38
welfare 960–62
winter feeding systems 37–8
dairy farming 22–53
Australia 1182
breeding 25, 47–9
breeds 25, 27–30
buildings 38–44
economics 50–52
efficiency measures 50–52
European trends 1151–2
farm assurance 52
grassland management 33–6
herd health schemes 52
herd replacements 59
herd size 24, 25
labour 47
management 25
milk purchase 25–6
milk utilization 26–7
New Zealand 1177
North America 1183–7
organic 52
overhead costs 52
public perceptions 955
Saudi Arabia 1172–6
UK structure 24–6
dairy heifers
age at calving 48, 54, 55
AI 59, 61–2
beef sire use 665
body condition 58–9, 63
breeding
controlled 61–2
policy 59
records 671–2
calf mortality 64, 66
calving time 55
competition effect on first lactation
65–6
cubicle training 63
dystokia 59, 60, 61, 63, 66
feeding 56, 58–9, 62
supplementary 58, 59
feedlots 78
female semen insemination 61
fertility 58–9, 61–2
control programme 665
fly prevention 63
fodder beet 125
forage 123
genetic merit accumulation 60
grazing systems 57–8
growth rate 54, 55, 56, 65, 123
optimum 56–7
pregnancy 62–3
growth targets 65
housing 55–6, 58
iodine deficiency 63–4

life expectancy 55
longevity 60–61
magnesium supplementation 64
maize silage 124
mammary growth 56–7
management
at calving 64, 65
first lactation 65–6
prior to calving 64
maximization of potential 54–5
milk yields 55, 56–7, 59, 63
minerals 63–4
pregnancy
growth rate 62–3
rate 61–2
production 48
puberty onset 481
rearing management 54–66
3–6 months 55–6
6–12 months 56–8
12–15 months 58–9
15–18 months 62
18–22 months 62
22–24 months 62–4
replacements 59, 60–61
Shorthorn 9, 28, 30
sire selection 59, 60–61
stocking rate 55, 58
stress 59, 63
survival rates 66
synchronized breeding 59, 61–2
trace elements 63–4
weighing 58
dairy ranching 75–6
dairy unit layout 39
Damalinia bovis 741, 880, 1031, 1032
Danish Red 459
danofloxacin 233, 245, 283, 1040–42
DCAB (dietary cationic anionic
balance) 787, 422
DCP *see* digestible crude protein
DDT 745, 746, 747
death, sudden 152–3
decoquinate 1030
deerflies 745–6, 762
degenerative arthritis 434–5, 458
degenerative joint disease (DJD) *see*
degenerative arthritis
dehorning 4, 1124–6
delactosed whey syrup 113, 114
deltamethrin 1031, 1032
Demodex spp 743, 881, 882
dentition 825
deoxycorticosterone acetate (DOCA)
1056
depopulation of buildings/sites 971–2,
977
Dermacentor spp 103, 744, 762, 775
dermatitis 886–7
digital 427–8, 430–31
interdigital 429
dermatophilosis 886–7
Dermatophilus congolensis 429, 886
dermatophytosis 878–80
dermoid formation 919
Devon 8

dexamethasone 245, 288, 795, 1049, 1056, 1057, 1059
Dexter cattle 162, 175
dextrose 831
diabetes mellitus 930
diagnosis 135–57
  clinical case approach 136–8
  description 137
  differential lists of syndromes 136
  history taking 136–7
  laboratory investigations 138
  preliminary inspection/examination 137
  presenting syndromes 138–57
  systematic examination 137–8
diaphragm
  defects 182
  hernia 145, 147, 848–9
diarrhoea 149–50, 850–53, 854, 855–8
acute 149
  calf 185–213
  causative mechanisms 185–8
  chronic peri-weaning 237–8
  effects 189–91
  epidemiology 206–7
  herd 149–50
  infectious agents 191–208
  intravenous fluid therapy 195–7
  investigation 206
  management 195–9, 200, 209–10
  mixed infections 207–8
  necrotic enteritis 213, 238
  oral rehydration 197–8
  osmotic 189
  secretory 188–9
  types 188–9
  see also bovine virus diarrhoea (BVD); scour/scouring
diazinon 743, 880, 881, 1032
dichloros 1032
Dicholobacter nodosus 425, 427
Dicrocoelium dendriticum 1026
Dictyocaulus viviparus 86, 239, 272–3, 1021, 1023, 1026, 1125
  vaccine 274, 1011, 1027
dietary cationic-anionic balance (DCAD) 787
diet, complete see total mixed rotations
diet formulation 120–21
  see also total mixed rations (TMR)
diethylamide copper oxyquinoline sulphonate 255
diethyl carbamzine citrate 1024, 1026, 1027
diffuse fibrosing alveolitis 865–6
digestibility of forages 101
digestibility valve 126
digestible crude protein (DCP) 31, 32, 71, 106–7, 108, 112, 123–31
digestible fibre 374
digestible undegraded protein (DUP) 109, 110, 113, 813
digestion optimization 99–100
digestion, speed of 101
digestive disorders in calves 231–8
digitalis 1086

digits
  amputation 1119–22
  dermatitis 427–8, 430–31, 888
dihydrostreptomycin 40, 72, 73, 245, 393, 394, 395, 400, 729, 735, 736, 849, 1036, 1037, 1039, 1040, 1043
1,25-dihydroxycholecalciferol 782
dimethyl phthalate 745, 746
dimethyl sulphoxide (DMSO) 261, 899–900, 1049
dimethyl tolomide 746
dimethicone 834
diminazene acetrate 760, 761, 1029
diphenoxyalkyl ethers 1020
diphtheria, calf 139, 250, 822, 1087
diprophylline 246
dipyrone 846
diseases
  Africa 1156–62
  biosecurity 987, 988
  endemic 989
  epizootic 1156–7
  genetics 168–9
  milk quality 377–8
  monitoring 1185
  notifiable 989
  patterns 136
  resistance 167–8
  statutory control/eradication 987
  susceptibility 975–7
  tropical cattle 70–71, 78
  see also infections/infectious disease; parasitic infections
disinfectants, chemical 977–80
disinfection/disinfection procedures 977–82
dislocations 447–51
distillers dark grains 112, 113, 114
dithiosemicarbazone 762, 764, 765
DJD see degenerative arthritis
DM see dry matter
DMI see dry matter intake
DNA analysis 165
DOCA (deoxycorticosterone acetate) 1056
doramectin 741–3, 747, 748, 1022, 1025, 1026, 1027, 1031
downer cow syndrome 151, 438, 439–41, 797–801
  hip dislocation 448
  hypophosphataemia 814
  learned helplessness 1146
  milk fever differential diagnosis 784
  muscle injuries 451
doxycycline 1036, 1037, 1040, 1041
draught cattle 68, 69, 74
dried grass 113, 114
dried Lucerne 113, 114
drooling 138–9
drought, tropical cattle 80
drug costs 83–4
dry cows, metabolic profiles 806, 810–11
dry cow therapy 399–402, 1044
dry matter (DM) in feeds 73, 113, 114, 117, 123, 124, 131

dry matter intake (DMI) 30–31, 32, 33, 37, 73, 100, 103, 123, 125
  enhancers 123
ductus arteriosus, patent 174
Dughe virus 772
dusty feed rhinotracheitis 860
DUP see digestable undegradable protein
dysentery, winter 852–3
dyspnoea 139, 155
dystokia 8, 9–10, 64, 121, 151, 1082, 1091, 1179
  avoidance 526–7, 545, 665
  dairy heifers 59, 60, 61, 63, 66
    management at calving 64, 65
  downer cow syndrome 439, 797–801
  endometritis 521
  flexor tendon contracture 452
  growth plate injuries 444–5
  magnesium supplementation 64
  ovarian cystic disease 556
  recto-vaginal fistula 859
  sire choice 59, 60, 61
  vertebral fractures 445–6

ear tags 6, 44
East coast fever (ECF) 77, 750–56, 1029, 1030, 1158, 1060
  vaccination 753
easy calving breeds 8, 9
EBL (enzootic bovine leukotis) 629, 630, 693–9, 700, 1079
  vaccination 753
EBV (estimated breeding value) 89, 658
East Coast fever 77, 750–56, 1029, 1030, 1158, 1160–61
Echinococcus granulosus 281–2, 1026, 1028
eclampsia 781–7
economic beef farming, 16
economic dairy farming 50–52
economic loss with genetic disease 162
ectoparasites 740–48, 992, 1030–33
  see also flies; lice; mites; ticks
ectopia cordis 173
ectopia lentis 923
eczema, facial 1180
effective rumen degradable protein (ERDP) 31, 108, 109, 110, 113
  feeds 113
  metabolizable energy 812–13
  suckler cows 816
egg transport interference 557, 567
Ehrlichia ondiri 763–5
Ehrlichia phagocyptophilia 586, 763
eicoasanoids 1047, 1048, 1050, 1056
Eimeria (coccidiosis) 282–3, 1029–30
Eizenmenger's syndrome 174
ejaculate 487, 488, 604–7
ejaculation failure 616–17
electrical currents, stray voltage 931
electrocution 152, 930–31
electrolyte solution 3, 852
electronic tagging 44
emaciation 150–51

embryo transfer 30, 48, 49, 570, 634–48
  advanced technologies 646–8
  closed herds 990
  disease control 644
  donors 637, 638, 640
  genetic defects 166
  hormone supplementation 645
  insemination 639–41
  legislation 645–6
  nutrition 638, 644
  procedures 634–7, 640, 641–8
  recipients 637–8, 644
embryonic death 559–62, 568–9, 577
emesis *see* vomiting
encephalitis 892, 895
  listerial 904–6
  tick-borne 770–71
encephalomyelitis 892, 895
  sporadic bovine 911–12
endectocides 1020
endocarditis
  bacterial 144, 726–8
  chronic vegetative 153–4
endocrine signal surges 476, 477
endometrial biopsy 512
endometritis 291, 500, 521–4, 569
  diagnosis 564
  embryonic death 560–61
  prognosis 571–2
  treatment 1063
endothelial dystrophy 922
endothelin 1 (ET-1) 496
endotoxaemia 1063
endotoxic shock 1052, 1059
endotoxins 561
energy
  feed levels 10, 11, 13, 31, 33, 104,
    112–13
    feed portionings 104
  requirements 33, 103–6, 657
  see also metabolizable energy (ME)
energy balance
  metabolic disease 1154
  metabolic profiles 807–11
  negative postpartum 525, 526, 801
  reproduction 477–8, 502–3
energy (Qi) flow 1093–4, 1095, 1096
enilconozole 879
enolic acids 1050
enrofloxacin 245, 248, 1040, 1041,
  1043
enteritis
  acute 140
  necrotic 213, 238
Enterobacter spp 327, 334, 391, 398
environment
  calf diarrhoea 210–13
  heat gain 89
  normality 135
  pneumonia 240–42
  see also humidity, environmental
environmental requirements of cattle
  974–5
environmental stress 70, 78, 1003
  embryonic death 559–60, 562
  tropical cattle 70, 78

enzootic bovine leukosis 629, 630,
  693–9, 700, 1079
enzootic haematuria 154, 946
enzootic hepatitis *see* rift valley fever
enzootic pneumonia 239–48
eosinophils 1045
ephemeral fever 741–3, 747, 1182
epididymis 487, 622
epididymitis 620–21
epilepsy, idiopathic 179
epitheliogenesis imperfecta 181
eprinomectin 1022, 1023, 1025, 1026,
  1027, 1031
ERDP *see* effective rumen degradable
  protein
erysipelas 1014–15
Erysipelothrix insidiosa 249, 455,
  1015–16
erythromycin 245, 286, 392, 393, 395,
  396, 428, 1036, 1037, 1041, 1042
Escherichia coli 4, 201–4, 249, 251, 455,
  457, 463, 725, 823, 901
  enterohaemorrhagic (EHEC) 189,
    191, 201, 204, 206, 208, 210
  enterotoxigenic (ETEC) 191, 198,
    201, 202–4, 206, 207, 208, 210
  immune response 383–4
  K99 antigens 1006
  mastitis 326, 327, 328, 334, 343, 383,
    384, 391, 392, 394, 396, 398
  verocytotoxin (VTEC) 201–2, 204,
    206, 210
essential oils 1102
estimated breeding value (EBV) 8, 9,
  658
etamiphylline camsylate 246
ethnoveterinary medicine 83–6
Eucalyptus grandis 84
Europe/European Union
  beef regime 15
  Common Agricultural Policy (CAP)
    23–4
  dairy farming trends 1151–2
  infectious diseases 1152–5
  milk production 22–4
  organic farming 52
  rabies 1165
evaporative cooling pads 92
evasive grazing strategy 1026
examination of animals 137–8
excrement disposal 42–4, 976, 986
exophthalmus with strabismus 181
extensive milk production 75, 79
eye
  enucleation 1126–7
  infections 63
  see also infectious bovine
    keratoconjunctivitis (IBKC);
    infectious bovine rhinotracheitis
    (IBR); ocular diseases
eyelid anomalies 918–19

F41 antigen 202
face abnormalities 176
facial eczema 1180
face fly 746, 1031

factor XI deficiency 175
faeces, bovine 334
famphur 1031
fan systems 92–3
FARAD 1040
farcy, bovine 885–6
farm assurance 38, 52
farm operations 962–3
farm size 971
farmer's lung, bovine 729, 821, 860,
  861–2, 1021, 1024, 1025, 1026
Fasciola (fasciolosis) 148, 150, 151,
  276–8, 1028
  Fasciola hepatica see fasciolosis
  Fasciola gigantas see fasciolosis
  Fascioloides magna see fasciolosis
fat 112
fat class (carcass) 14, 15
fat cow syndrome 151, 801–2
fat mobilization 801–2
fat necrosis 849
fats, dietary 375–6
  rumen fermentation 96
fattening, tropical beef production 81
fatty acids, free *see* non-esterified fatty
  acids (NEFA)
fatty liver syndrome 148, 801–2, 1154
febantel 1020, 1021, 1025, 1026, 1027
feed(s)
  alkali treated 117–18
  beef cattle 121
  budgets 121, 122
  cellulosic 112
  chopping 117
  classification 113
  composition 112–14
  constituents 373–5
  dry matter (DM) 113, 114
  drying 114
  dusty 866
  energy 104, 112–13
  ensiling 114–17
  ERDP 113
  FME 113
  intake 100–103, 120
  ME 113
  minerals 112–13
  non-cellulosic 112
  physical form 113–14
  preservation 114–17
  processing 117–18
  protein 112–13
  storage 38, 41–2
feeders, computerized out-of-parlour
  38, 119–20
feeding 118–22
  beef cattle 121
  buffer 119, 130, 377, 791
  changes and metabolic profiles 805
  complete diet 38
  dairy cows 25, 30–33, 37–8, 41, 121,
    124, 1151
  dairy heifers 56, 58–9, 62
  diet formulation 120–21
  flat rate 120
  food wagon 958

feeding (cont'd)
  frequency 119
  housed cattle 957
  machine 5
  metabolic disease 1153–5
  milk 11, 70
  milk composition 373–7
  selective 118
  strategies 32–3
  suckler cows 121
  systems 376–7
  tropical cattle 78
  winter 37–8
  see also nutrition
feeding barrier 38
feedlots, tropical cattle 80
femoral fractures 444
femoral nerve paralysis 437
femorotibial luxation/subluxation
    449–50
femur fractures 444, 445
fenbendazole 1020, 1021, 1025, 1026,
    1027
fenitrothion 1032
fenoterol 1073
fenthion 877, 1031
fenvalerate 1031, 1032
fermentable metabolizable energy
    (FME) 108, 113, 812–13
fermentation
  rumen 95, 96–100
  silage 114–17
fertility 572
  control programme 49, 50, 664–72
  dairy cows 49
  dairy heifers 58–9, 61–2, 530, 543,
    545
  heat stress 935
  herd management 49, 50, 652–75
    beef herds 652–62
    dairy herds 49, 50, 662–75
  herd problem 565–6
  monitoring 49, 50, 652–75, 1185–6
  nutrition 534
  pyometra 525
  retained fetal membranes 518–19
  see also infertility
fertilization failure 557–9, 567
fertilizers 34, 35, 42, 62
  see also nitrogen fertilizers
fetal death 524, 577–89
  examination 587, 589
  pathophysiology 577–8
  see also abortion
fetal membranes, retained 515–19, 1090,
    1091
  ecbolic drugs 517–18
  endometritis 522
  intrauterine antibiotics 518
  manual removal 516–17
fetlock joint 452
  subluxation 450–51
fever 151–2, 1091
fibre, dietary 97, 99
fibroblast 1046
fibrosing alveolitis, diffuse 860–61

field beans 113
fighting, beef cattle 960
financial records 47
finishing systems see beef finishing
    systems
firing 83
first calving age 48, 54, 55, 62, 63, 72
fish meal 96
'flabby bag' 735–7
flavivirus infections 770–71
flavomycin 1070
flexor tendons 451–3
flies 745–8, 768, 774, 775
  control 337–8, 370
  prevention 63
  see also tsetse flies
floor surfaces 423–4
flor de piedra 1086
floroquinolones 198, 245, 250, 393, 394,
    1036, 1038, 1040, 1041, 1043
florfenicol 245, 250, 288, 737, 1036, 1038,
    1040, 1041, 1043
flubenzdron 1031
fluid therapy 195–7, 209, 210, 398
flumethasone 245, 795, 1057
flumethrin 743, 1032
flunixin 246, 399, 867, 1051, 1053, 1056,
    1061, 1063
fluorosis 821, 949–50
fly traps 746
FMP see fermentable metabolizable
    energy
fodder banks 75
fodder beet 36, 124–5
  poisoning 151
fog fever 152, 866–7
foggers, high pressure 92
follicle
  cysts 555, 556, 566–7
  development 488–92, 502
  first dominant 502–3, 510, 512
follicle-stimulating hormone (FSH)
    473, 477
  oestrous cycle 489, 490, 491, 492, 493,
    494
  postpartum 509–10
  receptor binding 476
  Sertoli cell response 482, 484, 486
  superovulation 634, 638, 639
foma 776
food animal residue avoidance data
    (FARAD) 1042
food industry by-products 96, 131
food safety 1151–2
foot
  bones/bone disorders 413, 429–30
  claw size disparity 415
  deep infections 430
  dressings 431–2
  fissures 421, 425–6
  hardship lines 415, 421, 426
  lameness 413–32
  negative net growth 415
  skin disorders 426–9
  structure 411–13
  trimming 425

  weight-bearing surfaces 413, 414
  see also lameness
foot-and-mouth disease 138, 371,
    700–707, 822, 888, 987, 993, 994,
    1063, 1087, 1175
  Africa 1157
  anti-inflammatory therapy 1063
  biosecurity 988, 994
  congestive heart failure 928
  Europe 1152
  genetic component 168
  milk producers 24–5
  Saudi Arabia 1174–5
  transmission by semen 628, 629
  vaccination 704, 705, 706, 707,
    1016–17, 1175
footbaths 430–31
footblocks 432
foot rot 426–7
forage
  alternative 123–31
  beef finishing systems 14
  chopping 117
  conservation 35, 36, 95–6
  conserved for suckler calves 11
  crops for dairy cows 35–6
  digestibility 101
  energy contribution 809–10
  feeding 376
  intake 103
  maize 36, 123, 124
foramen ovale, patent 174
foreign bodies 139, 143, 425
  see also reticulitis/reticuloperitonitis
formaldehyde 880, 883
formulation, diet 120–21
foul foot 426–7, 737, 1041
fractures 441–7
  femoral 444
  first aid 442
  growth plate 444
  humeral 444
  jaw 824
  long bone 442–5
  pelvic 446–7
  tibial 444
    external fixation 442–4
    internal fixation 444–5
  open 443–4
  radiography 442–3
  vertebral 445–6
framycetin 392, 393, 851, 1036–41
freemartins 183–4, 545
free radical scavengers 1049
freeze branding 44
Friesian cattle 8, 9, 25, 27, 28, 29, 30,
    117, 458, 459, 1177
frenulum, persistent 615
fucidin 1036
Fulani cattle 74, 81
fungi
  mycotic infections 586, 823, 861–2,
    878–80, 932–4
  mycotoxins 117, 1180
  rumen fermentation 96
furazolidone 392, 1038, 1040

furazolidone poisoning 260–61
Fusobacterium necrophorum 148, 240, 241, 249, 250, 385, 426, 455, 737, 822, 823, 868, 888

GABA (γ-aminobutryic acid) 1023, 1024, 1032
galactopoiesis 320–21
gall bladder meridian (acupuncture) 1100
Galloway 9
Galloway tibial hemimelia 162, 176
gametes, aged 561
gametogenesis 481, 482
gamma benzene hydrochloride 880, 1031
gammexane poisoning 157
gas gangrene 152
gas intoxication 985–6
gastroenteritis, parasitic 70, 267–72, 1025–7
GE *see* gross energy
generation interval 665
genes
    deleterious major 161–2
    dominant 162, 164
    exhibiting good and bad effects 164–5
    frequency 164
    infertility 167
    penetrance 162, 164
    polygenic deleterious 166–7
    recessive 163, 164
    resistance 167–8
    semidominant 162–3
    sex-limited 163
    sex-linked 163
    susceptibility 167–8
genetic control 164–5
genetic counselling 166
genetic defects 166
genetic diseases 161–2, 165–6
genetic epidemiology 162, 164–5
genetic index, cow (CGI) 48
genetic merit 48
genetic polymorphism 163
genetics, clinical 161–71
genital tract
    haemorrhage/lacerations 513–14
    postpartum lesions 513–26
genomics 170–71
gentamicin 250, 392, 393, 395, 458, 851, 1036–8, 1040, 1041
gentian 456, 829
Germiston virus 772
gestation *see* pregnancy
glaucoma 925
globe anomalies 917–18
globidiosis 756
globulins, metabolic profile 813
Glossina spp 747, 756–61
glucocorticoids 398, 802, 1056–60, 1137, 1138, 1144–5
    stress counter-regulation 1141, 1142
glucose 795, 802
    blood 808, 810
    metabolic profiles 808

glutathione peroxidases 302, 303, 304, 814–15
glycerol 802
goitre, congenital 184, 302, 303
gonadotrophin-releasing hormone (GnRH) 473
    anoestrus treatment 526, 541–2, 543–4
    breeding synchronization 62
    embryo transfer 645
    exogenous 497
    follicular cyst treatment 567
    luteolysis induction 680
    oestrous cycle 489, 492
    ovulation induction 657, 658
    post-insemination treatment 569
    postpartum 502
    pregnancy establishment 685–6
    prostaglandin combination techniques 683
    pulse generator 480, 481, 492, 497
    pulses 477, 480, 497
    receptor binding 476
    receptors 477
    routine administration 546
    stress 1143–4
gonitis, idiopathic 45, 81
Governor vessel 1096
grain impaction 141
grain overload *see* acidosis
grains, moist 117
grass 101, 102, 112
    beef 20
    conserved 123
    digestibility 101
    feeding 32
    growth 35
    hay 78
    seed mixtures 33
    smallholder dairying in Kenya 76
    sward height 12, 18, 62, 118, 119
    tropical production 73–4
grass, finishing of beef cattle 17–18, 20–21
grass silage, bull beef 19
grass staggers *see* hypomagnesaemia
grass tetany *see* hypomagnesaemia
grassland
    conservation 11, 35, 36, 95–6
    ensiling 114–17
    management 12–13, 33–6, 73–4
    nitrogen fertilizers 33, 34–5
    production 33–5, 73
    utilization 35–6
grazing
    continuous 35, 58, 119
    crop residues 75
    dairy heifers 57–8, 64
    eighteen-month beef 20
    food intake 101–2
    grass finishing systems 17–18, 21
    kale 126
    leader–follower system 58
    root crops 125
    rotational 35, 58, 74, 119
    rye 129

stocking for 121
suckler cows 121
sward 33–4, 119
tropical cattle 72
white clover 128
zero 76, 77, 129
griseofulvin 879, 1036
gross energy (GE) 104
gross margin 47, 50
groundnut 70, 78, 80, 113
growth, energy requirements 104–5
growth hormone (GH) 57
    see also bovine somatotrophin (BST)
growth monitoring 72
growth plate injuries 444–5, 962, 1073, 1186
growth promoters 1067–75, 1191
    bovine somatotropin 962, 1073
    hormonal implants 1071–3
    in-feed additives 1067–71, 1072
    repartitioning agents 1073–5
growth rates *see* live weight gain
Guernsey cattle 28, 30, 101, 378, 459
Guinea corn 70
gut obstruction 140
gut tie 140
gut worms 267–72, 1025–7

Haemaphysalis spp 744, 749, 762, 775, 1030
Haematobia exigua 747
Haematobia irritans 747, 1031, 1032
Haematopinus spp 741, 888, 1023
Haematopota spp 745
haematuria 154–5
haemoglobinuria 155, 735, 748, 749, 780, 792
    bacillary 155, 719–21
    postparturient 155, 792–3
haemolytic anaemia 720, 735, 748, 749, 792
Haemonchus contortus 84
Haemonchus placei (haemonchosis) 275–6, 1024, 1026
Haemophilus somnus 239, 240, 241, 251, 731, 737, 907, 1010–11
    vaccination 731, 1010, 1011
haemorrhage, acute 152–3, 156, 1091
haemorrhagic septicaemia 632, 728–9
haemorrhagic shock 1059
halofuginone 1029, 1030
haloxon 1024
halquinol 1040, 1041
handling
    facilities 39
    lameness 424
    welfare 963–4
Harana virus 772
hardship lines 415, 421, 426
hare lip 177
hay 4, 35, 56, 78, 103, 112, 114, 119, 123
    additives 117
    buffer feeds 119
    chopping 117
head fly 746, 1031

health of cattle 49–50, 52, 971–2, 1178
  recording schemes 169
heart failure, congestive 928–9
heart meridian (acupuncture) 1100
heartwater 765–6
heat
  gain from environment 89
  loss from body 89, 92–3
  production by body 89
  tolerance 560
heat stress 78, 88–93, 935
  embryonic death 559–60, 562
heel/heel conditions 413, 419, 425
heel/horn erosion 425
heel necrosis 421
heifers 815
  beef 19–20, 661
  oestrous cycle problems 530, 543, 545
  rearing 54–67
  see also dairy heifers
hemicellulose 96
hepar sulphuris 1085, 1089, 1091
hepatic abscess 737
hepatic encephalopathy 156, 892
hepatitis 821
  enzootic 769
  infectious necrotic 729–31
heptenophos 1032
herbage intake 102
herbal medicine 1102
herd fertility management 652–75
  beef cattle 652–62
  control programmes 672–3, 674, 675
  dairy cattle 662–75
herds
  closed 990
  health schemes 52, 381
  incoming animals 991
  purchased stock introduction 990–91
  records 44–7, 511
  size 23, 25
herdsman 47
Hereford breed 8, 10, 30, 59, 1177
  AI bulls 59
  hip dysplasia 173
  osteopetrosis 176
  snorter dwarves 163
Hereford disease
  BVD 178
  see also hypomagnesaemia
Hereford x Friesian 6, 9, 20, 21
heritability estimate 166–7
hermaphroditism 183
herpes mammillitis, bovine 363–4, 888
heterosis 8, 9
hexachlorocyclohexane 1031
hexachlorophene 1024
high genetic merit (HGM) bulls 48
Highland 9
hip joint
  dislocation 447–8
  dysplasia 162, 173, 453–4
Hippobasum equina 747
Hippobasum maculata 747
Hippobasum rufipes 747
histamine 246, 1046, 1047

Histoplasma (histoplasmosis) 934
history taking 136–7
Holstein cattle 27, 62, 101, 175
Holstein x Friesian 6, 15, 16, 19, 20, 21,
    25, 30, 58, 59, 62, 124, 177, 459
homidium bromide 760, 761
homidium chloride 760, 761, 1029
homoeopathy 1081, 1082–91
  acupuncture combination 1102
  application 1085–8
  diagnosis 1096–8
  materia medica 1088
  remedies 1083–4, 1090–91
  treatment 1098–9, 1100, 1101–2
  veterinary application 1084–5
honey, ethnoveterinary use 83
hoof 411–13
  disorders 425–6
  fissures 421, 425–6
  overgrowth 413–15
  trimming 415–17
  wear 424
  wet 423
hoose see husk
hormonal implants 1071–3
hormones/hormone receptors 476–7,
    478
horn 411
horn cancer 887
horn flies 747, 1031, 1032
horse louse flies 747
horseflies 745–6, 762
houseflies 746, 762, 1031
housing 957–60, 972–4
  beef production 960
  calves 3
  controlled environment 972, 973
  dairy cows 37, 38, 40–41, 961
  dairy heifers 55–6, 58
  floor surfaces 423–4, 957–8
  gas dangers 985–6
  group size 972
  kennel accommodation 972, 973–4,
    985
  mastitis 331
  roof insulation 985
  suckler herds 7
  teat trauma prevention 369
  temperature control 975
  tropical calf rearing 70
  ventilation 984–5
HPA see hypothalamic pituary adrenal
  axis
HPG see hypothalamic pituary gonadal
  axis
HPO see hypothalamic pituary ovarian
  axis
HPT see hypothalamic pituary testicular
  axis
human chorionic gonadotrophin (hCG)
    566–7, 645, 685–6
human food chain, biosecurity 987, 988
humerus fractures 444
humidity, environmental 89, 240–41, 976
husk 272–4
hyaloid vessels, persistent 181

Hyalomma spp 744, 751, 753, 761, 762,
    771, 777, 1031
Hyalomma truncatum 776–7
hybrid vigour 8, 9
hydatid cysts 281–2
hydroallantois 1119
hydrocephalus 178
hydrocortisone 245, 1049, 1056, 1057
hydrophobia 1164
hydrops amnion/allantois 142
Hydrotaea irritans (cattle fly; sheep
    headfly) 334, 337–8, 339, 370,
    1031
β-hydroxybutyrate (BHB) 807, 808,
    810, 815
25-hydroxycholecalciferol 782
5-hydroxytryptamine 246, 1046, 1047
hygiene
  mastitis 332, 333, 403
  salmonellosis 227–8
  tropical cattle 78
hyosine butylbromide 264
hyperalgesia 1052
hypericum perforatum 1085, 1086, 1089
hyperpnoea 155
hypersensitivity reactions 1063
hypobiotic larvae 1021
hypocalcaemia 255, 514, 781–7, 814
  see also milk fever
Hypoderma (hypodermatosis) 740–41,
    875–8, 1023, 1031
  Hypoderma bovis see hypodermatosis
  Hypoderma lineatum see
    hypodermatosis
hypogammaglobulinaemia 212
hypoglycaemia 191, 794, 796
hypomagnesaemia 150, 151, 155, 157,
    178, 255–6, 439, 441, 787–91
  breed variation 168
  milk fever differential diagnosis 784
  predisposing factors 814
  suckler cows 816
  sudden death 152
hypomagnesaemic tetany of calves
    255–6
hypophosphataemia 463, 791–3, 814
hypothalamic–pituitary–adrenal (HPA)
    axis 478, 479, 1058, 1059
  stress 1134–5, 1136, 1137, 1139
hypothalamic–pituitary–gonadal (HPG)
    axis 471, 478–9, 489, 490
  stress 1143–4
hypothalamic–pituitary–ovarian (HPO)
    axis 502–3, 521
hypothalamic–pituitary–testicular
    (HPT) axis 484
hypothalamus 471–3, 477, 480, 495, 1045
hypothermia 784–5, 930
hypotrichosis, congenital 181
hypovitaminosis A 924, 925

Ibaraki virus 772
IBR 239, 286, 287, 289–92, 628, 629, 644,
    921, 922, 1007, 1009, 1010, 1153
IBRC 63, 917, 919–21, 1018
IBRI 138

ibuprofen 1051
ichthyosis, congenital 182, 888
identification of cattle 6, 44
IGF *see* insulin-like growth factors
ileum obstruction 140
ill treatment of animals 956–7
imidazothiazoles (group 2-LM)
    1020–22, 1023
imidocarb 749
immune response to pathogens 383–8,
    996
    generation 388
immune system 996–1003
    mastitis 479
    mucosal 388
    stress 1138, 1144–5
immunity
    acquired 996, 998–1001
    cell-mediated 1001–2
    cellular 996, 997–8, 1144–5
    disease susceptibility 977
    enhancement in mammary gland
        379–89
    humoral 388, 996, 997, 998–1001,
        1144–5
    innate 996, 997–8
    maternal 1002–3
    non-specific 321
    passive 3, 977
    specific 323
immunoglobulin(s) 210–12, 997,
        998–1001
    lacteal secretions 380
    mammary secretions 323–4
    specificity 1002–3
immunoglobulin A (IgA) 212, 324, 380,
        997, 1000, 1002
immunoglobulin D (IgD) 1001
immunoglobulin E (IgE) 380,
        1000–1001
immunoglobulin G (IgG) 211, 212, 324,
        380, 997, 999, 1002, 1061
    colostrum 999, 1002
immunoglobulin M (IgM) 324, 380,
        998–9, 1002, 1061
immunosuppression 1059, 1062
Improved Contemporary Comparisons
        (ICC), dairy bulls 47, 48
improvement schemes 168–9
in vitro fertilization (IVF) 647
inanition 784
inborn errors of metabolism 891
inbreeding depression 168–9
index of total economic merit (ITEM)
        48, 49
India, smallholder dairying 76
indigestion 829
    vagal 835–6
infections/infectious disease 1156–7
    abortion 578–86
    bacterial 580–84, 717–37, 895
    beef cattle reproductive performance
        654–5
    biosecurity 987, 988
    causal agent identification 1035–6
    conceptus 561

control in bulls 598
diarrhoea 191–208
differentiating genetic disease 165–6
embryo transfer 644
Europe 1152–5
infertility 560–61
intramammary 382–3
introduced animals 990–91, 992–3, 994
mycotic 586, 861–2, 932–4
neural pathogens 892, 895
routes of transmission 988–9
semen transmission 628, 629, 630–32
stress 1144–5
viral 578–80, 691–714, 767–74
    disinfection 978
    neural pathogens 892
see also abscess; parasitic infections;
        protozoa, infections
infectious bovine keratoconjunctivitis
        (IBKC) 63, 917, 919–21
    vaccination 921, 1018, 1087
infectious bovine penoposthitis 291
infectious bovine rhinotracheitis (IBR)
        239, 240, 241, 286, 287, 289–92
    bovine respiratory disease complex
        1007, 1009
    embryo transfer 644
    Europe 1153
    ocular involvement 921–2
    transmission by semen 628, 629
    vaccination 292, 644, 1010
infectious necrotic hepatitis 729–31
infectious pustular vulvovaginitis (IPV)
        290, 628, 629
infertility
    bulls 594–624
        investigation 598–610
    BVD 855
    genes 167
    infections 560–61, 596–8
    stress 1143–4
    see also conception failure
inflammation 1045–64
    anti-inflammatory drug therapy
        1060–64
    mediators/modulators 1046–8
    see also corticosteroids; non-steroidal
        anti-inflammatory drugs
        (NSAIDs); steroids
influential points (acupuncture) 1099
inheritance, modes of 162–4
inhibin 494
injection damage 1078–80
injection routes 1039
injection sites, intramuscular 1079
insect growth regulators 1033
insulin-like growth factor 1 (IGF-1)
        490–91, 494, 1071
intensification, tropical cattle 80
intensive dairy production (tropics) 76,
        79
interdigital dermatitis 429
interdigital hyperplasia 182
interdigital necrobacillosis 426–7
interdigital skin hyperplasia 429
interferon (IFN) 770, 997, 1052

interferon-τ (IFN-τ) 561
interleukins 1047, 1051
interservice intervals 531–2, 671
    conception failure 552
intestinal motility 187
intestine
    acute tympanitic fermentative colic
        141
    growth promoters 1069–71
    obstruction 140
        acute 845–9
        surgery 1113–15
    prolapse through mesentery 846–7
    Salmonella interactions 221–4
    torsion 846
    tympany 141
intoxication 937–8, 939
    see also poisoning
intra-articular injection 1039
intra-mammary insertion 1039
intra-muscular injection 1039, 1079
intra-peritoneal injection 1039
intra-pleural injection 1039
intra-vaginal devices 541–3, 1179
intravenous fluid therapy 195–7
    puerperal metritis 520
intravenous injection 1039
intussusception 140, 150, 847–8
    surgery 1114–15
iodide potassium 258, 823
iodide sodium 251, 258, 823, 879, 886
iodine
    biochemical indices 296
    deficiency 63–4, 249, 257–8, 301–2
    disorders 301–2
    supplementation 879, 880
    treatment 879, 880
iodism 253, 261, 302
ionophore 98, 1067
ion transport, altered 185–8, 187
Irish Bred Blue Grey 9
iron deficiency 258
iron dextran 258
iron supplementation 258, 721
ischaemic necrosis 797–8, 799, 801
isolation facilities 42, 972
isometamidium chloride 1029
isoprenaline 246, 1073
ITEM *see* index of total economic merit
ivermectin 741–3, 747, 748, 878, 881,
        1022, 1023, 1025, 1027, 1031, 1036
Ixodes spp 747, 749, 762, 763, 775, 1030,
        1031
Ixodidae family 744

Japanese encephalitis 771
jaw 824–5
    swellings 821
Jembrana disease 713, 766–7, 888
Jersey cattle 28, 30, 101, 378
    'loose shoulder' 451
Johne's disease 149, 150, 857–8, 988
    bulls 598
    Europe 1153
    transmission by semen 629, 631–2
    vaccination 1012–13

joint(s)
  contagious bovine pleuropneumonia
    871
  diseases 453–8
    anti-inflammatory therapy 1063
    degenerative 454–5
  hypermobility 178
joint ill 3, 249–50, 455–6, 1091
joint laxity dwarfism syndrome,
  congenital 175–6
Jos virus 772
jugular stasis 153–4

K99 antigens 195, 202, 204, 206, 1006,
  1007
kale 36, 112, 123, 125–6, 131, 792
  poisoning 155
kali chloratum 1086
kanamycin 1036, 1037, 1038, 1040, 1041
Kanwa mineral supplement 80
kennel accommodation 972, 973–4, 985
keratoconjunctivitis 746
  see also infectious bovine
    keratoconjunctivitis (IBKC)
keratogenesis imperfecta 181
ketone bodies 794
ketones 815
ketoprofen 399, 1050, 1051, 1056,
  1061–3
ketosis 150, 151, 156, 793–7
  see also acetonaemia; pregnancy
    toxaemia
kiddling 138, 139
kidney meridian (acupuncture) 1100
kidney worm 274–5
Klebsiella 327, 331, 334, 384–5, 391, 392,
  394, 396, 398
knopvelsiekte (lumpy skin disease)
  768–9, 887
Kodam virus 772
Kokobera virus 772
Kotonkan virus 773
Kowanyama virus 773
Kunjin virus 773
Kyasamar forest fever 770

laboratory examination 138
labour 47
lactamase-β 341–2, 391–2, 396, 397, 1038
lactate, sodium 843
lactation
  antimicrobial therapy for mastitis
    397–9
  calcium requirement 782
  energy requirements 105–6
  first, management 65
  heat stress 89
  manipulation 321
  mastitis 327
  metabolizable protein requirement
    111
  milk quality 377
  physiology 316–21
  transgenic techniques 321
lactation tetany see hypomagnesaemia
lactic acid 96, 114, 115, 117

Lactobacillus planterum 116
lactoferrin 211, 322, 379–80, 1003
lactogenesis 317–18
lactoglobulin 3
lactoperoxidase 211, 322
lactose 187–8, 318
laidlomycin 1057
lambdacyhalothrin 1032
lameness 150, 957–8
  above the foot 435–65
  ankylosing spondylitis 535
  anoestrus 462, 534
  bruised sole 1181
  conformation 425
  control 430–32
  dairy cattle 41, 960–61
  dairy heifers 63
  dislocations 447–51
  foot 409–11, 413–32, 737
  fractures 441–7
  globulin levels 813
  handling 424
  iatrogenic 465
  incidence 409–11
  joint diseases 453–8
  lesions 417–25
  muscle injuries 451
  nerve paralyses 436–9
  neuromuscular diseases 457–60
  New Zealand 1181
  nursing 431
  nutrition 422–3
  osteomalacia 462–3
  osteomyelitis 463–4
  physeal dysplasia 464–5
  prevalence 409–11
  rickets 462–3
  skin diseases 460, 461–2
  soft sole 424
  sole, foreign body penetration 425
  sole ulcer 41, 145, 150, 417–19
  stress 1142–3
  subcutis diseases 460–62
  subluxations 447–51
  tendon injuries 451–3
  treatment 430–32
  white line disease 41, 150, 424, 1181
  see also downer cow syndrome
laminitis 63, 150, 417–19, 420–25
  see also coriosis
Langot 770
large intestine 189
large intestine meridian (acupuncture)
  1100
lascalocid 1067
Lasiohelia spp 745
law of similars 1082, 1087
LDA (left displaced abomasum)
  839–42, 1109–12
lead poisoning 139, 149, 156, 789, 944–5
  hypomagnesaemia differential
    diagnosis 789
  neurological disease 892, 906
learned helplessness 1146
ledum 1085, 1091
legumes 74, 78, 80, 101, 102

legume seeds 112, 114
lens diseases 923–4
lentivirus 713
Leptospira (leptospirosis) 329, 335,
  580–81, 589, 734–5, 787, 990, 992
  bacillary haemoglobinuria differential
    diagnosis 720
  cooling ponds 93
  embryo transfer 644
  mastitis 329, 335
  transmission by semen 629, 631
  vaccination 581, 644, 736–7, 1015–16
Leptospira borgpetersenii serovar hardjo
  735–7
Leptospira hardjo (flabby bag) 735–7
Leptospira icterohaemorrhagiae 155
Leptospira interrogans serovar hardjo
  735–7
leukotrienes 1046, 1047, 1048
levamisole 1021, 1022, 1024, 1026, 1027
Leydig cells 485, 620
lice 741–2, 880–81, 1031, 1032
  biting 1031, 1032
  calves 3
  milk quality 378
  sucking 258, 1031, 1032
licking mania 139, 156
lightning strike 152, 789, 930–31
limb defects 176
Limousin breed 8, 30, 1177
Limousin x Friesian, beef finishing 19,
  20, 21
lincomycil 392, 393, 428, 1036, 1038,
  1040, 1041, 1043
Lincoln Red 8
lindane 1031
line breeding 165
liniosamides 393, 395
Linognathus spp 741, 880, 1023, 1031
linseed meal 113
linseed oil 834, 835
linseed poisoning 157
lipomatosis 849
lipopolysaccharide 383–4
lipoxin 1047, 1048
lipoxygenase (LO) 1048
lipoxygenase (LO) inhibitors 1048–9
liquid paraffin 845
Listeria monocytogenes (listeriosis) 156,
  251, 581–2, 789, 896, 900
  encephalitis 904–6
  hypomagnesaemia differential
    diagnosis 789
  uveitis 923, 1060
lithium antimony thiomalate 883
litter disposal 976
liver
  abscess 148, 150, 832, 868
  cholecystitis 148
  cirrhosis 148
  diagnosis of problems 147–8
  encephalopathy 156
  fatty 148, 801, 802, 1154
  foreign body penetration 146
  necrosis 148
  neoplasia 148

painful conditions 144
tuberculosis 148
see also fatty liver syndrome
liver fluke 148, 150, 151, 220, 276–8, 729, 821, 993, 1021, 1024, 1025, 1026, 1028
globulin levels 813
infectious necrotic hepatitis 729, 731
milk quality 377–8
liver meridian (acupuncture) 1100
livestock units (LU) 15
live weight gain 5, 12, 15, 17, 18, 20, 54, 56–8, 62, 64, 65, 71, 72, 81, 112
lochial discharge 509
Locus-Dolendi needling 1099
Lokern virus 773
Lolium perenne 1181
longevity in dairy cattle 47, 48, 54, 60–61, 65–6, 169, 665, 671
'loose shoulder' 451
louping ill vaccination 1014
LSD (lumpy skin disease) 768–9
LU *see* livestock unit
lucerne 36, 78, 116, 123, 126–7, 792
Lucilia spp 747
lumpy jaw 824–5
lumpy skin disease (LSD) 768–9, 887–8, 984
lung meridian (acupuncture) 1100
lungworm 13, 71, 56, 239, 272, 273, 993, 1021, 1023, 1025, 1026, 1027
lupinosis 452, 462
vaccination 274, 1011, 1027
lupins 113, 129, 177
luteinizing hormone (LH) 473, 485
male puberty 481
oestrous cycle 489, 490, 492, 493, 494–5
postpartum 509–10
ovulation induction 657, 658
ovulatory surge 488
postpartum 502–3, 509–10
receptor binding 476
receptors 477, 494
surge 480
luteolysis 492, 493, 494, 497
induction 678–80
success 543
timing 544
lymphatic system, congenital conditions 177
lymphocytes 323, 381, 1046, 1059
lymphosarcoma 693, 695–6
retrobulbar/periorbital 918
Lyperosia exigua 747
Lyperosia irritans 747, 1031, 1032
lysosomal storage disease 179, 892
lysozyme 379, 997
L-tryptophan 866–7, 1061
Lycopodium clavicum 1089, 1091
Lyssa virus 1164

mabuterol 1073
MACE *see* multiple trait across country evaluation
macrocyclic lactones 1022–4

macrolides 393–5, 1038, 1040, 1041, 1043
macrophages 1046
MADF *see* modified acid detergent fibre
machine feeding 5
magadu 777
magnesium 782, 788, 789, 1184
in feed 123–9, 131
metabolic profile 813–14, 1184
requirements 33
supplementation 64, 157, 790, 791
see also hypomagnesaemia
magnesium carbonate 8, 29, 831
magnesium chloride 831
magnesium hydroxide 831
magnesium oxide 256, 264
magnesium sulphate 790
magnesium tetany 157, 255–6
see also hypomagnesaemia
magnet 834
maize 78, 124
maize germ meal 113, 114
maize gluten 112, 113, 114, 124
maize gluten meal 113, 114
maize grain 113
maize silage 16, 36, 78, 103, 112, 123–4
beef production 16–17, 19–20
composition 117
spoiled 826
malabsorption, passive 187
male fern poisoning 925
malignant catarrhal fever (MCF) 138, 629, 630, 935–6
malignant oedema 724–5
malignant rickets 765–6
malt distiller's draff 112
malt distiller's dark grain 113
malt calms 113, 114
malt residual pellets 113, 114
malignant oedema 724–5
mammary growth
in dairy heifers 56–7
see also udder
mammary secretions
antimicrobial substances 322–3
immunoglobulins 323–4
see also lactation
mammillitis 363–4, 888
mammogenesis 311–13, 316–17
management of cattle 957–60
mandible abnormalities 176
manganese
biochemical indices 296
deficiency 305, 462
disorders 305
manioc (tapioca) 78, 113
metabolic profile 815
supplementation 63
mange 742–4, 881–2, 1027, 1031
control with ricin 83
mangels 125
mango fly 747
Mannheimia haemolytica 239, 240, 241, 286, 287, 727, 860, 865
antiserum 246, 288
vaccination 247, 288, 1008–9

mannosidosis 179
Mansonia spp 745
manure
storage 986
see also excrement disposal
maple syrup urine disease 180
Mapputta virus 773
marbofloxacin 245, 268, 1040, 1041, 1043
margin, gross 47
margin over purchased feed (MOPF) 51, 52
master points 1099
mast cells 1046
mastitis 150, 152, 326–36, 382–3, 1091
aetiology 332–5
anti-inflammatory drugs 1061–3
antimicrobial therapy 391–403
benefits 402–3
costs 403
dry period 399–402
infection reservoir elimination 403
during lactation 397–9
bulk milk testing 341–8
candidiasis 933
cattle housing 331
cell count 329, 330–31, 341
coliform 1016
contagious 328
control 330–31, 335–6, 361
cooling ponds 93
corium fragility 421
cryptococcosis 932–3
diagnosis 328–30
endotoxic 1061
environmental 328
globulin levels 813
immune response to pathogens 383–8
immune system effects 479
infection dynamics 326, 327
information analysis 349–50
milk fever differential diagnosis 784
milk quality 378
milking machines 331–2, 357–61
monitoring 348–51, 1185
pathogens 328
peracute 398–9
pyaemia 737
records 348–9
resistance genes 167
straw yards 41, 334
subclinical 329–30
summer 63, 334, 337–40, 370, 745
bacterial complex 385
transmission 746
teat trauma 368
transmission 328
vaccination 1016
welfare issues 961
maternal immunity 1002–3
ME *see* metabolizable energy
meat packers 1190
meclofenamic acid 246
Mediterranean coast fever 753–4
melilotus 1087
meloidosis 932
meloxicam 1051, 1053, 1056, 1061, 1063

meningitis 251–2, 892, 895
  tubercular 156
meningoencephalitis
  bacterial 194, 198, 209, 900, 901–2
  thromboembolic 198, 907
mercuralis cyanatus 1087, 1089
mercuralis solubilis 1089, 1091
mercurius corrosivus 1055, 1087
mercury poisoning 942
mesentery, common, torsion of
    caecum/colon 141
metabolic disease
  feeding management in Europe
      1153–5
  genetics 168
  stress 1144
metabolic fuel partitioning 1141
metabolic profiles 804–16, 1184
  blood test timing 805
  energy balance 807–11
  heifers 815
  metabolites measured 807
  on milk 815
  minerals 813–15
  protein 811–13
  selection of cows 805–6
  suckler cows 815–16
  trace elements 813–15
metabolizability (q) 104
metabolizable energy (ME) 10, 11, 73,
      78, 103, 104, 105, 113, 117, 121,
      123–31
  dairy cow feed 31
  dairy heifer feeding 58
  efficiency of use 104
  expected forage 809–10
  feeds content 113
  fermentable 108, 812–13
  lactating cattle 105–6
  silage 13
  tropical cattle 78
metabolizable protein (MP) 31, 107,
      108–10
  requirements 110–12
metamizole 827, 846, 850
methacillin 1040, 1041, 1038
methacycline 1036, 1037, 1040, 1041
methane 98, 1037
methionine 1037
metronidazole 427, 1037
3-methyl indole 867, 1061
methylprednisolone 1056, 1057
metriphonate 1024, 1032
metritis 150, 151, 559, 1091
  acute puerperal 519–21
  anti-inflammatory therapy 1063
  consequences 521
  corium fragility 421
  embryonic death 560–61
  globulin levels 813
  prognosis 571–2
  pyaemia 737
mhlosimge 777
MIC (minimum inhibitory
      concentration) 396, 398, 1008,
      1395

microbial protein 107–8
  crude (MCP) 108, 110
  true (MTP) 107, 110
microphthalmia 918
Middelburgh virus 773
middle ear infections 903
midges 745, 767
milbemycins 1020, 1022–4, 1023, 1032
milk
  antimicrobial substances 322–3
  bulk testing 341–8
  calf feeding 11, 70
  composition 319, 330, 331, 373–7
  discarded 403
  ejection 319–20
    reflex 472–3
  herd bulk cell count 343–5
  immunoglobulins 323–4
  iodine concentration 302
  metabolic profiles 815
  protein synthesis 318–19
  purchase 25–6
  in rumen 233, 234
  secretion/synthesis 318–19
  total bacterial counts 345–7
milk clot failure, abomasal 212, 231–2
  milk replacers 212, 232–3
milk composition 373–8
milk drop syndrome 736
milk fat 23, 24, 78, 130, 373–5
  content 319
  feeding systems 117, 376, 377
  milking intervals 378
  non-nutritional factors 377–8
  quota ceiling 24
milk fever 168, 441, 439, 527, 781–7,
      789
  downer cow syndrome 439
  hypomagnesaemia differential
      diagnosis 789
  licking mania 139, 156
  uterine prolapse 514
milk production
  antimicrobial therapy for mastitis
      402–3
  energy requirement 105
  EU 22–4, 1151
  intervention buying 24
  North America 1183
  super-levy 24
  tropical cattle 72, 75–7
  world 68, 69
milk production quotas 4, 22, 23, 24,
      376
  butterfat ceiling 24
  efficiency measures 51
  Europe 1151
milk protein 23, 375
  non-nutritional factors 377–8
milk quality 373–8
  age of cow 377
  antimicrobial therapy for mastitis 402
  genetic variation 378
  non-nutritional factors 377–8
milk records 45–7
milk recording 46

milk replacers 4, 5
  abomasal milk clot failure 212, 231–3
  diarrhoea 212
  hypomagnesaemic tetany of calves
      255
milk sales
  'gold top' 28
  liquid 26–7
  organic 52
  skim/semi-skim 27
milk tetany 791
milk unions 76
milk yields 11, 23, 51, 55, 57, 78, 89, 90,
      112, 130, 316, 1187
  dairy heifers 55, 56–7, 59, 63, 165
  drop 143, 736
  lifetime 48, 71
  ovarian cystic disease 555–6
  smallholder dairying in Kenya 76
  welfare of cattle 961–2
milking
  interval effects on milk fat 378
  milk ejection 320
milking machines 353–61
  automatic cluster removers 40
  automatic systems 358–9
  components 353–5
  maintenance 331–2, 335, 336
  mastitis 331–2, 357–61
  somatic cell count 342
  teat lesions 370
  technology development 357–61
  testing 355–6
milking parlour 38, 39–40
  abreast 39, 40
  automatic 39
  concentrate feeding 38
  herringbone 25, 39, 40
mineralocorticoids 1056–60
minerals
  dairy cows 33
  dairy heifers 56, 58, 63–4
  feeds 112–13
  metabolic profile 813–15
  supplements for tropical cattle 74, 80
minimum inhibitory concentration see
      MIC
mixer wagon 38
misters 92
mites 742–4, 881–2, 1031, 1032
modified acid detergent (MADFI)
      123–6, 129, 131
molassed sugar beet pulp 112
molasses 78, 80, 112, 113, 114, 124
molybdenum 298, 299, 300
  deficiency 465
  excess 814
monensin sodium 19, 1036, 1067–8,
      1070, 1072, 1181–2
Moniezia spp 280–82, 1021, 1024, 1026
Monilia spp 823
monocyte 1045
MOPF see margins over purchased feed
morantel 1022, 1026
Moraxella bovis see infectious bovine
      rhinotracheitis (IBR)

morbilliurius 707
mortality, calf 3, 4, 8, 64, 66
mosquitoes 745, 762
  viral disease spread 768, 769, 771–4
moulds 117, 123, 125
mounting
  beef cattle 960
  cows in oestrus 535
  failure by bull 610–12
  failure to locate vagina 615
mouth 821–4
  lesions 138
moxidectin 743, 1022, 1025, 1026, 1027, 1031
MP *see* metabolizable protein
MTP *see* microbial true protein
mucormycosis 932
mucosal disease 813, 822, 826, 853, 854, 855–7
  cerebellar hypoplasia 900
  mouth 822
mud fever 429
multiple trait across country evaluations (MACE) 49
multivitamin injection 3
Murray Valley encephalitis virus 773
Musca autumnalis 746, 1031
Musca domestica 746, 762, 1031
Musca fergusona 746
Musca hilli 746
Musca jorbens 746
Musca terraeregina 746
muscle abscess 1078
muscle fibrosis 1078
muscle injuries 451
muscular dystrophy 157, 451
muscular hypertrophy 178
muscular system, congenital defects 177–8
mutilations 962–3
Mycobacterium 251, 631
  Mycobacterium avium var *paratuberculosis* 857, 988
  Mycobacterium bovis 251, 862, 988
  Mycobacterium farcinogenes 885
  Mycobacterium johnei 857, 988
  skin diseases 885–6
  see also Johne's disease; tuberculosis
Mycoplasma 240, 241, 287, 327, 329, 334–5, 385, 391, 400, 1184
  Mycoplasma bovigentalium 334
  Mycoplasma bovis 240, 241, 327, 334, 385
  Mycoplasma canadase 334, 327
  Mycoplasma californicum 334
  Mycoplasm dispar 240, 241
  Mycoplasma mycoides subsp. mycoides 865, 868–74
  transmission by semen 629, 631
  see also contagious bovine pleuropneumonia (CBPP)
mycotic stomatitis 823
mycotoxins 117, 1180, 1186
myelitis 892, 895
myeloencephalopathy, bovine progressive degenerative 179

myiasis 747–8
myocardial abscess 154
myoclonus, inherited congenital 180, 891–2
myometrium/myometrial cells 501–2
myositis 723–5

nagana 757, 759, 1030
naphthanate, copper 880
naproxen 246
nasal polyps 933
natamycin 879, 1036
natural killer (NK) cells 998
natural law 1082
navel dipping 3
navel ill 3, 249–50, 1091
NDF *see* neutral detergent fibre
Near East encephalitis 771
necrobacillosis, laryngeal/oral 250–51
necrotic enteritis 213, 238
necrotic stomatitis 822
necrotic vaginitis 513
Neethling pox virus 857, 768–9
NEFA *see* non-esterified fatty acids
neglect of animals 956–7
nematodes 267–76, 895
Nematodirus (nematodirosis) 269, 1026
neomycin 392, 393, 394, 395, 458, 851, 1036, 1037, 1038, 1040, 1041, 1043
Neospora (neosporosis) 283, 584–5, 589, 989, 993
nerve paralyses, lameness 436–9
  fifth 139
  seventh 139
nervous syndromes 155–7
nervous system 891
netobimin 1020, 1021, 1025, 1026, 1029
neurodegenerative disease, inherited 179
neurological disorders 890–913
  biochemical causes 891–2
  congenital conditions 178–80
  genetic 892, 893–4
  micro-organisms 892, 895
  treatment 897–900
  see also named conditions
neurological examination 895–6
neuromuscular diseases 457–60
neurones 471–2, 473–4
neuropeptides 1047
neutral detergent fibre (NDF) 112, 117, 120, 123, 127, 129–31
neutrophils 324–5, 1045, 1051
Newbury agent 200
New Forest eye *see* infectious bovine keratoconjunctivitis (IBKC)
New Zealand 1177–82
nicofolan 1024, 1028
niclosamide 1024
nitrate/nitrite poisoning 950–51
nitrofurans 1038, 1040, 1041, 1043
nitrofurantoin 1037, 1038, 1040, 1041
nitrofurazone 1038, 1040, 1041
nitrogen
  lucerne growing 126, 127

lupin growing 129
  red clover growing 127, 128
  white clover growing 128
nitrogen fertilizers 12, 34, 35, 62, 126
  grassland 33, 34–5
nitrogen vulnerable zones (NUZ) 35
nitroxynil 1024, 1026, 1028
non-cellulosic feeds 112
non-esterified fatty acids (NEFA) 802, 807–8, 810, 1154
  metabolic profiles 807–8, 810
non-protein nitrogen 124
non-steroidal anti-inflammatory drugs (NSAIDs)
  bull fertility 621–2
  classification 1049
  diarrhoea 198
  lameness 458
  mastitis 334, 398, 1061–2, 1063
  mechanism of action 1049–50
  neurological disorders 899
  peracute mastitis 398–9
  pharmacokinetics 1052–5
  pneumonia 245–6
  reproductive tract trauma 513
  respiratory disease 245, 246, 288, 865, 867, 1060–61
  side effects/toxicity 1055–6
  uses 1051–2
Norcadia farcinica 885
Norgestomet 681–2
normality 135
North America
  beef production 1188–91
  dairy farming 1183–7
  rabies 1165–6
North Devon 8
nosode 1087
notebook 44
notifiable diseases 989
notkalersiekre 776
novobiocin 393, 737, 1040, 1041
NSAID *see* non-steroidal anti-inflammatory drugs
nuclear transplantation 648
nutrient gap 32
nutrition 95–122
  anoestrous prevention 546
  beef cattle 655–6
  bulls 611, 618
  calving 657
  calving season control 656
  conceptus survival 500, 505
  deprivation 478
  diarrhoea management 210, 212
  embryo transfer 638, 644
  fertility 58–9, 534
  lameness 422–3
  milk fever 781–2
  tropical calf rearing 70, 71–2
  see also calves, digestive disorders; feed(s); feeding
nutritional deficiency
  anoestrus 533–4
    postpartum 512–13
  conception failure 562, 563

nux vomica 829, 1086, 1087, 1089, 1095
nystagmus 918
nystatin 1036

O antigen 383, 384
oak poisoning 951–2
oats 78, 113
oat feed 113, 114
Obodhiang virus 773
obturator paralysis 438, 799
ocular defects, congenital 180–81
ocular diseases 917–25
  conjunctiva/cornea 919–22
  eyelids 918–19
  globe 917–18
  lens diseases 923–4
  optic nerve 924–5
  orbit 917–18
  retinal 924–5
  uveal tract 923
ocular squamous cell carcinoma 922
oedema 1045
oesophageal choke 139
oesophageal dilatation 139
oesophageal groove
  actinobacillosis 139
  dysfunction 233–4
  lesions 146, 837
oesophageal syndrome 828
oesophageal wall lesions 147
Oesophagostromum spp 1026
oesophagus/oesophageal conditions
  139, 147, 825–8
oestradiol 102, 490–91, 494, 1072, 1073
oestrogen 480, 492, 494, 782
  endometritis treatment 523–4
  ovarian cystic disease 556
  parturition 501, 502
    induction 687
  retained fetal membranes 517
oestrous cycle 471, 488–98
  calving to first service interval 530–31
  disturbance 530–48
  interservice intervals 531–2
  pattern 491–2
  pharmacological regulation 497–8,
    678–84
  phases 492–8
  postpartum 503–4, 509–10
oestrus 471, 488
  detection 534, 535, 543, 544, 546–8
    aids 547–8, 628
    rate 558
  synchronization of 59, 61–2, 497–8,
    543, 547, 573
    beef cattle 658–61
    embryo transfer 644
    luteolysis induction 678–82
    resynchronization of repeats 548
    'two plus two' technique 679, 680
  tropical cattle 71, 72
  unobserved 534–5, 542, 544
oilseed residues 114
oilseeds, whole 114
ol macheri 776
oleandomycin 1036, 1038, 1040, 1041

omasum impaction 145
omphalophlebitis 194
Omsk haemorrhagic fever 770
onchocerciasis 774, 888
ondiri disease 763–5
ondiritis 763–5
on-farm laboratory 601–2
oocyte harvesting 570
opsonins 325
optic nerve diseases 924–5
optic neuropathy 925
oral rehydration 197–8, 209–10
orbit anomalies/neoplasia 917–18
orbivirus 691
orchitis 620–21
organic farming
  clover growing 128
  dairy 52
  lucerne growing 127
  lupins 129
  sainfoin 129
organochlorines 881, 1031–2, 1158
  poisoning 942
organophosphates 741, 742, 743, 746,
    774, 877, 881, 882, 1020, 1024,
    1032
  poisoning 139, 892, 940, 944
oropharyngeal syndrome 828
osteoarthritis 176–7, 453
  hip 446–7
osteochondrosis 453
osteomalacia 462–3, 792
osteomyelitis 429, 463–4
  chronic 464
osteopetrosis 176
osteoporosis 446
Ostertagia (ostertagiosis) 267–9, 1021,
    1023, 1025
  Type II (ostertagiosis) 1025
otitis 252
OTMS 9, 14, 28, 29
  see also Over Thirty-Month Scheme
out-of-parlour feeders 38, 119–120
ovarian cysts 533, 554–5
  see also cystic ovarian disease
ovarian status assessment 536–40
ovary
  cycling 509–10
  oestrous cycle 495
overeating syndrome see acidosis
Over Thirty Month Scheme (OTMS) 9,
    14, 28, 29
ovulation 480, 492, 499
  delayed 557–8, 567
  failure after oestrus 554–7, 566–7
  first 481, 502–3
  induction in beef cattle 657–8
  pharmacological control 678–84
  silent 534–5, 540–41, 542, 544
  see also oestrus
ovum pick-up (OPU) 647–8
owners 135, 136, 137
  genetic counselling 166
oxfendazole 1020, 1021, 1025, 1026,
    1027
oxybendazole 800, 1020

oxyclozenide 1022, 1026
oxytetracycline 245, 250, 291, 394, 427,
    428, 753, 755, 762, 860, 861, 864,
    1036, 1037, 1040, 1041, 1043, 1061
oxytocin 319–20, 334, 396, 398, 472, 473,
    493
  corpus luteum 495, 524
  egg transport 557
  release 475
  retained fetal membranes 517
  uterine receptors 501
  uterine rupture 513

PAF (platelet activating factor) 1046,
    1047
pain 149, 1046
  anti-inflammatory therapy 1063–4
  see also abdominal pain
palm kernel 113
pancreatic extract 264
panfloxacacin 1041
Pangenia spp 745
papilloedema 924, 925
papillomatosis 365, 367, 881–2, 1091
  vaccination 1014
papillomatous digital dermatitis (PDD)
    428
papular stomatitis 822
paracetamol 1050
Parafilaria bovicola 1023
parainfluenza III virus (P13) 239, 240,
    247, 286, 289, 1007, 1009
parakeratosis, inherited 181–2
paralysis 100
  brachial 436
  femoral 203, 436
  obturator 438
  nerve 436–9
  peroneal 438
  suprascapular 436
  radical 436, 465
  scialie 439
  tibial 438
Paramphistomum (paramphistomosis)
    279, 1024
Paranaplasma caudatum 761
parapoxvirus 252, 364, 707
parasitic infections 774–5
  Africa 1157–61
  bronchitis 13, 56, 239, 272–4, 1011,
    1021, 1023, 1025, 1026, 1027
  gastroenteritis 13, 267–72, 1025–7
  genetic component 168
  skin 880–82
  tropical calf rearing 70
  see also ectoparasites; lice; mites
parasitic worms 13, 267–82, 895, 1028–9
  control programmes 18
  dairy heifers 57–8
  IgE reactions 1001
  milk quality 378
  tropical calf rearing 70–71
  see also anthelminthics; liver fluke
parathyroid hormone (PTH) 782, 783
paratuberculosis see Johne's disease
paresis, spastic 179–80, 458–9, 459

paromomycin 1036, 1037, 1038, 1040, 1041
parsnips 131
particle size (feed) 96
parturition 501–2
  caesarean section 1115–19
  calcium requirement 782
  coriosis 420–21
  delay 687–8
  'downer' cow 151
  hormonal control 501–2
  periparturient cow management 526–7
  pharmacological induction 686–8
  stretch receptors 475
  see also calving
parvaquone 753, 755, 1029
passage points (acupuncture) 1099
passports, cattle 6, 45
pastern paralysis, congenital 180
Pasteurella haemolytica see Mannheima haemolytia
Pasteurella multocida 200, 240, 241, 246, 249, 287, 289, 632, 728–9
pasteurellosis 286–8, 873
pastoralism 69, 70, 72, 75
pasture, grazed 101–2
patellar luxation 448–9
peanut (ground nut) 70
peanut oil 834
peas 113, 129, 130–31
pectin 199
pectin-extracted fruit 112, 113, 114
pedal bone 418, 419, 429–30
pediculosis 741–2
pedigree analysis 165
pelvis fractures 445, 446–7
pencthamale 393, 1036
penicillin 245, 250, 286, 291, 392, 393, 394, 395, 396, 398, 400, 427, 429, 443, 456, 458, 718, 721, 725, 726, 729, 733, 823, 825, 849, 851, 860, 864, 886, 1036, 1040, 1041, 1043
penicillinase 391–2, 1038
penile defects 612–16
penis abnormalities/conditions 614, 615–16
peptic ulcer, abomasal 146–7
Peptococcus indolicus 328, 385
pericarditis 153, 731–3, 928
pericardium meridian (acupuncture) 1100
perinatal weak calf syndrome 249
periople 411–12
peritoneum, tympany 141
peritonitis 150–51, 849–50
  acute diffuse 141, 146
  localized 143, 194
permethrin 881, 1031, 1032
peroneal nerve paralysis 438, 439
perosomus elumbis 180
petechial fever, bovine 763–5
PGE see parasitic gastroenteritis
phagocytic cells 324–5, 997–8
phagocytosis 325, 382

Phalaris staggers 296
phenols, substituted 1024
phenothrin 1032
phenoyl benzyl urea flubenzuron 1033
phenylbutazone 246, 399, 456, 460, 1050, 1051, 1053, 1055, 1056, 1062, 1063
phlegmonous stomatitis 823
Phosmet 741, 743, 877, 881, 1031
phosphate fertilizer 34, 62, 127
phosphate, inorganic 814
phosphoric acid 1089
phosphorus 63, 264, 462, 1086, 1089, 1091
phosphorus deficiency 253–4
  postparturient haemoglobinuria 792–3
  requirements 33
  see also hypophosphataemia
photosensitization 148, 884–5, 1180
  syndromes 139
  teats 140, 370, 371
phoxion 1032
phthalysulphonamide 1039
phylloerythrin 884–5, 1180
physeal dysplasia 464–5
Phytolacca americana 1090, 1091
pica 792
Picornaviridae 700
pilot points (acupuncture) 1099
PIN see production index number
piperazines 1020, 1024
pirlimycin 393
piroplasmosis 750
piroxicam 1050
Pithomyces chartarum 1180
pituitary gland 320, 472, 473
  oestrous cycle 495
placenta 500–501
  aborted 587
placentitis 578, 586, 932
  aspergillosis 934
platelet 1048, 1052
platelet activating factor (PAF) 1046, 1047
pleurisy 144, 146
pleuropneumonia
  contagious bovine 629, 631, 868–74
  peracute 865
  plumbum 1087
PLI see production plus lifespan index
pneumonia 144, 146, 152, 1091
  acute exudative 860
  aspiration 860–61
  calves 4, 239–48, 249, 274, 871
  candidiasis 933
  chronic suppurative 146, 864
  cuffing 239–48
  diagnosis 243–4
  environment 240–42
  enzootic 239–48
  epidemiology 239–40
  genetic component 167–8
  management 242
  prevention 247–8
  signs 242–3

  treatment 244–7
  tropical calf rearing 70
  vaccination 247–8
pneumovagina 519
poisoning 151, 153, 937, 941–3, 944–52
  diagnosis 937–9
  diarrhoea 149
  furazolidone 260–61
  neurological disorders 892
  plant 452, 1161–2
  tenesmus 150
  vomiting 826
  see also named toxicants and toxicoses
polioencephalomalacia see cerebrocortical necrosis
pollution control of slurry 42
poloxalene 834
polycythaemia, familial 184
polydactyly 176
polymorphonuclear neutrophil leucocytes (PMNs) 381, 382, 389, 395
polymyxin B 392, 393, 394, 1040, 1041, 1043
ponds, cooling 93
Pongola virus 773
pontomedullary syndrome 896
'poor man's grazing system' 1020
population, cattle see cattle population
porphyria, congenital 184, 919
post calving comfort 421–2
postpartum period 508–27
  anoestrus 525–6
  clinical examination 511–12
  enhancement 513
  genital tract lesions 513–26
  monitoring 511–12
  negative energy balance 525, 526
  shortening 513
  veterinary examination/treatment 545
post parturient haemoglobinuria 792–3
pot ale syrup 113, 114
potash fertilizer 34, 62, 127
potassium chloride 83, 441
potassium iodide 823
potassium, metabolic profile 814
potato waste 131
potatoes 113, 114, 131
potentiated sulphonamides 250, 252, 288, 292, 345, 393, 394, 395, 458, 737, 857, 860, 864, 1036, 1037, 1038, 1040, 1041, 1043
povidone-iodine 458
prairie meal (maize gluten) 112, 113, 114
praziquantel 1025, 1026, 1028
preconditioning 1190
predicted (production) transmitting ability (PTA) 49, 60
prednisolone 245, 1049, 1056, 1057
prednisone 1049, 1056, 1057
pregnancy 498–502
  diagnosis 569–70, 671
  energy requirement 105

pregnancy (cont'd)
  establishment 684–6
  heat stress 89
  hypomagnesaemia 150
  lengths 77
  local trauma 561–2
  maintenance 500–501
  management 526–7
  maternal recognition 499–500
  prolonged 183
  rate 572, 617–24
    embryo transfer 637–8
    pharmacological control of
      ovulation 61–2, 682
pregnancy toxaemia 784, 793, 796–7
preputial defects 612, 613–14
pressure syndrome 797–8, 799, 801
preventive grazing strategy 1026
Prevotella melaninogenicus 385, 425,
  426
prions 977, 1152
probenzimidazoles 1020–21, 1023
probing 827
procaine benzyl penicillin 288, 394, 458,
  1024
production index number (PIN) 48, 49,
  60
production monitoring 1186–7
production plus lifespan index (PLI) 49
production transfer ability (PTA) 49,
  60
profitable life index (PLI) 60
progestagen 497
  breeding synchronization 62, 659–60,
    683
  embryo transfer 645
  luteolysis induction 680–81
  repeat breeder cows 568
progesterone 488, 489, 492, 494, 1071,
  1073
  analysis 512
  anoestrus treatment 526
  assays 536, 538, 540, 548
    insemination 558
  embryo transfer 645
  maternal 561
  parturition 501
  postpartum 503
  pregnancy
    establishment 685
    maintenance 500–501
  prolonged low 558
  repeat breeder cows 568
progesterone-releasing intravaginal
  device (PRID) 541–2, 543, 1179
  follicular cyst treatment 567
  luteolysis induction 681
  ovulation induction 657–8
progressive retinal degeneration 925
prolactin 317
  postpartum 503–4
  serum levels 57
propetamphos 743, 1032
propionic acid 117
propoxus 1032
propylene glycol 795

prostaglandin(s)
  breeding synchronization 62, 497,
    659–60, 678–80
    asynchrony 682–3
  endometritis treatment 524
  eicosanoids 1047, 1051, 1052, 1061
  GnRH combination techniques 683
  luteolysis induction 678–80, 1051
  parturition induction 687
  uterine involution 504
prostaglandin 2_α 245, 398, 495
  anoestrus treatment 542, 543–4
  endometritis treatment 524
  luteolysis 492, 493
  oestrus synchronization 498
  parturition 501, 502
  pyometra treatment 524–5, 543
  retained fetal membranes 517, 518
  routine administration 546
  superovulation 634
  uterine receptors 501
prostaglandin E_2 (PGE$_2$) 1047, 1052
protein
  catabolism 1059
  degradation 96
  metabolic profiles 811–13
  milk 375, 377–8
  rumen degradable/undegradable 31,
    32
  total, blood 813
  see also metabolizable protein (MP);
    microbial protein
protein, dietary 106–13, 376, 1184–5
  conceptus survival 500, 505
  dairy cow feed 31–2
  degradation in rumen 96, 98, 99
  feed content 113
  quickly/slowly degradable proteins
    31, 108
  see also crude protein (CP); digestible
    undegraded protein (DUP);
    effective rumen degradable
    protein (ERDP); milk protein
proteomics 170–71
Protheca (achlorophyllic algae) 93, 327
protozoa 282–5
  infections 584–5, 1029–30
    neural 895
    tick-/louse borne 748–61
  rumen fermentation 96, 97, 98
pruritis/pyrexia/haemorrhagic syndrome
  (PPH) 884
pseudo-lumpy skin disease 887, 888
pseudocowpox 364–5, 371, 888
Pseudomonas spp 327, 334, 347, 391
  counts 347
Psorophora spp 745, 762
Psoroptes spp 742, 743, 881, 1023, 1031
PTA *see* predicted transmitting abilities
PTH *see* parathyroid hormone
puberty 72, 479–81
  delayed 530, 545
public health 987
public perceptions 955
pulmonary abscess 864
Pulsatilla nigricans 1086, 1089, 1091

pyaemia 737
pyelonephritis 144–5, 150, 154
  contagious bovine 725–6
pyloric obstruction 835
pyometra 524–5, 543
pyrantel 1022
pyrethrins/synthetic pyrethroids 881,
  1032
pyrexia of unknown origin 149, 151–2
pyrogenium 1089, 1091

QDP *see* quickly digestible protein
Q fever 586, 629, 632
quality assurance schemes 38, 52
quarantine of bulls 596
quickly degradable protein (QDP) 31,
  108
quinine 1082
quinolones *see* fluroquinolone

rabies 908–9, 1164–70
  clinical signs 1167–8
  control 1170
  diagnosis 1168–9
  epidemiology 1165–6
  pathogenesis 1167
  pathology 1168
  transmission 1166–7
  vaccination 1018, 1169–70
ractopamine 1073–5
radial nerve paralysis 436–7, 465
radiography of fractures 442–3
rafoxamide 1022, 1024
ragwort poisoning 148, 149, 150, 892,
  945–6
ranching
  dairy 75–6
  tropical cattle 78–80
range monitoring of tropical cattle 73
rape 36, 126
  poisoning 155, 156
rapeseed meal 113
rearing systems 3–5, 54–67
records
  breeding 45, 46
  cards 45
  dairy cattle 667–8, 672–3, 674
  embryo transfer 645
  financial 47
  health 169
  herd 44–7, 511
  mastitis 348–9
  milk 45–7
  reproductive 672–3
rectal palpation
  ovarian status assessment 537, 539
  repeat breeder cows 564
rectal prolapse 859
rectal tears 859
recto-vaginal fistula 859
recumbency 797–801
  see also downer cow syndrome
red gut 846
redwater 154–5, 748–50
rehydration, oral 197–8, 203–5, 209–10
relaxin 493, 502

remote sensing 73
Reoviridae 691
repartitioning agents 1073–5
repeat breeder cows 563–5, 568
  apparently normal 569
  prognosis 569–72
reproduction
  dairy cattle problems 961
  endocrine signals 476–9
  energy balance 477–8, 502–3
  feedback loops 474–6, 480
  female physiology 488–505
  male physiology 481–8
  neuro-immune reactions 479
  performance
    beef cattle 652–62
    dairy cattle 663–75
  pharmacological manipulation
    678–88
  physiology 471–506
  postpartum physiology 502–5
  puberty 479–81
  stress 478–9
reproductive system
  bovine herpes virus 1 infection 289,
    290–91
  congenital defects 182–4
retained fetal membranes *see* fetal
  membranes, retained
resistance genes 167–8
respiratory disease 860–74
  anti-inflammatory drugs 1060–61
  calves 239–48
  growing cattle 286–92
  vaccinations 1007, 1008, 1009–11
  see also pleuropneumonia;
    pneumonia
respiratory rate 155
respiratory syncytial virus *see* bovine
  respiratory syncytial virus
  (BRSV)
restraint
  injection damage 1079, 1080
  teat surgery 1127–8
reticular grunt 838
reticulitis/reticuloperitonitis, acute
  traumatic 140, 142–3, 145–6,
  837–9
  rumenotomy 1106
reticulo-rumen, gas escape obstruction
  147
reticulum injury 146
retinal diseases 924–5
retropharyngeal abscess 824
retro virus 694
Rhabdoviridae 710
rhinosporidiasis 933
rhinotracheitis, dusty feed 866
Rhipicephalus spp 747, 748, 751, 762,
  1030, 1036
rhododendron poisoning 139, 943
Rhus toxicodendron 1086, 1089, 1091
rice bran 78, 114
ricin 83, 1162
rickets 462–3, 792
rickettsia/rickettsial diseases 586, 761–7

ricobendazole 1020, 1021, 1025, 1026,
  1027
rifamycin 392, 393, 394, 395, 396
Rift Valley fever 745, 769–70, 1018
rinderpest 629, 630, 707–10, 989, 1156–7
  vaccination 710, 1013, 1156
Ringer's solution 836
ringworm 371, 878–80, 989, 993
  vaccination 880, 1017–18
robotic (automatic) parlours 39
root crops 36, 95, 96
rotavirus 188, 189, 191–9, 207, 208, 218
Rothera's test 795–6
roughage 101
  processing 117–18
  see also hay; straw
roundworms 267–9, 1021, 1023
rumen
  acidosis 119, 829–32
  acute tympany 141
  bacteria 96, 97
  bloat 234–6
  capacity 101
  cold water 147
  digestion optimizing 99–100
  diseases 828–39
  distension 835
  fermentation 95, 96–100
  growth promoters 1067–9
  impaction 140–41, 145, 236
  micro-organisms 96, 97, 98
  milk entering 233, 234
  outflow rate 109
  parakeratosis 832
  pH 97, 119, 120
  protozoa 97
  stasis 119
  tympany 127, 128, 129, 141, 145,
    146–7, 152, 828
  weak acids 96–7, 98
  see also bloat
rumen degradable protein (RDP) 31,
  32
rumen enhancers 19
rumen undegradable protein (UDP) 31,
  32
rumenotomy 827, 834, 836, 839, 1106–9
Russian spring-summer encephalitis
  770
Ruta graveolens 1054, 1086, 1091
Rwamba virus 773
rye 129
ryegrass staggers 1181

Sabina 1090, 1091
Sabo virus 773
sacroiliac luxation/subluxation 448
sadistic human behaviour 143, 150
safflower meal 113
Sahiwal x Friesian cattle 74, 77
Sahiwal 77
sainfoin 129, 835
salbutamol 1073, 1074
saler 9
salicylanilides 1020, 1024
salicyclate 399, 1053

saline, isotonic 197
saline, hypertonic 197, 334
saliva 97, 98, 108
salivation 822
  excess 138–9
Salmonella (salmonellosis) 4, 140, 152,
  178, 206, 207, 210, 215–30, 455,
  992, 1184, 1087
  abortion 582
  antibiotics 227, 229–30
    resistance 217–18
  calf scouring 4
  carrier state 219, 225, 226
  classification 216–17
  control measures 227–30
  diagnosis 226–7
  diarrhoea 850–52
  epidemiology 218–19
  hygiene 227–8
  intestinal interactions 221–4
  osteomyelitis 463
  pathogenesis 220–25
  persistence 224–5
  resistance 221, 224
  signs 225–6
  species 215, 216–18
  systemic spread 224–5
  vaccination 227, 228–9, 852, 1006, 1007
Salmonella Dublin 215–30, 992
Salmonella typhimurium 215–30, 992
Salmonella enteritidis 215
salpingitis 559
salt supplementation 80
sandcracks 425, 426
sandflies 745, 774
Sango virus 773
saponins 1080
Sarcocystis (sarcosporidiosis) 284–5
Sarcophaga 747
Sarcoptes spp 743, 881, 1023, 1031
Saudi Arabia 1172–6
scabies 743, 881–2
SCC *see* somatic cell counts
Schistosoma (schistosomosis) 279–80,
  1026, 1028
  Schistosoma reflexus 182
schwitzkrankheit 776
sciatic nerve paralysis 439, 799
scour/scouring
  calf 4, 70, 1006–7, 1063
  genetic component 167–8
  winter 13, 149
screw-worm flies 747–8
scrotal hernia 140
scrotal temperature 481–2
scrotum
  circumference 618–19
  sac disruption 620
SDP *see* slowly degradable protein
seasonal approach to managing mastitis
  (SAMM) 399–400, 401
seasons
  calving 656, 665, 667, 673, 675
  milk quality 377
  ovarian cystic disease 556
  postpartum acyclic period 657

seaweed meal 258
selection, genetic 169
selenate, barium 304
selenite, sodium 260
selenium
  biochemical indices 296
  deficiency 258–60, 302–3, 451, 1180
  disorders 302–5
  supplementation 63
  toxicity 305, 688
selenomethionine 304
Selenomonas ruminantium 97
semen
  collection 602–4
  pre-sexed 30, 48, 61, 648
  processing for AI 627
  quality 559, 617–18
  safety 632–3
  sexed 53, 61
  transmissible diseases 628, 629, 630–32
semi-intensive milk production 76
seminal plasma 488
seminal vesicle abnormalities 623
seminiferous tubules 482, 483
sensitivity testing, antibiotics 1036
sepia 109, 1090
septicaemia
  calves 194, 204, 209, 902
  haemorrhagic 632, 728–9
serotonin 1046, 1047
Serratia spp 398
Sertoli cells 482, 483, 484, 486, 620
service
  age at first 64
  failure to serve cow 559
  interservice intervals 531–2, 671
  natural 558–9, 594, 595
  observation 607–8
  per conception 50
  poor pregnancy rate 617–24
  return to 552–4, 562
  success rate 670–71
  see also artificial insemination (AI);
    conception failure
sesame meal 113
settled extensive cattle systems 69, 75
shade 90–91
shaker calf syndrome 179
Shamondu virus 773
shea nut meal 113
sheep headfly 337–8, 339
shiga-like toxin CSLT 201
shipping fever 286–9
shock, anaphylactic 1059
shock, endotoxic 1052, 1059
shock, haemorrhagic 1059
shorthorn, 8, 9
Shuni virus 773
sickness behaviour 1146
silage 35, 36, 103, 112, 119, 123, 124, 129,
    130
  acetonaemia 793–4
  additives 116–17
  analytical composition 37, 116, 117
  beef 19, 121
  big bale 35

buffer feeds 119, 791
dairy cow feeding 32, 33, 37, 121
dairy heifers 56
digestibility 101
feeding, beef 15, 18, 20
feeding, heifers 56
fermentation 114–16
flat-rate feeding 120
intake 121
listeriosis risk 582
maize 16–17, 19–20, 36, 123–4
  spoiled 826
making 13
mechanical feeding 37
peas 129
preservation 114–16
red clover 127
rye 129
sainfoin 129
self-feeding 37, 65, 66
storage 41–2
suckler herds 12, 13
whole crop 130
whole crop cereal with peas 130–31
whole wheat 130
silica 1090, 1091
silos 41–2
slurry 43–4
Simmental breed 7, 8, 30, 175, 1177
Simmental x Friesian 6, 19, 20, 21
Simuliidae family 745
Simulium spp 1031
Sindbis virus 773
skeletal defects, congenital 175–7
skimmed milk replacers 4
skin defects
  congenital 181–2
  foot 426–9
  interdigital hyperplasia 429
skin diseases 875–88
  cutaneous leukosis 698–9, 700
  lameness 460, 461–2
  lumpy skin disease 768–9
  mange 83, 742–4, 881–2
  see also named conditions
skin tuberculosis 886
slaughter age 14, 15, 20, 21, 81
slaughter of cattle 403, 963–4
slaughter weights 15, 17, 18, 20, 21, 81
slobbering 138–9
slowly degradable protein (SDP) 31,
    108
slurry compound, weepy-walled 44
slurry disposal 42–4
slurry heel 425
slurry pits/channels 986
slurry storage 39, 42, 43, 44, 988
small testes syndrome 618, 620
smallholders
  beef production 81
  dairying 76–7
small intestine meridian (acupuncture)
    1100
snails 276, 277, 278
sodium acetate 831
sodium acid phosphate 726, 792, 793

sodium bicarbonate 119, 203, 209, 829,
    831, 843, 1037
sodium chloride 831
sodium hydroxide 117–18
sodium iodide 251, 879
sodium in feed 123–9, 131
sodium lactile 843
sodium meclophenamate 246
sodium metabolic profile 814
sodium requirements 33
sodium selenite 260
soft sole syndrome 424
soil monitoring in tropics 73
solar radiation 90, 91, 92
sole
  bruising 1181
  foreign body penetration 425
  horn 413
  overgrowth 414
  soft 424
  ulcer 41, 145, 150, 417–19
Solenoptes spp 741, 880, 1023, 1031
solids not fats (SNF) 23, 24
somatic cell count 341–8
  interpretation 343–5
  late lactation 402
  mastitis 329, 330–31, 341, 399
  methods 342–3
somatotropin 320–21, 1073
source point (acupuncture) 1099
South America, beef ranching 77
South Devon 8
soya bean 112, 113, 124
soya bean oil 834
spasms, congenital 178
spastic paresis 179–80, 458–9
spastic syndrome 459–60
spasticity 180
spectinomycin 245, 288, 392, 395, 428,
    1040, 1041
sperm granulomas 622
spermatocele formation 622
spermatogenesis 481, 483–5
  disruption 620–22
  heat stress 935
spermatozoa 485, 487
  ageing 558
  capacitation 499
  morphology 605–607
  motility 604–605
  production 481
  storage interference 622
  transport 498–9
  interference 557, 567, 622
spinal cord lesions 912–13
spiramycin 245, 288, 392, 393, 394, 395,
    396, 398, 427, 1036, 1038, 1040,
    1041
spleen meridian (acupuncture) 1100
splints
  flexor tendon contracture 452
  fractures 443
  muscle injuries 451
spondylitis, ankylosing 462
sporadic bovine encephalomyelitis
    911–12

sporadic bovine leukosis 698–9, 700
sprayers, parlour exit lanes 93
sporidesmin 1180
sprinklers 92–3
stable fly 746–7, 762, 1031
staggers 296, 305, 1181
   see also hypomagnesaemia
stall feeding 81
standing, excessive 421
staphylococci 392, 347, 455, 457
   coagulase-negative 327, 328, 335
Staphylococcus aureus
   counts 347
   enterotoxins 386
   immune response 385–6
   mastitis 326–8, 330, 332–3, 343, 346,
      347, 382, 391, 392, 394, 396, 398,
      399, 400, 403
      antibiotics 396
   secondary infection of udder/teats
      363, 368, 888
   treatment 396, 1061, 1062
   virulence factors 385–6
starch
   dietary 374
   rumen fermentation 96, 98
starvation 150, 151
stephanofilariosis 774–5, 888
Stephanurus dentatus (stephanurosis)
   274–5
sterility 167
Sterner-Grymer closed suture technique
   842
steroidogenesis 481
steroids 1056–60
   administration 1058–9
   anabolic 621, 795–6
   contraindications 1060
   mastitis 1062–3
   mechanism of action 1057–8
   pharmacokinetics 1059
   side-effects 1059
   uses 1059–60
   see also corticosteroids
stifle joint luxation 448–50
stillbirth 249
stockers 1190
stocking rate 101, 121
   dairy cows 34, 35, 51
   dairy heifers 55, 58
   suckler herds 12, 15
stomach fluke disease 279
stomach meridian (acupuncture) 1100
stomatitis 822, 823
   stomatitis, mycotic 823
   stomatitis, necrotic 822
   stomatitis–nephrosis syndrome 777
   stomatitis, papular 822
   stomatitis, phlegmonous 823
Stomoxys calcitrans 746, 762, 1031
store cattle finishing 15–18
strabismus 918
straining *see* tenesmus
strangulated mesenteric hernia 140
strangulated scrotal hernia 140
strategic anthelmintic dosing 1020

straw 103, 112, 117, 118, 121, 123, 124,
   125
   calf feeding 4
   chopping 117
   dairy heifer feeding 56
   feeding 18, 56
straw yards 40, 41, 43, 44
   mastitis risk 41, 334
   post-calving 421–2
   space allowance 44
stray voltage 931
streptococci 96, 249, 450, 457
   aesculin-hydrolysing 333
   counts 347
   immune response 386–8
   mastitis 327–34, 343, 382
   meningoencephalitis 901
   secondary infection of udder/teats
      363, 368
   stomatitis 823
   virulence factors 386–8
Streptococcus agalactiae 326, 327, 328,
      332, 333, 343, 347, 387, 391, 399,
      403, 992
Streptococcus bovis 96
Streptococcus dysgalactiae 327, 328, 332,
      343, 346, 347, 385, 387–8
Streptococcus faecalis 333, 347
Streptococcus uberis 327, 329, 331, 332,
      343, 346, 347, 387, 391, 399
streptomycin 245, 250, 292, 392, 393,
      394, 395, 398, 400, 718, 729, 735,
      736, 823, 849, 851, 858, 860, 864,
      873, 886, 1036, 1037, 1038, 1039,
      1040, 1041, 1042
streptothricosis 886–7
stress 1133–47
   allostasis/allostatic load 1139–41,
      1142
   biological costs 1138
   clinical implications 1142–6
   coping strategies 1137–9, 1145–6
   counter-regulation 1136
   dairy cows 168
   dairy heifers 59, 63
   fertilization failure 558
   fetal 578
   metabolic responses 1136
   reproduction 478–9
   response 1134–6
   system 1134
   transition to pathology 1138–9
stressors 1133, 1137–8, 1146
Strongyloides spp 1026
stubble turnips 36, 123, 125
stunning 964
stunted growth 71
Stylosanthes fodder species 75
subconjunctival injection 1039
subluxations 447–51
Streptococcus uberis suboestrus, incidence 531
substituted phenols 1020, 1024
sucking lice 1023, 1031
suckled calves
   bull beef 16–17
   finishing 15–18

grass finishing 18
   management 11–12
   restricted suckling 71
   tropical cattle 70, 71
   worming 13
suckler cows
   anoestrus 534
   breed choice 8–9
   condition scoring 10, 11
   feed budgets 121, 122
   management 10–11
   metabolic profiles 815–16
   New Zealand 1177–8
   planning 7
   premiums 14
   stubble turnips 125
suckler feeding 12
   upgrading 117–18
suckler herds 7–13, 1117
   bulls 7–8, 594, 595
   calving period 12
   grassland management 12–13
   management 10–11
   New Zealand 1177–8
   performance targets 12, 13
   planning 7
   replacement heifer rearing 9–10
   reproductive performance 653–4
   stocking rates 12
suckling 3
   anoestrus 525, 535
   milk ejection 320, 472–3
   postpartum oestrous cycle 503–4, 512,
      656–7
   reflex 475
   restricted 71
sugar beet 792
sugar beet pulp 37, 113, 114, 115, 124
sugar cane tops 72
sugars
   ensiling process 114, 115
   rumen fermentation 96, 98, 245, 250,
      252, 398
sulphadiazine 245, 288, 292, 393, 394,
      851, 860, 864
sulphadimidine 245, 288, 292, 393, 860,
      861
sulphadoxine 245
sulphamethoxale 394
sulphamethoxypyradazine 245, 861
sulphanilamide 393
sulphonamides 154, 427, 737
sulphopyrazole 245, 291, 861
sulphur 33, 131
summer mastitis 63, 334, 337–45, 745
sunflower seed meal 183
super-levy 24
superovulation 49, 634–5, 638–9
supparative pneumonia, chronic 844–5
suprascapular nerve paralysis 436
suramin 1029
surgery 1105–30
   preparation of site 1105–6
   techniques 1106–30
   see also anaesthesia; named
      procedures

survival rates 66
susceptibility genes 167–8
Sussex 8
sustainable approach to disease
    treatment 84
sutures for uterine prolapse 515
swallowing interference 139
sward height 18, 62, 118, 119
sweating sickness 776
swedes 125
sweet fly 1031
sweetsiekte 776
sympathetic points (acupuncture)
    1099
sympathoadrenal (SA) axis 1134,
    1135–6, 1139
symphytum 109, 1086
syndromes
    differential lists 136
    presenting 138–57
synthetic pyrethroids 741, 742, 743, 745,
    763, 1032

T cells 323, 381, 1001–2
T helper cells 1145
Tabana disease see Jembrana disease
Tabanus spp 745, 762
Taenia saginata 280–81, 1020, 1028
tagging 44, 667
Taoism 1092
tapeworm 71, 280–82, 1021, 1024, 1026,
    1028
tapioca (manioc) 78, 113
tarsal cellulitis 460–61
tarsal bursitis 460
teat(s) 313–16
    antimicrobial substances 322
    burns 934
    chaps 369, 371
    chemical injury 369
    disinfection 333, 335
    environmental injury 369–70
    freezing/frost-bite 369
    immunology 321–5
    infectious lesions 363–7
    insect-induced lesions 370
    mastitis infection 327
    mechanical barrier function 322
    milking machine-induced lesions 370
    non-infectious lesions 367–70
    papillomatosis 365, 367, 371, 888
    photosensitization 140, 370, 371
    post-milking dipping 369
    skin lesion diagnosis 370–71
    stenosis 1128–9
    sunburn 369
    surgery 1126–30
    teat canal 313–14, 322
    traumatic lesions 368–9, 1128–30
    warts 365, 367, 371, 888
teat duct patency 322
Teatseal™ 400–401
teeth 825
    displaced cheek 177
    fluorosis 949–50
TEME 907

temperature, environmental 974–5
    ambient air 91–2
    breed susceptibility 560, 562
    critical 88–9, 974–5
    disease susceptibility 976
tendon contracture, multiple 178
tendon injuries 451–3
tenesmus 150, 858–9
tenotomy 458–9
terbutaline 1073
testes
    atrophy 618, 619–22
    degeneration 619–22
    hypoplasia 182, 618–19
    morphology 482–5
testosterone 1071, 1073
tetanus 145, 147, 733–4, 1005
    antitoxin 734
    vaccination 734, 1005
tetany
    hypomagnesaemic 157, 255–6
    transit 156
tetrachloruinphos 1032
tetracycline 392, 395, 762, 851
tetracyclines 392, 393, 395, 735, 737, 762,
    763, 764, 766, 767, 851, 1036,
    1037, 1040, 1041
tetrahydropyrimidines 1022, 1023
tetralogy of Fallot 174, 750–56
tetramisole 1021
Theileria (theileriosis) see also East
    Coast fever
    Theileria annulata 753
    Theileria lawreacei 751, 754
    Theileria mutans 751, 755
    Theileria parva 750, 751, 753
    Theileria sergenti 753
Thelazia rhodesii 775, 1023
thelaziosis 775, 1023
theleitis 368, 371
thermal comfort zone 88–9
thermoduric bacteria 347
thermoduric count 347
thermoregulation 88–9
thiabendazole 1019
thiamine deficiency 261, 904
thiamine hydrochloride 262
thiophanate 1020, 1025, 1026
Thogoto virus 773–4
thoracic pain, posterior 142–6
three day sickness 1182
thromboembolic meningoencephalitis
    (TEME) 907
thrombosis of caudal vena cava 867–8
thromboxane AL 1047, 1048, 1054, 1061
Thuja occidentalis 109, 1090
thyroxine (T₄) 301, 814
tiamulin 427, 428, 1040
tibial fractures 444
tibial nerve
    neurectomy 458, 459
    paralysis 438
tick-borne diseases 748–61
    Africa 1157–8, 1160–61
    encephalitides 770–71
    farcy 885–6

toxicosis 776–7
    viral 772–4
tick-borne encephalitides 770–71
tick-borne fever 586, 763
tick paralysis 775
ticks 77, 744–5, 1031
    resistance 1158
tilmicosin 288, 1041, 1043
tissue hydrostatic pressure 188
tissue salts 1103
TMR see total mixed ration
tocolysis 502
tocopherol acetate 259
toe ulcers 419, 424
tolfenamic acid 1051, 1056, 1061
tongue, smooth 33, 38, 177
total bacterial count 345–8
total mixed rations (TMR) 30, 32, 33,
    38, 120
    feeding barrier 38
    mineral/vitamin addition 33
total protein, blood 813
toxicoses 940, 941–3, 944–52
Toxoplasma gondii (toxoplasmosis) 284
trace elements
    biochemical indices 296
    dairy heifers 56, 63–4
    disorders 294–305
    hoof condition 422–3
    metabolic profile 813–15
tracing systems 6
traction injuries 151
transit fever 286–9
transit tetany 156
transketolase 261
transport of cattle 963
trauma
    eyelids 918–19
    genital tract 513–14
    oesophageal 826
    pericarditis 153
    reticulo-peritonitis 140, 142, 145–6
    teat injuries 368–9, 1128–30
traumatic flexon tendon injuries 452
trematodes 276–82, 1028
    see also liver fluke
Treponema spp 427
triamcinolone 245, 1049, 1056, 1057
tricarboxylic acid (TCA) cycle 794
trichlorphan 774
Trichophyton verucosum 878
Trichostrongylus spp 1026
triclabendazole 1020, 1026
triiodothyronine (T₃) 301
trimethoprim 245, 288, 392, 393, 394,
    395, 458, 737, 857, 860, 864, 1036,
    1037, 1038, 1040, 1041, 1043
triple heater meridian (acupuncture)
    1100
triticale 113, 130
Tritrichomonas fetus (trichomoniasis)
    560–61, 584, 992, 993, 1029
    abortion 584
    bovine genital 629, 632
    bulls 597
Trombicola spp 743

tropical cattle 68–81
  adult production 72–81
  AI 77
  beef production 77, 78–81
  calf management 69–72
  calving pattern 71, 77
  condition scoring 72
  diseases 70–71, 78
  environmental stress 70, 78
  ethnoveterinary medicine 83–6
  feeding 78
  health 78
  heat stress 88–93
  hygiene 78
  multi-purpose production 69
  numbers 68, 69
  production
    constraints 68
    strategy 69
    systems 74–7
  productivity 68
  range monitoring 73
  supplementation 79–80
  traditional systems 69, 70
  voluntary food intake maximization
    73–4
Trubanaman virus 773
Trypanosoma (trypanosomiosis) 745,
    756–61, 759, 1029, 1030
  Africa 1157, 1159–60
  Trypanosoma brucei 755, 757, 759
  Trypanosoma congolense 757, 758,
    759
  Trypanosoma evansi 757, 759
  Trypanosoma vivax 757, 758, 759, 761
trypanotolerance 761
L-tryptophan 866–7, 1061
tsetse flies 747, 756–61, 1157, 1158,
    1159, 1160
tuberculosis 143, 148, 150, 156, 862–4,
    993
  Africa 1157
  biosecurity 988
  intestine 149
  meningitis 156
  peritonitis 143
  skin 886
  transmission by semen 629, 631
tuberculin test 863
tumbu fly 747
turnips 292
  stubble 36, 125, 126
turpentine 834
twins, anomalous 184
TXA₂ *see* thromboxine A₂
tylosin 245, 288, 392, 393, 395, 427, 428,
    1036, 1038, 1040, 1041

udder
  adult 313–16
  anatomy 311–16, 379
  defence mechanisms 379–82
  development 311–13, 316–17
  disease dynamics 326, 327
  dry 327
  examination 151

growth 316–17
  immunity enhancement 379–89
  immunology 321–5
  infections 382–3
  mammary cells 381–2
  pathogens 328
  phagocytic cell mobilization 324–5
  phagocytosis 325, 382
  pharmacology 392–3
  skin lesion diagnosis 370–71, 989
  see also mastitis; teat(s); teat canal
UDP *see* rumen undegradable protein
UK
  beef sources 28–9
  bull use 595–6
  dairy cattle reproductive performance
    663–4
  dairy farming structure 24–6
  rabies control 1170
ulcer, heel and toe 419
ulcer, sole 41, 145, 150, 417–19
ultrasonography
  anoestrus detection 538–9
  postpartum 512
ultraviolet light electrocutor 746
umbilical abscess 456
umbilical hernia 182, 1122–4
undernutrition 71, 104, 121
unmolassed sugar beet pulp 112
unthrifty cow 150–51
urachus, pervious 184
uraemia 263
urban dairying in Africa 76
urea feeding 78, 124
urea, milk levels 815
urea-nitrogen, blood 98, 811–13
urea plasmas 240, 241
urea-treated feed 125
urea-treated whole crop 130
ureter, calculus passage 140
urinary tract
  congenital defects 184
  neoplasia 154
urine testing 1186
urolithiasis 140, 150, 154
  calves 263–4
urovagina 519
Urtica urens 1090, 1091
urticaria 883–4
USA
  beef finishing systems 14
  rabies 1165–6
  see also North America
uterus
  bacterial contamination elimination
    509
  bacterial infection/invasion 504, 505,
    509, 521
  caruncle sloughing 509, 516
  contractility 501–2
  cyclic ovarian activity 505
  dilatation 142
  epithelial regeneration 509
  examination 151
  flushing/fluid withdrawal 521
  involution 504–5, 508, 516

oestrus cycle 495
  prolapse 514–15
  prostaglandin 2α release 495–6
  rupture 513
  torsion 145, 1118–19
  see also endometritis; metritis
uveal tract diseases 923
uveitis 923

vaccination 1004–7, 1009–18
  anthrax 719, 1005
  bacillary haemoglobinuria 721
  blackleg 724
  bluetongue 1018
  botulism 722, 1005
  bovine respiratory disease 1007,
    1008–9, 288
  bovine respiratory syncytial virus
    1009–10
  bovine virus diarrhoea 644, 1011–12
  BPV teat warts 367
  brucellosis 1013–14
  clostridial infections 722, 724, 734,
    1005
  coliform mastitis 384
  contagious bovine pleuropneumonia
    1011
  East Coast fever 1161
  erysipelas 1014–15
  foot-and-mouth disease 704, 705, 706,
    707, 1016–17, 1175
  Haemophilus somnus 1010–11
  haemorrhagic septicaemia 729
  immune response generation 388
  immunity enhancement in mammary
    gland 379–89
  infectious bovine keratoconjunctivitis
    921, 1018
  infectious bovine rhinotracheitis 292,
    644, 1010
  infectious necrotic hepatitis 731
  Johne's disease 1012–13
  leptospirosis 581, 644, 736–7, 1015–16
  limitations 389
  louping ill 1014
  lungworm 56, 274, 1011
  malignant oedema 725
  mastitis 1016
  neonatal calf diarrhoea 1006–7
  papillomatosis 1014
  parasitic bronchitis 56, 274, 1011
  PI3 1007, 1009
  pneumonia 247–8
  rabies 1018, 1169–70
  respiratory disease 247–8, 1007, 1008,
    1009–11
  Rift Valley fever 770, 1018
  rinderpest 710, 1013, 1156
  ringworm 880, 1017–18
  salmonellosis 227, 228–9, 1006, 1007
  shipping fever 289
  Staphylococcus aureus 386
  tetanus 734, 1005
  tick-borne encephalidites 771
  tuberculosis 864
  vesicular stomatitis 712, 1018

vaccines 1004–7, 1008, 1009–18
vagal indigestion *see* vagus indigestion
vagina
 discharge 522
 examination in repeat breeder cow
  564, 565
  failure to locate 615
  stretch receptors 475
vaginitis 513, 519, 559
vagus indigestion 141, 146, 147, 835–6
vancomycin 1040, 1041
veal production 5–6
 calf welfare 959–60
 temperature sensitivity 975
 world production 68, 69
vegetable oils 834
vegetable waste 131
vena cava, caudal, thrombosis 867–8
venereal diseases 597
ventilation 982–6
 calf housing 3
 dairy cow housing 40–41, 43
 mechanical 984–5
 natural 983–4
 pneumonia 241–2
ventricular septal defects 173–4
vertebral cervical injury 145
vertebral column defects 176
vertebral fractures 445–6
vertebral malformation, complex 175
Verticillium spp 126, 128
vesicular stomatitis 366, 371, 710–13,
 989
 vaccination 712, 1018
vestibular syndrome 896, 903
veterinary clinicians 135–6
 clinical case approach 136–8
VFA *see* volatile fatty acids
virginiamycin 1070
virulence factors 383–8
viruses *see* infections/infectious disease,
 viral
vitamin(s) 33, 58
 hoof condition 422–3
vitamin A 3, 33, 247, 256, 257
 deficiency 126, 256–7, 462
 ocular defects 924, 925

vitamin B group 247, 831
vitamin B$_1$ 262
vitamin B$_{12}$ 258, 296, 297, 794, 815
vitamin C 256, 831
vitamin D 3, 33, 253–4, 460, 462–3, 782,
 791
vitamin E 3, 33, 126, 256, 259, 260,
 815
 deficiency 258–60, 303, 451
 supplementation 305
volatile fatty acids (VFA) 96, 1067
voluntary food intake 73
vomiting 139, 825–6
voursiekte 776

warbles/warble fly 740–41, 875–8, 989,
 993, 1023, 1031, 1032
warts *see* papillomatosis
wasting and diarrhoea syndrome
 828
water
 availability 71, 73, 78, 934–5
 cold 147, 155
 dairy cow requirement 38, 95
 food content 30
 requirement 95, 38
water flotation 800–801
water-soluble carbohydrate (WSC) 114,
 115, 116, 117
weak calf syndrome, perinatal 249
weaning 3–5
 suckler calves 11–12
 tropical calves 71
weaning weight, calf 8
weaver syndrome 179
weight gain *see* liveweight gain
weight loss 150–51
weight, mating 10, 11
weight, post calving 10, 11
weight, weaning 8, 12
welfare 955–64, 1152
 calves 958–60
 problem areas 956
Weybridge system 271
wheat 113
wheatbran 78, 113, 114
wheat distiller's dark grains 113

wheatfeed 112, 113, 114
whey 113, 114
whey-based milk replacers 4
white heifer disease 183, 557
white line 411, 412, 413
 axial wall fissures 426
 defects 417–20
white line disease 41, 150, 424, 1181
white muscle disease 258–60
white Shorthorn 9
wholecrop cereals 116, 130–31
wholecrop silage 130
whole-wheat silage 130
winter dysentery 852–3
winter finishing beef 15–17
winter scour 13, 149
winter store rations 18
wire 139, 140, 141, 142–3
 foreign body damage 145
 sudden death 152
 see also reticulitis/reticuloperitonitis
wooden tongue 823–4
World Trade Organization 22, 53
worm module disease 774
WSC *see* water soluble carbohydrate

yards
 covered 983–4, 985
 open-fronted 985
yeast 304
yeasts, mastitis 347
yew poisoning 947–8
yin/yang 1092–8

Zebu cattle (*Bos indicus*) 71, 72, 75–6,
 89
 calves 70
 disease resistance 167
zero-grazing 76, 77, 129
zilpaterol 1073, 1074
zinc
 biochemical indices 296
 deficiency 260, 305, 462
 disorders 305
 metabolic profile 815
 oxide 1180
zinc methionine 422

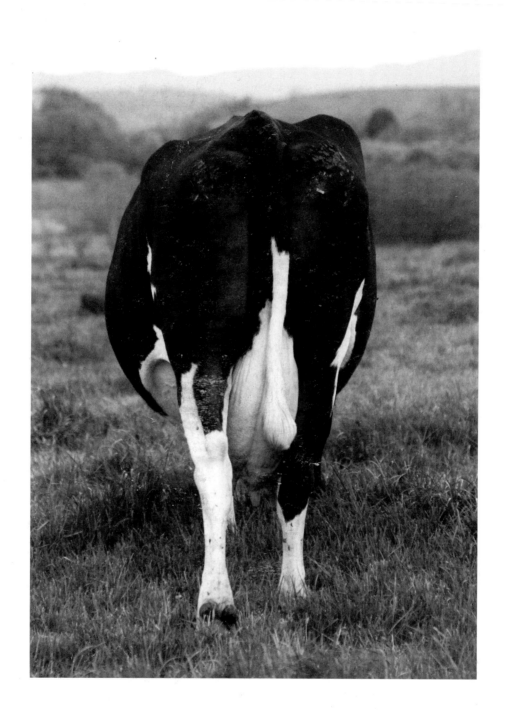